Medicine

Prep Manual for Undergraduates

Medicine
Prep Manual for Undergraduates

SEVENTH EDITION

K GEORGE MATHEW, MD
Associate Specialist in Orthogeriatrics
Torbay Hospital, Torquay, Devon
United Kingdom

Formerly Associate Professor, Department of Medicine
Kasturba Medical College, Manipal
Karnataka, INDIA

PRAVEEN AGGARWAL, MD, DNB (MEDICINE)
Professor and Head
Department of Emergency Medicine
All India Institute of Medical Sciences
New Delhi, INDIA

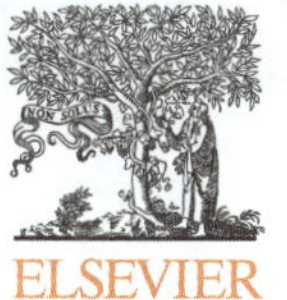

ELSEVIER

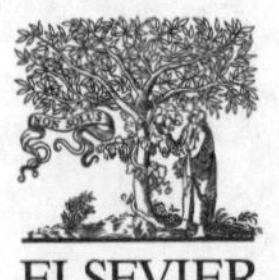

ELSEVIER

RELX India Pvt. Ltd.
Registered Office: 818, 8th Floor, Indraprakash Building, 21, Barakhamba Road, New Delhi 110001
Corporate Office: 14th Floor, Building No. 10B, DLF Cyber City, Phase II, Gurgaon-122002, Haryana, India

Medicine: Prep Manual for Undergraduates, 7e, K George Mathew and Praveen Aggarwal

ISBN: 978-81-312-6628-1
e-book ISBN: 978-81-312-6629-8

Notice

Practitioners and researchers must always rely on their own experience and knowledge in evaluating and using any information, methods, compounds or experiments described herein. Because of rapid advances in the medical sciences, in particular, independent verifi cation of diagnoses and drug dosages should be made. To the fullest extent of the law, no responsibility is assumed by Elsevier, authors, editors or contributors for any injury and/or damage to persons or property as a matter of products liability, negligence or otherwise, or from any use or operation of any methods, products, instructions, or ideas contained in the material herein.

Although all advertising material is expected to conform to ethical (medical) standards, inclusion in this publication does not constitute a guarantee or endorsement of the quality or value of such product or of the claims made of it by its manufacturer.

Please consult full prescribing information before issuing prescription for any product mentioned in this publication.

Content Strategist - Education Solutions: Mrinalini Bakshi
Content Project Manager: Anand K Jha
Sr Production Executive: Dhan Singh Rana
Sr Graphic Designer: Milind Majgaonkar

Typeset by GW India

Printed and bound at Sanat Printers, Kundli

To

My family

KGM

My parents, wife and children

PA

Preface to the Seventh Edition

Medicine: Prep Manual for Undergraduates, 7e by Mathew and Aggarwal is the premier and most-read manual by the undergraduates as it provides up-to-date information about various diseases. Since the field of Medicine is rapidly advancing, we proudly present the seventh edition of this top-selling book which has incorporated these advances in it.

The readers of this new edition will get updated and in-depth knowledge of medicine. For ease of reading, this edition is presented in two-column, full colour format. This edition has incorporated the most recent knowledge acquired in the field of medicine in the last couple of years. One of the major highlights of this edition is incorporation of more than 200 figures in full colour which will help the students to understand and then retain various disease conditions. This edition incorporates evidence-based guidelines in diagnosis and management of various medical conditions which will help the students in having an edge over others during theory, practical and even post-graduate entrance tests.

The previous style of question-answer format which helps the students in quick revision and self-assessment before examination has been retained in this edition also. As was true for previous editions, majority of the topics have been thoroughly revised to incorporate new knowledge. Every question has been closely reviewed and updated, with substantial revisions. Several new questions have been added. Questions on various aspects of SARS-CoV-2 infection have been added. Others include questions on monkeypox, porphyrias, mechanical ventilation, haemophagocytic lymphohistiocytosis, IgG4-related disease, immunodeficiency diseases, alopecia, spinal cord syndromes, Takotsubo cardiomyopathy, corrosive poisoning, psychiatric emergencies, immune checkpoint inhibitors, CAR T-cell therapy, rabies and genital ulcers. In view of specific medical issues related to the elderly population, a new chapter on Geriatrics has been added. An additional chapter on Clinical Pharmacology has also been added which will orient the students towards pharmacogenetics, pharmaceutical adverse effects as well as research methodology.

To make students understand the topics, previous figures have been updated wherever required while several new figures, flowcharts, boxes and tables have been added. We are very sure that this new edition will give the students necessary knowledge to come out with flying colours in the examinations.

Another feature of the current edition is that majority of the questions have been designed as per the latest Competency-Based Undergraduate Medical Curriculum for the subject of Medicine as prescribed by the National Medical Commission (erstwhile Medical Council of India). The competencies covered are mentioned prominently at the end of the question.

We would like to thank our families as without their extensive support, revision of this book would not have been possible. Our special thanks to the entire staff of RELX India Pvt. Ltd. for their constant help and support.

We sincerely hope that this new edition fulfills all the requirements of undergraduate medical students for the speciality of Medicine. As was true for the previous editions, we are sure that this seventh edition will also remain the most-trusted source of evidence-based content.

We appreciate and acknowledge any comments or suggestions for further improvements in the future editions of this book. Suggestions and comments from teachers and students can be emailed at indiacontact@elsevier.com.

K George Mathew
Praveen Aggarwal

Preface to the First Edition

The experience of teaching Medicine to a diverse group of undergraduate medical students made me realise the need for a manual in concise and tabular form to facilitate preparation of the students for the final examination.

I would like to very clearly emphasise that this is not a textbook. This is intended to be a companion to the textbook, an easy reference manual for the exam going undergraduates. Keeping this objective in mind, only important topics have been dealt with in detail. The rest have been given only cursory treatment. Interdisciplinary topics of marginal interest to the physician have been briefly dealt with. In the process of simplifying the subject, accuracy may have been compromised to a certain extent. The omission of topics from a postgraduate's point of view is deliberate. Standard textbooks in Medicine and its subspecialties have been used as reference in compiling this book.

A large number of people have helped me make this work possible. I wish to place on record the special help received from the following individuals.

This book would be incomplete if I did not place on record, the many contributions made by Dr N K Ravi Subramanya, Associate Professor, Department of Neurology, Kasturba Medical College, Manipal, starting from the specific chore of writing the chapter on Neurology, giving technical assistance, evaluating all the topics with a critical eye, he has been a great source of strength. I owe him for being a friend, philosopher and guide throughout.

I would also like to record my appreciation for Mr B V P Marianus, Director, information Systems, Manipal Academy of Higher Education, Manipal, for allowing access to the Computing Centre freely, for all the encouragement he gave me, and above all for being so patient for this seemingly long period of one year.

Mr Ashok Kumar, Computing Centre, Manipal Academy of Higher Education, Manipal deserves special praise, not just for having patiently composed the major part of the book, but also for being utterly meticulous and punctual. Thanks are due to him for making me realise the potential of a computer.

I would like to thank Dr Martin T Kurian, Assistant Professor, Department of Nephrology, Kasturba Medical College, Manipal, for writing the chapters on Nephrology and Fluid, Electrolyte and Acid-base disturbances. My thanks are also due to Dr Gayathri, Assistant Professor, Department of Radiodiagnosis, for the preparation on Radiology, Dr S Sujatha Sri and Dr Ramesh S Shenoy, Kasturba Medical College, Manipal, for their scientific expertise throughout.

I am grateful to Prof (Dr) G N Kundaje for his constant encouragement for the preparation of this book and for having written the foreword.

I welcome critical appraisal of the book and suggestions for the improvement, from the students.

K George Mathew, 1994

Competency Codes

COMPETENCY CODE	COMPETENCY DESCRIPTION	CORE (Y/N)	CHAPTER No.	PAGE NOS.
	GENERAL MEDICINE			
Topic: Anaemia				
IM9.1	Define, describe and classify anaemia based on red blood cell size and reticulocyte count	Y	1	9, 15
IM9.7	Describe and discuss the meaning and utility of various components of the hemogram	Y	1	9
IM9.8	Describe and discuss the various tests for iron deficiency	Y	1	11
IM9.12	Describe, develop a diagnostic plan to determine the aetiology of anaemia	Y	1	9
IM9.13	Prescribe replacement therapy with iron, B12, folate	Y	1	11, 18, 20
IM9.14	Determine the need for specialist consultation	Y	1	21
IM9.17	Describe the indications for blood transfusion and the appropriate use of blood components	Y	1	101
IM9.18	Describe the precautions required necessary when performing a blood transfusion	Y	1	101
Topic: Dermatology, Venereology & Leprosy				
DR11.1	Describe the etiology, pathogenesis and clinical features of the dermatologic manifestations of HIV and its complications including opportunistic infections	Y	3	262
Topic: HIV				
IM6.1	Describe and discuss the symptoms and signs of acute HIV seroconversion	Y	3	262
IM6.2	Define and classify HIV AIDS based on the CDC criteria	Y	3	262
IM6.3	Describe and discuss the relationship between CDC count and the risk of opportunistic infections	Y	3	262
IM6.4	Describe and discuss the pathogenesis, evolution and clinical features of common HIV related opportunistic infections	Y	3	262
IM6.5	Describe and discuss the pathogenesis, evolution and clinical features of common HIV related malignancies	Y	3	262
IM6.9	Choose and interpret appropriate diagnostic tests to diagnose and classify the severity of HIV-AIDS including specific tests of HIV, CDC	Y	3	262
IM6.11	Enumerate the indications and describe the findings for CT of the chest and brain and MRI	N	3	262
IM6.16	Discuss and describe the principles of HAART, the classes of antiretrovirals used, adverse reactions and interactions	Y	3	262
IM6.17	Discuss and describe the principles and regimens used in post exposure prophylaxis	Y	3	279
IM6.18	Enumerate the indications and discuss prophylactic drugs used to prevent HIV related opportunistic infections	Y	3	262

Continued

**Readers are advised to access full competency codes of Medicine on digital platform associated with this book.*

COMPETENCY CODE	COMPETENCY DESCRIPTION	CORE (Y/N)	CHAPTER No.	PAGE NOS.
Topic: HIV				
CT1.3	Discuss and describe the impact of co-infection with HIV and other co-morbid conditions. Like diabetes on the natural history of tuberculosis	Y	3	276
Topic: GI bleeding				
IM15.1	Enumerate, describe and discuss the aetiology of upper and lower GI bleeding	Y	5	371
Topic: Headache				
IM17.1	Define and classify headache and describe the presenting features, precipitating factors, aggravating and relieving factors of various kinds of headache	Y	5	337, 339
IM17.3	Classify migraine and describe the distinguishing features between classical and non classical forms of migraine	Y	5	337
Topic: Cerebrovascular accident				
IM18.2	Classify cerebrovascular accidents and describe the aetiology, predisposing genetic and risk factors pathogenesis of hemorrhagic and non hemorrhagic stroke	Y	5	348, 349
IM18.6	Distinguish the lesion based on upper vs lower motor neuron, side, site and most probable nature of the lesion	Y	5	314
Topic: Movement disorders				
IM19.2	Classify movement disorders of the brain based on distribution, rhythm, repetition, exacerbating and relieving factors	Y	5	365
IM19.8	Discuss and describe the pharmacology, dose, side effects and interactions used in the drug therapy of Parkinson's syndrome	Y	5	362
Topic: Psychiatry				
PS16.1	Enumerate and describe common psychiatric disorders in the elderly including dementia, depression and psychosis	Y	5	321, 322
Topic: Human Anatomy				
AN28.7	Explain the anatomical basis of facial nerve palsy	Y	5	332
AN56.2	Describe circulation of CSF with its applied anatomy	Y	5	325
AN62.6	Describe & identify formation, branches & major areas of distribution of circle of Willis	Y	5	348
Topic: Pathology				
PA35.1	Describe the etiology, types and pathogenesis, differentiating factors, CSF findings in meningitis	Y	5	371
Topic: Microbiology				
MI5.2	Describe the etiopathogenesis, clinical course and discuss the laboratory diagnosis of encephalitis	Y	5	375
Topic: Physiology				
PY3.13	Describe muscular dystrophy: myopathies	Y	5	406
Topic: Liver disease				
IM 5.1	Describe and discuss the physiologic and biochemical basis of hyperbilirubinemia	Y	6	426, 428
IM 5.2	Describe and discuss the aetiology and pathophysiology of liver injury	Y	6	437
IM 5.4	Describe and discuss the epidemiology, microbiology, immunology and clinical evolution of infective (viral) hepatitis	Y	6	432
IM 5.5	Describe and discuss the pathophysiology and clinical evolution of alcoholic liver disease	Y	6	444

COMPETENCY CODE	COMPETENCY DESCRIPTION	CORE (Y/N)	CHAPTER No.	PAGE NOS.
IM 5.6	Describe and discuss the pathophysiology, clinical evolution and complications of cirrhosis and portal hypertension including ascites, spontaneous bacterial peritonitis, hepatorenal syndrome and hepatic encephalopathy	Y	6	445, 450, 453, 456, 461, 463
IM 5.7	Enumerate and describe the causes and pathophysiology of drug induced liver injury	Y	6	431
IM 5.13	Enumerate the indications for ultrasound and other imaging studies including MRCP and ERCP and describe the findings in liver disease	Y	6	424, 425
IM 5.16	Describe and discuss the management of hepatitis, cirrhosis, portal hypertension, ascites spontaneous, bacterial peritonitis and hepatic encephalopathy	Y	6	432, 445, 450, 453, 456, 461, 463
IM 5.17	Enumerate the indications, precautions and counsel patients on vaccination for hepatitis	Y	6	432
Topic: GI bleeding				
IM 15.2	Enumerate, describe and discuss the evaluation and steps involved in stabilizing a patient who presents with acute volume loss and GI bleed	Y	6	453
Topic: Heart Failure				
IM 1.1	Describe and discuss the epidemiology, pathogenesis clinical evolution and course of common causes of heart disease including: rheumatic/ valvular, ischemic, hypertrophic inflammatory	Y	7	535
IM 1.3	Describe and discuss the aetiology microbiology pathogenies and clinical evolution of rheumatic fever, criteria, degree of rheumatic activity and rheumatic valvular heart disease and its complications including infective endocarditis	N	7	551
IM 1.4	Stage heart failure	Y	7	535
IM 1.5	Describe ,discuss and differentiate the processes involved in R Vs L heart failure, systolic vs diastolic failure	Y	7	535
IM 1.6	Describe and discuss the compensatory mechanisms involved in heart failure including cardiac remodelling and neurohormonal adaptations	Y	7	535
IM 1.7	Enumerate, describe and discuss the factors that exacerbate heart, dietary factors drugs etc.	Y	7	535
IM 1.8	Describe and discuss the pathogenesis and development of common arrythmias involved in heart failure particularly atrial fibrillation	Y	7	509
IM 1.9	Describe and discuss the clinical presentation and features, diagnosis, recognition and management of acute rheumatic fever	Y	7	551
IM 1.16	Generate a differential diagnosis based on the clinical presentation and prioritise it based on the most likely diagnosis	Y	7	639, 641, 642, 644
IM 1.18	Perform and interpret a 12 lead ECG	Y	7	499
IM 1.21	Describe and discuss and identify the clinical features of acute and subacute endocarditis, echocardiographic findings, blood culture and sensitivity and therapy	Y	7	574
IM 1.24	Describe and discuss the pharmacology of drugs including indications, contraindications in the management of heart failure including diuretics, ACE inhibitors, Beta blockers, aldosterone antagonists and cardiac glycosides	Y	7	535, 544, 546, 547, 548
IM 1.27	Describe and discuss the role of penicillin prophylaxis in the prevention of rheumatic heart disease	Y	7	551

Continued

COMPETENCY CODE	COMPETENCY DESCRIPTION	CORE (Y/N)	CHAPTER No.	PAGE NOS.
IM 1.28	Enumerate the causes of adult presentations of congenital heart disease and describe the distinguishing features between cyanotic and acyanotic heart disease	Y	7	627
IM 1.29	Elicit document and present an appropriate history, demonstrate correctly general examination, relevant clinical findings and formulate document and present a management plan for an adult patient presenting with a common form of congenital heart disease	Y	7	627, 629, 630, 631
Topic: Acute Myocardial Infarction/ IHD				
IM 2.1	Discuss and describe the epidemiology, antecedents and risk factors for atherosclerosis and ischemic heart disease	Y	7	580
IM 2.2	Discuss the aetiology of risk factors both modifiable and non modifiable of atherosclerosis and IHD	Y	7	580
IM 2.5	Define the various acute coronary syndromes and describe their evolution, natural history and outcomes	Y	7	586
IM 2.14	Discuss and describe the indications for admission to a coronary care unit and supportive therapy for a patient with acute coronary syndrome	Y	7	587, 595
IM 2.15	Discuss and describe the medications used in patients with an acute coronary syndrome based on the clinical presentation	Y	7	587, 595
IM 2.16	Discuss and describe the indications for acute thrombolysis, PTCA and CABG	Y	7	587
IM 2.17	Discuss and describe the indications and methods of cardiac rehabilitation	Y	7	587, 595
IM 2.19	Discuss and describe the pathogenesis, recognition and management of complications of acute coronary syndromes including arrhythmias, shock, LV dysfunction, papillary muscle rupture and pericarditis	Y	7	505, 587, 595
IM 2.20	Discuss and describe the assessment and relief of pain in acute coronary syndromes	Y	7	587, 595
IM 2.21	Observe and participate in a controlled environment an ACLS program	N	7	517
IM 2.22	Perform and demonstrate in a mannequin BLS	Y	7	517
IM 2.23	Describe and discuss the indications for nitrates, anti platelet agents, gpIIb IIIa inhibitors, beta blockers, ACE inhibitors etc in the management of coronary syndromes	Y	7	587, 595
Topic: Hypertension				
IM 8.1	Describe and discuss the epidemiology, aetiology and the prevalence of primary and secondary hypertension	Y	7	598
IM 8.2	Describe and discuss the pathophysiology of hypertension	Y	7	598
IM 8.4	Define and classify hypertension	Y	7	598
IM 8.6	Define, describe and discuss and recognise hypertensive urgency and emergency	Y	7	605
IM 8.8	Describe, discuss and identify target organ damage due to hypertension	Y	7	598
IM 8.14	Develop an appropriate treatment plan for essential hypertension	Y	7	598
IM 8.15	Recognise, prioritise and manage hypertensive emergencies	Y	7	605
Topic: Pathology				
PA 27.7	Describe the etiology, pathophysiology, pathology, gross and microscopic, features diagnosis and complications of pericarditis and pericardial effusion	Y	7	622, 624

COMPETENCY CODE	COMPETENCY DESCRIPTION	CORE (Y/N)	CHAPTER No.	PAGE NOS.
PA 27.9	Classify and describe the etiology, types, pathophysiology, pathology, gross and microscopic features, diagnosis and complications of cardiomyopathies	N	7	617
Topic: Dermatology, Venereology & Leprosy				
DR 16.2	Identify and distinguish Raynaud's phenomenon	Y	7	634
Topic: GI bleeding				
IM15.1	Enumerate, describe and discuss the aetiology of upper and lower GI bleeding	Y	8	661, 684
IM15.10	Enumerate the indications for endoscopy, colonoscopy and other imaging procedures in the investigation of Upper GI bleeding	Y	8	661
IM15.15	Describe and enumerate the indications, pharmacology and side effects of pharmacotherapy of acid peptic disease including Helicobacter pylori	Y	8	667
IM15.16	Enumerate the indications for endoscopic interventions and Surgery	Y	8	667
Topic: Diarrheal disorder				
IM16.1	Describe and discuss the aetiology of acute and chronic diarrhea including infectious and non infectious causes	Y	8	656, 657
IM16.2	Describe and discuss the acute systemic consequences of diarrhea including its impact on fluid balance	Y	8	657
IM16.3	Describe and discuss the chronic effects of diarrhea including malabsorption	Y	8	675
IM16.11	Enumerate the indications for stool cultures and blood cultures in patients with acute diarrhea	Y	8	657
IM16.14	Describe and enumerate the indications, pharmacology and side effects of pharmacotherapy for bacterial and viral diarrhea	Y	8	657
IM16.15	Distinguish based on the clinical presentation Crohn's disease from Ulcerative Colitis	Y	8	698
IM16.16	Describe and enumerate the indications, pharmacology and side effects of pharmacotherapy including immunotherapy	Y	8	691, 695
IM16.17	Describe and enumerate the indications for surgery in inflammatory bowel disease	Y	8	691
Topic: Rheumatologic problems				
IM7.3	Classify cause of joint pain based on the pathophysiology	Y	9	706
IM7.6	Discriminate, describe and discuss arthralgia from arthritis and mechanical from inflammatory causes of joint pain	Y	9	715
IM7.8	Determine the potential causes of join pain based on the presenting features of joint involvement	Y	9	706
IM7.15	Enumerate the indications for and interpret the results of : CBC, anti- CCP, RA, ANA, DNA and other tests of autoimmunity	Y	9	711, 727
IM7.19	Develop an appropriate treatment plan for patients with rheumatologic diseases	Y	9	706, 723
IM7.20	Select, prescribe and communicate appropriate medications for relief of joint pain	Y	9	712
IM7.21	Select, prescribe and communicate preventive therapy for crystalline arthropathies	Y	9	741
IM7.22	Select, prescribe and communicate treatment option for systemic rheumatologic conditions	Y	9	706, 723
IM7.23	Describe the basis for biologic and disease modifying therapy in rheumatologic diseases	Y	9	706

Continued

COMPETENCY CODE	COMPETENCY DESCRIPTION	CORE (Y/N)	CHAPTER No.	PAGE NOS.
Topic: Envenomation				
IM20.1	Enumerate the local poisonous snakesand describe the distinguishing marks of each	Y	10	748
IM20.2	Describe, demonstrate in a volunteer or a mannequin and educate (to other health care workers / patients) the correct initial management of patient with a snake bite in the field	Y	10	748
IM20.3	Describe the initial approach to the stabilisation of the patient who presents with snake bite	Y	10	748
IM20.7	Enumerate the indications and describe the pharmacology, dose, adverse reactions, hypersensitivity reactions of anti snake venom	Y	10	748
IM20.8	Describe the diagnosis, initial approach stabilisation and therapy of scorpion envenomation	N	10	752
Topic: Poisoning				
IM21.1	Describe the initial approach to thestabilisation of the patient who presents with poisoning	Y	10	744
IM21.2	Enumerate the common plant poisons seen in your area and describe their toxicology, clinical features, prognosis and specific approach to detoxification	Y	10	758
IM21.3	Enumerate the common corrosives used in your area and describe their toxicology, clinical features, prognosis and approach to therapy	Y	10	752, 754, 758
IM21.4	Enumerate the commonly observed drug overdose in your area and describe their toxicology, clinical features, prognosis and approach to therapy	Y	10	755, 756, 757
Topic: Obesity				
IM14.1	Define and measure obesity as it relates to the Indian population	Y	11	783
IM14.2	Describe and discuss the aetiology of obesity including modifiable and non-modifiable risk factors and secondary causes	Y	11	783
IM14.5	Describe and discuss the natural history of obesity and its complications	Y	11	783
IM14.11	Communicate and counsel patient on behavioural, dietary and lifestyle modifications	Y	11	783
IM14.13	Describe and enumerate the indications, pharmacology and side effects of pharmacotherapy for obesity	Y	11	783
IM14.14	Describe and enumerate the indications and side effects of bariatric surgery	Y	11	783
Topic: Nutritional and Vitamin Deficiencies				
IM23.3	Discuss and describe the aetiology, causes, clinical manifestations, complications, diagnosis and management of common vitamin deficiencies	Y	11	771, 776, 779, 780, 781
Topic: Geriatrics				
IM24.8	Describe and discuss the aetiopathogenesis, clinical presentation, identification, functional changes, acute care, stabilization, management and rehabilitation of osteoporosis in the elderly	Y	11	777
Topic: PharmacologyGeriatrics				
PH1.36	Describe the mechanism of action, types, doses, side effects, indications and contraindications of drugs used in endocrine disorders (diabetes mellitus, thyroid disorders and osteoporosis)	Y	11	777
Topic: Psychiatry				
PS4.1	Describe the magnitude and etiology of alcohol and substance use disorders	Y	12	800, 801
PS4.2	Elicit, describe and document clinical features of alcohol and substance use disorders	Y	12	800, 801

COMPETENCY CODE	COMPETENCY DESCRIPTION	CORE (Y/N)	CHAPTER No.	PAGE NOS.
PS4.3	Enumerate and describe the indications and interpret laboratory and other tests used in alcohol and substance abuse disorders	Y	12	800, 801
PS4.4	Describe the treatment of alcohol and substance abuse disorders including behavioural and pharmacologic therapy	Y	12	800, 801
PS4.6	Enumerate and describe the pharmacologic basis and side effects of drugs used in alcohol and substance abuse	Y	12	801
PS10.1	Enumerate and describe the magnitude and etiology of somatoform, dissociative and conversion disorders	Y	12	793
PS10.2	Enumerate, elicit, describe and document clinical features in patients with somatoform, dissociative and conversion disorders	Y	12	793
PS10.4	Describe the treatment of somatoform disorders including behavioural, psychosocial and pharmacologic therapy	Y	12	793
PS10.6	Enumerate and describe the pharmacologic basis and side effects of drugs used in somatoform, dissociative and conversion disorders	Y	12	806
PS16.1	Enumerate and describe common psychiatric disorders in the elderly including dementia, depression and psychosis	Y	12	788, 787, 790
Topic: Common malignancies				
IM13.12	Describe the indications and interpret the results of Chest X Ray, mammogram, skin and tissue biopsies and tumor markers used in common cancers	Y	13	811
Topic: Pediatrics				
PE32.9	Discuss the referral criteria and multidisciplinary approach to management of Turner Syndrome	N	14	832
Topic: Acute Kidney Injury and Chronic renal failure				
IM10.18	Identify the ECG findings in hyperkalemia	Y	15	846
IM10.20	Describe and discuss the indications to perform arterial blood gas analysis: interpret the data	Y	15	851
Topic: Mineral, Fluid Electrolyte and Acid base Disorder				
IM22.5	Enumerate the causes and describe the clinical features and the correct approach to the diagnosis and management of the patient with hyponatremia	Y	15	839, 841
IM22.6	Enumerate the causes and describe the clinical and laboratory features and the correct approach to the diagnosis and management of the patient with hyponatremia	Y	15	841
IM22.7	Enumerate the causes and describe the clinical and laboratory features and the correct approach to the diagnosis and management of the patient with hypokalemia	Y	15	845
IM22.8	Enumerate the causes and describe the clinical and laboratory features and the correct approach to the diagnosis and management of the patient with hyperkalemia	Y	15	846
IM22.9	Enumerate the causes and describe the clinical and laboratory features of metabolic acidosis	N	15	848
IM22.10	Enumerate the causes of describe the clinical and laboratory features of metabolic alkalosis	N	15	849
IM22.11	Enumerate the causes and describe the clinical and laboratory features of respiratory acidosis	N	15	850
IM22.12	Enumerate the causes and describe the clinical and laboratory features of respiratory alkalosis	N	15	850
IM22.13	Identify the underlying acid based disorder based on an ABG report and clinical situation	N	15	851

Continued

COMPETENCY CODE	COMPETENCY DESCRIPTION	CORE (Y/N)	CHAPTER No.	PAGE NOS.
Topic: Acute Kidney Injury and Chronic renal failure				
IM10.1	Define, describe and differentiate between acute and chronic renal failure	Y	16	867, 873
IM10.2	Classify, describe and differentiate the pathophysiologic causes of acute renal failure	Y	16	873
IM10.4	Describe the evolution, natural history and treatment of ARF	Y	16	873
IM10.5	Describe and discuss the aetiology of CRF	Y	16	868
IM10.6	Stage Chronic Kidney Disease	Y	16	867
IM10.7	Describe and discuss the pathophysiology and clinical findings of uraemia	Y	16	868
IM10.8	Classify, describe and discuss the significance of proteinuria in CKD	Y	16	855
IM10.9	Describe and discuss the pathophysiology of anaemia and hyperparathyroidism in CKD	Y	16	868
IM10.15	Describe the appropriate diagnostic work up based on the presumed aetiology	Y	16	868
IM10.17	Describe and calculate indices of renal function based on available laboratories including FENa (Fractional Excretion of Sodium) and CrCl (Creatinine Clearance)	Y	16	858
IM10.19	Enumerate the indications and describe the findings in renal ultrasound	N	16	858
IM10.24	Counsel patients on a renal diet	Y	16	868
IM10.26	Describe and discuss supportive therapy in CKD including diet, anti hypertensives, glycemic therapy, dyslipidemia, anaemia, hyperkalemia, hyperphosphatemia and secondary hyperparathyroidism	Y	16	868
IM10.27	Describe and discuss the indications for renal dialysis	Y	16	868
Topic: Fever and febrile syndromes				
IM4.3	Discuss and describe the common causes, pathophysiology and manifestations of fever in various regions in India including bacterial, parasitic and viral causes (e.g.Dengue, Chikungunya, Typhus)	Y	17	885, 902
IM4.6	Discuss and describe the pathophysiology and manifestations of malaria	Y	17	940
IM4.7	Discuss and describe the pathophysiology and manifestations of the sepsis syndrome	Y	17	885
IM4.8	Discuss and describe the pathophysiology, aetiology and clinical manifestations of fever of unknown origin (FUO) including in a normal host, neutropenic host, nosocomial host and a host with HIV disease	Y	17	882
Topic: Miscellaneous Infections				
IM25.8	Enumerate the indications for use of newer techniques in the diagnosis of these infections	N	17	884
Topic: Dermatology, Venereology & Leprosy				
DR9.1	Classify, describe the epidemiology, etiology, microbiology pathogenesis and clinical presentations and diagnostic features of Leprosy	Y	17	931
DR9.4	Enumerate, describe and identify lepra reactions and supportive measures and therapy of lepra reactions	Y	17	931
DR9.5	Enumerate the indications and describe the pharmacology, administration and adverse reaction of pharmacotherapies for various classes of leprosy based on national guidelines	Y	17	931
DR9.6	Describe the treatment of Leprosy based on the WHO guidelines	Y	17	931

COMPETENCY CODE	COMPETENCY DESCRIPTION	CORE (Y/N)	CHAPTER No.	PAGE NOS.
DR10.1	Identify and classify syphilis based on the presentation and clinical manifestations	Y	17	961
DR10.3	Enumerate the indications and describe the pharmacology, administration and adverse reaction of pharmacotherapies for syphilis	Y	17	961
DR10.4	Describe the prevention of congenital syphilis	Y	17	961
DR10.6	Describe the etiology, diagnostic and clinical features of non-syphilitic sexually transmitted diseases (chancroid, donovanosis and LGV)	Y	17	959, 960, 961
DR10.8	Enumerate the indications and describe the pharmacology, indications and adverse reactions of drugs used in the non-syphilitic sexually transmitted diseases (chancroid, donovanosis and LGV)	Y	17	959, 960, 961
DR10.9	Describe the syndromic approach to ulcerative sexually transmitted disease	Y	17	965
DR10.10	Describe the etiology, diagnostic and clinical features and management of gonococcal and non gonococcal urethritis	Y	17	958
Topic: Acute Myocardial Infarction/ IHD				
IM2.3	Discuss and describe the lipid cycle and the role of dyslipidemia in the pathogenesis of atherosclerosis	Y	18	1027
IM2.18	Discuss and describe the indications, formulations, doses, side effects and monitoring for drugs used in the management of dyslipidemia	Y	18	1028
Topic: Diabetes Mellitus				
IM11.1	Define and classify diabetes	Y	18	1001
IM11.2	Describe and discuss the epidemiology and pathogenesis and risk factors and clinical evolution of type 1 diabetes	Y	18	1002
IM11.3	Describe and discuss the epidemiology and pathogenesis and risk factors economic impact and clinical evolution of type 2 diabetes	Y	18	1002
IM11.4	Describe and discuss the genetic background and the influence of the environment on diabetes	N	18	1002
IM11.6	Describe and discuss the pathogenesis and precipitating factors, recognition and management of diabetic emergencies	Y	18	1013, 1015, 1016, 1019
IM11.9	Describe and recognise the clinical features of patients who present with a diabetic emergency	Y	18	1013, 1015, 1016
IM11.11	Order and interpret laboratory tests to diagnose diabetes and its complications including: glucoses, glucose tolerance test, glycosylated hemoglobin, urinary micro albumin, ECG, electrolytes, ABG, ketones, renal function tests and lipid profile	Y	18	1004, 1005, 1011, 1012
IM11.14	Recognise the presentation of hypoglycaemia and outline the principles on its therapy	Y	18	1016
IM11.15	Recognise the presentation of diabetic emergencies and outline the principles of therapy	Y	18	1013, 1015, 1016
IM11.16	Discuss and describe the pharmacologic therapies for diabetes their indications, contraindications, adverse reactions and interactions	Y	18	1006, 1009
IM11.18	Describe and discuss the pharmacology, indications, adverse reactions and interactions of drugs used in the prevention and treatment of target organ damage and complications of Type II Diabetes including neuropathy, nephropathy, retinopathy, hypertension, dyslipidemia and cardiovascular disease	Y	18	1020, 1021, 1022
IM11.22	Enumerate the causes of hypoglycaemia and describe the counter hormone response and the initial approach and treatment	Y	18	1016

Continued

COMPETENCY CODE	COMPETENCY DESCRIPTION	CORE (Y/N)	CHAPTER No.	PAGE NOS.
IM11.23	Describe the precipitating causes, pathophysiology, recognition, clinical features, diagnosis, stabilisation and management of diabetic ketoacidosis	Y	18	1013
IM11.24	Describe the precipitating causes, pathophysiology, recognition, clinical features, diagnosis, stabilisation and management of Hyperosmolar non ketotic state	N	18	1015
Topic: Thyroid dysfunction				
IM12.1	Describe the epidemiology and pathogenesis of hypothyroidism and hyperthyroidism including the influence of iodine deficiency and autoimmunity in the pathogenesis of thyroid disease	Y	18	978, 983, 986
IM12.3	Describe and discuss the physiology of the hypothalamopituitary - thyroid axis, principles of thyroid function testing and alterations in physiologic function	Y	18	969, 977
IM12.4	Describe and discuss the principles of radio iodine uptake in the diagnosis of thyroid disorders	Y	18	977
IM12.11	Interpret thyroid function tests in hypo and hyperthyroidism	Y	18	978, 983
IM12.12	Describe and discuss the iodisation programs of the government of India	Y	18	986
IM12.13	Describe the pharmacology, indications, adverse reaction, interactions of thyroxine and antithyroid drugs	Y	18	978
IM12.15	Describe and discuss the indications of thionamide therapy, radio iodine therapy and surgery in the management of thyrotoxicosis	Y	18	978
Topic: Physical Medicine & Rehabiliation				
PM8.4	Describe metabolic co-morbidities like SIADH, diabetes mellitus, insipidus and endocrine dysfunction following TBI	Y	18	975
Topic: Geriatrics				
IM24.2	Perform multidimensional geriatric assessment that includes medical, psycho-social and functional components	Y	19	1037
IM24.5	Describe and discuss the aetiopathogenesis clinical presentation identification, functional changes, acute care, stabilization, management and rehabilitation of depression in the elderly	Y	19	1042
IM24.7	Describe and discuss the aetiopathogenesis, clinical presentation, identification, functional changes, acute care, stabilization, management and rehabilitation of personality changes in the elderly	N	19	1039
IM24.13	Describe and discuss the aetiopathogenesis, clinical presentation, identification, functional changes, acute care, stabilization, management and rehabilitation of falls in the elderly	Y	19	1044
IM24.19	Enumerate and describe the social problems in the elderly including isolation, abuse, change in family structure and their impact on health.	Y	19	1052
IM24.22	Describe and discuss the aetiopathogenesis, clinical presentation, complications, assessment and management of nutritional disorders in the elderly	Y	19	1051

Brief Contents

Detailed Contents

1 Diseases of Blood

Q. Give a brief account of erythropoietin (EPO), recombinant human erythropoietin (rHuEPO) and darbepoetin alpha.

Q. What are the ectopic sources of EPO?

- EPO is a glycoprotein having a molecular weight of 36,000 dalton. It is primarily produced by the juxtatubular interstitial cells of the renal cortex. In foetus, liver is the primary site of production of EPO.
- Hypoxia is the most potent stimulus for EPO production. Kidneys respond to hypoxia by increased production of EPO. Another important stimulant is the presence of anaemia.
- EPO stimulates erythropoiesis by acting on the erythropoietic stem cells, stimulating their increased proliferation (Flowchart 1.1). It may also protect neuronal cells from noxious stimuli.
- Ectopic sources of EPO are given in Table 1.1.

RECOMBINANT HUMAN ERYTHROPOIETIN

- It has the same biological effects as endogenous erythropoietin.
- Available as erythropoietin-α and erythropoietin-β.
- Indications for use of recombinant human erythropoietin are given in Box 1.1.
- Not recommended in patients with heart failure having anaemia.

ADVERSE EFFECTS

- Hypertension, bleeding, increased risk of thrombosis, headache, arthralgia, cough, nausea, oedema, diarrhoea, hypertension, venous thromboembolism and progression of cancers. It can cause pure red cell aplasia in patients with chronic kidney disease.

DARBEPOETIN ALPHA

- An erythropoiesis-stimulating protein similar to EPO.
- Produced in Chinese hamster ovary cells by recombinant DNA technology.

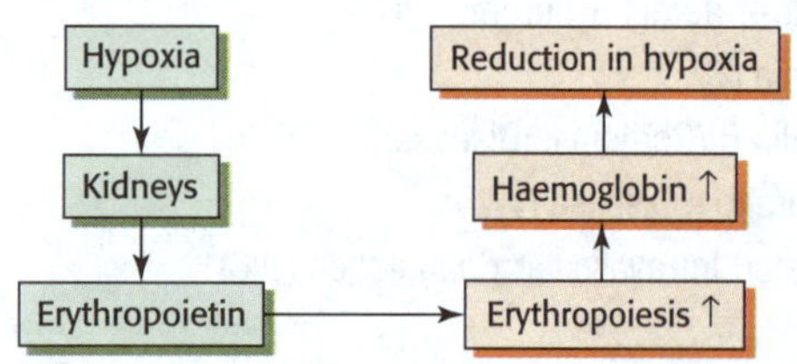

Flowchart 1.1 Erythropoietin Production and Its Action.

TABLE 1.1 Ectopic Sources of EPO

• Polycystic kidneys	• Renal carcinoma
• Cerebellar haemangioblastoma	• Hepatoma
• Uterine fibroma	• Phaeochromocytoma

BOX 1.1 Indications of Recombinant Human Erythropoietin

- Treatment of anaemia associated with chronic kidney disease; patients with normal or low iron stores need concomitant administration of iron to achieve an optimal erythropoietic response. Target is to maintain haemoglobin around 11–11.5 g/dL
- Chemotherapy-induced anaemia (haemoglobin <10 g/dL) in patients with cancer when intent of chemotherapy is noncurative
- Treatment of zidovudine-induced anaemia in HIV patients
- Treatment of anaemic patients (haemoglobin >10 to ≤13 g/dL) who are at high risk for perioperative blood loss from elective, non-cardiac, non-vascular surgery so as to reduce the need for allogeneic blood transfusions
- Patients of myelodysplastic syndrome with anaemia having low risk (low transfusion burden and low endogenous serum erythropoietin levels)

- Half-life approximately three times that of rHuEPO and hence needs to be given less frequently.
- Side effect profile and therapeutic value similar to rHuEPO; not approved for zidovudine-induced anaemia and for perioperative blood loss.

Q. Discuss briefly about haematopoietic growth factors (HGFs).

- HGFs act at different stages of haematopoietic cell differentiation.
- Some HGFs such as interleukin (IL)-1, IL-3, IL-6 exert their primary effects early in stem cell differentiation and are therefore important for the differentiation of multiple blood lineages.
- Others such as EPO, granulocyte colony-stimulating factor (G-CSF), granulocyte–macrophage colony-stimulating factor (GM-CSF) and thrombopoietin (TPO) exert their effects later in the differentiation cascade, and their effects are more lineage specific. Their recombinant forms are available for therapeutic use.

ERYTHROPOIETIN

- Discussed above.

GRANULOCYTE COLONY-STIMULATING FACTOR

- Promotes survival, stimulates proliferation of neutrophil progenitors and promotes their differentiation into mature neutrophils. In addition, it causes premature release of neutrophils from the bone marrow and enhances their phagocytic function.
- Normally, it is produced by endothelial cells, fibroblasts and macrophages.
- Also available as pegylated G-CSF which has longer duration of action.
- Indications of G-CSF are given in Table 1.2.

TABLE 1.2 Indications for Use of G-CSF

Indications	Comments
Primary prophylaxis (to reduce chances of febrile neutropenia following chemotherapy) for solid tumours and non-myeloid malignancies	If risk of febrile neutropenia is high (>20%) as determined by disease characteristics and myelotoxicity of drugs used ***OR*** If risk of febrile neutropenia is intermediate (10%–20%), age >65 years, presence of coexisting illnesses (including COVID-19) and poor performance status
Primary prophylaxis after autologous stem cell transplantation for non-myeloid malignancy following myeloablative chemotherapy	May be administered after allogeneic stem cell transplantation although there may be increased risks of severe graft-versus-host disease and transplantation-related death
For mobilising haematopoietic progenitor cells into the peripheral blood for peripheral stem cell transplantation	—
Secondary prophylaxis in patients with solid tumours and non-myeloid malignancies with a previous history of febrile neutropenia	Indicated only for those who require high-dose chemotherapy and any dose reduction may compromise treatment outcome (e.g. patients with oestrogen-receptor-negative breast cancer or non-Hodgkin's lymphoma)
May be administered in patients with febrile neutropenia who have high risk of infection-related complications, prolonged (>10 days) and severe neutropenia (<100/μL), hypotension, multiorgan dysfunction or invasive fungal infection	Not routinely recommended in all patients with neutropenia with or without and fever
Radiation-induced myelosuppression following nuclear/radiological incident	—

DOSE

- G-CSF is given in a dose of 5 μg/kg daily as subcutaneous injection. Pegylated G-CSF is given as a one-time dose of 6 mg subcutaneously for each cycle of chemotherapy.

ADVERSE EFFECTS

- Fever and bone and joint pains. Secondary myeloid tumours can occur in some patients as a late adverse effect.

GRANULOCYTE–MACROPHAGE COLONY-STIMULATING FACTOR

- It causes an increase in neutrophil, eosinophil, macrophage and sometimes lymphocyte counts.
- Usually administered as a daily subcutaneous injection of 250 μg/m^2.
- Both G-CSF and GM-CSF appear to have similar efficacy in the indications given above.

THROMBOPOIETIN

- It is the most potent cytokine promoting proliferation and maturation of megakaryocytes. It also primes the platelets to aggregate in response to subthreshold levels of thrombin, collagen and adenosine diphosphate (ADP).
- Normally produced by liver, skeletal muscles and kidneys.
- In cancer patients receiving chemotherapy, it has been shown to reduce the duration of postchemotherapy thrombocytopenia, though there is no increase in survival.
- However, many patients produce antibodies against TPO and these antibodies also cross-react with and neutralise endogenous TPO to produce a paradoxical thrombocytopenia.
- Indications of TPO are given in Table 1.3.

ADVERSE EFFECTS

- Adverse effects include headache, dizziness, muscle ache, nausea and rarely serious effects, such as vascular occlusions producing myocardial infarction, stroke and portal vein thrombosis. TPO-mimetics should be avoided in patients with thrombocytopenia associated with myelodysplastic syndrome (MDS) as they may increase the risk of progression to acute myeloid leukaemia.

Q. Define eosinophilia. What are the common causes of eosinophilia?

- Eosinophilia is an absolute eosinophil count exceeding 500/μL. Common causes of eosinophilia are given in Table 1.4.

Q. Discuss the abnormalities of red cells that can be seen on a peripheral blood smear examination. (IM 9.10)

- Common abnormalities in red blood cells on peripheral smear are given in Table 1.5 along with relevant figures.

TABLE 1.3 Indications of TPO

Disease Conditions With Thrombocytopenia	Approved TPO-receptor Agonists
Refractory immune thrombocytopenic purpura (ITP)	Eltrombopag, romiplostim, avatrombopag
Aplastic anaemia	Eltrombopag and romiplostim
Chronic liver disease about to undergo invasive procedures	Avatrombopag, lusutrombopag
Hepatitis C infection receiving interferon therapy	Eltrombopag

TABLE 1.4 Common Causes of Eosinophilia

- Helminthic infestations
- Loeffler's syndrome
- Tropical eosinophilia
- Eosinophilic pneumonia
- Allergic conditions
  - Hay fever
  - Atopic dermatitis
  - Allergic rhinitis
  - Asthma (including allergic bronchopulmonary aspergillosis)
  - Serum sickness
- Drugs (including drug reaction with eosinophilia and systemic symptoms [DRESS])
  - Antibiotics (sulphonamides, nitrofurantoin, cephalosporins, dapsone, penicillins, vancomycin)
  - Aspirin
  - Allopurinol
  - Anticonvulsants (carbamazepine, lamotrigine, valproic acid)
  - Antiretroviral agents (abacavir, nevirapine, raltegravir, efavirenz)
- Collagen vascular diseases
  - Rheumatoid arthritis
  - Eosinophilic granulomatosis with polyangiitis (Churg–Strauss syndrome)
  - Microscopic polyangiitis
- Malignancies
  - Hodgkin's lymphoma
  - Chronic myeloid leukaemia
  - Solid organ cancers
  - Eosinophilic leukaemia
- Idiopathic hypereosinophilic syndrome

TABLE 1.5 Common Abnormalities in Red Blood Cells

Abnormality	Description	Causes	Smear Findings
Anisocytosis	Variations in the size of red blood cells	Iron-deficiency anaemia, megaloblastic anaemia, moderate or severe thalassaemia, post-transfusion, sideroblastic anaemia	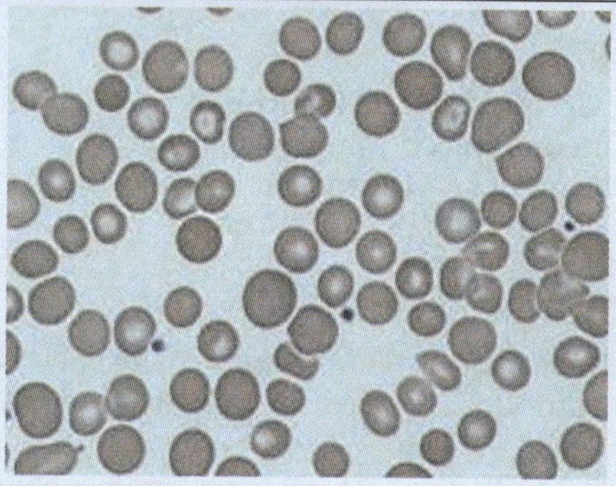
Poikilocytosis	Variations in the shape of red blood cells	Iron-deficiency anaemia, thalassaemia, sideroblastic anaemia	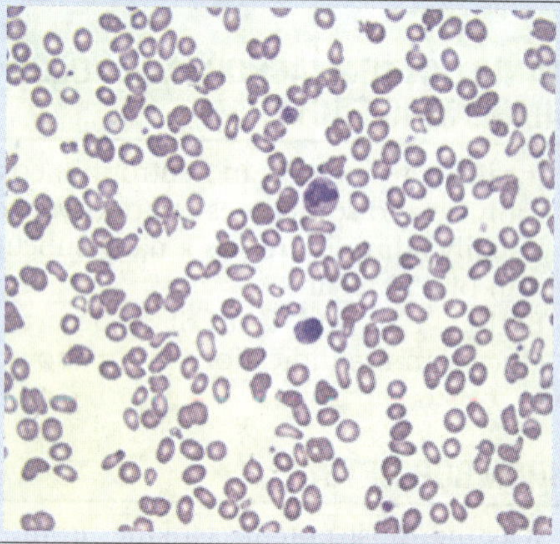
Microcytosis	Red blood cells smaller than their normal size (<75 fL)	Iron-deficiency anaemia, thalassaemia, sideroblastic anaemia	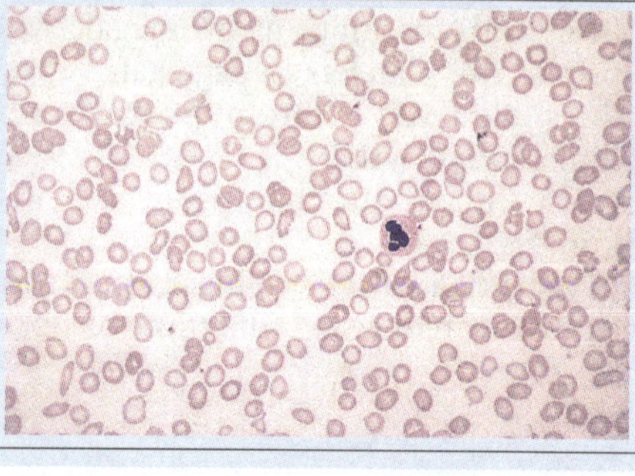

TABLE 1.5 Common Abnormalities in Red Blood Cells—cont'd

Abnormality	Description	Causes	Smear Findings
Macrocytosis	Red blood cells larger than 100 fL; may be oval or round	Oval macrocytes: megaloblastic anaemias, myelodysplasia Round macrocytes: liver disease, alcoholism	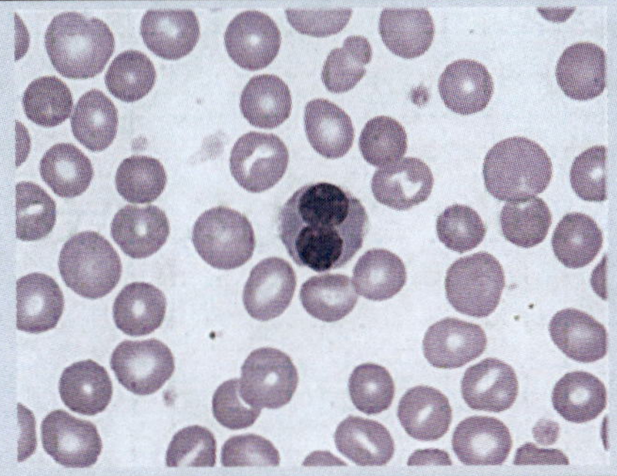
Hypochromia	Red cells having lower haemoglobin as judged by their appearance under microscopy with central pallor more than one-third the diameter of red cell	Iron-deficiency anaemia, thalassaemia, sideroblastic anaemia	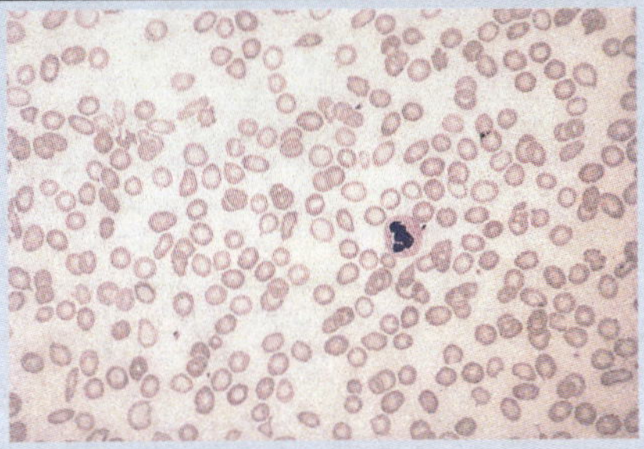
Polychromasia	Red blood cells show colour variability; some (usually the majority) are usual red coloured, while others are bluish	Reticulocytosis	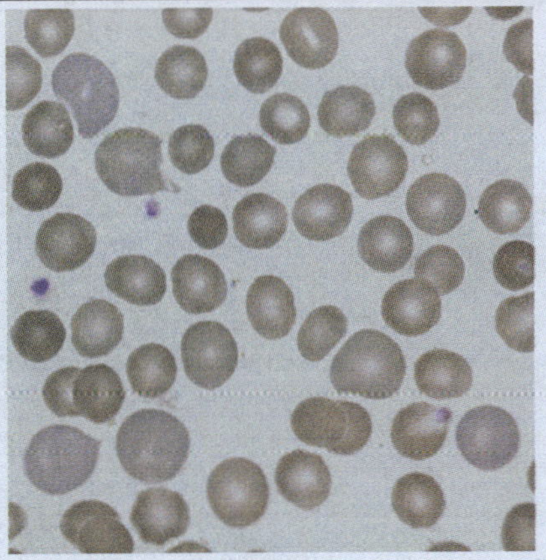
Basophilic stippling or punctate basophilia	Presence of scattered deep blue dots in the cytoplasm of red blood cells with Romanowsky staining; represent altered ribosomes	Pathologically damaged young red cells, seen in severe anaemia, β-thalassaemia, alcohol abuse, chronic lead poisoning, megaloblastic anaemia, sideroblastic anaemia, severe infections	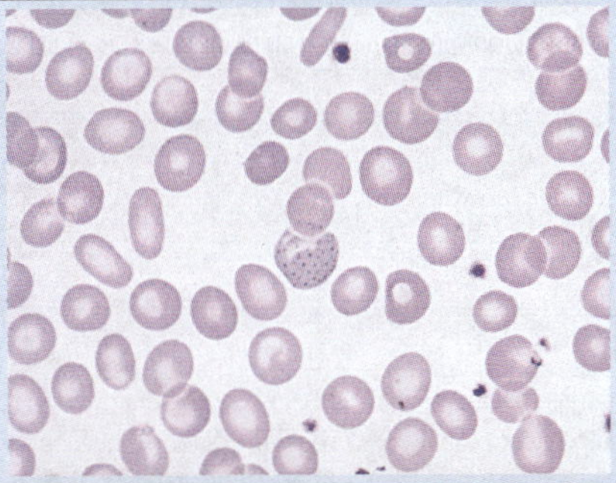
Target cells (codocytes)	Flat red cells with a central mass of haemoglobin (dense area), surrounded by a ring of pallor (pale area) and an outer ring of haemoglobin (dense area)	Chronic liver diseases, hyposplenism, haemoglobinopathies	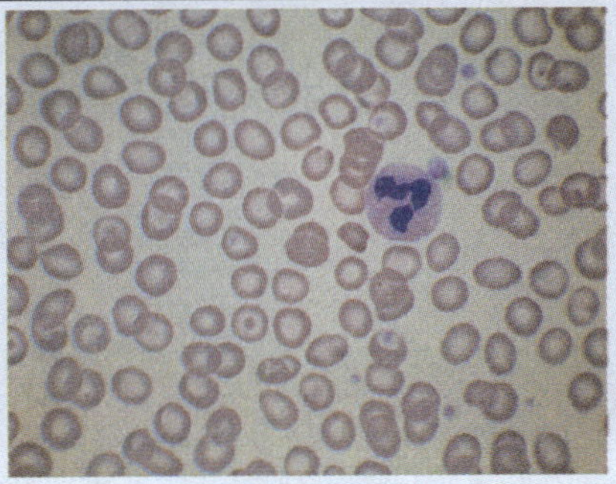

Continued

TABLE 1.5 Common Abnormalities in Red Blood Cells—cont'd

Abnormality	Description	Causes	Smear Findings
Tear drop cells (dacrocytes)	Appear like tear drops	Extramedullary haematopoiesis (e.g. primary myelofibrosis, thalassaemia)	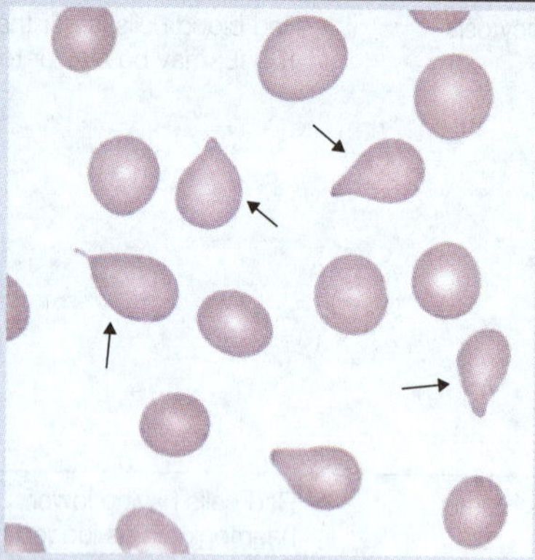
Howell–Jolly bodies	Remnants of nuclear material left in the erythrocyte after the nucleus is extruded; normally removed by the spleen. Appear as solitary round mass, relatively large within haemoglobinised portion of red blood cell; on Wright's stain, appear dark blue or purple	Non-functioning or absent spleen, megaloblastic anaemias	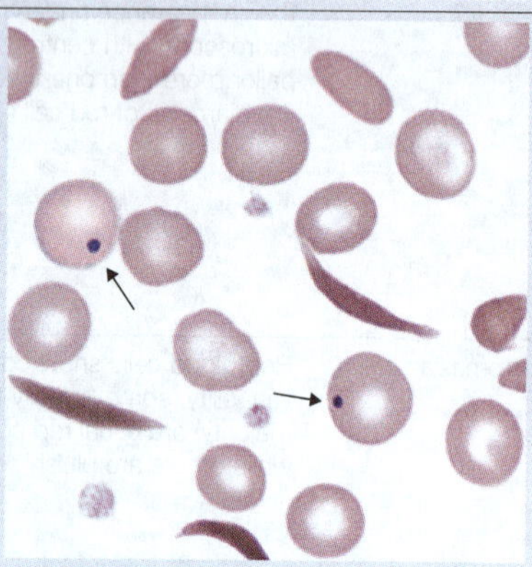
Heinz's bodies (Ehrlich's bodies)	Formed from denatured aggregated haemoglobin; appear as a submembranous, small round mass in red cells on supravital stain; not seen with routinely stained film	Thalassaemia, haemolysis in glucose-6-phosphate dehydrogenase (G6PD) deficiency, asplenia, chronic liver disease	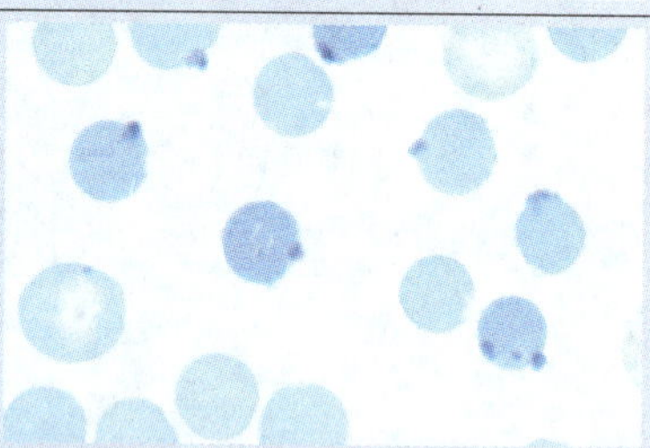
Spur cells (acanthocytes)	Red blood cells showing irregular spicules	Abetalipoproteinaemia, advanced liver disease, hyposplenism	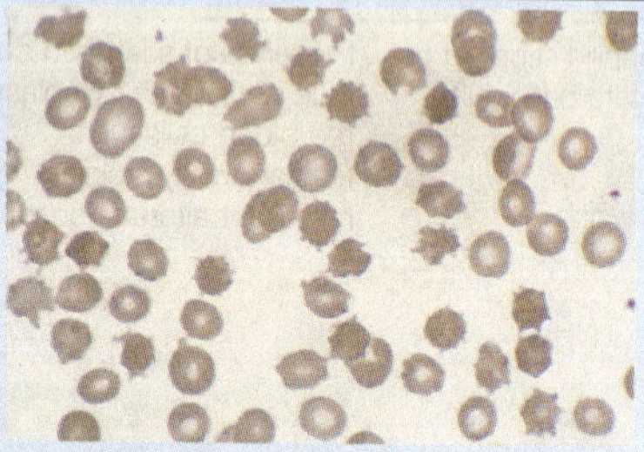
Burr cells (echinocytes)	Red blood cells showing regularly placed spicules; spicules are smaller in size compared to those in burr cells	Uraemia, post-transfusion	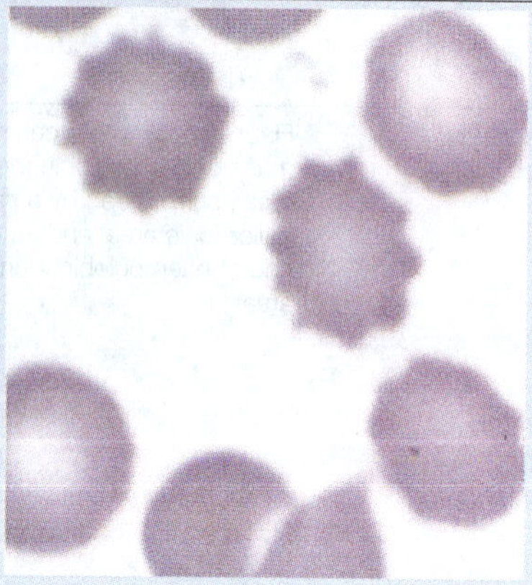

TABLE 1.5 Common Abnormalities in Red Blood Cells—cont'd

Abnormality	Description	Causes	Smear Findings
Schistocytes (helmet cells)	Fragmented red cells (with central pallor often missing)	Microangiopathic haemolysis (thrombotic thrombocytopenic purpura, disseminated intravascular coagulation)	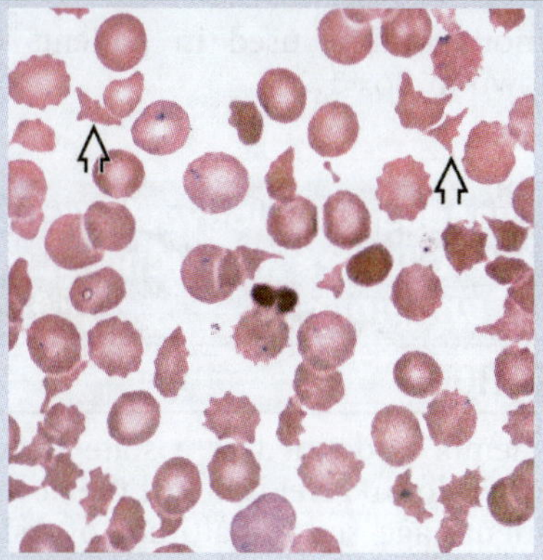
Spherocytosis	Small, densely packed red cells with loss of central pallor	Hereditary spherocytosis, immunohaemolytic anaemias	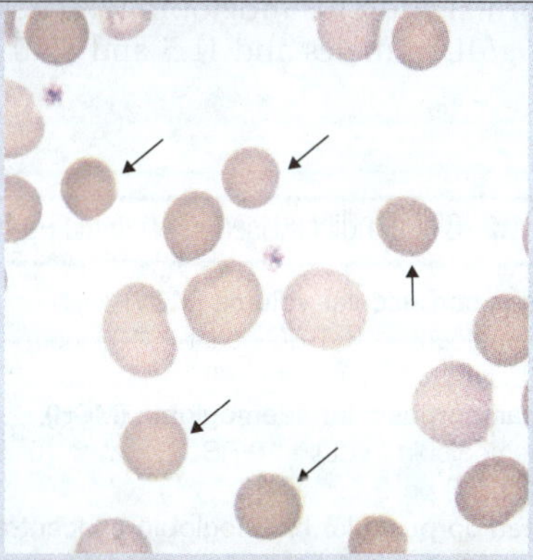
Microspherocytosis	Red blood cells are both hyperchromic and significantly reduced in size and diameter	Burns, microangiopathic haemolytic anaemia; occur in low numbers in patients with a spherocytic haemolytic anaemia	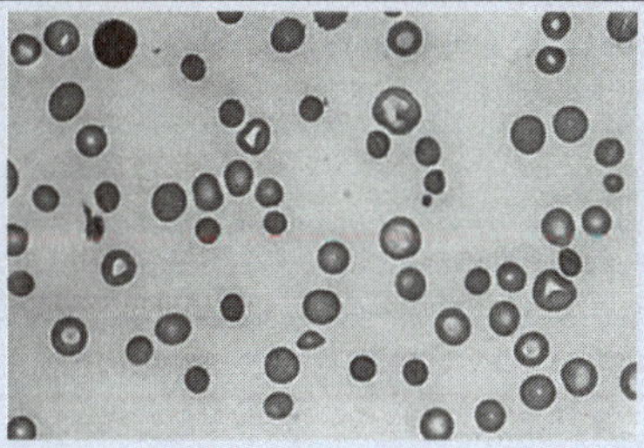
Sickle cells	Sickle-shape red cells	Sickle cell disease, haemoglobin SC disease	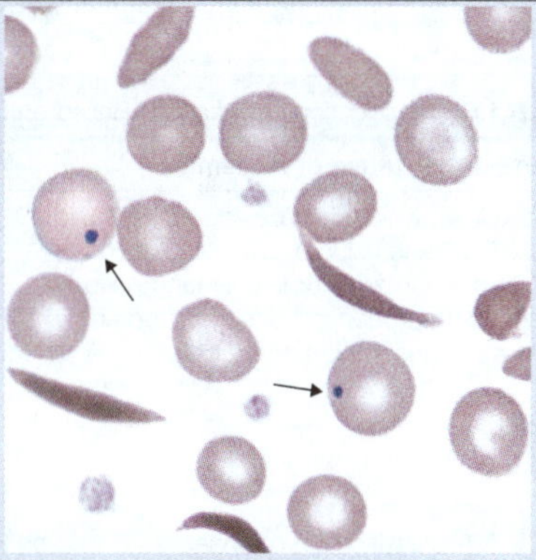

Q. Describe various blood indices used in patients with anaemia. (IM 9.7)

- Various indices used in patients of anaemia are shown in Box 1.2.

Q. Discuss aetiology, classification, clinical features and general management of anaemia. (IM 9.1, IM 9.12)

DEFINITION

- Anaemia is defined as a state in which the blood haemoglobin level is below the normal range for the patient's age, sex and altitude of residence.
- Normal adult haemoglobin level lies between 13 and 16 g/dL in males and 11.5 and 15.0 g/dL in females.

CLASSIFICATION

- Anaemias can be classified in two ways:
  1. Based on the cause of anaemia (Table 1.6)
  2. Based on the morphology of red cells (Table 1.6)
  3. Based on reticulocyte count (Table 1.7)

AETIOLOGY

- Various causes of anaemia are given in Table 1.8.

CLINICAL FEATURES

SYMPTOMS

- Fatigue, lassitude, dyspnoea, palpitation.
- Dizziness, headache, syncope, tinnitus, vertigo.
- Irritability, sleep disturbances, lack of concentration.

BOX 1.2 Blood Indices Used in Anaemic Patients

- **Mean corpuscular volume (MCV)**
  Haematocrit × 10/RBC count × 106 (normal range 90 ± 8 fL; fL stands for femtolitres)
- **Mean corpuscular haemoglobin (MCH)**
  Haemoglobin (g/dL) ×10/RBC count × 10^6 (normal range 30 ± 3 pg)
- **Mean corpuscular haemoglobin concentration (MCHC)**
  Haemoglobin (g/dL) × 10/haematocrit (normal range 33 ± 2%)
- **Red blood cell count**
  Males 4.5–5.5 × 10^6/mm^3; Females 4–4.5 × 10^6/mm^3
- **Reticulocyte count**
  Expressed as percent of red blood cell count (normal < 2.5%)
- **Corrected reticulocyte count (to adjust for severity of anaemia)**
  Expressed as % reticulocyte count × observed haematocrit/ normal haematocrit
- **Reticulocyte index or reticulocyte production index**
  Expressed as % reticulocyte count × observed haematocrit/ normal haematocrit × ½ (multiplication by ½ is to account for premature release of reticulocytes from bone marrow in anaemia) (normal range 0.5%–1.5%; a value >2% indicates normal bone marrow response in anaemic patient)
- **Red cell distribution width (RDW)**
  (Standard deviation of red cell volume ÷ mean cell volume) × 100 (normal 11–16) (an index of variation in cell volume within the red cell population)
  Increased in iron-deficiency anaemia, megaloblastic anaemia and myelodysplastic syndrome
  Normal in thalassaemias, anaemia of chronic disease and bone marrow aplasia

TABLE 1.6 Classification of Anaemias Based on Cause and Morphology of Red Cells

Based on the Cause of Anaemia	Based on the Morphology of Red Cells

• Blood loss, which may be acute or chronic
  • Acute (large volume over short period)
  • Chronic (small volume over long period)
• Inadequate production of normal red cells
• Excessive destruction of red cells
	• Normocytic (renal disease, haemolytic anaemia, autoimmune diseases, microangiopathic anaemia)
	• Microcytic (iron-deficiency, thalassaemias, anaemia of chronic disease, sideroblastic anaemia, lead intoxication)
	• Macrocytic (list given later)

TABLE 1.7 Classification of Anaemias Based on Reticulocyte Count

Low Reticulocyte Count	Normal Reticulocyte Count	High Reticulocyte Count
• Iron deficiency • Aplastic anaemia • Folate deficiency • Vitamin B_{12} deficiency • Chronic disease • Renal failure • Lead poisoning • Coeliac disease • Hypothyroidism	• Thalassaemia trait • Acute bleeding (early phase) • Sideroblastic anaemia	• Antibody-mediated haemolysis • Sickle cell disease • Hereditary spherocytosis • Thalassaemia intermedia and major • Glucose-6-phosphate dehydrogenase (G6PD) deficiency • Hypersplenism • Haemolytic uremic syndrome • Thrombotic thrombocytopenic purpura • Disseminated intravascular coagulation • Hypersplenism

TABLE 1.8 Causes of Anaemia

Due to blood loss	
• Acute blood loss	Trauma, postpartum bleeding, haematemesis, ruptured ectopic pregnancy, aortic aneurysm rupture
• Chronic blood loss	Hookworms, bleeding peptic ulcer, haemorrhoids, excessive menstrual loss
Due to inadequate production of normal red cells	
• Deficiency	Iron, vitamin B_{12}, folate, vitamin A
• Toxic factors	Chronic inflammatory and infective diseases, renal failure, hepatic failure, drugs leading to aplastic anaemia
• Endocrine deficiency	Hypothyroidism, hypoadrenalism, reduced erythropoietin due to renal failure, hypogonadism, hypopituitarism
• Marrow invasion	Leukaemias, fibrosis, secondary carcinoma
• Marrow failure	Hypoplastic or aplastic anaemia
• Maldevelopment	Sideroblastic anaemia, haemoglobinopathies like sickle cell disease and thalassaemias, neoplastic disorders of erythropoiesis
Due to excessive destruction of red cells (haemolytic anaemias)	
• Genetic disorders	Red cell membrane, haemoglobin or enzyme abnormalities
• Acquired disorders	Immune, toxic, mechanical and infectious causes, hypersplenism

- Throbbing in head and ears, paraesthesia in fingers and toes.
- Anorexia, indigestion, nausea, bowel disturbances.
- Angina, intermittent claudication, transient cerebral ischaemia.
- Symptoms of cardiac failure.
- Amenorrhoea, polymenorrhoea.

SIGNS

- Pallor of skin, palms, oral mucous membrane, nail beds and palpebral conjunctivae. The palmar creases become as pale as the surrounding skin when the haemoglobin is below 7 g/dL.
- Tachycardia, wide pulse pressure.
- Oedema.
- Cervical venous hum, hyperdynamic precordium.
- Ejection systolic murmur, best heard over the pulmonary area.
- Cardiac dilatation and later signs of cardiac failure.
- Hypotension, tachycardia, tachypnoea and altered mental status in severe acute blood loss.

Signs Suggesting a Specific Aetiology of Anaemia
(Table 1.9)

TABLE 1.9 Signs Suggesting a Specific Aetiology of Anaemia

• Jaundice	Haemolytic anaemia, chronic hepatitis, megaloblastic anaemia
• Angular cheilitis	Iron-deficiency anaemia
• Glossitis	Iron-deficiency anaemia, vitamin B_{12} deficiency, folate deficiency
• Splenomegaly	Malaria, chronic haemolytic anaemia, acute infection, leukaemia, lymphoma, portal hypertension, vitamin B_{12} deficiency
• Frontal bossing	Chronic haemolytic anaemia
• Neurological changes (dementia, ataxia)	Vitamin B_{12} deficiency

APPROACH TO DIAGNOSIS

- Flowchart 1.2 gives an approach to diagnose cause of anaemia.

GENERAL MANAGEMENT

- Blood transfusion:
  - In significantly symptomatic and severely anaemic patients.
  - In critically ill patients, transfuse if haemoglobin <7 g/dL, if haemodynamically stable.
  - For patients with cardiovascular disease, a transfusion threshold of 8 g/dL is recommended.
  - Packed cells are preferred.
  - Care has to be taken to avoid circulatory overloading, especially in elderly patients; intravenous frusemide 20 mg may be given prior to transfusion.
- Massive transfusion protocol:
  - Patients with trauma who are actively bleeding require massive transfusion protocol (MTP) to be activated if more than four units of packed red blood cells need to be given.
  - MTP involves infusion of packed red cells, plasma and platelet-rich plasma in the ratio of 1:1:1.
- Prompt treatment of infections and cardiac failure.

Q. Give a brief description about the anaemias due to blood loss.

- Anaemias due to blood loss could be acute (large volume over short period) or chronic (small volume over long period).

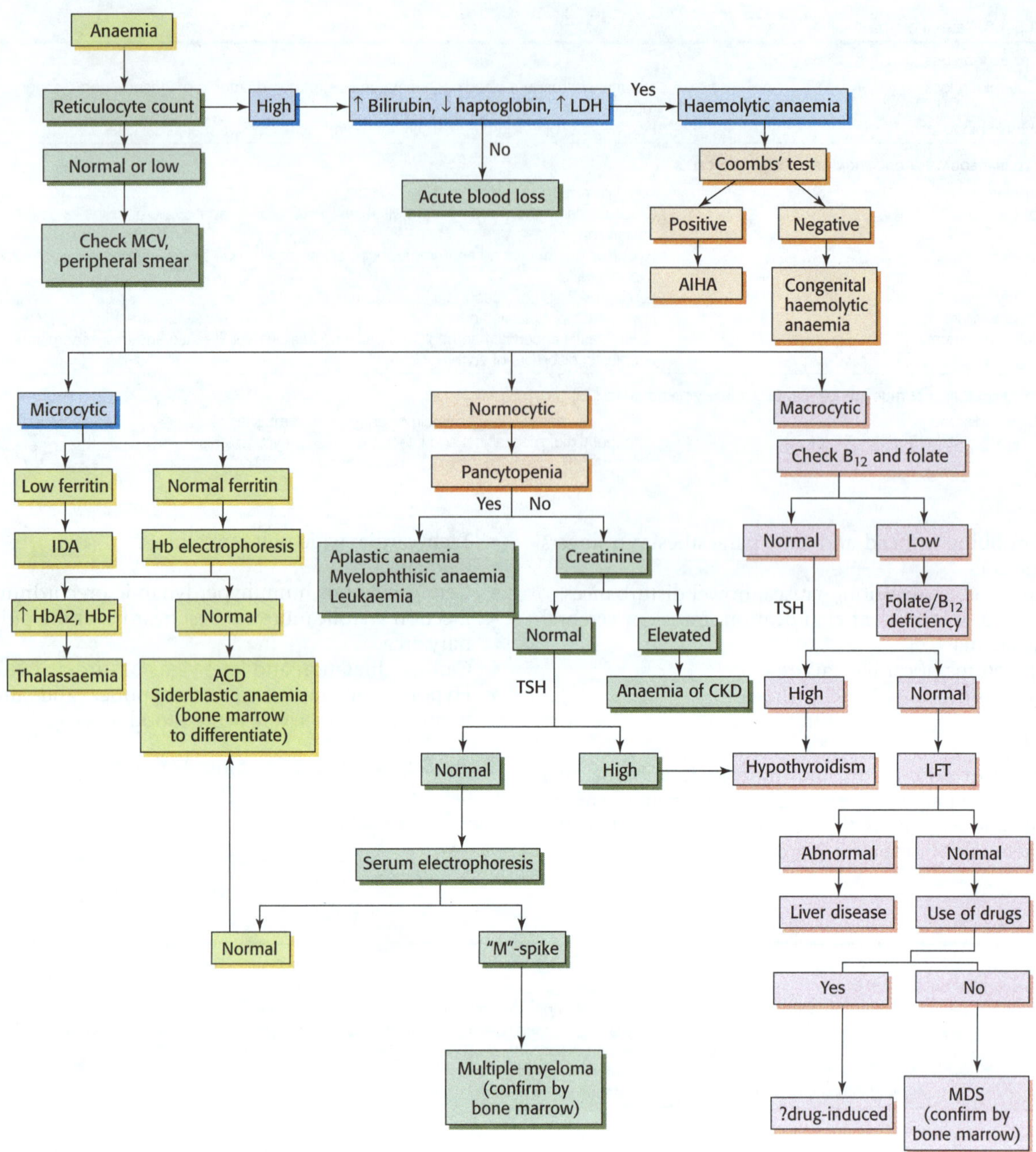

MCV, mean corpuscular volume; AIHA, autoimmune haemolytic anaemia; IDA, iron-deficiency anaemia; ACD, anaemia of chronic disease; TSH, thyroid stimulating hormone; CKD, chronic kidney disease; LFT, liver function tests; MDS, myelodysplastic syndrome

Flowchart 1.2 Approach to Diagnosis of Cause of Anaemia.

ANAEMIAS DUE TO ACUTE BLOOD LOSS

- A healthy adult can lose about 500 mL of whole blood without any ill effect, for example blood donation. When more is lost, compensatory mechanisms come into operation. The blood flow to skin and skeletal muscle is reduced, conserving the blood flow to vital organs like brain, kidney and heart. With continued blood loss, these compensatory mechanisms fail.

CLINICAL FEATURES

- In the initial stages, pulse rate rises and blood pressure is maintained though postural hypotension may be there (Box 1.3). Patient is pale, cold and sweating in severe bleeding.
- If bleeding gets arrested, production of plasma replenishes the volume loss, resulting in dilution of remaining red cells. Anaemia appears in 24–36 hours. This anaemia gets corrected in a few weeks, provided body iron stores are not depleted.

BOX 1.3 Earliest Signs of Blood Loss

Earliest signs to look for in a patient with suspected blood loss (especially internal bleeding) are postural hypotension and tachycardia.

- If bleeding continues, compensatory mechanisms fail and hypovolaemic shock ensues, which may result in death.

INVESTIGATIONS

- Haemoglobin and haematocrit are normal in early stages (before haemodilution).
- Anaemia (haemoglobin and haematocrit drop) develops in 24–36 hours due to haemodilution.
- A transient leucoerythroblastic blood picture may be seen in very early stages.
- Reticulocytosis occurs at a later stage.
- Elevated lactate and base deficit in case of cellular hypoperfusion.

TREATMENT

- If symptomatic, replace the blood loss by transfusion of packed cells.
- In trauma patients, use MTP with red cells, fresh frozen plasma and platelets in ratio of 1:1:1.

ANAEMIA OF CHRONIC BLOOD LOSS

- Compensatory mechanisms replenish the plasma volume and red cell loss. But if the blood loss continues, body iron stores are depleted and anaemia due to iron deficiency appears.

Q. Discuss the aetiology, clinical manifestations, diagnosis and management of iron-deficiency anaemia. (IM 9.13; IM 9.8)

Q. Write a short note on Plummer–Vinson syndrome (sideropenic dysphagia; Patterson–Kelly syndrome).

- Iron deficiency is the most common cause of anaemia.
- Most of the body iron is in haemoglobin (~2500 mg). Myoglobin has ~130 mg iron. Surplus iron is stored in the liver.
- Daily iron requirement in diet is 10–15 mg of which nearly 10% is absorbed in males and 15% in females.
- Children who consume large amounts of cow milk are particularly prone to iron deficiency:
  - Cow milk's iron is poorly absorbed.
  - Calcium present in milk inhibits iron absorption.
  - Cow's milk may cause protein allergy with GI bleeding (occult or gross).
- Approximately 20 mL of senescent red cells are cleared daily, and the 20 mg of iron in those cells is recycled for the production of new red cells.
- Postpartum, iron is lost as lactoferrin in breast milk. However, these losses are balanced by absence of menstruation in the lactating woman.

AETIOLOGY (CAUSES OF IRON DEFICIENCY) (Table 1.10)

- Iron-deficiency anaemia without other clinical clues of intestinal malabsorption is one of the most common extraintestinal manifestations of coeliac disease.
- High hepcidin levels occur in inflammatory conditions (including obesity and cancers) which produces sequestration of iron leading to functional iron deficiency. Later, inflammatory conditions can produce absolute iron deficiency due to decreased iron absorption signalled by high hepcidin levels.`

CLINICAL FEATURES

- Clinical features of iron-deficiency anaemia include the general symptoms and signs of anaemia (refer to clinical features of anaemia).
- Characteristic features of iron deficiency include the following:
  - Angular stomatitis.
  - Glossitis.
  - Brittle fingernails, platynychia, koilonychia.
  - Pica indicates a craving for nonnutritive and strange items like coal, earth (geophagia), tomatoes, greens, starch and ice (pagophagia; more specific for iron deficiency).
- Restless leg syndrome (compulsion to move limbs while at rest) may occur due to reduced brain iron levels.

TABLE 1.10 Causes of Iron-Deficiency Anaemias

• Physiological (increased iron demand)	Postnatal growth spurt, adolescent growth spurt, menstruation, pregnancy (2nd and 3rd trimester)
• Iron loss	Hookworm infestation, schistosomiasis, menorrhagia, postpartum haemorrhage, peptic ulcer, piles, neoplastic diseases, gastric erosions from anti-inflammatory drugs, malaria (intravascular haemolysis with subsequent loss of haemoglobin iron in urine; also suppresses erythropoiesis), haemolytic processes (e.g. autoimmune haemolytic anaemia, prosthetic valve, march haemoglobinuria, paroxysmal nocturnal haemoglobinuria), severe haemoptysis, haemodialysis
• Inadequate diet	Includes excessive consumption of cow milk in children
• Malabsorption (reduced iron absorption)	Inflammatory bowel disease, post-gastrectomy, coeliac disease, autoimmune gastric atrophy, *Helicobacter pylori* gastritis, bariatric procedures (particularly those bypassing duodenum), intestinal wall oedema in heart failure

- Iron deficiency during pregnancy may reduce foetal brain maturation, cognitive defects in child and maternal depression.
- **Plummer–Vinson syndrome** (sideropenic dysphagia; Patterson–Kelly syndrome) occurs in long-standing iron deficiency. The characteristic features are as follows:
  - Iron-deficiency anaemia.
  - Glossitis.
  - Koilonychia.
  - Postcricoid web resulting in dysphagia. The dysphagia is intermittent and is more for solids than liquids. The postcricoid web can be demonstrated endoscopically or by barium swallow. It may also be due to weakened oesophageal muscle contractions.
  - Increased risk of squamous cell carcinoma of pharynx and oesophagus.
  - Treatment of Plummer–Vinson syndrome is with iron. Dilatation of web in case of severe obstruction may be required.
  - Upper GI endoscopy may be required every year for the early diagnosis of cancers.

INVESTIGATIONS

- To confirm iron-deficiency anaemia.
- To determine the cause of iron deficiency.

TO CONFIRM IRON-DEFICIENCY ANAEMIA

- Haemoglobin is reduced.
- Mean corpuscular volume (MCV) is reduced (microcytosis) to below 80 fL.
- Peripheral smear study:
  - Microcytosis and hypochromia. Causes of microcytosis are given in Table 1.11.
  - Elliptical cells and poikilocytes are seen in severe cases.
- Reticulocyte count is normal; it is elevated if blood loss is the aetiology and the patient has enough iron stores or is on iron therapy.

TABLE 1.11 Common Causes of Microcytosis

• Iron deficiency	• Anaemia of chronic disease (some cases)
• Thalassaemia	• Lead poisoning
• Sideroblastic anaemia	

- Bone marrow study:
  - Moderate erythroid hyperplasia.
  - On Prussian blue stain, iron stores in erythroid precursors and macrophages are markedly reduced or absent. In contrast, in anaemia of chronic disease, increased stainable iron is seen in marrow macrophages but absent or reduced in erythroid precursors.
- Plasma iron is reduced and total iron-binding capacity (TIBC) is raised.
- Plasma transferrin saturation is reduced (<10%).
- Serum ferritin level is reduced (<15–30 μg/L; normal >100 μg/L); may be normal or elevated in presence of inflammation, liver disease or malignancy despite iron deficiency (Flowchart 1.3).

Other Tests

- Elevated red cell protoporphyrin (normal <30 μg/dL) reflecting the body's inability to complete haem production without iron; also elevated in lead poisoning.
- Serum-soluble transferrin receptor is increased. Unlike serum ferritin levels, it is not increased in the presence of inflammation.
- Hepcidin produced by the liver regulates iron concentrations and tissue iron distribution via inhibition of intestinal iron absorption, iron reclamation by macrophages and iron mobilisation from hepatic stores. It binds to its receptor, ferroportin, present on enterocytes and macrophages, thereby preventing iron export from these cells into the plasma (ferroportin is a transmembrane iron transporter). Hepcidin production is decreased in iron-deficiency anaemia and increased during inflammation and iron overloading.

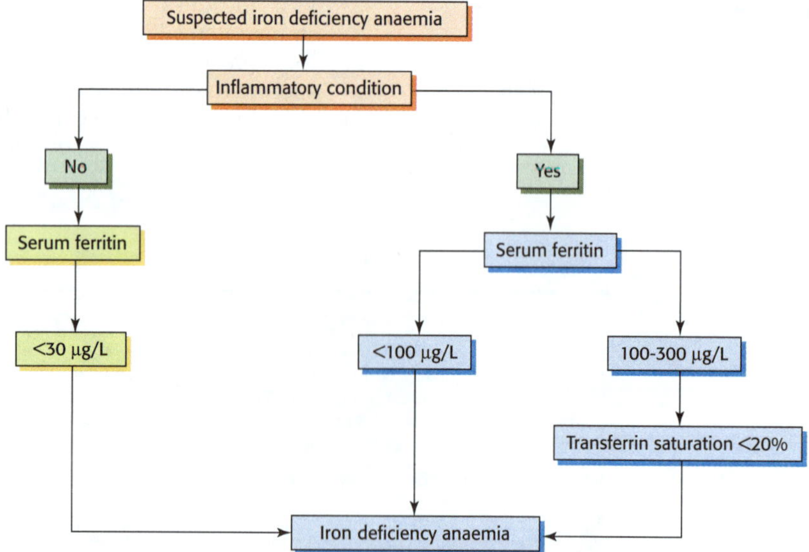

Flowchart 1.3 Workup for a Patient With Suspected Iron-Deficiency Anaemia.

TABLE 1.12 Investigations to Determine the Cause of Iron Deficiency

• Stool for occult blood and hookworm infestation • Sigmoidoscopy and colonoscopy • Upper gastrointestinal endoscopy • Barium meal and barium enema (less sensitive than colonoscopy and upper GI endoscopy)	• Investigations may be done for malabsorption if diarrhoea or steatorrhoea present or anaemia is refractory despite iron • Urine for schistosomiasis

TABLE 1.13 Important Causes of Failure to Respond to Oral Iron Therapy

• Not taking the tablets (check for grey- or black-coloured stools)	• Ingestion of certain drugs along with iron that reduce its absorption (antacids, H_2-receptor blockers, proton-pump inhibitors, tetracyclines)
• Continuing blood loss	• Concomitant inflammatory condition
• Severe malabsorption (including administration of oral iron with milk)	• Wrong diagnosis

TO DETERMINE THE CAUSE OF IRON DEFICIENCY

- The investigations chosen depend on the age, sex, history and physical findings. In the absence of any clear clue, investigations may be done, mainly to check for chronic blood loss from the GI tract (Table 1.12).

MANAGEMENT

- Treatment of underlying cause.
- Treatment of iron deficiency by oral iron therapy or parenteral iron therapy.

ORAL IRON THERAPY

- Most patients can be treated with oral iron.
- Commonly used salts of iron include ferrous sulphate, ferrous gluconate, ferrous fumarate, ferrous ascorbate, ferric maltol and others. Ferrous sulphate tablets contain 20% elemental iron; ferrous gluconate 12% elemental iron and ferrous fumarate 33% elemental iron. Ferric maltol absorption is good even in presence of inflammatory conditions of bowel.
- Dose is one tablet two to three times a day on empty stomach. It should not be given with food because phosphates, phytates and tannates in food bind iron and impair its absorption.
- Another form of iron is ferrous ascorbate. Iron absorption is greater as compared to other formulations of iron. Further iron absorption is not inhibited by food intake.
- Some patients develop side effects like dyspepsia, constipation or diarrhoea. This can be relieved by taking iron with food or by changing to a different iron salt or a controlled-release preparation or a liquid preparation.
- Response to oral iron therapy usually appears within 7–10 days. This is in the form of a reticulocyte response, usually not exceeding 10%.
- Some patients do not respond to therapy (Table 1.13).
- Duration of oral iron therapy:
  - Haemoglobin should return to normal range in 4–6 weeks, and if not, failure of response should be sought.
  - If haemoglobin has returned to normal, oral iron should be continued for at least 6 months or may be 1 year in order to replenish the body iron stores.
  - In those patients whose iron deficiency is recurrent (e.g. malabsorption, deficient intake, continuing blood loss), long-term iron supplements at a minimum dose are required.

PARENTERAL IRON THERAPY

- Parenteral iron therapy should be prescribed only if diagnosis of iron deficiency is definite, as otherwise therapy might result in iron overload.
- It should be avoided in patients with sepsis as iron can promote microbial growth.
- Indications for parenteral iron therapy are given in Box 1.4. Dose calculation is given in Box 1.5.

Iron Sorbitol

- Given intramuscularly but never intravenously.
- Recommended dose is 1.5 mg of iron/kg body weight daily, to a maximum of total dose calculated, but not exceeding 2.5 g.

BOX 1.4 Indications of Parenteral Iron Therapy

- Genuine gastrointestinal intolerance to oral iron
- Disorders of GI tract interfering with the absorption of iron, e.g. severe malabsorption, bariatric procedures like gastric bypass/resection or duodenal bypass
- When the rate of iron (blood) loss exceeds the rate at which iron can be absorbed
- When a gastrointestinal condition may worsen with oral iron (e.g. some cases with ulcerative colitis)
- For correction of severe anaemia associated with rheumatoid arthritis, late pregnancy and following major operations
- Non-compliance
- Anaemia (iron deficiency) associated with chronic renal failure (along with EPO) when oral iron does not produce expected rise in haemoglobin; also indicated in patients with anaemia and chronic renal failure who are on regular haemodialysis

BOX 1.5 Calculation of Total Dose of Intravenous Iron Required

Iron needed in mg = (normal haemoglobin – patient's haemoglobin) × weight in kg × 2.21 + 1000

- Normal haemoglobin in males is taken as 14 g/dL and females as 12 g/dL
- The addition of 1000 is to correct the deficit and replenish the body iron stores

Iron Dextran

- It may be given intramuscularly but is ideal for intravenous use.

Intramuscular

- Recommended dose is 100 mg daily until the total required dose is administered or to a maximum of 2 g. It should be administered deep intramuscularly into the buttocks using a 'Z-track technique'.

Intravenous

- Test dose of 25 mg IV over 5 minutes is required before administration of full dose.
- The total dose required is diluted in a solution of isotonic saline and infused over 4–6 hours.

Iron Sucrose

- Doses of 100–200 mg/day as an IV injection over 3–15 minutes or up to 500 mg over an infusion time of 3 hours.

Ferric Gluconate

- Maximum recommended daily dose is 125 mg IV due to potential for acute adverse reactions.

Newer Intravenous Preparations

- Iron ferumoxytol (510 mg over 15 minutes), ferric carboxymaltose (15 mg of iron/kg, maximum 1000 mg of iron in a single dose over 15 minutes) and ferric derisomaltoside (1000 mg infusion).

ADVERSE EFFECTS OF IRON THERAPY (Table 1.14)

TABLE 1.14 Adverse Effects of Parenteral Iron Preparations

• Pain and swelling at injection site	• Splenomegaly
• Tatooing due to extravasation	• Aseptic meningitis
• Arthralgias	• Anaphylactic reactions
• Fever	• Sarcomas at intramuscular injection sites
• Generalised urticarial rash	• Haemosiderosis
• Generalised lymphadenopathy	• Hypophosphataemia

Q. How will you differentiate various causes of hypochromic microcytic anaemias?

DIFFERENTIAL DIAGNOSES

- Differential diagnosis of hypochromic microcytic anaemia is given in Table 1.15.

Q. Give a brief account of sideroblastic anaemias.

- Sideroblastic anaemias are inherited or acquired disorders characterised by refractory anaemia, variable number of hypochromic red cells in peripheral smear, excess of iron and ring sideroblasts in the marrow and decreased production of mature red blood cells.

CAUSES

- Causes of sideroblastic anaemia are given in Table 1.16.

CHARACTERISTIC FEATURES OF NON-CLONAL CONDITIONS

- Iron overload.
- Characteristic ringed sideroblasts are seen in the bone marrow. The iron-laden mitochondria surround the nucleus and appear as the pathognomonic 'rings' with Prussian blue staining.

OTHER FEATURES

- Bone marrow erythroid hyperplasia and ineffective erythropoiesis.
- Microcytic and hypochromic red cells on peripheral smear.
- Marked increase in serum iron and transferrin saturation.
- Cardiac and liver MRI may show iron overload.

COMPLICATIONS

- Severe anaemia.
- Increased incidence of thrombosis particularly with MDS/MPN-RS-T.
- About 10% of the patients with sideroblastic anaemia develop acute myeloblastic leukaemia.
- Iron overload due to ineffective erythropoiesis and blood transfusions.

TREATMENT

- Some patients respond when the drugs, toxins or alcohol are withdrawn.
- In occasional cases, there is a response to pyridoxine or folic acid.
- Erythropoiesis stimulating agents (erythropoietin or darbepoetin) may reduce red blood cell transfusion need in

TABLE 1.15 Differential Diagnosis of Hypochromic Microcytic Anaemia

Laboratory Parameters	Iron-Deficiency Anaemia	β-Thalassaemia	Anaemia of Chronic Disease	Sideroblastic Anaemia
• Serum iron (normal 60–170 μg/dL)	<30 μg/dL	Normal to high	<50 μg/dL	Normal to high
• TIBC (normal 300–450 μg/dL)	>350 μg/dL	Normal	<300 μg/dL	Normal
• Saturation (%) (normal 20%–50%)	<10	30–80	10–20	30–80
• Serum ferritin (normal 15–300 μg/L)	<15 μg/L	50–300 μg/L	30–200 μg/L	50–300 μg/L
• Haemoglobin A_2 (normal <3%)	Reduced	Increased	Normal	Reduced

TABLE 1.16 Causes of Sideroblastic Anaemia

Non-clonal Conditions	Clonal Conditions (Stem Cell Disorders)
Hereditary sideroblastic anaemia • X-linked disorder ***Acquired sideroblastic anaemia*** • Drugs (e.g. isoniazid, cycloserine, chloramphenicol, busulphan, D-penicillamine, linezolid) • Alcohol abuse • Lead, arsenic or zinc toxicity • Pyridoxine or copper deficiency • Others (rheumatoid arthritis, carcinoma)	• Some myelodysplastic syndromes (MDS) and myeloproliferative neoplasms (MPN): • MDS with ring sideroblasts (MDS-RS) • MDS/MPN with RS and thrombocytosis (MDS/MPN-RS-T)

patients with MDS-RS and suboptimal endogenous erythropoietin response (erythropoietin <500 mU/L).

- Lenalidomide or luspatercept in MDS-RS or MDS/MPN-RS-T.
- Otherwise, treatment is supportive with transfusions and iron chelation to prevent organ damage from iron overload.

Q. Discuss the aetiology, diagnosis and management of megaloblastic macrocytic anaemias.

Q. Enumerate the causes of macrocytosis and its diagnostic workup. (IM 9.1)

MEGALOBLASTIC MACROCYTIC ANAEMIAS

- Megaloblasts are abnormal erythroblasts seen in the bone marrow of patients with deficiency of vitamin B_{12}, folate or both. Megaloblasts are abnormally large in size and nucleated. They are well haemoglobinised.
- Macrocytes are erythrocytes with increased MCV. Normal MCV ranges between 80 and 100 femtolitres (fL). It is calculated as:

$$\text{MCV (fL)} = [\text{Haematocrit (\%)} \times 10]/[\text{RBC count } (10^6/\ \mu\text{L})]$$

- Hence, the term megaloblastic macrocytic anaemia describes the outstanding feature (increased size of cells) of both the bone marrow and the peripheral blood. Some patients with macrocytosis and anaemia may not have megaloblasts in bone marrow. This is known as nonmegaloblastic macrocytic anaemia.
- Megaloblastic anaemias are characterised by macro-ovalocytes and hypersegmented neutrophils in the peripheral smear, which are absent in nonmegaloblastic macrocytic anaemia.

CONDITIONS RESULTING IN MACROCYTOSIS (Table 1.17)

TABLE 1.17 Causes of Macrocytosis

• Vitamin B_{12} deficiency • Folate deficiency • Antineoplastics (azathioprine, 6-mercaptopurine, 5-fluorouracil, cytosine arabinoside, imatinib, methotrexate, hydroxyurea) • Nitrous oxide abuse	• Liver disease • Alcohol • Aplastic anaemia • Myelodysplasia • Acyclovir, zidovudine, stavudine • Trimethoprim, pyrimethamine, metformin, phenytoin	• Myeloid leukaemia • Hypothyroidism • Sideroblastic anaemia • Spuriously elevated MCV by automated blood cell counter (hyperglycaemia, marked leucocytosis, cold agglutinins) • Pregnancy, newborn (physiological)

CONDITIONS RESULTING IN NON-MEGALOBLASTIC MACROCYTIC ANAEMIA (Table 1.18)

TABLE 1.18 Causes of Non-megaloblastic Macrocytic Anaemia

Physiological	Pregnancy, Newborn
Pathological	Alcohol, chronic liver disease, hypothyroidism, aplastic anaemia, sideroblastic anaemia, drugs (azathioprine, zidovudine, others), myelodysplasia, haemorrhage, haemolytic anaemia, erythropoietin treatment, copper deficiency

MECHANISM OF MEGALOBLASTIC ANAEMIA

- Most megaloblastic macrocytic anaemias are due to a deficiency of vitamin B_{12}, folate or both.
- Both vitamin B_{12} and folate are essential for DNA synthesis. Deficiency of one or both results in failure of DNA synthesis. This results in abnormal cell proliferation. The abnormality in cell proliferation mainly affects haemopoietic tissues (erythrocyte series, granulocyte series and megakaryocyte series) and gastrointestinal epithelial cells.
- Morphological changes in the erythrocyte series in the bone marrow are described as megaloblastic. When DNA synthesis is impaired, cell division is delayed, time between divisions increases, more cell growth occurs and cells become larger in size—'megaloblasts'. Synthesis of haemoglobin is unimpaired. The resultant mature erythrocytes derived from these megaloblasts are abnormally large (macrocytes) and abnormal in shape (usually oval) but well haemoglobinised.

- A large number of these megaloblastic erythroid cells are destroyed in the bone marrow (ineffective erythropoiesis):
  - This results in liberation of large amounts of lactate dehydrogenase (LDH) that rises to high levels in the blood.
- In the bone marrow, abnormal proliferation affecting the granulocyte series results in giant metamyelocytes, and the megakaryocyte series results in dysplastic megakaryocytes.

DIAGNOSTIC WORKUP FOR MACROCYTOSIS (Flowchart 1.4)

DIAGNOSIS OF MEGALOBLASTIC ANAEMIA (Table 1.19)

- Presence of macro-ovalocytes and hypersegmented neutrophils (Fig. 1.1) often indicate megaloblastic anaemia and a bone marrow examination may not be required. Round macrocytes generally indicate non-megaloblastic macrocytic anaemias.

MANAGEMENT

- Supportive therapy.
- Specific therapy:
  - Treatment of underlying cause of vitamin B_{12} or folate deficiency.
  - Vitamin B_{12} therapy.
  - Folate therapy.

SUPPORTIVE THERAPY

- Blood transfusions should be given in significantly symptomatic and severely anaemic patients. Adequate precautions are to be taken to avoid circulatory overloading, especially in elderly patients.

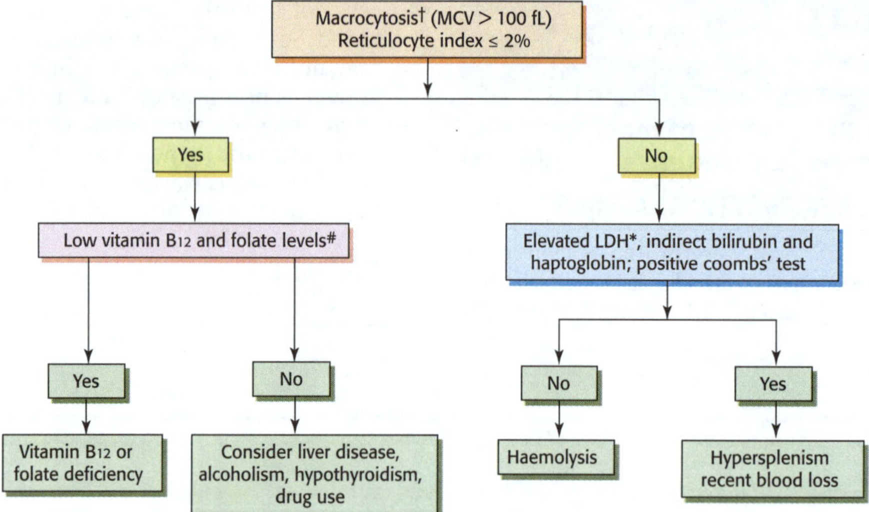

† Peripheral smear showing leucoerythroblastic picture indicates myelodysplastic syndrome and myelofibrosis
# Consider performing methylmalonic acid and homocysteine levels if vitamin B_{12} or folate levels are borderline low. Vitamin B_{12} deficiency produces elevated methylmalonic acid while folate deficiency produces elevated homocysteine level
* LDH = lactate dehydrogenase

Flowchart 1.4 Diagnostic Workup for Macrocytic Anaemia.

TABLE 1.19 Investigations for Megaloblastic Anaemia

INVESTIGATIONS

- Haemoglobin is reduced
- Mean corpuscular volume (MCV) is raised, usually more than 120 fL (macrocytes)
- RBC count is reduced
- Reticulocyte count is reduced
- Total leucocyte count is reduced
- Platelet count is reduced
- Peripheral smear study:
  - Oval macrocytosis
  - Poikilocytosis
  - Fragmented red blood cells
  - Hypersegmented neutrophils
- Indirect bilirubin is mildly elevated (due to increased breakdown of red cells in bone marrow)
- Serum iron is elevated
- Iron-binding capacity is reduced
- Serum ferritin level is increased
- Plasma lactate dehydrogenase is markedly increased
- Bone marrow study (not always required):
  - Hypercellular marrow
  - Megaloblastic erythroid cells
  - Giant metamyelocytes
  - Dysplastic megakaryocytes
  - Marrow iron stores increased
- Specific tests for B_{12}/folate deficiency:
  - Reduced serum B_{12}/folate
  - Plasma methylmalonic acid (MMA) elevated (in B_{12} deficiency)
  - Plasma homocysteine elevated
  - Plasma holotranscobalamin II reduced (in B_{12} deficiency)

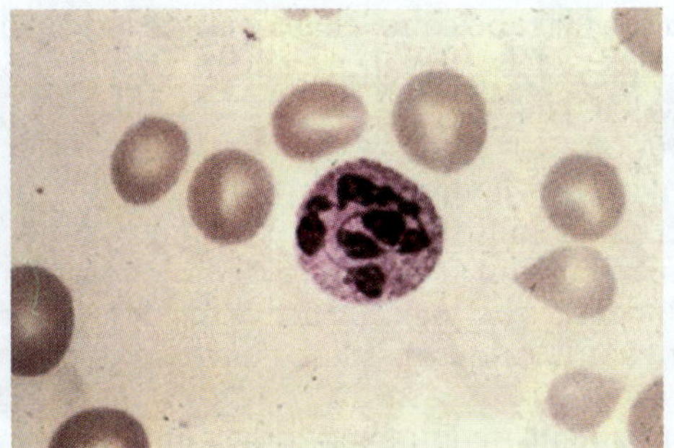

Fig 1.1 Hypersegmented neutrophil.

Intravenous frusemide, 20–40 mg may be given prior to transfusion.
- Treatment of infections.
- Treatment of cardiac failure.

Q. Discuss the aetiology, pathogenesis, clinical features, diagnosis and management of Addisonian pernicious anaemia.

- It is a megaloblastic macrocytic anaemia resulting from failure of secretion of intrinsic factor by the stomach not related to total gastrectomy. In the absence of intrinsic factor, dietary vitamin B_{12} is not absorbed and this results in vitamin B_{12} deficiency.

AETIOLOGY

- Autoimmune disease with permanent atrophy of gastric mucous membrane. Immune response is directed against gastric H^+/K^+-ATPase, which accounts for associated achlorhydria.

PATHOGENESIS

- Pathogenesis of pernicious anaemia is given in Flowchart 1.5.

CLINICAL FEATURES

- Both sexes equally involved.
- Usually occurs between 45 and 65 years of age.
- Higher incidence in people with blood group A.
- Onset and progression are often insidious.
- Clinical features are related to vitamin B_{12} deficiency (see below).
- Hypochlorhydria may lead to impaired gastric emptying that may produce dyspepsia, postprandial fullness and early satiety.
- Many patients have other autoimmune diseases including vitiligo, thyroid diseases, type 1 diabetes mellitus and Addison's disease (occur as part of autoimmune polyglandular endocrinopathy type 2).

INVESTIGATIONS

- Very low serum vitamin B_{12} levels.
- Antiintrinsic factor antibodies in the serum (in 70% of patients; highly specific). Must be tested >7 days after vitamin B_{12} injection to prevent false positive result.
- Antiparietal cell antibodies (in 85%–90%; less specific compared to antiintrinsic antibodies as also found at low frequency in other autoimmune diseases, e.g. Hashimoto's thyroiditis or type 1 diabetes, and in elderly subjects).
- Macrocytic blood picture.
- Megaloblastic bone marrow.
- Reticulocyte response to very small doses of parenteral vitamin B_{12}.
- Pentagastrin or histamine-fast achlorhydria.
- Elevated serum gastrin levels.
- Reduced serum pepsinogen I levels.
- Gastric biopsy showing mucosal atrophy.
- Low serum ferritin levels as iron deficiency is often present due to gastric atrophy.

TREATMENT

- Supportive therapy includes blood transfusion, treatment of infection and physiotherapy in nervous system involvement.

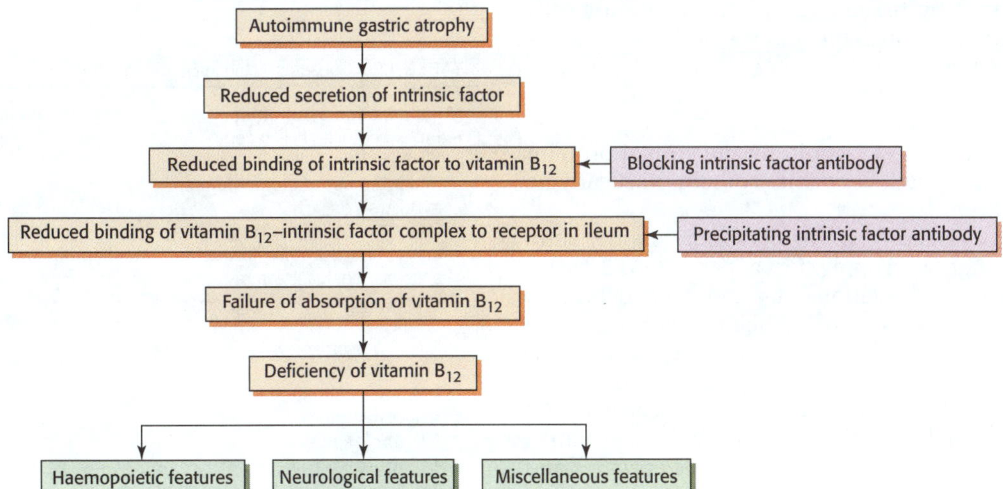

Flowchart 1.5 Pathogenesis of Addisonian Pernicious Anaemia.

- Vitamin B_{12} therapy:
  - Cyanocobalamin or hydroxocobalamin may be used. Another option is to use methylcobalamin, metabolically active form of vitamin B_{12}.
  - Initial dose of hydroxocobalamin is 1000 μg, deep intramuscularly once or twice every week for 4 weeks.
  - Maintenance dose is 1000 μg of hydroxocobalamin intramuscularly once in 2–3 months or 1000 μg of cyanocobalamin once in a month indefinitely.
  - An acceptable alternative is to give 1000–2000 μg of vitamin B_{12} orally daily for 1 month followed by 125–500 μg daily indefinitely. Absorption is by passive diffusion.
- Iron therapy with ferrous sulphate 200 mg thrice daily orally should be started soon after the commencement of vitamin B_{12} therapy if the patient has associated iron deficiency (dimorphic anaemia).

FOLLOW-UP

- Clinical and haematological examination once in 6 months.
- Early detection of carcinoma of stomach, which is three times more common in patients with pernicious anaemia. Gastric carcinoid is also more common in these patients as compared to general population.

Q. Write a short note on vitamin B_{12}.

Q. Discuss briefly the causes, manifestations and management of vitamin B_{12} deficiency. (IM 9.13)

VITAMIN B_{12}

- Vitamin B_{12} is essential for normal haemopoiesis and maintenance of normal integrity of the nervous system.
- Vitamin B_{12} belongs to the family of cobalamins. It is found only in trace amounts in tissues. It has to be converted to a biologically active form before it can be used by tissues. There are two biologically active forms of cobalamins in the body, both acting as coenzymes:
  1. Methylcobalamin
  2. Adenosylcobalamin
- The main sources of vitamin B_{12} are animal proteins and dairy products. Vegetables contain practically no vitamin B_{12}.
- Vitamin B_{12} is stored in the liver in a quantity sufficient enough to supply for a period of 3 years. Hence, the manifestations of vitamin B_{12} deficiency take at least 3 years to make their appearance.
- Acidic medium of the stomach and pepsin facilitate the breakdown of vitamin B_{12} that is bound to food proteins. The free B_{12} then binds to haptocorrins (HC) or R-factors released from salivary glands. In small intestine, HC is degraded by pancreatic enzymes and vitamin B_{12} binds to intrinsic factor secreted by gastric parietal cells. This complex is transported to the lower ileum where the complex dissociates and vitamin B_{12} is absorbed by the ileal cells. A small amount of ingested vitamin B_{12} can be absorbed by passive diffusion.
- In plasma, vitamin B_{12} is bound to two proteins, transcobalamin II and HC. Vitamin B_{12} attached to transcobalamin II is known as holotranscobalamin II. It denotes biologically active fraction that is transported to various tissues. Function of HC is not known.
- Normal daily requirement of vitamin B_{12} is 1–2 μg.

CAUSES OF VITAMIN B_{12} DEFICIENCY (Table 1.20)

- Approximately 10%–30% of patients on metformin have diminished B_{12} absorption due to calcium-dependent ileal membrane antagonism.
- Nitrous oxide inactivates cobalamin and its use in anaesthesia may precipitate haematologic and neurological deterioration in vitamin B_{12} deficient persons.

PATHOGENESIS OF NEUROLOGICAL INVOLVEMENT IN VITAMIN B_{12} DEFICIENCY

- Two mechanisms are responsible for neurologic complications of vitamin B_{12} deficiency:
  - Deficiency of methylcobalamin produces impairment in the conversion of homocysteine to methionine. Methionine is needed for the production of choline and choline-containing phospholipids. These are required by the neuronal cells.
  - Adenosylcobalamin, a B_{12}-containing cofactor, is required for the conversion of methylmalonyl-CoA to succinyl-CoA. Lack of this cofactor leads to increase in the levels of methylmalonyl-CoA and its precursor, propionyl-CoA. As a result, nonphysiologic fatty acids are synthesised and incorporated into neuronal lipids (Fig. 1.2).
- Severity of megaloblastic anaemia is inversely correlated with degree of neurologic dysfunction.

TABLE 1.20 Causes of Vitamin B_{12} Deficiency

Malabsorption syndromes	Inadequate intake

• Prolonged use of H_2-receptor blockers
• Prolonged use of proton-pump inhibitors
• Prolonged use of metfromin
• Lack of intrinsic factor (pernicious anaemia, postgastrectomy, gastric bypass surgery for obesity, atrophic gastritis)
• Ileal malabsorption
  • Crohn's disease
  • Coeliac disease
  • Ileal resection
  • Tropical sprue
  • Pancreatic insufficiency
• Infective causes (bacterial overgrowth, *Helicobacter pylori*, *Giardia*, tapeworm)
	• Alcoholics
	• Elderly
	• Pure vegetarians
	Defective transport
	• Transcobalamin II deficiency

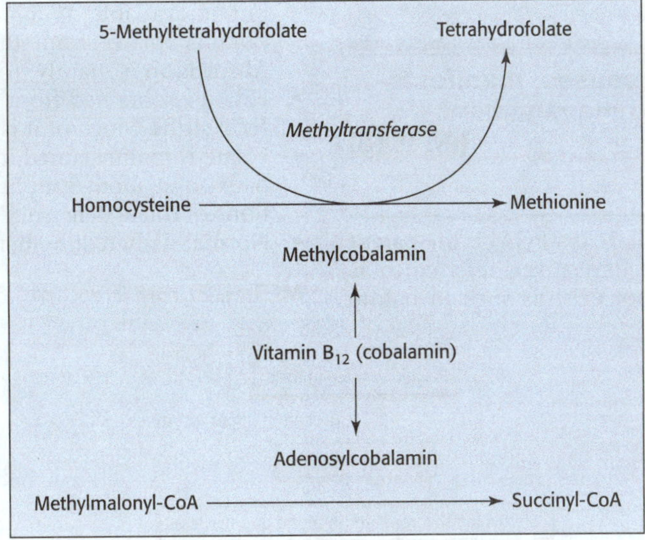

Fig. 1.2 Mechanism of neurological involvement in vitamin B_{12} deficiency.

MANIFESTATIONS (Fig. 1.3)

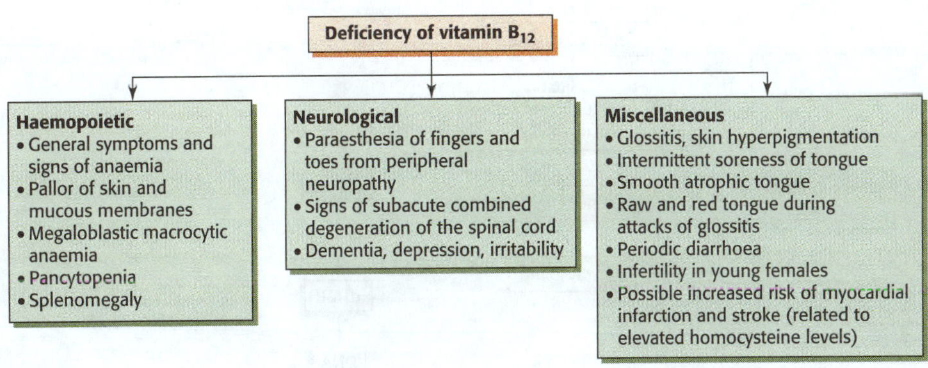

Fig. 1.3 Manifestations of vitamin B_{12} deficiency.

DIAGNOSIS

- Macrocytic anaemia.
- Hypersegmented neutrophils in peripheral smear.
- Pancytopenia. MDS and aplastic anaemia may also present with macrocytosis, reduced reticulocyte count and pancytopenia. In MDS, peripheral blood smear and bone marrow show dysplastic white blood cells while in aplastic anaemia, the marrow shows markedly reduced cellularity.
- Low serum vitamin B_{12} levels (<200 pg/μL). May be elevated if patient has associated myeloproliferative disorders, liver disease and intestinal bacterial overgrowth. Levels may be falsely low with folate deficiency, pregnancy and use of oral contraceptives.
- Elevated serum methylmalonic acid (MMA) and homocysteine levels. MMA is also elevated in the presence of renal failure.
- Low levels of holotranscobalamin II is a useful marker of early vitamin B_{12} deficiency. It can be used in patients with myeloproliferative disorders. Levels may be elevated in renal failure.
- Elevated LDH and indirect bilirubin due to ineffective erythropoiesis.

MANAGEMENT

- Treatment of underlying cause, whenever possible.
- Vitamin B_{12} therapy (cyanocobalamin, hydroxocobalamin or methylcobalamin may be used):
  - Initial dose of hydroxocobalamin is 1000 μg, deep intramuscularly once or twice a week for 4 weeks.
  - Maintenance dose is 1000 μg of hydroxocobalamin intramuscularly once in 2–3 months or 1000 μg of cyanocobalamin once in a month indefinitely (only when necessary).
  - An acceptable alternative is to give 1000–2000 μg of vitamin B_{12} orally daily for 1 month followed by 125–500 μg daily indefinitely (only when necessary).
  - Oral route is also used if patient does not have features of severe anaemia, neurological involvement or permanent alterations in gastrointestinal anatomy.
- Iron therapy with ferrous sulphate 200 mg thrice daily orally should be started soon after the commencement of vitamin B_{12} therapy if the patient has associated iron deficiency (dimorphic anaemia—macrocytosis and hypochromia).

Q. Give a brief account of folic acid.

Q. Discuss briefly the causes, manifestations, diagnosis and management of folate deficiency. (IM 9.13)

FOLIC ACID

- Folic acid (pteroylglutamic acid—PGA) is the parent compound of a group of derivatives, referred to as folates. Folic acid does not exist as such in nature but is available as a medicinal compound. Body obtains folates from the polyglutamates of food. Absorption is mainly from the jejunum.
- Folate is obtained from both vegetable and animal food stuffs. Much of it is destroyed by cooking.
- Folate is mainly stored in the liver. The stores are exhausted in about 3 months and hence the manifestations of folate deficiency appear in about 3 months.
- Normal daily requirement of folate is 100–200 μg.

METABOLISM (Flowchart 1.6)

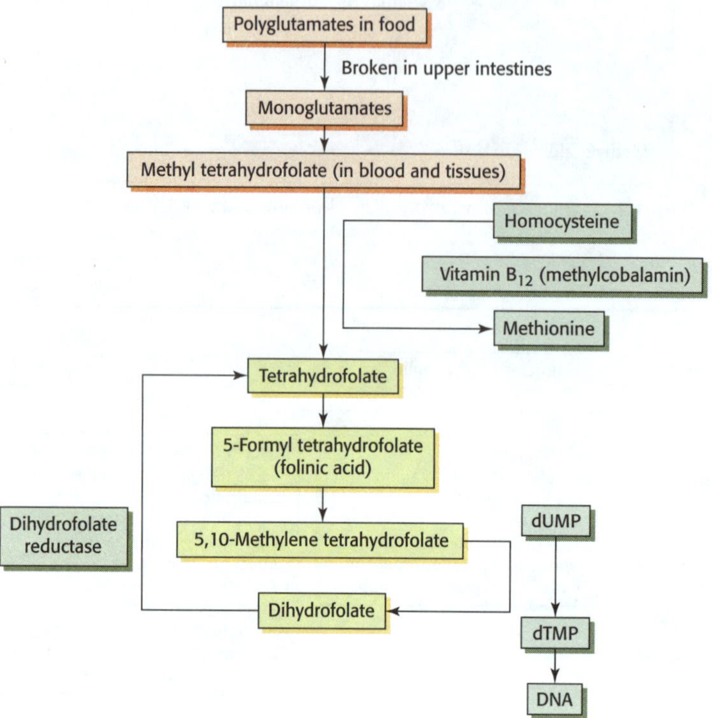

Flowchart 1.6 Metabolism of Folic Acid.

CAUSES OF FOLATE DEFICIENCY (Table 1.21)

TABLE 1.21 Causes of Folate Deficiency

• Inadequate intake or increased demand	Physiological—pregnancy, lactation, infancy Pathological—malignancies, haemolytic anaemias, chronic exfoliative skin disease, chronic inflammatory and infective diseases, haemodialysis
• Malabsorption	Diseases of upper small intestine like tropical sprue, coeliac disease, alcohol, phenytoin, primidone, metformin, cholestyramine, zinc deficiency
• Antifolate drugs	Methotrexate, trimethoprim, pyrimethamine, pentamidine, 5-fluorouracil, hydroxyurea, phenytoin, carbamazepine, valproate
• Increased loss	Vitamin B_{12} deficiency (loss in urine), chronic alcohol use (loss in bile)

CLINICAL MANIFESTATIONS OF FOLATE DEFICIENCY

- Features are similar to those seen with vitamin B_{12} deficiency.
- Glossitis, oral ulcers.
- Subacute combined degeneration of the spinal cord does not occur. However, some patients may develop neuropsychiatric features.
- Possible increased risk of myocardial infarction and stroke (related to elevated homocysteine levels).

DIAGNOSIS

- Low serum folate levels.
- Low red cell folate level.
- Macrocytic blood picture.
- Megaloblastic bone marrow.

- Normal or slightly reduced serum vitamin B_{12} levels.
- Elevated serum homocysteine level and normal MMA level.
- Elevated LDH and indirect bilirubin due to ineffective erythropoiesis.

MANAGEMENT

- Folic acid therapy:
  - An initial daily dose of 5 mg orally followed by a maintenance dose of 5 mg orally once a week.
  - All pregnant females should receive folic acid supplements (5 mg/day) by mouth.
  - Folic acid must never be given without vitamin B_{12} in Addisonian pernicious anaemia or other vitamin B_{12} deficiency anaemias. If given alone, the neurological features of vitamin B_{12} deficiency may be aggravated or precipitated.
- Folic acid deficiency from dihydrofolate reductase inhibitors (e.g. methotrexate) is treated with folinic acid (5-formyl tetrahydrofolate) as it is rapidly converted to the metabolically active form (tetrahydrofolate) without the need for dihydrofolate reductase.

Q. Describe the national programme for anaemia prevention. (IM 9.14)

- India is one of the countries with very high prevalence of anaemia in the world. Almost 58% of pregnant women in India are anaemic, and it is estimated that anaemia is the underlying cause for 20%–40% of maternal deaths in India. India contributes to about 80% of the maternal deaths due to anaemia in South Asia.
- Nutritional anaemia is a major public health problem in India and is primarily due to iron deficiency.
- The National Family Health Survey-3 (NFHS-3) data suggest that anaemia is widely prevalent among all age groups and is particularly high among the most vulnerable—nearly 58% among pregnant women, 50% among non-pregnant non-lactating women, 56% among adolescent girls (15–19 years), 30% among adolescent boys and around 80% among children under 3 years of age.
- The National Iron Plus Initiative for anaemia control is shown in Table 1.22.

Q. Enumerate the causes and management of normocytic anaemia.

- Normocytic anaemia is characterised by normal size of the red blood cells (MCV 70–110 fL).

CAUSES OF NORMOCYTIC ANAEMIA (Table 1.23)

TABLE 1.22 National Iron Plus Initiative for Anaemia Control

Age Group	Intervention	Regimen	Service Delivery
6–60 months	1 mL syrup containing 20 mg of elemental iron and 100 μg of folic acid	Biweekly Deworming of children >12 months of age	Inclusion in mother–child protection card Through Accredited Social Health Activist (ASHA)/Auxiliary Nurse Midwife (ANM)
5–10 years	Tablets of 45 mg of elemental iron and 400 μg of folic acid	Weekly and biannual deworming	In schools through teachers, and out-of-school children through Anganwadi Centres (AWC)
10–19 years	Tablets of 100 mg of elemental iron and 500 μg of folic acid	Weekly and biannual deworming	In schools through teachers, and out-of-school children through Anganwadi Centres (AWC)
Pregnant and lactating women	Tablets of 100 mg of elemental iron and 500 μg of folic acid	One tablet daily for 100 days starting after first trimester; to be repeated for 100 days after postpartum	Antenatal clinic, ASHA/ANM
Women in reproductive age group	Tablets of 100 mg of elemental iron and 500 μg of folic acid	Weekly	Through ASHA during house visit for contraception distribution

TABLE 1.23 Causes of Normocytic Anaemia

Decreased Red Cell Production	Increased Red Cell Loss or Destruction

• Anaemia of chronic disease
• Anaemia of critical illness
• Marrow hypoplasia or aplasia
• Myeloproliferative diseases
• Myelofibrosis
• Chronic kidney disease
• Chronic liver disease
• Sideroblastic anaemia
• Hypothyroidism
• Adrenal insufficiency
• Pituitary insufficiency
	• Acute blood loss
	• Hypersplenism
	• Haemolytic disorders
	  • Haemoglobinopathies (sickle cell disease)
	  • Hereditary spherocytosis
	  • Glucose-6-phosphate dehydrogenase (G6PD) deficiency
	• Microangiopathic anaemias (DIC—disseminated intravascular coagulopathy, thrombotic thrombocytopenic purpura/haemolytic-uraemic syndrome)
	• Autoimmune haemolytic anaemia
	• Paroxysmal nocturnal haemoglobinuria

Expansion of Plasma Volume	
• Pregnancy	

INVESTIGATIONS

- Peripheral blood smear (for type of anaemia, anisocytosis of red cells, leucoerythroblastic picture, spherocytes, target cells, basophilic stippling).
- Reticulocyte count—normal, low or high depending upon underlying cause.
- Total leucocyte count and platelet count.
- Other tests depending upon the possible aetiology.

MANAGEMENT

- Treatment is directed towards the underlying disease.

Q. Discuss briefly the anaemia of chronic disease.

Q. How will you differentiate anaemia of chronic disease from iron-deficiency anaemia?

- Also known as anaemia of inflammation.
- Most common cause of normocytic anaemia.
- In some patients, MCV may be low producing microcytic anaemia.
- Pathogenesis multifactorial: Several inflammatory markers like interleukin-, IL-6, IL-10, INF-γ and TNF-α are involved in pathogenesis.
  - Elevated hepcidin which decreases duodenal iron absorption and blocks iron release from macrophages and hepatocytes.
  - Bone marrow suppression.
  - Inadequate production of EPO.
  - Poor response of proerythroblasts to EPO.
  - Slightly shortened red cell survival.
- It occurs in a wide variety of chronic diseases including inflammatory conditions, neoplasms and various systemic diseases including rheumatoid arthritis, hepatitis, collagen vascular diseases, etc.
- The diagnosis of chronic disease is not usually applied to anaemias associated with renal, hepatic or endocrine disorders.

INVESTIGATIONS

- Haemoglobin generally between 8 and 10 g/dL.
- Peripheral smear showing normocytic normochromic red cells. Some cases show microcytic hypochromic picture.
- Most patients do not have associated leucopenia or thrombocytopenia.
- Reduced serum iron.
- Reduced TIBC.
- Reduced transferrin levels (due to down-regulation of transferrin synthesis as a result of an increase in ferritin).
- Elevated ferritin levels (does not exclude associated iron deficiency as ferritin may be elevated due to inflammation).
- Elevated inflammatory markers (CRP, ESR, IL-6).

DIFFERENCES BETWEEN ANAEMIA OF CHRONIC DISEASE AND IRON-DEFICIENCY ANAEMIA (Table 1.24)

TABLE 1.24 Anaemia of Chronic Disease Versus Iron-Deficiency Anaemia

Feature	Anaemia of Chronic Disease	Iron-Deficiency Anaemia
Underlying chronic disease	Yes	Uncommon
Haemoglobin concentration	>8 g/dL	May be <8 g/dL
Peripheral smear	Usually normocytic	Microcytic
Reticulocyte count	Low, normal or elevated	Low
Serum iron	Reduced	Markedly reduced
Serum ferritin	Normal or elevated	Reduced
Serum hepcidin level	Elevated	Reduced or normal
Serum erythropoietin level	Reduced	Normal

MANAGEMENT

- Treat the underlying chronic disease.
- Recombinant human erythropoietin may be tried if the anaemia is not corrected after treatment of the underlying disease. Its use is appoved in patients with cancers as well as with chronic kidney disease and HIV infection.
- Associated iron deficiency may require intravenous iron as elevated levels of hepcidin inhibit GI absorption of iron. However, oral iron with vitamin C may be tried initially.

Q. Discuss briefly anaemia of critical illness.

- Anaemia highly prevalent in critically ill and injured patients.
- Approximately 97% become anaemic by day 8 of illness.

PATHOGENESIS

- A shortened red blood cell circulatory life span:
  - Pathogen- and immune reaction-associated haemolysis.

- Losses from phlebotomy and invasive procedure sites.
- Oozing at injury sites.
- Gastrointestinal bleeding.
- Haemodilution from volume resuscitation.

- Diminished red cell production:
  - Nutritional deficiencies.
  - Anaemia of inflammation—impaired proliferation of red cell precursors, impaired iron metabolism, reduced EPO production.

MANAGEMENT

- Blood transfusion:
  - In most patients, transfuse RBC if Hb < 7 g/dL ('restrictive' strategy to maintain it between 7 and 8 g/dL). However, in patients with acute myocardial infarction, those who are very sick or when weaning from ventilator is difficult, blood transfusion may be given to achieve Hb >10 g/dL.
- Minimise blood loss (use of small-volume phlebotomy tubes, point-of-care testing and noninvasive testing and elimination of unnecessary laboratory studies).
- Erythropoietin is of little benefit in most cases.

Q. What are the causes of pancytopenia?

- Defined as a decrease in all three blood cell lines with haemoglobin <9 g/dL, WBC <4000/μL and platelets <100,000/μL.
- It can manifest with symptoms resulting from anaemia, leucopenia or thrombocytopenia; patients may, however, be asymptomatic.
- Various causes of pancytopenia are listed in Table 1.25.

TABLE 1.25 Causes of Pancytopenia

Pancytopenia With Cellular Bone Marrow	Pancytopenia With Hypocellular Bone Marrow
• Primary bone marrow diseases: • Myelodysplastic syndrome (MDS) • Myelofibrosis (initial phase) • Myelophthisis • Hairy cell leukaemia • Paroxysmal nocturnal haemoglobinuria • Systemic diseases: • Hypersplenism • Folate or vitamin B_{12} deficiency • Severe infection • Systemic lupus erythematosus • Tuberculosis • HIV, hepatitis B, hepatitis C • Malaria, kala-azar	• Aplastic anaemia • Aleukaemic leukaemia • Some myelodysplastic syndromes • Drugs (NSAIDs, chloramphenicol, cytotoxic drugs, antithyroid drugs) • Myelofibrosis (late phase)

Q. Define aplastic anaemia. Discuss the aetiology, clinical features, investigations and management of aplastic anaemia.

DEFINITION

- Aplastic anaemia is defined as a condition in which an acellular or markedly hypocellular bone marrow results in bicytopenia (in early stages) or pancytopenia (anaemia, granulocytopenia, thrombocytopenia), and there are no leukaemic or abnormal cells in marrow or blood.
- Patients with moderate cytopenia not requiring transfusions are referred to as hypoplastic anaemia.

CLASSIFICATION

- Classification of aplastic anaemia is given in Table 1.26.

AETIOPATHOGENESIS OF APLASTIC ANAEMIA (SECONDARY) (Table 1.27)

- Several drugs can produce aplastic anaemia either due to direct toxic effect (dose-dependent, predictable) or idiosyncratic reactions (dose-independent, unpredictable).
- There is strong evidence suggesting that aplastic anaemia is an immune-mediated disease. Genetic factors are also major contributors and it is believed that a predisposing genetics factor with certain environmental factors (damage induced by chemicals, drugs, viruses or antigens) leads to lymphocyte activation and immune reaction.

TABLE 1.26 Classification of Aplastic Anaemia

• Congenital	Fanconi's anaemia, Diamond–Blackfan anaemia
• Acquired	Primary or idiopathic (no definite cause) Secondary (definite or likely agent can be identified)

TABLE 1.27 Causes of Secondary Aplastic Anaemia

• Autoimmune	Antibody-induced, SLE, graft-versus-host disease (GVHD), eosinophilic fasciitis
• Drug-induced aplasia	
• Cytotoxic drugs	Alkylating agents, antimetabolites, others
• Antibacterial drugs	Chloramphenicol, sulphonamides, isoniazid, arsenicals
• Tranquilisers	Chlorpromazine, meprobamate, chlordiazepoxide, promazine, thioridazine
• Antirheumatic drugs	Oxyphenbutazone, phenylbutazone, indomethacin, gold salts, diclofenac, D-penicillamine
• Antidiabetic drugs	Tolbutamide, chlorpropamide
• Miscellaneous drugs	Chlorthiazide, mepacrine, hydralazine, acetazolamide, potassium perchlorate, carbamazepine, phenytoin, carbimazole, methimazole
• Chemicals	Benzene, lindane (gamma benzene hexachloride), DDT, glue vapours
• Radiation	Radiation accident, radiotherapy (whole body)
• Viral infections	Hepatitis viruses, Epstein–Barr virus, HIV, parvovirus, cytomegalovirus
• Miscellaneous	Vitamin B_{12} or folate deficiency, pancreatitis, paroxysmal nocturnal haemoglobinuria

CLINICAL FEATURES

- Clinical features of aplastic anaemia result from the complications of pancytopenia (anaemia, granulocytopenia, thrombocytopenia).
- Anaemia results in weakness, fatiguability, lassitude, dyspnoea on exertion and pallor.
- Granulocytopenia (neutropenia) results in various infections, sore throat, oral and pharyngeal ulcers, chronic skin infections, recurrent respiratory infections, pneumonia and sepsis.
- Thrombocytopenia results in various bleeding manifestations, when the platelet count is less than 20,000/μL. These include bleeding into skin (ecchymosis, petechiae), epistaxis, menorrhagia, bleeding from gums and gastrointestinal tract, retinal haemorrhage and cerebral haemorrhage.
- Physical examination characteristically shows that jaundice, splenomegaly and lymphadenopathy are absent. The presence of these should prompt one to search for an associated disease or alternate diagnosis.
- Aplastic anaemia may coexist or evolve to clonal disorders, like paroxysmal nocturnal haemoglobinuria (PNH), MDS or acute myeloid leukaemia.

FANCONI'S ANAEMIA

- Autosomal recessive.
- Congenital malformations—short stature, microphthalmia, cataracts, absence or hypoplasia of radius, micrognathia, ectopic kidney, horse-shoe kidney, patent ductus arteriosus, ventricular septal defect, pulmonic stenosis, coarctation of aorta, oesophageal or duodenal atresia, intestinal malrotation, microcephaly, hydrocephalus, micropenis, undescended testes, hypoplasia of uterus and vagina, prominent ears, deafness, café-au-lait spots.
- Progressive pancytopenia.
- Predisposition to both haematologic malignancies (MDS, acute myeloid leukaemia) and solid tumours (squamous cell carcinomas of head and neck and anogenital region).

DIAGNOSIS

- Haemoglobin is reduced.
- Corrected reticulocyte count is low.
- Leucopenia and thrombocytopenia.
    - In early stages, only one or two cell lines may be affected, producing monocytopenia and bicytopenia.
- Peripheral smear study:
    - Normocytic, normochromic anaemia; sometimes macrocytosis.
    - Neutropenia with relative lymphocytosis.
- Bone marrow study:
    - Aspirate of bone marrow has little yield ('dry tap'). Bone marrow biopsy is essential.
    - Markedly hypocellular or acellular marrow with no malignant infiltrates or fibrosis.
    - Haemopoietic cells are markedly reduced to absent.
    - Increase in fat cells.
    - Bone marrow iron stores are usually increased.
    - Serum iron and transferrin saturation are increased.
- Genetic testing with flow cytometry and fluorescence in situ hybridisation (FISH) useful to exclude haematologic malignancies responsible for pancytopenia.

DIAGNOSTIC CRITERIA (Box 1.6)

SEVERE APLASIA

- Criteria for severe aplasia are given in Box 1.7.

MANAGEMENT

- Removal of the causative agent wherever possible (see aetiology).
- Supportive therapy includes prevention and treatment of infections and haemorrhage and red cell transfusion for anaemia. Prophylactic platelet transfusions are given if platelet count is <10,000/μL. To reduce chances of transfusion-associated GVHD, irradiated blood products are used.
    - Multiple red blood cell transfusions may lead to iron overload and may require iron chelators (e.g. desferioxime, deferiprone and deferasirox).
- In severe aplastic anaemia, haematopoietic stem cell transplantation should be considered in patients younger than 40 years, who have HLA-identical donors. Patients older than 40 years have a high risk of graft-versus-host disease (Flowchart 1.7).
- Medical measures to stimulate haemopoiesis and promote marrow recovery are indicated in patients older than 40 years or when HLA-identical donor is not available:
    - Combination of horse antithymocyte globulin (ATG) along with cyclosporin is the standard medical treatment with 60%–70% response rate.
    - Cyclosporin alone if the patient cannot afford/tolerate ATG. The dose is 3–7 mg/kg/day in two divided doses for at least 1 year before tapering.
    - Eltrombopag, a TPO agonist, may be useful in some patients as it increases platelet counts

BOX 1.6 Diagnostic Criteria of Aplastic Anaemia

- Bone marrow hypocellular, with no abnormal cells and no fibrosis AND
- At least two among the following:
    - Haemoglobin <10 g/dL
    - Platelet count <50,000/μL
    - Absolute neutrophil count <1500/μL

BOX 1.7 Definition of Severe Aplastic Anaemia

- A marrow biopsy showing less than 25% of normal cellularity OR
- Marrow biopsy showing less than 50% normal cellularity in which fewer than 30% of the cells are haematopoietic and at least two of the following criteria:
    - Granulocyte count less than 500/μL (if granulocyte count <200/μL, it is known as very severe aplastic anaemia)
    - Platelet count less than 20,000/μL
    - Anaemia with corrected reticulocyte count less than 1%

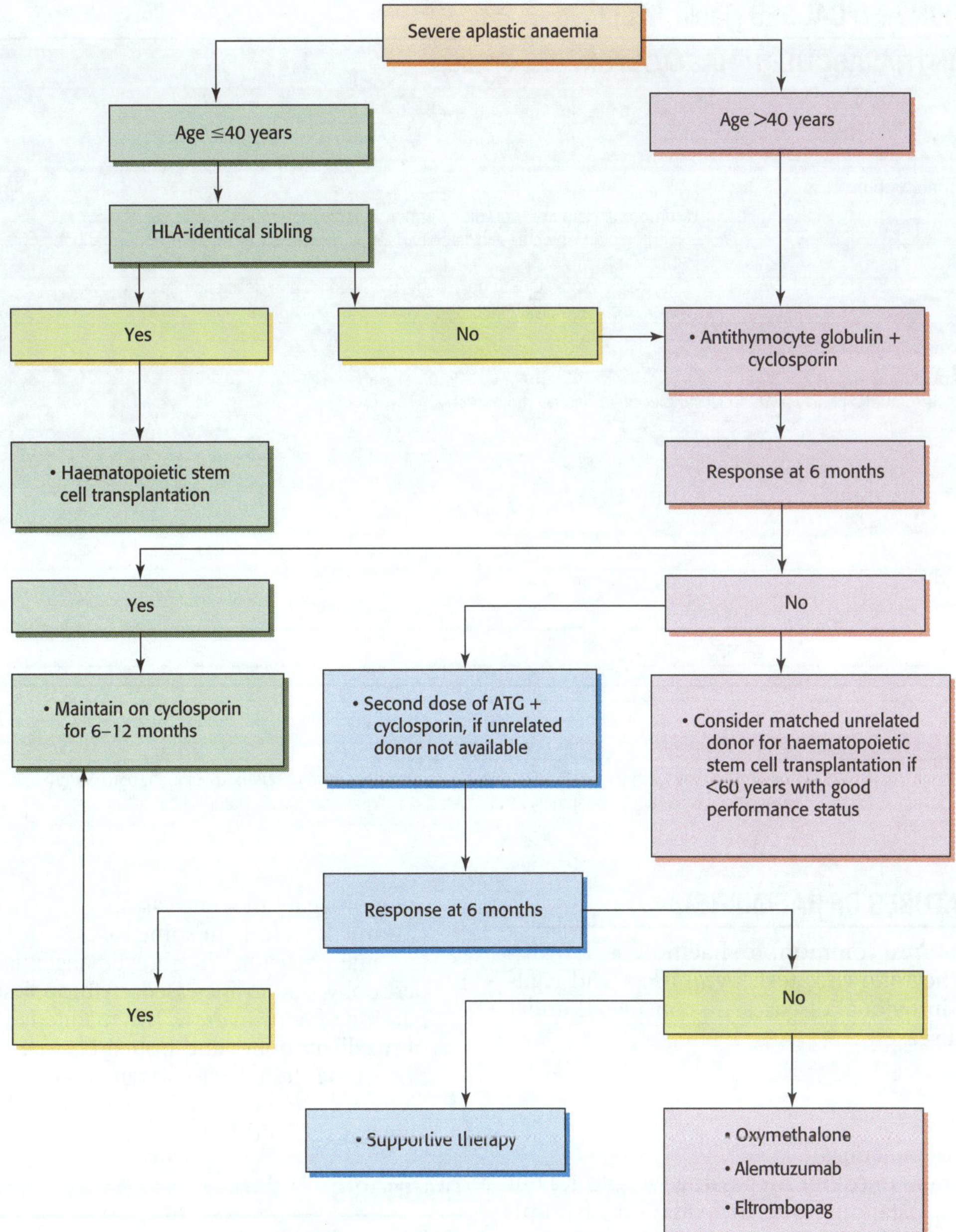

Flowchart 1.7 Management of Severe Aplastic Anaemia.

(and sometimes red blood cells and neutrophils as well) and activates intracellular signal transduction pathways to increase proliferation and differentiation of marrow progenitor cells. It may be combined with ATG and cyclosporin.

- Alemtuzumab, a monoclonal antibody against CD52 antigen which is found on the surface of many T-lymphocytes can be used to treat aplastic anaemia refractory to above treatment.
- Androgens (e.g. oxymetholone, danazol) are sometimes useful in moderate cases.
- Steroids have little role in aplastic anaemia but are useful in reducing side effects of ATG/ALG. However, steroids may be useful in children with congenital pure red cell aplasia (Diamond–Blackfan syndrome) and in some adults with pure red cell aplasia.
- Antifungal prophylaxis with voriconazole or posaconazole should be used in patients with severe neutropenia (absolute neutrophil count <500/μL)
- Antimicrobial prophylaxis with quinolone antibiotics may be used in very severe aplastic anaemia.

Q. Discuss the aetiology, classification, clinical features, diagnosis and management of haemolytic anaemias.

- Haemolytic anaemias result from an increased rate of red cell destruction. The life span of red cells (normal 90–120 days) is shortened.
- Marrow can compensate for increased red cell destruction by increased production of red cells (up to eight-folds).

CLASSIFICATION AND CAUSES (Table 1.28)

CAUSES OF INTRAVASCULAR HAEMOLYSIS (Table 1.29)

TABLE 1.28 Causes of Haemolytic Anaemias

Due to intraerythrocytic defects	
• Congenital	Membrane defects—hereditary spherocytosis, hereditary elliptocytosis Haemoglobin defects—sickle cell anaemia, thalassaemias, other abnormal haemoglobins (HbC, HbD, etc.) Enzyme defects—G6PD deficiency, pyruvate kinase deficiency
• Acquired	Paroxysmal nocturnal haemoglobinuria
Due to extraerythrocytic defects	
• Antibodies (autoimmune and alloimmune) • Mechanical (e.g. prosthetic heart valves, microangiopathic haemolytic anaemia) • Drugs (e.g. dapsone, primaquine) • Infections (e.g. malaria) • Inflammatory and neoplastic diseases • Mismatched blood transfusion	

TABLE 1.29 Causes of Intravascular Haemolysis

Toxins	Snake bite, copper toxicity, zinc toxicity
Infections	Malaria, babesiosis, Clostridium infection, leptospirosis
Mechanical causes	Prosthetic cardiac valves, disseminated intravascular coagulation, thrombotic thrombocytopenic purpura. haemolytic uraemic syndrome, march haemoglobinuria
Immunological causes	Some autoimmune haemolytic anaemias, paroxysmal nocturnal haemoglobinuria, paroxysmal cold haemoglobinuria, acute haemolytic transfusion reactions due to mismatched blood

CLINICAL FEATURES OF HAEMOLYSIS

- Clinical features common to haemolysis are discussed in the following text. Symptoms and signs specific for individual diseases are considered under respective diseases.

HISTORY

- Mild jaundice.
- Symptoms of anaemia.
- Urine is normal in colour on passing (acholuric) but turns dark on standing due to oxidation of urobilinogen to urobilin.
- Black urine ('black water') with haemoglobinuria in case of intravascular haemolysis (malaria, mismatched blood transfusion, G6PD deficiency).
- Symptoms of cholelithiasis may be present. Chronic haemolysis is associated with an increased incidence of pigmented gallstones.
- Acute crisis in many chronic haemolytic anaemias that produces sudden fall in haemoglobin and sometimes fever, joint pains and abdominal pain.
- Splenic pain from rapid enlargement of spleen or splenic infarction.
- Infections.
- Family history important in congenital haemolytic anaemias.

PHYSICAL FINDINGS

- Mild jaundice.
- Anaemia.
- Splenomegaly in some cases.
- Chronic leg ulcers in some cases.
- In some congenital haemolytic anaemias, skeletal hypertrophy due to increased erythropoiesis causing expansion of bone marrow. This manifests as enlargement of maxillary bones and frontal bossing and malocclusion of the teeth due to overgrowth of upper jaw.
- Signs of systemic diseases predisposing to haemolysis.
- Signs of cholelithiasis (cholecystitis or obstruction).

DIAGNOSIS

- Diagnosis of haemolytic anaemias can be considered under two headings: recognition of haemolysis and recognition of cause of haemolysis.

RECOGNITION OF HAEMOLYSIS

Evidence of increased erythrocyte destruction (Box 1.8)

BOX 1.8 Evidence of Increased Erythrocyte Destruction in Haemolysis

- Unconjugated hyperbilirubinaemia, usually less than 6 mg/dL (may not be present in all cases as it depends on the capacity of liver to conjugate and excrete bilirubin)
- Increased urobilinogen excretion in urine
- Decreased plasma haptoglobin and haemopexin
- Increased plasma LDH
- Demonstration of shortened red cell lifespan using ^{51}Cr-labelled red blood cells

Evidence of increased erythrocyte production (Box 1.9)

BOX 1.9 Evidence of Increased Erythrocyte Production in Haemolysis

- Increased reticulocyte count (reticulocytosis)
- Macrocytosis (due to increased reticulocyte count and folate deficiency), polychromasia and nucleated red cells in peripheral smear
- Spherocytes in hereditary spherocytosis and autoimmune haemolytic anaemia
- Marked anisopoikilocytosis, hypochromic red cells and target cells seen in thalassaemias
- Fragmented red cells in microangiopathic anaemias and prosthetic cardiac valve
- Erythroid hyperplasia of bone marrow
- Radiological changes in congenital haemolytic anaemias, e.g. 'hair-on-end' appearance in skull radiograph

Evidence specific to intravascular haemolysis (Box 1.10)

BOX 1.10 Evidence of Intravascular Haemolysis

- Haemoglobinaemia
- Haemoglobinuria
- Methaemoglobinaemia (in some cases)
- Haemosiderinuria (haemosiderin in urine) as demonstrated by Prussian blue staining; seen in chronic intravascular haemolysis

RECOGNITION OF CAUSE OF HAEMOLYSIS

- Dealt in details under individual diseases.
- However, the commonly done tests include one or more of the following:
  - Peripheral smear examination (sickle cells, spherocytes, red cell fragments).
  - Coombs' test.
  - Haemoglobin electrophoresis.
  - Heinz body preparation.
  - Osmotic fragility, sucrose lysis and Ham's test.
  - Measurement of enzyme activity.
- Evaluation of chronic haemolysis is shown in Flowchart 1.8.

TREATMENT

- Supportive therapy:
  - Blood transfusions.
  - Treatment of infections.
  - Treatment of leg ulcers.
  - Treatment of symptomatic cholelithiasis.
  - Splenectomy in selected cases.
- Specific therapies for individual diseases are dealt with under respective diseases.

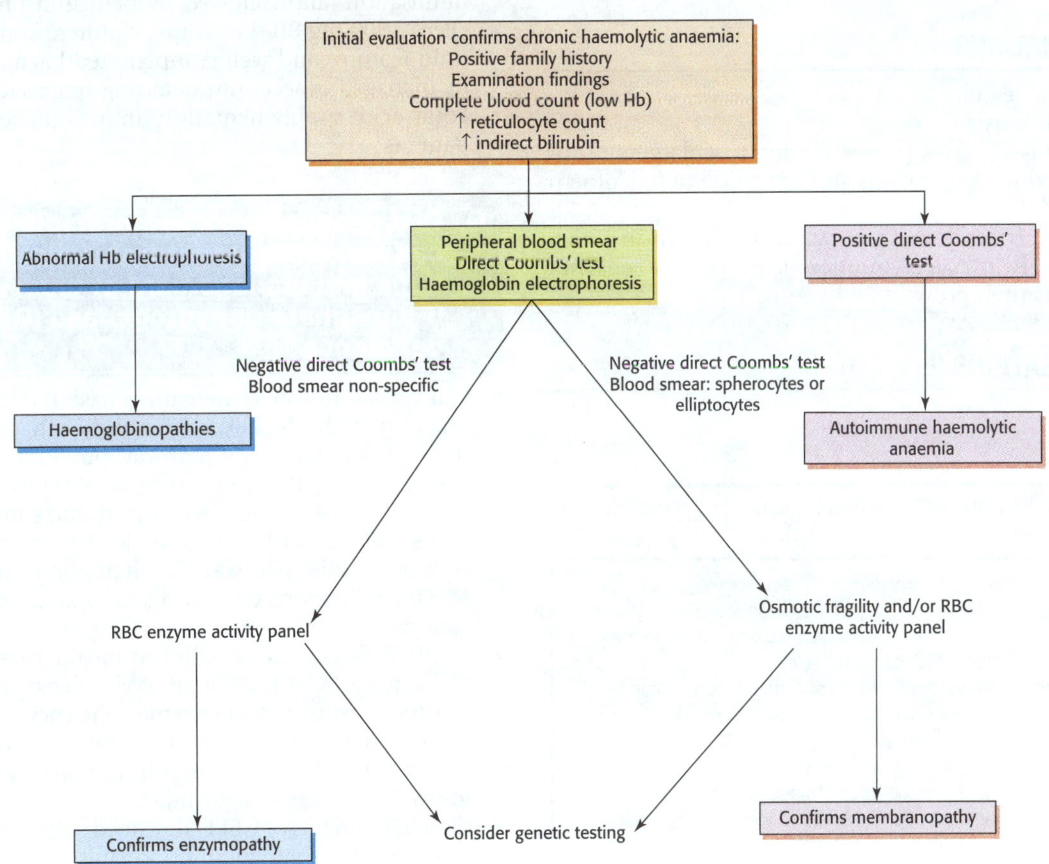

Flowchart 1.8 Evaluation of Chronic Haemolytic Anaemia. *(Adapted from Grace RF, Glader B. Red blood cell enzyme disorders. Pediatr Clin N Am 2018; 65:579–595.)*

Q. Briefly outline hereditary spherocytosis.

- Autosomal dominant inheritance in more than 75% cases.
- Characterised by deficiency of ankyrin, spectrin, band-3 or protein 4.2—transmembrane proteins that link the bilayer of red cells to the membrane skeleton.
- This results in spherical erythrocytes (spherocytes) that are more susceptible to osmotic lysis. However, the primary cause of anaemia is that the red cells with decreased membrane surface area are unable to effectively traverse the spleen; they are sequestered and removed from circulation by the spleen.

CLINICAL FEATURES

- Strong family history of anaemia, jaundice, splenomegaly and cholelithiasis.
- About 25% of the patients have mild compensated haemolysis, minimal spherocytosis, near normal haemoglobin levels, slight reticulocytosis (<6%) and mild splenomegaly.
- In children, growth retardation due to haemolysis and bone changes due to marrow hypertrophy.
- In adults, anaemia, intermittent jaundice and moderate splenomegaly.
- Regular blood transfusions in a small number of patients who have severe disease that is transmitted through autosomal recessive mechanism.

COMPLICATIONS

- Chronic leg ulcers.
- Cholelithiasis.
- Haemolytic crises (probably due to enlargement of spleen during infections and activation of reticuloendothelial system).
- Aplastic crises due to parvovirus B19 infection which selectively infects erythropoietic progenitor cells and inhibits their growth.

INVESTIGATIONS (Box 1.11)

BOX 1.11 Investigations in a Suspected Case of Hereditary Spherocytosis

- Demonstration of a haemolytic state (see above)
- Demonstration of spherocytes in the blood film (Fig. 1.4)
- Normal or reduced mean corpuscular volume (MCV) in most patients; reduced MCV in severe cases
- Increased mean corpuscular haemoglobin concentration (MCHC) (≥34.5 g/dL) due to relative cellular dehydration in more than 50% of patients
- Increased osmotic fragility (may be absent in mild cases; may be positive in autoimmune haemolytic anaemia)
- Reduced florescence of eosin-5-maleimide-labelled erythrocytes in flow cytometry-base analysis
- Negative Coombs' test
- Demonstration of same disorder in other family members

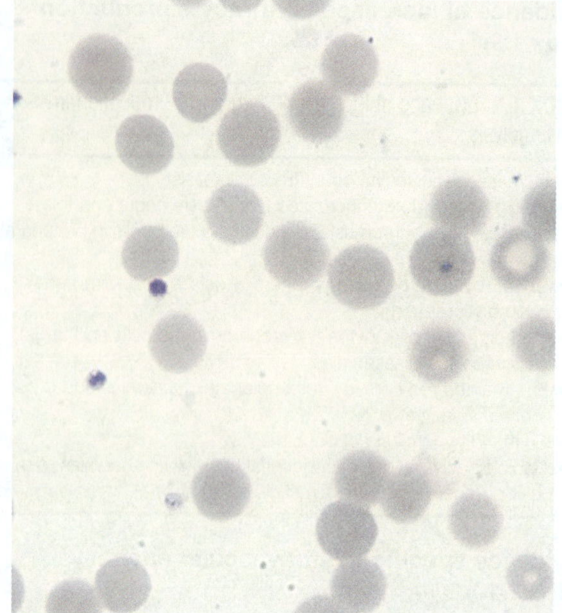

Fig. 1.4 Peripheral smear showing spherocytes which lack central pallor.

TREATMENT

- Splenectomy is the treatment of choice. It should not be done until the age of 6 years. It should be preceded by pneumococcal and *Haemophilus influenzae* immunisation, and followed by penicillin prophylaxis (Pen-V 500 mg BID) in young children. Patients with mild features and well-compensated haemolysis can be managed expectantly, deferring splenectomy.
- Folic acid supplementation in un-splenectomised patients.

Q. Discuss the aetiology, precipitating causes, clinical features, investigations and management of glucose-6-phosphate dehydrogenase (G6PD) deficiency.

- Glucose-6-phosphate dehydrogenase (G6PD) is the first enzyme in the hexose monophosphate shunt of the Embden–Meyerhof pathway, providing reducing power to all cells in the form of NADPH (reduced form of nicotinamide adenine dinucleotide phosphate). Since red blood cells do not contain mitochondria, this pathway is their only source of NADPH; therefore, defence against oxidative damage is dependent on G6PD.
- G6PD deficiency is an X-linked disorder resulting in G6PD variants with different levels of enzyme activity. It is the most common enzyme deficiency.
- Red cells deficient in G6PD are unable to keep glutathione in reduced state. This results in impaired response to oxidising drugs or toxic injury.
- Over 250 variants of G6PD described suggesting genetic heterogeneity. Three common variants are as follows:
    - G6PD (A-) seen in African black population; degree of deficiency mild and haemolysis self-limiting.

- G6PD (B-) or G6PD Mediterranean, seen in the Mediterranean area. It is the severe form of deficiency; most common variant seen in India (other variants reported from India include G6PD Kerala–Kalyan and G6PD Orissa).
- G6PD Canton seen in Chinese.

PRECIPITATING/AGGRAVATING CAUSES OF HAEMOLYSIS

- Precipitating causes of haemolysis in G6PD deficiency are given in Table 1.30.

DRUGS IN USUAL DOSES CONSIDERED SAFE IN G6PD DEFICIENT PATIENTS

- Table 1.31 gives a list of drugs considered safe in G6PD deficient patients.

CLINICAL FEATURES

- Most patients are asymptomatic unless any of the incriminated drugs or foods are ingested. The exposure is followed by haemolysis, rapid development of anaemia and haemoglobinuria (cola-coloured urine). Rarely anuria occurs due to acute kidney injury.
- Favism is haemolysis following ingestion of the broad bean, *Vicia faba*. It is a feature of the Mediterranean type.
- Neonatal jaundice is a feature of Mediterranean type. Haemolysis does not seem to contribute to it as much as impaired bilirubin conjugation and clearance by the liver. Severe neonatal jaundice if untreated could give rise to kernicterus.
- Chronic nonspherocytic haemolytic anaemia. Many such patients have a history of severe neonatal jaundice, chronic anaemia exacerbated by oxidative stress that typically requires blood transfusions, reticulocytosis, gallstones and splenomegaly. Haemolysis is mainly extravascular.
- In the African variety, growth of *Plasmodium falciparum* in red cells is markedly slow, and hence, these patients are protected from malaria.

TABLE 1.30 Precipitating Causes of Haemolysis in G6PD Deficiency

Drugs (haemolysis is dose-related)	Primaquine, dapsone, aspirin (high doses), sulphonamides[a] (particularly sulphanilamide, sulphacetamide, sulphapyridine, sulphamethoxazole), nitrofurantoin, L-dopa, quinidine, nalidixic acid, ciprofloxacin, ofloxacin, vitamin K*, phenacetin, phenazopyridine, cotrimoxazole, methylene blue, glibenclamide*, rasburicase
Toxins	Naphthalene
Viral and bacterial infections	Hepatitis A and B, *Salmonella*
Broad bean	*Vicia faba* (in Mediterranean variety)
Others	Diabetic ketoacidosis, myocardial infarction, strenuous exercise

[a]Haemolysis possible and therefore use carefully.

TABLE 1.31 Drugs Considered Safe in G6PD Deficient Persons

• Aspirin	• Para-aminosalicylic acid
• Ascorbic acid	• Paracetamol
• Chloramphenicol	• Phenytoin
• Chlororquine	• Procainamide
• Colchicine	• Pyrimethamine
• Diphenhydramine	• Quinine
• Isoniazid	• Streptomycin
• L-Dopa	• Trimethoprim

INVESTIGATIONS (Box 1.12)

BOX 1.12 Investigations in G6PD Deficient Haemolysis

- Evidence of intravascular haemolysis
- Anaemia that worsens until days 7–8
- Heinz bodies (denatured haemoglobin precipitates) in peripheral red blood cells
- Confirmation by estimating G6PD activity of the red cell[a]

[a]Estimation of G6PD should be done several days after the acute episode. Estimation of G6PD activity during or immediately after acute haemolysis may give a false normal value as the young red cells and reticulocytes have near-normal G6PD levels.

MANAGEMENT

- Removal of the offending agent and avoiding its further use.
- Supportive therapy for anaemia like blood transfusion.
- Treatment of infection.
- Phototherapy or exchange transfusion for neonal hyperbilirubinaemia.

Q. Describe the structure of normal haemoglobin.

- Haemoglobin consists of two pairs of polypeptide chains to each of which a haem is attached. Each polypeptide chain is composed of a number of amino acids. Iron is in the form of ferrous state (Fe^{2+}). Abnormalities resulting in conversion into ferric state lead to abnormal haemoglobin that is not capable of binding oxygen.
- Based on the number and sequence of amino acids, polypeptide chains are classified into several types (Table 1.32).
- There are three embryonic haemoglobins seen in the early embryonic period: Hb Portland I ($\zeta_2\gamma_2$), Hb Gower I ($\zeta_2\epsilon_2$), Hb Gower II ($\alpha_2\epsilon_2$). Later in foetal life, there is a switch to the production of α- and γ-chains, resulting in Hb-F. At birth, there is an additional switch from the production of γ-chains to the production of β- and δ-chains, resulting in Hb-A and Hb-A2.

TABLE 1.32 Classification of Polypeptide Chains of Haemoglobin

• Alpha chains (α)	• Beta chains (β)
• Alpha-like chain:	• Beta-like chains:
• (Zeta chain) (ζ)	• Gamma chains (γ)
	• Delta chains (δ)
	• Epsilon chains (ε)

- Haemoglobin A (Hb-A) that comprises about 97% of the haemoglobin of adult red cells consists of two alpha and two beta chains ($\alpha_2\beta_2$).
- Haemoglobin F (Hb-F) that accounts for about 70%–90% of foetal haemoglobin consists of two alpha and two gamma chains ($a_2\gamma_2$).
- The normal haemoglobins seen in the adult are Hb-A and Hb-A_2 ($\alpha_2\delta_2$) and the foetus are Hb-F and Hb-Bart's (γ_4).

Q. How do you classify haemoglobinopathies (hereditary disorders of haemoglobin; disorders of haemoglobin structure and synthesis)?

- Haemoglobinopathies are disorders that are due to structural abnormalities in the globin chains of haemoglobin (qualitative defect). However, in practice, this term applies to disorders that affect the structure, function or production of haemoglobin due to abnormalities in the formation of globin.

CLASSIFICATION (Table 1.33)

- Qualitative abnormality of haemoglobin results from alterations in the amino acid sequence of the polypeptide chains that produce structurally defective haemoglobins.
- Quantitative abnormality of haemoglobin results from impaired or absent polypeptide chain formation but amino acid sequence is normal.

INHERITANCE

- Subjects who inherit one normal and one abnormal gene are heterozygotes. The heterozygous state is usually referred to as the trait (e.g. sickle cell trait; Hb-S trait or Hb-AS).
- Subjects who inherit two identical abnormal genes are homozygotes. The homozygous state is usually referred to as the disease (e.g. sickle cell disease or Hb-S disease or Hb-SS).
- Subjects who inherit two different abnormal genes are double heterozygotes (e.g. Hb-SC; Hb-Sβ-thalassaemia).

TABLE 1.33 Classification of Haemoglobinopathies

Qualitative Haemoglobinopathies	Quantitative Haemoglobinopathies

• Haemoglobin S
• Haemoglobin C
• Haemoglobin D Punjab
• Altered oxygen affinity
  ◦ High-affinity haemoglobin
  ◦ Low-affinity haemoglobin
• Haemoglobins that oxidise easily
  ◦ Unstable haemoglobin
  ◦ M haemoglobin
	• Thalassaemias (α-, β-thalassaemia)
	Combined qualitative and quantitative haemoglobinopathies
	• Haemoglobin E[a]
	• Sickle cell β-thalassaemia
	Acquired haemoglobinopathies
	• Methaemoglobinaemia
	• Carboxyhaemoglobinaemia

[a]Results from a point mutation in the β-globin gene and behaves like a β+ mutation.

Q. Discuss the pathogenesis, clinical features, investigations and management of sickle cell anaemia.

- Sickle cell anaemia results from an abnormal haemoglobin known as haemoglobin-S (Hb-S) or sickle cell haemoglobin. The molecular lesion in Hb-S is the substitution of valine for glutamic acid at the sixth residue of the β-chain (Hb-S6$^{GLU\text{-}VAL}$).
- Sickle cell anaemia is the homozygous state for the Hb-S gene (*Hb-SS*). It is transmitted as an autosomal recessive disease.
- The heterozygous state (Hb-AS) is known as sickle cell trait.
- In India, it is common among certain tribes in South India, Assam, Bihar and Orissa.

PATHOGENESIS

- Deoxygenation causes the red cells containing Hb-S to become rigid and deformed, assuming a sickle or crescent shape (sickle-shaped cells). These changes are reversible with reoxygenation. However, the sickling may become permanent, and then the red cells are called irreversibly sickled.
- The consequences of sickling are the following:
  - Occlusion of microvascular circulation by the sickle cells leading to tissue ischaemia and infarction (infarction crisis or veno-occlusive crisis).
  - Destruction of the sickle cells by the reticuloendothelial system resulting in haemolysis (haemolytic crisis).

FACTORS PROMOTING SICKLING (Table 1.34)

- Haemoglobin F (Hb-F) strongly inhibits sickling. Sickle cell disease in India is associated with elevated Hb-F and hence is often not a severe disorder.
- Hb-S confers some protection against *P. falciparum* malaria so that these patients are relatively resistant to malaria.

CLINICAL FEATURES IN CHILDREN

- Clinical manifestations are absent in the first 6 months of life, since high Hb-F levels protect the red cells from sickling.
- Infections with *Pneumococcus, Meningococcus, Escherichia coli* and *H. influenzae* are common. Pneumococcal meningitis or pneumonia with septicaemia is particularly common.
- Hand–foot syndrome (dactylitis) due to micro-infarction of carpal and tarsal bones.
- Splenic sequestration syndrome—sudden pooling of blood within spleen resulting in splenomegaly, hypovolaemia and shock, requiring prompt blood transfusions.

TABLE 1.34 Factors Promoting Sickling

• Fever	• Hb-C and Hb-D
• Sluggish blood flow	• Increase in red cell 2,3-DPG
• Low oxygen tension	• Reduction in red cell water content
• Low pH (acidosis)	

TABLE 1.35 Clinical Features of Sickle Cell Anaemia in Adults

Anaemia	• Severe haemolytic type of anaemia • Secondary folate deficiency exacerbates anaemia • Results in fatigue, frequent infections, cardiomegaly and systolic murmur
Infarction crises (vaso-occlusive crisis)	• Most common—sudden attacks of bone pain and abdominal pain with or without fever • Bone pain due to ischaemia and infarction • Avascular necrosis of head of femur common • Mesenteric infarction results in acute abdominal pain • Splenic infarction and autosplenectomy (refer Clinical Features in Children) • Cerebral infarction results in hemiplegia • Acute chest syndrome (refer Clinical Features in Children) • Infarction of renal papillae results in haematuria • Retinal microinfarcts result in loss of vision
Aplastic crisis	• Results from temporary marrow suppression following infections, particularly with human parvovirus B19
Haemolytic crises	• Episodes of increased sequestration and destruction of red cells; an abrupt fall in haemoglobin and rapid enlargement of liver and spleen
Other manifestations	• Acute coronary syndrome, cardiac arrhythmias • Chronic leg ulcers • Cholelithiasis • *Salmonella* osteomyelitis • Proteinuria, pyelonephritis, renal failure • Priapism • Pulmonary hypertension • Frontal bossing of skull, prominent malar bones and protuberant teeth resulting from marrow hyperplasia • Iron overload due to repeated transfusions

- Splenomegaly is present throughout early childhood. But repeated episodes of splenic infarction ultimately lead to atrophy of the spleen (autosplenectomy). By about 8 years of age, spleen is no longer palpable and is reduced to a small fibrous remnant.
- Acute chest syndrome occurs in both children and adults. It indicates occurrence of a new pulmonary infiltrate on chest radiograph and can develop because of infection, fat embolism or vaso-occlusion of pulmonary vasculature. It is usually accompanied by pain in the chest, fever, respiratory distress and hypoxaemia. Typically, it presents 3 days after the start of a vaso-occlusive crisis.
- Others are acute coronary syndrome and stroke.

CLINICAL FEATURES IN ADULTS

- Clinical features of sickle cell anaemia in adults are given in Table 1.35.

INVESTIGATIONS

- Demonstration of a haemolytic state.
- Features of hyposplenism on peripheral blood (Howell–Jolly bodies, target cells and irregularly contracted red cells).
- Demonstration of sickling of the red cells when mixed with a solution of sodium metabisulphite ('sickle test').
- Haemoglobin solubility tests as a screening test
- Haemoglobin electrophoresis. There is no Hb-A, 80%–95% Hb-SS and 2%–20% Hb-F. In sickle cell trait (heterozygous state), Hb-S is 20%–40% and the rest is Hb-A.
- Before occurrence of stroke, transcranial Doppler can be done annually to detect stenosis of cerebral vessels.
- Tests for iron overload (serum ferritin levels, transferrin saturation, liver iron concentration using liver biopsy specimen, measurement of liver iron using MRI).
- Antenatal diagnosis by analysing DNA from amniotic fluid cells at 7–10 weeks of gestation.

BOX 1.13 Blood Transfusion in Sickle Cell Anaemia

- Transfusion required to increase oxygen carrying capacity, replace rigid, sickle-shaped red cells with normal, deformable cells, thereby reducing haemolysis and restoring blood flow. It also reduces HB-S production
- Indicated for severe anaemia due to aplastic crisis and acute splenic sequestration
- Exchange transfusion to reduce Hb-S to below 30% with increase in haemoglobin to more than 10 g/dL recommended for severe acute chest syndrome, severe sepsis and acute stroke
- Chronic transfusion to keep Hb-S below 30% is mainstay of secondary prevention of overt stroke

MANAGEMENT

- General measures:
  - Folic acid supplementation, 5 mg daily.
  - Avoidance of chilling, dehydration and hypoxia.
  - Prevention and prompt identification and treatment of infections with antibiotics.
  - Phenoxymethyl penicillin 250 mg daily starting at the age of 2 months and continued for 5 years.
  - Pneumococcal vaccination in young patients; also in adults who have hyposplenism.
- Blood transfusion (Box 1.13)
- Infarction crises are managed with hydration, oxygen, analgesics (NSAIDs, paracetamol, opioids) and transfusion with red cell concentrate in selected cases. Analgesics should be administered within 1 hour of arrival.
- Patients with acute stroke should be treated with simple transfusion (if Hb <8.5 g/dL) or exchange transfusion. Alteplase (tPA) may be considered based on criteria used for stroke patients but this should not delay transfusion therapy.
- Splenic sequestration crisis is treated with blood transfusions.

- Recurrent strokes (cerebral infarcts) are treated with chronic monthly exchange transfusions.
- Acute chest syndrome is treated with antibiotics, maintenance of arterial oxygenation and if required, exchange transfusion.
- Aplastic crisis is treated with red cell transfusions to maintain haemoglobin.
- Chronic leg ulcers are managed with elevation of limb, daily dressings with zinc sulphate and exchange transfusion in extreme cases.
- Drugs
  - Hydroxyurea (hydroxycarbamide) may be used in patients with severe symptoms. It increases production of Hb-F and reduces vaso-occlusive crisis.
  - Chronic use of large doses of glutamine orally has been found useful in reducing clinical features. It is an amino acid required in the production of NAD (nicotinamide adenine), a cofactor in the oxidation–reduction reactions.
  - Voxelotor binds to haemoglobin and increases its affinity for oxygen. This stabilises the sickle cell haemoglobin and prevents its polymerization. It can be used in patients resistant to hydroxyurea.
  - Crizanlizumab is a humanised monoclonal antibody that binds P-selectin. P-selectin is the primary mediator of the vaso-occlusive crisis in sickle cell disease.
- Management of iron overload using iron chelators (deferoxamine, deferiprone or deferasirox).
- Haemopoietic stem cell transplantation from HLA-matched donor is curative.
- Gene therapy is an emerging therapy

Q. Give a brief account of methaemoglobinaemia.

- Normal oxygen transport depends on the maintenance of haemoglobin in the reduced (Fe^{2+}) state. When haemoglobin is oxidised to methaemoglobin, the haem iron becomes Fe^{3+} and is incapable of binding oxygen. Normal red cells contain less than 1% methaemoglobin. An excess of methaemoglobin in the blood is termed methaemoglobinaemia. Clinically, when methaemoglobin level exceeds 1.5 g/dL, the patient develops cyanosis. At higher levels, they develop headache, weakness and breathlessness (due to hypoxia). At levels >40% coma, respiratory depression, convulsions, arrhythmias and death may occur.

CAUSES (Table 1.36)

TABLE 1.36 Causes of Methaemoglobinaemia

Congenital	Methaemoglobin reductase deficiency M haemoglobins (haemoglobin variants): Five variants are identified—Hb M Boston, Hb M Iwate, Hb M Saskatoon, Hb M Hyde Park and Hb M Milwaukee
Acquired	Exposure to certain drugs and toxins—nitrites, nitrates, primaquine, dapsone, phenacetin, phenazopyridine, benzocaine, metoclopramide, nitroglycerine, methylene blue

INVESTIGATIONS

- Blood is chocolate-coloured which does not change on exposure to air.
- Normal partial pressure of oxygen (PaO_2)
- Elevated saturation gap >10%. It is the difference between calculated arterial oxygen saturation given by blood gas machine and transcutaneous oxygen saturation measured by pulse oximeter.
- Co-oximetric measurement of fractions of hameoglobin gives levels of methaemoglobin.

TREATMENT

- Methaemoglobin reductase deficiency is treated with oral methylene blue or ascorbic acid.
- Severe methaemoglobinaemia is treated with intravenous methylene blue.
- M haemoglobins require no treatment though some patients require exchange transfusions.

Q. What are thalassaemias? What are the common forms and genetics of thalassaemias?

- The fundamental defect in thalassaemias is a reduction or absence of synthesis of one of the globin chains.
- There are two main groups of thalassaemias:
  - α-Thalassaemia, where the synthesis of α-chains is affected.
  - β-Thalassaemia, where the synthesis of β-chains is affected.

COMMON FORMS (Table 1.37)

CLASSIFICATION OF BETA-THALASSAEMIAS

- Classification of beta-thalassaemias is given in Table 1.38.

TABLE 1.37 Types of Thalassaemias

α-Thalassaemias	β-Thalassaemias
• α-Thalassaemia trait • Haemoglobin-H disease • Haemoglobin-Bart's hydrops fetalis	• β-Thalassaemia minor or trait (heterozygous state) • β-Thalassaemia intermedia • β-Thalassaemia major (Cooley's anaemia; homozygous state)

TABLE 1.38 Classification of Beta-Thalassaemias

• Transfusion-dependent β-thalassaemia:
  • β-thalassaemia major or severe HbE-β-thalassaemia
  • Require lifelong, regular transfusions for survival
	• Non-transfusion-dependent β-thalassaemia:
	  • β-thalassaemia intermedia or mild-to- moderate HbE-β-thalassaemia
	  • Require no transfusions OR
	  • Require occasional transfusions because of specific circumstances (e.g. surgery, pregnancy, acute infection) OR
	  • Require frequent transfusions only for a limited period (e.g. to support growth during childhood)

GENETICS

- In homozygous β-thalassaemia, either no normal β-chains are produced (β°) or β-chain production is markedly reduced (β^{+}). The excess α-chains combine with whatever β-, γ- and δ-chains are produced, resulting in increased quantities of Hb-A_2 and Hb-F, and at best, a small amount of Hb-A. Thalassaemia intermedia may be due to $\beta^{+}/\beta^{+\tilde{a}}$, β°/β^{+} or a combination of β^{+} and α-thalassaemia, where there is reduced α-chain precipitation and less ineffective erythropoiesis and haemolysis.
- There are four genes for α-chain, two on each chromosome (αα/αα). Deletion of one α-chain gene (-α/αα) produces silent carrier. Deletion of two genes (-α/-α or –/αα) produces α-thalassaemia trait. Deletion of three α-genes produces Hb H (β_4) due to excess β-chains. If all four genes are absent, there is no α-chain synthesis and only Hb-Bart's (γ_4) is present. It is incompatible with life. The infants are either stillborn at 28–40 weeks or die very shortly after birth. They are pale, oedematous and have large liver and spleen (hydrops fetalis). Hydrops fetalis requires treatment with in-utero transfusions in order to prevent foetal demise.

Q. Discuss the clinical features, salient investigations and management of beta-thalassaemia major (Cooley's anaemia).

- β-Thalassaemia major is the homozygous state of β-thalassaemia. β-Chain synthesis is absent or grossly reduced.
- In India, it is common among communities like Sindhi, Punjabi, Gujarati, Parsee; less common in South India.
- Anaemia occurs due to combined RBC destruction in the bone marrow (ineffective erythropoiesis) and spleen.
    - Free α-globin chains are unstable and generate cytotoxic reactive oxidant species and cellular precipitates that result in ineffective erythropoiesis and premature haemolysis of circulating red cells.
- Anaemia and poor tissue oxygenation stimulate increased kidney EPO production that further drives marrow erythropoiesis, resulting in increased ineffective marrow activity and the classic bony deformities.

CLINICAL FEATURES

- Severe anaemia (usually develops at 6–24 months of age) and its complications.
- Growth and development retardation, feeding problems, diarrhoea and irritability.
- Splenomegaly, at times massive (Fig. 1.5).
- Hepatomegaly.
- Bone marrow hyperplasia resulting in deformities of long bones of legs and craniofacial changes (bossing of the skull, prominent malar eminence, depression of bridge of nose, tendency to a mongoloid slant of the eye and hypertrophy of the maxillae, which tends to expose the upper teeth).

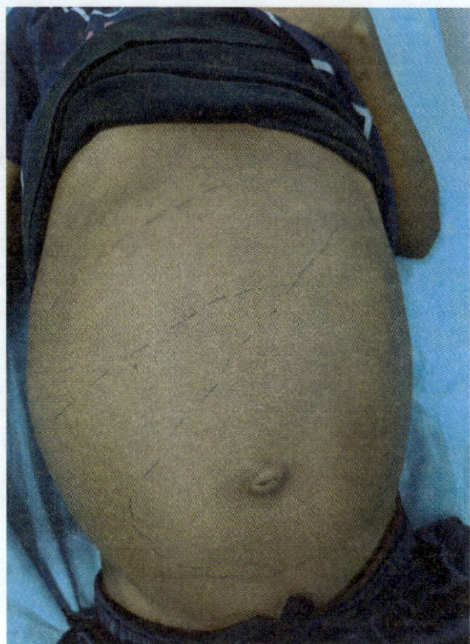

Fig. 1.5 Massive hepatosplenomegaly in a patient with thalassaemia major.

BOX 1.14 Causes of Increased Risk of Thrombosis in Thalassaemia Major

- Peripheral haemolysis causing red cells to express prothrombotic markers on their surface
- Platelet activation
- Iron-induced endothelial damage

BOX 1.15 Features Due to Haemosiderosis

- Pancreatic haemosiderosis resulting in type 1 diabetes
- Hepatic haemosiderosis resulting in cirrhosis and liver cancer
- Cardiac haemosiderosis resulting in arrhythmias, heart blocks and heart failure (primary causes of death)
- Renal deposition resulting in proteinuria and kidney failure
- Deposition of iron in various endocrine organs: growth hormone deficiency, delayed puberty, hypogonadotropic hypogonadism, osteopaenia, hypothyroidism and hypoparathyroidism

- Development of masses from extramedullary haematopoiesis. Paraspinal masses may produce cord compression.
- Increased risk of thrombosis particularly in patients who are non-transfused or infrequently transfused and in patients who are splenectomised. Various causes are given in Box 1.14.
- Deposition of iron in tissues (haemosiderosis) resulting in organ failure. This may be due to increased gastrointestinal absorption of iron as well as increased release from macrophages, as ineffective erythropoiesis and hypoxia lead to decreased production of hepcidin. Iron overload can occur even without exogenously administered iron (Box 1.15).
- Appropriately treated patients can survive beyond 40 years of age.

BOX 1.16 Investigations in Thalassaemia Major

- Severe microcytic, hypochromic anaemia with poikilocytosis (spiculated teardrop and elongated cells), target cells and nucleated red cells
- Osmotic fragility test shows increased resistance to haemolysis
- Markedly reduced or absent levels of haemoglobin A (Hb-A)
- Raised levels of haemoglobin F (>92%)
- Skull radiograph shows a 'hair-on-end' appearance and generalised widening of medullary spaces
- Evidence that both parents have thalassaemia minor

INVESTIGATIONS

- Relevant investigations in thalassaemia major are given in Box 1.16.

MANAGEMENT

- Folic acid supplementation.
- Repeated blood transfusions to maintain Hb of 9–10.5 g/dL. Regular transfusions suppress erythropoiesis preventing skeletal deformities and splenomegaly, and inhibiting increased gastrointestinal iron absorption.
- Desferrioxamine therapy to chelate iron and enhance iron excretion; indicated if serum ferritin >1000 μg/L or after transfusion of 10 units of red cells. Deferiprone and deferasirox are oral iron chelators.
- Luspatercept is a recombinant fusion protein which enhances erythroid maturation and is useful in patients with thalassaemia major.
- Splenectomy is indicated in children with massive symptomatic splenomegaly and those with progressively increasing transfusion requirements (above 200–250 mL/kg/year of packed red blood cells).
- Management of associated complications like heart failure and endocrinopathies.
- Allogenic haematopoietic stem cell transplantation in young patients is definite treatment.
- Gene therapy, betibeglogene autotemcel, has received conditional marketing authorisation in Europe for patients with transfusion-dependent β-thalassaemia who are >12 years but do not have a matched sibling haematopoietic stem cell donor.

Q. Discuss briefly thalassaemia minor (trait) and thalassaemia intermedia.

THALASSAEMIA MINOR

- Also called β-thalassaemia carrier or β-thalassaemia trait.
- It is due to β°/β or β^{+}/β.
- This common carrier state is usually asymptomatic.
- Anaemia mild or absent.
- Peripheral blood smear shows severely microcytic and hypochromic red cells with target cells.
- The red cell distribution (RDW) may assist in differentiating iron deficiency and sideroblastic anaemia from thalassaemia. RDW will be elevated in >90% of persons with iron deficiency but in only 50% of persons with thalassaemia. RDW is usually elevated in sideroblastic anaemia.
- Serum iron and ferritin are normal.
- Haemoglobin electrophoresis shows a raised Hb-A_2 (3.5%–7.5%) and often a raised Hb-F (0.5%–4.0%).
- Avoid iron unless iron deficiency has been documented.
- Genetic counselling important to prevent transmission of carrier state from both parents.
- Prenatal diagnosis in high-risk pregnancy by chorionic villi biopsy at 11 weeks.

THALASSAEMIA INTERMEDIA

- Patients generally have mild to moderate anaemia (Hb 7–9 g/dL).
- Patients may have mild splenomegaly, bone deformities, gallstones and chronic leg ulcers.
- Blood transfusions usually not required.
- Folic acid supplementation should be provided.
- Splenectomy is occasionally required if the patient develops growth retardation, leucopenia, thrombocytopenia, increased transfusion demand and symptomatic splenomegaly.
- A few patients will require iron chelation therapy.

Q. Give a brief account of paroxysmal nocturnal haemoglobinuria (PNH).

- An acquired nonmalignant clonal expansion of one or more haematopoietic stem cells.
- The stem cells and their progeny have deficient CD55 and CD59 proteins on their membrane (acquired membrane defect). This makes the red cells susceptible to complement-mediated, intravascular lysis through alternate pathway.
- Extravascular haemolysis also occurs in spleen and liver.

CLINICAL FEATURES

- Mainly seen in adults, usually in middle age. Both sexes equally affected.
- Presents with passage of dark-coloured urine, typically at night or in the morning; occurs intermittently.
- Dysphagia due to oesophageal spasm and abdominal pain in 10% cases.
- Mild jaundice and mild hepatosplenomegaly often present.
- Intravascular thrombosis frequent; may develop in cerebral, portal or mesenteric vessels. Most frequent cause of mortality.
- May begin as or progress to aplastic anaemia (due to cellular autoimmunity).

DIAGNOSIS

- Investigations show anaemia, reticulocytosis, varying degrees of thrombocytopenia and leucopenia, raised bilirubin and haemosiderinuria.
- Cellular bone marrow with erythroid hyperplasia.
- Diagnosis is confirmed by Ham's test and sucrose lysis test:
    - Ham test checks whether red blood cells become more fragile when they are placed in mild acid.

- In sucrose lysis test, patient's red cells are placed in low-ionic strength solution of sucrose and observed for haemolysis.
- These tests cannot reliably detect small populations of the affected red cells.
- Ham test can also be positive in congenital dyserythropoietic anaemia and the sucrose lysis test can be positive in megaloblastic anaemia and autoimmune haemolytic anaemia.
- Deficiency of CD57 and CD59 as shown by flow cytometric method is a rapid and sensitive test for diagnosis.

TREATMENT

- Mainly supportive with blood transfusions and control of infections.
- Iron therapy often required due to loss in urine.
- Steroids may be useful in some cases.
- Eculizumab and ravulizumab:
  - These are humanised monoclonal antibodies which bind to complement C5, preventing its activation to C5b and thereby inhibiting membrane attack complex (MAC—consists of C5b, C6, C7, C8 and C9), the cytolytic component of complement system.
  - Also reduce thrombotic episodes.
  - Most serious risk is infection with *Neisseria meningitidis;* such patients should be vaccinated against it.
- Heparin along with eculizumab or ravulizumab for acute thrombotic events.
- Stem cell transplantation is curative.

Q. Give a brief account of autoimmune haemolytic anaemias.

Q. What is the significance of Coombs' test?

Q. Discuss cold haemagglutinin disease (CHAD) in brief.

Q. Write briefly on paroxysmal cold haemoglobinuria (PCH).

Q. Write short note on drug-induced immune haemolytic anaemia.

AUTOIMMUNE HAEMOLYTIC ANAEMIAS

- A group of acquired disorders in which antibodies develop against red cell antigens. These antibodies cause destruction of red cells resulting in haemolytic anaemia.
- Autoimmune haemolytic anaemias (AIHA) may be classified in two ways:
  1. Based on the type of antibody (Table 1.39)
  2. Based on aetiology (Table 1.39).
- Warm AIHA is caused by antibodies that react with red cells at 37°C. Majority of them are of the IgG class. Red cells are coated with IgG or IgG plus C3d. The red cell destruction occurs extravascularly by two mechanisms:
- Erythrocyte phagocytosis mediated by antibody binding to tissue macrophage Fc receptors.
- Removal of a portion of the red cell membrane, resulting in microspherocytes which are trapped in the spleen.
- Cold AIHA is caused by antibodies that react with red cells at below 20°C (maximal at 4°C), and majority of them are of the IgM class. Red cells are usually coated with C3d only.

WARM ANTIBODY AUTOIMMUNE HAEMOLYTIC ANAEMIA

- Rhesus (Rh) polypeptides are the commonest targets for the autoantibodies in patients with warm AIHA.
- Most patients with idiopathic warm AIHA are women in their fourth or fifth decade of life.
- Clinical features include anaemia, jaundice, hepatosplenomegaly (20% cases) and manifestations of underlying disease. Acute cases present with intravascular haemolysis. Chronic cases occur more commonly and present with extravascular haemolysis. Venous thromboembolism may occur in many patients.
- Diagnosis is based on evidence of haemolysis, microspherocytes and macrocytes in peripheral blood and positive direct and indirect Coombs' tests. In some cases, autoimmune thrombocytopenia may also be present along with haemolysis (*Evan's syndrome*).
- Exclude underlying systemic lupus erythematosus, lymphoma and leukaemia.

TABLE 1.39 Classification of Autoimmune Haemolytic Anaemias

Based on Antibody Type	Based on Aetiology

• Warm antibody autoimmune haemolytic anaemia (warm AIHA)
  • Drugs (e.g. methyldopa, penicillins, quinidine)
  • Autoimmune disorders (SLE, others)
  • Idiopathic
  • Chronic lymphocytic leukaemia
  • Hodgkin's lymphoma
• Cold antibody autoimmune haemolytic anaemia (cold AIHA)
  • Cold haemagglutinin disease (CHAD)
  • Paroxysmal cold haemoglobinuria (PCH)
  • Associated with mycoplasma, chickenpox, lymphoma
  • Congenital or tertiary syphilis
	• Idiopathic or primary autoimmune acquired haemolytic anaemia (50%)
	• Secondary autoimmune acquired haemolytic anaemia (50%)
	  • Drugs—e.g. methyldopa, penicillins, quinidine
	  • Chronic lymphocytic leukaemia (CLL)
	  • Lymphomas
	  • *M. pneumoniae* infection
	  • Infectious mononucleosis
	  • SARS-CoV-2
	  • SLE and other connective tissue
	  • Nonlymphoid neoplasms (e.g. ovarian tumours) or certain chronic inflammatory diseases (e.g. ulcerative colitis)
	  • Solid organ transplantation
	  • Allogeneic stem cell transplantation

COOMBS' TEST (Box 1.17)

BOX 1.17 Direct and Indirect Coombs' Test

- Direct Coombs' test (direct antiglobulin test): Patient's red cells are washed and suspended in saline. Rabbit antihuman globulin is added. Agglutination of red cells indicates the presence of antibodies on the surface of red cells.
- Indirect Coombs' test: Normal red cells and rabbit antihuman globulin are added to the patient's serum. This produces agglutination of red cells if antibodies are present in the serum.

TREATMENT

- Blood transfusion is avoided as far as possible but may be used as a temporising measure in critically ill patients. Due to the presence of autoantibodies, it may be difficult to get cross-matched blood. In such situation, it is best to use ABO- and Rh-compatible blood under the cover of intravenous hydrocortisone.
- Prednisolone 1–2 mg/kg daily initially for first 2–4 weeks until achievement of haemoglobin >10 g/dL, followed by gradual tapering by 20 mg every week until a dose of 20 mg/day is reached. This is followed by a slower taper over 4–8 weeks.
- Patients with particularly rapid haemolysis may require intravenous methylprednisolone at a dose of 250–1000 mg/day for 1–3 days.
- Intravenous immunoglobulin for patients refractory to conventional therapy with corticosteroids; may also be used as a possible temporising measure before doing a splenectomy.
- Rituximab (Box 1.18).
- Splenectomy in patients who have not had a satisfactory response to initial corticosteroids, who relapse after having responded or who require the equivalent of more than 10–15 mg prednisone per day to maintain an acceptable haemoglobin level.
- Folic acid supplementation.
- Immunosuppression with azathioprine, cyclophosphamide, cyclosporin and others in patients unresponsive to rituximab and splenectomy.
- Table 1.40 summarises the treatment of warm antibody autoimmune haemolytic anaemia.

TABLE 1.40 Summary of Treatment of Warm Antibody Autoimmune Haemolytic Anaemia

First-line treatment	• Glucocorticoids (prednisolone or methylprednisolone) alone or in combination with rituximab
Second-line treatment	• Rituximab • Mycophenolate mofetil
Third-line treatment	• Azathioprine • Cyclosporin • Pulse dose cyclophosphamide
Fourth-line treatment	• Splenectomy

BOX 1.18 Rituximab in Warm Antibody Autoimmune Haemolytic Anaemia

- A humanised monoclonal antibody directed against CD20 on pre-B cells and mature B lymphocytes
- Useful in refractory cases and secondary type of warm AIHA
- May be combined with corticosteroids as first-line therapy
- Adverse effects: hypotension, fever, chills, rigors, hypertension, bronchospasm, pulmonary infiltrates, acute respiratory distress syndrome, myocardial infarction, cardiogenic shock
- Contraindicated in untreated hepatitis B infection

COLD HAEMAGGLUTININ DISEASE OR COLD AGGLUTININ DISEASE

- Cold haemagglutinin disease (CHAD) is characterised by haemolytic anaemia of varying severity. This results from autoantibodies that act as red cell agglutinins at low temperatures.
- After exposure to cold, the patient develops acrocyanosis as a result of red cell autoagglutination.
- CHAD is termed 'primary' if no malignant or infectious disease can be found by clinical and radiological assessment.
- Anti-I antibodies are associated with primary cold autoimmune haemolytic anaemia (cold agglutinin disease), as well as *Mycoplasma pneumoniae* and lymphoma. Anti-i is associated with haemolysis caused by infectious mononucleosis or lymphoma. I/i antigens are precursors of the ABH and Lewis blood group substances.
- Patients are advised to avoid cold exposure.
- Rituximab alone or in combination with bendamustine or fludarabine is the first-line treatment for severe disease. Chlorambucil and cyclophosphamide are useful in more severe chronic cases.
- Splenectomy and glucocorticoids are not much useful.
- Transfusion of red blood cells using warmer blood in severe symptomatic anaemia.
- Postinfectious cases are often self-limited.

PAROXYSMAL COLD HAEMOGLOBINURIA (DONATH–LANDSTEINER SYNDROME)

- PCH is characterised by attacks of acute haemolysis and haemoglobinuria on exposure to cold. This results from autoantibodies (IgG type) against P-antigen which lyse red cell at low temperatures. Other features include aching, abdominal cramps, headache, often followed by chills and fever. Rituximab alone or in combination with other drugs, especially bendamustine, is the first-line treatment for severe disease. Steroids can also be added if required.

DRUG-INDUCED IMMUNE HAEMOLYTIC ANAEMIA

- Drugs produce immune haemolysis by two mechanisms (Table 1.41).

TABLE 1.41 Mechanisms of Drug-Induced Immune Haemolytic Anaemia

• Drug-independent antibodies	• Drugs produce subtle alteration in red cell membrane resulting in production of antibodies and then extravascular haemolysis identical to warm AIHA • Direct Coombs' test is positive • Commonly occurs with α-methyldopa, cladribine and fludarabine • Can continue for several weeks after cessation of offending drug

• Drug-dependent antibodies	• Categorised into two subtypes:
	  • Hapten type which is due to non-covalent binding of drug to the RBC which is then targeted by autoantibody (e.g. penicillins)
	  • Drug-autoantibody immune (ternary) complexes leading to complement-dependent haemolysis (e.g. quinidine)

Q. What are myeloproliferative diseases or myeloproliferative neoplasms (MPN)?

Q. What are myelodysplastic syndromes (MDS)?

- Myeloproliferative neoplasms (MPN), previously called myeloproliferative diseases, occur due to clonal expansion of a multipotent haematopoietic progenitor cell with the overproduction of one or more of mature, functional elements of the blood (peripheral blood granulocytosis, thrombocytosis or erythrocytosis alone or in combination) with no dyserythropoiesis, granulocytic dysplasia or monocytosis. These conditions have an increased risk of thrombosis, bleeding and leukaemic transformation.
- MDSs are characterised by cellular dysplasia, variable degrees of peripheral blood cytopenias and bone marrow hyperplasia (or less often, hypoplasia). The paradox of proliferative bone marrow together with peripheral blood cytopenias in MDS may be explained by increased intramedullary myeloid precursor cell apoptosis. These are discussed separately.
- MDS/MPN include disorders that manifest both dysplastic and proliferative features. These include chronic myelomonocytic leukaemia (CMML), MDS/MPN with ring sideroblasts and thrombocytosis and others.
- Following conditions are included under the category of MPN:
  - Polycythaemia vera.
  - Idiopathic myelofibrosis or primary myelofibrosis (prefibrotic and fibrotic).
  - Essential thrombocytosis.
  - Chronic myeloid leukaemia or chronic myelogenous leukaemia (associated with *BCR-ABL1* genetic abnormality).
  - Others: Chronic neutrophilic leukaemia (CNL), chronic eosinophilic leukaemia-not otherwise classified (CEL-NOS), and MPN, unclassifiable (MPN-u).

Q. Classify myeloid neoplasms.

- The term 'myeloid' includes all cells belonging to the granulocytic (neutrophil, eosinophil, basophil), monocyte/macrophage, erythroid, megakaryocytic and mast cell lineages.
- Myeloid neoplasms include five major entities (Box 1.19).

BOX 1.19 Myeloid Neoplasms

- Acute myeloid leukaemia (AML)
- Myelodysplastic syndromes (MDS)
- Myeloproliferative neoplasms (MPN)
- Myelodysplastic/myeloproliferative neoplasms (MDS/MPN) overlap
- Myeloid neoplasms associated with eosinophilia and specific molecular abnormalities

Q. What is polycythaemia? How do you classify polycythaemia?

Q. What are the clinical manifestations of polycythaemia?

- Polycythaemia signifies an increase in the number of red blood cells above normal in the circulating blood. The increase may or may not be associated with an elevation in the total quantity of red blood cells in the body.
- In relative polycythaemia, the concentration of the red cells becomes greater than normal (but total red cell mass is normal) in the circulating blood. This occurs as a result of loss of plasma.
- In absolute polycythaemia, there is an increase in the total red cell mass. It is of two types:
  - Primary polycythaemia (erythraemia; polycythaemia vera; primary proliferative polycythaemia) denotes absolute polycythaemia of unknown aetiology. This is associated with decreased EPO levels.
  - Secondary polycythaemia (erythrocytosis) denotes absolute polycythaemia of known aetiology (which occurs in response to some known stimulus). This is associated with increased EPO levels.

CLASSIFICATION AND CAUSES

Relative polycythaemia (reduced plasma volume, normal red cell mass)
- Dehydration—low fluid intake, vomiting, diarrhoea, sweating, acidosis.
- 'Stress' polycythaemia.

Absolute polycythaemia (increased red cell mass)
- Primary polycythaemia (erythraemia; polycythaemia vera).
- Secondary polycythaemia (erythrocytosis)—causes given in Table 1.42.

TABLE 1.42 Causes of Secondary Polycythaemia

Increased Production of EPO as a Consequence of Central Hypoxia	Increased Production of EPO as a Consequence of Local Renal Hypoxia
• High altitude • Cyanotic congenital heart diseases (TOF—tetralogy of Fallot, Eisenmenger's complex) • Pulmonary diseases (e.g. COPD—chronic obstructive pulmonary disease) • Sleep apnoea syndrome • Chronic carbon monoxide poisoning • Smokers • Abnormal haemoglobins with high oxygen affinity	• Renal artery stenosis • End-stage renal disease • Hydronephrosis • Renal cysts (polycystic kidney disease) • Postrenal transplant erythrocytosis
Increased Production of EPO as a Consequence of Drugs	**Increased Production of EPO or EPO-like Substance by Tumours**
• EPO administration • Androgen administration	• Cerebellar haemangioblastoma • Renal tumours (carcinoma, adenoma, sarcoma) • Uterine myoma, hepatocellular carcinoma, phaeochromocytoma

CLINICAL FEATURES

- The clinical features of polycythaemia include a characteristic 'ruddy' cyanosis, dizziness, headache, epistaxis and an increased incidence of thrombotic complications. In addition, clinical manifestations of the underlying disease will be present in secondary forms.

Q. Discuss the clinical features, diagnosis and management of polycythaemia vera.

DEFINITION

- Polycythaemia vera is a clonal stem cell disorder characterised by an increased production of all myeloid elements; however, the disease is generally dominated by an elevated haemoglobin concentration.
- It is the most common MPN.

AETIOLOGY

- Unknown; however, hypersensitivity to interleukin-3 may play a role.

CLINICAL FEATURES

- Predominantly seen in people older than 40 years and more common in males.
- Neurological complaints related to increased viscosity and/or decreased cerebral perfusion (Table 1.43).
- Pruritus, particularly after bathing is frequent and may be disabling (occurs due to activated basophils).
- The patients often have a high colour, suffused conjunctivae, deep red palate, dusky red hands and retinal venous engorgement.
- Splenomegaly is very common and symptoms related to it may be present. Hepatomegaly occurs in 30% cases.
- Symptoms of peripheral vascular insufficiency and thrombotic and haemorrhagic complications.
- Incidence of peptic ulcer is five times higher in patients with polycythaemia vera.

TABLE 1.43 Neurological Features of Polycythaemia Vera

• Vertigo	• Ataxia
• Hearing loss or rushing in ears	• Chorea
• Tinnitus	• Syncope
• Fullness in the head	• Stroke
• Visual disturbances	• Seizures
• Paraesthesias	• Coma

- Bleeding manifestations like epistaxis, bleeding from peptic ulcer, intramuscular haemorrhages and bruising.
- Hyperuricaemia may result in the formation of urate stones and uric acid nephropathy.

DIAGNOSIS

- Haemoglobin concentration and haematocrit are markedly elevated. However, in many patients, the plasma volume is also elevated that results in near-normal haematocrit. Hence, it is important to determine the red cell mass.
- Increased red cell mass and blood viscosity. Red cell mass is reliably determined by isotope dilution using the patient's ^{51}Cr-tagged red cells.
- Total white cell count and platelet count are usually elevated.
- Absolute basophil count is increased to $>100/\mu L$ in majority.
- Leucoerythroblastic picture in many patients (immature cells of both myeloid and erythroid lineages).
- The arterial oxygen saturation is normal in contrast to hypoxic erythrocytosis where it is reduced. Patients with high-affinity haemoglobin also have normal oxygen saturation.
- Bone marrow shows either erythroid hyperplasia or panhyperplasia and depletion of iron stores.
- Urine and serum levels of EPO are reduced.
- Leucocyte alkaline phosphatase (LAP), LDH, serum vitamin B_{12} levels and B_{12}-binding capacity increased in majority.
- Abnormal liver function tests and increased urate levels.
- Janus kinase 2 (*JAK2*) mutations (seen in 95% patients with polycythaemia vera and in 50% cases of essential thrombocytosis and primary myelofibrosis).

JANUS KINASES

- A tyrosine kinase family comprising four members, JAK1, JAK2, JAK3 and TYK2, which are utilised by haematopoietic growth factors and cytokine receptors to phosphorylate tyrosine residues on specific intracellular proteins after the interaction of the receptor with its ligand.
- Located on chromosome 9.
- JAK2 is used by the EPO, TPO and G-CSF receptors to transmit signals and thus is integrally involved in haematopoiesis.
- JAK2 inhibitors may be useful for managing these patients.

DIAGNOSTIC CRITERIA (Table 1.44)

COMPLICATIONS (Table 1.45)

TREATMENT

- It has a very slow course. Aim of therapy is to maintain haematocrit below 45 in males and 42 in females.
- Repeated venesection (phlebotomy) is the treatment of choice. Urgent phlebotomy if features of hyperviscosity present (Flowchart 1.9).
- Alkylating agents and ^{32}P (phosphorus) should be avoided as these agents are leukaemogenic.
- Consider a cytotoxic agent if the patient is intolerant to venesection, thrombocytosis occurs, or symptomatic or progressive splenomegaly develops. Hydroxyurea is the agent of choice in all patients (Flowchart 1.9). Side effects of hydroxyurea include leg ulcers, mucocutaneous lesions, GI upset and fever. If it fails, ruxolitinib (an inhibitor of *JAK1* and *JAK2*) or pegylated interferon is used. Ruxolitinib may cause cytopenias, weight gain and skin cancer. In elderly patients (>75 years), ^{32}P or busulphan may still be useful.

TABLE 1.44 Diagnostic Criteria of Polycythaemia Vera

Major Criteria	Minor Criterion
1. Haemoglobin >16.5 g/dL (men) or >16.0 g/dL (women) OR haematocrit >49% (men) or >48% (women) OR elevated red cell mass >25% above mean normal predicted value 2. BM biopsy showing hypercellularity for age with trilineage growth (panmyelosis) including prominent erythroid, granulocytic, and megakaryocytic proliferation with pleomorphic, mature megakaryocytes (differences in size) 3. Presence of *JAK2V617F* (a mutation in *JAK2*) or similar mutation	Subnormal serum EPO level
Diagnostic criteria	
All three major criteria OR first two major criteria + minor criterion	

TABLE 1.45 Complications of Polycythaemia Vera

• Thrombotic episodes • Peptic ulcer • Hyperuricaemia • Sudden massive increase in splenic size	• Myelofibrosis • Acute myeloid leukaemia • Erythromelalgia

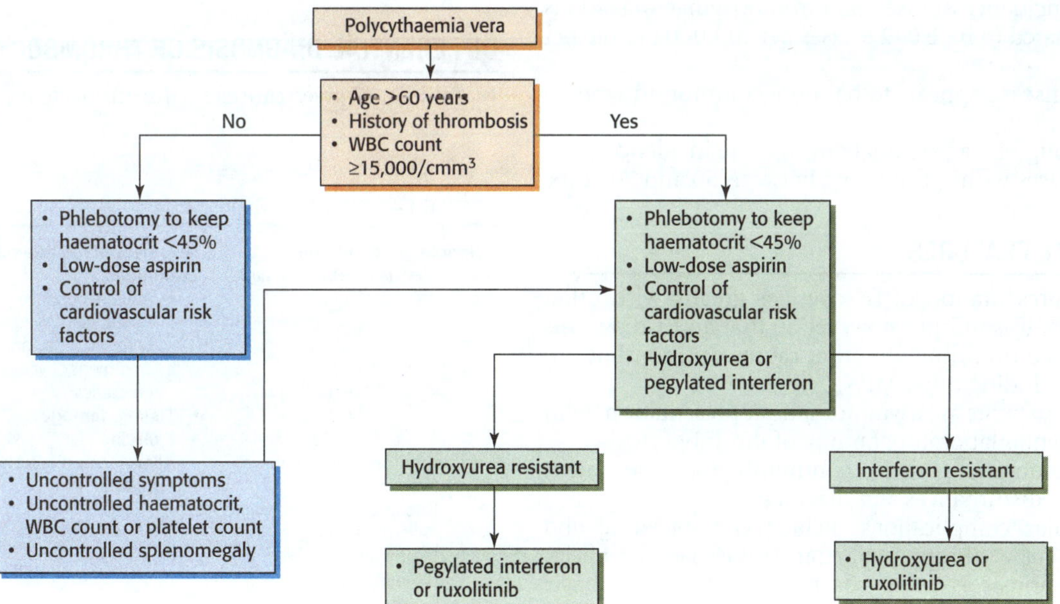

Flowchart 1.9 Management of Polycythaemia Vera.

TABLE 1.46 Differentiation Between Polycythaemia Vera and Secondary Polycythaemia With Hypoxia

Differentiating Feature	Primary	Secondary
• Oxygen saturation	Normal	Low
• Erythropoietin levels	Decreased	Increased
• Total white cell count	Increased	Normal
• Absolute basophil count	Increased	Normal
• Platelet count	Increased	Normal
• Leucocyte alkaline phosphatase (LAP)	Increased	Normal
• Vitamin B_{12} levels	Increased	Normal
• Bone marrow	Panhyperplasia	Erythroid hyperplasia
• Splenomegaly	Present	Absent

- Low-dose aspirin in all patients to reduce thrombotic episodes.
- Anagrelide (inhibitor of platelet aggregation) may be used if the patient continues to have thrombotic features despite above treatment.
- Asymptomatic hyperuricaemia does not require treatment unless chemotherapy is planned.
- Generalised pruritus should initially be treated with antihistamines. If these agents do not help, hydroxyurea, pegylated interferon and psoralens with UV light in 'A' range (PUVA) may be tried.

Q. How will you differentiate primary polycythaemia (polycythaemia vera) from secondary polycythaemia with hypoxia (e.g. chronic obstructive pulmonary disease [COPD])?

- Differentiating polycythaemia vera from secondary polycythaemia with hypoxia is shown in Table 1.46.

Q. Discuss briefly about essential thombocythaemia/thrombocytosis.

Q. What are the causes of thrombocytosis?

- The incidence of essential thrombocythaemia (ET) is estimated to be 1.0–2.5 cases per 100,000 people per year.
- The disease appears to be more common in women than men.
- Although it can occur at any age, the incidence of ET increases with age, peaking between 50 and 70 years.

CLINICAL FEATURES

- The presentation of ET overlaps greatly with other MPNs. It is unique, however, in that an ET diagnosis is based on ruling out other causes of thrombocytosis, including other MPNs.
- Most patients are asymptomatic at presentation, with incidental laboratory finding of thrombocytosis.
- Symptomatic patients commonly have headache, visual disturbances and dizziness.
- Vascular complications include easy bleeding and bruising, erythromelalgia, transient ischaemic attacks.
- Thrombosis is more common than haemorrhage. Arterial thrombosis is more common than venous thrombosis. Thrombotic episodes can produce stroke, pulmonary embolism, myocardial infarction, pulmonary hypertension and priapism.
- Mild splenomegaly develops in 50% cases.

DIAGNOSTIC CRITERIA (Box 1.20)

BOX 1.20 Diagnostic Criteria of Essential Thrombocytosis

Major Criteria:

1. Platelet count >450 × 10^9/L
2. Bone marrow biopsy showing proliferation mainly of the megakaryocyte lineage with increased numbers of enlarged, mature megakaryocytes with hyperlobulated nuclei. No significant left-shift of neutrophil granulopoiesis or erythropoiesis
3. Not meeting WHO criteria for BCR-ABL1+ chronic myeloid leukaemia, polycythaemia vera, primary myelofibrosis, myelodysplastic syndrome or other myeloid neoplasm
4. Presence of JAK2, CALR or MPL mutation

Minor Criteria:

1. Presence of a clonal marker (e.g. abnormal karyotype) or absence of evidence for reactive thrombocytosis

Diagnosis requires meeting all four major criteria or first three major criteria plus minor criterion

DIFFERENTIAL DIAGNOSIS OF THROMBOCYTOSIS

- Table 1.47 gives causes of thrombocytosis.

TABLE 1.47 Causes of Thrombocytosis

Neoplastic conditions: • Various myeloproliferative disorders • Myelodysplastic/ myeloproliferative neoplasm: • MDS/MPN with ring sideroblasts and thrombocytosis **Inflammatory conditions:** • Infections • Rheumatologic disorders • Vasculitides • Inflammatory bowel disease • Coeliac disease • POEMS syndrome	**Non-neoplastic haematologic conditions:** • Acute blood loss • Acute haemolytic anaemia • Iron-deficiency anaemia • Treatment of vitamin B_{12} deficiency • **Tissue damage** • **Exercise** • **Allergic/medication reactions** • **Asplenia**

TREATMENT

- The management of ET is very similar to that of PV. Main aims of treatment include treating the common vasomotor symptoms and preventing thrombotic complications.
- The mainstay of treatment is low-dose aspirin. In addition to microvascular symptoms, such as erythromelalgia, the use of low-dose aspirin is also useful in preventing thrombosis.
- Hydroxyurea is indicated in high-risk group of patients which include age >60 years, history of thrombosis, presence of a JAK2 mutation and the usual coronary artery disease risk factors (e.g. diabetes, smoking, hypertension).
- Anagrelide (inhibitor of platelet aggregation) may be used if the patient continues to have thrombotic features despite above treatment.

Q. Discuss the causes, clinical features and management of neutropenia.

- Normal absolute neutrophils count is greater than $1500/mm^3$.
- A reduction in number of circulating neutrophils below $1500/mm^3$ is known as neutropenia.
- Severe neutropenia means neutrophil count below $500/mm^3$ or is expected to decrease below this value over next 48 hours. These patients are at risk of developing serious infections.
- Agranulocytosis indicates neutrophil count below $100/mm^3$.

CAUSES OF NEUTROPENIA (Table 1.48)

TABLE 1.48 Causes of Neutropenia

Reduced Neutrophil Production	Increased Neutrophil Destruction
Marrow infiltration • Leukaemias • Myelodysplastic syndrome • Myelofibrosis • Granulomatous infiltration (e.g. tuberculosis, histoplasmosis)	• Hypersplenism • Severe sepsis • Autoimmune neutropenia • Systemic lupus erythematosus • Felty's syndrome • Medications (phenylbutazone, phenothiazines)
Marrow injury • Drugs (chloramphenicol, antithyroid drugs, nonsteroidal antiinflammatory drugs [NSAIDs], chemotherapeutic agents, sulpha drugs, penicillins, carbamazepine, clozapine, methimazole) • Infections (typhoid, malaria, viral hepatitis, kala-azar, infectious mononucleosis, measles, brucellosis, HIV) • Aplastic anaemia • Paroxysmal nocturnal haemoglobinuria • Radiation	**Miscellaneous causes** • Vitamin B_{12} deficiency • Folic acid deficiency • Copper deficiency • Cyclical neutropenia

CLINICAL FEATURES

- History of exposure to one of the agents.
- Sore throat, fever with chills and rigors.
- Necrotic ulcers in throat and mouth.
- Other infections include cellulitis, sinusitis, otitis, pneumonia, perirectal infections, etc. Bacterial infections generally involve *Staphylococcus aureus, Staphylococcus epidermidis*, streptococci, enterococci, *Pseudomonas aeruginosa* and other Gram-negative bacilli. Fungal infections usually arise from *Candida* or *Aspergillus* species.
- Toxaemia and sepsis later lead to death.
- Bleeding manifestations if the patient has associated thrombocytopenia or develops DIC due to sepsis.
- **'Cyclic neutropenia'**, most often an autosomal dominant disorder, is neutropenia occurring in cycles of 3–4 weeks. The neutropenia has a duration of 3–5 days. Though fatal infections are uncommon, recurrent fever and oropharyngeal/skin infections are common. Most patients respond to G-CSF.

INVESTIGATIONS

- Total leucocyte count is markedly decreased.
- Reduction or absence of neutrophils in the peripheral blood.
- In many, the bone marrow shows a virtual disappearance of the granular cells and their precursors.
- Evidence of other diseases, for example leukaemia and MDS.
- Vitamin B_{12} and folate levels.
- Cultures of various body fluids to find possible organisms causing infection.
- Radiographs and ultrasound to localise the site of infection.

TREATMENT

- General care:
  - Removal of offending agent.
  - Barrier nursing.
  - Maintain good oral hygiene.
  - Avoid rectal temperature measurements and rectal examinations.
  - Administer stool softeners for constipation.
- If febrile, initiate broad-spectrum antibiotics covering Gram-negative organisms within first hour of presentation. Monotherapy with piperacillin/tazobactam, meropenem or imipenem/cilastatin as initial empirical antibiotic treatment is recommended at present. Addition of vancomycin to cover for Gram-positive

organisms is usually not recommended empirically unless patient has a high risk (e.g. haemodynamic instability or other evidence of sepsis, pneumonia documented radiographically, clinically suspected catheter-related infection, skin or soft tissue infection at any site or severe mucositis).

- Role of granulocyte transfusions is controversial. Transfused granulocytes have a short life. They may form aggregates that can produce pulmonary compromise. Further, there is a possibility of CMV transmission.
- Recombinant G-CSF and granulocyte–monocyte colony-stimulating factor (GM-CSF) are useful in high-risk patients as they shorten the period of recovery and the duration of infection. These should not be used before or 24 hours after administering cytotoxic chemotherapy. Adverse effects include skin rash, acute respiratory distress syndrome and myalgias.

Q. How do you classify leukaemias?

- Leukaemias are classified as acute or chronic leukaemias (Tables 1.49, 1.50 and 1.51).

TABLE 1.49 Classification of Leukaemias

Acute	Chronic
• Lymphoid (lymphoblastic) • Myeloid (myelogenous)	• Lymphoid (lymphocytic) • Myeloid (myelocytic)

TABLE 1.50 Subclassification of Leukaemias: FAB (French–American–British) Classification

Acute Lymphoblastic	Acute Myeloid
• Common type (pre-B)—L1, L2 • T cell—L1, L2 • B cell—L3 • Undifferentiated (rare)	• M0—Minimally differentiated leukaemia • M1—Myeloblastic without maturation • M2—Myeloblastic with maturation • M3—Promyelocytic • M4—Myelomonocytic • M5—Monocytic • M6—Erythroleukaemia (Di Guglielmo's disease) • M7—Megakaryocytic
Chronic Lymphocytic	**Chronic Myelocytic (Myeloid)**
• B cell CLL—Common • T cell CLL (rare), e.g. T-cell granular lymphocytic leukaemia • Hairy cell leukaemia • B-cell prolymphocytic leukaemia (PLL)	• Ph[x] positive • Ph[x] negative, BCR[xx] positive • Ph[x] negative, BCR[xx] negative • Eosinophilic leukaemia

Ph[x], Philadelphia chromosome; BCR[xx], breakpoint cluster; L1—small cells with homogeneous chromatin, regular nuclear shape, small or absent nucleolus and scanty cytoplasm; L2—large and heterogeneous cells, heterogeneous chromatin, irregular nuclear shape and nucleolus often large (most common type); L3—large and homogeneous cells with multiple nucleoli, moderate deep blue cytoplasm and cytoplasmic vacuolisation that often overlies the nucleus.

TABLE 1.51 WHO Classification of Acute Myeloid Leukaemia and Acute Lymphoblastic Leukaemia

Acute Myeloid Leukaemia	Acute Lymphoblastic Leukaemia[a]

• AML with recurrent genetic abnormalities (includes acute promyelocytic leukaemia)
• AML with MDS-related changes
• Acute promyelocytic leukaemia
• Therapy-related myeloid neoplasms
• AML, not otherwise specified
  • AML with minimal differentiation
  • AML without maturation
  • AML with maturation
  • Acute myelomonocytic leukaemia
  • Acute monoblastic/monocytic leukaemia
  • Acute erythroid leukaemia
  • Acute megakaryoblastic leukaemia
  • Acute basophilic leukaemia
  • Acute panmyelosis with myelofibrosis
• Myeloid sarcoma
• Myeloid proliferations related to Down syndrome
	• B-cell lymphoblastic leukaemia/lymphoma with recurrent genetic abnormalities
	• T-cell lymphoblastic leukaemia/lymphoma
	• B-cell lymphoblastic leukaemia/lymphoma, not otherwise specified

[a]ALL and lymphoblastic lymphoma are the same disease entities at the morphologic and immunophenotypic levels and classified as either B- and T-cell lymphoblastic leukaemia/lymphoma.

Q. Discuss the aetiology of leukaemias.

- In majority of patients, the aetiology is unknown. However, in a minority of cases, some associations have been described (Table 1.52).
- For AML, preexisting MPNs are risk factors.

Q. Define acute leukaemia. Discuss the clinical features, investigations and management of acute leukaemias.

DEFINITION

- Acute leukaemia is characterised by a failure of cell maturation, proliferation of immature cells that fill up the bone marrow and ultimately spill over of these immature cells into the peripheral blood.

ACUTE LYMPHOBLASTIC LEUKAEMIA

- Also known as acute lymphoblastic leukaemia/lymphoma.
- Majority are B-cell leukaemias representing approximately 85% of all ALLs.
- T-cell ALL is found more typically in adolescents and the NK-cell ALLs are more common in adults.

ACUTE MYELOID LEUKAEMIA

- Occurs due to a somatic gene mutation in myeloid cells that results in the loss of control at one level of production. This loss of control then leads to increased, decreased or normal levels of production of that line and disturbed production of other cell lines resulting from crowding or inhibitory suppression in the bone marrow.
- Besides quantitative disturbances, function of cells can be affected.

CLINICAL FEATURES

- Both acute lymphoblastic (acute lymphocytic or acute lymphoid) and acute myeloblastic (acute myeloid) leukaemias share many clinical features in common. Patient often presents with nonspecific 'flu-like' symptoms.
- The symptoms and signs of acute leukaemias are due to one or more of the following:
  - Anaemia
  - Granulocytopenia
  - Thrombocytopenia
  - Expanding cell mass in bone marrow
  - Leukaemic infiltration of tissues
  - Others

ANAEMIA

- Pallor, tiredness, malaise.
- Cardiorespiratory symptoms in severe anaemia.

GRANULOCYTOPENIA

- Fever due to septicaemia.
- Infections at various sites, the common sites being skin, gingiva, lung, perirectal area and urinary tract.

THROMBOCYTOPENIA

- Thrombocytopenia results in bleeding. The common sites of bleeding include gum, nose (epistaxis), skin (purpura, ecchymoses, petechiae, easy bruising), buccal mucosa, fundus and per vaginam.
- Intracranial bleeding is a serious and fatal complication.

EXPANDING CELL MASS IN BONE MARROW

- Bone pains.
- Sternal tenderness.

LEUKAEMIC INFILTRATIONS

- Infiltrations of various tissues by leukaemic cells can occur. Common sites of leukaemic infiltration are as follows:
  - Leukaemic infiltration of liver, spleen and lymph nodes results in hepatosplenomegaly and generalised lymphadenopathy.
  - Involvement of the central nervous system (CNS) results in leukaemic infiltration of brain parenchyma, spinal cord parenchyma and meninges ('leukaemic meningitis'). Leukaemic meningitis starts as headache and nausea. Papilloedema, cranial nerve palsies, seizures and altered consciousness develop as disease progresses. The cerebrospinal fluid characteristically shows leukaemic blast cells, elevated proteins and reduced glucose.
  - Mediastinal masses with T-cell ALL.
  - Other areas of leukaemic infiltration include gums (gingival hypertrophy; particularly common with M4 and M5 types), skin (leukaemia cutis), testes, ovaries, eyes and bones. Extramedullary masses of neoplastic myeloid precursor cells are known as chloromas.

OTHERS

- Hyperleucocytosis (leucocyte counts $>100,000/mm^3$), usually seen in adult ALL and monocytic type of

TABLE 1.52 Causes of Leukaemias

Familial and genetic • Identical twins • Down's syndrome • Ataxia telangiectasia • Klinefelter's syndrome	**Drugs and toxins** • Cytotoxic drugs like alkylating agents, topoisomerase II inhibitors • Exposure to benzene • Chloramphenicol, phenylbutazone
Ionising radiation • Atomic bombing • Therapeutic irradiation • X-rays of foetus in pregnancy	**Retroviruses** • Human T-cell leukaemia lymphoma virus (human T-cell lymphotropic type I virus) **Immunological** • Immune deficiency states

AML, presents with fever, headache, blurred vision, stroke, intracranial haemorrhage, dyspnoea, chest pain, pulmonary infarction, acute respiratory distress syndrome or disseminated intravascular coagulation (DIC). Patient may present with tumour lysis syndrome even without chemotherapy and requires urgent leucopheresis.
- DIC in acute promyelocytic leukaemia.

INVESTIGATIONS

- Severe anaemia of normochromic type.
- MCV is normal or raised.
- Total leucocyte count is markedly raised but usually less than 100×10^9/L (range 1×10^9/L to 500×10^9/L). Leucopenia is also common particularly in AML.
- Peripheral smear shows numerous blast cells and other primitive cells.
- Auer rods in AML: Seen in peripheral smear within the leukaemic cells. They are seen as groups of rod-shaped red inclusions in the cytoplasm.
- Platelet count is markedly decreased.
- Bone marrow is hypercellular with replacement of normal elements by leukaemic blast cells (>20% lymphoblasts in ALL; >20% myeloid blasts in AML unless typical cytogenetic abnormalities are present). The presence of specific clonal cytogenetic abnormalities, such as t(8;21)(q22;q22), inv(16)(p13;q22), t(16;16)(p13;q22) and t(15;17)(q22;q12), also define AML irrespective of the blast count.
- Other routine investigations include liver function tests, renal function tests, coagulation studies, plasma LDH and plasma uric acid.
- In ALL, a lumbar puncture is necessary to rule out occult CNS involvement. In addition, computed tomography and gadolinium MRI are required to look for brain and spinal cord involvement, particularly if the patient has neurologic features.
- Immunophenotyping of leukaemic cells using flow cytometry is necessary for accurate diagnosis and to initiate risk-directed treatment. An extensive panel of monoclonal antibodies to cell surface 'cluster of differentiation' (CD) markers is used.
- Cytogenetic and molecular genetic analysis of leukaemia cells are important for prognosis and treatment outcome.

MANAGEMENT

- The first and major decision to be taken is whether to give specific therapy. If specific therapy is not desired, the patient is only given supportive therapy.

SUPPORTIVE THERAPY

- Treatment of anaemia with red cell concentrate.
- Treatment of thrombocytopenic bleeding with platelet transfusions.
- Identification of the organism and appropriate antimicrobial treatment in bacterial, fungal, protozoal and viral infections.
- Barrier nursing.
- Continuous monitoring of hepatic, renal and haemostatic functions.
- Maintenance of fluid and electrolyte balance. In patients undergoing rapid lysis of leukaemic cells following chemotherapy, the occurrence of hyperuricaemia, hyperkalaemia, hypocalcaemia and hyperphosphataemia (tumour lysis syndrome) can be prevented by close attention to hydration, urine alkalinisation and allopurinol/rasburicase before starting chemotherapy.
- For hyperleucocytosis, intravenous fluids are given followed by emergent reduction in leucocyte counts using chemotherapy or hydroxyurea and leucapheresis (removal of circulating cells with re-infusion of leucocyte-poor blood containing plasma, red cells and platelets). DIC and tumour lysis syndrome should be managed.
- Psychological support.

BONE MARROW TRANSPLANTATION

- Bone marrow transplantation has to be considered in young patients under 40 years with acute myeloblastic leukaemia in first remission, and ALL in first, second or subsequent remission, particularly in high-risk patients (Ph-positive ALL, elevated leucocyte count, CNS disease, high-risk gene rearrangements).

SPECIFIC THERAPY

Acute Lymphocytic Leukaemia

- Specific therapy involves remission induction, CNS-directed treatment and consolidation, re-induction and remission maintenance.
- The goal of induction therapy is to induce morphologic remission and to restore normal haematopoiesis and bone marrow showing normal cellularity with less than 5% blasts. Induction therapy consists of at least three systemic drugs—a glucocorticoid (usually dexamethasone or prednisolone), vincristine, L-asparaginase and daunorubicin (or idarubicin or doxorubicin) and intrathecal therapy (particularly in high-risk patient). It aims to induce complete morphologic response in 4–6 weeks. Toxicities of L-asparaginase include hepatotoxicity, pancreatitis and coagulation disorder.
- CNS-directed treatment and consolidation aim to prevent CNS relapses and to reduce systemic minimal residual leukaemic burden. CNS therapy involves weekly or biweekly intrathecal therapy (hydrocortisone, methotrexate and cytarabine) along with systemic drugs like high-dose methotrexate, asparaginase, cytarabine and 6-mercaptopurine.
- Re-induction or re-intensification (essentially similar to induction phase) is included in most regimens.
- Maintenance involves administering drugs for 2 years or more. It consists of daily 6-mercaptopurine and weekly methotrexate with monthly pulses of vincristine and dexamethasone. Periodic intrathecal therapy is continued.
- A subset of ALL patients is Philadelphia chromosome (Ph) positive (BCR-ABL1 fusion) and therefore, respond

to tyrosine kinase inhibitors like imatinib, dasatinib, nilotinib, ponatinib and bosutinib.

- Blinatumomab is a bispecific antibody with the ability to bind CD3 on T cells and CD19 receptors on B cells. It has been used in patients with relapsed/refractory B-cell ALL.
- Chimeric antigen receptor T cell (CAR-T) therapy targeting CD19 has shown remarkable results in young patients with relapsed/refractory B cell ALL.

Acute Myeloid Leukaemia

- Includes induction and maintenance (post-remission) therapy.
- Candidates for allogenic stem cell transplantation should be identified early during induction phase. These include patients younger than 70 years with high-risk karyotype (see section heading 'Poor Prognostic Factors' in the subsequent text) who are in first remission after induction phase.
- Induction therapy includes an anthracycline (e.g. daunorubicin or idarubicin) and cytosine arabinoside ± etoposide ± cladribine/fludarabine (along with G-CSF). Gemtuzumab ozogamicin (antibody against CD33–drug conjugate) may be added to the induction regimen to achieve better results.
- Patients achieving remission with induction therapy (blasts <5% in bone marrow, absolute neutrophil count >1000/mm^3, platelets >100,000/mm^3 and no extramedullary disease) should receive cycles of maintenance or postremission therapy or allogenic stem cell transplantation. In young patients (younger than 60 years), high-dose cytosine arabinoside alone or in combination with other drugs such as mitoxantrone, etoposide or amsacrine is recommended.

Acute Promyelocytic Leukaemia (M3)

- It is associated with severe coagulation complications (DIC) and represents a medical emergency because of risk of catastrophic bleeding.
- It has a better prognosis and responds well to combination of induction therapy (one of the anthracyclines) plus all-trans retinoic acid (ATRA; tretinoin). Treatment needs to be started as soon as diagnosis is suspected on the basis of presentation and bone marrow evaluation.
- Combination of ATRA and arsenic trioxide has been found to be as effective as ATRA + one of the anthracyclines.
- While receiving ATRA, differentiation syndrome may occur which is characterised by dyspnoea, fever, weight gain, hypotension, pulmonary infiltrates and pleural and pericardial effusion. Treatment is with dexamethasone.
- Granulocyte-colony stimulating growth factors (filgrastim, pegfilgrastim) should never be used in APL, as granulocyte growth factors may induce a drastic increase in APL progression and trigger fatal DIC.

SUMMARY

- Management of acute lymphocytic leukaemia and acute myeloid leukaemia is summarised in Flowcharts 1.10 and 1.11.

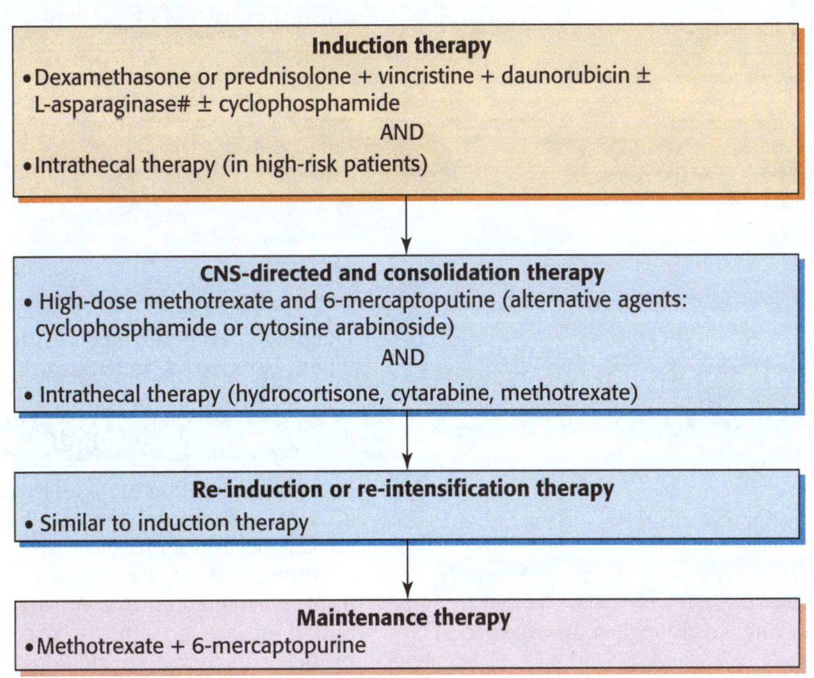

Flowchart 1.10 Management of Acute Lymphocytic Leukaemia.

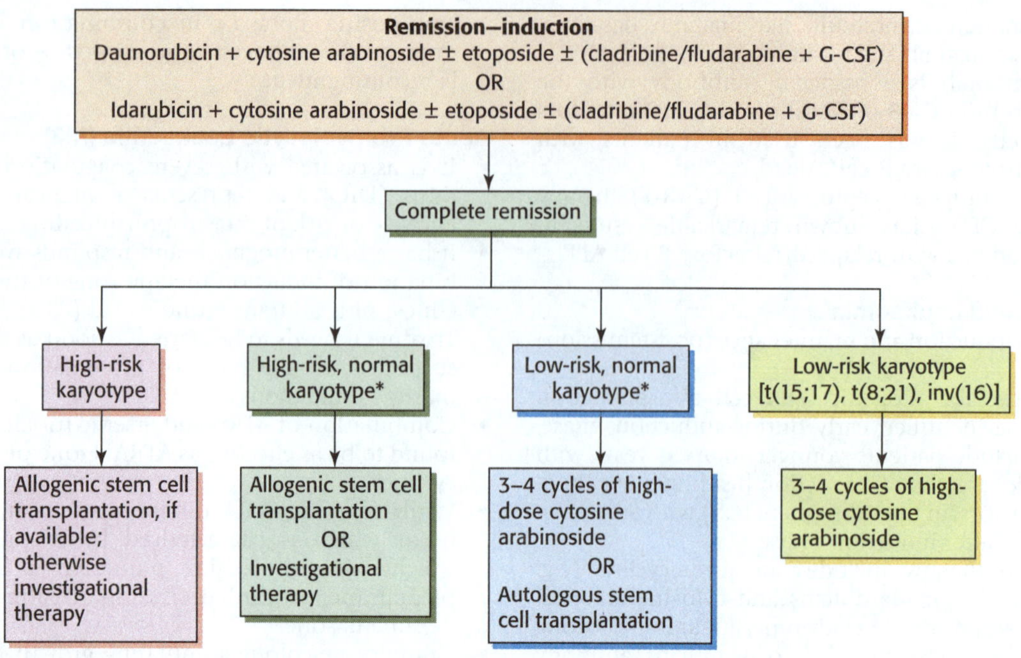

Flowchart 1.11 Management of Acute Myeloid Leukaemia.

POOR PROGNOSTIC FACTORS (Table 1.53)

TABLE 1.53 Poor Prognostic Factors in AML and ALL

AML	ALL
• Age >60 years • Secondary cause present • TLC >20,000/mm³ at presentation • Presence of DIC • French–American–British (FAB) type M0, M5, M6, M7 • Auer rod absent • Fibrosis on bone marrow examination • High-risk karyotype [t(6;9), inv(3)] • Therapy-related leukaemia	• Age >60 years (in adults); in children, age <1 year or >9 years • Male sex • TLC >50,000/mm³ for B-cell ALL and TLC >100,000/mm³ for T-cell ALL • Mediastinal mass • CNS involvement • L3 type • Pro-B or B-cell ALL (T-cell ALL in children) • Hypodiploidy (<45 chromosomes) • High-risk karyotype [t(9;22) and others]

Q. How do you differentiate acute lymphoblastic leukaemia from acute myeloblastic leukaemia?

- Table 1.54 gives differentiating points between ALL and AML.

Q. Describe subleukaemic leukaemia.

- In acute leukaemia, one would expect an increase in total leucocyte count.
- In a small percentage of patients with acute leukaemia, the total leucocyte count is normal or less than normal. Abnormal cells are seen in the peripheral blood. This is termed subleukaemic leukaemia.
- Diagnosis is confirmed from the bone marrow, which is replaced by leukaemic cells.

Q. Define aleukaemic leukaemia.

- In a patient with acute leukaemia, one would expect an increase in total leucocyte count and abnormal cells in peripheral blood.
- In about 10% of the patients with acute leukaemia, total leucocyte count is normal or less than normal and there are no abnormal cells in the peripheral blood. This is called aleukaemic leukaemia. Some patients may present with cutaneous involvement (aleukaemic leukaemia cutis).
- Diagnosis is confirmed from the bone marrow, which is replaced by leukaemic cells.

TABLE 1.54 Differentiation Between ALL and AML

Clinical Features	Acute Lymphoblastic Leukaemia	Acute Myelogenous Leukaemia
• Age group	Common in children	Common in adults
• Presentation as bleeding	Less common	More common (in 60%)
• Lymphadenopathy	More common	Less common
• Hepatosplenomegaly	In majority (50%–75%)	In minority
• CNS involvement	More common	Less common
• Gum involvement	—	Gum hypertrophy common in M5 type
• Testicular involvement	In 10%–20%	—
• Eye involvement	More common	Less common
• Skin involvement	Less common	More common
• Mediastinal involvement	More common	Less common
• Leukaemic involvement of CNS	More common	Less common
Investigations		
• Leukaemic blasts	Lymphoblasts (10–15 μm) are smaller than myeloblasts, with a thin rim of agranular cytoplasm and round or convoluted nucleus	Myeloblasts (12–20 μm) are larger than lymphoblasts, with discrete nuclear chromatin and multiple nucleoli
• Cytoplasmic Auer rods	Not present	Present in 10%–20% (diagnostic)
• Nuclear enzyme, terminal deoxynucleotidyl transferase (Tdt) in leukaemic blasts	In more than 90%	Rarely present
• Cytochemical staining		
• Myeloperoxidase	Negative	Positive
• Sudan black B	Negative	Positive
• Chloracetate esterase	Negative	Positive
• Periodic acid–Schiff (PAS)	Positive in >50% of cells	Positive in <25% of cells

Q. Discuss briefly about leukaemoid reaction.

- Total leucocyte count >50,000/μL is termed as leukaemoid reaction. It is usually due to excess of neutrophils and their precursors but sometimes can be due to lymphocytosis (lymphocytic leukaemoid reaction).
- It reflects the response of the normal healthy bone marrow to various stresses. The stresses include a number of infections (including tuberculosis), acute haemorrhage, acute haemolysis, drugs (e.g. steroids, growth factors), haematological and nonhaematological malignancies and various toxic states.

NEUTROPHILIC LEUKAEMOID REACTION

- Peripheral smear shows mix of neutrophils, myelocytes, metamyelocytes, promyelocytes and even a few myeloblasts.
- The bone marrow shows proliferation of all the normal myeloid elements; in contrast, in acute leukaemia, the most immature elements predominate.
- LAP score is normal or increased.
- No absolute eosinophilia or basophilia (vs CML—see in the subsequent text).
- Philadelphia chromosome or *ABL-BCR* negative.
- Treatment of underlying disorder corrects the blood picture.
- Differences between neutrophilic leukaemoid reaction and chronic myeloid leukaemia are given in Table 1.55.

Q. Define and classify stem cells. Discuss their clinical applications.

- Stem cells are undeveloped cells capable of proliferation, self-renewal, conversion to differentiated cells and regenerating tissues.

TABLE 1.55 Differentiating Neutrophilic Leukaemoid Reaction and Chronic Myeloid Leukaemia

Feature	Neutrophilic Leukaemoid Reaction	Chronic Myeloid Leukaemia
Total WBC count	Increased	Markedly increased
Differential leucocyte count	Few immature cells	Numerous immature cells
Toxic granulations in neutrophils	May be present	Absent
Leucocyte alkaline phosphatase	Increased	Reduced
Eosinophilia and basophilia	Usually absent	Present
Anaemia	Minimal or absent	May be present
Platelets	Normal or increased (due to acute phase reaction)	Normal or increased
Philadelphia chromosome	Absent	Present

- Three classes of stem cells: totipotent, pluripotent and multipotent:
  - A fertilised egg is considered totipotent because it has the potential to generate all the different types of cells in the body.
  - Pluripotent stem cells are those that can give rise to any type of cell in the body except those needed to develop a foetus. These cells give rise to cells derived from all three embryonic germ layers: endoderm, mesoderm and ectoderm.
  - Stem cells that can give rise to a small number of different cell types associated with different organs are called multipotent.
- Stem cells that are able to differentiate into cell types beyond those of the tissues in which they normally reside are said to exhibit plasticity. For example, stem cells from the bone marrow can give rise to three major types of brain cells: astrocytes, oligodendrocytes and neurons. The neural stem cells can differentiate into blood cells and muscle tissue.
- Two main types of stem cells are embryonic and non-embryonic.

EMBRYONIC STEM CELLS

- Embryonic stem cells (ESC) are pluripotent because they can differentiate into all cell types.
- Derived from the inner cell mass of a blastocyst, which forms several days after an egg is fertilised.
- An ESC line is created by placing the cells on a feeder layer of fibroblasts. The feeder layer assists in maintaining the ESC in an undifferentiated state or adult stem cells.

NON-EMBRYONIC (ADULT OR SOMATIC) STEM CELLS

- Non-embryonic stem cells (non-ESC) are also known as adult stem cells because the cells are obtained from adults. These are multipotent because their potential to differentiate into cell types is more limited.
- Two types of stem cells: haemopoietic (CD34 positive and are committed to differentiate into blood cells) and the less differentiated mesenchymal stem cells. Adult stem cells which undergo mesodermal lineage-specific differentiation to osteocytes, adipocytes and chondrocytes are named as mesenchymal stem cells.
- Adult stem cells (SC) such as haematopoietic stem cells (HSC) in bone marrow, peripheral blood or cord blood are currently the only types of SC commonly used to treat human diseases.

CLINICAL APPLICATIONS

THERAPEUTIC

- Only non-ESC have been used clinically so far.
- Beneficial for blood disorders such as leukaemia, multiple myeloma and lymphoma and disorders with defective genes such as severe combined immune deficiency.
- Other *possible* uses where clinical trials are ongoing are given in Table 1.56.

TABLE 1.56 Diseases With Potential for Stem Cell Transplantation

• Ischaemic heart disease	• Stroke
• Spinal cord lesions	• Parkinson's disease
• Nonunion of fractured bones	• Huntington's disease
• Type 1 diabetes	• Motor neuron disease
	• Alzheimer's disease
	• Muscular dystrophy
	• Multiple sclerosis

Q. Give a brief account of haematopoietic stem cells (HSC).

Q. Write a short note on peripheral blood stem cell transplantation.

- HSC transplantation refers to infusion of HSC from a donor to a recipient with the intention to re-populate or replace totally or partly the recipient's haematopoetic system.
- HSC are self-renewing cells that can re-populate all the cell lineages in the blood. Immature haematopoietic progenitor cells ($CD34^+$) are a surrogate measure of the stem cell dose in the transplant product.
- The major sources of HSC for transplantation include bone marrow (discussed in the subsequent text), peripheral blood (peripheral blood stem cells) and cord blood.
- Stem cells obtained from the recipient (same person) are called **autologous.** Immunosuppressives are not required. However, there is no graft-versus-tumour effect and therefore, increased risk of disease relapse or progression compared to allogenic graft. Further, graft may be contaminated with tumour cells.
- Stem cells obtained from someone other than the recipient are termed **allogenic**. Three types of allogenic donors are syngeneic, related and unrelated. When the donor is an identical twin, donation is termed syngeneic.
- The key to successful allogenic transplantation is finding an HLA-matched donor because it decreases the risk of graft rejection and graft-versus-host-disease (GVHD).

PERIPHERAL BLOOD STEM CELLS

- Peripheral blood stem cell transplantation is defined as transplantation of stem cells derived from the peripheral blood of a donor to a recipient (allogenic) or from the patient's own blood (autologous).
- HSC circulate in the peripheral blood but are in a very low concentration (<0.1% of all nucleated cells). To increase their numbers, haematopoietic growth factor (G-CSF or GM-CSF) is administered for 4–5 days to the donor (for allogenic transplant) or to the patient during recovery from intensive chemotherapy (for autologous transplant). Apart from increasing number of cells, G-CSF causes release of proteases that degrade proteins anchoring stem cells to the marrow stroma, thereby causing release of HCS into peripheral blood.

- If G-CSF fails, plerixafor, an HSC mobiliser may be used.
- After treatment with growth factors, stem cells are collected from the blood by pheresis and are infused in the recipient.
- The cells are engrafted in the recipient after variable period. Engraftment means recovery of neutrophil count to >500/mm^3 for three consecutive days.
- Compared to bone marrow transplant, use of peripheral blood stem cells results in more rapid haematopoietic recovery. However, the risks of GVHD are still similar to those associated with bone marrow transplantation.

CORD BLOOD STEM CELLS

- Cord blood is a good source of HSC with no risk to infant or mother. Contamination of cord blood with CMV and Ebstein–Barr virus is low due to poor transmission from placenta. However, the major limitation is that the number of cells that can be collected from cord blood is small and an adult might require multiple cord blood donors.
- The umbilical cord is rich in mesenchymal stem cells. One of the recent techniques is cord blood banking in which cord cells are cryopreserved immediately after birth, stored and may be used in therapies to treat future life-threatening diseases of a given person.

INDICATIONS

- Indications for haematopoietic stem cell transplantation are given in Table 1.57.

COMPARISON AMONG BONE MARROW, PERIPHERAL BLOOD AND CORD BLOOD STEM CELLS (Table 1.58)

TABLE 1.57 Indications for Haematopoietic Stem Cell Transplantation

Non-malignant conditions	
• Inherited metabolic disorders	Adrenoleucodystrophy, Hurler syndrome, metachromatic leukodystrophy, Gaucher's disease, osteopetrosis
• Inherited immune disorders	Severe combined immunodeficiency, Wiskott–Aldrich syndrome
• Inherited red cell disorders	Pure red cell aplasia, sickle cell disease, β-thalassaemia
• Marrow failure states	Severe aplastic anaemia, Fanconi's anaemia, paroxysmal nocturnal haemoglobinuria
• Autoimmune diseases (experimental)	Systemic sclerosis, severe systemic juvenile rheumatoid arthritis, lupus, multiple sclerosis
Malignant conditions	
• Selected cases of acute and chronic leukaemias	
• Plasma cell disorders	
• Myelodysplastic syndrome (MDS)	

TABLE 1.58 Comparison Among Various Types of Haematopoietic Cells

	Source		
Characteristic	**Cord Blood**	**Peripheral Blood**	**Bone Marrow**
• Stem cell content	Low	Good	Adequate
• Risk of tumour cell contamination	Not applicable	Low	High
• HLA matching	Less restrictive	Close matching	Close matching
• Engraftment	Slowest	Fastest	Medium
• Risk of acute graft-versus-host disease (GVHD)	Lowest	High	High
• Risk of chronic GVHD	Lowest	Highest	Medium

CONDITIONING REGIMENS

- Often required in recipient before transplantation.
- Can be myeloablative or nonmyeloablative (reduced intensity).
- Myeloablative regimens eliminate malignant cells so that transfused HSC can populate the bone marrow and grow.
- The aim of nonmyeloablative regimen is to induce immunosuppression in recipient so that graft of donor cells can take place. It is less toxic and can be performed in patients with mild organ dysfunction.
- Conditioning regimens can produce complications, generally within 30 days, and include infections, nausea, vomiting, alopecia, mucositis and interstitial pneumonia. Another important early complication is veno-occlusive disease of liver where patient develops jaundice, ascites and tender hepatomegaly.
- Conditioning regimens can also lead to late complications including infertility, ovarian failure and second malignancies (AML and solid organ malignancies).

Q. Briefly outline bone marrow transplantation.

- It is a type of haematopoietic stem cell transplantation (see above).

BONE MARROW TRANSPLANTATION

- Types of bone marrow transplantation are given in Box 1.21.

ALLOGENIC BONE MARROW TRANSPLANTATION

- Method of transplantation:
  - The recipient is suitably 'conditioned' with chemotherapy and radiotherapy. Conditioning ablates patient's haemopoietic and immunological tissues.
  - Healthy marrow from a donor (preferably histocompatible sibling) is injected intravenously into the conditioned patient. The injected cells 'home' to the marrow and produce erythrocytes, granulocytes and platelets. This usually takes 3–4 weeks. To regain good lymphocyte function and immunological stability, it takes longer time, even up to 3 years or more.
- Common complications of bone marrow transplantation are infections, GVHD, interstitial pneumonitis, veno-occlusive liver disease and graft failure.

COMPLICATIONS

Infections

- Infections may develop during three different phases after transplantation:
  - In the first phase, infections occur due to neutropenia and damage to gastrointestinal mucosal barrier produced by conditioning agents. Source of infection is oral, skin and gastrointestinal flora.
  - Second phase occurs during acute GVHD where T-cell function gets impaired. Patients are prone to develop opportunistic viral and fungal infections.
  - Third phase occurs due to chronic GVHD where both B-cell and T-cell functions are impaired. Therefore, patients are prone to develop bacterial (including encapsulated organisms), as well as opportunistic viral and fungal infections.

Graft Versus Host Disease (GVHD)

- GVHD results from the cytotoxic activity of donor T lymphocytes that become sensitised to their new host, which they regard as foreign.
- Occurs in 50%–80% of allogenic bone marrow transplantation and is the cause of high long-term morbidity and mortality. It can even occur in HLA-identical siblings.

BOX 1.21 Types of Bone Marrow Transplantation

- Syngeneic bone marrow transplantation, i.e. from identical twin donor
- Allogenic bone marrow transplantation, i.e. from non-identical donor
- Autologous bone marrow transplantation, i.e. the patient's own marrow is harvested to be given back again after intensive therapy

- GVHD can occur in two forms:
  - Acute GVHD occurs within first 100 days of transplantation. It occurs due to production of cytokines by Th1 cells. HLA mismatch is one of the most important risk factors for it. Main targets are skin, liver and gut. It causes diarrhoea, hepatitis, cholestasis and exfoliative dermatitis. Treatment includes methotrexate, cyclosporin, antithymocyte globulin, corticosteroids, tacrolimus, mycophenolate mofetil and monoclonal antibodies against T cells.
  - Chronic GVHD occurs more than 100 days after transplantation. It may arise independently or may follow acute GVHD. It occurs due to Th2 type cytokine production. It clinically resembles a connective tissue disorder and presents with dermatosis, liver injury, pulmonary fibrosis, alteration in gastrointestinal mucosa and reduced salivary and lacrimal flow. Treatment includes cyclosporin and corticosteroids.

Q. Discuss the natural course, clinical features and investigations of chronic myeloid leukaemia. Give a brief account of the treatment.

Q. Write a brief note on Philadelphia chromosome (Ph).

DEFINITION

- Chronic myeloid leukaemia is a myeloproliferative disease characterised by excessive proliferation of myeloid cells with fairly normal maturation.

CYTOGENETICS

- It is the result of a reciprocal translocation between the long arms of chromosomes 9 and 22 [t(9:22)]. The shortened chromosome 22 is cytogenetically evident as the Ph. About 5% patients are negative for Ph chromosome but have a complex translocation involving additional chromosomes but resulting in the same *BCR-ABL1* fusion gene.
- The fragment of chromosome 9 that joins the breakpoint cluster (*BCR*) of chromosome 22 carries Abelson (*ABL1*) protooncogene (9.22) (Fig. 1.6). This fusion gene (*BCR-ABL1*) codes for a protein with high tyrosine kinase activity. Increased and unregulated activity of tyrosine kinase can cause increase in tumour cell proliferation and growth, induce anti-apoptotic effects, and promote angiogenesis and metastasis.
- Ph chromosome is also found in about 20% of adults with acute precursor B-cell lymphoblastic leukaemia, 5%–10% of childhood ALL and about 1% of adult AML.

NATURAL COURSE

- The disease has three phases:
  - Chronic stable phase lasts for 3–5 years.
  - Accelerated phase.
  - Blast crisis phase in which it transforms into acute myeloid or lymphocytic leukaemia.

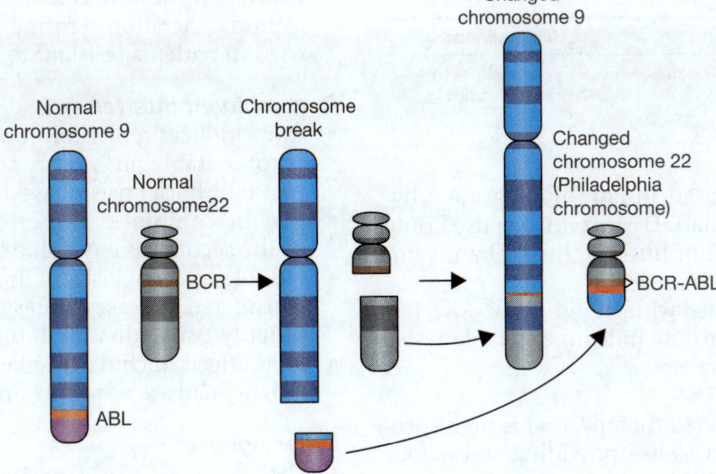

Fig. 1.6 Philadelphia chromosome.

- Approximately 20% of individuals progress directly from the chronic phase to blast crisis without any typical manifestation of accelerated phase.

CHRONIC STABLE PHASE

- Peak incidence in fourth and fifth decades; average age—55 years.

SYMPTOMS

- Many patients are asymptomatic early on and disease may be diagnosed on routine blood examination.
- Symptoms are due to massive splenomegaly like abdominal distension, postprandial fullness, reflux oesophagitis, dyspnoea and dragging discomfort in the left hypochondrium.
- Symptoms results from hypermetabolic state like fever, weight loss, sweating and heat intolerance.
- Symptoms of anaemia like fatigue, weakness and anorexia.
- Priapism.
- Bleeding tendencies, mainly due to platelet dysfunction occur late.

SIGNS

- Mild anaemia.
- Hepatomegaly.
- Moderate to massive, nontender splenomegaly; tenderness of spleen and splenic friction rub indicate splenic infarction.

INVESTIGATIONS IN CHRONIC STABLE PHASE

- Normocytic normochromic anaemia.
- Total leucocyte count is markedly raised, almost always more than 20,000/µL, often exceeding 200,000/µL.
- Peripheral smear (blood picture) examination:
  - Full range of granulocyte precursors ranging from myeloblasts, myelocytes, metamyelocytes to mature neutrophils are seen. The mature forms predominate.
  - Myeloblasts are less than 5%–10%, typically <2%.
  - Increase in basophils (<20%) and eosinophils.
  - Few nucleated red blood cells may be seen.
  - Platelet count may be normal, increased or decreased. Automated machines may give falsely elevated platelet counts due to disruption of granulocytes.
- Bone marrow study:
  - Although a diagnosis of CML can be made on peripheral blood examination, a bone marrow aspiration is needed to stage the patient and assess for additional chromosomal abnormalities.
  - Aspiration shows hypercellular bone marrow with marked proliferation of all granulocytic elements.
  - About 20%–30% of the patients have mild bone marrow fibrosis in late stages.
- Ph is positive in more than 95% of cases, in all three phases.
- In Ph-negative cases, evidence of translocation can be established by cytogenetics, reverse transcription-polymerase chain reaction (RT-PCR) and fluorescence in situ hybridisation (FISH).
- *BCR-ABL* rearrangement in peripheral blood or bone marrow.
- LAP score is very low, usually less than 5 (normal 20–100).
- Serum vitamin B_{12} levels are markedly raised due to increase in transcobalamin present in neutrophil granules.
- Serum LDH and uric acid levels are raised.
- Marked thrombocytosis may elevate serum potassium spuriously as platelets release potassium during clotting.
- Blood sugar may be falsely reduced due to glucose uptake and metabolism by leucocytes.

TREATMENT FOR CHRONIC STABLE PHASE

Chemotherapy

- The drugs available till the year 2000 did not produce cure (disappearance of Ph chromosome or *BCR-ABL*) in most patients.
- However, imatinib mesylate became available in 2001 and has been recommended in patients with chronic disease, accelerated phase and even in blast crisis.

TABLE 1.59 Drugs Commonly Used in CML

Drug	Induction	Maintenance
• Imatinib	300–400 mg/day	300–400 mg/day
• Hydroxyurea	0.5–2.0 g/day	0.5–2.0 g/day

- Other drugs that are used in chronic phase are hydroxyurea and busulphan. Hydroxyurea is used only to reduce leucocyte count initially. Busulphan is not often used.
- Chemotherapy is initiated with an induction dose, followed by a maintenance dose indefinitely (Table 1.59).

Imatinib Mesylate

- Imatinib provides targeted therapy, that is high specificity for the tumour cells, providing a broader therapeutic window with less toxicity.
- It is an inhibitor of tyrosine kinase activity of *BCR-ABL* proteins producing apoptosis of cancer cells.
- In chronic stable disease, imatinib can produce complete haematological response in >95% cases and complete cytogenetic response in as many as 75% cases.
- Despite complete cytogenetic response, residual disease remains detectable in majority of the cases, suggesting that it fails to eradicate the abnormal stem cells.
- Resistance to imatinib mesylate results from overexpression of the *BCR-ABL* gene or genetic alteration.
- Side effects include fluid retention, nausea, muscle cramps, diarrhoea, skin rash, liver toxicity, bleeding from mucous membranes, bone pains and myelosuppression. Therapy is stopped if severe neutropenia or thrombocytopenia develops; after recovery, dose reduction is considered.
- If a patient fails to respond to imatinib, other tyrosine kinase inhibitors (TKIs; dasatinib, nilotinib and bosutinib) may be used. These have also been used as first-line drugs in treatment of CML. One of the important adverse effects of dasatinib is occurrence of pleural effusion in as many as 30% cases. Ponatinib, a third-generation tyrosine kinase inhibitor, may be used in patients resistant to two or more TKIs.

Recombinant Interferon-α

- Can induce remission and maintain control in chronic stable phase. It is not effective in accelerated phase or blast crisis phase.
- May be combined with cytosine arabinoside or one of the second-line tyrosine kinase inhibitors.
- No role as a single agent in most patients; should be considered in cases unresponsive to imatinib and other tyrosine kinase inhibitors.
- Side effects include flu-like syndrome, weight loss, fatigue, nausea, vomiting and headache.

Other Agents

- Hydroxyurea (0.5–2.0 g/day) is a safe and effective agent to reduce initial leucocytic burden, as a temporary measure before definitive therapies, or in combination with TKIs to sustain complete haematologic or cytogenetic responses.
- Busulphan is often used in allogeneic stem cell therapy preparative regimens.

Splenectomy

- Splenectomy is done to relieve the symptoms resulting from the massive size of spleen and in repeated splenic infarctions.

Bone Marrow Transplantation

- Indicated in patients younger than 35 years who have a suitable donor and who do not respond to second-generation TKIs.
- Best results are obtained when the transplantation is done in early chronic stable phase.
- It can result in permanent disappearance of the Ph-positive clone and hence can cure CML in early stages.

SUMMARY OF TREATMENT (Table 1.60)

TABLE 1.60 Recommendations on Treatment

- Imatinib mesylate (400 mg/day) in newly diagnosed cases who are in chronic phase
- If response is suboptimal, consider a dose increase of imatinib, second-generation TKIs or allogenic haematopoietic stem cell transplantation or rINF-α with a TKI
- Failure is defined as:
  - No haematological response at 3 months
  - Incomplete haematological response at 6 months
  - No cytogenetic response at 6 months
  - Incomplete cytogenetic response at 12 months (Ph-positive >35%)

MONITORING OF THERAPY

- The first step is the haematologic response (WBC <10,000/μL, platelet count <450,000/μL, no immature granulocytes in peripheral smear and spleen nonpalpable) along with some cytogenetic response (Ph ≤35% and/or *BCR-ABL* ≤10%) within first 3 months.
- The second step is the complete cytogenetic response (no Ph+ metaphases and/or less than 1% *BCR-ABL* positive nuclei by FISH) at 6 months.
- The third step is the major molecular response (*BCR-ABL* ≤0.1%) on peripheral blood at 12 months.
- Once major molecular response has been achieved, response can be assessed by real-time quantitative polymerase chain reaction (RT-Q-PCR) every 3–6 months.

ACCELERATED PHASE AND BLAST CRISIS (Table 1.61).

TABLE 1.61 Accelerated Phase and Blast Crisis in CML

Accelerated phase of chronic myeloid leukaemia

If not treated, chronic myeloid leukaemia may transform itself to a blastic phase with or without going through an accelerated phase after 1–5 years of onset. Features of accelerated phase are the following:

- Development of anaemia
- Persistent or increasing splenomegaly, unresponsive to therapy
- Bone pain, skin infiltrates, lymphadenopathy
- Persistent or increasing leucocytes (>10,000/μL) unresponsive to therapy
- Increase in basophil count (>20%)
- Persistent thrombocytosis (>1,000,000/μL), unresponsive to therapy or persistent thrombocytopenia (<100,000/μL) unrelated to therapy
- About 10%–19% blasts in the blood and/or bone marrow
- Failure to achieve a complete haematologic response (leucocytes <10,000/μL, platelet count <450,000/μL, no immature granulocytes in the differential and spleen nonpalpable) to the first tyrosine-kinase inhibitor therapy
- Hydroxyurea along with one of the tyrosine kinase inhibitors are the most effective drug in accelerated phase
- Stem cell transplantation—once reversion to chronic phase or remission is achieved

Blast crisis phase of chronic myeloid leukaemia

Blast crisis phase represents the transformation of CML into an acute leukaemia

- 'Myeloid blast crisis' occurs in 70% when the disease transforms into acute myeloblastic leukaemia
- 'Lymphoid blast crisis' occurs in 30% when the disease transforms into acute lymphoblastic leukaemia

Features of blast crisis are the following:

- Refractoriness to treatment
- Abrupt increase in splenic size
- Bone pain and sternal tenderness
- Anaemia and bleeding tendencies
- Generalised lymphadenopathy
- Peripheral smear and bone marrow showing >20% blast cells simulating acute leukaemia
- Thrombocytopenia

Treatment of myeloid blast crisis is tyrosine kinase inhibitor with or without combination chemotherapy followed by stem cell transplantation in eligible patients

Treatment for lymphoid blast crisis is same as for acute lymphoblastic leukaemia

Q. Discuss the clinical features, investigations and management of primary myelofibrosis (agnogenic myeloid metaplasia, myelofibrosis with myeloid metaplasia).

Q. Define myelophthisis and discuss its causes.

DEFINITIONS

- Primary myelofibrosis is a MPN which has the worst prognosis among the Philadelphia chromosome-negative MPNs.
- Primary myelofibrosis is a clonal disorder of a multipotent haematopoietic progenitor cell characterised by increased fibrosis within the marrow, splenomegaly and extramedullary haemopoiesis. The extramedullary haemopoiesis can always be demonstrated in the spleen, usually in the liver and at times in lymph nodes, kidneys and adrenals.
- It can arise from antecedent polycythaemia vera or essential thrombocytosis (secondary myelofibrosis).

CLINICAL FEATURES

- Most cases occur after 60 years of age.
- A significant number of patients develop acute myeloid leukaemia.

SYMPTOMS

- Symptoms of anaemia like fatigue, weakness and anorexia.
- Symptoms due to massive splenomegaly like abdominal distension, postprandial fullness, reflux oesophagitis, dyspnoea and dragging discomfort in the left hypochondrium.
- Symptoms resulting from hypermetabolic state like fever, weight loss, sweating and heat intolerance.
- In late stages, bleeding tendencies due to thrombocytopenia.
- Death occurs due to portal hypertension and infections, with median survival around 5 years.

SIGNS

- Massive splenomegaly and hepatomegaly.
- Anaemia, lymphadenopathy, ascites, cardiac failure, jaundice and bleeding manifestations.
- Extramedullary haematopoiesis can also produce paraspinal masses with spinal cord compression, ascites and pleural and pericardial effusion.

INVESTIGATIONS

- Haemoglobin is normal in the early stages but markedly reduced in the late stages.
- Total leucocyte count may be normal, increased (early stages) or decreased (late stages).

BOX 1.22 Peripheral Smear in Primary Myelofibrosis

- Leucoerythroblastic blood picture (precursors of granulocytes and erythrocytes being present simultaneously)
- Many teardrop cells
- Anisocytosis and poikilocytosis
- Other features include many nucleated red blood cells, giant platelets with vacuoles, basophilic stippling and blasts up to 5%–10%

- Platelet count is elevated in the early stages but reduced in the late stages.
- Peripheral smear (Box 1.22).
- Bone marrow examination is diagnostic. Atypia of megakaryocyte proliferation even in the absence of overt reticulin fibrosis is diagnostic but the bone marrow findings are variable:
  - At one end of the spectrum (early stage or 'cellular phase' or 'prefibrotic phase'), the marrow is hypercellular with an increase in all three cell lines, particularly megakaryocytes. Fibrosis is minimal.
  - At the other end of the spectrum (late stage or 'hypocellular phase'), the marrow is hypocellular with reduction in all the three cell lines. The marrow is densely filled with fibrous tissue.
- LAP score is elevated.
- Philadelphia chromosome or BCR-ABL negative.
- Mutation in JAK2 gene (seen in 50%–60% cases).
- Serum vitamin B_{12} concentration is moderately elevated.
- Radiological examination reveals an increase in bone density of vertebrae and proximal ends of long bones.

DIAGNOSTIC CRITERIA (Box 1.23)

BOX 1.23 Diagnostic Criteria of Primary Myelofibrosis

Major Criteria:

1. Megakaryocyte proliferation and atypia accompanied by either reticulin and/or collagen fibrosis (grade 2 or 3)
2. Not meeting WHO criteria for BCR-ABL1+ chronic myeloid leukaemia, polycythaemia vera, essential thrombocytosis, myelodysplastic syndrome or other myeloid neoplasm
3. Presence of JAK2, CALR or MPL mutation or presence of another clonal marker or absence of evidence for reactive bone marrow fibrosis (due to infection, autoimmune disorder, chronic inflammatory conditions, hairy cell leukaemia or other lymphoid neoplasm, metastatic malignancy)

Minor Criteria:

Presence of one or more of the following confirmed in two consecutive determinations:

1. Anaemia not attributed to a comorbid condition
2. Leucocytosis ≥11 × 10^9/L
3. Palpable splenomegaly
4. Elevated LDH level
5. Leucoerythroblastic picture in peripheral smear

Diagnosis requires meeting all three major criteria and at least one minor criterion

TREATMENT

- Main goals of therapy are prolongation of survival and, if possible, cure by stem cell transplantation.
- If prolongation of survival or cure is not possible, symptom-orientated palliation is the main goal.

TREATMENT OF ANAEMIA (Box 1.24; Flowchart 1.12)

BOX 1.24 Treatment of Anaemia in Primary Myelofibrosis

- Correct other causes of anaemia
- Red cell transfusions
- Folic acid 5 mg daily
- Corticosteroids (prednisolone) to control any autoimmune haemolysis
- Erythropoiesis-stimulating agents (e.g. EPO) based on EPO level
- Danazol may be effective in controlling anaemia in some patients
- Thalidomide (50–200 mg/day) or lenalidomide (10 mg/day) with prednisolone; can control anaemia and splenomegaly in a substantial number of patients

TREATMENT OF SPLENOMEGALY

- Hydroxyurea is useful to control splenomegaly. It can lead to myelosuppression that further exacerbates underlying anaemia.
- Busulphan 2 mg daily in elderly patients with cellular bone marrow and marked leukocytosis who do not respond to hydroxyurea.
- Splenectomy in selected cases.
- Local radiotherapy to reduce splenic size. It is reserved for patients who cannot undergo splenectomy for any reason, but the efficacy of this therapy is poor, and subsequent cytopenias are often severe.
- Partial splenic artery embolisation.
- Intravenous cladribine in massive splenomegaly.
- Ruxolitinib, a *JAK1/2* inhibitor for patients with intermediate-/high-risk MF; also useful to reduce constitutional symptoms; may reduce bone marrow fibrosis as well. Adverse effects are anaemia, thrombocytopenia and increased risk of infections.

BONE MARROW TRANSPLANTATION

- Allogenic bone marrow transplantation is the only curative treatment. It can be performed only in a limited number of cases as most are above 60 years.

MISCELLANEOUS

- Allopurinol to control hyperuricaemia.
- Radiation therapy for symptomatic extramedullary haematopoiesis.
- Second line JAK inhibitors which may be used include momelotinib, fedratinib and pacritinib.

PROGNOSIS

- Median survival is 27 months to 135 months depending on the presence of poor prognostic factors.
- Poor prognostic factors include:
  - Age >65 years

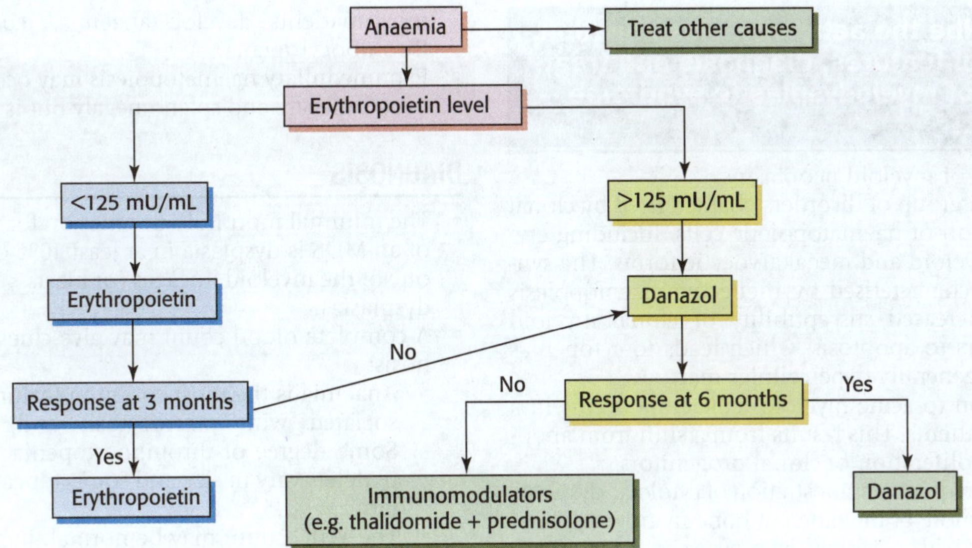

Flowchart 1.12 Management of Anaemia in Primary Myelofibrosis.

- Haemoglobin <10 g/dL
- Leucocytes $>25{,}000/\text{mm}^3$
- Circulating blasts $\geq 1\%$
- Platelets $<100{,}000/\text{mm}^3$
- Presence of constitutional symptoms

MYELOPHTHISIS

- Myelophthisis is infiltration of marrow by nonhaematopoietic or abnormal cells. Marrow fibrosis often occurs.
- Results in anaemia, leucopenia and thrombocytopenia. Splenomegaly may also develop.

CAUSES OF MYELOPHTHISIS OR OTHER CAUSES OF MYELOFIBROSIS (WHICH MAY ALSO PRODUCE SPLENOMEGALY)

(Table 1.62)

Q. How do you differentiate chronic myeloid leukaemia from myelofibrosis?

- Differentiating points between CML and myelofibrosis are given in Table 1.63.

TABLE 1.62 Causes of Myelophthisis

Malignant Conditions	Non-malignant Conditions
• Acute leukaemia (lymphocytic, myeloid) • Multiple myeloma • Chronic myeloid leukaemia • Hairy cell leukaemia • Polycythaemia vera • Carcinoma metastatic to marrow • Hodgkin's lymphoma • Non-Hodgkin's lymphoma • Essential thrombocytosis	• HIV infection • Tuberculosis • Exposure to thorium dioxide • Systemic lupus erythematosus • Renal osteodystrophy • Hyperparathyroidism • Radiation therapy • Gaucher disease

TABLE 1.63 Differences Between Chronic Myeloid Leukaemia and Myelofibrosis

Chronic Myeloid Leukaemia	Myelofibrosis
• Total leucocyte count markedly raised usually more than 20,000/μL • Peripheral smear shows full range of granulocyte precursors, predominantly mature forms • Nucleated red cells few or absent • Thrombocytopenia occurs late • Marrow fibrosis uncommon and minimal • LAP score is very low, usually <5 • Philadelphia chromosome positive • Very high vitamin B_{12} levels	• Total leucocyte count may be raised but usually less than 20,000/μL • Peripheral smear shows leucoerythroblastic blood picture, teardrop cells and anisopoikilocytosis • Nucleated red cells numerous • Thrombocytopenia common • Marrow fibrosis common and dense • LAP score is high, usually >100 • Philadelphia chromosome negative • Moderate elevation of vitamin B_{12} levels

Q. Describe the aetiology, classification, clinical features, diagnosis and treatment of myelodysplastic syndrome (MDS).

- A subtype of myeloid neoplasms.
- Refers to a group of disorders characterised by clonal proliferation of haematopoietic cells, including erythroid, myeloid and megakaryocytic forms. The syndrome is characterised by ineffective haemopoiesis due to increased susceptibility of clonal myeloid progenitors to apoptosis, which leads to cytopenias despite a generally hypercellular marrow.
- Progression to acute myeloid leukaemia occurs in a third of patients. This results from a shift from apoptosis to proliferation of clonal progenitors.
- Diagnosis requires demonstration of cytologic dysplasia in one or more of the different bone marrow cell lines in patients with persistent or progressive cytopenia or demonstration of increased myeloblasts (5%–19%).

AETIOLOGY

- The cause of MDS is unknown; however, exposure to radiation, certain pesticides and some chemotherapeutic (particularly alkylating agents and topoisomerase inhibitors) and nonchemotherapeutic agents may induce MDS.
- Another factor is aging. The median age of patients with MDS is 65 years.

CLASSIFICATION

- The disease can be classified by the WHO criteria given in 2016 (Table 1.64).

CLINICAL FEATURES

- The most significant features are due to failure of bone marrow to produce normal blood cells. Hence, most patients develop anaemia, leucopenia and thrombocytopenia.
- Extramedullary haematopoiesis may occur leading to hepatomegaly and splenomegaly but is uncommon.

DIAGNOSIS

- The minimal morphologic criterion for the diagnosis of an MDS is dysplasia in at least 10% of cells of any one of the myeloid lineages (or blasts <20% without dysplasia).
- A complete blood count may give clues to this diagnosis:
  - Anaemia is the most common feature, usually associated with macrocytosis and anisocytosis. Some degree of thrombocytopenia is usual. The platelets vary in size and some appear hypogranular.
  - The WBC count may be normal, increased or decreased. Neutrophils also show variation in size. Morphologic abnormalities are often observed in the granulocytes. These can include bilobed or unsegmented nuclei (pseudo-Pelger–Huet abnormality) or hypersegmented nuclei. Granulation abnormalities vary from an absence of granules to abnormal distribution inside the cytoplasm (Dohle bodies).
  - Immature myeloid cells are present.
- The bone marrow aspirate is hypercellular or normal in initial stages. It shows dysplastic features in one or several myeloid series. Myelofibrosis is occasionally present at diagnosis or may develop during the course of MDS. Bone marrow biopsy is useful when marrow is hypocellular as it helps in detecting fibrosis and also helps in differentiating it from aplastic anaemia or acute myeloid leukaemia.
- Cytogenetic study of the marrow is the most important test for establishing the diagnosis.
- In patients with megaloblastic features on bone marrow, serum vitamin B_{12} and folate levels should be measured.

TABLE 1.64 WHO Classification of Myelodysplastic Syndrome (2016)

	Dysplastic Changes	Cytopenias	Ring Sideroblasts	Blasts
MDS with single lineage dysplasia (MDS-SLD)	1	1 or 2	RS < 15%	PB < 1%; BM < 5%; no Auer rods
MDS with multilineage dysplasia (MDS-MLD)	2 or 3	1–3	RS < 15%	PB < 1%; BM < 5%; no Auer rods
MDS with ring sideroblasts (MDS-RS):				
MDS-RS with single lineage dysplasia (MDS-RS-SLD)	1	1 or 2	RS ≥ 15%	PB < 1%; BM < 5%; no Auer rods
MDS-RS with multilineage dysplasia (MDS-RS-MLD)	2 or 3	1–3	RS ≥ 15%	PB < 1%; BM < 5%; no Auer rods
MDS with excess blasts (MDS-EB)	0–3	1–3	None or any	PB 2%–19% or BM 5%–19% or Auer rods present
MDS, unclassifiable (MDS-U)	1–3	1–3	None or any	PB ≤ 1%; BM <5% Auer rods ±
MDS with defining cytogenetic abnormality (e.g. isolated del [5q])	0	1–3	RS < 15%	PB < 1%; BM < 5%; no Auer rods

Note: Cytopenias: Hb < 10 g/dL, platelet < 100,000/μL, leucocytes < 1800/μL, neutrophils < 1000/μL.
BM, bone marrow; PB, peripheral blood.

TREATMENT

- Therapy is supportive with packed cell transfusions for anaemia, platelet transfusions for bleeding associated with thrombocytopenia and antibiotic therapy for infections. Iron chelators are required to reduce iron overload from multiple transfusions.
- In some patients, EPO and G-CSF may be useful to ameliorate symptoms but survival benefit has not been shown.
- Antithymocyte globulin and cyclosporin in some hypoplastic MDS cases.
- Luspatercept is a recombinant fusion protein that binds transforming growth factor β superfamily ligands to enhance late-stage erythropoiesis. It may be useful in transfusion-dependent patients of MDS with ring sideroblasts who do not respond to erythropoiesis-stimulating agents.
- Other options include the use of thalidomide, lenalidomide (a derivative of thalidomide), 5-azacytidine and decitabine. 5-Azacytidine and decitabine (hypomethylating agents) have been shown to decrease blood transfusion requirements and to retard the progression of MDS to AML. Lenalidomide is beneficial in the MDS 5q-syndrome.
- Allogenic haematopoietic stem cell transplantation is the only potentially curative approach to MDS. However, it may be offered to less than 5%–10% of patients because MDS is most commonly diagnosed in patients in their seventh or eighth decade of life.

Q. Discuss the types, clinical features, investigations, clinical staging and management of chronic lymphocytic leukaemia (CLL).

DEFINITION

- CLL is characterised by excessive accumulation of mature-appearing lymphocytes in the peripheral blood, associated with infiltration of the bone marrow, spleen and lymph nodes.

TYPES

- More than 95% of the cases of CLL are due to the expansion of B lymphocytes. These express B-cell antigens (CD19, CD20 and CD24) and CD5 (aberrant expression), which is typically found on T cells.
- Less than 5% are due to the expansion of T lymphocytes.

CLINICAL FEATURES

- Most common form of chronic leukaemia.
- Common in patients older than 50 years; peak age around 65 years.
- More in males than in females (2:1).
- About 25% of the patients are asymptomatic.
- Generalised lymphadenopathy and hepatosplenomegaly.
- Slowly developing anaemia (due to immune haemolysis and bone marrow infiltration).
- Recurrent infections due to hypogammaglobulinaemia. *Streptococcus pneumoniae, Staphylococcus* and *H. influenzae* cause most of the infections; herpes zoster is also frequent.
- Bleeding manifestations extremely uncommon.
- May transform to prolymphocytic leukaemia (prolymphocytes >55%) or a large-cell lymphoma (Richter's syndrome).

INVESTIGATIONS

- Mild to moderate normocytic, normochromic anaemia.
- Total leucocyte count is raised to the range of 50,000–200,000/mm^3.
- Peripheral smear examination:
  - More than 95% of the cells are mature-appearing lymphocytes of the small variety.
  - Prolymphocytes may be present in varying proportions.
  - Platelets are normal or reduced in number (autoimmune thrombocytopenia).
- Bone marrow is hypercellular with infiltration of small- and medium-sized lymphocytes.
- Direct Coombs' test may be positive indicating an autoimmune haemolytic process.
- Lymph node biopsy shows well-differentiated, small, noncleaved lymphocytes.
- Immunoglobulin levels are normal or low
- Serum folic acid levels are low.

DIAGNOSTIC CRITERIA (Box 1.25)

BOX 1.25 Diagnostic Criteria for Chronic Lymphocytic Leukaemia

- At least 5 × 10^9 lymphocytes/L (5000/mm^3)
- Duration of lymphocytosis >2 months
- Atypical/immature cells ≤55% of lymphoid cells
- Low density of surface Ig (IgM or IgD) with k or λ light chains
- B-cell surface antigens (CD19, CD20, CD23)
- CD5 surface antigen

CLINICAL STAGING (Tables 1.65 and 1.66)

TABLE 1.65 Binet Staging of CLL

Stage	Features	Survival
A	No anaemia or thrombocytopenia Less than three areas of lymphoid enlargement	>10 years
B	No anaemia or thrombocytopenia Three or more areas of lymphoid enlargement	7 years
C	Anaemia (<10 g/dL) and/or thrombocytopenia (<100,000/mm^3) present, regardless of the number of areas of lymphoid enlargement	2 years

Lymphoid enlargement includes cervical, axillary and inguinal lymph nodes, and liver and spleen enlargement.

TABLE 1.66 Revised Rai Staging of CLL

Risk	Features	Survival
Low	Absolute lymphocytosis (>5000/mm^3) without adenopathy, hepatosplenomegaly, anaemia or thrombocytopenia	>10 years
Intermediate	Absolute lymphocytosis with lymphadenopathy with or without hepatosplenomegaly, without anaemia or thrombocytopenia	7 years
High	Absolute lymphocytosis and anaemia (haemoglobin <11 g/dL) or thrombocytopenia (<100,000/mm^3) with or without lymphadenopathy, hepatomegaly or splenomegaly	1.5–3 years

TREATMENT

- Indications of therapy (Box 1.26).
- Treatment options.
- Based on revised Rai (or Binet staging), treatment options are given in Table 1.67.

PURINE ANALOGUES

- Three purine analogues are currently used in CLL: fludarabine, cladribine and pentostatin. Fludarabine is the best studied agent of the three in CLL.

BOX 1.26 Indications of Therapy in CLL

- Fever (≥2 weeks) without evidence of infection, extreme fatigue, night sweats (≥1 month) without evidence of infection, weight loss (≥10% over 6 months)
- Increasing anaemia or thrombocytopenia due to bone marrow failure
- Bulky (≥10 cm) or progressive lymphadenopathy; massive (≥6 cm below costal margin) or progressive splenomegaly
- Autoimmune cytopenias not responsive to corticosteroids
- Rapidly rising lymphocyte count in peripheral blood (more than 50% increase over a 2-month period or doubling time <6 months)

TABLE 1.67 Treatment of CLL

• Low risk (or Stage A)	No specific treatment, but only reassurance
• Intermediate risk (or Stage B)	Asymptomatic: • No specific treatment Symptomatic, medically fit: • Fludarabine + cyclophosphamide + rituximab (age < 65 years) • Fludarabine + cyclophosphamide + rituximab and hyaluronidase human[a] • Bendamustine + rituximab (age > 65 years) • Fludarabine + rituximab (age > 65 years) • Obinutuzumab + chlorambucil (age > 65 years) Symptomatic, medically unfit: • Chlorambucil ± obinutuzumab • Bendamustine[b] Local radiotherapy to troublesome lymph nodes
• High risk (or Stage C)	• As for symptomatic intermediate risk (or Stage B) • Alemtuzumab + stem cell transplantation • Combination chemotherapy with cyclophosphamide, doxorubicin, vincristine and prednisolone (CHOP) in refractory cases • Packed cell transfusion for anaemia • Prednisolone for haemolytic anaemia and thrombocytopenia • Splenectomy for symptomatic splenomegaly

[a]Hyaluronidase human increases rate of dispersion and absorption of rituximab administered by subcutaneous injection.
[b]Bendamustine is an alkylating agent like chlorambucil.

- Fludarabine:
  - Dose—25 to 30 mg/m^2 intravenously daily for 5 days every 4 weeks.
  - Potential complications—autoimmune haemolytic anaemia; opportunistic infections including *Legionella pneumophila, Pneumocystis jiroveci, Listeria monocytogenes* and cytomegalovirus.

RITUXIMAB, OBINUTUZUMAB AND ALEMTUZUMAB

- Rituximab and obinutuzumab are monoclonal antibodies against CD20 while alemtuzumab is monoclonal antibody against CD52.
- CD20 present on normal and malignant B cells.
- CD52 present on all CLL cells.
- Side effects include fever, chills, myalgias, nausea and headache.

OTHER AGENTS

- These include Bruton's tyrosine kinase inhibitor (ibrutinib, acalabrutinib), BCL2 inhibitor (venetoclax) and phosphoinositide 3-kinase δ inhibitor (idelalisib) and are particularly useful in refractory/relapsed cases.

Q. Discuss the clinical features, investigations and management of hairy cell leukaemia.

CLINICAL FEATURES

- Hairy cell leukaemia is a malignant expansion of B lymphocytes.
- Common in patients older than 40 years with 4:1 male/female predominance.
- Symptoms are due to massive splenomegaly, pancytopenia and vasculitis (erythema nodosum and cutaneous nodules). Lymphadenopathy is uncommon.
- Hip pain due to bone lesions.
- Infections most common cause of death.
- Increased risk of secondary malignancies, particularly Hodgkin's lymphoma, non-Hodgkin's lymphoma and thyroid cancer.

INVESTIGATIONS

- Total leucocyte count normal or low. Pancytopenia, particularly monocytopenia in several patients.
- Peripheral smear shows the characteristic hairy cells. These are the malignant B lymphocytes. The hairy structures on the surface of the cell are cytoplasmic projections. They have an eccentrically placed nucleus and foamy cytoplasm. These hairy cells stain positively for tartrate-resistant acid phosphatase (TRAP).
- Bone marrow is difficult to be aspirated ('dry tap') and biopsy shows fibrosis with infiltration by mononuclear cells and hairy cells.
- LAP score is very high.

TREATMENT

- Follows an indolent course. The current recommendation is to initiate treatment if patient develops significant cytopenia (haemoglobin <11 g/dL; platelet count <100,000/μL; absolute neutrophil count <1000/μL), symptomatic splenomegaly or constitutional symptoms (e.g. fever, night sweats and fatigue).
- Treatment of infections with antibiotics.
- Treatment of choice is chemotherapy with one of the purine analogues (cladribine or pentostatin).
- Rituximab may be added to a purine analogue as a first-line therapy or in resistant cases.
- Corticosteroids and myelotoxic drugs are contraindicated in hairy cell leukaemia.

Q. How do you classify splenomegaly? Enumerate the common causes of splenomegaly.

CLASSIFICATION AND CAUSES (Table 1.68)

TABLE 1.68 Causes of Splenomegaly

• **Mild splenomegaly** (up to 5 cm)	
• Acute infections	Enteric fever, infectious hepatitis, infectious mononucleosis, brucellosis, septicaemia, cytomegalovirus, toxoplasmosis
• Subacute and chronic infections	Tuberculosis, infective endocarditis, syphilis, brucellosis, chronic bacteraemia, HIV
• Parasitic infestations	Malaria, kala-azar
• Others	Splenic sequestration syndrome in sickle cell disease; congestive heart failure
• **Moderate splenomegaly** (up to umbilicus)	Lymphomas, portal hypertension, acute leukaemias, chronic lymphocytic leukaemia, chronic myeloid leukaemia, chronic haemolytic anaemias, malaria, kala-azar, sarcoidosis
• **Massive splenomegaly** (below umbilicus)	Chronic myeloid leukaemia, kala-azar, myelofibrosis, hairy cell leukaemia, tropical splenomegaly, kala-azar, portal hypertension, (extrahepatic portal vein thrombosis), Gaucher's disease, thalassaemia major, lymphomas, cysts and tumours of spleen

Q. How will you investigate a patient with splenomegaly?

- Inevstigations which are required to evaluate a patient with splenomegaly are given in Table 1.69.

Q. Enumerate the causes of massive splenomegaly. Discuss the differential diagnosis.

- Causes of massive splenomegaly are given in Table 1.70.

TABLE 1.69 Investigations in a Patient With Splenomegaly

Investigations Often Required	Investigations Required in Some Patients
• Haematology: • Full blood count • Peripheral blood film • ESR	• Haematology: • Direct antiglobulin test • Reticulocyte count • Malaria blood film • Haemoglobin electrophoresis/HPLC
• Biochemistry: • Urea and electrolytes • Liver function tests • C-reactive protein • Serum LDH • Vitamin B_{12}, red cell folate	• Biochemistry: • Serum ACE • Serum protein electrophoresis • Urine Bence Jones protein
• Microbiology: • Monospot test • Serology: hepatitis B and C	• Microbiology • Blood cultures • Sputum microscopy, culture and AFB • Mantoux test • Serology: HIV, CMV, toxoplasmosis, brucella
• Radiology: • Plain chest radiograph • Ultrasound/CT abdomen	• Radiology: • Ultrasound abdomen with duplex-Doppler studies • CT chest, abdomen and pelvis • Transthoracic/transoesophageal echocardiogram
• Immunology: • Autoantibodies including ANA • Rheumatoid factor	• Others: • Malaria antibodies • Upper GI endoscopy • Bone marrow aspirate

TABLE 1.70 Causes of Massive Splenomegaly

Common Causes	Uncommon Causes
• Chronic myeloid leukaemia • Myelofibrosis • Hairy cell leukaemia • Tropical splenomegaly (hyperreactive malarial syndrome) • Kala-azar • Extrahepatic portal vein thrombosis	• Lymphomas • Gaucher's disease • Thalassaemia major • Cysts and tumours of spleen • Giant abscess

DIFFERENTIAL DIAGNOSIS (ALSO SEE INDIVIDUAL CONDITIONS)

CHRONIC MYELOID LEUKAEMIA

Clinical Features

- Peak age around 55 years.
- Symptoms of anaemia.
- Symptoms due to massive splenomegaly.
- Symptoms of hypermetabolic state.
- Occasional bleeding tendencies.
- Moderate to massive splenomegaly and hepatomegaly.
- Mild anaemia.

Investigations

- Normocytic normochromic anaemia.
- Total leucocyte count is markedly raised, always more than 20,000/mm^3.
- Platelet count is usually increased.
- Peripheral smear shows full range of granulocyte precursors ranging from myeloblasts to myelocytes to metamyelocytes to mature neutrophils. The mature forms predominate. Myeloblasts are less than 5%–10%. Nucleated red blood cells may be seen.
- Philadelphia chromosome is positive in more than 95% of cases.
- LAP score is very low.
- Vitamin B_{12} levels are markedly elevated.

MYELOFIBROSIS

Clinical Features

- May remain asymptomatic for many years.
- Symptoms resulting from anaemia, massive splenomegaly and hypermetabolic state.
- Massive splenomegaly and hepatomegaly.

Investigations

- Markedly reduced haemoglobin in the late stages.
- Total leucocyte count may be normal, reduced or increased. Usually, it is raised in the early stages to the range of 10,000–20,000/mm^3. Total leucocyte count is reduced in the late stages.
- Platelet count is raised in the early stages but reduced later.
- Peripheral smear examination:
  - Leucoerythroblastic blood picture.
  - Teardrop cells.
  - Anisopoikilocytosis.
  - Numerous nucleated red blood cells.
- Bone marrow study:
  - Usually a dry tap.
  - Increase in all three cells lines, hypercellularity and minimal fibrosis in early stages.
  - Decrease in all three cell lines, hypocellularity and dense fibrosis in late stages.
- Philadelphia chromosome is negative.
- LAP score is high.
- Increase in bone density of vertebrae and proximal ends of long bones.

HAIRY CELL LEUKAEMIA

Clinical Features

- May remain asymptomatic for years.
- Symptoms resulting from massive splenomegaly, infections and vasculitis.
- Hip pain due to bone lesions.
- Massive splenomegaly and hepatomegaly.

Investigations

- Total leucocyte count is normal or low.
- Peripheral smear shows the characteristic 'hairy cells' that stain positively for TRAP.
- Bone marrow shows numerous mononuclear cells and hairy cells.
- LAP score is very high.

TROPICAL SPLENOMEGALY SYNDROME

- Better termed as hyperreactive malarial syndrome (HMS).
- Due to abnormal immune response to repeated malarial infections.

Clinical Features

- Patient is usually a resident of malaria endemic area.
- Low-grade fever may be occasionally present.
- Massive splenomegaly and hepatomegaly.
- Features of hypersplenism.

Criteria for Diagnosis

- Residence of malaria endemic area.
- Chronic splenomegaly, often massive.
- Serum IgM at least 2 standard deviations (SD) above the local mean.
- High malarial antibody titre.
- Hepatic sinusoidal lymphocytosis.
- Clinical and immunological response to antimalarial prophylaxis.

Investigations

- Malarial parasite is absent in peripheral blood smear.
- High levels of antimalarial antibodies in blood.
- IgM levels are markedly raised (up to 20 times).
- Light microscopic examination of liver biopsy shows sinusoidal lymphocytosis.
- Immunofluorescence microscopy of liver biopsy shows IgM aggregates in reticuloendothelial cells.

KALA-AZAR (VISCERAL LEISHMANIASIS)

Clinical Features

- Patient is usually a resident of kala-azar endemic area.
- Fever with two peaks in 24 hours (camel hump fever) occurs in 10%–15% cases.
- Massive splenomegaly and hepatomegaly.
- Generalised lymphadenopathy (in patients from Bengal) and pigmentation of face.

Investigations

- Anaemia, granulocytopenia and thrombocytopenia.
- Low serum albumin and high serum globulin, especially IgG.
- Leishmania antigen and antibodies in blood.
- Demonstration of amastigotes (LD bodies) in aspirates of bone marrow, liver, spleen or lymph nodes.
- Culture of the aspirate for the organism.

EXTRAHEPATIC PORTAL HYPERTENSION

Clinical Features

- Relatively earlier age at presentation.
- Episodes of haematemesis and/or melaena, not accompanied by hepatic decompensation.
- Absence of jaundice, ascites and other signs of chronic liver cell disease.
- Normal size of liver.
- Moderate to massive splenomegaly and signs of portal hypertension.

Investigations

- Normal liver function tests, prothrombin time (PT) and liver biopsy.
- Ultrasonography of abdomen shows normal hepatobiliary system and evidence of portal hypertension.
- Upper gastrointestinal endoscopy and barium swallow reveal varices.
- Splenoportovenogram (SPV) can delineate the collaterals and feeders.

GAUCHER'S DISEASE

- Autosomal recessive, lysosomal storage disorder.
- Deficiency of the enzyme acid β-glucocerebrosidase results in the storage of glucosylceramide within lysosomes of the monocyte-macrophage system.
- Three forms of the disease exist:
  - Infantile form
  - Juvenile form
  - Adult form (type 1)
- Clinical manifestations of the adult form include massive splenomegaly, cytopenias, skeletal dysplasias, bone pain, pathological fractures, vertebral collapse and aseptic necrosis of femoral head.
- Investigations:
  - Increase in serum acid phosphatase.
  - Characteristic foam cells in the peripheral smear.
  - Characteristic 'Gaucher cells' in the bone marrow.
  - Enzyme assay establishes the diagnosis.

- Treatment:
  - Majority do not require any treatment.
  - Partial or total splenectomy in selected cases.
  - Enzyme replacement is currently the treatment of choice in significantly affected patients. Imiglucerase, velaglucerase alpha and taliglucerase alpha are recombinant DNA-produced analogues of human β-glucocerebrosidase and have proved highly efficacious in reducing hepatosplenomegaly and improving bone marrow involvement and haematological findings. Other form of therapy is to reduce substrate (i.e. glucocerebroside) for which an oral drug, eliglustat is available for adults with type 1 disease.

DIFFERENTIAL DIAGNOSIS (Tables 1.71 and 1.72)

TABLE 1.71 Differences Among CML, Myelofibrosis and Hairy Cell Leukaemia

Differentiating Feature	Chronic Myeloid Leukaemia	Myelofibrosis	Hairy Cell Leukaemia
• Total count	Markedly raised to >20,000/μL	Raised to 10,000–20,000/μL	Normal or low
• Differential count	Neutrophils > 95%	Normal	Neutropenia and lymphocytosis
• Peripheral smear	Full range of granulocyte precursors with mature forms predominating Myeloblasts <5%–10% Few nucleated red blood cells	Leucoerythroblastic blood picture Teardrop cells Anisopoikilocytosis Numerous nucleated red blood cells	'Hairy cells' that stain positively for tartrate-resistant acid phosphatase (TRAP)
• Bone marrow	Hypercellular Cells mainly of myeloid series, myelocytes being the predominant cells	Hypercellularity with increase in all three cell lines in early stages Hypocellularity with decrease in all three cell lines in late stages	Numerous mononuclear cells and 'hairy cells' with fibrosis
• Marrow fibrosis	Uncommon and minimal	Common and marked	Increase in marrow reticulin
• LAP score	Markedly lowered	Raised	Markedly raised
• Ph chromosome	Positive	Negative	Negative
• Vitamin B_{12} levels	Markedly raised	Raised	Normal

TABLE 1.72 Differences Among Tropical Splenomegaly Syndrome, Kala-azar and Extrahepatic Portal Hypertension

Differentiating Feature	Tropical Splenomegaly Syndrome	Kala-Azar	Extrahepatic Portal Hypertension
• Endemicity	Endemic	Endemic	Nonendemic
• Fever	Low grade	'Camel hump'	Absent
• GI bleeding	Absent	Absent	Present
• Immunoglobulins	IgM increased	IgG increased	—
• Antibodies	Antimalarial antibodies	Anti-*Leishmania* antibodies	—
• Bone marrow	Malarial parasites (rare)	LD bodies	Normal
• Liver biopsy	Light microscopy shows sinusoidal lymphocytosis Immunofluorescence microscopy shows IgM aggregates in reticuloendothelial cells	LD bodies, which are also seen in bone marrow, spleen and lymph nodes	Normal
• Evidence of portal hypertension on endoscopy, barium swallow and SPV[a]	Absent	Absent	Present

[a]SPV, splenoportovenography.

Q. Enumerate the causes, clinical features and treatment of hypersplenism.

- This is a term used to indicate anaemia, leucopenia and thrombocytopenia associated with prominent splenomegaly (due to any cause) and a normal or hypercellular bone marrow.
- No direct relation between splenic size and hypersplenism; however, hypersplenism is more common among those who have gross splenomegaly.
- Leucopenia and thrombocytopenia result from excessive sequestration of these cells in the large spleen.
- Anaemia is believed to be dilutional, resulting from an increase in total plasma volume.

COMMON CAUSES

- Common causes of hypersplenism are given in Box 1.27.

BOX 1.27 Common Causes of Hypersplenism

• Primary hypersplenism	No detectable cause of splenomegaly
• Secondary hypersplenism	Portal hypertension, malaria, kala-azar, tropical splenomegaly syndrome, myeloproliferative disorders, tuberculosis

CLINICAL FEATURES

- Symptoms related to the enlarged spleen such as abdominal fullness associated with feeling of heaviness and discomfort and pain in the left upper quadrant of the abdomen.
- Haematological symptoms: Symptoms related to thrombocytopenia, anaemia and leucopenia.
- Symptoms and signs of the underlying diseases.

TREATMENT

- Primary hypersplenism is treated by splenectomy or partial splenic embolisation.
- Secondary hypersplenism is managed by tackling the underlying cause.

Q. What are lymphomas? What are the common types of lymphomas?

- Lymphomas are a heterogeneous group of neoplasms arising from lymphoid cells and almost always present as solid tumours. Majority of lymphoid cells are present in lymph nodes, spleen, bone marrow, thymus and gastrointestinal tract.
- The major types of lymphomas are Hodgkin's lymphoma and non-Hodgkin's lymphoma. An uncommon lymphoma is mycosis fungoides.

Q. Discuss the pathological classification, clinical features, clinical staging, investigations and treatment of Hodgkin's lymphoma.

Q. Give a brief account of Read–Sternberg (RS) cell.

- Hodgkin's lymphoma (HL) is of B-cell origin.
- Bimodal age incidence with one peak in young adults (15–35 years) and the other in older adults (45–75 years).
- Infection by HIV is a risk factor for developing Hodgkin's lymphoma. Although the histologic features of Hodgkin's lymphoma are similar in HIV/AIDS and immunocompetent individuals, there are several clinical differences. Patients with HIV/AIDS have advanced stage disease at the time of diagnosis, an aggressive clinical course, poor response to conventional therapy, noncontiguous spread, frequent involvement of bone marrow and other extranodal sites and a strong association with Epstein–Barr virus (80%–100%).
- Association with Epstein–Barr virus demonstrated in 30%–50% immunocompetent patients also.

PATHOLOGICAL CLASSIFICATION

- WHO (2008) has divided Hodgkin's lymphoma into two types (Box 1.28). Prognosis varies depending upon the histological type.
  - Classic HL is characterised by presence of Reed–Sternberg cells in an inflammatory background.
  - Nodular lymphocyte predominant HL lacks Reed–Sternberg cells but is characterised by the presence of lymphocyte-predominant cells, sometimes termed as popcorn cells.
- Nodular sclerosis classical Hodgkin's lymphoma is more frequent in younger patients with mediastinal involvement.
- Mixed cellularity classical Hodgkin's lymphoma is usually found in older patients though in India, younger people are often involved. It is associated with Epstein–Barr virus and infra-diaphragmatic lymph nodal involvement, or bone or bone marrow disease.

CLINICAL MANIFESTATIONS

- Starts in one lymph node group (unifocal origin) and spreads in a predictable manner to the adjacent lymph node group (contiguous spread).
- The disease usually begins as painless enlargement of one group of cervical lymph nodes. Less commonly, the disease may start in the mediastinal or axillary nodes and rarely in the abdominal, pelvic or inguinal nodes. The involved nodes are discrete, nontender and 'rubbery' in consistency. Alcohol-induced discomfort in the lymph nodes is a common feature of Hodgkin's lymphoma. Sites that are rarely involved by Hodgkin's lymphoma include Waldeyer's ring and mesenteric, epitrochlear and popliteal nodes.
- Compression of various organs by lymph node masses or infiltration of various organs can produce clinical effects like dysphagia, dyspnoea, Horner's syndrome, hoarseness of voice, superior vena cava syndrome, inferior vena cava obstruction, jaundice and paraplegia. Mediastinal involvement is seen in 80% cases of nodular sclerosis classic Hodgkin's lymphoma, of which more than half have bulky mediastinal disease.
- Splenomegaly is uncommon in the beginning, but as the disease advances, hepatosplenomegaly becomes prominent.
- Involvement of extralymphatic organs is a late feature in Hodgkin's lymphoma.

BOX 1.28 WHO Classification of Hodgkin's Lymphoma

- Nodular lymphocyte predominant Hodgkin's lymphoma (<5%)
- Classic Hodgkin's lymphoma (>95%)
  - Nodular sclerosis classic Hodgkin's lymphoma
  - Mixed cellularity classic Hodgkin's lymphoma (most common type in India)
  - Lymphocyte-rich classic Hodgkin's lymphoma
  - Lymphocyte-depleted classic Hodgkin's lymphoma

- The 'B' symptoms or systemic symptoms that place the patient in the 'B' category are the following:
  - Unexplained weight loss of more than 10% of the body weight in the previous 6 months.
  - Unexplained fever above 38°C during the previous month.
  - Heavy night sweats during the previous month.
- The classical Pel–Ebstein fever is rarely seen. This fever occurs in a cyclical pattern, characterised by several days or weeks of fever alternating with afebrile periods.
- Pruritus is a common symptom and is troublesome at times.
- Nephrotic syndrome may occur from immune complex deposition in the kidneys.
- Hodgkin's lymphoma is associated with depressed cell-mediated immunity resulting in a higher risk of infections like herpes zoster, tuberculosis, cryptococcal infections, cytomegalovirus infections and infection with candida species.

CLINICAL STAGING (ANN ARBOR CLASSIFICATION) (Table 1.73)

- Lymphatic structures are defined as lymph nodes, spleen, thymus, Waldeyer's rings, appendix and Peyer's patches; liver and bone marrow are excluded.
- Each stage is further divided into A or B based on the absence or presence of systemic symptoms (B symptoms), respectively.
- In contrast to non-Hodgkin's lymphomas, the spleen is considered nodal in classical Hodgkin's lymphoma.

INVESTIGATIONS

- Haemogram:
  - Normocytic normochromic anaemia is common. In advanced disease, microcytic anaemia usually develops due to defective iron utilisation.
  - Total leucocyte count may be normal but is sometimes considerably raised with neutrophil leucocytosis.
  - Eosinophilia is present in about 20% of patients and thrombocytosis is seen in some cases.
  - In the terminal stages, there may be leucopenia and thrombocytopenia.
  - Erythrocyte sedimentation rate.
- Elevated serum alkaline phosphatase levels usually indicate bone marrow or liver involvement.
- Tissue biopsy, usually a lymph node biopsy, will establish the diagnosis. A fine needle aspiration is not recommended for diagnosis. Liver biopsy may provide the diagnosis in those with hepatomegaly.
- It is important to establish the extent of the disease. The investigations required for clinical staging include chest radiographs, liver function tests, renal function tests, abdominal ultrasound, bone marrow trephine and aspirate, CT scan (neck, chest, abdomen and pelvis) and/or PET/CT. Bone marrow biopsy is required only in presence of 'B' symptoms, clinically advanced disease or infra-diaphragmatic disease and in those with bone lesions, bone pain, hypercalcaemia or an elevated serum alkaline phosphatase. PET/CT may obviate the need for bone marrow biopsy as it is very sensitive for bone marrow involvement.
- PET scan is sensitive for evaluating the extent of disease and is an integral part of initial staging. The sensitivity of ^{18}FDG-PET and PET/CT is higher than that of CT in order to identify both nodal and extranodal disease. It is also very useful at the completion of therapy to document remission.
- Reed–Sternberg (RS) cell on histopathology are diagnostic (Box 1.29).
- Table 1.74 summarises investigations in a patient with suspected Hodgkin's lymphoma.

TABLE 1.73 Ann Arbor Classification of Staging of Hodgkin's Lymphoma

• Stage I	Involvement of a single lymph node region (I) or extralymphatic site (IE)
• Stage II	Involvement of two or more lymph node regions (II) or an extralymphatic site and lymph node regions on the same side (above or below) the diaphragm (IIE)
• Stage III	Involvement of lymph node regions on both sides of the diaphragm with (IIIE) or without (III) localised extralymphatic involvement or involvement of the spleen (IIIS) or both (IIISE)
• Stage IV	Diffuse involvement of one or more extralymphatic tissues (e.g. liver, bone marrow, pleura, lung, bone) with or without associated lymph node involvement; includes any involvement of the liver or bone marrow, lungs (other than by direct extension from another site) or cerebrospinal fluid

RISK STRATIFICATION (GERMAN HODGKIN STUDY GROUP)

- Risk stratification is based on risk factors as well as staging (treatment groups) of Hodgkin's lymphoma (Tables 1.75 and 1.76).

MANAGEMENT

RADIOTHERAPY

- Megavoltage radiotherapy to a dose of 3500–4000 cGy is given to the involved sites over a period of 4 weeks (involved-field radiotherapy).
- Radiotherapy given to an extended area that includes all lymph node-bearing areas above diaphragm is known as mantle field radiation. Sometimes periaortic lymph nodes and spleen (spade field) are also included.
- Inverted Y field radiotherapy includes periaortic iliac, hypogastric and inguinal lymph nodes and spleen.
- Indications for radiotherapy (combined with chemotherapy) are the following:
  - Stage I disease.
  - Stage II disease without any unfavourable features.
  - After chemotherapy to sites where there was originally bulk disease.
  - To lesions causing serious pressure problems.

BOX 1.29 Reed–Sternberg (RS) Cell

- The Reed–Sternberg (RS) cells are pathognomonic of Hodgkin's lymphoma. The presence of RS cells in histology specimen differentiates Hodgkin's lymphoma from non-Hodgkin's lymphoma (NHL). These cells are derived from lymphocytes.
- RS cells are presumed to evolve either due to viral infection or underlying immune derangement.
- They are giant cells with paired, mirror-imaged nuclei (binucleate) with large nucleoli in each nucleus ('owl's eye' cells).
- On immunophenotyping, these cells are usually $CD15^+$ and $CD30^+$. Nearly 40% are also $CD20^+$.
- In contrast to NHLs and other malignant tumours that are composed almost exclusively of malignant cells, RS cells comprise less than 1% of cells in the affected tissues.
- Uninucleate cells with cytologic features identical to those of RS cells are referred to as Hodgkin's cells. Hodgkin's cells by themselves are insufficient for a definitive diagnosis on the initial biopsy but are sufficient to establish a diagnosis of relapsed disease when the immunophenotype of these Hodgkin's cells is characteristic.

TABLE 1.74 Summary of Investigations

Diagnosis	• Lymph node biopsy (or a biopsy from another organ suspected to be involved)
Staging and risk stratification	• History and physical examination • Chest radiograph • Contrast-enhanced CT scan of the neck, chest and abdomen • PET scan • Full blood cell count and blood chemistry, ESR • HBV, HCV and HIV screening
Pretreatment examinations	• ECG • Echocardiography • Pulmonary function test • Reproductive counselling (in patients of reproductive age) • Urine pregnancy test (in female patients of reproductive age)

TABLE 1.75 Risk Factors in Hodgkin's Lymphoma

A: Large mediastinal mass (at least 33% as wide as the chest) B: Extranodal disease	C: Elevated ESR (>50 mm/h without B symptoms, >30 mm/h with B symptoms) D: ≥3 nodal areas

TABLE 1.76 Treatment Groups in Hodgkin's Lymphoma

Limited stage	• Stage I and II (without any risk factors)
Intermediate stage	• Stage I and IIA with ≥1 risk factors
	• Stage IIB with risk factors C and/or D but not A and B
Advanced stage	• Stage IIB with A and/or B risk factors
	• Stage III and IV

- For stages I and II A disease, radiotherapy is given to an extended area that includes all lymph node-bearing areas above diaphragm (mantle field) and sometimes including the periaortic lymph nodes and spleen (spade field).
- In stages II B and III A, standard chemotherapy with or without radiotherapy is given. In such case, radiotherapy involves mantle field as well as inverted Y field (periaortic iliac, hypogastric and inguinal lymph nodes and spleen).
- Involved-site radiotherapy (radiation field includes only the tumour plus a margin of healthy tissue) instead of involved-field radiotherapy (radiation field includes whole lymphatic region involved) has been found to be equally effective but with lesser side effects.

CHEMOTHERAPY

- Combination chemotherapy has been shown to be highly effective. The regimens commonly used are given in Table 1.77.
- These regimens are given on a 28-day cycle (21-day cycle for BEACOPP escalated for advanced disease) for a minimum of two pulses and up to nine, if necessary. Cure rates >75% can be achieved.

RECOMMENDATIONS ON TREATMENT

Limited Stage Classic HL

- Chemotherapy (ABVD for two to four cycles over 8–16 weeks or Stanford V for two cycles over 8 weeks) followed by involved-field radiotherapy OR chemotherapy for two cycles followed by evaluation by PET/CT and further treatment (Flowchart 1.13).

TABLE 1.77 Commonly Used Chemotherapeutic Regimens in Hodgkin's Lymphoma

Regimen	Drugs
• ABVD	Doxorubicin (Adriamycin), bleomycin, vinblastine, dacarbazine
• Stanford V	Doxorubicin, mechlorethamine (nitrogen mustard), vincristine, vinblastine, bleomycin, etoposide, prednisone
• BEACOPP escalated	Bleomycin, etoposide, adriamycin, cyclophosphamide, vincristine, procarbazine, prednisone in escalated dose
• MOPP	Mechlorethamine, vincristine, procarbazine, prednisone

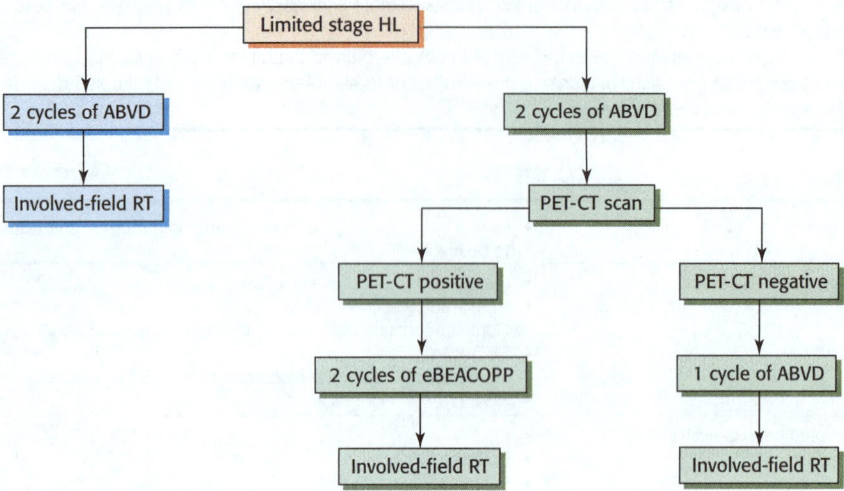

Flowchart 1.13 Treatment of Limited Stage Hodgkin's Lymphoma.

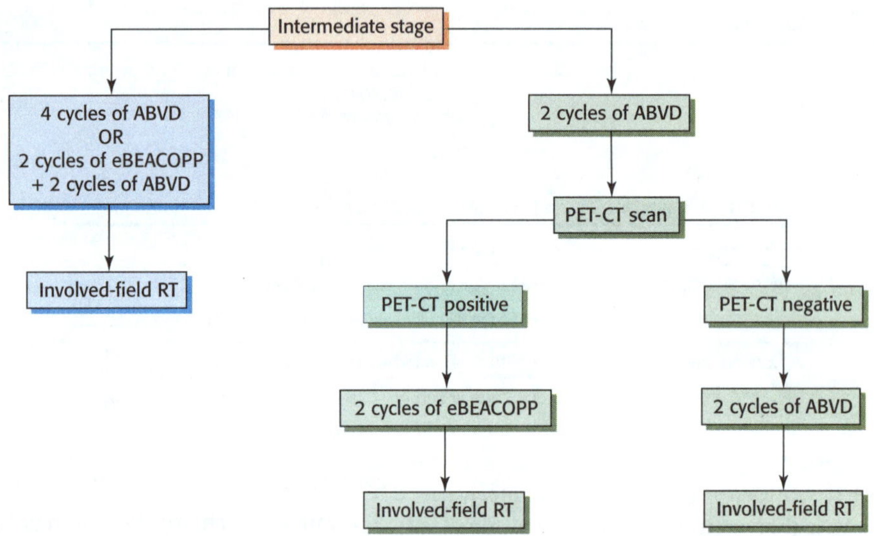

Flowchart 1.14 Treatment of Intermediate Stage Hodgkin's Lymphoma.

- Restaging is done at the completion of treatment.
- Cure rates (free of disease at 5 years) of about 80%–90% can be achieved with this therapy.

Intermediate-Stage Classic HL

- Four cycles of ABVD or two cycles each of ABVD and eBEACOPP followed by radiotherapy OR two cycles of ABVD followed by evaluation with PET-CT and further treatment (Flowchart 1.14).
- Another option is three cycles of Stanford V, followed by restaging and if complete or partial response occurs, involved-field radiotherapy.

Advanced Stage Classic HL

- Chemotherapy (ABVD, Stanford V or BEACOPP escalated) six cycles along with radiotherapy to initially bulky lymph nodes (>5 cm). Bleomycin should not be given for more than two cycles in patients >60 years (Flowchart 1.15).
- Overall survival is 75%–90% at 5 years.

BONE MARROW TRANSPLANTATION

- Salvage high-dose combination chemotherapy followed by autologous haematopoietic stem cell transplantation commonly represent the treatment

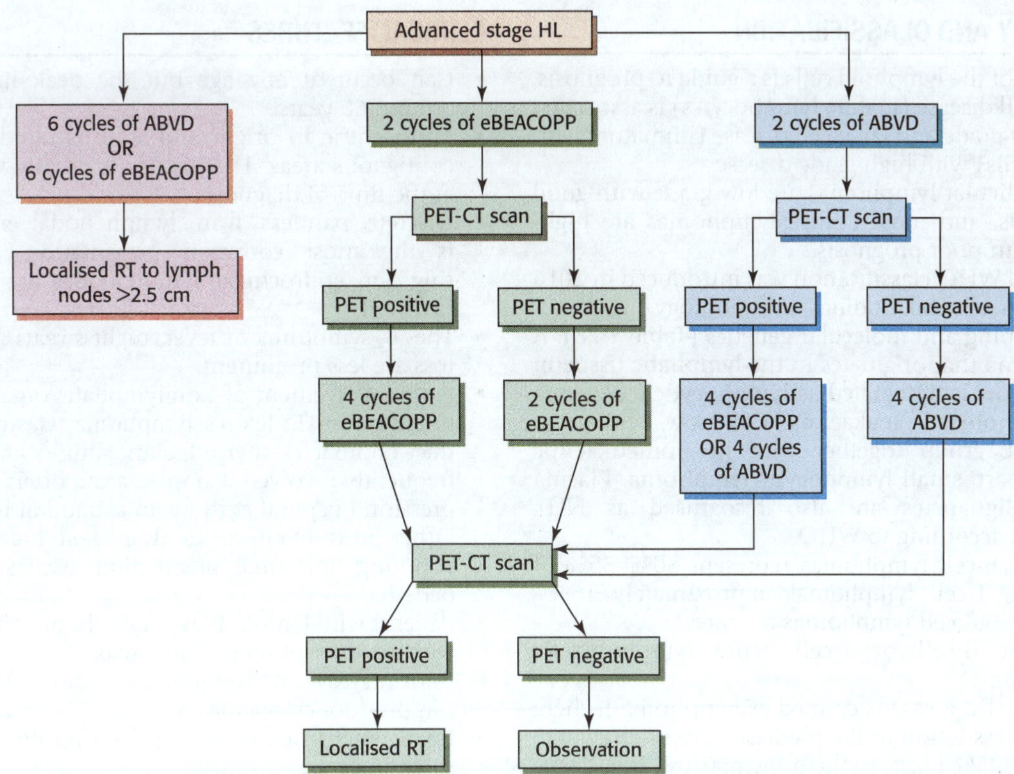

Flowchart 1.15 Treatment of Advanced Stage Hodgkin's Lymphoma.

of choice for patients with relapsed HL, curing about 50% of patients with relapsed HL.

NEW AGENTS

- Brentuximab vedotin (an anti-CD30 conjugated antibody-drug).
- Nivolumab and pembrolizumab (checkpoint inhibitors) block signalling through the programmed death-1 (PD-1) pathway, releasing inhibition of T cells and augmenting antitumour immune responses.

LATE COMPLICATIONS

- Occur due to high cure rates achieved with treatment.
- Second malignancies including acute leukaemia and solid organ cancers. Acute leukaemia generally occurs within 10 years of use of alkylating agents in combination with radiotherapy. Risk is greater with MOPP as compared to ABVD. Solid organ cancers usually occur more than 10 years after treatment and are associated with use of radiotherapy.
- Cardiac failure and accelerated coronary artery disease due to radiotherapy and use of doxorubicin.
- Pulmonary fibrosis (if bleomycin or radiation is used).
- Hypothyroidism.

Q. Discuss the pathological classification, clinical staging, clinical features, investigations and management of non-Hodgkin's lymphoma.

- In non-Hodgkin's lymphoma, there is a malignant monoclonal proliferation of lymphoid cells, the majority of cases (80%) originating in B cell, a minority in T cell (15%–20%) and rarely in natural killer cells.
- Non-Hodgkin's lymphomas merge with lymphoblastic/lymphocytic leukaemia.

AETIOLOGY (Box 1.30)

BOX 1.30 Aetiology of Non-Hodgkin's Lymphoma

- Unknown in most cases
- Associated with chronic inflammatory or autoimmune diseases such as Sjogren's syndrome, Hashimoto's thyroiditis and rheumatoid arthritis
- Associated with chronic infection (e.g. association between mucosa-associated lymphoid tissue lymphomas and *Helicobacter pylori* infection)
- Immune suppression as seen with solid organ transplantation and HIV infection

PATHOLOGY AND CLASSIFICATION

- The size of the lymphoid cells is a guide to prognosis. Small-cell disease (mature lymphocytes) is associated with low-grade and large-cell disease (immature lymphoid cells) with high-grade disease.
- Most follicular lymphomas are low-grade with good prognosis, and most diffuse lymphomas are high-grade with poor prognosis.
- A revised WHO classification was introduced in 2016 based on clinical findings, morphology, immunophenotyping and molecular genetics (Table 1.78). A lymphoma that originates in the lymphatic tissue in the marrow is designated as lymphocytic leukaemia or lymphoblastic leukaemia. CLL now belongs to the NHL group together with its nonleukaemic counterpart, small lymphocytic lymphoma. Plasma cell malignancies are also recognised as NHL subtypes according to WHO.
- In India, B-cell lymphomas represent 80%–85% of all cases, T-cell lymphomas approximately 15%–20% and NK cell lymphomas are rare.
- Precursor B-cell or T-cell acute lymphoblastic leukaemia:
  - Clinically, a case is defined as lymphoma if there is a mass lesion in the mediastinum or elsewhere and <25% blasts in the bone marrow. It is classified as leukaemia if there are >25% bone marrow blasts, with or without a mass lesion.
  - Precursor T-lymphoblastic leukaemia typically presents as a mediastinal mass in young men, whereas precursor B-lymphoblastic lymphoma is more likely to involve the lymph nodes, skin and bone.
- Follicular lymphoma and diffuse large B-cell lymphoma (DLBCL) are the two most common types and together account for more than 50% of cases. In AIDS patients, DLBCL, Burkitt lymphoma and primary CNS lymphoma are most commonly seen non-Hodgkin's lymphomas.

CLINICAL FEATURES

- Can occur at any age but the peak incidence is around 60 years.
- Multicentric in origin and spreads rapidly to noncontiguous areas. The disease is usually widespread at the time of diagnosis.
- Discrete, painless, firm, lymph nodal enlargement is the most common presentation. Waldeyer's ring and epitrochlear lymph nodes are frequently involved.
- The 'B' symptoms of fever, night sweats and weight loss are less prominent.
- Early involvement of extralymphatic organs is a feature of non-Hodgkin's lymphoma. Gastrointestinal tract (stomach), thyroid, skin, sinuses and CNS are frequently involved. Paraplegia can occur from compression of spinal cord by an extradural lymphoma. Other pressure effects are dysphagia, breathlessness, vomiting, intestinal obstruction, ascites and limb oedema.
- Patients with lymphoblastic lymphoma often present with an anterior mediastinal mass.
- Bone marrow involvement is common and early and can produce cytopenias.
- Involvement of liver and spleen results in hepatosplenomegaly.
- Bone involvement may manifest as pathological fractures with pain.
- Autoimmune haemolytic anaemia and immune thrombocytopenia.
- Burkitt's lymphoma typically disseminates to the bone marrow and meninges and involves extranodal sites.
- Paraneoplastic complications include polyneuropathy, Guillain-Barré syndrome, peripheral neuropathy, pemphigus, glomerulonephritis and dermatomyositis.

TABLE 1.78 WHO (2016) Classification of Lymphoid Malignancies (Important Categories)

B-cell Lymphoma	T-cell/NK Cell Lymphoma
Precursor B-cell Neoplasm	***Precursor T-cell Neoplasm***
• Precursor B-cell acute lymphoblastic leukaemia/lymphoma	• Precursor T-cell acute lymphoblastic leukaemia
Mature B Cell	***Mature T Cell/NK Cell***
• Chronic lymphocytic leukaemia and small lymphocytic lymphoma • B-cell prolymphocytic leukaemia • Splenic marginal zone lymphoma • Hairy cell leukaemia • Lymphoplasmacytic lymphoma (Waldenstrom macroglobulinaemia) • Extranodal marginal zone lymphoma of mucosa-associated lymphoid tissue • Nodal marginal zone lymphoma • Follicular lymphoma • Mantle cell lymphoma • Diffuse large B-cell lymphoma (DLBCL), not otherwise specified • Primary DLBCL of the CNS • Epstein–Barr virus (EBV)-positive DLBCL, not otherwise specified • Lymphomatoid granulomatosis • Primary mediastinal (thymic) large B-cell lymphoma • Burkitt lymphoma	• T-cell prolymphocytic leukaemia • T-cell large granular lymphocytic leukaemia • Adult T-cell leukaemia or lymphoma • Nasal-type extranodal NK–T-cell lymphoma • Enteropathy-associated T-cell lymphoma • Monomorphic epitheliotropic intestinal T-cell lymphoma • Hepatosplenic T-cell lymphoma • Mycosis fungoides • Sézary syndrome • Peripheral T-cell lymphoma, not otherwise specified • Angioimmunoblastic T-cell lymphoma • Anaplastic large-cell lymphoma

CLINICAL STAGING (ANN ARBOR CLASSIFICATION)

- Ann Arbor classification may be used to define patients into limited (stages I and II) and advanced (stages III and IV) lymphomas. However, it is more useful in Hodgkin's lymphoma rather than in non-Hodgkin's lymphoma. Further, 'B' symptoms are not included as they are not useful in predicting prognosis.

INVESTIGATIONS

- Haemogram:
  - Moderate degrees of anaemia may be seen when there is significant marrow involvement.
  - Blood counts are usually normal, but some patients show lymphocytosis. A leukaemic phase develops in 20%–40% of lymphocytic lymphomas. High-grade lymphomas may frequently be leukaemic.
  - Splenomegaly with hypersplenism or a complicating autoimmune haemolytic anaemia can result in low haemoglobin levels, reticulocytosis and positive Coombs' test.
- Bone marrow aspiration and trephine biopsy should be done early, since marrow involvement is common.
- Other investigations required are immunophenotyping of blood, lymph node and marrow lymphoid cells and estimation of serum immunoglobulin levels. Immunohistochemical study is essential for differentiating various subtypes of NHL and also to determine prognosis as these will influence the choice of therapy. It can be performed by flow cytometry and/or immunohistochemistry for B-cell markers CD79A and CD20, T-cell marker CD3 and the proliferative marker Ki67. Ki67 fraction >40% is highly suggestive of a high-grade lymphoma.
- In addition, serum levels of LDH, uric acid and β_2-microglobulin and serum protein electrophoresis are often included in the evaluation as these affect the prognosis.
- A diagnostic spinal tap directly combined with a first prophylactic instillation of cytarabine and/or methotrexate is indicated in high-risk patients, especially with involvement of CNS, orbit, bone marrow, testis, spine or base of the skull. It is also indicated in the case of HIV-associated lymphoma and highly aggressive lymphoma.
- The investigations required for staging the disease are the same as that for Hodgkin's lymphoma.

RISK FACTORS (Box 1.31)

BOX 1.31 Risk Factors in Non-Hodgkin's Lymphoma

- Age ≥60 years
- Elevated serum lactate dehydrogenase levels
- Performance status ≥2 (ECOG[a]) or ≤70 (Karnofsky)
- Ann Arbor stage III or IV
- >1 site of extranodal involvement

[a]ECOG: Eastern Cooperative Oncology Group.

MANAGEMENT

- Radiotherapy involves involved-field treatment which is given for localised disease.
- Chemotherapy can be given as a single drug therapy with chlorambucil or as a combination therapy with multiple drugs.
- In cases with high tumour load, special precautions (e.g. corticosteroid and alkaline diuresis) are required to avoid tumour lysis syndrome.
- Stem cell transplantation may be done if the disease relapses.
- The value of consolidative radiation therapy after immunochemotherapy has not been proved.

DIFFUSE LARGE B-CELL LYMPHOMA

- Constitutes about 30%–50% of all non-Hodgkin's lymphomas.
- AIDS-related DLBCL is the most common AIDS-related non-Hodgkin's lymphoma.
- Patients of all ages with stage I–II DLBCL and no adverse prognostic factors (nonbulky disease, age <60 years, serum LDH normal, performance status 2–4, extranodal involvement ≤1 site) should receive three to four cycles of chemotherapy (R-CHOP, i.e. rituximab plus cyclophosphamide, hydroxydaunorubicin or adriamycin, oncovin or vincristine and prednisolone) plus involved-field radiotherapy, or six to eight cycles of chemotherapy alone.
- All other patients should receive six to eight cycles of chemotherapy (R-CHOP).
- Patients at increased risk of CNS relapse (those with involvement of paranasal sinuses, testes, bone marrow involvement with large cells or having two or more extranodal sites with elevated LDH) should receive CNS prophylaxis with four to eight doses of intrathecal methotrexate.

FOLLICULAR LYMPHOMA

- Slow growing.
- Characterised by diffuse lymphadenopathy, bone marrow involvement and splenomegaly.
- Extranodal involvement is less common. Cytopenias are relatively common.
- Recurrence rate high after initial treatment.
- For stages I and II, local radiotherapy alone or observation (if significant morbidity expected from radiotherapy).
- For stages III and IV:
  - If asymptomatic patient, observation without any specific therapy is often recommended.
  - For symptomatic patient (symptomatic nodal disease, compromised end organ function, B symptoms, symptomatic extranodal disease or cytopenias), administer chemotherapy (R-CHOP or bendamustine plus rituximab).

RELAPSED/REFRACTORY B-CELL LYMPHOMAS

CHIMERIC ANTIGEN RECEPTOR T-CELL THERAPY

- Chimeric antigen receptor T-cell (CAR-T) therapy, a form of adoptive cellular therapies, has been used successfully in the treatment of relapsed B-cell lymphoid malignancies.

- Includes axicabtagene ciluecel, tisagenlecleucel, brexucabtagene autoleucel and lisocabtagene maraleucel.
- These drugs are directed against CD19.
- Produced from autologous T-cells obtained from patients via leucopheresis. This process typically involves autologous T-cell selection, gene transfer to express chimeric antigen receptor (CAR) on T-cells usually via a retrovirus, T-cell expansion and then infusion of the cells back to the patient.
- Acute toxicities include cytokine release syndrome and neurotoxicity, while chronic toxicities include cytopenias and hypogammaglobulinaemia.

Q. How do you differentiate Hodgkin's lymphoma from non-Hodgkin's lymphoma?

- Differentiating points between Hodgkin's lymphoma and non-Hodgkin's lymphoma are given in Table 1.79.

TABLE 1.79 Differences Between Hodgkin's Lymphoma and Non-Hodgkin's Lymphoma

Hodgkin's Lymphoma	Non-Hodgkin's Lymphoma
• Bimodal peak incidence, 15–35 years and 45–70 years	• Peak incidence around 60 years
• 'B' symptoms are more common	• 'B' symptoms are less common
• Alcohol-induced discomfort in lymph nodal region	• Not observed
• Usually well localised at the time of diagnosis	• Usually widespread at the time of diagnosis
• Unifocal origin and contiguous spread	• Multicentric origin and noncontiguous spread
• Involvement of extralymphatic organs is late	• Involvement of extralymphatic organs is early
• Waldeyer's ring involvement is uncommon	• Waldeyer's ring involvement is common
• Epitrochlear node involvement is rare	• Epitrochlear node involvement is common
• Early involvement of para-aortic lymph nodes	• Early involvement of mesenteric lymph nodes
• Mediastinal involvement is common	• Mediastinal involvement is uncommon
• Bone marrow involvement is late	• Bone marrow involvement is early

Q. Describe Burkitt's lymphoma/leukaemia.

- It is a high-grade, B-cell, non-Hodgkin's lymphoma having small noncleaved cells.
- Has the fastest doubling time among human tumours.
- Often presents with extranodal involvement or as leukaemia.
- Three variants: endemic, sporadic and immunodeficiency-associated BL.
- Endemic form mainly seen in tropical Africa and New Guinea.
- Epstein–Barr (EB) virus plays an important aetiological role.
- Majority of the cases occur in children.
- Nearly 80% cases have a translocation of *c-myc* from chromosome 8 to the immunoglobulin (Ig) heavy chain region on chromosome 14 [t(8;14)].

CLINICAL FEATURES

- Clinical features of various forms of Burkitt's lymphoma are given in Box 1.32.
- Mandible and maxillary bone involvement leads to deformity, loosening of teeth and extrusion of the eye with loss of vision.
- Abdominal involvement presents as tumours due to bilateral involvement of kidneys, adrenals, ovaries, bowel and lymph nodes.
- Other sites of involvement are CNS, long bones, salivary glands, thyroid, testes, heart, breast and bone marrow. CNS involvement is common in adults.

BOX 1.32 Clinical Features of Burkitt's Lymphoma

Endemic Form:
- Most commonly seen in young children (4–7 years)
- Frequent involvement of jaw, periorbital area and kidneys
- Sudden paraplegia may occur

Sporadic Form:
- Presents mainly with abdominal tumours
- One-fourth have ileocaecal disease and present with either a right lower quadrant mass or pain from intussusception
- Some cases classified as Burkitt's leukaemia, characterised by extensive marrow infiltration (more than 25% blasts), with possible bone pain as a presenting feature

Immunodeficiency Form:
- Associated with HIV infection
- Usually occurs with CD4 counts above 200/mm^3
- Presents with abdominal involvement

INVESTIGATIONS

- Imaging plays a critical role in initial detection, treatment response and potential complications.
  - Ultrasound and/or computed tomography to localise the tumour.
  - PET-CT.
- Histological examination shows presence of a monotonous infiltrates of medium-sized blastic lymphoid cells that show round nuclei with clumped chromatin and multiple, centrally located nucleoli. These are of B-cell lineage (CD20$^+$ and CD79a$^+$). The rate of proliferation and rate of death (apoptosis) are high, with the dead cells being taken up by pale histiocytic cells within the tumour that punctuate the low-power view, giving a 'starry sky' appearance.

- Chromosome analysis may show t(8:14) or in some cases, t(2:8) or t(8:22) translocation.
- Antibodies to EB viral capsid antigen may be detected (in most patients with endemic type, and in several patients with sporadic and HIV-associated tumours).

TREATMENT

- Treatment must be initiated urgently with adequate hydration and use of allopurinol or rasburicase to prevent tumour lysis syndrome.
- High-intensity, brief-duration chemotherapy is highly effective. Regimens include CHOP (cyclophosphamide, hydroxydoxorubicin or doxorubicin, vincristine, prednisolone) or rituximab plus EPOCH (etoposide, prednisolone, vincristine, cyclophosphamide and hydroxydoxorubicin) or CODOX-M/IVAC regimen (cyclophosphamide, vincristine, doxorubicin, methotrexate/ifosfamide, etoposide or VP-16, cytarabine or Ara-C).
- Prophylactic intrathecal methotrexate or cytarabine and hydrocortisone for meningeal prophylaxis is indicated in all patients.
- Cure rates as high as 70%–80%.

Q. Briefly discuss adult T-cell lymphoma/leukaemia.

- It is a type of non-Hodgkin's lymphoma that is caused by human T-cell lymphotropic virus-I (HTLV-I).
- Major routes of HTLV-I transmission are mother-to-child infections via breast milk, blood transfusion or sexual contact.
- Latency period between infection and development of disease is long (10–30 years).
- Four major presentations: acute, lymphomatous, chronic and smoldering.
- Most patients have an acute, aggressive disease characterised by peripheral blood lymphocytosis, lymphadenopathy, hepatosplenomegaly, skin infiltration, hypercalcaemia, lytic bone lesions and elevated LDH levels in blood. In these patients, median survival is 6 months. Opportunistic infections are commonly seen. Peripheral smear usually reveals characteristic, pleomorphic abnormal CD4+ cells with indented nuclei (called 'flower' or 'cloverleaf' cells). Bone marrow involvement is usually not prominent.
- About 20% patients have lymphomatous form associated with generalised lymphadenopathy without leukaemia and a median survival of approximately 1 year.
- The chronic subtype (15% of cases) may have a low-level absolute lymphocytosis in the peripheral blood associated with an exfoliative skin rash and a median survival greater than 2 years.
- The smoldering subtype (5% of cases) has a normal peripheral blood lymphocyte count and a small number of circulating tumour cells and skin rashes. There is no lymphadenopathy, hepatosplenomegaly or hypercalcaemia. Median survival is more than 2 years but less than 10 years.
- Treatment offered to acute and lymphomatous forms:
  - Treatment of hypercalcaemia and opportunistic infections.
  - Combination chemotherapy (CHOP) along with intrathecal drugs (methotrexate, cytarabine and hydrocortisone) may prolong life but usually does not produce remissions.
  - Combination antiretroviral drugs (zidovudine+interferon-α) may help some patients.

Q. Explain what is mucosa-associated lymphoid tissue (MALT) lymphoma or primary gastric lymphoma.

- It is a small-cell non-Hodgkin's lymphoma of B cells that is extranodal in origin.
- Gastric type of MALT lymphoma is associated with *Helicobacter pylori* infection. Salivary gland MALT is associated with Sjogren's syndrome.
- Mainly seen in elderly patients with median age of 60 years.
- May occur in the stomach, orbit, intestine, lung, skin, soft tissue, bladder, kidney, salivary gland and CNS.
- May present as a mass or be associated with local symptoms such as upper abdominal discomfort, dyspepsia and rarely upper GI bleed in gastric MALT lymphoma.
- Localised to the organ from which it arises in about 40% cases and to the organ and surrounding lymph nodes in 30% cases. Bone marrow involvement is uncommon and occurs in only 15% cases. Distant metastasis can also occur.
- Endoscopic features of gastric MALT often mimic benign conditions like chronic gastritis or a peptic ulcer. Multiple biopsies are required for establishing diagnosis.
- Endoscopic ultrasound (EUS) useful for staging of gastric MALT lymphoma.
- Prognosis is good in most cases with 5-year survival of 75%.

TREATMENT

- Treatment of MALT lymphoma is given in Box 1.33.

BOX 1.33 Treatment of MALT Lymphoma

- Antibiotic therapy aimed at the eradication of *H. pylori* for low-grade gastric MALT lymphoma
- Surgery, local radiotherapy or rituximab for localised MALT lymphoma
- Single agents like chlorambucil, cyclophosphamide, fludarabine or cladribine along with rituximab for extensive disease

Q. Write a short note on mycosis fungoides and Sezary syndrome.

- These are rare forms of T-cell non-Hodgkin's lymphoma that have an insidious onset.
- Derived from $CD4^+$ T cells of skin-associated lymphoid tissue.

CLINICAL FEATURES

- Classic presentation of mycosis fungoides is occurrence of patches and plaques on non-sun-exposed areas that may slowly evolve to tumours. The skin rash is usually itchy. Approximately 30% of patients present with skin tumours or erythroderma (erythrodermic mycosis fungoides) at disease onset.
- Sezary syndrome is an aggressive, leukaemic cutaneous T-cell lymphoma variant, characterised by a triad of circulating neoplastic T cells (Sezary cells), diffuse erythroderma and disabling pruritus, with/without associated lymphadenopathy. The circulating cells are malignant T cells with serpentine nuclei.
- Erythrodermic mycosis fungoides is differentiated from Sezary syndrome by absent/low circulating Sezary cell count and is regarded as a progression of mycosis fungoides, whereas Sezary syndrome typically arises de novo.

TREATMENT

- Local corticosteroid therapy most common therapy in early cases; also used as an adjunct for other therapies. Topical nitrogen mustard and phototherapy (narrow-band ultraviolet B or psoralen plus ultraviolet A) have similar efficacy.
- Electron beam radiotherapy along with the application of nitrogen mustard or corticosteroids locally is an effective treatment in refractory/relapsed extensive plaque.
- Single-agent systemic therapy using immunomodulators such as interferons and retinoids often used if skin-directed therapy is inadequate or in cases of advanced disease.
- Chemotherapy (e.g. methotrexate, fludarabine) and histone deacetylase inhibitors (vorinostat and romidepsin) generally reserved for treatment of refractory or rapidly progressive advanced cases.

Q. What are plasma cell disorders?

- Plasma cell disorders are monoclonal neoplasms developing from common progenitors in the B-lymphocyte lineage.
- These disorders are also known as monoclonal gammopathies, paraproteinaemias and plasma cell dyscrasias. Various disorders are shown in Table 1.80.

TABLE 1.80 Plasma Cell Disorders

• Multiple myeloma	• Plasma cell leukaemia
• Waldenstrom macroglobulinaemia	• Heavy chain disease
• Primary (AL) amyloidosis	• Monoclonal gammopathy of undetermined significance
• Solitary plasmacytoma of bone	• Smoldering multiple myeloma
• Extramedullary plasmacytoma	
• POEMS syndrome	

Q. Discuss the immunopathology, pathology, clinical features, investigations and treatment of multiple myeloma.

Q. Write a short note on POEMS syndrome.

- Multiple myeloma is a malignant proliferation of plasma cells derived from a single clone.
- Plasma cells are derived from B lymphocytes. Individual plasma cells produce immunoglobulins with only one type of light chain (k or λ).
- It is believed that most cases are preceded by a phase of monoclonal gammopathy of undetermined significance.

IMMUNOPATHOLOGY

- Multiple myeloma is 'monoclonal'—that is the tumour is derived originally from one cell by cloning. So, all the malignant cells produce the same immunoglobulin.
- The immunoglobulin produced is called a 'paraprotein' (M-protein). It appears on electrophoretic strip as a clear-cut band (M-band or M-component).
- In myeloma, the paraprotein produced belongs to one of the immunoglobulin types and has one or other of the two light chains—that is k or λ.
- In light-chain myeloma, only the light chains are produced in excess and not the whole immunoglobulin molecule. These excess light chains appear in the urine as Bence Jones proteinuria.
- Classification of myeloma is based on the type of paraprotein produced—that is IgG (55%), IgA (25%), IgD (uncommon), IgE (uncommon) and light chain disease (20%). In nonsecretory myeloma, there is no M-protein in the blood or urine but has bone marrow plasmacytosis and organ or tissue impairment.

POEMS SYNDROME

- Box 1.34 describes POEMS syndrome.

BOX 1.34 POEMS Syndrome

- A variant of multiple myeloma
- Acronym stands for polyneuropathy, organomegaly (adrenal, thyroid, pituitary, gonadal, parathyroid, pancreatic), endocrinopathy, M-protein (usually IgG or IgA λ light chain) and skin changes (hyperpigmentation, hypertrichosis, acrocyanosis, white nails, scleroderma-like changes, facial atrophy, flushing or clubbing)
- Other common features not included in this acronym include oedema, ascites, pleural effusion, osteosclerotic bone lesions, thrombocytosis, increased risk of arterial or venous thrombosis, papilloedema and a high level of serum vascular endothelial growth factor (VEGF)
- Treatment:
  - Autologous peripheral blood stem cells transplantation in younger patients
  - Melphalan and dexamethasone in older patients
  - Local radiation in localised disease without clonal plasma cells in bone marrow biopsy

PATHOLOGY AND PATHOGENESIS

- Bone marrow is infiltrated heavily with atypical plasma cells. Gradual replacement of the marrow by plasma cells results in anaemia, leucopenia and thrombocytopenia.
- In majority of patients, plasma cells are seen in the peripheral blood in small numbers. In a few patients, plasma cells are seen in the peripheral blood in significant numbers (more than 2000/mm^3), and this condition is known as 'plasma cell leukaemia'.
- Localised tumour formation results in punched-out lesions on radiographs of flat bones.
- Serum uric acid is elevated due to increased cell turnover.
- Osteoclasts are stimulated resulting in bone resorption and generalised osteoporosis.
- Mobilisation of calcium from bone results in hypercalcaemia, hypercalciuria and nephrocalcinosis.
- Bence Jones proteinuria, amyloidosis, hypercalcaemia and hyperuricaemia result in renal damage and renal failure.
- Hyperviscosity syndrome results from increased viscosity of blood and is more common in IgA subtype of multiple myeloma.

CLINICAL FEATURES

- Peak incidence is between 60 and 70 years, and males are more affected than females.
- Some patients are asymptomatic, and myeloma is accidentally detected during the preclinical phase.
- Plasmacytomas—some patients develop extramedullary masses of malignant plasma cell known as plasmacytomas. These may be present at the time of diagnosis of multiple myeloma or may develop later during its course. Para-skeletal soft tissue is the most common (80%) site of plasmacytoma. Other areas include gut, skin, airways, liver, kidneys, CNS and breast. In a patient with multiple myeloma, presence of plasmacytomas indicate poor prognosis. Palliative radiotherapy is indicated for controlling symptoms related to plasmacytomas. Lenalidomide (and not thalidomide) and bortezomib have some role in management of plasmacytomas.
- Patients with multiple myeloma may go onto develop primary amyloidosis, plasmacytomas, heavy-chain disease or plasma cell leukaemia.
- Clinical fearures of multiple myeloma are given in Table 1.81.

TABLE 1.81 Clinical Features of Multiple Myeloma

• Bone marrow involvement	Anaemia, leucopenia and thrombocytopenia
• Bone involvement	Localised bony swellings over vertebrae, skull, sternum, ribs and clavicle, bone pain due to pathological fractures and compressive myelopathy due to vertebral collapse and compression
• Renal involvement	Nephrocalcinosis, amyloidosis and progressive renal failure
• Immune system involvement	Increased susceptibility to infections, particularly of the respiratory system and urinary tract
• Hyperviscosity syndrome	Blurred vision with retinal venous congestion, papilloedema, headache, vertigo, nystagmus, postural hypotension and congestive cardiac failure
• Clotting problems	Purpura, epistaxis, gastrointestinal bleeding
• Neurological manifestations	Amyloid peripheral neuropathy, carpal tunnel syndrome, compressive myelopathy and radiculopathy

INVESTIGATIONS

- Haemogram usually shows anaemia, leucopenia, thrombocytopenia and raised ESR (often >100).
- Peripheral blood smear may show rouleaux formation.
- Bence Jones proteins may be present in the urine. Serum-free light-chain (FLC) assay is more sensitive than urine Bence Jones proteins.
- Urea, creatinine and electrolytes are used to assess renal function.
- Serum calcium level is usually raised.
- Serum uric acid level is elevated.
- Serum alkaline phosphatase is characteristically normal, in the absence of complications.
- Total serum protein level is increased, albumin is decreased and globulins are markedly increased.
- Serum immunoglobulin estimation reveals a reduction of normal immunoglobulins below normal levels.
- Serum β_2-microglobulin level may provide a useful assessment of prognosis. Higher levels indicate poor prognosis.
- Radiological examination reveals generalised osteoporosis. Radiographs of flat bones like skull, vertebral bodies, ribs and pelvis show the characteristic punched-out osteolytic lesions. Collapse of multiple vertebrae is a common radiological finding.
- Whole-body low-dose computed tomography is the new standard for diagnosis of lytic disease.
- Electrophoretic studies can demonstrate the paraprotein on the electrophoretic strip as the 'M-band'. Immunoelectrophoresis and immunofixation can determine the immunoglobulin type and confirm that the M-component is truly monoclonal.
- MRI and PET may detect bone involvement when skeletal survey is normal.
- Bone scan is not required as it is often negative (may show increased uptake if a fracture of bone develops).
- Bone marrow examination is important. Normal bone marrow contains 2%–10% plasma cells. In myeloma, the number of plasma cells is increased, and they are atypical in morphology.
- Confirmation of clonality of plasma cells in bone marrow by immunophenotyping with flow cytometry or immunohistochemistry.

DIAGNOSIS (Box 1.35)

- Light-chain multiple myeloma:
  - Same as MM except no evidence of Ig heavy-chain expression on immunofixation.
  - Around 20% of patients with myeloma produce only light chains in the serum and urine.
- Around 2% produce neither light chains nor a paraprotein and are termed non-secretors. In such cases, >30% monoclonal plasma cells in bone marrow are required to make a diagnosis of myeloma.

BOX 1.35 Diagnostic Criteria for Multiple Myeloma

Infiltration of bone marrow with malignant plasma cells ≥10% or biopsy-proven bony or extramedullary plasmacytoma AND any one or more of the following:

- Evidence of end organ damage which can be attributed to the underlying plasma cell proliferative disorder *(CRAB)*:
  - Calcium serum >11 mg/dL
  - Renal insufficiency: Creatinine clearance <40 mL/minute or serum creatinine >2 mg/dL
  - Anaemia: Haemoglobin <10 g/dL
  - Bone lesions: One or more osteolytic lesions on skeletal radiography, CT or PET-CT
- Any one or more of the following biomarkers of malignancy:
  - ≥60% clonal bone marrow plasma cells
  - Involved/uninvolved serum free light chain ratio ≥100
  - >1 focal lesion on MRI studies (each focal lesion must be ≥5 mm in size)

SMOULDERING OR ASYMPTOMATIC MULTIPLE MYELOMA

- Characterised by M-component >3 g/dL or urinary M-protein >500 mg per 24 hours and/or clonal bone marrow plasma cells ≥10%, without myeloma-related organ or tissue impairment.
- Progresses to multiple myeloma or AL amyloidosis at a rate of 10% per year in the first 5 years and at a lower rate after that.
- Serum protein electrophoresis, complete blood count, measurement of calcium and creatinine values and 24-hour urine collection for electrophoresis and immunofixation should be performed at diagnosis and in 2–3 months after the initial recognition. A skeletal survey and bone marrow are mandatory at baseline. If the results at 2–3 months are stable, the studies should be repeated every 4–6 months for 1 year and, if stable, evaluation can be lengthened to every 6–12 months.
- Risk factors for early progression to multiple myeloma are based on the 20–20–20 risk model. It includes serum M-protein (>20 g/L), involved to uninvolved serum free light chain ratio (>20) and bone marrow plasma cell infiltration (>20%). Patients with at least two risk factors have a 2-year progression rate of 46%.

STAGING (Table 1.82)

TABLE 1.82 Revised International Staging System for Multiple Myeloma

Stage	Definition	Median Survival
I	All of the following: • Albumin >3.5 g/dL • β_2-Microglobulin <3.5 mg/L • Normal serum LDH • No high-risk cytogenetics	60 months
II	Neither fitting in stage I nor in stage III	42 months
III	Both of the following: • β_2-Microglobulin >5.5 mg/L • High-risk cytogenetics OR elevated serum LDH	27 months

TREATMENT

- Median survival in patients with advanced myeloma is 7–8 months. With chemotherapy, this can be prolonged to 3–4 years. There is no cure available till now.
- Asymptomatic stage I patients are generally not given chemotherapy.
- Prognosis relies not only on staging but also to a large extent on the cytogenetic features.

GENERAL MEASURES (Box 1.36)

BOX 1.36 General Measures for Treatment of Multiple Myeloma

- Prompt treatment of infections
- Treatment of anaemia
- High fluid intake of about 3 L/day
- Oral sodium bicarbonate in patients with compromised renal function to make the urine alkaline
- Allopurinol 300 mg daily to reduce hyperuricaemia
- Analgesics for pain relief
- Expert orthopaedic assistance and skilled physiotherapy to improve the quality of life
- Renal failure to be treated medically and dialysis if necessary
- Rehydration and oral prednisolone for hypercalcaemia
  - Mithramycin highly effective in controlling hypercalcaemia but is highly toxic
  - Pamidronate (60 mg as slow infusion over 24 hours) is a better option
- Plasmapheresis for hyperviscosity syndrome

STEM CELL TRANSPLANTATION

- Treatment of choice in multiple myeloma in eligible patients.
- Induction therapy with one of the combinations as given in the box under section heading 'Treatment Regimens' followed by consolidation regimen using high-dose melphalan (200 mg/m^2) intravenously and then autologous stem cell transplantation is the standard treatment in young patients (<65 years) without renal failure.

DRUG THERAPY

- Currently, five classes of active agents are available: alkylating agents (melphalan and cyclophosphamide), anthracyclines (adriamycin and liposomal doxorubicin), corticosteroids (dexamethasone and prednisone), immunomodulatory drugs (thalidomide, lenalidomide and pomalidomide) and proteasome inhibitors (bortezomib and carfilzomib).
- Steroid (dexamethasone or prednisolone) use is pivotal in the treatment of multiple myeloma and is generally included in all treatment regimens.
- Bortezomib, a proteasome inhibitor, is usually included in all therapeutic regimens, particularly in patients with high-risk cytogenetic features.
- Immunomodulating drugs like thalidomide, lenalidomide and pomalidomide along with prednisolone or dexamethasone produce remission in about 60%–70% patients.

BOX 1.37 Treatment Regimens for Multiple Myeloma

STEM CELL TRANSPLANT ELIGIBLE
- Lenalidomide/dexamethasone
- Bortezomib/dexamethasone
- Bortezomib/lenalidomide/dexamethasone
- Bortezomib/cyclophosphamide/dexamethasone
- Bortezomib/doxorubicin/dexamethasone
- Bortezomib/thalidomide/dexamethasone

STEM CELL TRANSPLANT INELIGIBLE
- Melphalan or cyclophosphamide/bortezomib/dexamethasone or prednisolone
- Melphalan/thalidomide/dexamethasone or prednisolone
- Lenalidomide/bortezomib/dexamethasone or prednisolone
- Melphalan/prednisolone/lenalidomide

- Bortezomib, when combined with lenalidomide and dexamethasone may produce remission in >90% cases. Its side effects include thrombocytopenia, neutropenia, diarrhoea and sensory neuropathy. Reactivation of varicella zoster virus may occur and therefore, acyclovir is indicated for prophylaxis in patients receiving it.

TREATMENT REGIMENS

- Various treatment options in patients with multiple myeloma are given in Box 1.37.

RADIOTHERAPY

- Ideal for local problems like severe bone pain, pathological fractures and tumourous lesions.

MISCELLANEOUS

- Bisphosphonates (pamidronate, zoledronic acid, clodronate) and bone-stimulating agent (denosumab) reduce the incidence of vertebral fractures and ameliorate pain and should be considered in stages II and III disease. Bisphosphonates inhibit osteoclast recruitment and maturation, prevent development of monocytes into osteoclasts, induce osteoclast apoptosis and interrupt their attachment to the bone. However, they do not have any effect on overall survival or incidence of non-vertebral fractures. An important complication of bisphosphonates is osteonecrosis of jaw.
- Patients started on immunomodulatory treatment (thalidomide or lenalidomide) have increased risk of venous thrombosis. Hence, they should receive aspirin or low molecular weight heparin.
- Anti-CD38 antibodies (e.g. daratumumab), anti-SLAMF7 antibodies (e.g. elotuzumab) and anti-B cell maturation antigen (anti-BCMA) monoclonal antibody-drug conjugate (e.g. balantamab mafodotin) in combination with other drugs have been approved for refractory/relapsed patients. Daratumumab is also approved in combination with others as induction regimen before stem cell transplant as well as managing stem-cell transplant-ineligible patients.

SUMMARY OF TREATMENT OF MULTIPLE MYELOMA (Flowchart 1.16)

- Treatment of multiple myeloma is summarised in Flowchart 1.16.

Q. What are the causes of M-component on electrophoresis?

- Various conditions which can have M-component are shown in Table 1.83.

TABLE 1.83 Conditions That Can Have M-Component

Plasma cell disorders • Multiple myeloma • Waldenstrom macroglobulinaemia • Primary amyloidosis • Heavy chain disease • MGUS **Other lymphoid neoplasms** • Chronic lymphatic leukaemia • Lymphomas	**Non-lymphoid neoplasms** • Chronic myeloid leukaemia • Breast carcinoma **Non-neoplastic conditions** • Cirrhosis of liver • Sarcoidosis • Rheumatoid arthritis • Myasthenia gravis

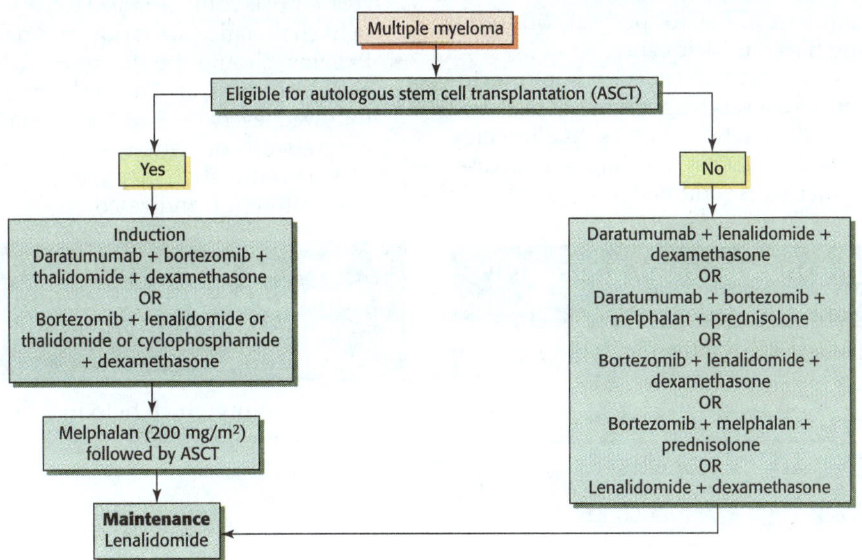

Flowchart 1.16 Treatment of Multiple Myeloma.

Q. What are the causes of renal failure in multiple myeloma?

- Frank renal failure is seen in about 25% of multiple myeloma patients.
- Some form of renal pathology can be observed in 50% of myeloma patients.
- Various factors responsible for renal failure are shown in Box 1.38.

BOX 1.38 Factors Contributing to Renal Failure in Multiple Myeloma

- Tubular damage (cast nephropathy) from excretion of light chains (Bence Jones proteinuria)
- Hypercalcaemia resulting in nephrocalcinosis and renal damage
- Glomerular deposition of amyloid (renal amyloidosis)
- Hyperuricaemia resulting in urate nephropathy
- Recurrent urinary infections
- Infiltration of the kidney by myeloma cells
- Hyperviscosity syndrome
- Use of nephrotoxic drugs (e.g. NSAIDs for bone pains)
- Monoclonal gammopathy of renal significance (MGRS)

Q. Briefly discuss monoclonal gammopathy of renal significance.

- MGRS is renal damage mediated by monoclonal immunoglobulin secreted by low-grade lymphoproliferative disorders, mainly monoclonal gammopathy of undetermined significance (MGUS); the kidney damage is induced by either monoclonal Ig deposition in renal tissues or by its activity as autoantibody.
- Kidney damage is characterised by:
    - Does not respond well to immunosuppressive regimens used in the treatment of autoimmune nephropathies.
    - A very high rate of recurrence after kidney transplantation (approximately 90%) if the monoclonal gammopathy is not eliminated before or immediately after transplantation.
    - Affected patients are at risk for progression to the corresponding haematologic cancer.
- Treatment involves substantial reduction in monoclonal immunoglobulin level by various agents. For plasma cell-based diseases, bortezomib-based therapy is indicated while for $CD20^+$ B-cell-based disease, rituximab-based therapy is indicated.

Q. What are the indicators of poor prognosis in multiple myeloma?

- Poor prognostic factors are shown in Table 1.84.

TABLE 1.84 Poor Prognostic Factors in Multiple Myeloma

• Low haemoglobin (<8.5 g/dL)	• Renal failure
• Serum calcium >12 mg/dL	• Thrombocytopenia
• Elevated β_2-microglobulin	• Advanced lytic bone lesions
• λ light chain secretors	• Elevated LDH
• High-risk karyotypes	• Plasma cell leukaemia

Q. Discuss the role of radiographic examination in the diagnosis of multiple myeloma.

- Radiographic findings which help in diagnosis of multiple myeloma are given in Table 1.85.

TABLE 1.85 Radiological Findings in Multiple Myeloma

• X-ray skull	Multiple punched out osteolytic lesions and osteoporosis
• X-ray chest	Pathological fractures of ribs, punched out lesions of ribs, clavicle and scapulae and osteoporosis
• X-ray spine	Collapse of multiple vertebrae and osteoporosis
• X-ray pelvis	Multiple punched out osteolytic lesions and osteoporosis
• X-ray KUB	Nephrocalcinosis

Q. What is monoclonal gammopathy of undetermined significance (MGUS)?

- Premalignant clonal disorder is characterised by M-component on electrophoresis but <3 g/dL, plasma cells <10% in bone marrow, no hypercalcaemia, renal impairment, anaemia, hyperviscosity, hepatosplenomegaly or osteolytic lesions, no light-chain amyloidosis or evidence of other B-cell neoplasms.
- Present in more than 3% of the general population older than 50 years.
- The most common immunoglobulin isotypes are immunoglobulin G (IgG) and kappa light chain.
- Progresses to multiple myeloma, Waldenstrom's macroglobulinaemia, primary AL amyloidosis or a lymphoproliferative disorder at a rate of 1%–1.5% per year.
- Risk of progression to multiple myeloma and related disorders depends upon size of M-component (risk of progression with an M-protein value of 1.5 g/dL almost twice that of a patient with an M-protein value of 0.5 g/dL), type of M-component (IgM and IgA increased risk compared to IgG) and an abnormal free light chain ratio (k:λ ratio—normal being 0.26–1.65).
- Patients should be followed with serum protein electrophoresis at 6 months and, if stable, can be followed every 1–2 years depending upon risk of progression or when symptoms suggestive of a plasma cell malignancy arise.
- No treatment is indicated.

Q. How do you differentiate between multiple myeloma and monoclonal gammopathy of undetermined significance?

- Various points which help in differentiating multiple myeloma from MGUS are given in Table 1.86.

TABLE 1.86 Differences Between Multiple Myeloma and MGUS

	Multiple Myeloma	MGUS
• M-protein level in serum	M-protein found in serum and/or urine except in patients with non-secretory myeloma	<3 g/dL with expression of intact immunoglobulin (e.g. IgG, IgM, IgA)
• Bone marrow	Clonal plasma cells ≥10% or Presence of plasmacytomas	Clonal plasma cells <10%
• Organ/tissue involvement	Presence of plasmacytomas At least one of the following: • Calcium (ionised) >5.5 mEq/L • Renal insufficiency (creatinine >2 mg/dL) • Anaemia (haemoglobin <10 g/dL) • Bone involvement—osteolytic bone lesions and/or osteopenia	No evidence of other B-cell proliferative disorders No hypercalcaemia, renal impairment, anaemia, bone involvement

Q. How do you differentiate between smoldering multiple myeloma and monoclonal gammopathy of undetermined significance?

- Various points which help in differentiating smoldering myeloma from MGUS are given in Table 1.87.

TABLE 1.87 Differences Between Smoldering Myeloma and MGUS

Parameter	Smoldering Multiple Myeloma	MGUS
Serum M-protein	≥3 g/dL	<3 g/dL
Urine M-protein	≥500 mg/day	—
Plasma cells in bone marrow	10%–60%	<10%
Progression rate to multiple myeloma	10% per year (initial 5 years) and then 3% per year (next 5 years)	1% per year

Q. Describe solitary plasmacytoma of bone.

- Localised accumulation of neoplastic monoclonal plasma cells to a single bone at presentation without a proof of a systemic plasma cell proliferative disorder.
- Represents 3% of plasma cell neoplasms.
- Primarily affects the axial skeleton, most commonly thoracic or lumbosacral vertebrae, causing localised bone pain or neurologic symptoms secondary to spinal cord or root compression.
- Nearly 70% eventually develop systemic disease at a median of 2–4 years despite radiation treatment.

DIAGNOSIS (Box 1.39)

- Low levels of serum or urine M-protein detectable in 24%–60% of patients by immunofixation.

TREATMENT

- Treatment is local radiotherapy.
- Overall median survival is 7–12 years.

BOX 1.39 Diagnosis of Solitray Plasmacytoma of Bone

- Solitary bone lesion confirmed by skeletal survey and MRI (or CT)
- Normal skeletal survey and MRI (or CT) of spine and pelvis (except for the primary solitary lesion)
- Plasma cell infiltration in the solitary lesion proven by biopsy
- Normal bone marrow biopsy (<10% plasma cells)
- Lack of myeloma-related organ dysfunction.

Q. What is solitary extramedullary (extraosseous) plasmacytoma?

- Occurs most commonly (85%) in head and neck region, followed by gastrointestinal tract.
- More than 75% of the tumours do not produce detectable serum M-protein.
- Diagnosis requires tissue biopsy indicating monoclonal plasma cell histology, bone marrow plasma cell infiltration <5% of all nucleated cells, absence of osteolytic bone lesions or other tissue involvement and lack of myeloma-related organ dysfunction.
- Nearly 15% of patients subsequently develop multiple myeloma.
- Low levels of serum or urine M-protein may be detectable in some cases.
- Treatment requires local removal. However, since most cases occur in head and neck area, surgery may not be a feasible option. In such cases, local radiotherapy is recommended.
- Median 10-year survival rate approximately 70% compared to 40% in solitary plasmacytoma of bone.

Q. Give a brief account of Waldenstrom macroglobulinaemia.

- It is a B-cell lymphoproliferative disorder characterised by a lymphoplasmacytic infiltration in the bone marrow or lymphatic tissue and a monoclonal immunoglobulin M-protein (IgM) in the serum.
- Classified as lymphoplasmacytic lymphoma under WHO classification of non-Hodgkin's lymphoma.
- Occurs in older adults.

CLINICAL FEATURES

- May be asymptomatic.
- Symptoms develop due to tumour infiltration (cytopenia, fever, night sweats, weight loss, lymphadenopathy, organomegaly) and/or monoclonal protein (hyperviscosity, cryoglobulinaemia, cold agglutinin, neuropathy and amyloidosis).
- Circulating IgM can be associated with type I cryoglobulinaemia or coagulation abnormalities due to coating of coagulation factors by IgM.
- Tissue deposition of monoclonal IgM is associated with systemic amyloidosis, macroglobulinaemia cutis, gastrointestinal symptoms (malabsorption, diarrhoea or bleeding) and glomerular injury.
- Monoclonal IgM can also produce haemolytic anaemia (due to cold agglutinin disorder), small vessel vasculitis and peripheral neuropathy.
- Hyperviscosity occurs due to large size of IgM molecule. It is most commonly manifested by bleeding (epistaxis, gingival bleeding), blurring or loss of vision, dizziness, headache, vertigo, nystagmus, hearing loss, ataxia, paraesthesias, diplopia, somnolence and coma.
- Peripheral neuropathy is present in near 20% patients. This is usually a distal, symmetric, chronic, demyelinating neuropathy, sometimes associated with abnormalities of proprioception and ataxia.
- Tumour cells can infiltrate organs and result in hepatomegaly, splenomegaly and lymphadenopathy in about 20% cases.

DIAGNOSIS

- Serum monoclonal protein detection by serum protein electrophoresis; samples may require warming to 37°C to avoid interference of cold agglutinins. Immunofixation is required to characterise monoclonal protein.
- Bone marrow aspirate and biopsy showing more than 10% lymphoplasmacytic cells (positive for CD19, CD20, CD22 and CD79a23).

TREATMENT

- The median survival for patients below 70 years of age is 10 years while for those above 80 years is 4 years.
- Plasmapheresis for severe hyperviscosity features.
- Disease incurable with currently available therapies but survival increased with rituximab and fludarabine or rituximab and bendamustine (Flowchart 1.17).
- Fludarabine may predispose to late myelodysplasia and large-cell lymphoma transformation.
- Very few patients are eligible for stem cell transplantation due to their age.

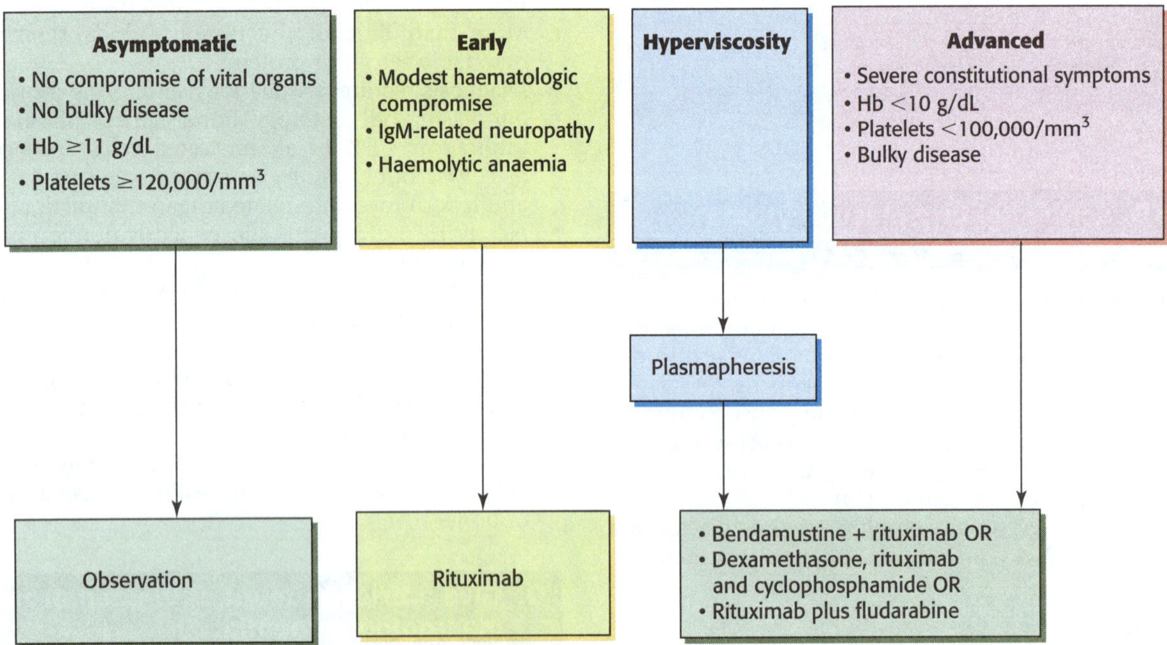

Flowchart 1.17 Treatment of Waldenstrom Macroglobulinaemia.

Q. Briefly outline the side effects, precautions and dosage of thalidomide.

- Introduced initially as sedative and for the treatment of morning sickness in pregnant females but was withdrawn in 1960s because of reports of teratogenicity associated with its use, particularly limb defects or phocomelia. The typical feature is defective, shortened limbs resulting in flipper hands and feet. In more severe cases, complete absence of limbs can occur. Additionally, foetus can develop external ear abnormalities, hypoplastic or completely absent bones, facial palsy, eye abnormalities and gastrointestinal and genitourinary tract malformations.
- Later, it was found to inhibit angiogenesis and possess immunomodulatory and antiinflammatory properties.
- Side effects of thalidomide are given in Table 1.88.

PRECAUTIONS

- It is important to remember that even a single dose of thalidomide can produce congenital malformations. Therefore, effective contraception must be used at least 4 weeks before beginning thalidomide therapy, during thalidomide therapy and for 4 weeks following discontinuation of thalidomide therapy.
- Once treatment has started, pregnancy testing should occur weekly during the first 4 weeks of use, then pregnancy testing should be repeated at 4 weeks in women with regular menstrual cycles. If menstrual cycles are irregular, the pregnancy testing should occur every 2 weeks.

DOSE

- Initially 200 mg/day, increased to 400–600 mg/day with increment of 100 mg/week.

USES

- Various uses of thalidomide are given in Table 1.89.

TABLE 1.88 Side Effects of Thalidomide

Side Effects	
• Peripheral nerves	Numbness, tingling, burning sensation
• Central nervous system	Tremors, confusion, fatigue, depression, somnolence, headache, bradycardia
• Gastrointestinal	Constipation, nausea, dry mouth, increased appetite
• Haematological	Deep vein thrombosis, neutropenia
• Skin	Skin rash, itching, red palms
• Endocrine	Hypothyroidism
• Pregnancy	Phocomelia

TABLE 1.89 Uses of Thalidomide

Established	Potential
• Multiple myeloma • Erythema nodosum leprosum • Myelofibrosis with myeloid metaplasia	• Some cases of myelodysplastic syndrome (MDS) • Waldenstrom's macroglobulinaemia • Solid organ tumours • Behcet disease • Pyoderma gangrenosum • Chronic graft-versus-host disease (GVHD)

Q. Discuss the mechanism of haemostasis.

Q. Write in brief about platelets and their functions.

Q. Briefly outline the natural inhibitors of coagulation.

Q. Describe fibrinolytic system.

- Haemostatic mechanism is responsible for prevention of blood loss from intact vessels, as well as for the arrest of bleeding from injured vessels.
- It is activated by damage to the vascular endothelium and exposure of subendothelial tissue to blood.

MECHANISM OF HAEMOSTASIS

- Three major components of the normal haemostatic mechanism—the vascular component, the platelet component and the coagulation component. The first two components are called primary haemostasis while the last component is called secondary haemostasis.
- A defect in any one of these three results in an abnormal tendency to bleed—that is bleeding disorder. The defect may be either quantitative (deficiency) or qualitative (functional).
- Venous thrombi, which form under low flow conditions, are predominantly composed of fibrin and red cell (red thrombi).
- Arterial thrombosis is usually initiated by spontaneous or mechanical rupture of atherosclerotic plaque, a process that exposes thrombogenic material in the lipid-rich core of the plaque to the blood. These thrombi form under high shear conditions and are primarily composed of platelet aggregates held together by fibrin strands (white thrombi).

VASCULAR COMPONENT

- This involves a reflex spasm of the injured vessel (vasoconstriction) that serves to minimise blood loss.

PLATELET COMPONENT

- Platelets are anucleate cells and have a discoid shape. The normal lifespan is about 10 days. The normal blood platelet count ranges from 150,000 to 450,000/μL. About 70% of the platelets are in circulation while 30% are in the spleen.

BOX 1.40 Storage Granules of Platelets

- α-Granules containing a variety of proteins like fibrinogen, von Willebrand factor, thrombospondin, platelet-derived growth factor (PDGF), platelet factor 4 and P-selectin
- Dense granules containing serotonin, ADP (which helps in platelet aggregation) and calcium
- Lysosomal granules containing acid hydrolases

- The cytoplasm of platelets contains three major types of storage granules (Box 1.40).
- The platelet component requires three critical events—platelet adhesion, release of granule contents and platelet aggregation.
- Following vessel constriction, platelets adhere to the vessel wall by platelet surface receptor—glycoprotein Ib/IX/V complex. This is facilitated by:
  - Factor VIII–von Willebrand factor released from damaged endothelial cells that form a link between platelet glycoproteins and exposed collagen.
  - Release of ADP and thromboxane A_2 (synthesised from arachidonic acid pathway).
- Platelet activation follows adhesion and results in the discharge of the granule content. Binding of collagen, epinephrine and thrombin to platelets also activates phospholipase A_2 and phospholipase C on the membrane of platelets which catalyses the release of arachidonic acid from two membrane phospholipids (phosphatidylinositol and phosphatidylcholine). The enzyme cyclooxygenase then converts arachidonic acid into endoperoxides. These are converted to thromboxane A_2 by thromboxane synthetase and to prostacyclin by prostacyclin synthetase (Flowchart 1.18). Thromboxane A_2 is a potent stimulant of platelet activation and aggregation while prostacyclin inhibits activation.
- Platelet aggregation (adhesion of activated platelets to each other) is facilitated by fibrinogen forming links among adjacent platelets via glycoprotein IIb/IIIa (GPIIb/IIIa).
- ADP binds to two G-protein coupled receptors, $P2Y_1$ and $P2Y_{12}$. Activation of $P2Y_1$ leads to calcium mobilisation, change in platelet shape and reversible aggregation. Activation of $P2Y_{12}$ leads to platelet secretion and more stable aggregation.

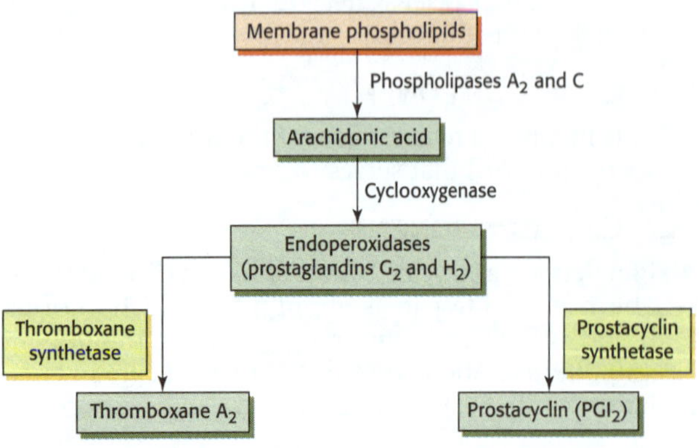

Flowchart 1.18 Arachidonic Acid Pathway.

- Platelet adhesion and platelet aggregation serve to form a platelet plug that seals off the vascular breach and arrests haemorrhage.

Functions of Platelets (Box 1.41)

BOX 1.41 Functions of Platelets

- Maintain vascular integrity
- Spontaneously arrest bleeding through platelet plug formation
- Participate in the intrinsic coagulation system
- Promote repair and healing through release of growth factors

COAGULATION COMPONENT (SECONDARY HAEMOSTASIS)

- During secondary haemostasis, the platelet plug is stabilised by the deposition of a network of fibrin formed through the activation of coagulation cascade.

COMPONENTS OF THE COAGULATION CASCADE

Coagulation Cascade

- Coagulation cascade can be conveniently considered under three 'pathways': the intrinsic pathway (contact activation pathway), the extrinsic pathway (tissue factor pathway) and the common pathway.
- Factors involved in coagulation cascade are shown in Table 1.90.
- Intrinsic pathway and extrinsic pathway are alternative routes to the production of factor Xa (activated X) with extrinsic pathway being the primary pathway.
- Common pathway is the process initiated by factor Xa leading to the production of fibrin.
- Intrinsic pathway is assessed in vitro by the activated partial thromboplastin time (aPTT).
- Extrinsic pathway is assessed by the PT.

Extrinsic Pathway

- 'Tissue factor' (a protein–phospholipid complex normally present on vascular cells and activated monocytes) converts factor VII into activated factor VII (VIIa) in presence of calcium.
- Activated tissue factor VII complex activates factors IX and X.

Intrinsic Pathway

- Initiation of the intrinsic pathway occurs when prekallikrein, high-molecular-weight kininogen and factor XII are exposed to a negatively charged surface (contact phase).

TABLE 1.90 Clotting Factors

Factor	Synonym
• I	Fibrinogen
• II	Prothrombin
• V	Proaccelerin
• VII	Proconvertin
• VIII	Antihaemophilic factor
• IX	Christmas factor
• X	Stuart–Prower factor
• XI	Plasma thromboplastin antecedent
• XII	Hageman factor
• XIII	Fibrin stabilising factor

- Prekallikrein is converted to kallikrein and factor XII becomes activated factor XII (XIIa).
- Factor XIIa converts factor XI into XIa.
- Factor XIa activates factor IX, and factor IXa with its co-factor FVIIIa activates X to Xa.

Common Pathway

- Factor Xa converts prothrombin to thrombin (factor IIa). This is greatly facilitated by factor Va.
- Thrombin enhances its own generation by:
  - Activating the factors V and VIII.
  - Activating factor XI, which generates more IXa and more XIa by positive feedback.
  - Encouraging platelet aggregation and disintegration.
- Factor IIa converts fibrinogen into fibrin monomers and also activates factor XIII to XIIIa that cross-links fibrin to fibrin polymers (Flowchart 1.19).

Inhibitors of Coagulation

- Natural inhibitors of coagulation provide a mechanism to limit clotting to the vicinity of tissue injury (Box 1.42).
- Antithrombin, a circulating serine protease inhibitor (serpin) inactivates thrombin, IXa, Xa and XIa. Its action is potentiated by heparin sulphate released from endothelium or given exogenously. It is also enhanced by heparan sulphate (found on endothelial surfaces), which contains a pentasaccharide sequence. Fondaparinux is pharmacologic version of this pentasaccharide sequence that mediates its binding to AT.
- Protein C, activated by the thrombin–thrombomodulin complex, inactivates Va and VIIIa in the presence of the activated cofactor protein S. Factor V Leiden is not susceptible to cleavage by activated protein C and is therefore inactivated more slowly, resulting in a hypercoagulable state.

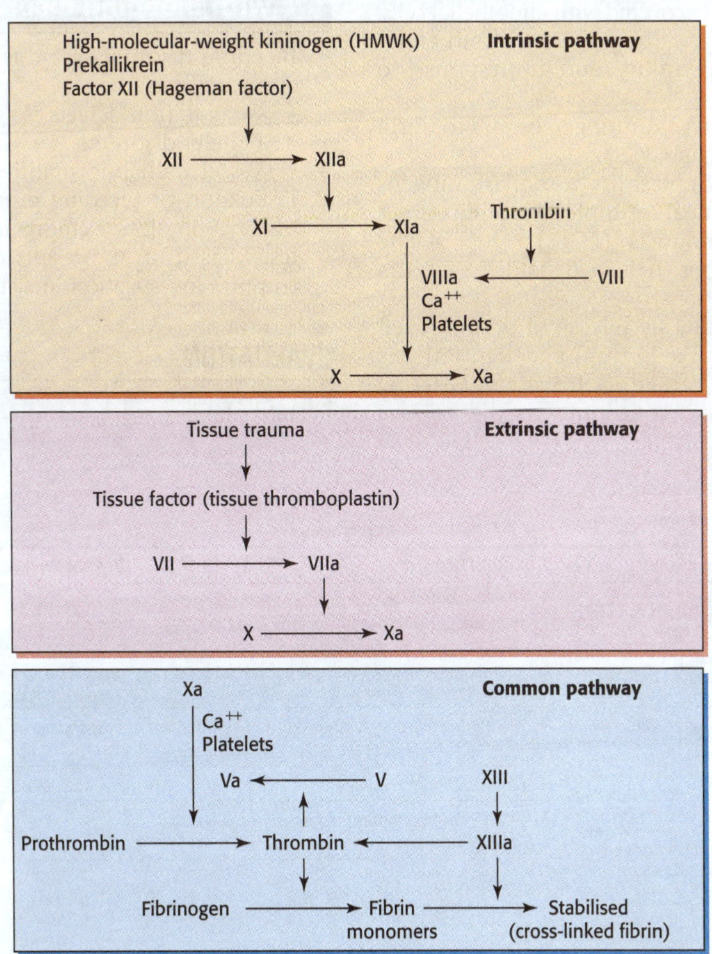

Flowchart 1.19 Coagulation Cascade (Intrinsic, Extrinsic and Common Pathways).

BOX 1.42 Inhibitors of Coagulation

- Antithrombin (AT)
- Heparin co-factor II
- α_2-Macroglobulin
- Protein C and protein S

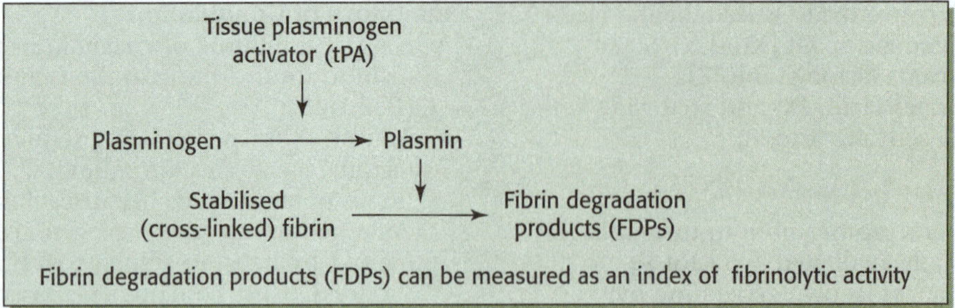

Flowchart 1.20 Fibrinolytic System.

- Endothelial cells also produce prostacyclin and nitric oxide that inhibit platelet aggregation.

FIBRINOLYTIC SYSTEM

- Physiological function of the fibrinolytic system is to digest deposits of fibrin (thrombi). The defect in the vessel wall then becomes covered with endothelial cells.
- Tissue plasminogen activator is released from endothelial cells following injury and in response to thrombin.
- It cleaves plasmin from plasminogen bound to fibrin within the clot (Flowchart 1.20).
- Kallikrein also activates plasmin from plasminogen.
- Plasmin degrades fibrin at multiple sites and releases fibrin degradation products (FDPs). One of the major FDPs is D-dimer. It also degrades Va, VIIIa and GPIb.
- Fibrinolysis is controlled by release of plasminogen activator inhibitor-1 (PAI-1) from platelets. PAI-1 is inhibited by activated protein C. Release of PAI-1 by activated platelets may contribute to the relative resistance of platelet-rich arterial thrombi to thrombolysis. Other inhibitors of fibrinolysis include α_2-antiplasmin and α_2-macroglobulin.

Q. Discuss the evaluation of a patient with bleeding disorder.

- Bleeding disorders are due to one of the following abnormalities:
  - Coagulation defects
  - Platelet disorders
  - Vessel wall abnormalities
- Evaluation of bleeding disorders includes a detailed history, physical examination and initial screening tests. Based on the results of these, some additional complex investigations may be necessary in some cases.

EVALUATION

HISTORY (Table 1.91)

TABLE 1.91 Differentiating Various Types of Bleeding Disorders Based on History

Coagulation Defects	Platelet Disorders	Vessel Wall Abnormalities
• Bleeding into viscera, muscles and joints; petechiae uncommon	• Bleeding into skin (purpura, petechiae), mucous membrane, GI system and central nervous system; epistaxis; prolonged bleeding from superficial cuts and petechiae common	• Bleeding into skin (purpura, petechiae); epistaxis; gingival bleeding; large bullous haemorrhages in the buccal mucosa; in case of a local vessel wall abnormality, recurrent bleeding at a single site
• Bleeding starts several hours after surgery or trauma	• Bleeding immediately after surgery or trauma	• Bleeding occurs immediately after trauma
• Local pressure ineffective	• Local pressure effective	• Local pressure effective
	• History of drug intake, especially nonsteroidal antiinflammatory drugs like aspirin	
Congenital defects • Lifelong history • Family history		
Acquired defects • Short duration • Evidence of liver disease, renal failure, disseminated intravascular coagulation (DIC)		

BOX 1.43 Physical Findings to Look for in a Patient With Bleeding Disorder

- Purpura, bruises and ecchymoses
- Telangiectasia in hereditary haemorrhagic telangiectasias
- Scars over elbows and knees in factor XIII deficiency
- Examination of joints, particularly knees, ankles and elbows for haemarthrosis
- Signs of liver cell disease
- Hepatosplenomegaly and lymphadenopathy
- Neurological signs

PHYSICAL EXAMINATION

- Physical examination should include a diligent search for various findings which point towards a specific cause of bleeding or complication (Box 1.43).

SCREENING TESTS (Table 1.92)

BLEEDING TIME

- Prolonged in thrombocytopenia, qualitative platelet abnormalities (e.g. uraemia), von Willebrand disease and severe fibrinogen deficiency.
- Ivy's method:
  - Tie a blood pressure cuff around the upper arm and inflate it to 40 mmHg to block venous return.
  - Clean the skin of the forearm and make two puncture marks using a lancet.
  - Soak the oozing blood every 15 seconds with a filter paper until bleeding stops.
  - Normal bleeding time <9 minutes.

PROTHROMBIN TIME

- Normal is within 3 seconds of control value (12–14 seconds).
- Prolonged in deficiency of fibrinogen (factor I) factors II, V, VII and X, liver disease, DIC, vitamin K deficiency, oral warfarin therapy and in presence of antiphospholipid syndrome.

ACTIVATED PARTIAL THROMBOPLASTIN TIME

- Normal PTT is 33–45 seconds.
- Prolonged in deficiency of factors I, II, V, VIII, IX, X, XI and XII, including haemophilia A and B, von Willebrand disease, DIC, heparin therapy and presence of lupus anticoagulant and acquired factor inhibitors.

TABLE 1.92 Screening Tests to Assess Coagulation Abnormalities

Screening Test	Components Assessed
• Peripheral smear	Platelets, leucocytes, red blood cells
• Platelet count (*N*: 150 to 350 × 10^3/mm^3)	Platelets
• Bleeding time (*N*: <9 minutes)	Platelet function, von Willebrand factor
• Prothrombin time (*N*: 12–14 seconds)	Extrinsic pathway, factors V, VII, X; factor I, II
• Activated partial thromboplastin time (*N*: 33–45 seconds)	Intrinsic pathway, factors V, VIII, IX, X, XI, XII; factors I, II
• Thrombin time (*N*: 12–16 seconds)	Common pathway, factors I, II
• Clot retraction	Platelets
• Fibrinogen concentration (*N*: 150–450 mg/dL)	Fibrinogen
• Fibrin degradation products (FDPs)	Lysis of fibrin

Q. Define thrombocytopenia. Enumerate the common causes, clinical manifestations, investigations and management of thrombocytopenia.

Q. Describe tourniquet test (capillary resistance test of Hess; Hess test).

Q. Enumerate the common conditions inhibiting platelet function or qualitative platelet disorders.

DEFINITION

- Thrombocytopenia is defined as a platelet count below 100,000/mm^3.

CAUSES

- Various causes of thrombocytopenia are given in Table 1.93.

GENERAL CLINICAL MANIFESTATIONS

- Bleeding into skin—purpura, petechiae, ecchymoses.
- Bleeding into mucous membranes—epistaxis, haemorrhagic bullae in oral mucosa, genitourinary bleeding, gastrointestinal bleeding.
- Fundal haemorrhage and intracranial bleeding occur in severe thrombocytopenia.
- Tourniquet test (capillary resistance test of Hess; Hess test) may be positive. The sphygmomanometer cuff applied around the upper arm is inflated to a pressure halfway between systolic and diastolic blood pressures. The cuff is deflated after 5 minutes. Count the number of petechiae in an area of 3 cm diameter, 1 cm below the cubital fossa. A number exceeding 20 is interpreted as positive Hess test. Positive Hess test indicates increased capillary fragility resulting from thrombocytopenia, defective platelet function, scurvy or primary vessel wall abnormality.
- Table 1.94 gives relationship between platelet counts and bleeding manifestations.

TABLE 1.93 Causes of Thrombocytopenia

Decreased production

- Marrow aplasia/hypoplasia, e.g. aplastic anaemia, congenital, cytotoxic drugs, alcohol, thiazides
- Marrow fibrosis, e.g. myelofibrosis
- Marrow infiltration, e.g. leukaemia, myeloma, carcinoma
- Vitamin B_{12} and folate deficiency
- Sepsis

Increased destruction

- Non-immunologic thrombocytopenia, e.g. vasculitis, DIC, thrombotic thrombocytopenic purpura (TTP), haemolytic-uraemic syndrome (HUS), HELLP (haemolysis, elevated liver enzymes, low platelets) syndrome of pregnancy, acute fatty liver of pregnancy, vascular prosthesis, sepsis
- Immunologic thrombocytopenia, e.g. idiopathic or immune thrombocytopenic purpura (ITP), viral and bacterial infections (including HIV, hepatitis C infection; *Helicobacter pylori*; transient in infections with dengue, cytomegalovirus, Epstein–Barr virus), drugs (penicillin, quinine, quinidine, methyldopa), SLE, heparin-induced thrombocytopenia (HIT), posttransfusion, sepsis
- Hypersplenism—portal hypertension, lymphomas, myeloproliferative disorders
- Dilutional—massive blood transfusion

TABLE 1.94 Platelet Counts and Bleeding Manifestations

Platelet count	Manifestation
• 150,000–450,000/mm³	• Normal
• Less than 100,000/mm³	• Thrombocytopenia
• Less than 50,000/mm³	• Post-traumatic bleeding
• Less than 20,000/mm³	• Spontaneous bleeding, fundal and intracranial bleeding

TABLE 1.95 Role of Peripheral Smear in Diagnosing Cause of Thrombocytopenia

Smear finding	Cause
• Platelet clumping	Pseudothrombocytopenia
• Giant platelets	Hereditary thrombocytopenia
• Macrocytosis	Vitamin B_{12} or folate deficiency
• Schistocytes	Haemolytic-uraemic syndrome/thrombotic thrombocytopenic purpura; disseminated intravascular coagulation
• Blasts, nucleated red cells	Probable primary bone marrow disorder
• Lymphocytosis, neutrophilia, toxic granules in neutrophils	Probable infection
• Isolated thrombocytopenia	Immune thrombocytopenic purpura, drug-induced thrombocytopenia, infections (HIV, hepatitis C, *Helicobacter pylori*), heparin-induced

INVESTIGATIONS

- Peripheral blood smear (Table 1.95).
- Platelet count is low. Clinical manifestations roughly correlate with the platelet count.
- Bleeding time is prolonged and it bears a close relationship to platelet count.
- Bone marrow with normal or increased number of megakaryocytes indicates increased platelet destruction, hypersplenism or ineffective platelet production.
- Bone marrow with decreased number of megakaryocytes indicates reduced production of platelets.
- Investigations to look for the cause of thrombocytopenia.

MANAGEMENT

- Management is essentially the treatment of underlying cause (see section heading 'Causes').
- Severe bleeding, life-threatening situations like fundal haemorrhages and threatening intracranial haemorrhage can be temporarily treated with platelet transfusions.

QUALITATIVE PLATELETS DEFECTS (Box 1.44)

- Platelet function is impaired but counts remain normal.
- Most commonly due to drugs, some of which may also produce thrombocytopenia.

BOX 1.44 Qualitative Platelet Defects

DRUGS INHIBITING PLATELET FUNCTION OR CAUSING THROMBOCYTOPENIA

- Nonsteroidal antiinflammatory drugs (NSAIDs)—aspirin, indomethacin
- Antibiotics—penicillins, cephalosporins, sulphonamides
- Heparin, dextran, β-blockers, quinidine, valproic acid, cimetidine

URAEMIA

CONGENITAL DISORDERS

- Disorders of membrane glycoproteins (Glanzmann thrombasthenia: deficiency or defect in GPIIb-IIIa; Bernard–Soulier syndrome: deficiency or defect in any of the components of GPIb/IX/V complex)
- Disorders of platelet secretion of ADP/prostaglandins (storage pool disorders)

Q. Discuss the pathogenesis, clinical features, investigations and management of immune (idiopathic) thrombocytopenic purpura (ITP).

DEFINITION

- Immune (idiopathic) thrombocytopenic purpura (ITP) is thrombocytopenia (platelets $<100,000/mm^3$) due to an autoimmune disorder which occurs due to presence of autoantibodies directed against platelet membrane glycoproteins mainly GPIIb/IIIa and GPIb/IX.
- Since every patient may not have purpura, the term ITP is redefined as immune thrombocytopenia.

PATHOGENESIS

- About 85%–95% of cases of ITP result from the presence of an antiplatelet antibody of IgG type. These antibody-bound platelets are removed and prematurely destroyed by macrophages in the spleen.
- These antibodies are produced by B cells. Helper T cells ($CD4^+$) are also important in production of antibodies.
- Impaired platelet production is also important in many cases. In adults, as many as 40% of ITP cases may have reduced platelet turnover reflecting inhibitory effect of platelet autoantibodies on megakaryopoiesis as well as due to cytotoxic T cell-mediated megakaryocytic damage.

CLINICAL FEATURES

- Three terms are used to describe ITP: newly diagnosed ITP (<3 months duration) that is more common in children; persistent ITP (3–12 months duration); and chronic ITP (>12 months) which is more common in adults (Table 1.96).
- Most cases are primary. Secondary ITP can occur in SLE, dengue, COVID-19 and chronic infections like HIV and hepatitis C, post-transfusion purpura and use of some drugs.
- Characteristically, the patient has no physical signs other than those due to bleeding and anaemia (occurs due to menorrhagia and epistaxis). Splenomegaly is characteristically absent in most patients (tip of spleen may be palpable in 10% case).
- May be associated with haemolysis (Evan's syndrome).
- More than two-thirds of patients with acute ITP recover within 6 months. More than one-third of remaining patients recover in next few months to years.

DIAGNOSIS

- Thrombocytopenia. Repeat platelet count using sodium citrate as anticoagulant so as to exclude pseudothrombocytopenia caused by platelet aggregation and clumping in the presence of EDTA anticoagulant.
- Peripheral smear to exclude other causes of thrombocytopenia.
- Positive tourniquet test (Hess test).
- Prolonged BT.
- Bone marrow examination characteristically shows normal or increased number and size of megakaryocytes. Bone marrow is not necessary in acute ITP with typical presentation if management involves observation or use of intravenous immunoglobulin or anti-RhD globulin.
- Antiplatelet antibodies may be demonstrated in blood. However, a negative test does not exclude ITP.
- In chronic ITP, exclude other causes like HIV, hepatitis C virus infection and lymphoproliferative disorders.

TREATMENT

- In acute and mild cases, no specific therapy will be necessary.
- Intervention is reserved for those who have overt haemorrhage and platelet counts below $20,000/mm^3$ or those who have organ- or life-threatening bleeding irrespective of the circulating platelet count.
- Active bleeding should be treated with platelet concentrates. Platelet have only transient effects for a few hours, and therefore the patient may need to undergo transfusions repeatedly. Platelets should be used in combination with intravenous immunoglobulin and glucocorticoids.
- The main therapeutic measures are corticosteroids and splenectomy.
- Immunosuppressive therapy, intravenous immunoglobulin, anti-RhD globulin and TPO receptor agonists are indicated in selected cases.

CORTICOSTEROIDS

- Indications of corticosteroids are given in Box 1.45.
- Dosage of corticosteroids:
  - Initial dose is 1–2 mg/kg of prednisolone/day.

TABLE 1.96 Differences Between Newly Diagnosed ITP and Chronic ITP

Newly Diagnosed ITP	Chronic ITP
• Most frequent in children (2–6 years)	• Most frequent in adults (20–40 years)
• Affects both sexes equally	• Females affected more than males (M:F ratio, 1:4)
• Commonly follows an antecedent upper respiratory viral infection	• Usually no preceding history of viral infection
• Usually a self-limiting disease	• Usually a chronic disease characterised by remissions and relapses
• Abrupt onset of haemorrhage into skin and mucous membranes, e.g. purpura, petechiae, ecchymoses, epistaxis, bleeding from oral cavity, gastrointestinal and genitourinary tracts	• Insidious onset of haemorrhage into skin and mucous membranes, e.g. purpura, petechiae, ecchymoses, epistaxis and menorrhagia; purpurae are more common in the distal parts of limbs
• Intracranial haemorrhage occurs rarely	• Intracranial haemorrhage occurs very rarely

BOX 1.45 Indication of Corticosteroids in ITP

- To induce remission
- Postoperatively, in failed splenectomy cases
- Pregnant females after the fifth month of pregnancy
- To maintain remission in chronic immune thrombocytopenic purpura

BOX 1.46 Indications of Splenectomy in ITP

- Chronic cases, especially in adults who have not responded to corticosteroids
- Unacceptably high doses of corticosteroids in maintaining remission
- Emergency measure in children and adults, when there is severe bleeding or threatening cerebral haemorrhage (despite adequate corticosteroid therapy)
- In the first 4–5 months of pregnancy, if steroids have failed to induce full remission

  - Initial dose is continued for at least 2 weeks or if necessary 3–4 weeks and then reduced slowly and stopped.

SPLENECTOMY

- Indications of splenectomy are given in Box 1.46.
- Mechanism of action of splenectomy:
  - Splenectomy removes the major site of platelet destruction.
  - Splenectomy brings down the concentration of circulating antiplatelet antibodies.

IMMUNOSUPPRESSIVE THERAPY

- Agents used are vincristine, vinblastine, azathioprine, cyclophosphamide, cyclosporin and mycophenolate mofetil.
- Indications of immunosuppressive therapy:
  - Refractory cases (i.e. those who have failed to respond to corticosteroids and splenectomy).
  - Those in whom corticosteroid therapy and splenectomy are contraindicated.

INTRAVENOUS IMMUNOGLOBULIN

- Transient blockade of Fc receptors on macrophages in the reticuloendothelial system, especially the spleen, is believed to play a major role in the immediate, and often dramatic, platelet responses observed after intravenous immunoglobulin.
- Dose: 1 g/kg.
- Indications of intravenous immunoglobulin are given in Box 1.47.
- It provides temporary effect only for 1–2 weeks.
- Adverse effects include nausea, vomiting, fever and headache. Uncommon side effects include neutropenia and haemolytic anaemia.

ANTI-RhD GLOBULIN

- Effective in patients with ITP.
- Should be given only if the patient is Rh-positive.

BOX 1.47 Indications of Intravenous Immunoglobulin in ITP

- Acute situations prior to surgery and child birth and in patients with intracranial bleeding
- Those in whom corticosteroid therapy and splenectomy are contraindicated
- Often used prior to splenectomy as a temporising measure

- Useful in patients who do not respond to steroids and may be tried before splenectomy. The effect is usually temporary and nearly 50%–75% patients relapse over variable period.
- Proposed mechanism is coating of Rh-positive red blood cells by anti-RhD antibodies, which are then preferentially destroyed by the reticuloendothelial cells with relative sparing of the antibody-coated platelets.
- Dose is 75 μg/kg intravenously.
- Side effects include nausea, vomiting, fever, chills and intravascular haemolysis.

THROMBOPOIETIN RECEPTOR AGONISTS

- Three TPO-RAs for refractory ITP patients: eltrombopag, avatrombopag and romiplostim.
- Eltrombopag and avatrombopag are orally administered. Important adverse effects of eltrombopag include headache, deep vein thrombosis and embolism and mild elevation in liver enzymes. Avatrombopag does not increase risk of thrombosis.
- Romiplostim is administered once a week subcutaneously.

OTHERS

- Danazol, an androgen with low virilising activity.
- Rituximab.
- Fostamatinib, an oral spleen tyrosine kinase (Syk) inhibitor.

EMERGENCY TREATMENT

- Required in case of life-threatening bleed.
- Intravenous administration of methylprednisolone (30 mg/kg, maximum dose 1 g) over 20–30 minutes plus platelet transfusion, followed by intravenous immunoglobulin (1 g/kg). Methylprednisolone is repeated daily for another 1–2 days.
- Antifibrinolytic treatment (tranexamic acid) can help to stop bleeding.

SAFE PLATELET COUNTS FOR VARIOUS INVASIVE PROCEDURES

- The platelet count for performing various invasive procedures is given in Table 1.97.

TABLE 1.97 Safe Platelet Counts for Various Invasive Procedures

Procedure	Threshold of Platelets Count
Insertion of central line	20,000/μL
Lumbar puncture	40,000/μL
Major surgery including vaginal delivery (without epidural)	50,000/μL
Insertion or removal of epidural catheter	80,000/μL
Neurosurgery or posterior eye surgery	100,000/μL

Q. Discuss thrombotic thrombocytopenic purpura.

Q. Discuss thrombotic microangiopathy.

THROMBOTIC MICROANGIOPATHY

- Thrombotic microangiopathy (TMA) is the term for diseases in which disseminated microthrombi composed of agglutinated platelets occlude arterioles and capillaries.
- Causes of TMA are given in Table 1.98.

THROMBOTIC THROMBOCYTOPENIA PURPURA

- Thrombotic thrombocytopenia purpura (TTP) is a severe microangiopathic haemolytic anaemia characterised by systemic platelet aggregation, organ ischaemia, profound thrombocytopenia (with increased marrow megakaryocytes) and fragmentation of erythrocytes.

AETIOLOGY

- TTP is caused by a deficiency of ADAMTS-13, a metalloprotease that cleaves ultra-large von Willebrand (vWF) factor multimers into smaller, less-adhesive multimers. Ultra-large vWF multimers cause extensive platelet aggregation and depletion of the circulating pool of platelets.
- Deficiency is often related to the presence of antibodies against this protease; rarely, it can be due to mutation in ADAMTS-13 gene (autosomal recessive).

TABLE 1.98 Causes of Thrombotic Microangiopathy

Primary	• Immune TTP (ADAMTS13 deficiency) • Haemolytic uremic syndrome (typical, atypical) • Drug-related TMA (mitomycin, cyclosporine, tacrolimus, quinine) • Disseminated intravascular coagulation
Secondary	• Systemic infection • Connective tissue diseases (lupus, scleroderma) • Tumour-related TMA (lymphomas, pancreatic cancer) • Transplant associated TMA • Malignant hypertension • HELLP syndrome

TABLE 1.99 Causes of Thrombotic Thrombocytopenic Purpura

- Medications (mitomycin C, cyclosporin, tacrolimus, quinidine, dipyridamole, ticlopidine, clopidogrel, gemcitabine, bevacizumab)
- Stem cell transplantation
- HIV infection
- Total body irradiation
- Pregnancy
- Autoimmune diseases
- Malignancy
- Idiopathic enzyme deficiency

- Several other causes can also produce deficiency of ADAMTS-13 and produce TTP (Table 1.99).

CLINICAL FEATURES

- The classic pentad of TTP is microangiopathic haemolytic anaemia with schistocytosis (at least 3 cells per 100 red blood cells), severe thrombocytopenia, fluctuating neurologic deficits secondary to CNS ischaemia, fever and renal abnormalities including haematuria and/or proteinuria.
- However, only a minority of patients have fever; renal involvement is also not required for the diagnosis.
- Neurologic features include headache, vertigo, confusion, seizures and focal deficits.
- Gastrointestinal features are common and include diarrhoea, nausea, vomiting and abdominal pain.

DIAGNOSIS

- Presence of thrombocytopenia, schistocytes and elevated serum LDH (out of proportion to the degree of haemolysis) are sufficient to suggest the diagnosis of TTP. Elevated LDH also occurs due to release from ischaemic tissues.
- Indirect hyperbilirubinaemia, decreased plasma haptoglobin level.
- PT, aPTT, fibrinogen and D-dimer are normal. FDPs may be normal or slightly elevated.
- Red cells, red cell casts and proteinuria on urine examination.
- Negative Coombs' test.
- Reduced activity of ADAMTS-13 below 5%–10% of normal. Most patients also have anti-ADAMTS13 antibodies.
- Troponin-I level, electrocardiogram and echocardiogram in suspected cardiac involvement.

TREATMENT

- Treatment of choice is daily plasma exchange (removing 40 mL/kg body weight of plasma and replacing it with equal volume of fresh frozen plasma); continued for at least 2 days after remission (defined as stabilisation of clinical symptoms and normalisation of platelet count and LDH levels along with rising haemoglobin). Plasma exchange removes antibodies against ADAMTS-13 as well as ultra-large vWF multimers:
  - Plasma exchange should be initiated as soon as possible, preferably within 4–8 hours, if a patient presents with a microangiopathic haemolytic anaemia and thrombocytopenia in the absence of any other identifiable clinical cause.

- Corticosteroids generally added to plasma exchange to suppress antibody production.
- Platelet transfusion contraindicated unless life-threatening bleeding occurs.
- Splenectomy in resistant cases. It removes antibody-producing cells.
- Rituximab, a monoclonal antibody against CD20, suppresses antibody-producing cells. It is used in patient's refractory to plasma exchange and corticosteroids. It may also be used along with plasma exchange if CNS or heart is significantly involved.
- Caplacizumab, a humanised anti-vWF antibody fragment, reduces the formation of microvascular thrombi by inhibiting the interaction between vWF multimers and platelets and may be used in combination with plasma exchange and steroids in refractory cases.
- Supportive care measures include packed red blood cell transfusion, strict blood pressure control and prophylaxis for deep vein thrombosis.

Q. Discuss the clinical features, investigations and treatment of haemolytic-uraemic syndrome (HUS).

- More often seen in children.
- Typical or diarrhoea-related HUS:
  - Preceded by haemorrhagic enterocolitis that is caused by cytotoxin-producing serotypes of *E. coli* (e.g. 0157:H7; 0104:H4) or *Shigella dysenteriae* type 1. Shiga toxins 1 and 2 produced by enterohaemorrhagic *E. coli* are the most frequent cause of diarrhoea-associated HUS.
  - Shiga toxins bind to globotriaosylceramide (GB3) membrane receptors present on endothelial cells of kidney and other target organs. This disrupts protein synthesis, causes endothelial cell death and damage, induces inflammatory and procoagulant cascades that promote microvascular thrombosis.
  - Usually occurs as a single episode, except in rare individuals who have a familial, recurrent type of the disease.
- Atypical or non-diarrhoea-related HUS (complement-mediated):
  - More severe than typical type and difficult to treat.
  - Can occur with diverse conditions, like pneumococcal infections, autoimmune disease, HIV, transplantation, irradiation and certain drugs.
- A number of drugs are implicated in development of HUS (Box 1.48).

BOX 1.48 Drugs Implicated in Development of HUS

- Calcineurin inhibitors: cyclosporine, tacrolimus
- Quinine
- Vascular endothelial growth factor inhibitors
- Quetiapine
- Drugs of abuse: cocaine, intravenous oxymorphone
- Chemotherapeutics: mitomycin C, cytosine arabinoside, cisplatin, gemcitabine
- Antiplatelet agents: ticlopidine, clopidogrel

CLINICAL FEATURES

- Most common in children between 1 and 5 years of age.
- Occurs within 2–12 days after initial episode of haemorrhagic enterocolitis.
- Classical presentation is with the triad of microangiopathic haemolytic anaemia, thrombocytopenia and renal failure.
- The commonest clinical presentation is acute pallor and oliguria, following diarrhoea or dysentery.
- Haematuria and hypertension common.
- Complications of fluid overload may result in pulmonary oedema and hypertensive encephalopathy. Despite thrombocytopenia, bleeding manifestations are rare.
- Neurological symptoms like irritability, encephalopathy and seizures may occur but are uncommon.

INVESTIGATIONS

- Anaemia, schistocytes on peripheral smear, elevated LDH and thrombocytopenia.
- Elevated blood urea and creatinine.
- Urine examination may show proteinuria and red blood cells.
- Normal PT and aPTT.
- Stool culture for enterohaemorrhagic *E. coli*; shiga toxin analysis in stools; PCR assay to detect shiga toxin genes in stool.

TREATMENT

- Therapy for diarrhoea-associated HUS is limited to supportive care for the renal and haematological complications. This involves meticulous fluid and electrolyte management after oligo-anuric renal failure develops, packed red blood cell transfusion, dialysis and control of blood pressure.
- Antibiotics should be avoided as they may worsen prognosis. It may be given if shigellosis is suspected. Azithromycin can safely be given.
- Eculizumab, monoclonal antibody to complement 5a, particularly in atypical HUS. A major risk is fulminant meningococcal infection. Meningococcal vaccination is mandatory, and the patients should take prophylactic antibiotics at least until 2 weeks after vaccination.

PROGNOSIS

- Acute mortality is estimated to be between 3% and 5%, with the primary causes of death being neurologic, cardiovascular or intra-abdominal catastrophe.
- Chronic kidney disease can develop in as many as 15% cases of which some may require renal replacement therapy.
- Hypertension and proteinuria may develop in 15% and 28% of cases on long-term follow up.
- CNS features include fatigue, headache and attention deficits.

Q. Discuss the aetiology, classification, clinical features, diagnosis and management of haemophilia A.

Q. Write a short note on acquired haemophilia A.

AETIOLOGY

- Haemophilia A is an X-linked genetic disorder of coagulation, affecting males. It results from a reduction of factor VIII (antihaemophilic factor).
- Antihaemophilic factor (factor VIII) is primarily synthesised by the liver. Plasma factor VIII has a half-life of 12 hours. In the plasma, it is carried bound to the von Willebrand's factor (vWF).
- Incidence of haemophilia A is 1 in 10,000 males.
- Acquired haemophilia A occurs due to presence of inhibitors (antibodies) against factor VIII and is unrelated to presence of congenital haemophilia A. It is more common in elderly patients. In about 50% cases, no underlying disease is present while in others, acquired haemophilia A is associated with autoimmune disorders, malignancies, pregnancy, various drugs (e.g. penicillin, sulphonamides, phenytoin) and dermatological diseases. Presentation is with acute onset of severe and life-threatening bleeding. Spontaneous subcutaneous, deep muscle and retroperitoneal bleeding represent the majority of events, but gastrointestinal, pulmonary and intracranial bleeding also occur. Trauma-related muscle bleeding and haemarthroses are uncommon.

GENETICS

- Haemophilia A is an X-linked recessive disorder.
- A haemophilic patient's daughters will all be carriers, but all his sons will be normal. A carrier female has a 50% chance of producing a haemophilic male or a female carrier.
- Females can be haemophilic if:
  - She is born to an affected father and a carrier mother (25% risk).
  - She has Turner's syndrome (45XO).
  - She has inactivation of normal X chromosome due to lyonisation (rare).
- The degree of factor VIII deficiency and severity of bleeding tend to be similar in all the affected members of the same family.
- Nearly 30% occur due to spontaneous mutation with no family history.

CLASSIFICATION

- Normal factor VIII level in the blood is 0.50–1.50 IU/mL. Haemophilia A can be classified based on the factor VIII activity in blood (Table 1.100).

TABLE 1.100 Classification of Haemophilia A

Severity of Haemophilia	Factor VIII Level	Occurrence of Bleeding
Mild	>5% of normal activity	After significant trauma
Moderate	1%–5% of normal activity	After mild trauma
Severe	<1% of normal activity	Frequent without trauma

CLINICAL FEATURES

- Haemophilia A is characterised by excessive bleeding. Virtually, no tissue is exempted from this. Spontaneous bleeding usually occurs after 6 months of age but in severe cases, it can occur in the first month also.
- When bleeding follows trauma, it is characteristically 'delayed'.
- Bleeding tendency may range from mild to severe.

BLEEDING INTO JOINTS (HAEMARTHROSES)

- Recurrent bleeding into large joints, especially knees, elbows, ankles, wrists and hips.
- Bleeding usually spontaneous or following minor trauma.
- In the acute stage, the affected joint is swollen, hot, tender and movements severely restricted. All these gradually subside over a period of days.
- Repeated haemarthroses eventually result in deformity, crippling and disuse atrophy of muscles around the joint.

BLEEDING INTO MUSCLES

- Muscle haematomas are common in calf and psoas muscles.
- Psoas haematomas may compress the femoral nerve resulting in sensory disturbances over thigh and quadriceps weakness. Often the patient is left with some residual weakness in the leg.
- Calf haematomas can result in contraction and shortening of the Achilles tendon.

OTHER BLEEDING MANIFESTATIONS

- Bleeding from wounds.
- Bleeding from sockets after dental extraction.
- Easy bruising.
- Retroperitoneal, mesenteric and intra-abdominal bleeding.
- Bleeding into muscles of tongue.
- Intracranial haemorrhage (subdural haematoma and intracerebral haemorrhage).
- Haematuria and ureteric colic due to passage of blood clots.

INVESTIGATIONS

- BT, PT and platelet counts are normal.
- aPTT is typically prolonged.
- Specific factor VIII assay can confirm the diagnosis.

ANTENATAL DIAGNOSIS

- Chorion villous sampling (CVS) at 8–9 weeks' gestation, sexing the foetus and using informative factor VIII probes.
- Sexing the foetus at 16 weeks' gestation by amniocentesis and, if male, a foetal blood sampling at about 19–20 weeks.
- The first technique is preferable to the second.

MANAGEMENT

- Routine immunisations, such as diphtheria-tetanus-pertussis or measles-mumps-rubella should be given subcutaneously using a thin needle.
- Given the risk of exposure to blood-derived products, patients should be vaccinated against hepatitis B by giving vaccine subcutaneously.

LOCAL TREATMENT

Wounds and Mucous Membrane Bleeding

- Local pressure may be applied digitally, with pressure bandages or sutures.
- Topical haemostatics like adrenaline and thrombin.
- Immobilisation of wounds by bandages, splinting, etc.

HAEMATOMAS AND HAEMARTHROSIS

- In acute stage, provide initial management [Rest, Ice, Compression and Elevation (RICE)] wherever the patient is. Ice pack should not be in direct skin contact and applied for 20 minutes once in 4–6 hours
- Pain is relieved by analgesics like acetaminophen or codeine. Drugs like aspirin affecting platelet function are contraindicated.
- Once acute stage is over, patient should be mobilised and should receive physiotherapy.

REPLACEMENT THERAPY

- Replacement therapy should start immediately and is aimed at rapid correction of deficiency of factor VIII. Desired levels of factor VIII are as follows:
  - For skin bleeding, epistaxis, oral bleeding: >30%
  - For gastrointestinal, genitourinary, joint bleeding: >50%
  - For CNS bleeding, preoperative: 100%
- Agents currently used for replacement therapy are cryoprecipitate, factor VIII concentrate and recombinant factor VIII given intravenously. Fresh frozen plasma is rarely used as the volume infused may produce fluid overload.
- Indications of replacement therapy:
  - Early treatment of spontaneous bleeding episodes.
  - Established severe or prolonged wound and tissue bleeding.
  - Control of bleeding during and after surgery and trauma.
- Prophylactic infusion (once every 2–3 days) is recommended at present in all patients with severe haemophilia so as to prevent arthropathy. Prophylaxis is superior to on-demand therapy in delaying or preventing the development of haemophilic arthropathy.
- One unit of factor VIII is that amount present in 1 mL of normal plasma. An individual with a plasma volume of 3000 mL would have 3000 units of clotting factor in the circulation. Each unit of cryoprecipitate contains about 100 units of factor VIII.
- Calculation of dose: For factor VIII, 1 unit/kg will raise blood level by 2%. In major bleeding, the aim is to raise factor VIII levels to at least 50% (presuming the initial level to be 0). This is maintained for 3–5 days. Volume of distribution for factor VIII is approximately 0.5 (i.e. half the plasma volume). The calculated dose is administered twice a day. The dose is calculated as:

$$\text{Dose of factor VIII} = \text{Desired factor level (\%)} \times \text{Weight (kg)} \times 0.5$$

- Complications of replacement therapy:
  - Transmission of infections (e.g. hepatitis B virus, delta virus, hepatitis C virus, HIV infection).
  - Development of antifactor VIII antibodies.

DESMOPRESSIN

- Causes release of stored vWF and factor VIII from endothelial cells into plasma.
- Desmopressin (DDAVP; 1-desamino-8-D-arginine vasopressin) can transiently raise factor VIII activities by three to five times. It is given intravenously at a dose of 0.3 μg/kg over 15 minutes. Intranasal route can be used for oral bleeding and before dental procedures. Patients should be advised to limit water intake to reduce chances of hyponatraemia.
- Indications are minor bleeding and minor surgery.

EPSILON AMINOCAPROIC ACID (EACA) AND TRANEXAMIC ACID

- These are antifibrinolytic agents that exert their effect by inhibiting the proteolytic activity of plasmin and, therefore, inhibiting fibrinolysis.
- When used concurrently with replacement therapy, these agents can reduce the factor VIII requirements.
- Indicated for control of oral and nasal bleeding and menstruation.
- Commonly used for dental extractions. Regimen is EACA taken orally in a dose of 5 g four times daily for 7 days, starting on the day of extraction. For tranexamic acid, dose is 10 mg/kg intravenously (or 15–25 mg/kg orally) 6–8 hourly.
- Contraindicated in presence of haematuria because of increased risk for intrarenal or ureteral thrombosis and in presence of DIC or thromboembolic disease.

EMICIZUMAB

- Emicizumab is a recombinant, humanised, bispecific monoclonal antibody that bridges activated factor IX and factor X to restore the function of missing activated factor VIII. It is administered as a once-weekly subcutaneous injection for prophylaxis in severe haemophilia.

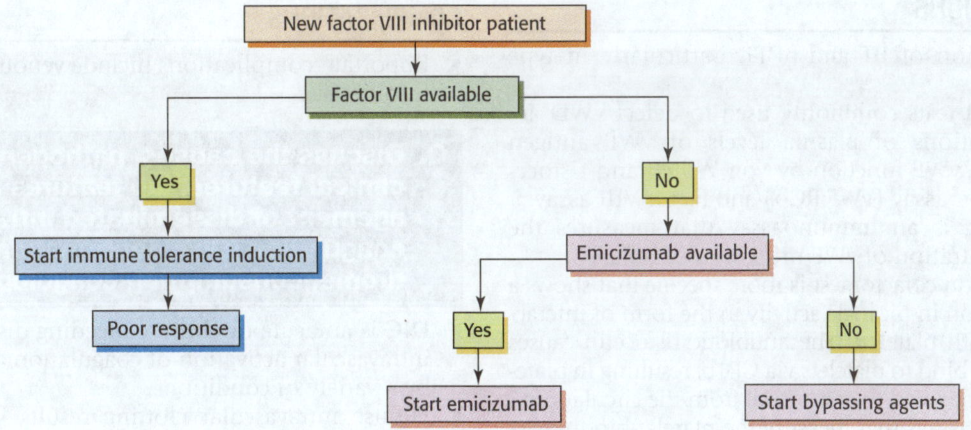

Flowchart 1.21 Treatment of Patients With Factor Inhibitors.

TREATMENT FOR PATIENTS WITH INHIBITORS AGAINST FACTORS

- Use of bypassing agents such as recombinant factor VIIa or activated prothrombin complex concentrates.
- Eradication of the inhibitor by means of immune tolerance induction:
  - Patients receive repetitive doses of factor VIII (or factor IX in haemophilia B), usually once a day, with or without associated immunosuppressive (immune tolerance therapy).
  - Typically, there is an initial rise in antibody titres as a result of anamnestic response.
  - Subsequently, however, a gradual reduction in titre is seen until in the end, the inhibitor becomes undetectable. This may take several months (Flowchart 1.21).
  - After successful immune tolerance, patients continue on regular factor infusions.
- Use of immunosuppressive agents (e.g. steroids, cyclophosphamide, rituximab).
- Emicizumab is also useful in presence of inhibitors against factor VIII.

Q. Briefly discuss haemophilia B (Christmas disease) and its management.

- It is an X-linked disorder resulting in deficiency of factor IX.
- Clinical features are indistinguishable from haemophilia A. Patients with severe disease present with muscle haematomas and haemarthroses progressing to crippling joint deformities.
- Diagnosis is established by factor IX assay.

MANAGEMENT

- Management is similar to that of haemophilia A.
- Desmopressin is not effective.
- Replacement therapy:
  - Fresh frozen plasma is used to treat mild to moderate bleeding.
  - Factor IX concentrate (prothrombin complex concentrates) is used to treat moderate to severe bleeding. Presently available factor IX concentrates are a mixture of factors II, VII, IX and X and proteins C and S. Hence, the replacement therapy carries an additional risk of thromboembolism.

Q. Discuss the aetiology, clinical features, investigations and treatment of von Willebrand's disease (vWD).

- Most common inherited bleeding disorder.
- vWD is characterised by the deficiency or dysfunction of von Willebrand factor (vWF).
- There are three major types of vWD: type 1 (partial quantitative deficiency), type 2 (qualitative defect—type 2A, 2B, 2M and 2N) and type 3 (complete absence of vWF).
- Type 1 is autosomal dominant. Type 2A and 2M are usually autosomal dominant, though a few cases may be autosomal recessive. Type 2N and type 3 are inherited as autosomal recessive.

VON WILLEBRAND FACTOR

- It is a protein synthesised by endothelial cells and megakaryocytes. It has two main functions:
  - vWF acts as a carrier protein for factor VIII. A deficiency of vWF hence causes a secondary reduction of factor VIII leading to a coagulation defect.
  - vWF plays an important role in platelet adhesion by forming bridges between platelets and subendothelial tissue. Hence, the deficiency of vWF results in a defect of platelet function.

CLINICAL FEATURES

- Clinical presentation can be very variable, ranging from a severe haemorrhagic disorder to an asymptomatic condition.
- Common clinical manifestations are epistaxis, easy bruising, menorrhagia, postpartum haemorrhage and haemorrhage following trauma, surgery and dental extraction.
- Less common clinical manifestations are haematuria, gastrointestinal bleeding and haemarthrosis. GI bleed can occur due to angiodysplasia in GI tract.

INVESTIGATIONS

- Prolongation of BT and aPTT, particularly in type 3 vWD.
- The initial tests commonly used to detect vWD are determinations of plasma levels of vWF antigen (vWF:Ag), vWF function by von Willebrand ristocetin cofactor assay (vWF:RCo) and factor VIII assay:
  - vWF:Ag is an immunoassay that measures the concentration of vWF protein in plasma.
  - Ristocetin cofactor test is more specific that shows a reduction in biologic activity in the form of interaction with platelets. The antibiotic ristocetin causes vWF to bind to platelets via GP1b, resulting in platelet clumps and their removal from the circulation.
  - Newer assays that measure the platelet-binding activity of vWF include vWF:GPIbM and vWF:GPIbR.
  - Remember, vWF is also an acute phase reactant and plasma levels may be high in conditions of stress, inflammation, exercise and pregnancy.

MANAGEMENT

- Mild bleeding is managed with desmopressin. Desmopressin is contraindicated in type 3 vWD because of a lack of efficacy and in type 2B vWD because of increased platelet binding with subsequent thrombocytopenia.
- Severe bleeding can be controlled by intravenous cryoprecipitate.
- If available, plasma-derived concentrates containing vWF and factor VIII is recommended in place of cryoprecipitate as the former are virus inactivated. Other new agents include plasma-derived vWF-only concentrate and recombinant vWF-only concentrate.
- For oral surgical procedures, EACA is given orally in a dose of 5 g four times daily for 7 days, starting on the day of procedure.
- Menorrhagia is managed with hormonal suppression. Tranexamic acid may be used to treat women with heavy menstrual bleeding who wish to conceive.

Q. Write briefly on recombinant factor VII activated.

- Recombinant factor VII activated (factor VIIa) is approved for management of patients with congenital factor VII deficiency and haemophilia A or B with inhibitors:
  - Presenting with episodes of severe haemorrhage.
  - During perioperative management of bleeding.
- Several other conditions where factor VIIa may be of use:
  - Trauma with massive bleeding.
  - Glanzmann's thrombasthenia.
  - Congenital factor VII deficiency.

MECHANISM OF ACTION

- rFVIIa binds to the surface of activated platelets and promotes factor X activation and thrombin generation on the activated platelet surface. Binding of factor VIIa to platelets involves the glycoprotein Ib/IX/V complex and anionic phospholipids expressed on activated platelets.

COMPLICATIONS

- Important complications include venous and arterial thrombosis.

Q. Discuss the causes, pathogenesis, clinical features, lab features and management of disseminated intravascular coagulation (DIC; defibrination syndrome; consumption coagulopathy).

- DIC is an acute or chronic bleeding disorder due to intravascular activation of coagulation and is caused by a variety of conditions.
- Diffuse intravascular clotting results in utilisation (consumption) of coagulation factors V, VIII and fibrinogen, and platelets, which in turn leads to bleeding. Derangement of coagulation and fibrinolysis in DIC is also mediated by several cytokines including tumour necrosis factor (TNF), IL-6 and IL-1.
- The cardinal clinical manifestations of DIC are bleeding and organ damage.

CAUSES

- Causes of DIC are given in Table 1.101.

PATHOGENESIS

- DIC is a form of consumptive coagulation characterised by an imbalance between coagulation and bleeding.
- The predisposing conditions result in expression of tissue factor on endothelial cells and circulating monocytes because of high levels of inflammatory cytokines, bacterial endotoxins and tissue damage.
- This process produces activation of factor VII via extrinsic pathway leading to excessive thrombin generation and widespread fibrin deposition in the microvasculature causing multiorgan dysfunction.
- Thrombin activates platelets and other coagulation factors such as factor VIII, IX, XI, which further augments the formation of fibrin thrombi.
- Excessive thrombin generation is also associated with a hyperfibrinolytic phase and severe bleeding.
- Platelets and coagulation factors are depleted as a result of the consumptive coagulopathy leading to bleeding (Flowchart 1.22).

CHRONIC DIC

- A compensated state that develops when blood is continuously or intermittently exposed to small amounts of tissue thromboplastin.
- There may be little obvious clinical or laboratory indication of the presence of DIC.

CLINICAL FEATURES

- There is a spectrum of thrombosis and haemorrhage in all cases of DIC; each or both may be encountered. Most cases present with haemorrhage.
- Classified as asymptomatic, organ failure (thrombotic), bleeding (hyperfibrinolysis) and massive bleeding (consumptive) types.

TABLE 1.101 Causes of Disseminated Intravascular Coagulation

Acute		
Infections	**Obstetric**	**Others**
• Sepsis • Gram-negative infections • Meningococcal infections • Malaria • Severe dengue • Rocky Mountain spotted fever • Fungal infections	• Abortions • Sepsis • Preeclampsia/eclampsia • Retained dead foetus • Amniotic fluid embolism • Acute fatty liver of pregnancy	• Snake bite • Major surgery or trauma • Major burns • Heat stroke • Neoplasms especially acute promyelocytic leukaemia • Cancer chemotherapy • Tumour lysis syndrome • Shock • Haemolytic transfusion reaction • Acute transplant rejection • Fat embolism • Near drowning • Aortic aneurysm • Shock • Acute pancreatitis • Catastrophic antiphospholipid syndrome
Chronic • Malignancies • Abruptio placentae • Giant haemangioma (Kasabach–Merritt syndrome)		

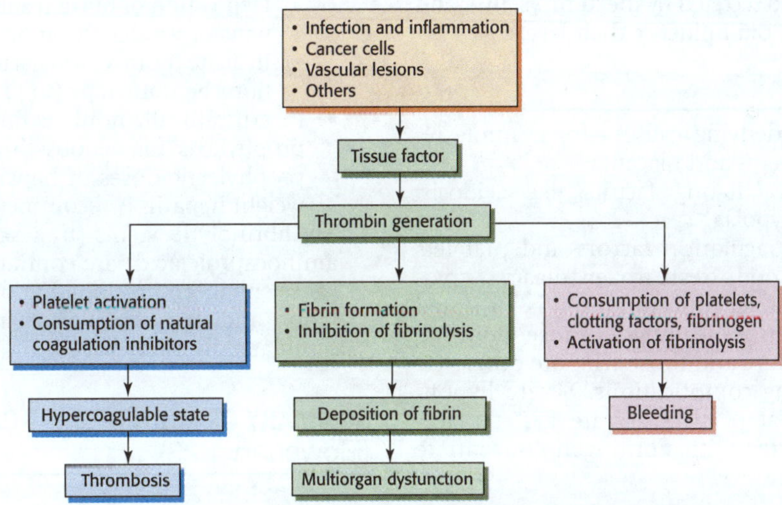

Flowchart 1.22 Pathogenesis of Disseminated Intravascular Coagulation.

ASYMPTOMATIC DIC

- It is an early stage of DIC characterised by presence of abnormal laboratory studies in the absence of clinical symptoms.

THROMBOTIC DIC

- It is more common in patients with severe infection/sepsis, wherein thrombosis of small and medium vessels leads to multiorgan dysfunction: digits (symmetric peripheral gangrene), kidneys (oliguria, anuria, haematuria), lungs (chest pain, dyspnea, tachypnea), liver (jaundice, coagulopathy) and brain (confusion, altered mental status, coma).
- Purpura fulminans, a severe form of DIC, is characterised by skin infarction and necrosis, which is commonly seen in patients with meningococcemia.
- Waterhouse–Friderichsen syndrome—an occult thrombosis of adrenal vein resulting in adrenal haemorrhage.
- In cancers, chronic DIC may lead to hypercoagulability. Migratory venous thrombosis is known as Trousseau sign.

BLEEDING-TYPE DIC

- Bleeding-type DIC is often seen in patients with leukemias, especially acute promyelocytic leukemia.
- Bleeding manifestations include oozing from various sites, petechiae, ecchymosis, and sometimes internal hemorrhage.

CONSUMPTIVE-TYPE DIC

- Consumptive-type is often associated with life-threatening massive bleeding that requires blood transfusions.

INVESTIGATIONS

- Low erythrocyte sedimentation rate (ESR) due to reduced fibrinogen.
- Thrombocytopenia.

- Microangiopathic haemolytic anaemia with increased reticulocytes.
- Schistocytes on peripheral smear.
- Prolongation of PT and aPTT. However, these tests may be normal in more than 40% cases; this is due to presence of circulating activated clotting factors, such as thrombin or Xa, which can accelerate the formation of thrombin.
- Reduced plasma fibrinogen level that correlates most closely with bleeding. However, fibrinogen is an acute phase reactant, and patients with conditions that cause elevation in acute phase reactants (e.g. inflammation, sepsis) may have normal serum values of fibrinogen. Further, in chronic DIC, fibrinogen and platelets may be normal.
- Elevated levels of FDPs.
- D-dimer (formed during fibrinolysis as a result of degradation of cross-linked fibrin by plasmin) levels are elevated in almost all cases of DIC. However, it is important to remember that many conditions other than DIC, such as trauma, recent surgery or venous thromboembolism, are associated with elevated FDPs including D-dimer. Also, because FDPs are metabolised by the liver and secreted by the kidneys, liver and kidney impairment can influence their levels.

MANAGEMENT

- Elimination of underlying causes—for example removal of a dead foetus and placenta.
- Correction of precipitating factors like acidosis, dehydration and hypoxia.
- Replacement of coagulation factors and platelets by fresh whole blood, fresh frozen plasma, cryoprecipitate and platelet concentrates. It is indicated in patients with active bleeding, in those requiring an invasive procedure and those who are otherwise at risk for bleeding complications. Severe hypofibrinogenaemia that persists despite FFP replacement may be treated with fibrinogen concentrate or cryoprecipitate.
- Dose:
  - Cryoprecipitate—1 unit/10 kg
  - Fresh frozen plasma—15–20 mL/kg
  - Platelet concentrates—1–2 units/10 kg
- Target is to achieve:
  - Fibrinogen level 100–150 mg/dL
  - Platelets >50,000/mm^3
  - Haemoglobin 6–10 g/dL
  - PT and aPTT of less than 1.5 times the control.
- Inhibition of coagulation process:
  - Role of heparin is controversial. However, it is often given in patients with thrombotic manifestations (e.g. arterial or venous thromboembolism, severe purpura fulminans associated with acral ischaemia or vascular skin infarct). Average requirement is 1000 units/hour by continuous intravenous infusion. It should be given after the correction of bleeding risk. Major indications of heparin are as follows:
    - Platelet counts or coagulation factors do not increase following replacement and patient continues to bleed
    - Retained dead foetus (before induction of labour)
    - Deposition of fibrin resulting in purpura fulminans or venous thromboembolism
    - In acute promyelocytic leukaemia, before induction chemotherapy (to prevent DIC)
  - In critically ill, nonbleeding patients with DIC, prophylaxis for venous thromboembolism with prophylactic doses of heparin or low-molecular-weight heparin is recommended.
- Antifibrinolytic agents (tranexamic acid and epsilon aminocaproic acid) are contraindicated as they may cause enhanced precipitation of fibrin in microcirculation and macrocirculation and lead to fatal disseminated thrombosis.

SUMMARY OF MANAGEMENT OF DIC (Flowchart 1.23).

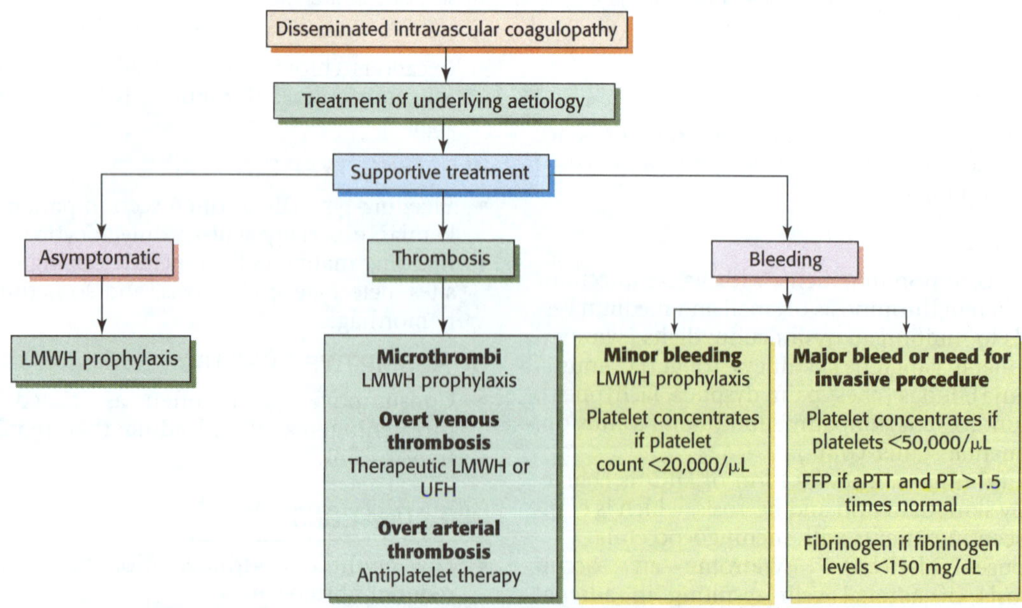

Flowchart 1.23 Treatment of Disseminated Intravascular Coagulation. LMWH = Low molecular wight heparin; UHF = Unfractionated heparin.

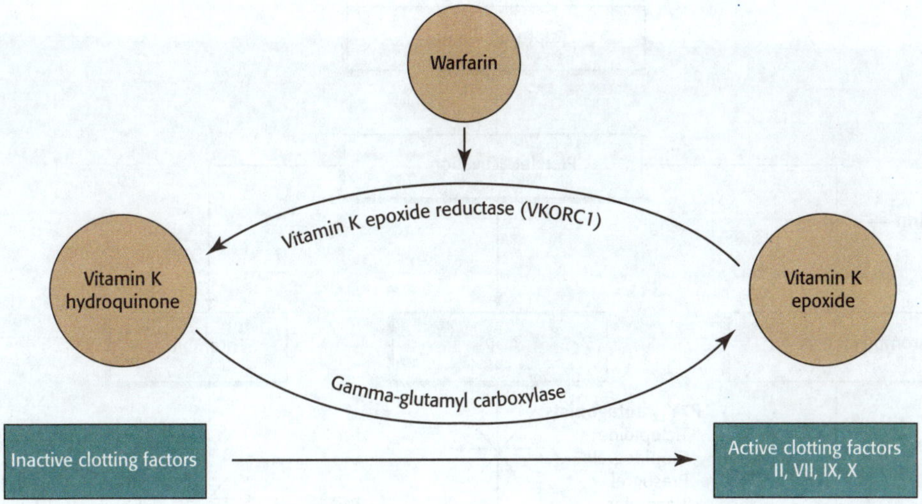

Fig. 1.7 Mechanism of action of Vitamin K.

Q. Give a brief account of vitamin K.

- Vitamin K is a fat-soluble vitamin and it exists in two forms:
  - Vitamin K_1 (phylloquinone) is present in vegetable oils and green leafy vegetables.
  - Vitamin K_2 (menaquinone) is synthesised by colonic bacteria.
- Vitamin K_3 (menadione) is a synthetic pro-vitamin that can be converted to menaquinone by the liver.
- Vitamin K is necessary for the posttranslational carboxylation of some coagulation factors synthesised in the liver. This is necessary for the functioning of these factors. These factors include II, VII, IX and X; protein C and protein S (Fig. 1.7).
- Warfarin-type anticoagulants inhibit carboxylation by preventing the conversion of vitamin K to its active hydroquinone form.
- Vitamin K deficiency occurs with diseases that interfere with fat absorption, long-term antibiotic therapy and warfarin therapy.
- Deficiency manifests as haemorrhagic stage.
- Deficiency is treated with daily injections of 10 mg of vitamin K. Vitamin K may not be effective in the presence of liver cell disease.

Q. Give a brief account of antiplatelet drugs.

- Prevent and/or reverse platelet aggregation in arterial thrombosis and inhibit thrombin formation. These are classified below:

CLASSIFICATION AND MECHANISMS OF ACTION

- Classification and mechanisms of action of antiplatelet drugs are given in Table 1.102 and Flowchart 1.24.

CYCLOOXYGENASE INHIBITORS

- Aspirin inhibits cyclooxygenase (both COX-1 and COX-2) that leads to prevention of synthesis of thromboxane A2 and impairment of platelet secretion and aggregation.
- Effects of aspirin on platelet function occur within an hour and last for the whole lifespan of platelets (7 days).
- Though the antiplatelet effects are seen with a low dose of 50 mg/day, the usual dose is 75–150 mg/day.
- Useful in acute coronary syndromes, stable angina, transient ischaemic attack, ischaemic stroke, following carotid artery surgery, atrial fibrillation (in selected cases to prevent thrombosis) and intermittent claudication.
- Important side effects are upper GI bleeding and renal function impairment.

TABLE 1.102 Classification of Antiplatelet Drugs Based on Mechanism of Action

Cyclooxygenase Inhibitor	Adenosine Reuptake/Phosphodiesterase Inhibitor
• Aspirin	• Dipyridamole • Cilostazol
Adenosine Diphosphate (ADP) Receptor Inhibitors	**Glycoprotein IIb/IIIa Inhibitors**
Irrevrsible • Ticlopidine • Clopidogrel • Prasugrel ***Reversible*** • Ticagrelor • Cangrelor	***Monoclonal antibody*** • Abciximab ***Synthetic*** • Eptifibatide • Tirofiban

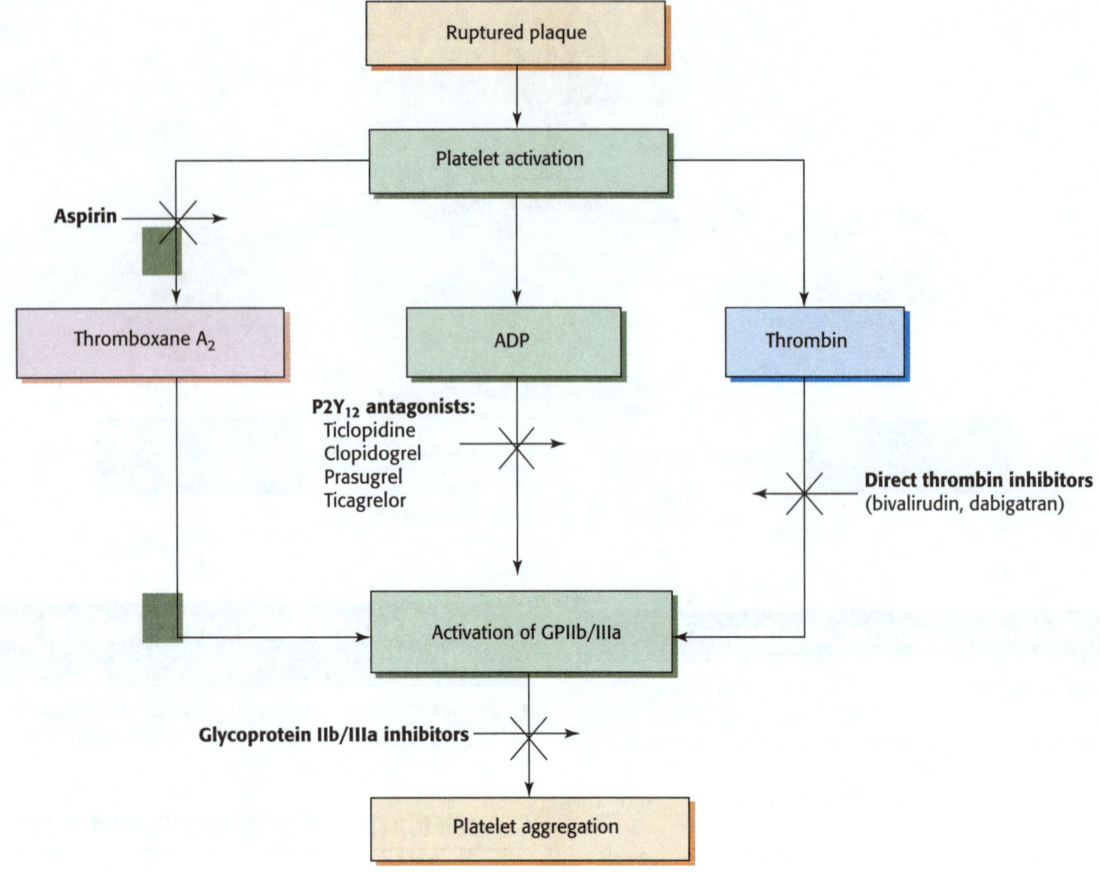

Flowchart 1.24 Classification and Mechanisms of Actions of Antiplatelet Drugs.

ADENOSINE REUPTAKE INHIBITORS OR PHOSPHODIESTERASE INHIBITORS

- Dipyridamole inhibits the cellular reuptake of adenosine into platelets leading to increased extracellular concentrations of adenosine. Adenosine interacts with the adenosine receptors to cause increased cAMP via cyclic adenylate cyclase. cAMP impairs platelet aggregation and also causes arteriolar smooth muscle relaxation.
- Used in coronary artery disease, cerebral ischaemia and in nuclear cardiac stress testing (where it acts as coronary vasodilator).
- Dose is 25–75 mg three to four times a day.
- Side effects include allergic reactions, vomiting, dizziness and headache. Due to vasodilatory property, it can lower the blood pressure.
- Rarely used at present due to dose inconvenience and side effects.

ADENOSINE DIPHOSPHATE RECEPTOR ANTAGONISTS (THIENOPYRIDINES) OR $P2Y_{12}$ ANTAGONISTS

- ADP, an important platelet agonist, has two types of receptors in the platelet plasma membrane: $P2Y_1$ and $P2Y_{12}$. $P2Y_{12}$ is a 7-transmembrane domain receptor linked to a G inhibitory protein. The end result of ADP signalling through its $P2Y_{12}$ receptor is an amplification of stable platelet aggregation and secretion.
- $P2Y_{12}$ ADP antagonists include ticlopidine, clopidogrel, prasugrel, ticagrelor and cangrelor which inhibit binding of ADP to platelet receptor $P2Y_{12}$, thereby inhibiting activation of the glycoprotein (GP) IIb/IIIa complex and platelet aggregation.
- One of the serious adverse effects of ticlopidine is occurrence of TTP. This side effect is less common with clopidogrel and others. Other side effects with ticlopidine include bone marrow suppression, thrombocytopenia and neutropenia.
- With clopidogrel, inhibition of platelet aggregation occurs within 2 hours while peak effect is after 5–6 hours. In patients with acute coronary syndrome, 600 mg loading dose is recommended in patients who will undergo angiography and possible revascularisation within 24 hours of diagnosis. If angiography is not planned, loading dose is 300 mg if age is less than 75 years. Loading dose is omitted in elderly above 75 years of age. The usual daily dose is 75 mg. The platelet functions return to normal about 7 days after the last dose. This can lead to bleeding problems when surgery particularly CABG surgery is done in patients on the drug. Clopidogrel needs to be discontinued at least 5 days before any major surgery.

About one-third of patients on clopidogrel are resistant and show only a low level of platelet inhibition.

- Prasugrel has a more rapid onset of action with its duration of action longer than that of clopidogrel. It is able to achieve higher degrees of platelet inhibition than clopidogrel. A loading dose of 60 mg prasugrel is generally recommended after angiography but may be given before it as well. Maintenance dose of prasugrel is 10 mg daily. Risk of bleeding is higher compared to clopidogrel. Avoid if age >75 years or weight <60 kg. It is contraindicated in patients with past stroke or transient ischaemic attack.
- Ticagrelor differs from clopidogrel and prasugrel in that it binds reversibly rather than irreversibly to $P2Y_{12}$ platelet receptor and has a more rapid onset but of shorter duration of action than clopidogrel. Loading dose is 180 mg followed by 90 mg twice a day. It is avoided in patients at risk for symptomatic bradycardia, including those with second- or third-degree atrioventricular block.
- Cangrelor is given intravenously and the onset of action is within seconds.
- Both clopidogrel and prasugrel can be used in patients with ischaemic stroke either alone (if aspirin resistance or intolerance is present) or in combination with aspirin.
- Resistance can be seen with clopidogrel and to some extent with prasugrel; not reported with ticagrelor.
- Where fibrinolytic therapy is planned for ST-elevation myocardial infarction, a 300 mg loading dose of clopidogrel should be used and prasugrel and ticagrelor avoided. In patients with ACS with planned revascularisation, aspirin can be combined with clopidogrel (600 mg loading dose), prasugrel (60 mg loading dose) or ticagrelor (180 mg loading dose).

GLYCOPROTEIN IIB/IIIA INHIBITORS

- This category includes abciximab, eptifibatide and tirofiban; given by intravenous route.
- Used in the setting of percutaneous coronary interventions for unstable angina and non-ST-elevation myocardial infarction (MI), if there is ongoing ischaemia or large thrombus or patient did not receive a $P2Y_{12}$ inhibitor.
- Abciximab is a chimeric monoclonal Fab fragment of murine and human immunoglobulin that binds to GPIIb/IIIa.
- Side effects include bleeding tendencies and thrombocytopenia. Eptifibatide may also produce hypotension.

Q. Classify anticoagulants. Give a brief account of the commonly used anticoagulants.

CLASSIFICATION

- Classification of anticoagulants is given in Table 1.103.

ANTICOAGULANT THERAPY

- When anticoagulation is required on an urgent basis and for long term, therapy is initiated with heparin along with oral anticoagulants which is followed by oral anticoagulants alone.
- When anticoagulation is needed for only brief periods, heparin alone is used.
- Indications for anticoagulants are given in Table 1.104.

TABLE 1.103 Classification of Anticoagulants

Parenteral, Rapidly Acting	Oral, Rapidly Acting	Oral, Slow Acting

• Heparin
  • Unfractionated heparin
  • Low-molecular-weight heparins (enoxaparin, dalteparin, tinzaparin, parnaparin, reviparin)
• Direct thrombin inhibitors (hirudin, lepirudin, desirudin, bivalirudin, argatroban
• Heparinoids (dermatan sulphate, danaparoid)
• Indirect factor Xa inhibitors (fondaparinux and idraparinux)
	• Oral direct factor Xa inhibitors (rivaroxaban, edoxaban, betrixaban and apixaban)
	• Direct thrombin inhibitors (dabigatran, ximelagatran)
		• Vitamin K antagonists
		  • Coumarin derivatives (warfarin sodium, dicoumarol, acenocoumarol, nicoumalone)
		  • Indandione deriva tives (phenindione, diphonindione)—not used clinically

TABLE 1.104 Common Indications for Anticoagulants

Purpose	Clinical Indications
Urgent and/or for long-term use	• Atrial fibrillation and cardiac disorders with thromboembolism (treatment and prevention) • Deep venous thrombosis (DVT) • Cerebral venous thrombosis • Recurrent transient ischaemic attacks • Pulmonary thromboembolism • Acute coronary syndromes—unstable angina, non-ST-elevation MI, ST-elevation MI (if indicated) • Prosthetic valves • Heart failure with low ejection fraction • Antiphospholipid syndrome
Brief period use	• Cardiac bypass surgery • Haemodialysis • DIC (if indicated) • Acute coronary syndrome (if indicated)

UNFRACTIONATED HEPARIN

- Heparin acts by binding to antithrombin, thereby potentiating its action. Though antithrombin complexes with and inhibits all activated clotting factors (except factor VIIa), its predominant action is to inhibit activated factor IIa (thrombin).
- Conventional heparin preparations are heterogeneous and unfractionated, with only 20% of the product biologically active. In addition, active heparin fractions may vary considerably in molecular weight.
- Heparin is given as an initial loading dose of 80–100 units/kg intravenously, followed by maintenance. For maintenance, any one of the following three regimens may be used:
  - Continuous intravenous.
  - Intermittent intravenous.
  - Intermittent subcutaneous.
- For total anticoagulation, continuous intravenous maintenance is preferred. Here, heparin is administered using an infusion pump at a rate of 18 units/kg/h.
- For low-dose heparinisation (e.g. prophylaxis of DVT), 5000 units 12 hourly or 8 hourly subcutaneously are preferred.
- Duration of therapy is variable but is usually 4–7 days. Overlapping therapy with warfarin should be started along with heparin.
- Heparin therapy is monitored with aPTT, which is maintained at 1.5–2 times the control value.
- Antidote of heparin is protamine sulphate. Fresh frozen plasma has little effect on bleeding associated with heparin, low-molecular-weight heparins and fondaparinux.
- Complications of heparin therapy include bleeding, thrombocytopenia, skin necrosis, osteoporosis, and osteomalacia (in long-standing therapy).
- Heparin-induced thrombocytopenia (HIT) is of two types: HIT type I and HIT type II.

Heparin-Induced Thrombocytopenia Type I

- HIT type I is a benign form which develops in the first few days (usually within 2 days) of initiation. Platelets generally do not fall below 100,000/mm^3. It often resolves despite continued heparin therapy.

Heparin-Induced Thrombocytopenia Type II

- HIT type II (also known as HIT) is due to platelet-activating IgG antibodies that recognise complexes of platelet factor IV bound to heparin, leading to activation of platelets, thrombocytopenia and risk of thrombosis. It presents 5–14 days after heparin exposure with thrombotic features (HIT and thrombosis syndrome). It can occur with all types of heparin.
- Risk factors and diagnostic criteria for HIT Type II are given in Tables 1.105 and 1.106.

Treatment of HIT Type II

- Immediately stop all types of heparins including 'flushes' of heparin.
- Do not give warfarin as it can lead to venous limb gangrene or classic skin necrosis. Vitamin K is recommended if a diagnosis of HIT is made after warfarin has recently been started. It repletes protein C and S stores, thereby reducing risk of thrombotic complications produced by depletion of proteins C and S.
- Start non-heparin anticoagulants (lepirudin—a recombinant hirudin, argatroban, danaparoid, fondaparinux and bivalirudin if parenteral administration is required, or apixaban, rivaroxaban or edoxaban if oral therapy is sufficient).
- Do not transfuse platelets even though severe thrombocytopenia is present.

TABLE 1.105 Risk Factors for HIT Type II

Characteristics	Relative Risk
Sex	• Females > males
Patient type	• Surgical (major surgery > minor surgery) > trauma > medical
Heparin type	• Unfractionated heparin > low-molecular weight heparins
Source of heparin	• Bovine > porcine
Duration of therapy	• 11–14 days > 5–10 days > 4 days
Dose	• Therapeutic > prophylactic
Route of administration	• Intravenous > subcutaneous

TABLE 1.106 Diagnostic Criteria for HIT Type II

Clinical
- At least one of the following:
  - Thrombocytopenia
  - Thrombosis (e.g. deep vein thrombosis, pulmonary embolism, adrenal haemorrhage, cerebral vein thrombosis, splanchnic vein thrombosis, limb artery thrombosis, stroke, myocardial infarction, mesenteric artery thrombosis)
  - Necrotising skin lesions at heparin injection sites
  - Acute anaphylactoid reaction (usually occurs 5–30 minutes after intravenous heparin bolus; rarely, after subcutaneous heparin)

Timing
- Above events bear temporal relation to a preceding heparin exposure

Pathologic
- Heparin-dependent, platelet-activating IgG:
  - Positive platelet activation assay (e.g. serotonin-release assay)
  - Positive anti-PF4/polyanion-IgG EIA

LOW-MOLECULAR-WEIGHT HEPARINS

- These are biologically active forms of conventional heparin with molecular weights ranging from 3000 to 8000 dalton.
- LMW heparins exert their anticoagulant effect primarily by inhibiting activated factor X (Xa) rather than activated factor II (IIa), which is preferentially inhibited by unfractionated heparin. Factor Xa inhibition is through binding to antithrombin.
- They have several advantages:
  - They can be administered subcutaneously once or twice a day.
  - Their pharmacokinetics is so predictable that aPTT monitoring is not necessary.
  - They are less immunogenic and are less likely to cause thrombocytopenia.
  - Many patients with deep vein thrombosis can be treated on an outpatient basis.
- If required (e.g. in patients with chronic kidney disease), anti-Xa is the gold standard for monitoring LMWH therapy, as aPTT is not significantly affected. It should be tested 4 hours after administration.
- The main disadvantage is their cost.
- Commonly available LMWH include enoxaparin, dalteparin and tinzaparin.

VITAMIN K ANTAGONISTS

- Warfarin and others acts by inducing a state analogous to vitamin K deficiency.
- Vitamin K is necessary for the posttranslational carboxylation of some coagulation factors synthesised in the liver. This is necessary for the functioning of these factors. These factors include factors II, VII, IX and X; protein C and protein S. Warfarin-type anticoagulants inhibit carboxylation by preventing the conversion of vitamin K to its active hydroquinone form.
- When short-term heparin followed by long-term warfarin is used, both anticoagulants must be started simultaneously.
- Heparin should be continued for a minimum of 4 days because the peak antithrombotic effect of warfarin is delayed for about 96 hours, independently of PT. The PT is particularly sensitive to factor VII deficiency. Factor VII has a short half-life of only 4–6 hours, and therefore, PT may get prolonged within a day of administration of warfarin. The goal is to inhibit all vitamin K-dependent factors; factor X and prothrombin have half-lives of less than 2 days.
- Along with warfarin, initial bridging therapy with heparins is necessary to avoid a potential hypercoagulable state induced by warfarin's effect on protein C, which has a short half-life of approximately 6 hours.
- Warfarin is started with an initial dose of 5 mg orally on the first day. Subsequent daily doses are adjusted according to PT, which is maintained at 1.5–3 times the control value. Usual maintenance dose varies from 2.5 to 7.5 mg/day.
- Duration of therapy is variable ranging from 3 months to lifelong.
- Warfarin and related coumarins are more efficacious than other oral anticoagulants in patients with prosthetic heart valves and recurrent thrombosis in the setting of antiphospholipid syndrome.
- Many drugs can interfere with warfarin therapy. This should be monitored by checking PT before and after stopping any other drug.
- Complications of warfarin therapy are bleeding and haemorrhagic skin necrosis. Venous limb gangrene can occur as a complication of warfarin therapy if an underlying hypercoagulable state (e.g. HIT type II) is present (although it can also occur without underlying HIT). The pathogenesis of skin necrosis and venous limb gangrene involves microthrombosis formation due to depletion of protein C in the setting of increased thrombin generation (e.g. from HIT). Skin necrosis involves skin and subcutaneous tissues at central (nonacral) sites, for example breast, abdomen, thigh and calf. In contrast, in venous limb gangrene, acral (distal) necrosis occurs in the affected limb. International normalised ratio (INR) is markedly elevated due to depletion of protein C.
- Antidotes of warfarin are injections of vitamin K1, 5 mg intravenously or fresh frozen plasma (FFP) or prothrombin complex concentrate (PCC). PCC is a human-derived blood product containing vitamin K-dependent clotting factors (II, VII, IX, X, protein C and protein S) and heparin. As it contains heparin, this product is contraindicated in patients with HIT.
- Contraindications:
  - Severe uncontrolled hypertension.
  - Severe renal or liver failure.
  - Preexisting haemostatic disorders.
  - Pregnancy as it crosses placenta and can cause foetal abnormalities.

International Normalised Ratio

- Thromboplastic reagents used for prothrombin test are derived from a variety of sources and give different PT results for the same plasma.
- Therefore, each thromboplastin is compared to an international reference preparation so that it can be assigned an international sensitivity index (ISI).
- INR is calculated as the ratio of the patient's PT to the mean PT for a group of normal people and then adjusted for ISI.
- Various limitations of warfarin are given in Table 1.107.

TABLE 1.107 Limitations of Warfarin and Related Drugs

Limitation	Consequences
• Slow onset of action	• Need of overlapping with heparin
• Genetic variation in metabolism	• Variable dose required in different patients
• Multiple drug and food interactions	• Frequent monitoring by INR
• Narrow therapeutic index	• Frequent monitoring by INR

HIRUDIN

- Hirudin is derived from a medicinal leech.
- It acts directly on thrombin.
- Monitoring is by measuring aPTT.
- Recombinant forms of hirudin available for use include lepirudin and desirudin. Bivalirudin is a synthetic analogue of hirudin.
- Lepirudin and bivalirudin are used in patients with HIT type II in whom anticoagulation is required to be continued. Bivalirudin is one of the preferred drugs for patients with unstable angina undergoing percutaneous intervention.

HEPARINOIDS

- Dermatan sulphate is a heparinoid that activates heparin cofactor II and inhibits factor X.
- Danaparoid is a mixture of anticoagulant glycosaminoglycans, predominantly low-sulphated heparan sulphate. Danaparoid has both antithrombin and anti-Xa activity, although the latter predominates (anti-Xa/antithrombin ratio ~22).
- Useful in HIT.

FACTOR Xa INHIBITORS

- Indirect factor Xa inhibitors include fondaparinux and idraparinux.
- Enhance the rate of factor Xa inactivation by binding to antithrombin, thereby blocking thrombin generation but have no effect on the rate of thrombin inhibition.
- Both agents have almost complete bioavailability after subcutaneous injection.
- Half-life of fondaparinux is 17 hours while that of idraparinux is 80 hours; the latter therefore can be given once a week.
- Fondaparinux approved for use in venous thromboembolic (VTE) prophylaxis in patients undergoing hip, knee or abdominal surgery, treatment of acute DVT or acute pulmonary embolism, immobilised medical patients who are at high risk for VTE, treatment of patients with non-ST-elevation acute coronary syndrome for whom urgent angiography is not indicated or treatment of patients with ST-elevation MI who are managed with thrombolytics.
- Useful in HIT type II.
- Oral direct factor Xa inhibitors (novel oral anticoagulants-NOACs; direct oral anticoagulant-DOACs) include rivaroxaban, edoxaban, betrixaban and apixaban. They directly inhibit free and prothrombinase-bound factor Xa. Andexanet alpha is the reversal agent for them. It is a modified, human recombinant factor Xa that is catalytically inactive but retains high-affinity binding to direct factor Xa inhibitors. If not available, prothrombin complex concentrate (PCC) can be used for reversal.

DIRECT THROMBIN INHIBITORS (DIRECT ORAL ANTICOAGULANTS)

- These agents directly act on thrombin leading to inhibition of conversion of fibrinogen to fibrin. They inhibit both fibrin-bound and free thrombin.
- DTIs do not interact with heparin-platelet-factor 4 antibodies and are thereby suitable for patients with HIT type II.
- Oral thrombin inhibitors include dabigatran etexilate and ximelagatran.
- Argatroban is another direct thrombin inhibitor that needs to be given intravenously. Others which have been discussed above include hirudin, lepirudin and bivalirudin.
- Oral direct factor Xa inhibitors are used for prevention of venous thrombosis after major orthopaedic surgery, prevention of stroke and systemic embolism in patients with nonvalvular atrial fibrillation and treatment and secondary prevention of symptomatic venous thrombosis.
- Advantages of oral direct thrombin and oral direct factor Xa inhibitors include:
  - Rapid onset of action and hence no need for overlapping with heparin.
  - Little to no food–drug interaction.
  - Limited drug–drug interactions.
  - No need for routine coagulation monitoring.
- Side effects include elevation in liver transaminases and possible increased rate of coronary artery disease.
- Reversing anticoagulation following major bleeding or for emergency surgery:
  - General measures: Fluid resuscitation, red blood cell transfusion, diagnostic and therapeutic procedures to identify the source of bleeding and application of local haemostatic measures.
  - Nonspecific pro-haemostatic agents: Recombinant factor VIIa (rFVIIa), PCC and FFP; can lead to thrombotic episodes.
  - Reversal agents: Idarucizumab, a humanised Fab antibody fragment that binds specifically and with high affinity to dabigatran.
  - Haemodialysis if idarucizumab not available.

Q. Give a brief account of fibrinolytic system and fibrinolytic agents.

Q. Briefly describe thrombolytics.

FIBRINOLYSIS

- Fibrinolytic system is important in normal haemostasis. Fibrinolysis is initiated by the release of either tissue plasminogen activator or pro-urokinase (pro-UK) from the endothelial cells. These agents activate plasminogen adsorbed onto fibrin clots producing plasmin. Plasmin then degrades fibrin polymers into small fragments.

COMMON INDICATIONS FOR FIBRINOLYTIC OR THROMBOLYTIC AGENTS

- Indications for fibrinolytic agents are given in Box 1.49.

FIBRINOLYTIC OR THROMBOLYTIC AGENTS

- Most fibrinolytic or thrombolytic agents are recombinant forms with plasminogen activator activity. They have different half-lives, fibrin specificity and infusion strategies. Common thrombolytics are listed below:
  - Streptokinase (STK) is obtained from β-haemolytic streptococci. On complexing with plasminogen, it

BOX 1.49 Indications for Fibrinolytic Agents

- Acute ST elevation myocardial infarction
- Acute peripheral artery occlusion
- Massive pulmonary embolism with hypotension
- Acute stroke (thrombotic or embolic)
- Thrombosed prosthetic cardiac valve

converts other plasminogen molecules into plasmin. It is not fibrin-selective as it produces lysis of both fibrinogen and fibrin. Since it is derived from bacteria, it can produce allergic reactions in nearly 5% of patients. It is used in acute ST-elevation myocardial infarction and pulmonary embolism.

- Urokinase (UK) is again not fibrin-selective. It activates plasminogen directly. It is useful in patients who received STK in the past 6 months and require a thrombolytic agent for MI or pulmonary embolism. It does not induce allergic reaction.
- Acyl-SK-plasminogen also activates both free and fibrin-bound plasminogen.
- Recombinant tissue plasminogen activator (rtPA) or alteplase is useful in acute thrombotic strokes (within 4.5 hours of onset) besides acute MI and pulmonary embolism. Though it is more fibrin specific compared to STK (it preferentially activates plasminogen bound to fibrin), bleeding complications with rtPA are similar with the two agents.
- Pro-UK, like rtPA, is also fibrin specific.
- Others are tenecteplase, reteplase and desmoteplase.

Q. Briefly discuss about tranexamic acid.

- Tranexamic acid is a synthetic derivative of lysine that blocks lysine binding sites on plasminogen molecules, thereby inhibiting interaction of plasminogen with formed plasmin and fibrin. Inhibition of plasminogen activation results in stabilisation of the preformed fibrin meshwork produced by haemostasis (anti-fibrinolysis).
- Tranexamic acid is six to ten times more potent in binding affinity to plasminogen and plasmin compared to epsilon-aminocaproic acid.
- It is available in intravenous, oral and topical formulation.

INDICATIONS

- Tranexamic acid is approved for reducing blood loss from various sites (Table 1.108).

TABLE 1.108 Indications for Tranexamic Acid

Established	Others
• Heavy menstrual bleeding	• Cardiovascular surgeries
• Postpartum haemorrhage	• Orthopaedic surgeries
• Major trauma with haemorrhage (within 3 hours)	• Haemoptysis
• Traumatic brain injury (within 3 hours)	• von Willebrand disease
• Haemophilia (tooth extraction)	• Hereditary angioedema
	• Melasma
	• Gastrointestinal bleed

DOSE

- 1 gm intravenously over 10 minutes thrice a day or 500–1.3 gm orally thrice a day.

ADVERSE EFFECTS

- Some of the adverse effects include headache, backache, abdominal pain, nausea, vomiting, diarrhoea and impaired colour vision.
- Serious adverse effects are rare and include anaphylaxis, deep vein thrombosis and pulmonary embolism.

Q. Discuss blood transfusion and blood component transfusion. (IM 9.17; IM 9.18)

Q. What are the complications of blood transfusion?

- Blood may be infused as whole blood or as component infusion. At present, almost all transfusions are in the form of transfusion of components.
- Important components of blood that are frequently used include packed red cells, platelets, fresh frozen plasma, cryoprecipitates and albumin.

PACKED RED CELLS

- Used when the primary aim is to increase the oxygen carrying capacity of blood.
- Can improve platelet function, particularly in uraemic patients.
- Stored between 1°C and 6°C in a solution containing citrate, phosphate, dextrose and adenine as well as nutrient additives, which confers a shelf life of 42 days.
- One unit of RBC can be expected to result in a rise of Hb of 1 g/dL in an adult.
- Indications for RBC transfusion are given in Box 1.50.

MASSIVE TRANSFUSION

- Generally defined as anticipated need for >10 units of packed red cells in 24 hours.
- Transfusions of isolated red blood cells can quickly lead to severe coagulopathies, which are often exacerbated by hypothermia, acidosis and other derangements that are common in the setting of trauma.
- A widely used practice is the transfusion of packed red cells, platelets and fresh frozen plasma in 1:1:1 ratio.

BOX 1.50 General Indications for RBC Transfusion

- Symptomatic anaemia in a euvolaemic patient
- Haemoglobin <7 g/dL in a critically ill patient with a target haemoglobin of 7–9 g/dL unless specific comorbidities or acute illness-related factors modify clinical decision-making
- Haemoglobin <8 or <9 g/dL in acute myocardial infarction, CHF, angina, TIA and syncope. Target is haemoglobin >9 g/dL
- Haemoglobin <8 g/dL in patients with thalassaemia
- Haemoglobin <10 g/dL in a patient with uraemic bleeding

- Common complications include hypocalcaemia, hyperkalaemia, metabolic alkalosis or acidosis and volume overload.

PLATELET-RICH PLASMA

- Required when bleeding occurs either due to reduced platelets or inadequate platelet function.
- One PRP bag generally increases the platelet count by 4000–8000/mm^3. Platelets are generally pooled from 4 to 6 donors (random donor platelets).
- Stored at 22°C and have a shelf life of 5–7 days.
- Because platelets express the same A and B antigens as red blood cells, it is best to issue platelets that are compatible with the recipient's naturally occurring anti-A or anti-B antibodies. For example, a recipient with blood group B has anti-A antibodies and therefore can receive platelets from donors with blood group of B. Infusion of ABO noncompatible platelets is an acceptable practice, in particular, when platelet concentrates are in short supply.
- Platelets can also be derived from a single donor (single donor platelets, SDP). The number of platelets that can be derived from SDR is 3×10^{11}. Apheresis platelets are indicated for patients with immune refractoriness when cross-matched or HLA-matched platelets have better posttransfusion survival.
- Indications for platelet transfusion are given in Box 1.51.

CONTRAINDICATION TO PLATELET TRANSFUSION

- Platelet transfusion is contraindicated in thrombotic thrombocytopenic purpura (TTP) and heparin-induced thrombocytopenia (HIT).
- Relatively contraindicated in immune thrombocytopenic purpura (ITP) or posttransfusion purpura (PTP) because the survival of transfused platelets is extremely brief.

AUTOLOGOUS PLATELET-RICH PLASMA

- Prepared from patient's own blood.
- Used in many conditions based on the fact that platelet growth factors support the wound healing.
- Various conditions in which it has been used include chronic non-healing wounds, osteoarthritis and tendinopathy refractory to standard conservative therapy, rotator cuff tears, ligament injuries and muscle tears.

BOX 1.51 General Indications for Platelet Transfusion

- Microvascular bleeding due to thrombocytopenia or platelet dysfunction
- Thrombocytopenia with significant risk of haemorrhage. Prophylactic platelet transfusion may be indicated if platelet count <10,000/mm^3. A higher threshold may be appropriate for patients with high fever, hyperleucocytosis, rapid fall in platelet count and coagulopathy (such as DIC)
- Central venous catheter placement if platelet count <20,000/mm^3
- Lumbar puncture, major surgery or interventional procedures if platelet count <50,000/mm^3
- Neurosurgery if platelet count <100,000/mm^3
- For massive transfusion in trauma patients with red blood cells, plasma and platelets in ratio of 1: 1: 1
- In patients with autoimmune thrombocytopenia, platelet transfusion reserved for patients with life-threatening bleeding

FRESH FROZEN PLASMA

- Fresh frozen plasma (FFP) contains all the coagulation factors including von Willebrand factor.
- Stored at –18° to –30°C and then thawed between 30°C and 37°C in a water bath under continuous agitation before transfusion.
- Plasma contains anti-A and anti-B antibodies depending upon blood group. Patients should only receive plasma which does not contain an antibody which could attack their own red cells. For example, a recipient with blood group A has anti-B antibodies and therefore can receive plasma from donors with blood group of either A or AB which has neither anti-A nor anti-B antibodies. Rh compatibility is not required.
- As FFP is not concentrated plasma, volume overload may occur if requirements are high.
- A dose of 10 mL/kg will typically provide sufficient coagulation factors to achieve haemostasis.
- Indications for FFP are given in Box 1.52.

COMPATIBILITY OF BLOOD COMPONENT TRANSFUSION

- Compatibility of blood component transfusion across various blood groups is shown in Table 1.109.

CRYOPRECIPITATE

- Concentrate of factor VIII, von Willebrand factor, fibrinogen and factor XIII.
- Does not require cross-matching before transfusion.
- Amount of various coagulation factors in cryoprecipitate is given in Table 1.110.
- Indications for cryoprecipitate transfusion are listed in Box 1.53.

Rh IMMUNE GLOBULIN

- It is indicated in:
  - Known or suspected inoculation of Rh-negative mother with unknown or Rh-positive foetal cells

BOX 1.52 General Indications for Fresh Frozen Plasma Transfusion

- Single coagulation factor deficiency particularly factors V and XI deficiency
- Consumptive coagulopathy such as DIC
- Dilutional coagulopathy due to massive transfusion
- Coagulopathy of liver disease
- Microangiopathic haemolytic anaemia including TTP, haemolytic-uraemic syndrome and HELLP syndrome
- Reversal of warfarin anticoagulation (prothrombin complex concentrate is preferred in urgent situations while vitamin K is preferable if reversal in not urgent)
- Massive transfusion in trauma patients with red blood cells, plasma and platelets in ratio of 1:1:1

TABLE 1.109 Compatibility of Blood Components

Recipient's Blood Group	Compatible Packed Red Cells	Compatible Fresh Frozen Plasma	Compatible Platelet-Rich Plasma		
			First Choice	Second Choice	Third Choice
O	O	O, A, B, AB	O	A, B	AB
A	A, O	A, AB	A	AB	B, O
B	B, O	B, AB	B	AB	A, O
AB	AB, A, B, O	AB	AB	A, B	O

TABLE 1.110 Factors in One Unit (10–15 mL) of Cryoprecipitate

Coagulation Factor	Amount Per Unit	Half-Life
• Fibrinogen	150–250 mg	100–150 hours
• Factor VIII	80–150 units	12 hours
• von Willebrand factor	100–150 units	24 hours
• Factor XIII	50–75 units	150–300 hours

BOX 1.53 General Indications for Cryoprecipitate Transfusion

- Factor VIII deficiency when factor VIII concentrate is not available
- von Willebrand's disease
- Hypofibrinogenaemia with fibrinogen <100 mg/dL (massive transfusion, congenital deficiency and DIC)
- Factor XIII deficiency
- May decrease bleeding due to uraemic platelet dysfunction

(threatened abortion, ectopic pregnancy, abortion, amniocentesis, abdominal trauma in second or third trimester, postpartum if newborn is Rh-positive).
- Also indicated following transfusion of Rh-positive cellular blood products (e.g. platelets) to an Rh-negative female of childbearing age or younger.
- Acute ITP resistant to steroids.

COMPLICATIONS OF BLOOD TRANSFUSION

IMMUNOLOGICAL REACTIONS

Acute Haemolytic Transfusion Reaction

- Occurs due to transfusion of incompatible donor red cells.

Clinical Features

- Early features are fever, chills, back pain, pruritus, burning sensation at the site of transfusion and centrally along the vein and chest pain.
- In an unconscious patient, more severe features like hypotension, shock, haemoglobinuria, oliguria and excessive bleeding due to DIC develop.

Management

- Stop the transfusion immediately if a transfusion reaction is suspected.
- Change the blood transfusion set and infuse normal saline to maintain high urine output.
- As soon as possible, check the identification details of the patient and the compatibility label of the component.
- Perform physical examination with special attention to the blood pressure, urine output and evidence of bleeding.
- Withdraw blood samples from the opposite arm. Send one sample to the blood bank for evaluation and centrifuge the other sample to look for any free haemoglobin in the supernatant.
- Get a coagulation screen including partial thromboplastin time, platelet count, fibrinogen levels and fibrin-degradation products to exclude DIC.
- Direct Coombs' test may become positive if tested before all the incompatible RBCs are destroyed.
- If hypotension develops, administer fluids and if required, vasopressors.
- Administer furosemide to maintain urine output.

Febrile Non-haemolytic Reactions

- Generally occur due to antileucocyte antibodies in a patient who has been pregnant or has been previously transfused. These antibodies react against leucocytes in the transfused blood.
- Can also occur due to cytokines in stored platelet concentrates.
- Generally occur towards the end of infusion or within hours of completing the transfusion.
- Features are fever, chills and rigors which are similar to acute haemolytic reaction.
- Management is to stop infusion immediately and investigate on the lines of acute haemolytic reaction before re-infusing same blood.
- Incidence can be reduced by leucoreduction in which WBCs are reduced in number through centrifugation or filtration.

Urticaria

- Due to the presence of antibodies in the recipient's blood to infused plasma proteins or infusion of allergens that react with IgE antibodies in the patient.

Anaphylaxis

- Occurs in patients who have antibodies against IgA and are often deficient in IgA. The antibodies react with IgA present in the donor blood.

Transfusion-Related Acute Lung Injury

- The donor plasma has antibodies to patient's leucocytes. Such antibodies are found most frequently in females after pregnancy and are not present in plasma of males unless they have been transfused.
- Patient develops an acute respiratory reaction with fever, cough, shortness of breath and typical appearance on chest X-ray. The reaction occurs during or soon after transfusion and may be life threatening.
- Treatment is supportive, with high-concentration oxygen therapy and ventilatory support if required.

Delayed Haemolytic Transfusion Reaction

- It occurs 3–21 days after transfusion with the incompatible blood. Patient has IgG antibodies to the red cell antigens such as Rh, Kidd, Kell, Duffy because of previous pregnancies or transfusions. The antibodies are undetectable during cross-match but further transfusion causes a secondary immune response resulting in delayed haemolysis.
- Direct Coombs' test will be positive if carried out while the patient is actively haemolysing. Later, only indirect Coombs' test may be positive.

Transfusion-Associated Graft-Versus-Host Disease (TA-GVHD)

- It occurs due to immune reaction of donor T cells against the recipient's cells, who is often immunodeficient, for example bone marrow allograft recipient, Hodgkin's lymphoma.
- Clinically, patient develops fever, skin rash, liver and renal failure and pancytopenia. It develops 4–30 days after transfusion and is often fatal.
- Prevention is by using gamma irradiation of cellular blood components.

Post-transfusion Purpura

- It is an immune-mediated thrombocytopenia that usually occurs in parous females.
- Antibodies against human platelet antigens (HPAs) are detectable in the patient's serum.
- It occurs 5–12 days after transfusion.
- Thrombocytopenia is usually severe and may cause bleeding.
- Platelet transfusions are usually ineffective and the treatment of choice is high-dose intravenous immunoglobulins (0.4 g/kg/day for 5 days).

NON-IMMUNE REACTIONS

- Transfusion associated circulatory overload (TACO), especially in patients with renal and cardiac failure. Table 1.111 outlines differences between TACO and TRALI.
- Adverse effects of massive transfusion—for example hyperkalaemia, ammonia and citrate toxicity and thrombocytopenia.
- Infections—for example viral infections (hepatitis, HIV, CMV), bacterial (syphilis, others), malaria. Bacterial infections more common with platelet transfusion since they are stored at a higher temperature. Features of bacterial infection may start within 2–3 hours after start of infusion.
- Air and fat embolism.
- Thrombophlebitis.
- Haemosiderosis as 1 unit of RBCs contains 200–250 mg of iron.

Q. Discuss the differential diagnosis of generalised lymphadenopathy in an adult.

ASSESSMENT OF THE EXTENT OF LYMPH NODAL ENLARGEMENT

- Clinical evaluation of lymph nodes should include the sites of enlargement, size, consistency, character, fixity, whether matted or not and presence or absence of tenderness. Associated other systemic abnormalities should be noted.
- Chest X-ray and CT scan of the thorax can detect mediastinal, hilar and paratracheal lymphadenopathy.
- Ultrasound scanning and CT scan of abdomen can detect intra-abdominal lymph nodes.
- PET scan can localise lymph nodes. It also indicates whether they are metabolically active.

TABLE 1.111 Differences Between TRALI and TACO

Features	TRALI	TACO
Patient characteristics	Can occur at any age	Most common in age >70 years
Implicated blood component	Usually plasma or platelets	Any
Onset	Usually within 2 hours of transfusion	Usually within 6 hours of transfusion
Blood pressure	Often low	Often high
Jugular venous pressure	Normal	Elevated
Chest radiograph	Bilateral perihilar and nodular shadowing; heart size normal	Enlarged heart and characteristics of pulmonary oedema
Echocardiogram	Normal	Abnormal
Fluid challenge	No change or improves	Worsens
Response to diuretics	Worsens	Improves

TABLE 1.112 Causes of Lymphadenopathy and Diagnostic Tests

Cause	Diagnostic Feature
• Lymphomas (Hodgkin's, non-Hodgkin's)	Histology of lymph node
• Leukaemias (ALL, CLL, CML in blast crisis)	Peripheral smear and bone marrow
• Disseminated tuberculosis	Caseating granulomas in lymph node; AFB positive
• Human immunodeficiency virus infection	ELISA and western blot
• Secondary syphilis	VDRL and TPHA
• Infectious mononucleosis	Monospot test and Paul–Bunnell test
• Brucellosis	Brucella agglutination test
• Systemic lupus erythematosus	ANA
• Rheumatoid arthritis	Rheumatoid factor, anti-CCP antibody
• Metastatic disease (head and neck cancers, lung and breast cancers, GIT malignancies)	Fine needle aspiration and biopsy
• Local infections (cellulitis, pharyngitis)	Local examination
• Plague	Inguinal lymph nodes; FNAC shows typical 'safety pin'-shaped bacteria

CAUSES OF LYMPHADENOPATHY AND REQUIRED DIAGNOSTIC TESTS

- Table 1.112 lists the causes of lymphadenopathy and required diagnostic tests.

MEDICATIONS CAUSING LYMPHADENOPATHY

- Box 1.54 gives a list of medications which can produce lymphadenopathy.

LYMPH NODE GROUPS, DRAINAGE AND DIFFERENTIAL DIAGNOSIS

- Lymph node groups in the head and neck area are shown in Fig. 1.8.
- Drainage of different lymph nodes and differential diagnosis of their enlargement is shown in Table 1.113.

DIFFERENTIAL DIAGNOSIS (ALSO SEE INDIVIDUAL CONDITIONS)

LYMPHOMAS (HODGKIN'S AND NON-HODGKIN'S)

Clinical Features

- Systemic symptoms like fever, weight loss and night sweats.
- Pel–Epstein type of fever uncommon.
- Pruritus.
- Alcohol-induced pain in the lymph nodes.

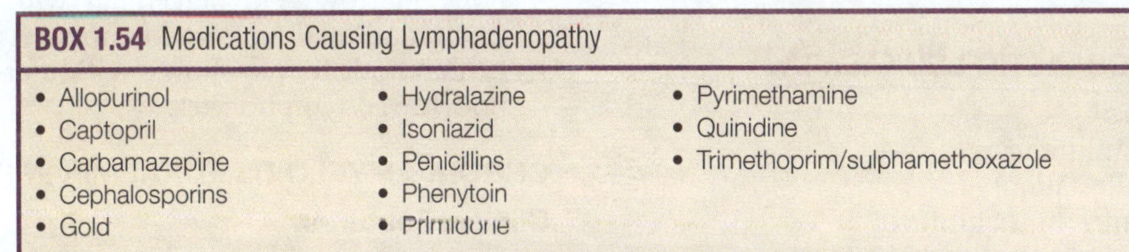

BOX 1.54 Medications Causing Lymphadenopathy

- Allopurinol
- Captopril
- Carbamazepine
- Cephalosporins
- Gold
- Hydralazine
- Isoniazid
- Penicillins
- Phenytoin
- Primidone
- Pyrimethamine
- Quinidine
- Trimethoprim/sulphamethoxazole

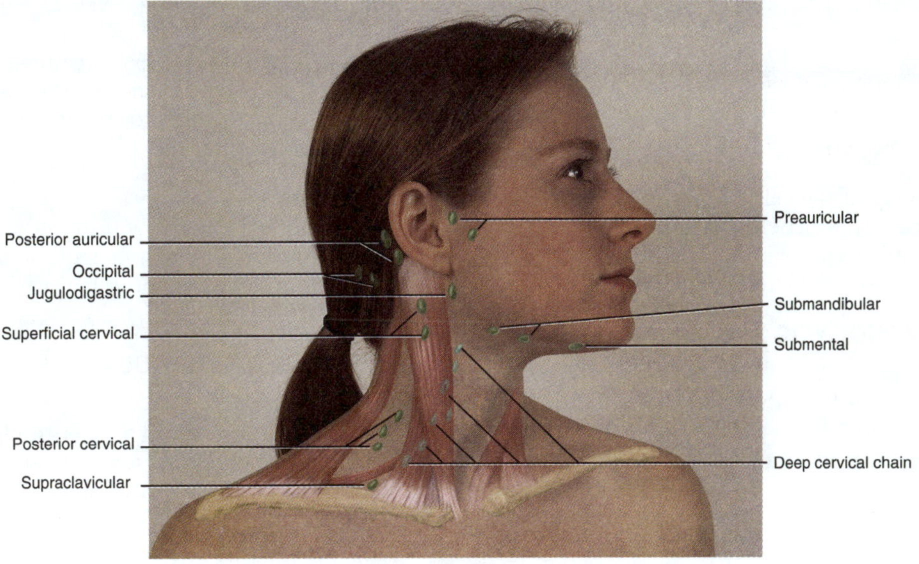

Fig 1.8 Location of Lymphnodes in Head and Neck.

TABLE 1.113 Lymph Node Groups: Drainage and Differential Diagnosis

Location	Drainage	Causes
Submental	Lower lip, floor of moth, tip of tongue, cheek	Dental diseases, infectious mononucleosis, cytomegalovirus, toxoplasmosis
Submandibular	Tongue, submandibular salivary gland, mouth, conjunctiva	Infections of head, neck, sinuses, ear, eye and pharynx, tuberculosis, dental diseases
Suboccipital	Scalp and head	Local infections
Postauricular	External auditory canal, pinna, scalp	Local infection
Preauricular	Eyelids, conjunctiva, pinna, temporal region	Local infection
Jugular	Tongue, tonsil, pinna, parotid	Pharyngitis, tuberculosis, rubella
Posterior cervical	Scalp and neck, upper chest, arms	Tuberculosis, lymphoma, head and neck malignancy
Right supraclavicular	Mediastinum, lungs, oesophagus	Tuberculosis, malignancy of right lung and lower lobe of left lung, GI malignancy
Left supraclavicular	Chest and abdomen (via thoracic duct)	Tuberculosis, lymphoma, malignancy left upper lobe, gastric malignancy, breast carcinoma
Axillary	Upper limb, chest wall, breast, parietal pleura	Tuberculosis, infections, lymphoma, breast carcinoma, cat-scratch disease
Epitrochlear	Ulnar aspect of forearm and hand	Infections, tuberculosis, lymphoma, sarcoidosis, HIV, kala-azar (West Bengal)
Inguinal	Penis, scrotum, vulva, vagina, perineum, gluteal area, lower abdominal wall	Tuberculosis, lymphoma, infections, sexually transmitted diseases (e.g. herpes simplex, gonococcal infection, chancroid, lymphogranuloma venereum), bubonic plague, pelvic malgnancy

- Clinical effects of pressure by lymph node masses on neighbouring structures.
- Painless, discrete, rubbery lymph nodes.

Lab Features

- Lymph node biopsy confirms the diagnosis.

ACUTE LYMPHOBLASTIC LEUKAEMIA

Clinical Features

- Common in children.
- Bleeding manifestations.
- Intermittent infections and fever.
- Severe anaemia.
- Bone pain and sternal tenderness.
- Hepatosplenomegaly.
- Frequent testicular, CNS and eye involvement.

Lab Features

- Blood examination shows severe anaemia of normochromic type, raised total leucocyte count, presence of lymphoblasts and other primitive cells and thrombocytopenia.
- More than 50% of the cells are periodic acid–Schiff (PAS)-positive on cytochemical staining.
- Bone marrow is hypercellular with the replacement of normal elements by leukaemic blast cells.

CHRONIC LYMPHOCYTIC LEUKAEMIA

Clinical Features

- More in males older than 50 years, with peak incidence around 65 years.
- Firm, rubbery, discrete, painless lymph nodes.
- Hepatosplenomegaly.

Lab Features

- Anaemia.
- Total leucocyte count is raised.
- More than 95% of the leucocytes in the peripheral blood are lymphocytes of small variety.
- Bone marrow is hypercellular with infiltration of small- and medium-sized lymphocytes.
- Lymph node biopsy shows well-differentiated, small, noncleaved lymphocytes.

CHRONIC MYELOID LEUKAEMIA IN BLAST CRISIS

Clinical Features

- Common in elderly people; average age around 55 years.
- The usual patient is one who had been diagnosed and treated for chronic myeloid leukaemia. Such a patient suddenly develops features of acute leukaemia, for example fever, bleeding manifestations, anaemia, bony tenderness, abrupt increase in splenic size and refractoriness to treatment.
- Massive splenomegaly.

Lab Features

- Blood and bone marrow findings are indistinguishable from acute leukaemia, with plenty of blast cells.
- Philadelphia chromosome is positive in more than 95% of the cases.

DISSEMINATED TUBERCULOSIS

Clinical Features

- Fever, weight loss, night sweats and loss of appetite.
- Usually the patient has toxic appearance.
- Hepatosplenomegaly may be present.

Lab Features

- Chest X-ray might show miliary mottling.
- Lymph node biopsy shows caseating granulomas and acid-fast bacilli.
- Liver biopsy may show granulomas.

HUMAN IMMUNODEFICIENCY VIRUS INFECTION

Clinical Features

- Common after heterosexual contact with HIV-positive person; also occurs in intravenous drug abusers, haemophiliacs (due to transfusion of blood from HIV-positive persons) and homosexuals.
- Generalised lymphadenopathy can occur in three situations:
  - Immediately after acquiring infection (within 2–3 weeks).
  - Persistent generalised lymphadenopathy (PGL) or AIDS-related complex (ARC).
  - As a part of full-blown AIDS.

Lab Features

- ELISA test for HIV antibody (screening test).
- Western blot test that identifies antibodies to specific viral proteins (confirmatory test).

SECONDARY SYPHILIS

Clinical Features

- Past history of exposure and primary syphilis (genital ulcers and inguinal lymphadenopathy).
- Generalised skin rashes.
- Condylomata lata.
- Mucous patches and snail track ulcers.
- Hepatosplenomegaly.
- Discrete, 'shotty' lymph nodes.

Lab Features

- Dark field microscopy can demonstrate *Treponema pallidum* in papules and mucous patches.
- Positive VDRL test.
- Positive *T. pallidum* haemagglutination test (TPHA).

INFECTIOUS MONONUCLEOSIS

Clinical Features

- Fever of short duration.
- Maculopapular rash.
- Petechial haemorrhages on palate.
- Hepatosplenomegaly.

Lab Features

- Atypical lymphocytes in the peripheral blood.
- Positive Monospot test.
- Positive Paul–Bunnell test.

BRUCELLOSIS

Clinical Features

- Common in veterinary surgeons and slaughterhouse workers handling cattle.
- Fever, polyarthritis, splenomegaly.

Lab Features

- Positive blood culture.
- Positive *Brucella* agglutination test.
- Positive complement fixation and antihuman globulin tests.

Q. Discuss briefly about porphyrias.

- The porphyrias are a group of rare inherited metabolic disorders that are caused by deficiencies of specific enzymes involved in the haeme biosynthetic pathway.
- All porphyrias are caused by decreased activity of one of the enzymes in the haeme biosynthetic pathway, with the exception of X-linked protoporphyria, which is a consequence of gain-of-function variants in a gene, leading to increased delta-aminolevulinic acid synthase activity.
- The symptoms observed in different types of porphyria result from excessive accumulation of porphyrins or haeme precursors in different tissues.
- Majority (~80%) of haeme synthesis occurs in erythroblasts in the bone marrow, while another ~15% in hepatocytes primarily for synthesis of cytochrome P450 enzymes.

HAEME BIOSYNTHESIS

- Haeme biosynthesis involves eight enzymatic steps in the conversion of glycine and succinyl-coenzyme A to haeme (Flowchart 1.25).
- The first and last three enzymes in the pathway are located in the mitochondrion, whereas the other four are in the cytosol.

CLASSIFICATION

- Based on the primary source of haeme precursor or porphyrin overproduction and accumulation, the porphyrias are classified as either hepatic or erythropoietic (Table 1.114).
- Porphyrin precursors, in particular aminolevulinic acid, are neurotoxins, whereas porphyrins are light-absorbing chemicals that act as photosensitizers, resulting in skin damage.
- The hepatic porphyrias commonly present with acute neurovisceral symptoms and include acute intermittent porphyria (AIP), hereditary coproporphyria (HCP) and variegate porphyria (VP). In addition, two types of hepatic porphyrias, porphyria cutanea tarda (PCT) and hepatoerythropoietic porphyria (HEP), present mainly with cutaneous symptoms and do not have neurovisceral involvement.
- Erythropoietic porphyrias include erythropoietic protoporphyria (EPP), X-linked protoporphyria (XLP) and congenital erythropoietic porphyria (CEP). These are characterised mainly by cutaneous manifestations due to phototoxicity.
- The excretion of the hydrophilic ALA, PBG and uroporphyrin is entirely in urine, whereas coproporphyrin is in both urine and faeces and protoporphyrin only in faeces.

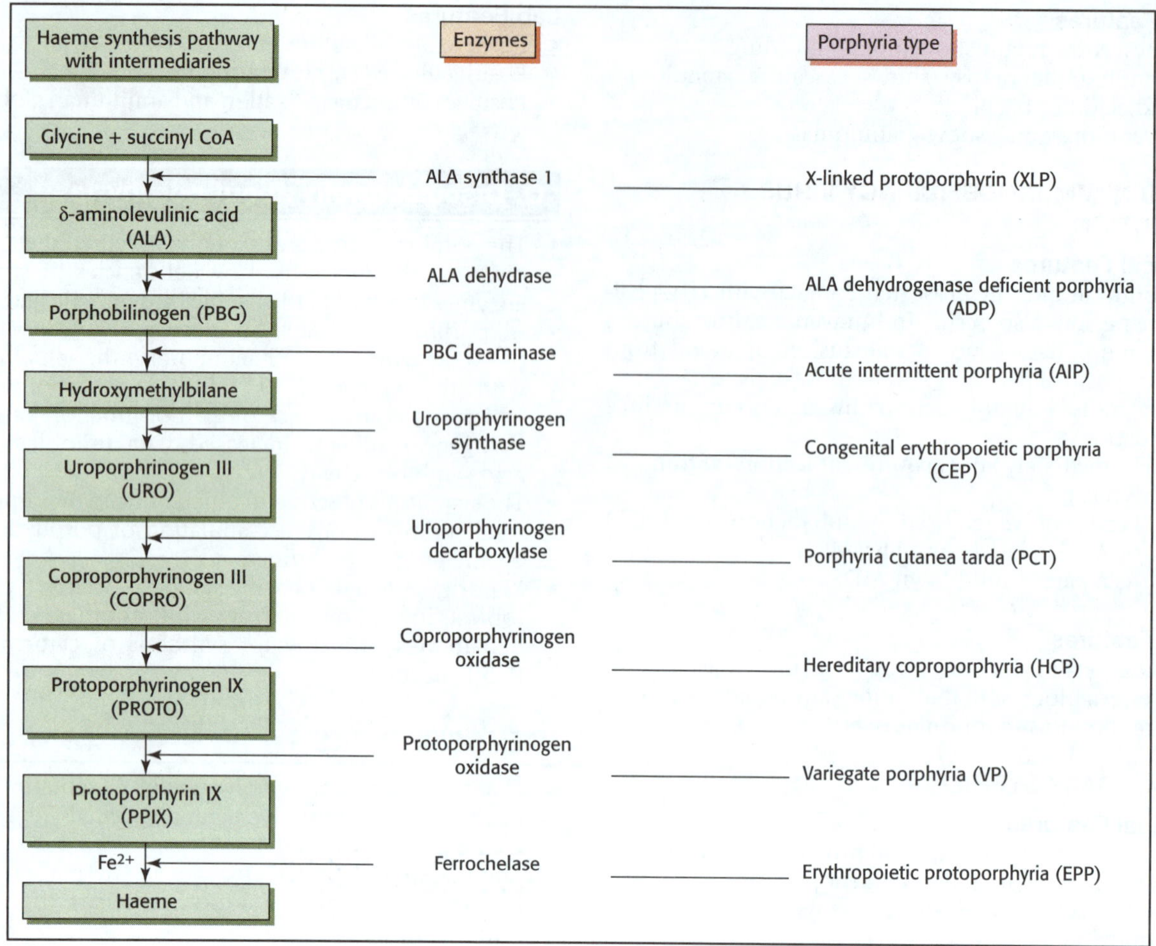

Flowchart 1.25 Haeme Biosynthesis and Associated Porphyrias.

TABLE 1.114 Major Porphyrias

Porphyria	Tissue Site of Porphyrin Origin	Enzyme Involved	Inheritance	Clinical Presentation	Biochemical Findings
ALA-dehydratase deficiency porphyria (ADP)	Hepatic	Delta-aminolevulinic acid dehydratase	Autosomal recessive	Acute neurovisceral	Urine: Aminolevulinic acid (ALA), coproprophrin III RBCs:Zn protoporphyrin
Acute intermittent porphyria (AIP)	Hepatic	Hydroxymethylbilane synthase	Autosomal dominant	Acute neurovisceral	Urine: Aminolevulinic acid (ALA), porphobilinogen, (PBG), uroporphyrin
Hereditary coproporphyria (HCP)	Hepatic	Coproporphyrinogen oxidase	Autosomal dominant	Acute neurovisceral and cutaneous	Urine: ALA, PBG, coproporphyrin (copro III) Faeces: copro III
Variegate porphyria (VP)	Hepatic	Protoporphyrinogen oxidase	Autosomal dominant	Acute neurovisceral and cutaneous	Urine: ALA, PBG, copro III Feces: copro III, protoporphyrin IX (PPIX)
Erythropoietic protoporphyria (EPP)	Erythropoietic	Ferrochelatase	Autosomal recessive	Cutaneous, rarely hepatic complications	Blood: PPIX
X-linked protoporphyria (XLP)	Erythropoietic	Increased activity of Delta-aminolevulinic acid synthase 2	X-linked	Cutaneous, rarely hepatic complications	Blood: PPIX and Zn-PPIX
Congenital erythropoietic porphyria (CEP)	Erythropoietic	Uroporphyrinogen III synthase	Autosomal recessive	Cutaneous, haemolytic anaemia	Blood and urine: uroporphyrin I, copro I Faeces: copro I
Porphyria cutanea tarda (PCT)	Hepatic	Uroporphyrinogen decarboxylase	Sporadic, autosomal dominant	Cutaneous	Urine: uroporphyrin, heptacarboxylporphyrin Faeces: iso-copro

CLINICAL FEATURES

ACUTE NEUROVISCERAL SYNDROME

- Approximately 90% of symptomatic patients are female and attacks typically begin only after the onset of menses and are rare after menopause.
- Attacks are characterised by diffuse abdominal pain accompanied by nausea, vomiting and constipation, back and chest pain, proximal muscle weakness and polyneuropathy.
- Tachycardia, hypertension and hyponatraemia are common.
- The symptoms buildup over the course of several days rather than hours. The physical examination is usually normal without abdominal guarding or rebound tenderness.
- Acute porphyria attacks can either occur as an isolated episode or become recurrent in some individuals.
- Triggering factors include fasting, alcohol and drugs like sulphonamides, anticonvulsants, oestrogen and progesterone.
- Long-term complications of AHP include hypertension, chronic pain, autonomic dysfunction, renal insufficiency and in rare cases, hepatocellular carcinoma.

CUTANEOUS PHOTOSENSITIVITY

- Cutaneous photosensitivity in EPP and XLP occurs due to protoporphyrin presence in the small blood vessels of the skin, leading to photoactivation upon sun exposure.
- Presents with swelling, itching, burning, erythema and severe pain in sun-exposed areas. Bullous skin lesions, skin fragility and hirsutism are absent. Symptoms resolve after several days of sun avoidance without scarring.
- In PCT, bullous skin lesions and fluid-filled vesicles occur on sun-exposed portions. These rupture easily and heal with crusting and scarring. Additional findings include skin fragility, hypertrichosis, hyperpigmentation and severe thickening of the skin.

DIAGNOSIS

- It depends on the pattern of porphyrins and its precursors in blood, urine and stool.
- Urine often gets reddish in colour on exposure to sunlight.

DIFFERENTIAL DIAGNOSIS

- Patients presenting with progressive weakness and neuropathy should be evaluated for Guillain-Barré syndrome (GBS). Some key differences include the lack of severe abdominal pain in GBS, and the lack of ascending paralysis in acute attacks. The most important difference is the presence of markedly elevated urine ALA and PBG, which are normal in GBS.
- In lead intoxication, excess lead inhibits the function of ALA dehydrase, the enzyme that is defective in ALAD porphyria. Biochemical testing shows isolated elevations of urine ALA but normal PBG, which helps distinguish it from AIP, VP and HCP attacks. Measuring the blood lead is definitive for diagnosis.

TREATMENT AND PREVENTION

- The treatment of acute porphyria attacks consists of symptomatic therapy, including medication for pain control and nausea, seizure control, correction of electrolyte disturbances, haemodynamic stabilisation and mechanical ventilation if indicated.
- To downregulate hepatic ALAS1 activity and subsequently decrease the production of ALA, PBG and porphyrin metabolites, carbohydrate loading, dextrose infusion and intravenous haematin administration are used during acute attacks
- The only curative treatment approach for AHP is orthotopic liver transplantation.
- For AIP, VP and HCP, givosiran is approved. It targets ALAS1, resulting in downregulation of ALAS1 and decreased production of haeme precursors ALA and PBG.
- For cutaneous photosensitivity, sun avoidance, sun-protective clothing and sunscreens are the mainstay of EPP/XLP management.
- For EPP and XLP, afamelanotide, a melanocyte stimulating hormone analogue is approved which leads to photoprotection.
- In PCT, reduction in iron stores and hepatic iron content is the mainstay of symptomatic treatment. This can be achieved by serial phlebotomies or oral iron chelator therapy. Antimalarial agents, such as hydroxychloroquine or chloroquine, at low doses are effective alternatives if phlebotomy is not an option.

MCQs

1. Eosinophilia is defined as absolute eosinophil counts of:
   A. $\geq 100/mm^3$
   B. $\geq 200/mm^3$
   C. $\geq 500/mm^3$
   D. $\geq 1000/mm^3$

Ans. C

2. Macrocytosis in peripheral smear is a feature of:
   A. Hereditary spherocytosis
   B. Thalassaemia intermedia
   C. G6PD deficiency
   D. Myelodysplastic syndrome

Ans. D

3. Target cells in peripheral smear are seen in all of the following conditions EXCEPT:
   A. Chronic liver diseases
   B. Hyposplenism
   C. Haemoglobinopathies
   D. Sideroblastic anaemia

Ans. D

4. Massive transfusion protocol involves infusion of packed red cells, plasma and platelet-rich plasma in the ratio of:
   A. 1:1:1
   B. 1:2:1
   C. 1:2:2
   D. 3:1:1

Ans. A

5. All of the following are typical features of Plummer-Vinson syndrome EXCEPT:
   A. Iron-deficiency anaemia
   B. Clubbing
   C. Increased risk of carcinoma of pharynx and oesophagus
   D. Post-cricoid web

Ans. B

6. Following statement is true regarding iron treatment in iron-deficiency anaemia:
   A. Ferrous sulphate tablets contain 34% iron
   B. Iron tablets should be taken empty stomach
   C. Reticulocyte response occurs by 3 weeks
   D. Tetracycline can be safely given along with iron

Ans. B

7. All of the following statements regarding pernicious anaemia are true EXCEPT:
   A. Anti-intrinsic factor antibodies are present
   B. Serum gastric levels are high
   C. Incidence of gastric carcinoma is high
   D. Treatment with vitamin B12 is for 1 year

Ans. D

8. Following is a typical feature of vitamin B12 deficiency:
   A. Hypersegmented neutrophils
   B. Severe microcytosis
   C. Heinz bodies in red cells
   D. High levels of holotranscobalamin II

Ans. A

9. All of the following are antifolate drugs EXCEPT:
   A. Methotrexate
   B. Trimethoprim
   C. Azithromycin
   D. Pyrimethamine

Ans. C

10. Following is a typical feature of anaemia of chronic disease:
    A. Serum ferritin is reduced
    B. Serum hepcidin is elevated
    C. Serum erythropoietin level is elevated
    D. Serum iron is elevated

Ans. B

11. Presence of all of the following excludes aplastic anaemia EXCEPT:
    A. Jaundice
    B. Lymphadenopathy
    C. Normocytic, normochromic anaemia
    D. Splenomegaly

Ans. C

12. The following are the features of chronic haemolytic anaemia EXCEPT:
    A. Normal coloured urine
    B. Jaundice
    C. Reticulocytosis
    D. Cholelithiasis

Ans. A

13. Following indicate increased erythrocyte destruction in haemolysis EXCEPT:
    A. Unconjugated hyperbilirubinaemia
    B. Reduced urobilinogen excretion in urine
    C. Decreased plasma haptoglobin
    D. Increased plasma LDH

Ans. B

14. Primary cause of anaemia in hereditary spherocytosis is:
    A. Red cells are more susceptible to osmotic lysis
    B. Sequestration and removal from circulation by the spleen
    C. Complement-mediated red cell lysis
    D. Abnormal haemoglobin chain

Ans. B

15. Following statement is true regarding G6PD deficiency:
    A. Estimation of G6PD should be done several days after the acute episode
    B. Haemolysis occurs mainly due to splenic sequestration
    C. Primaquine is an infrequent cause of haemolysis
    D. Urine colour remains normal during the episode of haemolysis

Ans. A

16. Following factors increase sickling in sickle cell disease EXCEPT:
    A. Fever
    B. Low oxygen tension
    C. Alkalosis
    D. Increase in red cell 2,3-DPG

Ans. C

17. One of the following statements is true regarding sickle cell anaemia
    A. Spleen becomes impalpable by the age of 15 years
    B. Infections with Pneumococcus and Meningococcus are common
    C. Clinical manifestations start by the age of 1 month
    D. Imatinib is the drug of choice

Ans. B

18. Methaemoglobinaemia is characterised by all of the following EXCEPT:
   A. Chocolate-coloured blood which becomes pink on exposure to air
   B. Normal partial pressure of oxygen
   C. Elevated saturation gap >10%
   D. CO-oximetric measurement is required to diagnose it

Ans. A

19. A 14-year old patient presents with massive splenomegaly and anaemia. On examination, there is bossing of the skull with prominent malar eminence. On investigations, he has microcytic anaemia with several tear drop cells. The likely diagnosis is:
   A. Thalassaemia major
   B. Extrahepatic portal vein thrombosis
   C. Kala-azar
   D. Primary myelofibrosis

Ans. A

20. Sucrose lysis test can be positive in the following EXCEPT:
   A. Megaloblastic anaemia
   B. Autoimmune haemolytic anaemia
   C. Paroxysmal nocturnal haemolysis
   D. Thalassaemia

Ans. D

21. Following is incorrect about warm antibody autoimmune haemolytic anaemia:
   A. Direct Coombs' test indicates presence of antibodies on the surface of red cells
   B. Indirect Coombs' test indicates presence of antibodies in the serum
   C. Blood transfusion is the treatment of choice as it restores haemoglobin
   D. Microspherocytes and macrocytes are seen in peripheral blood smear

Ans. C

22. All of the following are features of polycythaemia vera EXCEPT:
   A. Absence of splenomegaly
   B. Pruritus after bath
   C. Normal oxygen saturation
   D. Urate kidney stones

Ans. A

23. Following is a true statement regarding acute lymphocytic leukaemia
   A. Majority of ALL are of T-lymphocyte type
   B. Auer rods are present in about 40% of cases
   C. CNS involvement is rare
   D. Presence of mediastinal mass is a poor prognostic factor

Ans. D

24. All of the following are poor prognostic factors for AML EXCEPT:
   A. Absence of Auer rods
   B. Fibrosis on bone marrow examination
   C. Therapy-related AML
   D. Age >40 years

Ans. D

25. Following is a feature of chronic myeloid leukaemia:
   A. Vitamin B_{12} level is low
   B. Leucocyte alkaline phosphatase score is high
   C. Philadelphia chromosome is present in 70% cases
   D. Basophils are often increased

Ans. D

26. Late stage of primary myelofibrosis is characterised by:
   A. Thrombocytosis
   B. Leucoerythroblastic blood picture
   C. Low LAP score
   D. Hypercellular bone marrow

Ans. B

27. One of the following is NOT a typical feature of myelodysplastic syndrome
   A. Hypocellular bone marrow
   B. Can progress to acute myeloid leukaemia
   C. Anaemia
   D. Leuopenia

Ans. A

28. A 60-year old patient presents with history of recurrent infections. On examination he has generalised lymphadenopathy. His haemogram report shows total leucocyte count of 50,000/mm³. Serum albumin is 3.4 g/dL and globulin 2.0 g/dL. The likely diagnosis is:
   A. Multiple myeloma
   B. Leukaemoid reaction
   C. Chronic lymphocytic leukaemia
   D. Disseminated tuberculosis

Ans. C

29. All of the following are typical features of hairy cell leukaemia EXCEPT:
   A. Massive splenomegaly
   B. Generalised lymphadenopathy
   C. Pancytopenia
   D. Erythema nodosum

Ans. B

30. All of the following are true regarding Burkitt's lymphoma EXCEPT:
   A. Tumour lysis syndrome is common
   B. Has poor response to treatment
   C. Epstein–Barr (EB) virus plays an important aetiological role
   D. Majority of cases occur in children

Ans. B

31. Following is a typical feature of Hodgkin's lymphoma
    A. Involvement of extralymphatic organs is early
    B. Mediastinal involvement is uncommon
    C. Alcohol-induced discomfort in lymph nodal region
    D. Multicentric origin and noncontiguous spread

Ans. C

32. All of the following are typical components of POEMS syndrome EXCEPT
    A. Polycystic kidney disease
    B. Organomegaly
    C. Endocrinopathy
    D. M-protein

Ans. A

33. All of the following contribute to renal failure in patients with multiple myeloma EXCEPT:
    A. Hypocalcaemia
    B. Hyperuricaemia
    C. Amyloidosis
    D. Hyperviscosity

Ans. A

34. Following is a poor prognostic factor in multiple myeloma:
    A. Elevated beta2-microglobulin
    B. Serum calcium <10 mg/dL
    C. Normal LDH
    D. Kappa-light chain non-secretors

Ans. A

35. All of the following are features of Waldenstrom macroglobulinaemia EXCEPT:
    A. Hyperviscosity
    B. Neuropathy
    C. Warm antibody autoimmune haemolytic anaemia
    D. Vasculitis

Ans. C

36. Alpha granules of platelet contain:
    A. ADP
    B. von Willebrand factor
    C. Calcium
    D. Serotonin

Ans. B

37. All of the following are vitamin K-dependent factors EXCEPT:
    A. Factor II
    B. Factory V
    C. Factor VII
    D. Factor X

Ans. B

38. Following is a typical features of coagulation factor deficiency:
    A. Bleeding into skin
    B. Bleeding into muscles and joints
    C. Bleeding immediately after trauma
    D. Local pressure effective

Ans. B

39. Bleeding time checks for one of the following:
    A. Factors V
    B. Factor VII
    C. Factor X
    D. von Willebrand factor

Ans. D

40. All of the following are typical features of newly diagnosed ITP EXCEPT:
    A. Absence of splenomegaly
    B. Purpura
    C. Presence of an antiplatelet antibody
    D. Prolonged prothrombin time

Ans. D

41. The classic features of thrombotic thrombocytopenia purpura include all of the following EXCEPT:
    A. Liver failure
    B. Renal abnormalities
    C. Fever
    D. Neurologic deficits

Ans. A

42. Initial test which is done to detect von Willebrand disease is:
    A. Factor II assay
    B. Factor V assay
    C. Factor VIII assay
    D. Factor X assay

Ans. C

43. Clopidogrel is a:
    A. Adenosine diphosphate (ADP) receptor inhibitors
    B. Glycoprotein IIb/IIIa inhibitor
    C. Adenosine reuptake inhibitor
    D. Cyclooxygenase inhibitor

Ans. A

44. Antidote to reverse heparin-induced bleeding is:
    A. Fresh frozen plasma
    B. Protamine sulphate
    C. Cryoprecipitate
    D. Platelet-rich plasma

Ans. B

45. All of the following statements regarding HIT type II are correct EXCEPT:
   A. Generally occurs 5–14 days after initiation of heparin
   B. Characterised by bleeding from multiple sites
   C. Unfractionated heparin should not be replaced with low-molecular weight heparin
   D. Platelets should not be transfused even in presence of severe thrombocytopenia.

Ans. B

46. All of the following are true regarding blood components EXCEPT:
   A. Platelet rich plasma has a self-life of 5–7 days
   B. Packed red cells has a shelf-life of 42 days
   C. Fresh frozen plasma is stored at –18° to –30°C
   D. ABO and Rh compatibility is required for transfusing fresh frozen plasma

Ans. D

47. Cryoprecipitate contain all of the following EXCEPT:
   A. Factor VIII
   B. Factor V
   C. von Willebrand factor
   D. Factor XIII

Ans. B

48. All of the following porphyrias are caused by decreased activity of one of the enzymes in the haeme biosynthetic pathway EXCEPT:
   A. Acute intermittent porphyria
   B. X-linked protoporphyria
   C. Hereditary coproporphyria
   D. Porphyria cutanea tarda

Ans. B

2 Diseases of the Respiratory System

Q. Define a bronchopulmonary segment. Name the bronchopulmonary segments. (AN 24.3)

- Bronchopulmonary segment is a wedge of lung tissue supplied by one segmental bronchus along with the corresponding branches of pulmonary artery and pulmonary vein. Each segment is an independent unit and these units are separated from each other by fibrous septa.
- Figure 2.1 gives the major bronchial divisions and bronchopulmonary segments of lungs.
- Table 2.1 mentions the segmental bronchi and bronchopulmonary segments.

Q. Give the normal arterial blood gas (ABG) levels. (BI 6.8)

- Normal values of arterial blood are given in Box 2.1.

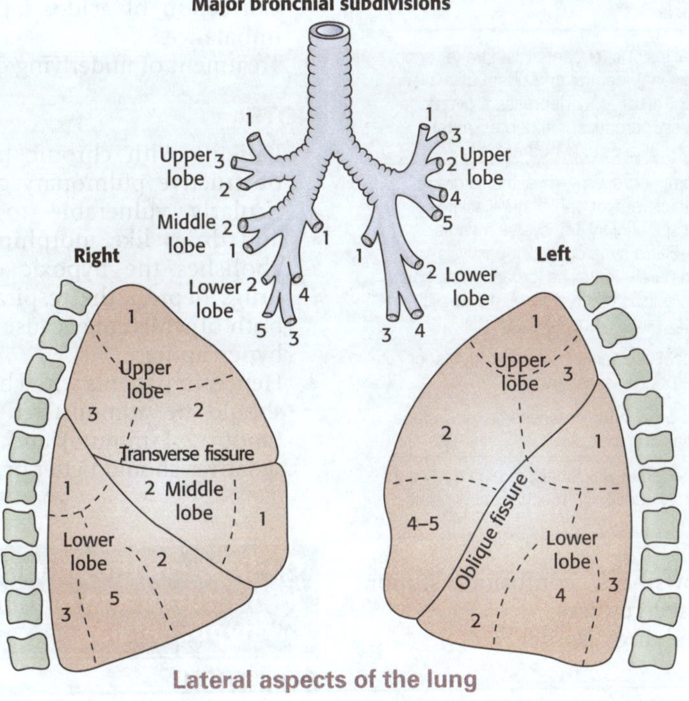

Fig. 2.1 Major bronchial subdivisions and bronchopulmonary segments. Bronchopulmonary segments. Right—*upper lobe*: 1, apical; 2, anterior; 3, posterior; *middle lobe*: 1, medial; 2, lateral; *lower lobe*: 1, apical; 2, anterior basal; 3, posterior basal; 4, medial basal; 5, lateral basal. Left—*upper lobe*: 1, apical; 2, anterior; 3, posterior; 4, superior (lingular); 5, inferior (lingular); *lower lobe*: 1, apical; 2, anterior basal; 3, posterior basal; 4, lateral basal.

TABLE 2.1 Segmental Bronchi and Bronchopulmonary Segments

Right Lung	Left Lung
• Upper lobe • Apical bronchus and segment • Anterior bronchus and segment • Posterior bronchus and segment • Middle lobe • Medial bronchus and segment • Lateral bronchus and segment • Lower lobe • Apical bronchus and segment • Anterior basal bronchus and segment • Posterior basal bronchus and segment • Medial basal bronchus and segment • Lateral basal bronchus and segment	• Upper lobe • Apical bronchus and segment • Anterior bronchus and segment • Posterior bronchus and segment • Superior (lingular) bronchus and segment • Inferior (lingular) bronchus and segment • Lower lobe • Apical bronchus and segment • Anterior basal bronchus and segment • Posterior basal bronchus and segment • Lateral basal bronchus and segment

BOX 2.1 Normal Arterial Blood Gas Values

• Arterial oxygen tension	PaO_2	95 ± 5 mmHg
• Arterial carbon dioxide (CO_2)	$PaCO_2$	40 ± 5 mmHg
• Arterial oxygen saturation	SaO_2	97 ± 2%
• Arterial blood pH	pH	7.40 ± 0.05
• Arterial bicarbonate	HCO_3	24 ± 2 mmol/L
• Base excess	BE	0 ± 2 mmol/L

Q. Discuss the causes, mechanisms, clinical features, investigations and management of hypercapnia/hypercapnic encephalopathy (carbon dioxide [CO_2] narcosis). (CT2.4)

DEFINITION

- Hypercapnia is defined as a $PaCO_2$ in excess of 45 mmHg (6 kPa) at rest.
- CO_2 narcosis may occur when $PaCO_2$ exceeds 90 mmHg (12 kPa).

CAUSES

- Causes of hypercapnia are given in Table 2.2.

MECHANISMS

- Decreased ventilatory drive ('won't breathe').
- Malfunction of the respiratory pump or increased airway resistance ('can't breathe').
- Inefficiency of gas exchange (increased dead space or V/Q mismatch).
- Increased CO_2 production.

CLINICAL FEATURES

- Intense headache that is generalised or bilateral frontal or occipital. It is especially severe on waking up.
- Intermittent drowsiness, indifference or inattention, reduction of psychomotor activity and forgetfulness in mild cases.

TABLE 2.2 Causes of Hypercapnia

Central (reduced respiratory drive)	• Cerebral lesions (encephalitis, stroke, brainstem lesions), central and obstructive sleep apnoeas, respiratory depressant overdose (sedatives, narcotics, antidepressants), metabolic alkalosis, hypothermia
Neuromuscular	• Peripheral neuropathy, myasthenia gravis, myopathies, amyotrophic lateral sclerosis, cervical spine injury, transverse myelitis, Guillain–Barré syndrome, tick paralysis, periodic paralysis, toxins (organophosphates, tetanus, botulism, strychnine), metabolic (hypokalaemia, hypomagnesaemia)
Chest wall	• Kyphoscoliosis, ankylosing spondylitis, chest trauma, pectus excavatum
Pulmonary	• Chronic bronchitis, emphysema, end-stage interstitial lung disease
Others	• Angio-oedema, epiglottitis, foreign body aspiration, malfunctioning mechanical ventilator

- Mental dullness, drowsiness, confusion, stupor, seizures and coma in severe cases.
- Manifestations of underlying disorder.

SIGNS

- Various signs of hypercapnia are shown in Box 2.2.

INVESTIGATIONS

- ABG studies confirm hypercapnia.
- Relevant investigations in relation to the underlying aetiology.

TREATMENT

- If oxygen saturation is <90%, administer oxygen. Use low-flow rate of 1–2 L/minute initially in patients with chronic obstructive lung disease.
- Mechanical ventilation with intermittent positive-pressure respirator.
- In a selected group of patients, noninvasive ventilation (NIV) may be tried (Box 2.3).

BOX 2.2 Signs of Hypercapnia

- Fast-frequency action tremor
- Flushed warm extremities
- Bounding peripheral pulses
- Flapping tremor (asterixis)
- Muscle twitching (fasciculations)
- Papilloedema
- Altered sensorium

BOX 2.3 Indications of Noninvasive Ventilation in Acute Hypercapnia

- Acute exacerbation of COPD
- Cardiogenic pulmonary oedema
- Obesity hypoventilation syndrome
- Weaning from mechanical ventilation
- Chest wall diseases
- Neuromuscular diseases
- Palliative care and do-not-intubate patients
- Miscellaneous (very old patients, pneumonia)

- Correction of acidosis (if severe) and electrolyte imbalance.
- Treatment of underlying disorder.

NOTE

- Patients with chronic hypercapnia (e.g. chronic obstructive pulmonary disease [COPD]) are particularly vulnerable to the effects of oxygen and drugs like morphine and sedatives. Oxygen abolishes the hypoxic drive to ventilation and drugs depress the respiratory centre in the brain, both of which may cause a disastrous worsening of hypercapnia.
- Hence, in patients with chronic hypercapnia, oxygen should be administered in a controlled manner (about 2 L/minute) and drugs like morphine and sedatives should better be avoided.

Q. Discuss the causes, clinical features and management of hypoxaemia. (CT2.4)

DEFINITION

- Hypoxaemia is defined as a PaO_2 of less than 80 mmHg (10.6 kPa) in a young healthy adult. However, the normal PaO_2 falls gradually as the age advances.
- Hypoxaemia indicates abnormally low PaO_2 while the term hypoxia indicates inadequate tissue oxygenation. These terms are not interchangeable. A person can be hypoxaemic without hypoxia and similarly a person can be hypoxic without hypoxaemia. For example, if a person is hypoxaemic but has polycythaemia, he/she may not have tissue hypoxia. Similarly, a severely anaemic patient may have tissue hypoxia without hypoxaemia.

CAUSES (Table 2.3)

- Hypoxaemia at rest is uncommon in conditions with reduced diffusion.

TABLE 2.3 Causes of Hypoxaemia

Ventilation–perfusion mismatching

- Chronic bronchitis
- Emphysema
- Acute asthma
- Interstitial lung diseases
- Pulmonary embolism

Right-to-left shunts

- Congenital cyanotic heart diseases
- Pulmonary atelectasis
- Pneumonia
- Acute respiratory distress syndrome
- Pulmonary AV malformations
- Hepatopulmonary syndrome

Hypoventilation[a]

Reduced inspired oxygen concentration

- High altitudes
- Malfunctioning of mechanical ventilators

[a]See causes of hypercapnia in Table 2.2 listed under the following categories: central, neuromuscular, chest wall and others.

CLINICAL FEATURES

- Acute hypoxaemia is characterised by impaired judgement, motor incoordination and a clinical picture closely resembling acute alcoholism.
- Long-standing hypoxaemia is characterised by fatigue, drowsiness, inattentiveness, apathy, delayed reaction time and reduced work capacity.
- Finally, centres in the brainstem are affected and death results from respiratory failure.

INVESTIGATIONS

- ABG studies confirm hypoxaemia.
- It is useful to calculate the alveolar–arterial oxygen ($PAO_2 - PaO_2$) gradient for differentiating various causes of hypoxaemia (see pulmonary function tests on page 119 and approach to respiratory failure on page 122). It is normal in patients with pure hypoventilation and reduced inspired oxygen concentration while elevated in others.

TREATMENT

- Treatment is that of the underlying disease or mechanism.

Q. Define clubbing. Enumerate the causes and give the mechanism of clubbing.

DEFINITION

- Clubbing is defined as a selective bulbous enlargement of distal segment of a digit due to an increase in soft tissue.
- Pseudoclubbing is increased in longitudinal curvature of the nail with loss of nail plate material and is seen in scleroderma, thyroid carcinoma and sarcoidosis. X-ray of fingers shows resorption of terminal tufts (acro-osteolysis) instead of an overgrowth of phalangeal tufts seen in clubbing. Finger involvement is asymmetrical as compared to clubbing.

MECHANISMS

- Humoral theory—an unidentified humoral substance causes dilatation of vessels of the fingertip.
- Persistent hypoxia causing opening up of deep arteriovenous fistulae of fingers.
- Reduced ferritin in systemic circulation causing dilatation of arteriovenous anastomoses and hypertrophy of terminal phalanx.
- Vagal theory—persistent vagal stimulation causing vasodilatation and clubbing.
- Recent studies—a possible role of platelets in the development of clubbing, particularly hypertrophic osteoarthropathy. It is postulated that circulating megakaryocytes and large platelet particles, normally destroyed by the lungs, reach distal extremities and interact with endothelial cells resulting in liberation of platelet-derived growth factor (PDGF), vascular endothelial growth factor and other factors which cause proliferation of connective tissue.

GRADING OF CLUBBING

- Grading of clubbing is shown in Table 2.4 and Figure 2.2.

COMMON CAUSES OF CLUBBING

- Table 2.5 shows common causes of clubbing.

TABLE 2.4 Grading of Clubbing

• Grade I	Increased fluctuation of the nail bed due to softening of nail bed
• Grade II	Obliteration of the angle between nail and nail bed (Lovibond angle; normal ≤ 160°)
• Grade III	Increased curvature of the nail resulting in a parrot beak or drumstick appearance
• Grade IV	Hypertrophic osteoarthropathy, characterised by digital clubbing, arthritis and periostitis of the long bones resulting in painful, tender swelling of wrists (most common), ankles, elbows and knees

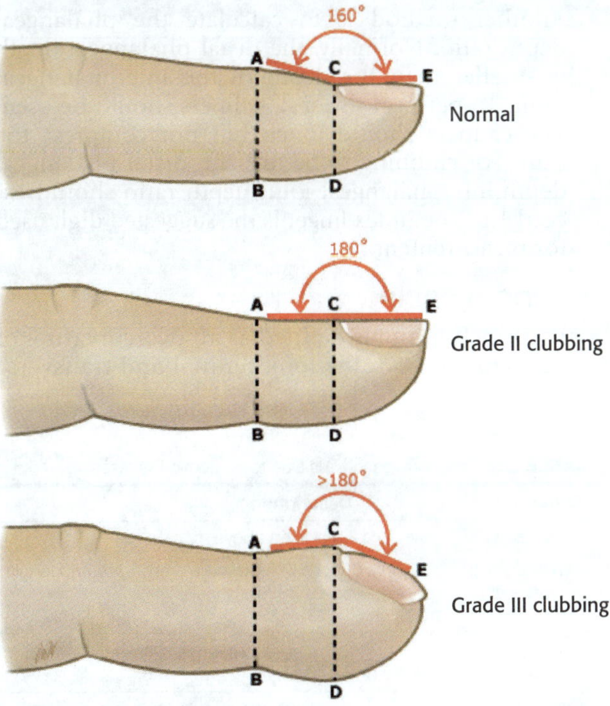

Fig. 2.2 Grading of clubbing.

TABLE 2.5 Common Causes of Clubbing

Respiratory causes	Alimentary causes
• Bronchogenic carcinoma • Bronchiectasis • Lung abscess • Empyema • Mesothelioma • Long-standing tuberculosis • Pulmonary AV fistula • Interstitial lung diseases **Cardiac causes** • Infective endocarditis • Congenital cyanotic heart diseases	• Ulcerative colitis • Crohn's disease • Cirrhosis of liver • Hepatoma **Miscellaneous causes** • Hereditary, idiopathic • Thyrotoxicosis • Acromegaly • HIV infection **Unilateral clubbing** • Pancoast's tumour, subclavian artery aneurysm, dialysis fistula, AV malformations and hemiplegia **Left-sided clubbing** • Presubclavian coartctation of aorta **Unidigital clubbing** • Repeated trauma, Takayasu's arteritis

EXAMINATION FOR CLUBBING

- Clubbing can be assessed by asking the patient to place dorsum of fourth finger of the opposite hands in opposition. Normally, an open diamond-shaped window is visible between the opposing nails due to the presence of Lovibond angle (Fig. 2.3A). Obliteration of this area indicates the presence of clubbing. This is known as Schamroth's sign (Fig. 2.3B).
- An objective measurement of finger clubbing can be made by determining diameter at the base of nail and at the distal interphalangeal joints of all 10 fingers and calculating the digit ratio for each finger. Clubbing is present when the sum of the individual digit ratio is greater than 10.
- Another method is to calculate the phalangeal depth ratio. Normally, the distal phalangeal depth is smaller than the depth of the interphalangeal joint. To perform this test, calipers should be used. The calipers should touch but not compress the skin. For clubbing to be present, distal phalangeal depth:interphalangeal joint depth ratio should exceed 1.0. The index finger is the suggested digit used for measurement.

PSEUDOCLUBBING

- Pseudoclubbing is defined as an overcurvature of the nails in both the longitudinal and transverse axes, with preservation of a normal Lovibond angle.
- Distributed asymmetrically in the fingers.
- Radiographically characterised by resorption of the terminal tufts (acro-osteolysis).
- It can develop in patients with secondary hyperparathyroidism, sarcoidosis, subungual haemangioma and scleroderma.

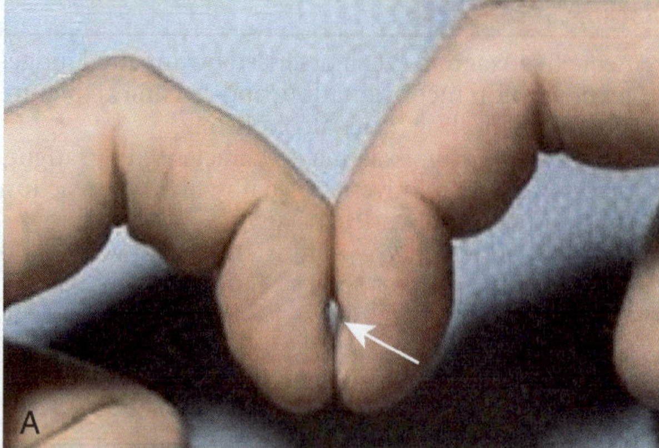

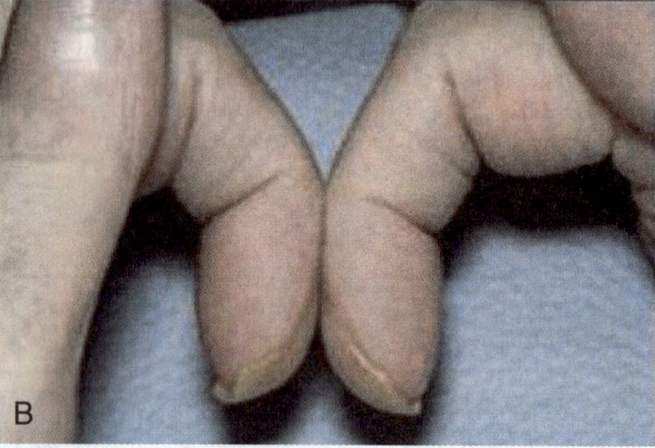

Fig. 2.3 (A) Lovibond angle. (B) Schamroth's sign.

Q. Describe abnormalities in nails due to systemic diseases.

- Table 2.6 describes nail abnormalities seen in systemic diseases.

TABLE 2.6 Abnormalities in Nails Due to Systemic Diseases

Abnormality	Description	Systemic Causes
• Clubbing	Discussed above	Discussed above
• Koilonychia/ platynychia	Spoon-shaped nails (transverse and longitudinal concavity) or flat nails	Iron-deficiency anaemia, haemochromatosis, Raynaud's disease, SLE, chronic exposure of hands to petroleum-based solvents, hypothyroidism or hyperthyroidism
• Pitting	Punctate depressions in nails	Psoriasis, Reiter's syndrome, sarcoidosis, pemphigus, lichen planus, alopecia areata, rheumatoid arthritis
• Onycholysis	Distal nail plate separated from nail bed, resulting in white discolouration of the affected part of the nail	Psoriasis, local infection, hyperthyroidism (Plummer's nail—onycholysis of fourth and fifth digits), sarcoidosis, amyloidosis, connective tissue disorders, pellagra

TABLE 2.6 Abnormalities in Nails Due to Systemic Diseases—cont'd

Abnormality	Description	Systemic Causes
• Onychomadesis	Proximal separation of nail plate from nail bed; often results in shedding of the nail	Trauma, drug sensitivity, poor nutrition, pemphigus vulgaris, Kawasaki disease, hand–foot–mouth disease
• Beau's lines	Transverse linear depressions over nails (occurring at same spot in most nails); move distally with the growth of nail. Reflects a transitory damage to the proximal matrix with a decrease in the keratinocyte mitotic activity	Severe systemic illness that disrupts nail growth, Raynaud's disease, pemphigus, chemotherapeutic drugs
• Yellow nails	Nail has a 'heaped-up' or thickened appearance, yellow in colour, with obliteration of lunula	Lymphoedema, pleural effusion, immunodeficiency, bronchiectasis, nephrotic syndrome, thyroiditis, tuberculosis, cancers, diabetes mellitus
• Terry's (white) nails	Most of the nail plate turns white with obliteration of lunula; all the nails uniformly affected	Liver failure, cirrhosis, diabetes mellitus, heart failure, hyperthyroidism, malnutrition, diabetes mellitus, HIV, pancreatic carcinoma, drugs (cyclophosphamide, itraconazole, vincristine)
• Half-and-half nails (Lindsay's nails)	Proximal portion of nail bed is white because of nail-bed oedema (half-brown, half-white appearance)	Renal failure, HIV infection, Crohn's disease, cirrhosis, malnutrition, drugs (androgens, chemotherapeutic agents)
• Mees' lines	Transverse white bands frequently affecting multiple nails; move distally with growth of nail	Arsenic and thallium poisoning, Hodgkin's disease, CHF, leprosy, malaria
• Muehrcke's lines	Pairs of transverse white lines; disappear on applying pressure; do not move with growth of nail	Hypoalbuminaemia due to any cause, high altitude
• Splinter haemorrhage	Longitudinal, thin, reddish, nonblanchable lines occurring beneath the nail plate	Bacterial endocarditis, SLE, rheumatoid arthritis, dermatomyositis, oral contraceptive use, pregnancy, psoriasis, trauma, trichinosis, scurvy, thrombocytopenia, thrombotic thrombocytopenic purpura, meningococcaemia, high altitude, tyrosine kinase inhibitors (sunitinib, sorafenib)
• Telangiectasia	Irregular, twisted and dilated vessels at the distal portion of cuticle covering the nail bed	Rheumatoid arthritis, SLE, dermatomyositis, scleroderma

Q. Enumerate the pulmonary function tests and give their clinical significance. (CT2.11)

- Various function tests are given in Box 2.4. Abbreviations used in pulmonary function tests are given in Box 2.5.

BOX 2.4 Pulmonary Function Tests

- Ventilatory capacity (FEV_1, FVC, PEF)
- Reversibility of airflow limitation (by administering inhaled bronchodilator)
- Flow–volume curves
- Airway resistance
- Gas transfer (diffusion)
- Lung volumes (TLC, RV)
- Blood gases
- Pulse oximetry
- Exercise tests
- Bronchoprovocative tests
- Exhaled nitric oxide

BOX 2.5 Abbreviations Used in Pulmonary Function Tests

FEV_1	Forced expiratory volume in 1 second	FRC	Functional residual capacity
FVC	Forced vital capacity	RV	Residual volume
VC	Vital capacity	DLCO	Diffusion capacity of the lungs for carbon monoxide
PEF	Peak expiratory flow		
TLC	Total lung capacity		

VENTILATORY CAPACITY

- Forced expiratory volume in 1 second (FEV_1), forced vital capacity (FVC) and vital capacity (VC) are recorded using a spirometer. The patient inhales fully and then forcibly exhales as fast as possible into the mouth piece of the spirometer until no more air can be expelled. A chart records the volume exhaled against time. From this, both FEV_1 and FVC can be measured.
  - FVC is the volume of air expired with a maximal effort after deep inspiration.
  - FEV_1 is the volume of air expired in the first second after deep inspiration.
  - VC is recorded separately by asking the patient to make a full but unhurried ('relaxed') exhalation into the spirometer.
- Two typical patterns of abnormalities can be found:
  1. Obstructive ventilatory defect, where there is narrowing of airways during expiration (e.g. bronchial asthma and chronic bronchitis). Here FEV_1 is markedly decreased, VC is decreased or normal and FEV_1/VC is decreased.
  2. Restrictive ventilatory defect, where FEV_1 and VC are decreased and FEV_1/VC is normal or increased.
- Peak expiratory flow (PEF) can be measured during forced expiration by a gauge or metre, which is simpler and cheaper than a spirometer. It measures the maximum flow generated during expiration performed with maximal force and started after a full

inspiration. Reduced values indicate airflow obstruction. It is of no use in restrictive ventilatory defect.

REVERSIBILITY OF AIRFLOW LIMITATION

- If an obstructive ventilatory defect is found, the responses to bronchodilators (salbutamol) can be measured.
- Reversibility of airflow obstruction is seen in bronchial asthma and, to some extent, in chronic obstructive pulmonary disease.

LUNG VOLUMES

- Values are obtained either by gas dilution methods (nitrogen washout and inert gas dilution) or using a whole body plethysmograph.
- Lung volumes include total lung capacity (TLC) and residual volume (RV). TLC is the amount of air in the lungs at the end of full inspiration. RV is the volume of air in the lungs at the end of full expiration.
- These measurements are not dependent on the effort (unlike spirometry methods).
- They are helpful in differentiating obstructive from restrictive lung diseases (Table 2.7).
- Both TLC and RV are increased in patients with obstructive lung disease while they are reduced in restrictive lung diseases due to parenchymal diseases. In extraparenchymal diseases with restriction during both inspiration and expiration (ankylosing spondylitis and kyphoscoliosis), RV is increased while TLC is reduced. Fig. 2.4 gives various lung volumes and capacities.

FLOW–VOLUME CURVES

- These curves measure flow rates against volume. This helps in analysing the site of obstruction within the lung.
- At the start of expiration, the site of maximum resistance is the large airways, which is reflected in the first 25% of the curve. As the lung volume reduces further, the smaller airways are responsible for most of the resistance. Therefore, calculation of flow rates at 50% and 75% of the VC may be disproportionately reduced in patients with early chronic obstructive airway disease.
- FEF25–75 is the maximal flow rate in the midportion of expiration, that is 25%–75%. It is a sensitive index of small airway function (Fig. 2.5).
- Figs. 2.6A to 2.6D give flow-volume curves in various conditions.

TABLE 2.7 Obstructive Versus Restrictive Patterns in Spirometry

Obstructive Disorders	Restrictive Disorders
FVC normal or reduced	FVC significantly reduced
FEV_1 significantly reduced	FEV_1 reduced
FEV_1/FVC reduced (<0.7)	FEV_1/FVC normal or increased
FEF25%–75% reduced	FEF25%–75% normal
TLC normal or increased	TLC reduced

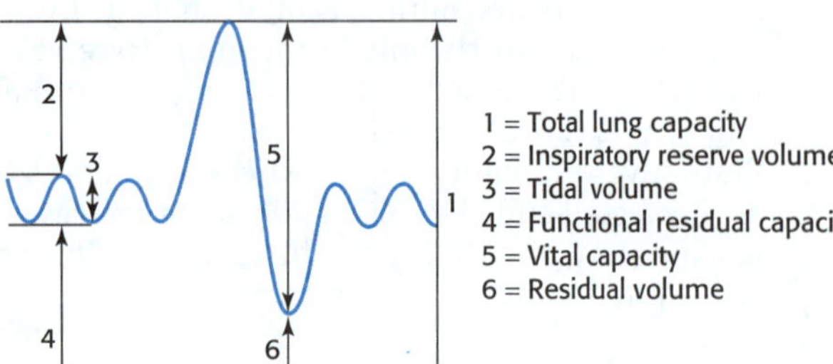

Fig. 2.4 Lung volumes and capacities.

ARTERIAL BLOOD GAS ANALYSIS

- Arterial blood gas (ABG) studies are done with automatic analysers. They measure PO_2, PCO_2 and H^+ concentration in the arterial blood. Oxygen saturation and bicarbonate concentration can be derived from the above-mentioned values.
- Studies are extremely useful in the management of respiratory failure, status asthmaticus and acute respiratory distress syndrome (ARDS).
- Alveolar-arterial oxygen ($PAO_2 - PaO_2$) or $P(A - a)$ O_2 gradient:
  - Useful to interpret PaO_2 when $PaCO_2$ is abnormal, which can occur due to hypoventilation or other reasons.

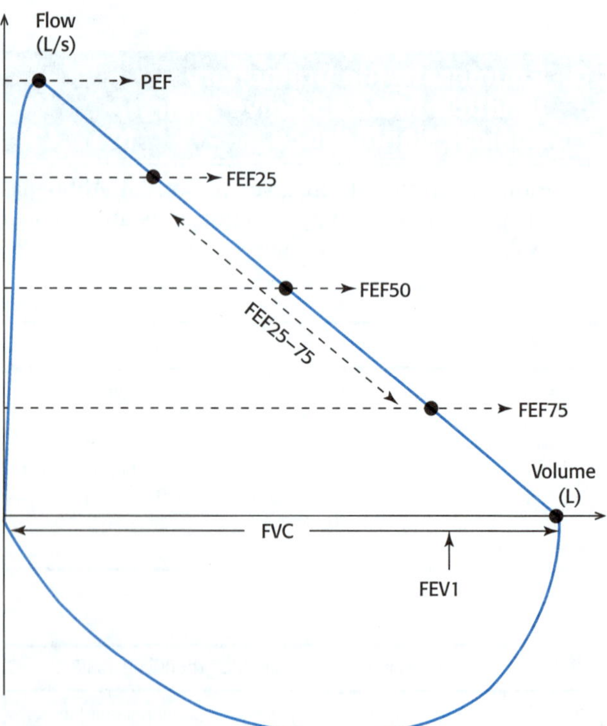

Fig. 2.5 Flow-volume curve. PEF = Peak expiratory flow; FVC = Forced vital capacity; FEV1 = Forced expiratory volume in 1 second; FEF25, 50, 75 = Forced expiratory flow at 25%, 50% and 75% exhalation of forced vital capacity; FEF25–75 = forced expiratiory flow between 25 and 75% of forced vital capacity

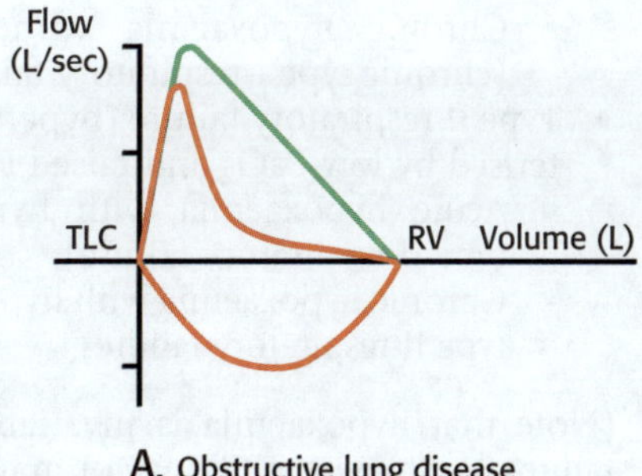

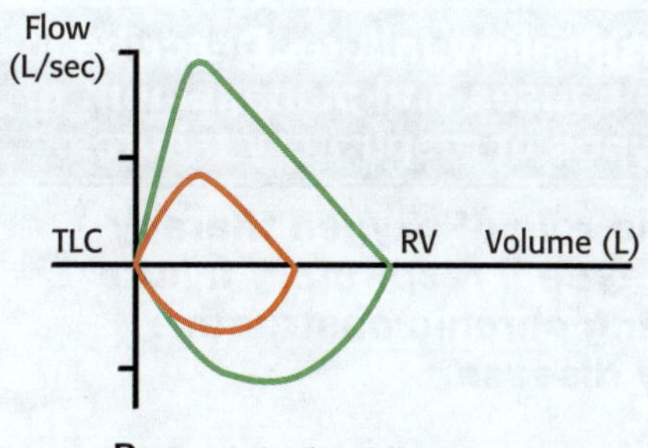

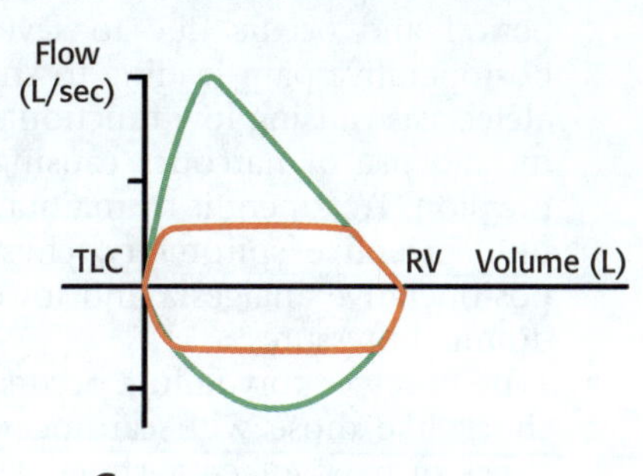

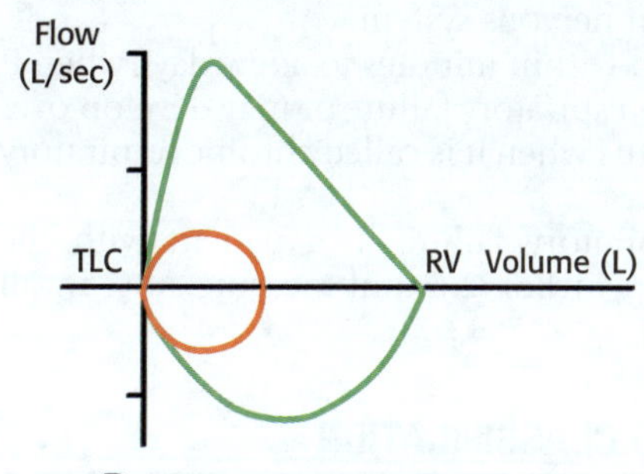

Fig. 2.6 Flow-Volume Curves. A–D: Dark green shows normal flow-volume loops while red shows abnormal flow-volume loops.

- $PAO_2 = FiO_2 \times (P_B - P_{H_2O}) - PaCO_2/R$, where FiO_2 is the oxygen fraction in inspired air (0.21 if breathing air), P_B is barometric pressure (760 mmHg at sea level), P_{H_2O} is water vapour pressure (47 mmHg when air is saturated with water) and R is respiratory quotient (the ratio of CO_2 production to oxygen consumption and is assumed to be 0.8). At sea level, $PAO_2 = 150 - (1.25 \times PaCO_2)$.
- Normal alveolar–arterial oxygen gradient is (age + 10)/4. For any age, this gradient is not more than 20 mmHg.
- A higher gradient in young person reflects impairment of alveolar oxygenation.

TABLE 2.8 Conditions Associated With Abnormal Diffusion Capacity

Reduced Diffusion Capacity	Elevated Diffusion Capacity
• Interstitial lung diseases • Sarcoidosis • Emphysema • Smokers • Anaemia • Pulmonary vascular diseases—chronic recurrent pulmonary emboli, idiopathic pulmonary arterial hypertension, pulmonary vascular involvement with connective tissue diseases (e.g. systemic sclerosis, systemic lupus erythematosus, rheumatoid arthritis) • Drugs—amiodarone, bleomycin, methotrexate	• Severe obesity • Asthma • Polycythaemia • Pulmonary haemorrhage • Left-to-right intracardiac shunting • Pregnancy

DIFFUSION CAPACITY OR TRANSFER FACTOR

- Diffusion capacity is estimated by measuring uptake of carbon monoxide from a single breath of air containing 0.3% carbon monoxide and 10% helium.
- It gives an estimate of matching of alveolar ventilation with pulmonary blood flow and not the diffusion of carbon monoxide. In effect, it gives an estimate of the ability of the lungs to exchange gases.
- Conditions associated with abnormal diffusion capacity are shown in Table 2.8.

EXERCISE TESTS

- Cardiac and respiratory response to bicycle or treadmill exercise can be measured.
- Simple method ('everyday' exercise test) is the measurement of distance that patient can walk in 6 minutes. During a 6-minute walk test, healthy subjects can typically walk 400–700 m.
- Exercise tests are useful in detecting exercise-induced asthma and exercise hypoxaemia, and in assessing disability due to respiratory diseases.

EXHALED NITRIC OXIDE

- Nitric oxide is produced by bronchial epithelium and its production is increased in asthma and airway diseases associated with inflammation.
- Measuring fractional exhaled nitric oxide (FeNO) helps to identify patients who are likely to respond to corticosteroids.

Q. Define respiratory failure. Describe in detail the causes and management of various types of respiratory failures.

Q. Discuss the role of oxygen therapy in chronic type II respiratory failure complicating chronic obstructive pulmonary disease.

- Respiratory failure is not a disease but a condition produced by several diseases.
- Respiratory failure may result from disorders of lungs, chest wall, diaphragm, neuromuscular apparatus or central nervous system.
- It may develop within minutes to a few days when it is called acute respiratory failure or may develop over weeks to months when it is called chronic respiratory failure.
- Consider respiratory failure in a patient with the features shown in Box 2.6 and measure ABG in all such patients.

DEFINITION AND CLASSIFICATION

- Respiratory failure is present when PaO_2 is <60 mmHg (8.0 kPa) with or without $PaCO_2$ >50 mmHg (6.5 kPa).
  - Type I respiratory failure (hypoxaemic) is characterised by low PaO_2 and low or normal $PaCO_2$.
    - Acute hypoxaemia without hypercapnia (acute type I respiratory failure).
    - Chronic hypoxaemia without hypercapnia (chronic type I respiratory failure).
  - Type II respiratory failure (hypercapnic) is characterised by low PaO_2 and raised $PaCO_2$.
    - Acute hypoxaemia with hypercapnia (acute type II respiratory failure).
    - Chronic hypoxaemia with hypercapnia (chronic type II respiratory failure).

(Note that hypoxaemia is invariable in respiratory failure, but hypercapnia may or may not be present.)

- Uncommon types of respiratory failure are type III and type IV.
  - Type III respiratory failure occurs in perioperative period and occurs due to several reasons like postoperative pain leading to shallow breathing, atelectasis causing low functional residual capacity and use of narcotics causing respiratory depression. Treatment is by maintaining sitting posture, incentive spirometry, chest physiotherapy, postoperative analgesia and lowering of intraabdominal pressure.
  - Type IV respiratory failure occurs in patients with shock like those with cardiogenic shock, septic shock or hypovolaemic shock. Due to shock, the oxygen delivery to respiratory muscles is reduced. In addition, the metabolic demand of body is increased.

BOX 2.6 Features Suggesting Respiratory Failure

- Breathlessness at rest
- Central cyanosis
- Raised respiratory rate
- Drowsiness, confusion or unconsciousness

MECHANISMS PRODUCING RESPIRATORY FAILURE (Table 2.9)

- Alveolar ventilation is tidal volume minus dead space multiplied by respiratory rate. Hypoventilation can, therefore, occur due to low tidal volume, increased dead space or reduced respiratory rate. In hypoventilation, $PaCO_2$ increases while PaO_2 decreases. Alveolar–arterial oxygen gradient is normal.
- V/Q mismatch is the most common cause of hypoxaemia. In V/Q mismatch, administration of 100% O_2

TABLE 2.9 Mechanisms Producing Respiratory Failure

• Decreased inspired oxygen concentration	High altitude—acute mountain sickness, chronic mountain sickness; mechanical ventilator failure
• Hypoventilation	Diminished ventilatory drive—drug overdose, primary alveolar hypoventilation, stroke Impaired neuromuscular transmission—Guillain–Barré syndrome, phrenic nerve injury, spinal cord lesion, amyotrophic lateral sclerosis, myasthenia gravis Muscle weakness—myasthenia gravis, muscular dystrophies, electrolyte disturbances, respiratory muscle fatigue Chest wall disorders—kyphoscoliosis, ankylosing spondylitis, flail chest, severe obesity Pleural disorders—pneumothorax, pleural effusion Parenchymal lung disease Airway obstruction—COPD, acute severe asthma, foreign body, vocal cord palsy
• Ventilation–perfusion (V/Q) mismatch	Interstitial lung disease Obstructive airway disease—chronic bronchitis, emphysema, bronchiectasis, asthma Alveolar diseases—pneumonia, acute respiratory distress syndrome (ARDS) Pulmonary vascular diseases—pulmonary embolism, pulmonary hypertension Decreased cardiac output
• Shunt	Intracardiac right-to-left shunts—tetralogy of Fallot, Eisenmenger's syndrome Intrapulmonary shunts—pulmonary arteriovenous shunts, alveolar collapse, pneumonia, pulmonary oedema, pulmonary haemorrhage
• Diffusion abnormality	Interstitial lung disease, ARDS, interstitial pneumonias

will markedly improve hypoxaemia. Alveolar–arterial oxygen gradient is elevated.

- If a shunt is present, deoxygenated blood bypasses ventilated alveoli and mixes with oxygenated blood to cause hypoxaemia. In shunts, hypoxaemia will persist even if patient is given 100% oxygen. Hypercapnia is not common and will occur when shunt fraction is more than 60%. Alveolar–arterial oxygen gradient is elevated.
- Impairment of diffusion is an uncommon cause of hypoxaemia. This is because blood has sufficient time to get oxygenated while passing through pulmonary capillaries. Impairment of diffusion is seen in interstitial lung diseases, ARDS and interstitial pneumonias but the major causes of hypoxaemia in these conditions are V/Q mismatch and shunts.
- In acute respiratory failure, pH of blood may drop to below 7.2 while in chronic, pH is near normal or slightly reduced and bicarbonate is elevated due to renal compensation. Due to associated hypoxaemia, patient with chronic respiratory failure may develop polycythaemia, pulmonary hypertension and cor pulmonale.

ACUTE TYPE I RESPIRATORY FAILURE

COMMON CAUSES (Box 2.7)

- These disorders typically have an abrupt onset, often in patients with previously normal lungs.

MANAGEMENT

- Treat the underlying condition.
- High concentrations (40%–60%) of oxygen through oronasal mask.
- Most patients recover with treatment of underlying disease and oxygen therapy, but a few very ill patients may require artificial ventilation.
- Prone position ventilation is helpful.
- Extracorporeal membrane oxygenation as a last resort.

CHRONIC TYPE I RESPIRATORY FAILURE

CAUSES (Box 2.8)

MANAGEMENT

- Treatment of the underlying causes wherever possible.
- Oxygen therapy, which may be intermittent or at times long term.
- Artificial ventilation may be tried, but in general the prognosis is poor.
- Venesection to reduce haematocrit in patients with severe secondary polycythaemia.
- Diuretics to reduce peripheral oedema.

ACUTE TYPE II RESPIRATORY FAILURE

CAUSES (Box 2.9)

MANAGEMENT

- Treatment of the underlying condition.
- Oxygen therapy to be started with 24% oxygen and adjusted further based on serial measurements of ABG levels.
- Removal of secretions by coughing or emergency bronchoscopic aspiration.
- Bronchodilators in severe airflow obstruction.
- Assisted ventilation (invasive or noninvasive) in selected cases.

CHRONIC TYPE II RESPIRATORY FAILURE

CAUSES (Box 2.10)

MANAGEMENT

- Treatment of the underlying causes.
- Oxygen therapy carries the risk of causing depression of ventilation if respiratory drive has been dependent

BOX 2.7 Common Causes of Acute Type I Respiratory Failure

- Pneumonia (including COVID-19)
- Pulmonary oedema
- Acute respiratory distress syndrome (ARDS)
- Diffuse alveolar haemorrhage
- Acute asthma
- Pulmonary embolism
- Pneumothorax

BOX 2.8 Common Causes of Chronic Type I Respiratory Failure

- Diseases associated with widespread pulmonary fibrosis
- Chronic pulmonary oedema
- Chronic chest wall or neuromuscular diseases
- Chronic pulmonary thromboembolism
- High altitude

BOX 2.9 Common Causes of Acute Type II Respiratory Failure

- Respiratory depressant drugs like diazepam, opiates and alcohol
- Brainstem damage from stroke, encephalitis and trauma
- Disorders of spinal cord, nerves and neuromuscular transmission like spinal trauma, transverse myelitis, acute GB syndrome, poliomyelitis, myasthenia gravis and botulism
- Disorders of muscle affecting respiratory muscles like acute polymyositis
- Severe airflow obstruction like severe acute asthma, laryngeal and tracheal obstruction, acute exacerbation of chronic obstructive pulmonary disease (COPD)
- Chest injuries resulting in tension pneumothorax, massive haemothorax and flail chest

BOX 2.10 Common Causes of Chronic Type II Respiratory Failure

- COPD (most common)
- Chest wall abnormalities like gross kyphoscoliosis, muscle weakness and gross obesity
- Amyotrophic lateral sclerosis, muscular dystrophy
- Central hypoventilation
- Sleep apnoea

on hypoxaemia. Correction of hypoxaemia will then cause a further rise in $PaCO_2$ resulting in confusion, drowsiness or loss of consciousness. Think carefully before prescribing oxygen to such patients. However, oxygen is indicated in selected cases. Note the following points on oxygen therapy:

- Measure ABG levels before oxygen therapy.
- Do not give more than 24% oxygen initially.
- Give oxygen continuously and not intermittently. It is preferable to give oxygen at a rate of 1–2 L/minute.
- Oxygen therapy should be monitored by serial ABG measurements and/or pulse oximetry. In selected cases, oxygen concentration can be increased to 28%–32%.
- Noninvasive or invasive ventilation for selected cases who fail to respond to all other measures.
- Supportive treatment includes antibiotics for respiratory infection, nebulised bronchodilators, clearing secretions by coughing, suction, chest physiotherapy, etc. and diuretics for oedema.

APPROACH TO RESPIRATORY FAILURE (Flowchart 2.1)

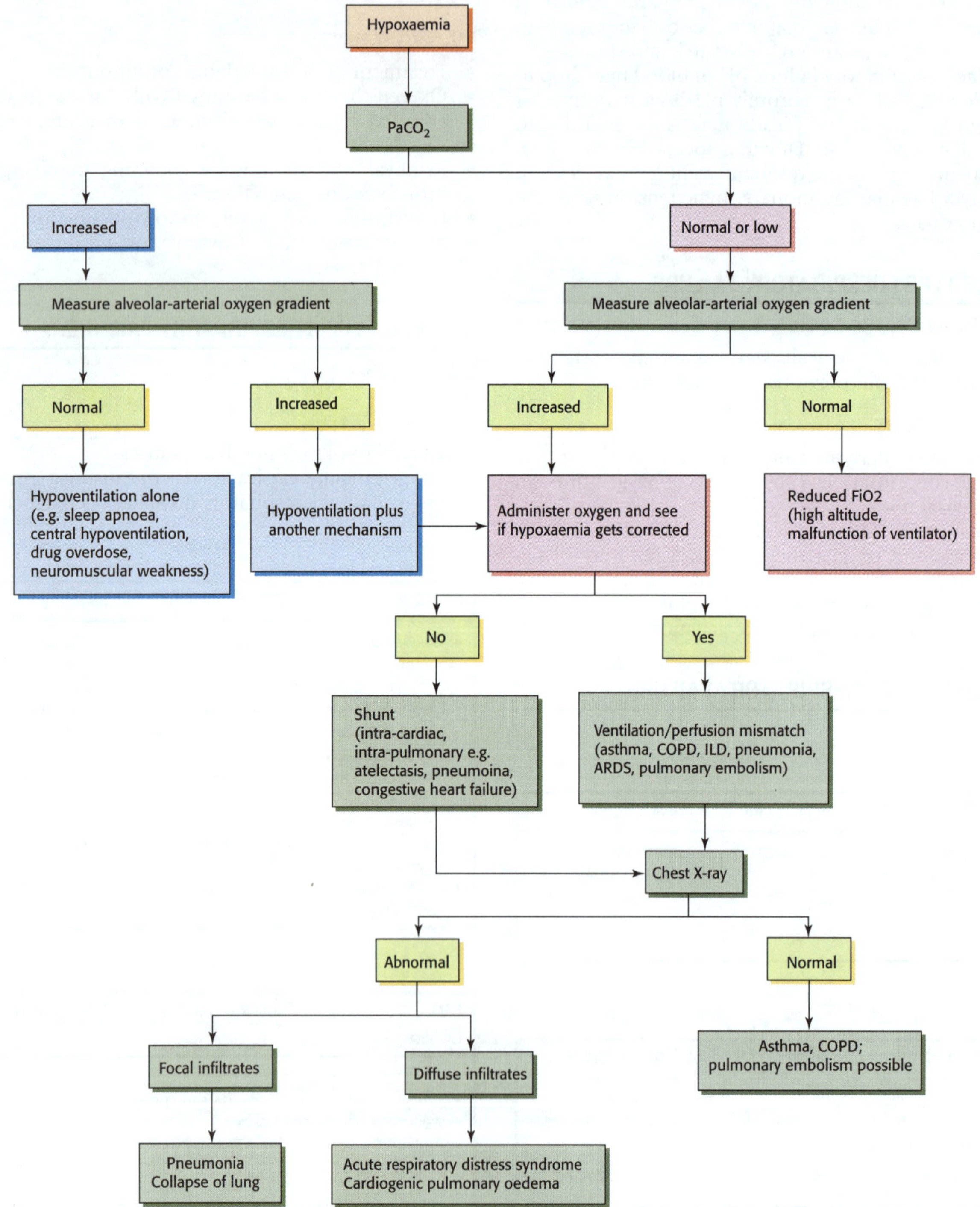

Flowchart 2.1 Approach to Respiratory Failure.

Q. What are sleep apnoea syndromes?

- Sleep apnoea is defined as an intermittent cessation of airflow in nose and mouth during sleep.
- Apnoea is defined as cessation of airflow for at least 10 seconds with a drop in oxygen saturation.
- Hypopnoea is a reduction in airflow to less than 30% for at least 10 seconds, which is followed by an EEG arousal from sleep or with a drop in haemoglobin oxygen saturation by at least 4%.
- Sleep apnoea is of two types:
  - Obstructive sleep apnoea (OSA).
  - Central sleep apnoea.

OBSTRUCTIVE SLEEP APNOEA

- This condition occurs most often in obese middle-aged males.
- Intermittent hypoxaemia leads to sympathetic nervous system overactivity, systemic inflammation and oxidative stress leading to endothelial dysfunction and, possibly, metabolic dysfunction.
- Associated with increased cardiovascular and cerebrovascular mortality and morbidity. Some of the cardiovascular conditions include hypertension, coronary heart disease, arrhythmias, aortic dissection, pulmonary hypertension and heart failure. Also increases risk of metabolic syndrome, type 2 diabetes mellitus and nonalcoholic fatty liver disease (Flowchart 2.2).

RISK FACTORS

- Risk factors for obstructive sleep apnoea are given in Box 2.11.

BOX 2.11 Risk Factors for Obstructive Sleep Apnoea

- Advancing age
- Sex (more common in males)
- Obesity
- Smoking and alcohol consumption
- Atrial fibrillation
- Stroke
- Heart failure
- Craniofacial abnormalities (e.g. retrognathia, tonsillar hypertrophy, enlarged tongue or soft palate, inferiorly positioned hyoid bone, maxillary and mandibular retroposition)
- Endocrine diseases (e.g. acromegaly, hypothyroidism)

PATHOPHYSIOLOGY AND CLINICAL FEATURES

- During sleep, apnoea follows obstruction of upper airway due to pharyngeal closure.
- When awake, this tendency is overcome by the action of opening muscles of the upper airway—the genioglossus and palatal muscles, which become hypotonic during sleep.
- Many patients commonly have anatomical abnormalities of the upper airway such as increased tongue size or enlarged tonsillar tissue, lateral pharyngeal walls and total soft tissue.
- Nonanatomical contributors include impaired pharyngeal dilator muscle function and premature awakening to mild airway narrowing (low respiratory arousal threshold).
- Apnoea leads to hypoxaemia and increasingly strenuous respiratory efforts until the patient overcomes the resistance. The combination of the effort and the central hypoxic stimulation wakes the patient from sleep. These awakenings are so brief that the patient remains unaware of them.
- This produces deprivation of night-time sleep with consequent daytime sleepiness and impaired intellectual performance.
- Many patients also develop hypertension secondary to chronic hypoxaemia.
- Nocturnal symptoms are sometimes apparent to the patient but generally are reported by a bed partner. Bed partners will report a sudden cessation of snoring followed by a loud snort and the resumption of snoring.
- Commonly reported features of obstructive sleep apnoea are mentioned in Table 2.10.

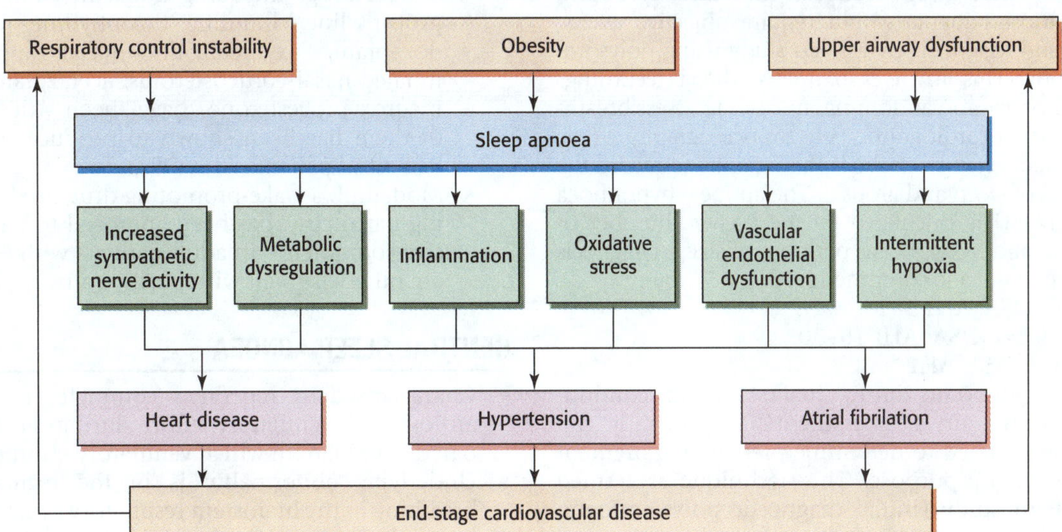

Flowchart 2.2 Potential Aetiological Risk Factors for Sleep Apnoea and the Downstream Consequences. *(Source: Adapted with permission from Javaheri S, et al. J Am Coll Cardiol 2017;69(7):841–58.)*

TABLE 2.10 Common Features of Obstructive Sleep Apnoea

Nocturnal Features	Daytime Features
• Loud snoring • Restless sleep • Nocturnal choking • Witnessed apnoea • Drooling • Gastro-oesophageal reflux • Vivid dreams • Nocturia	• Daytime sleepiness • Morning headache • Hypertension • Pedal oedema (due to pulmonary hypertension) • Reduced libido • Xerostomia • Impaired concentration (increased accidents) • Fatigue

- Pickwickian syndrome (also known as obesity hypoventilation syndrome) represents patients with morbid obesity (BMI > 30 kg/m^2) and daytime hypercapnia (arterial carbon dioxide tension ≥45 mmHg) who have chronic sleep-induced central hypoventilation and develop daytime somnolence. Disorders to be excluded include other disorders that may cause alveolar hypoventilation (severe obstructive or restrictive pulmonary diseases, chest wall disorders, neuromuscular diseases, severe hypothyroidism and congenital central hypoventilation syndrome). Many of these patients also have OSA while a few have sleep hypoventilation (an increase of at least 10 mmHg in $PaCO_2$ during sleep). These patients have daytime hypoxaemia (PaO_2 < 70 mmHg) and hypercapnia ($PaCO_2$ > 45 mmHg), and often develop polycythaemia, pulmonary hypertension and right-sided failure.

DIAGNOSIS

- In many cases, this can be made on the basis of good history supported by pulse oximetry demonstrating fall in oxygen saturation during apnoea. There are severe limitations to this technique, especially the inability to detect apnoeas or hypopnoeas not associated with oxygen desaturation. Furthermore, nocturnal oxygen desaturation may be related to sleep hypoventilation without upper airway obstruction, for example COPD, severe kyphoscoliosis, muscular dystrophy. Thus, most patients would require objective assessment and diagnosis by a sleep study using polysomnography. This involves oximetry, direct recordings from thoracic and abdominal muscles to assess breathing, electrocardiogram, electro-oculography (eye movement) and electroencephalography to record the patterns of sleep and arousal. The apnoea–hypopnoea index (AHI) is calculated by the average number of apnoeas and hypopnoeas per hour of sleep. Diagnosis of sleep apnoea is confirmed if AHI ≥ 5/hour.
    - Mild OSA: AHI 5–15
    - Moderate OSA: AHI 16–30
    - Severe OSA: AHI > 30
- If AHI of 40 occurs during the first 2 hours, continuous positive airway pressure (CPAP) therapy can then be initiated to determine pressure requirement for treatment purpose. This technique is termed split-night study (initial diagnostic polysomnography followed by CPAP titration during polysomnography on the same night).
- Daytime sleepiness can be assessed by various scales. One of the most commonly used scales is Epworth Sleepiness Scale (ESS).

TREATMENT

- Correction of treatable causes (obesity, acromegaly, hypothyroid, enlarged tonsils or adenoids) and removal of any respiratory depressants (alcohol and sedatives).
- Avoiding supine sleep may be all that is required in some patients, particularly those with mild apnoea.
- If these fail, the patient should be given CPAP during sleep. CPAP is initiated and titrated to the level required to eliminate all disordered breathing, snoring and flow limitation. CPAP maintains upper airway patency by creating a 'pneumatic splint'.
- Noninvasive positive-pressure ventilation (bilevel nasal positive pressure [BiPAP]) if CPAP fails.
- Obesity-hypoventilation syndrome:
    - Supplemental oxygen leads to reversal of hypoxic vasoconstriction and redistribution of blood flow to the poorly ventilated alveoli. This leads to an increase in dead space fraction, ultimately leading to worsening of hypercapnia. Therefore, administer oxygen only if oxygen saturation is below 88%.
    - Avoid treating peripheral oedema with diuretics as it can worsen underlying prerenal azotaemia as well as daytime hypercapnia (due to contraction metabolic alkalosis). If required, acetazolamide may be given.
    - Weight reduction and bariatric surgery.
- Oral appliances may be useful in some patients. These devices are designed to advance the mandible, thereby pulling the tongue structure forward and opening the pharyngeal airway.
- Another option is to activate upper airway muscles during sleep by delivering current to the muscles via direct stimulation or via stimulation of hypoglossal nerve.
- Surgery (uvulopalatopharyngoplasty) is required in some cases. It increases the pharyngeal lumen by resecting redundant soft tissue.
- Pharmacotherapy:
    - Several drugs including fluoxetine, mirtazapine, protriptyline, clonidine, theophylline, naloxone, doxapram, oxymetazoline nasal application, inhaled nasal corticosteroids, acetazolamide and medroxyprogesterone have been tried. None of them has been shown to produce consistent benefit in patients with OSA.
    - Modafinil, a wake-promoting drug used for treating narcolepsy, has been approved to treat excessive somnolence in adult patients with OSA who are otherwise well with positive airway pressure.

CENTRAL SLEEP APNOEA

- Characterised by repetitive, complete cessation of airflow and ventilatory effort during sleep (compared with OSA, in which ventilatory effort persists).
- Underlying abnormality is in the regulation of breathing in the brainstem respiratory centre: a modest rise in $PaCO_2$ during sleep results in hyperventilation due to increased chemosensitivity, driving

$PaCO_2$ below apnoeic threshold. At this point, neural drive to respire is too low to stimulate effective inspiration and an apnoea or hypopnoea ensues resulting in rise in $PaCO_2$; this cycle is repeated.

- Causes are a congenital central sleep apnoea (Ondine's curse) and a variety of neurological lesions leading to failure of respiratory drive. Common mechanisms include:
  - Primary central alveolar hypoventilation syndrome (patients have chronic hypoventilation even during daytime, which gets aggravated during sleep).
    - Unknown aetiology.
    - Probably due to high chemoresponsiveness of the respiratory system so that significant hypoxaemia and hypercapnia rarely develop during the course of the disease.
    - Apnoeas are terminated with an abrupt and large breath.
    - Daytime somnolence is less common than that in OSA.
  - High altitude.
  - Stroke, tumours and neurodegenerative diseases (e.g. Parkinson's disease and multisystem atrophy).
  - Left ventricular failure:
    - Associated with Cheyne–Stokes breathing.
    - Associated with the presence of at least 10 central apnoeas and hypopnoeas per hour of sleep in which the hypopnoea has a crescendo–decrescendo pattern of tidal volume accompanied by frequent arousals from sleep.
- Treatment:
  - Administration of oxygen during sleep.
  - Acetazolamide and theophylline may be tried, though effect is modest.
  - Nasal CPAP.
  - Noninvasive positive-pressure ventilation (BiPAP) in patients unresponsive to CPAP.
  - Treatment of heart failure.
  - β-Blockers useful in central sleep apnoea associated with heart failure.

Q. What are the common therapeutic indications of oxygen therapy in clinical practice? Add a note on the hazards of oxygen therapy. (CT 2.20)

THERAPEUTIC INDICATIONS

- Therapeutic indications of oxygen are given in Box 2.12.

BOX 2.12 Therapeutic Indications of Oxygen

- Pulmonary oedema
- COPD
- Respiratory paralysis
- To prevent development of severe pulmonary hypertension
- Carbon monoxide or cyanide poisoning
- Acute attack of bronchial asthma
- ARDS
- Anaerobic infections
- High altitude
- Pulmonary embolism
- Shock

HAZARDS OF OXYGEN THERAPY

- CO_2 narcosis occurs when high oxygen concentrations are administered to patients with ventilatory failure, who are dependent on hypoxic drive, for example COPD.
- Idiopathic epilepsy.
- Lung complications:
  - Irritation of respiratory tract.
  - Pulmonary oedema.
  - ARDS.
  - Consolidation.
  - Progressive decrease in lung compliance, ultimately leading to fibrosis.
- In premature infants and neonates:
  - Retrolental fibroplasia and blindness.
  - Bronchopulmonary dysplasia.

TECHNIQUES OF ADMINISTRATION

- Fraction of inspired oxygen (FiO_2) while inhaling 100% oxygen depends on rate of oxygen flow and minute ventilation of patient.
- Oxygen is humidified, either by passing it over warm water or through a nebuliser.

NASAL CANNULAE

- Double cannulae fit into the nostrils and do not interfere with eating, drinking and wearing of spectacles. They are particularly useful in long-term oxygen therapy.
- Low-flow nasal cannula can provide FiO_2 of 25%–40% depending on flow rate. A flow rate >4 L/minute is poorly tolerated.
- Preferred to a face mask for delivering oxygen to confused or delirious adults if saturation can be maintained.
- The resulting FiO_2 depends upon the patient's minute ventilation and how much room air is entrained. Thus it cannot be precisely controlled.

OXYGEN MASKS

- These are designed to produce a high inspired concentration with FiO_2 varying from 35% to 60% at flow rates of 10–15 L/minute.

VENTURI MASKS

- These are variable oxygen concentration, low to moderate flow devices.
- These air entrainment masks deliver 24%–50% oxygen through a jet-mixing device that causes a controlled entrainment of air and thus allows for deliver of precise oxygen.
- These masks are useful in patients with COPD in whom a precise titration of oxygen concentration may be desirable in order to minimise an increase in PCO_2.

NON-REBREATHER MASK

- A non-rebreather mask has an oxygen reservoir and can provide FiO_2 of 95%. It has a one-way valve that does not allow rebreathing of exhaled air.

HIGH-FLOW NASAL CANNULA

- High-flow nasal cannula oxygen therapy involves delivery of heated and humidified oxygen at rates up to 60 L/minute. Useful in patients with respiratory distress or failure without hypercapnia.
- HFNC provides a flow-dependent FiO_2 by reducing room air entrainment through a greater flow than inspiratory demand.
- It reduces the work of breathing by washing out the carbon dioxide from the upper airways, thereby diminishing the anatomical dead space.
- It also provides low-level positive pressure (~2 cm H_2O). The increase in end-expiratory lung volumes provides better alveolar recruitment and thereby reduces the risk of atelectasis and improves the oxygenation.
- It does not hinder with communication, oral intake and toileting of secretions.

THROUGH ENDOTRACHEAL TUBE

- When a patient cannot maintain adequate ventilation using cannula and mask, endotracheal intubation is required for administration of oxygen.

DEVICES FOR OXYGEN THERAPY (Fig. 2.7)

Device	Flow (L/min)	FiO_2	Advantages	Disadvantages
Nasal cannula (Fig. 2.7A)	1–6	0.24–0.40	• Comfortable • Low cost • No interference with oral feeding	• Limited flow rate • Epistaxis • Unreliable FiO_2
Face mask (Fig. 2.7B)	5–10	0.35–0.60	• Low cost • Can provide humidified oxygen	• Interferes with oral intake • Discomfort to patient
Venturi mask (Fig. 2.7C)	2–15	0.24–0.50	• Precise oxygen concentration • Can provide humidified oxygen	• Interferes with oral intake • Discomfort to patient
Nonrebreather mask	10–15	0.60–0.95	• Delivers high oxygen concentration	• Interferes with oral intake • Discomfort to patient
High-flow nasal cannula (Fig. 2.7D)	15–60	0.3–1.0	• Patient can eat, speak • Provides high minute ventilation • Provides small amount of PEEP • Provides washout of carbon dioxide from dead space	• Discomfort to patient due to high flow • Mucosal dryness and injury • Costly

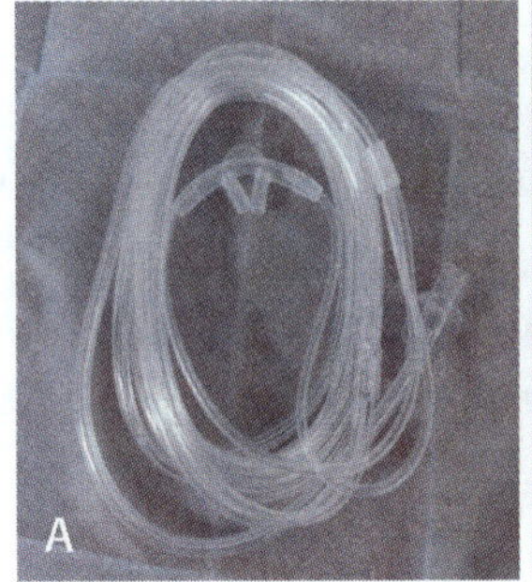

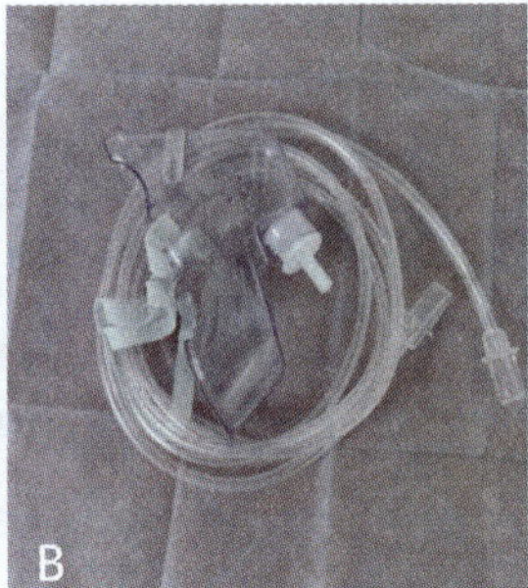

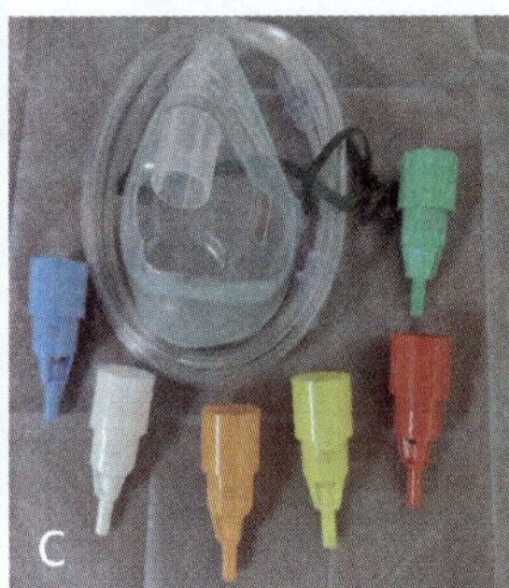

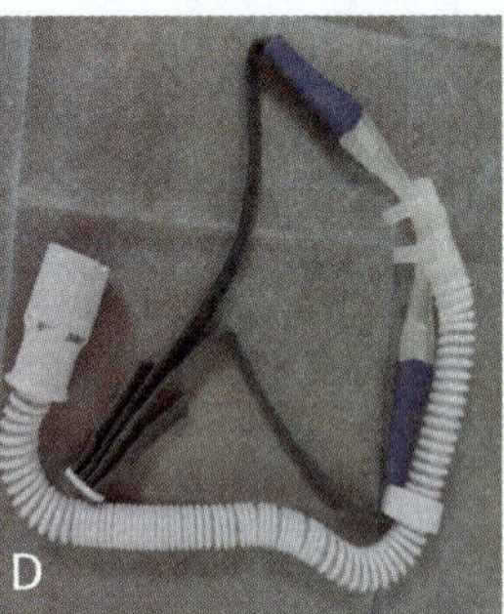

Fig. 2.7 (A) Nasal cannula, (B) face mask, (C) venturi mask, (D) high-flow nasal cannula.

Q. Write a short note on hyperbaric oxygen therapy.

- During hyperbaric oxygen therapy (HBOT), a patient inhales 100% pure oxygen greater than normal atmospheric pressure inside a highly pressured chamber. Inside this chamber, the oxygen pressure is usually 1.5–3 times than that at sea level.
- It increases amount of oxygen dissolved in plasma.
- In carbon monoxide poisoning, it hastens the removal from lungs.

INDICATIONS

- Indications of HBOT are given in Box 2.13.

BOX 2.13 Indications of Hyperbaric Oxygen

- Refectory osteomyelitis
- Carbon monoxide poisoning
- Gas gangrene
- Decompression sickness
- Crush injuries
- Delayed wound healing
- Necrotising bacterial soft tissue infection
- High altitude pulmonary oedema
- Air embolism
- Neuroblastoma stage IV
- Significant cyanide poisoning

CONTRAINDICATIONS

ABSOLUTE CONTRAINDICATION

- Presence of pneumothorax.

RELATIVE CONTRAINDICATIONS (Box 2.14)

BOX 2.14 Relative Contraindications of Hyperbaric Oxygen

- History of pneumothorax
- Uncontrolled hypothermia
- In claustrophobic individuals
- Epilepsy
- Sinusitis
- Otitis
- COPD and asthma
- Optic neuritis
- On bleomycin (increased lung toxicity)
- On insulin, thyroxin and sympathomimetics (increased risk of seizures)

ADMINISTRATION

- HBO therapy is given in chambers which are either monoplace or multiplace.
  - Monoplace chambers can accommodate only one patient at a time. The medical personnel monitor the patients from outside.
  - Multiplace chambers can accommodate multiple patients and a few medical personnel can be inside the chamber for monitoring.
- Generally, HBO therapy is given for 90 minutes with break of 5 minutes every 30 minutes.

COMPLICATIONS (Box 2.15)

BOX 2.15 Complications of Hyperbaric Oxygen

- Seizures
- Pneumothorax
- Tension pneumothorax
- Middle ear damage
- Tympanic membrane rupture
- Pulmonary oxygen toxicity

Q. Describe acute respiratory distress syndrome (ARDS).

Q. What is noncardiogenic pulmonary oedema?

- Acute respiratory distress syndrome (ARDS) is a serious disease characterised by damage to alveolar epithelium and pulmonary capillary endothelium. Alveolar spaces become flooded with oedema fluid of high protein content.
- Noncardiogenic pulmonary oedema is occurrence of pulmonary oedema due to various disorders in which factors other than elevated pulmonary capillary pressure are responsible for protein and fluid accumulation in the alveoli. ARDS is one form of noncardiogenic pulmonary oedema. Others include high-altitude pulmonary oedema, salicylate toxicity, neurogenic pulmonary oedema and re-expansion pulmonary oedema. In practice, terms ARDS and noncardiogenic pulmonary oedema are used interchangeably.

DEFINITION (BERLIN CRITERIA)

- Definition of ARDS is given in Box 2.16.

BOX 2.16 Definition of ARDS (Berlin Criteria)

- Onset within 1 week of a known clinical insult or new/worsening respiratory symptoms
- Partial pressure of arterial oxygen to FiO_2 ratio ≤300 mmHg, irrespective of PEEP
- Bilateral pulmonary infiltrates on chest radiograph not fully explained by effusions, lobar/lung collapse or nodules
- Respiratory failure not fully explained by cardiac failure or fluid overload; need objective assessment (e.g. echocardiography) to exclude hydrostatic oedema if no risk factor present

TABLE 2.11 Aetiology of ARDS

	Common Causes of ARDS
• Pulmonary infections	Viral, bacterial, fungal, *Pneumocystis jirovecii*, *Mycoplasma*
• Aspiration	Vomitus, water (near drowning)
• Inhalation	Ammonia, chlorine, nitrogen dioxide, ozone, oxygen, smoke
• Narcotic overdose	Heroin, methadone, morphine, dextropropoxyphene
• Nonnarcotic drugs	Barbiturates, thiazides, nitrofurantoin
• Systemic disorders	Shock, sepsis, uraemia, eclampsia
• Blood disorders	DIC, blood product transfusion, thrombocytopenic purpura, massive blood transfusion
• Lung emboli	Fat, air, amniotic fluid
• Miscellaneous	Acute pancreatitis, raised ICP, cardiopulmonary bypass, severe trauma with shock, Goodpasture's syndrome, SLE, burns

AETIOLOGY OF ARDS

- Occurs due to a primary lung disease or secondary to a number of systemic disease processes (Table 2.11).

PATHOPHYSIOLOGY

- Related to altered pulmonary capillary permeability and alveolar diffusion capacity, as well as increased intrapulmonary shunt (due to pulmonary vasodilation in nonventilated lung regions and vasoconstriction in ventilated areas).
- ARDS can be divided into three histopathological phases:
  - Exudative phase (1–6 days) is characterised by diffuse alveolar damage with necrosis of majority of type I pneumocytes, diffuse microvascular injury and influx of inflammatory cells and proteinaceous fluid into the interstitium. There is a complex interrelationship between cytokines and proinflammatory mediators that initiate and amplify the inflammatory response. The cellular response includes endothelial adhesion molecule expression, as well as margination and migration of neutrophils. The resulting acute inflammatory exudate inactivates surfactant leading to collapse and consolidation of distal airspaces with progressive loss of the lung's gas exchange surface area. Other responses include release of cytokines, lipid mediators, proteases, oxidants, growth factors, nitric oxide and nuclear factor-kB (NF-kB). Coagulation cascade abnormalities are characteristic in ARDS with an imbalance in both procoagulation and anticoagulation factors.

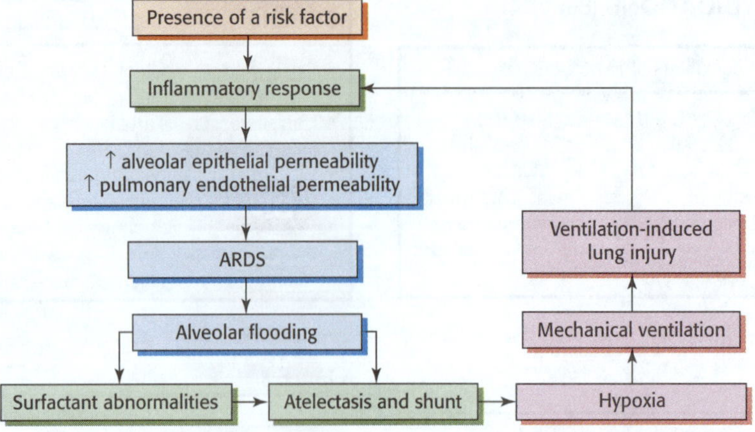

Flowchart 2.3 Pathophysiology of Acute Respiratory Distress Syndrome.

  - Proliferative phase (3–14 days) is characterised by prominent interstitial inflammation and early fibrosis.
  - Fibrotic phase occurs in some cases and is characterised by proliferation of fibroblasts resulting in lung fibrosis.
- Systemic manifestations are frequent due to underlying triggering conditions as well as release of various cytokines (including interleukin-1 [IL-1], IL-6 and tumour necrosis factor [TNF]).
- Multiorgan dysfunction syndrome (MODS) can occur.
- The major pathophysiological consequence of oedema in patients with ARDS is impaired gas exchange with intrapulmonary shunt, which manifests as profound hypoxaemia.
- Flowchart 2.3 depicts pathophysiology of ARDS.

CLINICAL FEATURES

- About 50% of patients who develop ARDS do so within 24 hours of the inciting event.
- The earliest sign is tachypnoea, shortly followed by dyspnoea. A few fine inspiratory crepitations may be audible.
- With progression, the patient becomes cyanotic, more dyspnoeic and tachypnoeic. Crepitations are more prominent and heard throughout both lung fields, especially over basal areas. Tubular breath sounds may be heard.
- Acute cor pulmonale develops in 8%–50% of all patients with ARDS and is associated with adverse haemodynamic and survival outcomes. Echo shows right ventricular dilatation and septal dyskinesia. Risk factors include pneumonia, hypercapnia, hypoxaemia, high airway pressures and concomitant pulmonary disease.
- With further progression, hypotension and worsening of blood gas abnormalities lead to death.

INVESTIGATIONS

- Chest radiography (Box 2.17).
  - Cardiac size is normal
  - Cardiomegaly, bilateral upper lobe vascular diversion and effusions are more suggestive of cardiac failure than ARDS.

BOX 2.17 Chest Radiographic Findings

- In early stages, chest radiograph may be normal or may demonstrate minimal scattered interstitial infiltrates
- Later, diffuse, extensive bilateral interstitial and alveolar infiltrates appear ('fluffy' or 'soft' shadowing). These are located more at the periphery of the lungs
- Air bronchograms are more commonly seen as compared to cardiac pulmonary oedema

BOX 2.18 Severity of ARDS (Based on PaO_2/FiO_2 Ratio)

SEVERITY	DEFINITION
• Mild	PaO_2/FiO_2 ≥200 to ≤300 mmHg with PEEP or CPAP ≥ 5 cm H_2O
• Moderate	PaO_2/FiO_2 ≥100 to ≤200 mmHg with PEEP ≥ 5 cm H_2O
• Severe	PaO_2/FiO_2 ≤100 mmHg with PEEP ≥ 5 cm H_2O

- ABG analysis:
  - In the early stages, the only abnormality is mild hypoxaemia (low PaO_2). As the disease progresses, hypoxaemia worsens and hypercapnia appears.
  - In the late stages, there occur severe hypoxaemia (low PaO_2) and severe hypercapnia (high $PaCO_2$).
  - Severity of ARDS based on ratio of PaO_2 and FiO_2 is given in Box 2.18.
- CT scan:
  - Predominant features of ARDS are diffuse consolidation with air bronchograms, bullae, pleural effusions, pneumomediastinum and pneumothorax.
  - Later, lung cysts may be evident.
- Ultrasound chest:
  - Lung ultrasonography can identify alveolar flooding as it shows bilateral B line patterns, (defined as three or more discrete vertical lines arising from the pleura in an intercostal space), spared areas, pleural line thickening, and subpleural consolidations.

DIFFERENTIATING ARDS FROM HEART FAILURE

- Features which help in differentiating ARDS from heart failure are shown in Table 2.12.

2

TABLE 2.12 ARDS Versus Heart Failure

Parameter	ARDS	Heart Failure
Pleuritic chest pain	May be present	Absent
Sputum production	May be present	Absent
Oedema	Absent	May be present
Jugular venous distension	Absent	Present
Third heart sound	Absent	Present
Bilateral infiltrates	Peripheral	Central (perihilar)
Cardiac enlargement	Absent	Present
Peribronchial cuffing	Uncommon	Common
Kerley lines	Absent	May be present
Pleural effusion	Uncommon	Common
Brain natriuretic peptide	Normal or elevated	Elevated
PaO_2/FiO_2 ratio <300	Present	Mostly absent
Response to diuretics	No	Yes

TABLE 2.13 Summary of ARDS Management

General	• Nutritional support • Prevention of stress ulcers and venous thromboembolism

Oxygenation	• Nasal cannula
	• High-flow nasal cannula
	• Continuous positive pressure ventilation
	• Mechanical ventilation:
	  • Tidal volume limitation—target 6 mL/kg
	  • Plateau pressure limitation < 30 cm H_2O
	  • PEEP titrated to oxygenation with plateau pressure < 30 cm H_2O
	  • Prone positioning (16 hours/day) in moderate to severe ARDS (PaO_2/FiO_2 < 150)
	• Veno-venous extracorporeal membrane oxygenation after prone positioning if PaO_2/FiO_2 < 80 for >6 hours with pH <7.25 and $PaCO_2$ >60 mmHg

Pharmacotherapy	• Early steroids for ARDS with COVID-19 • Conservative fluid strategy for patients not in shock

MANAGEMENT

- Supportive care:
  - Treatment of the underlying cause.
  - Avoiding secondary lung injury such as aspiration, barotrauma, nosocomial infections or oxygen toxicity.
  - Maintaining adequate oxygen delivery to end organs by minimising metabolic rate and optimising cardiovascular function and body fluid balance.
  - Nutritional support.
- Correction of hypoxaemia:
  - Initially, hypoxaemia may be correctable with supplemental oxygen and use of noninvasive ventilation including CPAP and high-flow nasal cannula.
  - In most patients, hypoxia is progressive and the patient often requires intubation and mechanical ventilation with low tidal volume (5–7 mL/kg) and positive end-expiratory pressure (PEEP) between 5 and 20 cm H_2O with a plateau pressure less than or equal to 30 cm H_2O. This strategy is called lung-protective ventilation as it minimises ventilator-induced lung injury. PEEP helps in redistribution of capillary blood flow resulting in improved ventilation–perfusion (V/Q) matching, and recruitment of previously collapsed alveoli and prevention of their collapse during expiration. The goal is to achieve PaO_2 of 55–80 mmHg and oxygen saturation of 88%–95%.
  - In severe ARDS (PaO_2/FiO_2 < 150 mmHg), ventilation in prone position for at least 12–16 hours a day has been shown to improve oxygenation. It optimises blood flow to dependent lung, reduces atelectasis, facilitates secretion drainage and increases functional residual capacity.
  - While on mechanical ventilator, the concentration of inspired oxygen should be kept as low as possible, the goal being maintaining oxygen saturation above 90%.
  - Permissive hypercapnia is a strategy to protect lungs. A gradual and modest increase in $PaCO_2$ (50–75 mmHg) with reasonable degree of acidosis (pH of 7.2–7.3) is achieved by adjusting tidal volume and respiratory rate.
- Optimise systemic perfusion by judicious use of fluids (fluid conservative strategy once shock is corrected), vasopressors, inotropic agents and PEEP.
- Routine stress ulcer prophylactic therapy.
- Role of steroids is controversial. Low-dose glucocorticoid treatment in early ARDS may be associated with reduction in duration of mechanical ventilation and ICU length stay but with no effect on mortality. Dexamethasone is recommended in hospitalised COVID-19 patients with ARDS who are on oxygen or mechanical ventilation.
- Experimental therapies:
  - Nitric oxide inhalation as it is a potent vasodilator that improves blood flow to well-ventilated areas.
  - Ulinastatin, an anti-inflammatory and antioxidant drug agent.
  - Bone marrow-derived multipotent mesenchymal stem cells can differentiate into alveolar epithelial/endothelial cells restoring the epithelial permeability, reduced inflammation and repair injured tissues.
  - Liquid ventilation by filling the lungs with a perfluorocarbon, a low-surface-tension fluid with a high affinity for oxygen and CO_2.
  - Inverse ratio ventilation (inspiration:expiration ratio of 1:1 to 3:1).
  - Extracorporeal CO_2 removal.
  - Extracorporeal membrane oxygenation of blood—utilising external membranes for oxygenation and removal of CO_2 from blood.
- Table 2.13 summarises the management of ARDS.

Q. Discuss noninvasive ventilation.

- Mechanical ventilation can be provided either by endotracheal intubation (invasive ventilation) or by a special mask (noninvasive ventilation [NIV]).

NONINVASIVE VENTILATION

- A tight-fitting full-face or nasal mask is required.
- Used to deliver either continuous positive-pressure ventilation (CPAP) or bilevel positive airway pressure (BiPAP—different levels of positive pressures during inspiration and expiration) ventilation. High-flow nasal cannula (HFNC) is also considered a type of NIV.
- CPAP is applied through a face mask or a nasal mask. During CPAP, pressure greater than atmospheric pressure is applied continuously to the airways. Its use averts airway collapse after expiration, thereby maintaining open alveoli. With CPAP, there is no inspiratory muscle unloading; in fact, tidal ventilation is completely dependent on the respiratory muscles.
- BiPAP, on the other hand, applies a pressure during the inspiratory phase greater than the pressure applied during exhalation. Thus, BiPAP unloads the respiratory muscles and can provide complete respiratory support.
- CPAP is most useful in patients who primarily have hypoxaemic respiratory failure. It is also useful in the final stages of weaning when patients are being observed without ventilatory support. BiPAP can be useful for patients with both hypercapnic and hypoxaemic respiratory failure.
- The patient should be cooperative and medically stable for NIV.

INDICATIONS FOR NONINVASIVE VENTILATION (Box 2.19)

BOX 2.19 Indications for Noninvasive Ventilation

- Acute exacerbation of COPD ($PaCO_2$ > 45 mmHg, pH < 7.35)
- Cardiogenic pulmonary oedema
- Obstructive sleep apnoea
- Others: Acute asthma, pneumonia, respiratory failure associated with blunt chest trauma, early stages of ARDS (PaO_2:FiO_2 ratio between 200 and 300 mmHg)

CONTRAINDICATIONS FOR NONINVASIVE VENTILATION (Box 2.20)

BOX 2.20 Contraindications of Noninvasive Ventilation

- Severe hypoxaemia (PaO_2:FiO_2 ratio < 75)
- Severe acidaemia
- Multiorgan failure
- Upper airway obstruction
- Anatomic abnormalities that interfere with gas delivery (e.g. facial burn and trauma)
- Respiratory arrest
- Cardiac arrest and haemodynamic or cardiac instability
- Uncooperative patient
- Encephalopathy with inability to protect airways and a high risk of aspiration
- Increased risk of aspiration: Copious secretions, vomiting or severe gastrointestinal bleeding
- Recent airway or gastrointestinal surgery
- Inability to fit mask

Q. Discuss various types and modes of mechanical ventilation.

- Mechanical ventilation can be provided either by endotracheal intubation (invasive ventilation) or by a special mask (noninvasive ventilation or NIV).
- Ventilators can be either volume-cycled, pressure-cycled or both volume- and pressure-cycled.
- In volume cycled ventilator, a tidal volume is delivered irrespective of the pressure generated. To protect the patient against high pressures and subsequent barotrauma, a pressure limit is set.

NONINVASIVE VENTILATION

- Discussed above.

INVASIVE VENTILATION

CONTROLLED MANDATORY VENTILATION

- It is the most basic form of positive pressure ventilation in which breaths are supplied at a constant rate with no provision for spontaneous or triggered breaths. A paralysed patient may be started on this mode.
- In the volume-targeted mode, breaths have a preset volume (volume-controlled CMV) while in the pressure-controlled mode, breaths are pressure-limited and time-cycled (pressure-controlled CMV).

ASSIST-CONTROLLED VENTILATION

- This mode allows patient to trigger a breath. A patient-initiated decrease in airway pressure that exceeds a preset threshold activates the ventilator to deliver a full positive pressure breath. The ventilator will use whatever pressure is required to deliver the volume, and patient's lungs and chest should accommodate that tidal volume. In addition, there is a basic back up rate which is reset after every spontaneous breath. If there is no spontaneous breath during this time limit, the ventilator delivers a preset tidal volume breath without patient's respiratory effort.
- This mode may be used in the immediate postintubation period; however, it is not a good mode for prolonged mechanical ventilation.

SYNCHRONISED INTERMITTENT MANDATORY VENTILATION

- At intervals predetermined by the set rate, the ventilator assists spontaneous ventilator efforts of the patient. Between these periods, the patient breathes spontaneously and if no spontaneous breaths are forthcoming, the ventilator delivers the requisite number of positive pressure breaths.
- Compared to CMV, SIMV is associated with a lower incidence of barotrauma.
- This mode is useful for weaning patients from ventilator.

CONTINUOUS POSITIVE AIRWAY PRESSURE

- CPAP is a mode in which the ventilator is only providing the positive end-expiratory pressure (PEEP),

FiO_2 and humidification but does not provide any mechanical breaths.

- CPAP is applied through a face mask or a nasal mask if patient is breathing spontaneously and is not intubated. It can also be applied through an endotracheal tube if patient is intubated. Its use averts airway collapse after expiration, thereby maintaining open alveoli.
- It is useful in patients with no ventilator difficulty who require PEEP to support oxygenation. It is also useful in the final stages of weaning when patients are being observed without ventilator support. It is also used in patients with obstructive sleep apnoea.

PRESSURE SUPPORT VENTILATION

- Strictly speaking, PSV is not a mode of mechanical ventilation; rather it is an adjunct to other modes.
- PSV is pressure-limited flow augmentation. During spontaneous inspiration, the flow is augmented until the desired pressure is achieved and maintained until patient demand decreases below a predetermined level. It results in improved tidal volumes, better patient tolerance of the ventilator, reduced work of breathing and reduced respiratory rates. However, absence of patient effort can result in apnoea.

Q. Discuss the common settings of various ventilatory parameters.

VENTILATOR SETTINGS

TRIGGER SENSITIVITY

- It indicates fall in circuit pressure required to trigger a ventilator. A trigger setting below 1–2 cm H_2O frequently causes ventilator autocycling while a high setting increases the work of breathing.

TIDAL VOLUME

- In ARDS, smaller tidal volumes (5–7 mL/kg) are recommended. With this tidal volume, a small rise in PCO_2 is permitted (permissive hypercapnia). However, the arterial blood pH should be kept above 7.2.

RESPIRATORY RATE

- Optimal respiratory rate depends on the mode of ventilation. With ACV mode, backup rate should be about four breaths less than the patient's spontaneous rate.

INSPIRATORY FLOW RATE

- In most patients on ACV, the initial inspiratory flow is set at 60 L/minute. However, in patients with COPD or with high respiratory drive, the flow rate is generally kept at 100 L/minute.

FRACTIONAL INSPIRED OXYGEN CONCENTRATION

- Initially, FiO_2 is set at 1.0 (i.e. 100%) to ensure adequate oxygenation. Thereafter, the lowest FiO_2 that achieves satisfactory arterial oxygenation should be selected. This helps in reducing oxygen toxicity. Usual target is a PaO_2 of 60 mmHg or oxygen saturation of 90%.

POSITIVE END-EXPIRATORY PRESSURE

- PEEP maintains a positive pressure at the end of expiration, thereby opening the closed alveoli. It improves oxygenation, enhances compliance and reduces works of breathing.
- Deleterious effects of PEEP include barotrauma and reduced cardiac output due to reduced venous return. In addition, myocardial function may be compromised as a result of increased afterload to right ventricle which in turn causes shift of interventricular septum to left side.
- PEEP has been used in patients with pulmonary oedema (both cardiogenic and noncardiogenic) and diffuse lung injury.
- Most initial setups include a PEEP of +3 to +5 cm H_2O. This is gradually increased to achieve the target results.
- Auto-PEEP is the difference between alveolar pressure and the set airway pressure at end-expiration. It is commonly observed with dynamic hyperinflation due to severe airway obstruction. It can be measured during ventilation as the difference between end-expiratory airway occlusion pressure (total PEEP) and the set level of PEEP. The lung distension caused by auto-PEEP increases the risk of barotrauma and may cause cardiovascular instability and increased work of breathing.

PRESSURE SUPPORT VENTILATION

- A pressure support of 8–10 cm H_2O can usually overcome the additional work imposed by the endotracheal tube and ventilator circuit, but higher values may substantially reduce dyspnoea.

Q. Discuss the aetiology, clinical features, investigations, complications and management of seasonal influenza. (IM3.19)

AETIOLOGY

- Influenza viruses type A and type B belong to the group of myxoviruses (RNA viruses). Another influenza virus type C generally causes mild respiratory illness, is associated with sporadic cases and minor localised outbreaks, only affects humans and is not believed to cause epidemics.
- Haemagglutinin and neuraminidase are the major antigenic determinants of influenza A viruses. There are 16 haemagglutinin (H1–H16) and 9 neuraminidase types (N1–N9).
- Since 1977, the circulating seasonal influenza A strains have been primarily of the H1N1 and H3N2 subtypes.
- Haemagglutinin mediates attachment and entry of the virus into host cells. It is also the main viral target of protective humoral immunity by neutralising antibody.
- Neuraminidase facilitates the spread of virions in the host and is the target of neuraminidase inhibitors.
- The M2 protein is a transmembrane proton channel protein responsible for acidifying the virion to allow replication.

- Immunity following infection is type-specific and of short duration.
- Minor antigenic changes periodically occur in either the haemagglutinin or the neuraminidase component or both. This phenomenon is called antigenic drift. It introduces viruses that are different enough from preceding strains and previously acquired immunity is not fully effective against them. This 'drift' contributes to yearly seasonal epidemics and is the basis for the yearly change in vaccine formulations.
- Antigenic shift results in a virus of distinctly different antigenic character to which most or all of the population is susceptible. Generally, such shifts occur only every few decades and are the basis for influenza pandemics.
- Influenza viruses also infect other species, including birds and pigs. At times, these animal strains infect humans and spread from person to person.
- Influenza B viruses also mutate periodically, but less dramatically; they drift but do not shift and thus are associated with seasonal epidemics but not with pandemics.

TRANSMISSION

- The most important transmission routes are through direct contact with infected individuals, contact with contaminated objects, and inhalation of virus-laden aerosols. Respiratory transmission through aerosols containing viral particles can happen during coughing, sneezing, speaking, singing, and even normal breathing.
- Following infection, viral shedding occurs about 24–48 hours before symptoms onset.

CLINICAL FEATURES

- Incubation period is 1–2 days.
- Clinical manifestations are sudden onset of fever (may be absent in infants, elderly patients or immunosuppressed patients), headache, generalised aches and pains, rhinitis, sore throat, anorexia, nausea, vomiting and a harsh unproductive cough. The fauces are hyperaemic and chest is usually clear.
- Ocular symptoms (photophobia, conjunctivitis, lacrimation and pain with eye movement) can also be present.
- In uncomplicated cases, the symptoms subside within 3–5 days.

INVESTIGATIONS (Box 2.21)

BOX 2.21 Investigations in Influenza

- Leucopenia
- Isolation of virus from nasopharyngeal aspirate
- Rapid antigen detection by direct fluorescent antibody or immunochromatogenic assay
- Molecular tests like RT-PCR to detect viral RNA
- Serological tests for specific antibodies

COMPLICATIONS

- Complications of influenza are given in Box 2.22.

BOX 2.22 Complications of Influenza

- Tracheitis, bronchitis, bronchiolitis and bronchopneumonia (primary influenza pneumonia)
- Secondary bacterial pneumonia
- Exacerbation of underlying asthma and COPD
- Myocarditis, worsening of underlying heart failure, myocardial infarction, arrhythmia, pericardial effusion
- Encephalitis, postinfluenzal demyelinating encephalopathy, Guillain–Barre syndrome, myositis, seizure, stroke
- Acute kidney injury, acute tubular necrosis, glomerulonephritis, haemolytic uraemic syndrome, myoglobinuria, rhabdomyolysis
- Postinfluenzal asthenia and depression

MANAGEMENT

- Bed rest till fever subsides.
- Paracetamol 0.5–1 g every 6 hours.
- Aspirin should be avoided, particularly in adolescents and children, because of its association with the Reye's syndrome.
- In influenza A infection, amantadine (100 mg twice a day) or rimantadine (100 mg twice a day) for 3–5 days reduces the average duration of illness by 1 day. Both are M2 inhibitors. Major side effects include central nervous system adverse effects (confusion, disorientation, mood alterations, memory disturbances, delusions, nightmares, ataxia, tremors, slurred speech, visual disturbances and delirium), gastrointestinal upset and antimuscarinic effects. Resistance to these drugs are common and, therefore, not recommended in most patients.
- Oseltamivir, zanamivir, peramivir (neuraminidase inhibitors) and baloxavir marboxil (endonuclease inhibitor) have been approved for the treatment of both influenza A and B. All are equally effective in reducing symptoms and duration of illness when taken within 48 hours of the onset of symptoms. Oseltamivir is given in a dose of 75 mg twice a day while zanamivir is administered by oral inhalation of dry powder at a dose of 10 mg twice a day. Duration of treatment is usually 5 days.
- Specific treatment of complications.

ADVERSE EFFECTS OF ANTI-INFLUENZA DRUGS

- Adverse effects of anti-influenza drugs are given in Table 2.14.

TABLE 2.14 Adverse Effects of Anti-influenza Drugs

Oseltamivir	Nausea, vomiting, abdominal pain, rash, delirium, anaemia
Zanamivir	Cough, headache, bronchospasm, nausea, vomiting, fever, myalgia
Peramivir	Diarrhoea, constipation, insomnia, hypertension
Baloxavir marboxil	Headache, nausea, diarrhoea, neuropsychiatric symptoms

TABLE 2.15 Categorisation of Infleunza Patients (Applicable to H1N1 Influenza as Well)

Category A	• Patients with mild fever plus cough/sore throat with or without body ache, headache, diarrhoea and vomiting • Do not require oseltamivir • Symptomatic treatment • Reassessed at 24–48 hours by the doctor • No tests for influenza • Patients should confine themselves at home and avoid mixing up with public and high-risk members in the family
Category B (i)	• In addition to all the signs and symptoms mentioned under Category A, patient has high-grade fever and severe sore throat • No tests for influenza • Patients should confine themselves at home and avoid mixing up with public and high-risk members in the family • May be given oseltamivir

Category B (ii)	• In addition to all the signs and symptoms mentioned under Category A, individuals having one or more of the following high-risk conditions:
	  • Children with mild illness but with predisposing risk factors
	  • Pregnant women
	  • Persons aged 65 years or older
	  • Patients with lung diseases, heart disease, liver disease, kidney disease, blood disorders, diabetes, neurological disorders, cancer and HIV/AIDS
	  • Patients on long-term cortisone therapy
	• No tests for influenza
	• Patients should confine themselves at home and avoid mixing up with public and high-risk members in the family
	• Treat with oseltamivir

Category C	• In addition to the above-mentioned signs and symptoms of Categories A and B, if the patient has one or more of the following:
	  • Breathlessness, chest pain, drowsiness, fall in blood pressure, sputum mixed with blood, bluish discolouration of nails
	  • Children with influenza-like illness who have a severe disease as manifested by the red flag signs (somnolence, high and persistent fever, inability to feed well, convulsions, shortness of breath, difficulty in breathing, etc.)
	  • Worsening of underlying chronic condition
	• Require testing, immediate hospitalisation and treatment

GUIDELINES TO PREVENT AND CONTAIN OUTBREAK OF INFLUENZA (APPLICABLE TO SWINE FLU AS WELL)

- All individuals seeking consultations for flu-like symptoms should be screened at healthcare facilities and categorised as shown in Table 2.15 to contain outbreak of influenza.

PREVENTION

VACCINATION

- Specific vaccination gives 70% protection.
- Two types of vaccines against seasonal influenza are commonly used: trivalent inactivated vaccine (injectable) and live attenuated influenza vaccine (nasal spray). Both vaccines contain three strains of influenza: an H3N2 virus, an H1N1pdm09 virus and an influenza B virus. Vaccine composition is adjusted yearly.
- Quadrivalent inactivated vaccine has two influenza B strains.
- A recombinant haemagglutinin influenza vaccine is also available for use above the age of 8 years.
- Annual winter vaccination is recommended for patients with chronic pulmonary, cardiac or renal disease. Also recommended for healthcare workers.
- Live attenuated influenza vaccine is approved only for healthy persons and nonpregnant females aged 2–49 years. The inactivated vaccine is approved for use in all persons older than 6 months. Both vaccines are produced in a process that uses chicken eggs and allergy to eggs is a contraindication to either vaccine.
- Live attenuated vaccine should not be given to persons with asthma, reactive airway disease or other chronic cardiopulmonary conditions. It is also contraindicated in persons with other medical conditions such as diabetes mellitus, renal dysfunction, haemoglobinopathies or immune deficiency. Other contraindications include pregnant women and those receiving antiviral drugs active against influenza.

DRUGS

- Amantadine and rimantadine are useful for prophylaxis of influenza A.
- Oseltamivir and zanamivir are helpful in influenza A and B prophylaxis.

Q. Discuss briefly about swine flu (H1N1 influenza) and prevention of human influenza pandemic.

- The pandemic of influenza labelled as H1N1pdm09 influenza or swine flu was reported for the first time in March 2009 from Mexico and then spread globally. Presently, H1N1 influenza is in postpandemic phase. Subsequently, the influenza activity in the world has declined.
- Despite its H1N1 designation, the currently circulating strain that seems to have originated in swine (pig) is entirely different from the H1N1 strains of seasonal influenza and thus triggered a pandemic. It has the genetic structure resulting from reassortment of genes from four influenza viruses, that is North American swine influenza, Asia/Europe swine influenza, human influenza and avian influenza

(non-H5). Reassortment is when two or more viruses infect the same host cell and then exchange genes during replication. The new virion has gene segments from each of its parent virus.

- Unlike yearly epidemics during the cold weather months, pandemics may begin and persist during the warmer months.
- In the H1N1 pandemic, mortality and morbidity is lower compared to that in seasonal influenza.
- Although regular flu is most serious in older persons, novel H1N1 seems to affect younger persons more than older persons, possibly as a result of preexisting immunity against antigenically similar influenza viruses in older people.
- Currently, H1N1pdm09 strain circulates along with typical seasonal influenza viruses and other influenza viruses (H3N2 and influenza B). The H1N1 pandemic was declared to be over in August 2010.

TRANSMISSION

- Like seasonal influenza, H1N1 is thought to be transmissible by three routes: contact exposure (when a contaminated hand is exposed to facial membranes), droplet spray exposure (when infectious droplets are projected onto mucous membranes) and airborne exposure (via inhalation of infectious airborne particles).
- Unlike other type A influenza viruses that are transmitted by small droplet nuclei, H1N1 virus is usually transmitted by large particle respiratory droplets and hence requires a less than 6-feet distance between the source and the susceptible individual to be present for effective spread.
- Indirect transmission from fomites and contaminated surfaces is possible and, therefore, all body fluids (e.g. stool and respiratory secretions) are potentially infectious.
- Infected persons start shedding virus 1 day before the onset of symptoms and shed it at least until symptoms resolve. Children and younger adults may shed the virus for as long as 10 or more days and immunosuppressed persons may shed the virus for weeks.

CLINICAL FEATURES

- The incubation period for the H1N1 virus has been estimated to be between 1 and 7 days, similar to that of seasonal influenza.
- Usually patients present with a mild disease characterised by fever (at least 100.4°F), cough and myalgias.
- Watery diarrhoea is common in H1N1 infection.
- Most patients recover with symptomatic treatment.
- Some cases may develop severe, rapidly progressive course. These patients develop dyspnoea, cyanosis, haemoptysis, chest pain, confusion and hypotension. Ventilatory support is often required in these patients.

COMPLICATIONS

- Similar to those of seasonal influenza (mentioned on page 134).

GROUPS AT HIGH RISK OF INFLUENZA-RELATED COMPLICATIONS (ALSO FOR SEASONAL INFLUENZA) (Box 2.23)

BOX 2.23 Groups at High Risk of Influenza-Related Complications

- Children <5 years
- Adults ≥65 years
- Women who are pregnant or postpartum (within 2 weeks after delivery)
- Persons with certain chronic medical conditions (asthma, COPD, cardiac, haematological, hepatic, neurological and metabolic diseases)
- Immunosuppressed patients
- Adolescents <19 years receiving long-term aspirin therapy

DIAGNOSIS

CASE DEFINITIONS

- These are utilised for reporting purpose.
- A suspected case of H1N1 virus infection is defined as a person with acute febrile respiratory illness (fever ≥ 38°C):
  - With onset within 7 days of close contact with a person who is a confirmed case of H1N1 influenza virus infection, or
  - With onset within 7 days of travel to areas where there are one or more confirmed H1N1 influenza cases, or
  - Who resides in a community where there are one or more confirmed H1N1 influenza cases.
- A probable case of H1N1 influenza virus infection is defined as a person with an acute febrile respiratory illness who:
  - Is positive for influenza A, but unsubtypable for H1 and H3 by influenza real-time polymerase chain reaction (RT-PCR) or reagents used to detect seasonal influenza virus infection, or
  - Is positive for influenza A by an influenza rapid test or an influenza immunofluorescence assay (IFA) plus meets criteria for a suspected case, or
  - Is an individual with a clinically compatible illness who died of an unexplained acute respiratory illness who is considered to be epidemiologically linked to a probable or confirmed case.
- A confirmed case of H1N1 influenza virus infection is defined as a person with an acute febrile respiratory illness and with laboratory-confirmed H1N1 influenza virus infection by one or more of the following tests:
  - RT-PCR, or
  - Viral culture or
  - Fourfold rise in H1N1 virus-specific neutralising antibodies.

DIAGNOSTIC TESTS

- For diagnosis of H1N1 influenza infection, respiratory specimen would generally need to be collected within the first 4–5 days of illness. However, some persons, especially children, may shed virus for 10 days or longer.

- Preferred respiratory samples include nasopharyngeal swab or aspirate, or oropharyngeal swab. In intubated patients, endotracheal aspirates or bronchoalveolar lavage (BAL) should be obtained.
- Clinical samples should be transported on dry ice.
- Available laboratory tests include:
  - Rapid antigen tests: Not as sensitive as other available tests; do not differentiate between various types of influenza A viruses. Detect influenza viral nucleoprotein antigen and can provide results within 30 minutes.
  - Real-time reverse transcription PCR.
  - Virus isolation.
  - Fourfold rise in H1N1 influenza virus-specific neutralising antibodies.
  - Other tests: Haematological and biochemical testing may suggest leucopenia, elevated lactate dehydrogenase and creatine kinase.
  - Chest X-ray abnormalities may be noted in seriously ill patients.

TREATMENT

DRUG THERAPY

- Drug resistance to amantadine and rimantadine has been reported widely and these agents are not recommended for H1N1 influenza.
- Oseltamivir and zanamivir, which inhibit viral release from cells are effective but only if used during the first 48 hours of illness. May improve outcome in critically ill or high-risk patients even if started late.
- Oseltamivir is recommended at a dosage of 75 mg twice daily for 5 days (for treatment) or 75 mg daily for 7–10 days (for postexposure prophylaxis). It can cause nausea and vomiting, rarely confusion, hallucinations and self-injury. Longer treatment is advisable for critically ill patients with respiratory failure.
- Zanamavir is recommended at two inhalations (10 mg) twice a day for similar periods. It is approved only for those without underlying pulmonary or cardiovascular disease.
- Peramivir (given intravenously) and laninamivir (given by inhalation), other neuraminidase inhibitors, may be useful for seriously ill patients.

SUPPORTIVE THERAPY

- Intravenous fluids, parenteral nutrition, oxygen therapy/ventilatory support in severe cases.
- Antibiotics for secondary infection.
- Symptomatic—paracetamol for fever, myalgia and headache; topical decongestants, saline nasal drops, throat lozenges and steam inhalation for sore throat.
- Corticosteroids avoided unless patient develops septic shock.
- Aspirin strictly contraindicated in any influenza patient due to its potential to cause Reye's syndrome.

PREVENTION

GENERAL MEASURES

- Avoid close contact with people who are having respiratory illness.
- Sick persons should keep distance from others. When the ill person is within 6 feet of others at home, the ill person should wear a face mask, if available, or handkerchief or tissues.
- Persons who develop influenza-like illness (fever with either cough or sore throat) should be strongly encouraged to stay at home for 7 days after the onset of illness or at least 24 hours after symptoms have resolved, whichever is longer. Such persons should contact their healthcare providers to report illness by telephone or other remote means before seeking care at a clinic or hospital. If ill persons must go into the community (e.g. to seek medical care), they should wear a face mask to reduce the risk of spreading the virus in the community. If a face mask is unavailable, ill persons should use a handkerchief or tissues to cover any coughing and sneezing.
- Cover your mouth and nose with a tissue or handkerchief when coughing or sneezing.
- If tissue or handkerchief is not available, avoid cleaning the nose with hands; instead, clean with the cuff of shirt or clothes.
- Frequent washing of hands with soap or alcohol-based hand wash (containing at least 60% alcohol) is recommended. Meticulous hand washing remains the cornerstone of effective infection control. Hands should be washed with soap and water for 20 seconds or more, or rubbed with alcohol gel, paying close attention to technique to ensure all areas of the hands and forearms are clean. Areas commonly missed are the web spaces and fingertips.
- Healthcare workers who are likely to come in contact with influenza patient should use surgical masks. N95 particulate respirator masks are recommended only during aerosol-generating procedures such as bronchoscopy or intubation.

DRUG PROPHYLAXIS

Indications

- All close contacts of patients need drug prophylaxis within 48 hours. A close contact is an individual/healthcare worker who has cared for or lived with a person who has confirmed, probable or suspected influenza infection, or who has been in a setting where there was a high likelihood of contact with respiratory droplets and/or body fluids of such a person, including having talked face to face with a person with suspected or confirmed influenza infection.

Drugs and Dosage

- Oseltamivir is the drug of choice. Prophylaxis provided till 10 days after last exposure (maximum period of 6 weeks). Dose is given in Table 2.16.

TABLE 2.16 Prophylactic Doses of Oseltamivir

• Infants younger than 3 months—not recommended
• Infants 3–5 months: 20 mg OD
• Infants 6–11 months: 25 mg OD
	• Older than 1 year:
	  • Weight < 15 kg: 30 mg OD
	  • Weight 15–23 kg: 45 mg OD
	  • Weight 24–40 kg: 60 mg OD
	  • Weight ≥ 40 kg: 75 mg OD

BOX 2.24 Priority Groups for Prophylactic Vaccination With Inactivated Influenza Vaccine

- Pregnant women (because they are at higher risk of complications and can potentially provide protection to infants who cannot be vaccinated)
- Household contacts and caregivers for children <6 months of age (because younger infants are at higher risk of influenza-related complications and cannot be vaccinated; vaccination of those in close contact with infants <6 months old might help protect infants)
- Healthcare and emergency medical services personnel (because they are at high risk for acquiring infection and can also be a potential source of infection for vulnerable patients; also, increased absenteeism in this population could reduce healthcare system capacity)
- All people from 6 months to 24 years of age
  - Children from 6 months to 18 years of age (because they are in close contact with each other in school, college and daycare settings that increases the likelihood of disease spread)
  - Young adults 19–24 years of age (because they often live, work and study in close proximity, and they are a frequently mobile population)
- Persons aged 25–64 years who have health conditions associated with higher risk of medical complications from influenza (cardiovascular disease, pulmonary diseases, diabetes, liver and kidney diseases, immunosuppressed individuals)

VACCINES

- Egg-based, inactivated and live attenuated vaccines (used intranasally) are available in India.
- Inactivated vaccines can be used in person older than 6 months. They are not given if person is allergic to eggs.
- Live attenuated vaccine is for people in the age group 2–49 years and is not meant for pregnant women and those with immunocompromised condition.
- Pandemic influenza vaccines are not expected to provide protection against other influenza viruses.
- The vaccine becomes effective approximately 14 days after vaccination.
- Groups considered to be high priority to receive prophylactic vaccination with inactivated vaccine are given in Box 2.24.

Q. Briefly discuss about avian influenza.

- A primary public health concern of the 21st century.
- Historically, several harmful influenza pandemics have originated from avian influenza viruses through genetic reassortment between human and avian influenza strains.
- Implicated strains of avian influenza at present include H5N1, H7N9, H6N1 and H5N6.
- Avian influenza viruses can be transmitted from their natural reservoir (ducks) to domestic poultry and subsequently to humans.
- Initially H5N1 was reported from China and Hong Kong, but later human cases have been recorded from other parts of the world. H7N9 was reported from China in 2013.
- No evidence of sustained human-to-human transmission, although several small clusters of infections reported.
- Mortality in humans is as high as 50% of the infected patients.

MODE OF TRANSMISSION

- Avian influenza A virus is shed in the faeces of healthy-appearing waterfowl (primarily ducks).
- This infects chickens and other poultry with which they come in contact (faeco-oral transmission).
- Mortality rates in chickens and other birds are high.
- Humans get infected primarily after direct contact of infectious secretions or excreta from infected birds or contaminated poultry products. The main infectious routes are via the upper respiratory tract and conjunctiva. In addition, gastrointestinal tract remains a possible means of entry. Eating cooked poultry poses no risk.
- Conditions for transmission and jumping species barriers often are ideal in Asia, where poultry, ducks, pigs and humans live in crowded conditions.

CLINICAL FEATURES

- History of exposure to infected birds is expected because sustained human-to-human transmission in community setting is not yet known to occur. Transmission can occur in healthcare setting.
- Symptom onset usually 2–5 days after exposure (longer than with human influenza infection).
- Characterised by fever (at least 100.4 °F), cough, rhinorrhoea and myalgias.
- Watery diarrhoea is fairly common particularly with H7N9 virus. Patients may also develop abdominal pain and vomiting.
- Usually followed by viral pneumonia with increasing respiratory distress and ARDS. Ventilatory support is often required. Mortality may be as high as 50%.

INVESTIGATIONS

- Leucopenia, thrombocytopenia.
- Elevated levels of hepatic aminotransferase, lactate dehydrogenase and creatine kinase.
- Chest X-ray shows infiltrates around 7 days after the onset of fever. Other findings may include lobar collapse and focal consolidation.
- Diagnosis is made by viral isolation or detection of H5-specific RNA. Pharyngeal swabs and specimens from lower respiratory tract are preferred for the diagnosis over nasal swabs because avian viral titres are greater in the throat and lower respiratory tract. Reverse transcriptase polymerase chain reaction (RT-PCR) assays are more sensitive in detecting H5N1 than commercial rapid antigen tests.

PREVENTION AND TREATMENT

- Avoid live animal markets and poultry farms in case of an outbreak.

DRUG TREATMENT

- Similar to H1N1 influenza.

Q. Write a short note on severe acute respiratory syndrome (SARS).

- SARS was described for the first time in 2002 from southern China and rapidly spread to several countries within less than a year. More than 8000 probable cases were reported in 29 regions with a death rate of nearly 10%. Presently, it has not been reported from any country. But given the possibility that human or animal reservoirs of the virus may still exist, there is concern that SARS may return.
- A novel coronavirus (SARS-CoV) was identified as the pathogen responsible for SARS. It is not closely related to any of the previously characterised coronaviruses.
- Spreads by close person-to-person contact via droplet transmission or fomite.

CLINICAL FEATURES

- Incubation period 2–10 days but may be as long as 16 days.
- Presents as prolonged influenza-like illness with persistent fever, chills/rigor, myalgia, malaise, dry cough, headache and dyspnoea. Less common symptoms include sputum production, sore throat, rhinorrhoea, nausea, vomiting and diarrhoea.
- About 20% of patients develop evidence of ARDS over a period of 3 weeks.
- Older subjects may present with decrease in general wellbeing, poor feeding, fall and, in some cases, delirium, without the typical febrile response.

LABORATORY INVESTIGATIONS

- Lymphopaenia occurs due to the destruction of both CD4 and CD8 lymphocytes.
- Features of low-grade disseminated intravascular coagulation (DIC) (thrombocytopenia, prolonged activated partial thromboplastin time and raised D-dimer).
- Elevated lactate dehydrogenase, liver transaminases and creatine kinase.
- Chest X-ray:
  - Predominant involvement of lung periphery and the lower zone, and absence of cavitation, hilar lymphadenopathy or pleural effusion.
  - Lesions progress from unilateral opacity to either multifocal or bilateral involvement.
  - Spontaneous pneumomediastinum in some patients.
  - Normal chest X-ray in about 25% of patients.
- Confirmation:
  - Detection of SARS-CoV in urine, nasopharyngeal aspirate and stool specimen using RT-PCR.
  - Quantitative measurement of SARS-CoV RNA in blood with RT-PCR technique.
  - Viral culture.

TREATMENT

- Supportive treatment includes fluid and electrolyte balance, oxygenation and, if required, ventilation with proper protection of healthcare workers.
- Others which have been tried and may be useful include high-dose methylprednisolone (0.5 g daily) if pneumonia or hypoxaemia develops, interferon-α combined with steroids, ribavirin, lopinavir/ritonavir and passive immunotherapy using convalescent phase human plasma.

Q. Write a short note on Middle East respiratory syndrome (MERS).

- Caused by a novel coronavirus (MERS-CoV).
- First case reported in 2012. Most cases have occurred within the Arab Peninsula and neighbouring countries with more than 70% from Saudi Arabia.
- Human-to-human transmission can occur, although spread may not be efficient. Unlike severe acute respiratory syndrome (SARS) coronavirus, MERS-CoV does not preferentially infect healthcare workers.
- Dromedary camels are the major reservoirs of MERS-CoV.
- Transmission occurs more readily if the patient is immunocompromised or has a comorbidity such as diabetes.
- Incubation period 2–14 days (mean 5.2 days).
- Clinical features include flu-like symptoms like cough and fever, followed by lower respiratory tract involvement and ARDS. Some patients may develop abdominal pain, vomiting and diarrhoea. Renal failure has also been commonly reported.
- Leucopenia, thrombocytopenia; elevated liver enzymes, LDH and creatine kinase.
- Chest X-ray shows unilateral or bilateral infiltrates or consolidation.
- Mortality ~50%.
- Diagnosis by RT-PCR.
- Treatment is symptomatic. No drug has been shown to be effective in reducing severity.

Q. Discuss the aetiology, classification, investigations, complications, indications for hospitalisation and treatment of pneumonia. (IM3.1; IM3.12; IM3.15; IM3.17; IM3.2; IM3.3; IM3.5)

Q. Describe suppurative pneumonias and necrotising pneumonias.

DEFINITION

- Pneumonia is defined as inflammation with exudative solidification of the lung parenchyma, generally acute. The term 'pneumonitis' is synonymous but is best avoided.

CLASSIFICATION

- Pneumonias can be classified in a number of ways. Three classifications are given as follows:

A. CLASSIFICATION BY SITE

- Table 2.17 gives classification of pneumonias based on the site of involvement.

B. CLASSIFICATION BY AETIOLOGY

- Pneumonias can also be classified into primary, secondary and suppurative pneumonias.

Primary Pneumonia

- Primary pneumonia is caused by a specific pathogenic organism. There is no preexisting abnormality of the respiratory system. The organisms causing primary pneumonia are given in Table 2.18.
- The term 'atypical pneumonia' has been used to describe pneumonia caused by agents such as *Mycoplasma, Legionella, Chlamydia* and *Coxiella*. Though there are a few symptoms that help in differentiating pneumonia caused by these organisms from pneumococcal pneumonia, there is a considerable overlap in the clinical presentation.

TABLE 2.17 Classification of Pneumonias by Site of Involvement

Alveolar or Air Space Pneumonia or Lobar Pneumonias

- The organism causes an inflammatory exudate that involves many contiguous alveoli. Segmental boundaries are not preserved and the bronchi remain patent. This results in a radiographic appearance of nonsegmental consolidation with air bronchograms. The typical example is pneumococcal pneumonia.

Interstitial Pneumonia

- The inflammation is confined to interalveolar septa. Radiographically, it gives a reticular pattern. *Mycoplasma pneumoniae, Pneumocystis jirovecii* and viruses cause interstitial pneumonia.

Bronchopneumonia

- Inflammation is restricted to the conducting airways, especially terminal and respiratory bronchioles, and the surrounding alveoli. Radiographically, atelectasis may be present and air bronchograms are absent.
- The typical example is staphylococcal pneumonia.

TABLE 2.18 Organisms Causing Primary Pneumonias

Common	Less Common
• *Streptococcus pneumoniae* (most common) • *Haemophilus influenzae* • *Moraxella catarrhalis* • *Staphylococcus aureus* • *Legionella pneumophila* • *Mycoplasma pneumoniae*	• *Klebsiella pneumoniae* • *Streptococcus pyogenes* • *Pseudomonas aeruginosa* • *Coxiella burnetii* (Q fever) • *Chlamydia pneumoniae* • *Chlamydia psittaci* • Viruses: H1N1 influenza virus, seasonal influenza virus, severe acute respiratory syndrome coronavirus-2 (SARS-CoV-2) • *Actinomyces israelii* • *Fungal: Histoplasma, Cryptococcus, Aspergillus*

Secondary Pneumonia (Including Aspiration Pneumonia)

- Secondary pneumonia (aspiration pneumonia) is characterised by absence of any specific pathogenic organism in sputum and the presence of some preexisting abnormality of respiratory system. The preexisting abnormality of the respiratory system predisposes to invasion of the lung by organisms of low virulence derived from upper respiratory tract or oropharynx.
  - Aspiration of pus from infected nasal sinuses.
  - Inhalation of septic matter during tonsillectomy or dental extraction under general anaesthesia.
  - Vomitus or the contents of a dilated oesophagus may enter the larynx and could be aspirated during general anaesthesia, coma or even sleep.
  - Aspiration of gastric contents in patients with gastro-oesophageal reflux disease (GERD).
  - In bronchiectasis and lung abscess, pus may be carried into the alveoli.
  - Ineffective coughing (posttraumatic, postoperative) and laryngeal paralysis predispose to aspiration.
  - Partial bronchial obstruction (e.g. by a tumour) causes stasis of secretions and secondary infection distal to the site of obstruction.

Suppurative Pneumonia (Necrotising Pneumonia)

- In most pneumonias (primary and secondary), with successful inactivation of the organism, complete resolution occurs and normal lung structure is restored. In some cases, complete healing does not occur. Here, the prominent features are destruction of lung tissue by inflammation, cavitation and abscess formation. More than 85% of patients also develop complications such as parapneumonic effusion, empyema or bronchopleural fistula. On healing, fibrosis and bronchiectasis are common. The term suppurative pneumonia (necrotising pneumonia) has been applied to this group of conditions.
- Causative organisms include *Staphylococcus aureus, Klebsiella pneumoniae* and, occasionally, *Haemophilus influenzae* and *Streptococcus pneumoniae*.
- Prolonged antibiotic therapy for more than 3–4 weeks along with drainage of parapneumonic effusion/empyema is required.

C. CLASSIFICATION BY MODE OF ACQUIRING PNEUMONIA

Community-Acquired Pneumonia

- It indicates pneumonia occurring in a person in a community (outside hospital). It is defined as an acute pulmonary infection in a patient who is not hospitalised or living in a long-term care facility 14 or more days before presentation and does not meet the criteria for healthcare-associated pneumonia (HCAP).
- The most common organisms producing CAP are *S. pneumoniae, H. influenzae, Moraxella catarrhalis, Legionella* sp. (Legionnaire's disease), *Mycoplasma pneumoniae* and *Chlamydia pneumoniae*. The first three organisms account for nearly 85% of all cases of CAP. This fact is important for selecting an antibiotic for treatment.

- This category includes both immunocompetent and immunocompromised patients as causative organisms are almost similar in both the cases.

Nosocomial Pneumonia or Hospital-Acquired Pneumonia

- Nosocomial pneumonia indicates the development of pneumonia after more than 48 hours of hospitalisation.
- Majority of cases of nosocomial pneumonia occur outside intensive care units. However, the highest risk is in the patients on mechanical ventilation (ventilator-associated pneumonia [VAP]).

Pneumonia in Immunocompromised Host

- Seen in immunocompromised patients like neutropenic patients, patients with HIV infection and malignancies and patients on immunosuppressives.
- May be caused by classical organisms, atypical organisms, *Mycobacterium tuberculosis* or *Pneumocystis jirovecii*.
- Symptoms are usually more than the signs.

Healthcare-Associated Pneumonia

- Defined as infection occurring within 90 days of a 2-day or longer hospitalisation; stay in a nursing home or long-term care residence in last 30 days; within 30 days of receiving intravenous antibacterial therapy, chemotherapy or wound care or after a hospital or haemodialysis clinic visit; or in any patient in contact with a multidrug-resistant pathogen.
- Patients with HCAP more closely resemble patients with nosocomial pneumonia and may require treatment accordingly.

PATHOLOGICAL STAGES IN DEVELOPMENT OF PNEUMONIA

- There are four pathological stages in development of pneumonia (Box 2.25).

CLINICAL FEATURES

HISTORY

- Classical features of CAP are sudden onset of rigors followed by fever, pleuritic chest pain, cough productive of purulent sputum and haemoptysis.
- Elderly patients often present with confusion, delirium, fatigue, lethargy, anorexia, tachypnoea, tachycardia and, less commonly, pleuritic pain, cough, fever and leucocytosis.

BOX 2.25 Pathological Stages in Development of Pneumonia

- Four stages; all stages may be seen at the same time in different areas:
  - Stage of congestion—just congestion of the vessels without alveolar exudation; fine crepitations may be heard
  - Stage of red hepatisation—intraalveolar exudation especially with RBCs; tubular bronchial breathing heard
  - Stage of grey hepatisation—the exudation is of mainly WBCs with minimal RBCs; tubular bronchial breathing heard
  - Stage of resolution—the exudate is absorbed or removed by macrophages and proteolytic enzymes; coarse crepitations heard

- Patients with atypical pneumonia may have a dry cough. These patients often have extrapulmonary features that include myalgias, arthralgias, prominent headache, mental confusion, abdominal pain and diarrhoea. Haemoptysis is uncommon in atypical CAP.

EXAMINATION

- Approximately 80% of patients are febrile, although this finding is frequently absent in older patients.
- Respiratory rate is high and this may be the most sensitive sign in the elderly.
- Tachycardia is common. However, relative bradycardia is a typical feature of Legionnaire's disease.
- Chest examination reveals crepitations in the involved area. About one-third have bronchial breathing.

INVESTIGATIONS

- Total and differential leucocyte count: Leucocytosis with a high percentage of polymorphonuclear leucocytes suggests bacterial pneumonia. In viral and atypical pneumonias, total leucocyte count is often less than 5000/mm^3.
- Blood culture: This may grow the causative organism, particularly in pneumococcal pneumonia. However, blood cultures are recommended only in hospitalised patients with severe pneumonia or those who are being empirically treated for MRSA or *Pseudomonas aeruginosa*.
- Respiratory secretions: Respiratory secretions should be subjected to microscopic examinations as well as culture. These are recommended only in hospitalised patients. Microscopic examination should include Gram staining and Ziehl–Neelsen staining. Culture (including anaerobic culture when indicated) and sensitivity testing should be done. A freshly obtained specimen of expectorated sputum is the ideal. An ideal sputum specimen can be distinguished from saliva by microscopic examination. An ideal sputum specimen from the lower respiratory tract will have polymorphonuclear leucocytes and alveolar macrophages, but very few oral squamous epithelial cells (a sputum specimen that has more than 25 polymorphonuclear neutrophils and less than 10 epithelial cells per low-power field represents a purulent specimen). If a patient is not able to expectorate, one of the following methods should be employed:
  - Attempt to induce sputum production by the administration of nebulised hypertonic saline.
  - Percutaneous transtracheal aspiration of secretions.
  - Fibreoptic bronchoscopy with BAL and brushings. A transbronchial biopsy of the lung tissue for culture and histology may be done in selected cases.
  - Percutaneous transthoracic needle aspiration, preferably under CT guidance.
- Serological and antigen detection tests: Pneumococcal antigens can be detected in the serum or urine in pneumococcal pneumonia. A fourfold rise in antibody titre over 10 days is useful in diagnosing recent

infection by *Mycoplasma*, *Chlamydia*, *Legionella* and viral infections.

- Radiological studies:
  - Chest radiograph is essential for the confirmation of diagnosis, follow-up and detection of complications like parapneumonic effusion and empyema. For the radiological features of various types of pneumonias, refer classification of pneumonias on page 140. Diagnosis of parapneumonic effusion is discussed on page 231.
  - Ultrasound of chest is more sensitive than chest radiograph. Findings include lung consolidation plus air bronchograms (scattered dotlike and branching hyperechoic dots) that are dynamic (centrifugal movements caused by breathing). Other findings can also be seen, such as the shred sign (or fractal sign), which is an irregular pattern seen in nontranslobar or small consolidations, and pleural effusion.
  - Computed tomography in selected patients.
- Oxygen saturation using a pulse oximeter in patients who are to be managed on outpatient basis.
- ABG analysis: The PaO_2, $PaCO_2$ and H^+ concentration levels are important in the management of seriously ill patients.
- Hyponatraemia, elevated liver enzymes and microscopic haematuria may occur in patients with Legionnaire's disease.
- C-reactive protein and procalcitonin may help distinguish between bacterial and nonbacterial pneumonia. CRP may also be elevated in patients with viral infections, although often not to the same extent as in bacterial infection.

COMPLICATIONS OF PNEUMONIA

- These include parapneumonic effusion, meningitis, arthritis, endocarditis, pericarditis, peritonitis, empyema, septicaemia and ARDS.
- Cavitation or abscess formation occurs in any severe pneumonia, but is more common in *S. aureus*, *Klebsiella* and aspiration pneumonia.
- Pneumothorax, especially in *Staphylococcus* pneumonia.
- Mortality rate of patients who require admission to hospital averages 12% overall but increases to 30%–40% for those with severe CAP who require admission to intensive care unit.

INDICATIONS FOR HOSPITALISATION (Table 2.19)

- The above-mentioned features may also be considered as bad prognostic features.
- The need to hospitalise a patient can also be decided using Pneumonia Severity Index (PSI), which combines several clinical and laboratory features and comorbid conditions, or **CURB-65** (**C**onfusion, **U**rea concentration > 40 mg/dL, **R**espiratory rate ≥ 30/minute, **B**lood pressure with systolic < 90 mmHg or diastolic ≤ 60 mmHg, and Age >65) score. Each parameter is assigned one point to get a severity score. The recommendations on the basis of CURB-65 scoring are: outpatient treatment for patients with a score of 0–1, hospital admission for a score of 2 and consideration for admission to ICU with a score of 3 or more.

TABLE 2.19 Indications of Hospitalisation in Patients With Pneumonia

Age over 65 years	**Signs**
Underlying diseases	• Respiratory rate >30/minute
• Diabetes	• Systolic blood pressure < 90 mmHg
• Renal failure	• Diastolic blood pressure < 60 mmHg
• Congestive heart failure	• Evidence of extrapulmonary involvement (meningitis, arthritis, etc.)
• Chronic lung disease	
• Alcoholism	**Laboratory parameters**
• Immunosuppression	• White blood cell count <4000 or >30,000/mm³
• Postsplenectomy	
• Malignancy	• PaO_2 < 60 mmHg on room air
Altered mental status	• Renal failure
	• Haematocrit <30%
	• Multilobar involvement on chest X-ray

TREATMENT

GENERAL MEASURES

- Check the airway, breathing and circulation.
- Treat shock with intravenous fluids initially.
- Correct hypoxia with oxygen inhalation. If hypoxia continues or patient develops increasing hypercapnia, ventilate the patient mechanically.
- Treatment of pleuritic pain with mild analgesics like paracetamol or codeine.

ANTIMICROBIAL THERAPY

Empirical Regimens

- Administer antibiotics as soon as feasible once the diagnosis of CAP is established.
- Empirical therapy for CAP is based on providing coverage against the most likely pathogens responsible for CAP.
- The antibiotic selected should therefore be active against common typical and atypical pathogens, unless one can clinically differentiate these organisms.
- Macrolides (erythromycin, clarithromycin and azithromycin) should not be used alone in moderately sick patients with CAP since nearly 25% of strains of *S. pneumoniae* are naturally resistant to macrolides.
- Newer fluoroquinolones like levofloxacin and moxifloxacin have better Gram-positive coverage than ciprofloxacin. These are effective against both typical and atypical pathogens and can be used as monotherapy, particularly if the patient is not severely ill. However, their use should be restricted as tuberculosis is always a possibility in patients with pneumonia and use of fluoroquinolones may produce partial response and lead to resistance of tubercular bacilli to these agents.
- Ceftriaxone has no activity against atypical pathogens and should not be used alone in moderately sick patients.
- Doxycycline remains effective against both typical and atypical pathogens and is an effective choice in patients with CAP.
- Daptomycin is not effective for MRSA pneumonia because it is inactivated by pulmonary surfactant.
- For pneumonia due to typical organisms without an underlying comorbidity, the usual duration of

therapy is 5–7 days. For *Mycoplasma* and *Chlamydia* pneumonia, and immunocompromised patients, the duration is 10–14 days. Patients initially treated with intravenous antibiotics can be switched to oral agents when afebrile.

- Lefamulin is the first pleuromutilin antibiotic approved for the treatment of CAP. Pleuromutilin antibiotics exert their action by binding to the peptidyl transferase centre of the 50S ribosome via several interactions, thereby preventing the binding of transfer ribonucleic acid (tRNA) for peptide transfer and inhibiting protein synthesis. Lefamulin exhibits both bactericidal and bacteriostatic activity against gram-positive (including MRSA), fastidious gram-negatives, atypical pathogens and some gram-negative anaerobes. It is an option for those who are intolerant to beta-lactams, fluoroquinolones and macrolides.
- The approach for empirical antibiotics is shown in Table 2.20.

CORTICOSTEROIDS

- For patients with severe CAP, corticosteroids may decrease the risk of ARDS and modestly reduce intensive care unit and hospital stays. Use of corticosteroids should be weighed against possible adverse effects.

RISK FACTORS FOR ANTIBIOTIC RESISTANCE

- Common risk factors for resistance to antibiotics are shown in Box 2.26.

BOX 2.26 Risk Factors for Antibiotic Resistance

- Age (either >65 or <5 years)
- Alcoholism
- Child attending a daycare centre
- Multiple comorbidities
- Prior exposure to an antimicrobial within last 3 months

UNRESOLVED PNEUMONIA

- Indicates persistent consolidation despite initial antibiotics and passage of more than 6 weeks.
- Important causes are:
  - Incorrect diagnosis (e.g. neoplasm, pulmonary embolism, systemic vasculitis and eosinophilic pneumonia).
  - Incorrect microbiological diagnosis (e.g. tuberculosis instead of classical organisms).
  - Bronchial obstruction causing partial or complete obstruction.
  - Immunocompromised state.
  - Nosocomial superinfection.
- Further evaluation in form of microbiological tests for the aetiological agent, CT chest, bronchoscopy, biopsy and other tests are required.

RECURRENT PNEUMONIA

- A number of conditions can produce recurrent pneumonias (Box 2.27).

TABLE 2.20 Empirical Antibiotic Therapy for Pneumonia

Type of Pneumonia	Antibiotic Treatment
• Uncomplicated pneumonia; patient not requiring hospitalization	Azithromycin (500 mg once a day) or clarithromycin (500 mg twice a day) orally alone[a] or in combination with cefuroxime (500 mg twice a day) or amoxicillin (1 gm thrice a day) Or doxycycline 100 mg 12 hourly Or fluoroquinolone (levofloxacin 750 mg once a day or moxifloxacin 400 mg once a day) Other alternatives: Amoxicillin/clavulanate, cefixime, cefpodoxime
• Outpatient adults with comorbidities such as chronic heart, lung, liver or renal disease, diabetes mellitus, alcoholism, malignancy or asplenia	Amoxicillin/clavulanate 500 mg/125 mg three times daily, or amoxicillin/clavulanate 875 mg/125 mg twice daily Or a cephalosporin (cefpodoxime 200 mg twice daily or cefuroxime 500 mg twice daily) PLUS a macrolide Or Respiratory fluoroquinolone as monotherapy (levofloxacin or moxifloxacin)
• Moderately sick patients requiring hospitalization	Ceftriaxone 2 g once a day IV or cefotaxime (1–2 g 8 hourly) or amoxicillin-clavulanic acid PLUS azithromycin or clarithromycin Fluoroquinolones alone
• Severely sick patients	Ceftriaxone or cefotaxime PLUS either azithromycin 500 mg IV once a day or levofloxacin 750 mg IV once a day If allergic to β-lactam, replace ceftriaxone with aztreonam If methicillin-resistant *S. aureus* (MRSA) is suspected,[b] add vancomycin or linezolid to the above-mentioned regimens
• Underlying diseases[c] (patient sick)	Piperacillin–tazobactam (4.5 g four times day) or cefepime (2 g thrice a day) or a carbapenem (meropenem 1 g thrice a day or imipenem/cilastatin 500 mg four times a day) or ceftazidime (2 g thrice a day) PLUS • A fluoroquinolone (ciprofloxacin or levofloxacin), or • An aminoglycoside

[a]Only in areas with pneumococcal resistance to macrolides <25%.
[b]Prior influenza-like illness, necrotising severe pneumonia or if a sputum Gram stain shows Gram-positive cocci in clusters.
[c]Bronchiectasis, use of steroids, repeated exacerbations of COPD, malnutrition, antibiotics for >7 days within 1 month increase risk of infection by *Pseudomonas*.

BOX 2.27 Causes of Recurrent Pneumonias

- Bronchial obstruction (e.g. foreign body, bronchial stenosis, compression of bronchus, endobronchial lesions)
- Bronchiectasis
- Sequestration of lung
- Immunocompromised state
- Ciliary dyskinesia
- Multiple myeloma and other lymphoreticular malignancies

Q. Discuss the aetiology, clinical features, diagnosis, complications and management of pneumococcal pneumonia (lobar pneumonia). (IM3.19)

AETIOLOGY

- It is the most common form of pneumonia and the causative organism is *S. pneumoniae* (i.e. pneumococcus, a Gram-positive, lancet-shaped diplococcus).
- The disease spreads by droplet infection.

PATHOLOGY

- Pneumococcal pneumonia is characterised by homogeneous consolidation of one or more lobes or segments. There are four stages in the natural course of the illness:
  1. Stage of congestion.
  2. Stage of red hepatisation.
  3. Stage of grey hepatisation.
  4. Stage of resolution.

RISK FACTORS FOR PNEUMOCOCCAL PNEUMONIA

- Risk factors for pneumococcal pneumonia are given in Box 2.28.

CLINICAL FEATURES

- Onset is often sudden with fever, chills and rigors and vomiting. Convulsions may occur in children. Fever is usually high grade (39 °C–40 °C).
- Nonspecific symptoms include loss of appetite, headache and aching pains in the body and limbs.
- Localised pleuritic chest pain develops at an early stage. It may be referred to the shoulder or abdominal wall.
- Cough is initially short, painful and dry but soon becomes productive.
- Sputum is characteristically rust coloured ('rusty' sputum) but occasionally frankly blood stained.
- Breathing is rapid and shallow due to pleuritic pain.
- Other features are tachycardia, hot and dry skin, herpes labialis, flushed face and, occasionally, central cyanosis.

PHYSICAL SIGNS IN THE CHEST

- In the first 2 days, physical signs are minimal. These include diminished respiratory movements, slight impairment of percussion note and pleural rub.
- Later, frank signs of consolidation appear. These are included in Box 2.29.

INVESTIGATIONS

- Marked neutrophil leucocytosis.
- Blood culture may show *S. pneumoniae*.
- Gram staining of the sputum may demonstrate pneumococci as Gram-positive and lancet-shaped diplococci.
- Sputum culture may show *S. pneumoniae*.
- Chest radiograph shows a homogeneous opacity localised to the affected lobe or segment, with air bronchograms.
- Associated parapneumonic effusion or empyema can be detected.
- Serological tests can detect pneumococcal antigen in serum, urine and sputum.
  - In urine, C-polysaccharide (part of pneumococcal cell wall) by an immunochromatography assay is quite sensitive. Urinary antigen remains positive for weeks after onset of severe pneumococcal pneumonia. However, it is often negative in mild infections.
  - Assays on sputum are based on detecting nucleic acids for pneumococci. However, these assays do not differentiate between colonisation and infection.
- In rare cases, fibreoptic, bronchoscopic aspiration or transthoracic needle aspiration is required.

COMPLICATIONS

- Complications of pneumococcal pneumonia are listed in Table 2.21.

TREATMENT

GENERAL MEASURES

- Oxygen in high concentrations should be administered to all hypoxaemic patients.

BOX 2.28 Risk Factors for Pneumococcal Pneumonia

- Younger than 2 years or older than 65 years
- Poverty and overcrowding
- Asplenia or hyposplenia
- Alcoholism
- Diabetes mellitus
- Antecedent influenza
- Defects in humoral immunity (complement or immunoglobulin)
- HIV infection
- Severe liver disease
- Chronic lung disease
- Use of inhaled corticosteroids or antipsychotics

BOX 2.29 Signs of Consolidation

- No mediastinal shift, diminished respiratory movements, dull percussion note, markedly increased vocal fremitus and vocal resonance and high-pitched tubular bronchial breathing. Bronchophony, aegophony and whispering pectoriloquy may be present. In early stages, numerous fine crepitations are audible, but later (during resolution) they become coarse.
- If parapneumonic effusion develops, additional signs of pleural effusion appear.

TABLE 2.21 Complications of Pneumococcal Pneumonia

Pulmonary	Pleural
• Delayed/incomplete resolution • Spread to other lobes (rare) • Necrotising pneumonia	• Sterile pleural effusion • Empyema
Cardiovascular	**Neurological**
• Acute circulatory failure • Acute pericarditis • Endocarditis (rare)	• Mental confusion • Meningism • Meningitis

- Treatment of pleuritic pain with mild analgesics like paracetamol. However, some patients require morphine 5–10 mg or fentanyl 50 µg intravenously.
- Assisted coughing in patients who suppress cough because of pleuritic pain.

ANTIBIOTIC THERAPY

- If patient is not seriously ill, the initial treatment should consist of one of the following:
  - Ampicillin 500 mg four times daily orally.
  - Erythromycin 500 mg four times daily orally or azithromycin 500 mg once a day.
  - Doxycycline 100 g twice a day orally.
- In moderate to severely ill cases, the treatment consists of the following:
  - Ceftriaxone 2 g IV once a day or cefotaxime 1–2 g 8 hourly.
  - Fluoroquinolone (e.g. levofloxacin 750 mg once a day).
  - Amoxicillin clavulanic acid 1.2 g 8 hourly intravenously.
- Total duration of therapy in an uncomplicated case is 5–7 days.

VACCINE

- Two types:
  - The pneumococcal polysaccharide vaccine (PPV) consists of 23 most common capsular serotypes that cause invasive pneumococcal disease in the developed world. Its effectiveness is hampered by poor responses in elderly people, immunocompromised patients and children younger than 2 years (precisely those at greatest risk for severe pneumococcal disease).
  - Second vaccine is polysaccharide–protein conjugate pneumococcal vaccine (pneumococcal conjugate vaccine [PCV]) that generally targets seven serotypes responsible for most of pneumococcal infections in children. It is approved for use mainly in children younger than 2 years and adults older than 50 years. It also induces herd immunity as it reduces the frequency of invasive pneumococcal disease infection in nonvaccinated siblings and even adult contacts. A 13-valent PCV is also available.

INDICATIONS

- Indications for pneumococcal vaccination are given in Box 2.30.

BOX 2.30 Indications of Pneumococcal Vaccine

- Age >65 years
- Patients with risk factors: Congestive heart failure, asthma, COPD, diabetes mellitus, chronic liver disease, alcoholism
- Splenectomised patients including patients with sickle cell anaemia
- Persons living in long-term care facilities
- Immunocompromised persons

TABLE 2.22 Recommendations on Use of Pneumococcal Vaccines

Persons ≥ 65 Years	
Not vaccinated previously	A single dose of PCV13 followed by a dose of PPV23 ≥ 1 year later
Vaccinated previously with PPV23	A single dose of PCV13 ≥ 1 year after receipt of PPV23
Persons between 19 and 65 years where pneumococcal vaccine is indicated	
Not vaccinated previously	A single dose of PCV13 followed by a dose of PPV23 ≥ 2 months later; a second dose of PPV23 recommended after 5 years
Vaccinated previously with PPV23	A single dose of PCV13 ≥ 1 year after receipt of PPV23 followed by one dose of PPV23 (≥2 months following PCV13 and ≥ 5 years after PPV23 dose)

RECOMMENDATIONS ON IMMUNISATION FOR PPV23 AND PCV13

- Table 2.22 gives current recommendations on the use of PPV23 and PCV13.

Q. Give a brief account of staphylococcal pneumonia.

- Caused by *S. aureus*.
- Common following influenza, in debilitated patients in hospital and in those with cystic fibrosis.
- Methicillin-resistant *S. aureus* (MRSA) is an important pathogen in nosocomial pneumonia.
- Recently, community-acquired MRSA (CA-MRSA) infections (skin and soft-tissue infections and necrotising pneumonia) occurring in previously healthy persons have emerged as a serious clinical concern.
- Abscess formation is very common. The abscesses are thin walled, multiple and often bilateral.
- Abscesses may rupture into pleura to produce pneumothorax or pyopneumothorax.
- Chest radiograph shows bronchopneumonia, often bilateral, with multiple thin-walled cyst-like lesions (pneumatocoeles).
- Sputum smear shows Gram-positive cocci in clumps.

ANTIBIOTIC THERAPY

- If the infection is not severe, second-generation cephalosporins (cefuroxime), amoxicillin-clavulanic acid, fluoroquinolones or macrolides (erythromycin, azithromycin, clarithromycin) are used.

- If the infection is severe, third- or fourth-generation cephalosporins (cefotaxime, ceftriaxone or cefepime) should be used.
- If methicillin-resistant organisms are suspected as in nosocomial infections or in locations where prevalence of CA-MRSA is significant, vancomycin (1 g IV twice a day) or linezolid (600 mg twice a day) should be given. Linezolid belongs to oxazolidinone group of antibiotics. It is useful in infections caused by Gram-positive organisms including MRSA, multiresistant strains of *S. pneumoniae* and vancomycin-resistant *Enterococcus faecium* (VRE).

Q. Give a brief account of Klebsiella pneumonia (Friedlander's pneumonia).

- Caused by *K. pneumoniae* (Friedlander's bacillus).
- Common in alcoholics and diabetics.
- Severe illness with a high mortality rate.
- Massive consolidation of one or more lobes, the upper lobes being most often involved. Abscess formation and pleural effusion are common.
- The sputum may be viscid, jelly like and blood stained (currant jelly sputum) but may be purulent or rusty.
- Chest radiograph shows an air space pneumonia, usually in one of the upper lobes, with abscess formation and pleural effusion. Bulging interlobar fissure is a characteristic finding.
- Sputum smear shows Gram-negative bacilli. *K. pneumoniae* can be isolated from the sputum.

ANTIBIOTIC THERAPY

- Gentamicin, ceftazidime or ciprofloxacin is given for a period of 2–3 weeks. In severe cases, piperacillin + tazobactam or meropenem should be given.
- Extended-spectrum β-lactamases (ESBL)–producing organisms have increasingly been reported. In such cases, treatment options include meropenem (or imipenem + cilastatin), amikacin and tigecycline. Polymyxin B can be considered against highly resistant strains.

Q. Discuss the aetiology, clinical features, investigations and treatment of atypical pneumonias.

Q. Give a brief account of Legionella pneumonia (Legionnaire's disease).

- Atypical pneumonias are caused by three organisms: *Legionella pneumophila*, *M. pneumoniae* and *C. pneumoniae*.
- Suspect an atypical organism as the cause of pneumonia if patient has four or more of the following:
  - Age <60 years
  - No underlying comorbid condition
  - Paroxysmal cough
  - No expectoration
  - Few clinical signs on chest examination
  - Total leucocyte count <10,000/mm^3

LEGIONELLA PNEUMONIA OR LEGIONNAIRE'S DISEASE

- Transmitted in water droplets originating in infected humidifier cooling systems and from stagnant water in cisterns and showerheads. Person-to-person spread has not been reported.
- Clinical features are fever with chills and cough with scanty mucoid sputum. Gastrointestinal symptoms like nausea, abdominal pain and diarrhoea, and mental confusion or delirium are common.
- Among cases of CAP with atypical causes, Legionnaires' disease has the most severe clinical course, and illness can become progressively more severe if the infection is not treated appropriately and early. Uncommon features include myocarditis, pericarditis and prosthetic valve endocarditis, as well as glomerulonephritis, pancreatitis and peritonitis.
- Chest radiograph shows parenchymal lesions progressing from patchy to lobar consolidation. Pleural effusion may be seen in more than one-third of patients. Complete clearing of infiltrates may take 1–4 months.
- Relative lymphopaenia, very high ESR, hyponatraemia, proteinuria and microscopic haematuria are common.
- The organism is not visible on Gram staining. Sputum and bronchoscopic specimens should be sent for culture. Direct fluorescent antibody test on sputum is highly specific but less sensitive than sputum culture.
- Specific diagnosis is often made by a fourfold or greater rise in indirect fluorescent antibody in the serum. Another moderately sensitive method is to demonstrate *Legionella* antigen in the urine.
- Another disease caused by *Legionella* is Pontiac fever, which is a self-limiting and flu-like illness.

MYCOPLASMA PNEUMONIA

- Caused by *M. pneumoniae*, an organism which lacks cell wall.
- It is the pathogen most often associated with atypical pneumonia.
- Onset is insidious, over several days to a week.
- Constitutional symptoms include headache exacerbated by cough, malaise, myalgias and sore throat. Cough is usually dry, paroxysmal and worse at night.
- Clinical course is usually mild and self-limited.
- Pulmonary complications include effusion, empyema, pneumothorax and acute respiratory distress syndrome.
- Extrapulmonary manifestations include skin manifestations (erythema multiforme, erythema nodosum, maculopapular and vesicular eruptions and urticaria), hepatitis, neurological involvement (aseptic meningitis, encephalitis, Guillain–Barré syndrome and transverse myelitis), myocarditis, pericarditis and pancreatitis.

- Production of cold agglutinins can result in haemolytic anaemia.
- Diagnosis:
  - Mild leucocytosis may be present.
  - Fourfold rise in antibody titres.
  - Nucleic acid amplification method for rapid detection in throat swab.
  - Cold agglutinins are nonspecific but help in diagnosis.

CHLAMYDIA PNEUMONIA

- *C. pneumoniae* is an obligate intracellular organism.
- Transmission results from contact with respiratory secretions.
- Incubation period is several weeks.
- More likely to occur in older patients with comorbid diseases than in those who are otherwise healthy.
- Presentation is usually with sore throat, headache, low-grade fever and cough that can persist for months.
- Chest radiographs tend to show less extensive infiltrates than are seen with other causes of pneumonia.
- Diagnosis is by serological studies and culture or PCR of respiratory tract samples.
- Another species of *Chlamydia* that can cause pneumonia is *C. psittaci*. It generally causes disease in birds. Occasionally, humans can get infected (psittacosis).
- Doxycycline is the drug of choice.

ANTIBIOTIC THERAPY OF ATYPICAL PNEUMONIAS

- Erythromycin or one of the other macrolides (clarithromycin or azithromycin) is the drug of choice.
- Doxycycline is also an effective drug.
- Fluoroquinolones have excellent activity against all three atypical organisms. In addition, fluoroquinolones have the advantage of once-daily dosing and excellent bioavailability, whether they are given intravenously or orally.
- β-Lactams are not effective.

Q. Give a brief account of actinomycosis.

- Caused by *Actinomyces israelii*, an anaerobic organism existing in the mouth as a commensal.
- When local defences are impaired, it can result in disease. Three forms of the disease are recognised:
  - Oral-cervicofacial actinomycosis with soft-tissue swelling, abscess and discharging sinuses.
  - Abdominal actinomycosis with discharging sinuses, abdominal mass or abscess.
  - Pulmonary actinomycosis with widespread suppurative pneumonia, empyema (often bilateral) and persistent discharging chest wall sinuses.
- Pus from the sinuses contains 'sulphur grains'.

ANTIBIOTIC THERAPY

- Benzylpenicillin 18–24 million units intravenously (in four divided doses) for 4–6 weeks followed by oral penicillin for 6–12 months.

Q. Give a brief description of pneumonias caused by viruses (viral pneumonias).

- Influenza, parainfluenza, measles, varicella (chickenpox), respiratory syncytial virus and SARS-CoV-2 (severe acute respiratory syndrome-coronavirus-2) are the commonly implicated pathogens.
- Other viral pneumonias include SARS and Middle East Respiratory Syndrome produced by novel *coronaviruses*.

CLINICAL FEATURES

- The clinical picture differs from that of bacterial pneumonias in a number of aspects.
- Fever and toxaemia usually precede respiratory symptoms by several days.
- Severe headache, malaise and anorexia are characteristic early features.
- Physical signs in the chest are absent or minimal, whereas radiological findings are striking.
- Splenomegaly may be present during the first week.
- Leucocyte count is usually normal and the condition may not respond to penicillins.
- Diagnosis is confirmed by isolation of virus, serological tests and RT-PCR.
- Viral pneumonias are usually self-limiting. Fever subsides in 5–10 days, followed by complete clinical recovery and radiographic resolution.
- Death occurs from complications like widespread extension of pneumonia or viral encephalitis.

TREATMENT

- Treatment is mainly supportive with oxygenation and cardiopulmonary support.
- Varicella can be treated with intravenous acyclovir or vidarabine.
- Treatment of influenza pneumonia includes use of oseltamivir, zanamivir, amantadine or rimantadine.
- Ribavirin is effective for respiratory syncytial virus infection.
- Dexamethasone is administered for hospitalised patients of SARS-CoV-2 infection requiring oxygen or mechanical ventilation.

Q. Give a brief account of acute bronchopneumonia.

- It is a type of secondary pneumonia, invariably preceded by bronchial infection. It is particularly common in patients with chronic bronchitis. The lesions are bilateral and patchy, often extensive in the lower lobes.
  - In children, it occurs as a complication of measles or whooping cough.
  - In adults, it occurs as a complication of acute bronchitis or influenza.
  - In elderly or debilitated patients, it is described as 'hypostatic pneumonia'.
- Viral pneumonias and 'atypical' pneumonias may also be present as bronchopneumonia.

CLINICAL FEATURES

- High fever, severe cough with purulent expectoration, breathlessness, tachycardia, tachypnoea and central cyanosis.
- In early stages, physical signs in the chest are those of acute bronchitis, but later crepitations become more numerous.
- Chest radiograph shows bilateral mottled opacities, predominantly in the lower zones.
- Neutrophil leucocytosis is common.

ANTIBIOTIC THERAPY

- Ampicillin or cotrimoxazole given orally is effective in mild bronchopneumonia.
- In serious cases, a third-generation cephalosporin along with a macrolide should be used.

Q. Describe eosinophilic pneumonias.

Q. Discuss in brief about pulmonary infiltrates with eosinophilia.

Q. Briefly discuss chronic eosinophilic pneumonia (Carrington's disease).

Q. What is tropical pulmonary eosinophilia? Explain.

- Pulmonary infiltrates with eosinophilia or eosinophilic pneumonias are characterised by eosinophilic pulmonary infiltrates and peripheral eosinophilia.
- Features include:
  - Peripheral blood eosinophilia with abnormal pulmonary imaging studies (chest X-ray and/or CT chest).
  - Eosinophilia in lung parenchyma in transbronchial or open lung biopsies.
  - Increased eosinophils in bronchoalveolar lavage (>10%).

PULMONARY INFILTRATES WITH EOSINOPHILIA—CAUSES

- Causes of pulmonary infiltrates with eosinophilia are listed in Box 2.31.

ASPIRIN-EXACERBATED RESPIRATORY DISEASE

- It is a syndrome characterised by severe asthma, eosinophilic chronic rhinosinusitis, nasal polyps and aspirin or nonsteroidal anti-inflammatory drug intolerance. Peripheral eosinophilia is common.
- Treatment is avoidance of aspirin and later, aspirin desensitisation using oral aspirin. Another method is intranasal ketorolac challenge and desensitisation followed by oral aspirin challenge.
- Omalizumab (anti-IgE monoclonal antibody) and dupilumab (anti-IL-4-receptor-α monoclonal antibody) improve symptoms.

BOX 2.31 Causes of Pulmonary Infiltrates With Eosinophilia

- Allergic bronchopulmonary aspergillosis (ABPA)
- Drug reactions (e.g. nitrofurantoin, sulphonamides, penicillins, allopurinol, thiazides, isoniazid, *para*-aminosalicylic acid, imipramine, chlorpropamide, daptomycin, vancomycin)
- Parasitic infestations (e.g. filaria, roundworm, hookworm)
- Aspirin-exacerbated respiratory disease
- Loeffler's syndrome
- Acute eosinophilic pneumonia
- Chronic eosinophilic pneumonia (CEP)
- Eosinophilic granulomatosis with polyangiitis (Churg–Strauss syndrome)
- Hypereosinophilic syndrome
- Tropical pulmonary eosinophilia

LOEFFLER'S SYNDROME

- A benign, acute eosinophilic pneumonia due to migrating larvae of *Ascaris lumbricoides, Ancylostoma duodenale, Necator americanus* and *Strongyloides stercoralis* through lungs.
- Migratory pulmonary infiltrates on imaging with minimal clinical features (an irritating, nonproductive cough and burning substernal discomfort). Uncommon features include dyspnoea, wheezing, fever and blood-tinged sputum containing eosinophil-derived Charcot–Leyden crystals.
- Diagnosis often requires detection of parasitic larvae in respiratory secretions, as stool examination for ova and parasites may be nondiagnostic, with the exception of strongyloidiasis.
- Specific therapy not required in most cases. Patients with strongyloidiasis should be treated with ivermectin mainly to reduce the risk of autoinfection and dissemination.

ACUTE EOSINOPHILIC PNEUMONIA

- Acute illness of unknown cause presenting with cough, fever and dyspnoea.
- Patient may develop acute respiratory failure.
- A recent history of cigarette smoking or exposure to smoke, fine sand, dust or e-cigarette use is often present.
- Basal crepitations on auscultation.
- Generally, illness lasts for <7 days. Some patients have symptoms for 4 weeks.
- Neutrophilic leucocytosis; peripheral eosinophilia rare at presentation but develops during the course of disease.
- Chest radiograph shows bilateral, diffuse pulmonary infiltrates; occasionally, pleural effusion.
- Bronchoalveolar lavage shows increased eosinophils (>25%).
- Diagnostic criteria are shown in Box 2.32.
- Treatment includes supportive care and mechanical ventilation. Steroids are life-saving.

CHRONIC EOSINOPHILIC PNEUMONIA (CARRINGTON'S DISEASE)

- Chronic eosinophilic pneumonia (CEP) is a disease of an unknown cause.

BOX 2.32 Diagnostic Criteria for Acute Eosinophilic Pneumonia

- Acute respiratory illness ≤1 month duration
- Pulmonary infiltrates on chest radiography or computed tomography
- Pulmonary eosinophilia (>25% eosinophils in BAL fluid) or eosinophilic pneumonia on lung biopsy
- Absence of other specific pulmonary eosinophilic diseases, including eosinophilic granulomatosis with polyangiitis, hypereosinophilic syndrome and allergic bronchopulmonary aspergillosis

- The hallmark of CEP is eosinophil accumulation in the lungs.
- Female preponderance with a peak incidence in the fifth decade.
- More common in nonsmokers.
- Onset is insidious with weight loss, cough, fever, dyspnoea, wheezing and night sweats.
- Asthma precedes or accompanies illness in 50%.
- Examination may reveal rhonchi and crepitations in some patients.
- Chest X-ray usually shows bilateral peripheral shadows (photographic negative of pulmonary oedema), which may be migratory. HRCT is more informative.
- Peripheral eosinophilia (>1000/mm^3) is usual.
- BAL reveals eosinophilia (eosinophils >25% of lavage fluid cells).
- Standard treatment is with oral steroids; however, relapses are common when daily steroid dose is reduced below 15 mg. Long-term oral steroids are often required.
- Treatment with inhaled steroids may be of some value.

HYPEREOSINOPHILIC SYNDROME

- A group of disorders with sustained overproduction of mature eosinophils (hypereosinophilia) with eosinophilic infiltration of organs causing their damage.

DIAGNOSTIC CRITERIA

- Diagnostic criteria for hypereosinophilic syndrome are shown in Table 2.23.

CLASSIFICATION

- Hypereosinophilic syndrome can be primary, secondary or idiopathic (Table 2.24).

CLINICAL FEATURES AND TREATMENT

- The most common presenting signs and symptoms are weakness, fatigue, cough, dyspnoea, myalgias, angioedema, rash, fever and rhinitis.
- Features of multiple organ involvement (e.g. cardiac involvement—myocarditis, endomyocardial fibrosis, tricuspid valve involvement; pulmonary involvement—dyspnoea, cough, parenchymal infiltrates, pleural effusion; skin involvement—eczema, dermographism, erythroderma, urticaria; CNS involvement—encephalopathy, thromboembolism, peripheral neuropathy, etc.).

TABLE 2.23 Diagnostic Criteria for Hypereosinophilic Syndrome

HYPEREOSINOPHILIA
• Presence of >1500 eosinophils/mm^3 in blood on two examinations separated in time by at least 1 month and/or tissue hypereosinophilia
TISSUE HYPEREOSINOPHILIA
• Bone marrow showing eosinophils >20% of all nucleated cells and/or • Tissue infiltration that is extensive in the opinion of a pathologist and/or • Marked deposition of eosinophil granule proteins in tissue (in the absence or presence of major tissue infiltration by eosinophils)
ORGAN DAMAGE
• Eosinophil-mediated organ damage and/or dysfunction, provided other potential causes for damage have been excluded

TABLE 2.24 Classification of Hypereosinophilic Syndrome

• Primary (or neoplastic) HES	An underlying stem cell, myeloid or eosinophilic neoplasm (clonal expansion)
• Secondary (or reactive) HES	Overproduction of eosinophilopoietic cytokines by other cell types (polyclonal). Examples include heavy parasitic infections, certain solid tumours and T-cell lymphoma
• Idiopathic HES	Underlying cause unknown despite thorough workup

- Treatment involves use of corticosteroids and hydroxyurea along with management of organ dysfunction.
- Those associated with myeloproliferative or lymphoproliferative diseases respond to imatinib.

TROPICAL PULMONARY EOSINOPHILIA

DEFINITION

- Tropical eosinophilia is a hypersensitivity response to microfilariae, particularly filarial parasite (*Wuchereria* and *Brugia*), trapped in lung.
- The syndrome is characterised by pulmonary manifestations and peripheral blood eosinophilia of more than 2000/mm^3.

CLINICAL FEATURES

- Tropical eosinophilia can present in various forms (Box 2.33).

BOX 2.33 Different Forms of Tropical Pulmonary Eosinophilia

- Asymptomatic form
- Respiratory form (commonest)
- Alimentary form
- A form with constitutional disturbances
- A form with generalised lymphadenopathy and hepatosplenomegaly

- The common respiratory form may be either acute or chronic.
  - The acute type presents with high-grade fever, exertional breathlessness and cough with scanty expectoration.
  - The chronic type presents with vague ill health, low-grade fever, exertional dyspnoea and cough with scanty expectoration.
  - Chest findings absent in majority; a few have bilateral rhonchi and crepitations, particularly basal.

INVESTIGATIONS

- Total leucocyte count is raised.
- Peripheral blood eosinophilia of more than 2000/mm^3.
- Raised serum IgE levels (>1000 units/mL).
- Raised filaria-specific IgG and IgE levels.
- Microfilariae are absent in peripheral smear.
- Sputum examination shows clumps of eosinophils and Charcot–Leyden crystals.
- Chest radiograph and CT chest (high-resolution) shows bilateral, diffuse, fine mottling in many patients, mimicking miliary tuberculosis. Some patients may show reticulo-nodular lesions on radiograph. Nearly 20% patients have normal chest radiograph.
- Pulmonary function tests show predominant restrictive defect with some evidence of obstructive ventilatory defects.

TREATMENT

- Diethylcarbamazine 6 mg/kg/day in divided doses for 3 weeks.
- Resistant cases are treated with prednisolone and bronchodilators. Pulmonary fibrosis can occur in long-standing cases.

Q. Give a brief account of aspiration pneumonia. (IM3.1)

- It occurs due to abnormal entry of fluid, particulate exogenous substances or endogenous secretions into the lower airways. It is of two types: chemical aspiration pneumonia (also known as aspiration pneumonitis) and bacterial aspiration pneumonia.
- Other aspiration syndromes include lung abscess and exogenous lipoid pneumonia.

PREDISPOSING FACTORS

- Box 2.34 lists common predisposing factors for aspiration pneumonia.

BOX 2.34 Predisposing Factors for Aspiration Pneumonia

- Reduced consciousness (including following anaesthesia).
- Dysphagia from neurological deficits.
- Disorders of the upper gastrointestinal tract including oesophageal disease, surgery involving the upper airways or oesophagus and gastric reflux.
- Mechanical disruption of the glottic closure or cardiac sphincter due to tracheostomy, endotracheal intubation, bronchoscopy, upper endoscopy and nasogastric feeding.
- Miscellaneous conditions such as protracted vomiting, large-volume tube feedings and feeding gastrostomy.

CHEMICAL ASPIRATION PNEUMONIA (ASPIRATION PNEUMONITIS)

- It occurs due to the aspiration of substances that are toxic to the lower airways, independent of bacterial infection. It includes chemical pneumonitis associated with the aspiration of gastric acid (Mendelson's syndrome).

CLINICAL FEATURES

- Abrupt onset of symptoms with low-grade fever and prominent dyspnoea.
- Examination reveals cyanosis and diffuse crepitations.
- Chest radiograph shows infiltrates involving dependent pulmonary segments that usually develop within 2 hours of aspiration.
- Some patients have a fulminant course and die shortly after aspiration, presumably from ARDS. Others have a rapid clinical improvement with clearing of the chest radiograph. Some patients have initial rapid improvement but then develop new expanding infiltrates on chest radiograph that probably represent secondary bacterial infection superimposed on the acid-injured lung.

TREATMENT

- Tracheal suction to clear fluids and particulate matter.
- Nasogastric aspiration.
- Flexible bronchoscopy for large-volume aspiration to clear the secretions.
- Support of respiration including mechanical ventilation, if required.
- Use of corticosteroids controversial.
- Antibiotics often given, though there is no evidence that bacteria are important in acute events.

BACTERIAL ASPIRATION PNEUMONIA

- The most common form of aspiration pneumonia is caused by bacteria that normally reside in the upper airways or stomach.
- Generally seen in hospitalised patients who have depressed gag reflex, impaired swallowing, or nasogastric or endotracheal tube. Also seen in elderly persons and patients with impaired consciousness due to drug and alcohol ingestion, stroke, etc.

CLINICAL FEATURES

- The presenting findings in aspiration pneumonia due to bacterial infection are highly variable and depend on the bacteria involved and status of the host.

- Most cases involve anaerobic bacteria that normally reside in the gingival crevices.
- Most patients present with the usual manifestations of pneumonia including cough, fever, purulent sputum and dyspnoea, but the process evolves over a period of several days or weeks instead of hours.
- Many patients have accompanying weight loss and anaemia caused by the chronic process.
- Oral examination may reveal periodontal disease.

DIAGNOSIS

- Presence of putrid discharge in sputum is regarded as diagnostic of anaerobic infection.
- Chest radiograph shows involvement of dependent pulmonary segments that are favoured in aspiration, the lower lobes when aspiration occurs in upright position and the apical segments of the lower lobes or posterior segment of the upper lobes when aspiration occurs in recumbent position.

TREATMENT

- Previously, antibiotic of choice for the treatment of aspiration pneumonia and lung abscess involving anaerobic bacteria was penicillin. However, approximately 25% of cases involve penicillinase-producing anaerobic bacteria.
- Clindamycin (600 mg 8 hourly IV followed by 300 mg 6 hourly orally) is now the preferred drug for anaerobic infections above the diaphragm, including pulmonary infections.
- Alternative regimens include amoxicillin-clavulanate or newer fluoroquinolones (levofloxacin and moxifloxacin).
- A combination of vancomycin and piperacillin–tazobactam for hospital-acquired aspiration pneumonia.
- Do not use metronidazole alone since monotherapy is associated with a failure rate of about 50%.

Q. What is meant by hospital-acquired pneumonia? How will you manage it?

Q. Write a short note on ventilator-associated pneumonia.

Q. What is nosocomial pneumonia? (IM3.1)

- Pneumonia developing in hospital in a patient who has been admitted for more than 48 hours should be considered as hospital acquired. The infection should not be in the incubation state at the time of admission.
- As per last update in 2016, hospital-acquired pneumonia (HAP) denotes an episode of pneumonia not associated with mechanical ventilation. Ventilator-associated pneumonia (VAP) is pneumonia occurring in patients who have been on ventilatory support for any reason for more than 48 hours. Both HAP and VAP are included under the term nosocomial pneumonia.

BOX 2.35 Risk Factors for Nosocomial Pneumonia

- Aspiration of oropharyngeal secretions
- Supine position in hospitalised patients
- Prolonged hospital stay
- Cigarette smoking
- Increasing age
- Uraemia
- Alcoholism
- Malnutrition
- Neutropenia
- Prior antibiotic use
- Endotracheal intubation
- Continuous sedation and use of paralytic agents
- Frequent ventilator circuit changes
- Stress ulcer prophylaxis using histamine blockers and proton pump inhibitors (PPI)

- The organisms causing HAP and VAP are different from those causing CAP, with predominance of Gram-negative bacteria like *Pseudomonas* species, *Escherichia* species, *Klebsiella* species, *S. aureus*, *Acinetobacter* species and *Enterobacter* species.

RISK FACTORS FOR NOSOCOMIAL PNEUMONIA

- Risk factors for nosocomial pneumonia are listed in Box 2.35.

DIAGNOSIS

- Nosocomial pneumonia is clinically diagnosed in patients who have been hospitalised for at least 48 hours and subsequently develop a new or progressive infiltrate, consolidation or cavitation on chest imaging, accompanied by at least two of the three systemic signs: fever, leucocytosis or leucopenia and purulent sputum.
- Other imaging modalities include lung ultrasound and low-dose computed tomography.
- Patients with HAP should have blood cultures and vigorous attempts, must be made to obtain sputum for identification of the organism and determining its sensitivity to antibiotics.
- Patients with VAP should have blood cultures and endotracheal aspirates for identification of organisms. Bronchoalveolar lavage or protected specimen brush is not recommended as a routine test.

TREATMENT

- Empirical therapy generally consists of a third-generation cephalosporin along with an aminoglycoside (gentamicin or amikacin).
- If multiantibiotic resistance is a problem in the hospital, then pneumonia due to Gram-positive organisms should be treated with vancomycin or teicoplanin or linezolid. For Gram-negative pneumonia, a β-lactam active against *Pseudomonas* (ceftazidime, cefoperazone, cefepime, piperacillin + tazobactam or meropenem) or a fluoroquinolone (ciprofloxacin or levofloxacin) + an aminoglycoside should be used.
- Another approach is 'de-escalation therapy' in which combination of antibiotics active against both Gram-positive and Gram-negative organisms is initiated keeping in mind the locally available data on resistance

pattern. The antibiotics are scaled down once the results of cultures are available.

- Novel antibiotics which may be used include ceftobiprole and ceftolozane/tazobactam (fifth generation cephalosporins), telavancin (against MRSA) and ceftazidime/avibactam (non-lactam-lactamase inhibitor).

PREVENTION OF VENTILATOR-ASSOCIATED PNEUMONIA (BUNDLES TO PREVENT INFECTION) (BOX 2.36)

BOX 2.36 Bundles to Prevent Ventilator-Associated Pneumonia

- Rigorous hand washing by caregivers
- Semirecumbent positioning (30°–45°) of the patient to prevent aspiration
- Adequate nutritional support
- Avoidance of gastric distention
- Maintenance of target pressure of endotracheal cuff at about 25 cm H_2O
- Chlorhexidine once daily to selectively decontaminate the oral cavity
- Early removal of endotracheal and nasogastric tubes
- Continuous subglottic suctioning
- Use of sucralfate and avoidance of proton-pump inhibitors (for stress ulcer prophylaxis)
- Avoidance of prophylactic antibiotic
- Minimise sedation and neuromuscular paralysis if possible

Q. How do you classify mycobacteria? Give an account of diseases produced by them.

Q. Describe mycobacteria other than tuberculosis (MOTT).

Q. Write a brief note on nontuberculous mycobacteria (NTM).

- Mycobacteria are divided into three groups:
  - *M. tuberculosis* complex (*M. tuberculosis*, *M. bovis* and *M. africanum*).
  - *Mycobacterium leprae*.
  - Atypical mycobacteria or NTM or mycobacteria other than tuberculosis (MOTT).
- MOTT or NTM are ubiquitous in the environment. Therefore, their isolation from a site that is not normally sterile (e.g. sputum, skin or urine) does not constitute proof of disease. Evidence of human-to-human transmission is present only in a few cases.
- In India, NTM disease prevalence is only about 0.8 per 100,000 population.
- Classical method for the isolation of mycobacteria is their culture on a solid medium (like LJ medium). However, this may take as long as 2–3 months.
- Culture in liquid broth using the radiometric BACTEC system or mycobacteria growth indicator tube (MGIT) shortens the time needed to culture mycobacteria.
- Methods like nuclear acid probes and polymerase chain reaction-restriction length polymorphism are now used for the rapid identification of some important species.

CLASSIFICATION

- Traditionally, based on growth rates and pigment production in the culture, NTM have been classified into four groups (Runyon classification): slow-growing NTM and fast-growing NTM (Group IV) (Flowchart 2.4). Slow-growing NTM are further subclassified based on pigment production in the culture:
  - Group I—Photochromogens (P) that are pigment producers in the presence of light.
  - Group II—Scotochromogens (S) that are pigment producers in the absence of light.
  - Group III—Nonchromogens (N) that do not produce any pigment.

RISK FACTORS FOR NTM DISEASE

- Risk factors for NTM disease are shown in Table 2.25.

DIAGNOSTIC CRITERIA FOR NTM-ASSOCIATED PULMONARY DISEASE

- Box 2.37 shows diagnostic criteria for NTM-associated pulmonary disease.

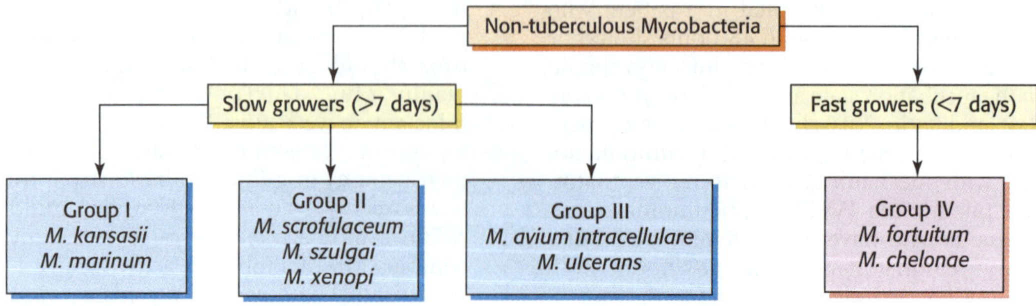

Flowchart 2.4 Classification of Nontuberculous Mycobacteria.

TABLE 2.25 Risk Factors for Nontuberculous Mycobacterial Infections

Pulmonary Disease	Extrapulmonary Disease
• Destroyed lungs due to TB or other diseases • Bronchiectasis • Chronic obstructive pulmonary disease • Cystic fibrosis • Alpha-1 antitrypsin deficiency • Lung cancer • Chronic aspiration	• Trauma (direct infection from environs) • Cosmetic surgeries • Prosthetic devices and implants • Organ transplantation • Dental procedures and surgeries • Intramuscular or intradermal injection
OTHERS	
• Immunodeficiency	

BOX 2.37 Diagnostic Criteria for NTM-Associated Pulmonary Disease

- Pulmonary symptoms, nodular or cavitary opacities on chest radiograph or high-resolution CT scan that shows multifocal bronchiectasis with multiple small nodules
- Positive culture results from at least two separate expectorated sputum samples or single-positive NTM culture from bronchoalveolar lavage or bronchial washing specimen from the affected lung segment of NTM suspect
- Other disorders such as tubercular and fungal infections must be excluded

TABLE 2.26 Diseases Caused by Various NTM and Their Treatment

		Localised Disease			
Agent	**Disseminated Disease**	**Lungs**	**Lymph Nodes**	**Skin**	**Treatment**
• *M. avium intracellulare* complex (N)	Yes; typical in AIDS with CD4 cells <50/ µL (fever, night sweat, diarrhoea, abdominal pain, weight loss with or without hepatosplenomegaly; blood and bone marrow cultures may be positive)	Cavities in cystic fibrosis and COAD; can occur with normal lungs also	Yes (accounts for 80% of cases of NTM-associated lymphadenitis)	Rare	Rifabutin, clarithromycin or azithromycin and ethambutol; add amikacin in severe cases; for lymphadenitis, complete excision of involved lymph node, if feasible
• *M. kansasii* (P)	Rare	Yes	Rare	Rare	Rifampicin, INH, ethambutol, streptomycin
• *M. marinum* (P)	Rare	–	Rare	Yes	Cotrimoxazole, ethambutol, rifampicin, clarithromycin, amikacin
• *M. ulcerans* (N)	Rare	–	–	Yes (Buruli's ulcer)	Debridement; rifampicin + clarithromycin or streptomycin
• *M. xenopi* (S)	Rare	Yes	–	–	Same as for *M. avium*
• *M. szulgai* (S)	Rare	Rare	–	Yes	Rifampicin, INH, ethambutol
• *M. scrofulaceum* (S)	Rare	Rare	Yes	Rare	Same as for *M. avium*
• *M. fortuitum* (group IV)	Rare	Rare	Rare	Yes	Imipenem, amikacin, ciprofloxacin, sulphonamides, clofazimine
• *M. chelonae* (group IV)	Rare	Rare	–	Yes	Debridement, clarithromycin, moxifloxacin, imipenem, clofazimine, amikacin, linezolid

DISEASES CAUSED BY VARIOUS NTM AND THEIR TREATMENT

- Table 2.26 gives diseases caused by various nontuberculous mycobacteria along with their treatment.

Q. Discuss the pathogenesis, pathology, clinical manifestations and diagnosis of primary pulmonary tuberculosis. (CT1.2)

Q. Write in brief about primary complex of Ranke and Ghon's complex.

PATHOGENESIS AND PATHOLOGY

- First infection of the lung with the tubercle bacillus is known as primary pulmonary tuberculosis.
- Mycobacteria are carried in airborne particles (droplet nuclei) of 1–5 µm in diameter. Transmission occurs when a person inhales droplet nuclei containing *M. tuberculosis* and the droplet nuclei traverse the mouth or nasal passages, upper respiratory tract and bronchi to reach the alveoli of the lungs.
- From this primary site of infection, bacilli are carried to the lymph nodes via lymphatics and the hilar nodes enlarge. This parenchymal lesion (Ghon's lesion) with its enlarged regional (hilar) lymph nodes and interconnecting lymphangitis is known as Ghon's complex.
- The parenchymal lesion is subpleural and is usually located in lower part of the upper lobe, upper part of the lower lobe or the middle lobe.
- Bacilli in alveoli also invade and replicate within alveolar macrophages that interact with T lymphocytes, resulting in differentiation of macrophages into epithelioid histiocytes. Epithelioid histiocytes and lymphocytes aggregate into small clusters resulting in granulomas. In the granuloma, $CD4^{+}$ T lymphocytes secrete cytokines, such as interferon-γ, which activate

macrophages to destroy the bacteria with which they are infected. CD^{8+} T lymphocytes (cytotoxic T cell) can also directly kill infected cells.
- The above-mentioned immunological reaction occurs after about 3–8 weeks of infection (by the time of tuberculin conversion), when the classical pathological features of tuberculosis may be found in varying proportions. This is a granulomatous lesion containing epithelioid cells derived from macrophages, Langhans' giant cells with multiple nuclei also derived from macrophages, lymphocytes and varying degrees of fibrosis. Later, a peculiar cheesy form of necrosis occurs in the centre, known as caseation. The caseous tissue may later become calcified. But if the lesion progresses, the caseous tissue may become liquefied to form purulent material. This material may be discharged into a bronchus resulting in cavitation of the lesion. Cavitation, however, is regarded as one of the manifestations of postprimary pulmonary tuberculosis.
- The pathological changes in the lymph nodes are similar to those of the parenchymal lesion.

CLINICAL MANIFESTATIONS

- Primary infection usually occurs in childhood. A history of contact with a case of active tuberculosis is present in many cases.

SYMPTOMS

- Vast majority are asymptomatic.
- A minority may experience a brief flu-like febrile illness, which lasts no more than 7–14 days. It occurs at the time of tuberculin conversion.
- If the infection is severe or the host resistance is low, child may appear to be vaguely unwell with reduced appetite, low-grade fever, fretfulness and failure to gain weight.
- Slight dry cough is occasionally present. Wheeze may be rarely present.

PHYSICAL SIGNS

- In vast majority, there are no abnormal physical signs.
- When the lesion is extensive, signs of general debility may be present. Child is thin, pale and fretful with less glossy hair and less elastic skin.
- Usually there are no abnormal physical signs in the chest. Sometimes, there may be a few crepitations over a large lung component of the primary complex. More extensive physical signs in the chest result from complications.
- Erythema nodosum may accompany primary pulmonary tuberculosis. These are bluish-red, raised, tender, cutaneous lesions on the shins and less commonly on the thighs. In some patients, it is associated with fever and polyarthralgia. Tuberculin reaction is strongly positive in this group. Erythema nodosum is also seen in other conditions like sarcoidosis, streptococcal infections and drug reactions.
- Symptoms and signs may result from progression of primary complex or complications of primary complex.

FATE OF THE PRIMARY COMPLEX

- In great majority, the primary focus heals completely with or without calcification. The Ghon's complex undergoes progressive fibrosis, often followed by radiologically detectable calcification (Ranke complex).
- In some cases, the primary focus is walled off by collagenous tissue, the tubercle bacilli cease to divide and the disease becomes dormant. However, these dormant lesions can re-activate later giving rise to active postprimary pulmonary tuberculosis.
- In a few individuals, primary lesion in the lung may be actively progressive from the beginning (progressive pulmonary tuberculosis or progressive primary pulmonary tuberculosis).
- In a few cases, healing, particularly in lymph nodes, is incomplete and viable tubercle bacilli may enter the bloodstream. As a result, haematogenous dissemination occurs resulting in tuberculous lesions elsewhere. The haematogenous forms can be of two types:
  - The acute form, which is more likely to occur in infants or young children, results in miliary tuberculosis or tuberculous meningitis.
  - The chronic form where tuberculous lesions develop in the lungs, bones, joints and kidneys. These lesions may develop months or even years after primary infection.
- In some cases, the infection may be carried by lymphatics from mediastinal lymph nodes to pleura or pericardium resulting in tuberculous pleurisy with effusion or tuberculous pericarditis with effusion.
- Bronchial complications resulting from primary complex are the following:
  - Enlarged mediastinal lymph nodes can compress a bronchus resulting in pulmonary collapse. Compression of middle lobe bronchus is especially common, leading to collapse consolidation and bronchiectatic changes. This may be present later as the 'middle lobe syndrome'.
  - Tuberculous lymph node may ulcerate through the bronchial wall and discharge caseous material into the lumen. This results in bronchial spread to the related lobe or segment.
  - Rarely, the bronchus is so compressed as to result in a valve action with air trapping. This leads to obstructive emphysema.
  - Calcification in a primary focus or lymph node may later be extruded into a bronchus as a 'broncholith', presenting as haemoptysis.
- Flowchart 2.5 shows pathogenesis of tuberculosis and its progression.

DIAGNOSIS

- History of contact with a case of active tuberculosis.
- Tuberculin test is very valuable in children. A positive test in a previously nonimmunised child strongly indicates the disease. A negative test makes the diagnosis very unlikely.
- Chest radiograph can visualise the primary complex as a peripheral parenchymal lesion and an enlarged hilar lymph node.

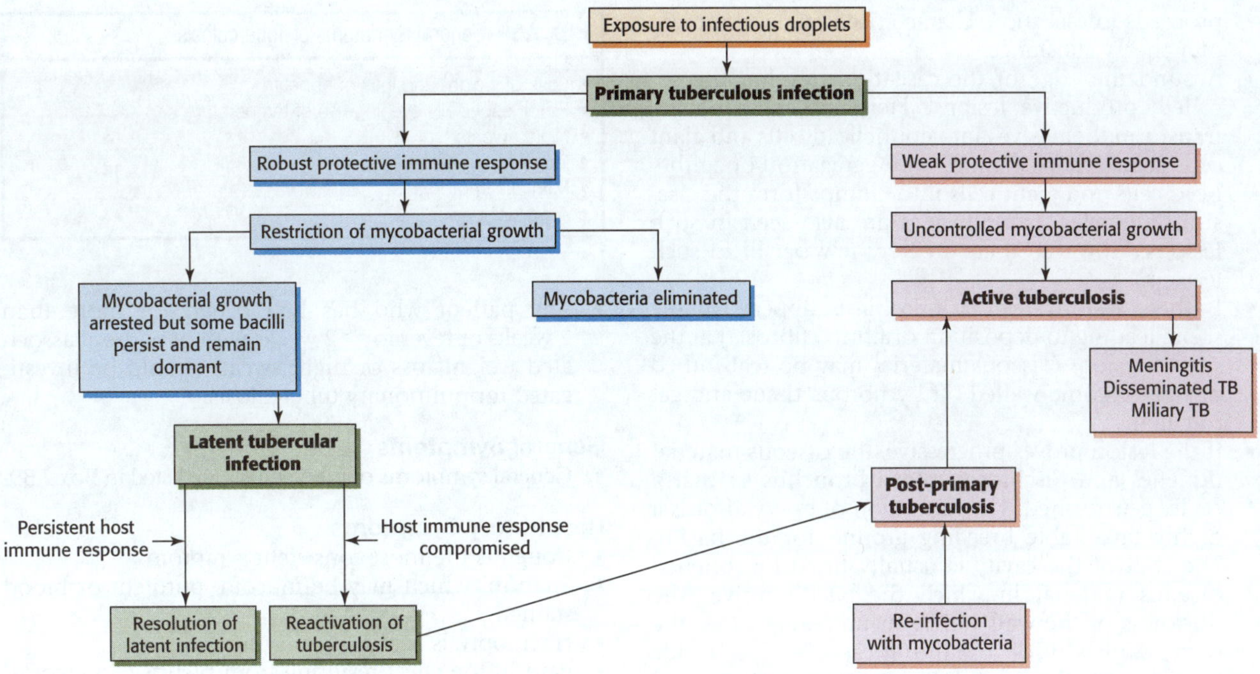

Flowchart 2.5 Pathogenesis of Tuberculosis and Its Progression.

- In children, glandular component (enlarged hilar lymph node) of the complex is more obvious than the pulmonary component.
- In adults, pulmonary component (peripheral parenchymal lesion) of the complex is more obvious than the glandular component.

- Bacteriological examination:
  - Sputum examination is preferable, but it is seldom available. Alternatively, three laryngeal swabs or fasting gastric washings can be examined.
  - Isolation of the tubercle bacilli by direct smear examination or culture confirms the diagnosis.

Q. Discuss the epidemiology, pathogenesis, pathology, clinical manifestations, complications and diagnosis of postprimary pulmonary tuberculosis. (CT1.1;CT1.12,CT1.3)

EPIDEMIOLOGY

- Globally, an estimated 10 million people developed tuberculosis in 2020 while 1.5 million people died from tuberculosis. Highest incidence is in India followed by Indonesia and Philippines.
- It is the 13th leading cause of death and the second leading infectious cause of death (first being COVID-19).
- In India, as per the data available, nearly 2.7 million cases are reported every year.

PATHOGENESIS

- Postprimary pulmonary tuberculosis may arise in any one of the following four ways:
  1. Direct progression of a primary lesion.
  2. Re-activation of a dormant primary lesion.
  3. Haematogenous spread to the lungs.
  4. Exogenous superinfection (re-infection).
- Postprimary pulmonary tuberculosis presents mainly as parenchymal disease with only minimal lymph node enlargement. The characteristic pathological feature is the tuberculous cavity which is formed when caseated and liquefied centre of a tuberculous pulmonary lesion is discharged into a bronchus.
- The common sites of involvement are apical and posterior segments of the upper lobe or apical segment of the lower lobe. This predilection may be due to good ventilation and decreased blood and lymphatic supply of these regions in the erect posture.

CONDITIONS THAT FAVOUR RE-ACTIVATION/ RE-INFECTION OF TUBERCULOSIS

- A number of conditions favour re-activation/re-infection of tuberculosis (Box 2.38).

PATHOLOGY

HISTOLOGICAL TYPES OF LESIONS

- An initial preexudate phase that is followed by an exudative phase. In most cases, exudative lesion

BOX 2.38 Conditions Favouring Re-Activation/Re-Infection of Tuberculosis

- Malnutrition
- Diabetes
- Immunosuppressive treatment (including steroids)
- HIV infection
- Haemophilia
- Chronic kidney disease
- Silicosis
- Malignancies

proceeds to caseation, characterised by development of a cheesy substance.

- Around the edge of the caseation develop the so-called 'productive lesions'. Here the macrophages transform themselves into epithelioid cells and giant cells (Langerhans giant cells). Aggregation of epithelioid cells and giant cells into clumps form the classical 'tubercles'. Lymphocytes are also seen in such lesions. However, there are very few bacilli in such lesions.
- If these lesions regress, fibroblasts appear on the scene leading to deposition of fibrin (fibrosis) at the site of lesion. Caseous material may be reabsorbed or may become walled off by fibrous tissue and get calcified.
- If the lesion proves progressive, the caseous material liquefies and discharges into a bronchus so that a cavity gets formed. The formation of cavity affords a highly favourable breeding ground for the bacilli. The wall of the cavity is usually lined by softened caseous material in which the bacilli thrive. The thickness of the wall varies. In untreated cases, the cavity wall is thick, the lining caseous layer inside is thicker and there may be an outer fibrous layer and superficial to it is a layer of alveolar atelectasis. In properly treated cases, the caseous elements gradually disappear and ultimately a thin-walled epithelialised cavity may be left over. At times, a check valve mechanism results from the involvement of the bronchial mucous membrane. This allows air to get into a cavity during inspiration but prevents its escape during expiration. This may result in a large thin-walled cavity. At times, necrotic material inside the bronchus may completely block the lumen, leading to reabsorption of air within the cavity and its closure.
- Secondary lesions may be seen around the main lesion or cavity or in other parts of both lungs. These may result from bronchial spillover or haematogenous spread.

MACROSCOPIC APPEARANCES

- If the lesions are limited, upper lobes are commonly involved. A whole lobe may be involved (tuberculous pneumonia).
- Large caseous areas and cavities are characteristic features of postprimary pulmonary tuberculosis. Cavities may be single or multiple, sometimes multilocular, of varying size with varying thickness of the walls. Sometimes, a pulmonary vessel may be seen running across a cavity.
- In chronic disease, there is gross fibrosis and distortion of lung architecture. In addition, there may be calcification and bronchiectasis.

CLINICAL FEATURES

SYMPTOMS

- Many patients are symptom-free, and tuberculosis may be detected on routine radiography.
- A characteristic feature of tuberculosis is the gradual onset of symptoms over weeks or months.

BOX 2.39 General Symptoms of Tuberculosis

- Loss of weight and loss of appetite
- Fever, especially evening rise of temperature
- Night sweats
- Tiredness, malaise
- Mental symptoms
- Amenorrhoea

- Any patient who has had cough for more than 2 weeks or fever for >2 weeks with or without associated weight loss or night sweats should be investigated for pulmonary tuberculosis.

General Symptoms

- General symptoms of tuberculosis are listed in Box 2.39.

Respiratory Symptoms

- Cough is the most consistent symptom.
- Sputum, which may be mucoid, purulent or blood stained.
- Haemoptysis is a classical symptom.
- Pain in the chest resulting from pleurisy, intercostal myalgia or cough fracture.
- Breathlessness is a feature of advanced and extensive disease.
- Localised wheeze resulting from local ulceration and narrowing of a major bronchus.
- Pneumonia (with acute presentation) that turns out to be tuberculous is another mode of presentation.

PHYSICAL SIGNS

- Pallor and cachexia in advanced cases.
- Fever, tachycardia and tachypnoea.
- Finger clubbing is unusual, but it may be present in chronic disease with purulent sputum.

Physical Signs in the Chest

- Often there are no abnormal signs.
- The most common sign is fine crepitations in the upper part (apices) of one or both lungs. These are heard particularly on taking a deep breath after coughing (posttussive crepitations). Later, there may be dullness to percussion or even bronchial breathing in the upper part. At times, there is a localised wheeze due to local tuberculous bronchitis or pressure by a lymph node on a bronchus. In chronic tuberculosis with fibrosis, evidence of volume loss and mediastinal shift may be present.
- Classical physical signs of consolidation, cavitation, collapse, fibrosis, bronchiectasis, pleural effusion or pneumothorax may be present.

COMPLICATIONS

- Complications of pulmonary tuberculosis are shown in Box 2.40.

INVESTIGATIONS

BLOOD EXAMINATION

- Moderate anaemia.

BOX 2.40 Complications of Pulmonary Tuberculosis

• Haemoptysis • Pneumothorax • Secondary infection of cavity • Pleural effusion • Empyema • Pulmonary fibrosis • Bronchiectasis	• Persistence of cavities even after treatment • Infection of cavities by *Aspergillus* (aspergilloma) • Scar carcinoma • Spread of tuberculosis to other organs • Respiratory failure and right heart failure • Amyloidosis • Anaemia

- White cell count is usually normal or below normal.
- ESR is usually raised.
- Hyponatraemia and hypokalaemia may be present in severe disease.
- Impaired liver function tests are occasionally seen.

RADIOLOGICAL EXAMINATION OF CHEST

- A normal chest radiograph for practical purposes excludes pulmonary tuberculosis. The radiological features of tuberculosis are given ahead in the chapter.
- CT chest may be useful in evaluating parenchymal lesions and lymph nodes.
- ^{18}F-FDG PET scans and ^{11}C-choline PET scans may be done in selected patients.

SPUTUM EXAMINATION

- Microscopic examination of sputum smear remains the most important investigation. WHO recommends that two sputum samples should be examined for screening of tuberculosis cases in places where a well-functioning external quality assurance system exists, where the workload is very high and human resources are scarce. Presence of at least one acid-fast bacillus in at least one sputum sample indicates sputum-positive pulmonary tuberculosis.
  1. A first spot specimen when the patient presents himself/herself.
  2. An early next-day morning specimen consisting of all sputum raised in the first 1–2 hours.
- If quality assurance system is not available, then three specimens of sputum should be examined:
  1. A first spot specimen when the patient presents himself/herself.
  2. An early next-day morning specimen consisting of all sputum raised in the first 1–2 hours.
  3. A second spot specimen when the patient returns with an early morning specimen.
     - A smear-positive pulmonary tuberculosis case is defined as one with:
       a. Two or more initial sputum smear examinations positive for acid-fast bacillus, or
       b. One sputum smear examination positive for acid-fast bacillus plus radiographic abnormalities consistent with active pulmonary tuberculosis as determined by a clinician, or
       c. One sputum smear positive for AFB plus sputum culture-positive for *M. tuberculosis*.
- Sputum culture for tubercle bacillus may be done, but results become available only in 4–8 weeks. Drug resistance tests should be done in selected cases. In all settings with an HIV prevalence of >1% in pregnant women or ≥5% in patients with tuberculosis, sputum culture should be performed in patients who are sputum smear-negative.

LARYNGEAL SWABS

- While taking a swab, the patient coughs and the swab catches some mucus. This is sent for culture.

GASTRIC ASPIRATION (GASTRIC LAVAGE OR GASTRIC WASHINGS)

- May be used in children as sputum is difficult to get from them. Early morning fasting (at least 4 hours in children and 3 hours in infants) gastric washings can show tubercle bacilli. For this, a sterile nasogastric tube is introduced into the stomach and 20 mL of sterile normal saline is injected. After 1 minute, aspirate out as much as possible.

BRONCHOALVEOLAR LAVAGE

- Bronchoalveolar lavage fluid gives more positive results, but it is reserved for selected cases.

TUBERCULIN TEST

- Tuberculin testing as a tool for diagnosis is much less valuable. This is partly because the test may be negative due to malnutrition or other diseases even when the patient has active tuberculosis. On the other hand, many people without active tuberculosis have positive tests.
- A strongly positive test is a point in favour of tuberculosis, but a negative test does not exclude tuberculosis.

T-CELL INTERFERON-γ RELEASE ASSAYS (IGRAS)

- T-cell-based interferon-γ (IFN-γ) assays are in vitro tests of cellular immunity. These assays measure cell-mediated immune response by quantifying IFN-γ released by T cells in response to stimulation by *M. tuberculosis* antigens.
- Currently two ex vivo assays are available: the ELISpot (T-SPOT™.TB) that directly counts the number of IFN-γ-secreting T cells and the whole-blood ELISA (QuantiFERON™-TB Gold In-Tube) that measures the concentration of IFN-γ secretion.
- Both the tests incorporate antigens that are more specific to *M. tuberculosis*. These specific antigens include early secretory antigenic target-6 (ESAT-6) and culture filtrate protein-10 (CFP-10). These antigens are not shared by any BCG strains, *M. bovis* or most nontuberculous mycobacteria (except *M. kansasii*, *M. marinum* and *M. szulgai*). Therefore, in comparison with the tuberculin skin test, T-cell responses to these antigens are not confounded by prior BCG vaccination and hence a more specific marker of TB infection.
- Compared to tuberculin skin test, IFN-γ-based tests do not show boosting effect on repeated tests.

However, these tests require high cost and trained personnel. Furthermore, like tuberculin test, a positive IFN-γ test does not indicate active infection as it is also positive in latent tuberculosis.

OTHER METHODS OF DIAGNOSIS

- In mycobacteria growth indicator tube (MGIT) method, growth is detected by a nonradioactive detection system using fluorochromes for detection and drug screening.
- BACTEC radiometric growth detection: In this method, ^{14}C-labelled palmitic acid is incorporated in a liquid culture medium. Growth of bacilli is detected by liberation of $^{14}CO_2$, produced as a result of metabolism of palmitic acid by viable mycobacteria. The growth can be detected in 4–8 days.
- Microscopic observation drug susceptibility (MODS) assay which detects *M. tuberculosis* bacilli on the basis of cording formation, as well as isoniazid and rifampicin resistance.
- *Molecular methods*: Nucleic acid amplification tests (NAAT) are rapid tests that can detect small amounts of genetic material (DNA or RNA target sequences) from the microorganism and are based on repetitive amplification of target sequences. If the target organism is not present in the sample, no amplification will occur. A variety of amplification methods may be used, including amplification of the target nucleic acid, such as the polymerase chain reaction (PCR), or amplification of a nucleic acid probe, such as a ligase chain reaction. These methods can detect mycobacteria in cultured material or in clinical sample directly.
  - Line probe assays and microfluidic PCR device (GeneXpert) allow both rapid detection of TB and drug resistance patterns. GeneXpert may give results within 2 hours and detects resistance to rifampicin (Xpert/RIF Ultra assay). Line probe assays detect resistance to both rifampicin and isoniazid.
- Mycobacterial-specific phages (reporter phages) to detect luciferase gene. Can be used to detect drug-resistant isolates.

Q. Enumerate the causes of haemoptysis in pulmonary tuberculosis.

HAEMOPTYSIS FROM A PULMONARY CAVITY

- Walls of the vessels traversing a cavity undergo atrophic changes due to inflammatory and necrotic degeneration.
- Over a period of time, these vessels develop aneurysmal dilatation. These aneurysms (Rasmussen's aneurysm) rupture resulting in haemoptysis.
- Occasionally, intense allergic response to antigens of tubercle bacilli damages the walls of the vessels in and around the cavities, which results in haemoptysis.

HAEMOPTYSIS FROM ENDOBRONCHIAL TUBERCULOSIS

- Endobronchial tuberculomas (tuberculous granulomas) are surrounded by vessels with small aneurysmal dilatation. Rupture of these aneurysms results in haemoptysis.
- Alternatively, as a result of secondary infection, part of the granuloma may slough out resulting in haemoptysis.

HAEMOPTYSIS AS A SEQUELA OF PULMONARY TUBERCULOSIS

- A cavity may persist despite complete epithelialisation following therapy. Such cavities are termed 'open-healed cavities'. The aneurysmal dilations would also persist in these open-healed cavities. These aneurysms can rupture resulting in haemoptysis.
- Bronchiectasis of the upper lobe is a common sequela of pulmonary tuberculosis ('post-tuberculous bronchiectasis'). This presents as bronchiectasis sicca or dry bronchiectasis, characterised by repeated attacks of haemoptysis without sputum production.
- Calcification in a primary focus or lymph node may later be extruded into a bronchus as a 'broncholith', which causes haemoptysis. Haemoptysis results from the broncholith eroding through blood vessels.
- Well-treated and 'healed' tuberculous cavities sometimes remain open and can be infected by the fungus *Aspergillus fumigatus*. This results in a fungal ball (aspergilloma), which can present as severe haemoptysis.

Q. Give a brief account of sputum smear examination for mycobacteria. (CT1.10)

Q. What are the common causes of false-positive and false-negative results of sputum examination?

COLLECTION OF SPUTUM

- Patient should be taught what constitutes 'sputum', and how to produce proper bronchial sputum from the 'depths of the chest'. Saliva and nasopharyngeal secretions are unsuitable for examination.
- If the patient discharges acid-fast bacilli in his/her sputum, these are more likely to be found in a specimen produced early morning than in one produced later during the day. Hence, the ideal sputum specimen is the one which is produced in early morning, before breakfast and before taking any medicaments. For convenience, three samples as stated above are collected on 2 days. However, at present, WHO recommends two samples for diagnosis when external quality assurance system is in place. Another recent move is to examine two samples on the same day ('same-day' diagnosis).
- The patient should rinse his/her mouth with pure water and clean his/her teeth (without using toothpaste or disinfectant) before coughing out the sputum specimen. If repeated attempts of coughing have failed, aerosol induction (should be done in a separate, well-ventilated room), gastric aspiration and bronchoscopy may be required.

STORAGE AND TRANSPORT OF SPUTUM AND STORAGE OF STAINED SPECIMENS

- The collected sputum should not be exposed to direct sunlight or excessive heat.
- While storing stained specimens, immersion oil on the slide should be removed with xylol.
- Fluorochrome will lose fluorescence with storage.

PREPARATION OF SMEARS

- If the quantity of sputum is sufficient, it is better to concentrate the specimen before preparing the smears. A solution of 4% sodium hydroxide is added to the sputum (two parts with one part of sputum) and incubated for 1 hour. Then it is concentrated by centrifugation. The supernatant is removed by pipette and the deposit is used for preparation of smears.
- If concentration is not done, select the suitable sputum particles for smear preparation. Tubercle bacilli are most likely to be found in little blobs ('lentils') of greenish-grey or yellowish matter of a thick, creamy consistency. Such blobs usually consist of dead caseous tissue eliminated from a cavity in the lung. These blobs have to be carefully separated from the rest of the sputum and transferred to a slide.
- The specimen is transferred to a new glass slide (with no scratches) with a wire loop of internal diameter 3 mm (WHO standard). The wire loop transfers roughly 0.01 mL of sputum. This sputum is spread over an area of 200 mm^2 (10 mm × 20 mm) (Fig. 2.8). The smear should be fixed by passing it over a Bunsen flame taking care not to overheat it.

STAINING TECHNIQUES

- Two methods of staining for tubercle bacilli are in common use.

ZIEHL–NEELSEN METHOD

- The fixed smears are kept on staining racks. Smears are covered with suitably cut filter papers. Carbol fuchsin is poured over the filter paper and gently heated till the smear steams. The smears are then washed under tap water. Next, 25% sulphuric acid is added on the smear and the smear is allowed to decolourise for 21/2 minutes. The smear is then washed twice in water and again decolourised with 95% alcohol for 2 minutes. It is again washed in water and counterstained with 0.1% methylene blue for 10 seconds and dried. The dried smear is examined under oil immersion.

FLUOROCHROME STAINING

- The fixed smear is covered with 0.3% auramine phenol for 15 minutes, and then washed with water and decolourised twice with 0.5% acid-alcohol for 2 minutes. The smear is then treated with 0.1% potassium permanganate solution for 30 seconds. The specimen is then washed and dried for examination under fluorescent microscope. It is more sensitive than conventional ZN stain and microscopy. Presently, it is recommended that conventional fluorescence microscopy be replaced by light-emitting diode (LED) microscopy while assessing auramine staining.
- The field observed through the fluorescent microscope is much larger than that observed through the oil immersion lens; hence, a larger area can be covered in a shorter duration.
- However, fluorescent microscope requires high cost and maintenance, advanced technical skill for operation and continuous electric supply with steady voltage.

FALSE-POSITIVE RESULTS

- Acid-fast particles other than tubercle bacilli can give false-positive results. These include some food particles, precipitates, other microorganisms, inorganic materials and artefacts. Besides mycobacteria, some other organisms may show some acid fastness (but not to 25% sulphuric acid) and include *Nocardia, Rhodococcus, Isospora, Cryptosporidium* and *Legionella*.

FALSE-NEGATIVE RESULTS

- Inadequate sputum collection.
- Inadequate storage of sputum specimens and stained smears.
- Failure to select suitable sputum particles for smear preparation.
- Inadequate preparation of smears or staining slides.
- Inadequate examination of the smear.

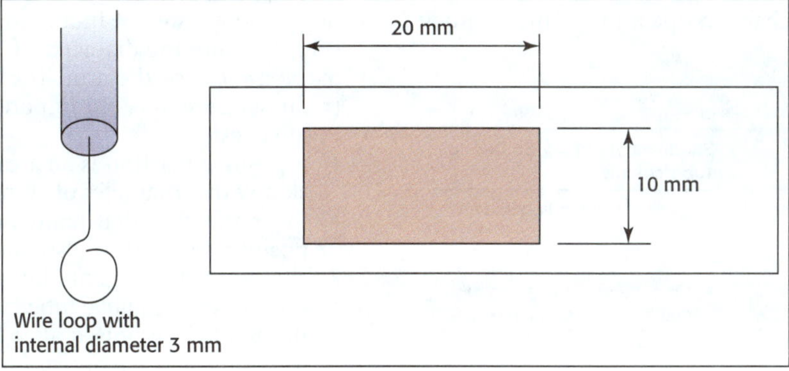

Fig. 2.8 Wire loop and slide used for the preparation of sputum smears.

Q. List down the radiological features of pulmonary tuberculosis.

- A normal chest radiograph for practical purposes excludes pulmonary tuberculosis.
- Table 2.27 lists radiological features of pulmonary tuberculosis.

CHARACTERISTIC RADIOGRAPHIC APPEARANCES

- Soft confluent shadows suggest exudative process.
- Linear shadows, especially if they produce distortion of fissures, trachea, mediastinum or diaphragm, suggest fibrosis.
- Tuberculomas—large solid-looking areas which contain caseation and productive lesions and measure 0.5–4.0 cm in diameter. Satellite nodules around the tuberculoma may be present in as many as 80% of cases. Because of active glucose metabolism by active granulomatous inflammation, tuberculomas may accumulate ^{18}F-FDG and produce hot-spots in PET scans (like malignant lesions).
- Very dense white shadows suggest calcification.
- Elongated translucent areas in the upper zones suggest bronchiectasis.
- CT is useful in demonstrating cavities, calcification, tuberculomas and lymph nodes. Enlarged nodes typically show central low attenuation, which represents caseous necrosis, and peripheral rim enhancement, which represents the vascular rim of the granulomatous inflammatory tissue. Another important finding on CT chest is 'tree-in-bud' sign—branching linear and nodular opacities; these reflect endobronchial spread and are due to the presence of caseous necrosis and granulomatous inflammation filling and surrounding terminal and respiratory bronchioles and alveolar ducts.
- Pleural effusion, empyema, aspergilloma, etc. may be seen on radiograph. These should be considered as complications of pulmonary tuberculosis.
- Cavitation can be made out only if the liquefied materials are coughed out and air gets into the cavity. Cavities may be single or multiple, small or large. The wall of the cavity may be thin or thick, regular or irregular.
  - In early stages, the cavity wall is thick and irregular. In the chronic phase, the wall is thin and regular.
  - During chemotherapy, the cavity wall becomes thinner and smoother.
  - Distended thin-walled cavity may result from a check valve mechanism operating in the draining bronchus.
  - A cavity may become 'blocked'. The draining bronchus may be obstructed and instead of the cavity collapsing, it may become filled with purulent or caseous material ('blocked cavity').

TABLE 2.27 Radiological Features of Pulmonary Tuberculosis

Shadows That Strongly Suggest Tuberculosis	Shadows That May Be Due to Tuberculosis
• Patchy or nodular shadows in the upper zone, on one or both sides	• Oval or round solitary shadow (tuberculoma)
• Cavitation, particularly if more than one cavity	• Hilar and mediastinal shadows due to enlarged lymph nodes
• Calcified shadows	• Diffuse small nodular shadows (miliary tuberculosis)

Q. Write a short note on tuberculin testing. (CT1.7)

Q. What is Mantoux test? (CT1.7)

- First infection with the tubercle bacillus leads to the development of sensitisation to the protein 'tuberculin'. When tuberculin (purified protein derivative [PPD]) is injected into the skin of an infected person, a delayed local reaction develops in 24–48 hours. This is mainly due to previously sensitised CD4+ lymphocytes.

TUBERCULINS

- There are two common tuberculins in present use:
  1. PPD-S has been adopted as the international standard for PPD of mammalian tuberculin.
  2. PPD-RT23 is widely used in epidemiological studies throughout the world. RT stands for Research Tuberculin. Tween 80 is a detergent added to tuberculin to prevent its adsorption on glass or plastic surface. It is most commonly used in India.
- PPD is a mixture of over 200 *M. tuberculosis* proteins.

MANTOUX TEST

- Tuberculin skin testing is performed via the Mantoux technique.
- It is ideal to begin the test with 5 IU PPD-S or 1 or 2 IU PPD-RT23.

METHOD

- Choose an area of skin at the junction of the mid- and upper-thirds of flexure surface of the left forearm. Clean the area with soap and water and allow it to dry. Using a tuberculin syringe and an intradermal needle, inject 0.1 mL of the tuberculin solution strictly intradermally. It should produce a papule in the skin 5–6 mm in diameter.

READING AND INTERPRETING THE RESULT

- The test is read after 48–72 hours. If a reaction has taken place, there will be an area of erythema (redness) and an area of induration (thickening) of the skin. Measure the diameter of induration across the *transverse axis* of the arm. The amount of erythema (redness) present is not important.
- Positive test:
  - A positive reaction is an area of induration of the skin with a diameter of 10 mm or more.
  - But remember that many normal people have a positive test and so also after previous BCG vaccination. Most infants immunised with BCG at birth have a negative tuberculin test by 1–2 years. In infants immunised after 1 year, the tuberculin reaction often remains positive for some years. A positive tuberculin test by BCG sensitisation can

be distinguished from latent tuberculosis by IGRAs.
  - It may also be positive in NTM infections.
  - However, a strongly positive test is particularly valuable in children, especially very young children.
- Negative test:
  - If the diameter is below 10 mm, the test is negative.
  - But a negative test does not exclude tuberculosis. A patient with active tuberculosis may have a suppressed tuberculin test (false-negative) due to a number of factors—for example malnutrition, viral infections, HIV infection, measles, chickenpox, glandular fever, cancer, severe bacterial infections (including overwhelming tuberculosis), use of immunosuppressive drugs (e.g. corticosteroids and similar drugs), recent live-virus vaccination (e.g. measles) and recent TB infection (within 8–10 weeks of exposure).

EFFECT OF REPEATING TUBERCULIN TEST

- A repeat tuberculin test does not have any effect on the size of induration, that is repeated testing does not sensitise individuals to tuberculin and there is no booster response.
- If the test is negative, it may be repeated on the other forearm in the following circumstances:
  - Close contacts of patients with untreated active pulmonary tuberculosis when initial test was done early before development of delayed hypersensitivity.
  - Individuals with ongoing potential exposure (often done annually).

BOOSTER RESPONSE

- If the exposure to BCG or NTM bacteria occurred several years ago, tuberculin reaction may become negative due to reduction in the number of sensitised T lymphocytes.
- Repeating tuberculin test 1–4 weeks after first negative test may become positive due to anamnestic recall of immunity. It occurs in the absence of new exposure.

Q. How do you make an assessment of activity of tuberculosis?

- A positive sputum, especially if repeated, certainly indicates activity.
- Presence of symptoms like cough, tiredness or weight loss is suggestive of activity.
- Detection of crepitations on auscultation, if persistent, is in favour of activity.
- There are certain radiological appearances that are suggestive of activity:
  - The presence of a cavity always indicates activity unless proved otherwise.
  - Soft shadows, even if very small, are suggestive of activity.
  - If shadows are extensive, activity is very probable.
  - Progression of shadows in serial X-rays suggests activity.
- A raised ESR may indicate an activity.
- A strongly positive tuberculin test is quite compatible with an active lesion, but a negative or weakly positive test is not very likely in the presence of activity.

Q. Describe latent tuberculosis infection.

- Latent tuberculosis infection is a condition in which a person is infected with *M. tuberculosis* but does not currently have active tuberculosis disease. During latent infection, the host immune system is able to contain the bacilli in a state of nonreplicating persistence.
- An estimated 2 billion persons worldwide have latent infection and are at risk for re-activation.

GROUPS OF PEOPLE AT HIGH RISK OF LATENT TUBERCULOSIS INFECTION (Box 2.41)

- Patients with latent tuberculosis are at risk of progressing to active tuberculosis. About 5%–10% is the lifetime risk of progression.
- Certain groups of people are at higher risk of progression to active tuberculosis (Box 2.42).

SCREENING FOR LATENT TUBERCULOSIS

- Tuberculin test.
- T-cell IGRAs.

BOX 2.41 People at High Risk of Latent Tuberculous Infection

- Employees of long-term care facilities, hospitals and medical laboratories
- Persons who have close contact with someone known or suspected to have active tuberculosis
- Residents and employees of congregate living facilities, including prisons and jails, nursing homes, hospitals and homeless shelters
- Some medically underserved, low-income populations

BOX 2.42 Groups at Increased Risk of Progression

- Children younger than 5 years
- Persons with HIV infection
- Persons infected with *Mycobacterium tuberculosis* within the past 2 years
- Injectable drug users
- Persons with a history of untreated or inadequately treated tuberculosis
- Silicosis
- Persons with immunocompromising conditions
  - Long-term use of corticosteroids or other immunosuppressants (including anti-TNF-α)
  - Chronic kidney disease
  - Diabetes mellitus
  - Malignancy

PROPHYLAXIS (TO PREVENT DEVELOPMENT OF ACTIVE TUBERCULOSIS)

- Persons deemed to have latent tuberculosis and who are at increased risk for progression to active TB should be considered candidates for preventive therapy.
- Treatment is not recommended for people with diabetes, people who engage in the harmful use of alcohol, tobacco smokers and underweight people unless they belong to the groups given below.
- WHO recommends prophylaxis in certain circumstances (Box 2.43).
- Please see tuberculosis prophylaxis on page 173.

BOX 2.43 Groups Where TB Prophylaxis Is Indicated

1. Adults and adolescents with HIV
2. Infants aged <12 months with HIV who are in contact with a person with TB
3. Children aged ≥12 months with HIV if they live in a setting with high TB transmission
4. Children aged <5 years who are household contacts of people with bacteriologically confirmed pulmonary TB
5. People who are initiating anti-TNF treatment, or receiving dialysis, or preparing for an organ or haematological transplant, or who have silicosis

Q. What do you understand by the terms 'bactericidal action' and 'sterilising action' in relation to antituberculous drugs?

- Bactericidal action is defined as the ability of antituberculous drugs to kill large numbers of actively metabolising bacilli rapidly.
  - Most of the antituberculous drugs with the exception of the bacteriostatic drugs such as thiacetazone and PAS have bactericidal action. Isoniazid is the most potent bactericidal drug.
  - Ethambutol is bacteriostatic at low doses and bactericidal at high doses.
- Sterilising action is defined as the capacity of antituberculous drugs to kill special populations of slowly or intermittently metabolising semidormant bacilli, the so-called 'persisters'. Rifampicin and pyrazinamide are the main sterilising drugs.

Q. What are antituberculous drugs and what are their dosages in adults? (CT1.14)

Q. Discuss modes of action of first-line drugs. (CT1.14)

- First-line drugs: Isoniazid, rifampicin, pyrazinamide, ethambutol, streptomycin.
- Table 2.28 gives dosage of various antituberculous agents according to weight.
- Other antituberculous drugs are given in Table 2.29.

MODE OF ACTION OF FIRST-LINE ANTITUBERCULOUS DRUGS

- In a tuberculous lesion, particularly a cavity, mycobacteria exist in several foci. These foci and the drugs acting on them are:
  - Extracellular, in alkaline medium—streptomycin.
  - Rapidly metabolising mycobacteria (generally in a cavity)—rifampicin.
  - Less actively multiplying bacilli in acidic and closed lesions—isoniazid.

TABLE 2.28 Antituberculous Drugs and Their Doses According to Body Weights

S. no.	Drugs	16–25 kg	26–45 kg	46–70 kg	>70 kg
1.	Rifampicin (R)	300 mg	450 mg	600 mg	600 mg
2.	Isoniazid (H)	200 mg	200 mg	300 mg	450 mg
3.	Ethambutol (E)	400 mg	800 mg	1200 mg	1600 mg
4.	Pyrazinamide (Z)	500 mg	1250 mg	1500 mg	2000 mg
5.	Streptomycin (S)	500 mg	750 mg	1000 mg	1000 mg
6.	Kanamycin (Km)	500 mg	500 mg	750 mg	1000 mg
7.	Capreomycin (Cm)	500 mg	750 mg	1000 mg	1000 mg
8.	Amikacin (Am)	500 mg	500 mg	750 mg	1000 mg
9.	Levofloxacin (Lfx)	250 mg	750 mg	1000 mg	1000 mg
10.	Moxifloxacin (Mfx)	200 mg	400 mg	400 mg	400 mg
11.	Ethionamide (Eto)	375 mg	500 mg	750 mg	1000 mg
12.	Prothionamide (Pto)	375 mg	500 mg	750 mg	1000 mg
13.	Cycloserine (Cs)	250 mg	500 mg	750 mg	1000 mg
14.	Terizidone (Trd)	250 mg	500 mg	750 mg	1000 mg
15.	*para*-Aminosalicylate sodium (PAS)	7.5 g	10 g	12 g	16 g
16.	High-dose INH (Hh)	400 mg	600 mg	900 mg	900 mg
17.	Clofazimine (Cfz)	100 mg	200 mg	200 mg	200 mg

TABLE 2.28 Antituberculous Drugs and Their Doses According to Body Weights—cont'd

S. no.	Drugs	16–25 kg	26–45 kg	46–70 kg	>70 kg
18.	Linezolid (Lzd)	300 mg	600 mg	600 mg	600 mg
19.	Amoxyclav (Amx-Clv)	875/125 mg BD	875/125 mg BD	875/125 mg two morning + one evening	875/125 mg two morning + one evening
20.	Clarithromycin (Clr)	250 mg BD	500 mg BD	500 mg BD	750 mg BD

Note: 1. Ethionamide, prothionamide, cycloserine, terizidone, PAS are bacteriostatic drugs.
2. Ethionamide, prothionamide, cycloserine, terizidone, PAS are given in two divided doses.
3. Pyridoxine in a dose of 10–20 mg/day is added to regimens containing isoniazid.

TABLE 2.29 Other Antituberculous Drugs

Drug	Dose
Bedaquiline	400 mg daily for 14 days followed by 200 mg thrice a week
Linezolid	600 mg daily
Delamanid	100 mg twice daily
Meropenem	1 g thrice a day
Imipenem–cilastatin	1 g thrice a day
Clavulanate	250 mg thrice a day

- Dormant bacilli (which cause a relapse)—pyrazinamide.

OTHER DRUGS

- A new drug approved for MDR tuberculosis is bedaquiline, which is a mycobacterial ATP synthase inhibitor. Dose is 400 mg/day for 2 weeks and then 200 mg thrice a week. Common adverse effects are cardiovascular including QTc prolongation, hepatotoxicity, central nervous system toxicity and musculoskeletal symptoms like myalgia and tendonitis.
- Another new drug approved is delamanid which inhibits synthesis of mycolic acids.
- Third drug is protamanid which is effective against both growing and nongrowing bacteria and acts by interfering in protein synthesis and formation of the lipids in the cell wall.

Q. Describe rifampicin-related antitubercular agents. (CT1.14)

RIFABUTIN

- It is active against *M. tuberculosis*.
- It is also active against some rifampicin-resistant strains of *M. tuberculosis* and is more active against *M. avium intracellulare* complex as compared to rifampicin.
- It is recommended in the treatment of tuberculosis in HIV-infected patients who are on protease inhibitors.
- Dose is 150 mg/day. Patients taking rifabutin also have discoloured (orange) body secretions.
- Adverse effects include GI distress, rash, myalgias and insomnia. Less common side effects are flu-like syndrome, anterior uveitis, leucopenia, skin discolouration and hepatitis.

RIFAPENTINE

- It is lipophilic and has a longer duration of action.
- Strains resistant to rifampicin are also resistant to this drug.
- Dose is 600 mg once or twice a week.
- It may be used in the treatment of pulmonary tuberculosis in place of rifampicin.
- Side effects are similar to those of rifampicin.

Q. What are the side effects of the commonly used antituberculous drugs? (CT1.14)

- Side effects of antituberculous drugs are given in Table 2.30.

TABLE 2.30 Side Effects of Antituberculous Drugs

Drug	Adverse Reactions
• Isoniazid	Uncommon—hepatitis, cutaneous hypersensitivity, peripheral neuropathy (preventable and treatable with pyridoxine) Rare—giddiness, convulsions, optic neuritis, mental symptoms, haemolytic anaemia, aplastic anaemia, agranulocytosis, lupoid reactions, arthralgia, gynaecomastia
• Rifampicin	Uncommon—hepatitis, cutaneous reactions, gastrointestinal reactions, thrombocytopenic purpura, febrile reactions (flu-like syndrome; more common with intermittent therapy which was given previously) Rare—shortness of breath, shock, haemolytic anaemia, acute renal failure
• Streptomycin and other aminoglycosides	Common—cutaneous hypersensitivity, giddiness, numbness, tinnitus Uncommon—vertigo, ataxia, deafness, hypokalaemia Rare—renal damage, aplastic anaemia, agranulocytosis

continued

TABLE 2.30 Side Effects of Antituberculous Drugs—cont'd

Drug	Adverse Reactions
• Pyrazinamide	Common—anorexia, nausea, flushing Uncommon—hepatitis (dose related), vomiting, arthralgia, cutaneous hypersensitivity Rare—sideroblastic anaemia, photosensitivity
• Ethambutol	Uncommon—retrobulbar neuritis (dose related), arthralgia Rare—cutaneous hypersensitivity, peripheral neuropathy
• Ethionamide	Common—anorexia, vomiting Uncommon—serious neurological reactions, hepatitis Rare—hypothyroidism
• Cycloserine[a]	Common—headache, somnolence Uncommon—psychosis, seizures, peripheral neuropathy, suicidal ideation
• Quinolones	Common—GI intolerance, skin rashes Uncommon—phototoxicity (with sparfloxacin), dizziness, headache, insomnia Rare—confusion, seizures, interstitial nephritis, vasculitis, acute renal failure, prolonged QT interval, hyperglycaemia, tendon rupture
• PAS	Common—gastrointestinal reactions Uncommon—hepatitis, cutaneous hypersensitivity, hypokalaemia Rare—acute renal failure, haemolytic anaemia, thrombocytopenia, hypothyroidism

[a]Terizidone may have less CNS side effects compared to cycloserine.

Q. Discuss regimen of antituberculous chemotherapy. (CT1.15)

- Commonly used antituberculous regimens are given in Box 2.44.
- Fixed drug combinations (FDCs) are preferred to have good compliance. The drug dosage of FDCs based on body weight is given in Table 2.31.

BOX 2.44 Antituberculous Regimen

Potent 6-Month Regimens

- When there is a low rate of initial drug resistance (recommended standard 6-month regimen)
  - 2HRZ/4HR
- When there is a high level of initial drug resistance (as in India)
  - 2HRZE/4HRE
  - 2SHRZ/4HRE

Note: The number used as prefix indicates the number of months of treatment.

TABLE 2.31 Fixed Drug Combinations Based on Body Weight

Weight Category	Number of Tablets (FDC) Intensive Phase	Continuation Phase	Streptomycin
	HRZE	HRE	
	75/150/400/275 mg	75/150/275 mg	Grams
25–39 kg	2	2	0.5
40–54 kg	3	3	0.75
55–69 kg	4	4	1.0
≥70 kg	5	5	1.0

Note: Streptomycin should be added in intensive phase for 2 months in the previously treated regimen of drug-sensitive patients. In patients older than 50 years, maximum dose of streptomycin should be 0.75 g.

Q. What is short-course chemotherapy? What are the advantages of short-course chemotherapy? (CT1.15)

- Short-course chemotherapy is now widely accepted as the treatment of choice for tuberculosis. It includes 6-month regimen (refer 'Antituberculous Regimen' in Box 2.44).
- Short-course regimens are divided into two phases: an initial or bactericidal phase and a continuation or sterilising phase.
- During the initial phase, majority of mycobacteria are killed, symptoms resolve and the patient becomes noninfectious.
- During continuation phase, the semidormant 'persisters' are eliminated.

ADVANTAGES OF SHORT-COURSE CHEMOTHERAPY

- This regimen is easy to take and produces fewer upsets in the patients.
- The patient feels better more quickly.
- The sputum becomes negative more quickly, 85% negative at 2 months compared to only 50% in older 12-month regimens.
- The relapse rate is low.
- If relapse does occur, the tubercle bacilli remain sensitive and the same treatment can be given again.

Q. What is the 'fall and rise' phenomenon?

- The 'fall and rise' phenomenon is observed in inadequately treated patients.
- Sputum smear is positive at the commencement of therapy. Thereafter, the sputum bacillary content declines, and it becomes negative on smear microscopy and positive only on culture—the 'fall'. Still later, the sputum bacillary content increases and the sputum smear becomes positive again—the 'rise'.

- What actually occurs in 'fall and rise' phenomenon is the 'fall' of drug-sensitive bacilli and the 'rise' of drug-resistant mutants of the strain. This is because the drug-resistant bacilli rapidly outgrow rest of the drug-sensitive bacilli. This results in the drug-resistant mutants completely replacing the drug-sensitive bacilli and finally the strain becoming fully resistant.

Q. How can the progress of antitubercular treatment be monitored and the treatment result assessed? (CT1.17)

- The main method of monitoring the progress of treatment and assessing the final result is bacteriological examination. Other less useful methods include radiological assessment, erythrocyte sedimentation rate (ESR) and body weight changes.

BACTERIOLOGICAL ASSESSMENT

- Bacteriological assessment is done by examining sputum by smear and culture. Serial sputum smear examinations alone would clearly indicate the progress and ultimate result. Culture examinations are merely confirmatory and are indicated only in selected cases.
- Sputum smear examination—see DOTS on this page.
- A treatment failure may be indicated by various patterns:
  - Persistence of sputum bacilli (no response).
  - An initial decline followed by a steady rise in sputum positivity ('fall and rise' phenomenon).
  - An initial decline and sputum negativity, followed much later by sputum positivity (relapse).

RADIOLOGICAL ASSESSMENT

- Serial chest radiographs can be used to assess progress and determine final result. Grossly, if serial radiographs show improvement, this may be considered as a favourable response.
- It is important to note that radiological assessment can be misleading many times. Patients with radiological improvement may still discharge tubercle bacilli. On the other hand, bacteriologically quiescent cases may show no radiological improvement or even worsening.

ERYTHROCYTE SEDIMENTATION RATE

- ESR is not a very satisfactory method of assessing the progress or activity of disease in patients on chemotherapy. However, a fall in ESR may be considered as a favourable response.

BODY WEIGHT CHANGES

- Body weight changes are also not very reliable. However, a gain in body weight may be considered as a favourable response.

Q. Discuss the directly observed treatment, short course (DOTS). (CT1.18)

Q. What is stop TB strategy?

Q. What is end TB strategy?

- Directly observed treatment, short-course or DOTS means administering potent antimycobacterial regimens to a patient with tuberculosis under direct supervision.
- Despite short-course therapy, tuberculosis remains the leading infectious cause of death in India, killing close to 370,000 people a year (i.e. roughly 1000 every day). India has far more cases of tuberculosis than any other country in the world—about 2.7 million new cases each year of which 800,000 are infectious. Daily therapy is excellent.
- DOTS is the backbone of Revised National Tuberculosis Control Programme (RNTCP) in India.
- The basic objectives of RNTCP are:
  - To treat successfully 85% of detected smear-positive cases.
  - To detect 70% of all such cases.
- DOTS is a five-point programme that can ensure effective TB control (Box 2.45).

PROGRESS UNDER RNTCP

- The RNTCP based on the DOTS strategy began as a pilot in 1993 and gradually expanded to cover a population of 20 million by mid-1998. Rapid RNTCP expansion began in late 1998. By the end of 2000, 30% of the country's population was covered, and by the end of 2002, 50% of the country's population was covered under the RNTCP. By the end of 2003, 778 million population was covered, and the coverage reached to 997 million at the end of year 2004. By December 2005, around 97% (about 1080 million) of the population had been covered, and the entire country has been covered under DOTS by 24 March 2006 (World TB Day).
- The National AIDS Control Programme and the RNTCP have developed a 'National Framework of joint TB/HIV Collaborative activities'. Nationwide coverage of services for programmatic management of drug-resistant TB, which began in 2007, has been achieved in March 2013.
- In 2012, the National Strategic Plan (NSP) under the RNTCP was released to achieve universal access to quality tuberculosis diagnosis and treatment by taking a detect–treat–prevent–build approach.
- To enhance notification of tuberculosis cases, private practitioners, private organisations, NGOs, professional

BOX 2.45 DOTS Programme

- Political and administrative support
- Diagnosis by sputum microscopy in patients attending health facilities
- Good drugs for short-course chemotherapy
- Directly observed treatment that should be accessible, acceptable and accountable
- Systematic monitoring and accountability

bodies like Indian Medical Association have been engaged.
- Complete geographical coverage for diagnostic and treatment services for MDR tuberculosis achieved in 2013, with a remarkable 93,000 persons with MDR-TB diagnosed and put on treatment till 2015.
- All healthcare providers mandated to notify every tuberculosis case diagnosed and/or treated to local authorities.
- Other initiatives include drug susceptibility test-guided treatment for drug-resistant patients, molecular techniques at antiretroviral treatment sites in five high TB/HIV burden states to detect MDR tuberculosis among people living with HIV and screening all tuberculosis patients for diabetes.

IMPLEMENTATION OF DOTS

- Patients with any one of the symptoms suggestive of tuberculosis—cough >2 weeks, fever >2 weeks, significant weight loss, haemoptysis or any abnormality in chest radiograph—are considered 'presumptive pulmonary tuberculosis case'.
- Such patients are encouraged to attend the nearest healthcare facility for chest radiograph (if available) and sputum examination over a 2-day period (one spot on the day of attending the health facility, second next-day morning sample collected at home and the third spot sputum when the patient comes to deposit the second sample). Only two sputum samples are advised in countries with active external quality assurance system, high workload and limited human resources, and if one is positive, it indicates active tuberculosis.
- Under the RNTCP, two methods of microscopy are currently being used—ZN stain-based microscopy using conventional microscope and light emitting diode-based fluorescent microscopy (LED FM).
- If one or two of the smears are positive for acid-fast bacilli, antituberculosis treatment is initiated.
- For DOTS, the patients with tuberculosis are categorised into three categories and treatment is given as per the recommendations.

CATEGORIES OF TUBERCULOSIS

- In 2009, WHO gave a new classification for tuberculosis patients:
  - New patients:
    - New case—patients have never had treatment for tuberculosis or have taken antitubercular drugs for <1 month. New patients may have positive or negative bacteriology and may have disease at any anatomical site.
    - New patients with pulmonary TB may receive a daily intensive phase followed by daily continuation phase (2HRZE/4HRE). Intermittent therapy is no longer recommended. Duration is for 6 months except for tuberculosis of meninges, bones and joints and lymph nodes, where duration may be 9–12 months.
    - A cartridge-based nucleic acid amplification test (CBNAAT) is performed on sputum-positive patients to rule out rifampicin resistance and categorised as microbiologically confirmed drug-sensitive TB or RIF-resistant TB.
    - If the first smear is negative and chest radiograph is suggestive of tuberculosis, second sputum sample is subjected to smear and cartridge-based nucleic acid amplification test (CBNAAT) simultaneously.
    - If both the sputum smear and chest radiograph are negative, the patient may be referred to a pulmonologist.
    - Follow-up sputum smear at completion of intensive phase and continuation phase. If smear is positive at any of these points, a culture should be done for drug sensitivity testing.
    - Chest radiograph if available at the end of treatment.
- Previously treated patients:
  - These are patients who have received 1 month or more of antitubercular drugs in the past. A culture and drug sensitivity test as well as a CBNAAT should be performed at the time of starting treatment; the latter is for rifampicin resistance. Further subdivided into:
    - Recurrent cases (cured initially with completed treatment and subsequently found to be microbiologically confirmed tuberculosis cases).
    - Failure patients (patients who have previously been treated for tuberculosis and whose treatment failed at the end of their most recent course of treatment).
    - Treatment after loss to follow-up cases (patients previously treated for tuberculosis for at least 1 month and were declared lost to follow-up in their most recent course of treatment and subsequently found microbiologically confirmed tuberculosis cases).
    - Other previously treated patients (those who have previously been treated for tuberculosis but whose outcome after their most recent course of treatment is unknown or undocumented).
- Transferred in patients (patients who have been received for treatment in a tuberculosis unit, after registered for treatment in another tuberculosis unit).

Note: As per a notification from the Ministry of Health and Family Welfare dated 18 December 2018, all previously treated TB should be initiated on standard first-line anti-tubercular regimen (2HRZE/4HRE) as prescribed for new TB patients. Drug susceptibility testing (DST) should be conducted for at least isoniazid and rifampicin before starting treatment and the most appropriate regimen should be prescribed as per the DST report. If resistance is detected, tests to find out fluoroquinolone resistance should also be carried out.

OPERATIONAL ASPECTS OF DOTS

- Specimens for culture and DST should be obtained from all previously treated TB patients at or before the start of treatment. Drug susceptibility test should be performed for at least isoniazid and rifampicin. Rapid molecular methods (e.g. GeneXpert) for detection of drug resistance should be used if available.

- For smear-positive pulmonary TB patients (both new and retreatment groups), sputum smear microscopy may be performed at completion of the intensive phase of treatment.
- In patients treated with the regimen containing rifampicin throughout treatment, if a positive sputum smear is found at completion of the intensive phase, the extension of the intensive phase is not recommended.
  - In new patients, if the specimen obtained at the end of intensive phase is smear-positive, sputum culture and DST should be performed.
  - In previously treated patients, if the specimen obtained at the end of the intensive phase (month 3) is smear-positive, sputum culture and DST should be performed.
- Sputum specimens for smear microscopy should be obtained at the end of continuation phase for all new pulmonary TB patients who were smear-positive at the start of treatment. Patients whose sputum smears are positive at that point of time should be re-registered as having failed treatment.
- Medications for both phases of treatment are kept in an individual box containing the entire course of treatment for a single patient. The drugs are in the form of fixed-drug combinations—two or more drugs are combined together in a single pill or tablet. For the intensive phase, patient is given 1-week supply of drugs while during combination phase, 1-month supply is provided.
- Under DOTS, the patient has to take the medication in front of a DOTS agent. The DOTS agent is usually a volunteer from the patient's community, and may be a family member.

STOP TB STRATEGY

- The vision of Stop TB Strategy is to free the world of tuberculosis.
- Its targets are:
  - Detect at least 70% of new sputum smear-positive TB cases and cure at least 85% of these cases by 2005.
  - Reduce prevalence of and death due to TB by 50% relative to 1990 by 2015.
  - Eliminate TB as a public health problem (<1 case per million population per year) by 2050.
- The new Stop TB Strategy by WHO in 2006 has the following components:
  - Pursue quality DOTS expansion and enhancement by improving the case finding and cure through an effective patient-centred approach to reach all patients, especially the poor.
  - Addressing TB/HIV.
  - Addressing MDR-TB by DOTS-Plus (providing drugs for MDR tuberculosis).
  - Health system strengthening by collaborating with other health programmes and general services.
  - Involvement of all care providers including NGOs and private doctors.
  - Engaging people with TB and affected communities.
  - Enabling/promoting research for developing new drugs, diagnostics and vaccines.

END TB STRATEGY

- Launched in 2014 with the goal of eliminating tuberculosis (<1 case per million population) by 2035.
- This vision stands on the growing awareness that tuberculosis cannot be eliminated from a single area unless all the countries collaborate together towards a shared objective and through a common strategic plan.
- Described under three pillars:
  - Pillar I: Activities focusing on integrated, patient-centred diagnosis, treatment and prevention of tuberculosis in adults and children, within close collaboration involving civil society, the social sector, local communities and other stakeholders.
  - Pillar II: Several socioeconomic and public health interventions, which are often under the responsibility of ministries other than the Ministry of Health and Family Welfare (e.g. economy, finance, interior or justice).
  - Pillar III: Intensified research activities and innovation.

SOME OF THE STANDARDS FOR DIAGNOSIS AND TREATMENT UNDER PILLAR I (Box 2.46)

BOX 2.46 Standards for Diagnosis and Treatment Under Pillar I of End TB Strategy

- All patients with signs and symptoms of pulmonary tuberculosis who are capable of producing sputum should have as their initial diagnostic test at least one sputum specimen submitted for Xpert MTB/RIF Ultra assay. A second Xpert MTB/RIF Ultra assay may be performed for all patients who initially test negative by Xpert MTB/RIF Ultra but whose signs and symptoms of TB persist.
- The Xpert MTB/RIF Ultra assay should be used in preference to conventional microscopy and culture as the initial diagnostic test for cerebrospinal fluid specimens from patients being evaluated for tuberculous meningitis. The Xpert MTB/RIF Ultra assay is recommended as a replacement test for usual practice (including conventional microscopy, culture or histopathology) for testing specific nonrespiratory specimens (lymph nodes and other tissues) from patients suspected of having extrapulmonary tuberculosis.
- Drug susceptibility testing using rapid tests should be performed for all TB patients prior to starting therapy, including new patients and patients who require retreatment. If rifampicin resistance is detected, rapid molecular tests for resistance to isoniazid, fluoroquinolones and second-line injectable agents should be performed promptly.
- Culture-based drug susceptibility testing for selected second-line antituberculous drugs should be performed for patients enrolled in individualised, longer-duration MDR tuberculosis treatment.
- While awaiting drug susceptibility testing results, patients with probable drug-susceptible tuberculosis and patients who have not been treated previously and do not have other risk factors for drug resistance should receive a WHO-recommended first-line treatment regimen using quality-assured anti-TB agents.

continued

BOX 2.46 Standards for Diagnosis and Treatment Under Pillar I of End TB Strategy—cont'd

- The initial phase should consist of 2 months of isoniazid, rifampicin, pyrazinamide and ethambutol. The continuation phase should consist of 4 months of isoniazid, rifampicin and ethambutol.
- Daily dosing (and not intermittent dosing) should be used throughout treatment.
- In patients who require retreatment, drug susceptibility testing should be conducted to decide treatment regimen.
- In patients with rifampicin-susceptible, isoniazid-resistant tuberculosis, 6 months of combination treatment with rifampicin, ethambutol, pyrazinamide and levofloxacin, with or without isoniazid, is recommended.
- Patients with MDR/rifampicin-resistant tuberculosis require second-line treatment regimens. They may be treated using a 9- to 11-month MDR-TB treatment regimen (the shorter regimen) unless they have resistance to second-line anti-TB agents or meet other exclusion criteria. In these cases, a longer (individualised) regimen with at least five effective antituberculous drugs in the intensive phase and four agents in the continuation phase is recommended for ≥20 months.
- Partial resection surgery has a role in treating MDR-TB.

Q. What is DOTS-Plus strategy? (CT1.18)

- Applicable to areas where prevalence of MDR tuberculosis is high. Outcome of the standard short-course regimen remains uncertain. Unacceptable failure occurs and resistance to additional agents may be induced. DOTS-Plus provides additional services in such areas to provide high cure rate and reduce transmission.
- DOTS-Plus launched in 2007.
- DOTS-Plus modified all the elements of the DOTS strategy:
  - Treatment may need to be individualised rather than standardised.
  - Laboratory services may need to provide facilities for on-site culture and drug-susceptibility testing.
  - Reliable supplies of a wide range of expensive second-line agents.
  - Operational studies required to determine the indications of modified treatment.
  - Financial and technical support from international organisations needed in addition to that obtained from local governments.
- By 2012, the DOTS-Plus service (now referred to as the 'Programmatic Management of Drug Resistant Tuberculosis') had been expanded across the whole country and by 2013, the service was available in all districts. The services were to be totally integrated into the main RNTCP services at local level.
- In 2014, India achieved complete geographical coverage for diagnostic and treatment services for multidrug-resistant tuberculosis.

Q. What are the forms of drug resistances encountered during antituberculous chemotherapy? (CT1.17)

Q. What are the common causes of drug resistance? (CT1.4)

PRIMARY DRUG RESISTANCE AND INITIAL DRUG RESISTANCE

- Primary drug resistance occurs in patients who have either not received any antituberculous chemotherapy before or received it for less than 1 month. It is caused by transmission of drug-resistant organisms from another patient with secondary resistance due to inadequate chemotherapy.
- When it is impossible to obtain a reliable history of previous chemotherapy from a new, drug-resistant patient, it is better to use the term initial drug resistance. This term would cover true primary as well as undisclosed acquired resistance.

SECONDARY OR ACQUIRED DRUG RESISTANCE

- Resistance to one or more drugs, often due to incorrect chemotherapy, is called secondary or acquired resistance.

NATURAL DRUG RESISTANCE

- Strains that have never been exposed to any antibacterial drug are termed 'wild strains'. A naturally drug-resistant strain is a wild strain resistant to a particular drug without ever coming in contact with it. Thus, neither the patient with naturally resistant bacilli nor his/her source of infection has had chemotherapy in the past.

MULTIPLE DRUG RESISTANCE OR MULTIDRUG-RESISTANT (MDR) STRAINS

- MDR tuberculosis is defined as resistance to isoniazid and rifampicin whether there is resistance to other drugs or not. It is therefore incorrect, by this definition, to classify a patient with a MDR disease if he/she has an infection with a bacterium susceptible to rifampicin but resistant to many other drugs.

EXTENSIVELY DRUG RESISTANCE

- XDR tuberculosis is defined as resistance to isoniazid and rifampicin along with any fluoroquinolone and at least one of the three injectable second-line drugs (capreomycin, kanamycin and amikacin).
- Worldwide, XDR-TB constitutes 9.7% of MDR-TB patients (WHO, 2015).
- In India, the prevalence of XDR-TB among MDR-TB patients varies from 0.3% to 60%.

EXTREMELY RESISTANT TUBERCULOSIS OR TOTALLY DRUG-RESISTANT TUBERCULOSIS

- Cases resistant to all available first-line drugs and second-line drugs.

CAUSES OF DRUG RESISTANCE (Box 2.47)

BOX 2.47 Causes of Drug Resistance in Tuberculous Bacilli

- Factors related to previous antituberculous treatment
  - Inadequate treatment regimen
  - Inadequate supervision of therapy
  - Use of poor-quality drugs
  - Poor absorption of drugs
  - Inadequate compliance
  - Development of adverse drug reactions
- Inadequate duration of treatment
- Infection due to organisms with primary resistance
- Lack of good laboratory facilities to monitor drug susceptibility
- Genetic factors

Q. What are the various methods for performing drug susceptibility tests for *M. tuberculosis*?

- Lowenstein–Jensen (LJ) culture for drug sensitivity testing takes about 6- to 8-week time.
- Radiometric methods (BACTEC radiometric method) give results within 10 days of inoculation.
- Mycobacteria growth indicator tube (MGIT) system is a rapid, nonradioactive method for detection and susceptibility testing of *M. tuberculosis*. The MGIT system relies on an oxygen-sensitive fluorescent compound contained in a silicone plug at the bottom of the tube which contains the medium to detect mycobacterial growth. The medium is inoculated with a sample containing mycobacteria and with subsequent growth, mycobacteria utilise the oxygen and the compound fluoresces.
- Nitrate reduction assays are based on the capacity of *M. tuberculosis* to reduce nitrate to nitrite, yielding a visually detected red colour after the Griess reaction. It is performed in the LJ medium. However, some strains of *M. tuberculosis* are nitrate-reductase negative.
- Ligase chain reaction (LCR) involves the use of an enzyme DNA ligase, which functions to link two strands of DNA.
- Luciferase reporter assay is a system for rapid determination of drug resistance. Luciferase is an enzyme identified as the light-producing system of fireflies. The luciferase gene is placed into a mycobacteriophage. Once this mycobacteriophage attaches to *M. tuberculosis*, the phage DNA is injected into it and the viral genes are expressed. If *M. tuberculosis* is infected with luciferase reporter phage and these organisms are placed in contact with antituberculous drugs, susceptibility can be tested by correlating the generation of light. It can detect resistant strains within 48 hours.
- PCR-based sequencing to detect mutations responsible for drug resistance.
- Line probe assays and GeneXpert to detect drug-resistant (particularly rifampicin-resistant) bacilli.

Q. How will you manage a patient with multidrug-resistant (MDR) tuberculosis? (CT1.17)

Q. How will you manage extensively resistant (XDR) tuberculosis? (CT1.17)

- The National Guidelines for Programmatic Management of Drug-Resistant Tuberculosis (PMDT) in India offer an integrated drug-resistant tuberculosis (DR-TB) treatment algorithm with standard treatment regimen for MDR-TB and XDR-TB designed in accordance with WHO guidelines for PMDT (2011 updates).
- Rifampicin-resistant tuberculosis (RR-TB) patients detected using WHO-endorsed rapid molecular tests are treated with the standard regimen for MDR-TB.
- In patients with confirmed rifampicin-susceptible, isoniazid-resistant tuberculosis, treatment with rifampicin, ethambutol, pyrazinamide and levofloxacin is recommended for a duration of 6 months. It is not recommended to add streptomycin or other injectable agents to the treatment regimen.
- The algorithm under PMDT also offers scope for modifying the standard regimen for MDR-TB in cases with additional resistance to fluoroquinolones or second-line injectable drugs based on second-line drug susceptibility testing at baseline.
- For managing MDR and XDR tuberculosis, drugs are categorised into three groups (Table 2.32).

TABLE 2.32 Antituberculous Drugs for Managing MDR/XDR Tuberculosis

Group	Drugs
A	Levofloxacin (Lfx) or moxifloxacin (Mfx) Bedaquiline (Bdq) Linezolid (Lzd)
B	Clofazimine (Cfz) Cycloserine (Cs) or terizidone (Trd)
C	Ethambutol (E) Pyrazinamide (Z) Delamanid (Dlm) Imipenem-cilastatin (Ipm-Cln) or meropenem (Mpm) along with clavulanic acid (Clv) Amikacin (Am) or streptomycin (S) Ethionamide (Eto) or prothionamide (Pto) Para-aminosalicylic acid (PAS)

Note: 1. Each dose of carbapenems (meropenem or imipenem-cilastatin) should be administered with amoxicillin-clavunate.
2. The commonly used second-line injectable drugs kanamycin and capreomycin are associated with worse outcomes, and are no longer recommended for the treatment of MDR-TB.

(*Source:* WHO Consolidated Guidelines on Tuberculosis. Module 4: Treatment. Drug-resistant Tuberculosis Treatment, 2020.)

BOX 2.48 Principles for Managing a Patient with MDR Tuberculosis

- Treatment should be in a specialised centre with standard laboratory facilities.
- An appropriate regimen for individual patient needs experience and skill.
- Initiation of MDR-TB treatment is devised on the following principles:
  - Preferably an oral treatment regimen for most patients.
  - Drug resistance to at least FQ and second-line injectables should be ruled out prior to initiating treatment, especially in shorter MDRTB regimen.
  - Close monitoring of these patients for adverse effects and treatment outcome is essential.
- WHO recommended an injection-free therapy (groups A and B drugs) at the initiation of MDR-TB treatment. Group C agents (oral and parenteral) should be administered when Groups A and B drugs cannot be used.
- A shorter all-oral bedaquiline-containing regimen of 9–12 months duration is recommended in eligible patients with confirmed multidrug- or rifampicin-resistant tuberculosis (MDR/RR-TB) who have not been exposed to treatment with second-line TB medicines used in this regimen for more than 1 month, and in whom resistance to fluoroquinolones has been excluded.
- The shorter regimen conditionally recommended of bedaquiline (used for 6 months), in combination with levofloxacin/moxifloxacin, ethionamide, ethambutol, isoniazid (high-dose; 15 mg/kg with maximum of 900 mg/day), pyrazinamide and clofazimine for 4 months (with the possibility of extending to 6 months if the patient remains sputum smear positive at the end of 4 months); followed by 5 months of treatment with levofloxacin/moxifloxacin, clofazimine, ethambutol and pyrazinamide.
- In MDR patients on longer regimens, all three Group A agents and at least one Group B agent should be included to ensure that treatment starts with at least four TB agents likely to be effective, and that at least three agents are included for the rest of treatment if bedaquiline is stopped.
  - If only one or two Group A agents are used, both Group B agents are to be included.
  - If the regimen cannot be composed with agents from Groups A and B alone, Group C agents are added to complete it.
  - Regimens containing amikacin or streptomycin, an intensive phase of 6–7 months is suggested for most patients
  - Performance of sputum culture in addition to sputum smear microscopy is recommended to monitor treatment response. It is desirable for sputum culture to be repeated at monthly intervals.
  - Total duration of therapy is 18–20 months
- A new 6- to 9-month regimen composed of bedaquiline, pretomanid and linezolid has been conditionally recommended for use in patients with MDR/RR-TB and additional fluoroquinolone resistance, who have either had no previous exposure to bedaquiline and linezolid or have been exposed for no more than 2 weeks.
- Community- or home-based directly observed treatment (DOT) is recommended over health facility-based DOT or unsupervised treatment.
- DOT administered by trained lay providers or healthcare workers is recommended over DOT administered by family members or unsupervised treatment.
- If resistance tests cannot be performed, treatment should be continued for a minimum of 18 months after culture conversion.
- Never add a single drug to a failing regimen.
- Surgical treatment should be considered as an adjunct to chemotherapy, wherever applicable, as results of chemotherapy are very unpredictable.

PRINCIPLES FOR MANAGING A PATIENT WITH MDR TUBERCULOSIS

- Guiding principles for managing a patient with MDR tuberculosis are given in Box 2.48.

TREATMENT OF XDR TUBERCULOSIS

- Antituberculous drugs are categorised as indicated for MDR tuberculosis.
- A drug is considered to be effective if the baseline drug susceptibility test (DST) shows susceptibility to that drug; however, if DST results are not available, a drug may still considered to be effective if not previously taken for at least 1 month.
- At least five drugs with proven susceptibility or which are most likely to be effective should be used.
- Both pyrazinamide and ethambutol should be used irrespective of DST.
- Another drug to be added is from group B. It is recommended to use an injectable agent that has never been used before (or consider designing the regimen without an injectable agent in case of reported resistance to all injectable agents). It can be given for 6–12 months based on culture conversion.
- Add one of the fluoroquinolones and one or two of group C drugs (that have not been used or less exposed in a previous regimen).
- Add one or more of group D2 and D3 drugs.
- High-dose isoniazid (H^h) may also be added.
- Localised disease should be considered for adjuvant surgery if possible.
- Indian guidelines recommend (6–12) Km/Am, PAS, Mfx, H^h, Cfz, Lzd, Amx-Clv followed by (18) PAS, Mfx, H^h, Cfz, Lzd, Amx-Clv for XDR tuberculosis.

Q. What are the indications of corticosteroids in the management of tuberculosis?

- Corticosteroids should always be given only in conjunction with antituberculous chemotherapy and never without ATT. They act by reducing the severity both of the local inflammatory reaction and of the associated systemic disturbances.

INDICATIONS

- Severe allergic reactions (hypersensitivity) to antituberculous drugs.
- Fulminating, life-threatening pulmonary tuberculosis (keeps the patient alive until the antituberculous drugs begin to act).
- Tuberculous pericardial effusion (reduces outpouring of fluid, reduces adhesions and reduces development of constrictive pericarditis).

- Tuberculosis of the eye, the larynx and ureteric obstruction in renal tuberculosis (reduces fibrosis and scar tissue formation).
- Tuberculous meningitis (reduces adhesions).
- Tuberculous adrenalitis with Addison's disease (replacement of corticosteroids).

DOSAGE

- In mild conditions, prednisolone is given 10 mg twice daily for 4–6 weeks, followed by a gradual tapering of 5 mg each week.
- In seriously ill patients, particularly tuberculous meningitis, the initial dose should be 60–80 mg daily, tapering gradually as above.

Q. What is extrapulmonary tuberculosis?

- The term extrapulmonary tuberculosis (EPTB) indicates isolated occurrence of tuberculosis at body sites other than the lung. Tuberculous intrathoracic lymphadenopathy (mediastinal and/or hilar) or tuberculous pleural effusion, without radiographic abnormalities in the lungs, constitutes a case of EPTB.
- However, when an extrapulmonary focus is evident in a patient with pulmonary tuberculosis, such patients are categorised as pulmonary tuberculosis.
- EPTB constitutes about 15%–20% of all cases of TB in immunocompetent patients.
- In HIV-positive patients, EPTB accounts for >50% of all cases of TB.
- TB lymphadenitis is seen in nearly 35% of EPTB cases. Cervical lymph nodes are the most common site of involvement and can occur with or without involvement of other lymphoid tissue. Cervical lymphadenitis is also referred to as scrofula. Antituberculous drugs are highly effective in treating lymph node tuberculosis. When lymph nodes are fluctuant, antigravity aspiration should be done.
- Scrofuloderma is a mycobacterial infection of the skin caused by direct extension of tuberculosis into the skin from underlying structures or by contact exposure to tuberculosis.
- Various forms of extrapulmonary tuberculosis are shown in Table 2.33.

TABLE 2.33 Extrapulmonary Tuberculosis

• Pleural	Pleural effusion
• Gastrointestinal	Ulcerations of the tongue, intestinal tuberculosis, tuberculous peritonitis
• Pericardium	Pericardial effusion and tamponade, constrictive pericarditis
• Genitourinary	Renal tuberculosis, salpingitis, tubal abscess, epididymal tuberculosis
• Nervous system	Tuberculous meningitis, tuberculous arteritis, cerebral tuberculoma
• Lymph nodes	Tuberculous lymphadenopathy (including mediastinal), nonhealing sinuses
• Skeletal system	Tuberculous osteomyelitis, cold abscess, vertebral tuberculosis, pyarthrosis
• Miscellaneous	Addison's disease (tuberculous adrenalitis), skin tuberculosis, phlyctenular keratoconjunctivitis, choroiditis, iritis

Q. Discuss the pathogenesis, types, clinical features, diagnosis and management of miliary tuberculosis in adults.

Q. Write in brief on cryptic miliary tuberculosis.

Q. Describe nonreactive miliary tuberculosis and disseminated nonreactive tuberculosis. Discuss their pathogenesis.

- Classified as pulmonary tuberculosis because there are lesions in the lungs.
- Results from widespread lymphohaematogenous dissemination of tubercle bacilli from a pulmonary or extrapulmonary focus.
- Most commonly involves liver, spleen, bone marrow, lungs and meninges.
- The tubercle bacilli may enter the bloodstream in various ways:
  - Spread to bloodstream from a recent primary infection. This may occur by way of lymph nodes and lymphatics or by a tuberculous lesion with erosion of a blood vessel.
  - Re-activation of an old tuberculous lesion with erosion of a blood vessel.
  - Spread into the bloodstream after a surgical operation on an organ containing a tuberculous lesion.

TYPES

- Clinically, the patients may be divided into three different types:
  1. Classical (acute) miliary tuberculosis.
  2. Cryptic (obscure) miliary tuberculosis.
  3. Nonreactive miliary tuberculosis.

CLASSICAL (ACUTE) MILIARY TUBERCULOSIS

- Can occur at any age, but children and young adults are more affected.
- Onset may be sudden or gradual. An insidious onset of fever, malaise and weight loss over weeks is the usual presentation.
- Systemic disturbances rapidly become profound, with high-grade fever, drenching night sweats and progressive pallor.
- Cough and breathlessness are occasionally present, but there may be no abnormal physical signs in the lungs. Widespread crepitations may be heard late in the disease.
- Hepatosplenomegaly may occur.
- Choroidal tubercles on ophthalmoscopy make the diagnosis certain. They are rare in the elderly.
- Tuberculous meningitis is a common complication. It manifests as neck stiffness and other signs of meningeal irritation.
- ARDS may complicate miliary tuberculosis.
- Without treatment, death occurs within days or weeks.
- Chest radiograph may show the characteristic 'miliary' mottling (size of millet seeds). Other causes of military shadows on chest radiograph include histoplasmosis, *Mycoplasma* pneumonia, sarcoidosis,

bronchoalveolar carcinoma, lymphangitis carcinomatosis, haemosiderosis (e.g. in long-standing rheumatic heart disease) and occupational lung diseases.
- Total leucocyte count is usually normal or low.
- Tuberculin test may be negative.

CRYPTIC (OBSCURE) MILIARY TUBERCULOSIS

- Usually occurs in the elderly.
- Often presents as lassitude, weight loss and general debility.
- Prolonged low-grade pyrexia is a common presenting manifestation.
- Anaemia is common and hepatosplenomegaly may occur. Chest is usually normal and choroidal tubercles are rare.
- Without treatment, patient slowly gets worse over months and eventually dies.
- Chest radiograph is usually normal. Miliary mottling may appear after weeks or months. The tuberculin test is usually negative.

NONREACTIVE MILIARY OR DISSEMINATED TUBERCULOSIS

- This condition is rare usually occurring in elderly with disease re-activation.
- It is an acute malignant form of tuberculous septicaemia, resulting in 'necrotic' lesions in various organs (no granuloma formation) containing massive number of bacilli.
- The patient is extremely ill and the diagnosis is often missed. If so, the patient dies rapidly.
- The chest radiograph may or may not show miliary mottling, and the tuberculin test is negative.
- Haematological abnormalities are very common. These include anaemia (often aplastic), pancytopenia (especially leucopenia or agranulocytosis) or leukaemoid reaction.

DIAGNOSIS

- Miliary tuberculosis should be suspected in any patient with prolonged fever, miliary mottling on radiograph and choroidal tubercles on fundoscopy.
- Chest radiograph may be virtually diagnostic if it shows the characteristic miliary shadows ('miliary mottling'). These are diffuse small shadows of 1–2 mm diameter. They are evenly distributed throughout both lung fields. Upper zones are always involved. The early lesions may be difficult to visualise. They are better visualised by one of the following methods:
  - Take an overpenetrated (dark) radiograph and shine a bright light behind the outer rib spaces.
  - Lateral chest film.
  - Underpenetrated anteroposterior radiograph.
  - High-resolution CT of chest.
- Positron emission tomography CT (PET-CT) using radiopharmaceutical ^{18}F-labelled 2-deoxy-D-glucose (FDG) may show 'hot' spots in areas of active tuberculosis. It can determine the activity of lesions, guide biopsy from active sites and detect occult distant foci.
- Sputum smear is usually negative but bronchoalveolar lavage and bronchial biopsy are likely to be positive.
- Bacteriological confirmation should be sought by culture of sputum, urine or bone marrow.
- Various haematological abnormalities may be seen, including anaemia, leucopenia, neutrophilic leucocytosis and leukaemoid reaction.
- DIC can develop in a minority of patients.
- Elevation of alkaline phosphatase and other liver enzymes may occur in severe hepatic involvement.
- Hyponatraemia occurs in about 50% of cases.
- Bone marrow biopsy may show miliary tubercles or tubercle bacilli on histology. Part of the specimen should be sent for culture for tubercle bacilli.
- Liver biopsy may show miliary tubercles on histology.
- Tuberculin test is only of limited value in the diagnosis of miliary tuberculosis.

MANAGEMENT

- Proved cases of acute and cryptic miliary tuberculosis should be treated with standard antituberculous chemotherapy. If the patient is desperately ill, prednisolone is given along with chemotherapy. This helps to reduce life-threatening toxicity and gives antituberculous drugs time to act.
- If the diagnosis is not proved in spite of strong clinical suspicion (e.g. cryptic miliary tuberculosis), give a therapeutic trial of antituberculous chemotherapy.

Q. Discuss the pathogenesis, clinical features, investigations and management of tuberculous pleural effusion. (CT1.11)

- Classically, tuberculous pleural effusion occurs in younger individuals in the absence of pulmonary tuberculosis. However, in one-third of cases, simultaneous pulmonary tuberculosis is present.

PATHOGENESIS

- Tuberculous pleural effusion results when the pleura is seeded with antigens released from *M. tuberculosis*. The pleural seeding may occur via lymphatics, bloodstream or by direct extension. There may be rupture of subpleural caseous focus into the pleural cavity. This results in development of delayed hypersensitivity reaction to tuberculous protein (produced by CD^{4+} cells). It causes increased permeability of pleural capillaries. There may also be some lymphatic block by fibrosis. Since pleural effusion develops as a result of hypersensitivity reaction, mycobacterial cultures of the pleural fluid from most patients with tuberculous pleural effusions are negative.
- Left untreated, the pleura may become very thick and fibrotic ('pleural fibrosis'), and pleural adhesions develop. This later results in a restrictive ventilatory dysfunction. Early treatment will prevent or reduce these sequelae.

CLINICAL FEATURES

- Classically, in an adolescent or young adult, the illness usually begins as an acute illness with dry cough, fever and pleuritic chest pain.
- Progressive breathlessness is another presentation.
- At times, the onset is less acute with mild chest pain, low-grade fever, nonproductive cough, weight loss and easy fatigability.
- Pleural friction rub may be audible in the early stages.
- Later, classical signs of pleural effusion develop. The physical signs of pleural effusion are discussed under 'pleural effusion'.

INVESTIGATIONS

- The total leucocyte count is usually normal, but the ESR may be raised.
- Tuberculin skin test is positive in 90% of cases.
- Sputum (spontaneous or induced) may be positive for acid-fast bacilli even when chest radiograph does not show a parenchymal lesion.
- Radiograph of the chest is characteristic. Large effusions are most dense at the base, obscuring the diaphragm. But the shadow thins out at the top. For a detailed description of the radiological features of pleural effusion, refer 'pleural effusion on page 226'. Approximately 20%–30% of patients with tuberculous pleural effusions have coexisting parenchymal disease on chest radiograph.

DIAGNOSTIC THORACENTESIS

- The fluid is usually amber coloured but sometimes haemorrhagic.
- The fluid is characteristically an exudate, with a high protein content (>3 g/dL) and predominant lymphocytosis. Patients with symptoms less than 2 weeks in duration are more likely to have predominantly polymorphonuclear leucocytes in their pleural fluid. If the pleural fluid contains more than 10% eosinophils, diagnosis of tuberculous pleuritis is unlikely unless the patient has a pneumothorax or has had a previous thoracentesis. Similarly, number of mesothelial cells is less than 5% of all cells.
- Films from the centrifuged deposit may rarely demonstrate the tubercle bacilli (<10% of immunocompetent cases).
- Cultures are positive in about 25% of cases.
- Adenosine deaminase (ADA) in pleural fluid:
  - In majority of patients with tubercular pleural effusion, the levels of ADA in the fluid are elevated (>40 units/L). This may be related to an increased activity of T lymphocytes (CD^{4+}) in the pleural fluid.
  - ADA levels may be low early in TB pleural disease. ADA levels may be falsely low in elderly patients and current smokers with TB pleurisy.
  - High levels of ADA are also reported in effusions due to rheumatoid arthritis, lymphoma, chronic lymphatic leukaemia, empyema, parapneumonic effusions and mesothelioma.
  - ADA exists as two isoenzymes: ADA1 and ADA2. ADA1 isoenzyme is found in all cells with the highest activity in lymphocytes and monocytes, whereas ADA2 isoenzyme appears to be found only in monocytes. In tuberculous pleural effusion, ADA2 isoenzyme is considered to be primarily responsible for total ADA activity, while in parapneumonic effusions, the ADA1 isoenzyme is the major isoenzyme of ADA.
- Other tests on pleural fluid:
  - Elevated LDH.
  - Marked elevation in the levels of soluble interleukin-2 (IL-2) receptors.
  - High levels of interferon-γ (INF-γ) and interleukin-27.
  - Detection of mycobacterial DNA by PCR.
  - Nucleic acid amplification assays (e.g. Xpert/RIF) to amplify *M. tuberculosis*—specific nucleic acid sequences with a nucleic acid probe. However, under RNTCP, it is not recommended as a routine test to diagnose pleural TB.
- Closed pleural biopsy reveals noncaseating granulomas in 80% of cases. It should also be stained with ZN stain and cultured for mycobacteria.

MANAGEMENT

- The treatment of tuberculous pleural effusion has three goals: (i) to prevent the subsequent development of active TB, (ii) to relieve the symptoms of the patient and (iii) to prevent the development of a fibrothorax.
- Spontaneous resolution is very common. However, 65% of patients with spontaneously resolved effusion develop active tuberculosis at extrapleural sites at a later time.
- Therapeutic aspiration of pleural fluid may be necessary in severely symptomatic cases.
- Antituberculous chemotherapy is the cornerstone of management.
- Corticosteroid drugs are useful in reducing the symptoms of toxaemia, but they do not reduce the incidence of pleural fibrosis. Prednisolone is given at a dose of 5 mg four times daily for 2–3 weeks followed by gradual tapering over the next 2–4 weeks.

Q. Write a short note on tuberculosis chemoprophylaxis.

- Two terms are used to describe two different sorts of chemoprophylaxis:
  1. Primary or infection prophylaxis where a drug is given to individuals who have not been infected in order to prevent development of disease (e.g. infants being breast-fed by a sputum-positive mother).
  2. Secondary or disease prophylaxis where the drug is used to prevent development of disease in people who have already been infected.
- Isoniazid is used for chemoprophylaxis at a dose of 5 mg/kg/day (but not exceeding 300 mg/day) orally for a minimum period of 9 months. Other options particularly for HIV patients are isoniazid plus rifampicin at 10 mg/kg daily for 3 months or isoniazid at

a dose of 15 mg/kg (adults 900 mg) plus rifampicin at a dose of 10 mg/kg twice weekly for 3 months or rifapentine (600 mg/day) plus isoniazid weekly for 3 months. Patients with HIV should receive daily isoniazid for 36 months.
- It is important to exclude active tuberculosis by history, physical examination, chest radiograph and, if necessary, other tests before commencing chemoprophylaxis.

INDICATIONS

- Breast-fed infants of sputum-positive mothers.
- Close contacts of aged 5 years or below who have a strongly positive tuberculin test—an age group liable to suffer from tuberculous meningitis or miliary tuberculosis.
- Newly infected patients as shown by recent change in tuberculin test from negative to positive.
- Certain clinical states in which tuberculosis is more likely to develop—for example HIV infection, Hodgkin's disease, prolonged treatment with prednisolone at a dose level exceeding 10 mg/day, leukaemias, severe diabetes mellitus and patients on antimalignancy drugs. If tuberculin test is ≥10 mm (in India), prophylaxis may be offered.

RISKS

- Isoniazid resistance can occur if tuberculosis develops despite preventive therapy. It is particularly likely to develop when preventive therapy with isoniazid is inadvertently given to patients with subclinical or unrecognised tuberculosis.
- Hepatotoxicity.

Q. What is bronchopulmonary aspergillosis? How do you classify bronchopulmonary aspergillosis?

- Bronchopulmonary aspergillosis includes the bronchopulmonary diseases caused by *Aspergillus* species, the most common being *A. fumigatus*. Others in the group include *A. clavatus*, *A. flavus*, *A. niger* and *A. terreus*.

CLASSIFICATION (Box 2.49)

BOX 2.49 Classification of Bronchopulmonary Aspergillosis

- Endobronchial saprophytic pulmonary aspergillosis
- Allergic bronchopulmonary aspergillosis (ABPA; asthmatic pulmonary eosinophilia)
- Extrinsic allergic alveolitis (hypersensitivity pneumonitis)
- Chronic pulmonary aspergillosis
- Chronic cavitary pulmonary aspergillosis
- Chronic fibrosing pulmonary aspergillosis
- Intracavitary aspergilloma
- Chronic necrotising aspergillosis
- Invasive pulmonary aspergillosis

Q. Discuss the aetiology, clinical features, diagnosis and management of intracavitary aspergilloma (fungal ball).

AETIOLOGY

- An 'aspergilloma' is a ball of *Aspergillus* fungus, the most common being of *A. fumigatus*. Occasionally other fungi (e.g. *Zygomycetes* and *Fusarium*) may also produce fungal ball.
- An intracavitary aspergilloma can develop in any area of damaged lung where there is a persistent cavity. The common predisposing lung conditions are tuberculous cavity (most common), abscess cavity, bronchiectatic cavity, bronchial cyst, emphysematous bulla, sarcoidosis and cavitated malignancy.
- Aspergilloma (fungus ball) is composed of fungal hyphae, inflammatory cells, fibrin, mucous and tissue debris.

CLINICAL FEATURES

- Usually no specific symptoms occur.
- At times, aspergilloma may be responsible for recurrent scanty to massive haemoptysis. Haemoptysis usually occurs from bronchial blood vessels, and may be due to local invasion of blood vessels lining the cavity, endotoxins released from the fungus or mechanical irritation of the exposed vasculature inside the cavity by the rolling fungus ball.
- Systemic features like lethargy and weight loss can occur.

DIAGNOSIS

- Chest radiograph shows a cavity with a tumour-like opacity inside. A crescentic air shadow separates the fungal ball from the upper wall of the cavity (Fig. 2.9). If the radiograph is repeated in a different position, this ball also moves to occupy the dependent portion of the cavity.

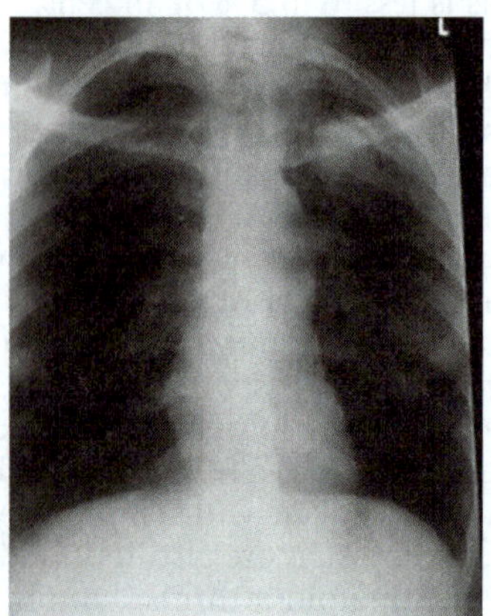

Fig. 2.9 Chest radiograph showing fungal ball in left apex. (From Ofori A, Steinmetz AR, Akaasi J, Asafu Adjaye Frimpong GA, Norman BR, Obeng-Baah J, Bedu-Addo G, Phillips RO. Pulmonary aspergilloma: An evasive disease. Int J Mycobacteriol. 2016 Jun;5(2):235-9.)

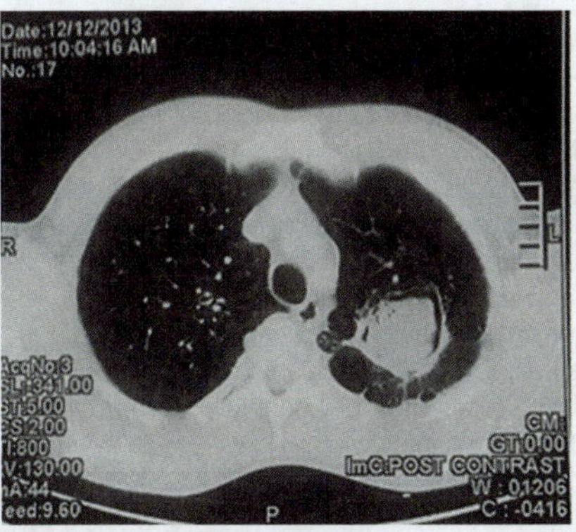

Fig. 2.10 Chest computed tomography scan showing left apical cavity with a solid intracavity mass with air crescent sign. (From Ofori A, Steinmetz AR, Akaasi J, Asafu Adjaye Frimpong GA, Norman BR, Obeng-Baah J, Bedu-Addo G, Phillips RO. Pulmonary aspergilloma: An evasive disease. Int J Mycobacteriol. 2016 Jun;5(2):235-9.)

- A CT scan is more sensitive in demonstrating the fungal ball (Fig. 2.10).
- Serum precipitins to *A. fumigatus* can be demonstrated in some patients.
- Microscopic examination of sputum may show fungal hyphae.
- Sputum culture may grow the fungus.

MANAGEMENT

- Surgical removal of the aspergilloma in suitable patients.
- If surgery cannot be performed, systemic antifungal therapy using itraconazole may be tried, although its value is doubtful.
- Ultrasound or CT-guided injection of amphotericin B into the cavity useful in some cases.
- Bronchial artery embolisation to control haemoptysis.
- Endobronchial removal using a thin bronchoscope may be tried in select cases.

Q. Discuss the aetiology, clinical features, diagnosis and management of invasive pulmonary aspergillosis.

AETIOLOGY

- Invasion of previously healthy lung tissue by *A. fumigatus*, usually in patients who are immunocompromised by either drugs or disease.

RISK FACTORS

- Risk factors for invasive pulmonary aspergillosis are given in Box 2.50.

BOX 2.50 Risk Factors for Invasive Aspergillosis

- Prolonged neutropenia (<500 cells/mm^3 for >10 days) most common
- Haematopoietic stem cell transplantation
- Solid-organ transplantation (particularly lung transplantation)
- Prolonged (>3 weeks), high-dose corticosteroids
- Haematological malignancies
- Cytotoxic therapy
- Advanced AIDS

CLINICAL FEATURES

- Severe systemic disturbances.
- Acute rapidly progressive consolidation, necrosis and cavitation of the lungs.
  - Copious amounts of purulent sputum, often blood-stained, due to multiple cavities.
  - Fever, dyspnoea and pleuritic pain.
  - Haemoptysis (mild to massive).
- May disseminate and spread haematogenously to other organs, most commonly brain (leading to seizures, ring-enhancing lesions, cerebral infarctions, intracranial haemorrhage, meningitis and epidural abscess). Less frequently, other organs such as skin, kidneys, heart and liver may be involved.

DIAGNOSIS

- Microscopic examination of sputum shows fungal hyphae.
- Positive culture of sputum.
- Demonstration of serum precipitins to *A. fumigatus*.
- Chest X-ray findings are nonspecific and include rounded densities, pleural-based infiltrates that are suggestive of pulmonary infarctions and cavitations. Pleural effusion is uncommon.
- Computed tomography of the chest is quite useful in suggesting this diagnosis particularly in neutropenic patients. It shows multiple nodules and the 'halo sign' (a zone of low attenuation due to haemorrhage surrounding the pulmonary nodule) in early stages. Another sign seen in late stages is the air crescent sign, which represents crescent-shaped lucency in the region of the original nodule secondary to necrosis.
- Bronchoscopy and BAL. Transbronchial biopsy is of little value and may produce complications.
- Detection of galactomannan antigen in serum. It is a polysaccharide cell-wall component that is released by *Aspergillus* during growth. Serum galactomannan can be detected several days before the presence of clinical signs, an abnormal chest radiograph or positive culture. Serial determination of serum galactomannan values may be useful in assessing the evolution of infection during treatment.
- Detection of (1→3)-β-d-glucan, a fungal cell wall constituent, in serum. Also positive in other invasive fungal infections.
- PCR to detect *Aspergillus* DNA in BAL fluid and serum.
- Biopsy may be required for confirmation.

MANAGEMENT

- Antifungal therapy with amphotericin (1.0–1.5 mg/kg/day) with or without flucytosine.
- Intravenous voriconazole is better tolerated and probably more efficacious than amphotericin B. The

most frequent adverse effect of voriconazole is visual disturbances, described as blurred vision, photophobia and altered colour perception.
- Intravenous echinocandin derivatives such as caspofungin, micafungin and anidulafungin for the treatment of refractory cases or if the patient cannot tolerate first-line agents.
- In less immunosuppressed patients, oral itraconazole (200 mg twice a day) is useful.

Q. Discuss the clinical features, diagnostic criteria and management of allergic bronchopulmonary aspergillosis (ABPA; asthmatic pulmonary eosinophilia).

- ABPA occurs in patients with preexisting bronchial asthma or cystic fibrosis.
- It results from hypersensitivity to *A. fumigatus*, though other species of *Aspergillus* and some other fungi can also cause it.
- The pathogenesis of ABPA is not completely understood. *Aspergillus*-specific IgE-mediated type I hypersensitivity reactions, specific IgG-mediated type III hypersensitivity reactions and abnormal T-lymphocyte cellular immune responses appear to play important roles in its pathogenesis.
- In ABPA, *Aspergillus* actually grows in the walls of the proximal bronchi and eventually produces proximal bronchiectasis. The patient also develops repeated episodes of eosinophilic pneumonia that is manifested by wheeze, cough, fever and expectoration with sputum containing fungal mycelia (expectoration of brownish mucus plugs).
- As a result of repeated pneumonic episodes, the chest radiographs show fleeting shadows of infiltrates. There may be transient areas of opacification due to mucoid impaction of the airways, which may present as band-like opacities emanating from the hilum with rounded distal margin (gloved finger appearance). The 'ring sign' and 'tram lines' are radiological signs on chest X-ray and represent thickened and inflamed bronchi. Eventually, the condition leads to central bronchiectasis and progressive pulmonary fibrosis.
- High-resolution computed tomography of chest delineates pulmonary changes better. The pathognomonic CT finding in ABPA is high-attenuation mucus (HAM), which is visually denser than the paraspinal skeletal muscle.
- Should be suspected in patients who have worsening asthma despite conventional therapy or require systemic corticosteroids.

DIAGNOSTIC CRITERIA FOR ABPA

- Diagnostic criteria for ABPA are given in Box 2.51.

BOX 2.51 Diagnostic Criteria for ABPA

(1) A predisposing underlying condition of either asthma or cystic fibrosis
(2) An elevated total IgE level greater than 1000 IU/mL AND either a positive *Aspergillus* skin test or detectable *Aspergillus fumigatus*-specific IgE
(3) At least two of the following three criteria:
- Serum precipitating or *Aspergillus*-specific IgG antibodies
- Characteristic radiographic findings
- Elevated total eosinophil count (>500/mm^3) in corticosteroid naive patients

MANAGEMENT

- Oral prednisolone 40 mg daily for 7–10 days followed by gradual tapering to a maintenance dose of 5–10 mg/day for long term (5–6 months). A 25% decline in serum total IgE along with clinical and/or radiological improvement indicates a satisfactory response to therapy.
- Bronchoscopic extraction of the casts in selected cases.
- Oral itraconazole (200 mg twice a day) is helpful in reducing exacerbations and requirement of steroids.
- Omalizumab, an anti-IgE recombinant humanised monoclonal antibody, is a promising agent particularly in patients who cannot tolerate high doses of steroids and antifungal therapy.

Q. Discuss the aetiology, clinical features, investigations and management of bronchial asthma. (CT2.16; CT2.18; CT2.22; CT2.7)

Q. How will you differentiate early-onset (atopic) asthma from late-onset (nonatopic) asthma?

Q. Discuss the clinical presentation and management of severe acute asthma (status asthmaticus). (CT2.19)

DEFINITION

- Bronchial asthma is a heterogeneous disease, usually characterised by chronic inflammatory disease of the airways. It is defined by history of dyspnoea, cough, chest tightness and wheezing, which vary over time and in intensity, together with variable expiratory airflow limitation.
- It results from narrowing of the airways produced by a combination of muscle spasm, mucosal oedema and viscid bronchial secretion. The airflow limitation is generally reversible spontaneously or with treatment but may later become permanent.
- Asthma is usually associated with bronchial hyperreactivity to several stimuli.
- Asthma–COPD overlap is characterised by persistent airflow limitation with several features usually associated with asthma as well as COPD. Outcomes (symptoms, quality of life, exacerbations, hospitalisations and mortality) are worse than with asthma or COPD alone. It is more common in smokers, but nonsmokers with asthma might have accelerated lung function decline and develop persistent airflow limitation despite a typical asthma profile.

- Some patients initially present with severe bronchospasm after taking aspirin or other nonsteroidal anti-inflammatory drugs. Aspirin-induced asthma is typically preceded by rhinitis and nasal polyposis.

CLASSIFICATION

- Bronchial asthma can be classified into two main groups or phenotypes (Table 2.34):
  1. Early-onset asthma (atopic, allergic and extrinsic).
  2. Late-onset asthma (nonatopic, idiosyncratic and intrinsic).
- Other groups of bronchial asthma include nonallergic asthma (often responds less to inhaled corticosteroids), asthma with persistent airflow limitation (which develops in some patients with long-standing asthma) and asthma with obesity (prominent respiratory symptoms with little eosinophilic airway inflammation).

AETIOPATHOGENESIS

- Pathogenesis of asthma involves two major factors:
  1. Bronchial hyperresponsiveness.
  2. Inflammatory reaction within bronchial wall.

ROLE OF ALLERGENS

- The allergens responsible for asthma enter the body through various routes:
  - Inspired air (house dust, pollen, feather, animal dander, fungal spores, etc.).
  - Ingestion (allergens in fish, egg, milk, yeast and wheat).
- Previous exposures to these allergens will have stimulated the formation of IgE. Hence, subsequent exposure to these specific allergens will result in an anaphylactic antigen–antibody reaction in the bronchi. This causes the release of pharmacologically active substances from cells in the bronchial wall, which provoke bronchial constriction and inflammatory reaction, leading to symptoms.

TABLE 2.34 Early-Onset Asthma Versus Late-Onset Asthma

Early-Onset (Atopic) Asthma	Late-Onset (Nonatopic) Asthma
• Early age of onset	• Late age of onset
• Atopic individuals	• Nonatopic individuals
• External allergens have strong role	• External allergens have no role
• Positive personal and/or family history of allergic diseases like rhinitis, urticaria and eczema	• Negative personal and/or family history of allergic diseases
• Increased levels of IgE in the serum	• Normal levels of IgE in the serum
• Positive skin hypersensitivity tests	• Negative skin hypersensitivity tests
• Positive response to provocation tests	• Negative response to provocation tests
• Responds well to inhaled corticosteroids	• Often requires higher doses of inhaled corticosteroids

Note that this classification is broad and by no means the features described are absolute. In fact, a great degree of overlap exists between these two types.

PATHOGENESIS

- Pathogenesis of asthma is complex and not fully understood. It involves a number of cells, mediators, nerves and vascular leakage. The airway inflammation is a chronic inflammation driven by CD^{4+} cells which leads to IgE synthesis through production of interleukin-4 (IL-4) and eosinophilic inflammation through IL-5.
- Mast cells:
  - Increased in both respiratory epithelium and surface secretions of asthmatics.
  - These cells can generate and release powerful mediators acting on smooth muscles and blood vessels. These mediators include histamine, prostaglandin D_2 (PGD_2) and cysteinyl leukotrienes (leukotriene C_4 [LTC_4], leukotriene D_4 [LTD_4] and leukotriene E_4 [LTE_4]) which cause the immediate asthmatic reaction.
  - Mast cells are activated by allergens through high-affinity IgE receptors as well as by osmotic stimulus (which account for exercise-induced asthma, more appropriately called exercise-induced bronchoconstriction—defined as transient narrowing of lower airway following exercise in the presence or absence of clinically recognised asthma).
  - They also release IL-4, IL-5 and IL-13. IL-4 and IL-13 help in switching of antibody production by B cells to IgE type. In addition, mast cells also secrete tumour necrosis factor-alpha (TNF-α), which may promote neutrophilia after allergenic stimulation. Conversely, mast cells also help limit airway damage. Mast cell-derived tryptase can cleave IgE, thereby preventing further mast cell activation and helping to contain the allergic response.
- Eosinophils release LTC_4 and basic proteins such as major basic protein, eosinophilic cationic protein and peroxidase that are toxic to epithelial cells. IL-5 has a key role in the modulation of eosinophil differentiation and promotion of eosinophil survival.
- Macrophages play a role in the initial uptake and presentation of allergens to lymphocytes. They are stimulated by low-affinity IgE receptors and release prostaglandins, thromboxane, LTC_4, LTB_4 and platelet-activating factor (PAF).
- T lymphocytes release IL-3, IL-4, IL-9 and IL-13, which activate mast cells. IL-3, IL-5 and other factors activate eosinophils. An increase in Th2 cell activity occurs in asthma.
- Basophils have a crucial role in initiating allergic inflammation through the binding of antigen-specific IgE antibodies.
- Dendritic cells sample allergens from the airways and migrate to regional lymph nodes where they stimulate production of Th2 cells from naïve cells.
- All these mediators lead to inflammation, oedema, hypertrophy of mucus-producing glands and bronchial constriction.
- A summary of cells and mediators involved in the pathogenesis of asthma are shown in Box 2.52 and Box 2.53 respectively. Some of the trigger factors for asthma are listed in Box 2.54. Flowchart 2.6 summarises pathogenesis of asthma.

BOX 2.52 Cells Involved in the Release of Mediators

Important	Less Important
• Mast cells	• Neutrophils
• Macrophages	• Platelets
• Eosinophils	• Epithelial cells
• Lymphocytes (Th2 lymphocytes)	

BOX 2.53 Mediators of Bronchial Hyperresponsiveness and Inflammation

- Histamine
- Prostaglandins (PGD_2, $PGF_{2}\alpha$ and PGE_2)
- Thromboxane
- Leukotrienes (LTB_4, LTC_4, LTD_4 and LTE_4)
- Platelet-activating factor (PAF)
- Bradykinin
- TNF-α, IL-4, IL-5, IL-13
- Adenosine
- Substance P
- Oxygen radicals
- Complement fragments
- Serotonin

BOX 2.54 Triggering Factors of Asthma

- Exercise (exercise-induced asthma)
- Hyperventilation
- Cold air
- Tobacco smoke
- Dust and acrid fumes including occupational sensitisers
- Respiratory viral infections
- Emotional stress
- Aspirin, β-blockers

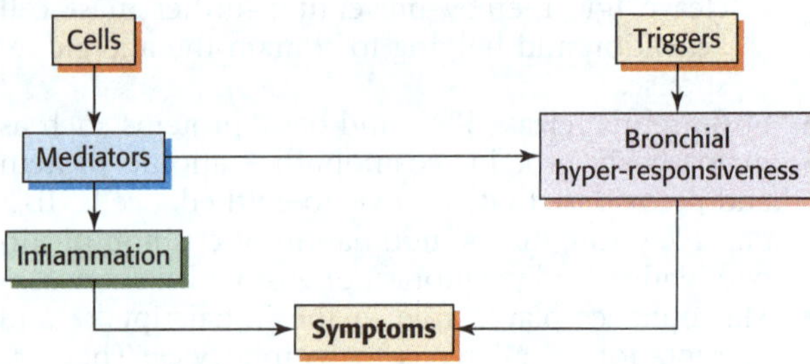

Flowchart 2.6 Pathogenesis of Asthma – Summary.

CLINICAL FEATURES

- Clinical features are conveniently discussed under four headings:
  1. Episodic asthma.
  2. Exacerbation of asthma.
  3. Severe acute asthma (status asthmaticus).
  4. Chronic asthma.

EPISODIC ASTHMA

- Occurs as episodes with asymptomatic intervening periods.
- Characterised by paroxysms of wheeze and dyspnoea with relatively sudden onset.
- Episodes may be spontaneous in onset or triggered by allergens, exercise or viral infections.
- Attacks may be mild or severe and may last for hours, days or even weeks.

EXACERBATION OF ASTHMA

- Episodes characterised by a progressive increase in symptoms of shortness of breath, cough, wheezing, chest tightness and progressive decrease in lung function.
- Represents a change from baseline status which requires intensification of treatment.

SEVERE ACUTE ASTHMA (STATUS ASTHMATICUS)

- It is a condition in which severe airway obstruction and asthmatic symptoms persist despite the initial administration of standard acute asthma therapy.
- Severe dyspnoea and unproductive cough.
- Patient adopts an upright position fixing the shoulder girdle to assist the accessory muscles of respiration.
- Physical signs on general examination include sweating, central cyanosis, tachycardia and pulsus paradoxus.

CHRONIC ASTHMA

- Symptoms are usually chronic unless controlled by appropriate therapy.
- Symptoms like chest tightness, wheeze and breathlessness occur on exertion.
- Episodes of spontaneous cough and wheeze occur during the night.
- Repeated attacks of 'severe acute asthma' are common.
- Chronic cough with mucoid sputum, punctuated by recurrent attacks of purulent expectoration from frank infection, is a common feature of chronic asthma. At times, it becomes difficult to distinguish it from chronic bronchitis.

PHYSICAL SIGNS IN THE CHEST

- During an attack of asthma, the following signs are detectable:
  - Respiratory rate is increased with the use of accessory muscles of respiration.
  - Breath sounds are vesicular in character with prolonged respiration.
  - Numerous high-pitched polyphonic expiratory and inspiratory rhonchi are audible.
  - During very severe attacks, the airflow may be insufficient to produce rhonchi. This results in a 'silent chest', which is an ominous sign.
- In between the attacks, the chest is clear and no abnormal physical signs may be detectable.
- Chronic asthmatics usually have some scattered rhonchi always persisting in their chest.

OTHER CAUSES OF WHEEZE

- A number of other conditions can also produce wheeze (Box 2.55).

INVESTIGATIONS

- Chest radiography:
  - In an acute attack, lungs appear hyperinflated.

BOX 2.55 Other Causes of Wheeze

- Cardiac asthma
- Chronic obstructive lung disease
- Recurrent pulmonary emboli
- Endobronchial lesions/foreign body
- Carcinoid tumours
- Eosinophilic pneumonia
- Pulmonary vasculitis

- In between attacks, lungs look normal.
- Long-standing cases have hyperinflated lungs indistinguishable from emphysema.
- Complications like pigeon chest, lobar or segmental collapse, pneumothorax and mediastinal and subcutaneous emphysema may be seen.

- Pulmonary function tests useful in bronchial asthma are FEV_1, VC and PEF.
    - Estimation of the degree of airflow obstruction.
    - To determine whether and to what extent the airflow obstruction can be relieved by bronchodilators. In adults, an increase in FEV_1 of >12% or >200 mL from baseline 10–15 minutes after inhalation of 200–400 μg of salbutamol is considered a positive bronchodilator reversibility test.
    - To confirm airflow obstruction provoked by exercise, hyperventilation and occupational exposure (fall in in FEV_1 of >10% or >200 mL from baseline).
    - To differentiate chronic asthma from chronic bronchitis. In asthma, there is a diurnal variation in PEF (average diurnal peak expiratory flow variability >10%), the lowest values being recorded in the mornings ('morning dipping').
    - Long-term monitoring of patients with poorly controlled disease.
    - Direct challenge tests: Histamine or methacholine provocation test (fall in FEV_1 by more than 20% after provocation with these agents) indicates presence of airway hyperresponsiveness and can be useful in patients in whom cough is the only symptom.
    - Pulmonary function tests should be done at diagnosis or start of treatment, after 3–6 months to assess response as well as patient's best FEV_1, and then periodically thereafter.
- ABG analysis shows hypoxaemia and hypocarbia during acute attack. In severe acute asthma, hypercarbia develops. ABG is done in patients with severe exacerbation with PEF or FEV_1 <50% of predicted, or those who are worsening despite treatment.
- Skin hypersensitivity tests check the development of a wheal and flare reaction to intradermal injections of common allergens. The chief value of this is to distinguish atopic from nonatopic subjects (though even this differentiation is not required for management).
- Sputum and blood eosinophilia.
- Elevated serum IgE levels.
- Fractional concentration of exhaled nitric oxide (FeNO) is of little value in diagnosing bronchial asthma.

MANAGEMENT OF BRONCHIAL ASTHMA

- Goals of asthma management are:
    - To achieve good control of asthma symptoms and maintain normal activities.
    - To minimise future risk of exacerbation, fixed airflow limitation and medication side effects.
- Management of bronchial asthma can be discussed under the following broad headings:
    1. Avoidance of allergens.
    2. Modification of risk factors for exacerbation.
    3. Desensitisation or immunotherapy.
    4. Drug therapy to control or suppress clinical manifestations.
    5. Bronchial thermoplasty.

AVOIDANCE OF ALLERGENS

- In cases where a single allergen is found responsible, it is easy to reduce or avoid the exposure to it.
- In cases where multiple allergens are found responsible, avoidance becomes a difficult task.

MODIFY RISK FACTORS FOR EXACERBATION

- Risk factors for asthma exacerbations are mentioned in Box 2.56. Some of them can be modified to control asthma.

DESENSITISATION OR IMMUNOTHERAPY

- Desensitisation is done by repeated subcutaneous injections of gradually increasing doses of the extracts of allergen(s). It can also be done by sublingual route. It may be useful in patients with allergic asthma but evidence is limited.

DRUG THERAPY

- The drugs useful in asthma can be grouped into seven major categories (Box 2.57). Often, a single drug may not be adequate.

BOX 2.56 Risk Factors for Asthma Exacerbations

- Uncontrolled asthma symptoms
- Smoking (both active and passive)
- Associated rhinitis
- Obesity
- Inadequate use of inhaled corticosteroids
- Overuse of inhaled short-acting beta-agonists (e.g. more than 1 canister of 200 doses/month)
- Ever intubated or ICU admission
- ≥Severe exacerbation in last 1 year
- Poor inhalation technique
- Major psychological problems.
- Other risk factors:
    - Low FEV1 especially below 60% of predicted
    - Sputum or blood eosinophilia
    - Gastro-oesophageal reflux
    - Ongoing exposure to allergens or irritants at home or occupation.

BOX 2.57 Classes of Drugs Used in Asthma

1. β-Adrenoreceptor agonists
2. Methylxanthines
3. Corticosteroids
4. Chromones
5. Anticholinergics
6. Leukotriene inhibitors
7. Miscellaneous agents

β-Adrenoreceptor Agonists

- Basically, there are two types of β-adrenoreceptors: β_1-adrenoreceptors and β_2-adrenoreceptors.
  - Stimulation of β_1-adrenoreceptors produces predominant effects on heart.
  - Stimulation of β_2-adrenoreceptors produces predominant effects on bronchial smooth muscles.

Catecholamines

- The useful catecholamines are adrenaline, isoprenaline and isoetharine. Adrenaline is the most commonly used agent in this group. However, it has the disadvantage of not being β_2-selective, which results in significant undesirable cardiovascular side effects. The usual dose is 0.3–0.5 mL of a 1:1000 solution administered subcutaneously which may be repeated thrice at an interval of 20 minutes. It is useful in children with acute exacerbation of asthma.

Salbutamol, Levosalbutamol, Terbutaline and Fenoterol

- These drugs are highly selective for β_2-adrenoreceptors with their predominant action on the respiratory tract. They are powerful and rapid but short-acting bronchodilators, which act by relaxing bronchial smooth muscles. They are active by all routes of administration (inhalation, oral, intravenous and subcutaneous), but the preferred route of administration is inhalation. Inhalation is extremely effective, since it rapidly reduces airflow obstruction. Intravenous administration of salbutamol and terbutaline offers no advantages over inhalation. For the same reason, other routes of administration are preferably avoided and reserved for selected indications. Levosalbutamol produces less tachycardia compared to salbutamol.
- For inhalational route, these are available as solutions (for nebulisation), aerosol (metered-dose inhaler [MDI]) and dry powder inhaler (DPI).
- Drugs in the MDIs can be dispensed as suspension in chlorofluorocarbons (CFC) or as solution in hydrofluoroalkanes (HFA). Because of impact of CFC on atmospheric ozone, CFC has been replaced by HFA.
- Dose:
  - Salbutamol is given in a dose of 2–4 mg thrice a day orally or two puffs of 100 µg each as required.
  - Terbutaline is given in a dose of 2.5–5 mg thrice a day or two puffs of 100 µg each as required.
  - Levosalbutamol is given in a dose of two puffs of 50 µg each as required.
- Main side effects are tremor and palpitation. These drugs can also produce hypokalaemia. Prolonged use of these β_2-adrenoreceptor agonists are preferably avoided as they worsen bronchial hyperresponsiveness.

Bambuterol

- It is a long-acting β_2-adrenoreceptor agent that gets converted into terbutaline in the body.
- Dose is 10–20 mg once in a day orally.
- Side effects are higher than those with inhaled β-agonists and include tachycardia, palpitations and tremors.

Salmeterol and Formoterol

- These are highly selective, potent and long-acting β_2-stimulants that need to be given once or twice a day by inhalation (as either aerosol or dry powder).
- These drugs are now routinely used in place of short-acting β_2-stimulants when the patient requires regular β_2-stimulant therapy. However, these drugs should not be used as monotherapy; instead, they may be given along with inhaled corticosteroids if response to inhaled corticosteroids is suboptimal.
- Salmeterol has a slow onset of action while formoterol has a rapid action. This makes formoterol suitable for immediate control of symptoms as well.
- Dose:
  - Salmeterol—two puffs of 25 µg each two to three times a day.
  - Formoterol—two puffs of 6 µg each one to three times a day.

Methylxanthines

- These agents have little role as monotherapy but may provide benefit as add-on therapy in patients not controlled with inhaled corticosteroids and long-acting inhaled β-agonists.

Theophylline

- Theophylline is a medium-potency bronchodilator, the exact mechanism of bronchodilatation being not clear. It improves the movement of airway mucus, improves diaphragm contractility and decreases the release of mediators.
- Can be given intravenously, orally or as suppository. Therapeutic plasma concentrations of theophylline lie between 10 and 20 µg/mL. However, the dose required to achieve this level varies from patient to patient.
- Acute attacks are treated with short-acting theophylline preparations. For maintenance therapy, long-acting theophylline preparations are used and are usually given once or twice a day. Single daily dose in the evening is effective in controlling nocturnal asthma.
- Usual dose is 100–200 mg (of plain preparation) three times a day, and 300 mg twice a day or 450–600 mg once a day for sustained-release preparation.
- Common side effects of theophylline preparations include nervousness, nausea, vomiting, anorexia and headache. Seizures and cardiac arrhythmias can occur when plasma levels are more than 30 µg/mL.
- Theophylline (and aminophylline) clearance is reduced in elderly, liver disease, congestive heart failure and with concurrent use of erythromycin, allopurinol and cimetidine. It is increased with concurrent use of phenytoin and phenobarbitone and in smokers.

Aminophylline

- Aminophylline is a bronchodilator, which is effective orally, intravenously and as a suppository. The preferred route of administration is intravenous.
- Aminophylline is given as a loading dose of 5 mg/kg slowly intravenously over 20 minutes. This is followed by a maintenance dose of 0.5 mg/kg/hour given as a continuous intravenous infusion. In those patients who are already receiving theophylline,

loading dose is preferably withheld or in extreme situations given in a reduced amount at 2.5 mg/kg.

- Rapid infusion of the bolus dose can result in sudden death from cardiac arrhythmias.
- At present, aminophylline or theophylline therapy is not recommended in the treatment of severe acute asthma as addition to SABA does not improve outcome compared to SABA alone.

Doxophylline (Doxofylline)

- Like theophylline, it also inhibits phosphodiesterase leading to increased cyclic 3′,5′-adenosine monophosphate (cAMP). It has reduced affinity for adenosine A1 and A2 receptors and, therefore, has a better safety profile compared to theophylline. It also inhibits PAF-induced bronchoconstriction and subsequent generation of thromboxane A2.
- It does not have significant drug–drug interactions as exhibited with theophylline.
- Dose is 400 mg twice a day.

Corticosteroids

- Corticosteroids are not bronchodilators, but they relieve or prevent airflow obstruction indirectly by their anti-inflammatory effect. They have a beneficial effect on bronchial inflammation and decrease bronchial hyperresponsiveness. They also reverse β_2-receptor downregulation induced by long-term use of β_2-agonists.
- The effects of corticosteroids in acute asthma are not immediate and may not be seen for 6 hours or more after the first dose. Consequently, it is mandatory to continue vigorous bronchodilator and oxygen therapy during this period.
- The vast majority of patients respond to corticosteroids. But there is a minority with little or no response to corticosteroids. They have been labelled corticosteroid-resistant cases.
- Common indications of corticosteroids in bronchial asthma are the following:
  - Acute illness, particularly when not responding to or even worsening despite optimal bronchodilator therapy.
  - Severe acute asthma (status asthmaticus).
  - Corticosteroid inhalers are now the first line of treatment in all patients who require some antiasthmatic drug regularly. This is because they have their main action on the basic pathophysiology, that is they reduce the hyperresponsiveness and inflammation of the bronchial tree.
- Hydrocortisone and methylprednisolone (intravenous) are useful in acute situations. Hydrocortisone is given as a loading dose of 4 mg/kg intravenously followed by 2–3 mg/kg every 6 hours. Methylprednisolone is administered in a dose of 40–125 mg every 6 hours.
- Oral prednisolone is equally effective as intravenous corticosteroids and is started as a single daily dose of 40–60 mg orally for 5–7 days.
- Beclomethasone dipropionate (200 µg), budesonide (200 µg) or fluticasone (125 µg) is given twice daily as aerosols or dry-powder form. Another inhalational steroid is ciclesonide that is given in a dose of 80–160 µg once a day. Others are flunisolide and mometasone. Higher doses may be necessary in severe illness but not beyond the maximum dose of 2000 µg beclomethasone, 1000 µg fluticasone and 1600 µg budesonide per day. They are relatively free from systemic side effects at the conventional doses. The common side effects are oropharyngeal candidiasis and a husky voice. This can be minimised by the use of a spacing device along with the MDI and gargling with water after use. Long-term use may produce osteoporosis, skin thinning and adrenal suppression.
- Budesonide is also available as a solution for nebulisation in a dose of 250–500 µg.

Doses of Inhaled Corticosteroids

- Table 2.35 gives doses of inhaled corticosteroids.

Chromones

- Sodium cromoglycate or cromolyn is not a bronchodilator. It inhibits degranulation of mast cells, thereby preventing mediator release. It is only of use in the prophylactic treatment of asthma.
  - Sodium cromoglycate is particularly useful in children with atopic asthma but may be of some value in a few patients with nonatopic asthma. Therapy is best initiated between attacks or in periods of relative remission. If no response is observed in 4–6 weeks, the drug can be discontinued.
  - Sodium cromoglycate is administered as an inhalation in a dose of 10 mg four times a day.
- Nedocromil sodium acts mainly by inhibiting release of mediators. It is given as an inhalation at a dose of 4 mg two to four times daily. It is of use in the prophylactic control of asthma.
- Ketotifen is not a chromone. It is an antihistamine that also inhibits release of mediators. It is useful in the prophylactic control of asthma at a dose of 1–2 mg twice daily by mouth. The main side effects are drowsiness and weight gain.

Anticholinergics

- The anticholinergic agents currently used are ipratropium bromide and tiotropium. These are nonabsorbable, quaternary ammonium compounds, relatively free from side effects. These are given as aerosol or in dry-powder form. Ipratropium is also available

TABLE 2.35 Doses of Inhaled Corticosteroids

Inhaled Corticosteroid	Total Daily Dose (mcg)		
	Low Dose	Medium Dose	High Dose
Beclomethasone (extrafine particles)	100–200	>200–400	>400
Beclomethasone (standard particle size)	200–500	>500–1000	>1000
Budesonide	200–400	>400–800	>800
Fluticasone	100–250	>250–500	>500
Ciclesonide	80–160	>160–320	>320

as nebulisation solution. These agents are particularly useful in two situations:

1. In patients with coexistent heart disease, in whom methylxanthines and β_2-adrenoreceptor agonists produce significant tachycardia.
2. In refractory cases, addition of ipratropium bromide or tiotropium enhances the bronchodilator action of β_2-adrenoreceptor agonists.

- Dose:
  - Ipratropium two puffs of 20 μg each four times a day.
  - Tiotropium two puffs of 9 μg each once a day.
  - Ipratropium 250–500 μg nebulisation; may be repeated if required.
- Side effects include dryness of mouth and bitter taste.

Leukotriene Modifiers

- Leukotriene receptor antagonists (montelukast, zafirlukast and pranlukast) and 5-lipoxygenase inhibitors (zileuton) are useful additive drugs in patients who do not respond to the conventional agents. They are also used in patients who require high doses of inhaled steroids. They can be used as a second-choice treatment to inhaled corticosteroids in mild persistent asthma.
- Dose of zafirlukast is 20 mg BID.
- Dose of montelukast is 10 mg once a day in the evening.
- Adverse effects are uncommon and include headache, abdominal pain, skin rashes, angio-oedema, pulmonary eosinophilia and arthralgia. Zileuton can produce liver toxicity.

Miscellaneous Agents

- Proton pump inhibitor (PPI) in patients with symptomatic gastro-oesophageal reflux disease and suboptimally controlled asthma.
- Anti-IgE therapy: Omalizumab, a recombinant humanised monoclonal antibody against IgE is useful in patients with allergic asthma. It blocks circulating IgE binding to receptors on mast cells and basophils and decreases release of mediators. It is given subcutaneously once every 2–4 weeks. In a small number of patients, it can produce anaphylaxis.
- Anti-IL5 therapy: Humanised monoclonal antibodies, mepolizumab and reslizumab (bind to IL-5) and benralizumab (binds to IL-5 receptors) are useful in resistant or severe asthma with persistent eosinophilia.
- Anti-IL4 therapy: Dupilumab is a fully humanised IgG4 monoclonal antibody directed against IL-4 receptor.

Note

- Avoid opiates, sedatives and tranquilisers in acutely ill asthmatics.
- Avoid β-blockers and parasympathetic agonists in asthmatics.
- Expectorants and mucolytic agents do not have any significant role in the management of bronchial asthma.

Use of an Inhaler and Spacer

- Use of an inhaler and spacer are shown in Box 2.58 and 2.59.

BOX 2.58 Use of an Inhaler

- The canister of inhaler is shaken well.
- The patient exhales till functional residual capacity (FRC), i.e. the end of normal expiration.
- The nozzle of inhaler is kept near the open mouth; it may also be kept inside the mouth.
- The patient activates the inhaler by pressing it and simultaneously inhales rapidly but smoothly till full inspiration.
- The breath is held for 10 seconds and then released.
- The patient rinses his/her mouth with plain water.
- The same steps are repeated after 2–5 minutes if the inhaler needs to be taken twice.

BOX 2.59 Use of a Spacer

- The spacer is conical in shape and is made of plastic or other materials.
- One end of this is attached to the inhaler (after the inhaler has been shaken) and the other end is kept in the mouth.
- The patient inhales after activating the inhaler.
- Spacers reduce the particle velocity so that less drug is deposited in the mouth; this increases the delivery of drug to the lower airway passages and also reduces the side effects (spacers are quite useful in reducing local side effects of steroids).
- Spacers also diminish the need of coordination between the activation of inhaler and inhalation.

Treatment of Exercise-Induced Asthma (Exercise-Induced Bronchoconstriction)

- Episodes can be prevented by inhalation of two metered doses of salbutamol or terbutaline a few minutes before exercise. However, regular use leads to relative loss of their efficacy.
- Regular treatment with sodium cromoglycate or leukotriene modifiers is often necessary.

BRONCHIAL THERMOPLASTY

- Controlled thermal energy is delivered to the airway wall during a series of bronchoscopies, resulting in a prolonged reduction in airway smooth muscle mass.

GOALS OF ASTHMA TREATMENT

- While managing a patient with asthma, it is important to achieve certain goals (Box 2.60).

BOX 2.60 Goals of Asthma Treatment

- Asthma is considered to be well controlled when in the last 4 weeks:
  - Daytime symptoms occur twice or less per week
  - No limitation of daily activities including exercise
  - No nocturnal awakening due to symptoms
  - Requirement of short-acting β-agonists twice or less per week
- No exacerbation or risk factors for exacerbation

TABLE 2.36 Global Initiative for Asthma (GINA) Severity Grades

Characteristic	Well-Controlled Asthma	Partly Controlled Asthma	Uncontrolled Asthma
• Daytime symptoms more than twice per week	No	Any one or two characteristics present	Any three or four characteristics present
• Limitation of activities due to asthma	No		
• Nocturnal symptoms/awakening due to asthma	No		
• Need for rescuer medicine more than twice per week	No		

ASTHMA SEVERITY

- Treatment depends on the severity of asthma (Table 2.36).

GUIDELINES ON THE MANAGEMENT OF ASTHMA

- Patient education regarding self-monitoring and correct use of inhalers is important.
- Stepwise management is given in Table 2.37.

BASED ON ASTHMA SEVERITY

- Once patient is on treatment for several months, asthma severity can be assessed using above-mentioned step-wise approach.
  - Mild asthma is well controlled with step 1 or step 2 treatment. Step 1 is for those patients who need inhaled corticosteroids + formoterol or SABA (former better than SABA) less than twice a month, or low dose inhaled corticosteroids, leukotriene receptor antagonists or chormones. There is no waking at night due to asthma symptoms in last 1 month and no risk factors for exacerbations (including no exacerbations in last 1 year).
  - Moderate asthma is one which is controlled with step 3 treatment.
  - Severe asthma is that which requires step 4 or 5 treatment to prevent it from becoming uncontrolled asthma or which remains uncontrolled despite these treatments. Azithromycin thrice a week for 6 months may be considered but sputum should be checked for atypical mycobacteria and ECG for long QTc interval.
- Once good symptom control is achieved, the doses of inhaled corticosteroids may be reduced to minimum dose which will maintain asthma control.

TREATMENT OF EXACERBATION OF ASTHMA

TREATMENT AT HOME

- High concentrations of oxygen through a mask.
- Bronchodilator therapy with one of the following:
  - Salbutamol (5 mg) or terbutaline (10 mg) by nebuliser every 20 minutes for three doses.
  - Salbutamol or terbutaline administered via MDIs (four to eight puffs with a spacer every 20 minutes for three doses) is as efficacious as nebulisation of these agents. These are followed by four to eight puffs every 2–4 hours.
- Oral prednisolone, 40–60 mg.
- If no response within 1 hour or patient becomes drowsy, shift to a hospital.

MANAGEMENT IN HOSPITAL

Initial Assessment and Management

- Take brief history and perform rapid examination.
- Controlled or titrated oxygen (35%–60%) to a target oxygen saturation of 93%–95%.

Assessment of Severity

- Severity of asthma exacerbation can be assessed using certain parameters as given in Box 2.61.

TABLE 2.37 Step-Wise Approach to Manage Asthma

Step-Wise Approach	Management
• Step 1 (only for intermittent symptoms)	• Low dose inhaled corticosteroids + formoterol combination on need basis (better than short-acting inhaled β_2-agonist in terms of risk of severe exacerbations). If not available, short-acting inhaled β_2-agonist (SABA) on need basis (required in all steps)
• Step 2	• Low dose inhaled corticosteroids + formoterol combination on need basis OR • Low-dose inhaled corticosteroids OR • Leukotriene modifiers (if patient develops side effects to inhaled corticosteroids)
• Step 3	• Low-dose inhaled corticosteroids plus long-acting β_2-agonist (LABA) OR • Medium- or high-dose inhaled corticosteroids OR • Low-dose inhaled corticosteroids plus leukotriene modifiers OR • Low-dose inhaled corticosteroids plus sustained-release theophylline
• Step 4	• Medium- or high-dose inhaled corticosteroids plus long-acting β_2-agonist • Add tiotropium (long-acting muscarinic antagonist [LAMA]) • May add leukotriene modifiers • May add sustained-release theophylline
• Step 5	• Add oral corticosteroids (lowest dose) • Consider anti-IgE treatment (omalizumab) and anti-IL5 treatment • Consider azithromycin (500 mg thrice a week)

BOX 2.61 Assessment of Severity of Exacerbation of Asthma

Mild-to-Moderate Exacerbation

- FEV_1 or PEF ≥ 50%
- Patient talks in sentences
- Pulse ≤ 120 beats/minute
- Minimal or no pulsus paradoxus
- SaO_2 ≥ 90%

Severe Exacerbation

- FEV_1 or PEF < 50%
- Patient talks in words but not sentences
- Pulse > 120 beats/minute
- Accessory muscles in use
- Respiratory rate > 30 breaths/minute
- Loud wheezes
- SaO_2 < 90% or PaO_2 < 60 mmHg

Life-Threatening Asthma

- Drowsy
- Silent chest

Treatment of Mild-to-Moderate Exacerbation

- Inhaled β-agonists (via inhaler or nebuliser) every 20 minutes for three doses as discussed above.
- Oral corticosteroids if no immediate response within 1 hour (Flowchart 2.7).
- Reassess every hour or earlier.

Treatment of Severe Exacerbation

- Controlled or titrated oxygen (35%–60%) as above.
- Salbutamol (5 mg) or terbutaline (10 mg) or levosalbutamol (1.25–2.5 mg) nebulised in oxygen should be administered immediately. This may be repeated after a few minutes if there is no response. Subcutaneous or intravenous administration of β_2-agonist is indicated in patients who are coughing excessively, too weak to inspire adequately or moribund. Terbutaline is given subcutaneously (0.25–0.5 mg) or intravenously (0.1–10 μg/kg/minute). Epinephrine (adrenaline) may be given in children and young adults. In adults, the dose is 0.2–0.5 mg as 1:1000 solution subcutaneously every 20

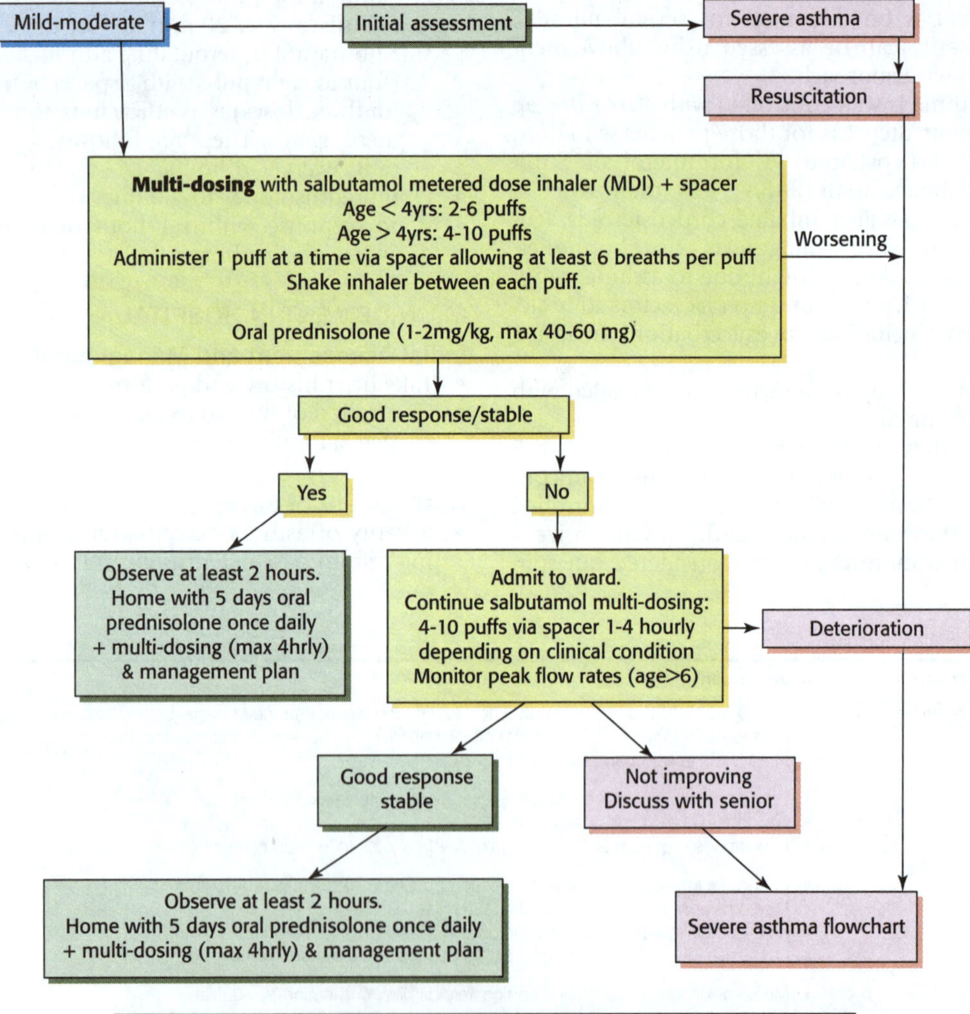

Flowchart 2.7 Mild-to-Moderate Asthma Management. Levin et al. Acute asthma management during SARSCoV2- pandemic 2020. World Allergy Organization Journal (2020) 13:100125 http://doi.org/10.1016/j.waojou.2020.100125.

minutes. However, it is not routinely indicated in adults unless angio-oedema or anaphylaxis is suspected.

- Add ipratropium bromide 0.5 mg nebulisation in those patients who do not respond within 15–30 minutes. Can be repeated every 20 minutes for three doses. It can also be given by MDI.
- Corticosteroids to be given within 1 hour:
  - Hydrocortisone sodium succinate 100 mg intravenously at presentation and then repeated 4–6 hourly in severely ill patients.
  - Oral prednisolone in a loading dose of 40–60 mg and thereafter 40–60 mg/day in a single dose. Total duration is 5–7 days. Patients receiving steroids before should also be given inhaled corticosteroids in high doses.
- High-dose inhaled corticosteroids within first hour of arrival reduces rate of hospitalisation if oral corticosteroids are not given. When given along with systemic corticosteroids, their role is controversial.
- Aminophylline should not be given due to poor efficacy and safety profile.
- Antibiotics are not indicated unless features of respiratory infection (fever or purulent sputum) are present.
- Role of magnesium sulphate administered intravenously or by nebulisation is controversial. It may be given if patient does not respond to initial treatment including corticosteroids.
- Endotracheal intubation and mechanical ventilation in patients who do not respond to above-mentioned measures. Indications for intubation include cardiac or respiratory arrest, severe hypoxia ($PaO_2 < 60$ mmHg), hypercapnia ($PaCO_2 > 50$ mmHg), acidosis (pH < 7.3), exhaustion or deterioration in mental status.
- NIV using continuous positive pressure or BiPAP machines and tight-fitting face mask helps in assisting breathing. It reduces the work of breathing without intubation. It is indicated in a cooperative and alert patient who has impending respiratory failure but does not need immediate intubation. However, the role of NIV in acute asthma is not clear.
- Treatment with 70%–80% helium with oxygen may be beneficial in severely ill patients not responding to initial treatment. This mixture reduces airway resistance and improves efficacy of bronchodilators.
- Response to treatment is assessed from patient distress, respiratory rate, FEV_1, heart rate, presence of pulsus paradoxus and serial ABG studies.
- Treatment of severe asthma is summarised in Flowchart 2.8.

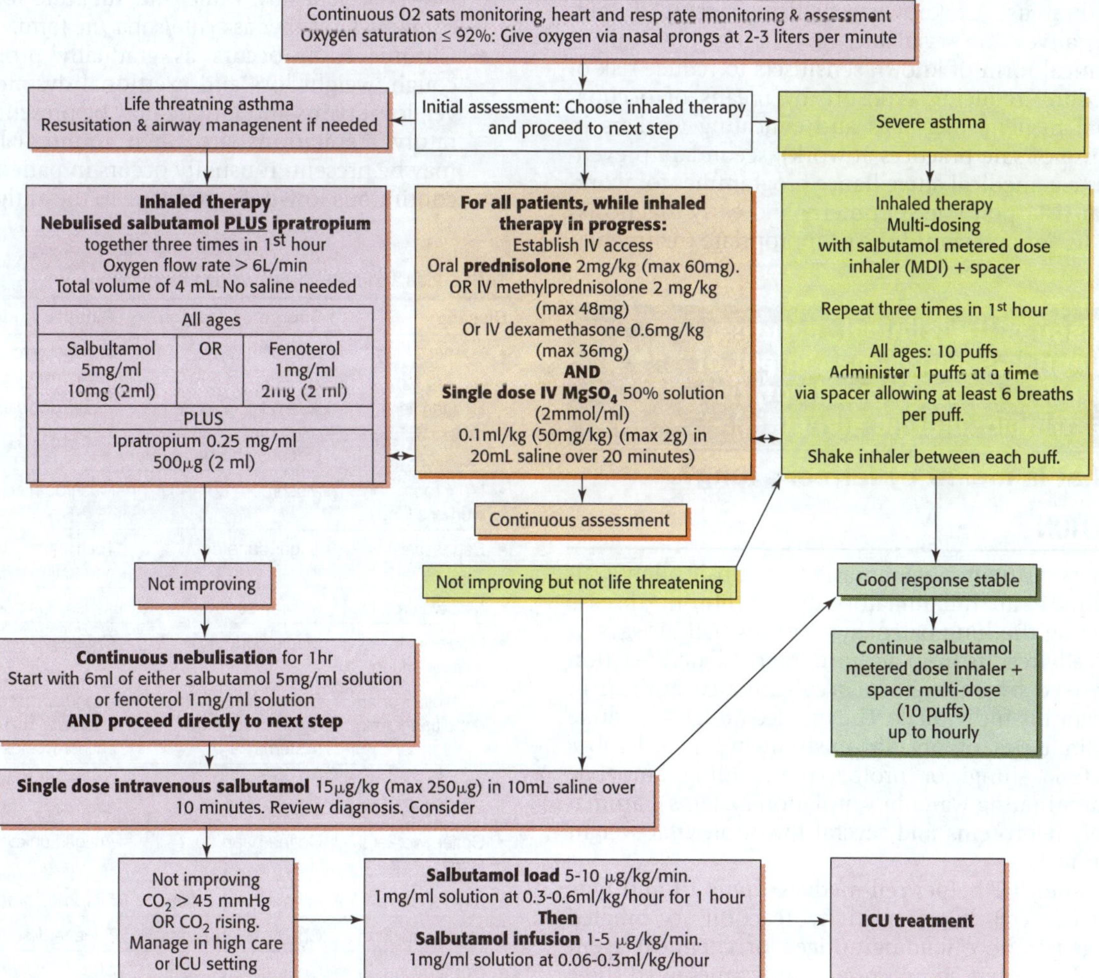

Flowchart 2.8 Management of Severe Asthma. Levin et al. Acute asthma management during SARSCoV2- pandemic 2020. World Allergy Organization Journal (2020) 13:100125 http://doi.org/10.1016/j.waojou.2020.100125.

Q. Write a short note on occupational asthma.

- Caused by a specific occupational sensitiser.
- Occupational sensitiser is usually a protein or a glycopeptide which can cause production of specific IgE antibodies and typical allergic responses.
- Examples of allergens include animal allergens, plants and plant products (e.g. natural rubber latex), cereals and grains, milk powder, fungi, diisocyanates (e.g. toluene diisocyanate), acrylic and drugs.
- Once a person is sensitised, very low exposures can induce asthma.
- A latency period ranging from weeks to years after the first exposure to the sensitiser is often seen before the initial onset of work-related symptoms.
- Symptoms begin variably—at the beginning of work shift, towards its end or even in the evening after working hours. They subside or improve during weekends and holidays.
- Often associated with allergic rhinitis and conjunctivitis.
- A subcategory of occupational asthma is irritant-induced occupational asthma. In this, occupational asthma occurs from exposure to agents which cause airway irritation with no airway sensitisation.
- Management includes primary prevention (e.g. avoiding use of known sensitising agents if safer alternatives are available, modifying physical or chemical form of known sensitisers to reduce risk of exposure, reducing exposure by means of occupational hygiene measures and educating workers in the use of safe practices at work), secondary prevention (e.g. medical-surveillance programmes for workers at risk, periodic spirometry and early diagnosis) and tertiary prevention (e.g. appropriate treatment).

Q. Discuss the clinical features, diagnosis and management of hypersensitivity pneumonitis (extrinsic allergic alveolitis).

Q. What is meant by farmer's lung?

DEFINITION

- Hypersensitivity pneumonitis or extrinsic allergic alveolitis is an inflammatory and/or fibrotic disease affecting the lung parenchyma and small airways. It typically results from an immune-mediated reaction provoked by an overt or occult inhaled antigen in susceptible individuals. The inhaled antigens include certain types of organic dusts including microbes (bacteria, fungi or protozoa, including amoebae contaminating water in ventilation systems), animal or plant proteins and several low-molecular-weight chemicals.
- It is due to T-helper cell-mediated type III and type IV (delayed) hypersensitivity reaction to inhaled antigens. The offending antigen or chemical agent initially triggers an immune complex-mediated (type III) hypersensitivity reaction after initial sensitisation. Continued exposure to the antigen shifts it to a delayed (type IV) hypersensitivity reaction which activates CD^{8+} cytotoxic T cells releasing chemokines that result in macrophage activation and granuloma formation. Later fibrosis develops.

EXAMPLES (Table 2.38)

- The most commonly implicated bacterial cause is thermophilic actinomycetes, which are Gram-positive filamentous bacilli that produce farmer's lung.

CLINICAL FEATURES

- Most patients (80%–95%) are nonsmokers.
- Most cases occur following months or years of continuous or intermittent inhalation of inciting agent.
- Clinical presentation can be acute, subacute or chronic.
  - Acute form presents as fever with chills, malaise, cough and dyspnoea occurring 6–8 hours after exposure to the antigen. It peaks at 6–24 hours and usually clears off within a few days if there is no further exposure. The physical examination may reveal inspiratory crackles but can be normal.
  - Subacute form appears more insidiously with cough, dyspnoea and cyanosis, lasting for weeks or months. However, generally, acute and subacute forms are combined together as acute/subacute form.
  - Chronic form occurs as gradually progressive cough, weight loss and exertional dyspnoea. Fever, joint pains and fatigue may be present. Inspiratory crepitations are often found. Clubbing may be present. It usually occurs in patients with continuous low-dose exposure to the antigen and

TABLE 2.38 Various Hypersensitivity Pneumonitis

Disease	Source of Antigen	Putative Antigen
• Farmer's lung	Mouldy hay	Thermophilic actinomycetes
• Bird fancier's lung	Avian droppings (most often droppings of pigeons and parakeets)	Protein in avian faeces, feathers
• Mushroom worker's lung	Mushroom compost	Mushroom spores
• Bagassosis	Sugar cane dust	Thermophilic fungi and actinomycetes
• Malt worker's lung	Mouldy barley	*Aspergillus* species
• Maple bark stripper's lung	Maple bark	*Cryptostroma* species
• Humidifier or air-conditioner lung	Contaminated water in air-conditioning systems	*Acanthamoeba*, *Naegleria*, thermophilic actinomycetes
• Woodworker's lung	Wood dust	Wood dust, *Alternaria* species
• Coffee worker's lung	Coffee bean dust	Antigen unknown
• Miller's lung	Infested wheat flour	*Sitophilus granarius*
• Isocyanate lung	Chemical industries	Toluene diisocyanate
• Hot tub lung	Contaminated hot tub water or outdoor water pool	*Mycobacterium* (usually *avium*)

is clinically indistinguishable from pulmonary fibrosis due to other causes.

- Another presentation is acute exacerbation of chronic disease which occurs without further exposure to offending antigen.
- Complications of long-standing disease are diffuse pulmonary interstitial fibrosis, pulmonary hypertension and cor pulmonale.
- At present, hypersensitivity pneumonitis is better classified as 'non-fibrotic' and 'fibrotic' hypersensitivity pneumonitis instead of acute, subacute and chronic forms. This is based on the presence or absence of fibrosis on high-resolution computed tomography (HRCT) of the chest. Acute and subacute presentations generally occur with non-fibrotic HP while chronic presentation occurs with both non-fibrotic and fibrotic forms.

INVESTIGATIONS

- Blood examination reveals raised ESR and neutrophilia, particularly in acute form. Eosinophil counts and IgE levels are typically normal.
- Precipitating antibodies of IgG type against offending microbe present in many patients, but their diagnostic utility is limited.
- Chest radiograph may show diffuse micronodular shadowing. Later, reticular shadows due to pulmonary fibrosis occur. In fibrotic HP, the fibrosing process may spare the most dependent lung bases or be more severe in the upper than lower lobes.
- Computed tomography with high resolution shows ground glass opacities, poorly defined centrilobular micronodules and mosaic attenuation or expiratory air trapping. When fibrosis develops, high-resolution CT usually demonstrates reticulation, mainly in the middle portion of the lungs or fairly evenly throughout the lungs but with relative sparing of the extreme apices and bases.
- Pulmonary function tests show a restrictive ventilatory defect with normal FEV_1:VC ratio and reduced diffusion for carbon monoxide. In farmer's lung, most common pattern on PFT is obstructive pattern.
- ABG studies show low PaO_2 and $PaCO_2$.
- Other investigations to confirm the diagnosis include provocation tests, BAL and lung biopsy.
    - Provocation test: Appearance of respiratory or systemic findings, especially fever, 4–10 hours after exposure, leucocytosis, diminished diffusion capacity, diminished VC, or both, increased radiographic abnormalities and worsening alveolar–arterial oxygen pressure difference indicate a positive response.
    - BAL typically shows an increase in the number of T lymphocytes, though some patients may show elevated neutrophils, particularly during acute and subacute stages. BAL lymphocytosis is present when lymphocytes exceed 30% of all cells in nonsmokers and 20% in current smokers. Most often, CD4:CD8 ratio is <1 (normal is about 1.8) but it may be as high as 4 which is also seen in patients with sarcoidosis.
    - Lung biopsy (transbronchial, cryobiopsy or surgical) may show chronic inflammatory cells and poorly defined noncaseating granulomas. In late stages, fibrosis is visible.

TREATMENT

- Identification and avoidance of the causative antigen.
- Oxygen therapy in severely hypoxaemic patients.
- Prednisolone 1 mg/kg/day orally for 1–2 weeks, followed by gradual tapering over the next 4–6 weeks. Corticosteroids hasten recovery from acute stage but have no beneficial effects on long-term prognosis.
- Mycophenolate mofetil and azathioprine may be used as steroid-sparing agents and may be useful in fibrotic disease
- Role of antifibrotic agents (pirfenidone, nintedanib) is not clear.

Q. Discuss the causes, clinical presentation and management of bronchial obstruction.

CAUSES

- Various causes of bronchial obstruction are given in Box 2.62.

CLINICAL FEATURES

- Clinical manifestations of bronchial obstruction depend on the following:
    - Whether the obstruction is complete or partial.
    - Presence or absence of secondary infection.
    - Effect on pulmonary function.
    - Cause of obstruction.

CLINICAL FEATURES RELATED TO DEGREE OF OBSTRUCTION

Complete Obstruction

- Air distal to the obstruction is absorbed, alveolar spaces close and the affected lung tissue becomes collapsed and solidified.
- Physical signs are mediastinal shift to the side of collapse, dull percussion note and absent or diminished breath sounds over the collapsed part of lung.
- Radiological features include mediastinal shift to the same side, elevation of the diaphragm on the same

BOX 2.62 Causes of Bronchial Obstruction

• Tumours	Bronchial carcinoma, bronchial adenoma
• Enlarged tracheobronchial lymph nodes	Malignant, tuberculous
• Inhaled foreign bodies	—
• Bronchial casts or plugs	Inspissated mucus, blood clots
• Ineffective expectoration	Collection of mucus or mucopus in the bronchus
• Rare causes	Congenital bronchial atresia, posttuberculous bronchial stricture, aortic aneurysm, giant left atrium, pericardial effusion

side and a dense pulmonary opacity. Other features include compensatory hyperinflation and hyperlucency of the remaining aerated lung, and obscuration or silhouetting of the structures adjacent to the collapsed lung (e.g. diaphragm and heart borders).
- If the collapse involves a small portion of the lung, mediastinal displacement and abnormal physical signs may be absent, but a characteristic opacity will be seen on the radiograph.

Partial Obstruction

- Results in less resistance to the airflow during inspiration than during expiration. The difference in airflow resistance is accentuated by coughing. The end result is air trapping distal to the obstruction, leading to overdistension of the part of the lung distal to the obstruction (obstructive emphysema).
- Percussion note over such a lesion is hyperresonant and breath sounds are diminished.
- Radiological examination shows hypertranslucency of the affected part of lung.

CLINICAL FEATURES RELATED TO SECONDARY INFECTION

- Secondary bacterial infection of the lung distal to the obstruction is common. This is usually of low virulence, but in some cases, pulmonary suppuration and lung abscess follow.
- Can present with recurrent pneumonia in the same segment/lobe.

CLINICAL FEATURES RELATED TO IMPAIRED PULMONARY FUNCTION

- Symptoms usually follow obstruction of a main or lobar bronchus.
- Sudden occlusion can result in severe breathlessness and hypoxaemia.

CLINICAL FEATURES RELATED TO THE CAUSE OF OBSTRUCTION

Tumours

- Bronchial carcinoma produces pulmonary collapse at an early stage. Secondary bacterial infection and empyema are common.
- Bronchial adenoma grows less rapidly and hence complete obstruction and pulmonary collapse are late features. Obstructive emphysema may be seen in the early stages of partial bronchial obstruction.

Enlarged Tracheobronchial Lymph Nodes

- May compress or invade the bronchial wall.
- Clinical manifestations are similar to those seen in tumours.
- Commonest cause is bronchial carcinoma, but less common causes are tuberculosis, Hodgkin's lymphoma and other lymphomas.

Foreign Bodies

- Inhaled foreign body usually gets lodged in the right main, intermediate or lower lobe bronchus. Common foreign bodies inhaled are nuts, peas, beans, small pieces of toys, articles of food and fragments of tooth during dental extractions under general anaesthesia.
- Initial presentation is either as obstructive emphysema or as lobar collapse, with a persistent low-pitched rhonchus (fixed rhonchus).
- Later, there is development of suppurative pneumonia in the collapsed lobe, manifested as high fever, cough with purulent expectoration, pleural pain, pleural rub and signs of either collapse or consolidation.
- Radiological examination may reveal obstructive emphysema or collapse or consolidation.

Bronchial Casts or Plugs

- Mucus plugs cause bronchial obstruction in patients with asthma or pulmonary eosinophilia. Secondary bacterial infection of the collapsed lung may occur.
- Blood clots produce bronchial obstruction following severe haemoptysis.

Retained Secretions

- Bronchial obstruction by retained mucus or mucopus occurs in patients who are unable to cough effectively for some reason.
- Secondary bacterial infection is common and occurs early.

MANAGEMENT

- Identification of the cause by chest radiograph, bronchoscopic examination and biopsy, and CT chest.
- Bronchoscopic removal of the foreign bodies, bronchial casts, plugs and secretions.
- Treatment of the underlying cause.

Q. Define chronic obstructive pulmonary disease (COPD), chronic obstructive lung disease (COLD) or chronic obstructive airway disease (COAD). (CT2.1)

Q. What are small airways diseases?

DEFINITION

- Chronic obstructive pulmonary disease (COPD), COLD or COAD, is a preventable and treatable disease characterised by persistent respiratory symptoms and airflow limitation that is due to airway and/or alveolar abnormalities usually caused by significant exposure to noxious gases and particles and influenced by host factors including abnormal lung development. The chronic airflow limitation is caused by a mixture of small airways disease and parenchymal destruction, the relative contributions of which vary from person to person.
- The most common respiratory symptoms are dyspnoea, cough and/or sputum production.
- The obstruction is not relieved (improvement $<15\%$ of baseline) with bronchodilators.
- Chronic inflammation is hallmark of COPD which causes structural changes, narrowing of small airways and destruction of lung parenchyma which leads to reduced lung elastic recoil.

TABLE 2.39 Indicators for Considering a Diagnosis of COPD

Dyspnoea	• Progressive over time • Worse with exercise • Persistent
Chronic cough	• May be intermittent
Chronic sputum production	• Any pattern of sputum production
History of risk factors	• See under 'Chronic Bronchitis'
Family history of COPD	—

- COPD forms a spectrum with pure chronic bronchitis at one end and pure emphysema at the other end.
- Chronic bronchitis and emphysema are pathologically distinct but usually coexist in the same patient in varying proportions.
- Small airways diseases include COPD and asthma. Others include hypersensitivity pneumonitis, bronchiolitis and mineral dust pneumoconiosis.
  - Small airways are defined as noncartilaginous airways with an internal diameter <2 mm. These airways are located from approximately the eighth generation of airways down to the terminal bronchioles and respiratory bronchioles.
  - Normally, small airways contribute only a little to total airway resistance.

INDICATORS FOR CONSIDERING A DIAGNOSIS OF COPD

- Table 2.39 lists the indicators for considering a diagnosis of COPD when spirometry is indicated.

Q. Discuss the aetiology, pathology, clinical features, course, prognosis and treatment of chronic bronchitis. (CT2.2; CT2.20; CT2.3; CT2.6; CT2.7)

Q. Discuss the pathogenesis of the complications of chronic bronchitis.

Q. How do you manage a case of acute exacerbation of chronic bronchitis?

Q. Discuss briefly about Global Initiative for Chronic Obstructive Lung Disease (GOLD).

DEFINITION

- Chronic bronchitis is defined as a condition associated with excessive tracheobronchial mucus production to cause cough with expectoration for at least 3 months of the year, for more than 2 consecutive years in a patient in whom other causes of chronic cough (e.g. bronchiectasis) have been excluded.

INCIDENCE

- Various factors related to incidence of chronic bronchitis are listed in Box 2.63.

BOX 2.63 Incidence of Chronic Bronchitis/COPD

- Middle and late adult life
- More in males than in females
- More in smokers than in nonsmokers
- More in urban than in rural dwellers

BOX 2.64 Abnormalities in Respiratory System Produced by Smoking

- Sluggish ciliary movement
- Bronchoconstriction (through smooth muscle constriction)
- Hypertrophy and hyperplasia of mucus-secreting glands. The ratio of thickness of the submucosal glands to that of the bronchial wall is expressed as Reid index (normal 0.44 ± 0.09; in chronic bronchitis >0.51)
- Release of proteolytic enzymes from polymorphonuclear leucocytes
- Release of inflammatory mediators in lungs
- Inhibition of the function of alveolar macrophages

AETIOLOGY (RISK FACTORS)

- Cigarette smoking is the most important risk factor for the development of COPD. However, only about 15%–20% of smokers develop clinically significant COPD, suggesting that genetic predisposition and environmental factors play a role in the pathogenesis of the disease. Pipe, cigar and water-pipe smokers have increased risk of COPD, although lower than that with cigarette smoking. Cigarette smoking is associated with a variety of abnormalities of the respiratory system which predispose to the development of chronic bronchitis (Box 2.64).
- Air pollution with dust, smoke and fumes, sulphur dioxide and particulate matter.
  - Indoor air pollution, especially from burning biomass fuels (wood, animal dung and crop residues) and coal in confined spaces, is associated with increased risk of COPD.
- Occupational hazards as with exposure to dust, smoke and fumes, toluene diisocyanate in plastic industry and carding room workers in cotton mills.
- Familial and genetic factors influence the development of chronic bronchitis.
  - Genetic predisposition (e.g. hereditary deficiency of α1-antitrypsin).
  - Smokers who are siblings of a patient with severe COPD.
  - Passive smoking (also known as environmental tobacco smoke).
  - Natural gas used for cooking.
- Previous tuberculosis.
- Low socio-economic status.
- Preexisting asthma.
- Increased risk of COPD in HIV-positive patients.
- Infections with rhinovirus, *S. pneumoniae*, *H. influenzae* and *M. catarrhalis* can cause exacerbations of chronic bronchitis.
- Exposure to dampness, fog and sudden changes in temperature can cause exacerbations of chronic bronchitis.

PATHOGENESIS

- Chronic bronchitis and emphysema occur as a result of an inflammatory process involving the airways and distal airspaces.
- Increased activity of oxidants combined with reduced activity of antioxidants has been implicated in the development of inflammation and COPD.
- Cigarette smoke produces high concentration of oxygen free radicals (reactive oxygen species [ROS]) including superoxide, hydrogen peroxide and hypochlorous acid. These are responsible for tissue damage and activation of eosinophils and neutrophils. Inflammatory response is initiated through the activation of transcription factors (nuclear factor-kB [NF-kB] and activator protein-1 [AP-1]) and gene expression of proinflammatory mediators.
- Furthermore, cigarette smoke, various oxidants and activated neutrophils damage α1-antitrypsin that is required to prevent degradation of elastin. All these result in various changes seen in patients with chronic bronchitis and emphysema.
- Various inflammatory mediators involved in COPD include leukotriene B_4 (which attracts neutrophils and lymphocytes), interleukin-8 (which attracts neutrophils and monocytes), TNF-α, IL-1β and IL-6 (which amplify inflammatory response and may be responsible for systemic effects) and transforming growth factor-β (which may induce fibrosis in small airways).
- Pulmonary hypertension develops due to vascular remodelling in COPD, which results from combined effects of hypoxia, inflammation and in severe emphysema, loss of capillaries.

PATHOLOGICAL CHANGES

- Pathological changes seen in a patient with chronic bronchitis are given in Box 2.65.

BOX 2.65 Pathological Changes in Chronic Bronchitis

- Hypertrophy and hyperplasia of the mucus-producing glands
- Goblet cell hyperplasia
- Reduction in the ciliated cells
- Mucosal oedema and intraluminal mucus plugs
- Increased smooth muscle
- Reduction in the calibre of the air passages

CLINICAL FEATURES

HISTORY

- The most striking features are an impressive history of cough with sputum production for many years and a relatively late onset of breathlessness.
- Initially, the cough is present only in the winter seasons ('winter cough' or 'smoker's cough'), especially in the mornings ('morning cough'). Over years, cough increases in frequency, severity and duration until it is present all round the year.
- The sputum is usually scanty, mucoid and more in the mornings. Sputum is occasionally blood-stained (haemoptysis) and occasionally frankly purulent ('mucopurulent relapse').
- Breathlessness is relatively late in onset in chronic bronchitis. It is due to airflow obstruction and is aggravated by infection, excessive smoking and adverse atmospheric conditions.
- Other symptoms include fever during mucopurulent relapses, wheezing and tightness in the chest.

Modified Medical Research Council Scale for Dyspnoea (Table 2.40)

PHYSICAL SIGNS

- Usually the patient is overweight.
- At rest, there is no respiratory distress. Respiratory rate is normal and accessory muscles of respiration are not acting.
- Percussion note is normally resonant over the lungs. Liver dullness and cardiac dullness are normal in position.

Auscultation

- Vesicular breath sounds with prolonged expiration.
- Inspiratory and expiratory rhonchi.
- Crepitations that either disappear or change in location and intensity after coughing.

Systemic Features

- Decreased fat-free mass.
- Impaired systemic muscle function and muscle wasting.
- Normocytic anaemia.
- Osteoporosis.
- Depression.
- Increased risk of angina, acute myocardial infarction and heart failure.
- Metabolic syndrome.

INVESTIGATIONS

- Blood eosinophil count—a biomarker for estimating the efficacy of inhaled corticosteroids (ICS) for the prevention of exacerbations.
- Radiological examination:
  - Chest radiograph does not show any characteristic abnormality but is useful in excluding other diseases.
- Electrocardiography may show features of right atrial and ventricular hypertrophy (tall P waves—P-pulmonale; right bundle branch block; RSR′ pattern in V_1).

TABLE 2.40 Modified Medical Research Council (mMRC) Scale for Dyspnoea

Grade	Description
Grade 0	Gets breathless only on strenuous exercise
Grade 1	Gets breathless when hurrying on level or walking up a slight hill
Grade 2	Walks slower than people of same age on the level because of breathlessness or has to stop for breath while walking at his/her own pace on the level
Grade 3	Stops for breath after walking 100 m or after a few minutes on the level
Grade 4	Too breathless to leave the house or gets breathless while dressing or undressing

BOX 2.66 Pulmonary Function Tests in Chronic Bronchitis/COPD

- FEV_1 is reduced
- FVC is decreased
- Ratio of FEV_1 to FVC is subnormal. Presence of *postbronchodilator* FEV_1/FVC < 70% confirms diagnosis. It should be repeated on a separate occasion if the ratio is between 60% and 80%
- PEF is reduced
- RV is increased
- FRC is increased
- TLC is increased
- Gas transfer (diffusion) may be normal or mildly reduced

- Pulmonary function tests (Box 2.66):
- ABG studies in patients with FEV_1 < 50% of predicted, or those with respiratory failure or cor pulmonale.
  - PaO_2 is markedly reduced (hypoxaemia).
  - $PaCO_2$ is markedly raised (hypercarbia).
- Exercise testing:
  - Six-minute walk test used to assess disability and effectiveness of pulmonary rehabilitation.

COMPLICATIONS

MUCOPURULENT RELAPSES

- Due to secondary bacterial infection with *S. pneumoniae, H. influenzae* or *M. catarrhalis* in 70%–75% of cases.
- Presents as fever with increased sputum production, which is frankly purulent.

CARBON DIOXIDE NARCOSIS

- Persistent CO_2 retention (hypercarbia; high $PaCO_2$) manifests itself as clouding of consciousness, altered behaviour, drowsiness, headache and papilloedema.

RESPIRATORY FAILURE

- Type I respiratory failure (low PaO_2, normal $PaCO_2$) occurs in mild to moderate disease.
- Acute or chronic type II respiratory failure occurs in severe disease.
- Patient is deeply cyanotic, oedematous and stuporous with respiratory failure.

SECONDARY POLYCYTHAEMIA

- This results from hypoxaemia stimulating erythropoiesis.

PULMONARY HYPERTENSION AND RIGHT VENTRICULAR FAILURE (COR PULMONALE)

- Pulmonary hypertension results in a chronic afterload on the right ventricle, which hypertrophies and ultimately fails (right ventricular failure; cor pulmonale).
- Manifestations of pulmonary hypertension like visible and palpable pulmonary artery pulsations, sustained left parasternal heave, epigastric pulsations and a palpable and loud second heart sound may be present.
- Manifestations of right ventricular failure include peripheral oedema, raised JVP, tender hepatomegaly and a third heart sound of right ventricular origin.
- Functional tricuspid regurgitation occurs as a late phenomenon. The manifestations include distended neck veins with large *v* waves and a rapid descent, and a pansystolic murmur accentuated during inspiration.
- Because of cyanosis (blue) and oedema (bloated up), such patients are referred to as blue bloaters.

PATHOGENESIS OF COMPLICATIONS (Flowchart 2.9)

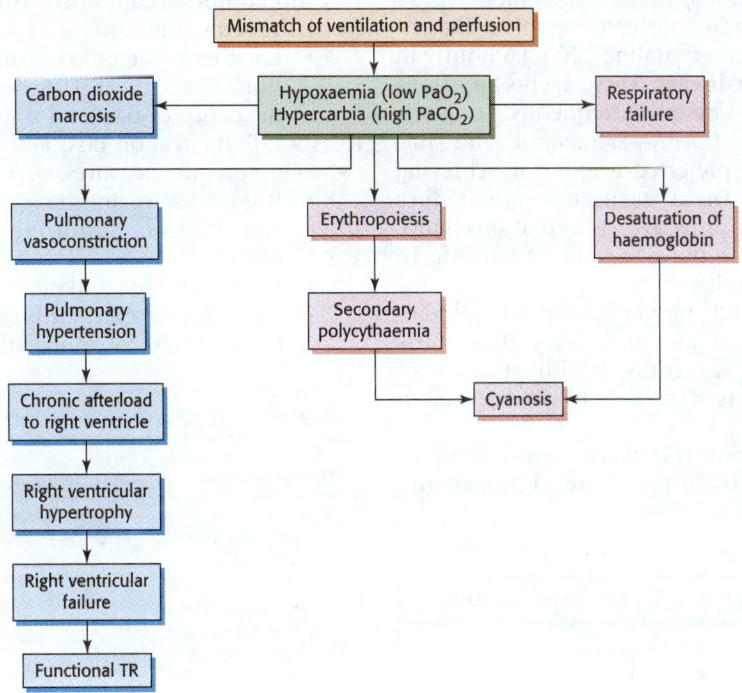

Flowchart 2.9 Pathogenesis of Complications.

COURSE AND PROGNOSIS (NATURAL HISTORY)

- Chronic bronchitis is a progressive disease characterised by exacerbations and remissions.
- Eventually leads to respiratory and cardiac failure (cor pulmonale).
- Repeated episodes of respiratory and cardiac failure occur, from which prompt recovery occurs with proper treatment.
- Some patients may survive for a few years, while others for many years.

DIFFERENTIAL DIAGNOSIS

- Some of the differential diagnoses are listed in Box 2.67.

MANAGEMENT

- Regular exercises and nutritional management.
- Weight reduction in obese patients.
- Reduction of bronchial irritation:
  - Stop smoking completely.
  - Dusty and smoke-laden atmospheres should be avoided.
- Treatment and prevention of respiratory infections:
  - Purulent sputum is treated with oral tetracycline or ampicillin 250 mg 6 hourly or cotrimoxazole 960 mg 12 hourly for 10 days.
  - In the absence of response, sputum culture and sensitivity is done and the antibiotic is changed accordingly.
  - Vaccination with pneumococcal, influenza and COVID-19 vaccines.
- Bronchodilator and steroid therapy: None of the existing medications for COPD have been shown to reduce the rate of decline of lung functions. These reduce frequency and severity of exacerbation and improve health status and exercise tolerance.
  - Inhalation of β_2-adrenoreceptor agonists like salbutamol 200 μg or terbutaline 250 μg 6 hourly in mild to moderate disease. These agents are short-acting and need to be taken frequently. Long-acting β-stimulants (LABA—salmeterol and formoterol) are the preferred agents for achieving bronchodilation. These agents may also reduce the incidence of infective exacerbations since these drugs reduce the adhesion of bacteria to airway epithelial cells.
  - Indacaterol (75–300 μg via inhalation), olodaterol and vilanterol are once-a-day β_2-agonists (ultra-long-acting β_2-agonists) with duration of action for 24 hours. They should not be used in asthma.
  - Anticholinergic bronchodilator drugs, ipratropium bromide (40–80 μg 6 hourly), tiotropium bromide (18 μg once a day) or aclidinium bromide (400 μg 12 hourly) should be added in severe disease. Long-acting muscarinic antagonists (LAMA) have greater effect on exacerbation reduction as compared to LABAs.
  - Combination of LAMA and LABA increases FEV_1 and reduces symptoms as well as exacerbations as compared to monotherapy with either of them.
  - ICS (beclomethasone, budesonide, fluticasone, ciclesonide) seem to reduce exacerbations, improve airway reactivity and respiratory symptoms and should be added in moderately severe cases. Unlike asthma, they should not be used alone. In addition, their regular use increases the risk of pneumonia especially in those with severe disease. COPD patients with the highest pneumonia risk are those with low body mass index, advanced age, male gender and greater airflow obstruction.
    - Patients with blood eosinophil counts <100/mm³ generally do not show any significant response to ICS. Patients with blood eosinophil counts >300/mm³ generally show the greatest likelihood of benefit with ICS.
    - Factors which should be considered before starting inhaled corticosteroids are given in Table 2.41.
  - Triple therapy with ICS/LAMA/LABA improves lung functions and reduces exacerbations compared to ICS/LABA or LAMA/LABA.
  - Oral theophylline or doxophylline may be beneficial in selected cases as add-on therapy.
- Roflumilast, a phosphodiesterase 4 inhibitor, can be given once a day in combination with inhaled β-agonists, anticholinergics and corticosteroids in patients with severe COPD and a history of acute exacerbation. Weight loss, diarrhoea, headache and sleep disturbances are significant side effects. It should not be combined with theophylline.
- Long-term antibiotics:
  - Long-term use of azithromycin reduces exacerbations over 1 year. However, it leads to increased incidence of bacterial resistance, prolongation of QTc interval on ECG and hearing impairment.
- Symptomatic measures:
  - Regular use of antitussives is not recommended.
  - Hot drinks or steam inhalations to liquefy sputum.
  - Mucolytic agents like bromhexine, *N*-acetylcysteine, carbocysteine, ambroxol and erdosteine may be tried. Use of mucolytics is associated with a

BOX 2.67 Differential Diagnosis of Chronic Bronchitis/COPD

- Asthma
- Congestive heart failure
- Bronchiectasis
- Tuberculosis
- Interstitial lung disease

TABLE 2.41 Considerations for Initiating Inhaled Corticosteroids

Recommended	May Be initiated	Should Be avoided
• History of hospitalisation due to acute exacerbation • ≥2 exacerbations/year despite use of LAMA/LABA • Blood eosinophils ≥300/μL • Concomitant asthma	• 1 exacerbation/year • Blood eosinophils 100–300/μL	• History of tuberculosis • Blood eosinophils <100/μL • History of repeated pneumonias

small reduction in acute exacerbations and a reduction in total number of days of disability but does not alter loss of lung function.
  - Chest physiotherapy.
- Long-term domiciliary oxygen therapy:
  - Long-term, low-dose (2 L/minute) oxygen therapy (goal to maintain oxygen saturation ≥90%) through nasal cannulae for at least 15 hours a day in patient with:
    - Daytime PaO_2 ≤ 55 mmHg at rest or oxygen saturation ≤ 88% with or without hypercapnia confirmed twice over a period of 3 weeks OR
    - Daytime PaO_2 between 56 and 59 mmHg or oxygen saturation >88% with the evidence of hypoxic organ damage (including right heart failure, pulmonary hypertension or polycythaemia with haematocrit >55%).
  - This decreases pulmonary hypertension and prolongs life in hypoxaemic patients who have developed right heart failure. Other benefits include reductions in polycythaemia, pulmonary artery pressures, dyspnoea, hypoxaemia during sleep and reduced nocturnal arrhythmias.
- Treatment of pulmonary hypertension involves long-term oxygen therapy. Drugs approved for treatment of primary pulmonary hypertension are not recommended for COPD-induced pulmonary hypertension. Use of synthetic prostacyclin (epoprostenol), prostacyclin analogues, endothelin-1 receptor antagonists and phosphodiesterase-5 inhibitors for pulmonary hypertension due to COPD is experimental.
- Management of associated comorbidities (e.g. CAD, heart failure, cardiac arrhythmias, hypertension, osteoporosis, anxiety or depression, diabetes, GERD and obstructive sleep apnoea) as they contribute to hospitalisation and mortality.
- Pulmonary rehabilitation:
  - The primary goal of pulmonary rehabilitation is to reverse muscular and cardiovascular dysfunction through an individually designed programme.
  - It includes breathing techniques, chest physical therapy, postural drainage, exercise conditioning (upper and lower extremity) and activities of daily living. Also included are evaluation and advice on nutritional needs and psychological and vocational counselling.

SEVERITY IN COPD (BASED ON POSTBRONCHODILATOR FEV_1 WITH PREBRONCHODILATOR FEV_1/FVC <0.70)

- GOLD (Global Initiative for Chronic Obstructive Lung Disease) is the global strategy for the diagnosis, management and prevention of COPD.
- Spirometry remains key in diagnosis, prognostication and treatment including nonpharmacological therapies (e.g. lung volume reduction and lung transplantation).
- Current therapy as per GOLD guidelines is based on patient needs in terms of symptom reduction and/or exacerbation prevention.

TABLE 2.42 Classification of Airflow Limitation Severity in COPD (Based on Postbronchodilator FEV_1) in Patients With FEV_1/FVC <0.70

Mild COPD (GOLD 1)	FEV_1 ≥80% of predicted
Moderate COPD (GOLD 2)	FEV_1 50% to <80% of predicted
Severe COPD (GOLD 3)	FEV_1 30% to <50% of predicted
Very severe COPD (GOLD 4)	FEV_1 <30% of predicted

- Based on spirometric classification, the patient is graded as mild, moderate, severe, very severe COPD (Table 2.42).

EXACERBATIONS OF COPD

- Acute exacerbations are defined as mild (treated with short-acting bronchodilators), moderate (treated with short-acting bronchodilators with antibiotics and/or oral corticosteroids) and severe (requiring hospitalisation or visit to an emergency room).

THERAPY OF COPD PATIENTS

- Patient's symptoms and exacerbations in the past 1 year help in guiding therapies in COPD.
- Based on mMRC scale and history of moderate or severe exacerbation in past 1 year, the patient is treated with LAMA or LABA or LAMA + LABA or ICS + LAMA or ICS + LAMA + LABA.

SUMMARY OF TREATMENT (Table 2.43)

TABLE 2.43 Summary of Treatment of COPD

Exacerbation History	mMRC Grade of Dyspnoea	Pharmacological Treatment
0 or 1 (Not needing hospitalisation)	0–1	A bronchodilator (short- or long- acting)
0 or 1 (Not needing hospitalisation)	≥2	A long-acting bronchodilator (LAMA or LABA)
≥2 or ≥1 Needing hospitalisation	0–1	LAMA
≥2 or ≥1 Needing hospitalisation	≥2	LAMA or LAMA + LABA or LABA + ICS (if blood eosinophil count >300/μL

ACUTE EXACERBATIONS

- COPD exacerbation is an acute event characterised by worsening of respiratory symptoms with worsening beyond day-to-day variation and leads to change in medication.
- Indicates a combination of increased sputum volume, sputum purulence and increasing dyspnoea.
- Mainly triggered by viral infections, although bacterial infections and environmental factors may also initiate it.
- Exacerbations increase rate of decline in lung function, deterioration in health status and risk of death.
- Classified as:
  - Mild (treated with short-acting bronchodilators only).

- Moderate (treated with short-acting bronchodilators along with antibiotics with or without oral corticosteroids).
- Severe (require treatment in a hospital).

TREATMENT OF SEVERE ACUTE EXACERBATIONS

OXYGEN

- Initial therapy should focus on maintaining oxygen saturation at 90% or above.
- This can be achieved by administering oxygen by a nasal catheter or through a face mask equipped to control the inspired oxygen fraction. Venturi masks are the preferred means of oxygen delivery because they permit a precise fraction of inspired oxygen (FiO_2).
- One should be careful while administering oxygen as high flow rates can worsen hypercapnia. Mechanisms proposed to explain this phenomenon are:
  - Increased dead space due to aggravation of ventilation/perfusion mismatch resulting from the release of hypoxic vasoconstriction.
  - Loss of hypoxic respiratory drive.
  - CO_2 binding capacity decreases as haemoglobin oxygen saturation increases (Haldane effect).
- High-flow oxygen therapy through nasal cannula is an alternative to standard oxygen therapy or NIV in patients with acute hypoxaemic respiratory failure.

BRONCHODILATORS

- Use of nebulised β-adrenergic agonists (salbutamol 2.5 mg every 20 minutes for initial 1–2 hours) and anticholinergic agents (ipratropium bromide 0.5 mg) improves airflow during acute exacerbations. Both the agents can be combined if required.

ANTIBIOTICS

- Indicated in patients with increased dyspnoea, increased sputum volume and increased sputum purulence or those requiring mechanical ventilation.
- Most common organisms during exacerbations include *S. pneumoniae*, *H. influenzae* and *M. catarrhalis*. Risk factors for *P. aeruginosa* infection include recent hospitalisation, frequent use of antibiotics (four or more courses in last 1 year) and severe exacerbation.
- For outpatient management, doxycycline, cotrimoxazole or amoxicillin-clavulanate can be given. Patients older than 65 years should also be prescribed one of the newer fluoroquinolones (levofloxacin, moxifloxacin).
- Hospitalised patients should receive intravenous antibiotics (azithromycin or fluoroquinolone or a third-generation cephalosporin like ceftriaxone or cefotaxime).
- In severe exacerbations, treatment should include a third-generation cephalosporin plus a fluoroquinolone or an aminoglycoside.

CORTICOSTEROIDS

- Intravenous or oral corticosteroids should be administered for 5–7 days as they shorten recovery time and improve lung functions (FEV_1) and hypoxaemia.

DIURETICS

- Diuretics are administered in patients with gross right ventricular failure.

NONINVASIVE POSITIVE AIRWAY PRESSURE VENTILATION

- Noninvasive positive-pressure ventilation using tight-fitting face mask to deliver BiPAP should be tried when there is a need for ventilatory assistance. It is indicated if patient develops:
  - Acute respiratory acidosis (pH < 7.3 and/or $PCO_2 > 45$ mmHg) and/or
  - Severe dyspnoea with clinical signs suggestive of respiratory muscle fatigue, increased work of breathing or both, such as use of accessory muscles of respiration, paradoxical motion of abdomen or retraction of intercostal spaces.
- The patient should be cooperative and medically stable for NIV.

INVASIVE VENTILATION

- If NIV fails or cannot be given, the patient should be intubated for mechanical ventilation (Box 2.68).
  - Use low tidal volume and prolonged expiration.
  - Apply moderate PEEP.
  - Do not attempt to normalise arterial carbon dioxide.

ADMISSION

- Indications for admitting a patient with acute exacerbation are given in Box 2.69.

BOX 2.68 Indications of Invasive Ventilation

- Unable to tolerate NIV or failure of NIV
- Postrespiratory arrest
- Postcardiac arrest
- Altered level of consciousness
- Recurrent vomiting
- Inability to manage respiratory or oral secretions
- Severe haemodynamic instability despite vasopressors
- Uncontrollable cardiac arrhythmias

BOX 2.69 Indications for Admission

- Marked increase in symptom intensity (e.g. resting dyspnoea)
- New physical findings (e.g. cyanosis and peripheral oedema)
- Severe underlying COPD
- Presence of important comorbidities (e.g. cardiac disease)
- New arrhythmias
- Older age
- Failure to respond to initial medical treatment
- Diagnostic uncertainty
- Insufficient home support

Q. What is emphysema? What are the various types of emphysema?

Q. Describe mediastinal emphysema.

Q. What is subcutaneous emphysema?

Q. Discuss compensatory emphysema.

- The word 'emphysema' means inflation or distension with air.
- Emphysema can be classified based on the anatomical site:
  - Pulmonary emphysema.
  - Mediastinal emphysema.
  - Subcutaneous emphysema.

PULMONARY EMPHYSEMA

- A detailed description of generalised bilateral pulmonary emphysema is given later. Compensatory emphysema is a form of pulmonary emphysema that is localised.

COMPENSATORY EMPHYSEMA

- It is a condition where the normal lung tissue undergoes hypertrophy as a compensatory mechanism for an extensive damage to the other lung or to a part of the same lung.
- Being a compensatory phenomenon, this is asymptomatic.
- Physical findings in compensatory emphysema include reduced respiratory movements, hyperresonant percussion note and reduced intensity of the breath sounds.
- On chest radiograph, one lung will be hyperinflated (Fig. 2.11).

MEDIASTINAL EMPHYSEMA

- Mediastinal emphysema occurs as a result of escape of air rapidly into the mediastinum following rupture of overdistended alveoli in severe bronchial asthma, rupture of emphysematous bulla and rupture of oesophagus.

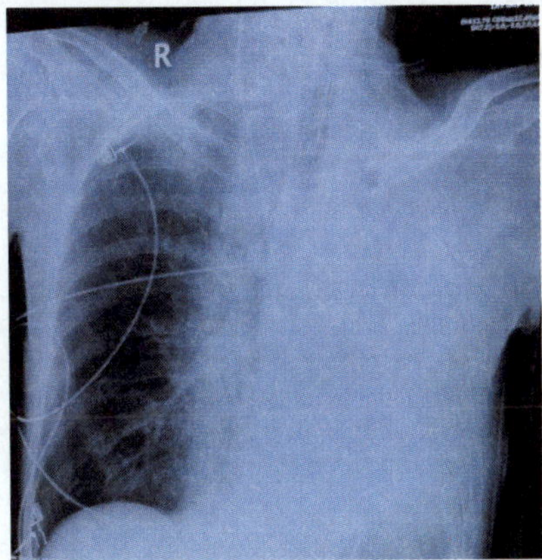

Fig. 2.11 Left lung collapse with compensatory emphysema of right lung (you can count 11 ribs posteriorly).

- Air usually tracks upwards into the subcutaneous tissues of the neck where it manifests as 'subcutaneous emphysema'.
- If severe, mediastinal emphysema may produce cardiac tamponade.
- Auscultation may reveal a crunching sound ('mediastinal crunch' or Hamman crunch).

SUBCUTANEOUS EMPHYSEMA

- Subcutaneous emphysema is due to the presence of air in the subcutaneous tissues.
- Common causes are penetrating chest injuries, fracture of ribs and intercostal tube introduction.
- Clinically, subcutaneous emphysema imparts a characteristic crepitation or crackling sensation on palpation.
- No treatment is generally indicated as the air will get absorbed slowly. In severe cases, subcutaneous incisions may be made to relieve pressure.

Q. Discuss the aetiology, pathology, clinical features, investigations, complications and management of pulmonary emphysema.

Q. What is α1-antitrypsin deficiency? (CT2.5)

Q. Give a brief account of pulmonary bullae.

DEFINITION

- Emphysema is defined as a distension of the air spaces distal to the terminal bronchiole with destruction of alveolar septa but without obvious fibrosis.

AETIOLOGY

- Smoking:
  - Alveolar macrophages accumulate around the terminal bronchioles and release proteolytic enzymes. Leucocytes release enzymes such as elastase.
  - These enzymes cause enzymatic digestion and destruction of alveolar walls, resulting in emphysema.
- Occupational causes—furnace blowers, goldsmiths, exposure to cadmium.
- α1-Antitrypsin deficiency:
  - Connective tissue of the lung is digested by the proteolytic enzyme 'protease' released from leucocytes. α1-Antitrypsin is a protease inhibitor (antiprotease), preventing this proteolytic digestion. Hence, a deficiency or absence of α1-antitrypsin results in the proteolytic destruction of lung, eventually leading to emphysema.
  - α1-Antitrypsin deficiency is an autosomal recessive disorder.
  - Pathologically, these patients develop severe panacinar emphysema, predominantly at the lung bases.
  - This type of emphysema is rare and occurs in young adults. It manifests as progressive dyspnoea and minimal cough.

- Other conditions associated with its deficiency include bronchiectasis, hepatic cirrhosis, vasculitis and panniculitis.

PATHOLOGY

- Pathologically, emphysema can be classified into three types according to the pattern of involvement of acini:
  1. Centriacinar (centrilobular) emphysema, where distension and destruction are limited to the respiratory bronchiole and the alveoli closely related to them (central involvement of the acinus with sparing of the periphery). It is the primary pathological subtype associated with cigarette smoke-induced COPD. This pattern of emphysema is typically more prominent in the upper lung zones.
  2. Panacinar emphysema, where there is generalised destruction of alveoli (both central and peripheral portions of the acinus involved). It is classically associated with α1-antitrypsin deficiency and is more prominent in the lower lung zones.
  3. Paraseptal emphysema, where distension involves only the distal acinus. It is found near the pleura and may cause spontaneous pneumothorax.

CLINICAL FEATURES

HISTORY

- The most striking feature is steadily progressive exertional breathlessness with minimal cough and expectoration.
- Breathlessness is insidious in onset, initially only exertional, but gradually and steadily progressive, ultimately ending in breathlessness on trivial exertion and even at rest.
- Cough with expectoration of scanty mucoid sputum is characteristically minimal.
- Weakness, anorexia, lethargy and weight loss can occur with advanced disease.

PHYSICAL FINDINGS

Inspection and Palpation

- Body build is asthenic.
- Neck is short and thick.
- Neck veins may distend during expiration, but they collapse briskly during inspiration.
- Patient sits leaning forwards, extending the arms to brace himself/herself.
- Patient appears distressed and tachypnoeic.
- Accessory muscles of respiration (sternomastoid and scalene muscles) are hypertrophied. They lift the sternum in an anterosuperior direction during inspiration.
- Prolonged expiration through pursed lips ('pursed lip breathing').
- Expiration begins with a grunting sound.
- Exaggerated tracheal descent during inspiration (Campbell's sign).
- Reduction in the length of trachea above the suprasternal notch.
- Apical impulse is usually invisible or feeble.
- Excavation of the suprasternal and supraclavicular fossae during inspiration.
- Indrawing of the costal margins during inspiration.
- Chest appears cylindrical or barrel-like ('barrel-shaped chest'). Anteroposterior diameter of the chest is markedly increased, and the normal ratio of anteroposterior to transverse diameter of 5:7 is altered.
- Whole of the chest is in a fixed state of full inspiration.
- Sternum is arched forwards and angle of Louis is unduly prominent.
- Subcostal angle is widened (normal: 70°).
- Ribs are placed more horizontally and widely.
- Kyphosis of the thoracic spine.
- Chest expansion is symmetrically diminished.

Percussion

- Hyperresonant percussion note over the lungs.
- Cardiac dullness is reduced or obliterated.
- Liver dullness is pushed down or absent.

Auscultation

- Intensity of the breath sounds is diminished.
- Breath sounds are vesicular in character with prolonged expiration.
- Scattered, faint, high-pitched, end-expiratory rhonchi may be audible.

INVESTIGATIONS

- Radiological features of pulmonary emphysema on chest radiograph PA view are given in Box 2.70.
- Chest radiograph lateral view may show a large retrosternal translucency.
- Computed tomography of the chest can detect emphysema with certainty.
- Pulmonary function tests are given in Box 2.71.
- ABG studies usually reveal a slightly reduced PaO_2 and normal or mildly elevated $PaCO_2$.

BOX 2.70 Radiological Features of Pulmonary Emphysema

- Bullae
- Low-set, flat diaphragm
- Unusually translucent lung fields
- Loss of peripheral vascular markings
- Widely placed and horizontal ribs
- Long and narrow heart ('tubular heart')
- Prominent pulmonary artery shadows at the hilum

BOX 2.71 Pulmonary Function Tests in Pulmonary Emphysema

- FEV_1 is decreased
- FVC is decreased
- FEV_1: FVC ratio is reduced
- PEF is reduced
- TLC is increased
- RV is increased
- RV:TLC ratio is increased
- Gas transfer factor for carbon monoxide (diffusion) is reduced

COMPLICATIONS

PULMONARY BULLAE

- Bullae are inflated thin-walled spaces created by the rupture of alveolar walls.
- Bullae may be single or multiple, large or small.
- They are usually located subpleurally and along the anterior borders of lungs.
- A subpleural bulla can rupture causing spontaneous pneumothorax.
- Large bullae can interfere with pulmonary ventilation.

RESPIRATORY FAILURE

- Type I and type II respiratory failure can occur as a late complication of emphysema.

PULMONARY HYPERTENSION AND RIGHT HEART FAILURE

- These are late complications in emphysema.
- The occurrence of right ventricular failure in emphysema is usually a terminal event.

WEIGHT LOSS

- Severe weight loss leading to emaciation can occur. This is probably due to impaired testosterone secretion.

COURSE AND PROGNOSIS (NATURAL HISTORY)

- Pulmonary emphysema progresses steadily and gradually as breathlessness with minimal cough and expectoration. Patients are less prone to mucopurulent relapses. Right-sided heart failure and hypercapnic respiratory failure are often terminal events. In the absence of such events, the clinical course is characterised by severe and progressive dyspnoea for which little can be done.

TREATMENT

- There is no specific treatment for established generalised emphysema. At the most, one can prevent its further progression and treat the aggravating factors and complications.
- Prevention of progression of emphysema includes cessation of smoking and avoidance of occupational exposure.
- Treatment of aggravating factors and complications include prompt treatment of infections, respiratory failure and right heart failure.
- A trial with inhaled bronchodilators and steroids is given, though it may not be successful in patients with pure emphysema.
- Physiotherapy aids in relaxation of cervical muscles and helps the patients to exhale slowly and steadily through the pursed lips. It can also facilitate expectoration.
- Surgical ablation of giant bullae may bring about dramatic improvement in pulmonary function.
- Lung volume reduction surgery reduces hyperinflation of one or both lungs by surgical and/or laser resection. This makes respiratory muscles more effective pressure generators due to improved efficiency.
- Bronchoscopic lung volume reduction procedures include endobronchial valves (EBV), lung volume reduction coils and bronchoscopic thermal vapor ablation. EBV blocks inspiration of air into severely diseased pulmonary segments while allowing egress of air to produce atelectasis of the target segment or lobe.
- Heart and lung transplantation may be considered in young patients with severe emphysema due to α1-antitrypsin deficiency.
- For patients with α1-antitrypsin deficiency, intravenous replacement therapy using α1-antitrypsin derived from pooled human plasma is being used but its efficacy is not clear.

Q. What are blue bloaters?

- This is a distinctive clinical pattern seen in chronic bronchitis.
- Marked cyanosis ('blue') and peripheral oedema ('bloated') are dominant.
- These patients have prominent cough with expectoration, mucopurulent relapses, repeated episodes of right ventricular failure and respiratory failure, arterial hypoxaemia (low PaO_2) and hypercapnia (high $PaCO_2$).

Q. What are pink puffers?

- This is a distinctive clinical pattern seen in pulmonary emphysema.
- They have marked dyspnoea ('puffer') and no cyanosis (hence 'pink').
- The clinical course is characterised by steadily progressive dyspnoea. They maintain a near-normal PaO_2 and $PaCO_2$. The occurrence of respiratory failure and right heart failure is late and often terminal.

Q. What are the differentiating features of emphysema and chronic bronchitis?

- Table 2.44 gives differentiating features between emphysema and chronic bronchitis.

TABLE 2.44 Emphysema Versus Chronic Bronchitis

Feature	Emphysema	Chronic Bronchitis
Clinical features		
• Dyspnoea	Severe	Mild
• Cough	After dyspnoea starts	Before dyspnoea starts
• Sputum	Scanty, mucoid	Copious, purulent
• Mucopurulent relapses	Less frequent	More frequent
• Cyanosis	Absent	Present
• Pulmonary hypertension	Late and mild	Early and severe
• Right ventricular failure	Late and often terminal	Repeated episodes
• Respiratory failure	Late and often terminal	Repeated episodes
Investigations		
• Haematocrit	Normal	Increased
• PaO_2	Normal to low	Low
• $PaCO_2$	Normal	High
• Diffusion capacity	Reduced	Normal
• Chest X-ray	Features of hyperinflation, bullae and tubular heart	Increased bronchovascular markings and cardiomegaly

TABLE 2.45 Asthma Versus COPD

Feature	Asthma	COPD
• Age of onset	Generally, children and young adults	Generally, older people
• Risk factors	Family history of allergies Allergen exposure Occupational sensitisers	Smoking Occupational exposure Atmospheric pollution α1-Antitrypsin deficiency
• Respiratory symptoms	Wheezing, cough, dyspnoea Symptoms vary from time to time and even over hours or days May be triggered by exercise, dust or exposure to allergens Often shows improvement spontaneously or with optimal treatment	Chronic dyspnoea, productive cough Usually continuous symptoms Chronic symptoms usually unrelated to triggers Slowly progressive symptoms despite therapy
• Comorbidities	Generally not present	Often present (e.g. depression, metabolic syndrome, coronary heart disease, osteoporosis, muscle wasting)
• Chest X-ray	Chest X-ray normal	Shows hyperinflation and other changes
• Spirometry	Reversibility of airway obstruction Normal between symptoms	FEV_1 may improve with bronchodilators but $FEV_1/FVC < 0.7$ persists Persistent airflow limitation
• Computerised tomography (if performed)	May show bronchial thickening	Emphysema
• Response to bronchodilators	Reversible	Partially reversible
• Treatment response with inhaled corticosteroids	Positive	Nil/mild

Q. What are the differentiating features of asthma and chronic obstructive pulmonary disease?

- Table 2.45 gives differentiating features between asthma and COPD.

Q. Describe various components of cigarette smoke.

Q. Name the diseases caused by smoking.

Q. Discuss smoking cessation. (CT2.21)

- Cigarette smoke is a complex aerosol composed of gaseous and particulate compounds.
- Smoke consists of mainstream smoke and sidestream smoke components.
  - Mainstream smoke is produced by inhalation of air through the cigarette and is the primary source of smoke exposure for smokers.
  - Sidestream smoke is produced from smouldering of the cigarette between puffs and is the major source of environmental tobacco smoke or second-hand smoke.
- There are more than 4000 chemical constituents of cigarette smoke: 95% of the weight of mainstream smoke comes from more than 400 gaseous compounds; rest of the weight is made up of more than 3500 particulate components.
- Primary determinant of tobacco addiction is nicotine; tar is the total particulate matter of cigarette smoke after nicotine and water have been removed.
- Exposure to tar seems to be a major component of lung cancer risk.

BOX 2.72 Diseases Caused by Smoking

- Cancers: Lung, oropharynx, oesophagus, stomach, pancreas, bladder, kidney, cervix, possibly colon and acute myeloid leukaemia
- Respiratory diseases: COPD, chronic cough and infections
- Cardiovascular diseases: Coronary artery disease, cerebrovascular disease, peripheral artery disease, abdominal aortic aneurysm
- Reproductive: Miscarriage, prematurity, low birth weight
- Gastrointestinal: Gastro-oesophageal acid reflux, peptic ulcer and Crohn's diseases
- Others: Poor oral and skin health, cataract, fire-related injuries

- Mainstream smoke contains many potential carcinogens, including polycyclic aromatic hydrocarbons, aromatic amines, *N*-nitrosamines and other organic and inorganic compounds, such as benzene, vinyl chloride, arsenic and chromium.
- Diseases caused by smoking are mentioned in Box 2.72.

SMOKING CESSATION

- Behavioural interventions:
  - Counselling.
- Pharmacotherapy:
  - Nicotine replacement therapy (by gum, transdermal patch or inhaler). Contraindicated in recent myocardial infarction and stroke.
  - Bupropion—a noradrenergic antidepressant.
  - Varenicline—a nicotinic acetylcholine receptor partial agonist which reduces nicotine withdrawal symptoms.

- Electronic cigarette (e-cigarette):
  - Battery-operated device popularised to help reducing cigarette smoking.
  - Contains a liquid of nicotine which is vapourised by heat. Therefore, it acts like nicotine replacement therapy while the person has satisfaction of smoking.
  - Found to have several adverse effects due to associated harmful chemicals and is at present, its role is controversial.

Q. Briefly discuss e-cigarette or vaping product use associated lung injury (EVALI).

- Inhalation of aerosolised products created by using different electronic devices is called vaping.
- The process involves heating the liquid or wax containing different products including cannabis, tetrahydrocannabinol (THC), nicotine, flavours, vitamin E acetate and glycerol.
- EVALI is an acute or subacute respiratory illness in people who had used e-cigarettes (vaping) in the last 90 days. Additional requirements include radiographic abnormalities and exclusion of alternative specific diagnoses.
- Vitamin E acetate and THC are implicated for the lung injury.

CLINICAL FEATURES IN EVALI

HISTORY

- Table 2.46 mentions symptoms of EVALI.

EXAMINATION

- Examination may reveal bilateral crepitations in some patients.

INVESTIGATIONS

- Approximately 25% of patients have a pulse oxygen saturation below 88% at the time of presentation.
- Other findings include mild leucocytosis with a neutrophil predominance, normal or mildly elevated procalcitonin, elevated CRP and elevated ESR.

TABLE 2.46 Symptoms of EVALI

Constitutional symptoms	• Fever • Chills • Weight loss • Fatigue
Respiratory symptoms	• Dyspnoea • Chest pain • Pleuritic pain • Cough • Haemoptysis
Gastrointestinal symptoms	• Nausea • Vomiting • Abdominal pain • Diarrhoea

- Chest radiograph and CT chest show bilateral ground-glass opacities.
- Bronchoscopy is indicated mainly to exclude specific suspected alternative diagnoses.

DIFFERENTIAL DIAGNOSIS

- Other possibilities like pneumonia (viral and bacterial), hypersensitivity pneumonitis, diffuse alveolar haemorrhage, eosinophilic pneumonia and lung involvement due to autoimmune diseases should be excluded.

TREATMENT

- Treatment is mainly supportive with supplemental oxygenation to maintain a target pulse oxygen saturation of 88%–92%; this can be achieved through high flow nasal cannula if nasal cannula alone is insufficient. In some cases, mechanical ventilation is required.
- In severe cases, a short course of corticosteroids may be given.

Q. Discuss air pollution briefly. (CT2.6)

- Air pollution consists of hazardous biological, chemical and particulate matter (PM) present in the air.
- Rural air is contaminated by burning biomass (either wood or dung for cooking or burning crops in fields) and urban air is contaminated by vehicular exhaust, industrial contaminants, construction material and coal-based power stations.
- The air pollutants associated with significant health adverse effects include PM, nitrogen dioxide (NO_2), other oxides of nitrogen, ozone (O_3), sulphur dioxide, carbon monoxide and lead.
- The particulate matter adversely affects human health; its inhalation leads to increased morbidity and mortality.
- There are numerous particles which remain suspended in air and can be grouped as 'total suspended particles (TSP)'. These particles have a diameter <100 µm.
- The depth of absorption into the human lung varies as per the size of PM. The PM can be divided into:
  - PM larger than 10 µm gets deposited in the nose and upper airways.
  - PM with size <10 µm settle in the bronchi.
  - Fine PM (PM2.5) with a particle size <2.5 µm can reach up to the alveoli.
  - Ultrafine PM have size <0.1 µm and reach alveoli; they may cross over to the bloodstream.
- The PM exert their toxicity both directly and indirectly by initiating free radical reactions in the cells and tissues. Prolonged exposure also leads to oxidative stress, telomere erosions leading to chronic diseases and increased mortality. Their toxicity is enhanced by concomitant pollutants such as NO_2, O_3 and host factors determining the site of deposition.
- Various diseases which are associated with atmospheric pollution are given in the Table 2.47.

TABLE 2.47 Diseases Associated With Air Pollution

Lungs: • COPD • Lung cancer • Asthma • Interstitial lung disease	Reproductive system: • Preterm birth • Low birth weight • Foetal growth retardation • Poor quality sperm • Preeclampsia
CNS: • Impact on neurological development and on mental health • Neurodegenerative disorders • Stroke	Endocrine: • Insulin resistance • Diabetes mellitus
Cardiovascular: • Myocardial infarction • Arrhythmias • Heart failure • Hypertension	Miscellaneous: • Increased mortality • Early skin aging

Q. Discuss the aetiology, classification, clinical features, investigations, complications and management of bronchiectasis.

DEFINITION

- Bronchiectasis is defined as a permanent abnormal dilatation of one or more bronchi due to the destruction of elastic and muscular components of the bronchial wall.

CLASSIFICATION (Fig. 2.12)

1. Saccular (cystic) bronchiectasis:
   - This occurs in the proximal large bronchi.
   - The bronchi show marked dilatation, ending in large sacs.
2. Cylindrical (fusiform) bronchiectasis:
   - This involves the airways from 6th to 10th generation.
   - The bronchi look cylindrical or beaded, and end squarely and abruptly.
3. Varicose bronchiectasis:
   - This is intermediate between saccular and cylindrical changes.
   - The bronchi resemble varicose veins.

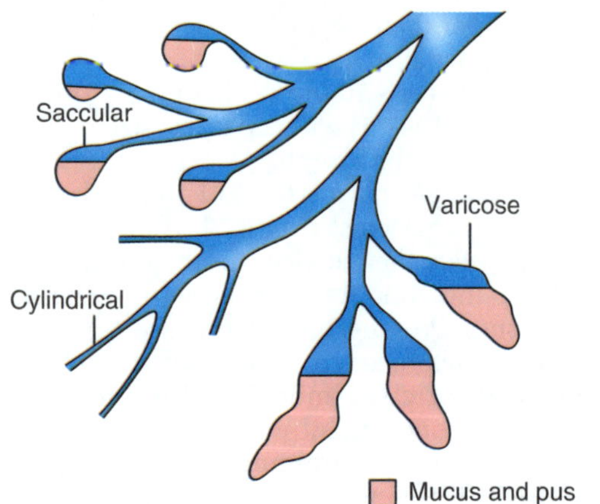

Fig. 2.12 Types of bronchiectasis.

TABLE 2.48 Aetiology of Bronchiecatsis

• Congenital	Bronchial cysts, α1-antitrypsin deficiency, cystic fibrosis, primary hypogammaglobulinaemia, ciliary dyskinesia syndromes (e.g. Kartagener's syndrome), atopic bronchial asthma, pulmonary sequestration
• Acquired (children)	Necrotising pneumonias (measles, whooping cough, *Staphylococcus*, adenovirus and influenza), primary tuberculosis, foreign bodies
• Acquired (adults)	Pulmonary tuberculosis, suppurative pneumonias, postobstructive bronchiectasis (endobronchial tumours or foreign bodies, enlarged hilar lymph nodes or tumour masses and bronchostenosis following endobronchial tuberculosis), allergic bronchopulmonary aspergillosis (ABPA), repeated aspiration of gastric fluid, inhalation of toxic gas (ammonia), long-standing asthma and COPD, HIV infection, rheumatoid arthritis, inflammatory bowel disease, Sjogren's syndrome, interstitial lung fibrosis (traction bronchiectasis), radiation fibrosis, sarcoidosis, chronic hypersensitivity pneumonitis

AETIOLOGY

- Various causes of bronchiectasis are given in Table 2.48.

PATHOLOGY

- Characteristic feature of bronchiectasis is multiple 'bronchiectatic cavities'.
- Left lung is involved more frequently than the right lung.
- Bronchiectasis can affect any part of the lung, but lower lobes are involved more commonly than upper lobes due to more efficient drainage of the upper lobes by gravity.
- Common sites of involvement are lower lobes, lingula and middle lobe.

CLINICAL FEATURES

- The hallmarks of bronchiectasis are chronic cough with sputum production, haemoptysis and recurrent pneumonias.
- Cough is chronic and worse in the mornings. It is brought about by postural changes.
- Sputum is characteristically copious, purulent and foul-smelling due to anaerobic infections. Sputum production varies with posture and is maximum in the first 2 hours after waking up.
- If sputum is collected in a conical flask and allowed to stand for some time, it separates into three layers ('three-layered sputum'), a mucoid layer on the top, a mucopurulent layer in the middle and a purulent layer at the bottom.
- Haemoptysis is due to rupture of the thin-walled vessels on the walls of dilated bronchi. It is often recurrent and may vary from slight blood-streaked sputum to massive fatal bleeding.
- Chest pain, which may be pleuritic, is present in 20%–30% of patients.
- In widespread bronchiectasis, dyspnoea and wheezing may occur.
- In some cases, the patient is asymptomatic or has nonproductive cough ('bronchiectasis sicca'). It commonly occurs following upper lobe tuberculosis.

- Systemic symptoms include fever, weight loss, anaemia, night sweats and weakness.
- Situs inversus in 50% of cases of ciliary dyskinesia.
- Acute exacerbation is characterised by increase of sputum with cough, increased dyspnoea, fever, increased wheezing, fatigue and radiological signs of infection.
- Recurrent pneumonias are characterised by fever with chills and rigors, night sweats, increased quantity and purulence of the sputum, neutrophil leucocytosis in the blood and radiographic evidence of pneumonia.

PHYSICAL FINDINGS

- General examination may reveal anaemia, clubbing of the digits (2%–3% of cases), fever, halitosis and sinusitis.
- Respiratory signs may be unilateral but are usually bilateral and basal.
- Presence of large amounts of secretion is responsible for the characteristic 'bilateral, basal, coarse, leathery crepitations' of bronchiectasis.
- If the bronchiectatic cavities are dry, there may be no abnormal physical signs.

INVESTIGATIONS

- Blood picture shows anaemia, raised ESR and leucocytosis indicating suppuration.
- In advanced and chronic cases, urine examination may show proteinuria due to renal amyloidosis.
- Sputum studies should include Gram stain, Ziehl–Neelsen staining for acid-fast bacilli and culture and sensitivity. The culture usually grows normal nasopharyngeal flora. Other commonly grown organisms are *S. pneumoniae, H. influenzae* and *P. aeruginosa* in cystic fibrosis.
- Chest radiograph is usually normal. Cystic or saccular bronchiectasis may be diagnosed by multiple 1- to 2-cm cystic-appearing lesions with or without fluid levels ('honeycomb' appearance or 'bird's-nest' appearance). Less often, the chest film shows linear streaks (tram tracks), end-on thickened bronchi or signet ring deformity and groups of small curvilinear shadows called grape clusters.
- Electrocardiogram is usually normal, but evidence of right ventricular hypertrophy develops with cor pulmonale.
- Bronchoscopy does not establish the diagnosis. It is indicated in selected situations like identifying the source of secretions, identifying the site of bleeding in patients with haemoptysis and therapeutically to remove secretions.
- High-resolution computed tomography in which the images are only 1 mm thick is diagnostic.
  - Specific criteria include:
    - Internal diameter of the bronchus is larger than that of its accompanying vessel, or
    - Bronchus fails to taper in the periphery of the chest.
  - Besides, some features on CT scan may suggest the aetiology of bronchiectasis (e.g. proximal bronchiectasis suggests ABPA).
- Pulmonary function tests may show obstruction, but a restrictive pattern evolves with advanced disease.
- ABG studies may show respiratory alkalosis or hypoxaemia.
- Measurement of chloride concentrations in sweat is useful in cystic fibrosis. Two sweat chloride levels >60 mmol/L are diagnostic of cystic fibrosis.
- Immunological survey is important if primary hypogammaglobulinaemia is suspected.
- Assessment of ciliary function may be done in a number of ways:
  - Assessment of the time taken for a small pellet of saccharin placed in the anterior chamber of the nose to reach the pharynx, where patient can taste it. Normally, it is less than 20 minutes. A prolongation of this time to more than 60 minutes is seen in patients with ciliary dysfunction.
  - Measurement of ciliary beat frequency using biopsies taken from the nose.
  - Electron microscopic study of the ciliary ultrastructure.
  - Study of the sperms.

COMPLICATIONS

- Complications of bronchiectasis are listed in Box 2.73.

MANAGEMENT

GOALS OF TREATMENT

- Treatment of the underlying problems.
- Drainage procedures to improve clearance of tracheobronchial secretions.
- Antibiotics for infections.
- Reversal of airflow obstruction.
- Surgery.

DRAINAGE PROCEDURES

- Nebulisation with 7% hypertonic saline in conjunction with chest physiotherapy.
- Postural drainage consists of adopting a position in which the lobe to be drained is uppermost. Postural drainage should be performed for a minimum of 5–10 minutes twice a day.
- Gentle percussion of the chest wall with cupped hands aids dislodgement of sputum.
- Bronchoscopic removal of inspissated secretions is rarely required.

ANTIBIOTIC THERAPY

Antibiotics for Eradication of Bacteria

- *Pseudomonas* and MRSA should be eradicated on first identification with a course of antibiotics.

BOX 2.73 Complications of Bronchiectasis

• Haemoptysis	• Septicaemia	• Aspergilloma
• Pneumonia	• Osteomyelitis	• Cor pulmonale
• Lung abscess	• Amyloidosis	• Respiratory failure
• Empyema	• Brain abscess	• Hypoproteinaemia

- For *Pseudomonas*, oral ciprofloxacin 750 mg twice daily or intravenous combination therapy with ceftazidime and an aminoglycoside for 2 weeks followed by nebulised colistin/tobramycin/gentamicin for 3 months is given.
- For eradication of other pathogenic bacteria in stable patients, antibiotics are given for 5–10 days.

Suppressive Antibiotics

- The goal is to reduce bacterial burden for patients in whom eradication of the organism is not successful so as to reduce frequency of exacerbations.
- Inhaled antibiotics are safe and effective in reducing sputum bacterial load of *Pseudomonas*. Tobramycin, gentamicin and colistin are antibiotics that are commonly used for nebulisation.

Antibiotics for Acute Exacerbation

- Choice of the antibiotic should primarily be based on the results of culture and sensitivity.
- When no specific pathogen is identified and the patient is not seriously ill, an oral agent like amoxicillin, ampicillin, tetracycline, cotrimoxazole, one of the fluoroquinolones (if tuberculosis has been excluded) or a fixed combination of amoxicillin and clavulanic acid should be used. More seriously ill patients with pneumonitis should be given parenteral antibiotics including antipseudomonal coverage.
- Duration of therapy is variable. A 10- to 14-day course is usually sufficient.

INHIBITION OF INFLAMMATION

- Inhaled corticosteroids:
  - Have possible benefit in patients with bronchiectasis.
- Macrolides:
  - Have immunomodulatory action.
  - Azithromycin 500 mg thrice a week has been shown to reduce exacerbations particularly in those with three or more exacerbations in a year. However, infection with NTM should be excluded before initiating macrolides. Also there is a concern for development of resistant bacteria. Azithromycin may prolong QT interval and may cause hearing impairment.

REVERSAL OF AIRFLOW OBSTRUCTION

- Bronchodilators to improve obstruction and aid clearance of secretions are particularly useful when some element of reversible airway obstruction is present.
- Inhaled corticosteroids may also be of some use.

PULMONARY REHABILITATION

- May benefit patients with exertional dyspnoea.

SURGICAL TREATMENT

- The procedure involved is resection of areas of bronchiectatic lung. Indications of surgery in bronchiectasis are the following:
  - Children or young adults with localised lesions, who do not respond to medical treatment.
  - Recurrent haemoptysis.
  - Recurrent localised pneumonias.
- Lung transplantation in patients with extensive disease and respiratory failure.

OTHER MEASURES

- Cigarette smoking should be interdicted.
- A programme of graded exercise, routine deep breathing and maintenance of good nutrition forms essential parts of general management.
- Expectorants and mucolytic agents like carbocysteine and *N*-acetylcysteine may be of some value in reducing excerbations.
- Episodes of sinusitis should be treated promptly.
- Complicated ABPA should be treated with prednisolone and itraconazole.
- Primary hypogammaglobulinaemia should be treated with human immune globulin.
- Complicated cases may require nasal oxygen on a chronic basis to maintain adequate oxygenation.
- Aerosolised recombinant DNase has been tried with some success in cystic fibrosis–related bronchiectasis. It reduces the viscosity of sputum by breaking down DNA released from neutrophils.

PREVENTION OF BRONCHIECTASIS

- Adequate treatment and prophylaxis of childhood whooping cough, measles and primary tuberculosis.
- Early recognition and removal of bronchial obstruction.
- Genetic counselling in cystic fibrosis.

Q. What is pseudobronchiectasis?

- A 'true' bronchiectasis is not reversible, whereas 'pseudobronchiectasis' is reversible.
- The bronchographic abnormalities displayed by atelectasis and tracheobronchitis with ulcerations of the bronchial mucosa simulate cylindrical bronchiectasis. But re-expansion of the collapsed lung in atelectasis and regeneration of the mucosa in tracheobronchitis result in reversibility of the bronchographic appearance. This is known as pseudobronchiectasis.

Q. What is postobstructive bronchiectasis?

- Postobstructive bronchiectasis is bronchiectasis developing distal to a bronchial obstruction.
- Obstruction of a bronchus results in collapse of the lung and accumulation of secretions distal to obstruction. Secondary bacterial infection supervenes and this results in permanent damage to the distal bronchi resulting in bronchiectasis.
- Since bronchial obstruction is usually confined to one part of bronchial system, postobstructive bronchiectasis is of the localised variety.
- Postobstructive bronchiectasis results from obstructions due to endobronchial tumours and foreign bodies, enlarged hilar lymph nodes or tumour masses and bronchostenosis resulting from endobronchial tuberculosis.

Q. What is bronchiectasis sicca (dry bronchiectasis)?

- This is a condition where bronchiectasis presents with repeated episodes of haemoptysis without sputum production.
- This usually occurs in upper lobe bronchiectasis of the post-tuberculous variety.

Q. What is atelectasis? Discuss it briefly.

- The term 'atelectasis' describes incomplete expansion or complete collapse of part of the lung parenchyma. This part of lung does not contribute to ventilation and perfusion.

CLASSIFICATION

- Obstructive atelectasis (also known as resorptive atelectasis):
  - Most common type.
  - Results from absorption of gas from the alveoli when communication between the alveoli and major airways is obstructed.
  - Intrabronchial obstruction can be exogenous (as in foreign body aspiration, or recurrent aspiration of either gastric or oral contents due to a swallowing disorder) or endogenous (as with tumours, mucus plugging or tracheomalacia or bronchomalacia).
- Nonobstructive atelectasis:
  - Compression atelectasis:
    - Caused by compression of the lung.
    - Results from any space-occupying lesion of the thorax (e.g. tumours, cysts, enlarged lymph nodes, cardiomegaly), chest wall defects (e.g. scoliosis), neuromuscular diseases and emphysematous bulla compressing on adjacent lung.
  - Relaxation or passive atelectasis:
    - Contact between parietal and visceral pleurae is lost resulting in passive loss of lung volume. Examples include pleural effusion and pneumothorax.
    - Generally, atelectasis is due to combined effects of compression and relaxation.
  - Fibrotic or cicatrisation atelectasis:
    - Reduction in volume as a result of parenchymal scarring.
- Atelectasis due to surfactant deficiency or dysfunction (adhesive atelectasis):
  - Causes increased alveolar surface tension as well as failure to maintain small airway patency.
  - Results from ARDS (particularly in preterm neonates and meconium aspiration) and pneumonia in elderly.
- Plate-like atelectasis:
  - Occurs in regions of the lung which are hypoventilated or close to linear scars.
- Rounded atelectasis (folded lung, Blesovsky's syndrome):
  - Associated with pleural disease, particularly following asbestos exposure. Others include hydrothorax associated with cirrhosis of liver, sequela of infection, congestive heart failure, uraemia, pulmonary infarct and interstitial lung disease.
  - Round or pseudomass shape with volume loss, subpleural location and presence of converging bronchovascular markings or 'comet tail' sign.

CLINICAL FEATURES

- Depend on the underlying cause, the degree of volume loss within the lung and how quickly the volume loss develops.
- A slowly developing atelectasis of a lobe may produce no symptoms.
- A large atelectatic area of lung may produce features like tachypnoea, tachycardia and cyanosis.
- Chronic atelectasis of any aetiology can become a nidus of chronic purulent infection with bronchial wall damage leading to bronchiectasis.
- Examination may show reduced chest movement during breathing on the involved side, deviation of trachea and apex beat towards affected side, dullness over the involved area and diminished or absent breath sounds.

INVESTIGATIONS

- Chest radiograph and CT chest.
  - Opacification of collapsed lobe/segment.
  - Displacement of fissure.
  - Ipsilateral loss of volume with shift of mediastinum and trachea, and elevation of diaphragm and crowding of ribs.
  - Compensatory hyperinflation (visible as hyperlucency) of the remaining lobes.
- Arterial blood gas may show hypoxaemia. Hypocapnia may occur due to tachypnoea.
- Bronchoscopy to look for any obstruction. It also helps in removing mucous plug.

Q. Discuss middle lobe bronchiectasis (middle lobe syndrome or Brock's syndrome).

- Classically, the term middle lobe syndrome is applied to recurrent or chronic atelectasis of the right middle lobe without any endobronchial lesion. However, at present, atelectasis due to endobronchial lesion is also included under this term.
- Deep fissure of middle lobe (also of lingula) is a barrier for collateral ventilation.
- The most common cause is obstruction of the middle lobe bronchus produced by tuberculous lymph nodes. This is a type of postobstructive bronchiectasis. Other causes of obstruction include tumours (both benign and malignant), histoplasmosis, sarcoidosis and aspirated foreign bodies.
- The most common symptoms are chronic or recurrent cough, dyspnoea, chest pain, and fever and chills related to obstructive pneumonia. These symptoms are often intermittent and recurrent.
- Physical examination is often normal. Patients with partial obstruction may have a localised wheeze on forced expiration.

- Due to repeated episodes of atelectasis, bronchiectasis and fibrosis of right middle lobe develops.
- The posteroanterior chest radiograph may be normal or may show obscuring of the right cardiac border (silhouette sign) because the medial segment of middle lobe is contiguous with the right atrium. Lateral radiograph may show a triangle of increased density between the minor fissure and the lower half of the major fissure. This is due to volume loss.
- High-resolution CT, bronchoscopy and endobronchial ultrasound are helpful in diagnosis.

Q. Enumerate the clinical features, diagnosis and treatment of ciliary dysfunction syndromes (ciliary dyskinesia syndromes).

Q. Describe primary ciliary dyskinesia (PCD).

Q. What are Kartagener's syndrome and Young's syndrome?

- Ciliary dysfunction syndromes or primary ciliary dyskinesia are a group of genetically determined disorders characterised by dysfunction of cilia of the respiratory tract epithelium, sperms and other cells, causing impairment of mucociliary clearance, left–right body asymmetry and impaired sperm motility. Majority are autosomal recessive disorders. Acquired ciliary defects may occur due to infection and inflammation.
- Kartagener's syndrome is one of the ciliary dysfunction syndromes. It is characterised by recurrent sinusitis, bronchiectasis, dextrocardia or situs inversus and infertility.
- Young's syndrome is characterised by recurrent sinopulmonary infections and obstructive azoospermia.

CLINICAL FEATURES OF PRIMARY CILIARY DYSKINESIA

- Clinical features of primary ciliary dyskinesia are given in Table 2.49.

TABLE 2.49 Clinical Features of Primary Ciliary Dyskinesia

Organ	Clinical Manifestations
• Lung	Respiratory distress in neonates Recurrent infections Bronchiectasis
• Sinus	Chronic sinusitis
• Ear	Otitis media Hearing loss Cholesteatoma
• Genitourinary tract	Male infertility Reduced fertility in females; ectopic pregnancy
• Organ laterality	Situs inversus totalis Polysplenia or asplenia Complex congenital heart disease
• Central nervous system	Vascular anomalies Hydrocephalus (rare)

DIAGNOSIS

- Screening tests:
  - Low exhaled nasal nitric oxide (less than 100 nL/min).
  - Saccharin test—a microtablet of saccharin is placed on the inferior turbinate and the time taken for the subject to taste it is recorded. An abnormal test is any length of time greater than 60 minutes.
- Measurement of nasal nitric oxide (nNO) is an accurate and immediate screening tool for patients >5 years of age. nNo is elevated in cilicary dyskinesia. It is not elevated in cystic fibrosis.
- Electron microscopic analysis of respiratory cilia in samples of nasal or airway mucosa reveals defects in the outer or inner dynein arms of the cilia in nearly 70% of cases.
- Another test is immunofluorescent antibody staining of ciliary proteins.

TREATMENT

- No specific treatment.
- General treatment of bronchiectasis.
- Cough suppressants should be avoided because cough is the only intact mechanism for mucociliary clearance in these patients.

Q. Define lung abscess. Discuss the aetiology, clinical features, investigations, complications and management of lung abscess. (PA 26.2)

DEFINITION

- Lung abscess is defined as a circumscribed necrotic area of lung parenchyma containing purulent material.

AETIOLOGY

- Aspiration of nasopharyngeal or oropharyngeal contents (aspiration abscess) is the most common cause.
  - Depression of cough reflex favours aspiration. This occurs during sleep, anaesthesia, alcohol intoxication, epilepsy and coma.
  - Aspiration also occurs in achalasia cardia, carcinoma of oesophagus, hiatus hernia, gastro-oesophageal reflux disease and large-volume tube feed.
  - Pre-existing sources of infection for aspiration include sinusitis, dental sepsis, gingivitis, periodontal infection, etc.
  - Dominant organisms in aspiration abscess include anaerobic organisms (e.g. *Peptostreptococcus, Prevotella, Bacteroides, Fusobacterium*), streptococci and *H. influenzae*.
  - Because of relatively more vertical course of right main bronchus, aspiration abscesses are more common in the right lung.
  - Aspiration abscess cavities are located in those bronchopulmonary segments that are most dependent at the time of aspiration. Aspiration in supine position results in abscess in posterior segment of the upper lobes or superior segments of

the lower lobes. Aspiration in the upright position results in abscess in the basilar segments.

- Pulmonary tuberculosis is an important cause of lung abscess.
- Necrotising pneumonias, especially due to *K. pneumoniae*, *S. aureus* and streptococci may produce abscess.
- Bronchial obstruction by foreign body, tumour or bronchostenosis may lead to abscess formation distally.
- Haematogenous spread of the organisms to the lung results from bacteraemia, right-sided endocarditis and septic thrombophlebitis. This often leads to multiple lung abscesses.
- Secondary infection of cavitary malignancy or pulmonary infarct.
- Rupture of amoebic liver abscess into lung.
- Rare causes include pulmonary fungal infections, infected cysts (including hydatid cyst) and vasculitis.

CLINICAL FEATURES

HISTORY

- Lung abscess can have two modes of presentations: acute (<1 month of symptoms) and chronic (>1 month of symptoms).
    - In acute presentation, the disease starts acutely with high-grade fever, chills and rigors, pleuritic chest pain and dry cough. After a few days, when the abscess cavity ruptures into a patent bronchus, the patient suddenly starts expectorating large quantities of sputum. The sputum is large in volume, purulent, foul-smelling and often blood-tinged. The expectoration varies with posture.
    - Lung abscess due to aspiration is often chronic in presentation with insidious onset of low-grade fever, cough, malaise, weight loss, anorexia and a deep-seated chest discomfort. Sputum has putrid smell in many cases.

PHYSICAL FINDINGS

- General examination reveals anaemia, fever, finger clubbing, halitosis and oronasal sepsis.
- Respiratory system examination may be normal in the early stages. Later, frank signs of consolidation like dullness on percussion, increased vocal fremitus and vocal resonance, bronchial breathing, crepitations and pleural rub appear. Once the abscess cavity opens into a bronchus, signs of cavitation like cavernous or amphoric bronchial breathing and coarse posttussive crepitations appear.

INVESTIGATIONS

- Anaemia, leucocytosis and raised ESR.
- Sputum studies should include Gram stain, Ziehl–Neelsen staining for acid-fast bacilli, aerobic and anaerobic cultures and sensitivity and cytological examination for malignant cells.
- Chest radiograph often shows radiolucency in an opaque area of consolidation. The wall or the border of the cavity completely surrounds the lucent area and an air–fluid level may be seen. Acute lung abscess is usually circumscribed with not so well-defined surrounding to lung parenchyma. Chronic lung abscess is usually irregular star-like shape with well-defined surrounding to lung parenchyma.
- Bronchoscopy is indicated to exclude malignancy, obtain specimens for studies and for removal of secretions.
- CT scan of thorax can detect lung abscess with certainty.

DIFFERENTIAL DIAGNOSIS

- Box 2.74 gives differential diagnosis of lung abscess.

COMPLICATIONS

- Complications of lung abscess are listed in Box 2.75.

TREATMENT

- Postural drainage and chest physiotherapy.
- Antibiotic therapy should be based on sensitivity reports. However, certain broad guidelines are:
    - Antibiotic therapy of aspiration abscess is similar to that of aspiration pneumonia.
    - Majority of the patients with lung abscess will respond to oral treatment with amoxicillin–clavulanic acid 625 mg three times daily, or cotrimoxazole 960 mg twice daily or clindamycin 300 mg three times a day.
    - In anaerobic bacterial infection (e.g. those with foul-smelling sputum), oral metronidazole 400 mg 8 hourly should be added. It should never be used as a single agent due to polymicrobial flora.
    - Aminoglycosides are not recommended since they poorly pass through fibrous pyogenic membrane of chronic abscess.
    - Seriously ill patients will require parenteral antibiotic therapy in the form of imipenem, meropenem, ampicillin–sulbactam or clindamycin (600 mg thrice a day) plus metronidazole.
    - Duration of antibiotic therapy is variable. Some patients may require prolonged treatment for 4–6 weeks.
- In large abscess, percutaneous aspiration and placement of pigtail catheters under ultrasound or CT-guidance

BOX 2.74 Differential Diagnosis of Lung Abscess

- Cavitating bronchial carcinoma
- Tuberculous cavity
- Localised pleural empyema
- Infected emphysematous bullae
- Cavitary pneumoconiosis
- Hiatus hernia
- Pulmonary haematoma
- Hydatid cyst of lung
- Cavitary infarcts of lung
- Polyangiitis with granulomatosis (Wegener's granulomatosis)

BOX 2.75 Complications of Lung Abscess

- Haemoptysis
- Pleural effusion, empyema
- Pneumothorax, pyopneumothorax and bronchopleural fistula
- Metastatic cerebral abscess
- Amyloidosis
- Aspergilloma
- Residual fibrosis and bronchiectasis

play an important role. The usage of intracavitary fibrinolytic agents (streptokinase, urokinase) is not recommended due to possibility of development of bronchopulmonary or bronchopleural fistula.
- Resectional surgery is indicated only in selected situations:
  - Massive haemoptysis.
  - Rupture of abscess in pleural cavity resulting in pyopneumothorax/empyema.
  - Localised malignancy.
  - Associated symptomatic bronchiectasis.
  - Persistent abscess cavity.
  - Abscess greater than 6 cm in size with poor response to antibiotics.
  - Minimal invasive surgical procedure (video-assisted thoracoscopy) is the method of choice for peripherally localised lung abscess.

Q. Discuss briefly about diffuse alveolar haemorrhage (DAH).

- DAH presents with features of acute- or subacute-onset cough, haemoptysis, diffuse radiographic pulmonary infiltrates, anaemia and hypoxaemic respiratory distress.
- Should be differentiated from localised pulmonary haemorrhage (e.g. due to chronic bronchitis, bronchiectasis, tumour or localised infection).

CAUSES OF DAH

- Can be divided into three groups: those associated with inflammation of the small pulmonary capillaries (capillaritis), those associated with alveolar damage and those without capillaritis or alveolar damage (Table 2.50).

CLINICAL FEATURES

- Haemoptysis may develop suddenly or over a period of days to weeks. It may be absent in nearly 30% of cases.
- Dyspnoea.
- Some patients present with severe acute respiratory distress requiring mechanical ventilation.

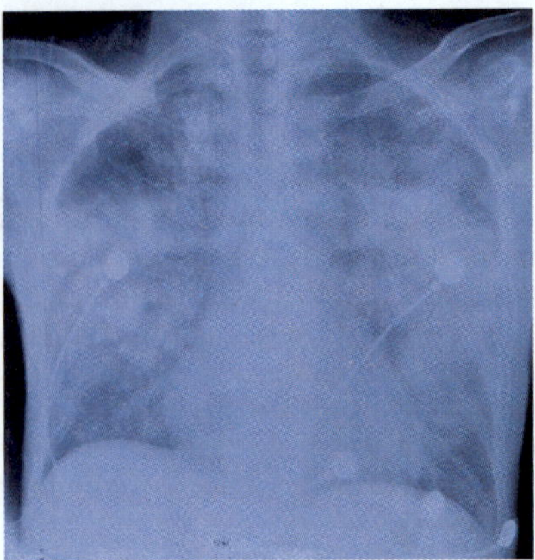

Fig. 2.13 Chest radiograph showing diffuse alveolar haemorrhage.

- Unexplained anaemia.
- Clinical features of associated diseases may be present.

DIAGNOSIS

- Hypoxaemia due to impairment of oxygen transfer.
- Elevated diffusion capacity of the lung for carbon monoxide (DL_{CO}).
- Chest radiography shows diffuse alveolar opacities (Fig. 2.13). Recurrent episodes of haemorrhage may produce reticular interstitial opacities due to pulmonary fibrosis.
- CT chest shows bilateral ground glass opacities or consolidation.
- Bronchoalveolar lavage reveals several haemosiderin-laden macrophages which usually appear 24–48 hours after the DAH has started.
- Various blood tests to establish aetiology (e.g. antineutrophil cytoplasmic antibodies, antinuclear antibodies, antiglomerular basement membrane antibodies, antiphospholipid antibodies). Other relevant blood tests include platelet count, prothrombin time and partial thromboplastin time.
- Urine may show abnormalities where the disease also involves kidneys (e.g. Goodpasture's syndrome, vasculitides).
- In selected cases, transbronchial, video-thoracoscopic or open lung biopsy for histopathology.

TABLE 2.50 Causes of Diffuse Alveolar Haemorrhage

With Pulmonary Capillaritis	Without Pulmonary Capillaritis and Alveolar Damage	Diffuse Alveolar Damage
• Wegener granulomatosis • Microscopic polyangiitis • Eosinophilic granulomatosis with polyangiitis • Systemic lupus erythematosus[a] • Antiphospholipid syndrome • Mixed cryoglobulinaemia • Behcet's syndrome • Henoch–Schönlein purpura • Acute lung transplant rejection • Goodpasture's syndrome[a] • Rheumatoid arthritis • Drugs (e.g. carbimazole, retinoic acid)	• Idiopathic pulmonary haemosiderosis • Goodpasture's syndrome[a] • Systemic lupus erythematosus[a] • Mitral stenosis • Coagulopathy • Haemangiomatosis • Infections (e.g. influenza, malaria, dengue, leptospirosis) • Thrombocytopenia (idiopathic thrombocytopenic purpura, thrombotic thrombocytopenic purpura, haemolytic uraemic syndrome) • Acute promyelocytic leukaemia	• Any infection causing ARDS • Polymyositis • Lymphangioleiomyo-matosis • Tuberous sclerosis • Drugs (e.g. amiodarone, cocaine, nitrofurantoin, penicllamine) • Pulmonary infarction • Any cause of ARDS

[a]Can cause DAH due to capillaritis and also without it.

TABLE 2.51 Classification of Primary Bronchial Tumours

Benign Tumours (5%)	Malignant Tumours (95%)

• Pulmonary hamartoma
• Others (chondroma, lipoma)
	• Non-small-cell carcinoma (85%)
	  • Squamous or epidermoid carcinoma
	  • Large-cell carcinoma
	  • Adenocarcinoma
	• Neuroendocrine tumours (15%)
	  • Small-cell carcinoma (oat cell carcinoma)
	  • Large-cell neuroendocrine carcinoma
	  • Typical carcinoid
	  • Atypical carcinoid
	• Others
	  • Mucoepidermoid carcinoma
	  • Adenoid cystic carcinoma
	  • Pulmonary blastoma

Note: Even though carcinoids are sometimes classified as benign tumours, some carcinoids behave like low-grade malignant tumours.

TREATMENT

- Establish the underlying diagnosis and treat it.
- Provide respiratory support.
- Prevent progression of microcirculation damage, typically with corticosteroids and immunosuppressive agents.

Q. Classify primary bronchial tumours.

PRIMARY BRONCHIAL TUMOURS

- Table 2.51 shows classification of primary bronchial tumours.

Q. Discuss the aetiopathogenesis, histopathological features, clinical features, investigations and management of bronchial carcinoma (bronchogenic carcinoma).

Q. What are the paraneoplastic syndromes associated with bronchogenic carcinoma?

- Bronchial carcinoma is the most common primary malignant tumour of the lung arising from bronchial epithelium or mucous glands.

INCIDENCE

- More common in males than in females.
- Most frequent in 50- to 75-year age group.
- More in urban than in rural dwellers.
- More in smokers than in nonsmokers.

AETIOLOGY (Box 2.76)

- Cigarette smoking is the most important cause.
  - The risk is directly proportional to the amount smoked and the tar content of the cigarettes.
  - Cigarette pack-years is calculated by multiplying the number of packs of cigarettes (each containing 20 cigarettes) smoked per day by the number of years the person has smoked.
- Smokers are 40–70 times more prone than nonsmokers. Bidi smoking may be more dangerous than cigarette smoking in predisposing to lung cancer. Cigar smoking and pipe smoking are almost as likely to cause lung cancer as cigarette smoking.
- With comparable amount of smoking, women have higher chances of developing lung cancer than men.
- The chance of developing lung cancer decreases with cessation of smoking but may never return to the nonsmoker level.
- Second-hand smoke exposure (passive smoking) is also a risk factor.
- Adenocarcinoma is not related to smoking in many cases. In nonsmokers with adenocarcinoma, possibility of other primary sites should be considered.

BOX 2.76 Aetiological Factors in Bronchogenic Carcinoma

- Cigarette smoking
- Atmospheric pollution
- Occupational exposure (mining of arsenic, chromium, uranium and nickel and exposure to vinyl chloride and asbestos)
- Radiation exposure (radon—a gaseous radioactive decay product of uranium, thoracic radiation therapy)
- Household coal combustion
- Preexisting nonmalignant lung diseases (e.g. COPD, idiopathic pulmonary fibrosis, tuberculosis)
- Others: Familial, HIV infection, dietary supplementation of beta-carotene *in smokers*

GENETIC MUTATIONS FOUND IN BRONCHOGENIC CARCINOMA

- Mutation in epidermal growth factor receptor (EGFR) tyrosine kinase domain in adenocarcinoma.
- Anaplastic lymphoma kinase (ALK) mutations resulting in its fusion with echinoderm microtubule-associated protein-like 4. The expression of PD-1 (programmed cell death protein 1) and PD-L1 (programmed cell death 1 ligand 1) on the surface of tumour cells in NSCLC is a predictive biomarker and is used to guide treatment decisions with anti-PD-1 or anti-PD-L1 antibodies.

PATHOLOGY

- To facilitate treatment and prognostic decisions, lung cancer is categorised as neuroendocrine tumours (mainly small-cell lung carcinoma—SCLC; 15% of total bronchogenic cancers) or non-small-cell lung carcinoma (NSCLC; 85% of total bronchogenic cancers). On the basis of microscopic examination, four major types can be recognised with the first three under the category of non-small-cell carcinomas (see classification given in Table 2.51).

1. Squamous (epidermoid) carcinoma.
2. Adenocarcinoma.
3. Large-cell carcinoma. A subtype is large cell neuroendocrine carcinoma which behaves like SCLC.

4. Small-cell (oat cell) carcinoma.
   Note: A classification given in 2021 has subclassified lung adenocarcinoma into several types. The term bronchioloalveolar carcinoma was eliminated in 2015 classification.

- Squamous cell and small-cell carcinomas are generally centrally placed tumours while large-cell and adenocarcinoma are generally peripherally placed.
- Neuroendocrine tumours of the lung arise from Kulchitsky cells of the bronchial mucosa and comprise typical carcinoid, atypical carcinoid, small-cell lung cancer and large-cell neuroendocrine carcinoma.
- Treatment decisions are based on whether histologically the tumour is SCLC or one of the NSCLC varieties.

CLINICAL FEATURES

- Some of the adenocarcinomas may present with profuse mucoid sputum (bronchorrhoea).
- Clinical manifestations of bronchial carcinoma can be considered under the following headings.

MANIFESTATIONS DUE TO A CENTRAL OR ENDOBRONCHIAL GROWTH

- Cough with haemoptysis
- Wheeze and stridor
- Dyspnoea
- Pneumonitis manifesting as fever and productive cough

MANIFESTATIONS DUE TO A PERIPHERAL GROWTH

- Chest pain from pleural or chest wall involvement
- Cough and dyspnoea
- Symptoms of lung abscess from tumour cavitation

MANIFESTATIONS OF REGIONAL SPREAD IN THE THORAX

- The regional spread of tumour in the thorax may occur by direct extension or by metastasis to regional lymph nodes.
  - Haematogenous, lymphatic or direct spread to pleura resulting in malignant pleural effusion
  - Superior vena caval (SVC) obstruction resulting in SVC syndrome
  - Tracheal obstruction leading to stridor and dyspnoea
  - Oesophageal obstruction leading to dysphagia
  - Recurrent laryngeal nerve involvement with resultant hoarseness of voice and 'bovine' cough
  - Phrenic nerve involvement resulting in dyspnoea and diaphragmatic paralysis
  - Sympathetic chain involvement leading to Horner's syndrome
  - Pancoast's syndrome from superior sulcus tumour (refer page 212)
  - Direct extension to chest wall resulting in rib pain, pathological fractures and intercostal neuralgia
  - Lymphangitic spread (lymphangitis carcinomatosis) resulting in dyspnoea and hypoxaemia
  - Pericardial and cardiac involvement with resultant tamponade, arrhythmias or cardiac failure

MANIFESTATIONS OF EXTRATHORACIC METASTASIS

- Brain metastases with headache, vomiting, neurological deficits, seizures and confusion
- Bone metastases with pain, pathological fractures or raised alkaline phosphatase
- Bone marrow involvement with cytopenias or leucoerythroblastosis
- Liver metastases resulting in biochemical liver dysfunctions, anorexia, biliary obstruction and pain
- Lymph node metastases in the supraclavicular region (scalene node)
- Epidural and bone metastases resulting in spinal cord compression syndromes

PARANEOPLASTIC SYNDROMES

- Paraneoplastic syndromes are not due to local presence of cancer cells but usually due to humoral factors (hormones or cytokines) secreted by tumour cells or by an immune response against the tumour. They are often relieved by successful treatment of the primary tumour. Sometimes, these syndromes may be present before a tumour is diagnosed.
- These are common with neuroendocrine tumours, particularly small-cell carcinoma (Table 2.52).

Lambert–Eaton Syndrome

- An immune-mediated disorder of neuromuscular junction.
- Associated with presynaptic voltage-gated calcium channel (VGCC) antibodies.

TABLE 2.52 Paraneoplastic Syndrome Associated With Bronchogenic Carcinoma

• **Systemic**	Anorexia, cachexia, weight loss, fever
• **Endocrine**	Syndrome of inappropriate secretion of antidiuretic hormone resulting in hyponatraemia (small-cell carcinoma), ectopic ACTH secretion resulting in hypokalaemia rather than full-blown Cushing's syndrome (small-cell carcinoma), ectopic production of parathyroid hormone or parathyroid hormone-related peptide resulting in hypercalcaemia and hypophosphataemia (usually squamous cell carcinoma or adenocarcinoma)
• **Skeletal**	Digital clubbing (usually NSCLC), hypertrophic pulmonary osteoarthropathy (usually adenocarcinoma)
• **Neuromyopathic**	Lambert–Eaton syndrome, limbic encephalitis and retinal blindness (small-cell carcinoma); peripheral neuropathy, subacute cerebellar degeneration, cortical degeneration and polymyositis (all types of lung cancers)
• **Haematological**	Migratory venous thrombophlebitis (Trousseau's syndrome), marantic endocarditis, disseminated intravascular coagulation (DIC), anaemia, granulocytosis, leucoerythroblastosis, eosinophilia, thrombocytosis
• **Cutaneous**	Dermatomyositis, acanthosis nigricans
• **Renal**	Nephrotic syndrome, glomerulonephritis

- Majority of cases (50%–60%) associated with small-cell lung cancer.
- Clinical triad typically consists of proximal muscle weakness (starting from lower limb and extending to upper limb and later involvement of bulbar and ocular muscles), autonomic features (dry mouth, erectile dysfunction, constipation, orthostatic hypotension) and areflexia. A characteristic phenomenon present in 40% of cases is postexercise facilitation, a short-term return of tendon reflexes and muscle strength to normal after muscle contraction.
- Treatment includes use of 3,4-diaminopyridine, which increases duration of presynaptic action potential by blocking potassium efflux, thereby prolonging the activation of VGCC and increasing calcium entry into nerve terminals.

INVESTIGATIONS

- Liver function tests (including alkaline phosphatase and gamma-glutamyl transpeptidase) to look for liver or bone metastasis; hypercalcaemia (may be due to paraneoplastic manifestation or bone metastasis).
- Plain radiograph of the chest may reveal several findings (Box 2.77).
- Computed tomography of chest and abdomen is an important investigation for diagnosis and staging of carcinoma. It is useful in several ways:
  - Evaluation of tumour size.
  - Evaluation of mediastinal or hilar lymph node involvement (however, nodal involvement, if seen on CT, should be confirmed by histopathology if the finding will influence therapeutic decisions).
  - To detect pleural extension.
  - To detect occult abdominal disease (e.g. liver and adrenals).
  - For CT-guided biopsy of suspected lesions.
  - To assess the response to treatment.
- Cytological examination of the following specimens may be positive for malignant cells:
  - Sputum.
  - Bronchial washings and brushings.
  - Percutaneous needle aspiration biopsy from a peripheral tumour.

BOX 2.77 Chest Radiographic Findings of Bronchogenic Carcinoma

- Peripheral pulmonary opacity with or without cavitation (squamous cell carcinoma may cavitate)
- Unilateral enlargement at hilum resulting from a central tumour or hilar glandular enlargement or a peripheral tumour in the apical segment of the lower lobe
- Adenocarcinomas can present as a single mass, as a diffuse, multinodular lesion or as fluffy infiltrate
- Pleural effusion
- Collapse of the whole lung, lobe or segment
- Mediastinal widening due to mediastinal invasion
- Elevation of haemidiaphragm due to pulmonary collapse or phrenic nerve paralysis
- Rib destruction from direct extension of tumour or blood-borne metastasis

  - Fine needle aspiration of lymph node, skin or liver in patients with metastasis.
- Bronchoscopy:
  - Bronchoscopy permits visualisation and biopsy of an intrabronchial tumour.
  - Collection of bronchial washings from the suspicious segments.
- Other investigations useful in diagnosis and staging of disease in appropriate patients are:
  - Scalene node biopsy.
  - Mediastinoscopy.
  - Pleural aspiration and biopsy.
- Endoscopic ultrasound-guided fine needle aspiration of mass or lymph node.
- Endobronchial ultrasound-guided transbronchial needle aspiration (EBUS-TBNA) helpful in diagnosis of mediastinal, paratracheal and peribronchial lesions, as well as in lymph node staging for lung cancer.
- Liquid biopsy (testing on a variety of cancer biomarkers, such as circulating tumour DNA, microRNA and circulating tumour cells) in blood may be useful in diagnosis particularly if tissue-biopsy is not feasible.
- Ultrasonographic examination of liver and adrenal glands.
- Bone scans and bone biopsy if metastasis is suspected.
- Brain CT if metastasis is suspected.
- PET scan is often used to detect both intrathoracic and metastatic diseases. Though CT may be used for mediastinal structures, staging is enhanced by PET. Integrated CT/PET scanners are better than CT or PET alone.
- Molecular testing for EGFR mutations and ALK fusions to guide treatment.

STAGING

- Involves extent of tumour (anatomic staging) and assessment of a patient's ability to withstand various treatments (physiological staging).

STAGING OF NON-SMALL CELL CARCINOMA

- The non-small-cell carcinoma is staged into stages I–IV depending on the size and location of primary tumour, involvement of lymph nodes and distant metastasis (TNM International Staging System) (Table 2.53).
- Based on TNM classification, the non-small-cell carcinoma can be divided into various stages (Table 2.54).

STAGING OF SMALL-CELL CARCINOMA

- The small-cell carcinoma is staged into limited-stage and extensive-stage disease based on whether the known tumour can be encompassed within a tolerable radiation therapy port (Table 2.55).

FUNCTIONAL EVALUATION

- Evaluation of performance (Karnofsky Performance Status; Eastern Co-Operative Oncology Group Performance Status) and pulmonary status before discussing the treatment options.
- Pulmonary function tests, specifically FEV_1 and diffusion capacity, helpful in predicting morbidity and mortality in patients undergoing lung resection.

TABLE 2.53 Staging of Non-Small-Cell Carcinoma (TNM Classification)

TNM	Description
T0	No primary tumour
Tis	Carcinoma in situ
T1	Tumour ≤3 cm in diameter; surrounded by lung or pleura
T1mi	Minimally invasive adenocarcinoma
T1a	Superficial spreading tumour of any size but confined to tracheal or bronchial wall
T1a	Tumour ≤1 cm
T1b	Tumour >1 but ≤2 cm
T1c	Tumour >2 but ≤3 cm
T2	Tumour >3 but ≤5 cm or tumour involving: visceral pleura, main bronchus (but not carina), atelectasis or obstructive pneumonitis extending to hilum
T2a	Tumour >3 but ≤4 cm
T2b	Tumour >4 but ≤5 cm
T3	Tumour >5 but ≤7 cm or invading chest wall, phrenic nerve or pericardium; or separate tumour nodule(s) in the same lobe
T4	Tumour >7 cm or tumour invading: mediastinum, diaphragm, heart, great vessels, recurrent laryngeal nerve, carina, trachea, oesophagus, spine; or tumour nodule(s) in a different ipsilateral lobe
Nx	Regional nodes cannot be assessed
N0	No nodal metastasis
N1	Involvement of ipsilateral peribronchial or hilar nodes and intrapulmonary nodes
N2	Involvement of ipsilateral mediastinal or subcarinal nodes
N3	Involvement of contralateral mediastinal, hilar nodes or any supraclavicular nodes
M0	No distant metastasis
M1a	Malignant pleural or pericardial effusion, or pleural or pericardial nodules or separate tumour nodule(s) in a contralateral lobe
M1b	Single extrathoracic metastasis
M1c	Multiple extrathoracic metastases (1 or >1 organ)

M, distant metastasis; N, regional lymph nodes; T, primary tumour.

(*Source*: *J Thorac Cardiovasc Surg* 2018;155:357, Table 1. Copyright 2017, published by Elsevier Inc. on behalf of the American Association for Thoracic Surgery.)

TABLE 2.54 Stages of Non-Small-Cell Carcinoma

Stage	Description
Occult carcinoma	TxN0M0
0	TisN0M0
IA1	T1aN0M0
IA2	T1bN0M0
IA3	T1cN0M0
IB	T2aN0M0
IIA	T2bN0M0
IIB	T1aN1M0, T1bN1M0, T1cN1M0, T2aN1M0, T2bN1M0, T3N0M0
IIIA	T1aN2M0, T1bN2M0, T1cN2M0, T2aN2M0, T2bN2M0, T3N1M0, T4N0M0, T4N1M0
IIIB	T1aN3M0, T1bN3M0, T1cN3M0, T2aN3M0, T2bN3M0, T3N2M0, T4N2M0
IIIC	T3N3M0, T4N3M0
IVA	T1–T4N0–N3M1a, T1–T4N0–N3M1b
IVB	T1–T4N0–N3M1c

TABLE 2.55 Staging of Small-Cell Carcinoma of Lung

Stage	Description
• Limited stage	Disease confined to one hemithorax and regional lymph nodes (including mediastinal, contralateral hilar and ipsilateral and contralateral supraclavicular) which can be encompassed within a tolerable radiation port
• Extensive stage	Disease with metastasis beyond ipsilateral hemithorax (including malignant pericardial or pleural effusion)

TREATMENT

NON-SMALL-CELL CARCINOMA

- Surgical resection of the tumour is possible but only in a few selected cases (stages IA, IB, IIA, IIB and selected IIIA) (Flowchart 2.10).
    - Video-assisted thoracoscopic surgery (VATS) is increasingly used as an alternative to open thoracotomy.
    - Image-guided percutaneous lung ablation is an alternative to surgical removal in patients with early-stage non-small-cell lung carcinoma. Available

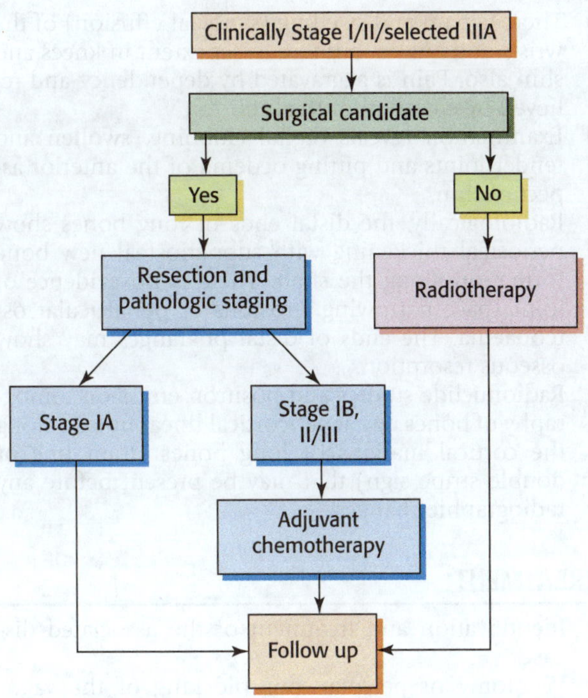

Flowchart 2.10 Management of Early NSCLC.

ablative modalities include radiofrequency ablation, microwave ablation and cryoablation.

- Postoperative chemotherapy (adjuvant therapy) is often given to most patients in stages IIA, IIB, IIIA and selected IB (Flowchart 2.10).
- Preoperative chemotherapy (neoadjuvant chemotherapy) improves survival in stage IIIA patients.
- Drugs commonly used are cisplatin/carboplatin and paclitaxel. Bevacizumab (an antiangiogenesis drug) should not be used in squamous cell carcinoma because of risk of severe bleeding. It can be added in nonsquamous cell non-small-cell carcinoma.
- Treatment for unresectable non-small-cell carcinoma (stages IIIB, IIIC and IV) involves radiotherapy and chemotherapy. First-line drugs include either cisplatin or carboplatin and one of the taxanes (paclitaxel or docetaxel) or gemcitabine or a vinca alkaloid.
- Targeted therapies, specifically the epidermal growth factor receptor (EGFR) tyrosine kinase inhibitors (afatinib, gefitinib, erlotinib and osimertinib) in patients with EGFR mutations may increase survival. Others include ALK tyrosine kinase inhibitors like crizotinib, alectinib, brigatinib and ensartinib. These are used in stage III and IV disease. Immune checkpoint inhibitors (ICIs) like atezolizumab, nivolumab and durvalumab have been approved as neoadjuvant and adjuvant (postoperative) therapy in select group of patients.
- Radiotherapy is much less effective than surgical therapy. Patients with stage III disease as well as stage I and II disease, who refuse surgery or are not the candidates for pulmonary resection, should be considered for radiation therapy with curative intent. Palliative radiotherapy is indicated in the following situations:
  - SVC obstruction.
  - Recurrent haemoptysis.
  - Painful skeletal metastasis.
  - Tracheal and main bronchial obstruction (neodynamic-YAG [yttrium–aluminium–garnet] laser therapy administered through a flexible bronchoscope can also provide palliation in such patients).
  - Pain caused by chest wall invasion.
  - Pancoast's tumour is usually treated with combined radiotherapy and surgery.

SMALL-CELL CARCINOMA

General Plan of Treatment

- Limited stage with good performance status of patient—combination chemotherapy with radiotherapy.
- Limited stage with poor performance status—modified chemotherapy and/or palliative radiotherapy.
- Extensive stage with good performance status—combination chemotherapy + local radiotherapy.
- Extensive stage with poor performance status—modified chemotherapy and/or palliative radiotherapy.
- If the patient responds, prophylactic radiotherapy is given to brain. High-dose radiotherapy to the whole brain is also given to patients with documented brain metastasis producing significant symptoms.

Chemotherapeutic Regimens

- Commonly used drugs include cisplatin, carboplatin, etoposide, cyclophosphamide, ifosfamide, doxorubicin, vincristine, topotecan, irinotecan and paclitaxel.
- Commonly used combinations include cisplatin or carboplatin plus etoposide (most often used); ifosfamide, carboplatin and etoposide with or without vincristine; cyclophosphamide, doxorubicin and vincristine; cyclophosphamide, doxorubicin and etoposide; or etoposide, cisplatin and paclitaxel.
- Anti-PD-1 or anti-PD-L1 antibodies (atezolizumab or durvalumab) have been shown to improve survivor in extensive disease.

SCREENING

- Annual low-dose CT in high-risk patients (e.g. heavy smokers) reduces lung cancer-related mortality.
- Screening for lung cancer by chest radiograph and/or sputum cytology is not recommended.

PREVENTION

- Avoidance of risk factors.
- Chemoprevention—use of dietary or pharmaceutical interventions to slow or reverse the progression of premalignancy to invasive cancer. At present, it is in experimental stages.
  - Primary chemoprevention is preventing cancer in healthy individuals who are at increased risk.
  - Secondary chemoprevention is blocking the development of cancer in individuals in whom a precancerous lesion has been detected.
  - Tertiary chemoprevention is in patients who had a previous lung cancer in an effort to prevent the development of a second primary tumour.
  - Various agents being studied include inhaled corticosetroids, low-dose aspirin, retinoids, iloprost

TABLE 2.56 Neurological Manifestations of Bronchial Carcinoma

Regional Effects	Remote Effects (Paraneoplastic)
• Horner's syndrome • Recurrent laryngeal nerve paralysis • Phrenic nerve paralysis • Pancoast's syndrome • Intercostal neuralgia **Metastatic effects** • Brain • Spine	• Polyneuropathy • Myelopathy • Cerebellar degeneration • Cortical degeneration • Polymyositis and dermatomyositis • Lambert-Eaton syndrome • Limbic encephalitis • Opsoclonus-myoclonus-ataxia • Encephalomyelitis • Autonomic neuropathy

(a long-acting oral prostaglandin analogue) and cyclooxygenase oxidase (COX) inhibitors (e.g. celecoxib). Two agents, vitamin E and β-carotene, actually increase the risk of lung cancer in heavy smokers.

Q. What are the neurological manifestations of bronchial carcinoma?

- Neurological manifestations of bronchial carcinoma are given in Table 2.56.

Q. Briefly discuss hypertrophic osteoarthropathy (hypertrophic pulmonary osteoarthropathy).

- Also known as Pierre–Marie–Bamberger syndrome, hypertrophic osteoarthropathy is characterised by periosteal new bone formation, clubbing of digits and arthritis.
- Possible mechanisms suggested invoke stimulation of vagal neural arc and circulating vasodilators, hormones and immune complexes (see 'Clubbing' on page 117).

CAUSES

- Any disease producing clubbing can lead to this condition. However, common causes are given in Table 2.57.

CLINICAL FEATURES

- Most commonly involved are the distal parts of the long bones of wrists (radius and ulna) and ankles (tibia and fibula).

TABLE 2.57 Common Causes of Hypertrophic Osteoarthropathy

Primary or hereditary (autosomal dominant)	Secondary
	• Bronchial carcinoma • Chronic suppurative lung diseases (bronchiectasis, lung abscess) • Chronic liver diseases • Metastases to the lung • Pleural mesothelioma • Cyanotic congenital heart diseases • Cystic fibrosis

- There is pain and swelling (synovial effusion) of the wrists and ankles, but to a lesser extent in knees and shin also. Pain is aggravated by dependency and relieved by elevation of the limb.
- Examination reveals digital clubbing, swollen and tender joints and pitting oedema of the anterior aspect of shin.
- Radiologically, the distal ends of long bones show periosteal thickening with subperiosteal new bone formation along the shaft. There is no evidence of joint space narrowing, erosions or periarticular osteopaenia. The ends of distal phalanges may show osseous resorption.
- Radionuclide studies and positron emission tomography of bones reveal pericortical linear uptake along the cortical margins of long bones (tram line or double stripe sign) that may be present before any radiographic changes.

TREATMENT

- Identification and treatment of the associated disease.
- Vagotomy or percutaneous blocking of the vagus nerve provides relief in some patients.
- Aspirin or other nonsteroidal anti-inflammatory drugs and analgesics.

Q. Describe Pancoast's syndrome (Pancoast's tumour; superior sulcus tumour syndrome, Pancoast–Tobias syndrome).

- Pancoast's tumour or Pancoast–Tobias tumour is a tumour of lung apex (superior sulcus tumour). Anatomically, pulmonary sulcus is synonymous with the costovertebral gutter, which extends from the first rib to the diaphragm. The superior pulmonary sulcus describes the uppermost extent of this recess.
- Most cases are NSCLC.
- Local extension of the tumour involves the eighth cervical (C8) and first thoracic (T1) nerves.
- Pancoast's syndrome comprises:
  - Shoulder pain that radiates to neck, axilla, anterior chest wall and medial aspect of scapula, and in the ulnar distribution of arm, that is along the C8, T1 distribution. Pain is attributed to invasion of parietal pleura, endothoracic fascia, bony skeleton and brachial plexus.
  - Wasting of the small muscles of the hand from C8, T1 nerve involvement.
  - Pain and tenderness over the first and second ribs and radiological evidence of rib destruction resulting from local invasion by tumour.
  - Horner's syndrome due to involvement of the sympathetic pathway as it passes through T1 root.
  - Upper arm oedema due to invasion and partial or complete occlusion of subclavian vein.
- Cough, dyspnoea and haemoptysis occur less frequently.
- Investigations include Chest X-ray (Fig. 2.14), CT scan, fine needle aspiration and MRI. MRI is the

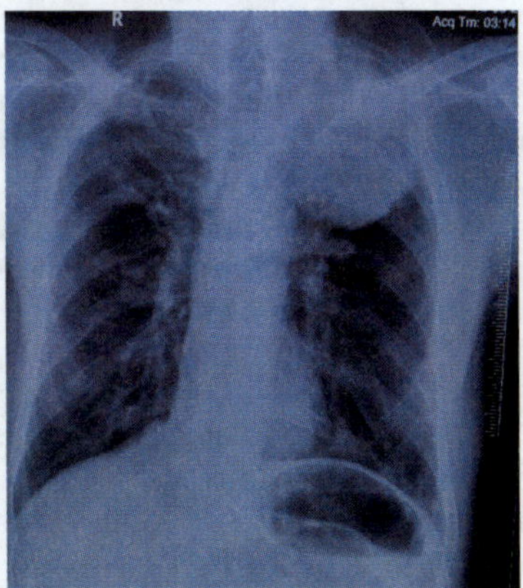

Fig. 2.14 Left-sided Pancoast's tumour.

modality of choice for imaging structures of the thoracic inlet, including brachial plexus, subclavian vessels, spine and neural foramina.
- Treatment is generally combined chemoradiotherapy and surgery. Preoperative radiotherapy along with chemotherapy (cisplatin and etoposide) is given followed by an en bloc resection of the tumour and involved chest wall 3–6 weeks later.

Q. Discuss the clinical manifestations and treatment of carcinoid tumours (bronchial adenomas).

- Carcinoid tumours (typical and atypical) occur more often in the younger age group, affecting females more than males.
- At present, these tumours are classified as malignant tumours, thus requiring their surgical removal.
- There are two histological types of bronchial adenoma: typical and atypical depending on the number of mitoses.
- Recurrent haemoptysis is the most common presentation. Other manifestations include recurrent bronchopulmonary infections and physical signs of collapse. Carcinoid syndrome (cutaneous flush, bronchospasm, diarrhoea and valvular lesions, particularly tricuspid regurgitation) is unusual with bronchial carcinoid; it can occur if hepatic metastasis occurs. On the other hand, this tumour may secrete ACTH causing full-blown Cushing's syndrome.
- Imaging:
  - CT scan.
  - Somatostatin-receptor-based imaging techniques—somatostatin receptor scintigraphy (octreotide scan) or gallium Ga-68 DOTATATE positron emission tomography (PET) scan.
- Diagnosis can be confirmed by bronchoscopy, biopsy and histology.
- Ideal treatment is surgical resection. When surgical resection is not possible, laser therapy may be tried.
- Medical therapy for metastatic or advanced carcinoids includes somatostatin analogues (e.g. octreotide and lanreotide), mammalian target of rapamycin (mTOR) inhibitors (everolimus) and cytotoxic chemotherapy (cisplatin and etoposide).

BOX 2.78 Boundaries of Mediastinum

- Thoracic inlet—above
- Diaphragm—below
- Mediastinal pleura—laterally
- Paravertebral gutter and ribs—posteriorly
- Sternum—anteriorly

Q. Define mediastinum. What are its various compartments? (AN 21.11)

- Mediastinum is the region between the pleural sacs.
- It is anatomically defined by the structures given in Box 2.78.

COMPARTMENTS

- Based on the lateral chest radiograph, mediastinum can be divided into four compartments:
  1. Superior mediastinum—bounded above by the plane of the first rib and below by an imaginary line drawn anteroposteriorly from the sternal angle to the inferior margin of forth thoracic vertebra.
  2. Anterior mediastinum—in front of the heart (extends from sternum anteriorly to pericardium and brachiocephalic vessels behind).
  3. Posterior mediastinum—behind the heart (bounded by pericardium and trachea anteriorly and vertebral column posteriorly).
  4. Middle mediastinum—between the anterior and posterior mediastinum.
- The contents of various compartments of mediastinum are given in boxes 2.79-2.82.

BOX 2.79 Contents of Superior Mediastinum

- Trachea
- Upper oesophagus
- Thymus gland
- Thoracic duct
- Superior vena cava (SVC)
- Arch of aorta and its branches
- Phrenic nerve
- Vagus nerve
- Left recurrent laryngeal nerve
- Lymph nodes

BOX 2.80 Contents of Anterior Mediastinum

- Thymus gland
- Anterior mediastinal lymph nodes
- Internal mammary artery and vein
- Fatty tissue

BOX 2.81 Contents of Middle Mediastinum

- Heart
- Ascending aorta
- Arch of aorta
- Vena cavae
- Brachiocephalic arteries and veins
- Phrenic nerves
- Trachea
- Main bronchi
- Hilar lymph nodes
- Pulmonary arteries and veins

BOX 2.82 Contents of Posterior Mediastinum

- Descending aorta
- Oesophagus
- Thoracic duct
- Azygos vein
- Sympathetic chain
- Lymph nodes

Q. Discuss the causes, clinical features and management of superior vena cava (SVC) syndrome.

- SVC syndrome results from obstruction of SVC secondary to compression and/or invasion by superior mediastinal tumours or other lesions and/or thrombosis of SVC.

CAUSES OF SVC OBSTRUCTION (Box 2.83)

- Note that all the causes listed in the Box 2.83 other than bronchial carcinoma and lymphoma are extremely rare.

CLINICAL FEATURES

- Clinical features due to involvement of other structures of mediastinum may be present (refer to Table 2.60 on page 215).
- Clinical features due to involvement of SVC are the following:
  - Headache, visual disturbances and alteration in the state of consciousness (due to raised intracranial pressure).
  - Orthopnoea may occur since a supine position will increase the amount of blood flow to the upper torso.
  - Conjunctival oedema, suffusion and subconjunctival haemorrhage.
  - Oedema, swelling and cyanosis of face, neck and upper limbs due to reduced venous flow.
  - Hoarseness, cough, stridor, dyspnoea and dysphagia due to oedema of larynx or pharynx.
  - Distended nonpulsatile neck veins.
  - Dilated veins on the upper thorax and upper limbs.

FEATURES BASED ON LOCATION OF SVC OBSTRUCTION

Preazygos or Supraazygos

- Obstruction of blood return above the entrance of azygos vein into the SVC results in venous distension and oedema of the face, neck and upper extremities.

BOX 2.83 Causes of Superior Vena Cava Obstruction

- Bronchial carcinoma (75%)
- Lymphomas (20%)
- Metastatic tumours
- Tuberculosis
- Fibrosing mediastinitis
- Retrosternal goitre
- Thymoma
- Parathyroid tumour
- Aortic arch aneurysm
- Central venous catheter, causing thrombosis

Postazygos or Infraazygos

- Obstruction below the entrance of azygos vein into the SVC results in retrograde flow through the azygos via collaterals to the inferior vena cava, resulting in not only the symptoms and signs of preazygos disease but also dilation of the veins over the abdomen. This is usually more severe and poorly tolerated than preazygos obstruction.

DIAGNOSIS

- It is based on clinical features.
- Chest radiograph shows widening of the superior mediastinum, most commonly on the right side. Pleural effusion may be seen in 25% of cases. Rarely, the chest radiograph may be normal, particularly when the syndrome is due to SVC thrombosis.
- CT of the chest provides the most important view of the mediastinum.
- MRI and MR angiography.
- Invasive procedures like bronchoscopy, percutaneous needle biopsy, mediastinoscopy and thoracoscopy for tissue diagnosis, though there is some danger of bleeding.

MANAGEMENT

- Tracheal obstruction, if it occurs, is an indication for emergency radiotherapy.
- Diuretics, head elevation and oxygen may provide temporary symptomatic relief in some patients.
- Radiotherapy (elective) is the treatment of choice for non-small-cell tumours of lung and metastatic tumours causing SVC syndrome.
- Chemotherapy is useful in some tumours like small-cell carcinoma of lung or lymphoma.
- If the patient is seriously ill (e.g. presence of hypotension, coma, stridor), empirical corticosteroids and cyclophosphamide may be given intravenously for temporary relief.
- Endovascular stent placement.
- Local, catheter-directed thrombolytic agents for SVC thrombosis.

Q. What are the common mediastinal masses? Discuss briefly the clinical features, investigations and management of mediastinal tumours.

AETIOLOGY

- Common mediastinal masses are listed in Table 2.58. Based on location, mediastinal masses are listed in Table 2.59.

CLINICAL FEATURES

- Germ cell tumours and lymphoma/leukaemias are more common between 20 and 40 years of age.
- Clinical features are due to the involvement of the structures of mediastinum (Table 2.60). The mediastinal structures are involved by compression and/or

TABLE 2.58 Common Mediastinal Tumours, Cysts and Masses

• Benign	Retrosternal goitre, thymoma, aortic aneurysm, neurogenic tumours, dermoid cysts, pericardial cysts, developmental cysts, lipoma
• Malignant	Lymph node metastases (especially from bronchial carcinoma), lymphomas, leukaemias, malignant thymoma, mediastinal teratoma, seminoma, nonseminomatous germ cell tumours

TABLE 2.59 Common Mediastinal Masses According to Location

• Superior mediastinum	Thymoma, thymic cyst, lymphoma, retrosternal goitre, aneurysm involving arch of aorta, thyroid malignancies
• Anterior mediastinum	Thymoma, very large retrosternal goitre, lymphoma, germ cell tumours (teratoma, seminoma, nonseminomatous tumours)
• Middle mediastinum	Cysts (bronchogenic, oesophageal, pericardial), metastatic lymphadenopathy (from lung, oesophageal, and head and neck cancers), benign lymphadenopathy (tuberculosis, sarcoidosis, histoplasmosis, Castleman's disease)
• Posterior mediastinum	Neurogenic tumours (schwannoma, neurofibroma, neuroblastoma, ganglioneuroma), aneurysm of descending aorta, Pott's spine

TABLE 2.60 Clinical Features of Mediastinal Masses

Structure Involved	Effects
• Oesophagus	Dysphagia
• Trachea and main bronchi	Stridor, dyspnoea, cough and lung collapse
• Phrenic nerve	Diaphragmatic paralysis and dyspnoea
• Left recurrent laryngeal nerve	Paralysis of left vocal cord resulting in hoarseness of voice and 'bovine' cough
• Sympathetic trunk	Horner's syndrome
• SVC	SVC syndrome
• Pericardium	Pericarditis and/or pericardial effusion, cardiac tamponade

invasion (infiltration). Benign tumours compress but do not invade, whereas malignant tumours compress and invade the vital structures of mediastinum.

INVESTIGATIONS

- Sputum examination for malignant cells.
- Radiological studies:
  - Plain radiograph of chest can give certain clues. A benign tumour appears as a sharply circumscribed opacity situated mainly in the mediastinum but often encroaching on one or both lung fields. A malignant tumour has ill-defined margins and often presents as a generalised widening of the mediastinal shadow.
  - Fluoroscopic examination for paradoxical movement of the diaphragm, in diaphragmatic paralysis.
  - Barium swallow for oesophageal involvement.
- CT scan of thorax.
- Magnetic resonance imaging (MRI) is helpful for evaluating cystic lesions.
- Positron emission tomography (PET).
- α-foetoprotein and β-human chorionic gonadotropin levels in any male with an anterior or superior mediastinal mass (elevated in nonseminomatous tumours).
- Antiacetylcholine receptor antibodies in some patients with thymic tumours.
- Technetium scan for suspected substernal goitre.
- Bronchoscopy, mediastinoscopy and thoracotomy to obtain tissue for diagnosis.

MANAGEMENT

- Benign mediastinal tumours should be removed surgically.
- SVC obstruction should be treated as outlined before (refer SVC syndrome on page 214).
- Lymph nodal metastases from bronchial carcinoma should be treated by radiotherapy and/or chemotherapy.
- Malignant thymoma is treated by radiotherapy.
- Treatments of lymphomas and leukaemias are discussed elsewhere.

Q. Discuss briefly about solitary pulmonary nodule (SPN).

DEFINITION

- A single, discrete pulmonary opacity <3 cm in size and surrounded by normal lung tissue without associated lymphadenopathy or atelectasis.
- SPN of >3 cm is almost always malignant.

CLINICAL FEATURES

- Most are discovered as an incidental finding on a chest radiograph.
- Some may have symptoms related to underlying cause

DIFFERENTIAL DIAGNOSIS

- Differential diagnosis of SPN is given in Table 2.61.

INVESTIGATIONS

- Sputum cytology is highly specific but insensitive for detecting malignant nodules.

TABLE 2.61 Differential Diagnosis of Solitary Pulmonary Nodule

Benign tumours	Noninfectious granulomas
• Hamartoma	• Sarcoidosis
• Lipoma	• Rheumatoid nodule
Malignant tumours	• Wegener's granulomatosis
• Bronchogenic carcinoma	Miscellaneous
• Carcinoid	• Lung abscess
• Pulmonary lymphoma	• Hydatid cysts (before rupture)
• Metastatic cancers	• Pulmonary infarction
Infectious granulomas	• Arteriovenous malformation
• Tuberculosis	• Bronchogenic cyst
• Histoplasmosis	• Pseudotumour (loculated fluid in a fissure)
• Coccidiodomycosis	

TABLE 2.62 Computed Tomography Findings in Malignant Versus Benign Lesions

CT Features Suggestive of Malignancy	CT Features Suggestive of a Benign Lesion
• Spiculations or a peripheral halo • Sparse stippled or eccentric calcifications • Thick-walled (>16 mm) cavitary lesions	• Smooth, well-defined margins • Dense central or laminar calcifications

- Chest radiograph. The doubling time of malignant lesions is generally between 30 and 300 days while for an infective lesion, it is less than 30 days. For benign lesions, doubling time is >465 days.
- Computed tomography (Table 2.62).
- PET/CT improves the differential diagnosis among benign and malignant pulmonary nodules.
- Transthoracic needle aspiration, bronchoscopic biopsy or biopsy using video-assisted thoracoscopic surgery may be done.

TREATMENT

- If diagnosis is not made, excision is required in suspicious nodules.

Q. What are the types of pulmonary fibrosis?

Q. Enumerate the causes of interstitial fibrosis.

Q. Discuss the clinical features, radiological features and management of replacement fibrosis.

- A wide variety of pulmonary disorders heal by laying down fibrous tissue. This results in pulmonary fibrosis. There are two types of pulmonary fibrosis.

REPLACEMENT FIBROSIS

- Fibrous tissue replaces the lung parenchyma damaged by suppuration or infarction.
- Common causes of replacement fibrosis include pulmonary tuberculosis, bronchiectasis, lung abscess, pulmonary infarcts, pneumoconiosis and necrotising pneumonias.
- The extent of fibrosis may vary from small nodular lesions (focal fibrosis) to extensive areas.
- Common causes of focal fibrosis include coal worker's pneumoconiosis (CWP), asbestosis and silicosis.

INTERSTITIAL FIBROSIS

- This is diffuse fibrosis of lung parenchyma, which is the end result of interstitial lung diseases.
- Common causes of interstitial lung disease are listed in Box 2.84.

BOX 2.84 Common causes of interstitial lung disease

- Connective tissue disorders
- Radiation injury to lung
- Cryptogenic fibrosing alveolitis
- Extrinsic allergic alveolitis
- Idiopathic pulmonary haemosiderosis
- Drugs like nitrofurantoin, amiodarone, gold, bleomycin, busulfan and methotrexate

CLINICAL FEATURES OF REPLACEMENT FIBROSIS

- The most common cause of replacement fibrosis is pulmonary tuberculosis. Upper lobes are affected most frequently. Fibrosis is usually associated with bronchiectasis.
- History is characterised by cough with or without expectoration and dyspnoea. Sputum may be blood-tinged.

PHYSICAL FINDINGS IN THE CHEST

- Inspection and palpation reveal shift of the mediastinum towards the affected side (shift of trachea and apex beat), drooping of the shoulder, retraction and flattening of the chest (supraclavicular hollowing, infraclavicular flattening and suprascapular wasting), crowding of the ribs, diminished movements of the chest wall and scoliosis of the spine. On measurement, the affected hemithorax is smaller with diminished expansion and spinoscapular distance. Vocal fremitus is variable and it may be increased or decreased.
- Percussion note is impaired over the affected areas.

Auscultation

- In extensive fibrosis, the intensity of breath sounds is diminished and they are vesicular in character with prolonged expiration. Vocal resonance is diminished and coarse crepitations are heard.
- If a major bronchus or trachea lies subjacent to the fibrotic area (which is usually the situation because of the shift of trachea due to the pulling by fibrosis), the intensity of breath sounds is increased, breath sounds are low-pitched, bronchial in character, vocal resonance is increased and coarse crepitations are heard.

RADIOLOGICAL FINDINGS OF REPLACEMENT FIBROSIS

- Findings of replacement fibrosis on a chest radiograph are listed in Box 2.85.

MANAGEMENT OF REPLACEMENT FIBROSIS

- Symptomatic measures like expectorants, breathing exercises.

BOX 2.85 Radiological Findings of Replacement Lung Fibrosis

- Shift of the mediastinum towards the affected side
- Affected hemithorax is smaller than the other
- Crowding of the ribs
- Fibrous bands in the lung fields
- Hilum is pulled upwards
- Diaphragm is raised on the affected side (tenting)

- Treatment of intercurrent infections with antibiotics.
- Specific treatment of the underlying causes (e.g. tuberculosis).
- Supplemental oxygen in hypoxaemic patients.
- Resectional surgery or lung transplantation in selected cases.

Q. Discuss briefly about interstitial lung diseases.

DEFINITION

- Interstitial lung diseases (also known as diffuse parenchymal lung diseases [DPLD]) are noninfectious and nonmalignant, usually chronic conditions that diffusely involve the lungs but predominantly the interstitial tissue of the lungs—the space between epithelial and endothelial basement membranes of the alveoli.
- These diseases often involve the alveoli, the capillary endothelium, as well as the perivascular and lymphatic tissues.
- Many of these can produce fibrosis in the interstitium (interstitial pulmonary fibrosis).

AETIOLOGY

- A number of diseases can produce interstitial lung disease. Some of the common diseases are classified as shown in Table 2.63.

TABLE 2.63 Aetiology of Interstitial Lung Diseases

ILD Due to Known Causes	ILD Due to Unknown Causes
Nongranulomatous interstitial inflammation	**Nongranulomatous interstitial inflammation**

• Drugs—antibiotics, gold, busulfan, bleomycin, methotrexate, D-penicillamine, nitrofurantoin, amiodarone
• Asbestos
• Fumes and gases
• Radiation
• Aspiration pneumonitis
• Residual of ARDS
• Toxins (e.g. paraquat)
	• Idiopathic interstitial pneumonias (IIPs)
	• Connective tissue diseases—systemic lupus erythematosus, rheumatoid arthritis, ankylosing spondylitis, systemic sclerosis, Sjogren's syndrome
	• Diffuse pulmonary haemorrhage
	• Goodpasture's syndrome
	• Idiopathic pulmonary haemosiderosis
	• Lymphocytic interstitial pneumonia (seen in HIV)
	• Pulmonary alveolar proteinosis
	• Eosinophilic pneumonias
	• Amyloidosis
	• Lymphangioleiomyomatosis (LAM)
	• Inherited disorders
	  • Neurofibromatosis
	  • Tuberous sclerosis
	• Graft-versus-host disease
	• Gastrointestinal/liver diseases
	  • Chronic liver disease
	  • Primary biliary cirrhosis
	  • Ulcerative colitis

Granulomatous interstitial inflammation	**Granulomatous interstitial inflammation**
• Hypersensitivity pneumonitis • Silicosis • Berylliosis	• Sarcoidosis • Pulmonary Langerhans cell histiocytosis • Wegener's granulomatosis • Eosinophilic granulomatosis with polyangiitis (Churg–Strauss syndrome)

- Idiopathic pulmonary fibrosis (IPF; a type of idiopathic interstitial pneumonia), pulmonary fibrosis associated with connective tissue diseases and sarcoidosis are the most common types of ILDs.

CLINICAL FEATURES

ACUTE PRESENTATION

- Acute presentation is uncommon but can occur with drugs, acute idiopathic interstitial pneumonia and 'non-fibrotic' hypersensitivity pneumonitis.
- Patient presents with cough, dyspnoea and occasionally fever.
- Chest radiograph shows diffuse alveolar opacities and therefore can be confused with 'atypical' pneumonia.

SUBACUTE PRESENTATION

- Patient presents with gradually increasing symptoms of cough and dyspnoea over weeks to months.
- This type of presentation can occur with all types of interstitial lung diseases, especially sarcoidosis, drug-induced ILDs and SLE-associated ILD.

CHRONIC PRESENTATION

- This is the most common presentation where the symptoms are present for months to years.
- Common symptoms and signs are shown in Boxes 2.86 and 2.87.

CAUSES OF RESPIRATORY FAILURE

- Patients with ILD may develop respiratory failure. Various causes are listed in Box 2.88.

BOX 2.86 Common Symptoms of Interstitial Lung Diseases

- Shortness of breath, especially with exertion
- Fatigue and weakness
- Loss of appetite
- Loss of weight
- Dry cough
- Chest pain and haemoptysis are unusual
- Sudden dyspnoea due to spontaneous pneumothorax with lymphangioleiomyomatosis (LAM), pulmonary Langerhans cell histiocytosis, tuberous sclerosis and neurofibromatosis
- Frank haemoptysis with diffuse pulmonary haemorrhage, LAM and tuberous sclerosis
- Wheezing in eosinophilic granulomatosis with polyangiitis and sarcoidosis

BOX 2.87 Examination Findings in Interstitial Lung Diseases

- Tachypnoea
- Clubbing
- Cyanosis
- Bilateral superficial leathery crepitations (end-inspiratory)
- Features of right-sided heart failure in late stages
- Signs of underlying aetiologies

BOX 2.88 Causes of Respiratory Failure in ILD Patients

- COPD
- Obstructive sleep apnoea
- Lung cancer
- Congestive heart failure
- Worsening of underlying ILD
- Pulmonary embolism
- Pulmonary hypertension

INVESTIGATIONS

BLOOD

- Blood investigations include total leucocyte count, ESR, urinalysis, renal and liver functions, antinuclear antibodies, rheumatoid factor and circulating immune complexes. The last three tests may be positive in some patients with IPF without underlying connective tissue disease.
- Serum precipitins in suspected hypersensitivity pneumonitis.
- Angiotensin-converting enzyme levels are elevated in most patients with sarcoidosis.
- Antineutrophil cytoplasmic antibodies and antibasement membrane antibodies if Wegener's granulomatosis and Goodpasture's syndrome, respectively, are suspected.

CHEST RADIOGRAPHY

- It often shows a bibasilar reticular or linear pattern.
- Mixed nodular pattern (of alveolar filling) along with reticular pattern.
- Nodular opacities (in some cases of sarcoidosis, chronic hypersensitivity pneumonitis, silicosis, rheumatoid arthritis).
- Ground glass appearance in early cases.
- Honeycombing (small, 0.5–2.0 cm, thick-walled cystic lesions) in long-standing conditions. These represent dilated and thickened terminal and respiratory bronchioles.
- Basal fibrosis with pleural thickening and pleural plaques suggest asbestosis.

COMPUTED TOMOGRAPHY

- High-resolution CT of chest is superior to chest radiography for early detection and confirmation of suspected interstitial lung disease.
- It demonstrates the extent and distribution of disease.
- Shows coexistent pathology (e.g. lymph node involvement).

PULMONARY FUNCTION TESTS

- Restrictive defect (reduced FVC, reduced FEV_1, normal or elevated FEV_1: FVC ratio, reduced total lung capacity and reduced diffusion capacity).
- Many ILDs are associated with an obstructive pattern in addition to restrictive pattern because of their bronchiolocentric propensity. These include sarcoidosis, hypersensitivity pneumonitis, LAM, tuberous sclerosis and neurofibromatosis.

EXERCISE TESTS

- Exercise tests may help evaluation of disease severity. The 6-minute walk test records oxygen saturation before, during and after 6-minute walk and measures the total distance walked.

ARTERIAL BLOOD GAS

- Hypoxaemia and respiratory alkalosis.
- Hypercapnia is rare until end stage.
- Increased alveolar–arterial oxygen gradient ($PAO_2 - PaO_2$).

BRONCHOSCOPY

- In some cases, analysis of BAL may be useful in narrowing down the possibilities among various types of interstitial lung diseases.
  - In sarcoidosis and hypersensitivity pneumonitis, BAL fluid shows T-cell lymphocytosis (increased CD4 cells in sarcoidosis and CD8 cells in hypersensitivity pneumonitis).
  - In IPF, neutrophils, eosinophils and macrophages predominate in BAL.
  - In pulmonary alveolar proteinosis, BAL is milky containing foamy macrophages and PAS-positive material.
  - In diffuse pulmonary haemorrhage, BAL shows red blood cells and haemosiderin-laden macrophages.
- Transbronchial lung biopsy or transbronchial cryobiopsy of lung may help in diagnosis.

LUNG BIOPSY (OPEN OR VIDEO-ASSISTED)

- Confirmation of diagnosis.
- Assessment of activity.

TREATMENT

- Treatment of the underlying causes if possible.
- Removal of offending agent.

DRUGS

- Corticosteroids are the mainstay of treatment, though they are not effective in majority of the patients, particularly those with significant fibrosis. Dose is 1 mg/kg for 6–12 weeks, which is then tapered to a maintenance level if the patient improves.
- If the patient does not respond to steroids, another immunosuppressant (cyclophosphamide or azathioprine) is added.
- Other drugs include colchicine and cyclosporin.
- *N*-acetylcysteine is often combined with other medicines and has been found useful in some studies.
- Pirfenidone (an antifibrotic agent due to its transforming growth factor-β inhibition properties) and nintedanib (a tyrosine kinase inhibitor) have been found to be useful in some patients with idiopathic lung fibrosis.

- Dose of pirfenidone is 801 mg (three capsules of 267 mg) three times daily. The most commonly reported adverse events include nausea, dyspepsia, anorexia, vomiting, rash and photosensitivity reaction.
- The targeted nintedanib dose is 150 mg twice daily. The most frequent adverse event is diarrhoea.
- Anti-gastro-oesophageal reflux agents (as prevalence of gastro-oesophageal reflux is high in these patients).

MISCELLANEOUS

- Oxygen therapy if $PaO_2 < 55$ mmHg.
- Treatment of pulmonary hypertension and cor pulmonale.
- Lung transplant.
- Experimental therapies include interferon-γ-1b, etanercept and infliximab (anti-TNF-α), anticoagulants, bosentan (a dual endothelin-receptor antagonist) and imatinib mesylate.

Q. What are idiopathic interstitial pneumonias?

Q. Discuss the clinical features, investigations and treatment of idiopathic pulmonary fibrosis.

- Idiopathic interstitial pneumonias (IIPs) are a subset of acute and chronic lung disorders (collectively referred to as interstitial lung diseases or diffuse parenchymal lung diseases) which have no known aetiology. These disorders involve the lung parenchyma by varying combinations of fibrosis and inflammation.
- Based on clinicopathological criteria, these are further subdivided into eight types (Box 2.89.
- AIP is an acute form (Hamman–Rich syndrome) which occurs in a small proportion of patients and is rapidly fatal.
- Smoking-related IIPs include RB-ILD and DIP.

BOX 2.89 Types of Idiopathic Interstitial Pneumonias

- Usual interstitial pneumonia (UIP) or idiopathic pulmonary fibrosis (IPF)
- Desquamative interstitial pneumonia (DIP)
- Respiratory bronchiolitis-associated interstitial lung disease (RB-ILD)
- Acute interstitial pneumonia (AIP)
- Cryptogenic organising pneumonia (COP)
- Nonspecific interstitial pneumonia (NSIP)
- Lymphoid interstitial pneumonia (LIP)
- Idiopathic pleuroparenchymal fibroelastosis (IPPFE)

IDIOPATHIC PULMONARY FIBROSIS

- Also known as UIP.
- Risk factors include smoking, exposure to antidepressants, chronic aspiration and exposure to toxic dust and fumes.
- Patients have an increased risk of lung carcinoma.
- A focused history, physical examination and investigations should be performed to identify disorders that are known to cause interstitial lung disease. These include chronic hypersensitivity pneumonitis, connective tissue diseases, drugs and pneumoconiosis.

CLINICAL FEATURES

- Middle-aged patients (generally 55–75 years); more common in males.
- Progressive dyspnoea and dry cough which over years eventually lead to cyanosis, respiratory failure, pulmonary hypertension and cor pulmonale.
- The median survival is about 4 years.
- Examination reveals gross clubbing, cyanosis and bilateral superficial crepitations (end-inspiratory and velcro crepitations).
- Late features include peripheral oedema, pulmonary hypertension and cor pulmonale.
- Acute worsening of symptoms may occur due to infections, pulmonary embolism, pneumothorax or heart failure.
- Another reason for acute deterioration is acute exacerbation of IPF, defined as a clinically significant respiratory deterioration developing within typically less than 1 month, accompanied by new radiological abnormalities and absence of other obvious clinical causes like fluid overload, left heart failure or pulmonary embolism. It can be triggered by infection or various procedures on lung or drug toxicity, or may be idiopathic. HRCT shows new bilateral ground glass opacities and/or consolidation superimposed on a reticular pattern or honeycombing. Therapy includes high-dose steroids, antibiotics and noninvasive ventilation. Nearly 75% of patients with acute exacerbation of IPF die despite ventilatory support.
- Extrapulmonary features include coronary artery disease, gastro-oesophageal reflux, diabetes mellitus, osteoporosis and many other chronic diseases.

INVESTIGATIONS

- ESR is raised.
- Antinuclear antibodies and rheumatoid factor are present in nearly 30% of cases.
- Chest radiograph shows irregular reticulonodular shadows, more in the lower zones.
- High-resolution CT scan of the chest shows peripheral subpleural and basal reticular opacities with honeycomb appearance (typical UIP pattern; absence of honeycombing indicates possible UIP pattern). Ground glass appearance is uncommon.
- Pulmonary function tests show a restrictive pattern.
- Blood gas analysis shows hypoxaemia with normal or low CO_2.

BOX 2.90 Diagnostic Criteria for Idiopathic Pulmonary Fibrosis

1. Exclusions of other possible causes of interstitial lung disease
2. Specific findings of usual interstitial pneumonia (UIP) on HRCT chest OR a combination of possible UIP findings on HRCT chest and UIP findings on lung biopsy

BOX 2.91 Summary of Treatment of Idiopathic Pulmonary Fibrosis

- Antifibrotic medications
- Smoking cessation
- Management of comorbidities (obesity, obstructive sleep apnoea, COPD, GERD)
- Regular exercises
- Supplementary oxygen
- Update vaccinations
- Symptom management
- Nutrition
- Management of acute exacerbations
- Transplant referral

- BAL shows increased number of cells, particularly neutrophils (>5%), eosinophils (>2%) and macrophages. Lymphocytosis is not usual.
- Histological confirmation, if required, can be done by lung biopsy (transbronchial, video-assisted or open).

DIAGNOSIS

- Based on presence of the criteria given in Box 2.90.

TREATMENT

- See treatment of interstitial lung disease on page 218.
- Currently, the only approved treatments that slow lung function decline in IPF patients are nintedanib and pirfenidone.
- Response to steroids and immunosuppressives is poor and in fact may be harmful and these agents should be avoided.
- Lung transplantation.
- Summary of treatment is given in Box 2.91.

Q. Enumerate the common occupational lung diseases and give their aetiologies.

Q. Write a note on pneumoconiosis.

- Strictly speaking, the term 'pneumoconiosis' includes those occupational lung diseases which are due to exposure to inorganic or mineral dust that is retained in the lung parenchyma and incites fibrosis. In contrast, other occupational lung diseases which occur due to organic dust are not associated with such accumulation of particles within the lungs and are believed to have an immunological pathogenesis. However, generally, both the terms are used interchangeably.

AETIOLOGY

- Table 2.64 gives various causes of occupational lung diseases.
- Siderosis and stannosis are nonfibrotic forms of occupational lung diseases.

TABLE 2.64 Aetiology of Occupational Lung Diseases

Aetiology	Diseases
• Diseases due to mineral dusts (pneumoconiosis)	
• Coal	Coal worker's pneumoconiosis (CWP)
• Silica	Silicosis
• Asbestos	Asbestos-related diseases
• Iron oxide	Siderosis
• Tin dioxide	Stannosis
• Beryllium	Berylliosis
• Diseases due to organic dusts	
• Cotton, flax or hemp dust	Byssinosis
• Mouldy hay, grain, silage	Farmer's lung
• Mouldy barley	Malt worker's lung
• Mushroom compost	Mushroom worker's lung
• Contaminated bagasse (sugar cane)	Bagassosis
• Diseases due to gases and fumes	
• Irritant gases, cadmium, isocyanates	Occupational asthma, bronchitis, ARDS
• Platinum salts	Occupational asthma
• Diseases due to biological substances	
• Proteolytic enzymes, animal and insect excreta, contaminated grain dust	Occupational asthma, bronchitis
• Diseases due to chemicals and radioactive substances	
• Polycyclic hydrocarbons, radon	Bronchial carcinoma

Q. Give a brief account of the asbestos-related diseases of lungs and pleura.

- The main types of asbestos are white asbestos (chrysotile), blue asbestos (crocidolite) and brown asbestos (amosite). All fibre types have the potential to cause asbestos-related diseases.
- Occupational exposure is highest with mining and milling of asbestos, manufacturing processes involving asbestos and demolition and shipyard workers. It can also occur in automobile and railroad workers and those involved in electrical wire insulation.
- There are six asbestos-related diseases (Box 2.92).
- Of all asbestos-related effects, highest dose is required to cause asbestosis.

BENIGN PLEURAL PLAQUES

- These are localised or diffuse areas of pleural thickening which are often calcified.
- Common sites are diaphragm and anterolateral pleural surfaces.

BOX 2.92 Asbestos-Related Diseases

- Benign pleural plaques
- Benign pleural effusion
- Asbestosis (progressive pulmonary fibrosis)
- Bronchial carcinoma
- Mesothelioma of pleura
- Mesothelioma of peritoneum (rare)

- Clinically, the patients are asymptomatic. The disease is usually identified on a routine chest radiograph.
- May lead to a significant decrease in total lung capacity, forced expiratory volume in 1 second and forced vital capacity (restrictive pattern).

BENIGN PLEURAL EFFUSION

- Benign (nonmalignant) and self-limiting disease; may be bilateral.
- Associated with pleuritic pain, fever and leucocytosis.
- Pleural fluid is often haemorrhagic.
- Common complication is pleural fibrosis.
- Exclude pleural mesothelioma by thoracoscopy and biopsy.

ASBESTOSIS

- Moderate to severe exposure for at least 10 years.
- Pathologically characterised by progressive pulmonary fibrosis.
- Clinically characterised by progressive exertional breathlessness, finger clubbing and end-inspiratory crepitations over lung bases.
- Radiologically (chest X-ray and HRCT) characterised by mottled shadows with some streaky opacities and sometimes 'honeycombing' in the mid and lower zones. On plain chest radiograph, many do not manifest pleural disease; however, CT picks up pleural disease in more than 90% of cases.
- Pulmonary function tests show reduced carbon monoxide transfer factor, decreased lung volumes and a restrictive ventilatory defect.
- Lung biopsy may show asbestos bodies.
- Complications of asbestosis include respiratory failure, right ventricular failure and bronchial carcinoma.

BRONCHIAL CARCINOMA

- Either squamous cell carcinoma or adenocarcinoma.
- Minimum lapse of 15–20 years between exposure and development of carcinoma.
- Multiplicative effect of smoking (risk more than additive effect of smoking and asbestos).

MESOTHELIOMA

- Mesothelioma is a primary malignant tumour of pleura, most commonly caused by blue asbestos.
- In contrast to bronchial carcinoma, development of mesothelioma is not related to smoking.
- Relatively short period of exposure (even 1–2 years) that occurred more than 20–30 years ago is required.
- Clinically, the patient presents with chest pain, breathlessness and haemorrhagic pleural effusion.
- Although approximately 50% of mesotheliomas metastasise, the tumour is locally invasive and death usually occurs due to local invasion. On chest radiograph, the mediastinum is either not shifted or shifted to the same side (a point to differentiate from other effusions).
- Diagnosis is confirmed by closed pleural biopsy.

Q. Give a brief account of coal worker's pneumoconiosis (CWP).

Q. What is progressive massive fibrosis (PMF)?

Q. Write a short note on Caplan's syndrome (rheumatoid pneumoconiosis).

- Coal worker's pneumoconiosis (CWP) is seen in coal miners with a prolonged history of inhalation of coal dust. More common in anthracite coal miners as compared to in bituminous miners.
- Chronic obstructive pulmonary disease is often associated with CWP.
- CWP is subdivided into two:
  1. Simple CWP.
  2. Progressive massive fibrosis (PMF).

SIMPLE COAL WORKER'S PNEUMOCONIOSIS

- Develops after prolonged exposure (15–20 years) to coal dust.
- Does not progress if the miner leaves the industry.
- There is considerable dispute whether simple CWP can produce significant symptoms, though many patients have cough and dyspnoea. Some patients do develop COPD which is independent of smoking status.
- Depending on the site and extent of the nodulation, simple CWP is radiologically divided into three categories:
  1. Category 1: Few small round opacities.
  2. Category 2: Numerous small round opacities but normal lung markings still visible.
  3. Category 3: Numerous small round opacities and the normal lung markings partly or fully obscured.
- The importance of simple CWP is that categories 2 and 3 can advance to PMF.

PROGRESSIVE MASSIVE FIBROSIS

- This condition progresses even after the miner leaves the industry.
- Characterised by single or multiple nodules (>1 cm in size to large dense masses in the upper lobes, which may cavitate).
- Clinically characterised by cough with blackish expectoration (melanoptysis) and progressive breathlessness.
- Complications of PMF include pulmonary tuberculosis, respiratory failure, right ventricular failure and Caplan's syndrome. Some patients may develop bronchogenic carcinoma.

CAPLAN'S SYNDROME

- Caplan's syndrome is PMF coexisting with seropositive rheumatoid arthritis.
- Rounded fibrotic nodules of 0.5–5 cm diameter without a background of smaller opacities are seen mainly in the periphery of the lung fields. These opacities may regress, in contrast to the lesions of classic CWP.
- Rheumatoid factor is positive.
- This syndrome is also seen in a number of pneumoconioses (e.g. silicosis) other than CWP.

TREATMENT

- Workers with advanced radiographic or physiologic abnormalities should be asked to discontinue working in the mine.
- Treatment is generally directed at specific disease manifestations, such as the use of bronchodilators for obstructive lung disease or supplemental oxygen for hypoxaemia.
- Stop smoking.
- Pulmonary rehabilitation.
- Regular follow-up to monitor for development or progression of disease.
- Lung transplantation.

PREVENTION

- Dust control measures.
- Use of respiratory personal protective equipment.
- Medical surveillance programmes to detect early lung disease.

Q. Give a brief account of silicosis.

- Silicosis (silica-induced lung disease) is caused by inhalation of silica dust or quartz particles.
- Occupations with high risk include mining, quarrying, dressing of sandstone and granite, pottery and ceramics industry, boiler scaling, sandblasting, etc. Silica is highly fibrogenic and causes development of hard nodules that coalesce as the disease advances.
- Tuberculosis commonly complicates silicosis (silicotuberculosis). The increased risk of both pulmonary and EPTB is lifelong even if exposure ceases. Chemoprophylaxis using INH for 9 months is recommended if latent tuberculosis is diagnosed with a positive tuberculin test or, where possible, interferon-gamma releasing assay (IGRA) testing.
    - Tuberculosis is suspected in presence of typical features of pulmonary TB such as persistent cough, fever, weight loss or haemoptysis.
    - Diagnosis of active tuberculosis superimposed on silicosis is often difficult, particularly in initial phases, as radiological alterations can be indistinguishable from those due to the preexisting silicosis.
    - Radiologically, rapid appearance of new opacities, and the finding of pleural effusion should raise the suspicion.
- Silica exposure increases the risk for developing lung cancer, chronic kidney disease and autoimmune diseases, particularly scleroderma, rheumatoid arthritis and Wegener's granulomatosis. It can also produce chronic airway obstruction similar to COPD.
- Silicosis can present in three forms: chronic, acute or accelerated.

CHRONIC OR SIMPLE SILICOSIS

- It is the most common form of silicosis which occurs after many decades of exposure to relatively low levels of silica.
- This form of silicosis is characterised by gradually progressive dyspnoea and dry cough. It is often compatible with normal life.
- The radiological features of silicosis are variable and range from diffuse fine rounded regular nodulation resembling miliary tuberculosis through coarse irregular nodules to extensive fibrosis resembling PMF. In early stages, upper zones of the lungs are more commonly involved as compared to the lower zones. The involvement of lymph nodes by chronic silicosis is fairly characteristic, with a tendency towards peripheral calcification, which produces the so-called egg shell appearance. Other causes of lymph node calcification include sarcoidosis, radiation-treated Hodgkin's disease, scleroderma and histoplasmosis.
- Pulmonary function tests typically reveal a mixed pattern of obstruction and restriction with a reduced diffusion capacity.
- No specific treatment available.

ACUTE SILICOSIS

- It occurs after exposure to a very high concentration of dust over a few months and is usually rapidly fatal within years.
- Characterised by pulmonary oedema, interstitial inflammation and accumulation of proteinaceous fluid rich in surfactant within the alveoli.
- Chest radiograph may show military infiltration or areas of consolidation. HRCT chest may show a characteristic 'crazy paving' pattern.
- Whole lung lavage via multiple bronchoscopies may slow progression.

ACCELERATED SILICOSIS

- It occurs after a few years of exposure to silica and is associated with rapidly progressive features of dyspnoea and pulmonary fibrosis. Involvement of middle and lower zones of the lungs is more frequent as compared to that in chronic silicosis.

TREATMENT

- Symptomatic treatment.
- Experimental therapies include aluminium citrate (acts by coating silica particles within the lung, thus, reducing their solubility) and polyvinylpyridine-N-oxide (by concentrating silica particles inside the cell, acting as a hydrogen acceptor and coat surface of silica particles).

Q. Discuss the clinical features, investigations and management of sarcoidosis.

Q. Describe Lofgren's syndrome.

Q. Give a brief account of Heerfordt–Waldenstrom syndrome.

DEFINITION

- Sarcoidosis is a multisystem, chronic granulomatous inflammatory disorder of unknown aetiology. It is characterised by the accumulation of T lymphocytes and mononuclear phagocytes and noncaseating epithelioid granulomas in the affected organs.

AETIOLOGY

- Aetiology of sarcoidosis is unknown.
- The disease probably results from an exaggerated cellular immune response to an infectious or noninfectious environmental agent in a person genetically susceptible to develop sarcoidosis. Probable infectious agents include *Propionibacterium acnes*, atypical mycobacteria, and a *M. tuberculosis* protein. Noninfectious agents include insecticides, moulds and metals (e.g. beryllium, zirconium and aluminium).

PATHOLOGY

- Sarcoidosis can affect any part of the body. The most frequently involved organ is lung. The other organs commonly involved are lymph nodes, eyes, skin, parotid glands, liver, spleen and kidneys.
- The characteristic histological feature of sarcoidosis is noncaseating epithelioid granulomas. Tuberculosis, on the other hand, is characterised by caseating epithelioid granulomas with tubercle bacilli.

CLINICAL FEATURES

- Sarcoidosis can manifest in three forms:
  1. Asymptomatic form (30%–45%).
  2. Acute or subacute form (10%–15%).
  3. Chronic form (40%–60%).
- Asymptomatic form is usually detected incidentally on a routine chest film.
- Acute or subacute form develops abruptly over a period of few weeks. Patients have constitutional symptoms like fever, fatigue, malaise, anorexia and weight loss. Respiratory symptoms are cough, dyspnoea and retrosternal chest discomfort. Two syndromes have been identified in the acute group:
  1. Lofgren's syndrome characterised by acute onset of fever, erythema nodosum, migratory polyarthritis and radiographic evidence of bilateral hilar adenopathy. Uveitis may occur in some patients. It resolves over 6 months to 2 years with NSAIDs or colchicine.
  2. Heerfordt–Waldenstrom syndrome or uveoparotid fever characterised by anterior uveitis, parotid enlargement, fever and facial palsy.
- Chronic form develops over months, characterised by respiratory complaints (dry cough, dyspnoea and chest discomfort) without significant constitutional symptoms. Clubbing and haemoptysis are uncommon. The disease keeps waxing and waning over many years with nearly 60% of patients recovering spontaneously over 10 years. Pulmonary hypertension may occur due to pulmonary fibrosis; other causes include granulomatous infiltration of the pulmonary arteries and direct compression by lymphadenopathy. Patients with chronic form of sarcoidosis have increased risk of developing lymphoproliferative disorders (Hodgkin's and non-Hodgkin's lymphomas).

PULMONARY MANIFESTATIONS

- Pulmonary feature of sarcoidosis are given in Box 2.93.

EXTRAPULMONARY MANIFESTATIONS

- Patients with sarcoidosis can present with several extrapulmonary features (Table 2.65).

Lupus Pernio

- Skin lesions around nose, eye and cheeks.
- These lesions are often disfiguring and can erode into cartilage and bone, especially around the nose.
- Involvement of the upper respiratory tract, bones (most commonly fingers and toes) and severe arthropathy are common
- Associated with poor prognosis of sarcoidosis.

INVESTIGATIONS

- Blood examination shows lymphocytopenia, anaemia, eosinophilia, raised ESR, hyperglobulinaemia and elevated serum alkaline phosphatase.
- Hypercalcaemia and hypercalciuria due to increased production of 1,25-dihydroxyvitamin D by the granuloma occur uncommonly.
- Plasma level of angiotensin-converting enzyme (ACE) is elevated in about 70% of cases with acute disease

BOX 2.93 Pulmonary Manifestations of Sarcoidosis

- Interstitial lung disease
- Atelectasis
- Cavitation (may develop aspergilloma)
- Unilateral pleural effusion
- Pulmonary nodules

TABLE 2.65 Extrapulmonary Manifestations of Sarcoidosis

• Lymph nodes	Hilar adenopathy (70%–90%), paratracheal and generalised lymphadenopathy
• Skin	Erythema nodosum, plaques (Fig. 2.15), papular eruptions (Fig. 2.16), subcutaneous nodules, lupus pernio, keloid, infiltration of previous scars and tattoos by granuloma
• Eyes	Uveitis, iridocyclitis, retinitis, phlyctenular conjunctivitis, lacrimal gland involvement (dry eyes), optic neuritis
• Salivary glands	Parotid gland enlargement
• Heart	Myocarditis, pericarditis, papillary muscle dysfunction, CHF, conduction defects, arrhythmias
• Liver and spleen	Hepatosplenomegaly, hypersplenism, portal hypertension
• Nervous system	Seventh nerve, cerebral, meningeal and peripheral nerve involvement, optic neuritis, diabetes insipidus due to hypothalamic involvement, seizures
• Kidneys	Nephrocalcinosis, nephrolithiasis, tubuloglomerular and renal artery disease
• Musculoskeletal	Arthralgias, arthritis, phalangeal cysts, polymyositis, chronic myopathy
• Endocrine	Diabetes insipidus, anterior pituitary dysfunction, Addison's syndrome, hypercalcaemia

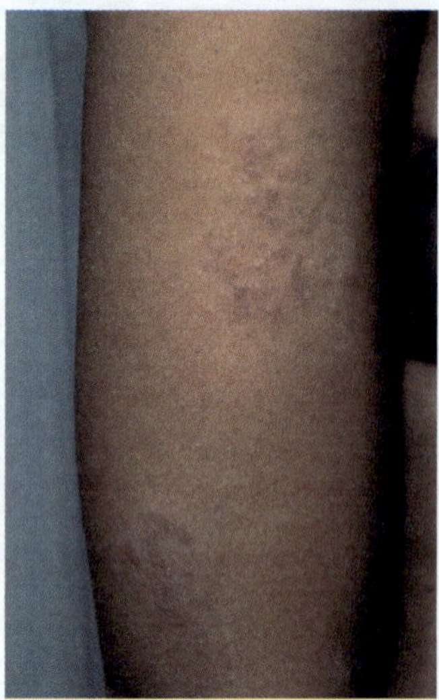

Fig. 2.15 Plaque sarcoidosis.

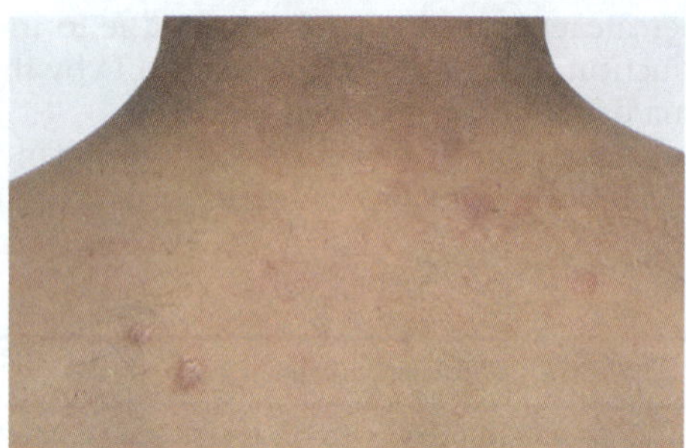

Fig. 2.16 Papular sarcoidosis on the back of a patient.

and only 20% of with chronic disease. It may also be elevated in several other diseases including tuberculosis, leprosy and hyperthyroidism. In lymphoma, ACE level is usually lower than normal range.

- Skin sensitivity to tuberculin is depressed or absent because activated T cells are sequestered in the lung, leading to peripheral depletion. So, Mantoux test is a useful screening test. A strongly positive reaction virtually rules out sarcoidosis.

BOX 2.94 Chest Radiographic Features of Sarcoidosis

- Hilar adenopathy, usually bilateral (70%–90%)
- Reticulonodular shadows in lung fields (usually upper lobes)
- Paratracheal lymph nodal enlargement
- Egg shell calcification of hilar nodes (unusual)
- Pleural effusion (very uncommon)
- Large nodules
- Cavitation
- Atelectasis
- Cardiomegaly

TABLE 2.66 Radiological Staging of Sarcoidosis

• Stage 0	Normal chest radiograph
• Stage I	Bilateral hilar adenopathy with no parenchymal abnormalities (50% of cases)
• Stage II	Bilateral hilar adenopathy with diffuse parenchymal infiltrates (30% of cases)
• Stage III	Diffuse parenchymal infiltrates without hilar adenopathy (10% of cases)
• Stage IV	Evidence of diffuse pulmonary fibrosis (Fig. 2.17)

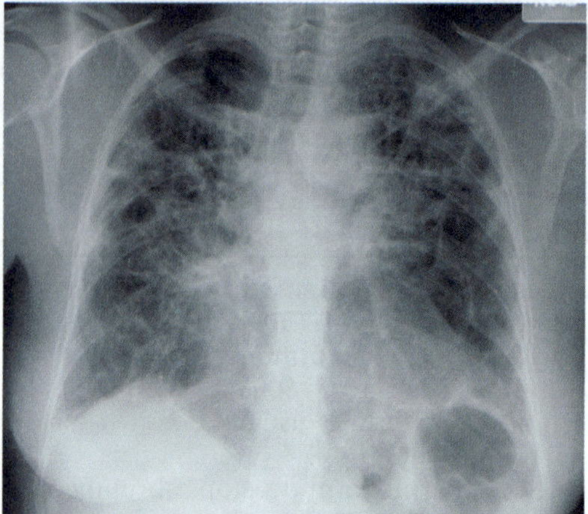

Fig. 2.17 Stage IV sarcoidosis (chest X-ray shows extensive parenchymal fibrosis, most marked in the upper parts of the lungs and in the perihilar regions). From Ungprasert P, et al. Clinical Manifestations, Diagnosis, and Treatment of Sarcoidosis. Mayo Clin Proc Inn Qual Out 2019;3(3):358-375.

RADIOLOGICAL FEATURES OF SARCOIDOSIS

Chest Radiography

- Features of sarcoidosis on chest radiography are given in Box 2.94.
- Scadding's staging based on classic radiographic patterns of pulmonary sarcoidosis is shown in Table 2.66.
- In addition to sarcoidosis, upper lobe involvement occurs with tuberculosis, *Pneumocystis* pneumonia, hypersensitivity pneumonitis, silicosis and Langerhans cell histiocytosis.

Computed Tomography

- Computed tomography of the chest (contrast-enhanced) is helpful in better delineation of the hilar and mediastinal lymph nodes. These lymph nodes are homogeneous and do not show any evidence of necrosis or rim enhancement (features typically seen in tubercular involvement of mediastinal nodes).
- HRCT shows reticular shadows and nodules. Confluence of numerous interstitial granulomas can result in large, irregular, mass-like opacities (alveolar sarcoid). Small satellite nodules are often present at the periphery of these large nodules, termed the 'galaxy sign' (a collection of stars). Honeycombing is uncommon.
- Airway involvement results in nodular bronchial wall thickening, small endobronchial lesions and obstructive small airways disease. Bronchi can be seen to be obstructed by either endobronchial granulomas or extrinsic compression by enlarged lymph nodes, leading to atelectasis, particularly of the right middle lobe.

OTHER TESTS

- The pulmonary functions tests reveal a typical restrictive pattern. Occasionally, obstructive pattern may be seen.

TABLE 2.67 Causes of Pulmonary Granulomas

Infectious Diseases	Noninfectious Diseases

• Mycobacterial infections
  • *Mycobacterium tuberculosis*
  • Nontuberculous mycobacteria (NTM)
• Fungal infections
  • *Histoplasma*
  • *Cryptococcus*
  • *Coccidioides*
  • *Blastomyces*
  • *Pneumocystis*
  • *Aspergillus*
• Other infections
  • *Brucella*
• *Chlamydia*
	• Sarcoidosis
	• Lymphoma
	• Chronic beryllium disease
	• Hypersensitivity pneumonitis
	• Wegener's granulomatosis
	• Eosinophilic granulomatosis with polyangiitis
	• Talc granulomatosis
	• Rheumatoid nodule

- The gallium-67 scan shows diffuse uptake. However, it may become negative within a few days of start of corticosteroids and is not done routinely to diagnose sarcoidosis.
- PET scan using radiolabelled fluorodeoxyglucose is more useful than gallium-67 scan to detect both pulmonary and extrapulmonary sites with active inflammation, thereby indicating possible sites of biopsy.
- Bone marrow examination may show granulomas in about 30% of cases.
- BAL shows increased proportion of lymphocytes, most of which are activated Th1 (subset of CD^{4+} cells) cells.
- Transbronchial biopsy may show noncaseating granulomas with epithelioid cells and multinucleated giant cells. There are several causes of pulmonary granulomas (Table 2.67).
- Mediastinoscopic biopsy/endoscopic ultrasound-guided biopsy/endobronchial ultrasound-guided biopsy of mediastinal or hilar lymph nodes.
- MRI may be useful in brain and cardiac involvement.

TREATMENT

- Sarcoidosis is divided into four stages based on chest radiograph and clinical manifestations.
- Stage I disease usually resolves spontaneously and does not require treatment unless patient is significantly symptomatic.
- Symptomatic or progressive stages II and III of pulmonary disease and sarcoidosis involving vital structures are treated with corticosteroids. Prednisolone is given 20–40 mg daily for 4 weeks, followed by tapering to a maintenance dose of 7.5–10 mg daily for 6–18 months.
- Azathioprine and methotrexate as steroid-sparing agents that are given if patient cannot be maintained on prednisolone dose of 10 mg/day or less.
- Hydroxychloroquine for skin, bone and joint involvement, and those with hypercalcaemia.
- Other agents used include mycophenolate, leflunomide, infliximab and adalimumab (TNF-alpha antagonists).

POOR PROGNOSTIC FACTORS

- Poor prognostic factors in sarcoidosis are given in Box 2.95.

BOX 2.95 Poor Prognostic Factors in Sarcoidosis

- Age at onset >40 years
- Females
- Presence of hypercalcaemia
- Extrathoracic disease
- Lupus pernio
- Splenomegaly
- Stage III and IV sarcoidosis
- Chronic uveitis
- Cystic bone lesions
- Cardiac involvement (except pericarditis)

TABLE 2.68 Sarcoidosis Versus Tuberculosis

Features	Sarcoidosis	Tuberculosis
ACE level	• Elevated in 50%–80%	• Usually normal
Hypercalcaemia	• Uncommon	• Rare
Mantoux test	• Negative in majority	• Positive in majority
BAL findings	• $CD4^+/CD8^+$ ratio >3.5 • BAL negative for mycobacteria	• $CD4^+/CD8^+$ ratio not markedly elevated • BAL positive for mycobacteria by smear, culture or PCR
Histopathology	• Noncaseating granulomas	• Caseating granulomas with mycobacteria positivity
Chest radiograph and CT scan of chest	• Bilateral, symmetrical hilar lymphadenopathy • Non-contrast-enhancing lymph nodes • Bilateral reticulonodular opacities • Cavitation rare	• Usually, unilateral hilar lymphadenopathy • Contrast-enhancing lymph nodes • Tree-in-bud appearance • Cavitation common
Treatment	• Immunosuppressants like corticosteroids	• Antituberculous drugs

Q. How will you differentiate sarcoidosis from pulmonary tuberculosis?

- Features which help in differentiating sarcoidosis from tuberculosis are given in Table 2.68.

Q. Discuss the causes, clinical features, investigations and management of pleural effusion.

Q. How will you differentiate transudative pleural effusions from exudative pleural effusions? (CT1.11)

Q. Describe phantom tumour.

Q. What is Grocco's sign?

DEFINITION

- Abnormal accumulation of fluid between parietal pleura and visceral pleura is called pleural effusion. Accumulation of purulent fluid is called empyema. Normally, the pleural space contains a small amount of fluid (about 0.26 ± 0.1 mL/kg) which allows the lungs to inflate and deflate with minimal friction.
- A minimum of 500 mL of fluid is necessary for clinical detection of pleural effusion.

PATHOPHYSIOLOGY

- The mean rate of both the production and the absorption of pleural fluid is normally 0.2 mL/kg/hour which implies that the entire volume of the pleural fluid normally turns over within 1 hour.
- The parietal side of the pleura accounts for most of the production of pleural fluid, and for most of its resorption as well except in heart failure where most of the fluid comes from visceral pleura.
- Pleural fluid is resorbed via lymphatics in the parietal pleura. This reabsorption can increase by a factor of 20 if more than the usual amount of pleural fluid is produced.
- The volume of the pleural fluid is determined by the balance of the hydrostatic and oncotic pressure differences present between the systemic and pulmonary circulation and the pleural space.
- Transudate is an ultrafiltrate of plasma, resulting from increased hydrostatic pressure or decreased serum oncotic pressure. This is essentially an effusion with normal pleura. Transudative effusions are also called hydrothorax, although some use this term for any pleural effusion.
- Exudate resembles plasma and is rich in proteins. This results from increased capillary permeability. This is essentially an effusion with diseased pleura.

CLASSIFICATION AND CAUSES

- Table 2.69 gives classification and causes of pleural effusion.
- Drugs which can produce pleural effusion are listed in Box 2.96.

CLINICAL FEATURES

- Symptoms and signs of pleurisy may precede the development of pleural effusion.
- Breathlessness may occur, the severity of which is related to the size and rate of accumulation of fluid.
- Some patients complain of a dry cough which can be explained as a manifestation of pleural inflammation or lung compression due to a large effusion.

TABLE 2.69 Classification and Causes of Pleural Effusion

• Transudates	Congestive heart failure, cirrhosis of liver, nephrotic syndrome, severe malnutrition, peritoneal dialysis, hypothyroidism, constrictive pericarditis, Meigs' syndrome (benign ovarian tumours with ascites and pleural effusion), superior vena cava obstruction
• Exudates	Tuberculosis, malignancy (primary or metastatic), pneumonia, pulmonary infarction, rheumatoid arthritis, pancreatitis, systemic lupus erythematosus, drug-induced effusion, benign asbestos-related effusion, Dressler's syndrome, intraabdominal abscess, Meigs' syndrome (can be transudative as well), uraemia, ruptured amoebic liver abscess, chylous pleural effusion

BOX 2.96 Drugs Producing Pleural Effusion

- Nitrofurantoin
- Dantrolene
- Methysergide
- Dasatinib
- Amiodarone
- Procarbazine
- Methotrexate
- Clozapine

PHYSICAL FINDINGS IN THE CHEST

- Inspection and palpation will disclose shift of trachea and mediastinum (shift of apex beat) to the opposite side (depending on size of effusion), reduction in the chest movements on the affected side, bulging of the intercostal spaces, fullness of the affected chest and markedly reduced vocal fremitus. Measurements reveal diminished chest expansion, increase in the size of the affected hemithorax and an increase in spinoscapular distance.
- Percussion reveals a stony dull note over the fluid. Upper level of the dullness is highest laterally in the axilla and is lower anteriorly and posteriorly (Ellis S-shaped curve). A small pleural effusion on the left side may be detectable only by the obliteration of Traube's space on percussion. Likewise, a small effusion on the right side may be detectable only by tidal percussion (percuss down the back or front until the normal hyperresonance of the lungs becomes dull over the liver/diaphragm; then ask the patient breath in and out deeply while continuing to percuss; normally, the percussion sound should wax and wane).
- On auscultation, intensity of the breath sounds is markedly diminished-to-absent over the fluid. Adventitious sounds are not audible, although pleural rub may be heard in some cases. Vocal resonance is markedly diminished over the fluid. Occasionally, aegophony, whispering pectoriloquy and a tubular bronchial breathing may be audible just above the level of a pleural effusion.

Grocco's Sign (Grocco's Triangle; Paravertebral Triangle of Dullness)

- In moderate- to large-sized pleural effusions, a triangular area of dullness or impaired note can be percussed over the back of chest on the contralateral side or opposite side of the effusion. This is probably due to shift of the posterior mediastinum to the opposite side by effusion.
- The Grocco's triangle is bounded medially by the mid-spinal line from the upper level of effusion down to the level of the 10th thoracic vertebra. It is bounded below by a horizontal line of about 3–7 cm extending laterally from the 10th thoracic vertebra, along the lower limit of lung resonance. It is bounded laterally by a curved line connecting the above-mentioned two lines.

INVESTIGATIONS

CHEST RADIOGRAPH

- Chest radiograph (posteroanterior view) in the erect posture can detect pleural effusion. A minimum of 200 mL of fluid is required for detection in this view.
- Chest radiograph (anteroposterior view) in the supine posture needs even larger amounts for detection. Here, the fluid layers are out posteriorly and give a

generally hazy shadow (ground glass appearance) with preserved vascular shadows. This is the usual radiological appearance in bedridden patients.

- Chest radiograph (lateral decubitus view) with the affected side down can detect an effusion as small as 100–150 mL. However, only 50 mL of pleural fluid can produce detectable posterior costophrenic angle blunting on a lateral chest X-ray.
- Loculated effusions are typically seen in conditions which cause intense pleural inflammation (e.g. tuberculosis, parapneumonic effusion, empyema and haemothorax). However, even malignancy, pulmonary embolism and congestive heart failure may also produce loculated effusion.
- In heart failure, loculated fluid within lung fissure may give the appearance of an intraparenchymal mass which disappears with diuretic therapy (phantom tumour or vanishing tumour).

Radiological Features of Pleural Effusion in an Erect Chest Film

- Radiological features of pleural effusion on chest film are given in Box 2.97.

ULTRASONOGRAPHY

- Can detect as little as 5 mL of but a minimal volume of 20 mL is more reliably detected.
- It is useful in differentiating loculated pleural effusion from pleural tumour or pleural thickening.
- It detects septations within pleural fluid with greater sensitivity than CT scanning.
- Useful in localisation of an effusion prior to aspiration and biopsy.
- Detection of solid pleural abnormalities may suggest pleural malignancy.

PLEURAL ASPIRATION AND FLUID ANALYSIS

- At diagnostic aspiration, at least 50 mL of pleural fluid should be withdrawn. The fluid is collected in separate containers for microbiological examination including culture for mycobacteria, cytological examination including malignant cells and biochemical examination.
- Exudative fluid can be differentiated from transudative fluid as per Table 2.70.

BOX 2.97 Radiological Features of Pleural Effusion

- Tracheal shift to the opposite side.
- Mediastinal (apex of heart) shift to the opposite side (Fig. 2.18).
- Obliteration of costophrenic angle.
- A dense uniform opacity in the lower and lateral part of hemithorax.
- Upper border of the opacity is concave upwards and is highest laterally.
- Wider than normal interlobar fissure in 'interlobar effusion'.
- Encysted interlobar effusion may be seen as a rounded opacity resembling solitary pulmonary nodule (phantom tumour).
- Encysted effusion in the presence of adhesions between contiguous pleural surfaces (loculated effusion).
- Shift of mediastinum towards the side of effusion in a patient with massive effusion indicates either an endobronchial obstruction or a mediastinum encasement by tumour (e.g. mesothelioma).

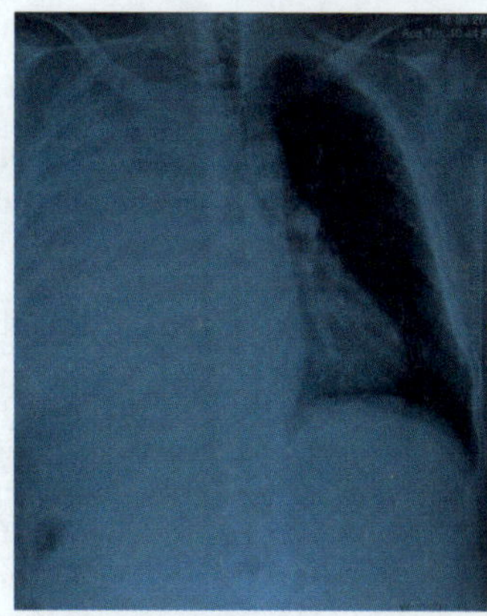

Fig. 2.18 Massive right pleural effusion with mediastinal and tracheal shifts to opposite side.

TABLE 2.70 Pleural Fluid Analysis

Test	Transudate	Exudate
• Appearance	Clear	Clear, cloudy or haemorrhagic
• Protein		
• Absolute value	<3.0 g/dL	>3.0 g/dL
• Pleural fluid:serum ratio	<0.5	>0.5
• Lactic dehydrogenase		
• Absolute value	<200 IU/L	>200 IU/L
• Pleural fluid:serum ratio	<0.6	>0.6
• Glucose	>60 mg/dL (usually same as in blood)	<60 mg/dL (variable)
• Leucocytes		
• Total leucocytes	<1000/mm³	>1000/mm³
• Differential leucocytes	>50% lymphocytes or mononuclear cells	>50% lymphocytes (tuberculosis, malignancy) >50% polymorphs (acute inflammation)
• Erythrocytes	<500/mm³	Variable

Note

- A low pleural fluid glucose concentration (<60 mg/dL) suggests complicated parapneumonic effusion, empyema, malignancy or tuberculosis. Very low levels (<15 mg/dL) are characteristic of rheumatoid effusions.
- Pleural fluid eosinophilia (>10% of all cells) may be seen in resolving infections (especially viral pneumonias and acute bacterial pneumonias), drug-induced effusion (e.g. nitrofurantoin, bromocriptine, amiodarone and phenytoin), hydropneumothorax, benign asbestos-related effusion, pancreatitis and trauma. It is uncommon in patients with cancer or tuberculosis unless the patient has undergone repeated thoracenteses.
- Pleural fluid erythrocyte counts exceeding 100,000/mm^3 are most often seen in malignancy and pulmonary embolism.
- Pleural fluid pH is a very unreliable guide to differentiate between transudates and exudates. However, a pleural fluid pH below 7.2 in a patient with a

parapneumonic effusion indicates the need for drainage of the fluid.

- Pleural fluid amylase is elevated in patients with malignancies, pancreatic diseases and oesophageal rupture. However, routine amylase estimation is not recommended unless the clinical features suggest any of the three diseases.
- Pleural fluid triglycerides help in diagnosis of chylothorax.
- Pleural fluid determination of antinuclear antibody titres or rheumatoid factor levels adds little diagnostic information and is not indicated in most cases.
- Other special characteristics of pleural fluid in relation to various diseases are discussed along with individual diseases (ADA estimation discussed under 'tuberculous pleural effusion').

Light's Criteria

- Light's criteria are used to differentiate exudative from transudative fluid. These include one or more of the features given in Box 2.98.
- These criteria are highly sensitive for identifying exudative fluid but have lower specificity, that is some patients with transudative effusion will be classified as exudative fluid using these criteria. Therefore, if clinical findings suggest a transudative effusion but the pleural fluid appears to be an exudate on Light's criteria, the difference between the albumin level in serum and pleural fluid should be measured. Almost all patients with transudative effusion have a serum albumin level that is more than 1.2 g/dL higher than the pleural fluid albumin level (serum-effusion albumin gradient).
- Of note, a large percentage of exudates will be misclassified if serum-effusion albumin gradient is used as the only method of differentiating between transudates and exudates.
- Diuretics given to treat congestive heart failure can increase the concentrations of protein, LDH, and lipids in pleural fluid which can lead to the incorrect identification of fluid as an exudate.

Lymphocytic Pleural Effusion

- Causes of lymphocytic pleural fluid are given in Box 2.99.

BOX 2.98 Light's Criteria to Differentiate Exudative From Transudative Pleural Fluid

- Ratio of pleural fluid protein to serum protein level >0.5
- Ratio of pleural fluid LDH to serum LDH > 0.6
- Pleural fluid LDH level >2/3rd of the upper level of serum LDH levels

BOX 2.99 Causes of Lymphoytic Pleural Effusion

- Malignancy (primary or secondary)
- Tuberculosis
- Lymphoma
- Congestive heart failure (long standing)
- Rheumatoid effusion
- Chylothorax
- Uraemic pleuritis

PLEURAL BIOPSY

- Usually indicated in some exudates that are undiagnosed.
- Closed pleural biopsy can be performed with Abrams or Cope or Tru-Cut needle. It should be done under ultrasound guidance when the effusion is small or loculated.
- The needle should be inserted through an intercostal space at the area of maximum dullness on percussion and at the site of maximum radiological opacity or at a site determined by ultrasonography. It should be inserted just above the upper border of the rib.

OTHER INVESTIGATIONS IN PLEURAL EFFUSION

- Pleural fluid tumour markers like carcinoembryonic antigen (CEA), cancer antigen 125 (CA-125), cancer antigen 15-3 (CA 15-3) and cytokeratin 19 fragments (CYFRA) do not have any role in routine investigations of pleural effusion. However, immunocytochemical markers (e.g. epithelial membrane antigen, CEA, calretinin) can be performed on the atypical cells seen in the effusion.
- Blood examination for total and differential leucocyte counts, ESR, proteins, sugar, LDH, amylase, rheumatoid factor and antinuclear factor.
- Sputum examination for tubercle bacilli and malignant cells.
- In a massive effusion, a repeat radiograph after removal of a large volume of fluid may reveal an underlying parenchymal lesion.
- CT scan of chest.
- Bronchoscopy and biopsy.
- Thoracoscopy (video-assisted or open surgical) and biopsy of pleura.

MANAGEMENT OF PLEURAL EFFUSION

- Treatment of the underlying causes.
- Therapeutic aspiration may be necessary to relieve dyspnoea. Not more than 1-1.5 L should be removed at a sitting because pulmonary oedema (refer below) may follow removal of large volumes.
- Insertion of chest tube if rapid reaccumulation of fluid occurs.
- Pleurodesis for malignant effusion using bleomycin or talc powder.

EVALUATION OF A PATIENT WITH PLEURAL EFFUSION

- Flowchart 2.11 summarises evaluation of a patient with pleural effusion.

Q. Discuss briefly about re-expansion pulmonary oedema.

- Occurs in a small number of patients who undergo rapid inflation of the lung (e.g. evacuation of >1-1.5 L of air/fluid) after a prolonged period of collapse (generally >3 days) produced by either pneumothorax or pleural effusion.
- More common in young patients.

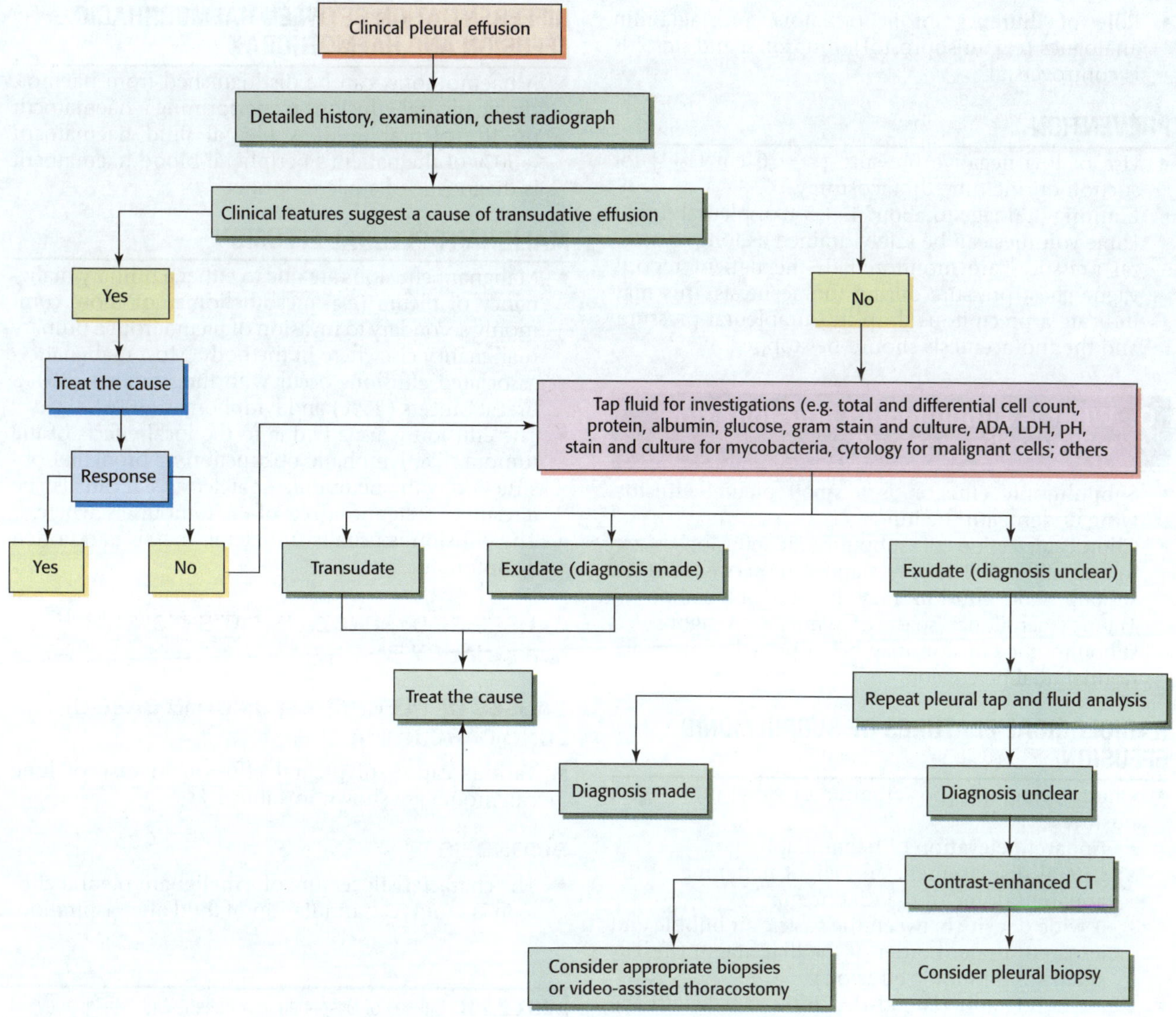

Flowchart 2.11 Evaluation of a Patient With Pleural Effusion.

PATHOGENESIS

- Exact reason for development of re-expansion pulmonary oedema is not known.
  - Ventilation and reperfusion of a previously collapsed lung may lead to an inflammatory response, with production of reactive oxygen species and superoxide radicals, which results in increased capillary permeability.
  - Increased pulmonary hydrostatic pressure caused by enhanced venous return.
  - Pressure-induced mechanical disruption of alveolar capillaries.
  - Decreased levels of functional surfactant.
  - Increased pressure across the capillary–alveolar membrane from bronchial obstruction.
  - Altered lymphatic clearance.

CLINICAL FEATURES

- Onset of symptoms usually within 24 hours, with nearly two-thirds of patients having onset within 1–2 hours after lung re-expansion.
- Chest discomfort, persistent severe cough, production of frothy sputum and dyspnoea.
- Signs include tachypnoea, tachycardia and crackles on the affected side of the lung.
- Oedema generally affects the entire re-expanded lung. Occasionally, it may affect a single lobe or the contralateral lung, or it may be a bilateral process.
- A chest radiograph shows features of pulmonary oedema on one side.
- CT shows ipsilateral ground glass opacities, septal thickening, consolidation and persistent areas of atelectasis.
- Mortality is about 20%.

TREATMENT

- Most patients completely recover within 5–7 days with supportive treatment that includes oxygen administration in mild cases to mechanical ventilation in severe cases.
- Patient should lie on his or her unaffected side to help reduce perfusion, oedema and intrapulmonary shunting.

- Role of diuretics, bronchodilators, prostaglandin analogues (e.g. misoprostol), ibuprofen and steroids is controversial.

PREVENTION

- Use of low negative pressure (<-20 cm H_2O) for suction during tube thoracostomy.
- Limiting drainage to about 1–1.5 L of pleural fluid.
- Large volumes can be safely drained as long as pleural pressures are monitored. If the patient reports vague chest pressure during thoracentesis, this may indicate a precipitous drop in intrapleural pressure, and the thoracentesis should be stopped.

Q. What is subpulmonic effusion? How will you diagnose it?

- Subpulmonic effusion is a small pleural effusion lying underneath the lung.
- Clinical detection of subpulmonic effusion is extremely difficult. The only manifestation of a left-sided subpulmonic effusion may be the obliteration of Traube's semilunar space of tympany. A right-sided subpulmonic effusion may be suspected with an abnormal tidal percussion.

RADIOLOGICAL FEATURES OF SUBPULMONIC EFFUSION

- Chest radiograph (posteroanterior view) in the erect posture:
    - Apparent elevation of haemidiaphragm.
    - Lateral displacement and slight flattening of the apparent dome of the diaphragm.
    - A wide density between the gastric air bubble and apparent upper border of the diaphragm (in left-sided subpulmonic effusion).
- Chest radiograph (lateral decubitus view) with the affected side down will show the pleural fluid layering out along the lateral chest wall.
- Ultrasonographic examination can detect a subpulmonic effusion with certainty.

Q. What are the common causes of haemorrhagic pleural effusion? Give a brief account of malignant pleural effusion.

CAUSES OF HAEMORRHAGIC PLEURAL EFFUSION

- Box 2.100 gives some of the causes of haemorrhagic pleural effusion.

BOX 2.100 Causes of Haemorrhagic Pleural Effusion

- Malignancy (including mesothelioma)
- Pulmonary infarction
- Benign asbestos-related pleural effusion
- Tuberculosis (uncommonly)
- Postcardiac injury effusion

DIFFERENTIATION BETWEEN HAEMORRHAGIC EFFUSION AND HAEMOTHORAX

- A haemothorax can be distinguished from haemorrhagic pleural effusions by performing a haematocrit on the pleural fluid. A pleural fluid haematocrit >50% of the patient's peripheral blood haematocrit is diagnostic of a haemothorax.

MALIGNANT PLEURAL EFFUSION

- Malignant effusions are due to either a primary malignancy of pleura (e.g. mesothelioma) or more commonly secondary to invasion of pleura from a primary malignancy elsewhere in the body. Most malignancy-associated effusions occur with lung cancers (35%), breast cancers (25%) and lymphomas (10%).
- The effusion is usually due to the local effects of the tumour, like lymphatic obstruction or bronchial obstruction with pneumonia or atelectasis. It can also be a result of systemic effects of the tumour elsewhere.
- The effusion is usually unilateral, massive and often symptomatic.

CAUSES OF DYSPNOEA IN PATIENTS WITH MALIGNANCY (Box 2.101)

CAUSES OF PLEURAL EFFUSION IN CASE OF LUNG CARCINOMA

- Various causes of pleural effusion in case of lung carcinoma are shown in Table 2.71.

DIAGNOSIS

- The characteristic feature of a malignant pleural effusion is rapid reaccumulation of fluid after aspiration.

BOX 2.101 Causes of Dyspnoea in a Patient With Malignancy

- Pleural effusion
- Lymphangitis carcinomatosis
- Airway obstruction
- Radiation pneumonitis
- Chest wall invasion
- Direct effects of a tumour mass on the lung
- Underlying lung disease
- Pulmonary vascular disease (e.g. pulmonary emboli)
- Cardiac compromise
- Pericardial disease

TABLE 2.71 Causes of Pleural Effusion in Lung Carcinoma

• Local effects of tumour	• Lymphangitis carcinomatosis • Bronchial obstruction producing distal pneumonia • Chylothorax • Superior vena cava syndrome
• Systemic effects of tumour	• Pulmonary embolism • Hypoalbuminaemia
• Miscellaneous	• Metastasis to pleura • Radiation therapy • Chemotherapy

- The pleural fluid is often haemorrhagic, with a high erythrocyte count (>100,000/mm^3). It shows the characteristics of an exudate, like high protein content (>3.0 g/dL), high LDH levels (>200 IU/L), low glucose levels (<60 mg/dL) and a total leucocyte count exceeding 1000/mm^3. The predominant cells in the pleural fluid are lymphocytes (>50%). Clumps of malignant cells may be seen in the pleural fluid on cytological examination.
- Closed pleural biopsy can demonstrate malignancy in about 40% of the cases.

TREATMENT

- Asymptomatic effusions do not require any treatment specific to effusion.
- Mildly symptomatic cases are treated by repeated aspirations.
- Severely symptomatic and recurrent effusions are treated by pleurodesis. This involves instillation of tetracycline hydrochloride, talcum powder, bleomycin or inactivated *Corynebacterium parvum* into the pleural cavity after drainage of fluid through tube thoracostomy. This induces an intense inflammatory reaction in the pleura, followed by extensive pleural adhesions. Talc is more effective than other agents.
- Alternatively, thoracotomy with pleurectomy or pleural abrasion may be tried.

Indwelling Pleural Catheter

- It is a silicone tube that is inserted percutaneously. It has a one-way valve.
- It maintains lung expansion by intermittently draining pleural fluid.
- It is as effective as pleurodesis.
- It can achieve spontaneous pleurodesis in 46%–70% of patients which is caused by local inflammation induced by the tumour or the catheter.

Q. Describe parapneumonic effusion (synpneumonic effusion and post-pneumonic effusion).

- Parapneumonic effusion is a pleural effusion complicating pneumonia or lung abscess.
  - It is more frequent with bacterial pneumonias, especially Gram-negative and pneumococcal. Here, the effusion is large and predominant cells are polymorphs.
  - It is less frequent with viral pneumonias. Here the effusion is small and predominant cells are lymphocytes.
- Parapneumonic effusions have three stages that represent a continuous spectrum. Most patients do not progress beyond the stage of simple parapneumonic effusion.
  1. Benign, simple or sterile parapneumonic effusion forms when lung interstitial fluid increases during pneumonia and moves across the adjacent visceral pleural membrane. It is exudative with influx of neutrophils and is characterised by pH > 7.20, glucose > 60 mg/dL, negative Gram stain and LDH less than three times the normal serum LDH. It resolves with resolution of pneumonia.
  2. Complicated or infected parapneumonic effusion develops when there is bacterial invasion of the pleural space which leads to an increased number of neutrophils, pH < 7.20 and glucose < 60 mg/dL. Pleural fluid cultures are often positive. Deposition of a dense layer of fibrin on both visceral and parietal pleurae can lead to pleural loculation.
     - Another form of complicated parapneumonic effusion is empyema in which the fluid is grossly purulent or shows bacteria on Gram stain.
  3. The third and final stage of pleural infection is the organising, fibrotic phase. During this fibrotic response, pleural space may become focally or massively obliterated and is accompanied by the formation of dense fibrous adhesions. This process eventually results in a thick pleural peel that restricts chest mechanics and often necessitates a surgical decortication so as to address restrictive impairment.

TREATMENT

- Patients with benign parapneumonic effusion may be observed and a repeat tap is done if it persists or increases. If the free fluid separates the lung from the chest wall by >1 cm, a therapeutic thoracentesis should be performed.
- Treatment of underlying pneumonia should proceed on usual lines. Empirical anaerobic antibiotic cover is generally advised, as there may be an anaerobic coinfection. Choices in community-acquired empyema include amoxicillin with clavulanic acid or a combination of a second-generation cephalosporin (e.g. cefuroxime) and metronidazole. Clindamycin monotherapy is an effective alternative for patients with a β-lactam allergy. Patients with nosocomial empyema need adequate Gram-negative cover. Possible choices include carbapenems, antipseudomonal penicillins (e.g. piperacillin/tazobactam), or third- or fourth-generation cephalosporins (e.g. ceftazidime and cefepime) with metronidazole. Vancomycin or linezolid may have to be added for suspected or proven methicillin-resistant *S. aureus* infections. Aminoglycosides demonstrate poor pleural penetration and reduced efficacy in acidic environments and should thus be avoided.
- Complicated parapneumonic effusion (empyema) should be treated by aspiration or thoracotomy tube drainage. If the fluid cannot be completely removed by thoracentesis, a thrombolytic agent (streptokinase—250,000 IU in 100–200 mL saline daily for up to 7 days, or tissue plasminogen activator—10 to 25 mg twice a day for 3 days) may be instilled into the pleural cavity to break the fibrous septa.
- Addition of deoxyribonuclease (DNase) to thrombolytic agents gives better results.
- Decortication should be considered in patients with empyema who do not respond to conservative management.

Q. Write a brief note on chylous pleural effusion (chylothorax).

- Chylous pleural effusion results from leakage of chyle (thoracic duct lymph) into the pleural space. This is commonly associated with lymphomas, lung cancer with mediastinal spread, mediastinal fibrosis and following trauma (Box 2.102).
- The pleural fluid appears milky (Fig. 2.19) and shows the characteristics of an exudate. Sudan III staining of the fluid shows fat globules. Total triglyceride level is more than 110 mg/dL. The cholesterol concentration is very low. Presence of chylomicrons also confirms the diagnosis of a chylothorax.
- Occasionally an empyema can be sufficiently turbid to be confused with chyle. It can be distinguished by centrifugation that leaves a clear supernatant in empyema while chylous effusion remains milky. However, in starved patients, chyle may not appear milky.
- In the absence of trauma, a contrast-enhanced CT for mediastinal structures and a lymphangiogram are required.
- Lymphangiography, lymphoscintigraphy and magnetic resonance lymphangiography are alternative imaging techniques to visualise the lymphatic system.
- Treatment includes chest tube drainage, medium-chain triglycerides in the diet and use of octreotide.
    - Long-chain triglycerides are taken up in the mucosal membrane of intestinal lacteals and the thoracic duct; whereas, absorption of medium-chain triglycerides occurs through the portal vein bypassing the lymphatic system.
    - Octreotide binds to somatostatin receptors and reduces chyle production, lymph flow and intestinal fat absorption.
    - Long-term tube drainage may produce malnutrition and immune deficiency. Therefore, if patient does not respond, a pleuroperitoneal shunt may be tried.
- Other measures include thoracic duct ligation, thoracic duct embolisation or disruption and pleurodesis.

BOX 2.102 Causes of Chylous Pleural Effusion

• Lymphomas	• Lymphangioleiomyomatosis	• Sarcoidosis
• Lung cancer with mediastinal spread	• Lymphangiectasis	• Tuberculosis
• Mediastinal fibrosis	• SVC thrombosis	• Filariasis
• Trauma	• Yellow nail syndrome	

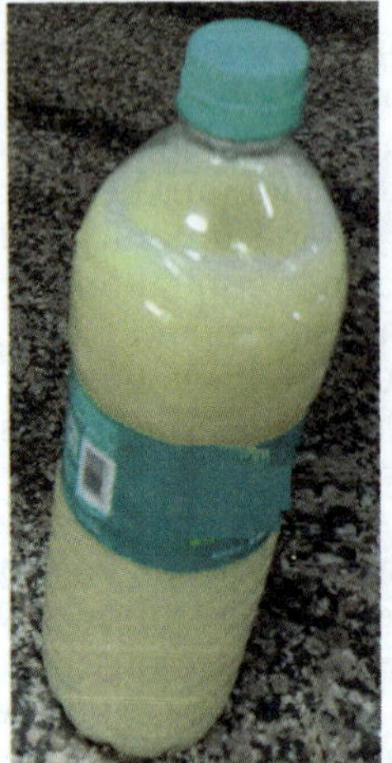

Fig. 2.19 Chylous pleural fluid.

Q. Describe pseudochylous pleural effusion (pseudochylothorax).

- This is a rare condition where the pleural fluid appearance is similar to that of chylous effusion (milky).
- It is seen in long-standing benign pleural effusions—for example tuberculous effusion, rheumatoid effusion.
- The pleural fluid appears milky. Cholesterol content of the fluid is very high (>200 mg/dL), which gives the fluid a milky appearance. Cholesterol crystals can be demonstrated in the fluid. Sudan III staining of the fluid does not show fat globules.

Q. Discuss the aetiology, clinical features, investigations, complications and management of empyema thoracis.

Q. Discuss the management of nontuberculous empyema.

DEFINITION

- Empyema thoracis is a condition in which pus and fluid from infection collects in the pleural cavity. It usually involves whole of the pleural space. If only a part of the pleural space is involved, it is called encysted or loculated empyema.

AETIOLOGY

- Infection of pleural space from neighbouring structures—for example bacterial pneumonias, bronchiectasis, lung abscess, rupture of subphrenic abscess, oesophageal perforation and infection of haemothorax.
- Infection of pleural space from a distant source—for example bacteraemia.
- Infection of pleural space from external source—for example penetrating chest injury, chest tube placement and thoracic surgery.
- The common organisms involved are *Pneumococcus, Streptococcus, Staphylococcus, Pseudomonas, M. tuberculosis, H. influenzae* and anaerobes.

CLINICAL FEATURES

- Patients with aerobic bacterial infection often present with acute onset of symptoms while immunocompromised or elderly patients or those with anaerobic infections present with chronic features.
- Systemic symptoms like high-grade, remittent fever with chills and rigors, malaise and weight loss.

- Respiratory symptoms like pleuritic chest pain, breathlessness and dry cough. Copious and purulent sputum indicates the presence of a bronchopleural fistula.
- Digital clubbing, oedema of the chest wall, intercostal tenderness and signs of fluid in the pleural space.

INVESTIGATIONS

- Polymorphonuclear leucocytosis and raised ESR.
- Chest radiographic findings are similar to those of pleural effusion.
- Aspiration and examination of the pus.
  - The pus may vary from very thin to very thick in consistency.
  - The pus contains large numbers of polymorphonuclear leucocytes.
  - Gram staining may identify the organism.
  - The causative organism may be cultured from the pus.
  - Tubercle bacilli may be seen and culture for tubercle bacilli may be positive in tuberculous empyema.

COMPLICATIONS

- As a rule, complications occur in neglected cases where the pus is not fully removed from the pleural space at an early stage.
- The common complications of empyema are:
  - 'Empyema necessitans'—the pus may track through and point on the chest wall.
  - Rupture through the chest wall forming a sinus.
  - Rupture into a bronchus may result in a bronchopleural fistula and pyopneumothorax.
  - Pleural fibrosis.
  - Metastatic brain abscess.
  - Amyloidosis.

MANAGEMENT OF EMPYEMA THORACIS

NONTUBERCULOUS EMPYEMA

Acute

- Antibiotics should be administered based on the sensitivity of the organism. Empirical anaerobic coverage is often given. Treatment should be aimed at Gram positive aerobes as well as anaerobes, as these organisms have a much lower positive culture yield. Most antibiotics have good pleural penetration except aminoglycosides. Treatment should be continued for at least 4 weeks.
- The pus in the pleural cavity should be drained. Daily aspiration of the fluid with a wide-bore needle can be attempted in an early and small empyema with thin fluid. Tube drainage is required in most cases. If this fails, limited thoracotomy or thoracoscopy is done. Thoracotomy involves resection of a small segment of the rib, clearing the empyema cavity and introducing a wide-bore tube for prolonged drainage.
- Intrapleural administration of fibrinolytic agents (e.g. streptokinase) is done in the case of presence of multiple septae.

Chronic

- Resection of an empyema sac in toto is the procedure of choice in a chronic empyema where no drainage procedure has been attempted before.
- Decortication is the procedure in a chronic empyema which has not responded to open drainage. The procedure involves stripping of whole of the grossly thickened visceral pleura. Thoracotomy allows the lung to re-expand and obliterate the pleural space.

TUBERCULOUS EMPYEMA

- Antituberculous chemotherapy.
- Repeated aspiration through a wide-bore needle or tube drainage.
- Rarely, surgical treatment may be necessary.

Q. Discuss the aetiology, clinical features, types and management of pneumothorax.

Q. Describe tension pneumothorax.

Q. Write a short note on catamenial pneumothorax.

Q. What is clicking pneumothorax? Explain.

DEFINITION

- Presence of air in the pleural cavity is known as pneumothorax.

AETIOLOGY

- Primary (simple) spontaneous pneumothorax:
  - Commonly affects tall, slender males between the ages of 20 and 40 years who are smokers.
  - It is believed to be due to rupture of subpleural blebs at the lung apices.
  - The gradient of negative pleural pressure increases from the lung base to the apex so that alveoli at the lung apex in tall individuals are subject to significantly greater distending pressure than those at the base of the lung and this predisposes to development of apical subpleural blebs.
- Secondary spontaneous pneumothorax occurs in patients with known lung disease (Box 2.103).
- Catamenial pneumothorax (refer to page 236).
- Traumatic pneumothorax:

BOX 2.103 Causes of Secondary Pneumothorax

- Rupture of emphysematous bullae
- Rupture of a subpleural tuberculous focus
- Rupture of a lung abscess, especially staphylococcal
- Bronchial carcinoma
- Pulmonary infarction
- Bronchial asthma
- ARDS
- Chest trauma
- Rare causes—sarcoidosis, *Pneumocystis jirovecii* pneumonia, lymphangioleiomyomatosis [LAM], Marfan's syndrome, cystic fibrosis

- Blunt and penetrating injuries to the chest wall, bronchi, lung or oesophagus.
- Iatrogenic pneumothorax:
  - Following diagnostic or therapeutic interventions (e.g. secondary to transthoracic and transbronchial biopsy, central venous catheterisation, pleural biopsy and thoracentesis).

CLINICAL FEATURES

- A small pneumothorax may be asymptomatic with no abnormal physical signs in the chest.
- Sudden-onset chest pain and dyspnoea are the most common symptoms.
- Patients with secondary pneumothorax are more likely to be symptomatic because of the underlying lung disease.

PHYSICAL SIGNS

- General examination may reveal cyanosis, rapid thready pulse, pulsus paradoxus and signs of peripheral circulatory failure in severe cases.
- Inspection and palpation of respiratory system reveals tachypnoea, shallow breathing, accessory muscles of respiration in action, shift of trachea and mediastinum (apex beat) to the opposite side, fullness of the chest on the affected side, diminished chest movements and markedly diminished vocal fremitus on the affected side. Measurements show a reduction in total chest expansion, increase in the size of the affected hemithorax, diminished expansion of the affected hemithorax and increased spinoscapular distance. Subcutaneous emphysema may be present.
- Percussion note is hyperresonant over the affected hemithorax. In right-sided pneumothorax, liver dullness is obliterated and cardiac dullness is shifted to the opposite side.
- Auscultation reveals markedly diminished-to-absent breath sounds, absence of adventitious sounds and markedly diminished vocal resonance. In an open pneumothorax with a bronchopleural fistula, amphoric bronchial breathing may be heard. Coin test may be positive. Two coins when tapped on the affected side produce a tinkling resonant sound that is audible on auscultation.

RADIOLOGICAL FINDINGS ON CHEST RADIOGRAPH

- Standard erect chest radiograph in inspiration is recommended for the initial diagnosis of pneumothorax rather than expiratory films. The findings are given in Box 2.104.

BOX 2.104 Radiological Findings of Pneumothoarx

- Mediastinal shift to the opposite side
- Sharply defined edge of the deflated lung (Fig. 2.20)
- Complete translucency and absence of bronchovascular markings in the area between the edge of the lung and chest wall
- Presence or absence of a complicating pleural effusion
- Presence or absence of underlying lung lesion

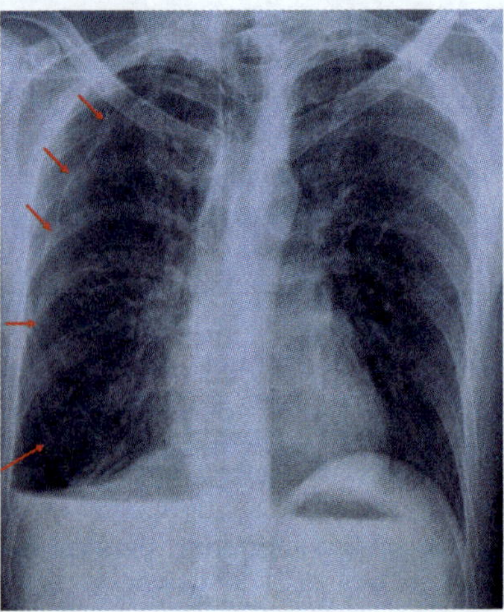

Fig. 2.20 Right-sided hydropneumothorax (arrows show lung margin; horizontal level seen due to presence of both air and fluid).

ULTRASONOGRAPHY

- It provides a rapid, sensitive and specific tool for the diagnosis of pneumothorax. The signs on ultrasound include absence of the pleural sliding, the stratosphere sign and the lung point.

TYPES OF PNEUMOTHORAX

- There are three types of spontaneous pneumothorax (Fig. 2.21):
  1. Closed spontaneous pneumothorax.
  2. Open spontaneous pneumothorax.
  3. Tension (valvular) pneumothorax.

CLOSED SPONTANEOUS PNEUMOTHORAX

- The communication between pleura and lung seals off and does not reopen. Air can neither enter nor leave the pleural space. The trapped air is slowly reabsorbed and the lung re-expands completely in 2–4 weeks.
- Clinically, closed pneumothorax manifests most often as trivial breathlessness that gradually abates over a few days. Pleural space infection is uncommon.

Treatment

- Asymptomatic or slightly breathless patients with small pneumothorax (<2–3 cm from chest wall) need no treatment, but only serial radiographic monitoring is required till the lung re-expands. Spontaneous reabsorption of pneumothoraces has been estimated at 1.25%–1.8% (about 50–70 mL) of the total volume of air in the pleural space per day. Administration of supplemental oxygen reduces the partial pressure of nitrogen in the pleural capillaries and increases air reabsorption from the pleural space.
- If the patient is breathless and the pneumothorax is large, it should be treated actively by one of the following methods:
  - Evacuation of the air using a syringe and needle, a three-way tap and an underwater seal system.

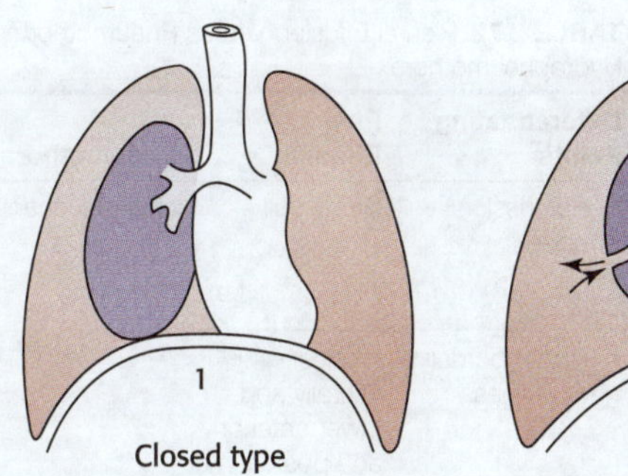

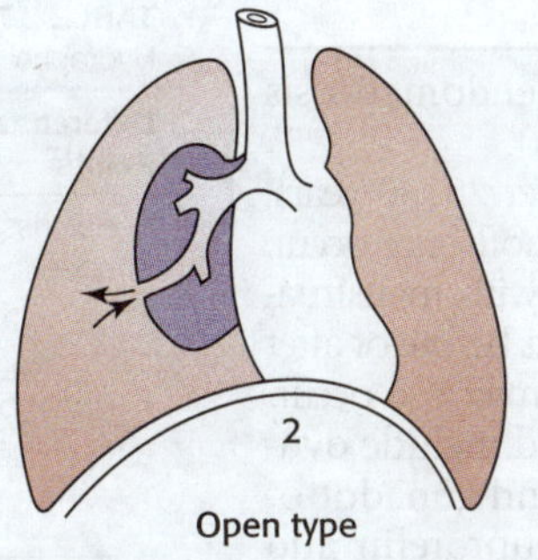

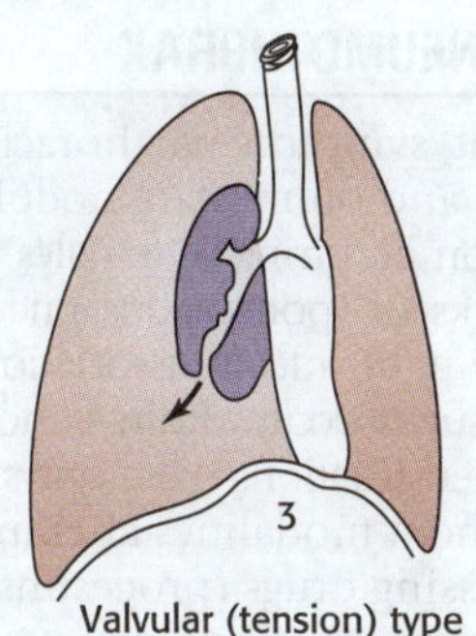

Fig. 2.21 Types of spontaneous pneumothorax.

- Inserting a chest tube into the pleural cavity and connecting it to a water seal drainage system or a nonreturn valve.
- Recurrence rates can be as high as 50% in spontaneous pneumothorax and can be reduced if an agent such as talc is instilled through a chest tube or through thoracoscopy.

OPEN SPONTANEOUS PNEUMOTHORAX

- The communication between bronchus and pleura does not seal off and remains patent, resulting in a 'bronchopleural fistula'. Since air can freely flow through the bronchopleural fistula, intrapleural pressure and atmospheric pressure remain the same throughout the respiratory cycle. This prevents re-expansion of the collapsed lung. In addition, bronchopleural fistula facilitates spread of infection into the pleural space resulting in empyema. Penetrating trauma of chest can produce open, secondary pneumothorax with communication to atmosphere (open 'sucking' wound).
- Open pneumothorax usually follows rupture of an emphysematous bulla, a small pleural bleb, a tuberculous cavity or a lung abscess into the pleural space.
- Clinically, the patient presents with breathlessness. If pleural space infection sets in, fever and systemic disturbances ensue. The physical signs are those of air and fluid in the pleural space (hydropneumothorax).

Treatment

- This form of pneumothorax usually requires surgical closure, though a trial with chest tube insertion with low-pressure suction may be tried. Various modalities of surgical closure are the following:
  - Cauterisation of the opening.
  - Video-assisted thoracoscopic surgery (VATS) may be used for cutting and release of adhesions that prevent the closure of the fistula.
  - Open thoracotomy and direct closure of the fistula.
- Open 'sucking' chest wound is treated initially with a three-sided occlusive dressing to prevent occurrence of tension pneumothorax, following which tube thoracostomy is required.

TENSION (VALVULAR) PNEUMOTHORAX

- The communication between pleura and lung persists. It acts as a one-way valve allowing air to enter the pleural space during inspiration, coughing, sneezing and straining but not allowing it to escape. Large amount of air gets 'trapped' in the pleural space and the intrapleural pressure becomes much higher than the atmospheric pressure.
- The high intrapleural pressure results in compression of the underlying lung, as well as gross shift of the mediastinum to the opposite side with consequent compression of the opposite lung also. It also reduces venous return by compressing the vena cavae.
- Clinically, these patients present with rapidly progressive breathlessness, central cyanosis, rapid thready pulse and signs of peripheral circulatory failure. Frank signs of pneumothorax are present. Jugular venous distention is present. Death can occur within few minutes from asphyxia.
- Typical clinical situations where a tension pneumothorax may develop include the following:
  - Ventilated patients (invasive or noninvasive).
  - Traumatic chest injuries.
  - During cardiopulmonary resuscitation.
  - Lung disease, especially acute presentations of asthma and COPD.
  - Blocked, clamped or displaced chest drains.
  - Patients undergoing hyperbaric oxygen treatment.

Treatment

- Tension pneumothorax is an acute medical emergency.
- Emergency treatment is the introduction of a wide-bore plastic cannula in the fifth intercostal space (in mid-axillary line) attached to a long rubber tubing, the end of which is placed underwater in a bottle.
- If patient is not haemodynamically compromised, alternative is the introduction of an intercostal catheter connected to a water seal drainage system.
- If nothing is available, simple stab on chest wall is sufficient to release pressure.

RECURRENT SPONTANEOUS PNEUMOTHORAX

- Recurrent episodes of pneumothorax are common in patients with emphysematous bullae. The episodes usually occur on the same side. They can also occur with LAM.
- The treatment includes obliteration of the pleural space by artificial pleurodesis. This can be accomplished by intrapleural instillation of an irritant like tetracycline hydrochloride or talc powder. Alternatively, pleural abrasion or parietal pleurectomy may be attempted.

CATAMENIAL PNEUMOTHORAX

- Most frequent symptom is thoracic endometriosis (haemoptysis and pulmonary nodules).
- A rare condition occurring in females over 25–30 years. Repeated attacks of spontaneous pneumothorax occur, usually on the right side, in association with menstruation. Attacks usually occur within 48 hours before or after the onset of menstruation. Haemoptysis may also occur.
- Various treatment modalities attempted include ovulation-suppressing drugs (progestins and gonadotropin-releasing hormone analogues—leuprorelin and triptorelin), surgical exploration and pleurodesis.

CLICKING PNEUMOTHORAX

- A small left-sided pneumothorax may get localised in front of the pericardium. This may alter the heart sounds to make them sound loud and resonant ('clicking').

Q. What are the physical signs of hydropneumothorax?

- Fig. 2.22 shows hydropneumothorax with bronchopleural fistula which allows air entry and exit during inspiration and expiration
- Inspection and palpation:
  - Tracheal and mediastinal shift (apex beat) to the opposite side.
  - Fullness of chest on the affected side, with bulging of lower intercostal spaces.
  - Diminished chest movements and vocal fremitus on the affected side.
  - Affected hemithorax is usually bigger than the other.
  - Expansion of the affected hemithorax is reduced.
  - Spinoscapular distance is increased on the affected side.
- Percussion:
  - Percussion note is hyperresonant over the upper air-containing part and stony dull over the lower fluid-containing part.
  - The upper border of the stony dullness is horizontal or straight. Shifting dullness can be elicited.
- Auscultation:
  - Breath sounds are absent over the entire hemithorax if there is no bronchopleural communication.
  - If a bronchopleural fistula is present, breath sounds are audible over the upper air-containing part. However, the intensity of breath sounds is diminished and it usually has an amphoric character.
  - Metallic crepitations may be heard over the upper air-containing part.
  - Vocal resonance is reduced over the entire affected hemithorax.
  - Coin test is positive over the upper air-containing part.
  - Succussion splash can be elicited on the affected side.

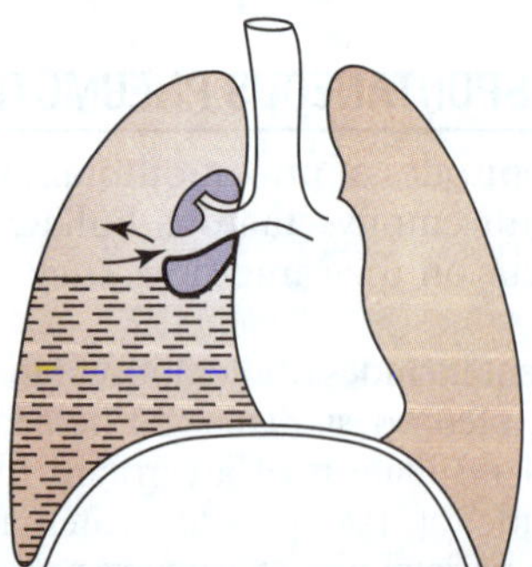

Fig. 2.22 Hydropneumothorax with bronchopleural fistula.

TABLE 2.72 Pleural Effusion Versus Pneumothorax Versus Hydropneumothorax

Differentiating Points	Pleural Effusion	Pneumothorax	Hydropneumothorax
• Percussion note	Stony dull	Hyperresonant	Hyperresonant over upper part, stony dull over lower part
• Upper border of dullness	Highest laterally and lower anteriorly and posteriorly	—	Straight or horizontal
• Shifting dullness	Absent	—	Present
• Bronchial breathing	Tubular (above the level of effusion)	Amphoric (with BP fistula)	Amphoric (with BP fistula)
• Coin test	Negative	Positive	Positive
• Succussion splash	Absent	Absent	Present
• Aegophony and whispering pectoriloquy	Present above the level of effusion	Absent	Absent

Q. How can you clinically differentiate pleural effusion from pneumothorax and hydropneumothorax?

- Features which help in differentiating pleural effusion, pneumothorax and hydropneumothorax are given in Table 2.72.

Q. How will you differentiate haemoptysis from haematemesis?

- Features which help in differentiating haemoptysis from haematemesis are shown in Table 2.73.

TABLE 2.73 Haemoptysis Versus Haematemesis

Haemoptysis	Haematemesis
• Prodrome of tingling in the throat or a desire to cough	• Prodrome of nausea and abdominal discomfort
• Blood is coughed out	• Blood is vomited out
• Blood mixed with sputum	• Blood mixed with food particles
• Bright red and frothy blood	• Magenta-coloured blood
• pH is normal as of blood	• pH is acidic
• Symptoms and signs of respiratory disease	• Symptoms and signs of gastrointestinal disease
• Confirmed by bronchoscopy	• Confirmed by upper GI endoscopy

2

Q. Define haemoptysis. What are the common causes of haemoptysis?

Q. Outline the management of a case of haemoptysis.

Q. Discuss the management of massive (potentially lethal) haemoptysis.

DEFINITION

- Haemoptysis is defined as the expectoration of blood or bloody sputum.
- 'Potentially lethal' or 'massive' haemoptysis is defined as greater than 600–800 mL blood in 24 hours. A more clinical and practical definition of massive haemoptysis is any bleeding that results in a threat to life because of airway or haemodynamic compromise by bleeding.

PATHOPHYSIOLOGY

- The lungs receive their blood supply via the pulmonary arterial circulation and the systemic bronchial arteries.
- More than 90% of cases of haemoptysis result from disruption of branches of bronchial arteries.
- Bronchial artery neovascularisation is the most common pathway for haemoptysis and generally results from diseases that cause pulmonary arteriole occlusion from hypoxic vasoconstriction, thrombosis or vasculitis.
- In bronchitis or fungal infections, acute or chronic inflammation creates tortuous ectatic vessels through neovascularisation that are prone to rupture.
- Pulmonary parenchymal necrosis from necrotising pneumonia or infarction of lung from pulmonary embolism, and inflammatory and immunological vasculitides can also lead to haemorrhage by exposing the capillary bed.
- Haemoptysis in tuberculosis has been discussed elsewhere.

CAUSES (Table 2.74)

- Bevacizumab, a vascular endothelial growth factor angiogenesis inhibitor, if used in the treatment of central squamous carcinomas of the lung may result in massive haemoptysis.

TABLE 2.74 Causes of Haemoptysis

Common Causes	Uncommon Causes
• Pulmonary tuberculosis • Bronchial carcinoma • Chronic bronchitis • Bronchiectasis • Lung abscess • Pneumonia (particularly *Klebsiella*) • Fungal infections (aspergilloma and invasive aspergillosis) • Pulmonary contusion/ laceration (traumatic)	• Pulmonary thromboembolism • Left ventricular failure • Mitral stenosis • Bronchial carcinoid • Pulmonary arteriovenous malformations • Primary pulmonary hypertension • Goodpasture's syndrome • Wegener's granulomatosis • Idiopathic pulmonary haemosiderosis • Haemorrhagic diathesis (disseminated intravascular coagulation, thrombocytopenia, von Willebrand disease, platelet dysfunction) • Drugs and toxins (bevacizumab, cocaine, nitrofurantoin, anticoagulants, antiplatelets) • Aortic aneurysm (aortobronchial fistula) • Penetrating or blunt chest trauma

INVESTIGATIONS

- In massive haemoptysis, initial diagnostic tests must begin in concert with efforts to stabilise the patient and control the bleeding.
- Blood should be examined for haemoglobin level, total and differential leucocyte counts, erythrocyte sedimentation rate (ESR) and blood group. In addition, clotting screen including platelet count should be done if a haemorrhagic diathesis is suspected.
- Urine should be examined by microscopy for red cells and red cell casts in suspected haemorrhagic diathesis and Goodpasture's syndrome.
- Sputum should be examined in all cases by microscopy and culture.
  - Ziehl–Neelsen staining may show acid-fast bacilli in pulmonary tuberculosis.
  - *K. pneumoniae* may be isolated from the sputum in *Klebsiella* pneumonia.
  - Cytological examination for malignant cells in suspected bronchial carcinoma.
  - Sputum studies may be helpful in identifying the pathogenic organism in acute exacerbations of chronic bronchitis, bronchiectasis and lung abscess.
- Chest radiographs, both posteroanterior and lateral views, can provide important diagnostic clues.
  - Presence of cystic lesions, ring shadows, tram tracks and grape clusters favours the diagnosis of bronchiectasis.
  - A distinct air–fluid level in a cavity is diagnostic of lung abscess.
  - Fibrotic bands, bronchiectatic changes, cavity formation or fluffy shadows in the upper lobes suggest pulmonary tuberculosis.
  - Rarely, an intracavitary aspergilloma is visible on chest radiograph as a cavity with a tumour-like opacity inside. A crescentic air shadow separates the fungal ball from the upper wall of cavity.
  - Upper lobe consolidation with bulging interlobar fissure is characteristic of *Klebsiella* pneumonia.
  - Bronchial carcinoma may manifest as central or peripheral pulmonary opacity, mediastinal widening, collapse of a lung or a lobe, or consolidation.
  - Chest radiographs can be useful at times in pulmonary thromboembolism, mitral stenosis, primary pulmonary hypertension and pulmonary haemosiderosis.
- Computed tomography of the chest is useful in delineating lesions that are not seen on a plain radiograph. It also better defines the lesions seen on radiograph.
- Electrocardiogram may be useful in unsuspected mitral stenosis, pulmonary thromboembolism and pulmonary hypertension.
- Bronchoscopy is the most important diagnostic procedure. Rigid bronchoscopy permits visualisation of

the more central airways, whereas fibreoptic bronchoscopy permits visualisation of the more peripheral airways. In addition to localising the site of bleeding, bronchoscopy provides definitive visual, biopsy or cytological information.
- CT pulmonary angiography if pulmonary embolism is suspected.
- CT bronchial angiography if bleeding site is not detected using a CT chest.

TREATMENT

MINOR HAEMOPTYSIS

- Minor haemoptysis, which is scanty, will stop spontaneously without specific therapy. Treatment is aimed at the underlying cause. Tranexamic acid can be given in mild to moderate haemoptysis.
- Substantial haemoptysis should be treated by keeping the patient calm, instituting complete bed rest and suppressing the cough. However, intubation and suction equipment should be ready at the bedside.

POTENTIALLY LETHAL OR MASSIVE HAEMOPTYSIS

- Position the patient so that the side of the chest from which bleeding is arising is lowermost. This is to prevent asphyxiation due to aspiration of blood into the normal lung. If the location of bleeding is undetermined or the patient prefers, an upright position is also acceptable during this initial phase of management.
- Set up an intravenous infusion and collect blood for grouping and cross-matching. Maintain a chart of vital signs including blood pressure, pulse rate, respiratory rate and urine output.
- Administer oxygen.
- Blood transfusions are given according to the usual clinical guidelines of quantity of blood lost, haematocrit, blood pressure, pulse rate and urine output.
- Strong sedatives should be avoided, but mild sedatives may be given to relieve anxiety.
- Distressing cough may be suppressed with linctus codeine 15 mL thrice daily.
- Consider endotracheal intubation if the patient has poor gas exchange, has rapid ongoing haemoptysis, is haemodynamically unstable or has severe shortness of breath.
- An alternative strategy is to place an endotracheal tube into either the right or left mainstem bronchus. This is easier to achieve with bleeding from the left lung when selective intubation of the right mainstem bronchus is required.
- Double-lumen endotracheal tube allows the two lungs to be isolated and ventilated separately.
- Correction of coagulopathy.
- Role of tranexamic acid, an antifibrinolytic agent, is controversial, though most physicians would use it intravenously in massive haemoptysis.
- Consider emergency bronchoscopy if the bleeding is torrential.
  - The rigid bronchoscope is preferred as it enables blood to be aspirated more easily.
  - The fibreoptic bronchoscope may be used for cold saline lavage, which may sometimes arrest bleeding. The iced saline is instilled in 50–100 mL aliquots followed by suctioning and repeated until there is noticeable improvement. Other techniques used to control bleeding include:
    - Topical thrombin or fibrinogen.
    - Topical coagulation with laser photocoagulation (Nd:YAG).
    - Argon plasma coagulator.
    - Endobronchial brachytherapy in high doses (10–12 Gy/hour for a total of 500–4000 Gy).
    - Endobronchial cryotherapy.
  - A balloon catheter passed through the bronchoscope can be inflated proximally in the bleeding bronchus. This will isolate the source of bleeding from the rest of the lung and the contralateral lung, preventing asphyxiation by blood flooding.
- Bronchial arterial catheterisation and embolisation can at least temporarily arrest bleeding. Embolisation is performed using absorbable gelatin sponge or polyvinyl alcohol particles between 325 and 500 μm. The most important complication is spinal cord ischaemia.
- Surgical intervention is indicated in selected cases. Emergency resection of the lobe or lung, which is bleeding, may be necessary.

Q. Discuss briefly the differential diagnosis of acute-onset dyspnoea.

- Dyspnoea, defined as an uncomfortable awareness of breathing, is a subjective sensation for which there is no accurate objective measurement.
- Acute dyspnoea is defined as dyspnoea arising over the course of a few minutes to 24–48 hours.

COMMON CAUSES

- Common causes of acute onset dyspnoea are given in Box 2.105.

DIFFERENTIAL DIAGNOSIS

CARDIOGENIC PULMONARY OEDEMA

- History: A history of long-standing hypertension, ischaemic heart disease or valvular heart disease may be present. The characteristic symptoms of heart failure like exertional dyspnoea, orthopnoea, paroxysmal

BOX 2.105 Common Causes of Acute Onset Dyspnoea

- Cardiogenic pulmonary oedema
- Acute bronchial asthma
- Spontaneous pneumothorax
- Acute pulmonary embolism
- ARDS
- Laryngeal obstruction
- Hysterical hyperventilation syndrome
- Sympathetic crashing acute pulmonary oedema (SCAPE)
- Others: Guillain–Barré syndrome, myasthenia gravis, neurotoxic snake bite (krait, cobra), acute poisoning (organophosphate, hydrocarbon, botulism, carbon monoxide, toxin-related metabolic acidosis)
- Acute anaemia

nocturnal dyspnoea and nocturia may precede the attack of acute breathlessness by days or weeks. Acute dyspnoea is usually associated with cough and pink frothy expectoration.
- Physical findings: Acute breathlessness is associated with profuse sweating, cyanosis, tachypnoea, tachycardia and pulsus alternans. There may be cardiomegaly with the apex beat shifted downwards and outwards, third heart sound (S_3) or a summation gallop. Examination of lungs reveals bilateral fine crepitations, predominantly basal. Other clinical evidences of long-standing hypertension (fundal changes and loud A_2 component of second heart sound), ischaemic heart disease (dyskinetic segment at or around cardiac apex, murmur of mitral regurgitation due to papillary muscle dysfunction and arrhythmias) or valvular heart disease (murmurs) may be present.
- The diagnosis can be confirmed by electrocardiogram, chest radiography, echocardiography, lung ultrasound, N-terminal pro-brain natriuretic peptide (NT-proBNP) and angiography.

ACUTE BRONCHIAL ASTHMA

- History: Usually, previous history of similar attacks may be present. There may be family history of bronchial asthma, chronic eczema or allergic rhinitis in atopic individuals. A precipitating event like exposure to cold air or dust, respiratory infections, exercise, emotional stress, or intake of drugs like aspirin or propranolol may be identified.
- Physical findings: A severe attack is usually associated with cyanosis, tachycardia, tachypnoea and pulsus paradoxus.
- Examination of the respiratory system may reveal a hyperresonant percussion note and extensive bilateral rhonchi. A very severe attack may be associated with a 'silent chest'.

SPONTANEOUS PNEUMOTHORAX

- History: The usual history is sudden onset of chest pain and dyspnoea, usually following strenuous exertion or coughing. History related to a predisposing disease like emphysema, lung abscess, bronchial asthma, pulmonary tuberculosis or bronchial carcinoma may be present.
- Physical findings: The patient is usually severely dyspnoeic and tachypnoeic, with cyanosis, sweating, tachycardia, rapid thready pulse and signs of peripheral circulatory failure. Physical signs of pneumothorax include mediastinal shift (apex beat and trachea) to opposite side, fullness of the affected hemithorax, diminished respiratory movements and diminished vocal fremitus and vocal resonance. The percussion note is hyperresonant and cardiac dullness is shifted to the opposite side. Auscultation reveals markedly diminished to absent breath sounds. Physical signs related to the predisposing disease may be evident.
- Diagnosis of tension pneumothorax is clinical and one should not wait for chest radiography and ABG studies.

ACUTE PULMONARY EMBOLISM

- History: A characteristic clinical setting such as prolonged immobilisation, recent surgery, congestive heart failure or recent trauma may be present. Oral contraceptives, sickle cell anaemia and polycythaemia are associated with increased incidence of pulmonary embolism. The usual history is acute-onset breathlessness and chest pain, occasionally associated with blood-tinged sputum.
- Physical findings: Respiratory findings include crepitations over the involved area, a pleural friction rub and evidence of pleural effusion. Cardiac findings include signs of right ventricular failure, including a right-sided third heart sound, early diastolic murmur of pulmonary regurgitation or increased intensity of the pulmonary component (P_2) of second heart sound.
- Diagnosis can be confirmed by electrocardiogram, chest radiography, echocardiography, lung scans and pulmonary arteriography.

ACUTE RESPIRATORY DISTRESS SYNDROME

- History: Characteristic history is acute breathlessness in a patient with an underlying disease. The usual underlying causes are pneumonias, inhalation and aspiration of toxic and irritant substances, septicaemia, eclampsia, DIC, lung embolism, trauma, certain drugs and acute pancreatitis.
- Physical findings: Dominant features are those of the underlying disease. There will be hypotension, hypoxaemia and bilateral crepitations, especially basal.
- Diagnosis can be confirmed by chest radiography and ABG studies.

LARYNGEAL OBSTRUCTION

- Acute laryngeal obstruction may follow anaphylactic reactions to drugs (penicillin, foreign proteins, etc.) and foreign body inhalation. Foreign bodies produce a picture of acute asphyxia characterised by cyanosis, stridor, violent but ineffective inspiratory efforts and indrawing of intercostal spaces. If untreated, the patient may progress to coma and death.
- Foreign body should be removed by direct laryngoscopy.

HYSTERICAL HYPERVENTILATION SYNDROME

- History: This commonly occurs in young females, often associated with a recent emotional upset. In addition to acute dyspnoea, patients usually complain of tingling sensation around the mouth (circumoral paraesthesia), fingers and toes. Carpopedal spasms may occur.
- Physical findings: Physical examination reveals no evidence of cardiopulmonary disease. Tachypnoea and occasionally tachycardia may be present.

SYMPATHETIC CRASHING ACUTE PULMONARY OEDEMA

- Severe acute heart failure which presents with dramatic onset and rapid progression of symptoms of pulmonary oedema (flash pulmonary oedema).
- A subset of hypertensive heart failure.
- Occurs due to sudden increase in sympathetic tone.
- Presents with abrupt onset of dyspnoea which progresses over minutes to hours.
- Develops over minutes producing life-threatening pulmonary oedema.

- Blood pressure is elevated (usually above 180/120).
- Treatment includes noninvasive ventilation with careful monitoring, high-dose intravenous nitroglycerine (NTG) and, if required, invasive ventilation. Typical dose of NTG is 500 µg over 2 minutes followed by 100 µg/minute as infusion till systolic blood pressure is reduced to less than 140 mmHg. Then infusion dose is rapidly reduced. Close haemodynamic monitoring is required.
- No role of diuretics.

Q. What are the borders of Traube's space? How is it clinically significant?

- Traube's space is a semilunar area of tympanitic note, located at the left lower chest anteriorly. It is bounded by the normal lung resonance above, costal margin below, spleen on left side and left lobe of the liver on right side.
- Surface marking:
    - Draw two vertical lines, one passing through the sixth rib in the midclavicular line and the next passing through the ninth rib in midaxillary lines.
    - Now draw a smooth curving line with convexity upwards from the sixth rib in midclavicular line to ninth rib in midaxillary line.
    - Draw another straight line passing through the costal margin from sixth rib to ninth rib.
- Traube's space is normally occupied by the fundus of stomach with air inside, which gives the tympanitic note on percussion (done from medial to lateral side).
- Traube's space is obliterated in pericardial effusion, left pleural effusion, fundal tumours and enlargement of left lobe of liver or spleen. Also obliterated when patient is full stomach.
- A left lung mass lesion/consolidation alone never produces impairment as lung does not extend to Traube's space.

MCQs

IM3.2|PA26.1

1. A 65-year-old man with a history of cigarette and alcohol consumption for 30 years has fever, cough, chest pain, nausea, vomiting and diarrhoea. Among the laboratory's findings are a hyponatraemia and a hypophosphataemia at their limit. Chest X-ray is more compatible with atypical pneumonia. Test for detection of *Legionella pneumophila* antigen in urine is positive. Which of the following is the characteristic of intracellular parasitism of *L. pneumophila*?

Options:

A. Escape from the phagosome and transfection by polymerisation of the host cell
B. Phagocytosis by rolling up with recruitment of cellular organelles
C. Apoptosis of macrophages
D. Multiplication within the lysosomes
E. Prevention of phagolysosome acidification

Ans: B. Phagocytosis by rolling up with recruitment of cellular organelles

This is in fact the type of phagocytosis characteristic of *L. pneumophila*. Macrophages swallow microorganisms in a rolled-up vesicle that does not acidify. The bacterium can also prevent the fusion of the phagosome with the lysosome.

A is incorrect. This is the immune system evasion mechanism used by *Listeria monocytogenes* and some species of *Shigella*.

C is incorrect. *Salmonella* can induce programmed cell death of macrophages. In addition, the microorganism can block fusion of the phagosome with the lysosome, a frequent way to prevent intracellular death.

D is incorrect. This is a characteristic of the intracellular survival of *Leishmania*.

E is incorrect. The *Mycobacterium tuberculosis* uses this strategy to evade the host immune system and avoid being lysed by macrophages.

IM7.1

IM7.10

2. A 64-year-old woman presented with a mild increase in shortness of breath. She had a 10-year history of limited cutaneous systemic sclerosis. She was positive for anticentromere antibody. She was otherwise well. On cardiovascular examination, there was nothing abnormal to find.

Investigations: Forced vital capacity 95% of predicted (unchanged over 1 year), forced expiratory volume in 1 second 97% of predicted (unchanged over 1 year), diffusing capacity for carbon monoxide 68% of predicted (89% 1 year previously). What is the most likely cause for her breathlessness?

A. Pulmonary fibrosis
B. Pulmonary arterial hypertension
C. Chest wall constriction
D. Multiple small pulmonary emboli
E. Central airway obstruction from cartilage degeneration

Ans: B. Pulmonary arterial hypertension

Around 10%–15% of patients with systemic sclerosis develop pulmonary arterial hypertension, often late in the disease, and the patient is at increased risk of this condition as there is anticentromere antibody positivity. The key factors here are the falling diffusing capacity for carbon monoxide but normal forced vital capacity (a common finding in pulmonary arterial hypertension), and the fact that she was well otherwise with nothing to find on examination.

IM3.7

3. A 32-year-old woman presented to the emergency department. She was 14 weeks pregnant and reported a 2-day history of shortness of breath, sharp right-sided chest pain, fever and chills. On examination, her heart rate was 130 beats/minute, blood pressure 89/44 mmHg, respiratory rate 22 per minute and oxygen saturation 91% on air. Her temperature was 37.8 °C. On auscultation of the chest, there

were some crackles at the right base. Which imaging modality should be performed next?
A. CT pulmonary angiogram
B. Doppler studies of the legs
C. Nuclear medicine perfusion scan
D. Chest X-ray
E. Echocardiogram

Ans: D. Chest X-ray

This patient has symptoms and signs of pneumonia, and a Chest X-ray is the most appropriate form of imaging to confirm this. She has features of sepsis and needs prompt assessment and treatment.

CT1.2, CT1.10

4. A 53-year-old man presented with back pain and night sweats. He was originally from Kenya. On clinical examination, there was tenderness over the lower thoracic region of the back. X-rays of the spine showed nonspecific changes; MR scan of the spine showed an epidural abscess with no spinal cord compromise. Aspirate from the abscess showed *M. tuberculosis* bacilli. What is the most appropriate investigation to assess for infectivity?
A. Chest X-ray
B. Tuberculin test
C. Interferon-γ release assay
D. Early-morning urine specimens for acid-fast bacilli (AFB)
E. Sputum specimens for AFB

Ans: E. Sputum specimens for AFB

It is always important to check for pulmonary TB in anyone diagnosed with extrapulmonary tuberculosis as TB can be present at more than one site, and pulmonary disease has infection control implications.

5. A 65-year-old man is being preassessed for an open abdominal aortic aneurysm repair. He has a past history of chronic obstructive pulmonary disease (on inhalers), hypertension and type 2 diabetes mellitus. What is the best measure available to assess the efficiency of oxygen uptake and transport in this patient?
A. Spirometry
B. Cardiopulmonary exercise testing
C. Haemoglobin saturation
D. Stress echocardiography
E. Resting heart rate

Ans: B. Cardiopulmonary exercise testing

This is a dynamic test of oxygen transport and delivery which also gives some data on functional capacity.

IM24.10

6. A 67-year-old man is admitted to the emergency department complaining of a 2–3 day history of breathlessness. His admission SpO2 is 80% on room air. On examination, he has central cyanosis with grade 2 clubbing. He has a barrel-shaped chest and auscultation reveals expiratory wheeze. His cardiac examination is normal. His respiratory rate is 28 breaths/min and only medication is codeine 30 mg thrice a day for back pain. What is the most likely cause for his desaturation?
A. Opiate-mediated respiratory depression
B. Eisenmenger's syndrome
C. Pulmonary fibrosis
D. Chronic obstructive pulmonary disease
E. Basal atelectasis

Ans: D. Chronic obstructive pulmonary disease

This is due to mismatch of hypoxic areas and blood flow following progressive airway dilation and gas trapping in response to inflammation.

IM24.10

7. A 59-year-old man presents with a chronic cough and shortness of breath. He has a 30 pack-year history of smoking. A diagnosis of chronic obstructive pulmonary disease is suspected and he is sent for respiratory function tests. Which finding would support this diagnosis?
A. Reduced FEV1 and FVC with normal ratio
B. Reduced total lung capacity (TLC)
C. Increased residual volume (RV)
D. Increased FEV1:FVC ratio
E. Decreased residual volume of lung (RV)

Ans: C. Increased residual volume (RV)

Typical of COPD where there is increased lung compliance (decreased elastic recoil) and gas trapping related to dynamic pressure-dependent airway closure.

CT1.9

8. A previously healthy 12-year-old girl who recently arrived from Afghanistan as a refugee is seen for a chronic cough, which has been going on for a year. The cough is productive, and she has noticed blood in her sputum on occasion. She has also been waking up drenched in sweat. Her mother is concerned about her weight loss. Sputum samples sent for acid-fast bacilli screening have come back positive. A chest radiograph was also requested. Which of the following is most likely to be seen on the chest radiograph?
A. Cavities
B. An ill-defined mass
C. Cardiomegaly
D. Collapse of the right upper lobe
E. Bullae

Ans: A. Cavities

This girl has active pulmonary tuberculosis; she is infectious and requires treatment. The fever, night sweats and weight loss are typical. Haemoptysis is suggestive of disease affecting the lung parenchyma, with a possible consequence of cavitating lesions.

IM24.10

9. A 55-year-old heavy smoker presents to his GP requesting antibiotics for his cough. It is noted that he is a frequent attendee for the same problem. Upon further questioning, he admits to having occasional wheezing episodes and exertional dyspnoea. On examination, he has a barrel chest and quiet breath sounds throughout both lung fields and a PEFR of 200 L/min. He is sent for

lung function tests which showed a reduced FEV1 and VC. What is the most likely diagnosis?
A. Sarcoidosis
B. Asthma
C. Asbestosis
D. Alpha-1 antitrypsin deficiency
E. Chronic obstructive pulmonary disease (COPD)

Ans: E. Chronic obstructive pulmonary disease (COPD)

The clinical features of COPD are essentially productive cough, breathlessness and, in some patients, respiratory failure and cor pulmonale. Chronic bronchitis is defined clinically as chronic cough and sputum for at least 3 months each year for 2 consecutive years. Spirometry will show the following: reduced FEV1 and VC, reduced FEV1:VC ratio (i.e. the FEV1 is more reduced than the VC).

IM1.8

10. A 78-year-old woman presents with a 4-hour history of a unilateral acutely painful, pale, cold lower leg. On examination, no popliteal or foot pulses are palpable, and she is unable to move the foot or toes. An ECG shows atrial fibrillation. You diagnose an acute ischaemic limb. What is the most appropriate management?
A. Angioplasty
B. Below knee amputation
C. Systemic thrombolysis
D. Embolectomy
E. Femoral-popliteal bypass

Ans: D. Embolectomy

Embolectomy via a Fogarty catheter is the treatment of choice in this situation.

IM7.1

11. A 50-year-old woman presents with symptoms of fatigue and tiredness. She has also experienced prolonged constipation and shortness of breath on exercise. Auscultation of her chest reveals fine inspiratory crackles over the upper zones. Her relevant investigations revealed total calcium of 11.8 mg/dL and Chest X-ray showed bilateral hilar lymphadenopathy. What is the most likely diagnosis?
A. Multiple myeloma
B. Carcinoma of the bronchus
C. Parathyroid adenoma
D. Sarcoidosis
E. Hyperthyroidism

Ans: D. Sarcoidosis

Sarcoid is a multisystemic noncaseating granulomatous disorder. Macrophages within the granuloma activate vitamin D, resulting in increased activated vitamin D levels, leading to hypercalcaemia.

IM7.1

12. A 59-year-old man complains of increasing dyspnoea over 18 months and an itchy, painful rash over the legs and ankles for one week. On examination, there is parotid gland enlargement and hepatosplenomegaly. Chest X-ray shows bilateral hilar lymphadenopathy. Serum calcium is 11.2 mg/dL. What is the most appropriate diagnosis?
A. Hyperparathyroidism
B. Multiple myeloma
C. Paget's disease
D. Sarcoidosis
E. Squamous cell carcinoma

Ans: D. Sarcoidosis

Sarcoidosis has hilar lymphadenopathy on Chest X-ray with or without parenchymal lung lesions. Hypercalcaemia is due to macrophage production of 1,25 dihydroxyvitamin D.

3 Immunological Factors in Disease

Q. What are the body's defence mechanisms?

- The first line of defence against pathogens is the epithelial barrier—skin and mucosa. Other first-line defences include commensal flora and acidic gastric contents.
- The second line of defence system is provided by the immune system. Cells of immune system originate from the stem cells in bone marrow. Immune system is divided into two functionally distinct systems:
  1. Innate or nonspecific immune system.
  2. Adaptive or specific immune system.
- Table 3.1 lists the defence mechanisms in humans.
- Fig. 3.1 summarises innate and adaptive immune systems.

TABLE 3.1 Defence Mechanisms in Humans

First Line of Defence	Second Line of Defence: Innate or Nonspecific Defence	Second Line of Defence: Adaptive or Specific defence
• Skin • Mucous membranes • Commensal flora on various parts of body • Acidic gastric contents	• Phagocytic cells • Inflammatory response • Antimicrobial peptides	• T Lymphocytes • B lymphocytes (antibodies)

Q. Discuss briefly about innate or nonspecific immunity. (MI 1.8)

- Refers to inborn resistance to pathogens that does not require activation of immune system or adaptation upon exposure to them. The resistance is static, that is it does not improve with repeated exposure.
- Provides almost immediate protection against invading pathogens.
- Limited capacity to distinguish one microbe from another. Response is mostly focused on a limited set of microbial determinants shared by a large number of pathogens.

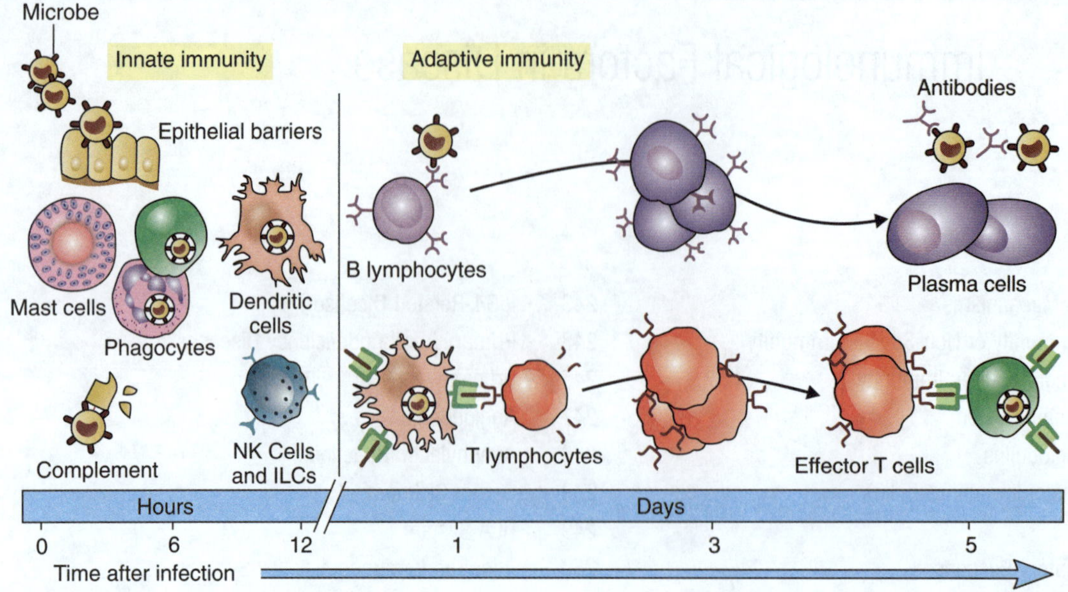

Fig. 3.1 Innate and adaptive immunity. *From* Abbas AK, Lichtman AH, Pillai S. Basic Immunology: Functions and Disorders of the Immune System. 6th ed. Philadelphia, PA: Elsevier; 2020:4.

- Also plays a role in the induction of specific immune responses (e.g. release of cytokines and activation of complements that stimulate specific immunity).
- Recognises molecular patterns common to many classes of pathogens known as pathogen-associated molecular patterns (PAMP).
- Recognises PAMP using a group of proteins termed as pathogen-recognition receptors (PRR). These are present on several cells.
- Toll-like receptors (TLRs)
  - An important group of PRR expressed on both innate immune cells and on cells in various tissues including endothelial cells, epithelial cells and fibroblasts.
  - TLRs expressed on cell surface recognise mostly bacterial products, while TLRs localised to intracellular compartments recognise mostly viral products and nucleic acids.
  - Binding of TLR to their microbial ligands leads to the activation of phagocytes and direct killing of pathogens, as well as to the release of pro-inflammatory cytokines and antimicrobial peptides (AMPs).
  - In addition, these molecules activate dendritic cells and are therefore important in the initiation of adaptive immune responses.
- Other innate immune PRRs include retinoic acid-inducible gene-I-like receptors (RLRs) and nucleotide binding and oligomerisation domain (NOD)-like receptors (NLRs).
- Due to limited diversity of PRRs, pathogens displaying a high mutation rate can easily escape recognition by the innate immune system. Moreover, ability of intracellular TLRs to kill several pathogens such as viruses is limited. Adaptive immunity is required for efficient immune response.

COMPONENTS OF INNATE IMMUNITY (Box 3.1)

BOX 3.1 Components of Innate Immunity

Cells	Complement Components
• Monocytes/macrophages	**Cytokines**
• Dendritic/Langerhans cells	**Host Defence Peptides**
• Follicular dendritic cells	**(Antimicrobial Peptides)**
• Large granular lymphocytes/ natural killer cells (NK cells)	• Defensins • Cathelicidins
• Neutrophils	
• Eosinophils	
• Mast cells	
• Basophils	

CELLULAR COMPONENTS OF INNATE IMMUNITY

Monocytes/Macrophages

- Monocytes arise from bone marrow and circulate in the blood.
- Macrophages arise from monocytes migrating to tissues.
- Their main functions are:
  - Binding to lipopolysaccharides released by bacteria.
  - Presentation of antigen to T lymphocytes.
  - Secretion of cytokines such as interleukin-1 (IL-1), tumour necrosis factor (TNF) and interleukin-6 (IL-6) that help in the activation of T and B cells.
  - Destruction of antibody-coated bacteria.

Dendritic/Langerhans Cells

- These are derived from bone marrow.
- These cells possess both human leucocyte antigen (HLA) class I and class II molecules on the surface

(see HLA system) and are the most potent antigen-presenting cells (APCs) for T lymphocytes (both CD4 and CD8).

Follicular Dendritic Cells

- These are antigen-presenting cells for B lymphocytes.

Large Granular Lymphocytes/Natural Killer Cells

- Large granular lymphocytes (LGLs) are divided into two major components—natural killer (NK) cells and CD3+ T cells.
- LGLs mediate both antibody-dependent cellular toxicity and NK activity.
- NK cells circulate in the blood but do not enter thymus to mature. NK cells do not have antigenic surface markers of T or B lymphocytes. They recognise and kill cells which become coated with antibodies such as tumour cells or cells infected with microbes. Their action does not require major histocompatibility complex (MHC) molecules and is therefore less specific than cytotoxic T cells. NK cells are part of both innate and adaptive immune systems.
- Upon stimulation, NK cells secrete large amounts of cytokines including interferon-γ (IFN-γ), tumour necrosis factor-α (TNF-α), granulocyte-macrophage colony-stimulating factor (GM-CSF) and several other chemokines.

Neutrophils, Eosinophils, Mast Cells and Basophils

- These cells produce inflammatory response to infection.
- They also phagocytose the microbial agents and cause their death. Efficient elimination of pathogens through phagocytosis requires rapid recruitment of effector cells to the infection site and this process is often referred to as the inflammatory response.

COMPLEMENTS

- These are a family of proteases produced by the liver and macrophages that circulate in inactive forms.
- These can be sequentially activated when bound to antigen–antibody complexes (classical pathway) or to the surface of a pathogen (alternative pathway).
- They damage cell membranes of pathogens and enhance recognition and killing by other immune system cells.

CYTOKINES

- These are soluble proteins secreted by a wide variety of cells. These are critical for both innate and acquired immune responses.
- Their functions include regulation of growth, development and activation of immune system cells and mediation of inflammatory responses.
- They may act in three manners: autocrine (action on the same cell that secretes them), paracrine (action on cells nearby to the cells producing them) and endocrine (action on distally located cells).
- Examples of cytokines in innate immunity are interleukins (IL-1, IL-6, IL-12), interferons (INF-*a*, INF-*b*), TNF-*a* and others.

HOST DEFENCE PEPTIDES (ANTIMICROBIAL PEPTIDES)

- Short peptides (8–50 amino acids) which exhibit broad-spectrum antimicrobial activity to directly kill bacteria, yeasts, fungi, viruses and even cancer cells.
- Able to traverse cell barriers to reach the target components in the cytoplasm of the cells.
- Paneth cells are the major source of AMPs in the small intestine.

Q. Describe the acquired immunity (specific or adaptive immunity). (MI 1.8)

- Specific, acquired or adaptive immunity is characterised by antigen-specific responses to foreign antigens that take a few days to weeks to develop.
- It is mediated by T and B lymphocytes.
- Foreign substances that induce specific immune responses are called 'antigens'.
- Organs of immune system are lymphoid organs.
    - Lymphocytes are generated in primary lymphoid organs. These are bone marrow and thymus.
    - In secondary lymphoid organs, adaptive immune responses are initiated. These secondary lymphoid organs include lymph nodes, spleen and mucosa and gut-associated lymphoid tissues (MALT and GALT), that is tonsils, adenoids, appendix and Peyer's patches of small intestine.

DEVELOPMENT OF LYMPHOCYTES

- All lymphocytes are derived from bone marrow stem cells.
- Lymphocytes enter the blood and are distributed either to thymus or to bone marrow. T lymphocytes are produced in the thymus while B lymphocytes (bursa-equivalent) are produced in the bone marrow.
- B lymphocytes differentiate into plasma cells when stimulated by antigen. Plasma cells produce immunoglobulins or antibodies that bind to the foreign antigen with high specificity.
- T lymphocytes recognise foreign antigens on the surface of host cells that include infected host cells and specialised host cells called APCs.

ANTIBODY OR HUMORAL IMMUNE RESPONSE

- B lymphocytes mature in bursa of Fabricius in birds, hence named bursa derived. In humans, they mature in bone marrow (bone marrow derived).
- B lymphocytes are derived from stem cells in the bone marrow. The maturing pre-B cells remain in the marrow and express surface immunoglobulins (Ig).
- A process of selection then identifies the B cells with surface immunoglobulins that recognise self-antigens and these cells are disabled or eliminated. The surviving cells that will recognise foreign antigens

enter the circulation and migrate to the lymphoid tissues.

- The B cells that are not exposed to a foreign antigen are naive cells. When these cells encounter an antigen, they are stimulated to undergo clonal expansion and become activated B cells. These cells release antibodies or immunoglobulins.
- B lymphocytes can bind foreign proteins, polysaccharides, lipids and other chemicals in extracellular or cell-associated forms.
- B cells are also APCs which present antigenic peptides to T cells after processing the antigen.
- Although antibodies allow immune system to react with a large variety of antigens, these large molecules cannot cross the plasma membrane and are therefore unable to bind and destroy intracellular pathogens such as viruses.

PRIMARY AND SECONDARY RESPONSE

- When an individual is exposed to an antigen for the first time, there is a lag of several days before specific antibody becomes detectable. Initially, this antibody is of IgM class. After another few days, IgG antibody is formed.
- Some cells from the activated clone become memory cells that circulate in the blood and remain dormant until they are re-activated by the same antigen.
- If at a later date the individual is exposed to the same antigen, there is a rapid appearance of much greater amount of IgG antibody (sometimes IgE or IgA). This is called secondary response. Thus, secondary response requires the phenomenon known as class switching of antibodies.
- Table 3.2 gives differences between primary and secondary immune responses.

CELL-MEDIATED IMMUNE RESPONSE

- Cell-mediated immunity is important in the elimination of intracellular infections and neoplastic cells. It is involved in graft rejection as well as cellular autoimmune responses. T cells (part of cell-mediated immunity) activate innate immune cells such as phagocytic cells to become more effective at killing pathogens such as fungi.
- T lymphocytes develop from stem cells in the bone marrow but these cells migrate to thymus for maturation, hence are named T cells.
- In thymus, T cells proliferate and mature, acquiring a variety of cell-surface markers including T-cell receptor (TCR) and coreceptors (CD4, CD8 and others). In the thymus, T cells that recognise self-antigens are eliminated or disabled.

TABLE 3.2 Primary Response Versus Secondary Response

Primary Response	Secondary Response
• Slow in onset	• Rapid in onset
• Low in magnitude	• High in magnitude
• Short lived	• Long lived
• IgM antibody formed	• IgG (or IgA or IgE) antibody formed

- Mature but naive T cells leave the thymus and migrate to secondary lymphoid follicles where they are exposed to antigens and become reactive T cells. T cells comprise 70%–80% of circulating lymphocytes.
- T lymphocytes recognise only short peptide sequences in protein antigens that are present on the surfaces of other cells, bound to class I or II MHC proteins.
- TCR differ from B-cell receptors. They are never secreted, existing instead on the cell surface as heterodimers of $\alpha\beta$ or $\gamma\delta$ subunits.
- These cells are classified into several subtypes based on their functions:
    - Cytotoxic T cells (T8 cytotoxic cells or CD8+ cells) comprise 25% of circulating T cells. They destroy host cells harbouring viruses and other foreign microbes.
    - Helper T cells (T4 helper cells or CD4+ cells) synthesise and secrete hormones called cytokines that activate the immune response in local populations of cytotoxic T cells, macrophages and B cells.
    - Regulatory T cell (Treg) or T-suppressor cells (generally CD4+) repress the immune response by inhibiting other T cells and B cells and are important for maintenance of tolerance. These cells may contribute to disease through inappropriate downregulation of protective immune responses.
    - T-memory cells are clonal populations of T cells that have been exposed to antigen but do not become activated until subsequent exposure.
- T-helper cells have been further classified on the basis of cytokines they secrete:
    - Th1 cells respond to microbes and activate macrophages and NK cells and secrete IFN, IL-2, TNF and IL-10. These are efficient at activating macrophages and stimulating cytotoxic T cells, thereby inducing cell-mediated immunity. These cytokines may suppress Th2 response, though INF-γ can stimulate Th2 response and antibody production. Th1 responses are prominent in the defence against pathogens that replicate intracellularly (viruses and intracellular bacteria).
    - Th2 cells respond to worms and allergens and secrete IL-3, IL-4, IL-5, IL-10 and IL-13. These cytokines activate B cells producing humoral response particularly production of IgE and IgG4, and stimulate eosinophil development.

MECHANISM OF CELL-MEDIATED IMMUNE RESPONSE

- The first step is processing of antigens by APCs followed by presentation of processed antigens on the surface of these cells using the MHC on the cell surface.
- There are two distinct classes of MHC molecules:
    - Class I MHC molecules are expressed by most nucleated host cells. The class I proteins on the surface of infected host cells display foreign antigen (as peptide) and this is recognised by TCR of cytotoxic T cells that destroy the infected host

cells. The TCR is very similar to immunoglobulin in structure, although it is encoded by a distinct set of genes. The diversity of TCRs is such that a given TCR is able to specifically react to a given peptide/MHC combination.
- Class II MHC molecules are expressed by the APCs that include B cells and macrophages. These cells endocytose foreign proteins that are processed and then displayed on cell surface using the class II MHC. Helper T cells recognise the foreign antigens displayed by class II molecules and release cytokines that signal B cells to make antibodies against the foreign antigen and activate macrophages to destroy the ingested microbes.

- Other markers on the surface of T cells include coreceptors that increase the recognition of the MHC proteins. These include:
  - CD4 (CD—cluster of differentiation) is expressed on the surface of helper T cells and binds to class II MHC proteins on the APCs. It also functions as the receptor for human immunodeficiency virus (HIV).
  - CD8 is expressed on the surface of cytotoxic T cells and binds to class I MHC proteins on host cells. It is also expressed on T-suppressor cells.

ROLE OF OTHER CELLS AND PROTEINS IN IMMUNE RESPONSE

- After lymphocytes are activated by antigens, several other cells and components, including those of innate immunity, get activated to enhance the immune response. These are:
  - Enhancing phagocytosis by macrophages and neutrophils.
  - Lysis and enhancing phagocytosis of microbes by complements.
  - Enhancing phagocytosis and stimulating further inflammatory responses by cytokines.

CARDINAL FEATURES OF IMMUNE RESPONSES

- Specificity: Immune responses are specific for different antigens and in fact, for different structural components of a single protein, polysaccharide or other antigens. The portions of such antigens that are specifically recognised by individual lymphocytes are called determinants or epitomes. The total number of antigenic specificities of lymphocytes in an individual is called lymphocyte repertoire or repertoire of the immune system.
- Diversity: The lymphocyte repertoire is very large in an individual. It is due to an extreme variability in the structures of antigen-binding sites of lymphocytes. Therefore, body can respond to an extremely large number of antigens. This is known as diversity of immune system.
- Memory: As discussed above, secondary response occurs after re-exposure to the same antigen. This property of immune system is known as immunologic memory. Each exposure to an antigen expands the progeny of a particular antigen-responsive lymphocyte, that is it expands the clone of a lymphocyte specific for a particular antigen. These memory cells survive for long periods. The immune response of memory cells is rapid, larger and more efficient compared to the previous exposure.
- Self-tolerance: One of the important properties of immune system is its ability to respond only to foreign antigens (nonself) while not reacting to body's own antigens (self). This tolerance to self is discussed separately. A breakdown in this self-tolerance may lead to autoimmune diseases.

Q. Write a short note on the complement system.

- The complement system consists of a series of plasma proteins (β-globulins). These are proteases in nature that play an important role in both inflammation and immunity.
- Complements are present as inactive forms in plasma (C1–C9).
- Complement system is a major constituent of the innate immune defence system that is also involved in the initiation of adaptive immunity.
- The major source of most circulating complement components is the liver. C1q production is mainly by bone marrow-derived cells like macrophages and dendritic cells.
- Three different pathways of complement activation:
  - Classical pathway.
  - Alternative pathway.
  - Lectin pathway.
- These three pathways converge at the central component of the complement system, C3. The common pathway finally leads to the formation of a protein complex named the membrane attack complex.

CLASSICAL PATHWAY

- Activated via binding of C1q to immunoglobulins (IgG1, IgG3 and IgM), acute phase proteins, charged molecules, and apoptotic or necrotic cell debris.
- This results in activation of serine proteases C1r and C1s.
- C1s activates C4 and C2 leading to the formation of the C4b2a complex (C3 convertase) that leads to the activation of C3.

ALTERNATIVE PATHWAY

- C3 produced in the liver is cleaved into C3a and C3b by enzymes in the blood.
- If there is no pathogen in the blood, C3a and C3b protein fragments will be deactivated.
- If there is a nearby pathogen, some of the C3b is bound to plasma membrane of the pathogen and will then bind to factor B.
- This complex is then cleaved by factor D into C3bBb, which is the alternative pathway C3 convertase.
- This convertase is stabilised by properdin and can subsequently activate C3.

- Activated C3 can bind with factor B and the subsequent activation of factor B leads to the formation of a more active C3 convertase, C3bBb.
- Alternative pathway does not require antibody or prior contact with a microbe to function and serves as a part of innate immunity.

LECTIN PATHWAY

- Activation occurs in response to the recognition of mannose-binding lectin (MBL) and ficolins (L-ficolin and H-ficolin) of various carbohydrate ligands instead of C1q as in classical pathway.
- This pathway is activated by binding of MBL to mannose residues on the pathogen surface, which activates the MBL-associated serine proteases (MASP), MASP-1 and MASP-2. These then split C4 into C4a and C4b, and C2 into C2a and C2b. C4b and C2a then bind together to form C3 convertase.

TERMINAL PATHWAY

- Incorporation of C3b molecule in the C3 convertases leads to the formation of C5 convertase.
- C5 is activated and subsequent binding of C6, C7, C8 and C9 results in the formation of the membrane attack complex C5b–C9.
- During complement activation, cleavage fragments of complement components are generated that include anaphylotoxins—C3a, C4a and C5a. These low-molecular-weight peptides have the ability to bind to mast cells and basophils and release histamine and other highly active peptides. These peptides increase permeability of the vascular walls allowing neutrophils to migrate into the area.
- C5a is a potent chemotactic (attractant) factor.
- C4b and C3b can opsonise particles by binding to the surface leading to the recognition of these particles by phagocytes.

SUMMARY OF COMPLEMENT SYSTEM

- Figure 3.2 summarises three pathways of complement activation.

COMPLEMENT SYSTEM IN DISEASES

- Complement system might play a role in many diseases with an immune component, such as asthma, lupus erythematosus, membranoproliferative glomerulonephritis, multiple sclerosis and inflammatory bowel disease.
- Deficiencies of the terminal pathway predispose to both autoimmune diseases and infections. More than 90% of C1q-deficient individuals develop SLE and they may also have recurrent bacterial infections. C3 deficiency predisposes to life-threatening pyogenic infections and early death. A deficiency of a component of the membrane attack complex (C5–C9) is associated with infection by *Neisseria meningitidis*.

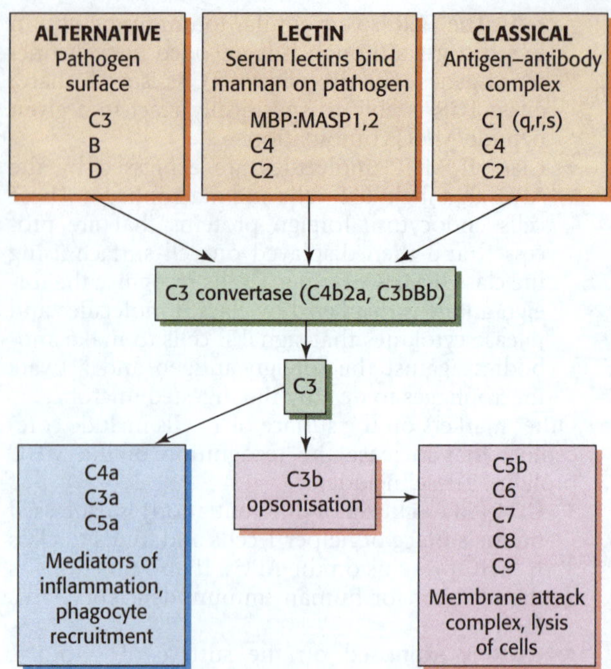

Fig. 3.2 Three different pathways of complement activation.

Q. Briefly discuss immunoglobulins.

- Immunoglobulins are end products of plasma cells that develop on the stimulation of B lymphocytes by an antigen. They are humoral mediators of immunity.
- Antibodies or immunoglobulins bind to a specific portion of antigen called epitome. Thus, an antibody recognises one epitome rather than whole antigen.
- Various immunoglobulin classes are IgG, IgA, IgM, IgD and IgE.
- There are four subtypes of IgG: IgG1, IgG2, IgG3 and IgG4.
- Immunoglobulin molecule has two subunits—two light chains and two heavy chains that are linked by disulphide bonds (S–S).
- Light chains exist in two classes, lambda (λ) and kappa (κ). Each antibody molecule has either λ or κ chains, not both.
- There are five different heavy chains (α, γ, δ, ε and μ). The type of heavy chain determines the class or isotype of the antibody molecule, that is IgA, IgG, IgD, IgE and IgM antibodies.
- IgA exists in monomeric and dimeric forms, whereas IgM exists in pentameric form. Additionally, IgA molecules receive a secretory component from the epithelial cells into which they pass.
- The enzyme papain cleaves the Y-shaped immunoglobulin molecule at the hinge region into two parts:
  - Fab region—antigen binding site.
  - Fc region—binds to surface Fc receptors of macrophages, neutrophils and eosinophils.
- The heavy and light chains are each made up of variable (V) and constant (C) regions (e.g. VH, CH—variable and constant regions of heavy chain; VL, CL—variable and constant regions of light chain) (Fig. 3.3).

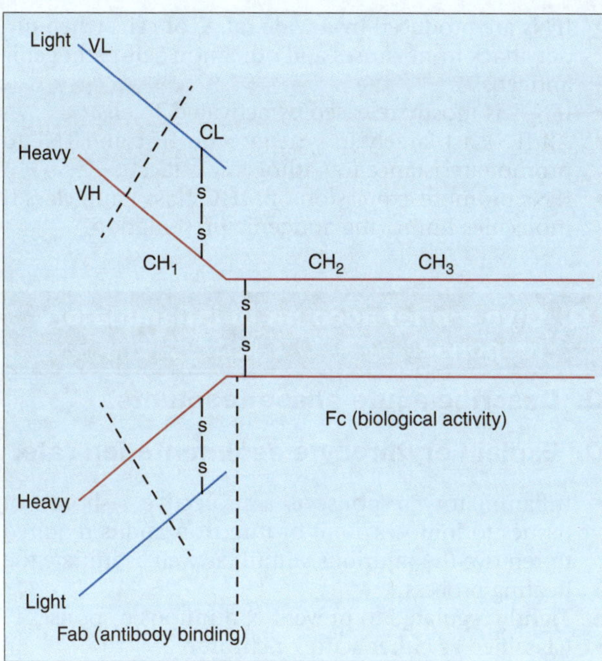

Fig. 3.3 Structure of immunoglobulin molecule.

VARIOUS IMMUNOGLOBULINS (Table 3.3)

TABLE 3.3 Various Immunoglobulins

• **IgG—70%**	Found in serum and ECF; opsonisation of antigens for phagocytosis, complement fixation by activating classical pathway, antibody-dependent cell killing by NK cells and macrophages and blocks viral entry into cells; directed against proteins; transplacental transfer
• **IgA—20%**	Secretory type involved in mucosal and epithelial defence
• **IgM—10%**	Macromolecular, having complement fixing activity; binds foreign antigens to initiate antibody production; produced in response to polysaccharide antigens; secreted during primary response
• **IgD—<0.5%**	Lowest level in serum; exact function not known
• **IgE—<0.5%**	Considerable affinity to mast cells and basophils; involved in immediate (anaphylactic) hypersensitivity and plays a role in immune response to parasites

Q. Describe the functions of immunoglobulins. (MI 1.8; PA 9.1)

- **Processing antigen:** Antibodies present on B cells help in interiorisation of antigen and further processing it for presentation to other cells.
- **Agglutination:** Antibodies help in agglutination of particulate matter including bacteria and viruses. IgM is particularly suitable for this function.
- **Opsonisation:** It implies coating of bacterial surface for which the Fab region of antibody has specificity. This facilitates subsequent phagocytosis by cells possessing Fc receptor (e.g. neutrophils).
- **Neutralisation:** Some antibodies neutralise the toxins released by bacteria. Some antibodies can hinder the ability of viruses to attach to receptors on host cells.
- **Immobilisation:** Antibodies against bacterial cilia or flagella hinder their movement and ability to escape the phagocytic cells.
- **Complement activation:** IgG and IgM antibodies can activate the complement system by classical pathway. The terminal components of complement pathway cause death of microbes. These components also help in phagocytosis.
- **Mucosal protection:** This is provided by IgA.
- **Immune complex formation:** Depending upon the ratio of antigen to antibody, immune complexes of varying sizes are formed. Larger complexes can be removed by the phagocytic cells.
- **Antibody-dependent cell-mediated cytotoxicity (ADCC):** Here antibodies bind to microbes via their Fab region. LGLs (NK cells) attach via Fc receptors of bound antibodies and kill these organisms by release of toxic substances called perforins.
- **Transplacental passage:** By this mechanism, antibodies confer immunity to the newborn.

Q. What are cytokines?

- Cytokines are small polypeptides secreted by several cells of immune system.
- They promote proliferation and differentiation of T cell as well as other cells. They also play a critical role in many pathophysiological processes such as allergic responses, infectious and autoimmune diseases, angiogenesis, inflammation, tumour growth and haematopoietic development.
- These may act on the same cells (autocrine), other cells surrounding the cell where they are produced (paracrine) or on cells present at a distant site (endocrine).
- Cytokines have been named based on the presumed target or based on presumed functions. Those cytokines that are thought to primarily target leucocytes are termed as interleukins, that is cytokines which mediate communication between leucocytes. Those involved in chemotaxis of inflammatory cells are termed chemokines.
- Cytokines belong to four major families: the four-*a*-helix bundle family, the IL-1 family, the IL-17 family and chemokines. Another important cytokine family is TNF family.
- The four-*a*-helix bundle family has three subfamilies each with several cytokines:
  - IL-2 subfamily: IL-2, IL-3, IL-4, IL-5, IL-6, IL-7, IL-9, IL-11, IL-12, IL-13, IL-15, IL-21, IL-23, granulocyte-macrophage colony-stimulating factor, erythropoietin, etc.
  - Interferon subfamily: IFN-β and IFN-α.
  - IL-10 subfamily: IL-10, IL-19, IL-20, IL-22, IL-24 and IL-26.
- All chemokines signal through seven transmembrane domain and G-protein-coupled receptors. To date, more than 40 distinct chemokines have been well characterised. Important chemokines include granulocyte chemotactic protein 2 (GCP-2), stromal

cell-derived factor 1 (SDF-1), neutrophil activating peptide 2 (NAP-2), macrophage inflammatory protein 1 (MIP-1), monocyte chemoattractant protein (MCP-1, MCP-2, MCP-3, MCP-4), macrophage inflammatory protein (MIP) and RANTES (regulated on expression, normal T cell expressed and secreted).

- Interleukin-1 (IL-1), interleukin-2 (IL-2), interferons (IFNs) and TNF are the key groups of cytokines that carry out the most important functions.
- Other cytokines include granulocyte-macrophage colony-stimulating factor, platelet-derived growth factor and fibroblast growth factor.

INTERLEUKINS

- Predominant actions of various interleukins are given in Table 3.4.

TUMOUR NECROSIS FACTOR-α

- TNF-α is produced by macrophages in response to infection by bacteria and other microbes. Its functions are as follows:
  - It promotes the production of more cytokines including IL-1.
  - It enhances stimulation of T and B cells and other immune system cells to make a response to antigenic challenge more potent.
  - It also increases the expression of MHC class I and class II molecules and so improves antigen presentation.
  - It is an antiviral cytokine.
  - It has antitumour properties.
  - It can adversely affect endothelial cells which can produce ARDS, disseminated intravascular coagulation (DIC) and acute renal failure.

INTERFERONS

- Interferons include interferon-alpha (IFN-α), interferon-beta (IFN-β) and interferon-gamma (IFN-γ).
- IFNs are produced by a wide range of cells when under attack from viruses and other non-self-pathogenic antigens.
- IFN-γ is mostly released by activated T cells.
- All IFNs act largely in synergy with IL-1 and TNF to promote resistance to pathogenic attack.
- IFNs promote expression of MHC class I and class II molecules improving antigenic presentation.

Q. Give a brief account of inflammatory response.

Q. Describe acute phase reactants.

Q. Explain erythrocyte sedimentation rate.

- Inflammatory response is a protective response of tissues to injury, irritant or infection and is required to remove the injurious stimuli as well as initiate the healing process.
- Tightly regulated to prevent continuous response.
- Classified as either acute or chronic.
- Acute inflammation.
  - Initial response of the body to harmful stimuli.
  - Involves local vascular system, immune system and various cells within the injured tissue that results in infiltration of phagocytic cells and increase in enzymes (e.g. cyclo-oxygenase, inducible nitric oxide) within the tissues. These result in release of leucotrienes, prostaglandins, histamine, kinins and nitric oxide, producing vasodilatation and increased local vascular permeability. In addition, cytokines like IL-1, IL-6 and TNF-*a* produced at the site of inflammation have systemic effects including the production of acute phase reactants.
  - Acute inflammation is characterised by classic local signs of inflammation—swelling, redness, pain, heat and loss of function.
  - Systemic features occur due to release of cytokines and are shown in Table 3.5.
  - Outcomes of acute inflammation:

TABLE 3.4 Interleukins

Interleukin	Main Cells of Origin	Predominant Actions
Interleukin-1	Macrophages, large granular lymphocytes, B cells, endothelium, fibroblasts	Lymphocyte activation, macrophage stimulation, fever due to hypothalamus stimulation, release of acute phase proteins by the liver, B-cell proliferation and antibody production, production of IL-2 by T cells
Interleukin-2	T cells	T-cell proliferation and differentiation, increased cytokine synthesis, proliferation and activation of NK cells and B-cell proliferation and antibody synthesis
Interleukin-3	T cells and stem cells	Differentiation of multipotent haematopoietic stem cells into myeloid progenitor cells
Interleukin-4	CD4+ T cells (Th2)	Stimulation of B cells, IgE and IgG1 isotype selection, Th2 differentiation and proliferation, inhibition of IFN gamma-mediated activation of macrophages
Interleukin-5	CD4+ T cells (Th2)	B-cell growth factor and differentiation and IgA selection, eosinophil activation
Interleukin-6	T and B lymphocytes, fibroblasts and macrophages	B-cell differentiation and stimulation of acute phase proteins
Interleukin-12	Monocytes	Induction of Th1 cells, induction of interferon gamma production by T lymphocytes and NK cells

TABLE 3.5 Systemic Features Produced by Cytokines

CNS • Fever, sweating (due to change in hypothalamic set point) • Headache • Confusion • Anorexia **Liver** • Increased synthesis of acute phase reactants **Cardiovascular** • Tachycardia • Hypotension	**Respiratory** • Tachypnoea **Endocrine** • Increased secretion of catecholamines • Increased secretion of glucocorticoids • Increased secretion of insulin **Others** • Increased production of neutrophils • Flushing • Enlarged draining lymph nodes

- Complete resolution.
- Fibrosis.
- Abscess formation.
- Chronic inflammation.

- Chronic inflammation:
  - Progressive shift in the type of cells that are present at the site of inflammation.
  - Characterised by simultaneous destruction and healing of the tissue.
  - Inflammatory cells include lymphocytes, macrophages and plasma cells.
  - Exudation of fluid is not significant.
  - Continued tissue necrosis may occur.
  - Granulomatous inflammation occurs in context of foreign materials and infectious agents resistant to phagocytosis.
  - Typically seen in tuberculosis and leprosy.

INVESTIGATIONS

- Leucocytosis, increased platelet counts.
- Elevated erythrocyte sedimentation rate (ESR).
- Elevated acute phase reactants or proteins.
- Normocytic and normochromic anaemia in chronic inflammation.

ERYTHROCYTE SEDIMENTATION RATE

- Measures the rate of fall of red blood cells through plasma and is an indirect measure of acute phase reactants.
- Normally, red cells do not aggregate because of their repellent negative charge. Plasma proteins that are positively charged neutralise the surface charge of red cells. Elevation in plasma proteins, particularly fibrinogen, causes aggregation of red cells forming rouleaux. Rouleaux have a higher mass/surface area ratio than single erythrocyte and thus fall faster, leading to elevated ESR.
- ESR is elevated in acute inflammation where levels of acute phase reactants are increased. Due to increased levels of fibrinogen, ESR is elevated in pregnancy, old age and chronic renal failure. It is also elevated in many other conditions where there is no alteration in acute phase reactants. For example, ESR is increased in conditions associated with monoclonal (multiple myeloma) or polyclonal (chronic infections) increase in immunoglobulins. In systemic lupus erythematosus (SLE), ESR is elevated while CRP may be normal.
- ESR may be low if plasma proteins are low or red cell morphology is abnormal, thereby making rouleaux formation impossible. Examples include hereditary spherocytosis, sickle cell anaemia and microcytic anaemia.

ACUTE PHASE REACTANTS

- Defined as proteins produced by liver whose serum concentrations increase or decrease by at least 25% during both acute and chronic inflammatory states.
- Associated with a wide variety of disorders, including infection, trauma, infarction, inflammatory arthritides and other systemic autoimmune and inflammatory diseases, and various neoplasms.
- Play an important role in host defence and stimulate repair and regeneration.
- Major inducers of acute phase reactants are IL-6, IL-1 beta, TNF-α and INF-γ.
- Include C-reactive protein (CRP), fibrinogen, *a*-1 antitrypsin, haptoglobin, ceruloplasmin, manganese superoxide dismutase, iron-binding proteins (ferritin, transferrin, lactoferrin), procalcitonin, serum amyloid A and serum amyloid P.
- In chronic inflammation, these proteins may contribute to the development of amyloidosis.

C-Reactive Protein

- Levels increase within 6 hours of acute inflammation and fall within a few days after inflammation subsides.
- Therefore, sequential measurement is useful in monitoring the disease activity.
- Some inflammatory diseases are associated with normal or slightly elevated levels of CRP. These include SLE, scleroderma and ulcerative colitis. However, concurrent infection in these conditions produces significant elevation of CRP levels.

Procalcitonin

- It is a peptide and is a sensitive marker of bacterial infections.
- Levels of procalcitonin can be used to guide progression of infections and antibiotic therapy.

Ferritin

- Levels of ferritin increase during infections.
- Pseudomonas infections cause reduced levels of ferritin because of presence of virulence factors siderophores (pyoverdine and pyocyanin) which chelate and import iron.

Haptoglobin

- Its levels increase during infection but reduce during haemolysis.

Q. What is tolerance? Explain briefly.

- It is an active physiological process producing immunological unresponsiveness to an otherwise immunogenic substance (self-antigens) present in body. It involves both humoral- and cell-mediated immunity.
- Possible mechanisms are given in Box 3.2.

BOX 3.2 Possible Mechanisms of Tolerance

- Elimination of self-reacting T and B cells
- Disabling self-reacting T and B cells
- Presence of T-suppressor cells that are antigen specific
- Presence of antibodies that alter self-antigen such that they are no longer susceptible to an immune response
- Sequestration of antigens

BOX 3.3 Postulated Mechanisms of Autoimmunity

- Failure of suppression of self-reacting T and B cells
- Tissue damage resulting in the release of sequestered antigens
- Tissue damage altering the antigenic structure
- Shared immunologic epitope with a microbe and the host (molecular mimicry)
- Infection altering cell-surface markers in a genetically susceptible individual
- Persistent viral infections leading to immune-mediated injury due to constant presence of viral antigen driving the immune response
- Decline in T-suppressor cells

Q. Describe autoimmunity.

- It indicates development of immune reaction against self-antigens.
- Postulated mechanisms of autoimmunity are given in Box 3.3.

Q. What are the different types of immune reactions/hypersensitivity reactions? (MI 1.10)

- Immunologically mediated reactions are of five types that may result in tissue damage. They are summarised in Table 3.6.

Q. Write a short note on monoclonal antibodies.

- A monoclonal antibody (mAb) is directed against a specific epitome of an antigen.
- Used for treatment of immunologic diseases, diagnosis and treatment of malignancies and reversal of drug effects.

NOMENCLATURE

- The name of an mAb consists of:
  - A prefix ('random') which provides a unique name to it.
  - Two substems: The first defines the target of mAb—molecule, cell or organ (e.g. 'tu' in old classification and 'ta' in new classification for tumour, 'ci' for cardiovascular, 'o' for bone) and the second the species on which the immunoglobulin sequence of the mAb is based (e.g. 'u' for human, 'o' for mouse), as well as modifications ('-xi-' for chimeric—e.g. rituximab, '-zu-' for humanised—e.g. trastuzumab). The second substem of source has been eliminated in the 2017 classification for those mAb produced after this revision.
  - The suffix for all mAbs is 'mab'.
  - Fab indicates fragment, antigen-binding (one arm).
  - F(ab')2 indicates fragment, antigen-binding, including hinge region (both arms).
  - Fab' indicates fragment, antigen-binding, including hinge region (one arm).

MODIFICATIONS

- A risk with mouse-derived mAb is that some patients can develop an immune response to the mouse antibody sequence. This led to changes in mAb molecule producing a chimeric antibody (Fc part or constant

TABLE 3.6 Various Immune/Hypersensitivity Reactions

Type	Prototype Disorder	Immune Mechanism
I. Anaphylactic type or immediate hypersensitivity type	Anaphylaxis, urticaria, angioedema, bronchial asthma, allergic rhinitis	• Formation of IgE antibody leading to release of vasoactive amines and other mediators from basophils and mast cells; not all type I reactions are anaphylactic • Very small amounts of an allergen seem to be sufficient to allow interaction and cross-linking of receptor-bound IgE molecules
II. Cytotoxic type	Autoimmune haemolytic anaemia, Goodpasture's syndrome	• Formation of IgG (occasionally IgM) antibodies that bind to antigen on target cell surface (red cells, leucocytes, platelets, etc.) and activate complement system via classical pathway, leading to phagocytosis or lysis of target cell; this reaction is also known as antibody-dependent cellular cytotoxicity (ADCC)
III. Immune complex type	Serum sickness, vasculitis, Arthus reaction, SLE, Henoch–Schönlein purpura, immune-complex type of glomerulonephritis, transfusion reactions	• Antigen–antibody complex (immune complex) deposition in microcirculation → complement activation → neutrophil chemotaxis → release of lysosomal enzymes and other toxic moieties → tissue destruction
IV. Cell-mediated (delayed) type	Tuberculosis, transplant rejection, DRESS syndrome, Stevens–Johnson syndrome/toxic epidermal necrolysis, contact dermatitis	• Sensitised T lymphocytes → release of cytokines, T cell-mediated cytotoxicity; independent of antibody production; reaction appears in 18–24 hours with maximal response at 48–72 hours
V. Stimulatory antibody mediated	Graves' disease	• Long-acting thyroid stimulator (LATS)

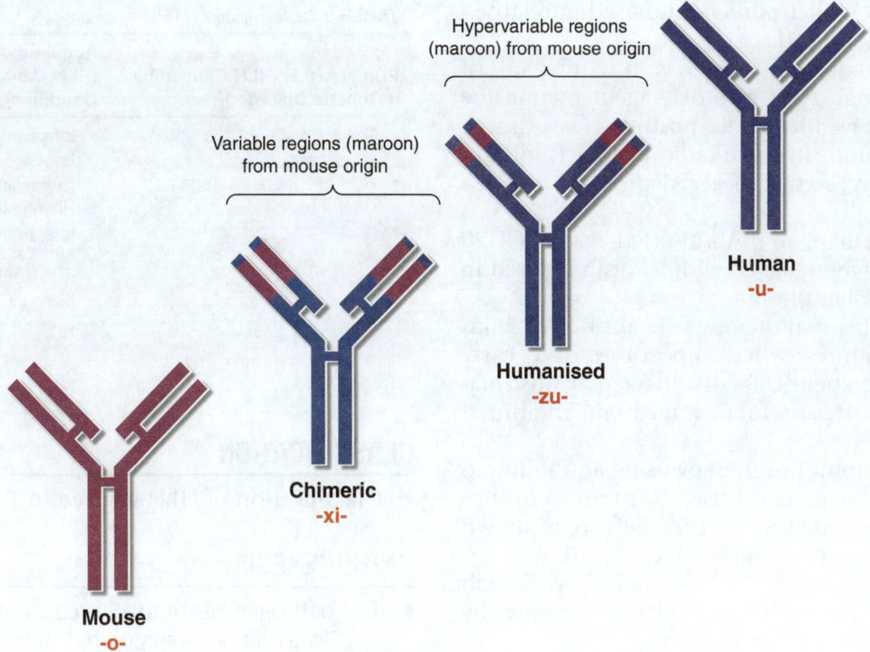

Fig. 3.4 Humanisation of monoclonal antibodies.

region of the immunoglobulin molecule is of a human sequence but variable region is of mouse sequence) and humanised antibody (by engineering amino acid substitutions making them more similar to the human sequence) or creating fully human sequence-derived antibody molecules (Fig. 3.4).

- The use of antibody fragments instead of full-length antibodies may enhance pharmacokinetic (PK) properties and/or the efficiency of penetration into tissues or tumour masses.

ADVERSE EFFECTS

- Infusion reaction occurs within 1–2 hours of starting infusion. The reactions range from mild local irritation to severe anaphylaxis. These occur due to development of antibodies against nonhuman mAbs.
- Cytokine release syndrome occurs due to progressive increase in inflammatory cytokines by T lymphocytes. The incidence is higher with increased tumour cell load. Clinical features include fever, headache, hypotension, rash, chills, dyspnoea, tachycardia, and in some cases, hepatic injury and DIC.
- Infections and autoimmunity due to reduced immune function.

APPLICATIONS

- **Reversal of drug effects:**
  - Some mAbs are used against drugs, for example idarucizumab for reversal of dabigatran effects and digoxin Fab fragment for digoxin overdose.
- **Effects on cellular receptors:**
  - Abciximab is Fab antibody fragment derived from a chimeric human-murine mAb that binds to platelet IIb/IIIa receptors thereby inhibiting platelet aggregation and used in percutaneous coronary stent placement.
  - Alemtuzumab acts on CD52 and is used in multiple sclerosis.
- **Autoimmune and other immune-related diseases:**
  - Adalimumab, certolizumab and infliximab bind to TNF and are useful in autoimmune diseases like rheumatoid arthritis, Crohn's disease, ulcerative colitis, ankylosing spondylitis, psoriasis, etc.
  - Basiliximab and daclizumab inhibit IL-2 on activated T cells and help prevent acute rejection of kidney transplants.
  - Omalizumab inhibits IgE and is useful in treating moderate-to-severe allergic asthma.
- **Treatment of malignancies:**
  - Unconjugated (naked) mAbs directly affect the signalling pathways by binding to tumour cell receptors, kill the tumour cells directly. These may also indirectly stimulate host defence mechanisms such as antibody-dependent cellular cytotoxicity.
    - Rituximab binds CD20 and is useful for lymphomas.
    - Trastuzumab binds to HER2 receptors and is useful in HER2-positive breast cancer.
    - Bevacizumab acts on vascular endothelial growth factor, blocking its action of proliferation of blood vessels. It is useful in nonsmall cell lung carcinoma (nonsquamous) and colorectal carcinoma.
  - Conjugated mAb is conjugated with toxins derived from plants or bacteria (immunotoxins) or cytotoxic agents so that the toxin is directed to the tumour cells by the bound mAb.
    - Gemtuzumab ozogamicin is an anti-CD33 antibody conjugated with a cytotoxic antitumour

antibiotic, calicheamicin and used in relapsed or refractory AML.
    - Trastuzumab emtansine is a conjugate of trastuzumab with cytotoxic agent mertansine and approved for HER2-positive breast cancer.
  - mAbs are conjugated to a radio-isotope (radioimmunotherapy) so that local radiation can be given to tumour cells.
    - Tositumomab, an mAb directed against CD20 antigen, when tagged with I^{131}, can be used in refractory lymphomas.
  - Immunoliposomal therapy uses antibody-conjugated liposomes where liposomes can carry drugs or therapeutic agents directed against malignant cells. It is useful in some brain and breast cancers.
  - Checkpoint inhibitor therapy using antibodies to circumvent the defences used by tumours to suppress the immune system. Each defence is known as a checkpoint. Examples include CTLA-4 targeted by ipilimumab, PD-1 targeted by nivolumab and pembrolizumab, and PD-L1 targeted by atezolizumab and durvalumab.
- **Diagnostic applications:**
  - Can be used for diagnosis of primary malignancies and metastatic lesions. For it, mAb specific for a tumour-associated membrane antigen is attached to a radioactive compound which can then be detected. Examples include I^{131}-labelled mAb for detection of regional lymph nodes in patients with breast carcinoma.
  - Pregnancy rapid test kit which detects presence of beta-hCG by using mAb against it.
- **Miscellaneous applications:**
  - Emicizumab binds to two coagulation factors (factor IXa and factor X), taking the place of activated factor VIII (factor VIIIa) in the coagulation cascade. This mAb is available for prophylaxis against bleeding in certain individuals with haemophilia A.
  - Casirivimab plus imdevimab and sotrovimab have been given emergency use authorisation (a mechanism to facilitate the availability and use of medical countermeasures during public health emergencies) for treatment of mild-to-moderate COVID-19.

Q. Describe haemophagocytic lymphohistiocytosis

Q. Describe macrophage activation syndrome.

- Haemophagocytic lymphohistiocytosis (HLH) is a cytokine storm which may be fatal.
- Macrophage activation syndrome (MAS) falls under the umbrella of haemophagocytic lymphohistiocytosis and is applied when it occurs due to underlying systemic juvenile chronic arthritis or other rheumatological diseases.
- HLH is characterised by uncontrolled activation and proliferation of T cells and macrophages, leading to a storm of inflammatory cytokines, resulting in cytokine-mediated tissue injury and multiorgan dysfunction.

TABLE 3.7 Classification of Haemophagocytic Lymphohistiocytosis

Primary HLH (HLH Caused by a Genetic Disorder)	Acquired or Secondary HLH (HLH Caused by Another Condition)
• Familial haemophagocytic lymphohistiocytosis • HLH associated with genetic disorders	• Infection-associated HLH (e.g. Epstein-Barr virus, influenza, SARS-CoV2) • Rheumatologic HLH or MAS (e.g. systemic juvenile chronic arthritis, SLE, Adult-onset Still disease, Kawasaki disease) • Malignancy-associated HLH • Chemotherapy-associated HLH

CLASSIFICATION

- Classification of HLH is given in Table 3.7.

PATHOGENESIS

- The pathogenesis of MAS is complex and multifactorial, causing a dysregulated immune response to various stimuli with consequent hypercytokinaemia which is self-propagating in the absence of normal downregulation.
- Due to overactivation of the immune response, an inapt activation of T lymphocytes and histiocytes occurs, which causes these hyperactive immune cells to start attacking the blood cells, bone marrow, spleen and other organs. Inflammatory cytokines are also produced in excess, creating a 'cytokine storm' which results in clinical symptoms such as fever and rash.

CLINICAL FEATURES

- Patients present with high, nonremitting fever due to the excess interleukins.
- Hepatosplenomegaly and lymphadenopathy occur because of tissue infiltration
- Coagulopathy manifesting as haemorrhage, petechiae, ecchymosis, purpura and DIC.
- Gastrointestinal symptoms include diarrhoea, nausea, vomiting, jaundice and abdominal pain.
- CNS features include seizures, meningismus, cranial nerve involvement, ataxia, dysarthria, lethargy and encephalopathy.
- Cardiopulmonary involvement can lead to hypotension and respiratory failure requiring vasopressor and ventilator support.

LABORATORY FEATURES

- Pancytopenia secondary to the TNF and interferon surge coupled with phagocytosis
- Low fibrinogen because of excess plasminogen activator from macrophages leading to increased plasmin which cleaves fibrinogen with consequent coagulation disorder
- Sharply raised ferritin levels consequent to secretions from activated macrophages
- Raised triglycerides because of decreased lipoprotein lipase
- Haemophagocytes in bone marrow

BOX 3.4 Diagnostic Criteria (HLH-2004)

- Fever
- Splenomegaly
- Cytopenias (affecting minimum two lineages in peripheral blood)
  - Haemoglobin <9 g/dL
  - Platelets < 100,000/μL
  - Neutrophils <1000/μL
- Hypertriglyceridemia (fasting triglycerides >265 g/dL) or hypofibrinogenaemia (fibrogen <150 mg/dL)
- Ferritin >500 ng/mL
- Haemophagocytosis in bone marrow, spleen or lymph nodes
- Low or absent NK cell activity
- Elevated soluble CD25 (i.e. sIL2R)

DIAGNOSTIC CRITERIA (HLH-2004)

- Five out of the eight criteria are required to diagnose HLH (Box 3.4).

TREATMENT

- Supportive care—packed red cells, platelets, fresh frozen plasma.
- Suppression of the uncontrolled inflammation is the primary aim of therapy in MAS.
- HLH-94 protocol (etoposide and dexamethasone along with intrathecal methotrexate) and HLH-2004 protocol (cyclosporin, etoposide and dexamethasone along with intrathecal hydrocortisone and methotrexate) are widely used for the treatment of HLH.
- Rituximab, an anti-CD20 monoclonal antibody that destroys B cells is useful in EBV-associated HLH.
- The IL-1 receptor blocking agent, anakinra to achieve rapid remission when conventional therapy fails.
- IL-1 neutralising antibody or soluble decoy receptors, namely canakinumab and rilonacept, respectively, in resistant cases, have now been approved.
- Haematopoietic stem cell transplantation is the treatment of choice in familial HLH FHL and recurrent secondary HLH.

Q. Write a brief note on IgG4-related disease.

- IgG4-related disease (IgG4-RD) is an immune-mediated condition of unknown aetiology that can cause fibro-inflammatory lesions in nearly any organ.
- Patients may present with involvement of a single organ or with multiple organs involved at the same time.
- In untreated patients, different organs may be involved sequentially; this is termed metachronous involvement.

CLINICAL FEATURES

- IgG4-RD typically presents in an indolent fashion and is sometimes discovered incidentally. This is in contrast to infectious diseases, which generally present in acute or subacute fashion.
- Symptomatic patients present due to mass effect or injury caused by the inflammatory lesion.
- Constitutional symptoms such as fatigue and arthralgias may occur in a few patients.

SYMPTOMS RELATED TO IGG4-RELATED DISEASE IN THE CHEST

- More than 50% are asymptomatic and are discovered on routine investigations. When present, symptoms include cough, shortness of breath and chest pain.

SYMPTOMS RELATED TO GASTROINTESTINAL INVOLVEMENT

- The most common gastrointestinal organ affected by IgG4-RD is the pancreas followed by bile ducts.
- Autoimmune pancreatitis is the most common manifestation and the patient may present with jaundice, and hyperglycaemia and steatorrhoea due to endocrine and exocrine pancreatic deficiency respectively.

OTHER ORGAN INVOLVEMENT

- Orbital involvement produces periorbital swelling and proptosis secondary to lacrimal gland enlargement (dacryoadenitis).
- Painless, firm bilateral enlargement of two or more sets of salivary glands (Mikulicz disease).

INVESTIGATIONS

- Elevated ESR and globulins.
- Elevated IgG4 levels in more than 70% cases.
- Chest radiograph is not sensitive enough to diagnose IgG4-RD of chest.
- CT chest may show symmetrical, contrast-enhancing lymphadenopathy involving neck, axillae, hila and mediastinum. Airway changes are characterised by smooth or nodular thickening of the airway wall. Consolidation, ground glass opacities, pulmonary nodules and/or small pleural effusion are the most frequent intrapulmonary manifestations. Cardiac features include coronary artery pseudotumours and aneurysms. Periaortitis manifests as a soft-tissue formation around the aorta and other vessels.
- CT abdomen may show diffusely enlarged pancreas, focal pancreatic mass or ductal dilatation.
- Histopathologic evaluation of the affected tissue shows dense lymphoplasmacytic infiltration, storiform fibrosis (an irregularly cartwheel-like fibrotic pattern) and obliterative phlebitis. Immunohistochemistry shows the presence of IgG4-positive plasma cells. Prominent neutrophilic infiltration, granuloma and necrosis exclude the diagnosis of IgG4-RD.

DIAGNOSTIC CRITERIA

- Diagnostic criteria for IgG4-RD are shown in Table 3.8.

TREATMENT

- Patients with symptoms and organ impairment should be treated with glucocorticoids.
- Azathioprine, methotrexate and rituximab may be useful in select group of patients.
- Significant fibrosis and damage can lead to obstruction and this can be alleviated with stents.

TABLE 3.8 Diagnostic Criteria for IgG4-Related Disease (2020)

Item 1	Clinical and radiological features: • One or more organs show diffuse or localised swelling or a mass or a nodule characteristic of IgG4-RD. In single organ involvement, lymph node swelling is omitted
Item 2	Serological diagnosis: • Serum IgG4 levels greater than 135 mg/dL
Item 3	Pathological diagnosis: • Positivity for two of the following three criteria: • Dense lymphocyte and plasma cell infiltration with fibrosis • Ratio of IgG4-positive plasma cells/IgG-positive cells greater than 40% and the number of IgG4-positive plasma cells greater than 10 per high power field • Typical tissue fibrosis, particularly storiform fibrosis, or obliterative phlebitis
Definite: 1+2+3; Probable: 1+3; Possible: 1+2	

Q. Describe primary immunodeficiency diseases (MI 1.10)

- Primary immunodeficiency disorders (PIDs) are a group of heterogeneous immune disorders that affect distinct components of the adaptive and innate immune system.
- The clinical presentation is variable and includes increased susceptibility to infections, autoimmunity and malignancy.
- It can present in the neonatal period or as late as adulthood depending upon the severity of the immune defect.

CLASSIFICATION OF PRIMARY IMMUNODEFICIENCY DISEASES (Box 3.5)

BOX 3.5 Classification of Primary Immunodeficiency Diseases

- Immunodeficiencies affecting cellular and humoral immunity
- Combined immunodeficiencies with associated or syndromic features (includes Wiskott-Aldrich syndrome)
- Predominantly antibody deficiencies
- Diseases of immune dysregulation
- Congenital defects of phagocyte number or function
- Defects in intrinsic and innate immunity
- Autoinflammatory disorders
- Complement deficiencies
- Phenocopies of inborn errors of immunity

WARNING SIGNS OF PRIMARY IMMUNODEFICIENCY DISORDERS (Box 3.6)

BOX 3.6 Warning Signs of Primary Immunodeficiency Disorders

- ≥4 ear infections in 1 year
- ≥2 serious sinus infections in 1 year
- ≥2 pneumonias in 1 year
- Recurrent, deep skin or organ abscesses
- Persistent thrush in mouth or fungal infection on skin
- ≥2 deep-seated infections including sepsis
- ≥2 months on antibiotics with little effect
- Need for intravenous antibiotics to clear infections
- Failure of an infant to gain weight or grow normally
- Family history of primary immunodeficiency

BOX 3.7 Disorders of Antibody Deficiency

- X-linked agammaglobulinaemia
- Common variable immunodeficiency
- IgA deficiency
- IgG-subclass deficiency
- Others

- The 10 warning signs do not take into account the fact that PIDs include diseases that present with sporadic infections, autoimmunity, autoinflammation and malignancy.

PREDOMINANTLY ANTIBODY DEFICIENCIES

- Constitute 70% of all PIDs.
- Presentation with recurrent pyogenic infections starting after the age of 6–12 years.
- Various disorders are listed in Box 3.7.

X-LINKED AGAMMAGLOBULINAEMIA (BRUTON AGAMMAGLOBULINAEMIA)

- Occurs due to deficiency of Bruton tyrosine kinase (Btk), which is required for the growth and maturation of B-cell precursors.

Clinical Features

- Described as 'little boys with big infections'.
- Symptoms appear at the age of 6–12 months, that is after the loss of maternal immunoglobulins.
- Presentation is with infections of skin, mucous membranes, ear (ototis media), lungs (pneumonia), blood (sepsis), gut (giardia) and meninges.
- Tonsils are small and lymph nodes are not palpable.
- Typical bacterial infections include *Haemophilus influenzae* and *Streptococcus pneumoniae*.
- Malignancy can develop in older patients.
- Prevention of infection is by avoidance measures, vaccination, prophylactic antibiotics and administration of immunoglobulins.

COMMON VARIABLE IMMUNODEFICIENCY

- Usually presents in the second or third decade of life with increased infections.
- The estimated prevalence is one in 20,000 to one in 50,000.
- Patients with common variable immunodeficiency (CVID) typically have normal total B cells, but many will have low memory B cells.
- Presents with chronic lung infections, chronic giardiasis, intestinal malabsorption, atrophic gastritis and pernicious anaemia.
- CVID can also present with noninfectious sequelae, such as autoimmune disease.
- Increased risk of lymphoreticular and gastrointestinal malignancies.

IGA DEFICIENCY

- Presents with recurrent respiratory infections and chronic diarrhoea.
- May be associated with ataxia-telangiectasia.

HYPER-IGE SYNDROME (JOB SYNDROME)

- Presents with recurrent abscesses, eczema, eosinophilia and high serum IgE levels.

COMBINED HUMORAL AND CELLULAR IMMUNITY DEFICIENCIES

SEVERE COMBINED IMMUNODEFICIENCY

- In one of the types of severe combined immunodeficiency (SCID), the enzyme adenosine deaminase is deficient.
- Presents in the neonatal period with infections including opportunist infections (e.g. *Pneumocystis jirovecii*), chronic thrush and chronic diarrhoea.
- Lack of lymphoid tissue including thymus, tonsils and lymph nodes.
- Profound lymphopaenia (<500/µL) and absence of thymus shadow on chest radiograph.
- In ADA-deficient SCID, chest radiograph shows cupping at the ends of the ribs. Other abnormalities include chondro-osseous dysplasia with abnormalities in vertebrae.
- Treatment is prophylaxis for *Pneumocystis* with sulphamethoxazole-trimethoprim, immunoglobulin therapy and enzyme replacement therapy using polyethylene glycol ADA (PEG-ADA).
- Patients should not receive any live vaccines
- Blood products for transfusion should be irradiated.

ATAXIA-TELANGIECTASIA

- An autosomal recessive disorder.
- Patients present with progressive cerebellar ataxia, abnormal eye movements, oculo-cutaneous telangiectasia and immune deficiency. They often have recurrent sinopulmonary infections and bronchiectasis.
- Associated endocrine abnormalities include gonadal dysgenesis, testicular atrophy and diabetes mellitus
- There is IgA and IgG2 deficiency with variable depression of T cell functions
- Elevated serum alpha-foetoprotein is diagnostic.
- There is an increased risk of malignancies including lymphoma, leukaemias and breast cancer.

WISKOTT-ALDRICH SYNDROME

- It is an X-linked disorder.
- Patients have low IgM, normal IgA and IgG, and high IgE.
- Patients present with immunodeficiency, thrombocytopenia with small platelets (microplatelets) and eczema.

PHAGOCYTE DEFICIENCIES

- These include DiGeorge syndrome, chronic granulomatous disease (CGD), Chediak-Higashi syndrome and cyclic neutropenia.

DIGEORGE SYNDROME

- In this syndrome, there is defective development of thymus and parathyroid glands which develop from third and fourth pharyngeal pouch.

Clinical Features (CATCH)

- **C**ardiac abnormalities (interrupted aortic arch, truncus arteriosus, tetralogy of Fallot)
- **A**bnormal facies with low set ears
- **T**hymic aplasia
- **C**left palate
- **H**ypocalcaemia (due to hypoparathyroidism)

CHRONIC GRANULOMATOUS DISEASE

- X-linked recessive transmission in 50% of cases while rest are autosomal recessive.
- White blood cells do not produce hydrogen peroxide, superoxide and other activated oxygen compounds because nicotinamide adenine dinucleotide phosphate oxidase activity is deficient. This leads to defective intracellular phagocytic activity. Bacteria and fungi are not killed despite normal phagocytosis.
- Presents with recurrent abscesses during early childhood although the onset may be delayed in some patients.
- Multiple granulomatous lesions occur in the lungs, liver, lymph nodes, and gastrointestinal and genitourinary tracts.
- Treatment is prophylactic antibiotics and usually antifungals. Haematopoietic stem cell transplantation is curative.

CHEDIAK-HIGASHI SYNDROME

- It is an autosomal recessive condition, characterised by oculocutaneous albinism, easy bruisability, abnormal function of natural killer cells and recurrent pyogenic infections.
- Giant lysosomal granules develop in neutrophils and other cells. The abnormal lysosomes cannot fuse with phagosomes, so ingested bacteria cannot be lysed normally.
- In about 80% of patients, an accelerated phase occurs, causing fever, jaundice, hepatosplenomegaly, lymphadenopathy, pancytopenia, bleeding diathesis and neurologic changes.
- Most patients die of infections by age 7 years.
- Treatment is supportive care using antibiotics, interferon gamma and sometimes corticosteroids. Haematopoietic stem cell transplantation is curative.

CYCLIC NEUTROPENIA

- It is usually transmitted in an autosomal dominant fashion.
- It is characterised by regular, periodic oscillations in the number of peripheral neutrophils. The mean oscillatory period is 21 ± 3 days. Cycling of other blood cells is also evident in most cases.
- Patients may develop infections at the nadir of neutrophil count.

COMPLEMENT DEFICIENCIES

- Complement deficiencies are rare (≤2%); they include isolated deficiencies of complement components or inhibitors.

- Hereditary deficiencies are autosomal recessive except for deficiencies of C1 inhibitor, which is autosomal dominant, and properdin deficiency, which is X-linked.
- The deficiencies result in defective opsonisation, phagocytosis and lysis of pathogens, and in defective clearance of antigen–antibody complexes.
- The most serious consequences are recurrent infections due to defective opsonisation, and autoimmune disorders (e.g. systemic lupus erythematosus, glomerulonephritis) due to defective clearance of antigen–antibody complexes.
  - Deficiency of C5, C6, C7, C8, C9 (membrane attack complex) causes recurrent *N. meningitidis* and disseminated *N. gonorrhoeae* infections.
  - Deficiency of C1, C2 and C4 is associated with development of SLE
- A deficiency in C1 inhibitor causes hereditary angioedema.

Q. Explain urticaria or hives. (DR14.1, DR14.5)

- Formation of 'wheal-and-flare' cutaneous lesions involving only the superficial portions of the dermis. This results in circumscribed wheals with erythematous, raised and serpiginous borders with blanched centres.
- The lesions vary in size from 1 mm to several centimetres.
- Fresh lesions may appear as the older ones fade.
- Almost always pruritic and usually last for a few to 24 hours. When individual lesions last more than 36–48 hours and leave postinflammatory hyperpigmentation or palpable purpura, diagnosis of urticarial vasculitis is more likely.
- Some lesions may last for several weeks. Those lasting up to 6 weeks are classified as acute urticaria while those persisting beyond 6 weeks are classified as chronic urticaria.
  - Acute urticaria has many causes, with the most common being viral infections and food.
  - Chronic urticaria can be idiopathic, cold-induced or cholinergic (results from an increase in body temperature, such as when sweating, exercising or taking a hot shower).
- May be associated with headache, dizziness, nausea, vomiting, abdominal pain, diarrhoea and arthralgias. In most severe form, it may be associated with anaphylaxis.
- Pathogenesis involves degranulation of mast cells, which may be induced by immunologic or nonimmunologic mechanisms, and subsequent release of histamine and various cytokines leading to oedema. Non-immunological mast cell activation may occur via substances such as neuropeptides (e.g. substance P), drugs (e.g. morphine, codeine, vancomycin), foods (e.g. strawberries) and radiocontrast media.
- Types of urticaria (based on aetiopathogenesis) are shown in Box 3.8.
- Cold urticaria is a common form of chronic-inducible urticaria characterised by the development of wheals, angioedema or both in response to cold exposure.

BOX 3.8 Types of Urticaria

Immunologic
- IgE dependent
- Autoimmune
- Immune complex mediated
- Contact
- Complement dependent

Nonimmunologic
- Direct mast cell-releasing agents
- NSAIDs, ACE inhibitors

Physical
- Dermatographism
- Delayed pressure
- Cold
- Localised heat
- Cholinergic

Idiopathic

TREATMENT

ACUTE URTICARIA

- Long-acting, nonsedating antihistamines (e.g. cetirizine, levocetirizine, fexofenadine).
- Avoidance of trigger if identified.

CHRONIC URTICARIA

- Additional treatment is omalizumab if required.

Q. Discuss the clinical features and treatment of angioedema. (DR14.1, DR14.5)

- An IgE-mediated reaction to a variety of allergens presenting as well-demarcated oedema involving the deeper layers of skin as well as subcutaneous and submucosal tissues.
- May occur at any age but most commonly affects young adults.
- Acute angioedema lasts for up to 6 weeks; chronic angioedema beyond 6 weeks.
- Most cases are idiopathic. It may occur due to insect sting, drug reaction, food allergy and exposure to other biological products. It can also occur due to direct release of histamine from the mast cells. Rarely, angiotensin-converting enzyme (ACE) inhibitors can cause angioedema (bradykinin-mediated).
- Hereditary angioedema, an autosomal dominant disorder, is due to the deficiency of production of C1-esterase inhibitor, a complement protein that inhibits spontaneous activation of classical complement pathway. Angioedema occurs either spontaneously or following infection or injury particularly dental injury. Urticaria does not occur. Onset is usually in early childhood but it can begin during adulthood also. The attacks become worse at puberty and usually decrease in frequency and severity after the age of 50 and may even disappear totally. Diagnosis confirmed by low levels of C1-esterase inhibitor (in 85% cases) or dysfunctional C1-esterase inhibitor (in 15% cases). C4 levels are also low while C1q levels are normal.
- Acquired C1-esterase inhibitor deficiency can present very similar to the hereditary angioedema, but the onset occurs in the fifth and sixth decades of life.

Both C1-esterase inhibitor and C1q levels are low. It may occur with B-cell lymphoma, multiple myeloma, Waldenstrom's macroglobulinaemia and chronic lymphocytic leukaemia.

- ACE inhibitors usually produce angioedema due to increased bradykinin levels which is normally metabolised by ACE. Most cases occur within 3 weeks of starting treatment but can occur at any time during treatment. It usually affects the face and oral mucosa and can cause serious breathing difficulty.

CLINICAL FEATURES

- Presents with well defined, nonpitting swelling, usually nonpruritic.
- In a large proportion of patients, it is associated with urticarial lesions.
- May involve any area of the body and may occur as single or multiple lesions. Characteristically, the peri-orbital, peri-labial (Fig. 3.5) and genital areas are involved.
- Involvement of tongue and pharynx may produce dysphagia.
- Stridor, hoarseness, dysphagia and drooling indicate impending airway compromise.
- Angioedema of intestines may produce severe abdominal pain.

TREATMENT

- Remove the offending agent if possible.
- Control an acute attack with epinephrine.
- Administer high doses of antihistamines to control the lesions, for example diphenhydramine in a dose of 50 mg four times a day.
- Observe the patient for any evidence of airway obstruction. Manage patients with features of airway obstruction in a fashion similar to those with anaphylaxis.
- In patients with chronic angioedema not responding to antihistamines used in maximal dosages, glucocorticosteroids and other immunomodulating agents (e.g. methotrexate, cyclosporin and intravenous immunoglobulins) may be considered.

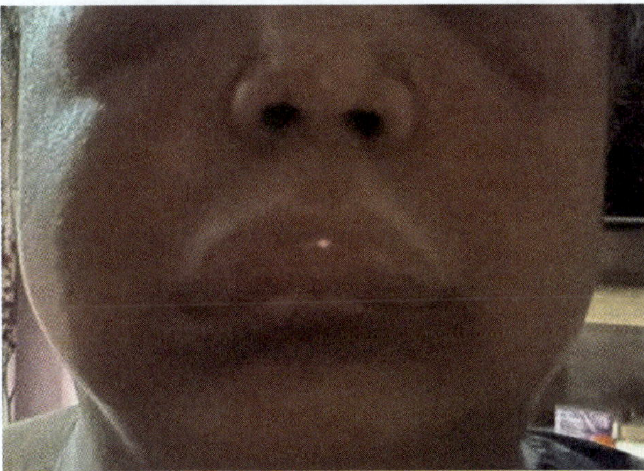

Fig. 3.5 Peri-labial angioedema.

HEREDITARY ANGIOEDEMA

- During severe attacks of hereditary angioedema, fresh frozen plasma (or plasma-derived C1-esterase inhibitor concentrate) is life-saving as it provides C1-esterase inhibitor. Another option is solvent/detergent-treated plasma. Recombinant C1-esterase inhibitor is available in some countries and is used for both treatment and prophylaxis. Ecallantide, a kallikrein inhibitor and icatibant, a bradykinin-receptor antagonist, are also approved for treatment of acute attack. Antihistamines and steroids are not effective. Danazol is useful to prevent episodes of hereditary angioedema.

ACE-INDUCED ANGIOEDEMA

- Treatment is still controversial. Corticosteroids and antihistamines do not show efficacy.
- Use of fresh frozen plasma or C1 inhibitor concentrate may be beneficial.

Q. What are anaphylactic reactions?

Q. Discuss briefly anaphylactoid reaction.

- Anaphylactic reaction is a prototype example of a type I hypersensitivity immunologic reaction that is IgE mediated. It is defined as a severe, life-threatening, rapidly evolving, generalised or systemic hypersensitivity reaction.
- Prior sensitisation to inciting antigen, either alone or in combination with a hapten, is required. This initial event results in the synthesis of specific IgE, which attaches to mast cells and basophils. Subsequent exposure to the antigen produces IgE-induced degranulation of mast cells and basophils resulting in the liberation of a number of active substances (Box 3.9).
- The release of these mediators of inflammation is responsible for the pathogenesis of an anaphylactic reaction.
- In addition, myocardial depression also develops which contributes to hypotension and relative bradycardia.
- Anaphylactic reactions have three patterns: uniphasic, biphasic and protracted reactions.
    - A uniphasic reaction occurs as an isolated reaction producing signs and symptoms typically within 30 minutes of exposure to an offending allergen and resolving usually within 1–2 hours.
    - In biphasic reaction, initial reaction is followed by occurrence of second wave of symptoms after

BOX 3.9 Active Substances Released From Mast Cells and Basophils

- Histamine
- Leucotrienes (LTC_4, LTD_4, LTE_4)
- Prostaglandins
- ECF-A (eosinophil chemotactic factor of anaphylaxis)
- Kinins
- NCF (neutrophil chemotactic factor)
- Platelet-activating factor
- Heparin

resolution (spontaneously or with treatment) of the first phase. Most biphasic reactions occur within 8 hours of the first symptoms.
  - A protracted reaction may last for a prolonged period of time.
- Anaphylactoid reactions (pseudo-allergic reactions) are indistinguishable from anaphylactic reactions. However, these reactions involve IgG and IgM antibodies and not IgE antibodies. These antibodies activate the complement system through classical pathway that results in the formation of activated complements. Further, there may be direct release of preformed mediators from mast cells and basophils. Reaction may occur on first exposure to an agent. The radiographic contrast reactions are typically anaphylactoid reactions. Other causes of anaphylactoid reaction include use of opiates, aspirin, vancomycin, plasma expanders and quinolones, exposure to cold and exercise. Since manifestations are similar to anaphylaxis, the term anaphylactoid is no longer recommended.
  - Intravenous (IV) vancomycin's classic side effect, red man syndrome (upper body—erythema and pruritus), is a predictable pharmacologic side effect of nonspecific mast cell activation and histamine release that can be managed by slowing the infusion rate (e.g. 10 mg/min or 1 g over 100 minutes) and treatment with H_1 antihistamines.

CLASSIFICATION AND CAUSATIVE AGENTS

- Anaphylaxis classified into four categories:
  - Immunologic IgE-mediated anaphylaxis.
  - Immunologic non-IgE-mediated anaphylaxis.
  - Nonimmunologic anaphylaxis.
  - Idiopathic anaphylaxis.
- Various causes of anaphylaxis are listed in Table 3.9.

CLINICAL FEATURES

- Within minutes to hours of antigenic exposure, several clinical symptoms may occur due to anaphylaxis (Box 3.10).
- Insect stings:
  - Yellow wasps do not lose their stinger and the sting site frequently becomes infected. On the other hand, honeybees lose their stinger that may be implanted at the site of a sting.
  - Clinical features of anaphylaxis induced by insect sting are similar to the ones produced by other causes.
  - The most common reaction to insect stings is local reaction (erythema, itching, pain and swelling). Multiple stings (50–100 simultaneously) may produce toxic reaction in the form of nausea, vomiting, diarrhoea, light-headedness and syncope but without urticaria, bronchospasm and angioedema.
  - Occasionally, haematological, renal and neurological features are also seen after the insect sting but these are not related to IgE-mediated reactions.
  - Delayed reaction can occur in three forms: early delayed reaction (urticaria, arthritis and pedal oedema) within 6–24 hours, reaction within 24–72 hours (skin rash and urticaria) and serum sickness after 10–14 days.

TABLE 3.9 Causes of Anaphylaxis According to Its Category

Category	Causative Agents
Immunologic IgE-mediated anaphylaxis	Food allergens (peanuts, fish, egg, milk, soy products) Airborne allergens (animal dander, aerosolised foods, pollen) Latex Insects (honey bee, wasp, yellow jacket, hornet) Antibiotics (penicillins, cephalosporins, tetracyclines, trimethoprim-sulphamethoxazole, vancomycin, nitrofurantoin) Chemotherapeutic agents Other medications (insulins, vitamin B1 and folic acid, diuretics and β-blockers, suxamethonium, propofol) Biologicals (blood and its components, tetanus, rabies and diphtheria antitoxins, antithymocyte globulin, vaccines, cytokine inhibitors, omalizumab)
Immunologic non-IgE-mediated anaphylaxis	Radiocontrast agents Intravenous immunoglobulin Aspirin and NSAIDs ACE inhibitors Dialysis membranes Dextrans High-molecular-weight iron (injectable) Biologicals
Nonimmunologic anaphylaxis	Opiates Physical (heat, cold, exercise, sunlight) Radiocontrast agents
Idiopathic	–

BOX 3.10 Clinical Features of Anaphylaxis

Mucocutaneous
- Pruritus
- Flushing
- Urticaria
- Angioedema
- Conjunctival injection

Respiratory
- Bronchospasm resulting in chest tightness, dyspnoea and wheeze
- Laryngeal oedema resulting in stridor
- Pulmonary oedema

Gastrointestinal
- Nausea, vomiting
- Abdominal cramps
- Diarrhoea

Cardiovascular
- Tachycardia
- Hypotension
- Arrhythmias
- Shock and collapse

DIAGNOSIS

- Diagnostic criteria for anaphylaxis are given in Box 3.11.

TREATMENT

- Epinephrine is the first treatment to be given to patients with anaphylaxis. 0.2–0.5 mL of a 1:1000 solution epinephrine is given intramuscularly (lateral aspect of thigh) and repeated at 5–10 minutes intervals if response is inadequate. In severe cases, 1 mL of 1:100,000 of solution is given intravenously over 2–10 minutes.

BOX 3.11 Diagnosis of Anaphylaxis

- With unknown allergen or an acute onset of illness with:
  - Development of mucocutaneous features (pruritus, flushing, urticaria, angioedema) with one of the following:
    - Respiratory compromise (wheezing, stridor, hypoxaemia/cyanosis)
    - Reduced blood pressure or end-organ dysfunction (e.g. collapse, syncope, incontinence)
- After exposure to known or likely allergen, rapid occurrence of ≥2 of:
  - Development of mucocutaneous features
  - Respiratory compromise
  - Reduced blood pressure (systolic blood pressure <90 mmHg or greater than a 30% decrease in systolic blood pressure from the patient's baseline) or end-organ dysfunction (e.g. collapse, syncope, incontinence)
  - Persistent gastrointestinal features (abdominal pain, nausea, vomiting)
- After exposure to known allergen:
  - Rapid fall in blood pressure

- IV line.
- Oxygen 4–6 L/minute.
- Remove allergen if still present (e.g. honeybee sting).
- Endotracheal intubation or tracheostomy with intermittent positive pressure ventilation, if laryngeal oedema is severe and patient shows signs of asphyxiation and hypoxaemia.
- Hypotension is managed with intravenous fluids (30 mL/kg over 1 hour or faster) and if required with noradrenalin.
- Bronchodilators—nebulised salbutamol.
- Glucagon if anaphylaxis develops in patients taking β-blockers.
- Hydrocortisone 200 mg IV stat (not effective for the acute event as it takes 4 hours to act; but may be considered for persistent bronchospasm and hypotension).
- Diphenhydramine (H_1-blocker), 50–100 mg IM/IV mainly for associated urticaria.
- Ranitidine (H_2-blocker), 50 mg IV.
- Fig. 3.6 summarises treatment of a patient with anaphylaxis.

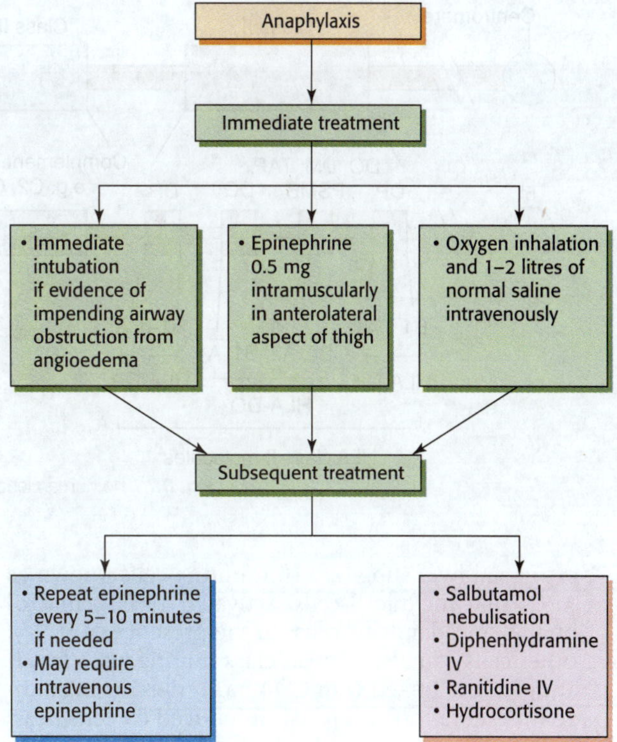

Fig. 3.6 Treatment of anaphylaxis.

Q. What is meant by serum sickness?

- This is a type III hypersensitivity immune reaction where IgG is produced in response to the injection of foreign antigen in large quantities. These form soluble immune complexes that result in fever, vasculitis, glomerulonephritis, arthritis and cardiac involvement. At the local site of injection, there would be urticaria and enlargement of lymph nodes. This is an immune complex deposition mediated disease.
- Develops 1–3 weeks after exposure to the antigen.

Q. Explain the HLA system.

- The HLA (human leukocyte antigens) system plays a central role in intercellular recognition and discrimination between self and nonself.
- The term 'tissue rejection' connotes a type IV immune reaction that leads to the destruction of a transplant by a recipient who is genetically nonidentical to the donor. Here the recipient lymphoid system recognises foreign (nonself) antigens in the donor tissue. These cell surface antigens that evoke rejection of transplants are called HLA. The genes that code for HLA are called HLA genes or histocompatibility genes.
- The HLA genes are clustered and located on the short arm of chromosome 6, identified as HLA complex or the MHC (major histocompatibility complex). MHC refers to a genetic region containing hundreds of genes, including the HLA genes.
- The HLA genes code for cell-surface glycoproteins called HLA or human leucocyte antigens.
- The HLA genes that are involved in the immune response fall into two main classes: class I and class II.

CLASS I GENES

- Three common class I genes are HLA-A, -B and -C. These genes produce class I molecules or antigens that are expressed by most somatic cells except erythrocytes and trophoblasts. Class I molecules interact with CD8+ T cells during antigen presentation and therefore, are involved in mainly driving cytotoxic reactions. Since this class of molecules is present on all nucleated cells, nearly all cells can present to cytotoxic cells.

CLASS II GENES

- Class II genes are HLA-D with several families (DR, DQ and DP are the major ones). These genes are

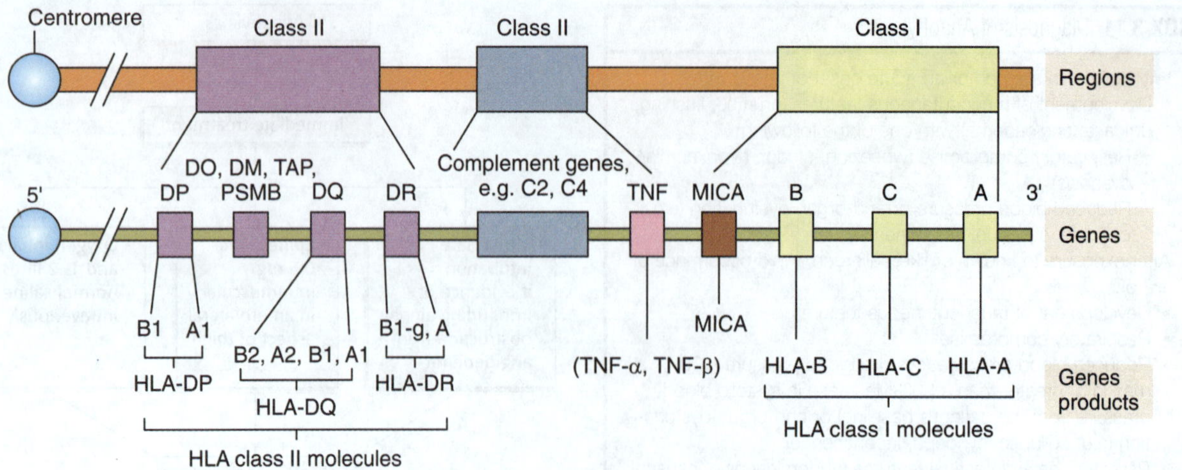

Fig. 3.7 The human leucocyte antigen (HLA) system.

expressed by a subgroup of immune cells known as APCs that include B cells, activated T cells, macrophages and dendritic cells. In the presence of IFN-γ, other cells can also express class II antigens. Class II antigens are linked with CD4 molecules during antigen presentation and reaction induced by cells bearing this class of molecules is of helper type.

OTHER GENES

- Besides class I and class II genes, another group of genes, that is class III is present between class I and class II regions and include genes for TNF-α, TNF-β, the complement components C2, C4 and Bf and the enzyme 21-hydroxylase. These are non-HLA genes. (Fig. 3.7).

HLA GENES AND IMMUNE FUNCTIONS

- The main function of both the classes of genes is to present pathogen-derived peptides to T cells. The antigen must be presented to the T cells as a peptide fragment within the groove of the HLA molecules on the APCs. Free antigen will have no effect. Antigen expressed with class I is endogenous, that is the molecules are produced within the cell, such as viral proteins and tumour antigens. On the other hand, cells bearing class II molecules take up exogenous antigen by endocytosis and degrade it intracellularly. The processed antigen is then re-expressed on the cell surface with class II molecules.

SIGNIFICANCE OF HLA SYSTEM

- HLA typing is prerequisite in selecting appropriate donor and recipient combinations for transplantation.
- Regulation of cell-to-cell interaction in the immune response (immune response Ir genes).
- Role in host defence against viral infections.
- Association of HLA with disease.
  - Individuals who possess HLA-B27 antigen have an 87-fold greater risk of developing ankylosing spondylitis than do individuals lacking this antigen. HLA genes are therefore related to disease susceptibility. Other diseases associated with HLA-B27 include acute anterior uveitis, Reiter syndrome, reactive arthritis and psoriatic arthritis.
  - HLA-DR3 is associated with coeliac disease and IgA deficiency.
- Drug-induced hypersensitivity may also be related to HLA system:
  - HLA-B*15:02 with carbamazepine-induced Stevens–Johnson syndrome/toxic epidermal necrolysis (SJS/TEN) in Southeast Asian populations.
  - HLA-B*57:01 with abacavir hypersensitivity.

Q. What is acquired immunodeficiency syndrome? Discuss the staging, aetiology, transmission, clinical manifestations, laboratory diagnosis and management. (DR11.1, IM6.1, IM6.11, IM6.16, IM6.18, IM6.2, IM6.3, IM6.4, IM6.5, IM6.9)

- Worldwide over 38.4 million people are seropositive for HIV, and more than 1.5 million people acquired HIV (2021 data).
- In India, estimated number of HIV-positive cases is 2.401 million (2021 data). Maharashtra had the highest number of HIV persons followed by Andhra Pradesh. HIV incidence was estimated at 0.05 per 1000 uninfected population. In 2021, India had 62,970 new HIV infections compared to 150,000 in 2005. Nearly 42,000 people died of HIV infection in 2021 compared to 150,000 in 2005.
- AIDS is caused by a single-stranded RNA human retrovirus known as HIV. It possesses the RNA-dependent DNA polymerase [reverse transcriptase (RT) enzyme].

DEFINITION

- An individual infected with HIV is known as HIV-infected individual.

- AIDS is the most advanced stage of HIV infection and is defined as symptomatic HIV infection as defined below in clinical stage 4 or CD4+ count <200/mm³.

STAGING

- WHO clinical staging of HIV infection is shown in Table 3.10.

AETIOLOGY

- Human retroviruses belong to two distinct groups: Human T-lymphotropic viruses (HTLV-I and HTLV-II) and human immunodeficiency viruses (HIV-1 and HIV-2).

TABLE 3.10 WHO Clinical Staging of HIV Infection

Primary HIV Infection	Asymptomatic A cute HIV Infection
Clinical stage 1	Asymptomatic Persistent generalised lymphadenopathy (PGL)
Clinical stage 2	Moderate unexplained weight loss (<10% of presumed or measured body weight) Recurrent respiratory tract infections (sinusitis, tonsillitis, otitis media, pharyngitis) Herpes zoster Angular cheilitis Recurrent oral ulceration Seborrhoeic dermatitis
Clinical stage 3	Fungal nail infections Unexplained severe weight loss (>10% of presumed or measured body weight) Unexplained chronic diarrhoea for longer than 1 month Unexplained persistent fever (above 37.6°C intermittent or constant for >1 month) Persistent oral candidiasis Oral hairy leucoplakia Pulmonary tuberculosis Severe bacterial infections Acute necrotising ulcerative stomatitis, gingivitis or periodontitis Unexplained anaemia (<8 g/dL), neutropenia (<500/μL) or chronic thrombocytopenia (<50,000/μL)
Clinical stage 4	HIV wasting syndrome *Pneumocystis* pneumonia Recurrent severe bacterial pneumonia Chronic herpes simplex infection Oesophageal candidiasis Extrapulmonary tuberculosis Kaposi's sarcoma Cytomegalovirus infection Central nervous system toxoplasmosis HIV encephalopathy Extrapulmonary cryptococcosis including meningitis Disseminated nontuberculous mycobacterial infection Progressive multifocal leucoencephalopathy Chronic cryptosporidiosis (with diarrhoea) Chronic isosporiasis Disseminated mycosis (coccidiomycosis or histoplasmosis) Recurrent nontyphoidal *Salmonella* bacteraemia Lymphoma (cerebral or B-cell non-Hodgkin) or other solid HIV-associated tumours Invasive cervical carcinoma Atypical disseminated leishmaniasis

- HIV has an icosahedral structure containing numerous external spikes formed by two major envelope proteins, gp120 and gp41.
- HIV-1 comprises several subtypes with different geographic distribution.
- There are three main groups of HIV-1: group M (major), group O (outlier) and group N (new). The M group comprises nine subtypes or clades designated A, B, C, D, F, G, H, J and K as well as four major circulating recombinant forms (AE or simply E, AG, AGI and AB). Subtype C is the major clade of HIV in India.
- HIV RNA has three structural genes: *gag*, *pol* and *env*.
  - The *gag* gene encodes the structural proteins of the core (p24, etc.).
  - The *env* gene encodes the viral envelope glycoproteins, gp120 and gp41.
  - The *pol* gene encodes for enzymes crucial for viral replication. These are the RT that converts viral RNA into DNA, the integrase that incorporates the viral DNA into host chromosomal DNA and the protease that cleaves large *gag* and *pol* protein precursors into their components.

REPLICATION CYCLE OF HIV

- HIV can infect a number of different cells, including CD4-bearing macrophages, T-helper lymphocytes and dendritic cells within the host.
- HIV attaches to the target cells through binding of surface glycoprotein gp120 to cell surface CD4 molecules.
- Binding to another coreceptor, CCR5 or CXCR4, produces conformational changes on viral surface exposing gp41 that allows it to fuse with the cell membrane. Inhibition of this binding will inhibit viral replication.
- T-cell tropic HIV strains mainly use CXCR4 as a coreceptor and are called X4 strains, whereas macrophage-tropic strains responsible for host-to-host transmission use CCR5 as a coreceptor and are referred to as R5 strains. The significant role of CCR5 in this process is borne out by the observation that individuals homozygous for mutations within CCR5 gene are resistant to infection by HIV-1.
- After the virus invades a macrophage or T lymphocyte, RT enzyme initiates copying of the viral RNA into single-stranded DNA and then a complimentary copy of DNA is created producing a double-stranded DNA.
- The viral DNA migrates and enters the host cell nucleus and becomes integrated into the cell DNA with the help of the enzyme integrase. The provirus can then remain latent or be active, generating products for the generation of new virions.
- Transcription and translation of viral DNA produces viral RNA. The HIV genes, *gag* and *pol*, produce large polypeptides. Before budding of virus, these polypeptides undergo processing by the enzyme protease (Fig. 3.8).
- Once infection is systemic, HIV preferentially targets CCR5/CD4 memory T lymphocytes in the gastrointestinal tract, a crucial element in host defence in the gut.
- The average time from HIV acquisition to a CD4 cell count <200 cells/mm³ is approximately 8–10 years.

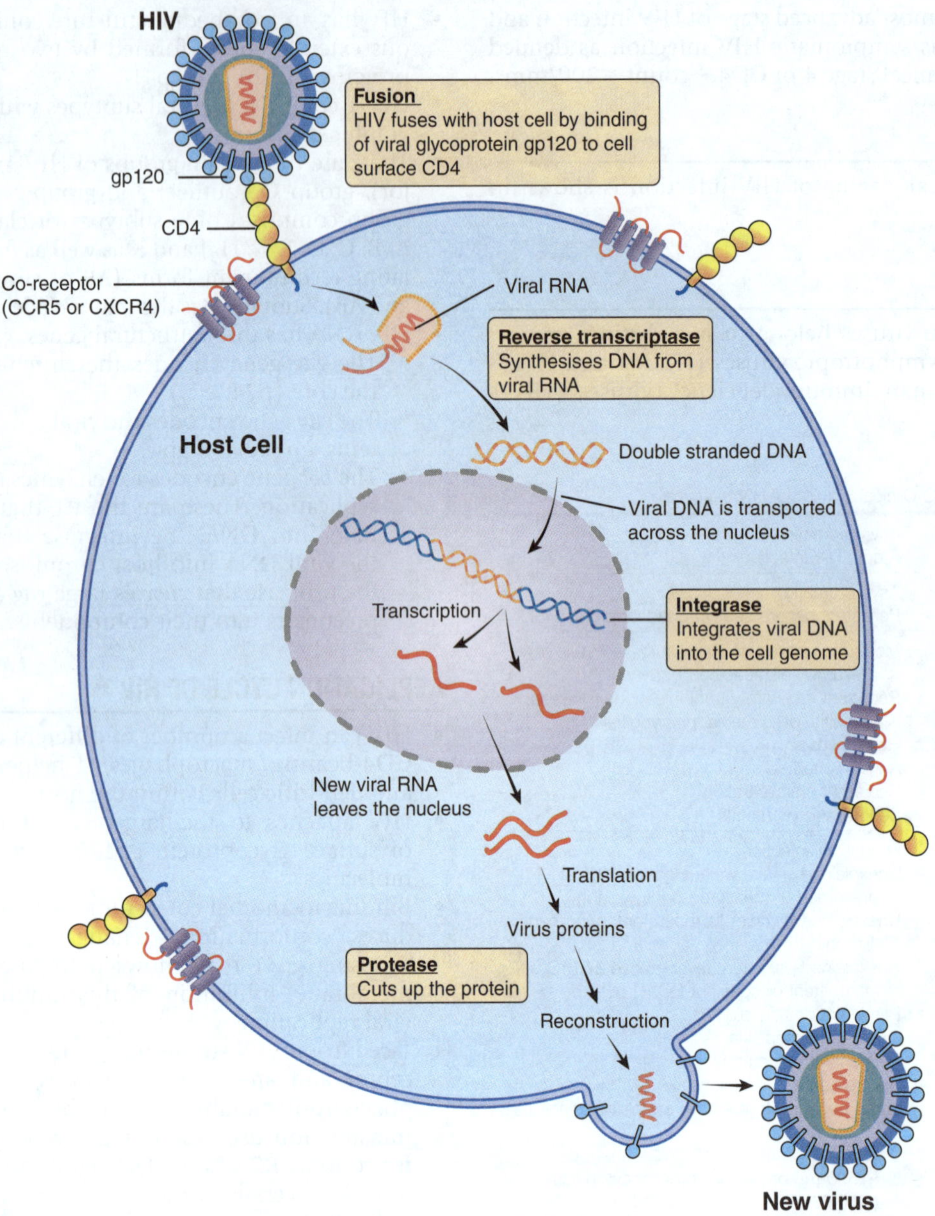

Fig. 3.8 Lifecycle of HIV.

TRANSMISSION

- Table 3.11 lists routes of transmission of HIV while Table 3.12 lists routes not involved in transmission of HIV.

CLINICAL MANIFESTATIONS OF HIV/AIDS

- The seroconversion occurs within 3 weeks to 3 months after exposure.
- Spectrum of HIV/AIDS is shown in Box 3.12.

ACUTE SEROCONVERSION

- In about 15% of cases acquiring HIV infection, an acute viral illness develops about 6 weeks after exposure.
- Features of acute seroconversion are shown in Table 3.13.
- This illness is self-limiting and lasts for 2–3 weeks.
- Usually, the person is in the 'window period' and hence seronegative but during the recovery phase HIV antibody test often turns positive.
- When diagnosis is not made in acute phase, it is often delayed for years until opportunistic infections develop.
- Diagnosis can be made by detecting HIV RNA or p24 antigen. HIV-specific antibodies are not detectable. The period from the time the virus enters the host until detectable levels of HIV-specific antibodies appear is called the 'window period' or 'acute infection phase'.
- Antiretroviral therapy (ART) should be started in these individuals. It helps in preserving immune function and reduces infectiousness.

TABLE 3.11 Routes of Transmission of HIV

Parenteral	Sexual
• Transfusion of blood and blood products • Needle sharing (including intravenous drug users) • Needle stick injuries • Injections with unsterile needles • Splash of body fluids on mucosa (mouth, nose and eyes)	• Homosexuals • Heterosexuals **Perinatal** • Vertical transmission from mother to foetus • Peripartum • Breastfeeding

TABLE 3.12 Routes Not Involved in Transmission of HIV

- Close personal contact including kissing
- Household contact
- Contact at school, swimming pool
- Sharing of utensils and insect bites

BOX 3.12 Spectrum of HIV Infection/AIDS

- Acute seroconversion illness
- Chronic HIV infection:
  - Asymptomatic viral carriage (with or without abnormal cell-mediated immunity)
  - Persistent generalised lymphadenopathy
  - Early symptomatic HIV infection (previously known as AIDS-related complex (ARC) [also known as HIV-associated neurocognitive disorders—HANDs] and HIV constitutional disease)
  - AIDS characterised by a CD4+ cell count <200 cells/mm^3 or the presence of any AIDS-defining condition (opportunistic infections, malignancies) regardless of CD4+ cell count
  - Advanced HIV infection characterised by a CD4+ cell count <50 cells/mm^3

TABLE 3.13 Clinical and Laboratory Features of Acute Seroconversion

Clinical Features	Laboratory Features
• Fever • Fatigue • Pharyngitis • Headache • Myalgia/arthralgia • Urticaria, skin rash • Lymphadenopathy • Aseptic meningitis, encephalitis, cranial nerve palsies	• Thrombocytopenia • Leucopenia • Elevated liver enzymes

ASYMPTOMATIC CARRIER STAGE

- The individual is asymptomatic but is potentially infectious for others.
- This stage may last for 5–10 years.
- Laboratory abnormalities may include anaemia, leucopenia, lymphopaenia, reduced CD4+ counts and cutaneous anergy.

PERSISTENT GENERALISED LYMPHADENOPATHY

- Though asymptomatic, some HIV carriers develop PGL.
- It is characterised by lymph node enlargement at two or more extrainguinal sites that are noncontiguous that persist for more than 3 months in the absence of any other illness. The lymph nodes are more than 1 cm in size.
- Biopsy reveals nonspecific lymphoid hyperplasia.

EARLY SYMPTOMATIC HIV INFECTION (HIV CONSTITUTIONAL DISEASE AND AIDS-RELATED COMPLEX)

- Within an average of 7–8 years, sometimes earlier (particularly in children), the patient develops features of early HIV infection. The patient has at least two of the following clinical symptoms and signs along with two or more abnormal laboratory features that persist for more than 3 months:
  - Fever more than 38°C (intermittent or continuous).
  - Weight loss of more than 10% of body weight.
  - PGL.
  - Diarrhoea.
  - Fatigue and night sweats.
  - Lymphopaenia, leucopenia and thrombocytopenia.
  - Reduced helper cells.
  - Cutaneous anergy.
- The condition of ARC with minor opportunistic infections like oral or vulvovaginal candidiasis was known as constitutional disease.
- Other features in early phase include oral hairy leucoplakia, seborrhoeic dermatitis, bacterial folliculitis and infections with herpes simplex virus, varicella zoster virus and human papillomavirus virus.

FULL-BLOWN AIDS

- Within a few months to years of showing features of early symptomatic HIV infection, the CD4+ count drops below 200/mm^3 and the patient develops a number of life-threatening infections and cancers (Table 3.14). The patient may also develop several neurological features. Clinical features of full-blown AIDS can be categorised into certain well-defined patterns (described below).
- There is a relation between CD4+ cell count and common illnesses in HIV patients (Table 3.15).

PULMONARY DISEASES

- In a patient with AIDS, three common causes of lung involvement are tuberculosis, bacterial pneumonia and *P. jirovecii* pneumonia (PCP). Other causes of lung involvement include CMV, toxoplasma and fungal infections, and Kaposi's sarcoma.
- Presentation of bacterial pneumonia is similar to that in immunocompetent people.

TABLE 3.14 List of Important Infections and Cancers in AIDS

Infections	Cancers
• *Pneumocystis jirovecii* • *Candida (invasive)* • *Cryptococcus* • *Toxoplasma* • Typical/atypical mycobacteria • Amoebiasis	• Kaposi's sarcoma • B-cell lymphoma of brain • Others

TABLE 3.15 Relation Between CD4+ Cell Count and Common Illnesses in HIV Patients

CD4+ Count	Illnesses
• 200–350/mm³	• Herpes simplex • Tuberculosis • Oral and vaginal thrush • Herpes zoster
• 100–200/mm³	• *Pneumocystis jirovecii* pneumonia • *Candida* oesophagitis
• 50–100/mm³	• Cryptococcal meningitis • AIDS dementia • Toxoplasma encephalitis
• <50/mm³	• Progressive multifocal leucoencephalopathy • *Mycobacterium avium* complex • Cytomegalovirus infection

PNEUMOCYSTIS JIROVECII INFECTION

- *P. jirovecii* (previously known as *Pneumocystis carinii*) is a fungus.
- Three stages in life cycle: cysts, trophozoites (outside cyst) and sporozoites (inside cyst). Methenamine silver stains the cyst wall while Giemsa stain is taken by the wall of the trophozoites and sporozoites. Trophozoites are in plenty in the lungs.

Clinical Features

- PCP presents with subacute onset of progressive dyspnoea, fever and nonproductive cough that gradually lead to respiratory distress and cyanosis. Acute onset is uncommon. Examination reveals crepitations; findings of consolidation are unusual.
- Extrapulmonary sites may be involved rarely; sites include skin, meninges, brain, eyes, heart, liver, spleen and kidneys. It is usually associated with the use of aerosolised pentamidine prophylaxis.

Diagnosis

- Arterial blood gas:
  - In mild cases, room air arterial oxygen (pO_2) > 70 mmHg or alveolar–arterial O_2 difference <35 mmHg.
  - In moderate to severe cases, $pO_2 < 70$ mmHg or alveolar–arterial O_2 difference > 35 mmHg.
- Chest radiograph shows a ground glass appearance or bilateral infiltrates (Fig. 3.9) but in some patients, it may be normal.
- Unusual patterns on X-ray include nodular shadows, cystic lesions, pneumothorax, lobar consolidation and apical involvement (in patients on pentamidine prophylaxis). Pleural effusion, cavitation and mediastinal lymphadenopathy are rare.
- Serum shows elevated LDH levels.
- Pulmonary functions show restrictive pattern with reduced diffusion capacity.
- CT chest shows patchy ground glass appearance (Fig. 3.10).
- Gallium-67 scan shows diffuse pickup even when the radiograph is normal.
- Diagnosis is established by demonstration of organisms in sputum (spontaneously expectorated or induced by hypertonic saline nebulisation) using methenamine silver or toluidine blue stain (Fig. 3.11). Other modes include bronchial lavage and transbronchial biopsy.

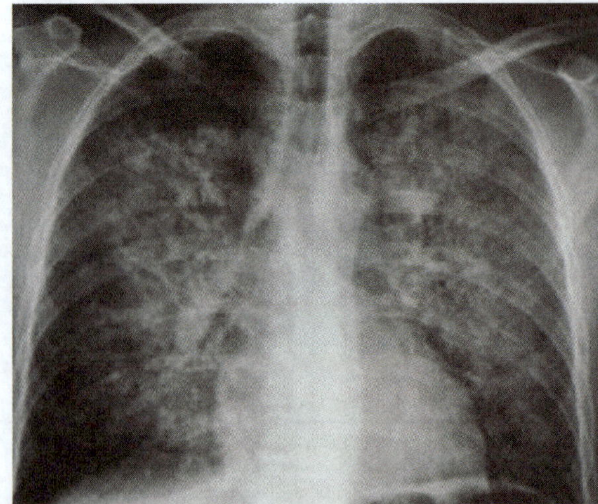

Fig. 3.9 Chest radiograph showing bilateral perihilar infiltrates.

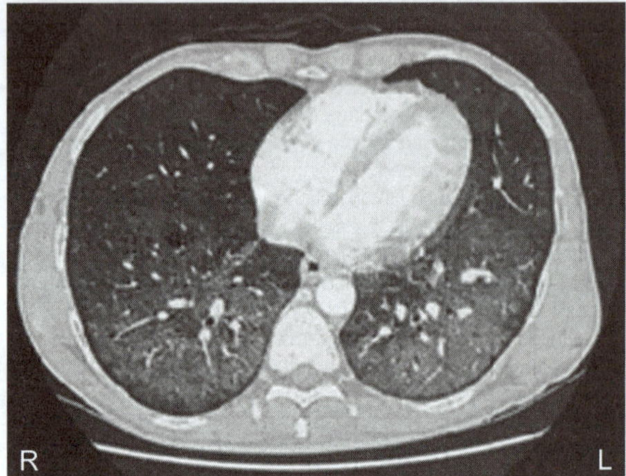

Fig. 3.10 CT scan of the chest demonstrating ground-glass opacity in a patient with *Pneumocystis jirovecii* pneumonia.

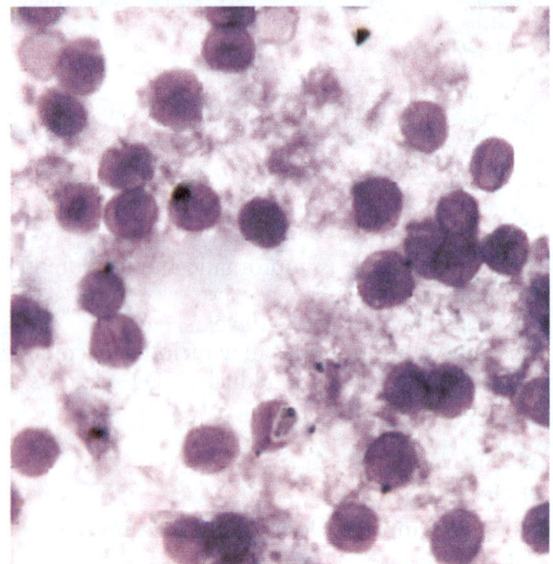

Fig. 3.11 Toluidine blue stain showing numerous *Pneumocystis jirovecii* cysts. *From* DP: Infectious Diseases.

TABLE 3.16 Treatment of Pneumocystis *jirovecii* Pneumonia

Mild Cases	Moderate to Severe Cases (PaO_2 < 70 mmHg)
• Trimethoprim 5 mg/kg 6 hourly + sulphamethoxazole 25 mg/kg 6 hourly orally OR • Trimethoprim 5 mg/kg 6 hourly + dapsone 2 mg/day OR • Pentamidine 4 mg/kg/day IV OR • Atovaquone 750 mg tid	• Trimethoprim 5 mg/kg 6 hourly + sulphamethoxazole 25 mg/kg 6 hourly IV OR • Pentamidine 4 mg/kg/day IV OR • Clindamycin (600 mg qid) + primaquine (30 mg od) • In all cases, add prednisolone 40 mg bid for 5 days, then 40 mg/day for 5 days and then 20 mg/day for 11 days

- Polymerase chain reaction is an alternative method for diagnosing PCP; however, it cannot reliably distinguish colonisation from disease.
- 1,3-β-D-glucan (a component of the cell wall of *Pneumocystis* cysts) is often elevated.

Management

- The drug of choice is trimethoprim/sulphamethoxazole combination for 21 days.
- Treatment is shown in Table 3.16.

Prophylaxis

- Primary prophylaxis (preventing first episode) is indicated in patients with CD4 cell count <200/mm³ (NACO recommends CD4 cell count <350/mm³) or if patient is in WHO clinical stage 3 or 4. Secondary prophylaxis is indicated in all patients who have recovered from PCP.
  - Trimethoprim 160 mg + sulphamethoxazole 800 mg/day, that is one single-strength tablet daily (TMP–SMX at a dose of one double-strength tablet daily confers cross-protection against toxoplasmosis also) OR
  - Aerosolised pentamidine 300 mg once a month OR
  - Dapsone 50 mg bid.
  - Others include atovaquone (1500 mg od), or dapsone (200 mg) plus pyrimethamine (75 mg) plus leucovorin (25 mg) all once a week.
- Primary and secondary *Pneumocystis* prophylaxis may be discontinued if the patient responds to ART with an increase in CD4+ counts from <200 cells/mm³ to >200 cells/mm³ for >3 months.

GASTROINTESTINAL DISEASES

CAUSES OF DIARRHOEA (TABLE 3.17)

- Acute infection with various bacterial agents usually produces abdominal pain, fever, diarrhoea and bloody stools.
- Standard antibiotic therapy is recommended; however, patients with AIDS are more likely to have protracted illness and suffer recurrences.
- Protozoal, CMV and mycobacterial infections tend to produce protracted diarrhoea and fluid and electrolyte imbalance.

TABLE 3.17 Causes of Diarrhoea in HIV/AIDS

Bacterial • *Salmonella* • *Campylobacter* • *Mycobacterium avium complex* • *Mycobacterium tuberculosis* • *Clostridioides difficile* • *Shigella* • Small bowel bacterial overgrowth **Protozoal** • *Microsporidium* • *Cryptosporidium* • *Cystoisospora belli* • *Giardia lamblia* • *Entamoeba histolytica* • *Cyclospora*	**Viral** • Cytomegalovirus • Herpes simplex • Rotavirus • Norwalk • HIV **Malignancies** • Lymphoma • Kaposi's sarcoma **Fungal** • Coccidioidomycosis • Histoplasmosis **AIDS enteropathy** **Antiretroviral drugs**

- ART is indicated in all patients with opportunistic infections including cryptosporidium, microsporidium and isospora infections as immune restoration often leads to eradication of infections. Nitazoxanide is the treatment of choice for *Cryptosporidium* infection. TMP–SMX is the antimicrobial agent of choice for treatment of isosporiasis. No specific therapeutic agent is available for microsporidium.

OESOPHAGITIS

- Oesophagitis is encountered in as many as 90% of the patients with AIDS. It is usually due to *Candida*, CMV and *Herpes simplex* virus.

MUCOCUTANEOUS DISEASES

- These include candidiasis, warts, molluscum contagiosum, herpes simplex, varicella-zoster and Kaposi's sarcoma.
- Kaposi's sarcoma can involve virtually any site in the body; however, cutaneous disease is most common. It presents as red or purple, flat or raised skin lesions. Involvement of lymph nodes, oral mucosa and viscera is quite common. Human herpes virus-8 is aetiologically associated with Kaposi's sarcoma. Treatment is chemotherapy in combination with ART. Liposomal doxorubicin and paclitaxel have comparable response rates. Importantly, concurrent use of corticosteroids should be avoided. Curettage of single nodules followed by topical application of hydrogen peroxide (to achieve haemostasis) is a safe, effective and simple method for lesion control.

NEUROLOGICAL DISEASES

ACUTE MENINGITIS

- During acute seroconversion, CNS invasion occurs in more than 90% cases. The clinical spectrum varies from a silent CSF pleocytosis, aseptic meningitis, an infectious mononucleosis-like syndrome, multiple cranial nerve palsies to acute encephalopathy. CSF shows lymphocytosis along with raised proteins (<200 mg/dL). CT is normal and recovery is usually complete.

AIDS DEMENTIA COMPLEX (ADC) OR HIV-ASSOCIATED NEUROCOGNITIVE DISORDERS

- It precedes the diagnosis of AIDS in about 25% of cases and can occur at any stage of AIDS.
- Includes three categories: asymptomatic neurocognitive impairment, mild neurocognitive disorder (MND) and HIV-associated dementia (HAD).

VACUOLAR MYELOPATHY

- It involves the white matter of lateral and posterior columns of the spinal cord resulting in spastic paraparesis and sensory ataxia. The onset is subacute.

VIRAL INFECTIONS

- Progressive multifocal leucoencephalopathy (PML) is caused by the polyoma virus (JC virus [JCV]) and is characterised by focal neurological abnormalities including blindness, aphasia, haemiparesis and ataxia that progress to altered sensorium and death within 6 months. Focal or multifocal nature of PML is responsible for distinct focal symptoms and signs rather than a more diffuse encephalopathy or dementia. CT scan shows nonenhancing, focal hypodense lesions. MRI confirms distinct white matter lesions in areas of the brain corresponding to clinical deficits. Confirmation is by PCR to identify JCV DNA in CSF. Treatment is mainly by starting ART immediately.
  - Also seen with lymphoproliferative disease and use of natalizumab in multiple sclerosis patients.
- Herpes simplex encephalitis may have an insidious onset as compared to an immunocompetent host. Despite treatment with acyclovir, the prognosis is poor.
- Herpes zoster may also produce myelitis or radiculitis.
- Cytomegalovirus may present with slowly progressive encephalitis or with myelitis and retinitis (retinal haemorrhage resulting in blindness). Other features include colitis and oesophagitis. Treatment involves lifelong use of intravenous ganciclovir (or oral valganciclovir) and foscarnet, either alone or in combination. For CMV retinitis, intravitreal ganciclovir plus oral valganciclovir is superior to once daily IV ganciclovir.

FUNGAL INFECTIONS

- Cryptococcal meningitis may present with headache and fever. However, meningismus may be present in only a minority of cases and fever may be absent in 10%–30% of episodes. The CSF may not show pleocytosis or raised proteins in some cases, thus complicating the diagnosis. However, cryptococcal antigen and culture are usually positive, both in serum and CSF. India ink staining on CSF may show the organisms (Fig. 3.12).
- Treatment is by administering amphotericin B (0.7 mg/kg/day) and flucytosine (25 mg/kg qid) for 2 weeks (induction phase) followed by flucytosine (400 mg/day) for 8–10 weeks (consolidation phase). Relapse rates are high and therefore, continuous therapy with flucytosine (200 mg/day) is recommended for at least 1 year to prevent relapse (maintenance phase).

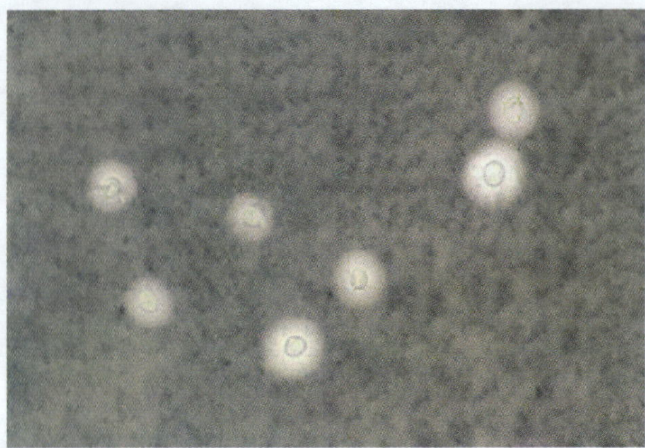

Fig. 3.12 India ink preparation of cerebrospinal fluid showing encapsulated yeast forms of *Cryptococcus neoformans*.

BACTERIAL INFECTIONS

- Tuberculous meningitis, common in AIDS patients, may present in a manner similar to cryptococcal meningitis. CSF usually reveals elevated cell counts and protein along with low glucose. CT scan may show multiple ring lesions suggestive of tuberculomas.
- Syphilis may progress rapidly to late manifestations including neurosyphilis. Manifestations include optic neuritis, uveitis, meningitis, encephalitis and cerebral infarction.

PROTOZOAN INFECTIONS

- The most common opportunistic infection of CNS is caused by *Toxoplasma gondii*. Toxoplasma encephalitis presents with headache, confusion, seizures, ataxia and focal deficits. A contrast CT or MRI is required for making a presumptive diagnosis of toxoplasma infection as the lesions appear as single or multiple contrast enhancing lesions often with surrounding hypodensity due to oedema, mainly in basal ganglia. Patients are seropositive for antitoxoplasma IgG antibodies. Brain biopsy is generally reserved for patients who fail to respond to specific therapy. Treatment is by a combination of pyrimethamine + sulphadiazine + leucovorin for at least 6 weeks.

Prophylaxis

- Prophylaxis indicated in toxoplasma-seropositive patients with a CD4+ count <100 cells/mL. One double-strength tablet of TMP–SMX daily is the preferred regimen.
- If patients cannot tolerate TMP–SMX, alternative is dapsone + pyrimethamine + leucovorin.

MISCELLANEOUS CNS MANIFESTATIONS

- Primary CNS lymphoma occurs in about 5% of cases and may present with encephalopathy, focal deficits, seizures or lymphomatous meningitis. CT scan shows multiple hypodense lesions with homogeneous or ring enhancement.
- Polyneuropathy.
- Central nervous system immune reconstitution syndrome (IRIS) is a significant complication of

anti-retroviral initiation with the most common causes due to cryptococcus, tuberculosis and progressive multifocal leukoencephalopathy.

OCULAR DISEASES

- Cotton wool spots are seen in 40%–60% of patients with AIDS and are benign in nature.
- Retinitis due to CMV is the most serious infection of the eyes. This may lead to a painless visual loss. Fundus may reveal cotton wool spots similar in appearance to the benign spots. More commonly, there are fluffy white retinal lesions with areas of haemorrhage. CMV can also produce colitis and oesophagitis.
- Another cause of retinitis in AIDS patients is infection with toxoplasma that presents with visual loss, photophobia and floaters.
- Herpes zoster may lead to ocular pain, conjunctival injection and corneal opacification.

OTHERS

MYCOBACTERIUM AVIUM COMPLEX

- Usually occurs if CD4+ <50/μL.
- Often presents with disseminated multiorgan infection (hepatomegaly, splenomegaly, lymphadenopathy) along with fever, night sweats, weight loss, fatigue, diarrhoea and abdominal pain.
- Localised manifestations occur among persons who are receiving and have responded to ART. Localised syndromes include cervical or mesenteric lymphadenitis, pneumonitis, pericarditis, osteomyelitis, skin or soft tissue abscesses, genital ulcers or CNS infection.
- Anaemia and raised alkaline phosphatase are common.
- Blood, bone marrow or lymph node aspirate may grow the organisms.
- Chemoprophylaxis against disseminated mycobacterium avium complex (MAC) disease is indicated if CD4+ count <50/μL. Azithromycin or clarithromycin are the preferred prophylactic agents.
- Treatment includes use of clarithromycin + ethambutol + rifabutin.

CARDIOVASCULAR DISEASES

- Increased risk for cardiovascular (CV) diseases (e.g. coronary artery disease, cardiomyopathy, myocarditis and arrhythmias).
- Increased risk of CAD and CHF due to several factors (Box 3.13).
- Myocarditis may be due to infections (e.g. fungal—*Candida, Histoplasma, Cryptococcus, Aspergillus*; viral—herpes simplex, cytomegalovirus; bacterial—tuberculosis; toxoplasmosis; and HIV infection itself).

SUMMARY OF TREATMENT OF OPPORTUNISTIC INFECTIONS IN HIV/AIDS

- Table 3.18 summarises treatment of opportunistic infections in patients with HIV/AIDS.

BOX 3.13 Risk Factors for CAD in HIV Patients

- Traditional risk factors (e.g. hypercholesterolaemia/atherogenic dyslipidaemia, high blood pressure, smoking, proatherogenic diet, obesity, diabetes, low physical activity)
- Decreased apolipoprotein B
- Increased level of proatherogenic 'small dense LDL'
- Increased LDL cholesterol, particularly small dense LDL during treatment
- Hypertriglyceridaemia due to PI drugs
- Increased blood pressure and insulin resistance due to ART
- Elevated inflammatory parameters (e.g. d-dimer, interleukin-6, CRP)
- Direct damage to coronary arterial wall by HIV

LABORATORY DIAGNOSIS OF HIV INFECTION

- By days 8–10 of infection, virus can be detected by a nucleic acid amplification test (NAAT). Viral proteins (p24 antigen) can be detected between days 13 and 20. IgM antibodies are detectable by day 20, and IgG antibodies by day 30 (Fig. 3.13).
- Testing begins with a fourth-generation combination immunoassay that detects HIV-1 and HIV-2 antibodies and HIV-1 p24 antigen. No further testing is required for specimens that are nonreactive on the initial immunoassay.
- Specimens with a reactive antigen/antibody combination immunoassay result is tested with an antibody immunoassay that differentiates HIV-1 antibodies from HIV-2 antibodies.
- Specimens which are reactive on the initial antigen/antibody combination immunoassay and nonreactive or indeterminate on the HIV-1/HIV-2 antibody differentiation immunoassay should be tested with an HIV-1 nucleic acid test (NAT).
- A reactive HIV-1 NAT result and nonreactive HIV-1/HIV-2 antibody differentiation immunoassay result indicate laboratory evidence for acute HIV-1 infection.
- A reactive HIV-1 NAT result and indeterminate HIV-1/HIV-2 antibody differentiation immunoassay result indicate the presence of HIV-1 antibodies confirmed by HIV-1 NAT.
- A negative HIV-1 NAT result and nonreactive or indeterminate HIV-1/HIV-2 antibody differentiation assay result indicate a false-positive result on the initial immunoassay (Fig. 3.14).
- Other findings include lymphopaenia, leucopenia, thrombocytopenia and decrease in T4-helper cells (CD4+ counts).
- Another test is polymerase chain reaction (PCR) for measuring the amount of viral particles (HIV RNA) in the blood (viral load).

DIAGNOSTIC STRATEGY AS PER NATIONAL AIDS CONTROL ORGANIZATION (NACO)

All persons should undergo pretest and posttest counselling and confidentiality should be maintained while disclosing the results.

For Diagnosis in Symptomatic Patients

- Serial testing strategy is configured as two tests algorithm and refers to the use of one screening test

TABLE 3.18 Summary of Treatment of Common Opportunistic Infections in AIDS

Opportunistic Infection	First-Line Treatment	Alternate Treatment
• *Pneumocystis jirovecii*	See text	See *Pneumocystis jirovecii* infection
• *Toxoplasma*	Pyrimethamine 50–100 mg/day + Sulphadiazine 1–1.5 g qid + leucovorin 25 mg od	Pyrimethamine 50–100 mg/day + Clindamycin 600 mg qid OR Trimethoprim (160 mg) + sulphamethoxazole (800 mg) qid
• *Cryptococcus*	Amphotericin 0.7 mg/kg/day + Flucytosine 25–37 mg/kg qid	Liposomal amphotericin 3–4 mg/kg/day
• *Isospora (Cystoisospora) belli*	Trimethoprim (160 mg) + sulphamethoxazole (800 mg) qid	–
• *Candida* (mucosal)	Clotrimazole 200–600 mg OR Fluconazole 50–100 mg/day	Ketoconazole 200 mg/day
• *Candida* (systemic)	Amphotericin 0.7 mg/kg/day	–
• *Cytomegalovirus*	Ganciclovir 5 mg/kg bid IV OR Valganciclovir 900 mg orally bid OR Foscarnet 60 mg/kg tid IV	Cidofovir 5 mg/kg/week IV
• *Herpes simplex* (oral or genital)	Acyclovir 200–400 mg five times/day	Valacyclovir 1 g bid Famciclovir 500 mg bid
• *Herpes simplex* (encephalitis)	Acyclovir 10 mg/kg tid IV	–
• *Herpes zoster* (local)	Valacyclovir 1 g tid OR Famciclovir 500 mg tid	Acyclovir 800 mg five times a day
• *Herpes zoster* (disseminated)	Acyclovir 10 mg/kg tid	–
• *Mycobacterium avium* complex	Clarithromycin 500 mg bid + ethambutol 15 mg/kg od	Azithromycin 500 mg od + ethambutol 15 mg/kg od

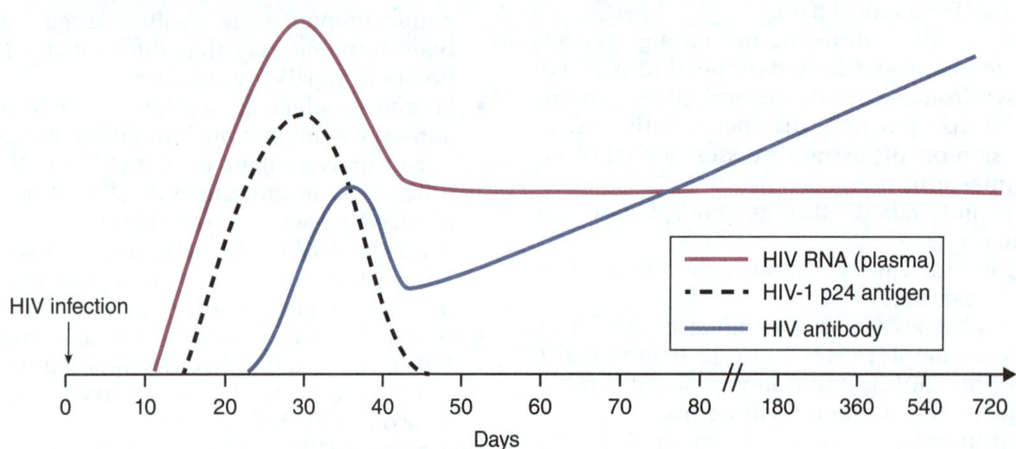

Fig. 3.13 Detection of HIV RNA, HIV p24 and HIV antibodies after HIV infection.

(rapid kit test or ELISA test) followed by *another* ELISA/rapid tests, depending on the results of the first.

- A nonreactive result from the initial screening test completes the testing, that is report is given out as HIV negative.
- If the initial test is reactive, it is followed by a single test for resolution. In case a specimen is reactive with the first test kit and nonreactive with the second test kit, the specimen is subjected to a third tiebreaker test. If the third test is reactive, the specimen is reported as indeterminate and follow-up testing is undertaken after 2–4 weeks or sample can be sent for confirmation by western blot test. In case the third test is nonreactive, the specimen is reported negative.

For Diagnosis in Asymptomatic Patients

- It is similar to above except that a positive test by initial two tests is confirmed by a third test.
- If the specimen gives a reactive result with two tests and nonreactive result with the third assay, it is reported as 'indeterminate' and the patient is called again for repeat testing after 2–4 weeks.

MANAGEMENT OF A PATIENT WITH HIV INFECTION

GENERAL MEASURES

- These include balanced diet, quitting smoking and intake of alcohol, adequate rest and practice of safer sex so as to avoid infection of partner and also to

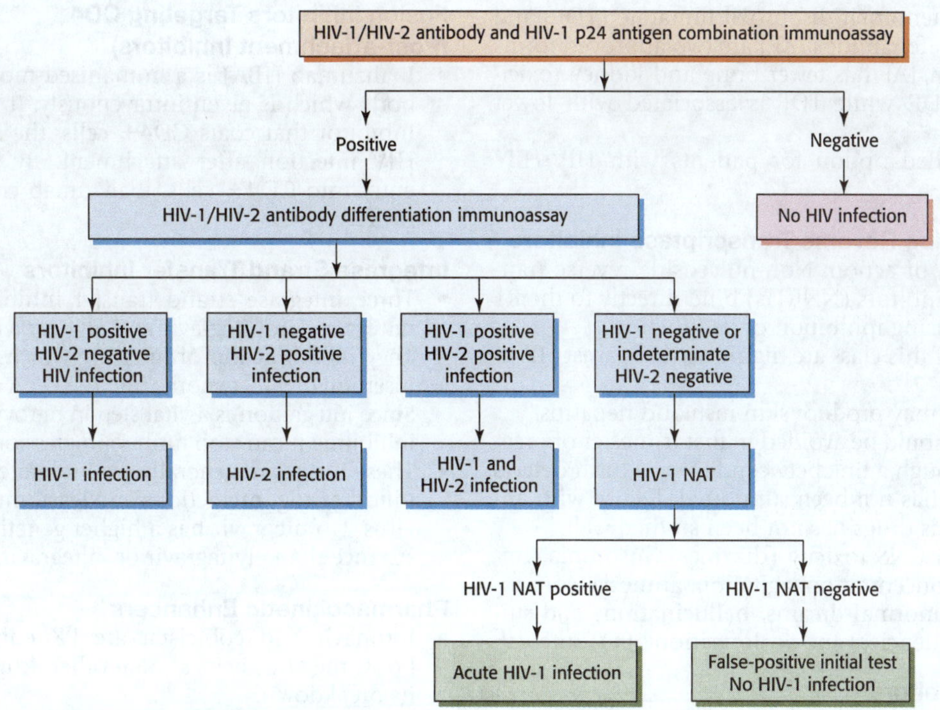

Fig. 3.14 Recommended laboratory HIV testing algorithm. (*Source*: Centers for Disease Control and Prevention and Association of Public Health Laboratories. Laboratory Testing for the Diagnosis of HIV Infection: Updated Recommendations; Figure 12, June 27, 2014.)

avoid infection with other organisms that may hasten the progress of the disease.

- An important aspect of treatment is counselling and proper education of the patient.

ANTIRETROVIRAL DRUGS

- Based on the action at various sites during HIV replication cycle and structure of drugs, several classes of drugs are presently available for treatment of HIV infection (Table 3.19).

Nucleoside Reverse Transcriptase Inhibitors

- Mechanism of action: These agents diffuse into the infected cells and are converted to their active triphosphate forms by cellular kinases. These active nucleosides are incorporated into the growing viral DNA and cause premature chain termination.
- Fatty change in the liver (hepatic steatosis) and lactic acidosis are two important adverse effects of nucleoside reverse transcriptase inhibitors (NRTIs) (particularly with zidovudine, stavudine and didanosine) that occur due to their effect on cellular mitochondria.
- Zidovudine can produce neutropenia and anaemia.
- Zalcitabine and stavudine may produce peripheral neuropathy.
- Didanosine may lead to pancreatitis.
- Zidovudine and stavudine can produce lipoatrophy.
- Abacavir can cause an increased risk of cardiovascular events and is associated with a serious hypersensitivity reaction in patients who are HLA-B*5701 positive.

Nucleotide Reverse Transcriptase Inhibitors

- This category includes nucleotide analogues that inhibit reverse transcriptase inhibitor.

TABLE 3.19 Classification of Antiretroviral Drugs

Nucleoside Reverse Transcriptase Inhibitors (NRTIs)	**Entry Inhibitors**
• Zidovudine[a] (AZT, ZDV)	***Fusion Inhibitors***
• Didanosine (ddI)	• Enfuvirtide (T20)
• Zalcitabine (ddC)	***CCR5 Inhibitors***
• Stavudine (d4T)	• Maraviroc (MVC)
• Lamivudine[a] (3TC)	***Fusion Inhibitors Targeting CD4 (postattachment inhibitors)***
• Abacavir[a] (ABC)	• Ibalizumab (IBA)
• Emtricitabine (FTC)	**Protease Inhibitors (PIs)**
Nucleotide Reverse Transcriptase Inhibitors (NtRTIs)	• Indinavir (IDV)
• Tenofovir disoproxil fumarate[a] (TDF)	• Ritonavir[a] (RTV)
• Tenofovir alafenamide (TAF)	• Saquinavir (SQV)
Non-nucleoside Reverse Transcriptase Inhibitors (NNRTIs)	• Nelfinavir (NFV)
• Nevirapine[a] (NVP)	• Amprenavir (APV)
• Delavirdine (DLV)	• Lopinavir/ritonavir[a] (LPV/r)
• Efavirenz[a] (EFV)	• Atazanavir[a] (ATV)
• Etravirine (ETR)	• Fosamprenavir (FPV)
• Rilpivirine (RPV)	• Tipranavir (TPV)
• Doravirine (DOR)	• Darunavir[a] (DRV)
	Integrase Strand Transfer Inhibitors (INSTIs)
	• Raltegravir[a] (RAL)
	• Dolutegravir (DTG)
	• Elvitegravir (EVG)
	• Bictegravir (BIC)
	• Cabotegravir (CAB)
	Pharmacokinetic Enhancer (PK)
	• Ritonavir (RTV or r)
	• Cobicistat (COBI or c)

Note: Lamivudine, emtricitabine and tenofovir also have activity against hepatitis B virus.
[a]Available under National Programme.

- At present, tenofovir disoproxil fumarate (TDF) and tenofovir alafenamide (TAF) are two approved forms of tenofovir. TAF has fewer bone and kidney toxicities than TDF, while TDF is associated with lower lipid levels.
- Recommended option for patients with HIV/HBV coinfection.

Non-Nucleoside Reverse Transcriptase Inhibitors

- Mechanism of action: Non-nulceoside reverse transcriptase inhibitors (NNRTIs) bind directly to the RT enzyme causing inhibition of its function.
- Members of this class are highly active against HIV-1 but not HIV-2.
- Nevirapine may produce skin rash and hepatitis.
- Efavirenz should be avoided in first trimester of pregnancy although a link between EFV and birth defects in humans has not been supported. Its use with antituberculous drugs has not been studied well.
  - It causes CNS toxicity (dizziness, insomnia, impaired concentration, agitation, amnesia, somnolence, abnormal dreams, hallucinations and suicidal tendencies) and prolongation of QT interval.

Protease Inhibitors

- Mechanism of action: These drugs inhibit enzyme protease and therefore, inhibit the final assembly of virus before release from infected cells.
- Protease inhibitors (PIs) have been associated with body fat redistribution that manifests physically as thinning of arms, legs and face and/or deposition of fat in the abdominal and shoulder regions along with lipomas (lipodystrophy). It occurs in 6%–80% of patients and develops after several months of therapy. The effects on fat metabolism may lead to raised levels of serum cholesterol and triglycerides, insulin resistance and rarely elevated blood glucose levels, which may increase cardiovascular risk.
- Some PIs, especially indinavir may produce hyperglycaemia.
- PIs have several drug interactions that need to be kept in mind while prescribing other drugs to patients taking PIs.
- Ritonavir is a potent inhibitor of the P450CYP3A enzyme and is typically used at low doses to boost the concentrations of other PIs since most are heavily metabolised by the P450 system. Hence, PIs are often used in combination with ritonavir ('ritonavir boosting').

Fusion Inhibitors

- This group contains agents that block the initial fusion of HIV with cell-surface receptors.
- Enfuvirtide (T20) is being used from this class of drugs. It is given by subcutaneous route. It does not inhibit HIV-2.

CCR5 Inhibitors

- Maraviroc is a CCR5 inhibitor that binds to the host cells through CCR5 receptors. It is only active in patients who do not have virions that use CXCR4 for cell entry. A specialised assay is therefore needed to screen for coreceptor tropism which will determine if a patient's virus will respond to this medication.

Fusion Inhibitors Targeting CD4 (Post-attachment Inhibitors)

- Ibalizumab (IBA) is a humanised monoclonal antibody which is given intravenously. It is a viral-entry inhibitor that coats CD4+ cells, the main target of HIV infection after attachment. By blocking viral entry into CD4+ cells, ibalizumab creates a barrier for HIV entry.

Integrase Strand Transfer Inhibitors

- Three integrase strand transfer inhibitors (INSTIs), raltegravir, dolutegravir and elvitegravir are in use.
- They inhibit action of integrase which is required for insertion of viral genome into the DNA of the host cell. Since integration is a vital step in retroviral replication, inhibiting it can stop further progression of disease.
- These drugs are generally well tolerated with no significant drug interactions and least initial resistant of virus. Dolutegravir has a higher genetic barrier to resistance than elvitegravir or raltegravir.

Pharmacokinetic Enhancers

- Ritonavir and cobicistat are PK enhancers which boost the effectiveness of another drug by inhibiting its breakdown.
- These drugs inhibit CYP3A4, with cobicistat being a more specific CYP inhibitor than ritonavir. Unlike ritonavir, cobicistat does not have antiretroviral (ARV) activity.
- Nearly all PIs and elvitegravir require a PK enhancer in order to achieve therapeutic plasma concentrations at the desired dose and frequency.

DOSES, ADVERSE EFFECTS AND SPECIAL PRECAUTIONS OF ANTIRETROVIRAL DRUGS

- Doses and adverse effects of antiretroviral drugs are given in Table 3.20.

GOALS OF ANTIRETROVIRAL THERAPY

- Eradication of HIV infection cannot be achieved with the currently available ARV regimens. This is due to the establishment of a pool of latently infected CD4+ cells during the earliest stages of acute HIV infection that persists with an extremely long half-life.
- The goals of treatment are given in Box 3.14.

INDICATIONS FOR ANTIRETROVIRAL THERAPY

- ART is recommended for all patients with HIV (including acute HIV infection) irrespective of CD4+ counts.
- Deferring ART until CD4+ decline puts patient at risk of both AIDS-defining and certain serious non-AIDS conditions. Furthermore, the magnitude of CD4+ count recovery is directly correlated with CD4+ count at ART initiation.
- Initiation of ART is urgently required in certain subgroups as shown in Box 3.15.

EVALUATION BEFORE INITIATING ART

- Complete history and physical examination.
- Ophthalmologic examination.
- Complete blood count, blood sugar, chemistry profile, urine analysis, creatinine clearance and lipid profile.

TABLE 3.20 Doses, Adverse Effects and Special Precautions of Commonly Used Antiretroviral Drugs

Drug	Dose	Adverse Effects	Remarks
Zidovudine (ZDV, AZT)	300 mg bid	Anaemia, neutropenia, bone marrow suppression, GI intolerance, headache, insomnia, myopathy, lactic acidosis, skin and nail hyperpigmentation	Monitor blood glucose and LFTs Monitor CBC every 4–8 weeks
Lamivudine (3TC)	150 mg bid or 300 mg od	Minimal toxicity; peripheral neuropathy, skin rash uncommon	Do not administer with emtricitabine or zalcitabine
Emtricitabine (FTC)	200 mg od	Skin discolouration in palms and soles, hepatotoxicity in hepatitis B coinfected persons who discontinue drug	Do not administer with lamivudine
Didanosine (ddI)	400 mg od	Peripheral neuropathy, pancreatitis, hepatitis	Evaluate for neuropathy every 2 months Avoid stavudine, zalcitabine and allopurinol
Stavudine (d4T)	40 mg bid	Peripheral neuropathy, pancreatitis, hepatitis, lipodystrophy	Evaluate for neuropathy every month Avoid zidovudine, didanosine and zalcitabine
Abacavir (ABC)	300 mg bid or 600 mg od	Hypersensitivity reaction (may be fatal), fever, rash, vomiting, sore throat, cough, shortness of breath	Get HLA B*5071 testing prior to initiation Avoid alcohol Avoid in persons with high risk of cardiovascular disease
Tenofovir disoproxil fumarate (TDF)	300 mg od	Glycosuria, proteinuria, elevation in creatinine, bone demineralisation	Creatinine at baseline, at 2–6 weeks and then every 3–6 months Urinalysis for glucose and protein Avoid atazanavir
Tenofovir alafenamide (TAF)	25 mg od	Renal toxicity (less than TDF), bone demineralization, hepatotoxicity	Avoid if eGFR <30/mL/min/1.73 m^2 Creatinine at baseline, at 2–6 weeks and then every 3–6 months Urinalysis for glucose and protein
Efavirenz (EFV)	600 mg od at bed time	Dizziness, somnolence, insomnia, hallucinations, agitation, abnormal dreams, personality change, skin rash (less common than nevirapine)	Avoid elvitegravir/cobicistat, etravirine, indinavir
Nevirapine (NVP)	200 mg od for 14 days and then 200 mg bid	Skin rash (may progress to Stevens-Johnson syndrome and toxic epidermal necrolysis), hepatitis, hepatic failure	Avoid atazanavir, elvitegravir/cobicistat, etravirine
Bictegravir (BIC)	50 mg od	Diarrhoea, nausea, headache	One of the first line integrase strand transfer inhibitors
Raltegravir (RAL)	400 mg bid	Rhabdomyolysis, myalgia, diarrhoea, fever, skin rash (including Stevens-Johnson syndrome and toxic epidermal necrolysis), hepatitis	May be used in place of dolutegravir if women is concerned about neural tube defect with latter drug Resistance develops in many persons
Dolutegravir (DTG)	50 mg od	Insomnia, headache, hypersensitivity reaction, hepatitis (patients with history of hepatitis B or hepatitis C infection may have increased risk of developing new or worsening liver problem), very low risk of neural tube defect when taken in first trimester of pregnancy	Resistance is uncommon with continuation
Elvitegravir (EVG)	85–150 mg od	Diarrhoea, rash, hepatitis	85 mg with atazanavir/ritonavir or lopinavir/ritonavir 150 mg with others Avoid efavirenz and nevirapine
Atazanavir/ritonavir (ATV/r) or Atazanavir/cobicistat[a] (ATV/c)	300 mg atazanavir + 100 mg ritonavir od or 300 mg atazanavir + 150 mg cobicistat	Unconjugated hyperbilirubinaemia, lipid abnormality, hyperglycaemia, lipodystrophy, nephrolithiasis, cholelithiasis, prolongation of PR interval on ECG	Avoid in severe hepatic insufficiency
Lopinavir/ritonavir (LPV/r)	400 mg lopinavir + 100 mg ritonavir bid	Diarrhoea, vomiting, abnormal lipid profiles, glucose intolerance, skin rash, hepatitis	

Continued

TABLE 3.20 Doses, Adverse Effects and Special Precautions of Commonly Used Antiretroviral Drugs—cont'd

Drug	Dose	Adverse Effects	Remarks
Darunavir/ritonavir (DRV/r) or Darunavir/cobicistat[a] (DRV/c)	600 mg darunavir + 100 mg ritonavir bid or 800 mg darunavir + 150 mg cobicistat od	Hepatotoxicity, skin rash (10%), diarrhoea, headache, hyperlipidaemia, hyperglycaemia	Avoid in persons with sulpha allergy
Enfuvirtide (T20)	90 mg subcutaneously bid	local pain, increased risk of pneumonia	—
Maraviroc (MVC)	150–300 mg bid	Cough, fever, rash, hepatitis, myalgias	Avoid in presence of severe renal insufficiency Viral tropism test to be done before initiation (cannot be used for CXCR4-tropic virus as it is CCR5 inhibitor)
Ibalizumab (IBA)	2000 mg loading followed by 800 mg every 2 weeks IV	Diarrhoea, skin rash	—

[a]Cobicistat does not have antiretroviral activity; used as a boosting agent. May falsely increase creatinine level.

BOX 3.14 Goals of Antiretroviral Therapy

- Maximally and durably suppress plasma HIV RNA
- Restore and preserve immunologic function
- Reduce HIV-associated morbidity and prolong the duration and quality of survival
- Prevent HIV transmission

BOX 3.15 Indications for Initiating ART Urgently

- Pregnancy
- AIDS-defining conditions, including HIV-associated dementia and AIDS-associated malignancies
- Acute opportunistic infections excluding cryptococcal and tubercular meningitis (risk of development of immune reconstitution inflammatory syndrome is high if ART is started before initiating treatment for these diseases)
- CD4+ counts below 200/mL
- Acute/early infection
- Coinfection with hepatitis B or hepatitis C
- Serodiscordant couples and prevention of transmission

- CD4+ cell count and percentage; measurement of CD8 cell count is unnecessary.
- Quantitative plasma HIV RNA.
- Drug resistance with an HIV genotype test strongly recommended.
- Coreceptor tropism testing if use of a CCR5 antagonist is being considered.
- HLA-B*5701 testing before initiating abacavir therapy as patients positive for this HLA type are prone to develop severe hypersensitivity reaction.
- Others tests including VDRL, Mantoux test, toxoplasma IgG serology, chest radiography and serology for hepatitis C and B.

INITIAL TREATMENT OF HIV PATIENTS

ANTIRETROVIRAL REGIMENS

- An ARV regimen for a treatment-naive patient generally consists of two NRTIs in combination with a third active ARV drug from one of three drug classes: an NNRTI, an INSTI or a PI with a PK enhancer (cobicistat or ritonavir).
- While initiating therapy, consideration should also be given to the number of pills per day, frequency of dosing, food requirements, toxicity and drug interactions with other drugs being used by the patient.
- INSTI-based regimens are recommended as initial therapy for most people with HIV as they achieve high rates of virologic suppression and often have greater tolerability than PI-based or NNRTI-based regimens.
- When starting ART, all drugs should be started simultaneously at full dose with the exception of ritonavir and nevirapine where dose escalation is recommended.
- Initial ART regimens recommended are shown in Table 3.21.

COMBINATIONS AND DRUGS NOT RECOMMENDED AS INITIAL TREATMENT

- Certain combinations and drugs are not recommended as initial treatment due to inferior efficacy or increased toxicity compared to recommended regimens (Table 3.22).

FACTORS AFFECTING RESPONSE TO ART

- To maximise the benefits of ART following factors should be ensured:
  - Adherence to the drug regimen.
  - Adequate serum levels of ARV drugs.
  - Rational sequencing of ARV drugs to preserve future treatment options for as long as possible.

TABLE 3.21 Recommended Initial ART Regimens

Integrase Inhibitor-Based Regimens (INST Plus 2 NRTIs):

- Bictegravir + Tenofovir alafenamide + Emtricitabine
- Dolutegravir + Tenofovir alafenamide (or Tenofovir disoproxil fumarate) + Emtricitabine (or Lamivudine)
- Dolutegravir + Abacavir + Lamivudine (or Emtricitabine) only for patients who are HLA-B*5701 negative
- Raltegravir + Tenofovir + Emtricitabine (or Lamivudine)
- Elvitegravir/cobicistat + Tenofovir + Emtricitabine (or Lamivudine)

INSTI Plus 1 NRTI:

- Dolutegravir + Lamivudine, except for individuals with HIV RNA >500,000 copies/mL, HBV coinfection, or in whom ART is to be started before the results of HIV genotypic resistance testing for reverse transcriptase or HBV testing are available

Alternative regimens for certain categories of patients (e.g. those with plasma HIV RNA **<100,000 copies/mL; resource-limited settings)—in addition to above-mentioned regimens:**

Nucleoside/nucleotide reverse transcriptase inhibitors + non-nucleoside reverse transcriptase inhibitor-based regimen (2 NRTIs Plus 1 NNRTI):

- Efavirenz + Tenofovir + Lamivudine (or Emtricitabine)[#]
- Efavirenz + Abacavir + Lamivudine (or Emtricitabine) only for patients who are HLA-B*5701 negative and abnormal creatinine value[#]
- Rilpivirine + Tenofovir + Emtricitabine (or Lamivudine) only for patients with CD4 count >200 cells/mm^3
- Doravirine + Tenofovir + Emtricitabine (or Lamivudine)

Boosted protease inhibitor–based regimens (PI + 2 NRTIs)— patients with uncertain adherence or in whom treatment needs to begin before resistance testing results are available (e.g. during acute HIV infection, pregnancy and in the setting of certain opportunistic infections):

- Atazanavir/ritonavir or Atazanavir/cobicistat + Abacavir + Lamivudine (or Emtricitabine) only for patients who are HLA-B*5701 negative
- Darunavir/ritonavir or Darunavir/cobicistat + Tenofovir + Emtricitabine (or Lamivudine)
- Atazanavir/ritonavir or Atazanavir/cobicistat+ Tenofovir + Lamivudine (or Emtricitabine)
- Darunavir/ritonavir or Darunavir/cobicistat + Abacavir + Emtricitabine only for patients who are HLA-B*5701 negative
- Tenofovir + Lamivudine + Lopinavir/ritonavir

Note:

1. Recommended regimen by National AIDS Control Organisation is Tenofovir disoproxil fumarate (300 mg) + Lamivudine (300 mg) + Dolutegravir (50 mg) in a single pill once a day.

[#]Alternate regimens by NACO.

2. The main advantages of tenofovir over abacavir are its activity against hepatitis B virus and the fact that HLA-B*5701 testing is not required for their use.
3. The main advantages of abacavir over TDF are that it does not require dose adjustment in patients with renal insufficiency and has less nephrotoxicity and less deleterious effects on bone mineral density than TDF.

TABLE 3.22 Combinations/Drugs Not Recommended as Initial Treatment

Combinations	Drugs
• Stavudine + Zidovudine	• Delavirdine
• Stavudine + Lamivudine	• Nevirapine (in ARV-naive women with CD4+ <250/mL or in ARV-naive men with CD4+ <400 cells/mL—increased risk of symptomatic, and sometimes life-threatening liver injury)
• Stavudine + Didanosine	• Nelfinavir
• Tenofovir + Didanosine	• Darunavir (unboosted)
• Zidovudine + Lamivudine[a]	• Atazanavir (unboosted)
• Didanosine + Tenofovir	• Fosamprenavir (boosted or unboosted)
• Didanosine + Lamivudine	• Indinavir (boosted or unboosted)
• Abacavir + Zidovudine + Lamivudine	• Ritonavir (as sole PI)
• Abacavir + Zidovudine + Lamivudine + Tenofovir	• Saquinavir (boosted or unboosted)
• Atazanavir + Indinavir	• Saquinavir (hard gel capsules)
• Emtricitabine + Lamivudine	
• Etravirine + Unboosted protease inhibitor	
• Lopinavir + 2 NRTIs	
• Triple NRTIs	
• Two NNRTIs	
• Maraviroc + Raltegravir	
• Maraviroc + Boosted protease inhibitor	

[a]Unless patient is already on this combination (along with one NNRTI) with HIV infection under control.

MONITORING OF THERAPY

- After initiation of ART, HIV RNA should be measured at 2–8 weeks to assess the efficacy of treatment. If detectable, repeat every 4–8 weeks until viral load is suppressed to undetectable level. Thereafter, repeat every 3–6 months. It should be suppressed by 16–20 weeks. Optimal viral suppression is defined generally as a viral load persistently below the level of detection (HIV RNA <20–75 copies/mL, depending on the assay used). As per National Programme, virological suppression means a viral load of less than 1000 copies/mL after at least 6 months on ART.
- A significant increase in CD4+ cell count is an increase of >30% from baseline for absolute cell numbers within 3–6 months. Therefore, monitor CD4+ count every 3–6 months till it is above 300–500 when the frequency can be reduced to once in 1–2 years.

STEM CELL TRANSPLANTATION IN HIV/AIDS

- Long-term control of HIV is possible with CCR5-delta-32 mutation stem cell transplantation. It is to be considered only if patient has another indication for stem cell transplantation (e.g. leukaemia or lymphoma).
- CCR5 delta-32 mutation on CD4+ T-cells are almost immune to HIV infection.
- At least four patients have been cured of HIV infection using this type of transplantation:
  - Berlin patient: He had HIV for 12 years but developed acute leukaemia for which he received chemotherapy. He had a relapse of leukaemia and then a stem cell transplant was done from a donor having CCR5 delta-32 mutation. After transplantation, he was able to stop all antiretroviral treatment and is free of disease.

- London patient: He had HIV for a decade but developed lymphoma for which he received chemotherapy followed by a stem cell transplant from a donor having CCR5 delta-32 mutation. After transplantation, he was able to stop all antiretroviral treatment and is free of disease.
- Brazil patient: A third patient of acute myeloid leukaemia received cord blood transplantation (with CCR5 delta-32 mutation) and is free of HIV for more than 14 months.
- 'City of Hope' patient: He had HIV since 1988 and got a stem cell transplant for treatment of acute leukaemia from a donor having CCR delta-32 mutation. He has been free of HIV for more than 3 years.

Q. Discuss tuberculosis in HIV infection. (CT 1.3)

- Leading cause of morbidity and mortality in HIV infection.
- About 25%–65% persons with HIV infection have tuberculosis.
- Estimated annual risk of reactivation among those coinfected with HIV and TB is about 5%–8% with a cumulative lifetime risk of 30% or more compared to a cumulative lifetime risk of 5%–10% in HIV-negative adult patients.
- Course of HIV infection is accelerated subsequent to the development of TB.
- Prevalence of multidrug resistant TB is higher in HIV-positive compared to HIV-negative persons. However, this is not caused directly by HIV infection.

CLINICAL FEATURES

- Active TB occurs throughout the course of HIV disease.
- Clinical presentation of TB in HIV-infected persons depends on the level of immunosuppression resulting from HIV infection. In patients with relatively intact immune function (CD4+ count >200/mm^3), pulmonary TB is more frequently seen than extrapulmonary TB.
- With CD4+ counts >200 cells/μL, HIV-related TB generally resembles TB among HIV-uninfected persons with common chest radiographic manifestations of upper lobe infiltrates with or without cavitation. Sputum smears are often positive for acid-fast bacilli. In patients with CD4 counts <200 cells/mL, the chest radiographic findings of pulmonary TB are markedly different with infiltrates showing no predilection for the upper lobes, and cavitation is uncommon.
- As immunosuppression progresses, extrapulmonary tuberculosis becomes increasingly common. The disease is often disseminated.

DIAGNOSIS

- Please see topics of pulmonary and extrapulmonary tuberculosis (Chapter 2).
- A nucleic acid amplification tests is recommended on at least one sputum or other tissue specimen.
- Screening for HIV in those with possible TB.
- There has been a switch from voluntary counselling and testing (VCT) to provider-initiated testing and counselling (PITC) in patients with diagnosed tuberculosis. With PITC, all patients undergo routine testing unless they specifically opt out.
- It is recommended to expand PITC to include all patients being investigated for TB regardless of whether or not TB is diagnosed.

TREATMENT CONSIDERATIONS

- Incidence of relapse and/or failure among patients treated with intermittent TB therapy throughout was two to three times higher than that in patients who received a daily intensive phase. Hence, daily therapy with antitubercular drugs is recommended in HIV-positive patients.
- PIs and NNRTIs are ARV agents that may inhibit or induce cytochrome P-450 isoenzymes (CYP450). Rifampicin induces CYP450 and may substantially decrease blood levels of the ARV drugs. It should also not be used with PIs, elvitegravir, etravirine, rilpivirine, bictegravir or TAF.
- NRTIs are not metabolised by CYP450. Concurrent use of NRTIs and rifampicin is not contraindicated and does not require dose adjustments.
- Rifampicin can be used for the treatment of active TB in patients on NNRTI efavirenz and two NRTIs. It should not be used in patients on PIs.
- Rifabutin is preferred to rifampicin due to lesser degree of drug interactions with PIs and NNRTIs. It may be used in a dose of 300 mg/day in patients on NRTIs and NVP. However, its dose should be reduced to 150 mg per day when it is administered to patients taking ritonavir or ritonavir/lopinavir. On the other hand, its dose should be increased to 450–600 mg daily when it is used concurrently with efavirenz.
- Simultaneous initiation of treatment for tuberculosis and HIV should be avoided as risk of immune reconstitution inflammatory syndrome (IRIS) is more if both are started together or baseline CD4+ count >50/mm^3.
  - If CD4+ counts are <50/mm^3, ART should be started as soon as possible but within 2 weeks of TB treatment.
  - If CD4+ counts ≥50 cells/mm^3 with patient having tuberculous meningitis, ART should be delayed by about 2 months of starting TB treatment. Many experts, however, recommend initiating ART early in settings where close monitoring of drug-related toxicities and central nervous system adverse events is feasible.
  - If CD4 counts ≥50 cells/mm^3 with patient not having severe disease, ART may be initiated within 8 weeks of starting TB treatment. This is to reduce confusion about overlapping toxicities, drug interactions and occurrence of paradoxical reactions or IRIS.

TUBERCULOUS PARADOXICAL REACTION

- It is a long-recognised feature in the course of TB treatment where there is a brief paradoxical worsening of symptoms after initiating TB treatment. This is independent of rapid immune recovery caused by ART.

LATENT TUBERCULOSIS

- Testing by tuberculin skin test or IGRA is not a requirement for initiating preventive treatment in people living with HIV but is often used.
- Various options for prevention are:
- Isoniazid (INH) daily for 9 months.
- INH (900 mg in adults) plus rifapentine (900 mg in adults) once weekly for 12 weeks (directly observed).
- Rifampicin (or rifabutin) daily for 4 months.

Q. Describe the management of HIV/AIDS during pregnancy.

- ART in pregnant females should not be withheld unless the risk of adverse effects outweighs the possible benefits. ART is considered the standard of care for pregnant women with HIV, both to treat HIV infection and prevent perinatal transmission of HIV.
- ART initiation should not be delayed in pregnant women pending genotypic resistance testing results.
- Preferred regimens should include two NRTIs (abacavir + lamivudine or TDF + emtricitabine [or with lamivudine]). Dolutegravir (DTG) is the preferred integrase inhibitor while atazanavir/ritonavir or darunavir/ritonavir are preferred PIs to be added to two NRTIs.
- Alternate regimen include zidovudine + lamivudine which is given with dolutegravir. Alternate PI is lopinavir (boosted). NACO recommends TDF + lamivudine + Efavirenz.
- Drugs not recommended for initial use because of toxicity (stavudine, didanosine and full-dose ritonavir) should be stopped in women who present during pregnancy while taking these medications. Efavirenz should be avoided in the first trimester.
- If maternal HIV RNA is $\geq$1000 copies/mL (or unknown) near delivery, intravenous infusion of zidovudine during labour is recommended regardless of the mother's antepartum regimen and resistance profile, and the mode of delivery. Administration of combination ART should continue during labour and before a caesarean delivery.
- All women who have HIV RNA levels >1000 copies/mL or presumed >1000 copies/mL near the time of delivery should be offered a scheduled caesarean delivery at 38 weeks, which may significantly reduce the risk of transmission.
- If the mother cannot afford drugs, cannot tolerate triple-drug regimens or does not want to take the possible risks to the baby, ARV prophylaxis should be offered to reduce the chances of perinatal transmission (previously known as mother-to-child transmission or MTCT; now called parent to child transmission). For this, oral ZDV throughout antenatal period (at least from 28 weeks onwards), intravenous ZDV during intranatal period and oral ZDV to the newborn should be given for 6 weeks.
- If mother is found to be HIV-positive at the time of labour, intravenous ZDV during intranatal period and three-drug ART medications to the newborn should be given for 6 weeks. Although intrapartum/neonatal ARV medications will not prevent perinatal transmission that occurs before labour, most transmission occurs near to or during labour and delivery.
- ARV drugs to newborns.
  - Newborns of mothers who were on ART throughout the pregnancy with sustained viral suppression should receive zidovudine for 6 weeks.
  - Newborns of mothers who received neither antepartum nor intrapartum ART or those who received only intrapartum HIV drugs, should receive daily nevirapine prophylaxis for 12 weeks. An alternative is to start empiric ART consisting of zidovudine, lamivudine and nevirapine at least for 6 weeks unless the virologic test (HIV RNA or HIV DNA nucleic acid) of newborn is positive.

BREASTFEED

- Breast milk transmission contributes significantly to PTCT rates.
- The WHO recommends that where replacement feeding is 'acceptable, feasible, affordable, sustainable and safe' ('AFASS' criteria), HIV-infected women should avoid breastfeeding.
- In resource-limited situations, breastfeeding is still recommended.
- Daily newborn nevirapine, lamivudine, lopinavir/ritonavir or nevirapine plus zidovudine can reduce the risk of postnatal infection during breastfeeding.

Q. Give a brief account of immune reconstitution inflammatory syndrome.

- IRIS is a clinical condition caused by ART-induced restoration of pathogen-specific immune responses to opportunistic infections, resulting in either the deterioration of a treated infection (paradoxical IRIS) or a new presentation of a previously subclinical infection (unmasking IRIS).
- Thus, in IRIS, there is occurrence or worsening of clinical and/or laboratory parameters despite a favourable outcome in CD4 cell count and plasma viral loads.
- Both infective (clinical or subclinical) and noninfective conditions can act as triggering factors for precipitating IRIS.
- A variety of fungal, parasitic, mycobacterial and viral opportunistic infections are associated with manifestations of IRIS.
- The risk factors for IRIS include CD4 count <50 cells/mm^3, a high viral load, a rapid decline in viral load, active or subclinical infection by opportunistic pathogens, initiation of ART in close proximity to the diagnosis and initiation of treatment for an opportunistic infection.
- Noninfectious IRIS may present with cutaneous involvement (papular urticaria, eosinophilic folliculitis, Reiter's syndrome, sarcoidosis and SLE) or without cutaneous involvement (autoimmune thyroiditis, Guillain–Barre syndrome, myopathy, radiculopathy, acute porphyria, non-Hodgkin's lymphomas and Castleman's disease).

- The infectious syndromes occur with various opportunistic infections with tuberculosis being the most common. IRIS in tuberculosis typically occurs 1–6 weeks after the patient begins ART. The signs and symptoms of tuberculous IRIS may include high fever, new or worsening lymphadenopathy (mediastinal or peripheral), worsening of pulmonary symptoms and infiltrates, or new or increasing pleural effusion. Lymph node abscesses usually occur during the first weeks on ART. CNS tuberculosis IRIS may present with headache, neck stiffness, confusion, new-onset seizures, paraparesis, disconjugate eye movements, aphasia, and decreased vision.
- Differential diagnoses include failure of ART, toxicity of ART, active opportunistic infection and failure of antimicrobial therapy.
- Treatment includes continuation of primary therapy against the offending pathogen in order to decrease the antigenic load, continuation of effective ART and judicious use of antiinflammatory agents. In severe cases, a short course of steroids may be indicated. Procedures including lymph node aspiration, pericardiocentesis, paracentesis and thoracentesis are sometimes required to alleviate symptoms or manage complications.

Q. Discuss briefly about preexposure prophylaxis (PrEP) for HIV infection.

- PrEP is indicated for people who are at risk of HIV infection.
- A high risk of HIV infection has been associated with:
  - unprotected receptive anal intercourse
  - a history of sexually transmitted infections, particularly anorectal gonorrhoea and chlamydia
  - use of illicit drugs, particularly crystal methamphetamine because of its effect on behaviour.
  - sex workers
  - people who use intravenous drugs
- At the initial visit, patients should be advised that while PrEP is highly effective in preventing HIV infection, it does not protect against other sexually transmitted infections and condom use is encouraged.
- Tenofovir disoproxil fumarate 300 mg (or tenofovir alafenamide 25 mg) plus emtricitabine 200 mg as a combined pill should be taken with food once a day. It should be continued as long as the risk of infection persists. Individuals with eGFR <60 mL/min/1.73 m^2 should not be given tenofovir disoproxil fumarate.
- Regular monitoring is done every 3 months for adherence, potential adverse reactions and, with the patient's agreement, for development of sexually transmitted infections and HIV infection.
- On-demand or intermittent use of PrEP has demonstrated effectiveness for men who have sex with men. Two pills of tenofovir disoproxil/emtricitabine are taken 2–24 hours before sex, followed by a single pill 24 hours and 48 hours after the initial dose ('2-1-1' PrEP). Not recommended in transgender women and heterosexual males and females. Also should not be used in persons with chronic hepatitis B infection.
- Dapivirine (a novel nonnucleoside reverse transcriptase inhibitor) vaginal ring for women at substantial risk of HIV has shown encouraging results.

Q. Write a short note on HIV vaccines.

- Despite advances in drug treatment of HIV, no vaccine has been approved for use to prevent HIV infection.

CHALLENGES

- HIV mutates rapidly. The high rate of mutation of HIV is due to the error-prone viral reverse transcriptase and has been estimated to lead to 1–10 mutations per genome per replication cycle. This mutation rate mostly leads to changes within the *Env* glycoprotein, allowing glycan shielding so the virus can evade the immune system.
- Lack of animal model. Although the standard animal model widely accepted today is macaque monkeys, this standard accepted animal model is only a model and may not reflect the disease pathology and immune response in humans.
- HIV can be transmitted by cell-free or cell-associated virus.
- The virus integrates itself into the genome of human cell and is not exposed to immune system.
- The virus has developed multiple mechanism to evade the body's defences. The virus targets CD4+ cells which are the cells involved in defence to viral infections.

VACCINES

- Currently there is no safe and effective vaccine approved for prevention of HIV infection.
- A large number of vaccine candidates have been studied since 1987.
- The first vaccine candidates targeted gp120 or gp160 producing neutralising antibodies. However, results in term of protection were poor.
- The second approach was based on administering a viral vector to induce a CD8+ cell response. However, again the vaccine candidates provided no efficacy and did not decrease viral load in participants who contracted HIV.
- The current approach is to utilise a heterologous prime-boost to elicit humoral and cell-mediated immune responses. A homologous prime-boost is utilised for diphtheria, tetanus, and pertussis (DTP) and involves administering the same vaccine at intervals to boost the previous responses. The heterologous prime-boost utilises the same antigens in different types of vaccines and has been proven to be more immunogenic than the homologous series.

Q. Discuss transmission of HIV to healthcare workers.

- Major hazard to a healthcare worker (HCW) is from various body fluids of a patient. These fluids include

blood and fluids from eyes, nose and mouth. Intact skin and mucous membranes of an HCW are important defences against HIV.
- Following percutaneous exposure to a needle contaminated with HIV-infected blood, the risk of transmission of HIV to an HCW is 0.13%–0.5%, which is 45–120 times less than the risk of hepatitis B virus infection following similar exposure.
- Splashes of infectious material to mucous membranes or broken skin may also transmit HIV infection (estimated risk per exposure, 0.09%).
- The major risk of transmission of HIV infection to a HCW is from a patient with unknown HIV status particularly when the 'universal precautions' (now called 'standard precautions') are ignored.

UNIVERSAL PRECAUTIONS (STANDARD PRECAUTIONS)

- Standard precautions apply to the care of all patients, irrespective of their disease state. These precautions apply when there is a risk of potential exposure to:
  - Blood.
  - All body fluids, secretions and excretions (except sweat), regardless of whether they contain visible blood.
  - Nonintact skin.
  - Mucous membranes.
- The precautions include the use of hand hygiene and personal protective equipment (PPE).
- For preventing transmission of HIV:
  - Gloves should be worn whenever there is likelihood of contact with body fluids.
  - During procedures (in which there may be splashing of blood), eyes, nose and mouth should be protected with mask and protective glasses. Further, rest of the body should be protected by suitable gowns.
  - Needles should not be re-capped.

Q. What are the recommendations on postexposure care of a healthcare worker? (IM6.17)

MANAGEMENT OF THE WOUND

- Wound and skin should be washed with soap and water.
- The area exposed should be soaked in povidone-iodine 10% or alcohol.
- 'Squeezing out' needlestick injuries or wounds is to be avoided as it may promote hyperaemia and inflammation at the wound site, potentially increasing systemic exposure to HIV if present in the contaminating fluid.
- In case of exposure to a mucous membrane, it should be flushed with water. Topically applied povidone–iodine 10% is well tolerated by the ocular and oral mucous membranes and can be used in cases of suspected mucous membrane inoculation. However, topical alcohol on mucous membranes should be avoided.

DETERMINE RISK ASSOCIATED WITH EXPOSURE

- Exposures that may warrant postexposure prophylaxis (PEP) include:
  - Parenteral or mucous membrane exposure (sexual exposure and splashes to the eye, nose or oral cavity) from following bodily fluids: blood, visibly blood-stained fluid, blood-stained saliva, breast milk, genital secretions and cerebrospinal, amniotic, rectal, peritoneal, synovial, pericardial or pleural fluids.
- Exposures that do not require PEP include:
  - When the exposed individual is already HIV-positive.
  - When the source is established to be HIV-negative.
  - Exposure to bodily fluids that do not pose a significant risk: tears, non-blood-stained saliva, urine and sweat.
  - Exposure of intact skin to infectious fluids.
- A known source patient should be tested for anti-HIV, HBsAg and anti-HCV.

PEP REGIMENS

- A regimen for PEP for HIV with three drugs is recommended.
- Tenofovir (300 mg od) plus lamivudine (300 mg od) (or emtricitabine 200 mg od) are the two preferred drugs as backbone for prophylaxis.
- Lopinavir/ritonavir boosted (400 mg/100 mg bid) or atazanavir/ritonavir boosted (300 mg/100 mg od) or darunavir/ritonavir boosted (800 mg/100 mg od) is the preferred third agent. NACO recommends efavirenz as the third drug if lopinavir/ritonavir boosted is not available.
- If available, raltegravir (400 mg bid) or dolutegravir (50 mg od) should be preferred to ritonavir-boosted PIs as the third agent.
- Agents not recommended for PEP include nevirapine, delavirdine, abacavir and zalcitabine.

TIME TO START HIV PEP

- PEP should be initiated promptly, preferably within 1–2 hours of postexposure.

DURATION OF PROPHYLACTIC TREATMENT

- PEP is continued for 4 weeks.

MONITORING THE EXPOSED HEALTHCARE WORKER

- HCW should be monitored for any serious side effects of the ARV drugs.
- Complete blood counts and renal and hepatic function tests should be done at baseline and then 2 weeks after initiating chemoprophylaxis.
- Baseline HIV-antibody test and tests for hepatitis B and C infections should be done that are repeated at 4–6 weeks, 12 weeks and 6 months postexposure.

MCQs

1. During prenatal screening, a 30-year-old woman with a known allergy to penicillin is found to have syphilis. The patient undergoes desensitization with increasing doses of intravenous penicillin. The reason for this treatment is to induce the production of which one of the following immunoglobulins?
   A. IgA
   B. IgD
   C. IgE
   D. IgG
   E. IgM

Ans: D. IgG

During desensitization, increasing amounts of an allergen (penicillin in this case) are injected at regular intervals to induce the production of specific IgG antibodies. During subsequent exposures, the allergen will be neutralised by IgG before it has a chance to bind to IgE located on the surface of mast cells. (A) is incorrect. IgA antibodies are found on various mucosal surfaces. They cannot be induced by specific antigens and therefore do not intervene in immunotherapy. (B) is incorrect. IgD antibodies are found in small amounts in the blood, peritoneum, and pleura. They are present on the surface of many B lymphocytes, but their precise function is unclear. They may be involved in allergic reactions to milk and some medications. Increased IgD titre would not prevent allergic reactions. (C) is incorrect. IgE antibodies mediate immediate hypersensitivity. The goal of immunotherapy is to reduce the amount of IgE antibodies. (E) is incorrect. IgM antibodies are produced in the first phase of the immune response. They bind to antigens and effectively activate the complement, neutralising and binding. IgM antibodies do not participate in the prevention of allergic reactions.

2. A 12-month-old infant receives an inactivated flu vaccine in October. The infant's immune system is likely to produce one of these elements:
   A. Specific cytotoxic T lymphocytes (CTLs) against the influenza virus
   B. CD8+ T lymphocytes specific against the influenza virus
   C. Specific NK lymphocytes against the influenza virus
   D. Specific antibodies and T-helper lymphocytes the against influenza virus
   E. Specific antibodies and CTLs against the Influenza virus but not T-helper lymphocytes

Ans: D.

Specific antibodies and T-helper lymphocytes the against influenza virus

As this is a vaccine of dead or inactivated viruses, its components will be processed as exogenous antigens in the antigen-presenting cells (APCs) and presented to T-helper lymphocytes with MHC class II molecules. A TH2 response will be induced resulting in stimulation of B lymphocytes so that they differentiate and produce antibodies. (A) is incorrect. This would happen if the child received a live attenuated influenza vaccine (LAIV). Virus-infected cells would be recognised by CTLs through class I MHC-viral peptide complexes expressed on cell surfaces. (B) is incorrect. CD8+ lymphocytes are CTLs which do not participate in antigen recognition when a dead virus vaccine is used. (C) is incorrect. NK lymphocytes kill virus-infected cells in the same way as CTLs. (E) is incorrect. CTLs do not participate when a dead virus as vaccine is given.

4 Diseases of Skin

Q. Describe various primary and secondary skin lesions.

PRIMARY AND SECONDARY SKIN LESIONS

- Figures 4.1 and 4.2 depict and describe various primary and secondary skin lesions.

EXAMPLES OF PRIMARY SKIN LESIONS

- Table 4.1 gives a list of commonly seen primary skin lesions.

Q. What are the various types of eczema? Briefly outline their clinical features and general management. (DR12.1, DR12.3, DR12.4, DR12.5)

Q. Give a brief account of dermatitis.

- The terms eczema and dermatitis are used synonymously. Eczema is not a specific disease entity but a characteristic inflammatory response of the skin to both exogenous and endogenous agents.

TYPES OF ECZEMA

EXOGENOUS

- Irritant contact eczema is due to detergents, alkalis, acids, solvents and abrasive dust. Strong irritants often cause acute eczema, whereas weak irritants often cause chronic eczema.
- Allergic contact eczema is due to delayed hypersensitivity reaction following contact with antigens or haptens. Previous exposure to the allergen is required for sensitisation.
  - Common allergens include metals (nickel, gold, silver, cobalt), fragrances, surfactants, topical antibiotics and preservatives.
  - The eczema occurs wherever the allergen contacts the skin.
  - During the acute phase, lesions are marked by oedema, erythema and vesicle formation. As the vesicles rupture, oozing ensues and papules and plaques appear.

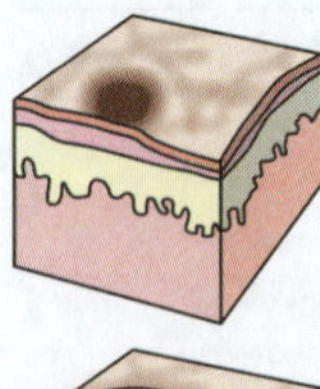

Macule

Flat area of colour change (no elevation or depression)
Example: Freckles

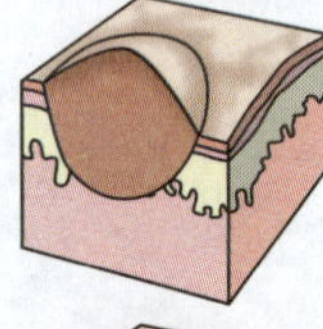

Papule

Solid elevation less than 0.5 cm in diameter
Example: Naevi, warts

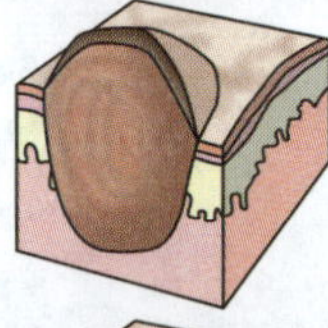

Nodule

Solid elevation 0.5 to 1 cm in diameter
Extends deeper into dermis than papule
Example: Allergic eczema

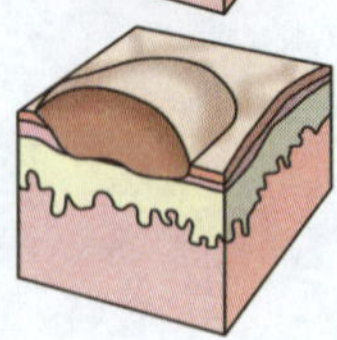

Plaque

Flat elevated surface found on skin or mucous membrane
Example: Psoriasis

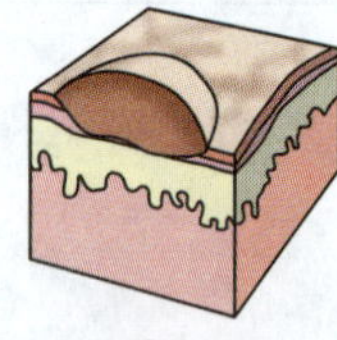

Wheal

Type of plaque. Result is transient oedema in dermis
Example: Urticaria

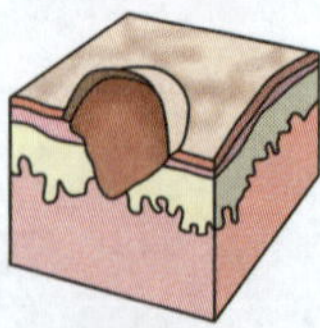

Vesicle

Small blister—fluid within or under epidermis
Example: Herpesvirus infection

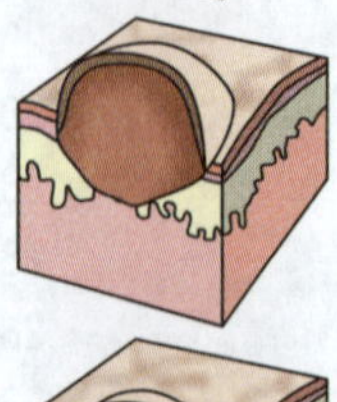

Bulla

Large blister (greater than 0.5 cm)
Example: Pemphigoid

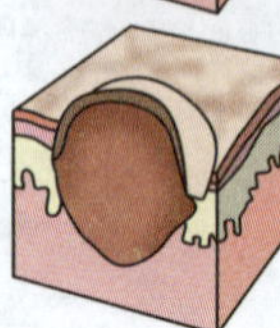

Pustule

Vesicle filled with pus
Example: Folliculitis

Fig. 4.1 Common primary skin lesions—a schematic representation.

SECONDARY LESIONS (Modification of Original Appearance)

DAMAGED OR DIMINISHED SKIN SURFACE

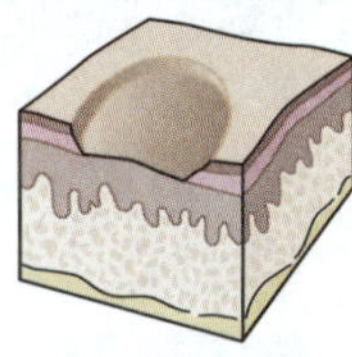

Erosion: Loss of epidermis that does not extend into dermis. **Example:** Ruptured chickenpox vesicle.

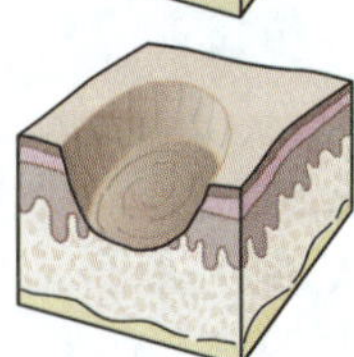

Ulcer: Loss of skin through the epidermis; healing results in scar formation. **Example:** Stasis ulcer.

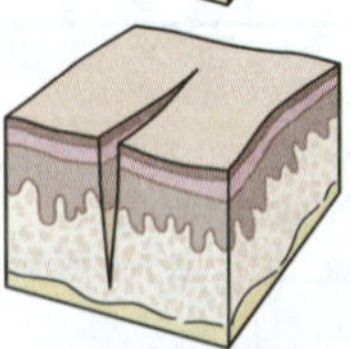

Fissure: A split in all epidermal layers of skin. **Example:** Athlete's foot.

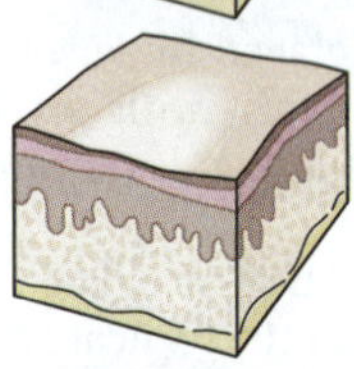

Atrophy: Diminution of epidermal surface; skin looks thinner and more translucent than normal; atrophy of the dermal layers may result in wasting or depression of the skin surface. **Example:** Arterial insufficiency.

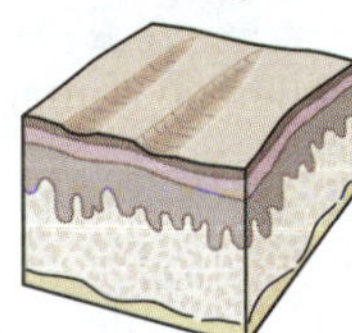

Excoriation: Loss of outer skin layers from scratching or rubbing. **Example:** Scratched insect bite.

AUGMENTED OR INCREASED SKIN SURFACE

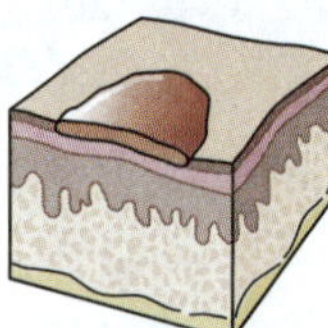

Crust: A collection of serous exudate and debris on the surface of damaged or absent outer skin layers. **Example:** Impetigo.

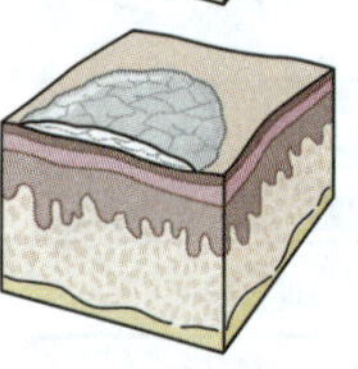

Scale: A compact portion of desquamating stratum corneum; may vary in size, thickness, and consistency. **Examples:** Psoriasis scale (compact and thick), pityriasis rosea scale (thin and small).

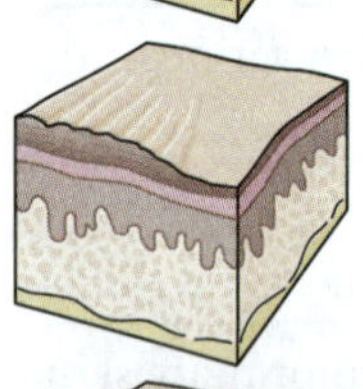

Lichenification: Epidermal thickening and roughening of the skin with increased visibility of skin surface furrows. **Example:** Chronic atopic dermatitis.

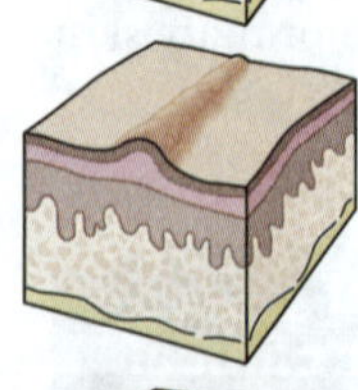

Scar: A collection of fibrous tissue that forms to replace lost epidermal and dermal tissue. **Examples:** Surgical scar, acne scar.

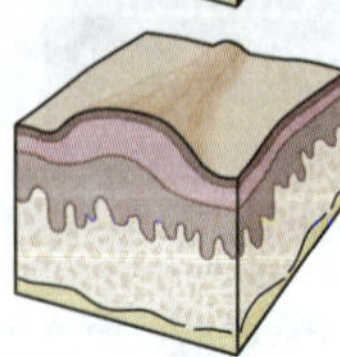

Keloid: Augmentation of scar tissue, creating a significant elevation on the skin surface after healing. **Examples:** Postsurgical scar, postacne scar.

Fig. 4.2 Common secondary skin lesions—a schematic representation.

TABLE 4.1 Common Examples of Primary Skin Lesions

Lesion Morphology	Differential Diagnosis
Macule	Drug eruption, nevus, tattoo, secondary syphilis, viral exanthema, toxic or infectious erythema, external trauma (ecchymosis), vitiligo, tinea versicolor
Papule	Acne, melanoma, nevus, warts, molluscum contagiosum, eczema, insect bites, vasculitis, scabies, erythema multiforme, varicella (early), gonococcaemia
Plaque	Eczema, pityriasis rosea, tinea corporis, psoriasis, seborrhoeic dermatitis, secondary syphilis
Nodule	Basal cell carcinoma, squamous cell carcinoma, melanoma, erythema nodosum, lipoma, warts
Wheal	Urticaria, angioedema, insect bites, erythema multiforme
Vesicle	Herpes simplex, herpes zoster, varicella, impetigo, thermal burn, toxic epidermal necrolysis, bullous pemphigoid, pemphigus vulgaris, monkeypox
Bulla	Bullous impetigo, thermal burn, toxic epidermal necrolysis, bullous pemphigoid, pemphigus vulgaris
Pustule	Acne, folliculitis, gonococcaemia, herpes simplex, herpes zoster, varicella, impetigo

- In the chronic stage, scaling, lichenification and excoriations predominate.
- Face, neck and hands are the most common body parts involved.
- Forehead and ears are commonly affected by hair dyes and shampoos; ears are susceptible to metals from earrings; eyelids are particularly affected by airborne allergens and nail polish; cheeks and lips are prone to react to facial cosmetics.
- Diagnosis can be confirmed by a patch test.

ENDOGENOUS

- Atopic eczema (or atopic dermatitis) is due to a genetic predisposition to form excessive IgE antibodies to inhaled, injected or ingested antigens.
  - Patients with atopic eczema have a tendency to develop other allergic diseases like asthma, allergic rhinitis, hay fever, urticaria, food and other allergies. Many have family history of allergic disorders.
  - More than 95% of cases develop before the age of 5 years.
  - The cardinal features of atopic eczema are itch, erythema, xerosis, oedema, oozing, crusting and lichenification. Pruritus is the hallmark of it.
  - The area of skin covered by a child's diaper is also frequently involved.
  - Primarily flexural (antecubital and popliteal fossae) in its distribution in older children and adults, but facial and truncal involvement predominates in infants (Fig. 4.3).
  - Usually chronic or relapsing.
  - In severe atopic dermatitis, areas of eczema coalesce into larger regions of generalised redness of the skin (erythroderma).
  - Associated clinical signs include rarefaction of the lateral eyebrows (Hertoghe's sign) and increased density and depth of palmar creases (hyperlinear palms).

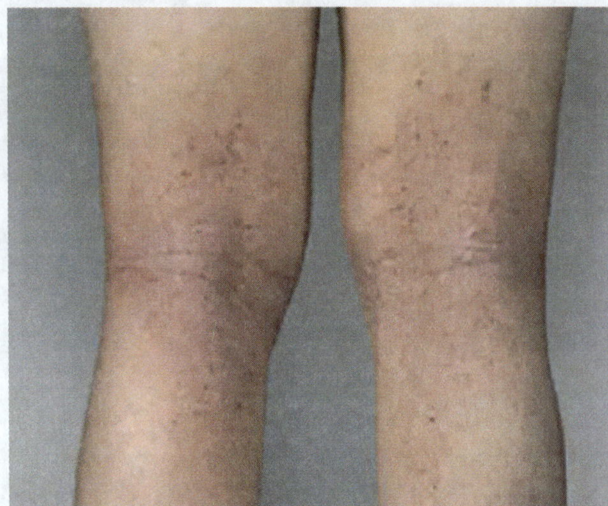

Fig. 4.3 Atopic dermatitis (involvement of popliteal fossae).

  - There is an increased incidence of infections due to skin barrier defects, suppression of cutaneous innate immunity and *Staphylococcus aureus* colonisation.
  - By adulthood, 40%–80% of patients will experience either a decrease or complete resolution of their disease.
- Seborrhoeic eczema often runs in families and is associated with a tendency to dandruff.
  - Possibly due to excessive growth of fungi of the genus *Malassezia* (formerly called *Pityrosporum*).
  - Not a disorder of sebaceous glands.
  - High prevalence in HIV-infected persons particularly if CD4 cell count is $<400/mm^3$.
  - Patient has characteristic 'seborrhoeic look'—oily skin with patulous, prominent follicular orifices.
  - Involves areas rich in sebaceous glands—scalp, retroauricular folds, eyebrows, nasolabial folds (Fig. 4.4), beard area, interscapular and presternal regions, axillae, pubic region, groin, umbilicus and folds under pendulous breasts.

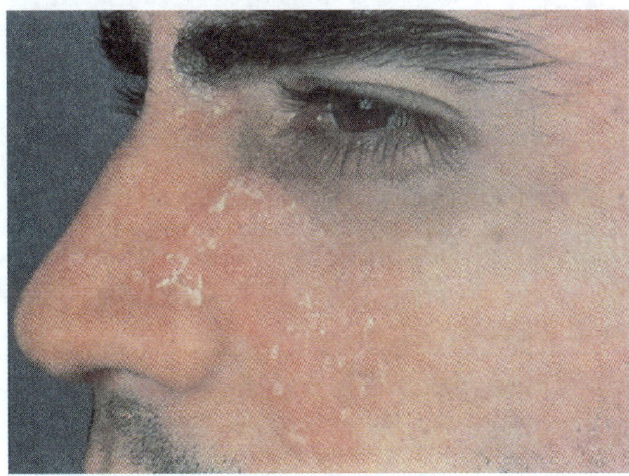

Fig. 4.4 Seborrhoeic dermatitis.

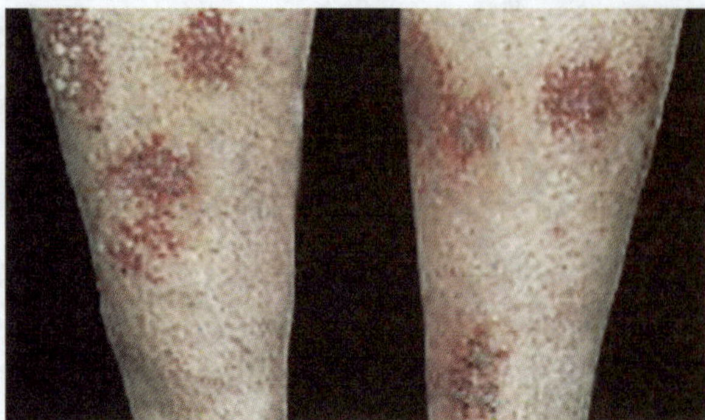

Fig. 4.5 Discoid eczema of lower legs.

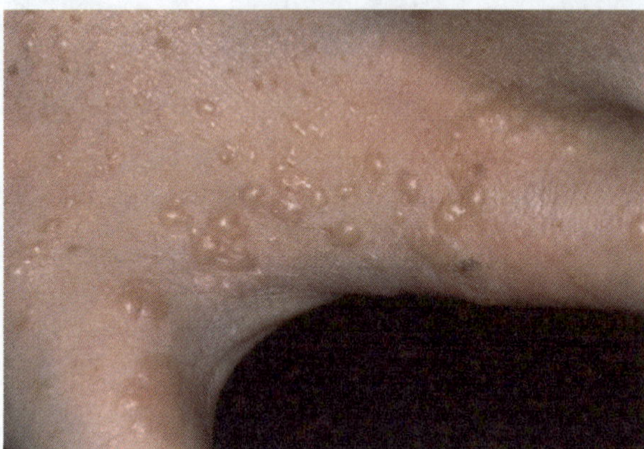

Fig. 4.6 Pompholyx.

- Scalp area—diffusely involved with greasy scales on a dull red background.
- Intertriginous areas—erythematous scaly lesions or exudative crusted lesions.
- Eyebrows—fine scaling of eyelid margins.
- An infantile form, which usually involves the scalp (cradle cap), the face and the diaper area, affects as many as 70% of newborns during the first 3 months of life but usually disappears by 1 year of age.

- Discoid eczema (nummular eczema) is seen most often on the limbs of elderly males, and is of uncertain aetiology. Coin-sized eczematous patches are seen (Fig. 4.5).
- Asteatotic eczema is commonly seen on the lower legs in hospitalised elderly patients.
- Gravitational (stasis) eczema occurs on the lower legs and is often associated with signs of venous insufficiency.
- Pompholyx (dyshidrotic eczema) describes a form of eczema in which bouts of recurrent vesicles or bullae affect the palms, fingers and soles (Fig. 4.6).

MANAGEMENT

GENERAL

- Emollients and moisturisers are helpful for moisturising the skin. Ointments are preferred over creams because creams may contain potentially sensitising preservatives and mildly irritating emulsifiers.

CONTACT DERMATITIS

- Avoidance of suspected allergen.
- For active lesions, topical steroids may be used.

ATOPIC ECZEMA

- Explanation, reassurance and encouragement.
- Avoidance of heat, dryness and contact with irritants.
- Oral antihistamines.
- Topical moisturisers with a hydrophilic base.
- Topical steroids should be used judiciously. The various preparations available are 1% hydrocortisone (mildly potent), clobetasone butyrate (moderately potent), betamethasone valerate (potent) and 0.05% clobetasol propionate (very potent) and their use depends on severity of lesions.
- Topical calcineurin inhibitors (tacrolimus and pimecrolimus)—topical immunomodulators, are useful if steroids are not effective.
- Crisaborole, a phosphodiesterase-4 inhibitor, is indicated for mild to moderate cases above 2 years of age.
- For moderate eczema, ultraviolet phototherapy (narrow-band ultraviolet B and medium-band ultraviolet A1) can be used in adults. It can produce skin cancer if used in children and young adults.
- Dupilumab, a monoclonal antibody that binds IL-4α receptor and blocks both IL-4 and IL-13, for adults with moderate to severe eczema. It is administered as a subcutaneous injection.

SEBORRHOEIC ECZEMA

- Ordinary shampooing in mild cases with scalp involvement.
- In severe cases, medicated shampoos containing selenium sulphide (2.5%), zinc pyrithione (1%) or ketoconazole (2%). For facial lesions, topical ketoconazole cream (2%) or topical calcineurin inhibitors may be used.
- Topical lithium succinate and lithium gluconate are effective alternative agents for the treatment of seborrhoeic eczema in areas other than the scalp.
- In acute stage, topical steroids of low potency to control erythema and itching.

Q. Discuss aetiology and management of xerostomia.

- Daily production of saliva in healthy adults is approximately 1500 mL.
- Xerostomia—a subjective complaint of dry mouth, which may result from a decrease in the production of saliva.
- Effects of xerostomia:
  - Symptoms may be minor for some, while for others they may hamper activities of daily living.
  - May cause burning sensation in mouth, difficulty in eating, chewing and swallowing.
  - May cause serious health problems, such as tooth decay, bad breath, *Candida* infection, viral infections (e.g. herpes simplex) and bacterial sialadenitis.

AETIOLOGY OF XEROSTOMIA

- Various causes of xerostomia are given in Box 4.1.
- The causes of xerostomia in haemodialysis patients are multifactorial: Use of antihypertensives, diabetes mellitus, restricted fluid intake, water removal during dialysis, salivary gland fibrosis and changes in salivary composition.

DIAGNOSIS

- Salivary function tests where saliva volume <0.1 mL/minute is considered as low salivary flow.
  - Unstimulated salivary flow: Patients are instructed to spit the contents of the mouth into a receptacle at 1-minute intervals for 5 minutes.
  - Stimulated salivary flow: Patients are instructed to chew an unflavoured gum base at a rate of 60 chews/minute for at least 2 minutes. A stimulated saliva flow rate less than 0.5–0.7 mL/minute is considered significant.

MANAGEMENT

- Stop the offending drug if possible.
- Oral hygiene including chlorhexidine rinses.
- Frequent sips of water and teeth brushing.
- Artificial salivary substitutes—intended to act as a replacement of lubricative and protective function of the natural saliva and not as substitutes for digestive and enzymatic actions. Examples include sodium carboxymethylcellulose, potassium dihydrogen orthophosphate and sorbitol.
- Cholinergic agonists (sialogogues).
  - Pilocarpine (5 mg tid) and cevimeline (30 mg tid).
  - Cautious use in patients with cardiovascular disease and chronic respiratory conditions.
  - Side effects include excessive sweating, cutaneous vasodilatation, emesis, nausea, diarrhoea, persistent hiccup, bronchoconstriction, hypotension, bradycardia, increased urinary frequency and vision problems.
  - Contraindicated in patients with uncontrolled asthma, angle-closure (narrow-angle) glaucoma and liver disease.

BOX 4.1 Causes of Xerostomia

• Anticholinergic drugs (reduce volume of saliva)	Anticholinergics, antidepressants, antiemetics, antihistamines, antihypertensives (ACE inhibitors, diuretics), antiparkinsonian drugs, antipsychotics, antispasmodics, diuretics
• Sympathomimetic drugs (produce viscous saliva)	Amphetamines, appetite suppressants (e.g. sibutramine), bronchodilators, decongestants
• Systemic causes	Addison's disease, Alzheimer's disease, alcoholic cirrhosis, diabetes mellitus, HIV/AIDS, radiation to head and neck area (e.g. for cancer therapy), salivary gland infection, severe dehydration, Sjogren's syndrome
• Others	Elderly persons, sleep-related xerostomia (due to mouth breathing during sleep), haemodialysis

Q. Discuss briefly about pruritus.

- Defined as a cutaneous sensation that provokes the desire to scratch. It is intended to serve a protective function to remove pruritogenic stimuli.

PATHOPHYSIOLOGY

- Pruritus originates in the terminal nerve endings within the skin and can be elicited by inflammation, dryness, contact exposure and allergic responses.
- In allergic responses, histamine is the mediator in many cases.
- In some conditions such as chronic kidney disease, cholestasis and lymphoma, serotonin may play a role. It excites nociceptive C-fibres, which in turn produce itching.

AETIOLOGY (Table 4.2)

- Can be due to a dermatological or systemic cause.
- Localised itching is rarely caused by a systemic process.
- Pruritus may precede the development of a systemic disease by several years.

COMPLICATIONS OF PRURITUS

- Lichen simplex chronicus (localised skin thickening due to intense scratching).
- Prurigo nodularis (variant of lichen simplex chronicus where nodules develop at the site of itching).
- Local infection.

TABLE 4.2 Causes of Pruritus

Dermatological causes:	Systemic causes:

• Xerosis
• Atopic dermatitis
• Contact dermatitis
• Seborrhoeic dermatitis
• Folliculitis
• Psoriasis
• Scabies
• Urticaria
• Drug eruption (e.g. angiotensin-converting enzyme inhibitors, salicylates, chloroquine and calcium channel blockers)
Psychogenic causes (e.g. delusions of parasitosis, formication):
• Obsessive-compulsive disorder
• Depression
• Anxiety
• Psychosis
Drug-induced causes
Unknown cause:
• Senile pruritus
	• Hepatic diseases:
	  • Cholestasis
	  • Hepatitis
	• Renal disease:
	  • Chronic kidney disease
	• Haematological diseases:
	  • Polycythaemia vera
	  • Iron-deficiency anaemia
	• Endocrine diseases:
	  • Hyperthyroidism and hypothyroidism
	  • Carcinoid syndrome
	• Malignant diseases:
	  • Solid tumours
	  • Lymphomas
	  • Leukaemias
	• Others:
	  • HIV

TREATMENT

GENERAL MEASURES

- Controlling xerosis with moisturisers and humidification of indoor environment.
- Use of antihistamines like diphenhydramine.

SPECIFIC MEASURES

- Treatment of underlying cause (e.g. atopic dermatitis).
- Ursodeoxycholic acid (UDCA) in cholestasis.
- Cholestyramine, rifampicin and opioid antagonists (e.g. naltrexone) in primary biliary cirrhosis.
- Ultraviolet B phototherapy, gabapentin and ondansetron in uraemic patients.
- Corticosteroids in patients with Hodgkin's disease.
- Paroxetine, a selective serotonin reuptake inhibitor, is useful in itching produced as a paraneoplastic manifestation. It may also be used in other causes of pruritus.
- Indomethacin for HIV-associated itching.

Q. Briefly outline the clinical manifestations and management of psoriasis. (DR3.1, DR3.3)

- The main abnormality in psoriasis is the increased epidermal proliferation due to excessive division of cells in the stratum basale and a shorter cell cycle. In association with the basal cell hyperplasia, there is enhanced metabolism and accelerated synthesis and degradation of nucleoproteins, resulting in hyperuricaemia. There is proliferation of the subepidermal vasculature, which is responsible for the 'Auspitz's sign'. T-lymphocytes are important in the pathogenesis.
- Commonly presents before the age of 35 years. It is equally common in both males and females.
- May be a presenting sign of HIV infection.
- Characteristic lesions are pink–red, sharply demarcated papules and rounded plaques, covered by silvery scales (plaque psoriasis) (Fig. 4.7).

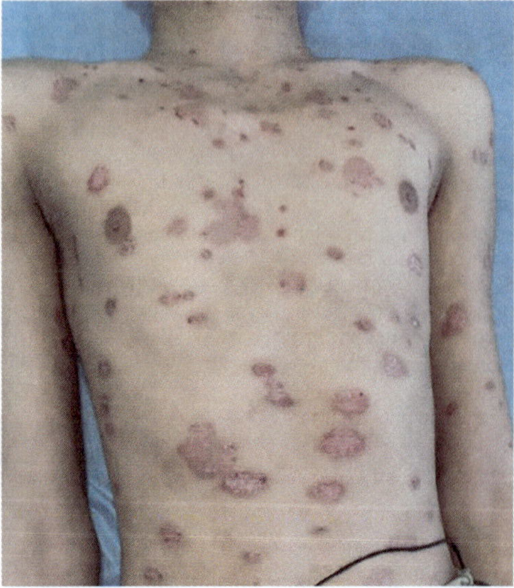

Fig. 4.7 Plaque psoriasis.

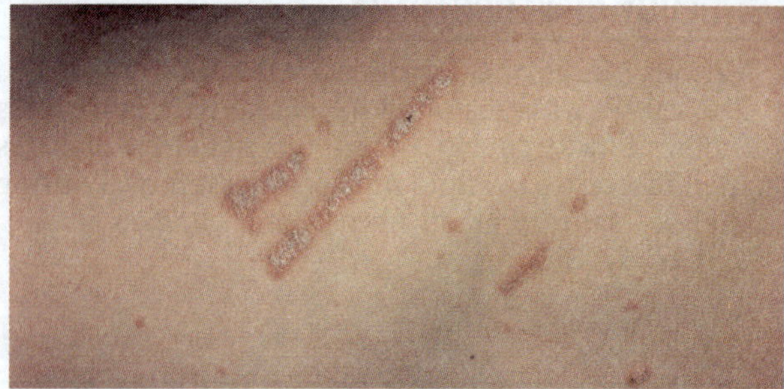

Fig. 4.8 Koebner's phenomenon in a patient with psoriasis.

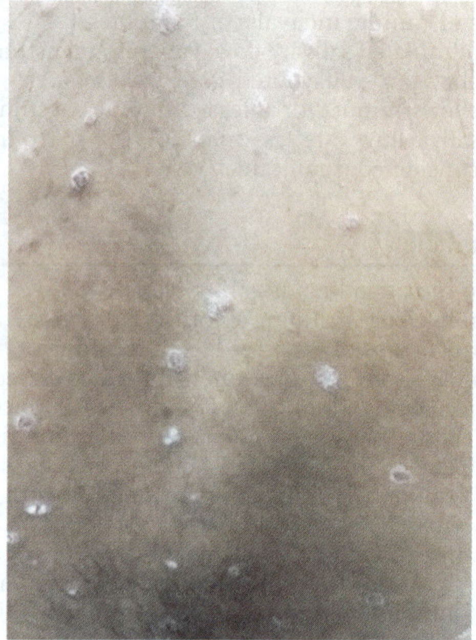

Fig. 4.9 Guttate psoriasis.

- The most common areas of involvement are extensor body areas (elbows and knees), gluteal cleft and scalp. Trunk is also commonly involved. Traumatised areas are often involved (Koebner's or isomorphic phenomenon—Fig. 4.8) and this explains common involvement of elbows and knees.
- Besides typical lesions described above, the skin lesions can range from small drop-shaped papules (guttate psoriasis—frequently affects children and adolescents following a streptococcal infection or an upper respiratory tract infection—Fig. 4.9) to pustules (pustular psoriasis—multiple tender, sterile pustules with an underlying, blotchy and erythematous base), to generalised erythema and scales (erythrodermic psoriasis—develops if existing psoriasis is poorly controlled, systemic medication are withdrawn suddenly, reaction to a drug such as lithium or presence of an underlying systemic infection—Fig. 4.10).
- Another type of psoriasis is inverse psoriasis characterised by lesions in the skin folds (Fig. 4.11). Due to its occluded location, this form is shiny, red and does not present the characteristic scaling seen in plaque disease. Another type is sebopsoriasis which occurs on

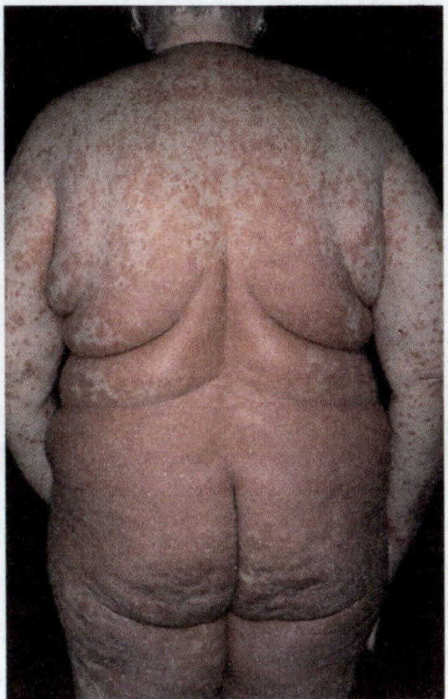

Fig. 4.10 Erythrodermic psoriasis.

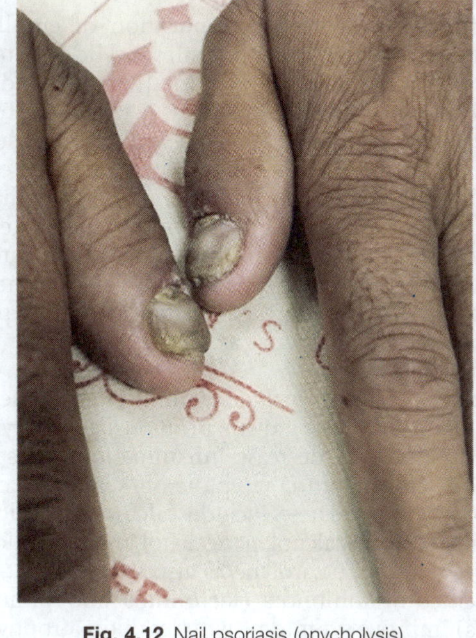

Fig. 4.12 Nail psoriasis (onycholysis).

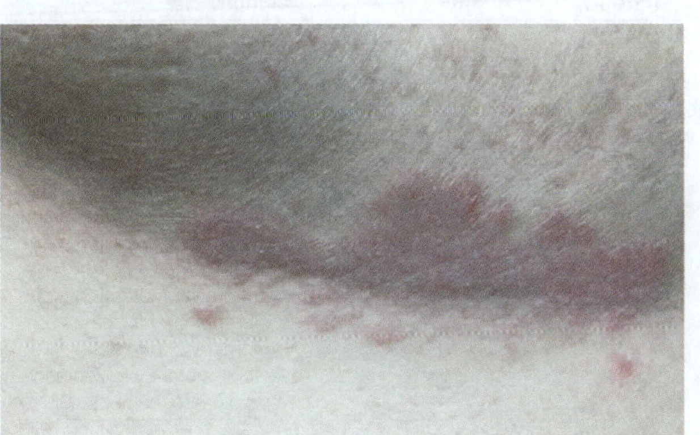

Fig. 4.11 Inverse psoriasis.

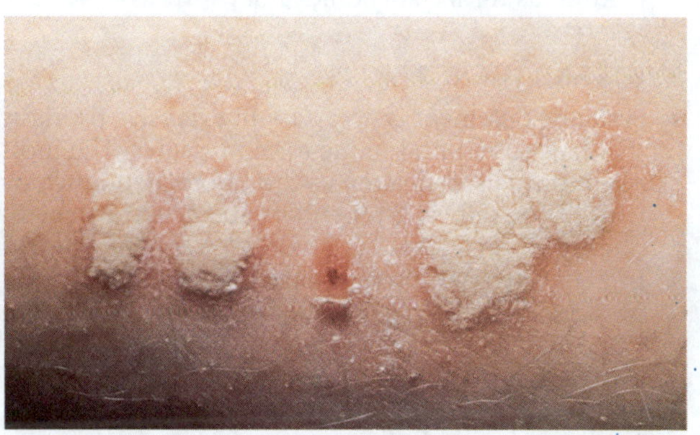

Fig. 4.13 Auspitz's sign.

the scalp, seborrhoeic regions of the face (e.g. eyebrows and nasolabial folds), and postauricular and presternal areas.

- About half of the patients have fingernail involvement. The characteristic nail changes are punctate pitting, onycholysis (separation of nail from the nail bed) and subungual hyperkeratosis (Fig. 4.12). Ten pits in one nail or >50 pits on all nails are regarded as proof of psoriasis.
- On scrapping a psoriatic lesion with a microscopic slide, silvery scales come out first. After that, pinpoint bleeding appears at the base of the lesion. The latter is known as Auspitz's sign (Fig. 4.13).
- Psoriatic arthritis is seen in 5%–10% of psoriatic patients and usually occurs several years after appearance of skin lesions. It is a form of seronegative spondyloarthropathy.
- Medical comorbidities: Some of the comorbidities associated with psoriasis include ulcerative colitis, Crohn's disease, coronary artery disease, metabolic syndrome and lymphoma.

DIFFERENTIAL DIAGNOSIS

- Pityriasis rosea: It appears like guttate psoriasis but has collarette scales and a larger—herald patch—a week or two before the main rash.
- Atopic dermatitis: There is no clear demarcation from uninvolved skin; lesions are quite itchy and are more on flexural areas.
- Seborrhoeic dermatitis: It appears like sebopsoriasis, but scales tend to be greasy and adherent.
- Secondary syphilis: It appears like guttate psoriasis, but its unique features include orange, pink, or violaceous macules on the palms and soles.
- Tinea corporis: Scales are not silvery and Auspitz's sign is negative.

TREATMENT

- Most patients with psoriasis have skin lesions limited to localised areas. For these patients, topical therapy remains a part of their therapeutic regimen.

LOCAL TREATMENT

- Local measures include application of emollients, coal tar preparations, dithranol, salicylic acid, topical steroids and ultraviolet radiation [narrow-band UVB, and psoralens with ultraviolet A (PUVA)]. Topical steroids range in strength from weak steroids such as 1% hydrocortisone to superpotent corticosteroids, such as clobetasol propionate and betamethasone dipropionate. Side effects of topical corticosteroids, especially those that carry the superpotent categorisation, include cutaneous atrophy, development of striae and formation of telangiectasia. Hypothalamic–pituitary–adrenal axis suppression can occur with prolonged use.
- Other local agents include vitamin D analogues that inhibit keratinocyte growth, promote keratinocyte differentiation and decrease inflammation in psoriatic lesions via vitamin D receptors on keratinocytes and T-lymphocytes. These include calcipotriol, calcitriol, tacalcitol, maxacalcitol, paricalcitol and becocalcidiol.
- Local retinoid, tazarotene, is also useful.
- Calcineurin inhibitors (tacrolimus and pimecrolimus) improve symptoms with less skin atrophy than topical corticosteroids and are considered first-line treatments for facial and flexural psoriasis.

SYSTEMIC TREATMENT

- Systemic treatment is necessary in extensive psoriasis that fails to respond to the local measures. The most commonly used treatments are photochemotherapy with PUVA, retinoids (etretinate and acitretin), methotrexate and cyclosporin.
- In PUVA therapy, after ingestion or local application of a psoralen preparation, patients are exposed to UVA that activates the psoralens. Once activated, psoralens cross-link DNA strands preventing replication of keratinocytes and induce death of activated T-cells in skin. In India, an alternative to UVA light is to ask the patient to sit in the sunlight. However, long-term PUVA treatment may lead to an increased risk of squamous cell carcinoma and possibly malignant melanoma.
- Methotrexate is one of the most effective treatments for psoriasis and psoriatic arthritis. However, it has a number of side effects including bone marrow toxicity, nausea, aphthous stomatitis and development of megaloblastic anaemia. Chronic administration of methotrexate has been associated with the development of hepatic fibrosis.
- Etretinate has a long half-life; therefore, it should not be prescribed to females of child-bearing potential due to the risk of long-term teratogenicity. Acitretin, the active metabolite of etretinate, has a shorter half-life and, therefore, can be given to females as long as they are not planning a pregnancy for 3 years after discontinuing its use.
- Cyclosporin (2.5–5 mg/kg for 10–12 weeks) is highly effective oral therapy for psoriasis. The side effects include hypertension, nephrotoxicity, hypomagnesaemia, hyperkalaemia, hyperuricaemia, elevation of liver transaminases, development of paraesthesias and hypertrichosis.

BIOLOGICAL THERAPY

- Includes drugs to target specific points of inflammation cascade, including antibodies against cell surface markers, cytokines and adhesion molecules.
- Indicated in patients with severe disease not responding to other measures.
- Includes alefacept (causes apoptosis of T-cells), efalizumab (inhibits T-cell activation), and etanercept, infliximab, adalimumab and certolizumab (TNF inhibitors).
- Others include ustekinumab and guselkumab (anti-IL-12/IL-23), secukinumab (anti-IL-17A), ixekizumab (anti-IL-17A) and brodalumab (anti-IL-17 receptor).

SUMMARY OF TREATMENT OF PSORIASIS (Table 4.3)

TABLE 4.3 Summary of Treatment Options for Psoriasis

Type of Therapy	Agents	Examples
Local therapy	Dithranol Salicylic acid Coal tar	
	Topical glucocorticoids	Low potency (hydrocortisone, betamethasone valerate, clobetasol butyrate) Medium potency (fluocinolone, triamcinolone, desoximetasone) High potency (betamethasone dipropionate, fluticasone, mometasone furoate) Ultrahigh potency (clobetasol propionate, halobetasol)
	Vitamin D analogues	Calcipotriol Maxacalcitol Paricalcitol Becocalcidiol Tacalcitol
	Calcineurin inhibitors	Tacrolimus Pimecrolimus
	Local retinoid	Tazarotene
	Phototherapy	Ultraviolet B
Systemic therapy	Methotrexate Cyclosporin	
	Retinoids	Etretinate Acitretin
	Phototherapy	Psoralen and ultraviolet A (PUVA)
Biological therapy	TNF-alpha inhibitors	Etanercept Infliximab Adalimumab Certolizumab
	Anti-IL-12/IL-23	Ustekinumab Guselkumab
	Anti-IL-17	Secukinumab Ixekizumab
	Anti-IL-17 receptor	Brodalumab

Q. Discuss the aetiology, clinical features, diagnosis and treatment of erythema nodosum.

- Erythema nodosum is inflammation of subcutaneous fat (panniculitis) of skin.
- It develops as a result of a nonspecific cutaneous reaction to a variety of antigens, with many immune-mediated mechanisms implicated including immune-complex-mediated reaction and type IV delayed hypersensitivity response to antigens.

AETIOLOGY (Box 4.2)

BOX 4.2 Causes of Erythema Nodosum

COMMON CAUSES

- Idiopathic (most common)
- Infections: Streptococcal pharyngitis, mycobacterial (tuberculosis—usually primary, leprosy), Mycoplasma, *Chlamydia*, *Yersinia*, histoplasmosis
- Sarcoidosis
- Drugs: Antibiotics (e.g. sulphonamides, penicillin, amoxicillin, cephalosporins, nitrofurantoin), oral contraceptives, phenytoin, carbamazepine
- Pregnancy
- Inflammatory bowel disease: Ulcerative colitis, Crohn's disease, coeliac disease
- Rheumatological diseases: Behçet's disease, Reiter's syndrome, systemic lupus erythematosus, rheumatoid arthritis, ankylosing spondylitis, granulomatosis with polyangiitis, adult Still's disease

RARE CAUSES

- Viral infections: Herpes simplex virus, Epstein–Barr virus, hepatitis B and C viruses, human immunodeficiency virus
- Bacterial infections: Syphilis, *Campylobacter* spp., rickettsiae
- Parasitic infections: Amoebiasis, giardiasis, toxoplasmosis, taeniasis, ascariasis
- Miscellaneous: Lymphoma, other malignancies

CLINICAL FEATURES

- More common in females (male-to-female ratio, 1:6).
- Can occur at any age with peak incidence between 20 and 30 years.
- A prodrome commonly occurs before the onset of erythema nodosum regardless of aetiology. It lasts for 3–6 days. Features of prodrome include weight loss, malaise, low-grade fever, cough and arthralgia with or without arthritis (knee and ankle). Arthralgias may persist for several months after resolution of erythema nodosum.
- Presents with painful, symmetrical, erythematous nodules and plaques ranging in size from 1 to 10 cm. Nodules are poorly demarcated due to their subcutaneous location and are most commonly located on the anterior aspect of legs, particularly shins, ankles and knees (Fig. 4.14). Within a few days, the nodules become livid red or purplish colour. Finally, they exhibit a yellow or greenish appearance often taking on the look of a deep bruise (erythema contusiformis).

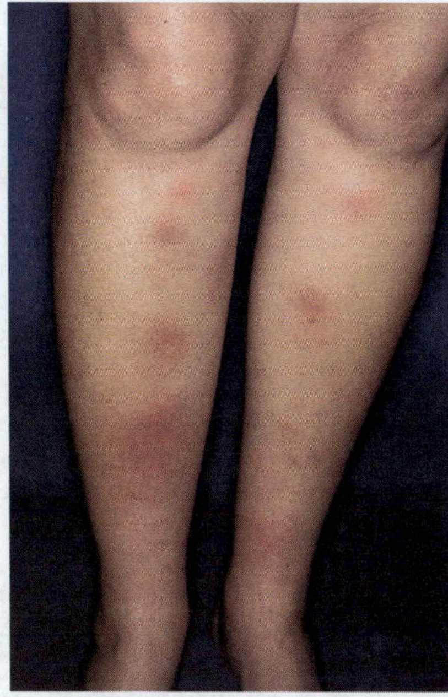

Fig. 4.14 Erythema nodosum.

This contusiform colour evolution is quite characteristic of erythema nodosum and allows a specific diagnosis in late-stage lesions. Ulceration is never seen and the nodules heal over several weeks without atrophy or scarring.

- Less frequent clinical manifestations associated with erythema nodosum are lymphadenopathy, hepatomegaly, splenomegaly and pleuritis.

DIAGNOSIS

- Most often, diagnosis is based on clinical presentation.
- If required, a deep biopsy should be obtained for best results. It shows an inflammation of the septa in the subcutaneous fat tissue (septal panniculitis). Erythema nodosum is not associated with vasculitis, although small vessel inflammation and haemorrhage can occur.
- Diagnosis of cause of erythema nodosum:
  - Complete blood count with differential, erythrocyte sedimentation rate and C-reactive protein level.
  - Evaluation for streptococcal infection (i.e. throat culture for group A streptococci, rapid antigen test, antistreptolysin-O titre and polymerase chain reaction assay).
  - Chest radiograph for tuberculosis and sarcoidosis.
  - Stool examination for ova and parasites in patients with gastrointestinal symptoms.
  - Consider evaluation for inflammatory bowel disease if symptoms are present.

TREATMENT

- Treat any underlying disorders.
- Compression bandages and limb elevation for oedema and pain relief.

- Rest and analgesics with NSAIDs for pain control. However, NSAIDs should be avoided in treating erythema nodosum secondary to Crohn's disease because they may trigger a flare-up of the underlying Crohn's disease.
- Potassium iodide is given orally (300–900 mg/day) for symptomatic relief if NSAIDs do not relieve pain or the lesions persist. It is contraindicated during pregnancy.
- Colchicine mainly for patients with erythema nodosum and Behçet's disease.
- Other drugs include dapsone, hydroxychloroquine and thalidomide.
- Systemic steroids may be given if underlying infection and malignancy have been excluded.
- Tumour necrosis factor-α inhibitors such as etanercept, adalimumab and infliximab in patients with recalcitrant disease.

Q. Briefly outline the aetiology, clinical features and management of acne vulgaris. (DR1.1, DR1.2, DR1.3)

- This is a disorder characterised by chronic inflammation of blocked pilosebaceous follicles. It predominantly affects teenagers.

AETIOPATHOGENESIS

- There is an increase in sebum excretion, which is probably androgen mediated.
- Increased and abnormal keratinisation at the exit of the pilosebaceous follicle causes obstruction to the flow of sebum.
- The sebum of patients with acne contains an excess of free fatty acids that may be responsible for triggering the inflammatory process.
- Colonisation by pathogenic *Cutibacterium acnes* (previously called *Propionibacterium acnes*) causing inflammation at a later stage of the disease.
- Important endocrine causes of acne are given in Box 4.3.
- Pathophysiology is summarised in Box 4.4.
- A number of drugs can produce acne. In such cases, the lesions are usually on the trunk rather than on face. Some of the commonly implicated drugs are listed in Box 4.5.

BOX 4.3 Endocrine Causes of Acne Vulgaris

- Polycystic ovarian syndrome
- Cushing's syndrome
- Congenital adrenal hyperplasia
- Androgen-secreting tumours of adrenals, ovary and testis
- Acromegaly

BOX 4.4 Pathophysiology of Acne Vulgaris

- Abnormal keratinocyte proliferation and desquamation which leads to obstruction of ducts of sebum glands
- Androgen-driven increase in sebum production
- Proliferation of *Cutibacterium acnes*
- Inflammation

BOX 4.5 Drugs Causing Acne Vulgaris

• Glucocorticoids	Systemic and local agents
• Anabolic	Danazole, stanozolol
• Antiepileptics	Phenytoin, carbamazepine, topiramate, gabapentin
• Antidepressants	Amitriptyline, lithium, sertraline
• Antitubercular	Isoniazid, rifampicin
• Chemotherapeutic agents	Dactinomycin, pentostatin, gefitinib
• Antiviral	Ritonavir, ganciclovir
• Vitamins	B_6, B_{12}

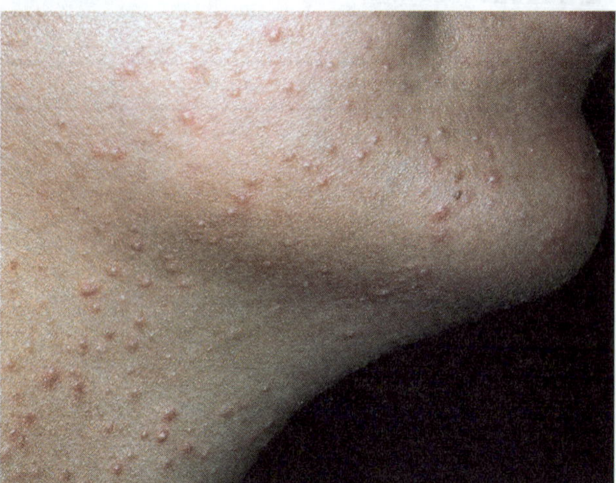

Fig. 4.15 Closed or whitehead comedones of acne.

CLINICAL FEATURES

- Lesions are limited to the face, shoulders, upper chest and back.
- Seborrhoea (greasy skin) is often present.
- Acne formation starts when sebum and keratinous material shed from the skin clog up a pore and trigger bacterial colonisation, leading to a closed or whitehead comedone (Fig. 4.15).
- With more accumulation of sebum and keratinous material, the follicular orifice opens and forms an open or blackhead comedone (Fig. 4.16). The black colour is the result of oxidised lipids and the skin pigment melanin.
- Later in the course, inflammatory lesions occur that tend to lead to more scarring. The lesions may include papules, pustules, nodules and cysts, and any combination of these. Severe forms of inflammatory acne include nodular cystic disease with all its potentially destructive sequelae.

MANAGEMENT

- Given the current data, no specific dietary changes are recommended in the management of acne.
- General measures:
  - Regular washing with soap and water.
  - Antibacterial skin cleansers containing chlorhexidine.

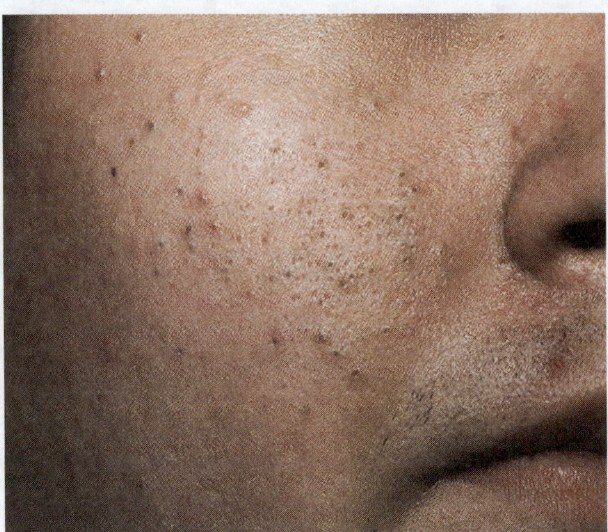

Fig. 4.16 Open or blackhead comedones of acne.

- Local measures:
  - Keratolytics include α- and β-hydroxy acid (like salicylic acid), azelaic acid and retinoids. Tretinoin is the most potent keratolytic agent. Other retinoids include isotretinoin (less effective), adapalene (less irritating), tazarotene and trifarotene. Topical retinoids may produce skin irritation, sun sensitivity and initial flaring of acne.
  - Reducing infection by *C. acnes* by using benzoyl peroxide and local antibiotics. Benzoyl peroxide has mild but significant keratolytic effect. It inactivates topical retinoic acid when used concurrently and may cause skin bleaching. Topical antibiotics include clindamycin and erythromycin.
  - Usually, topical benzoyl peroxide or antibiotic is applied in the morning and a keratolytic preparation at night.
  - Combining adapalene and benzoyl peroxide may be more effective than either of them alone.
  - Another topical agent is clascoterone which has antiandrogen and anti-inflammatory properties.
- Systemic measures:
  - Long-term antibiotic therapy with doxycycline, minocycline or erythromycin/azithromycin for duration of 3 months (occasionally for 2 years). Erythromycin/azithromycin is less effective due to development of resistance in *C. acnes* but is used if tetracyclines cannot be used.
  - Another antibiotic approved for moderate to severe acne in patients aged 9 years and older is sarecycline. It is a modified tetracycline that binds to 30S ribosomes but does not bind to aminoacyl-tRNA.
  - Isotretinoin (13-*cis*-retinoic acid) given orally in a 4-month course can reduce sebum excretion and may be required in severe acne. Oral isotretinoin is a potent teratogen and may be associated with development of mood disorders, depression, suicidal ideation, hepatotoxicity and hypertriglyceridaemia. Other adverse effects include secondary skin infections, myalgia, arthralgia, mucocutaneous dryness and cheilitis. It is contraindicated during pregnancy due to its teratogenic effects.
  - Hormonal treatment:
    - Androgen receptor blockers:
      - Spironolactone, cyproterone acetate, drospirenone and flutamide.
      - Cyproterone acetate is combined with oestrogen and is given in courses as an oral contraceptive.
    - Inhibitors of adrenal androgen production:
      - Low-dose glucocorticoids in acute and severe acne.
    - Inhibitors of ovarian androgen production:
      - Oral contraceptives containing oestrogen in the form of ethinyl oestradiol combined with a progestin.
- Physical measures:
  - Incision and drainage of cysts.
  - Intralesional injections of triamcinolone acetonide.
  - Light (blue light with wavelength of 407–420 nm) and laser treatment.
  - Photodynamic therapy using aminolevulinic acid or indocyanine green dye application.

Q. Briefly outline the precipitating causes, clinical manifestations and management of erythema multiforme.

Q. Give a brief account of target lesions, iris lesions and bull's-eye lesions.

Q. Write a short note on Stevens–Johnson's syndrome.

Q. Briefly outline toxic epidermal necrolysis.

- Erythema multiforme (EM) is an acute, self-limiting and sometimes recurring skin condition considered to be a hypersensitivity reaction associated with certain infections and medications.
- Previously, EM was thought to be part of a clinical spectrum of disease that included erythema minor, erythema major [often equated with Stevens–Johnson's syndrome (SJS)] and toxic epidermal necrolysis (TEN).
- Although SJS and TEN may represent the same process with differing severity, EM with its minimal mucous membrane involvement and less than 10% epidermal detachment is now accepted as a distinct condition.

CAUSES

- EM as well as SJS/TEN can be induced by a variety of inciting agents which are shown in Box 4.6.
- The most common cause of SJS and TEN is medications. These are T-cell-mediated diseases with drug-specific CD8+ cells acting as the major mediator of keratinocyte death. *Fas*-mediated keratinocyte apoptosis is also implicated.

BOX 4.6 Causes of Erythema Multiforme, Stevens–Johnson's Syndrome and Toxic Epidermal Necrolysis

Infections
- Herpes simplex virus (most common)
- Cytomegalovirus
- Dengue
- Mycoplasma pneumoniae
- Epstein–Barr virus
- Hepatitis C virus
- Influenza virus

Vaccines
- Measles, mumps and rubella
- Hepatitis B
- Meningococcal
- Pneumococcal
- Varicella
- Influenza

Drugs
- Antibiotics
  - Sulphonamides
  - Penicillins
  - Fluoroquinolones
  - Macrolides
  - Tetracyclines
  - Nitrofurantoin
- Antiepileptics
  - Phenytoin
  - Barbiturates
  - Carbamazepine
  - Lamotrigine
- Abacavir
- Nevirapine
- Nonsteroidal antiinflammatory drugs
- Tumour necrosis factor-α inhibitors

Others
- Inflammatory bowel disease
- Malignancy
- Menstruation

- HLA-B*1502 and HLA-B*5701, respectively, implicated in carbamazepine- and abacavir-induced SJS/TEN.

CLASSIFICATION OF SJS/TEN (Table 4.4)

TABLE 4.4 Classification of Stevens–Johnson's Syndrome and Toxic Epidermal Necrolysis

Diagnosis	Skin Detachment Area
SJS	<10%
SJS/TEN overlap	10%–30%
TEN	>30%

CLINICAL FEATURES

ERYTHEMA MULTIFORME

- Usually occurs in adults 20–40 years of age.
- A self-limited eruption with usually mild or no prodromal symptoms.
- Patients may experience burning at the site of the eruption; itching is minimal.
- Individual lesions begin acutely as numerous, sharply demarcated, red or pink macules that then become papular. The papules may enlarge gradually into plaques several centimetres in diameter. The central portion of the papules or plaques gradually becomes darker red, brown, dusky or purpuric. Crusting or blistering sometimes occurs in the centre of the lesions.
- The characteristic 'target' or 'iris' lesion, less than 3 cm in diameter, has a regular round shape and three concentric zones: a central dusky or darker red area, a paler pink or oedematous zone and a peripheral red ring (Fig. 4.17). Atypical lesions may only have two zones of colour and may have poorly defined borders.

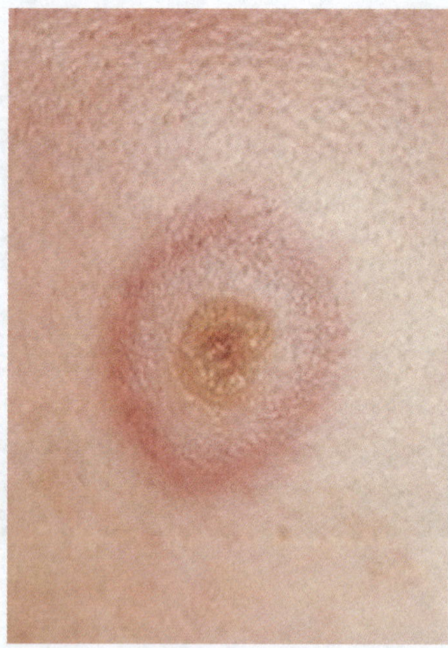

Fig. 4.17 Target lesion of erythema multiforme.

- Common sites of involvement are hands, extensor part of forearms, palms, soles (acral distribution) and mucous membranes of mouth, nose, eyes and genitalia.
- Mucosal lesions may occur in about 30%–50% of cases but are mild and usually limited to the oral cavity. Lesions vary from diffuse oral erythema to multifocal superficial ulcerations. Initially, vesicles or bullae may also be present. Although the oral mucosa is the most commonly involved, genital and ocular mucosa also may develop lesions.
- The lesions resolve spontaneously in 3–5 weeks without sequelae, but may recur. Recurrent EM may occur because of the reactivation of HSV. Persistent EM is a rare condition which has been associated with inflammatory bowel disease, malignancies and infections.

STEVENS–JOHNSON'S SYNDROME

- Risk factors include HIV infection (100-fold increased risk), autoimmune disease such as systemic lupus erythematosus (50-fold increased risk), and active malignancy (particularly haematologic) (30- to 60-fold increased risk).
- Characterised by skin and ≥2 mucous membranes involvement.
- Begins with a prodrome of fever and flu-like symptoms lasting 1–3 days, followed by photophobia, conjunctival itching, dysphagia and skin tenderness.
- Skin involvement is characterised by painful, confluent purpuric macules, sometimes blisters, on the face and trunk (axial distribution) (Fig. 4.18). Target lesions are not seen and the epidermal detachment

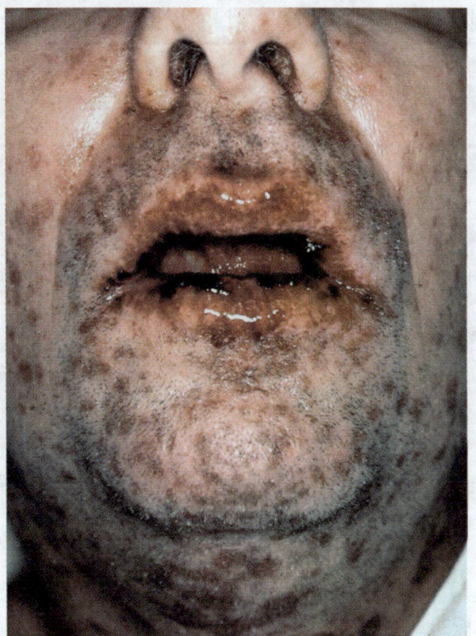

Fig. 4.18 Stevens–Johnson's syndrome with involvement of face and oral mucosa.

does not involve >10% of the surface area. Nikolsky's sign is often positive.
- Involvement of oral and/or mucous membranes may be severe enough that patients may not be able to eat or drink (Fig. 4.18).
- Usually, it is accompanied by severe constitutional symptoms in the form of fever, tachycardia and hypotension. Electrolyte imbalance is frequent.
- Patients with genitourinary involvement may complain of dysuria or an inability to void.
- Severe ophthalmic involvement may lead to permanent scarring and blindness.
- Epidermal sloughing of the bronchial epithelium can occur and patients may require mechanical ventilation.
- Epithelial loss results in vulnerability to bacterial infections and predisposes to sepsis.
- Mortality approximately 5%–10%.

SJS/TEN OVERLAP

- Skin involvement is between 10% and 30%.
- Systemic features are present.

TOXIC EPIDERMAL NECROLYSIS (LYELL'S SYNDROME)

- Begins with severe mucosal erosions and progresses to diffuse, generalised detachment of the epidermis. Nikolsky's sign is often positive.
- Target lesions are not seen.
- More than 30% of skin is involved.
- Mortality as high as 30%.

MANAGEMENT

- Management of the primary causes (discontinuation of medications and treatment of infection).

ERYTHEMA MULTIFORME

- Mild cases do not require any specific treatment. Antihistamines and local corticosteroids may provide symptomatic relief.
- Severe cases of EM may require systemic corticosteroids.
- Oral acyclovir early in herpes-associated outbreaks of EM is useful to lessen the number and duration of lesions, and recurrences. However, in cases of established herpes-associated EM, there is no evidence that antiviral therapy improves the time to lesion resolution.

SJS/TEN

- Due to the severity of SJS/TEN, including the potential for rapid progression and the need for complex nursing care, all patients should be managed initially in an ICU or burn unit.
- Fluid and electrolyte balance must be maintained. Environmental temperature is maintained at 30°C–32°C to prevent hypercatabolic state by reducing caloric losses through the skin. Oral lesions are managed with mouthwashes. Topical anaesthetics as well as nonsteroidal antiinflammatory drugs and opioids are useful in reducing pain and allowing the patient to take fluids. Areas of denuded skin must be covered with compresses of saline. Barrier nursing and sterile handling of the patient is required to prevent infection.
- Women must be monitored for vulvar ulceration, synechiae of the vulva and vagina, and vaginal stenosis. Vaginal dilators and potent topical corticosteroids have a role in preventing stenosis in some patients.
- Ocular involvement is treated with aggressive lubrication, judicious use of topical corticosteroid eye drops, prevention of infection with antibiotic eye drops, and if required, amniotic membrane transplantation.
- Antibiotic treatment should be given when cutaneous infection is clinically suspected.
- Role of systemic steroids, intravenous immunoglobulins, cyclosporin and plasmapheresis is controversial.

PROGNOSIS

- The severity-of-illness Score for TEN (SCORTEN) is widely used to predict mortality for SJS/TEN. SCORTEN should be assessed within the first 24 hours after admission and again on Day 3. SCORTEN is based on seven independent risk factors, each given one point. The more risk factors that are present, the higher the mortality rate (Box 4.7).

BOX 4.7 Score of Toxic Epidermal Necrosis (SCORTEN)

- Age >40 years
- Heart rate >120/minute
- Presence of cancer or haematologic malignancy
- Epidermal detachment area involving body surface area >10%
- Blood urea nitrogen >28 mg/dL
- Blood glucose >252 mg/dL
- Bicarbonate <20 mEq/L

Q. Describe the aetiology, clinical features and management of staphylococcal toxic shock syndrome.

- Toxic shock syndrome (TSS) can be caused by staphylococci (staphylococcal TSS) and streptococci (streptococcal TSS).
- TSS is a toxin-mediated disease characterised by rapid onset of generalised erythema with desquamation, fever, hypotension and potential multisystem failure.

AETIOLOGY

- Occurs due to exotoxin produced by *S. aureus*.
- Common in women using menstrual tampons of high absorbency and in patients with superficial skin or surgical wound infections.
- *S. aureus* elaborates TSS toxin-1 and other exfoliative toxins. These are known as superantigens as they can directly activate T-cells by bypassing certain steps of the antigen-mediated immune response sequence. This causes a massive, uncontrolled T-cell activation, resulting in the release of a substantial amounts of cytokines. This leads to recruitment and further activation of additional T- and B-cells, thereby causing fever, hypotension and multiorgan failure.

CLINICAL FEATURES

- After a 2- to 3-day prodrome period of malaise, patients typically present with fever, chills, nausea and abdominal pain.
- A diffuse erythematous, nonpruritic, maculopapular or petechial rash initially appears on the trunk and spreads peripherally to involve palms and soles. It desquamates in 1–3 weeks (Fig. 4.19).
- Mucosal involvement includes conjunctival–scleral haemorrhage and hyperaemia of the vaginal and oropharyngeal mucosa. In more severe cases, superficial ulcerations occur on the mucous membranes.
- Multisystem involvement includes cardiac arrhythmias, hepatic and renal failure, disseminated intravascular coagulation and acute respiratory distress syndrome. Diarrhoea is common.

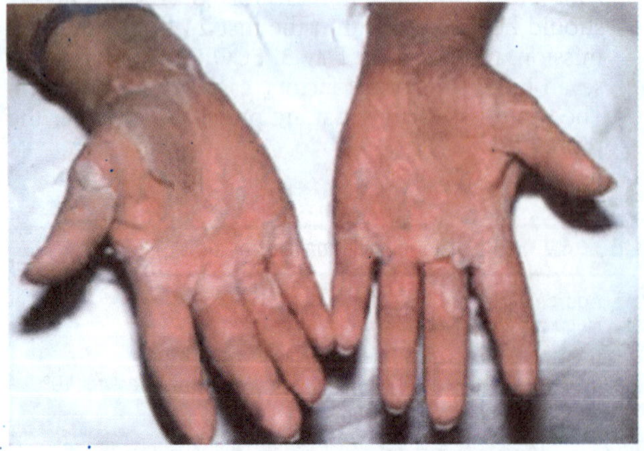

Fig. 4.19 Desquamation after staphylococcal toxic shock syndrome.

DIAGNOSTIC CRITERIA (Table 4.5)

TABLE 4.5 Diagnostic Criteria for Staphylococcal Toxic Shock Syndrome

Clinical criteria:	
Fever	Temperature ≥38.9°C
Rash	Diffuse macular rash
Desquamation	1–2 weeks after onset of illness, particularly on palms and soles
Hypotension	Systolic blood pressure of ≤90 mmHg
Multisystem Involvement (3 or More of the Following Organ Systems):	
Gastrointestinal	Vomiting or diarrhoea at onset
Muscular	Severe myalgia or CPK >twice normal
Mucous membranes	Vaginal, conjunctival or oropharyngeal hyperaemia
Renal	Blood urea or creatinine >twice normal or pyuria (≥5 leucocytes per high power field) in the absence of urinary tract infection
Haematologic	Platelet count <100,000/mm^3
Hepatic	Bilirubin, AST and ALT >twice normal
Central nervous system	Disorientation or altered consciousness without focal neurologic deficit when fever and hypotension are absent
Laboratory diagnostic criteria if obtained:	
Negative	Blood, throat or CSF culture (except *S. aureus*)
Negative	Serologic tests for Rocky Mountain spotted fever, leptospirosis or measles

Case classification:
- Probable: ≥4 clinical criteria + laboratory criteria met
- Confirmed: 5 clinical criteria + laboratory criteria met, including desquamation (unless death occurs prior to desquamation)

MANAGEMENT

- Removal of inciting factors, including removal of tampon and drainage of focus of infection.
- Aggressive treatment of hypotension and of potential multiorgan failure.
- Antistaphylococcal antibiotic therapy (e.g. clindamycin + vancomycin initially). Clindamycin also inhibits its toxin production.
- β-Lactamase inhibitor (e.g. piperacillin-tazobactam) or a carbapenem (e.g. meropenem) is often added as it may be difficult to differentiate this condition from other organisms causing septic shock.
- Role of intravenous immunoglobulins (IVIg) is controversial.

Q. Briefly outline keloid and hypertrophic scar.

- More commonly observed in Asians and dark-skinned races; this association is less commonly seen with hypertrophic scars.
- May follow local skin trauma or inflammatory skin disorders like laceration, tattoos, burns, injections, ear piercing, vaccination, bites, acne, abscess or surgery.
- Occur due to uncontrolled synthesis and deposition of dermal collagen.

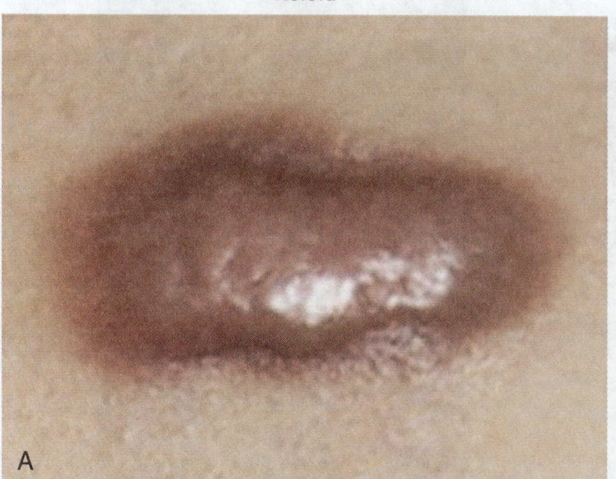

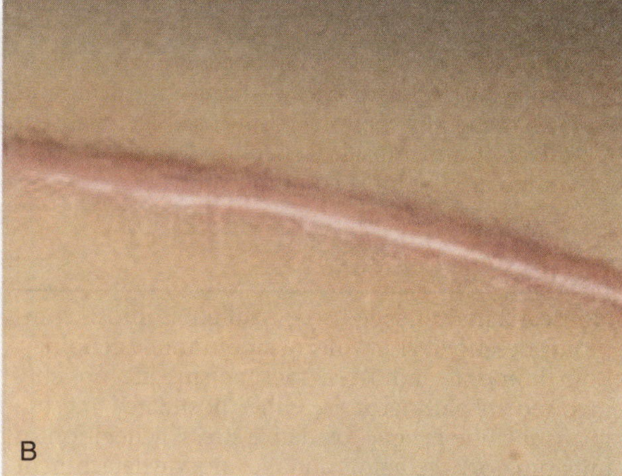

Fig. 4.20 (A) Keloid, (B) hypertrophic scar.

- Wounds subjected to tension due to motion, body location or loss of tissue are at increased risk of scar hypertrophy and keloid formation.
- Hypertrophic scar usually appears within a month of injury, whereas keloids may take 3 months or even years to develop.

CLINICAL FEATURES

- A keloid extends beyond the borders of the original wound, does not regress spontaneously, grows in pseudotumour fashion with distortion of the lesion and tends to recur after excision. Itching and pain are common. It has a firm and inflexible texture, a shiny appearance and is usually flesh coloured, but may be erythematous or hyperpigmented (Fig. 4.20).
- Hypertrophic scars remain confined to the borders of the original wound and most of the times retain their shape. Itching may occur (Fig. 4.20).

DIFFERENCES BETWEEN KELOID AND HYPERTROPHIC SCAR (Table 4.6)

TABLE 4.6 Keloid Versus Hypertrophic Scar

Keloid	Hypertrophic Scar
• Thick, unevenly organised	• Thin, well organised
• Associated with dark skin colour	• Not associated with dark skin colour
• Generally develops months after injury	• Develops within a month of injury
• Does not regress with time	• Generally regresses with time
• Extends beyond borders of original wound	• Remains confined to borders of wound
• No association with contracture	• Associated with contracture
• Highly vascularised dermis	• Less vascularised dermis
• Commonly occurs on sternal skin, shoulders, upper arms, earlobes and cheeks	• Arises in any location but usually on extensor surfaces of joints
• Worsened by surgery	• Improves with surgery

TREATMENT

- Treatment modalities include compression garments, radiation, excision, intralesional injections, cauterisation, cryotherapy, laser surgery and silicone gel dressings.
- Excision of keloid with scalpel, electrosurgery or laser surgery will result in almost 100% chances of recurrence. Keloids over areas like earlobes are less likely to recur.
- Surgical excision of hypertrophic scars may be efficacious in selected cases but requires meticulous adherence to the surgical principles and adjunctive measures like radiation, intralesional interferon or topical imiquimod.
- Intralesional injections are useful in the treatment. Various agents used for injection include triamcinolone, 5-fluorouracil, bleomycin and interferon-α-2b.
- Freezing the lesions of keloid with liquid nitrogen (cryotherapy) helps to soften the lesions, which makes the intralesional administration of medication easier.

SURGICAL COMBINATION THERAPIES

- These include surgical excision + triamcinolone, surgical excision + radiation, surgical excision + pressure therapy (in auricular keloid), surgical excision + cryotherapy and surgical excision + mitomycin C.

Q. Write briefly about the aetiology, clinical features and treatment of vitiligo. (DR2.1, DR2.2)

- Occurs due to selective destruction of the skin melanocytes that results in development of unsightly depigmented patches.
- Onset before the age of 18 years in more than 50% of cases.
- Vitiligo can be separated into segmental and nonsegmental (vitiligo vulgaris).

- Segmental vitiligo has important differences in aetiology, prevalence of associated illnesses and therapy compared to other forms of vitiligo.
- Various forms of nonsegmental vitiligo include acrofacial (lesions in acral—hands and feet, and face—generally perioral), mucosal, generalised, universal and mixed. Generalised and acrofacial vitiligo are the most common subtypes.

AETIOLOGY

- Nonsegmental (generalised) vitiligo is most commonly described as having an autoimmune aetiology. Both humoral and T-cell mechanisms are possibly involved in pathogenesis. Other postulated mechanisms include genetic, oxidative stress, generation of inflammatory mediators and melanocyte detachment mechanisms.
- Segmental vitiligo is possibly due to some chemical mediators released from peripheral nerve endings that cause decreased production of melanin (neural theory).
- Therapy of cancers using checkpoint inhibitors may produce vitiligo as a side effect. These drugs target PD-1 (pembrolizumab and nivolumab) or CTLA4 (ipilimumab and tremelimumab).

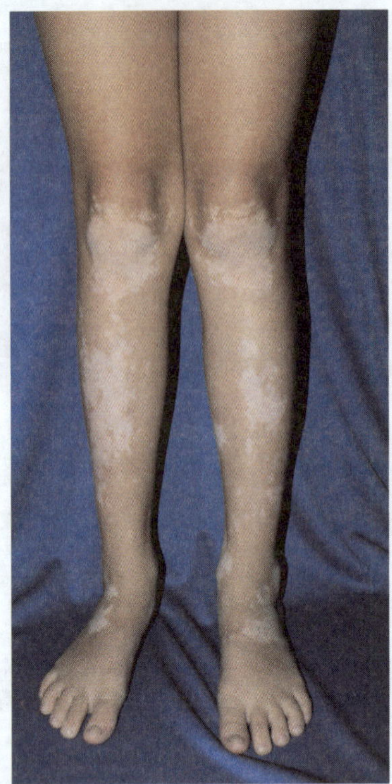

Fig. 4.21 Nonsegmental vitiligo.

CLINICAL FEATURES

- Presents as small, depigmented lesions which may enlarge and coalesce into larger patches.
- Vitiligo is most striking around the body orifices: eyes, nostrils, mouth, nipples, umbilicus and genitalia.
- Can affect melanocytes in the hair roots resulting in patches of white hair. Depigmentation can affect mucosal areas such as in the mouth or genitalia.
- In nonsegmental vitiligo, lesions are usually symmetrical (Fig. 4.21) and new patches may appear throughout the patient's life. It may be either generalised or localised. The overlying hair may remain pigmented or turn white. This type of vitiligo is often associated with a number of immune system aberrations. Frequently associated with a number of autoimmune disorders, including alopecia areata, diabetes mellitus, pernicious anaemia, Addison's disease and Hashimoto's thyroiditis.
  - Vitiligo universalis refers to complete or nearly complete depigmentation of the skin (80%–90% of body surface). It is usually preceded by nonsegmental vitiligo that gradually progresses to complete or near complete depigmentation of the skin and hair.
- Segmental vitiligo usually has unilateral involvement and a dermatomal distribution (Fig. 4.22). Without treatment, the depigmentation spreads within the segment over a period of 6–24 months. After initial rapid spreading in the affected dermatome, the patch most often remains stable. It is typically associated with leucotrichia (white hair). The most commonly involved dermatome is that of the trigeminal nerve. Segmental vitiligo has no association with autoimmune thyroiditis and is in fact rarely associated with any autoimmune disease.

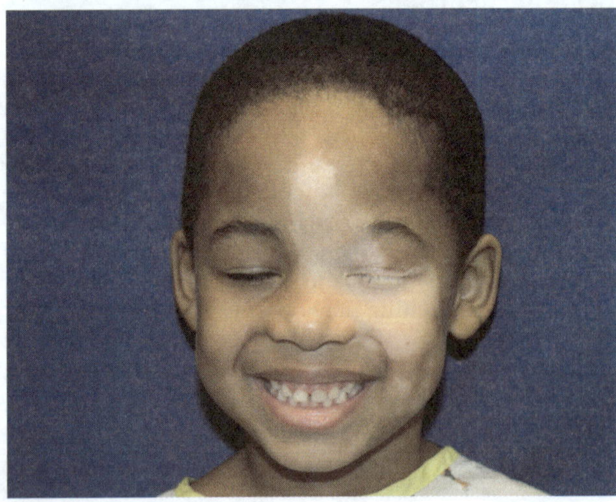

Fig. 4.22 Segmental vitiligo.

- Koebner's phenomenon: Nonsegmental vitiligo can spread by Koebner's phenomenon. Other skin conditions that can also spread by Koebner's phenomenon include psoriasis and lichen planus. Koebner's phenomenon is the initiation of new lesions that occur as a result of trauma, particularly mechanical trauma such as scratching.
- Use of a Wood's lamp with UV light in the range of 320–400 nm can greatly assist in locating areas of pigment disruption. It can detect areas of depigmentation that may not be visible to the naked eye, particularly in pale skin. Under the Wood's light, the vitiligo lesions emit a bright blue-white fluorescence

and appear sharply demarcated. A complete examination should include inspection of the genitalia and areas of skin folds as these areas can be easily overlooked.
- Dermoscopy can be used to differentiate vitiligo from other depigmenting disorders. Vitiligo typically shows residual perifollicular pigmentation and telangiectasia, which are absent in other hypopigmentation disorders. It can also be useful in assessing disease activity in vitiligo and the stage of evolution.

TREATMENT

- Topical psoralen plus ultraviolet A (UVA) phototherapy (PUVA therapy) is a well-established treatment for nonsegmental vitiligo (less effective in segmental vitiligo). Topical application of psoralen is followed half an hour later by exposure to long UV rays (320–400 nm) from sunlight or artificial light sources. However, it is effective in only about half of the patients and has a high relapse rate. Common side effects include darkening of normal skin, erythema, scaling and pruritus. Less common side effects include phototoxic effects, photoallergic reactions, hyperkeratosis of lesional skin and, rarely, skin malignancies. Another less toxic agent is khellin which is used with UVA.
- Narrow-band UVB (NB-UVB) phototherapy is the treatment of choice for patients with active, spreading lesions or those with generalised (>20% of body surface area) vitiligo. Cosmetic results are better and side effects are less with this therapy compared to those with PUVA.
- Local application of corticosteroids with or without UVA exposure is effective in many patients.
- Targeted phototherapy using the excimer laser is useful in treating localised vitiligo. The targeted exposure of this strategy spares the normal skin from potentially harmful radiation.
- Local application of calcineurin inhibitors (pimecrolimus and tacrolimus) is also effective.
- Systemic corticosteroids given twice a week for up to 6 months can be effective in halting progression of unstable vitiligo.
- Surgical modalities are quite effective in treating certain types of vitiligo. Autologous skin grafting and noncultured epidermal suspension grafting, also known as a melanocyte keratinocyte transplant procedure, are the methods of choice for treating stable and focal vitiligo.
- Extensive vitiligo may be treated with removal of pigment from the remaining normally pigmented skin. Bleaching creams used for this purpose include monobenzyl ether of hydroquinone and 4-methoxy-phenol. Another option is to give oral psoralen after a meal followed 2–3 hours later by exposure to long UV rays.

PLATELET-RICH PLASMA

- Local injection of autologous platelet-rich plasma (PRP) has been tried with some success in patients with stable vitiligo. Secretion of platelet's alpha granules increases the release of growth factors, adhesion molecules and chemokines, which interacting with the local environment, promote cell differentiation, proliferation and regeneration. It is often combined with NB-UVB or fractional CO_2 laser.
- It is also used in other dermatologic conditions like androgenic alopecia, facial skin rejuvenation, healing of refractory cutaneous ulcers and even acne scar management.

Q. Name a few conditions which can cause hypopigmentation.

- Conditions which can cause hypopigmentation are listed in Table 4.7.

Q. Name a few conditions which can cause hyperpigmentation.

- Conditions which can produce skin hyperpigmentation are listed in Box 4.8.

Q. What is café au lait? Explain.

Q. Write a short note on McCune–Albright's syndrome.

- Café au lait lesions are well circumscribed, evenly pigmented, light-brown-coloured macules ranging

TABLE 4.7 Aetiology of Skin Hypopigmentation

Postinflammatory	Others
• Pityriasis alba • Atopic dermatitis • Allergic contact dermatitis • Psoriasis • Lichen planus • Toxic drug reactions • Posttraumatic hypopigmentation (scar) • Phototherapy and radiotherapy induced **Chemically induced leukoderma (occupational)** • Phenols and other derivatives • Chloroquine and hydroxychloroquine	• Vitiligo • Leprosy • Topical drug-induced depigmentation • Mycosis fungoides • Pityriasis versicolor • Tuberous sclerosis • Cutaneous leishmaniasis • Melanoma-associated leukoderma • Systemic lupus erythematosus • Syphilis, yaws and pinta

BOX 4.8 Aetiology of Skin Hyperpigmentation

- Ephelides (freckles)
- Melasma (chloasma)
- Acanthosis nigricans
- Fixed drug eruptions
- Café au lait spots
- Peutz–Jeghers' syndrome
- Mongolian spots
- Lichen planus pigmentosus
- Discoid lupus erythematosus
- Drug-induced melanosis (e.g. clofazimine, minocycline, antimalarial induced)
- Agyria
- Ochronosis
- Postinflammatory pigmentation
- Lichen planus
- Pellagra
- Haemochromatosis
- Cirrhosis of liver
- Chronic kidney disease

in size from 1 to 2 mm to greater than 20 cm. The size of the macule has no greater or lesser significance.

- Histologically, increased melanin content of both melanocytes and basal keratinocytes is seen. There is no increase in the number of melanocytes in the area.
- Morphologically, these spots may be either oval and smooth bordered, resembling the 'coast of California' (Fig. 4.23), or with jagged contours resembling the 'coast of Maine' (Fig. 4.24).
- Café au lait with smooth borders is more typical of the café au lait spots seen in neurofibromatosis type 1 (NF-1), whereas those with jagged borders are more indicative of the café au lait spots seen in McCune–Albright's syndrome, although variations are common. Multiple café au lait spots (≥6 in number, each >5 mm in size) raise the suspicion of NF-1.
- Solitary café au lait spots are a common birthmark. Although most café au lait spots are present at birth, they may also manifest within the first few years of life. In general, it is unusual for additional sporadic café au lait to develop after the age of 6 years; in NF-1, however, new café au lait spots may continue to develop throughout childhood and adulthood.
- In fair-skinned infants, they may be difficult to perceive on routine physical examination, but may be accentuated with examination under a Wood's lamp.
- Café au lait spots may develop anywhere on the body, although they more commonly occur on the torso, buttocks and lower extremities and are uncommon on the face.

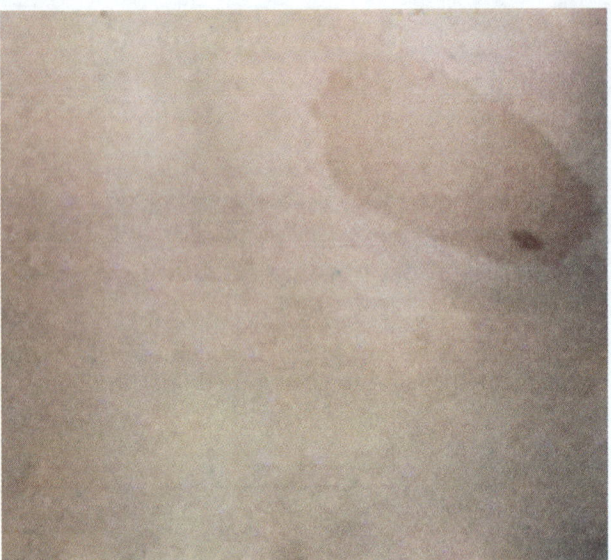

Fig. 4.23 Café au lait spots ('coast of California').

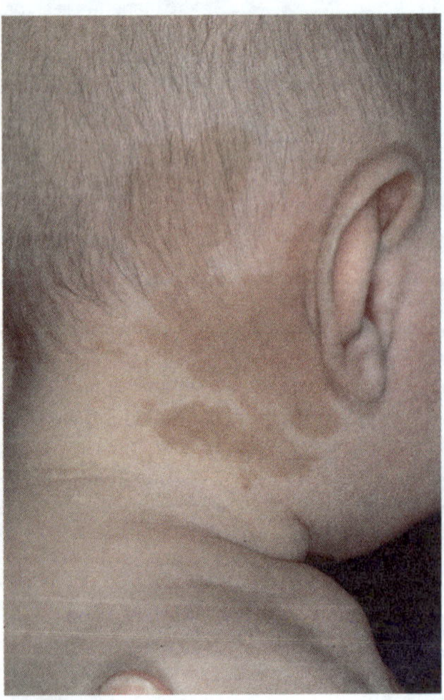

Fig. 4.24 Café au lait spots ('coast of Maine').

McCUNE–ALBRIGHT'S SYNDROME

- A rare disorder which occurs due to mutation occurring in early embryogenesis.
- Cardinal features include polyostotic fibrous dysplasia (commonly presenting with fracture, deformity and/or bone pain), precocious puberty and other endocrinopathies (e.g. hyperthyroidism, hyperparathyroidism and acromegaly), and large and irregular segmental (not crossing midline) café au lait that typically involve the torso or buttocks (Fig. 4.25). Two of these features are required for diagnosis.
- Males must be followed for testicular lesions (macroorchidism) on physical examination and ultrasonography, and females require more stringent breast cancer screening.

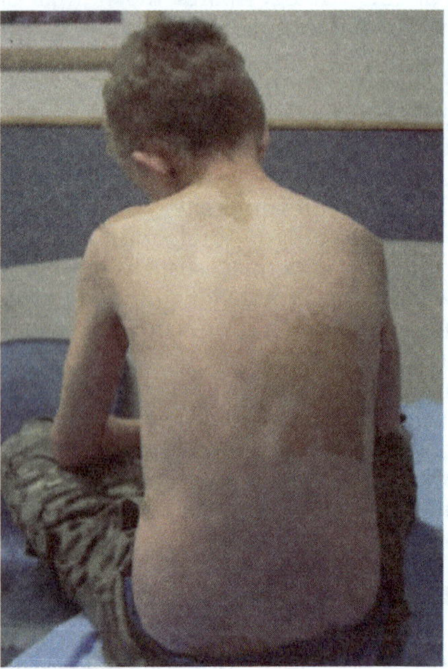

Fig. 4.25 Characteristic appearance of a café au lait spot in a patient with McCune–Albright's syndrome.

- Girls with precocious puberty can be managed with the aromatase inhibitor letrozole, which is effective in decreasing frequency of vaginal bleeding and improving final adult height. If letrozole monotherapy is ineffective, oestrogen receptor modulators such as tamoxifen and fulvestrant may be considered.
- Boys with precocious puberty are treated with testosterone receptor blockers, such as bicalutamide or spironolactone, used in combination with an aromatase inhibitor to prevent bone age advancement.

Q. Write a short note on alopecia.

Q. Write a short note on alopecia areata.

ALOPECIA

- Alopecia is defined as absence or loss of hair due to disorders of hair follicle, hair shaft or scalp.

CAUSES OF ALOPECIA

- Alopecia can be associated with scarring or can occur without scarring. In addition, alopecia can be localised or diffuse.
- Various causes of alopecia are given in Table 4.8.

ANDROGENIC ALOPECIA

- Also known as male-pattern baldness. It is defined as thinning of the hair to an almost transparent state in both men and women. It is hereditary in nature.
- Linked to excess of androgens around the hair follicles.
- Women tend to develop androgenic alopecia after menopause when they have less of female hormones.

INVESTIGATIONS FOR ALOPECIA

- Complete blood counts, serum ferritin, blood glucose, liver and renal function tests, hormonal assays (T4, TSH, LH and testosterone), vitamin B12 and vitamin D.
- Trichometric analysis: Folliscope magnifies images to give a detailed look at hair, hair follicles and the scalp.
- Fungal smear and culture.
- At times, punch biopsy is required.

TREATMENT OF ALOPECIA

- Many cases of hair loss are temporary, for example due to chemotherapy, or the loss is due to natural process of ageing for which no treatment is required.
- Spontaneous recovery is common for patchy alopecia areata.
- Intralesional and topical steroids and short courses of systemic steroids.
- Topical 1% anthralin cream.
- Five percent topical minoxidil.
- Finasteride acts by preventing conversion of testosterone to dihydrotestosterone as the latter causes hair follicles to shrink.
- PUVA therapy.
- Low-level laser therapy (LLLT).
- Psychological support.
- Hair transplantation: It is a technique to remove hair follicles from one part of the body (donor site) and transplant them to a bald part. It is primarily used to treat male type of baldness. The two more accepted techniques for hair transplants are the follicular unit transplantation (FUT) (also known as the strip technique) and the follicular unit extraction (FUE).
  - FUT technique requires the excision of hair-bearing strips from a donor and dissecting into small follicular units.
  - The FUE technique uses small individual follicular grafts extracted through manual or motorised punches.
  - The FUE technique has some advantages over FUT, for example less scarring, shorter recovery time and have minimal risk of nerve injury.
- Experimental: Stem cell therapy.

ALOPECIA AREATA

- It is defined as acute onset of nonscarring hair loss in one or more sharply defined round or oval patches, most commonly on scalp, bearded area, eyebrows and eyelashes.
- Some patients lose hair in only a small patch, while others have more extensive or less frequently diffuse involvement.

PATHOGENESIS

- It is an autoimmune disease mediated by T-cells and macrophages.
- The hair follicle is an immune-privileged site with low levels of major histocompatibility complex (MHC) expression. It is assumed that alopecia areata

TABLE 4.8 Causes of Alopecia

Localised (Nonscarring)	Localised (Scarring)	Diffuse
• Alopecia areata • Syphilitic alopecia • Androgenetic alopecia or androgenic alopecia • Triangular alopecia • Tinea capitis • Traction alopecia • Trichotillomania	• Acne • Tinea capitis • Cutaneous lupus erythematosus • Discoid lupus erythematosus • Others	• Alopecia areata • Telogen effluvium • Hair breakage • Unruly hair • Hereditary vitamin-D-resistant rickets • Androgenic alopecia • Associated with other diseases (hypothyroidism, hyperthyroidism, diabetes mellitus, hypopituitarism, iron deficiency, chronic liver disease) • Drug induced (chemotherapy, retinoids) • HIV infection • Discoid lupus erythematosus • Radiotherapy • Postpartum

results from a breakdown in immune privilege with the subsequent assault on the follicle by CD8+ T-lymphocytes.
- Genetic factors are often present with HLA-DQ3, a susceptibility allele.

CLINICAL FEATURES

- Rapid and complete loss of hair in one or more patches which are 1–5 cm in size.
- The skin within the patches is inconspicuous, and hair follicles are intact.
- Towards the periphery of the area of active hair loss, one can usually note characteristic, smaller 3 to 4-mm exclamation mark hairs and/or black dots (Fig. 4.26). They represent dystrophic hairs that have fractured tips due to an inhibition of cell division in the hair matrix at the level of the hair bulb. Severe inhibition leads to fracturing of the hair shaft before emergence from the scalp and then appears as a black dot. This exclamation mark appearance describes a damaged strand of hair that is thicker at its distal end and notably thinner proximally as it enters the scalp. These are pathognomonic of alopecia areata.
- Nail involvement may occur in the form of nail pitting (Fig. 4.27) with nail plate appearing rough, lustreless.
- *Alopecia totalis* is a more advanced form of alopecia areata in which there is total loss of hair on the scalp.
- *Alopecia universalis* is the most advanced form of alopecia areata in which there is total loss of all hair on the body including eyebrows and eyelashes.
- *Alopecia barbae* is alopecia areata localised to the beard area. It can be a single bald patch or may involve whole of the beard area.
- *Ophiasis* is a form of alopecia areata characterised by the loss of hair in the shape of a wave at the circumference of the head.
- Sisaipho is an extensive hair loss in the central scalp, while the periphery of the scalp is not significantly involved.

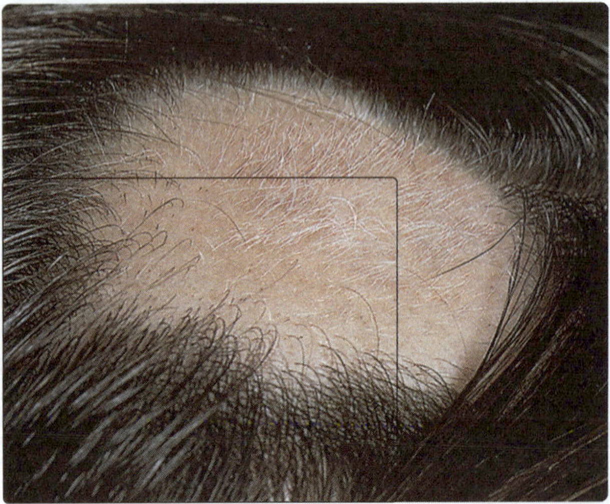

Fig. 4.26 Alopecia areata showing some exclamation mark (!) hair.

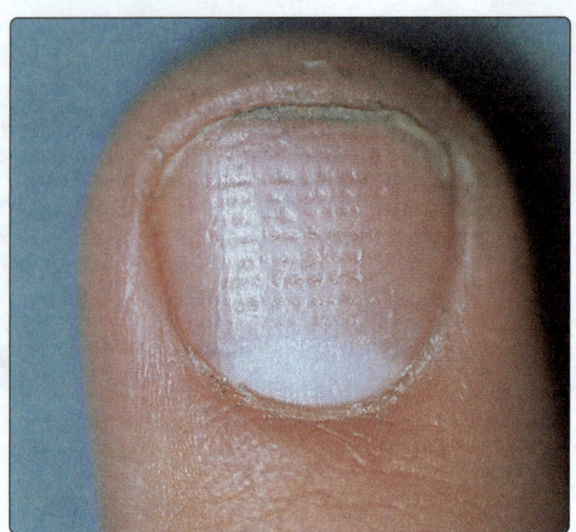

Fig. 4.27 Nail pitting in a patient with alopecia areata.

CLINICAL COURSE

- Spontaneous remission rates are 30%–50% within the first 6–12 months of disease onset, and 66% of the patients will show complete regrowth of hair within 5 years.
- However, relapses occur in as many as 85% of cases.

ASSOCIATED DISEASES

- Several comorbidities have been found to be associated with alopecia areata. These include atopic dermatitis, thyroid disease, lupus erythematosus, vitiligo, psoriasis, inflammatory bowel disease and rheumatoid arthritis.

TREATMENT

- Despite lack of evidence, topical steroids and immunotherapy are being used to treat patients with alopecia areata.
- Single patches of AA are best treated with topical or intralesional corticosteroids.
- Acute and widespread alopecia areata (>30% surface area) are best treated with systemic corticosteroid therapy, either orally or intravenously as pulse therapy.
- Topical immunotherapy with allergic contact sensitisers like squaric acid dibutyl ester (SADBE) and diphenyl cyclopropenone (DPCP).
- Topical anthralin, a contact irritant is also used particularly in children as an alternative to corticosteroids due to its low risks.
- Topical minoxidil acts mainly to promote hair growth, and is therefore used in combination with other treatment modalities.
- Experimental therapies include Janus kinase (JAK) inhibitors (tofacitinib, ruxolitinib), laser therapy and platelet-rich plasma (PRP) therapy.
    - PRP contains and releases through degranulation several growth factors and cytokines. These include platelet-derived growth factor, TGF-beta, fibroblast growth factor, vascular endothelial growth factor, epidermal growth factor and keratinocyte growth factor.

Q. Give a brief account of scabies. (DR5.1, DR5.3)

Q. What is Norwegian or crusted scabies?

- An intensely itchy dermatosis caused by the mite *Sarcoptes scabiei* var. *hominis*.
- Occurs at all ages but particularly in children.

MODE OF TRANSMISSION

- Highly contagious and person-to-person spread occurs via direct contact with the skin. It takes approximately 15–20 minutes for the mite to transfer between people.
- Transfer from clothes and bedding if contaminated by infested people.

PATHOGENESIS

- Infestation occurs when the pregnant female mite burrows into the skin and lays eggs.
- After 2 or 3 days, the larvae emerge and dig new burrows. They mature, mate and repeat this cycle every 2 weeks.
- The main symptoms of scabies are probably a result of the host immune reaction to the burrowed mites and their products.

CLINICAL FEATURES

- Incubation period is 3 weeks. In cases of reinfestation, symptoms develop in 1–3 days.
- Patients with scabies complain of itching, which is most severe at night.
- Other skin manifestations include papules, blisters, nodules and eczematous changes (Fig. 4.28).
- These lesions commonly involve web spaces, flexor surface of wrists, axillae, waist, feet, ankles, lower portions of buttocks and genital areas.
  - In females, itching of the nipples associated with generalised pruritic papular eruption is characteristic.
  - In males, itchy papules on the scrotum and penis are virtually pathognomonic.
  - In infants and young children, scabies often affects face, head, neck, scalp, palms and soles and there is often generalised skin involvement.
- The pathognomonic sign is burrow, the linear tunnel in which the mites live. These occur as short, wavy, scaly, grey lines on the skin surface (Fig. 4.29) and are most easily found on hands and feet, particularly in the finger web spaces, thenar and hypothenar eminences, and on the wrists. They are often missed if the skin has been scratched, has become secondarily infected or if eczema is present.
- Secondary infection can occur with *Staphylococcus*, *Streptococcus* or both.

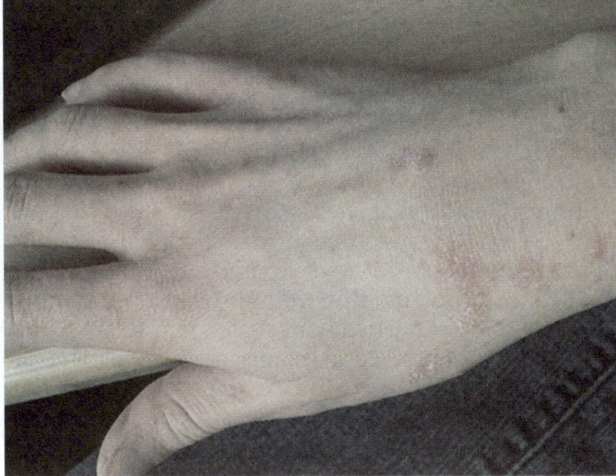

Fig. 4.28 Papular lesions of scabies.

CRUSTED OR NORWEGIAN SCABIES

- Crusted scabies, also known as Norwegian scabies (because of its initial description in Norwegian patients with leprosy), occurs in patients with neurological disorders or immunosuppression including HIV.
- The number of mites escalate rapidly due to impaired immune response, lack of pruritus or patient's physical inability to scratch.
- Presents with marked thickening and crusting of the skin, particularly on the hands, although the entire body including the face and scalp is often involved (Fig. 4.30).
- Nails often show hyperkeratosis.

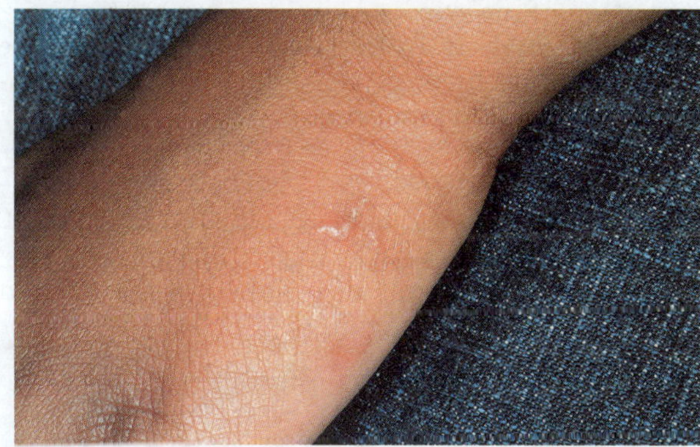

Fig. 4.29 Curvilinear burrow on the lateral part of hand in a patient with scabies.

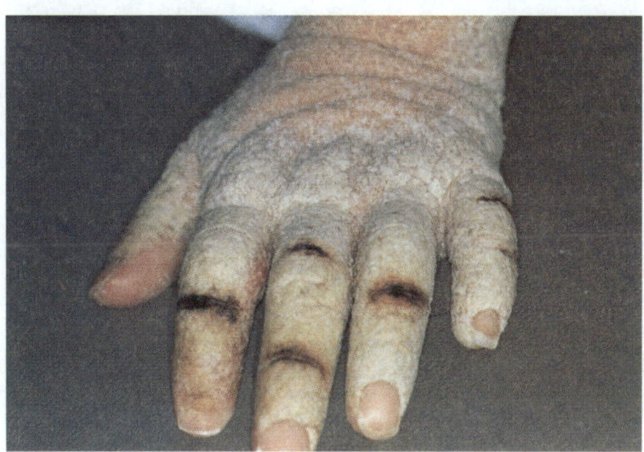

Fig. 4.30 Norwegian scabies.

- Transmission via fomites is possible as mites survive on the sloughed skin in the environment.

DIAGNOSIS

- Scabies is usually diagnosed on history and examination.
- Definitive diagnosis relies on microscopic identification of mites or eggs from skin scrapings of a burrow.
- Burrow ink test: Papules are marked with ink and wiped off with an alcohol swab to remove ink from the surface of lesion. Positive burrow ink test is when a dark, zigzagged line can be seen with the naked eye after wiping with alcohol. This occurs due to tracking down of ink into the burrow.
- Other noninvasive tests include videodermoscopy, dermoscopy, reflectance confocal microscopy and optical coherence tomography. These tests are rapid, useful for mass screening and posttherapeutic follow-up, with no physical risk.
- The diagnostic criteria as per International Alliance for the Control of Scabies is given in Table 4.9.

COMPLICATIONS

- Secondary bacterial infection including impetigo, cellulitis, furunculosis, ecthyma, lymphangitis and sepsis primarily by *S. aureus* or *Streptococcus pyogenes*. Poststreptococcal glomerulonephritis, scarlet fever and acute rheumatic fever may follow streptococcal infection of the skin.
- Pruritus may lead to sleep disturbance/somnolence with resulting tiredness, reduced ability to concentrate and reduced productivity.

TREATMENT

- Oral antihistamines can be used to alleviate pruritus.
- It is important to treat all members of the affected household at the same time.

TABLE 4.9 2020 International Alliance for the Control of Scabies Criteria for the Diagnosis of Scabies

A. Confirmed scabies	At least one of: • Mites, eggs or faeces on light microscopy of skin samples • Mites, eggs or faeces visualised on an individual using a high-powered imaging device • Mite visualised on an individual using dermoscopy
B. Clinical scabies	At least one of: • Scabies burrows • Typical lesions affecting male genitalia • Typical lesions in a typical distribution and two history features
C. Suspected scabies	One of: • Typical lesions in a typical distribution and one history feature • Atypical lesions or atypical distribution and two history features
History features: • Itch • Positive contact history	

- All clothes and bed linen should be washed at temperatures above 50°C. Items that cannot be laundered may be kept in a sealed plastic bag for at least 48–72 hours or in a freezer at −20°C for 72 hours.

TOPICAL TREATMENT

Sulphur

- It is the oldest antiscabietic that is used as an ointment (2%–10%).
- After a bath, sulphur ointment is applied and thoroughly rubbed into the skin over the whole body for three consecutive nights.
- Topical sulphur ointment is messy and malodorous, stains clothing and may lead to irritant dermatitis in hot and humid climate.
- It has the advantage of being cheap. It is also a safe alternative for the treatment of scabies in infants, children and pregnant females.

Benzyl Benzoate

- Benzyl benzoate is used as a 25% emulsion and the contact period is 24 hours.
- It should be applied below the neck three times within 24 hours without an intervening bath.
- It can also cause irritant dermatitis on the face and scrotum.
- It should be avoided in children younger than 2 years. Although no adverse effects have been noted during pregnancy, it should be used if sulphur or permethrin is not available.

Crotamiton

- Crotamiton is used as 10% cream or lotion.
- It is applied twice daily for 5 consecutive days after bathing and changing clothes.
- The success rate varies between 50% and 70%.
- It has some antipruritic effects.
- Uncommon adverse effect includes methaemoglobinaemia.

Malathion

- Malathion is an organophosphate insecticide that irreversibly blocks the enzyme acetylcholinesterase.
- It is rarely used because of the potential for severe adverse effects.

Lindane

- Lindane, also known as gamma benzene hexachloride, acts on the central nervous system of insects and leads to increased excitability, convulsions and death.
- A single 6-hour application of 1% cream is effective in treatment of scabies.
- It can rarely cause CNS toxicity, convulsions and death. To reduce its adverse effects, it should be applied on a cool, dry skin for only 6 hours after which whole body is washed with soap and water.
- It should not be used in infants, pregnant patients or if the skin is inflamed and excoriated.

Permethrin

- Permethrin is a synthetic pyrethroid and potent insecticide.

- Permethrin 5% dermal creams are applied overnight once a week for 2 weeks to the entire body, including the head in infants. The contact period is about 8 hours.
- It can be safely used in children older than 2 months and is considered as a treatment of choice. However, it is the most expensive of all the topical scabicides.

ORAL THERAPY

Ivermectin

- Ivermectin is an effective scabicide. It suppresses conduction of nerve impulses in the nerve–muscle synapses of insects by stimulation of gamma-aminobutyric acid from presynaptic nerve endings and enhancement of binding to postsynaptic receptors.
- Two doses of ivermectin (200 μg/kg body weight 2 weeks apart) are effective.
- The toxic effect of iverme-ctin after a single dose for scabies appears to be insignificant. It is relatively safe after a single dose with side effects such as headache, pruritus, pains in the joints and muscles, fever, maculopapular rash and lymphadenopathy rarely reported.
- It is contraindicated in patients with an allergy to ivermectin and CNS disorders. It is also not indicated during pregnancy, lactation and in children younger than 5 years.

SUMMARY OF TREATMENT OF SCABIES

- Flowchart 4.1 summarises treatment of a patient with scabies.

Q. Write a short note on pediculosis. (DR6.1)

- Caused by lice infestation.
- Common in school children, homeless people and refugees.

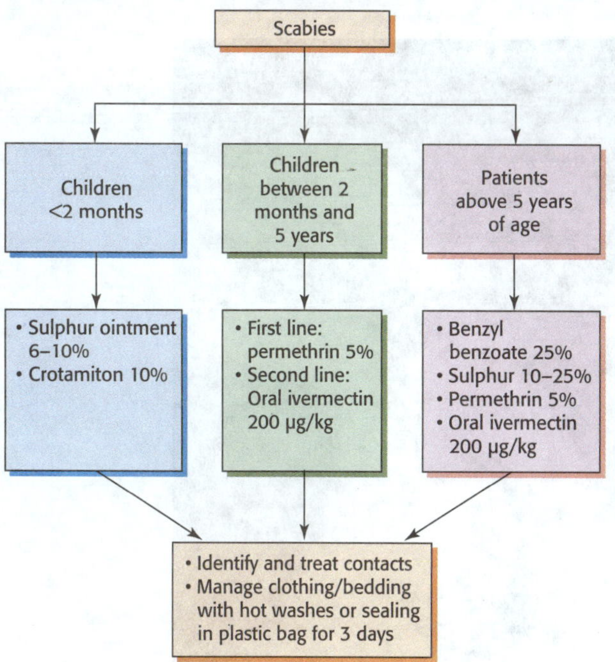

Flowchart 4.1 Summary of Treatment of Scabies.

- Diagnosis by clinical inspection for nits (eggs; look like whitish shells; found attached to the base of hair strands near the scalp), nymphs (young lice) and adult parasites; combing can help in this regard.

HEAD LOUSE (PEDICULUS HUMANUS CAPITIS)

- Transmission occurs person-to-person and indirectly through hats, clothes or pillow covers.
- Presents with rash and pruritus.
- Persistent infection is often associated with secondary infection of the scalp and is an important cause of impetigo.
- Because of pruritus and subsequent sleep disturbances and difficulties in concentration, infested children may perform poorly in school.
- Wood's light and dermoscopy can be used to aid diagnosis.

BODY LOUSE (PEDICULUS HUMANUS CORPORIS)

- Transmission occurs person-to-person through infested clothes.
- A vector for epidemic typhus, relapsing fever and trench fever.
- By stinging the skin, the louse causes pruritus, leading to erythematous macules, papules, scabs and abrasions, mainly seen on the trunk, armpits and buttocks. Secondary infection, hyperpigmentation and lichenification may occur.

PUBIC LOUSE (PTHIRUS PUBIS)

- Infests pubic hair and occasionally other hairy areas, such as eyelashes.
- Usually transmitted during sexual intercourse.
- Treatment must therefore include the patient's partner.

TREATMENT

- Physical removal by wet combing (every 1–3 days for at least 2 weeks) is suboptimal.
- Topical occlusive agents include synthetic compounds (e.g. silicone oils) and natural oils (e.g. coconut oil). They are believed to either coat and block the excretory system of the lice, causing osmotic stress which results in the rupture of internal organs or prolonged immobilisation, or cause suffocation or respiratory asphyxiation of the lice and eventual death. Topical occlusive agents require two to three applications since they have little ovicidal activity.
- Topical application of neurotoxic agents like lindane, malathion (0.5%), permethrin (shampoo 1% or cream 5%), benzyl alcohol and spinosad. Oral ivermectin is also effective. Available treatments destroy lice, but do not reliably destroy eggs. Repeat treatment for 7–10 days later is required for complete eradication.
- For body lice, use of a pediculicide is not required because improvements in hygiene, including showering and laundering clothing in hot water, often eradicate the infestation.
- Treatment of secondary bacterial infection.

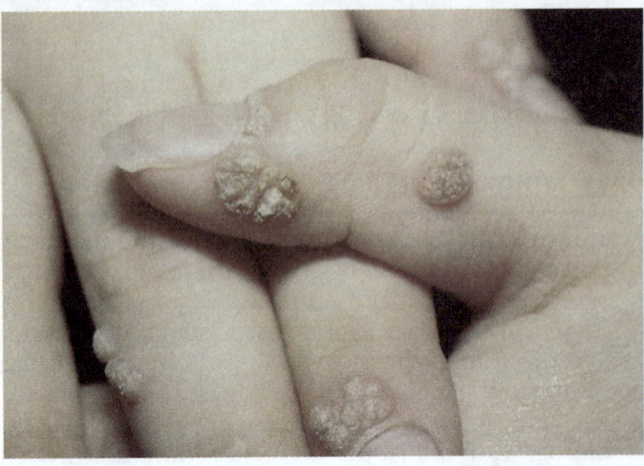

Fig. 4.31 Common warts.

Q. What are warts? Discuss their treatment. (DR8.4)

- Warts are the cutaneous manifestations of human papillomavirus (HPV) infection.
- Approximately two-thirds of lesions resolve spontaneously within 2 years without treatment.
- Warts may exist in different forms:
  - Common warts (*verruca vulgaris*) appear as firm, irregular, verrucous surfaced papules that vary in size, shape and number (Fig. 4.31). These are distributed anywhere on the body and are asymptomatic.
  - Plantar warts (*verruca plantaris*) occur on the plantar aspects and are painful keratotic plaques with a central depressed area.
  - Flat or planar warts (*verruca plana*) are smooth, skin-coloured and flat-topped papules that are more frequently seen on the face or hands of children.
  - Warts located in anogenital region are due to sexual transmission of virus and are known as venereal or genital warts. They are caused by multiple strains of HPV. They can vary from flesh coloured to white, pink or brown. The locations involved in women can be the cervix, vagina, vulva, urethral meatus and perianal region. In men, the scrotum, penis shaft, corona and under the foreskin, and perianal region can be involved (Figs. 4.32A and B).
  - *Condyloma acuminata* is a type of venereal wart that shows vegetative or cauliflower-like growth.

TREATMENT

- Indications for treatment include pain, discomfort, recurrent bleeding and cosmesis. Early treatment is also important to prevent spread to close contacts.
- No single therapy has been proven effective at achieving complete remission in every patient.
- These can be destroyed by local application of salicylic acid (10%–20%) or imiquimod (5% cream), cryotherapy with liquid nitrogen (at −196 °C), chemical cauterisation (50%–100% trichloroacetic acid or phenol), electric cauterisation or surgical removal.
- Using cryotherapy with liquid nitrogen, warts are frozen until a 1 to 2 mm ice halo forms around the target area. This may take 10–30 seconds of application. The most common side effects of cryotherapy are pain and blistering.
- Salicylic acid (10%–20%), a keratolytic agent, is a useful topical agent for cutaneous warts. The recommended use is once to twice daily. Overnight occlusion with a tape after application is recommended.
- Sinecatechins are derived from green tea leaves of the *Camellia sinensis* species containing the active ingredient epigallocatechin gallate (EGCG). It is available as 10% cream and 15% ointment and can

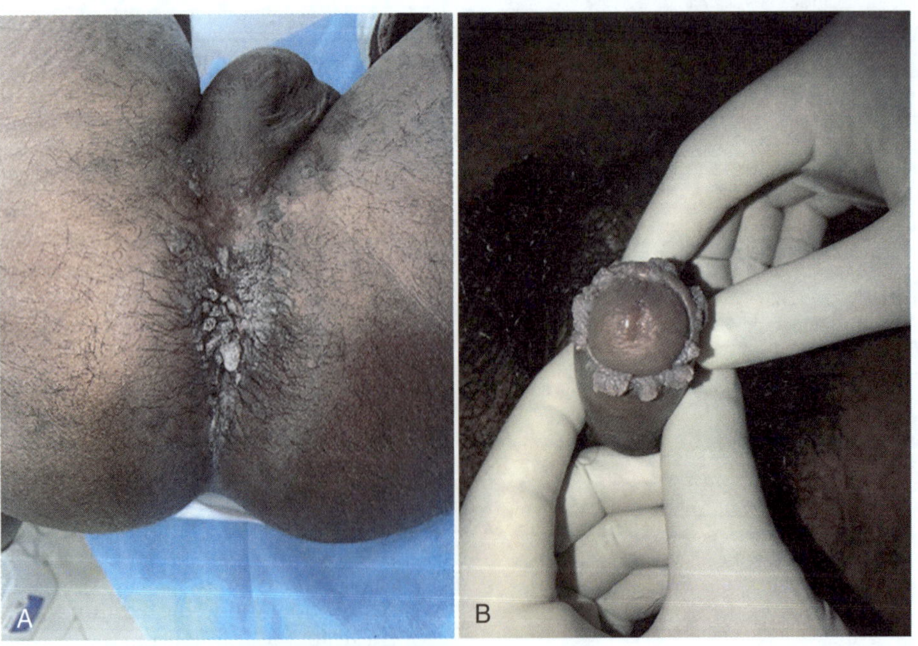

Fig. 4.32 (A and B) Genital warts.

be applied by the patient for treatment of external genital warts and perianal warts.
- Podophyllin resin 25% (active ingredient podophyllotoxin) in alcohol is effective in condyloma acuminata.
- Bleomycin injection into the wart may be used as a second-line agent if others fail.
- Systemic retinoids have the ability to alter keratinisation and accelerate clearing of warts by inducing an irritant dermatitis.

IMMUNOTHERAPY

- Topically applied immunotherapy includes diphenylcyclopropenone (DPCP) and squaric acid dibutylester (SADBE).
- Intralesional immunotherapy includes candida antigen, MMR (measles, mumps, rubella) vaccine, tuberculin purified protein derivative (PPD) and BCG vaccine.
- These treatments are thought to stimulate the cellular immune system to increase clearance of HPV.

Q. Discuss the aetiology, clinical features, diagnosis and treatment of pemphigus vulgaris.

Q. What is Nikolsky's sign?

- Pemphigus vulgaris (PV) is a chronic vesicular and erosive disease characterised by intraepithelial blister formation. It may lead to systemic features due to fluid exudation or infection.
- PV affects both sexes equally.
- The disease is most prevalent between the fourth and sixth decades of life.
- Most patients with PV express HLA-DRB1*04:02 or HLA-DQB1*05:03.

AETIOLOGY

- While the precise aetiology of PV is not clear, it is known to involve an autoimmune mechanism with IgG antibodies that alter the epithelial intercellular junctions. These antibodies target desmoglein 3, and later desmoglein 1. Desmogleins belong to a subfamily of cellular adhesion molecules found within desmosomes which are cell–cell adhesion structures that connect neighbouring keratinocytes. Patients with pemphigus foliaceus have only antidesmoglein 1 antibodies.
- Most patients with PV express HLA-DRB1*04:02 or HLA-DQB1*05:03 indicating role of genetic factors in aetiopathogenesis.
- Pemphigus can also be drug induced. Some known PV-inducing agents are sulphonamides, penicillins, antiepileptic drugs, penicillamine, captopril. Other factors include exposure to pesticides, metal vapour, ultraviolet light and ionising radiation.

CLINICAL FEATURES

- In most cases (75%), oral lesions are the first manifestation of the disease. In pemphigus foliaceus, mucous membranes are generally spared as desmoglein 1 is expressed only in skin and not in mucous membranes.

ORAL CAVITY

- The lesions at first comprise small asymptomatic blisters that are very thin walled and easily rupture giving rise to painful and haemorrhagic erosions.
- While the lesions can be located anywhere within the oral cavity, they are most often found in areas subjected to friction trauma, such as cheek mucosa, tongue, palate and lower lip.
- The lesions within the mouth may persist for a number of months before progressing to the skin and other mucosal membranes (nose, pharynx, larynx, oesophagus, vulva, penis or anus).

SKIN LESIONS

- The primary lesion of PV is a flaccid blister filled with clear fluid that arises on normal skin or on an erythematous base.
- The blisters are fragile; therefore, intact blisters may be sparse (Fig. 4.33).
- The contents soon become turbid or the blisters rupture producing painful erosions which is the most common skin presentation.
- Erosions are often large because of their tendency to extend peripherally with the shedding of the epithelium (Fig. 4.34).
- Nikolsky's sign is positive—apply pressure to the blister or rub sideways the perilesional skin or normal skin with a cotton swab or finger; a positive response is indicated by extension of the blister (direct Nikolsky's sign) and/or removal of epidermis in the area immediately surrounding the blister or normal skin (indirect Nikolsky's sign). It is also positive in patients with TEN, staphylococcal scalded skin syndrome, bullous impetigo and epidermolysis bullosa. This sign is usually negative in bullous pemphigoid.
- Skin lesions heal without scarring.

DIAGNOSIS

- Confirmation is provided by the histological biopsy study that shows the presence of intraepithelial blisters, acantholysis and acantholytic cells (Tzanck cells). Tzanck cells can also be demonstrated in a smear taken from the base of a blister or oral erosion. These are rounded epidermal cells with large dense nuclei,

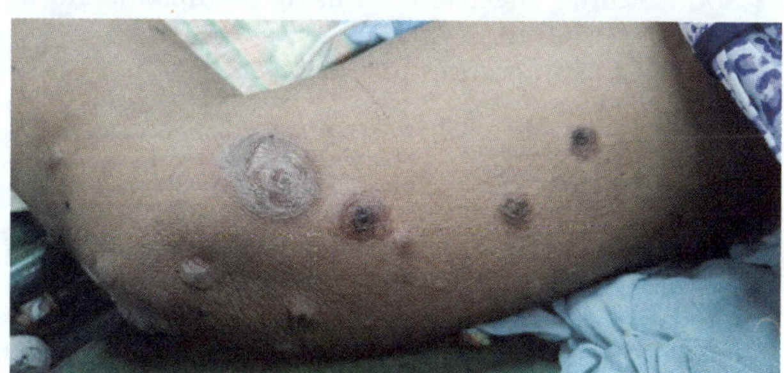

Fig. 4.33 Pemphigus vulgaris.

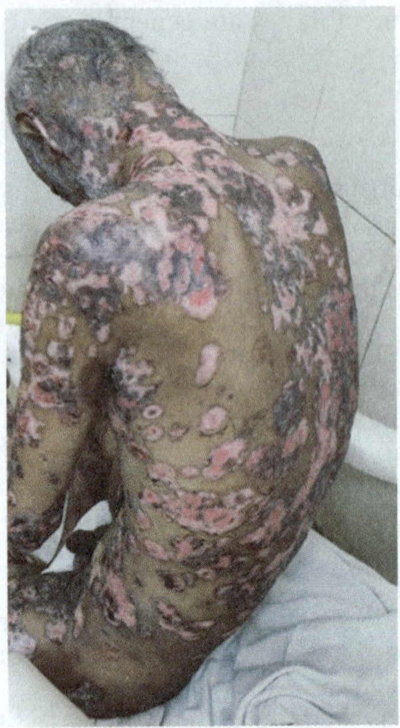

Fig. 4.34 A patient with extensive pemphigus vulgaris.

hazy or absent nucleoli, and abundant basophilic cytoplasm. Tzanck cells are also seen in chickenpox and herpes zoster vesicles. In pemphigus foliaceus, blisters occur in the superficial layers of the epidermis.
- Direct immunofluorescence evaluation of fresh lesion specimens reveals IgG (or occasionally IgA) and complement fragments in the intercellular space.

TREATMENT

- Fluid and electrolyte balance, and nutritional support may be required.
- Anaesthetic mouth lozenges may reduce the pain of mild to moderate mouth ulcers.
- Antibiotics may be required to control infections.
- To inhibit production of the aggressor antibodies, moderate doses of corticosteroids via oral or intravenous route are required.
- Immunosuppressors such as azathioprine, methotrexate, cyclosporin or mycophenolate mofetil can be used if steroids do not help.
- Rituximab, an anti-CD20 monoclonal antibody, intravenous immunoglobulin and immunoadsorption help in treatment-refractory PV.
- First-line use of rituximab plus short-term prednisone is more effective than using prednisone alone, with fewer adverse events.
- Table 4.10 summarises treatment of PV.

TABLE 4.10 Summary of Treatment of Pemphigus Vulgaris

First-Line Therapy	Adjunctive Therapy	Other Therapy
Corticosteroids alone Corticosteroids + rituximab	Azathioprine Methotrexate Cyclosporin Mycophenolate mofetil	Intravenous immunoglobulin Immunoadsorption

Q. Define bullous pemphigoid or pemphigoid. Briefly outline its aetiology, clinical features, diagnosis and treatment.

- Bullous pemphigoid (BP) or pemphigoid is a chronic, autoimmune, subepidermal and blistering skin disease that uncommonly involves mucous membranes.
- It primarily affects elderly individuals in the fifth to seventh decades of life with an average age of 65 years at onset.

AETIOLOGY

- BP is characterised by the presence of IgG autoantibodies specific for the hemidesmosomal antigens (BP180 and BP230) present in the basement membrane.
- BP may be precipitated by ultraviolet irradiation, X-ray therapy and exposure to some drugs (furosemide, ibuprofen and other nonsteroidal antiinflammatory agents, captopril, penicillamine and antibiotics).
- It may develop shortly after vaccination, particularly in children.
- It is occasionally associated with systemic malignancies.

CLINICAL FEATURES

- The patient often presents with generalised bullous lesions on erythematous or urticarial background.
- Tense bullae arise on any part of the skin surface with a predilection on the flexural areas of the skin. Face and neck are generally unaffected. The bullous lesions usually have clear fluid but may also contain haemorrhagic fluid (Fig. 4.35).
- Severe pruritus is present in most cases.
- Oral and ocular mucosa involvement occurs uncommonly, and when seen, it is of minor clinical significance. Nasopharyngeal mucosal membranes are almost always unaffected.
- The bullae usually heal without scarring.
- Relapses occur less frequently than PV.
- About 30%–50% of patients have associated neurological diseases including major cognitive impairment,

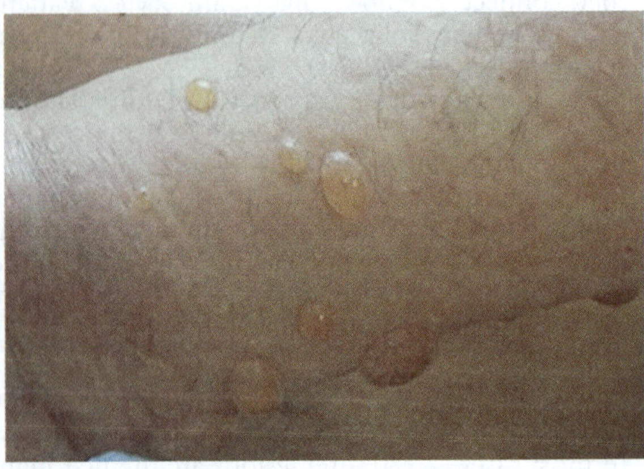

Fig. 4.35 Bullous pemphigoid.

Parkinson's disease, stroke, epilepsy and multiple sclerosis.

DIAGNOSIS

- Direct immunofluorescence studies demonstrate deposits of antibodies and complements in a linear band at the dermal–epidermal junction.
- Indirect immunofluorescence and ELISA show presence of circulating IgG autoantibodies in the serum.

TREATMENT

- The most commonly used medications are antiinflammatory agents (e.g. corticosteroids, tetracyclines and dapsone) and, if required, immunosuppressants (e.g. azathioprine, methotrexate, mycophenolate mofetil and cyclophosphamide). Doxycycline is an alternative to steroids.

Q. Differentiate pemphigus vulgaris from bullous pemphigoid.

- Differentiating features between PV and bullous pemphigoid are shown in Table 4.11.

Q. Discuss briefly about lichen planus. (DR4.1, DR4.2)

- Lichen planus (LP) is a chronic inflammatory disorder that most frequently involves the skin and/or oral mucosa. Compared with cutaneous disease, oral LP tends to be more chronic, with a mean age at onset in the fifth to sixth decades.
- Up to 60% of patients with cutaneous LP have oral disease while only 15% of patients with oral disease develop cutaneous lesions.
- Lesions occur because of a T-cell-mediated reaction directed against epithelial basal cells. This leads to apoptosis of basal keratinocytes.
- Implicated factors include psychological stress, local and systemic inducers of cell-mediated hypersensitivity, and infections.
- Acute exacerbation of oral LP has been linked to psychological stress.
- Lesions on skin are violaceous papules, sometimes polygonal, and often covered by a network of fine white lines (Wickham striae) (Fig. 4.36). These lesions appear mainly on the flexural aspect of the wrists and ankles and in the lumbar region. Genitalia may also be involved. The lesions are characteristically pruritic. These generally remit in 1 to 2 years. Koebner's phenomenon is seen. On healing, hyperpigmentation occurs.
- Oral lesions are bilaterally symmetrical and involve buccal mucosa, gingiva and tongue. These may present as reticular (white striations or Wickham striae), ulcerative or papular, plaque and bullous lesions (Fig. 4.37). They are severely painful.

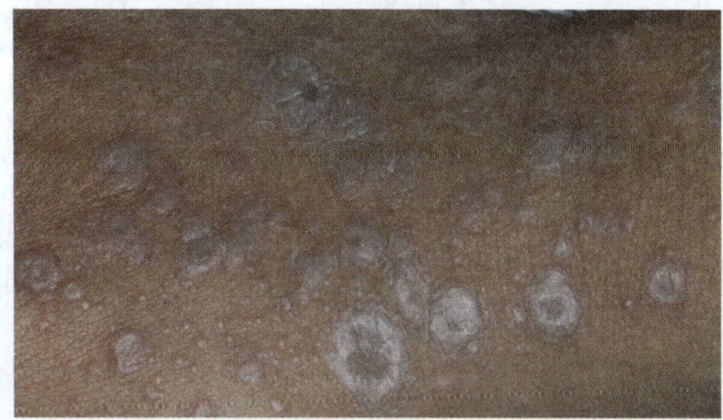

Fig. 4.36 Shiny, flat-topped, polygonal, violaceous papules of lichen planus. Note the Wickham striae (linear, whitish-grey streaks) on the surface.

TABLE 4.11 Pemphigus Vulgaris and Bullous Pemphigoid: Differentiating Features

	Pemphigus Vulgaris	Bullous Pemphigoid
Age group	• 50–60 years most common	• Above 60 years most common
Pathogenesis	• Autoantibodies against desmoglein 3 (present at epithelial intercellular junctions)	• Autoantibodies against hemidesmosome (present in basement membrane of epidermis)
Blister features	• Superficial, intraepidermal • Fragile and rupture easily • Flaccid • Face and neck involvement common • Less itchy • More painful • Nikolsky's sign present	• Subepidermal • Do not rupture easily • Tense • Face and neck involvement uncommon • Intensely itchy • Less painful • Nikolsky's sign absent
Mucosal involvement	• Common and often begins in oral mucosa • Nasopharyngeal mucosa often involved	• Not common • Nasopharyngeal mucosal membrane almost never affected
Infection rate	• High	• Low
Associated neurological diseases	• Uncommon	• Associated with neurological diseases in 30%–50% of cases
Histopathology	• Acantholysis and acantholytic cells (Tzanck cells) present	• Acantholysis and acantholytic cells absent
Direct immuno-fluorescence of fresh lesion specimens	• IgG (or occasionally IgA) and complement fragments in the intercellular space of epidermis	• Deposits of antibodies and complements at the dermal–epidermal junction

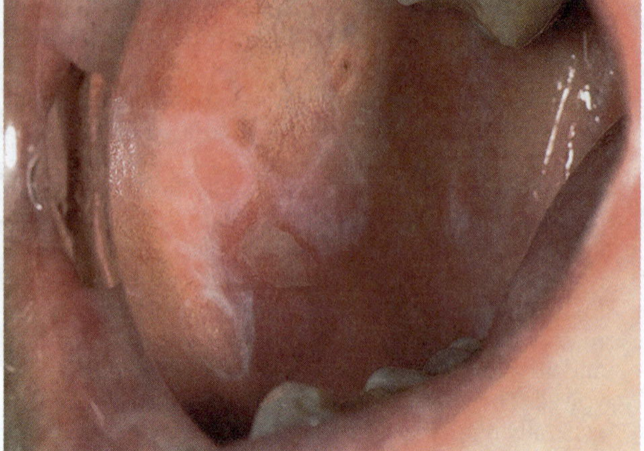

Fig. 4.37 Lichen planus in oral cavity showing reticular lesions.

- Diagnosis is clinical. Histopathological changes include hyperkeratosis, basal cell degeneration and T-lymphocyte infiltration at the dermal–epidermal junction.
- Management of oral lesions is mainly symptom relief. Patients may benefit from elimination of local factors that may trigger or exacerbate symptoms. These factors include sharp or rough teeth or ill-fitting dentures.
- For refractory and symptomatic localised ulcerative lesions, intralesional injections of triamcinolone acetonide can be used. Alternatively, corticosteroids and tacrolimus can be used topically. Topical retinoids (tretinoin or isotretinoin) can also be considered as second-line treatment.
- Oral prednisolone may be considered in case of refractory disease.

Q. Write a short note on DRESS syndrome.

- DRESS (drug reaction with eosinophilia and systemic symptoms) syndrome or drug-induced hypersensitivity reaction (DIHS) is a potentially life-threatening adverse reaction to a number of drugs.
- Characterised by a long latency (2–8 weeks) between drug exposure and disease onset and a prolonged course with frequent relapses despite discontinuation of the culprit drug.

AETIOLOGY

- Common causes include dapsone, allopurinol, phenytoin, carbamazepine, lamotrigine, sulphonamides, phenobarbital, abacavir and nevirapine. Immunosuppression may predispose individuals to develop this condition, especially when accompanied by a primary or reactivation of human herpesvirus, particularly HHV-6, Epstein–Barr virus and cytomegalovirus.

CLINICAL FEATURES

- It presents as morbilliform cutaneous eruption with fever, lymphadenopathy, haematologic abnormalities and multiorgan manifestations (e.g. hepatic, renal, pulmonary, cardiac, neurologic, gastrointestinal and endocrine abnormalities). Fever generally precedes cutaneous eruptions by several days, with temperatures ranging from 38°C to 40°C and may last for several weeks. Skin rash progresses rapidly to a diffuse, confluent and infiltrated erythema. Facial oedema develops in approximately 50% cases. Paradoxical worsening of clinical symptoms may occur 3 to 4 days after withdrawal of the causative drug.
- The liver is the most common extra-cutaneous organ involved. The most commonly observed hepatic abnormality is a transaminitis, but a small subset of patients go on to develop fulminant hepatic failure.
- Myocarditis is a rare but fatal complication.
- Atypical lymphocytosis is common. Leucocytosis occurs in 90% while eosinophilia in 50%.
- A marked decrease in serum immunoglobulin levels is typically observed in the acute phase.
- Patients with DRESS are at risk for systemic autoimmune sequelae, which can appear months after resolution of the cutaneous eruption and acute systemic involvement.

BOX 4.9 Diagnostic Criteria for DRESS

1. Maculopapular rash developing >3 weeks after starting with a limited number of drugs
2. Prolonged clinical symptoms after discontinuation of the causative drug
3. Fever (>38°C)
4. Liver abnormalities (ALT>100 U/L) OR other organ involvement
5. Leucocyte abnormalities (at least one present)
   a. Leucocytosis (>11,000/mm^3)
   b. Atypical lymphocytosis (>5%)
   c. Eosinophilia (>1500/mm^3)
6. Lymphadenopathy
7. HHV-6 reactivation

The diagnosis is confirmed by the presence of the seven criteria above (typical DRESS) or of five of the seven (atypical DRESS).

DIAGNOSIS

- Diagnostic criteria for DRESS are shown in Box 4.9.

DRESS VERSUS SJS/TENS (Table 4.12)

TABLE 4.12 Differentiating Features Between DRESS and SJS/TEN

Feature	DRESS	SJS/TEN
Onset	Delayed (>2 weeks)	Acute (within 1 to 2 weeks)
Rash	Generally, morbilliform with facial oedema	Denuded skin, blisters
Immunoglobulins	Reduced	Normal
Histology	No epidermal change	Severe epidermal injury
Virus activation	Usually present for human herpesvirus	No
Complications	Delayed autoimmune disease	Fluid and electrolyte disturbances, local infection, others

TREATMENT

- Mortality is about 10% and is usually due to fulminant hepatic failure.
- Treatment is discontinuation of the offending drug, supportive and use of corticosteroids.

Q. What are the common dermatophytoses? Briefly describe them. (DR7.1)

Q. What is id reaction?

- Dermatophytosis, also known as ringworm or tinea, is a chronic infection of the skin, hair or nails by dermatophytes (a group of fungi that invade the superficial layer of the epidermis and survive on the keratin of skin, hair and nails). Species of *Trichophyton*, *Microsporum* and *Epidermophyton* are called dermatophytes.

TYPES

- Dermatophytosis of the glabrous skin is called tinea corporis. The lesions are circinate (hence the term 'ringworm'), and erythematous pruritic papules that enlarge to form a ring. The borders are irregular, raised and active. The centre is relatively normal (Fig. 4.38).
- In tinea cruris, the lesions start at the apex of the groin and extend to the inner aspect of the thighs, genitalia, perineum or gluteal regions (Fig. 4.39).
- Dermatophytosis of the foot is called tinea pedis (athlete's foot). This may present as fissuring of the toe webs (Fig. 4.40), scaling of the plantar surfaces or vesicles around the toe webs and soles.
- Scalp dermatophytosis is known as tinea capitis. This commonly presents as circular areas of alopecia and scaling. The 'kerion' type is characterised by intense inflammatory reaction. In the so-called 'endothrix infection', the hair shaft breaks off at the skin surface, leaving the hairs visible as black dots on the scalp.
- Dermatophytosis of the bearded area is known as tinea barbae.
- Tinea unguium (onychomycosis) presents as white or yellow, discoloured nails, or thickened and chalky crumbling nails. Subungual hyperkeratosis may be present (Fig. 4.41). Risk factors for developing onychomycosis (fungi causing nail involvement) include atopy, diabetes mellitus, immunosuppression,

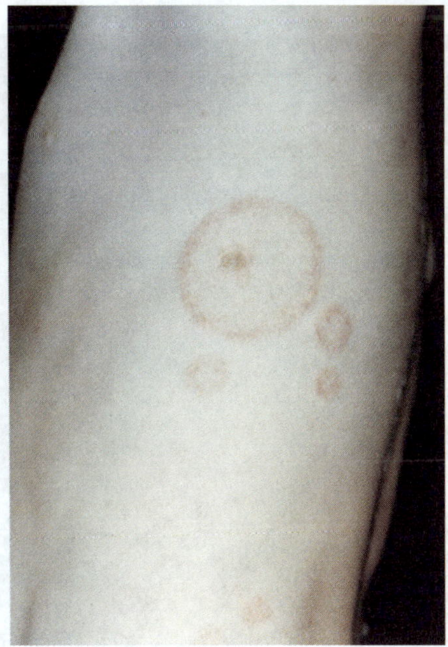

Fig. 4.38 Tinea corporis.

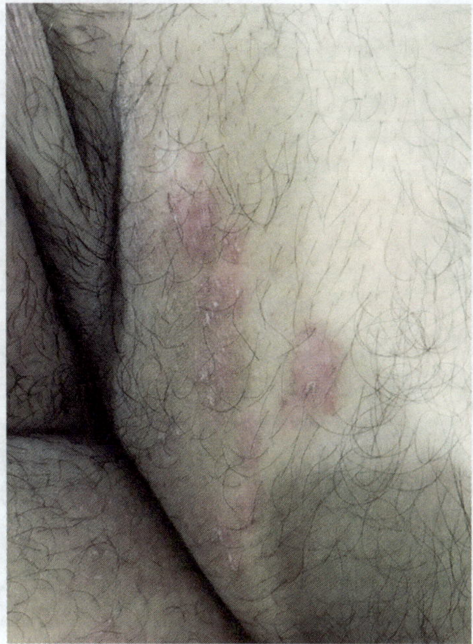

Fig. 4.39 Tinea cruris.

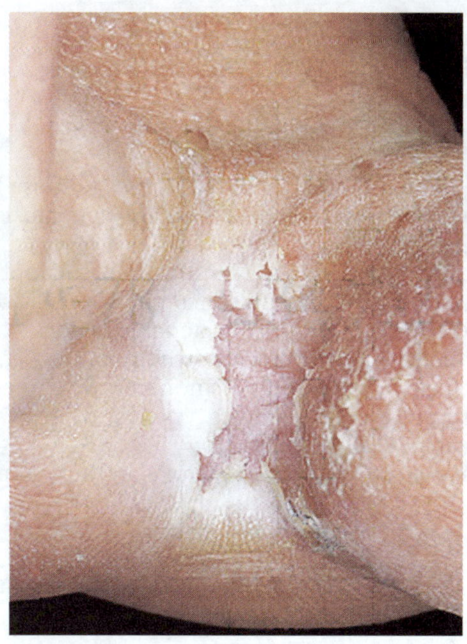

Fig. 4.40 Tinea pedis.

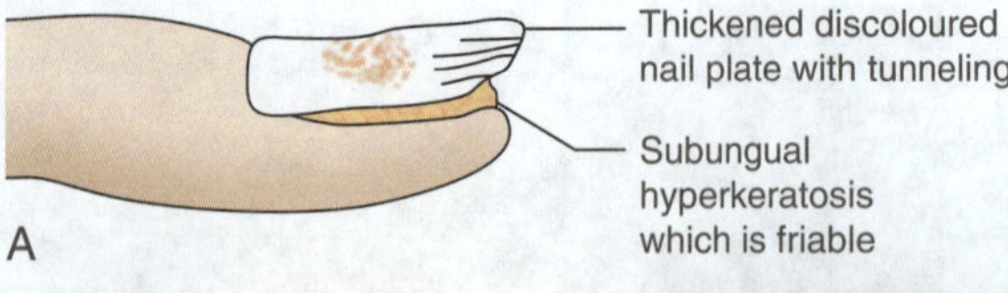

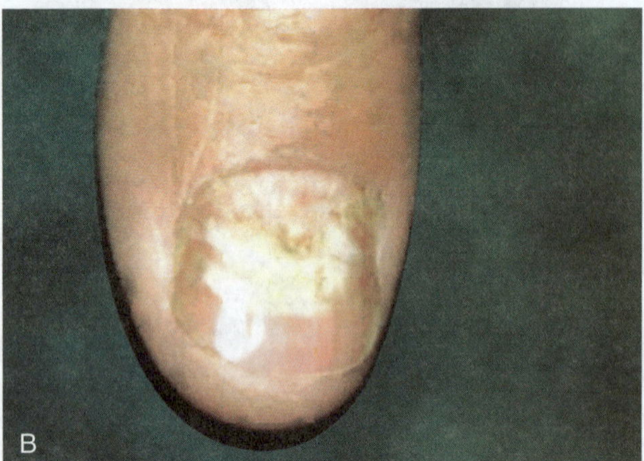

Fig. 4.41 Tinea unguium.

peripheral vascular insufficiency, occlusive footwear and nail trauma.

ID REACTION

- The dermatophytid or id reaction is a diffuse hypersensitivity response to a primary dermatosis elsewhere on the body.
- Frequently occurs in the setting of a dermatophytosis but may also occur with concomitant allergic contact dermatitis or superficial bacterial infection.
- Hallmark features include itching and generalised, symmetric distribution of monomorphic juicy papules (and even, sometimes, vesicles), which can last several weeks or longer.
- Treatment includes topical steroids and antihistamines.

DIAGNOSIS

- Based on history and characteristic cutaneous findings.
- Confirmed by potassium hydroxide (KOH) microscopy, fungal culture and skin or nail biopsy.
- Wood's lamp examination useful in confirming a hair infection with zoophilic dermatophytes (e.g. *Microsporum*) that produce blue-green fluorescence.
- Polymerase chain reaction (PCR) a highly specific, sensitive and accurate diagnostic tool.

TREATMENT

- Topical therapy is effective in mild or moderately severe lesions. Seldom effective in tinea unguium and tinea capitis.
- For tinea capitis and barbae, ketoconazole cream or shampoo can be used as an adjunct. Systemic therapy is often required.
- For tinea corporis, cruris and pedis, topical therapy using clotrimazole, ketoconazole or miconazole applied twice a day for 4 weeks.
- For distal tinea unguium, amorolfine 5%, tioconazole 28% or ciclopirox olamine 8% may be tried.
- More severe and unresponsive lesions are treated with griseofulvin 500–1000 mg daily, fluconazole 400 mg daily, itraconazole 200 mg daily or terbinafine 250 mg daily. The period of treatment is 6–12 weeks. Fluconazole can also be given in a dose of 150–300 mg once a week for 6–12 months.

Q. Write a short note on tinea versicolor or pityriasis versicolor.

- Tinea versicolor is caused by a nondermatophyte fungus, *Malassezia furfur* (also known as *Pityrosporum ovale*), which is a normal inhabitant of the skin. Infection is promoted by heat and humidity.
- The typical lesions consist of oval scaly macules, papules and patches concentrated on the chest, shoulders and back and rarely on the face. On dark skin, they appear as hypopigmented areas (Fig. 4.43), while on light skin they are slightly hyperpigmented. The pink and brown tonality is more frequent in covered areas while in exposed areas, the most frequent are whitish lesions.
- Underlying diseases include Cushing's syndrome, hyperhidrosis and altered immune status such as HIV.
- A KOH preparation from scaling lesions will demonstrate characteristic short, cigar-butt hyphae, and spores in clusters resembling spaghetti and meatballs.
- Wood's lamp shows some pigment still evident in areas of tinea versicolor; in vitiligo, there is a total loss of pigment in the affected areas.

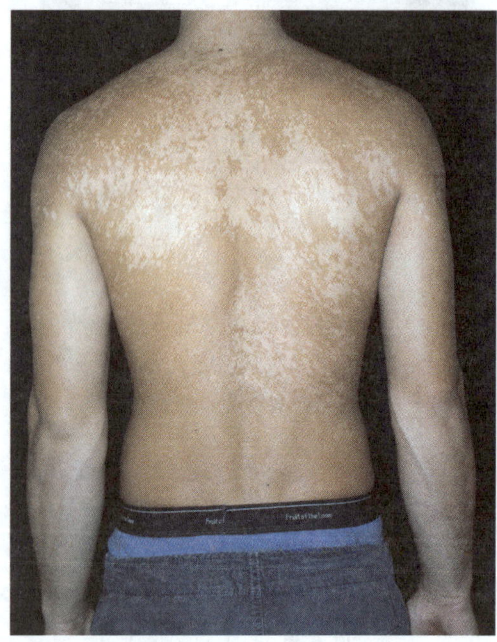

Fig. 4.42 Tinea versicolor.

- Treatment includes topical application of solutions containing sulphur and salicylic acid, or selenium sulphide, or propylene glycol or zinc pyrithione or imidazoles (miconazole, clotrimazole and ketoconazole) or triazoles (fluconazole and itraconazole):
  - Selenium sulphide lotion is liberally applied to affected areas of the skin for 2 weeks; each application is allowed to remain on the skin for at least 10 minutes prior to being washed off. In resistant cases, overnight application can be helpful.
  - Topical imidazole or triazole antifungals can be applied every night for 2 weeks.
- Oral therapy is also effective for tinea versicolor and is often preferred by patients because it is more convenient and less time consuming. Ketoconazole (200 mg daily for 10 days), fluconazole (300 mg stat and repeat after 2 weeks, or 150–300 mg weekly for 2–4 weeks) and itraconazole (200 mg daily for 7 days or 400 mg once only) are the preferred oral agents.

Q. Describe acanthosis nigricans.

- Presents with symmetric, darkened areas of skin that are thickened and described as 'velvety' in texture, and located in areas of creases such as the axillae, neck and groin.
- Other locations include the face, elbows, knees and hands.
- Acanthosis nigricans can be divided into three types:
  - Type I is associated with malignant diseases, particularly adenocarcinoma of stomach and lung; may develop acutely.
  - Type II is familial, inherited as autosomal dominant and is usually apparent at birth or may develop later in childhood.
  - Type III is the most common form and is associated with obesity, insulin-resistant disorders and other endocrine disorders, including diabetes mellitus, Cushing's disease, Addison's disease, pinealoma, and hyperandrogenic and hypogonadal states. Some medications have been linked to the development of acanthosis nigricans including oral contraceptives, insulin, glucocorticoids, nicotinic acid and methyltestosterone.

DIAGNOSIS

- Diagnosis is mostly clinical.
- Occasionally histopathological assessment may be needed. Usual histopathologic findings include epidermal hyperkeratosis and mild acanthosis, and projection of dermal papillae into thinned epidermis causing papillomatosis. No inflammatory infiltrate is usually present in dermis.

TREATMENT

- Treat the underlying disease.
- Reduce weight in obesity-related acanthosis nigricans.
- Some patients may benefit from medications such as metformin, oral isotretinoin, topical retinoic acid, topical salicylic acid, topical calcipotriol (vitamin D analogue) and oral fish oil.

Q. Briefly discuss the common skin malignancies.

SKIN MALIGNANCIES

- Skin malignancies are listed in Table 4.13.

BASAL CELL CARCINOMA

- At least three times more common than squamous cell carcinoma.
- Usually occurs on sun-exposed areas of skin. Sun exposure between 10 a.m. and 4 p.m. is thought to be most harmful.
- Nose is the most frequent site.
- High-risk areas for tumour recurrence include periorbital region, eyelids, nasolabial fold, postauricular region, pinna, ear canal, forehead and scalp.
- Most characteristic presentation is the asymptomatic nodular or nodular-ulcerative lesion that has a pearly quality and contains telangiectatic vessels (Fig. 4.43). Crusting and bleeding in the centre of the tumour frequently develops.
- Has a tendency to be locally destructive.
- Noninvasive approaches for diagnosis include dermoscopy, reflectance confocal microscopy and optical coherence tomography.

TREATMENT

- Basal cell carcinoma rarely metastasises and, thus, a metastatic workup is usually not necessary.
- Options for treatment include Mohs micrographic surgery (using microscopic control to evaluate the extent of tumour invasion before surgical excision),

TABLE 4.13 Various Skin Malignancies

Common	Uncommon
• Basal cell carcinoma (most common form of skin cancer) • Squamous cell carcinoma • Bowen's disease	• Malignant melanoma • Cutaneous T-cell lymphomas (e.g. mycosis fungoides) • Kaposi's sarcoma • Apocrine carcinoma of the skin • Metastatic malignancies

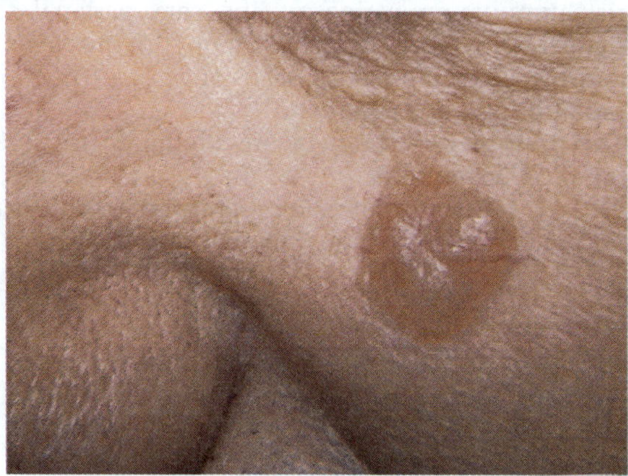

Fig. 4.43 Basal cell carcinoma. From Bolognia, J. L., Schaffer, J. V., & Cerroni, L. (2018). Dermatology (Vol. 1, 4th ed.). Elsevier.

cryosurgery, radiation therapy, electrodesiccation and curettage, and simple excision. These methods have cure rates ranging from 85% to 95%.

- Other options include topical application of imiquimod, 5-fluorouracil, intralesional interferon-α and photodynamic therapy using photosensitisers like aminolevulinic acid and its methylated ester, and methyl aminolevulinate.
- In advanced cases, Hedgehog pathway inhibitors (e.g. vismodegib) may be used.

SQUAMOUS CELL CARCINOMA

- Also tends to occur on sun-exposed portions of the skin such as ears, lower lip and dorsal aspect of hand.
- Chronic sun damage, sites of prior burns, chronic arsenic exposure, chronic cutaneous ulcers and sites of previous radiotherapy predispose to development of squamous cell carcinoma.
- Actinic keratosis, which appears as red scaly patches on areas of chronically sun-exposed skin (face and dorsal aspects of hands), is a potential precursor of squamous cell carcinoma. High-risk population to develop actinic keratosis include the elderly and people receiving immunosuppressive therapy and psoralen plus ultraviolet A therapy, and arsenic exposure. As many as 5% of actinic keratosis will evolve into locally invasive carcinoma.
- Squamous cell carcinomas are also frequently associated with HPV.
- Chronic inflammatory conditions may also result in keratinocyte transformation to squamous cell carcinoma. These conditions include chronic venous ulcers, discoid lupus erythematosus lesions, erosive LP and lymphoedema.
- Presents commonly as a red, scaling, thickened patch on sun-exposed skin. Ulceration and bleeding may occur. If not treated, it may develop into a large mass.
- Squamous cell carcinoma in situ, also known as Bowen's disease, also has invasive malignant potential. These lesions present clinically as pink, well defined, erythematous papules and plaques anywhere on the body including the trunk, eyelids, hands, feet, face and genital area. The lesions may have scale and may bleed.

MANAGEMENT

- In squamous cell carcinoma, regional lymph nodes should be routinely examined particularly for high-risk tumours appearing on lips, ears, perianal and perigenital regions, or if the tumour arises at sites of chronic ulceration, burn scars or sites of previous radiation therapy treatment.
- The options for treatment are similar to those for basal cell carcinoma.
- Anti-PD1 drug cemiplimab is approved for advanced and metastatic squamous cell carcinoma.

MALIGNANT MELANOMA

- Risk factors include sun sensitivity, white skin, fair hair, light eyes, tendency to freckle, family history of melanoma (8–12 times increased risk), dysplastic naevi and immunosuppression.
- Solar ultraviolet exposure is the most important environmental risk factor.

BOX 4.10 Significant Changes in Melanocytic Naevus (Mole) Suggesting Development of Melanoma

- Itching
- Increase in size
- Reduced or increased pigmentation
- Bleeding
- Ulceration
- Change in shape or colour
- Irregularity of surface or margin

- Melanocytic naevi (moles) are also risk factors for the future development of melanoma. Total nevus count more than 100 naevi increases the risk for melanoma sevenfold.
- Nearly 60% present initially as superficially expanding, irregularly pigmented macule or plaque. Some present as nodular growth.
- In a patient with a pigmented lesion, important clinical features suggesting a diagnosis of malignant melanoma are ABCDE:
  - Asymmetrical lesion.
  - Border irregular.
  - Colour irregular.
  - Diameter greater than 6 mm.
  - Elevation irregular.
- Since nearly 30% of melanomas develop in preexisting moles, a change in any naevus should be considered suspicious of malignant transformation (Box 4.10).
- Diagnosis is by full-thickness biopsy including the underlying subcutaneous tissue and 1 to 2 mm clear borders. If lesion is large, incisional or punch biopsies may be performed.

TREATMENT

- For local disease, surgical excision is curative.
- Patients with nonulcerated melanoma <1 mm deep are unlikely to have nodal metastasis and do not require further surgical evaluation of the lymph nodes.
- Sentinel lymph nodal biopsy is important in patients diagnosed with a melanoma with intermediate thickness (1–4 mm) and clinically negative nodes. In this technique, draining lymph node is identified by injecting radioisotope adjacent to the primary tumour. The node is then identified using radioscintigraphy and then removed to look for any histological evidence of metastasis.
- Patients with metastatic tumour in the sentinel lymph node and those who have clinically evident nodal metastasis should undergo lymph node resection with postsurgical adjuvant therapy (interferon-α-2b) as an optional therapy.
- Patients with advanced melanoma may also be offered systemic therapy like interleukin-2, vemurafenib (kinase inhibitor), dacarbazine, temozolomide, paclitaxel and combination therapy. Others include ipilimumab (targets CTAA-4—cytotoxic T-lymphocyte associated protein 4), pembrolizumab and nivolumab (PD-1 inhibitor—programmed cell death protein 1 inhibitor) and atezolizumab (PD-L1 inhibitor—programmed cell death ligand 1 inhibitor). These are all immune checkpoint inhibitors.

5 Diseases of the Nervous System

Q. Discuss the signs of upper motor and lower motor neuron lesions. (IM 18.6)

- Upper motor neurons are corticospinal interneurons which arise from the motor cortex and descend in the spinal cord, mostly in lateral part (lateral corticospinal tract) where they synapse with lower motor neurons.
- Lower motor neurons start from the anterior horn cells where upper motor neurons synapse and go to the effector organs (mainly muscles and glands).
- Table 5.1 mentions differences between upper motor neuron and lower motor neuron lesions.

Q. Describe plantar reflex and extensor plantar reflex.

Q. What are the alternative methods to elicit plantar reflex?

- Plantar reflex is a superficial reflex subserved by S1 segment of the spinal cord. It is a nociceptive reflex.
- Described in detail first by Babinski.
- The afferent fibres travel in the tibial nerve, which is a branch of the sciatic nerve, to relay in the L5 to S1 cord segments. The efferent fibres from the spinal cord travel back in the sciatic nerve which divides into tibial and peroneal nerves. Fibres supplying the toe flexors travel in the tibial nerve, while those supplying the toe extensors travel in the peroneal nerve to reach the foot.
- Method of elicitation:
  - Position of patient—supine with hip and knee extended (an up-going toe response may not occur with knee flexed).
  - Stimulus—mildly nociceptive by gentle but firm pressure with tip of a key.
  - Site—stimulus directed on outer aspect of heel forwards towards the little toe, and on reaching the foot pad, directed transversely across metatarsal pad from the base of the little toe to the base of the great toe. The stimulus should stop short of the base of the great toe.

TABLE 5.1 Upper Motor Neuron Versus Lower Motor Neuron Lesions

Sign	Upper Motor Neuron	Lower Motor Neuron
• Weakness	• Voluntary movements are disturbed; distal predominant	• Paralysis of muscles supplied by that segment or nerve; proximal predominant
• Tone	• Hypertonia (clasp-knife spasticity)	• Hypotonia
• Reflex (tendon)	• Increased, ±clonus	• Decreased or absent
• Reflex (superficial)	• Absent or decreased	• Absent or decreased
• Plantar response	• Extensor	• Flexor or absent
• Muscle atrophy	• Disuse atrophy	• Marked atrophy
• Fasciculations	• Absent	• Often present
• Bilateral movements (eyes, face, jaw, neck)	• Spared	• Affected
• Reaction of degeneration	• Absent	• Present
• Nerve conduction	• Normal	• Abnormal

Note: Hyporeflexia and flaccid (hypotonia) paralysis may occur with acute central lesions (spinal shock), with hyperreflexia and spasticity developing later.

- Normal response is characterised by the following:
  - Flexor—consists of flexion of great toe at metatarsophalangeal joint with adduction of other toes.

ABNORMAL RESPONSES

- Absent—no response is seen.
  - Causes—thick sole, lower motor neuron or first-order sensory neuron lesions.
- Extensor—extension (dorsiflexion) of the great toe with or without fanning of other toes (abduction). This is called Babinski's sign. Fanning of toes without great toe extension is of little significance. The fully developed response is also accompanied by dorsiflexion of ankle and flexion of hip and knee joint and slight abduction of thigh, leading to withdrawal of leg on plantar stimulation.
  - Causes—infants and children up to 1 year of age (physiological, due to immature or unmyelinated corticospinal tracts), during deep sleep, lesions of corticospinal tract above S1 segment, deep coma, under general anaesthesia, alcohol intoxication, hypoglycaemia and postictal stage (when it is pathological).
  - Never use the term 'negative Babinski's sign' for a normal response; flexor plantar response is the appropriate description.
- Withdrawal—in sensitive soles, voluntary withdrawal may occur resulting in difficulties of interpretation.

PHYSIOLOGY

- Plantar response is a spinal reflex. It is a part of spinal flexor reflex and consists of shortening of the limb on exposure to nociceptive stimulus. With maturation of nervous system and mainly due to myelination of corticospinal tract, this response is modified to typical normal response under supraspinal control. With interruption of corticospinal influence, infantile pattern re-emerges.

ALTERNATIVE METHODS TO ELICIT PLANTAR REFLEX

- The method described above is probably the most reliable method for elicitation of plantar reflex; however, at times, it may fail to do so or produce an equivocal response. Other methods can then be used to elicit the response.
  - Chaddock's sign—stimulus is applied along the lateral and dorsal aspect of the foot, below the lateral malleolus.
  - Oppenheim's reflex or sign—firm pressure is applied along the shin (medial part) of the tibia from below the knee up to the ankle with the knuckles of the examiner's index and middle fingers.
  - Gordon's sign—calf muscle is squeezed.
  - Schaefer's sign—Achilles tendon is squeezed.

Q. How will you differentiate rigidity from spasticity?

- Muscle tone is defined as 'the tension in the relaxed muscle' or 'the resistance, felt by the examiner during passive stretching of a joint when the muscles are at rest'.
- Clonus is defined as the regular, repetitive, rhythmic contractions of a muscle subjected to sudden, maintained stretch. Clonus sustained for five or more beats is considered as clinically abnormal.
- Differentiating features between spasticity and rigidity are shown in Table 5.2.

Q. Discuss hemiplegia in an elderly male. Give the differential diagnosis, investigations and treatment.

- Hemiplegia is paralysis of one side of the body (hemiparesis indicates weakness of one side of body).
- Paraparesis indicates weakness of both legs, and quadriparesis is weakness of all four limbs.

TABLE 5.2 Spasticity Versus Rigidity

Feature	Spasticity	Rigidity
Location of lesion	• Pyramidal tract	• Extrapyramidal tract
Character	• Clasp-knife type (initial resistance on extending or flexing muscles of a joint which gives way abruptly to allow easy flexion or extension)	• Lead pipe (uniform resistance on extending or flexing a muscle around a joint) or cogwheel type (passive movement of the limbs elicits ratchet-like start-and-stop movements through the range of motion of a joint)
Muscle tone	• More in antigravity group of muscles than in gravity-assisted group of muscles	• Increased in both antigravity and gravity-assisted muscles
Resistance to movement	• In one direction (flexion or extension)	• In both directions
Deep tendon reflexes	• Exaggerated	• Normal or reduced
Plantar reflex	• Extensor	• Flexor
Abdominal reflex	• Absent	• Normal
Clonus	• Often present	• Absent

CAUSES (Table 5.3)

- The most common cause of hemiplegia in elderly is cerebral infarct. Next common cause is neoplasm, either primary or metastatic. Most common primary tumour is glioblastoma, whereas most common metastasis is from lung.
- Slow-growing tumours and granulomas are relatively more common in younger age group.
- Spinal cord lesions rarely cause hemiplegia. Brown-Sequard lesion of cord can cause hemiplegia.

CLINICAL EVALUATION

- Ask about onset and progression of hemiplegia, any associated symptoms related to cardiovascular or other systems.
  - In thrombotic stroke, onset of hemiplegia often occurs during sleep followed by stepwise worsening over a short period; consciousness is generally preserved.
- Ask about headache, loss of consciousness, memory impairment, affection of sensory impairment and meningeal signs.
- Ask about use of oral antidiabetic drugs, insulin or seizures before onset of hemiplegia.
- Examine for fundus, cranial nerves, motor weakness, sensory impairment, meningeal signs and reflexes. Look for cortical signs such as aphasia, neglect, agnosia or apraxia.
- Based on examination, the lesion can be localised as shown in Table 5.4.

INVESTIGATIONS

- Most useful initial investigation is CT scan. In acute hemiplegia, neuroimaging is required as early diagnosis and treatment are crucial in patients with acute stroke.
- A blood glucose should be done in acute or subacute hemiparesis.
- Others that are useful or may be necessary include the following:
  - Angiogram.
  - Magnetic resonance imaging (MRI) provides a more detailed view of anatomical and pathological changes, as well as enabling noninvasive imaging of intracranial vessels. Diffusion-weighted MR sequences are able to detect ischaemia within 30 minutes of onset.
  - Histopathology of mass lesion.

TABLE 5.3 Causes of Hemiplegia in an Elderly

Onset	Cause
• Acute	
• Stroke	Cerebral infarct (thrombotic, embolic), intracerebral haemorrhage (hypertensive), subarachnoid haemorrhage (SAH) with intracerebral haemorrhage or ischaemia
• Trauma	Epidural haematoma, subdural haematoma, cerebral contusion
• Others	Meningitis, encephalitis, brain abscess, postseizure (Todd's paralysis), cerebral venous thrombosis, hemiplegic migraine (usually in younger patients), bleeding into a brain tumour, drug abuse (cocaine, amphetamine), hypertensive encephalopathy (rare)
• Subacute	Cerebral metastasis, subdural haematoma, rapidly growing malignant neoplasms (malignant glioma), granulomas (tubercular, fungal), pyogenic abscesses (metastatic infection, post-traumatic), multiple sclerosis, hypoglycaemia
• Chronic	Slow-growing neoplasms (lymphoma, glioma), Mill's hemiplegic variant of motor neuron disease

TABLE 5.4 Site of Lesion

Site	Features
• Cortical lesion	Unequal weakness in upper and lower limbs, facial involvement, cortical sensory deficit, focal seizure, other features of involvement of various lobes of brain; visual fields normal (unless occipital lobe is also involved)
• Subcortical lesion	Unequal weakness of upper and lower limbs, sensory loss, visual field defects, absence of seizure and speech disturbances
• Internal capsule lesion	Dense hemiplegia with UMN facial palsy, sparing of speech, absence of seizure
• Thalamic lesion	Hemiparesis, hemianopia, hemisensory deficit, hyperpathia
• Brainstem lesion	Hemiplegia with involvement of ipsilateral cranial nerves (crossed hemiplegia)
• Spinal cord (rare)	Hemiplegia without facial involvement (in hemisection of cord below C4 level), posterior column sensory and motor loss on the side of lesion, pain and temperature loss on the opposite side, lower motor neuron (LMN) type of weakness and hyperaesthesia at the level of involvement

TREATMENT

- Stroke is managed with supportive measures, antioedema measures and care of risk factors unless patient presents early when thrombolytic therapy or endovascular thrombectomy may be considered.
- Intracerebral haemorrhage (ICH) and aneurysmal subarachnoid haemorrhage (SAH) may or may not require surgery.
- Infective conditions will require appropriate antimicrobial therapy with or without surgery (for decompression or histological diagnosis).
- Neoplasms will require surgery for decompression and radiotherapy/chemotherapy, if they are malignant.

Q. Write a short note on apraxia.

DEFINITION

- Disorder of learnt motor act in the absence of weakness, akinesia, incoordination, sensory loss, abnormal tone, movement disorders (e.g. tremors or chorea), intellectual deterioration or failure to comprehend commands.
- It appears as if the person has forgotten to perform a motor act that he/she is expected to do without difficulty.
- Apraxia occurs in frontal and parietal lobe lesions and is seen in a variety of neurological disorders such as dementia, stroke and parkinsonism.

TYPES

- Ideomotor apraxia is the inability to carry out a motor command in the absence of motor weakness, incoordination, sensory loss or aphasia, for example miming the brushing of teeth and lighting a cigarette with a matchstick. The person is able to carry same motor movement automatically (voluntary-automatic dissociation). This is seen with left parietal lobe lesions.
- In dressing apraxia, the person is unable to wear his/her dress. This is seen with right parietal lobe lesions.
- In constructional apraxia, the person is unable to copy simple diagrams or build simple blocks. This is seen with right parietal lobe lesions.
- Ideational apraxia is the inability to create a plan for a specific movement, for example 'pick up this pen and write down your name' or 'mailing a letter'. This is commonly associated with confusion and dementia. Seen with bilateral parietal lesions.

Q. What is agnosia? Give a brief account.

- Failure to recognise objects, persons, sounds, shapes or smells despite intact sensory, visual and auditory pathways.
- Agnosia results from lesions that disconnect and isolate visual, auditory and somatosensory input from higher level processing.

TACTILE AGNOSIA OR ASTEREOGNOSIS

- Inability to recognise known objects, while holding in hands in the presence of intact sensory system and without problems in memory or intellectual decline. It occurs due to lesions of contralateral parietal lobe.

VISUAL AGNOSIA

- Inability to recognise what is seen with eyes in the presence of intact visual pathways. The person can describe the shape, colour and size without naming it. It occurs due to damage in posterior occipital or temporal lobes.

PROSOPAGNOSIA

- A type of visual agnosia with inability to identify familiar faces, sometimes even including their own. Patients can identify facial parts, recognise a face as a face but with no recognition of the person. It occurs due to parieto-occipital lesions.

SIMULTANAGNOSIA

- Inability to perceive more than one object at a time. It occurs due to bilateral lesions of the junction between parietal and occipital lobes.

ALEXIA

- Also known as pure word blindness in which there is impairment in reading words and letters. The patient can copy words and letters and in the act of copying the words or tracing out the letters, will recognise the word or letter. The patient can write to dictation but is unable to read back what has been written.

Q. Describe anosognosia.

- Lack of awareness of the paralysed left limb.
- Although the term anosognosia was initially used to describe only lack of awareness for left hemiplegia, it has now been used to describe the lack of subjective experience for a wide range of neurological and neuropsychological disturbances (e.g. anosognosia for visual loss, anosognosia for aphasia and anosognosia for memory loss).
- Anosognosia with hemiplegia occurs predominantly, though not exclusively, with nondominant (right) parietal lesions.

Q. What are aphasia, dysphasia, dysarthria and aphonia?

Q. What is sensory aphasia? What is Wernicke's aphasia?

Q. What is motor aphasia? What is Broca's aphasia?

- Aphasia is a loss or impairment of verbal communication which occurs as a consequence of dysfunction of dominant hemisphere.
- A mild form of aphasia is termed dysphasia.
- Dysarthria is a motor dysfunction due to disrupted innervation to the face, tongue or soft palate which results in impairment of articulation but intact fluency and comprehension.
- Aphonia is impairment of voice.

CLASSIFICATION OF APHASIA (Flowchart 5.1)

FLUENT APHASIA

- Person is able to produce connected speech; the sentence structure is relatively intact but lacks meaning.
- It is divided into two types: language comprehension impaired (sensory aphasia) and language comprehension relatively intact.

Sensory Aphasia

- Sensory aphasia is fluent aphasia with impaired language comprehension. Sensory aphasia denotes dysfunction in the afferent area, that is failure to comprehend verbal or written messages. Lesions in the dominant posterior perisylvian areas (i.e. parietal and temporal lobes) are responsible. Signs consist of poor comprehension of spoken speech and inability to read, though person is able to hear and see. Patient's spoken speech is fluent, and consists of inappropriate choice of words (paraphasia), and misses substantive elements. Answers given seem to be totally irrelevant, though he/she is verbose. Various types of sensory aphasias are as follows:
  a. Wernicke's aphasia (repetition of words/phrases is defective).
  b. Transcortical sensory aphasia (repetition of words/phrases is preserved; occasionally may repeat the question rather than answering it—echolalia).

Conduction Aphasia

- It is a fluent aphasia with language comprehension relatively intact. The person finds it difficult to repeat phrases.

Anomic Aphasia

- It is a fluent aphasia with language comprehension relatively intact. Repetition of words/phrases is good but word finding is difficult; uses generic filters (e.g. 'things') or circumlocution.

NONFLUENT APHASIA

- In this type of aphasia, speech production is halting and effortful; grammar is impaired. Speech is hesitant and slow with many pauses.
- It is divided into two types: language comprehension relatively intact (motor aphasia) and language comprehension impaired (global aphasia).

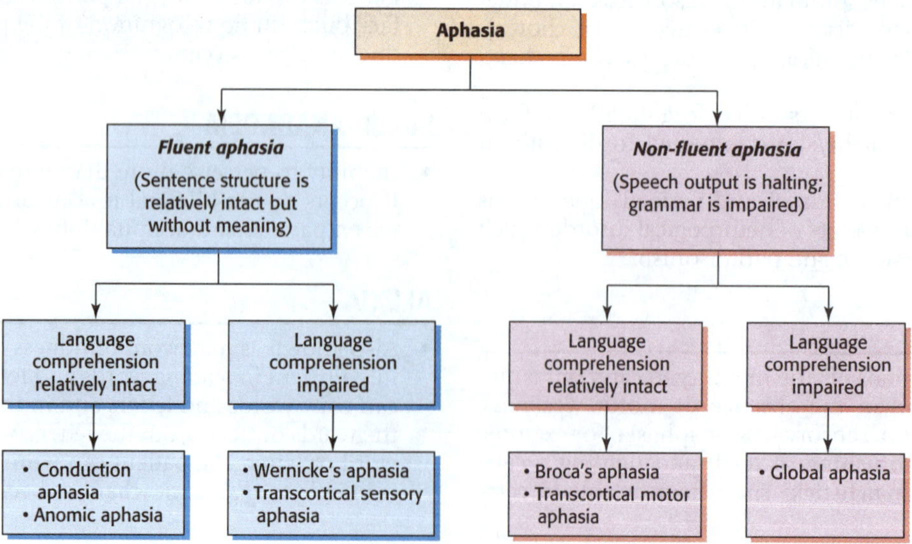

Flowchart 5.1 Classification of Aphasia.

Motor Aphasia

- Motor aphasia is a disorder in the efferent area. Lesions responsible are located in the anterior perisylvian area (e.g. inferior lateral frontal lobe). Comprehension is relatively well preserved. Spoken speech is nonfluent. Word output is reduced, effortful, dysarthric and monosyllabic. There is a loss of normal grammatical structure (agrammatic speech). Patient is able to communicate to some extent as speech is rich in substantive elements, though it lacks the usual melody. Types of motor aphasia are as follows:
  a. Broca's aphasia (repetition of words/phrases is abnormal).
  b. Transcortical motor aphasia (repetition of words/phrases is preserved). Occurs due to damage to the dominant hemisphere outside the speech area.

Global Aphasia

- In it, there is severe expressive and receptive language impairment. Person may be able to communicate using facial expressions, intonation and gestures.

Q. Discuss the normal lobar functions and their abnormalities.

- In most people, the left side is the dominant hemisphere.
- Lobes of brain are shown in Fig. 5.1.

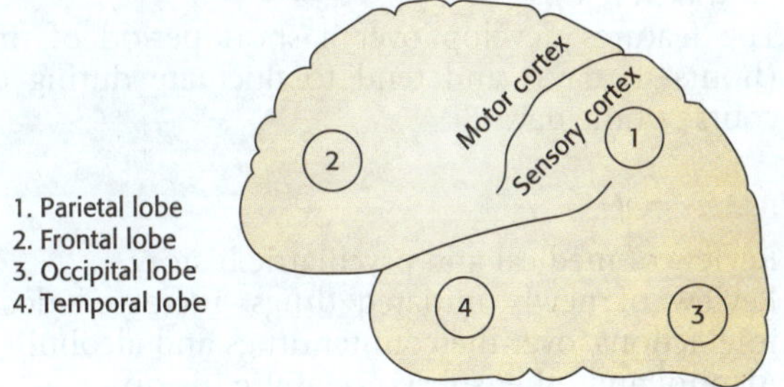

Fig. 5.1 Lobes of the brain.

FEATURES OF LOCALISED CEREBRAL LESIONS (Table 5.5)

- A patient with hemispatial neglect tends to ignore the spatial world on the contralateral side (usually the left side of visual space) as the lesion is in nondominant parietal lobe. For example, they may draw a clock with the numbers 1–12 all on the right side of the circle or they may draw an object, but leave out features on the left side. In severe cases, patients can be unaware that the left side of their body belongs to them.
- A patient with hemispatial extinction does not notice a visual or tactile stimulus on their affected side (usually the left) when simultaneously presented with a similar stimulus on both sides, but they are able to notice it when presented alone.

Q. What is organic brain syndrome?

Q. Discuss briefly about delirium.

- Organic brain syndrome (OBS) is an abnormal mental state with changes in orientation, memory, judgement and affect. It results from diffuse impairment of brain tissue.
- The two most important types of OBS are delirium and dementia.

DELIRIUM

- Delirium, also known as acute confusional state, is characterised by an acute change (usually over hours to days) in mental status along with global cognitive impairment that shows fluctuation over a period of observation.
- Predisposing factors include age >70 years, underlying dementia, functional disabilities, male gender, and poor vision and hearing (Box 5.1).
- Often precipitated by a medical illness, substance intoxication/withdrawal or medication effect (Box 5.2).

TABLE 5.5 Features for Localising Cerebral Lesions

Parietal Lobe			
Dominant Side		**Nondominant Side**	
Function	**Lesions**	**Function**	**Lesions**
Calculation Language Planned movement Appreciation of size, shape, weight, texture Visual	Dyscalculia Dysphasia Dyslexia Apraxia Agnosia Homonymous hemianopia	Spatial orientation Constructional skills Visual	Neglect of contralateral side and hemispatial extinction Spatial disorientation Constructional apraxia Dressing apraxia Homonymous hemianopia
Frontal Lobe		**Occipital Lobe**	
Function	**Lesions**	**Function**	**Lesions**
Personality Emotional response Social behaviour Intelligence Micturition Primitive reflex Smell	Disinhibition Lack of initiative Antisocial behaviour Impaired memory Incontinence Grasp reflexes Anosmia	Analysis of vision	Homonymous hemianopia Visual agnosia Impaired face recognition (prosopagnosia) Visual hallucinations (lights, lines, zig-zags)

Continued

TABLE 5.5 Features for Localising Cerebral Lesions—cont'd

Temporal Lobe			
Dominant side		**Nondominant Side**	
Function	**Lesions**	**Function**	**Lesions**
Auditory perception	Impaired	Auditory perception	Impaired
Speech, language	Sensory aphasia Dyslexia	Music, tone sequences	Loss of musical skills
		Nonverbal memory (faces, shapes, music)	Poor nonverbal memory
Verbal memory	Poor memory		
Olfaction	Complex hallucinations (smell, sound, vision)	Olfaction	Complex hallucinations
Visual	Homonymous hemianopia	Visual	Homonymous hemianopia

BOX 5.1 Common Predisposing Conditions

- Pre-existing cognitive impairment
- Multiple comorbid conditions, including depression
- Polypharmacy
- Impaired sensation (e.g. vision, hearing)
- Impaired functional ability (i.e. diminished activities of daily living)
- History of alcohol misuse and/or malnutrition
- Anaemia

CLINICAL FEATURES

- It is acute in onset and is transient in course with disturbances in attention and memory.
- Deficits in attention are characterised by ease of distractibility with a reduced ability to focus, sustain or shift attention, resulting in difficulty in following commands. Patients may have trouble maintaining conversations, may repeatedly ask same questions or give different replies to same question.
- Memory impairment usually involves recent memory (e.g. forgetting about meals, medicines, visitors).
- Patients may be disoriented to time or place but only rarely to person.
- Perceptual disturbances that may occur include misinterpretations, illusions or hallucinations (often visual hallucinations).
- Agitation (e.g. try to get out of bed repeatedly, wander around in the ward, try to pull out the tubes/catheters repeatedly—hyperactive delirium) or apathy (hypoactive delirium).
- More common is hypoactive form which often goes unrecognised, and is associated with higher rates of complications and mortality.
- Other features:
  - Speech and language disturbances (incoherent or irrelevant speech, pressure of speech, naming things incorrectly or inability to understand what is being said).
  - Sleep disturbance (not able to sleep at night, interrupted sleep, daytime sleepiness, reversal of sleep–wake cycle).
- The features develop over a short period of time (hours to days) and tend to fluctuate during the course of the day.

EVALUATION

- Review of medical and psychiatric history.
- Review of newly initiated drugs, increased doses, interactions, over-the-counter drugs and alcohol.
- Alcohol and other substance abuse history.
- Physical examination to assess systemic causes and effects.

BOX 5.2 Common Causes (Mnemonic—DELIRIUM)

Drugs (including poisoning)	Alcohol, anticholinergic agents, amphetamines, benzodiazepines, barbiturates, lithium, psychotropic drugs, steroids, carbon monoxide
Electrolytes, metabolic and endocrine	Electrolyte imbalance (sodium, magnesium, calcium), hypoglycaemia, hyperosmolar hyperglycaemic state, diabetic ketoacidosis, liver failure, renal failure, Wernicke's encephalopathy, hypopituitarism, myxoedema, thyrotoxicosis, hypoparathyroidism, hyperparathyroidism, Addison's disease, Cushing's syndrome, hypothermia, hyperthermia, porphyria
Lack of drugs (including drug withdrawal)	Alcohol, benzodiazepines, poor pain control
Infections	Urinary tract, respiratory tract, SARS-CoV-2, soft-tissue and other infections
Reduced sensory input	Reduced hearing, reduced vision
Intracranial lesions	Infection, haemorrhage, stroke or tumour
Urinary and faecal disorders	Urinary retention (cystocerebral syndrome), faecal impaction
Myocardial and pulmonary disorders	Myocardial infarction, arrhythmia, heart failure, hypotension, severe anaemia, exacerbation of chronic obstructive pulmonary disease, hypoxia, hypercapnia
Miscellaneous	Hospitalisation (particularly in elderly)

BOX 5.3 Confusion Assessment Method (CAM)

Presence of features 1 and 2, and either 3 or 4

- Acute change in mental status with a fluctuating course (feature 1)
- Inattention (feature 2)
- Disorganised thinking (feature 3)
- Altered level of consciousness (feature 4)

- Evaluation of cognition by Mini-Mental State Examination (MMSE—a 30-item instrument that includes tests of orientation, memory and concentration) or Confusion Assessment Method (CAM) (Box 5.3).
    - Inattention can be assessed by asking the patient to name the months backwards from December to July.
    - Disorganised thinking is assessed by asking some questions like:
        - Will a stone float on water?
        - Are there fish in the sea?
        - Does 1 kg weigh more than 2 kg?
        - Ask him to hold up two fingers after showing it with your hand; then ask him to do so with the other hand without showing him yourself.
    - Altered level of consciousness can be assessed by Richmond Agitation-Sedation Scale (Table 5.6)
- Serum electrolytes, blood sugar, liver and kidney function tests, complete blood count, blood alcohol, thyroid-stimulating hormone, pulse oximetry and arterial blood gas.
- Cultures of blood, urine and sputum, if indicated.
- Chest radiograph, CT head and cerebrospinal fluid analysis in some patients.

MANAGEMENT

- Potentially life-threatening causes, including hypoxia, hypotension, hypoglycaemia, electrolyte imbalance and hyperthermia or hypothermia, should be treated.

TABLE 5.6 Richmond Agitation-Sedation Scale

Score	Term	Description
+4	Combative	Overtly combative, aggressive, danger to the staff
+3	Very agitated	Pulls tubes and catheters
+2	Agitated	Frequent nonpurposeful movements, fights ventilator
+1	Restless	Anxious but movements not aggressive or vigorous
0	Alert and calm	
−1	Drowsy	Sustained awakening to voice (≥10 seconds)
−2	Light sedation	Briefly awakens with eye contact to voice (<10 seconds)
−3	Moderate sedation	Movement or eye opening to voice but no eye contact
−4	Deep sedation	No response to voice but movements or eye opening to physical stimulus
−5	Unarousable	No response to voice or physical stimulus

BOX 5.4 Principles of Verbal De-escalation

- Listen closely to what the patient is saying
- Do not be provocative
- Agree or agree to disagree
- Establish verbal contact
- Be concise and use simple language
- Identify the patient's wants and feelings
- Ensure patients have their vision glasses and hearing aids
- Allow people who are familiar to the patient to be at the bedside
- Use easily visible clocks and calendars

- Underlying cause of delirium should be treated.
- Supportive treatment is instituted so as to prevent any harm to the patient, while being investigated.
- The verbal de-escalation techniques, turning off the lights and minimising ambient noise can reduce agitation in some patients. Some of the principles of verbal de-escalation are given in Box 5.4.
- If there is a potential danger of injury to the patient due to violent behaviour, physical restraints or chemical restraints may be used.
- Chemical agents include first generation antipsychotics, second generation antipsychotics and benzodiazepines.
- First generation antipsychotics include haloperidol and droperidol. Haloperidol is given in a dose of 1 to 2 mg orally; if no response, 1 to 2 mg is given intramuscularly or intravenously; some patients may require 5-10 mg. Droperidol is given in a dose of 2.5–5 mg intramuscularly or intravenously.
- Atypical or second generation antipsychotics (olanzapine—5 to 10 mg intramuscularly; and risperidone—1 to 2 mg) are also useful and have lower incidence of side effects compared to haloperidol.
- Benzodiazepines (diazepam or lorazepam) are the treatment of choice when delirium is due to alcohol, benzodiazepine or barbiturate withdrawal, or patient is agitated. Otherwise, they may produce excessive sedation.
- Some patients require combination of benzodiazepines and antipsychotic agents.
- Most patients will require admission for further management.

Q. Discuss the aetiology, clinical features, investigations and management of dementia. (PS 16.1)

Q. Describe mild cognitive impairment.

DEFINITION

- Dementia is a global deterioration of the higher mental functions. It is characterised by problems with memory and at least one other cognitive function (learning, reasoning, language, spatial ability and orientation, and handling complex tasks) which are severe enough to interfere with occupational, domestic or social functioning.

COMMON CAUSES (Table 5.7)

TABLE 5.7 Causes of Dementia

Dementia without Additional Neurological Deficits	Dementia with Additional Neurological Deficits
Neurological disorders • Alzheimer's disease • Frontotemporal dementia (Pick's disease) **Metabolic disorders** • Dialysis dementia • Hypothyroidism • Hyperparathyroidism • Uraemia • Hepatic encephalopathy • Porphyria • Vitamin B_{12} deficiency • Adrenal insufficiency • Cushing's syndrome • Chronic hypoglycaemia **Toxic causes** • Heavy metal poisoning • Chronic substance abuse (e.g. alcohol) **Others** • Vasculitides (primary vasculitis of the central nervous system, Behçet's disease, SLE-related)	• Vascular dementia (multi-infarct dementia, small-vessel ischaemic disease, chronic/subacute subdural haematomas, hypoxic/ischaemic encephalopathy) • Parkinson's disease dementia • Wilson's disease • Chronic infections (tuberculosis, fungal, HIV, progressive multifocal leucoencephalopathy, syphilis) • Hydrocephalus (obstructive and non-obstructive) • Normal pressure hydrocephalus • Chronic subdural haematoma • Dementia with Lewy bodies • Frontotemporal dementia • Multiple system atrophy • Brain neoplasms

CLINICAL FEATURES

- Mild cognitive impairment (MCI): Memory complaints (preferably qualified by an informant) and memory impairment relative to the patient's age and education, but preserved general cognitive function and intact activities of daily living (ADL). On MMSE, the patients generally score in the range of 26–28. It is the precursor to several types of dementia, including neurodegenerative dementia (e.g. Alzheimer's disease, Parkinson's disease and dementia with Lewy bodies), vascular dementia and dementia caused by neoplasms, normal-pressure hydrocephalus and metabolic factors.
    - MCI may also represent a reversible condition in the setting of depression, as a complication of certain medications, or during the recovery from an acute illness.
- Progression of dementia varies with the cause. Early symptoms include lapses in memory, reasoning and judgement. Mood disorders like sadness, anger and frustration are common. Gradually, deficits in all higher mental functions become evident. Deficits occur in the following:
    - Retaining new information (e.g. trouble remembering events)
    - Handling complex tasks (e.g. balancing a chequebook)
    - Reasoning
    - Spatial ability and orientation (e.g. getting lost in familiar places)
    - Language (e.g. word finding)
- Later, dysphasia, apraxia, agnosia, urinary incontinence and focal neurological deficits occur. In later stages, deterioration in personality, personal hygiene and self-care becomes evident. The person requires to be looked after by others. In advanced stages, the person is mute, lies on bed and succumbs to intercurrent infections.
- The normal cognitive decline associated with ageing consists primarily of mild changes in memory and rate of information processing. However, compared to dementia, deficits are generally not very progressive and usually do not affect daily function.

INVESTIGATIONS (Box 5.5)

BOX 5.5 Investigations in a Case With Dementia

- Liver function tests
- Renal function tests
- Endocrine evaluation, particularly thyroid profile
- Serum vitamin B_{12} estimation
- VDRL } for syphilis if clinically indicated
- TPHA } for syphilis if clinically indicated
- HIV
- CSF analysis
- EEG
- CT scan
- MRI
- PET

TREATMENT

- Treat the underlying cause wherever possible.

Q. Differentiation between delirium, dementia and psychosis. (PS 16.1)

- Differences between delirium, dementia and psychosis are tabulated in Table 5.8.

Q. Give a brief account of nuclear magnetic resonance (NMR) and MRI.

- MRI is an imaging technique used primarily in medical settings to produce high-quality images of the inside of the human body. It is based on the principles of NMR of atoms in the tissue, a spectroscopic technique used by scientists to obtain microscopic, chemical and physical information about molecules. The technique was called MRI, rather than nuclear magnetic resonance imaging (NMRI), because of the negative connotations associated with the word nuclear.
- Presently, hydrogen atom in the tissue is selected, as it is present in every tissue, though other atoms can also be chosen. Changes in the energy state are measured under the influence of powerful fixed external magnetic field with pulses of radiofrequency waves.
- Normally, magnetic axes of multiple protons within tissues are randomly aligned. When surrounded by a strong magnetic field, as in an MRI machine, the magnetic axes align along the field. Application of a radiofrequency pulse causes the axes of all protons to momentarily align against the field in a high-energy state. Then the field is suddenly reduced. Some protons then relax back to their baseline state within the magnetic field. The magnitude and rate of energy release that occurs with return to baseline alignment (T_1 relaxation) and with the wobbling (precession) of

TABLE 5.8 Differences Between Delirium, Dementia and Psychosis

Feature	Delirium	Dementia	Psychosis
• Onset	• Rapid	• Slow	• Variable
• Pattern	• Fluctuating	• Stable; occasionally fluctuating	• Stable
• Speech	• Incoherent	• Preserved	• Rapid, pressured
• Attention	• Impaired	• Normal	• Poor due to delusions
• Consciousness	• Marked fluctuation	• Clear till late stages	• Generally no impairment
• Orientation	• Disoriented	• Oriented	• Usually oriented
• Memory	• Short-term memory impaired	• Both short- and long-term memory impaired	• Selectively impaired

protons during the process (T_2 relaxation) are recorded as spatially localised signal intensities by a coil (antenna). These intensities are used to produce images.

- Magnetic strength of MRI is measured in tesla.
- A T_1-weighted sequence accentuates substances that contain fat, while a T_2-weighted sequence accentuates substances that contain water.
- In the brain, T_1-weighted images show the nerve connections of white matter to appear white (hyperintense), and the congregations of neurons of grey matter to appear grey, while cerebrospinal fluid appears dark. This is reversed in T_2-weighted imaging.
- MRI is preferred to CT when soft-tissue contrast resolution is important, for example to evaluate intracranial, spinal or spinal cord abnormalities, or to evaluate suspected musculoskeletal tumours, inflammation, trauma or internal joint derangement.

CONTRAST MRI

- The most frequently used intravenous contrast agents are based on chelates of gadolinium, which have magnetic properties that affect proton relaxation times.
- Contrast may be used to highlight vascular structures (magnetic resonance angiography) and to help characterise inflammation and tumours.
- Can cause headache, nausea, pain and sensation of cold at the injection site, taste distortion, dizziness, vasodilation and reduced threshold for seizures. Anaphylactoid reactions are rare.
- Another rare but important complication of gadolinium is nephrogenic systemic fibrosis that involves fibrosis of dermis, joints and internal organs including lungs and heart. It usually occurs in patients with underlying chronic kidney failure; most of these patients are on dialysis. Because of this reason, gadolinium-enhanced MRI is contraindicated in patients with acute or chronic renal insufficiency, with a glomerular filtration rate <30 mL/minute/1.73 m^2.

SPECIAL FORMS OF MRI

- Diffusion MRI measures the movement or diffusion of extracellular water molecules. Diffusion is restricted in areas of damage from such causes as trauma, stroke or some tumours. Diffusion-weighted imaging is highly sensitive to diagnose early ischaemic stroke. It is also used to differentiate active from dormant plaques in multiple sclerosis.
- Magnetic resonance angiography is used to generate pictures of the arteries in order to evaluate them for stenosis or aneurysms. It is often used to evaluate the arteries of the neck and brain, the thoracic and abdominal aorta and the renal arteries.
- Magnetic resonance spectroscopy combines the spatially addressable nature of MRI with the spectroscopically rich information obtainable from MRI. It allows for the detection of amount and spatial distribution of various molecular compounds that are involved in the metabolism of pathological and healthy tissue. The most important metabolites are creatine, choline, *N*-acetylacetate, citrate, lactate and lipids. Magnetic resonance spectroscopy is used to study metabolic changes in brain tumours, strokes, seizure disorders, Alzheimer's disease and depression.
- Functional MRI (fMRI) measures signal changes in the brain that are due to changing neural activity. It collects functional information on blood oxygenation or flow changes, perfusion or diffusion. fMRI studies are strongly recommended for the preoperative diagnostics of brain tumour patients to delineate functionally important neuronal tissue, which should be preserved during surgery.

USES IN NEUROLOGY

- Imaging section in any desired plane is possible.
- Clearly differentiates grey from white matter.
- Eliminates bone artefacts, for example at posterior fossa, spinal column and craniovertebral junction.
- Particularly useful in recognising demyelinating plaques and early gliomas.
- Magnetic resonance angiography is another application of magnetic resonance. The fast-flowing arterial blood does not produce any signal, while slower flowing blood in veins or distal to an arterial block or stenosis shows a signal. By varying the magnetic resonance parameters, both qualitative and quantitative data about blood flow can be assessed. This can be used to assess extracranial portion of carotid artery, intracranial major vessels and renal arteries.

OTHER USES

- Cardiovascular MRI is the 'gold standard' for quantifying ventricular volumes, ejection fraction and myocardial mass.
- Useful in orthopaedic diseases like disc prolapse, etc.

COMPLICATIONS

- MRI is a quite safe procedure. However, serious injuries have been described if a metal is present nearby, which gets attracted to strong magnets of MRI and can act as a missile.
- Similarly, ferromagnetic metal clips used to clip an aneurysm may come off and cause bleeding.
- Implanted cardiac pacemakers are a contraindication to MRI. Other contraindications include vagus nerve stimulators, implanted cardio-defibrillators (ICD), cochlear implants and deep brain stimulators, although some of them may be MRI-compatible.

ADVANTAGES AND DISADVANTAGES OF MRI (Table 5.9)

TABLE 5.9 Advantages and Disadvantages of MRI

Advantages	Disadvantages
• No radiation exposure • Excellent differentiation of substances in the brain that cannot be differentiated on CT • Best detailed view of soft tissues of extremities • Detailed and accurate evaluation of breast cancers • Good for evaluating medullary bone	• Expensive and time-consuming • Spatial resolution not as good as CT • Requires experienced reader • Not good for evaluation of bone cortex • Less effective than CT at seeing air (lungs) or gas (as in infection or bowel perforation) • Makes loud knocking, tapping and other noises • Claustrophobic for some patients

Q. What is the significance of xanthochromia in cerebrospinal fluid (CSF) analysis?

- Xanthochromia is the yellowness of CSF.
- It is always pathological. Xanthochromia is seen in the following conditions:
  - SAH (within 4–12 hours in 90% of cases) where it is due to breakdown of haemoglobin into bilirubin.
  - Jaundice (bilirubin >10 mg/dL).
  - Excess protein in CSF.
  - Carotene excess.
  - Froin's syndrome (spinal subarachnoid block, pronounced xanthochromia and great excess of protein).

Q. List down the indications and contraindications of lumbar puncture.

- Indications, contraindications and complications of lumbar puncture are given in Table 5.10, Box 5.6 and Box 5.7.

Q. What are the features of normal cerebrospinal fluid? (BI 11.15)

- Composition of normal CSF is given in Table 5.11.

TABLE 5.10 Indications of Lumbar Puncture

Diagnostic Indications	Therapeutic Indications
Absolute • Meningitis • Encephalitis • SAH (if CT normal) • Guillain–Barre syndrome (GB syndrome) • Acute demyelinating diseases • Acute disseminated encephalomyelitis • Transverse myelitis (TM) • Unexplained coma • Unexplained dementia • Meningeal carcinomatosis **Relative** • Multiple sclerosis • Pyrexia of unknown origin • Neurosyphilis	• Methotrexate and steroids in leukaemia • Spinal anaesthesia • Benign intracranial hypertension [to reduce intracranial pressure (ICP)]

BOX 5.6 Contraindications of Lumbar Puncture

- Raised ICP
- Spinal deformity
- Local infections
- Coagulation disorders (platelets <40,000/mm^3, use of anticoagulants)

BOX 5.7 Complications of Lumbar Puncture

• Brain herniation	• Meningitis
• Traumatic tap	• Headache
• Spinal epidural haematoma or spinal subdural haematoma	• Diplopia (due to unilateral or bilateral sixth nerve palsy; lowered CSF pressure causes the sixth nerve to stretch as it courses over the petrous bone)

TABLE 5.11 Normal Composition of CSF

Colour	Clear
Opening pressure	50–200 mm H_2O
RBC count	Nil
WBC count	0–5 (up to 30 in neonates)
WBC types	Lymphocytes
CSF proteins	15–40 mg/dL
CSF glucose	50–80 mg/dL (two-thirds of blood glucose)
Microbial examination	No microorganism

Q. Discuss the value of CSF analysis. (BI 11.15, IM 17.19)

- Analysis of CSF is of diagnostic value. Disorders of central nervous system and some peripheral nervous system may be made out by CSF examination. Major causes of CSF abnormalities are listed in Table 5.12.
- In infections of central nervous system, pathogens can be isolated from CSF by staining techniques (Gram stain, Ziehl–Neelsen stain, India ink preparation, etc.) or cultures.

TABLE 5.12 Major Causes of Abnormalities in CSF

Physical abnormalities	
• High CSF pressure (normal 60–200 mm H_2O)	Raised ICP
• Blood stained	Traumatic puncture, SAH
• Xanthochromia	SAH, Froin's syndrome (spinal block), high serum bilirubin level, high carotene
• Turbidity	Increased cellularity
• Cobweb formation	Tuberculous meningitis (TBM)
Chemical abnormalities	
• Low sugar (normal two-thirds of blood glucose)	Pyogenic, tuberculous, fungal and carcinomatous meningitis, rheumatoid arthritis, neurosarcoidosis
• Raised protein (normal <40 mg/dL)	Nonspecific—reflects break in blood–brain barrier; occurs in inflammatory, infective, neoplastic and ischaemic disorders, GB syndrome, certain other peripheral neuropathies
Cytological abnormalities	
• Increase in cell count (normal <5 WBCs/mm^3)	Inflammatory disorders
• Polymorphonuclear reaction (normal <1–2/mm^3)	Acute inflammation, mainly pyogenic meningitis
• Lymphocytic reaction	Chronic infective disorders like TBM and fungal meningitis
• Other abnormal cellular elements	Immunological disorders like demyelinating diseases
	Carcinomatous meningitis
	Meningeal seedling of intracranial neoplasms

- Serological tests are available for many bacterial, mycobacterial and fungal infections, for example Venereal Disease Research Laboratory (VDRL) and treponema pallidum haemagglutination (TPHA) in neurosyphilis.
- Oligoclonal immunoglobulin bands in multiple sclerosis (on paired samples).

Q. Discuss the formation of CSF and its functions. (AN 56.2)

- CSF is formed from mainly the choroid plexuses of lateral third and fourth ventricles. Some may originate as tissue fluid formed in the brain substance. It leaves the ventricular system through the apertures in the roof of the fourth ventricle and flows through the cerebral and spinal subarachnoid spaces. It is reabsorbed in the arachnoid villi, located along the superior sagittal and intracranial venous sinuses, and around the spinal nerve roots.

FUNCTIONS

- Serves as a cushion between the CNS and surrounding bones, thus protecting CNS against mechanical trauma.
- Serves as a reservoir and assists in the regulation of intracranial volume as a buffer, for example if brain volume or blood volume increases, the CSF volume decreases as skull is a rigid structure. Monro–Kellie doctrine states that sum of volumes of brain, CSF and intracranial blood is constant. An increase in one should cause a decrease in one or both of the remaining two.
- Nourishment of the nervous tissue.
- Removal of products of neuronal metabolism.

Q. What is Froin's syndrome?

Q. Describe Queckenstedt's test.

- Froin's syndrome describes the CSF findings in cases of spinal subarachnoid block. Xanthochromia, elevated CSF protein and hypercoagulable CSF forms the triad of Froin's syndrome.
- Various CSF findings below the block are given in Box 5.8.
- Common causes of Froin's syndrome are listed in Box 5.9.

BOX 5.8 CSF Findings in Froin's Syndrome

- CSF pressure is reduced.
- Queckenstedt's test suggests a block.
- Physical—xanthochromic; coagulum may form.
- Chemical—protein levels are grossly elevated, sugar levels are normal or occasionally reduced if the cause is tuberculous meningitis (TBM).
- Cytology—normal; increased cells if the cause is TBM.

BOX 5.9 Common Causes of Froin's Syndrome

- Total block due to any obstruction in CSF pathway in the spinal column.
- Tumours (intraspinal).
- Vertebral diseases with compression.
- Chronic spinal arachnoiditis.

QUECKENSTEDT'S TEST

- The test is performed by putting bilateral pressure on the jugular veins during the course of a lumbar puncture. Normally, there is a sharp rise in the pressure of spinal fluid in the lumbar region within 10–12 seconds and then a sharp fall when the pressure is released. If there is no rise in the pressure, it is a sign of blocking of the subarachnoid channels.

Q. Enumerate the causes of papilloedema.

- Strictly speaking, the term papilloedema is applied to optic disc swelling due to raised intracranial pressure

(ICP). However, it is often applied to swollen optic disc produced by any cause.
- On fundoscopy, an early finding is loss of spontaneous venous pulsations. Later, the optic disc becomes elevated with obliteration of cup, and the disc margins become obscured.
- In papilloedema, central visual acuity is typically spared (at least initially) compared to other causes of optic nerve oedema (e.g. optic neuritis).

CAUSES (Table 5.13)

TABLE 5.13 Causes of Papilloedema

Orbital	Intracranial
Ocular Venous Drainage Block: • Central retinal venous block • Cavernous sinus thrombosis **Local Lesions:** • Optic neuritis • Ischaemia of the nerve head • Toxins (methanol) • Infiltration of the disc by glioma, sarcoidosis and lymphoma **Systemic disorders affecting retinal vessels:** • Hypertension, vasculitis, chronic hypercarbia, COPD, polycythaemia	**Raised ICP:** • Tumours • Abscesses, granulomas • Intracranial haemorrhage • Hydrocephalus, diffuse brain oedema • Intracerebral haemorrhage • Benign intracranial hypertension • Cerebral venous sinus thrombosis • Meningitis • Steroid withdrawal • Hypervitaminosis A • Superior vena cava obstruction • Anoxia • Sleep apnoea syndrome

TREATMENT

- Correction of underlying cause.
- Correction of raised ICP by mannitol and hypertonic saline.
- Lumboperitoneal shunt (LPS) or ventriculoperitoneal shunt (VPS).
- Optic nerve sheath fenestration for stabilising visual loss and protecting the optic nerve from further damage.

Q. What is ptosis? List down its causes. (OP 2.1)

- Inability to open an upper eyelid.
- Occurs in third nerve palsy and Horner's syndrome (always partial).
  - The third nerve supplies levator palpebrae superioris, which when affected results in ptosis. Other signs of third nerve palsy will be present.
  - Horner's syndrome occurs due to weakness of Muller's muscle, innervated by sympathetic nerves. Ptosis is mild, usually 1 to 2 mm.
- Relation between ptosis and pupillary size is given in Box 5.10.

BOX 5.10 Ptosis and Pupillary Size

- Ptosis with a small pupil suggests Horner's syndrome.
- Ptosis with a large pupil suggests third nerve palsy.
- Ptosis with normal pupillary size may suggest infarction of the third nerve, myasthenia gravis, myopathies or GB syndrome.

Note: Pupillary fibres of the third nerve are located peripherally in the optic nerve; a compressive lesion causes early loss of pupillary reflex, while an ischaemic lesion causes pupillary sparing.

CAUSES (Table 5.14)

TABLE 5.14 Causes of Ptosis

Third nerve palsy	• Diabetes mellitus • Multiple sclerosis • Meningovascular syphilis • Cerebral aneurysm • Cavernous sinus thrombosis or infection • Brainstem stroke • False localising sign in increased intracranial pressure (due to brain displacement) • Wernicke's encephalopathy (occurs due to vitamin B_1 deficiency)
Neuromuscular junction or muscle involvement (produces bilateral ptosis)	• Myasthenia gravis • Ocular myopathies • Neuroparalytic snake bites • Botulism
Horner's syndrome	• Various causes listed later

Q. Discuss the visual pathway. Illustrate the field defects produced at various levels. (OP 8.5)

- Visual sensory system begins at the retina, inner layer of which contains light-sensitive receptor cells (rods and cones). The highest concentration of cones is in the central macular area, the fovea.
- As a result of the convex lens in the eye, objects located in the temporal visual field stimulate the nasal retina and those located in the superior visual field stimulate the inferior retina.
- More than 90% of retinal nerve fibres arise from the macula to form papillomacular bundle that pass to the optic nerve, taking up its central core. Lesions of this bundle (either in the retina or in the optic nerve head) produce central scotomas.
- Retinal nerve fibres temporal to the macula arc above or below form the papillomacular bundle to enter the optic disc. Lesions of these arcuate bundles produce arcuate scotomas.
- Nasal fibres pass directly to the nasal border of disc. Lesions of nasal retinal axons cause temporal field defects.
- In the optic nerve, macular fibres are in a central position with the superior retinal fibres above and the inferior retinal fibres below. Temporal and nasal fibres retain these positions within the optic nerve.
- At optic chiasma, the nasal fibres cross to other side, while temporal fibres continue on the same side.

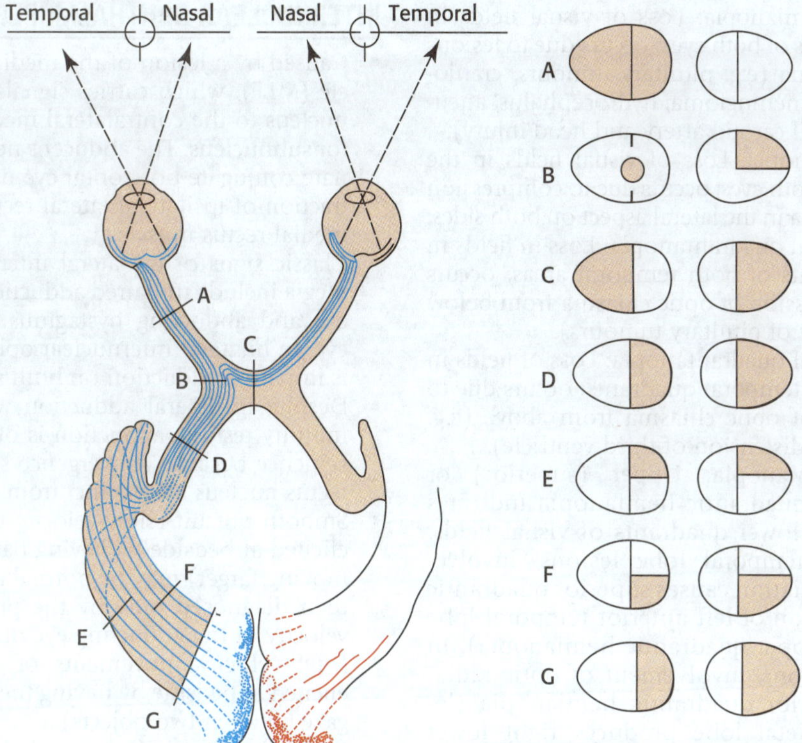

Fig. 5.2 Effects on the fields of vision produced by lesions at various points along the optic pathway. (A) Complete blindness in left eye. (B) The usual effect is a left junction scotoma in association with a right upper quadrantanopia. The latter results from interruption of right retinal nasal fibres that project into the base of the left optic nerve (Wilbrand's knee). A left nasal hemianopia could occur from a lesion of this point, but is exceedingly rare. (C) Bitemporal hemianopia. (D) Right homonymous hemianopia. (E and F) Right upper and lower quadrant hemianopia. (G) Right homonymous hemianopia.

Thus, visual information from the left hemifields of both eyes continues through the visual pathway towards the right occipital cortex, while that from right hemifields towards the left occipital cortex.

- The crossed nasal fibres once joined with uncrossed temporal fibres proceed as the optic tract.
- These fibres in the optic tract then pass to the lateral geniculate nucleus of the thalamus.
- From the lateral geniculate nucleus, optic radiations pass posteriorly to the visual cortex. Nerve fibres originating from the superior retina (i.e. lower visual field) travel directly to the visual cortex through the parietal lobe while those from the inferior retina (superior visual field) pass through the temporal lobe (Fig. 5.2).
- The primary visual cortex lies along the superior and inferior sides of the calcarine fissure. It contains a large macular projection area in the occipital pole.

VISUAL FIELD DEFECTS (Fig. 5.2)

CENTRAL SCOTOMA

- Loss of vision confined to central field of vision.
- Unilateral scotoma commonly due to diseases of choroid, retina and optic nerve demyelination (as seen with multiple sclerosis) or compression.
- Bilateral scotoma due to vitamin B_{12} deficiency and alcohol.

HEMIANOPIA

- Loss of vision in one-half of the vision.
- Homonymous hemianopia: Loss of nasal field in one eye and temporal field in the other eye. Occurs due to lesion in optic tract (left optic tract lesion produces right homonymous hemianopia).
  - It is complete when the visual field defect respects the vertical meridian, has macular splitting and involves the entire hemifield on the affected side (e.g. complete lesions anywhere along the retrochiasmal visual pathway). Others are called incomplete which may be incongruous or congruous.
  - Congruous hemianopia: The outlines of visual field defect in both eyes are similar in size and shape (e.g. lesions of occipital cortex).
  - Incongruous hemianopia: The outlines of visual field defect in both eyes are different (e.g. lesions of optic tract or chiasma or radiation).
- Homonymous hemianopia with macular sparing: Loss of nasal field in one eye and temporal field in the other eye with sparing of central vision in both the eyes; occurs due to lesion in occipital cortex (lesion in left occipital cortex produces right homonymous hemianopia with macular sparing).
- Heteronymous hemianopia: Loss of either the nasal or the temporal fields in both eyes.

  - Bitemporal hemianopia: Loss of visual fields in temporal halves of both eyes; occurs due to lesions of optic chiasma (e.g. pituitary tumours, craniopharyngioma, meningioma, hydrocephalus, aneurysm of internal carotid artery and head injury).
  - Binasal hemianopia: Loss of visual fields in the nasal parts of both eyes; occurs due to compression of optic chiasma in the lateral aspect on both sides.
  - Upper temporal quadrantanopia: Loss in fields in upper quadrants of both temporal areas; occurs due to compression of optic chiasma from below (e.g. early stage of pituitary tumours).
  - Lower temporal quadrantanopia: Loss of fields in bilateral lower temporal quadrants; occurs due to compression of optic chiasma from above (e.g. early stages of distension of third ventricle).
- Quadrantic hemianopia: Upper (superior) or lower (inferior) quadrantic hemianopia indicates loss of upper or lower quadrants of visual fields, respectively. In temporal lobe lesions, involvement of optic radiation causes superior quadrantic hemianopia (lesion of left anterior temporal lobe produces right upper quadrantic hemianopia). In parietal lobe lesions, involvement of optic radiation causes inferior quadrantic hemianopia (lesion of left parietal lobe produces right lower quadrantic hemianopia).

Q. Give a brief account of diplopia.

- Diplopia indicates double vision.
- Uniocular or monocular (diplopia with one eye closed) and binocular (diplopia when both eyes are open).
- Uniocular diplopia occurs due to uncorrected refractory error, astigmatism, corneal opacity, corneal defect induced by laser eye surgery, lenticular opacity, ectopic lens, ill-fitting contact lens, keratoconus and macular defects. If none of these is present, it indicates hysterical cause.

CAUSES OF BINOCULAR DIPLOPIA (Table 5.15)

TABLE 5.15 Causes of Binocular Diplopia

• Third nerve palsy	Refer above (Table 5.14)
• Fourth nerve palsy	Isolated lesion is rare (trauma), almost always associated with third or sixth nerve palsies
• Sixth nerve palsy	Carotid artery aneurysm, increased intracranial pressure, diabetes
• Neuromuscular junction abnormalities	Myasthenia gravis, botulism
• Extraocular muscle involvement	Thyroid-associated ophthalmopathy, extraocular muscle injury, congenital myopathies, muscular dystrophy
• Central nervous system diseases	Ischaemia, haemorrhage, tumour, vascular malformations, multiple sclerosis (causing internuclear ophthalmoplegia), hydrocephalus, Wernicke's encephalopathy, neurodegenerative diseases (e.g. supranuclear palsy, Parinaud's syndrome)

INTERNUCLEAR OPHTHALMOPLEGIA

- Caused by a lesion of the medial longitudinal fascicle (MLF), which carries signals from the abducens nucleus to the contralateral medial rectus oculomotor subnucleus. The abducens nerve and MLF coordinate conjugate horizontal eye movements with contraction of ipsilateral lateral rectus and contralateral medial rectus muscles.
- Classic signs of unilateral internuclear ophthalmoplegia include impaired adduction of the ipsilesional eye and abducting nystagmus of the contralateral eye. In bilateral internuclear ophthalmoplegia, there is impaired adduction on both sides (Fig. 5.3).
- Despite ipsilateral adduction weakness with direct motility testing, adduction is often intact with convergence because convergence signals to the medial rectus nucleus are distinct from the MLF.
- Smooth pursuit (slow-velocity tracking movements; elicited at bedside by having patient follow a slowly moving target) may be normal and this condition is then diagnosed only by the presence of decreased velocity of the adducting eye during saccadic testing (high-velocity movements of varying amplitudes; elicited at bedside by having the patient rapidly shift gaze between two objects).
- Multiple sclerosis (commonly bilateral) and microvascular brainstem ischaemia (commonly unilateral) are the most common causes. Other causes include trauma, brainstem and fourth ventricle tumours, and meningoencephalitis.
- A partial third nerve palsy with prominent medial rectus weakness may be confused with internuclear ophthalmoplegia. Distinguishing features include other third nerve deficits (weakness of elevation, ptosis, pupillary dilatation), impaired convergence and absence of the contralateral abduction nystagmus.

SUPRANUCLEAR PALSIES

- Result from dysfunctional cerebral, cerebellar and brainstem afferent connections to the ocular motor nuclei.
- A clinical hallmark is disproportionate involvement of saccades. Vestibular eye movements are typically spared. In contrast, nuclear and infranuclear lesions impair saccades, smooth pursuit and vestibular eye movements equally.
- Examples include progressive supranuclear palsy (a degenerative condition that initially affects vertical

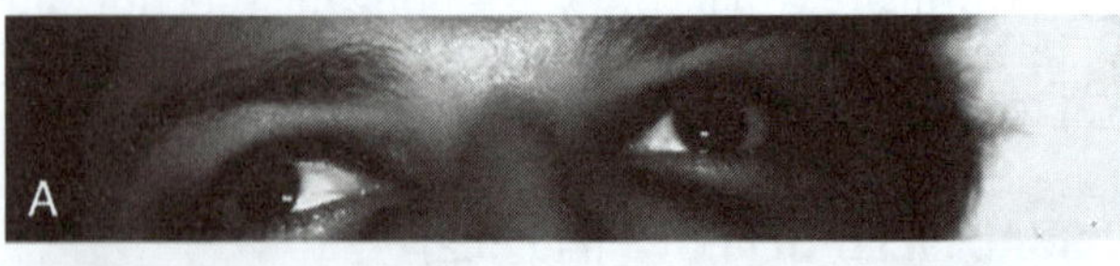

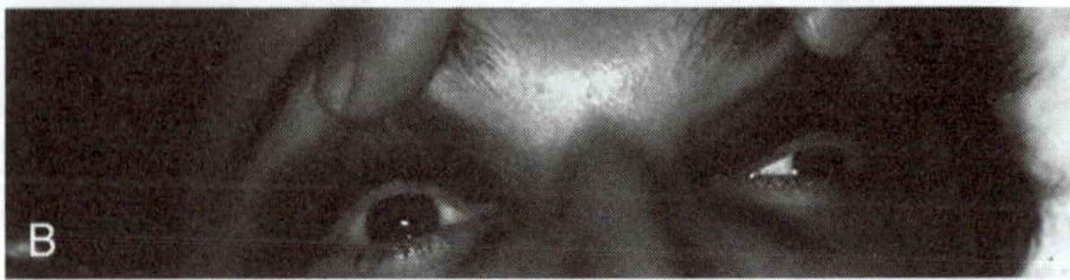

Fig. 5.3 Bilateral internuclear ophthalmoplegia (note impaired adduction in both eyes).

gaze to a greater extent than horizontal, and is accompanied by progressive dysphagia, cognitive decline and falls) and Parinaud's syndrome (comprises supranuclear upgaze palsy, convergence nystagmus, lid retraction, and dissociation of papillary light and accommodation reflex; occurs due to pineal gland lesions and hydrocephalus).

Q. Briefly outline the clinical features and treatment of trigeminal neuralgia (tic douloureux).

- Occurs in elderly; aetiology is unknown in many; may be due to vascular compression at root entry zone of the fifth nerve.

CAUSES (Box 5.11)

BOX 5.11 Causes of Trigeminal Neuralgia

- Idiopathic
- Vascular compression at root entry zone of the fifth nerve
- Multiple sclerosis (bilateral in many cases)
- Basilar artery aneurysm
- Cerebral tumour (especially neurofibroma of the fifth nerve or epidermoid at cerebellopontine angle)
- Syringobulbia
- Brainstem infarction

CLINICAL FEATURES

- Paroxysmal, sharp, shooting and electric shock-like pain confined to the distribution of the nerve.
- Maxillary and mandibular divisions are commonly affected. Ophthalmic division is rarely affected.
- Each paroxysm lasts only a few seconds, and may be followed by a dull ache.
- Pain is precipitated by touching trigger zones, for example cold wind blowing on face, washing face, chewing or talking. Touch and vibration seem to trigger more attacks than pinprick. Trigger zones are small areas around face, nose and lips. There is often a refractory period when the pain cannot be triggered.
- A patient experiencing a trigeminal neuralgia attack typically freezes in place with hands slowly rising to the area of pain on the face but not touching it. The patient then grimaces or quirks the face in a tic (tic douloureux) and then either remains in this position or cries out in pain.
- Paroxysms are followed by remission; later, periods of remission become shorter.
- No abnormalities of fifth nerve function are seen on physical examination. Presence of sensory loss warrants investigations to exclude other conditions like multiple sclerosis and basilar artery aneurysm.
- Hearing loss is absent.
- The pain of trigeminal neuralgia differs from the pain following reactivation of the varicella zoster virus, which typically is seen in older people. When the varicella zoster virus involves the face, it has a predilection for ophthalmic division of the trigeminal nerve.

DIAGNOSTIC CRITERIA (Table 5.16)

TABLE 5.16 Diagnostic Criteria of Trigeminal Neuralgia (International Classification of Headache Disorders, 2018)

A. Recurrent paroxysms of unilateral facial pain in the distributions of one or more divisions of the trigeminal nerve, with no radiation beyond, and fulfilling criteria B and C
B. Pain has all of the following characteristics: 1. Lasting from a fraction of a second to 2 minutes 2. Severe in intensity 3. Electric shock-like, shooting, stabbing or sharp in quality
C. Precipitated by innocuous stimuli within the affected trigeminal distribution
D. Not better accounted for by another diagnosis

TREATMENT

- Treatment of trigeminal neuralgia is given in Table 5.17.

TABLE 5.17 Treatment of Trigeminal Neuralgia

- Carbamazepine—start with 100–200 mg/day, increase in 2 to 3 weeks to 200–400 mg TID; or oxcarbazepine—10 to 20 mg/kg/day (most effective drugs)
- Phenytoin—100 mg TID
- Lamotrigine—start with 25 mg/day, increased by 25 mg every third day, up to 400 mg a day
- Gabapentin—300 to 900 mg TID; or pregabalin—75 to 150 mg BID
- Microvascular decompression—compressing blood vessels are separated from the trigeminal nerve root in the posterior fossa
- Botulinum toxin type A—a nonablative, local treatment
- Phenol or alcohol injection into particular branch of the nerve
- Radiofrequency thermal rhizotomy—heat lesion of trigeminal ganglion or nerve
- Injection of glycerol into Gasserian ganglion if whole nerve is involved
- Gamma knife radiosurgery—using stereotactic imaging of the trigeminal nerve root entry zone, radiation is delivered to trigeminal nerve, usually 2–4 mm anterior to the brainstem
- Sectioning of the sensory part of the fifth nerve or its descending tract in the medulla
- Posterior cranial fossa exploration and removing compressive lesions (typically arteries or veins from trigeminal root—microvascular decompression)

Q. What are the causes of pinpoint pupil?

- Causes of pinpoint pupils are given in Box 5.12.

BOX 5.12 Causes of Pinpoint Pupils

- Pontine haemorrhage
- Poisoning—organophosphorus and carbamate insecticides, opium and opioids, clonidine, barbiturates (constricted but not pinpoint)
- Pilocarpine instillation in eyes
- Thalamic haemorrhage (occasionally)
- Horner's syndrome (unilateral)

Q. Draw a diagram showing oculosympathetic pathways relevant to Horner's syndrome.

Q. Write a brief note on Horner's syndrome.

OCULOSYMPATHETIC PATHWAY

- Sympathetic neurons originate in the hypothalamus, pass through the brainstem and cervical spinal cord, and terminate in ciliospinal centre located between C8 and T2 in the spinal cord.
- Preganglionic sympathetic neurons exit the spinal cord via the ventral nerve roots from C8 to T2 and travel within the sympathetic chain over the lung apex and up the carotid sheath, terminating in the superior cervical ganglion which is located near the common carotid artery bifurcation.
- Postganglionic neurons emerge from the superior cervical ganglion and ascend along the internal carotid artery to form sympathetic plexus which innervate the pupillary dilators through long ciliary nerve and also Muller's muscle (smooth muscles in the upper and lower eyelids). It also sends sudomotor fibres to the ipsilateral face which produce sweating.
- Fig. 5.4 shows the oculosympathetic pathways.

HORNER'S SYNDROME

- Horner's syndrome is produced by damage to the sympathetic pathway.
  - Preganglionic sympathetic fibres after they exit from C8 to T2 spinal roots.
  - Sympathetic fibres through the third nerve innervate superior tarsal muscle of eyelid (Muller's muscles).
  - Sympathetic fibres through nasociliary nerve supply the blood vessels of eye.
  - Sympathetic fibres through long ciliary nerve innervate pupil.
- Damage to sympathetic pathway causes abnormalities in all the above-mentioned structures.

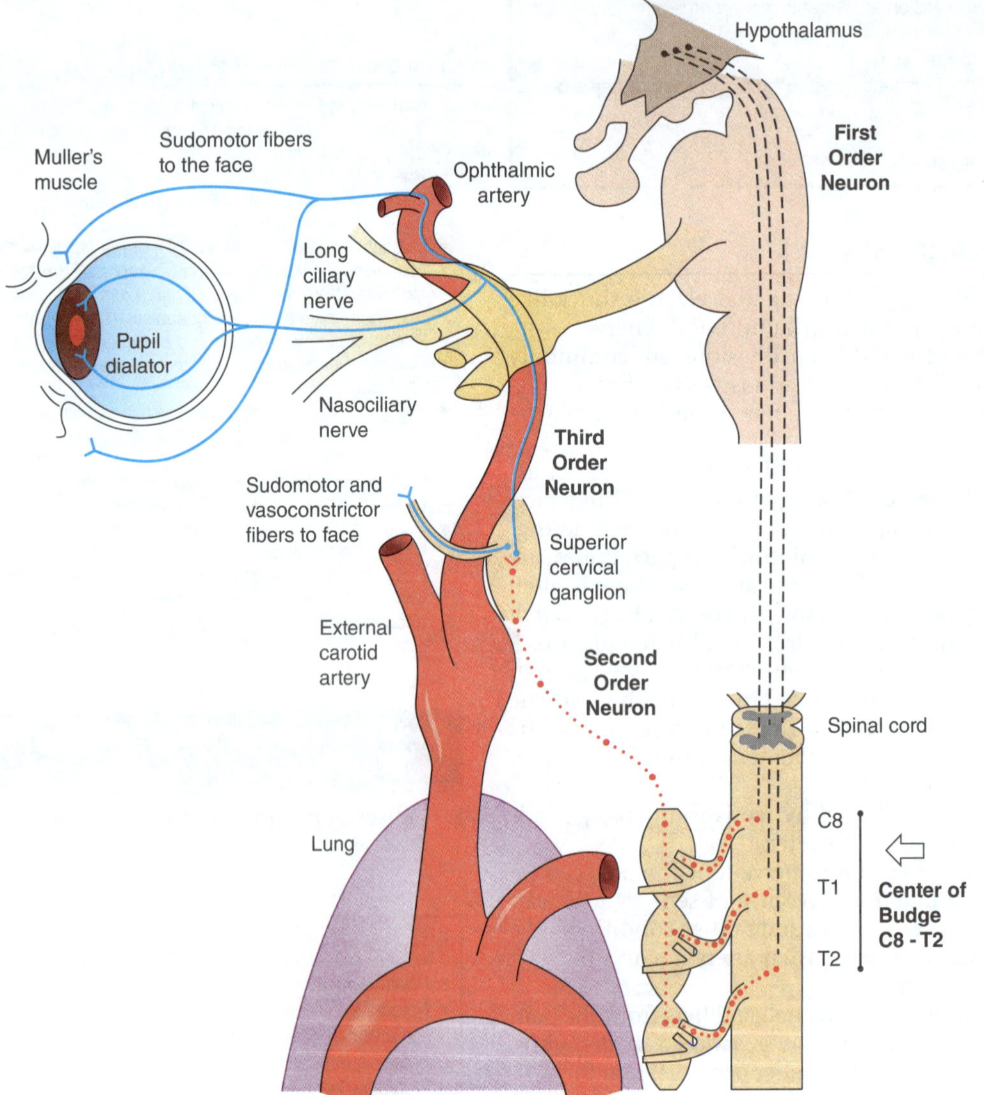

Fig. 5.4 Anatomy of oculosympathetic pathways.

COMPONENTS (Box 5.13)

BOX 5.13 Components of Horner's Syndrome

- Miosis due to reduced pupillodilator activity
- Ptosis of eyelid
- Bloodshot conjunctiva due to loss of vasoconstrictor activity
- Enophthalmos
- Anhidrosis of ipsilateral half of face due to involvement of sudomotor fibres to face
- Loss of ciliospinal reflex

CAUSES (Box 5.14)

BOX 5.14 Causes of Horner's Syndrome

- Hemispherical lesions—hemispherectomy or massive infarction
- Brainstem lesions—lateral medullary syndrome (vascular), multiple sclerosis, pontine glioma, brainstem encephalitis
- Cervical cord lesions—syringomyelia, glioma, ependymoma
- D_1 root lesions—primary and metastatic tumour of lung apex (Pancoast's tumour), cervical rib, Klumpke's paralysis
- Sympathetic chain—neoplastic infiltration, surgery of larynx or thyroid, malignant disease near foramen lacerum or carotid canal, carotid artery dissection
- Miscellaneous—congenital Horner's syndrome, Raeder paratrigeminal neuralgia

Q. Discuss the aetiology, pathology, clinical features, differential diagnosis and management of Bell's palsy. (EN 4.18)

- Aetiology is not definitely known. Herpes simplex virus and herpes zoster are suspected.
- Pathologically, oedema and swelling of the nerve occur within the facial canal, often at stylomastoid foramen. Severity in a given case varies from simple conduction block to severe axonal degeneration.

CLINICAL FEATURES

- Onset is acute (over a day to a week or so; often reaches maximum severity in 72 hours). Sometimes history of exposure to cold is present. Mild pain at stylomastoid foramen for a few days may precede the palsy. Examination shows isolated lower motor neuron facial paralysis with or without loss of taste sensation at anterior two-thirds of tongue and hyperacusis.

FEATURES OF LOWER MOTOR FACIAL NERVE PALSY

- Paralysis of all the muscles of facial expression on the side of palsy.
- Drooping of corner of mouth, effacement of creases and skin fold on the affected side.
- Weakness of frowning and eye closure as the upper facial muscles are weak.
- Drooling of saliva from angle of mouth.
- On asking the patient to show his/her teeth, the angle of mouth deviates away from the side of lesion.
- On attempted closure of the eyelid, the eye on the paralysed side rolls upwards (Bell's phenomenon).
- Corneal ulceration due to inability to close the eye during sleep.

DIFFERENTIAL DIAGNOSIS

- Herpes zoster of the seventh nerve (Ramsay Hunt syndrome).
- Middle ear disease with seventh nerve compression.
- Trauma.
- Occasional case of intracanalicular seventh nerve neuroma.
- Diabetic mononeuropathy.
- Upper motor neuron seventh nerve palsy as in cerebrovascular accident (frontalis is spared, normal furrowing of the brow is preserved, and eye closure and blinking are not affected).

INVESTIGATIONS

- No specific confirmatory diagnostic procedure.
- Electrophysiological tests [electromyography (EMG)] may help in prognostication.
- To rule out alternate diagnosis, appropriate diagnostic procedures may be necessary.

TREATMENT

- If patient is seen early (within 3 days), a short course of prednisolone may be given. Usually, prednisolone is given at 1 mg/kg/day for the first week, with the dosage tapering off over the second week.
- Addition of acyclovir does not alter recovery.
- Adhesive tape to keep the eye closed so as to prevent corneal ulceration.
- Surgical decompression in complete paralysis with >90% nerve degeneration on electrodiagnostic studies.

PROGNOSIS

- Majority recover very well (by more than 90%) if recovery starts within a few days. Poor prognosis is seen in elderly who show delayed recovery, those with hyperacusis or loss of taste sensation, and when severe axonal degeneration is suggested on electrophysiological studies. If no signs of recovery are seen at the end of 3 months, alternate diagnosis will have to be considered (seventh nerve neuroma).
- Those who recover may show signs of anomalous reinnervation resulting in 'crocodile tears' (tears when eating; occur due to misdirection of regenerating gustatory fibres destined for the salivary glands so that they become secretory fibres to the lacrimal gland and cause ipsilateral tearing while the patient is eating), 'jaw-winking' (involuntary mouth movement during voluntary eye closure), etc.

OTHER CAUSES OF LOWER MOTOR NEURON (LMN) FACIAL NERVE PALSY (Box 5.15)

BOX 5.15 Causes of LMN Facial Palsy Other Than Bell's Palsy

- Infections—varicella zoster virus (VZV), human immunodeficiency virus, Lyme disease
- Otitis media
- Benign and malignant tumours—parotid tumours, squamous cell carcinoma metastatic to the parotid gland, perineural tumour extension from minor salivary gland neoplasm, facial nerve schwannomas
- Autoimmune/inflammatory processes such as sarcoidosis
- Amyloidosis
- Guillain–Barre syndrome
- Trauma

WHAT IS NOT BELL'S PALSY IN LMN SEVENTH NERVE LESION? (Box 5.16)

BOX 5.16 Features Against Diagnosis of Bell's Palsy

- Progression at beyond 15 days
- Severe pain (herpes zoster)
- Any other associated neurological findings
- Evidence of ear disease
- Presence of diabetes
- No evidence of any recovery at 3 months
- Bilateral facial palsy at onset

Q. Describe the aetiology, clinical features and treatment of Ramsay Hunt syndrome (geniculate herpes).

AETIOLOGY

- Reactivation of herpes zoster of geniculate ganglion.

CLINICAL FEATURES

- Onset is with severe pain in external ear, followed by appearance of vesicles in the external auditory meatus, and occasionally on tongue and pharynx, along with ipsilateral LMN facial paralysis (Box 5.17). Eighth nerve palsy may be associated leading to nausea, vomiting, vertigo, nystagmus, tinnitus and hearing loss. Cranial nerves V, IX and X may also be involved.
- Complete recovery is less likely than in Bell's palsy.

TREATMENT

- Analgesics.
- Oral acyclovir 800 mg five times a day is useful if started early (within 72 hours) along with corticosteroids.

BOX 5.17 Triad of Ramsay Hunt Syndrome

- Ipsilateral facial paralysis
- Ear pain
- Vesicles in the auditory canal

- Other agents are famciclovir (500 mg three times a day) and valaciclovir (1 g three times a day).
- Prednisolone (1 mg/kg) is often added to antiviral agents.
- Idoxuridine (5% solution) may be applied over the vesicles in early stages.

Q. Briefly outline the course of facial nerve. What are the various levels at which facial nerve can get damaged? How will you clinically differentiate between the lesions at different sites? (AN 28.7)

COURSE OF FACIAL NERVE

- Fig. 5.5 depicts the course of facial nerve along with its supranuclear connections in the opposite cortex.

FEATURES OF FACIAL NERVE LESIONS AT VARIOUS SITES (Table 5.18)

Q. Write a brief note on Argyll Robertson pupil.

- Describes the pupillary change where accommodation reflex is present but light reflex is impaired.
  - Pupils are small, irregular and unequal in size.
  - Atrophy and depigmentation of iris is seen.
  - Light reflex is absent for direct (always) and consensual (usually) stimulus.
  - Accommodation reflex is intact.
  - Ciliospinal reflex is absent.
- Tropicamide often has little or no effect on pupillary size; phenylephrine, which actively stimulates the iris dilators, is often required for pupillary dilatation.
- Site of lesion is believed to be at tectum of the midbrain or peripherally in the branch of the third nerve.
- Causes are given in Box 5.18.

Q. What is Adie's pupil or tonic pupil?

- Common cause of anisocoria or unequal pupils.
- Reaction to light is absent or greatly diminished when tested in the routine examination; however, Adie's pupil does react slowly with prolonged maximal stimulation.
- Reacts better to accommodation (near response), such that the initially larger Adie pupil becomes smaller than the other normal pupil. Once the Adie's pupil constricts to accommodation, the pupil tends to remain tonically constricted and dilates very slowly.
- Instillation of pilocarpine causes rapid constriction (cholinergic supersensitivity).
- Caused by parasympathetic denervation due to ciliary ganglion destruction. Most cases are idiopathic.
- Patients may have decreased deep tendon reflexes in the complete Holmes–Adie syndrome.
- Most patients with a tonic pupil do not require any treatment.

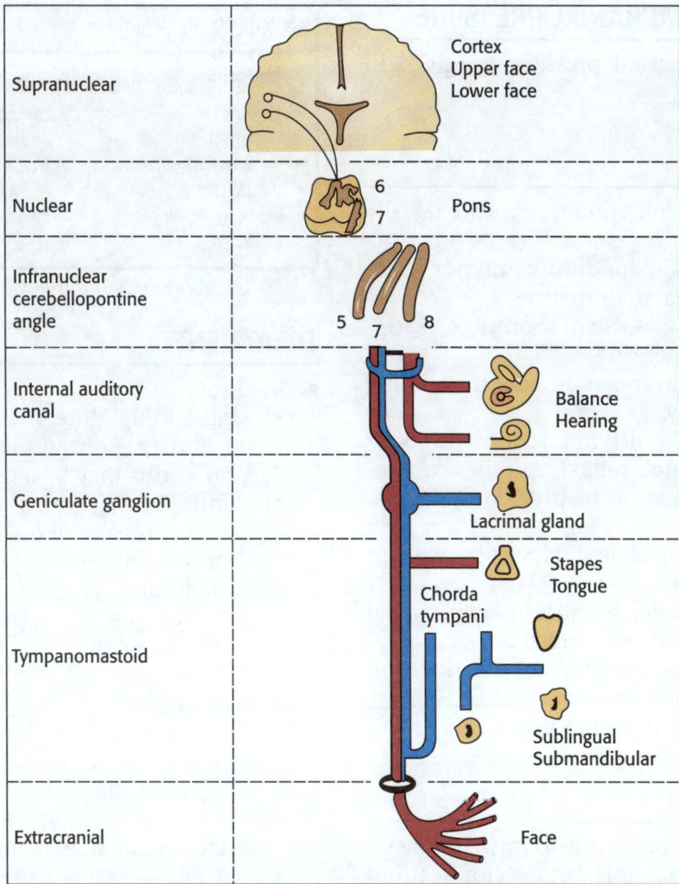

Fig. 5.5 Topographical anatomy of the facial nerve.

TABLE 5.18 Features of Facial Nerve Lesions at Various Sites

Site of Lesion	Clinical Manifestation
• Supranuclear	Contralateral upper motor neuron facial palsy and hemiparesis
• Nuclear	Ipsilateral lower motor neuron facial palsy and contralateral hemiparesis
• Cerebellopontine angle	Ipsilateral lower motor neuron facial palsy, sensorineural deafness, loss of corneal reflex (involvement of ophthalmic division of trigeminal nerve) and ipsilateral cerebellar signs
• Internal auditory canal	Lower motor neuron facial palsy, sensorineural deafness, tinnitus or dizziness
• Tympanomastoid	Lower motor neuron facial palsy with loss of taste at anterior two-thirds of tongue, with or without conduction deafness and hyperacusis
• Extracranial	Lower motor neuron facial palsy with intact taste sensation

BOX 5.18 Causes of Argyll Robertson Pupil

- Neurosyphilis (mainly in tabes dorsalis)—pupillary changes generally bilateral
- Diabetes
- Sarcoidosis
- Multiple sclerosis
- Tumours of pineal region

Q. Describe briefly the manifestations of raised intracranial pressure and its management.

Q. Discuss various brain herniation syndromes.

- Skull encloses tightly the brain tissue, CSF-containing spaces and blood in vessels. It is incompressible and, therefore, volume inside the cranium is fixed. Any increase in volume of one of the cranial constituents must be compensated by a decrease in volume of another. Initially, ICP does not rise due to compensatory decrease in other two components. However, after this limit is crossed, the ICP rises sharply leading to reduction in cerebral perfusion and displacement/compression of brain tissue. This is known as Monro–Kellie doctrine or hypothesis.
- Normal ICP is <15 mmHg.
- Cerebral perfusion pressure (CPP) depends on mean systemic arterial pressure (MAP) and ICP. An increase in ICP results in decrease in CPP. Through normal regulatory process (autoregulation), brain is able to maintain a normal cerebral blood flow (CBF) with a CPP ranging from 50 to 150 mmHg.

CAUSES OF RAISED INTRACRANIAL PRESSURE

- Causes of raised intracranial pressure are given in Table 5.19.

CLINICAL FEATURES

- Signs and symptoms of underlying cause are usually evident.
- Features due to raised ICP are diffuse anterior headache, vomiting and visual disturbances.
  - Headache—classically worse in mornings, exacerbated by coughing/sneezing.
  - Vomiting—typically in mornings and may relieve headache temporarily.
- If ICP has risen acutely, pulse rate is slower and BP may be elevated (Cushing's reflex). Another component is respiratory depression or irregularity (Cushing's triad).
- Raised ICP of more than a few days will result in papilloedema.
- Diplopia due to cranial nerve palsies—sixth cranial nerve particularly vulnerable to stretch.
- Other features are drowsiness, mental deterioration and seizures.
- Features of raised ICP are listed in Box 5.19.

HERNIATION SYNDROMES

- Herniation of brain can occur due to raised intracranial tension (ICT) and patients can develop features due to these syndromes (Table 5.20).
- Supratentorial herniations occur above the meningeal layer of the tentorium cerebelli and include central, uncal and subfalcine herniation.
- Infratentorial herniation occurs due to infratentorial lesions that may result in upward herniation of brainstem through tentorium (upward transtentorial herniation) or downward displacement of cerebellar tonsils through foramen magnum (tonsillar herniation).

INVESTIGATIONS

- Relevant to possible underlying pathology.
- CT head may show midline shift and compressed basal cisterns.
- ICP monitoring in selected cases (e.g. those with Glasgow Coma Scale ≤8 with CT scan showing haematoma, contusion, oedema, herniation or compressed basal cisterns).

BOX 5.19 Clinical Features of Raised Intracranial Pressure

Symptoms	Signs
• Headache • Vomiting • Drowsiness • Visual disturbances including diplopia • Seizures	• Depressed level of consciousness (lethargy, stupor, coma) • Papilloedema • Sixth cranial nerve palsy • Cushing's triad (hypertension, bradycardia and irregular respiration)

TREATMENT

- Medical:
  - Maintaining mean arterial pressure above 90 mmHg. Be cautious about treating hypertension as this may be a Cushing's response.
  - Administering normal saline to achieve a central venous pressure of 8–10 mmHg.
  - Osmotic diuretics or other diuretics.
    - Mannitol—1 g/kg/dose.
    - Glycerol—30 mL orally 6 or 8 hourly (only in mild cases).
    - Frusemide—20 mg 8 hourly (along with mannitol).
    - A total of 7.5% hypertonic saline (4 mL/kg) over 15–30 minutes (with monitoring of serum sodium).
  - Sedation and analgesia using short-acting benzodiazepines, fentanyl and propofol.
  - Steroids—dexamethasone 4 mg 6 hourly. Helps only in reducing vasogenic oedema around tumour, abscess or subdural haematoma. Routine administration of steroids should be avoided in patients with traumatic brain injury and raised ICP.
  - Elevation of head by 15°C–30°C, keeping it in midline to maximise cerebral venous drainage.
  - Anticonvulsant therapy should be instituted if seizures are suspected.
  - Barbiturate coma in refractory cases. It lowers ICP by lowering the rate of the body's metabolic process, oxygen consumption and carbon dioxide production. However, its efficacy is controversial.
  - Cooling to about 32°C–34°C may be helpful in refractory cases, although evidence is lacking.
  - Assisted ventilation to correct hypoxia and hypercarbia. Short durations of mild hyperventilation (PCO_2 30–35 mmHg) may be acceptable as a temporising measure until other methods of managing ICP are available. Prolonged hyperventilation has

TABLE 5.19 Causes of Raised Intracranial Pressure

Primary or Intracranial Causes	Secondary or Extracranial Causes
• Brain tumour • Trauma (epidural and subdural haematoma, cerebral contusion) • Nontraumatic intracerebral haemorrhage • Ischaemic stroke • Hydrocephalus (due to tumours or adhesions obstructing CSF flow) • Idiopathic or benign intracranial hypertension or pseudotumour cerebri • Major sinus vein occlusion • Other (e.g. pneumocephalus, abscess) • Postneurosurgery	• Hypoxia or hypercarbia (hypoventilation) • Hyperpyrexia • Seizure • Drug and toxins (e.g. tetracycline, valproate sodium, lead intoxication) • Hepatic failure • Reye's syndrome • High-altitude cerebral oedema • Hypertensive encephalopathy

TABLE 5.20 Herniation Syndrome

Herniation Syndrome	Mechanism	Features
Subfalcine herniation	Herniation of ipsilateral cingulate gyrus underneath the falx cerebri; caused by mass effect in the ipsilateral cerebral hemisphere	• Medial frontal lobe dysfunction producing abulia, emergence of frontal release signs and loss of initiative • In severe cases, unilateral or bilateral compression of the anterior cerebral arteries, leading to unilateral or rarely bilateral leg weakness, and acute urinary retention
Central transtentorial herniation	Brain swelling or an expanding space-occupying lesion that displaces medial temporal lobes along the brainstem through tentorial notch, resulting in compression and lengthening of the diencephalon	• Initial—alteration in consciousness, Cheyne–Stokes respiration, bilateral small pupils, normal oculovestibular reflexes, decorticate posture (occur due to compression of diencephalon) • Later—hyperventilation, midpositioned and fixed pupils, abnormal oculovestibular reflex, decerebrate posture in response to noxious stimulation (occur due to compression of midbrain and pons) • Terminal—ataxic breathing, coma and death (occur due to dysfunction of pons and medulla)
Uncal herniation	An expanding mass lesion in a temporal lobe or lateral part of the cranial vault (including epidural and subdural haematomas) that forces uncus of the temporal lobe downwards and over the edge of the tentorium	• Initial—ipsilateral pupillary dilatation with sluggish reaction (occurs due to compression of outer pupillary part of the third cranial nerve) • Later—complete third nerve palsy, abnormal oculovestibular reflex, hyperventilation and decorticate or decerebrate posturing; ipsilateral hemiparesis (due to compression of contralateral cerebral peduncle against the edge of the tentorium; a false localising sign known as Kernohan's notch) • Terminal—hyperventilation, dilated and fixed contralateral pupil, absent oculovestibular reflex (due to compression of midbrain and upper pons), death
Upward transtentorial herniation	Infratentorial lesions that result in upward herniation of cerebellum through tentorium resulting in compression of midbrain	• Early—hyperventilation, decorticate and decerebrate posturing, vomiting, small fixed pupils, and absent vertical doll's eye movements with brisk horizontal responses • Later—dilated, fixed pupils, coma • Terminal—death
Tonsillar herniation	Cerebellar tonsils herniate downward through foramen magnum compressing on medulla and upper cervical cord	• Early—headache, neck stiffness • Later—flaccid paralysis, reduced consciousness, respiratory failure • Terminal—coma, sudden death

been associated with exacerbation of cerebral ischaemia. Should be avoided in patients with stroke or brain injury.
  - Medical therapy should also include management of underlying cause wherever applicable.
- Surgical management:
  - Management of underlying cause.
  - Removal of space-occupying lesion.
  - External ventricular drainage, ventriculoatrial or ventriculoperitoneal shunting in hydrocephalus.
  - Decompressive craniectomy.

Q. Write a short note on cerebellopontine angle tumours.

Q. What is acoustic neuroma?

CEREBELLOPONTINE ANGLE

- Cerebellopontine (CP) angle is the area of lateral cistern containing CSF, arachnoid tissue, cranial nerves and their associated vessels. The borders of CP angle are as follows:
  - Medial border—lateral surface of the brainstem.
  - Lateral border—petrous bone.
  - Superior border—middle cerebellar peduncle and cerebellum.
  - Inferior border—arachnoid tissue of lower cranial nerves.
  - Posterior—cerebellar peduncle.

BOX 5.20 Various Cerebellopontine Angle Mass Lesions

- Acoustic neuroma or schwannoma (more than 80%)
- Meningioma
- Seventh or fifth nerve neuromas
- Epidermoid tumour
- Giant basilar aneurysm
- Cerebellar glioma
- Pontine glioma
- Nasopharyngeal tumour extension
- Metastatic tumours (very rare)
- Cholesteatoma
- Epidermoid cyst

VARIOUS CP ANGLE TUMOURS

- CP angle tumours are the most common posterior fossa tumours (Box 5.20). Majority are benign.

CLINICAL FEATURES OF CP ANGLE TUMOURS

- Combination of involvement of eighth, seventh and ophthalmic branch of fifth, with or without ipsilateral cerebellar signs, is the hallmark of CP angle lesion.
- Common presenting features are ipsilateral hearing loss, tinnitus, vertigo, unsteadiness and facial hypoaesthesia. The Weber and Rinne tests may be useful in suggesting asymmetric sensorineural hearing impairment.
- Facial weakness is uncommon.
- Tumours later will result in raised ICP by displacing brainstem and obstructing CSF flow.

- Large tumours can compress cerebellum resulting in ipsilateral ataxia.
- In some cases, there may be signs of brainstem compression, particularly contralateral hemiparesis.
- May result in IX and X nerve palsies when tumour is very large.

ACOUSTIC NEUROMA

- Acoustic neuroma (or vestibular schwannoma) is a benign primary intracranial tumour of the myelin-forming cells called 'Schwann cells' of the eighth cranial nerve.
- May occur sporadically, or in some cases occurs as part of von Recklinghausen neurofibromatosis in which case it may take on one of the following two forms:
    - Neurofibromatosis type I occurs usually in adult life and may involve the eighth nerve or any other cranial nerve or the spinal root. Bilateral acoustic neuromas are rare in this type.
    - Neurofibromatosis type II usually occurs before the age of 20 years. Bilateral acoustic neuromas are the hallmark. This type shows autosomal dominant inheritance.

INVESTIGATIONS

- Radiograph of skull—periorbital view for internal acoustic canal or foramen.
- Audiometry and brainstem auditory evoked responses (BAER).
- CT scan (with IV contrast).
- MRI with gadolinium enhancement.

TREATMENT

- Surgical excision.
- Stereotactic radiosurgery (gamma knife—multiple convergent beams to deliver a single, high dose of radiation) is used in small tumours or in elderly or sick patients who are unable to tolerate brain surgery. Others include stereotactic radiotherapy (focused doses of radiation given over a series of treatment sessions) and proton beam therapy.

Q. Mention the causes of intracranial space-occupying lesions and describe the signs and symptoms of such lesions.

CAUSES

- Intracranial space-occupying lesions can develop acutely within days or more slowly (Table 5.21).

TABLE 5.21 Causes of Intracranial Space-Occupying Lesions

Acute to subacute lesions (developing within days and weeks):	
• Subdural haematoma • Glioblastoma • Metastatic brain tumours • Cerebral abscess and granulomas	
Chronic lesions:	

Extracerebral
• Meningioma
• Neurofibroma
• Pituitary adenoma
• Craniopharyngioma
• Base of the skull tumours
• Pinealoma (children)
Intraventricular
• Ependymoma
• Colloid cyst
• Meningioma
	Intracerebral
	• Gliomas
	  • Astrocytoma
	  • Oligodendroglioma
	  • Glioblastoma
	• Haemangioma
	• Medulloblastoma (children)
	• Lymphoma
	• Large aneurysms
	• Tuberculoma
	• Neurocysticercosis

CLINICAL FEATURES

- Rapidly growing tumours produce nonlocalising features in the form of apathy, clouding of consciousness, global deterioration in intellect with or without features of raised ICP and seizures.
- Subacute or chronic lesions produce the following features:
    - Specific syndromes due to the lesion compressing on adjacent neural structures include the following:
        - Cerebellopontine angle syndrome.
        - Sellar, suprasellar and parasellar syndromes (bitemporal hemianopia, scotomas, ophthalmoplegia, hypogonadism, hypothyroidism, temperature dysregulation, sleep disorders, diabetes insipidus and features of raised intracranial tension).
        - Orbital fissure syndrome (proptosis, reduced acuity, pupillary changes and limited eye movements).
        - Foster–Kennedy syndrome (papilloedema in one eye and optic atrophy in the other; results from simultaneous raised ICP and optic nerve compression secondary to tumour—meningioma of the olfactory groove or sphenoid wing).
        - Intracerebral tumours result in hemiparesis, aphasia, hemianopia, cerebellar signs and brainstem signs depending on their location.
    - Features of raised ICP are headache, vomiting and papilloedema. Tumours located close to ventricular system produce early rise in ICP by blocking CSF flow even when the size of the tumour is small. Elsewhere, tumours have to be large enough to produce raised ICP.
    - False localising signs appear after raised ICP occurs. They are the following:
        - Sixth nerve palsy (unilateral or bilateral).
        - Pyramidal disturbances (ipsilateral or contralateral side).
        - Third nerve palsy.
        - Rarely seventh and eighth nerve palsy.
- Seizures occur in supratentorial lesions.
    - Low-grade gliomas present more frequently with seizures than high-grade primary brain tumours or metastases.
    - Cortical tumours more likely cause seizures than infratentorial, deep grey or white matter lesions.
- If the tumour is metastatic, features of primary neoplasm are evident. Common primary tumours resulting in brain metastasis are from lung, bowel, kidney, breast and thyroid.

- If the space-occupying lesion is inflammatory, source of infection may be evident (middle ear disease, lung abscess, bronchiectasis, abscess elsewhere in the body, cyanotic heart disease, tuberculosis elsewhere in the body, etc.).
- Risk of deep venous thrombosis and pulmonary embolism is increased in patients with tumours.

INVESTIGATIONS

- Skull radiography:
  - It shows features of raised ICP at sella with shift of calcified pineal gland. Calcification within tumours may be seen.
- CT scan:
  - It allows localisation of the tumour, its size, characters, etc., allowing identification of nature of underlying pathology in most of the cases.
- MRI:
  - Detects early gliomas and posterior fossa tumours by eliminating bone artefacts (a disadvantage with CT scan).
- Angiography:
  - Occasionally required to study vascularity of tumour or to rule out giant aneurysms that mimic or act as space-occupying lesions.
- Investigations to look for primary site of malignancy when metastatic tumour is suspected.
- PET scan.
- Single-photon emission computed tomography (SPECT) scan using various tracers (e.g. 99m-Tc-glucoheptonate) to differentiate neoplastic intracranial lesions from non-neoplastic ones. Also useful to distinguish tumour recurrence from tumour necrosis that can occur with radiotherapy.

TREATMENT

- Seizure control.
- Control of raised ICP.
- Surgical removal to the extent possible.
- Radiotherapy is indicated in all malignant and some benign lesions.
- Chemotherapy in malignant neoplasm. Temozolomide is the most often used agent.
- Antibacterial agents in infective lesions.
- Prophylaxis with heparin/oral anticoagulants for patients who have lower limb immobility.

Q. What are primary and secondary headaches? (IM 17.1)

- A primary headache has no known underlying cause while a secondary headache is the result of another condition causing traction on or inflammation of pain-sensitive structures.
- The most common primary headaches include migraine, tension-type headache and cluster headache.
- Headaches related to infection, vascular disease, trauma, substance withdrawal, giant cell arteritis, etc., are common causes of secondary headache.

Q. Discuss the classification, pathogenesis, clinical features and management of migraine. (IM 17.3)

- Migraine is characterised by periodic headaches, typically unilateral, often associated with visual disturbance and vomiting.

CLASSIFICATION (Box 5.21)

BOX 5.21 Classification of Migraine

CLASSICAL MIGRAINE:
- Visual or sensory symptoms precede or accompany the headache

COMMON MIGRAINE:
- No visual or sensory features
- Headache, nausea, vomiting and photophobia occur

BASILAR MIGRAINE:
- Occipital headache, preceded by vertigo, diplopia and dysarthria, ±visual and sensory symptoms (brainstem symptoms)

HEMIPLEGIC MIGRAINE:
- Prolonged headache lasting hours or days
- Aura consisting of fully reversible hemiparesis and at least one of the following: fully reversible visual symptoms; fully reversible sensory symptoms; fully reversible dysphasic speech disturbance

TYPICAL AURA WITHOUT HEADACHE:
- Presence of migraine aura without headache (visual aura most common)

RETINAL MIGRAINE:
- Repeated attacks of monocular visual disturbance, including scintillations, scotomata or blindness associated with or followed by migraine headache

PATHOGENESIS

- Multiple environmental and genetic factors combine to induce cerebral electrical and vascular changes. Many neurotransmitters seem to be involved (e.g. serotonin, noradrenaline and substance P).
- Initiated by spreading waves of depolarisation from either cortex or brainstem. These central processes generate meningeal neurogenic inflammation and vasodilation, which in turn activates nociceptive afferents that carry the pain signals through the trigeminal ganglion to trigeminal nucleus caudalis in the trigeminocervical complex.
- Meningeal neurogenic inflammatory changes include the release of calcitonin gene-related peptide (CGRP), a profound endogenous vasodilator, and initiation of the arachidonic acid cascade.
- Aura is also thought to be caused by cortical spreading depression. It is associated with a localised reduction in blood flow followed by an increase in blood flow and characteristically affects the parieto-occipital cortex.

PRECIPITATING FACTORS

- 'Anything under the sun including sun' can precipitate an attack, but each person has his/her own triggering factors.

- Commonly, these are stress, exposure to bright light, loud noises, smoke or strong scents, menstruation, lack or excess of sleep, cheese, caffeine, alcohol, chocolate, citrus fruit and food additives such as monosodium glutamate, vasodilators, exercise and contraceptive pills.
- Familial tendency is usual.

CLINICAL FEATURES

- Attacks are episodic and start at puberty and continue till late middle life with variable degree of spontaneous remissions. Frequency, duration and severity of attacks vary in the same individual.
- Headache is typically hemicranial, throbbing in character, and associated with nausea and vomiting.
- In classical migraine, headache is preceded by an aura that is a focal neurological disturbance manifesting as visual aura (flashing lights or scintillating spots that may cross visual field over minutes, scotoma), sensory aura or language aura.
  - Both sensory and visual auras have a slow migratory or spreading quality in which symptoms slowly spread across the affected body part or the visual field, followed by a gradual return to normal function in the areas first affected after 20–60 minutes. In contrast, in an ischaemic event, neurological deficits tend to appear somewhat suddenly and tend to be equally distributed within the relevant vascular territory.
  - In migraine aura, different neurological symptoms tend to occur sequentially (e.g. visual aura followed by sensory aura). In contrast, simultaneous manifestation of multiple types of neurological symptoms is quite common in cerebral ischaemia.
  - In migraine aura, positive features (e.g. scintillations) are followed by negative symptoms (e.g. scotoma) instead of occurring simultaneously.
- Allodynia (production of pain from normally non-painful stimuli) is an extremely common phenomenon in migraine, occurring in about two-thirds of patients.
- Severe attacks are associated with photophobia and prostration. The attack spontaneously terminates after a few hours or sleep.

DIAGNOSTIC CRITERIA (Box 5.22 and Box 5.23)

BOX 5.22 Diagnostic Criteria for Common Migraine

Repeated attacks (at least five attacks) of headache lasting 4–72 hours that have the following features:

- Normal physical examination
- No other reasonable cause for the headache
- Headache has at least two of the following:
  - Unilateral pain
  - Throbbing or pulsatile pain
  - Aggravation by or causing avoidance of routine physical activity (e.g. walking or climbing stairs)
- At least one of the following during headache:
  - Nausea or vomiting
  - Photophobia and phonophobia

BOX 5.23 Diagnostic Criteria for Classical Migraine

Repeated attacks (at least two attacks) of headache lasting 4–72 hours that have the following features:

- Normal physical examination
- No other reasonable cause for the headache
- Aura consisting of at least one of the following, but no motor weakness:
  - Fully reversible visual symptoms including positive features (e.g. flickering lights, spots or lines) and/or negative features (e.g. loss of vision)
  - Fully reversible sensory symptoms including positive features (e.g. pins and needles) and/or negative features (e.g. numbness)
  - Fully reversible dysphasic speech disturbance
  - Brainstem features
  - Retinal symptoms
- At least three of the following:
  - At least one aura symptom developing gradually over ≥5 minutes
  - Two or more aura symptoms occurring in succession
  - Each aura symptom lasting >5 and ≤60 minutes
  - At least one unilateral aura symptom
  - At least one positive aura symptom
  - Headache begins during aura or follows aura within 60 minutes

BOX 5.24 Dangerous Features of Headache in a Patient Known to Have Migraine

- Rapidly increasing frequency of headache
- Abrupt onset of severe headache
- Marked change in headache pattern
- Headache awakening the patient from sleep
- Triggered by Valsalva manoeuvre, cough, exertion or sexual activity
- Associated incoordination
- Presence of focal neurological signs or symptoms
- Associated fever, neck stiffness
- Associated with tenderness over temporal artery
- Associated with altered sensorium, seizures

DANGEROUS FEATURES OF HEADACHE IN A PATIENT KNOWN TO HAVE MIGRAINE ('RED FLAGS')

- Certain features associated with headache require special attention if they occur in a patient known to have migraine (Box 5.24).

TREATMENT

- Explain that headache has no sinister prognosis (significance).
- Trigger factors like bright light and dietary precipitants are avoided. Keeping a headache diary can help in this regard.

DRUGS USEFUL IN ACUTE MIGRAINE (Table 5.22)

- Initiate with an NSAID.
- Use a triptan, if no relief with an NSAID previously.
- Avoid use of opioids.
- Medication-overuse headache can occur with overuse of drugs used in acute migraine.

TABLE 5.22 Drugs Useful in Migraine

Drug	Dose	Remarks
• Paracetamol/aspirin/ibuprofen/naproxen	1 g/600 mg/600 mg/500 mg	Should be initial line of treatment
• Ketorolac	30–60 mg IM	Nonsedating; can produce GI bleed
• Ergotamine	1 mg orally; can be repeated to a maximum of 3 mg/day and 5 mg/week	Use at the beginning of headache/prodrome Contraindications: Pregnancy and coronary or peripheral vascular disease Avoid if neurological defects are present Avoid using on 2 consecutive days
• Dihydroergotamine	1 mg SC, IM or IV; can be repeated to a maximum of 3 mg/day and 5 mg/week	Same as ergotamine
• Prochlorperazine	12.5 mg IM	Effective in nearly 75% of cases; can produce extrapyramidal features
• Metoclopramide	10–20 mg IV slowly	Also has antiemetic properties; can produce extrapyramidal features
• Sumatriptan (also available in combination with naproxen)	50–100 mg orally, 6 mg SC, 20 mg nasal spray	See 'Triptans' in text
• Zolmitriptan	2.5–5 mg orally, 5 mg nasal spray	See 'Triptans' in text
• Rizatriptan	5–10 mg	See 'Triptans' in text
• Dexamethasone	4–8 mg IM/IV	Nonsedating
• Magnesium	1 g IV	Works best for patients with aura
• Rimegepant	75 mg orally	Antagonist of the CGRP receptor; can produce nausea, somnolence, dry mouth, hypersensitivity reactions, hepatic impairment
• Ubrogepant	50–100 mg orally	See 'Rimegepant' above
• Lasmiditan	50–100 mg orally	Serotoninergic agonists with specific affinity towards 5-HT1F receptors (5-HT1F agonist); can produce dizziness, somnolence, impaired driving, tingling or numb sensation on the skin, fatigue

Triptans

- There are seven different triptans—almotriptan, eletriptan, frovatriptan (slower onset), naratriptan (slower onset), rizatriptan, sumatriptan and zolmitriptan.
- These are 5-HT1B/1D receptor agonists that work via the serotonin 1D receptors to inhibit CGRP and inflammatory peptide release in the meninges and prevent the pain signal from returning from the periphery to the trigeminal nucleus caudalis. They also work via the 5-HT1B receptor to constrict vessels dilated by CGRP. Because there are some 5-HT1B receptors in coronary and other arteries, triptans are contraindicated in patients who have vascular disease.
- All triptans are available for oral use. Sumatriptan can also be given parenterally as well as by nasal spray. Zolmitriptan is also available as nasal spray.
- Should be given at the onset of headache to achieve maximum efficacy. A second dose should not be given within 2 hours if first dose is not effective.
- Side effects include tingling, flushing and sensations of warmth, heaviness, pressure or tightness in different parts of the body including the chest and neck, shortness of breath and palpitations. Triptans can constrict the coronary arteries and in rare instances may cause myocardial ischaemia.
- They are contraindicated in patients with ischaemic heart disease, uncontrolled hypertension, cerebrovascular disease, peripheral vascular disease, or hemiplegic or basilar migraine. Also contraindicated in pregnancy.
- They are compatible with most other medications. However, avoid ergotamine within 24 hours of their use.

NONINVASIVE NEUROMODULATORY APPROACHES

- Noninvasive neuromodulatory approaches for aborting an acute attack include single-pulse transcranial magnetic stimulation (s-TMS), external trigeminal nerve stimulation (e-TNS), noninvasive vagus nerve stimulation and remote electrical neuromodulation.

DRUG PROPHYLAXIS

INDICATIONS (Box 5.25)

- Prophylaxis may be attempted with any of the drugs listed in Table 5.23.

Q. Write a short note on cluster headache. (IM 17.1)

- Usually occurs in young adult males.
- Precise mechanism not known; cluster headache is associated with trigeminovascular activation, and neuroendocrine and vegetative disturbances. Involvement of hypothalamus may explain the cyclic aspects of cluster headache.

BOX 5.25 Indications of Drug Prohylaxis in Migraine

- Recurring migraine that significantly interferes with a patient's quality of life and daily routine despite acute treatment
- Four or more attacks per month
- Failure of, contraindication to or troublesome side effects from acute medications
- Frequent, extremely long or uncomfortable auras

TABLE 5.23 Drugs Useful in Prophylaxis of Migraine

Drug	Dose	Comments
• Propranolol	40–60 mg TID	May be avoided in migraine with aura
• Metoprolol	25–100 mg BID	May be avoided in migraine with aura
• Atenolol	25–100 mg OD	May be avoided in migraine with aura
• Pizotifen	0.5–2 mg at bedtime	Can produce weight gain, drowsiness
• Amitriptyline	25–100 mg at bedtime	Sedating but effective
• Flunarizine	5–10 mg OD at bedtime	Can produce weight gain, somnolence, dry mouth, dizziness, hypotension, exacerbation of depression
• Cyproheptadine	2–8 mg OD	Used in children
• Gabapentin	900–3600 mg/day	Sedating particularly in elderly
• Valproate	400–600 mg BID	Weight gain
• Topiramate	25–100 mg BID	Do not use in pregnancy
• Verapamil	80 mg TID	Useful in presence of prolonged aura
• Methysergide	1 to 2 mg TID	Used in resistant cases Prolonged use may produce retroperitoneal and mediastinal fibrosis
• Erenumab	70 mg SC once monthly	Monoclonal antibody that targets calcitonin gene-related peptide (CGRP) receptor Contraindicated in coronary heart disease, cerebrovascular disease, inflammatory bowel disease
• Eptinezumab	100 mg or 300 mg IV once quarterly	Monoclonal antibody that targets CGRP
• Galcanezumab	240 mg SC initial loading dose and then 120 mg SC once monthly	Monoclonal antibody that targets CGRP
• Fremanezumab	225 mg SC once monthly or 675 mg once quarterly	Monoclonal antibody that targets CGRP

- Familial in about 10% of cases. Having a first-degree relative with cluster headache increases the risk 14-fold to 40-fold.
- Two types:
    - Chronic: At least one cluster period lasting at least 1 year, with no remission or remission of less than 3 months.
    - Episodic: At least two cluster periods of at least 1 week but less than 1 year, with remission for at least 3 months.

CLINICAL FEATURES

- Characterised by recurrent, short-lasting attacks (15–180 minutes) of excruciating unilateral periorbital pain.
- Often accompanied by ipsilateral autonomic signs (lacrimation, nasal congestion, ptosis, miosis, lid oedema, forehead and facial sweating, and redness of the eye).
- Circadian periodicity with attacks being clustered in bouts that can occur during specific months of the year.
- Alcohol, strong odours and napping may trigger headache.
- Attacks may happen at precise hours, especially during the night.

DIAGNOSTIC CRITERIA (Box 5.26)

BOX 5.26 Diagnostic Criteria for Cluster Headache

A. At least five attacks fulfilling B through D listed next
B. Severe or very severe unilateral orbital, supraorbital and/or temporal pain lasting 15–180 minutes if untreated
C. Headache is accompanied by at least one of the following:
  1. Ipsilateral conjunctival injection and/or lacrimation
  2. Ipsilateral nasal congestion and/or rhinorrhoea
  3. Ipsilateral eyelid oedema
  4. Ipsilateral forehead and facial sweating
  5. Ipsilateral miosis and/or ptosis
  6. A sense of restlessness or agitation
D. Attacks have a frequency from one every other day to eight per day

TREATMENT

- Treatment is not curative:
    - Acute treatment by subcutaneous sumatriptan, intranasal zolmitriptan and high-flow oxygen (7–15 L/minute).
    - Prophylaxis by verapamil, lithium, melatonin, prednisone, topiramate, greater occipital nerve

block and noninvasive vagus nerve stimulation. Prednisone and greater occipital nerve block are also used as bridging therapy while prophylactic treatment takes its effect.
- Galcanezumab, a humanised monoclonal antibody against CGRP is approved for preventive treatment of episodic cluster headache.
- Deep brain stimulation in refractory cases.

Q. Classify epilepsy. Discuss the aetiology, clinical features, diagnosis and management of idiopathic epilepsy.

Q. Describe petit mal epilepsy and its treatment.

Q. What is Jacksonian epilepsy?

DEFINITION OF EPILEPSY

- Epilepsy is a brief recurrent disorder of cerebral function that is usually associated with disturbance of consciousness and accompanied by a sudden, excessive electrical discharge of cerebral neurons. Electroencephalography (EEG) is of high voltage relative to the background.
- Clinically, epilepsy is defined as a condition characterised by any of the following conditions:
  - At least two unprovoked seizures occurring >24 hours apart.
  - One unprovoked seizure and a probability of further seizures similar to the general recurrence risk (at least 60%) after two unprovoked seizures, occurring over the next 10 years.
  - Diagnosis of an epilepsy syndrome (types of epilepsy in which a clear demographic, seizure type(s), EEG pattern, and prognosis are known).

CLASSIFICATION (INTERNATIONAL LEAGUE AGAINST EPILEPSY, 2017)

- Epilepsy is classified based on the onset: focal or generalised (Table 5.24).
- In focal onset seizure (previously known as partial seizure), the seizure activity starts focally in the cerebral cortex and may or may not spread to rest of the brain. In focal onset aware seizure (simple partial seizures), awareness is retained while in focal onset impaired awareness seizure (complex seizures), awareness is impaired.
- In primary generalised onset seizure, the seizure activity appears abruptly and involves entire brain simultaneously. There is no aura. EEG shows synchronous bilateral discharges.

TABLE 5.24 Classification of Epilepsy

Focal Onset	Generalised Onset	Unknown Onset
AWARE/ IMPAIRED AWARENESS		
Motor onset	**Motor**	**Motor**
• Automatism	• Tonic–clonic	• Tonic–clonic
• Atonic	• Clonic	• Epileptic spasms
• Clonic	• Tonic	**Nonmotor**
• Epileptic spasms	• Myoclonic	• Behaviour arrest
• Hyperkinetic	• Myoclonic–tonic–clonic	
• Myoclonic	• Myoclonic–atonic	
• Tonic	• Atonic	
Nonmotor onset	• Epileptic spasms	
• Automatic	**Nonmotor (absence)**	
• Behaviour arrest	• Typical	
• Cognitive	• Atypical	
• Emotional	• Myoclonic	
• Sensory	• Eyelid myoclonia	
FOCAL TO BILATERAL TONIC–CLONIC		

(*Source: Epilepsia*, 58(4):531–542, Figure 2, Wiley Periodicals, Inc., 2017.)

AETIOLOGY

- Epilepsy is due to a population of abnormal hyperexcitable neurons. Such neurons are subject to excitatory and inhibitory influences from other sources. Excitatory transmitters depolarise and inhibitory transmitters hyperpolarise the neuronal membrane. The discharge is governed by the balance between these two opposing factors.
  - Acetylcholine is the excitatory transmitter.
  - GABA is the inhibitory transmitter.
- Epilepsies may be primary or secondary (symptomatic).

PRIMARY

- In majority of cases, epilepsy is idiopathic and the cause is not known. There may be a positive family history; onset is often in childhood and has a genetic background.

SECONDARY (SYMPTOMATIC)

- Any intracranial disease like cerebral tumours, head injury, cerebrovascular accidents and CNS infections.
- Hypoglycaemia, hyperglycaemia, hyponatraemia.
- Uraemia, heart block.
- Ingestion or withdrawal of alcohol or drugs.

CLINICAL FEATURES

GENERALISED ONSET SEIZURES (PRIMARY GENERALISED SEIZURES)

- Electrical abnormality occurs simultaneously over the entire cerebral cortex and is recognised clinically and electroencephalographically.

Tonic–Clonic Seizures

- There is an altered consciousness at the onset that may be associated with an epileptic cry. Fit starts simultaneously with generalised tonic state that lasts for few seconds to minutes. Patient is unconscious and cyanosed, does not breathe (as glottis is closed and respiratory muscles are in tonic contraction) and pupils are dilated. Heart rate changes and may even stop. This is followed by clonic state where rhythmic jerks appear and last for 1 to few minutes. Tongue may be bitten and urinary or bowel incontinence may occur. (Tonic state occurs during continuous

discharge from the cortex when synchronous continuous excitatory activity starts. Clonic phase indicates appearance of inhibitory influence that breaks the continuous discharges to intermittent pattern.)
- This is followed by postictal phase where patient passes off into sleepy state and may have headache and vomiting. During initial few minutes, he/she is not arousable and may be totally flaccid. Plantar response is extensor and heart rate may be slow. On gradual recovery, he/she may be confused and show automatic behaviour. Whole phase may last from a few minutes to 1 to 2 hours.

Absence Seizures (Previously Called Petit Mal)

- Characteristic EEG pattern is synchronous generalised spike and slow-wave complex occurring at a frequency of 3/second.
- Three types of clinical manifestations are seen:
  1. Commonest variety (classical absence) is characterised by transient loss of consciousness. An interruption occurs in current activity and patient may stare blankly ahead. It lasts for 15–20 seconds only; being so brief, it may pass unnoticed. It invariably starts in childhood and may persist into adulthood. Attacks are frequent and up to 100 attacks per day may be seen. Most often there is spontaneous remission during adulthood. However, at times, absence seizure ceases and gives way to tonic–clonic seizures in adulthood.
  2. Brief loss of consciousness associated with myoclonic jerking of arms.
  3. Least common is called 'akinetic seizure'. Patient falls to ground, loses consciousness, recovers and rises up immediately.

Juvenile Myoclonic Epilepsy

- Juvenile myoclonic epilepsy (JME) is an idiopathic generalised epileptic syndrome characterised by myoclonic jerks, generalised tonic–clonic seizures (GTCSs) and sometimes absence seizures.
- Onset is around adolescence.
- Common precipitating factors include sleep deprivation and psychological stress.
- About 17%–49% of patients have a family history of epilepsy.
- The seizures usually occur shortly after awakening.
- Myoclonic jerks occur as the only seizure type in approximately 17% of patients with JME; the rest have additional GTCSs (80%) or absence seizures or both.
- Patient gets bilateral, single or repetitive, arrhythmic, irregular myoclonic jerks and predominantly in the arms. Jerks may cause some patients to fall suddenly. No disturbance of consciousness is noticeable.
- Intelligence remains normal.
- Patients usually require lifelong treatment with anticonvulsants. Valproic acid or lamotrigine is useful.

FOCAL ONSET SEIZURES (PARTIAL SEIZURES)

- Partial or focal onset seizure is a term used to describe abnormal electric activity only in a localised part of the brain.
- The patient may be fully aware (focal onset aware seizures—elementary symptoms occur with no change in consciousness) or may have impaired awareness (symptoms at onset are complex and are associated with altered awareness of the surroundings; this does not mean that patient will lose consciousness). These attacks may terminate as focal seizures or may develop into secondary bilateral, generalised tonic–clonic fits.

Focal Onset Aware Seizures (Simple Focal or Partial Seizures)

- Symptoms at onset may be motor (jerking of muscles at one area, head turning), sensory (paraesthesia), visual (flashes of light), auditory (ringing sound), gustatory, olfactory or autonomic. Further symptoms depend on the spread of seizure activity.

Jacksonian Seizures

- March of symptoms occurs where if it is motor, clonic jerking starts at a point, say face, and spreads to upper limb, then to lower limb and then on to opposite side to become a generalised fit. This denotes the path of spread of the epileptic activity and is called Jacksonian spread.

Focal Onset Impaired Awareness Seizures (Complex Partial Seizures)

- Complex symptoms at onset and is associated with altered awareness of the surroundings. Patients appear awake but do not meaningfully interact with people around them or respond normally to instructions or questions. Instead, patients seem to stare off into space and either remain still or demonstrate abnormal repetitive movements. Various features include the following:
  - Psychomotor (automatic, repetitive and nonpurposeful behaviour such as blinking, lip smacking, chewing, grunts, repetition of words or phrases, walking—automatism).
  - Psychosensory (complex formed sensory hallucinations).
  - Cognitive (altered perception of reality like depersonalisation, derealisation, e.g. déjà vu—the feeling of being familiar with particularly new situations or settings).
  - Affective (change in mood, euphoria, sadness, anger, etc.).
  - Consciousness (unawareness of surroundings).
- Typically, last for less than 3 minutes.
- May or may not progress to bilateral tonic–clonic (secondary generalised) seizures.

Focal to Bilateral Tonic–Clonic Seizures (Secondary Generalised Seizures)

- Attack starts with an aura (which actually denotes the site of onset of seizure discharge) that may be simple or complex, and is soon followed by loss of consciousness and GTCSs or generalised clonic seizures.
- Seizures with focal onset may have focal deficit during postictal period in the form of weakness on one side, focal sensory deficit, hemianopia, etc., which clears off over next few minutes to 1 to 2 hours. Presence of postictal focal deficit always suggests a focal

TABLE 5.25 Seizure Versus Syncope

Feature	Seizure	Syncope
• Circumstances	None	Prolonged standing, alcohol, heat, pain, cough, micturition
• Aura/prodrome	Variable	Visual blurring, tinnitus, nausea, dizziness, pallor, sweating
• Duration	1–5 minutes	10–30 seconds
• Muscle tone	Usually hypertonic	Hypotonic
• Motor features	Tonic/clonic, focal progressing to generalised movements	Myoclonic/clonic jerks may be present
• Tongue bite	Frequent	Rare
• Urine/faecal incontinence	Common	Uncommon
• Cardiovascular	Tachycardia	Bradycardia and hypotension
• Postictal confusion	Lasts for >1 minute	Lasts for a few seconds
• Postictal headache	Common, may be severe	Uncommon, short lasting
• Serum lactate	Elevated (within 2 hours of seizure)	Normal

onset of seizure activity. Postictal motor paralysis is called Todd's palsy.

REFLEX EPILEPSY

- At times, an epileptic attack may be precipitated by a sensory stimulus and may be easily reproduced. Common examples are the following:
  - Television epilepsy (occurs while watching television at close quarters).
  - Musicogenic (certain musical tones bring about the attack).
  - Eating.
  - Hot water (pouring hot water only over vertex).

DIAGNOSIS OF EPILEPSY

- Attempt should be made to find out:
  - Whether an attack is really an epileptic fit or some other brief disorder of consciousness or disorder of CNS, for example syncope, migraine, transient ischaemic attack, psychogenic nonepileptic spells (also known as psychogenic nonepileptic episodes; previously known as pseudoseizure), sleep disorders and movements disorders.
  - Differentiation of seizure from syncope is given in Table 5.25.
  - Psychogenic nonepileptic seizure—an observable abrupt paroxysmal change in behaviour or consciousness that resembles an epileptic seizure, but that is not accompanied by electrophysiological changes that accompany an epileptic seizure or clinical evidence of epilepsy, and for which no other evidence is found for other somatic causes of the seizures, whereas there is positive evidence or a strong suspicion for psychogenic factors that may have caused the seizure. Differentiation of seizure from psychogenic nonepileptic seizure is given in Table 5.26.
  - Type of fit—primary generalised, focal or secondary generalised (presence of aura, change in consciousness and details of the fit by a reliable observer).
  - Cause of epilepsy (primary or symptomatic) by type of fit, age of onset, family history, presence or absence of neurological deficit, systemic abnormalities and by laboratory investigations, as and when necessary.

TABLE 5.26 Seizure Versus Psychogenic Nonepileptic Seizure

Feature	Seizure	Psychogenic nonepileptic seizure
Duration	Generally <10 minutes	Generally >10 minutes
Occurrence during sleep	Yes	No
Aura	Difficult to describe	Factual description
Asynchronous movements	No	Yes
Clenching of jaw	Occurs during tonic phase	Does not occur during tonic phase
Eyes	Open	Closed
Heart rate	Increased	Normal
Tongue biting	Yes	No
Faecal and urinary incontinence	Yes	No
Postictal phenomenon	Yes (including headache)	No
Occurrence of vocalisation	At the beginning	During or after episode
Recollection of items during seizure	No	Yes

ROLE OF EEG

- Helps in differentiating primary generalised attacks from focal epilepsies.
- Confirms the clinical diagnosis (by showing spikes and sharp waves), but normal record may occur in about 60% of cases with one seizure and 40% of cases with established epilepsy. If first EEG is normal, it should be repeated with the patient sleep deprived, although the test may still be normal.
- Video EEG: Prolonged EEG-video monitoring provides information about electrographic seizures and seizure activity (actual events recorded on video). It helps in making a definitive diagnosis of epilepsy.
- Ambulatory EEG is analogous to Holter monitor for cardiac arrhythmias. However, unlike video EEG, it does not permit correlation between electrographic seizures with actual events.

- A portable EEG can be done in patients with convulsive status epilepticus who do not regain consciousness as expected, so as to exclude an ongoing nonconvulsive status epilepticus.

DETERMINING THE CAUSE OF EPILEPSY

- Any person having a fit with focal onset or a fit starting for the first time after the age of 25 years (late onset) or having two or more fits should be investigated for symptomatic epilepsy.
- Causes of seizures vary according to age (Table 5.27).

TABLE 5.27 Common Causes of Epilepsy Based on Age of Onset

Infancy: • Anoxia (or postanoxic) • Hypocalcaemia • Hypoglycaemia • Hyponatraemia • Fever (febrile seizures) • Meningitis, birth trauma • Intracranial haemorrhage • Genetic disorders **Early childhood:** • Genetically determined metabolic disorders of brain • CNS infections • Idiopathic **Late childhood and adolescence:** • Idiopathic (genetically determined) • Sequelae of previous injury • Infections • Drugs and toxins including lead poisoning	**Adult life:** • Tumours • Current or previous brain injury (traumatic or postoperative) • CNS infections, including HIV • Metabolic • Drugs and toxins (cocaine, amphetamines, theophylline, alcohol, organophosphates); alcohol or benzodiazepine withdrawal • Idiopathic **Late life:** • Metabolic • Tumours • Current or previous brain injury (traumatic or postsurgical) • Ischaemia to the brain • Drugs and toxins

- Procedures:
  - CSF examination (if an infection is suspected).
  - Metabolic parameters like blood sugar, sodium, calcium, urea, creatinine, acid–base balance and magnesium.
- Neuroimaging:
  - Required in almost all cases of epilepsy unless a cause is obvious.
  - MRI is superior to CT scan for the detection of cerebral lesions associated with epilepsy.
  - When an acute intracranial pathology is suspected, an emergency CT scan is recommended. Common indications for emergency CT scan are listed in Box 5.27.

BOX 5.27 Indications for an Emergency CT Scan in a Patient With Seizures

- Age over 40 years
- Partial-onset seizure
- Persistent altered mental status or headache postictally
- Presence of fever
- History of recent trauma
- History of cancer
- History of anticoagulation
- Immunodeficiency
- Focal deficits on examination

  - Use of newer MRI methods [e.g. fluid-attenuated inversions recovery (FLAIR)] has increased the sensitivity for detection of abnormalities of cortical area.
- Functional imaging procedures such as PET and SPECT are useful in the evaluation of patients who are refractory to medical treatment.

TREATMENT

- A first seizure provoked by an acute brain disturbance is unlikely to recur (3%–10%), whereas a first unprovoked seizure has a recurrence risk of 30%–50% over the next 2 years.
- A first seizure mandates individual counselling about the risk of recurrence, pros and cons of the drug treatment and the impact on lifestyle.
- General guidance which should be given to the patients are given in Box 5.28.

BOX 5.28 General Guidance to Be Provided to a Patient With Epilepsy

- Tide over the stigma by proper explanation
- Avoid cycling on public roads and swimming
- Adopt an occupation at which neither the patient nor society is put to risk
- Avoid exposure to moving machinery and working at heights
- Driving only as per regulations (free of attacks for 2 years)
- Adequate sleep
- Avoid hyperpyrexia, flickering lights and emotional disturbances

DURING A FIT

- Protect from injury by moving the patient away from fire, sharp and hard objects.
- Padded gag inserted within teeth (*only if can be done easily*).

ANTIEPILEPTIC DRUGS FOR CHRONIC USE

- In general, for partial epilepsies, carbamazepine (alternatives oxcarbazepine and lamotrigine) is recommended initially, whereas for generalised epilepsies, the first-line choice is usually valproate (alternatives lamotrigine, topiramate or levetiracetam).
- Phenytoin is no longer widely used because of long-term toxicity concerns, but retains a place in terms of the ease of once-daily usage and low cost.
- The new antiepileptic agents include lamotrigine, gabapentin, topiramate, tiagabine, levetiracetam, oxcarbazepine, vigabatrin and pregabalin. These are effective for partial epilepsies and some (particularly lamotrigine, topiramate and levetiracetam) are also effective in generalised epilepsies. However, in new-onset patients, none have been shown to be superior to the 'older' drugs in terms of efficacy. Broadly, the newer agents have advantages of lower risk of side effects, less drug interactions and less enzyme induction. Because of their higher cost, these are advised as second-line agents.
- General instructions:
  - Better to use one drug rather than combination.
  - If no control is obtained with maximum doses of first drug, a second first-line drug is initiated and

the first drug is tapered. If partial control is achieved, then a second drug should be added.
- If single drug does not control, at least three single drugs should be tried before combination.
- Phenytoin may be combined with phenobarbital or carbamazepine.
- Primidone and phenobarbital should not be given together because primidone is partially converted to phenobarbital.
- Phenytoin, carbamazepine, gabapentin, pregabalin and vigabatrin can worsen nonmotor generalised onset (absence) seizures.
- Therapeutic drug monitoring is useful in only few situations, including breakthrough or refractory seizures, to assess compliance, for diagnosis of clinical toxicity or with use of phenytoin, which has dose-dependent pharmacokinetics.

- Osteomalacia and osteoporosis may occur with chronic use of phenobarbital, primidone, phenytoin and carbamazepine.
- Folic acid deficiency may occur due to phenytoin, carbamazepine, phenobarbital, primidone, oxcarbazepine and lamotrigine.
- Phenobarbital, primidone, phenytoin and carbamazepine induce metabolism of lipid-soluble drugs, such as the combined oral contraceptive pill, cytotoxic agents, antiretrovirals, statins, warfarin and antiarrhythmics.
- Side effects of primidone and phenobarbital are listed in Box 5.29.
- Side effects of phenytoin are listed in Box 5.30.
- Valproate can produce weight gain, tremors, hair loss and thrombocytopenia. Occasionally, can produce hyperammonaemic encephalopathy.
- Side effects of carbamazepine are listed in Box 5.31.
- Levetiracetam is a broad-spectrum antiepileptic drug. It inhibits calcium channels, and also reduces calcium release from intraneuronal stores. It is safe for patients with liver disease. Its side effects are listed in Box 5.32.
- Teratogenic effect is maximum with phenytoin (foetal hydantoin syndrome—mental retardation, craniofacial anomalies including microcephaly, growth retardation, hypoplasia of distal phalanx of fingers and toes, nail hypoplasia, cleft lip/palate and rib anomalies) and valproate (foetal valproate syndrome—central nervous system dysfunction, spina bifida, development delay, intrauterine growth retardation and cardiac anomalies). Carbamazepine is the safest drug in females of reproductive years, though it can also produce teratogenicity.
- Antiepileptic therapy can gradually be withdrawn if patient is totally seizure free for 3–5 years depending on the seizure type, age of the patient and previous seizure control.

BOX 5.29 Side Effects of Primidone and Phenobarbital

• Drowsiness, ataxia	• Rickets/osteomalacia
• Decreased libido	• Folate deficiency leading to megaloblastic anaemia
• Depression	• Fibrosing disorders (e.g. reflex sympathetic dystrophy, shoulder–hand syndrome, frozen shoulder, Dupuytren's contracture)
• Skin rashes	• Teratogenic effect

BOX 5.30 Side Effects of Phenytoin

- Drowsiness and ataxia
- Rickets/osteomalacia
- Folate deficiency leading to megaloblastic anaemia
- Teratogenic effect
- Gingival hyperplasia
- Coarsening of features, hirsutism
- Lymphadenopathy
- Syndrome mimicking systemic lupus erythematosus

BOX 5.31 Side Effects of Carbamazepine

- Ataxia
- Dizziness
- Diplopia
- Vertigo
- Hyponatraemia
- Bone marrow suppression
- Hepatotoxicity
- GI irritation
- Stevens–Johnson syndrome (most often in individuals with HLA-B*1502 allele)

BOX 5.32 Side Effects of Levetiracetam

- Anorexia
- Headache
- Behavioural disturbances
- Somnolence
- Dizziness
- Fatigue

TREATMENT OF VARIOUS TYPES OF EPILEPSIES

- Drug treatment of various types of epilepsies is given in Table 5.28.
- Second generation antiepileptic agents are described in Table 5.29.

SURGERY

- Surgical treatment is an option for epilepsy when an underlying brain abnormality such as where a benign tumour can be identified and removed.
- In other cases, surgery is usually offered only when epilepsy has not been controlled by adequate attempts with multiple medications.
  - Drug resistance is when two well tolerated, appropriately selected drugs (used singly or in combination) fail to achieve sustained freedom from seizures.
- The most common form of resective surgical treatment for epilepsy is to remove the front part of either the right or left temporal lobe.
- Palliative surgery for epilepsy is intended to reduce the frequency or severity of seizures. Examples are callosotomy or commissurotomy to prevent seizures from generalising.
- Hemispherectomy is a drastic operation in which most or all of one-half of the cerebral cortex is removed. It is reserved for people suffering from the most catastrophic epilepsies.

TABLE 5.28 Treatment of Various Types of Epilepsies

Type of Epilepsy	First-Line Drugs	Alternative Drugs
• Primary generalised tonic–clonic epilepsy	Valproic acid (400–3000 mg/day in two to three divided doses) Phenytoin (200–400 mg/day as single dose) Carbamazepine (600–1800 mg/day in two to three divided doses)	Phenobarbital (60–180 mg/day as single dose) Lamotrigine (150–500 mg/day in two divided doses) Topiramate (400 mg/day in two divided doses) Felbamate (2400–3600 mg/day in three to four divided doses)
• Focal onset epilepsy	Carbamazepine Phenytoin Oxcarbazepine (0.6–2.4 g/day in two to four divided doses) Lamotrigine Levetiracetam (in elderly)	Phenobarbital Gabapentin (as adjunct; 900–2400 mg/day in three divided doses) Topiramate (as adjunct; 400 mg/day in two divided doses) Brivaracetam (second-line agent; 50–200 mg in two divided doses)
• Absence epilepsy	Ethosuximide (750–1250 mg/day as single dose) Valproic acid	Lamotrigine Clonazepam (1–12 mg/day in one to three divided doses)
• Atypical absence, myoclonic and atonic epilepsy	Valproic acid	Lamotrigine Clonazepam Topiramate (as adjunct)

TABLE 5.29 Second-Generation Antiepileptic Agents

Drug	Side Effects	Dose
• Brivaracetam	Somnolence, dizziness, fatigue, ataxia, constipation	50–200 mg/day (in two divided doses)
• Clobazam	Somnolence, fever, drooling, aggression, vomiting, insomnia, ataxia, constipation	10–40 mg/day (in two divided doses)
• Felbamate	Substantial risk for aplastic anaemia or liver failure, drowsiness, headache, nausea, constipation	1.2–3.6 g/day (in three to four divided doses)
• Gabapentin	Dizziness, ataxia, somnolence, GI irritation	0.9–2.4 g/day (in three divided doses)
• Lacosamide	Dizziness, blurring of vision, vomiting, ataxia, vertigo	150–200 mg/day (in two divided doses)
• Lamotrigine	Headache, dizziness, ataxia, skin rash, GI irritation, hepatotoxicity, Stevens–Johnson syndrome	Monotherapy 300–500 mg/day With valproic acid: 100–150 mg/day
• Levetiracetam	Somnolence, incoordination, irritability, mood swings, psychosis	1–3 g/day (in two divided doses)
• Oxcarbazepine	Ataxia, dizziness, diplopia, blurred vision, vertigo, rash, bone marrow depression, GI irritation, hepatotoxicity, hyponatraemia	0.6–2.4 g/day (in two to four divided doses)
• Pregabalin	Drowsiness, dizziness, oedema, impaired concentration, blurred vision, weight gain, ataxia	150–600 mg/day (in two divided doses)
• Tiagabine	Somnolence, paraesthesia, psychosis, tremors	Without enzyme-inducing drugs 15–30 mg/day (in two to four divided doses)
• Topiramate	Somnolence, speech problem, paraesthesia, weight loss, renal calculus, metabolic acidosis, angle-closure glaucoma	With enzyme-inducing drugs 30–45 and 200–400 mg/day (in two divided doses)
• Vigabatrin	Headache, drowsiness, skin rash, constipation, depression, weight gain	Maximum 800 mg/day 2 to 3 g/day (maximum 3 g/day)

MISCELLANEOUS

- Direct brain stimulation has been shown to be effective in some cases.
- Ketogenic diet—a stringently controlled high-fat and low-protein/carbohydrate diet given with/without a restricted fluid intake to maintain ketosis on a long-term basis—in refractory cases where surgery cannot be performed. Adverse effects include GI disturbances, acidosis, increased susceptibility to infections, drowsiness, weight loss and nutritional deficiencies.
- Vagus nerve stimulator is used as an adjunctive therapy with partial-onset seizures that are resistant to antiepileptic drugs.

Q. What is status epilepticus? How will you manage a case of status epilepticus?

- Status epilepticus denotes sustained epileptic activity, and is clinically diagnosed with one of the following two:
  - Two fits occur without recovery of consciousness in between.
  - A single fit lasting longer than 30 minutes with or without loss of consciousness.
- However, currently, status epilepticus is defined as either convulsions lasting for more than 5 minutes (as patients with seizures that last more than 5 minutes

are not likely to improve spontaneously) or when two seizures occur between which there is incomplete recovery of consciousness.

- Condition is fatal or results in severe morbidity if not treated rapidly.

CLASSIFICATION

- Status epilepticus can be classified into: focal and generalised.
  - Generalised status epilepticus is further divided into: convulsive status epilepticus (tonic-clonic being the commonest) and nonconvulsive status epilepticus (characterised by slowness in behaviour and mentation, confusion and sometimes stupor, and accompanied by generalised epileptic discharges). The latter includes absence status.
  - Focal status epilepticus includes focal motor status (associated with characteristic march of motor symptoms), focal sensory status, focal status with impaired consciousness and epilepsia partialis continua (focal motor seizures without a march).

CAUSES (Box 5.33)

BOX 5.33 Causes of Status Epilepticus

- Sudden antiepileptic withdrawal
- Infections—encephalitis and meningitis
- Alcohol or benzodiazepine withdrawal
- Overdose—organophosphates, tricyclic antidepressants, isoniazid, sympathomimetics, cocaine, camphor, amphetamines, methylxanthines (theophylline, caffeine), phencyclidine (PCP), lead, lithium, lidocaine, lindane
- Metabolic disorders—hypoglycaemia and hyponatraemia, hepatic encephalopathy, uraemia, hypocalcaemia
- Brain tumour or trauma, stroke
- Prior head injury or neurosurgery, arteriovenous malformations

TREATMENT

- Priority should be to control seizures as fast as possible, along with identification of an underlying cause and its correction.

STEP A (FIRST 20 MINUTES)

- Maintain airway.
- Secure a proper IV line, and draw blood for metabolic parameters. Check for blood sugar on bedside.
- Elicit a brief history from the relatives about any previous seizures, diabetes, hypertension, drug exposure or withdrawal, and head injury.
- Conduct a rapid examination to determine presence of focal signs, obvious medical illness, increased intracranial tension and associated injuries.
- Simultaneously, administer diazepam (10–20 mg IV over 1 to 2 minutes; may be repeated every 10 minutes) or lorazepam (2–4 mg IV over 2 minutes) or midazolam (10 mg IV over 2 minutes) followed by loading dose of phenytoin (18–20 mg/kg) at a rate of not more than 50 mg/minute in adults and 25 mg/minute in children. Otherwise, hypotension or bradyarrhythmia may occur. Total dose should not exceed 1000 mg. Phenytoin will precipitate if infused using any fluid containing dextrose.
- An alternate agent is fosphenytoin, which is a prodrug of phenytoin that gets converted into phenytoin following intravenous administration. A dose of 1.5 mg of fosphenytoin is equivalent to 1 mg of phenytoin. Dose is 15–20 mg PE/kg at 100–150 mg/minute (where PE is phenytoin equivalent). Risk of hypotension is less compared to phenytoin.
- The second alternative to phenytoin is levetiracetam (40 mg/kg over 5–10 minutes; maximum of 3 g).
- These measures should control seizures in 20 minutes; *if no*, go to step B.

STEP B (20–60 MINUTES)

- Phenobarbital (20 mg/kg IV at a rate of 50 mg/minute) or diazepam infusion (2–4 mg/hour in adults). Both may require assisted ventilation.
- Since use of phenobarbital is associated with serious adverse reactions, alternatives include valproic acid and levetiracetam. Either of them can also be used as a first-line drug in place of phenytoin.
- Valproic acid is given in a dose of 30 mg/kg over 2–5 minutes, followed by infusion at 1–5 mg/kg/hour. Another 10 mg/kg may be given 10 minutes after initial dose. Adverse effects include hypotension, dizziness, thrombocytopenia and, rarely, valproic acid encephalopathy.
- Levetiracetam is given in a dose of 2 to 3 g over 15 minutes. Both phenytoin and levetiracetam are equally effective in terminating status epilepticus.
- ***If not controlled, go to step C.***

STEP C

- General anaesthesia using pentobarbital or thiopental infusion is tried ***under continuous EEG monitoring***. Other drugs include midazolam and propofol:
  - Midazolam—0.1 to 0.2 mg/kg loading followed by 0.1–2.0 mg/kg/hour.
  - Propofol—1 to 2 mg/kg loading followed by 1–10 mg/kg/hour. Rarely, it can cause propofol infusion syndrome (lactic acidosis, rhabdomyolysis, renal failure and heart failure),
  - Thiopental—5 to 7 mg/kg IV followed by 50 mg boluses every 2 to 3 minutes till seizure control and then 3–5 mg/kg/hour.
  - Pentobarbital—5 to 15 mg/kg loading dose over 10 minutes followed by infusion at 0.5–5 mg/kg/hour.
- Simultaneously, blood pressure, acidosis, ventilation and electrolyte balance are taken care of. Underlying cause should be rectified appropriately.
- Aim should be to control seizures within 1 hour after admission. Otherwise, chances of residual morbidity or mortality rise steeply as duration of status gets prolonged.

SUMMARY OF MANAGEMENT OF CONVULSIVE STATUS EPILEPTICUS (Table 5.30)

TABLE 5.30 Summary of Management of Convulsive Status Epilepticus

Minutes of Arrival	Action
• 0–5	• Maintain airway, breathing and circulation • Administer oxygen • Insert an IV line • Obtain blood samples for glucose, urea, electrolytes, bilirubin, haemogram, acid–base analysis, toxicology screen • Administer glucose (and thiamine) if hypoglycaemic • Elicit brief history and conduct brief examination
• 5–10	• Administer diazepam or lorazepam
• 5–20	• Administer phenytoin or fosphenytoin • Repeat diazepam if seizures persist • Evaluate for intubation
• 20–60	• Administer phenobarbital/valproate/levetiracetam • Support of respiration often required • Conduct detailed examination
• >60	• Intubate and ventilate (if not done before) • Administer general anaesthetic agents (midazolam, propofol, thiopental) with EEG monitoring • Admit in intensive care unit

COMPLICATIONS OF GENERALISED CONVULSIVE STATUS EPILEPTICUS (Box 5.34)

BOX 5.34 Complications of Generalised Convulsive Status Epilepticus

- Metabolic—anion gap metabolic acidosis, respiratory acidosis
- Pulmonary—upper airway obstruction, aspiration, neurocardiogenic pulmonary oedema
- Cardiac—stress-induced cardiomyopathy, cardiac arrythmias, myocardial ischaemia
- Infections—pneumonia, urinary tract infection
- Renal—acute kidney injury (secondary to rhabdomyolysis and myoglobinuria)
- Musculoskeletal—fractures, dislocation (posterior dislocation of shoulder common), tendon injuries
- CNS—brain damage (after prolonged seizure)

Q. Describe the circle of Willis. (AN 62.6)

- Circle of Willis is shown in Fig. 5.6.
- The circle of Willis is supplied by two internal carotid arteries and basilar artery formed by joining of two vertebral arteries.
- This anastomotic pathway is crucial to preservation of brain function in the event of a major flow disruption in one of the major feeding vessels. As a result, most of the stroke syndromes occur from occlusion distal to the circle of Willis or in areas that receive blood supply from arteries that originate prior to the connection with the circle.
- Patency of communicating arteries is variable and is based on developmental and degenerative changes in a particular individual.

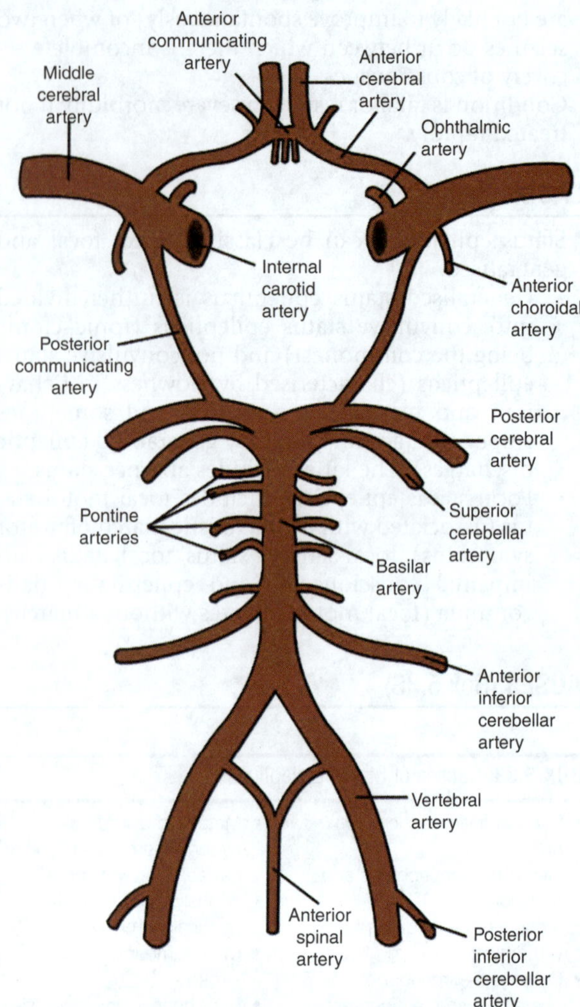

Fig. 5.6 Arteries contributing to the circle of Willis and their major branches.

Q. Give an account of different types of cerebrovascular accidents and their pathophysiology. (IM 18.2)

- Cerebrovascular accident or stroke is defined as abrupt-onset neurological disorder of vascular aetiology.
- Strokes may be haemorrhagic or ischaemic in nature.
- Ischaemic strokes can be due to embolism or thrombosis.

TYPES OF HAEMORRHAGIC STROKES

- Primary intracranial haemorrhage (ICH).
- Subarachnoid haemorrhage (SAH).
- Primary intraventricular haemorrhage.

TYPES OF ISCHAEMIC STROKES

- Thrombotic stroke.
- Embolic stroke.
- Lacunar infarcts.
- Watershed infarcts, also known as border zone infarcts, develop from relative hypoperfusion in the

most distal arterial territories and can produce bilateral symptoms. Frequently, these occur perioperatively or in situations of prolonged hypotension.

- In addition to these, multifocal small infarcts or ischaemia may result in slowly progressive neurological disorders, causing multi-infarct dementia and subcortical arteriosclerotic encephalopathy (Binswanger's disease).

PATHOPHYSIOLOGY

- The two main developments in stroke are the delineation of the ischaemic penumbra in ischaemic stroke and the observation of haematoma growth in ICH.

ISCHAEMIC STROKE

- The severity of an acute ischaemic stroke depends on the degree of impairment of cerebral blood flow (CBF) and the time to reperfusion. As the ischaemic process evolves, most commonly due to thromboembolic arterial occlusion, there is a progressive decrease in CBF. When it falls from normal levels of approximately 50 to <10 mL/100 g brain tissue/minute, neuronal cell death occurs rapidly.
- However, between the ischaemic core and the normally perfused brain at the periphery lies the ischaemic penumbra, a zone of moderately reduced CBF.
- Within the ischaemic penumbra, the neurons are hypoxic, functionally inactive, but still viable. In the penumbra, the brain tissue will undergo necrosis over hours due to perfusion failure, and a secondary cascade of damaging biochemical events. These neurotoxic processes include release of glutamate, activation of *N*-methyl-D-aspartate (NMDA) and other cell receptors, influx of sodium and calcium into cells, release of free radical species and ultimately cellular destruction.
- A limited therapeutic window of opportunity underlies the concept that 'time is brain'.

INTRACEREBRAL HAEMORRHAGE

- ICH is also a dynamic process and substantial haematoma growth (greater than one-third increase in volume) can occur within the first 3 hours with most of the growth in the first 1 hour. This expansion is probably due to continued bleeding or rebleeding. Haematoma expansion is an important cause of early neurological deterioration, the severity of which depends on original haematoma size and subsequent expansion rate. This observation is the basis of giving haemostatic therapy in ICH that could reduce the volume of the haematoma and possibly result in improved outcomes.
- Another cause of deterioration is development of perihaematoma brain oedema that may evolve over many days. It is the primary cause of neurological deterioration after the first day of bleed. Perihaemorrhagic tissue damage is primarily related to the inflammatory and cytotoxic response and not due to ischaemia produced by oedema.

Q. What are the risk factors for stroke? (IM 18.2)

- Risk factors for stroke based on age groups are shown in Table 5.31.

TABLE 5.31 Risk Factors for Stroke

Risk Factors in Patients of All Age Groups	Additional Risk Factors That Are More Common in Young Patients
High risk: • Hypertension (including isolated systolic) • Diabetes mellitus • Atrial fibrillation with or without valvular heart disease • Smoking • Use of cocaine or amphetamines • Vasculitis (polyarteritis nodosa, Wegener's, Takayasu's arteritis, primary CNS vasculitis, vasculitis related to meningitis) • Dilated cardiomyopathy • Endocarditis ***Low risk:*** • Migraine • Use of oral contraceptives or alcohol • Patent foramen ovale • Recent myocardial infarction • Prosthetic valve	• Protein C and S deficiencies • Antithrombin deficiency • Antiphospholipid syndrome • Factor V Leiden • Sickle cell anaemia • Hyperhomocysteinaemia • Thrombotic thrombocytopenic purpura • Arterial dissection • Infections (e.g. syphilis, HIV)

Q. Define transient ischaemic attack. Discuss its mechanism, clinical features, investigations and management.

DEFINITION

- Abrupt-onset focal neurological deficit of presumed vascular aetiology not lasting longer than 24 hours. Many episodes last for a few seconds to minutes and rarely up to 24 hours. Defining transient ischaemic attack (TIA) with a 24-hour maximum duration has the potential to delay the initiation of effective stroke therapies.
- A more recent definition of TIA is a brief episode of neurological dysfunction caused by focal brain or retinal ischaemia without neuroimaging evidence of acute infarction. Therefore, without diagnostic imaging, it is not possible to make a distinction between TIA and stroke. This definition underscores the urgency of recognising TIA as an important warning of impending stroke and facilitating rapid evaluation and treatment of TIA to prevent permanent brain ischaemia. There is no reliable way to determine whether the abrupt onset of neurological deficits represents reversible ischaemia without subsequent brain damage or whether ischaemia will result in permanent damage to the brain (e.g. stroke).

MECHANISM

- Various causes of TIAs are given in Box 5.35.

BOX 5.35 Causes of Transient Ischaemic Attacks

Mechanism	Common Examples
Large artery atherosclerosis	Carotid stenosis, vertebrobasilar disease, aortic atherosclerosis
Cardioaortic embolism	Atrial fibrillation, valvular disease, left ventricle thrombus
Small artery occlusion	Intracranial small-vessel disease from long-standing hypertension, intracranial atherosclerosis
Others	Arterial dissection, hypercoagulable states

- Usually, TIAs occur due to a platelet thrombus getting dislodged from an atherosclerotic plaque to cause short-lasting obstruction at a distal branch. Embolus gets broken down resulting in re-establishment of perfusion with clearance of neurological deficit.

SYMPTOMS AND SIGNS

- Most TIAs resolve in less than 30 minutes. If symptoms of cerebral ischaemia do not resolve by 1 hour or rapidly improve within 3 hours, complete resolution is rare.
- TIA implies an active plaque in the major feeding artery and is a warning sign of a major stroke. The risk of recurrence and stroke is about 10% within the first 7 days of a TIA, with most of them occurring within 48 hours. More than 30% of patients with recurrent TIAs will suffer from completed stroke if untreated.

CAROTID TERRITORY

- Ipsilateral monocular blindness (amaurosis fugax), contralateral hemiparesis, hemianaesthesia, dysarthria and rarely hemianopia, monoparesis, isolated facial weakness or sensory symptoms in face or limbs alone may occur.
- Reduced common carotid or superficial temporal pulsation, and bruit over carotid artery in the neck or over orbit may be heard.
- Occasionally, cholesterol crystals may be seen in the retinal vessels on fundoscopy.

VERTEBROBASILAR TERRITORY

- Ataxia, dysarthria, hemianopia, diplopia, sudden fall (drop attacks), weakness on both sides or on one side, paraesthesia on both sides, difficulty in swallowing, vertigo and tinnitus may occur. More than one symptom may occur simultaneously and vertigo is a common symptom.

INVESTIGATIONS (Table 5.32)

TABLE 5.32 Investigations in a Case of Transient Ischaemic Attack

Routine tests for TIA:	Additional tests:
• Full blood count, ESR • Serological tests for syphilis • Blood glucose, urea, proteins • Chest X-ray, ECG **In younger patients:** • Antinuclear factor • Lipid profile • Coagulation studies (anticardiolipin antibodies, proteins C and S, antithrombin III)	***In vertebrobasilar TIAs*** • Lying and standing BP • 24-Hour ECG monitoring • X-ray of cervical spine • MRI angiography ***In carotid TIAs*** • CT scan or diffusion-weighted MRI of brain • Carotid Doppler study • Arteriography, CT or MR angiography

Note: Neuroimaging should be done as soon as possible but within 24 hours of suspected TIA. If available, magnetic resonance imaging (MRI) with diffusion-weighted imaging (DWI) is the preferred imaging modality.

DIAGNOSIS

- TIA will have to be differentiated from focal seizures, hypoglycaemia and migraine.
- TIA typically has a rapid onset, and maximal intensity usually is reached within minutes.
- Younger age, previous history of migraine (with or without aura), and associated headache, nausea or photophobia are more suggestive of migraine than TIA. In general, migraine aura tends to have a marching quality; for example symptoms such as tingling may progress from the fingers to the forearm to the face. Migraine aura also is more likely to have a more gradual onset and resolution with a longer duration of symptoms than in a typical TIA.
- Workup in a case of TIA should include evaluation for risk factors for stroke. They are the following:
  - Hypertension.
  - Diabetes.
  - Hyperlipidaemia.
  - Arterial disease affecting the heart and limbs.
  - Cardiac disease (valvular and ischaemic).
  - Smoking.

RISK ASSESSMENT FOR OCCURRENCE OF STROKE

- Calculate ABCD2 score; risk of stroke is high if ABCD2 score ≥4 points (Box 5.36).
- At present, it is recommended not to use any risk-prediction scoring system, but refer the patients as early as possible so that imaging is not delayed.

BOX 5.36 ABCD2 Score in a Patient With Transient Ischaemic Attack

- **A**ge >60 years, 1 point
- **B**P >140/90 mmHg, 1 point
- **C**linical features
  - Speech disturbance, 1 point
  - Unilateral weakness, 2 points
- **D**uration
  - ≥10 minutes, 1 point
  - ≥1 hour, 2 points
- **D**iabetes, 1 point

TREATMENT

- Positioning the patient with the head of the bed flat so as to increase blood flow to brain.

- Patients who score 4 and above on ABCD2 are at high risk of recurrent stroke and should be given immediate aspirin (after CT scan to exclude haemorrhage) and referred to a higher centre within 24 hours of symptom onset for assessment and investigation.
- If the ABCD2 score is <4, start aspirin and have specialist assessment within 7 days. People with crescendo TIA (two or more TIAs in a week) should be treated as being at high risk of stroke.
- Antiplatelet agents—aspirin in doses ranging from 75 to 300 mg/day reduces the chances of stroke by 25% and death by 30%. If there is gastric intolerance, dose may be reduced to 75 mg/day or clopidogrel (75 mg) should be given. If ABCD2 score is ≥4, combination of aspirin and clopidogrel may be given for initial 3 weeks followed by aspirin alone after that. Antiplatelet agents should be given after a CT scan has excluded haemorrhage.
- Correction of risk factors—this includes treatment of hypertension, diabetes and hyperlipidaemia, correction of valvular heart diseases and cessation of smoking. However, BP should not be lowered acutely unless it is above 220 mmHg systolic or 120 mmHg diastolic when it should be lowered gradually.
- Anticoagulants—role of anticoagulants in TIA has not been properly assessed but these agents are given if aspirin fails or if there is a definite cardiac source of embolism (e.g. atrial fibrillation).
- Surgery—once a carotid territory TIA is diagnosed, carotid imaging should be performed, and if it shows >70% stenosis, patient should be immediately referred for carotid endarterectomy. If stenosis >50%, refer within 2 weeks. Carotid artery stenting is another option in place of carotid endarterectomy. Medical treatment is continued.
- Flowchart 5.2 summarises treatment of a patient with transient ischaemic attack.

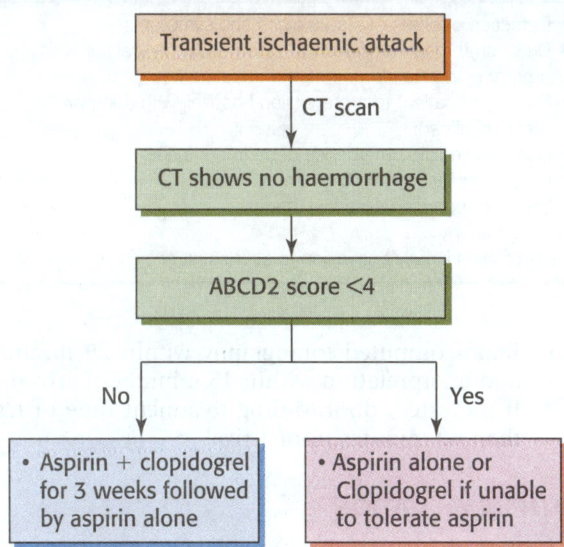

Flowchart 5.2 Management of Transient Ischaemic Attack.

TABLE 5.33 Signs Seen in Wallenberg's Syndrome (Lateral Medullary Syndrome)

Ipsilateral Signs	Contralateral Signs
• Facial numbness and impaired sensation (VII) • Diplopia (VI) • Ataxia (cerebellar) • Horner's syndrome • Palatal palsy (IX and X nerve lesions)	• Analgesia over trunk and extremities (spinothalamic) • Nystagmus (fast component towards contralateral side) • Hemiparesis (*mild, unusual*)

Q. Discuss briefly about Wallenberg's syndrome (lateral medullary syndrome).

- It is a type of vertebrobasilar ischaemic syndrome.
- It is due to an infarct that is located at dorsolateral medulla and occurs due to occlusion of posterior inferior cerebellar artery, its branch or parent vertebral artery itself. Symptoms consist of sudden-onset vertigo, vomiting, dysphagia and ataxia. At times, syndrome is incomplete and various partial combinations may be seen.
- Various signs seen are listed in Table 5.33.

Q. How do you differentiate between haemorrhagic, thrombotic and embolic strokes?

- Features which may help in differentiating haemorrhagic, thrombotic and embolic strokes are given in Table 5.34.
- In a given case, it is not possible to differentiate with absolute certainty as none of the features mentioned in Table 5.34 are exclusive and there is marked overlap.

Q. Discuss clinical features and management of cerebral infarct.

- Caused by embolism, thrombosis or due to severe hypotension/hypoperfusion of brain.
- Thromboembolism is characterised by sudden or rapid onset of focal neurological signs. Preceding TIAs may have occurred. Neurological examination shows signs attributable to a brain region supplied by a single cerebral or posterior circulation artery.

CLINICAL FEATURES

- In the prehospital phase, Cincinnati Prehospital Stroke Scale is a popular scale to detect stroke early. It can be remembered by acronym 'FAST'—*F*acial asymmetry, *A*rm drift (while holding arms in front of body), *S*peech abnormality (dysarthria or aphasia) and *T*ime of onset.
- Various features of ischaemic stroke are related to the artery blocked by embolus or thrombus (Box 5.37).

TABLE 5.34 Haemorrhagic Versus Thrombotic Versus Embolic Stroke

Feature	Haemorrhagic	Thrombotic	Embolic
• Time of onset	During activity	In sleep	Any time
• Progression	Over minutes and hours	On waking up or over hours	Within seconds
• TIAs	Absent	Present	Present
• Vomiting	Recurrent	Absent or occasional	Absent or occasional
• Headache	Prominent	Mild or absent	Mild or absent
• Early resolution (within minutes or days)	Unusual	Variable	Possible
• Meningeal irritation	May be present	Absent	Absent
• Carotid bruit (and absent pulse)	Not seen	Highly supportive	Possible
• Valvular heart disease and atrial fibrillation	Not seen	Unusual	Highly supportive
• CT scan	Haemorrhage	Pale infarct (normal in early stage)	Pale infarct (normal in early stage), haemorrhagic infarct in some cases

BOX 5.37 Features of Cerebral Infarction Based on Artery Involved

- Left anterior circulation (supplied by left internal carotid artery and its anterior cerebral and middle cerebral branches)—right hemiparesis, hemisensory loss, hemianopia, aphasia
- Right anterior circulation (supplied by right internal carotid artery and its anterior cerebral and middle cerebral branches)—left hemiparesis, hemisensory loss, hemianopia; left neglect, decreased awareness of the deficit, abnormal drawing and copying
- Middle cerebral artery—global aphasia if dominant hemisphere is involved and contralateral hemispatial neglect if nondominant hemisphere is involved; motor and sensory deficits of the side opposite to the occlusion involving the face and arm, and, to a lesser extent, the leg; deviation of eyes towards the side of occlusion; may have homonymous hemianopia
- Anterior cerebral artery—contralateral motor and sensory deficits, more prominent in the leg than in the arm (face and tongue usually spared); lack of concern and disinhibition; incontinence; primitive frontal lobe reflexes (grasp and suck)
- Vertebrobasilar circulation involving brainstem and cerebellum—vertigo, diplopia, crossed motor or sensory signs (one side of the face and the contralateral body), ataxia, bilateral motor or sensory signs
- Left posterior cerebral artery territory—right hemianopia, alexia without agraphia; right hemisensory symptoms
- Right posterior cerebral artery territory—left hemianopia, left hemisensory symptoms, topographic disorientation (inability to orient to surroundings)
- Basilar artery—pontine localisation with impaired lateral gaze, horizontal diplopia and disconjugate gaze, nonlocalised hemiparesis, dysarthria; 'locked-in syndrome' with bilateral pontine infarction (intact vertical eye movements, anarthria, quadriplegia)

WAKE-UP STROKE

- Wake-up stroke (WUS) is a subgroup of ischaemic stroke in which patients show no abnormality before sleep but wakes up with neurological deficits.
- MRI—mismatch between diffusion-weighted image and FLAIR images indicates an acute ischaemic lesion within 4.5 hours of onset and it strongly suggests that the patient is amenable to thrombolytic therapy.

MANAGEMENT

- Successful care of acute stroke patients relies on 'Stroke Chain of Survival' that has eight Ds (Box 5.38).
- Initial investigations, monitoring and treatment are carried out simultaneously.
- In the emergency department, the following should be observed so as to maximise the chances of thrombolysis:
  - Emergency physician evaluation within 10 minutes of arrival.
  - Stroke team notification within 15 minutes of arrival.
  - Brain-computed tomography within 25 minutes and interpretation within 45 minutes of arrival.
  - If indicated, door-to-drug treatment time of less than 60 minutes from arrival.

BOX 5.38 Stroke Chain of Survival

- Detection of onset of stroke signs and symptoms
- Dispatch through activation of emergency medical services and prompt response
- Delivery of patient to a prenotified hospital, with appropriate prehospital care
- Door (immediate emergency department triage)
- Data compilation including head CT scan
- Decision regarding potential therapies
- Drug therapy
- Disposition (timely admission to stroke unit or transfer)

INITIAL EVALUATION

- Cardiovascular status: Blood pressure, cardiovascular examination and ECG.

- Degree of neurological deficit (by Neurological Institutes of Health Stroke Scale—NIHSS) and vascular territory involved.
- Metabolic status:
  - Blood sugar.
  - Presence or absence of hypoxia.
  - Renal functions.
  - Electrolyte status.
- Haematological parameters.
  - Haemoglobin.
  - Coagulation parameters.

Note: Except for blood sugar, other tests may be done but should not delay initiation of thrombolytic therapy if indicated.

OTHER INVESTIGATIONS

- CT scan—to confirm infarct and to rule out haemorrhage, tumour and subdural haematoma. In case of an infarction, there is a period of 1 to 2 days before a focal area of hypodensity appears on CT scan. Only large infarcts with oedema can be visualised during the first few hours of stroke. Another finding which may be seen on CT is dense middle cerebral artery (Fig. 5.7). The main role of CT scan, if the patient comes within 3–4.5 hours of onset of symptoms, is to exclude an intracranial haemorrhage so as to decide about thrombolytic therapy.
- MRI scan—diffusion-weighted imaging is most sensitive and specific for acute ischaemic stroke.
- CT angiography and MR angiography—if either intra-arterial fibrinolysis or mechanical thrombectomy is contemplated for management but it should not delay intravenous recombinant tissue plasminogen activator (rtPA) if indicated.

MONITOR (IN ALL PATIENTS)

- Neurological and cardiovascular status frequently.
- Metabolic parameters daily.

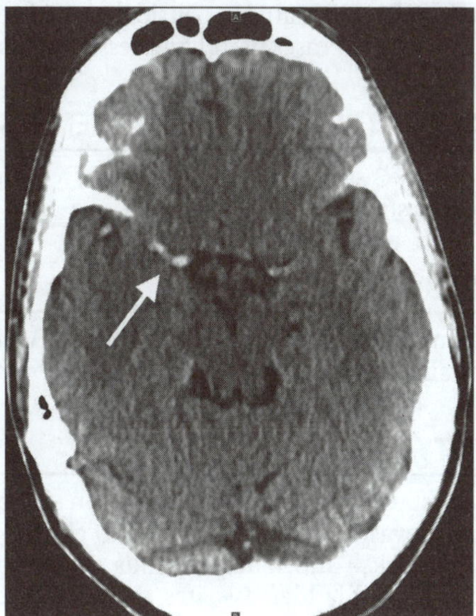

Fig. 5.7 'Dense MCA sign' on noncontrast enhanced CT of brain.

TREATMENT

- An organised protocol (including stroke team) for the emergency evaluation of patients with suspected stroke is recommended.

General

- Maintain adequate airway with periodic clearance of secretion and chest physiotherapy in unconscious patients.
- Administer oxygen if oxygen saturation is below 94%.
- Treat hypoglycaemia with 50% dextrose; treat hyperglycaemia with insulin, if serum glucose >180 mg/dL.
- Continuous cardiac monitoring for ischaemic changes or atrial fibrillation.
- Infuse normal saline at 50 mL/hour unless otherwise indicated.
- Avoid hyperthermia.
- Skincare by changing position once in 2 hours to prevent bedsore.
- Nil per orally initially. Nasogastric tube (if unable to swallow) to maintain adequate fluid balance or to prevent vomiting by keeping stomach empty and depending on the need.
- Bladder catheterisation, if incontinence or retention has occurred.
- Passive movements of limbs to prevent contractures, oedema of the limb, venous stasis and pulmonary embolism.

Specific Measures

- BP—many show reactive hypertension. A rapid reduction in BP can increase the size of infarct:
  - Urgent reduction is required only if systolic BP is above 220 mmHg, diastolic pressure is above 120 mmHg or mean arterial pressure is above 130 mmHg.
  - If BP is not elevated to that extent but the patient has pulmonary oedema, renal failure, acute myocardial infarction, etc., antihypertensives are required. Otherwise, BP is gradually reduced over several days.
  - In patients who are candidates for thrombolytic therapy, antihypertensives are recommended if systolic BP >185 mmHg or diastolic BP >110 mmHg.
  - Drugs most often used include intravenous labetalol, enalapril or sodium nitroprusside.
- Antioedema measures—large infarcts will show significant oedema that may be reduced by antioedema measures. However, hypovolaemia must be avoided:
  - Mannitol 20% IV over 20 minutes (0.25–1 g/kg) three to four times a day.
  - Glycerol 30 mL orally three to four times a day.
  - Frusemide 20 mg IV three times a day.
  - These agents at best may only be life-saving by preventing brain herniation, and do not reduce the severity of morbidity. They are not necessary in smaller infarcts, where they may actually result in unnecessary dehydration and electrolyte imbalance.
- Measures to reduce the size of cerebral infarct by attempts to salvage tissue at ischaemic penumbra:
  - By avoiding reduction in cerebral perfusion through preventing rapid reduction of BP.

- Maintain normal blood sugar levels (avoid infusion of dextrose if blood sugar is normal).
- Avoid raised body temperature (using antipyretics and cooling blankets).
- Avoid hypoxia.
- Maintain haemoglobin levels above 9 g/dL.
- Thrombolysis.
- Intra-arterial devices for clot extraction or clot maceration.

Anticoagulants

- Role of heparin in acute stage is controversial and at present not recommended. Anticoagulants are recommended only when mild cerebral ischaemic event occurs in the presence of:
  - Recent myocardial infarction where anticoagulants are recommended for a period of 3 months.
  - Previous myocardial infarction with ventricular akinetic segment or ventricular aneurysm.
  - Presence of other cardiac conditions as noted above.
  - Presence of prosthetic valves.
  - Thrombotic stroke as indicated by progressive stroke (though use of heparin is still controversial in this setting).
- Not recommended for patients with moderate to severe strokes because of an increased risk of serious intracranial haemorrhagic complications.
- Subcutaneous administration of anticoagulants is recommended for treatment of immobilised patients to prevent deep vein thrombosis.

Intravenous Thrombolytic Therapy

- Intravenous rTPA and tenecteplase have been shown to be beneficial when initiated within the first 3–4.5 hours of an ischaemic stroke in a patient older than 18 years. However, there is a significant risk of intracerebral bleeding in stroke patients treated with thrombolytic agents.

Eligibility

- Box 5.39 gives eligibility criteria for thrombolysis within 3 hours of onset of stroke.
- Eligibility criteria for thrombolytic treatment between 3 and 4.5 hours after acute stroke onset are similar to those for treatment before 3 hours, with any of the exclusion criteria given in Box 5.40.

BOX 5.39 Eligibility Criteria for Thrombolysis Within 3 Hours of Onset of Stroke

- Age >18 years
- Measurable neurologic deficit
- Platelet count >100,000/mm[a]
- Current anticoagulant use but INR <1.7 or PT <15 seconds or aPTT <40 seconds[a]
- Blood pressure below 185/110 mmHg
- Therapeutic doses of low molecular weight heparin received >24 hours ago

[a]Thrombolytic therapy should not be delayed while results are pending. Thrombolysis should be discontinued immediately, if results are abnormal.

BOX 5.40 Exclusion Criteria for Thrombolysis Between 3 and 4.5 Hours of Onset of Stroke

- Age >80 years
- All patients on oral anticoagulants regardless of INR
- Patients with baseline National Institutes of Health Stroke Scale (NIHSS) score >25
- Patients with imaging evidence of ischaemic damage to more than one-third of the middle cerebral artery territory
- Patients with a history of stroke as well as diabetes

Contraindications (Box 5.41)

BOX 5.41 Contraindications of Thrombolytic Therapy

- Blood on CT scan
- Possible SAH
- A large hypodense lesion in a distribution consistent with the neurological examination
- Active internal bleeding
- Bleeding diathesis
- Presentation consistent with infective endocarditis
- Systolic pressure >185 mmHg and diastolic pressure >110 mmHg
- Major neurosurgery or head injury within 3 months
- History of intracranial haemorrhage or AV malformation
- Stroke known or suspected to be associated with aortic arch dissection

Dose

- Dose of rTPA: 0.9 mg/kg (maximum 90 mg) with 10% of total dose as bolus and rest over 1 hour.
- Dose of tenecteplase is 0.25 mg/kg IV over 2 minutes.
- Aspirin should be delayed until 24 hours after thrombolysis.

Intra-arterial Thrombolysis

- Intra-arterial (through carotid artery) rTPA is an experimental therapy in selected patients and can be given up to 6-9 hours after onset.

Other Treatment Options

- Intra-arterial thrombectomy using mechanical devices or stent retrievers can be considered within 16–24 hours in selected cases with large vessel occlusion.

SUMMARY OF TREATMENT OF ISCHAEMIC STROKE

- Flowchart 5.3 summarises treatment of a patient with iscahemic stroke.

SECONDARY PROPHYLAXIS

- It is similar to the primary prevention. Antiplatelet agents should be started within 24–48 hours.

MORTALITY

- In the first week—mortality depends on size of infarct and cardiovascular status (difficult to control).
- In later weeks—mortality depends on infections of lung, urinary bladder, IV sites or metabolic disturbances like water and electrolyte imbalance (easy to prevent and correct).

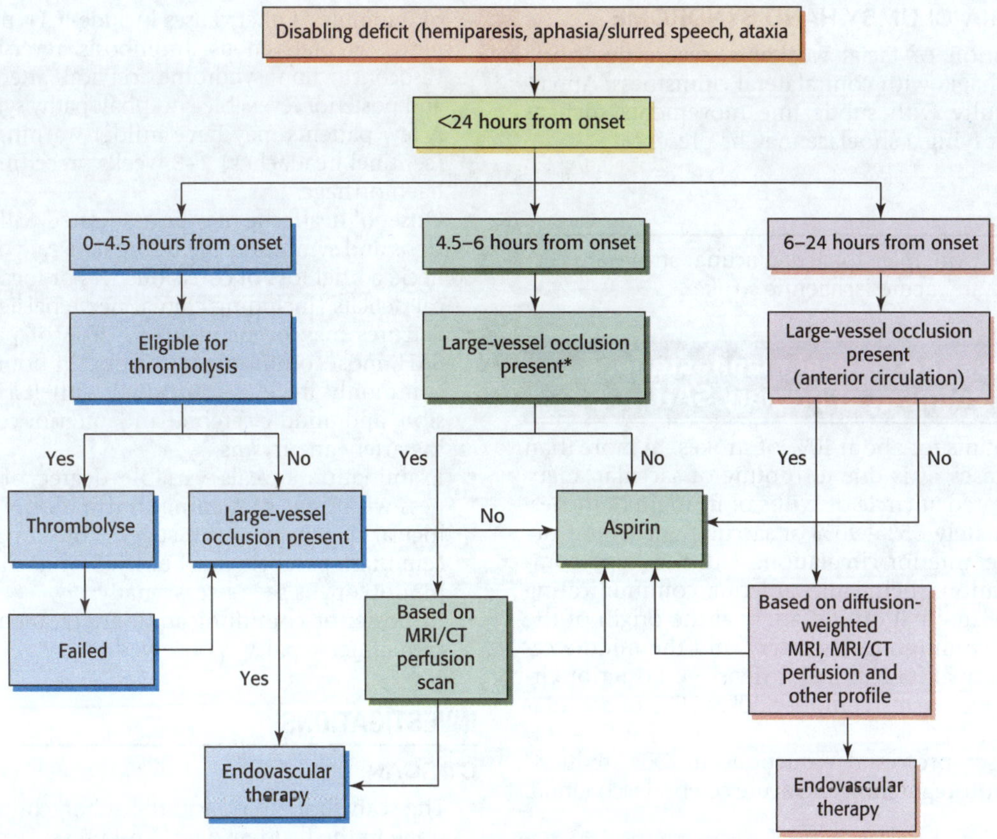

Flowchart 5.3 Management of Ischaemic Stroke *ALBERTS >6 (Alberta Stroke Programme Early CT Score).

- Later management includes rehabilitation, adequate control and maintenance of risk factors. Rehabilitation should involve family members, and includes motor, sensory, cognitive and psychological measures, and attempts at occupational rehabilitation.

Q. Discuss briefly about lacunar infarction.

- Lacunar infarctions are caused by occlusion of small deep perforating branches of the cerebral vessels from the circle of Willis, including branches from the middle cerebral artery, anterior cerebral artery, posterior cerebral artery or the basilar artery.
- Their size varies from 3 to 15 mm in dimension.
- May or may not present with symptoms or signs.
- The occlusion may be due to microatheroma and lipohyalinosis that are associated with hypertension, smoking and diabetes, or due to microembolism from the heart or carotid arteries.

CLINICAL FEATURES

PURE MOTOR STROKE

- Occurs due to lesion in the posterior limb of internal capsule (which carries descending corticospinal and corticobulbar tracts) or basis pontis.
- Clinical course is often stuttering, with the symptoms developing in a stepwise fashion over several hours.
- Hemiparesis or hemiplegia typically affects face, arm and leg equally.
- Motor aphasia also present, if lesion in genu and anterior limb of internal capsule.
- Occurs due to involvement of lenticulostriate artery, a branch of middle cerebral artery.

ATAXIC HEMIPARESIS

- Second most frequent lacunar syndrome.
- Combination of cerebellar and motor symptoms, including weakness and clumsiness on the ipsilateral side of the body.
- Usually affects the leg more than the arm.
- The most frequent sites of infarction are the posterior limb of the internal capsule, basis pontis and corona radiata.

PURE SENSORY STROKE

- Persistent or transient numbness and/or tingling on one side of the body.
- Occasionally, pain, burning or other unpleasant sensations.
- The most frequent site is thalamus.

MIXED SENSORIMOTOR STROKE

- Hemiparesis or hemiplegia with ipsilateral sensory impairment.
- The infarct is usually in the thalamus and adjacent posterior internal capsule.

DYSARTHRIA-CLUMSY HAND SYNDROME

- Combination of facial weakness, severe dysarthria and dysphagia with contralateral clumsiness. Apparent difficulty with subtle fine movements such as writing or tying a shoelace may be present.

TREATMENT

- Treatment principles for acute lacunar stroke are very similar to any acute ischaemic stroke.

Q. Discuss the clinical manifestations and treatment of primary SAH.

- SAH accounts for about 10% of strokes. In more than 80% of cases, it is due to rupture of saccular aneurysms located at circle of Willis or its main branches.
- Approximately 85%–90% of saccular aneurysms occur in the anterior circulation, with the most common locations being the anterior communicating artery, the internal carotid artery at the origin of the posterior communicating artery, and the middle cerebral artery at its first major division. Posterior circulation aneurysms comprise 10%–15% of saccular aneurysms.
- SAH causes profound reductions in CBF, reduced cerebral autoregulation and acute cerebral ischaemia.

CAUSES OF SAH

- Various causes of SAH are given in Box 5.42.

BOX 5.42 Causes of Subarachnoid Haemorrhage

- Aneurysm
- Arteriovenous malformations
- Extension from intracerebral bleed
- Trauma
- Mycotic aneurysms
- Anticoagulant therapy
- Bleeding diathesis

RISK FACTORS

- Important risk factors include alcohol consumption, smoking and hypertension. Use of sympathomimetic drugs, including cocaine and phenylpropanolamine, is also a risk factor.
- Certain genetic syndromes have also been associated with an increased risk of SAH. These include autosomal dominant polycystic kidney disease and type IV Ehlers–Danlos syndrome.

CLINICAL FEATURES

- The characteristic is abrupt severe headache (thunderclap headache) with or without associated vomiting. Onset may be associated with any activity that results in rise in BP. Consciousness may be lost and a seizure may occur.
- Thunderclap headache is severe headache peaking within 1 minute of the onset and lasting for a minimum of 5 minutes. Other causes include ICH, pituitary apoplexy, cerebral venous thrombosis, reversible cerebral vasoconstriction syndrome, cervical artery dissection and posterior reversible encephalopathy syndrome.
- A few patients may have milder warning headaches (sentinel headaches) 2–8 weeks preceding the major haemorrhage.
- Onset of headache may be associated with additional signs and symptoms including nausea, vomiting, stiff neck, a brief loss of consciousness or focal neurological deficits (including cranial nerve palsies).
- Seizures may occur in up to 20% of patients after SAH, most commonly in the first 24 hours and more commonly in SAH associated with ICH, hypertension, and middle cerebral and anterior communicating artery aneurysms.
- Examination reveals variable degree of consciousness with signs of meningeal irritation. Focal neurological deficits at onset suggest bleeding into adjacent brain parenchyma. Subhyaloid haemorrhage on fundoscopy is seen occasionally.
- In posterior communicating artery aneurysm, third cranial nerve palsy is observed.

INVESTIGATIONS

CT SCAN

- The scan shows blood in the subarachnoid space (if done in the first few days) and presence of intracerebral haematoma, hydrocephalus, associated brain ischaemia and occasionally location of aneurysm itself (Fig. 5.8).

LUMBAR PUNCTURE

- It should be done if clinical suspicion is high but CT scan fails to show subarachnoid blood, and there is no mass effect. CSF will be uniformly blood stained

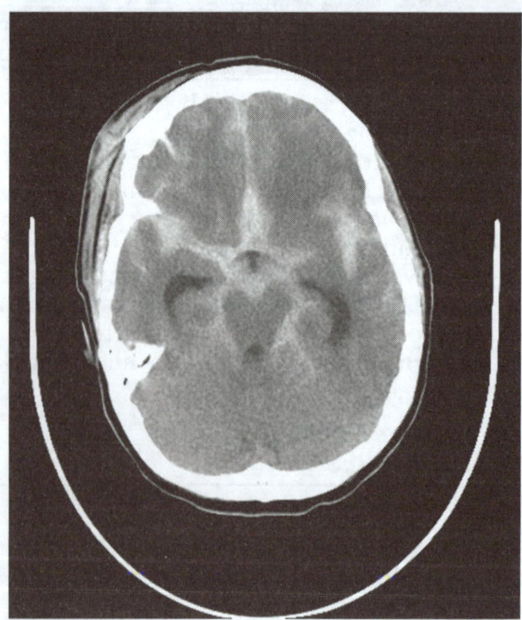

Fig. 5.8 CT scan showing subarachnoid haemorrhage (blood is hyperdense).

in the initial hours and becomes xanthochromic in later days (first appears after 4–6 hours of the bleed).

DIGITAL SUBTRACTION ANGIOGRAPHY

- It is needed to locate the site of aneurysm which has bled, and other details that neurosurgeon needs to know in order to ligate the aneurysm adequately.
- It should be performed in all patients fit for surgery (age <65 years, not in coma) and is the standard for diagnosis.

MR ANGIOGRAPHY (MRA)

- It can demonstrate aneurysms >5 mm in size with great accuracy. However, due to lack of easy availability and time required for performing it, MRA has not replaced conventional angiography.

CT ANGIOGRAPHY

- A rapid, readily available, less invasive alternative to catheter angiography and is equivalent to conventional angiography for demonstrating larger aneurysms.
- May be considered when conventional angiography cannot be performed in a timely fashion.

MANAGEMENT

- Immediately shift the patient to a centre where neurosurgical care is possible unless patient is too ill to be shifted. Rebleed is usual in the first 2 weeks, which is often fatal. There is at least a 3% to 4% risk of rebleeding in the first 24 hours and then a 1% to 2%/day risk in the first month. A longer interval from haemorrhage to admission and treatment, higher initial BP and worse neurological status on admission have been related to recurrent haemorrhage in the first 2 weeks after SAH.
- In properly chosen patient with proper timing of surgery, clipping of aneurysm is followed with very good results. Endovascular coiling to ablate aneurysm is also used in centres with experience and gives better results compared to coiling.
- Medical treatment of patients with aneurysmal SAH is directed towards the prevention and management of neurological complications (e.g. aneurysm rebleeding, hydrocephalus, cerebral vasospasm and ischaemia, and seizures) and systemic complications (e.g. hyponatraemia, cardiac arrhythmia and myocardial damage, and neurogenic pulmonary oedema).
- Immediate administration of antifibrinolytic agent tranexamic acid (1 g IV, followed by 1 g every 6 hours) may be useful to reduce the rate of early aneurysm rebleeding. In some cases, it may worsen cerebral ischaemia.
- Pain management, sedation and control of hypertension (goal of achieving systolic arterial pressure ~ 160 mmHg) are also important in the prevention of aneurysm rebleeding.
- In conscious patients without evidence of raised ICP, active hypertension treatment is indicated. A target mean arterial pressure of 110 mmHg (systolic ~ 160 mmHg) is recommended, if it is elevated beyond this value. Agents used include labetalol, esmolol or nicardipine. Sodium nitroprusside should be avoided as it may elevate ICP.
- Strict avoidance of hypovolaemia, hypotension, hyperthermia, hyperglycaemia and hyponatraemia is important in preventing delayed cerebral ischaemia.
- Raised intracranial pressure should be aggressively treated with head of bed elevation, sedation, analgesia, hyperosmolar therapy, normal ventilation, cerebrospinal fluid drainage and, in refractory cases, barbiturate sedation or decompressive craniectomy.
- Calcium blocking agent nimodipine (60 mg orally every 4 hours) provides a modest but significant improvement in outcome by reducing cerebral arterial vasospasm.
- Anticonvulsants are recommended for prophylaxis.
- Absolute bed rest for 4 weeks is advised followed by gradual resumption of physical activities.

Q. Briefly outline the risk factors, clinical features, diagnosis and management of ICH.

- Occurs secondary to hypertension where penetrating branches undergo degeneration and develop microaneurysms within the brain. Common sites of bleeding in order of frequency are as follows:
  - Putamen.
  - Thalamus.
  - Frontal or parietal lobes.
  - Pons.
  - Cerebellum.

RISK FACTORS

- Incidence of ICH increases exponentially with age and is higher in males than in females.
- Most spontaneous haematomas are attributed to chronic arterial hypertension.
- Other risk factors are ageing (which produces cerebral amyloid angiopathy), alcohol consumption, anticoagulant treatment and antiplatelet therapy.
- Use of amphetamines or cocaine, cigarette smoking and diabetes mellitus are also associated with increased risk.
- Coagulation disorders and bleeding tendency (e.g. thrombocytopenia) are rare causes of ICH.
- Other conditions that may complicate haemorrhage include brain tumours, dural venous sinus thrombosis, vascular malformations, etc.

CLINICAL FEATURES

- Clinical features are often indistinguishable from ischaemic stroke, and a CT scan is often required.
- Patients present with a smooth onset of focal neurological deficit over minutes to hours often accompanied by headache and vomiting due to increased ICP.
- More than 90% of patients present with acute hypertension, hyperventilation, tachycardia or bradycardia, central fever and hyperglycaemia. Clinical deterioration occurs in 30%–50% of patients, usually within the first

24 hours, and may be attributable to any combination of haematoma expansion, perihaematoma oedema, hydrocephalus and seizures.
- Involvement of putamen often presents with hemiparesis along with some depression of consciousness.
- Thalamic haemorrhage commonly produces hemianaesthesia more prominently than hemiparesis along with impaired upward gaze.
- A significant haemorrhage into pons is usually a catastrophe as it leads to coma, pinpoint pupils, quadriparesis and a dysconjugate ocular mobility disorder.
- Lobar haemorrhage, depending on the size and location, produces unilateral hemiparesis and hemisensory deficits along with speech impairment.
- Cerebellar haemorrhage presents with sudden onset of headache, vertigo, vomiting, ataxia and sometimes paralysis of conjugate gaze to one side. Initially, no change in the level of consciousness occurs; however, a mass effect produces brainstem compression later and leads to coma.

CONSEQUENCES

- Expansion of haematoma that occurs over several hours.
- Hydrocephalus.
- Cerebral oedema (may produce delayed worsening).

DIAGNOSIS

- CT scan (Fig. 5.9) or MRI brain.
- Cerebral angiography in young patients with no obvious risk factors for intercerebral haemorrhage.

MANAGEMENT

- Management is on similar lines as in infarcts but thrombolysis is contraindicated.
- Patients with Glasgow Coma Scale <8 often require intubation and ventilation.

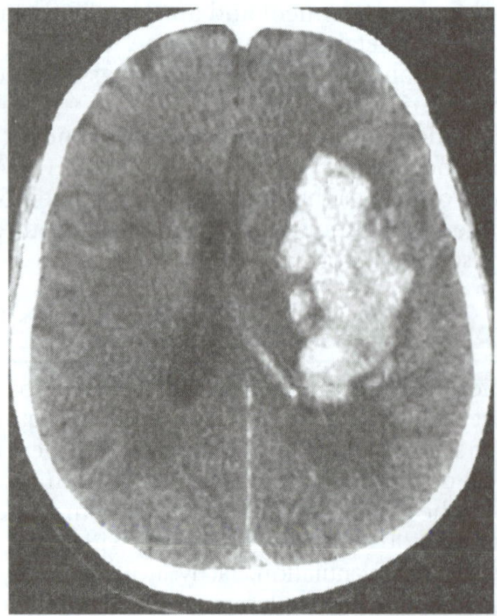

Fig. 5.9 Left intracerebral haemorrhage.

- Control of raised ICP (do not give steroids).
- Administer phenytoin if seizures develop.
- BP should be reduced to 140 mmHg systolic.
- Certain intracerebral haematomas are amenable for surgical evacuation, for example patients with cerebellar haematoma who are deteriorating neurologically or who have brainstem compression and/or hydrocephalus should undergo surgical evacuation of haematoma. Patients with lobar haematoma who are gradually worsening neurologically may also be considered for evacuation.
- If the patient presents within 3 hours of onset, recombinant activated factor VII (rFVIIa) or tranexamic acid may be administered but their role in reducing haematoma expansion, residual neurologic deficit and mortality is controversial. Potential adverse effects include increased incidence of arterial thromboembolism.

Q. How will you prevent occurrence of first episode of stroke?

Q. Discuss in brief the primary prevention of stroke.

- Lifestyle modifications include healthy diet, weight loss, regular physical activity and reduce alcohol.
- Stopping smoking.
- Control of diabetes.
- Lowering systolic BP by 10 mmHg is associated with a reduction in the risk of stroke by about one-third, irrespective of baseline blood pressure levels. Long-acting dihydropyridine calcium channel blockers, angiotensin-converting enzyme inhibitors or angiotensin II receptor blockers are possibly more effective than other classes of antihypertensive drugs.
- Reducing LDL cholesterol to 100 mg/dL using statins.
- Prophylactic aspirin is not recommended as it carries an increased risk of cerebral haemorrhage as well as major bleeding.
- Avoiding routine use of hormonal replacement therapy as its use is associated with increased risk of stroke.
- For asymptomatic patients who are detected to have carotid artery stenosis of 60%–99%, carotid endarterectomy may be considered.
- Anticoagulants in patients with atrial fibrillation and high risk of embolism.

Q. Give a brief account of cerebral venous thrombosis.

- Cerebral venous thrombosis (CVT) is an important cause of stroke in young adults caused by occlusion of the major cerebral venous sinuses (cerebral venous sinus thrombosis) or the smaller feeding cortical veins (cortical vein thrombosis).
- CVT is the cause of approximately 1% to 2% of strokes in young adults.
- Superior sagittal sinus is most commonly involved. Thrombus may extend into transverse and sigmoid sinuses.

- Deep venous system thrombosis (e.g. thrombosis of internal cerebral veins and vein of Galen or straight sinus) is less common.

CAUSES (Table 5.35)

TABLE 5.35 Causes of Cerebral Venous Thrombosis

Local causes:	Systemic causes:
• Trauma to the dural sinuses • Infection in structures adjacent to the dural sinuses (ears, sinuses, mouth, face, neck) • Otitis media • Mastoiditis • Sinusitis • Tonsillitis • Invasion or compression of venous sinuses by neoplastic processes	• Hypercoaguable states • Oral contraceptive use • Pregnancy • Malignancy • Protein C or protein S deficiency • Presence of lupus anticoagulant • Dehydration

PATHOPHYSIOLOGY

- Cerebral venous thrombosis results in elevated cerebral venous pressure that produces decline in cerebral perfusion pressure.
- If reduction of cerebral perfusion pressure is severe enough and prolonged enough, venous infarction occurs and haemorrhage may ensue.

CLINICAL FEATURES

- Unlike arterial thrombosis, symptoms tend to develop slowly or subacutely.
- Most patients develop generalised neurological symptoms with headache as a common first clinical symptom.
- Nausea and vomiting are common.
- Papilloedema due to elevated ICP.
- Some patients develop seizures, or focal sensory or motor deficits. However, unlike arterial thrombosis in the setting of cerebrovascular accident, localisation to one vascular territory is often absent.
- Cranial nerve palsies may occur particularly when there is involvement of petrous sinuses.
- In some cases, coma or death.
- Classical picture of superior sagittal sinus thrombosis is bilateral or alternating deficits and/or seizures. Cavernous sinus thrombosis presents with chemosis, proptosis and painful ophthalmoplegia.

DIAGNOSIS

- CT or MR venography.
- CT or MRI to detect secondary parenchymal lesions.
- CSF examination in appropriate clinical context to rule out meningitis or SAH.
- Coagulation studies in appropriate patients.

TREATMENT

- Supportive measures such as hydration, appropriate antimicrobials, control of seizures with anticonvulsants and control of ICP. Prophylactic antiepileptics are not indicated.
- Intravenous heparin to halt progression of thrombosis. Can be given even if haemorrhage is present.
- Intradural thrombolysis in patients whose clinical status worsens while on anticoagulation.
- Mechanical thrombectomy.

Q. What are the causes of stroke in young?

- Stroke in young is defined as occurrence of stroke in persons between the ages of 15 years and 45 years (some keep the upper age below 40 years or 50 years).
- Various causes of stroke in young are listed in Table 5.36.

Q. Describe the pathogenesis, clinical features and management of Alzheimer's disease.

- Alzheimer's disease is a progressive neurodegenerative disease resulting in decline in cognitive functions together with declining ADL and behavioural disturbances.
- It is the most common cause of cognitive impairment in elderly persons. From the age of 60 years onwards up to 80 years, incidence and prevalence of Alzheimer's disease increases exponentially with age, doubling every 5 years.

PATHOLOGY

- The pathological process consists principally of neuronal loss, principally in the temporoparietal cortex but also in the frontal cortex, together with an inflammatory response to deposition of senile plaques and neurofibrillary tangles.
- Senile plaques and neurofibrillary tangles are regarded as hallmark of Alzheimer's disease, though they may also be present with normal ageing.
- Senile plaques consist of extracellular deposition of congophilic, insoluble material that is amyloid-β (Aβ). It is derived from the enzymatic cleavage of a larger membrane protein, the amyloid precursor protein (APP).
- Neurofibrillary tangles represent intracellular-paired helical filaments of hyperphosphorylated protein known as tau protein. Tau protein is expressed in neurons and normally acts to stabilise microtubules in the cells.
- Other pathological features include synaptic degeneration, accumulation of abnormal lysosomes and mitochondria, neuronal loss and glia-mediated inflammation.

AETIOLOGY

- The exact aetiopathogenesis is not known.
- Three hypotheses include cholinergic hypothesis (reduced acetylcholine), amyloid hypothesis and tau hypothesis.

TABLE 5.36 Causes of Stroke in Young

Ischaemic Stroke	Haemorrhagic Stroke	Venous Thrombosis
• Cardioembolic ◦ Rheumatic heart disease ◦ Bacterial endocarditis ◦ Prosthetic valves • Atrial fibrillation • Arterial dissection • Infections • Atherosclerotic vascular disease • Patent foramen ovale • Atrial myxoma • Mitral valve prolapse • Prothrombotic states ◦ Antiphospholipid antibody syndrome ◦ Protein C deficiency ◦ Protein S deficiency ◦ Antithrombin deficiency • Sickle cell disorder • Paroxysmal nocturnal haemoglobinuria • Vasculitis ◦ Polyarteritis nodosa ◦ Takayasu's arteritis ◦ Systemic lupus erythematosus ◦ Giant cell arteritis • SARS-CoV-2 infection	• Arterio-venous malformations • Saccular aneurysms • Moya Moya syndrome • Septic arteritis • Mycotic aneurysms • Bleeding disorders • Anticoagulants • Cocaine abuse • Intracerebral tumours	• Cortical venous thrombosis ◦ Pregnancy ◦ Postpartum ◦ Dehydration • Oral contraceptive use • Prothrombotic states • Connective tissue disease

- Genes that increase the probability of sporadic Alzheimer's disease include the allele ϵ4 of apolipoprotein E (*APOE*) and the sortilin-related receptor 1 (*SORL1*) gene (which is involved in cholesterol transport, amyloid-β formation and APP processing).
- Carriers of the protective APOE ϵ2 allele have an estimated two times decreased lifetime risk of Alzheimer's disease compared with noncarriers.
- Early onset of Alzheimer's disease (onset <60 years) is uncommon and is usually autosomal dominant. Three gene mutations have been identified: *APP* gene, and the presenilin-1 (*PS1*) and presenilin-2 (*PS2*) genes.
- Moderate consumption of red wine, increased dietary intake of fruits and vegetables, and the use of nonsteroidal anti-inflammatory drugs are associated with a lower risk.
- Potential acquired risk factors for Alzheimer's disease are given in Box 5.43.

BOX 5.43 Risk Factors for Alzheimer's Disease

- Ageing
- Family history of Alzheimer's disease
- Reduced reserve capacity of brain
- Low educational and occupational attainment
- Low mental ability in early life
- Reduced mental and physical activity during late life
- Diet
- Reduced consumption of fish
- Increased consumption of dietary fat
- Head injury
- Risk factors associated with vascular disease
- Hypercholesterolaemia
- Hypertension
- Smoking
- Obesity
- Diabetes

CLINICAL FEATURES

- It is an insidious-onset disease with symptoms in three domains: cognitive, behavioural and functional. Mild cognitive impairment is transitional stage between normal ageing and Alzheimer's disease.
- The patient has disturbances of memory, language and visual skills:
  - There is an impaired ability to learn new things and recall previously learnt information. An inability to retain recently acquired information is typically the initial symptom, whereas memory for remote events is relatively spared until late. Episodic memory impairment (memory for personally experienced events in a particular temporal and spatial context) is an important cognitive deficit. This can be tested by the three-word recall item and the orientation items of the MMSE.
  - Impairment of semantic memory (knowledge of public events, words and the associations between concepts), working memory (ability to manipulate short-term memory representations) and executive functions (coordination of multiple cognitive processes) is often present.
  - A decline in language function and increased difficulty with names and understanding what is being said (nominal and comprehensive dysphasia). The first manifestations of language dysfunction usually include word-finding difficulties, circumlocution and reduced vocabulary in spontaneous speech and anomia.
  - An impaired ability to carry out motor activities despite intact motor function (dyspraxia).
  - Failure to recognise or identify objects despite intact sensory function (agnosia).
- There is a gradual decline in ADL that ultimately leads to profound disability and dependence on others.

- Other features include behavioural problems, psychotic symptoms and depression. Psychotic symptoms are not the presenting features but develop later during the course of disease. Occurrence of psychosis during the initial stages of dementia suggests other diagnoses such as dementia with Lewy bodies. Persecutory delusions occur in nearly 50% of the patients.
- It is important to differentiate between Alzheimer's disease and other treatable causes of dementia (see under 'dementia' on page 321).
- Pneumonia is a common cause of death because aspiration is common due to impaired swallowing mechanisms in the later stages. Other common causes of death include complications from urinary tract infections and falls.

LABORATORY INVESTIGATIONS

- These are carried out to exclude a treatable cause of dementia (see 'dementia' on page 321).
- Common investigations are blood chemistry, a complete blood count, tests for syphilis, serum levels of vitamin B_{12} and thyroid functions.
- A CT head is usually done to exclude an intracranial pathology. An MRI may show atrophy in the hippocampus, mesial and lateral temporal, isthmus cingulate and orbitofrontal areas. It can help exclude normal-pressure hydrocephalus. Focal frontal or anterior temporal atrophy suggests a diagnosis of frontotemporal dementia. Large white matter abnormalities indicate a vascular dementia, particularly if the history is one of a stepwise decline in cognitive function.
- High-resolution functional MRI may distinguish Alzheimer's disease from normal ageing.
- Cerebrospinal fluid is normal but may show slight elevation in protein content. There is an increase in total tau and phosphorylated tau but a decrease in Aβ.
- Functional neuroimaging studies such as PET and SPECT scans can provide a supporting role in diagnosis. PET shows decreased FDG uptake in hippocampus, parietotemporal cortex and posterior cingulate cortex bilaterally. Amyloid PET imaging shows cortical amyloid β deposition while tau PET using the tau tracer flortaucipir is also helpful for diagnosis.
- Biomarkers are being increasingly used to diagnose Alzheimer's disease. These include amyloid, phosphorylated tau and neurodegeneration (measured by total tau) in CSF and blood.

DIAGNOSIS

- Criteria for a diagnosis of clinically probable Alzheimer's disease are the presence of an episodic memory deficit in combination with impairment of at least one other cognitive domain. Frequently affected domains at an early stage are executive functions and word finding. There must be a significant impact on ADL with no alternative explanations (delirium, medication, comorbidity and depression).
  - MMSE is useful in the initial evaluation of patients with suspected dementia.

BOX 5.44 Criteria for Probable Alzheimer's Disease (National Institute on Aging and the Alzheimer's Association)

- Presence of dementia and the following:
  - Interference with ability to function at work or at usual activities
  - A decline from a previous level of functioning and performing
  - Not explained by delirium or major psychiatric disorder
  - Cognitive impairment established by history-taking from the patient and a knowledgeable informant; and objective bedside mental status examination or neuropsychologic testing
  - Cognitive impairment involving a minimum of two of the following domains:
    - Impaired ability to acquire and remember new information
    - Impaired reasoning and handing of complex tasks, poor judgement
    - Impaired visuospatial abilities
    - Impaired language functions
    - Changes in personality, behaviour or comportment
  - Other core clinical criteria include:
    - Insidious onset
    - Clear-cut history of worsening
    - Initial and most prominent cognitive deficits are one of the following: amnestic presentation (i.e. impairment in learning and recall of recently learned information) or nonamnestic presentations (including either a language presentation, with prominent word-finding deficits; a visuospatial presentation, with visual cognitive deficits; or a dysexecutive presentation, with prominent impairment of reasoning, judgement, and/or problem solving)
  - No evidence of substantial concomitant cerebrovascular disease, core features of dementia with Lewy bodies (DLB), prominent features of behavioural variant frontotemporal dementia (FTD) or prominent features of semantic or nonfluent/agrammatic variants of primary progressive aphasia (PPA), or evidence of another concurrent, active neurologic or nonneurologic disease or use of medication that could have a substantial effect on cognition

  - Cognitive ageing (age-related cognitive decline) refers to age-related decline that selectively affects specific cognitive processes, including delayed recall, processing speed and executive functions. Familiarity of past objects and persons is usually not affected in age-related cognition decline.
- As per the National Institute on Aging and the Alzheimer's Association, the criteria for probable Alzheimer's disease are given in Box 5.44.

MANAGEMENT

GENERAL

- Combined healthy balanced nutrition, physical exercise, cognitive training and social activities, and vascular and metabolic risk management show benefits on cognition.
- Role of omega-3 fatty acids is controversial.

COGNITIVE DEFICITS

- Cholinesterase inhibitors provide modest improvement in symptoms and reduction in the rate of cognitive decline. They inhibit acetylcholinesterase, the enzyme that degrades acetylcholine in the synaptic cleft, thereby increasing the availability of acetylcholine.

These drugs include donepezil, rivastigmine and galantamine. Common side effects include nausea, vomiting, diarrhoea and weight loss.
  - Donepezil is started at a dosage of 5 mg daily at bedtime and increased to 10 mg daily after 1–4 weeks.
  - Galantamine is started at a dosage of 4 mg twice daily and gradually titrated to 12 mg twice daily with step-ups at 1-week to 4-week intervals.
  - Rivastigmine is started at a dosage of 1.5 mg twice daily and titrated over 1–3 months to 6 mg twice daily.
- In moderate to severe cases, memantine, an NMDA antagonist, may be added to cholinesterase inhibitors. It is believed to protect neurons from glutamate-mediated excitotoxicity.
- Other agents include vitamin E, statins and NSAIDs, though their exact role is not clear.

DISEASE-MODIFYING DRUGS

- Aducanumab, an amyloid beta-directed monoclonal antibody is approved for use as disease-modifying drug.

COMORBID CONDITIONS

- Optimal management should be provided for any comorbid conditions including visual or hearing deficits, dental problems and other common medical illnesses.

BEHAVIOURAL PROBLEMS

- Treatment of associated behavioural problems by nonpharmacological and pharmacological interventions (psychotropic agents) should be prescribed. Atypical antipsychotic drugs (risperidone and olanzapine) are preferred for the management of psychosis. For depression, serotonin reuptake inhibitors (e.g. citalopram, escitalopram and sertraline) are used.

EDUCATION

- Education of caregiver is very important in patients with Alzheimer's disease.

Q. Describe the aetiology, clinical features and diagnosis of Parkinson's disease. (IM 19.8)

Q. What is parkinsonism? How would you classify parkinsonism? Discuss the management of idiopathic parkinsonism.

PARKINSONISM

- Parkinsonism is a clinical syndrome involving bradykinesia, plus at least one of the following three features: tremor, rigidity and postural instability. All patients with Parkinson's disease have parkinsonism, but not all patients with parkinsonism have Parkinson's disease.

BOX 5.45 Classification of Parkinsonism

PRIMARY PARKINSONISM:
- Paralysis agitans or Parkinson's disease or idiopathic parkinsonism

SECONDARY (SYMPTOMATIC):
- Postencephalitic (postencephalitis lethargica)
- Toxins—for example methyl-phenyl-tetrahydropyridine (MPTP), manganese, carbon monoxide
- Drugs—for example reserpine, phenothiazines, butyrophenones (including haloperidol), α-methyldopa, metoclopramide
- Ischaemic (vascular parkinsonism)
- Tumours in basal ganglion
- Punch-drunk syndrome in boxers
- Infections—for example HIV, influenza
- Normal-pressure hydrocephalus

PARKINSONISM PLUS (DEGENERATIVE DISORDERS WITH PROMINENT ADDITIONAL NEUROLOGICAL FEATURES):
- Progressive supranuclear palsy, multiple system atrophy (MSA) (striatonigral degeneration, Shy–Drager syndrome, sporadic olivopontocerebellar atrophy), diffuse Lewy body disease

HEREDODEGENERATIVE PARKINSONISM:
- Spinocerebellar ataxia, Wilson's disease, juvenile-onset Huntington's disease

- Two environmental factors are recognised to lower the risk for Parkinson's disease—cigarette smoking and coffee drinking.

CLASSIFICATION (Box 5.45)

- Parkinsonism plus is a group of degenerative disorders that have additional neurological signs other than those of parkinsonism. For example, multiple system atrophy (MSA) includes variable combination of parkinsonism (poor response to L-dopa), cerebellar, pyramidal and autonomic degeneration. MSA encompasses three syndromes: a predominance of parkinsonian features (MSA-P subtype), Shy–Drager syndrome and predominance of cerebellar ataxia (MSA-C subtype). Autonomic dysfunction results in urinary symptoms (urge incontinence and incomplete bladder emptying), erectile dysfunctions in males, orthostatic hypotension and chronic constipation.

PATHOLOGY OF PARKINSON'S DISEASE (PARALYSIS AGITANS)

- There is loss of pigmented cells and deposition of Lewy bodies in locus coeruleus followed by substantia nigra. This results in degeneration of nigrostriatal pathway. These cells normally synthesise dopamine. With degeneration of these cells, dopamine level in the striatum gets depleted; this is the major chemical pathology in Parkinson's disease. Degeneration of nondopaminergic neurons also occurs, but it usually occurs later in the course of the disease. The loss of nondopaminergic neurons contributes to the non-motor features.

CLINICAL FEATURES

- Affects both sexes equally and starts usually during sixth decade and later. Occasionally, it may appear during fifth decade. Initial symptoms may be easy tiredness or muscular aches, usually unilaterally. Mild slowness of activity or depression may be present. Later, classical combination of tremor, rigidity and hypokinesia appears.

TREMOR

- It is classically a tremor at rest and is compound (called pill-rolling tremor) occurring at wrist and fingers on one side first that decreases with action. At times, action or postural tremor may also be present. Tremor may also occur at head, jaw or lower limbs.

RIGIDITY

- Hypertonia is due to rigidity. When tremor is present, it adds cog-wheeling character to the basic lead-pipe hypertonia (cogwheel rigidity). It is unilateral in the beginning of disease.

HYPOKINESIA/AKINESIA

- It is difficulty in initiating the motor acts. This results in delay or slowness of motor act after intention to start.

BRADYKINESIA

- It is the paucity or slowness of movements. Some physicians consider hypokinesia under the term bradykinesia when it is defined as slowness of initiation of voluntary movement with progressive reduction in speed and amplitude of repetitive actions. There is reduced movement in acts like getting up, adjusting posture and walking. Two common features are reduced arm swing on one side (which is often misinterpreted by patients and physicians as an orthopaedic problem) and slowness of repetitive supination/pronation of hands. Face looks blank and expressionless ('mask-like face'). Amplitude of writing declines near the end of a sentence.

DISTURBED POSTURAL REFLEXES

- Occurs about 5 years after the onset of disease.
- Results in stooped or bent posture with tendency to fall easily, and difficulty in maintaining equilibrium while sitting or standing.
- Muscle strength and tendon jerks remain normal. Glabellar tap becomes positive. Primitive reflexes get released.
- Speech is of low volume and is monotonous. Micrographia is present with a tendency to tail off at the end of a line. Stance is stooped, gait becomes shuffling (festinant), associated arm swinging is absent, and turning about becomes slow and laborious.
- With advancing disease, patient assumes fixed flexed postures, and remains curled in bed, unable to move. Death occurs due to infection (bronchopneumonia and septicaemia).

OTHERS (NONMOTOR FEATURES) (Box 5.46)

BOX 5.46 Other (Nonmotor) Features of Parkinson's Disease

- Autonomic dysfunction
  - Orthostatic hypotension
  - Urinary incontinence
  - Impotence
  - Constipation
  - Sialorrhoea
  - Anhidrosis
- Neuropsychiatric symptoms
  - Depression
  - Psychosis
  - Dementia
  - Anxiety
  - Panic attacks
- Sensory problems
  - Reduced smell
  - Pain
  - Sleep disorders
  - Restless legs
  - Insomnia
  - Daytime somnolence

EXCLUSION CRITERIA FOR PARKINSON'S DISEASE (Box 5.47)

BOX 5.47 Exclusion Criteria for Parkinson's Disease

- Repeated strokes with stepwise progression
- Repeated head injury
- Antipsychotic or dopamine-depleting drugs
- Definite encephalitis and/or oculogyric crises
- More than one affected relative
- Strictly unilateral features after 3 years
- Other neurological features: Supranuclear gaze palsy, cerebellar signs, early severe autonomic involvement, Babinski's sign, early severe dementia with disturbances of language, memory or praxis
- Exposure to known neurotoxin
- Presence of cerebral tumour or communicating hydrocephalus on neuroimaging

PARKINSON'S DISEASE VERSUS PARKINSONISM PLUS SYNDROMES (Table 5.37)

TABLE 5.37 Parkinson's Disease Versus Parkinsonism Plus Syndromes

Features	Parkinson's Disease	Parkinsonism Plus Syndrome
• Pattern of onset	Asymmetrical	Usually symmetrical
• Rigidity	More in peripheral parts	More in axial parts
• Tremors	Resting	Absent or atypical
• Associated features (e.g. dysautonomia, early dementia, cerebellar signs, pyramidal signs)	Usually absent	Some of them are often present
• Response to L-dopa	Good to excellent	Mild to moderate response initially only
• Progress	Slow	Relatively rapid

DIAGNOSIS

- It is purely clinical and there is no definitive diagnostic test to confirm Parkinson's disease. The four cardinal features of Parkinson's disease can be grouped under the acronym TRAP: *T*remor at rest, *R*igidity, *A*kinesia (or bradykinesia) and *P*ostural instability.
- If clinical features are not strictly within the syndrome or if the disease occurs in earlier life, Wilson's disease will have to be ruled out by estimating serum copper, ceruloplasmin and urinary copper levels.
- Symptoms that suggest a diagnosis other than Parkinson's disease include lack of response to levodopa, hallucinations, prominent and early dementia, early postural instability, severe and early autonomic dysfunction, upward gaze paralysis and involuntary movements other than tremors.
- CT scan or MRI is required if these additional signs are present.
- In atypical cases, PET and SPECT.

MANAGEMENT

- If any offending drug was used, it should be withdrawn. Patient should be seen by a physiotherapist and occupational therapist to help him/her live well with the disability by modifying home surroundings intelligently.

DRUG THERAPY

Anticholinergics

- Trihexyphenidyl (benzhexol) and orphenadrine are useful in controlling tremors but do not help in other disturbances. They can cause urinary retention, worsen glaucoma and cause confusion in elderly. Hence, they are rarely used as first-line drugs unless patient has severe tremors. They should be avoided if the patient is older than 65 years.

Amantadine

- Potentiates endogenous dopamine (presynaptic agonist) and has mild antiparkinsonian effect. It is useful early in the disease or in conjunction with L-dopa replacement.
- Important adverse effects include psychosis, oedema and livedo reticularis in the lower limbs.

L-Dopa

- Highly effective in treating motor symptoms of bradykinesia and hypokinesia.
- Orally administered L-dopa after absorption crosses blood–brain barrier and gets metabolised to dopamine within the brain. But large amount gets metabolised peripherally to dopamine by decarboxylation. Dopamine cannot cross the blood–brain barrier. By combining a peripheral decarboxylase inhibitor (e.g. carbidopa and benserazide) with L-dopa, this can be overcome.
- The currently used combinations are given as follows:
    - L-Dopa + carbidopa (4:1 or 10:1 ratio).
    - L-Dopa + benserazide (4:1 ratio).
- Drug is started at a low dose (50 mg/dose). Requirement is titrated for frequency per day and strength per dose, slowly. Increments are made once in 2 weeks. Full therapeutic effect may take 4–8 weeks. Maximum dose is 800–1000 mg of L-dopa per day (with peripheral decarboxylase inhibitor). At higher doses, dose-related side effects like dyskinesias and hallucinations occur frequently.
- Over a period of time (after 3–5 years) with progression of disease, control becomes poor and fluctuations in symptoms occur frequently. These fluctuations include wearing-off effect (transient deterioration shortly before the next dose is due), peak-dose dyskinesias (appearance of choreic movements of the trunk, arms and neck during the period of maximum therapeutic efficacy of dopaminergic drugs) and the 'on–off' phenomenon (abrupt and transient deterioration occurring frequently without an obvious relation to the dosage schedule). Catechol-*O*-methyltransferase (COMT) inhibitors (see the subsequent text) are useful to reduce these response fluctuations. For dyskinesias, amantadine, dopamine receptor agonists and COMT inhibitors are useful.
- Levodopa–carbidopa intestinal gel (LCIG) is an approved therapy for patients with advanced PD. LCIG is delivered continuously by a percutaneous endoscopic gastrojejunostomy tube through a portable infusion pump.

Dopamine Receptor Agonists

- Postsynaptic dopamine agonists may be classified as ergot derived (bromocriptine, pergolide and cabergoline) or nonergot derived (apomorphine, pramipexole, ropinirole and rotigotine).
- Ergot-derived dopamine agonists should not be used as first-line treatment for Parkinson's disease as they may produce moderate to severe cardiac valvulopathy and serosal fibrosis (pleural, pericardial and retroperitoneal).
- Nonergot dopamine agonists are preferable to ergot dopamine agonists and are used as an alternative or an addition to levodopa therapy.
- All types of dopamine agonists can produce impulse control disorders (including pathological gambling, binge eating and hypersexuality) and daytime somnolence.

MAO-B Inhibitors

- Selegiline, rasagiline and safinamide are MAO-B inhibitors, and have dual role to play.
    - They reduce the metabolism of dopamine and thereby reduce the dose and frequency of administration of L-dopa at all stages.
    - They can slow down the degeneration in substantia nigra and are recommended to be used in all patients from early stages of the disease (selegiline 5 mg BD; rasagiline 1 mg OD). However, they can produce serious side effects and drug interactions.

Catechol-O-Methyltransferase Inhibitors

- This category of drugs includes tolcapone, entacapone and opicapone that enhance the benefits of levodopa therapy by reducing the conversion of levodopa to 3-*O*-methyldopa (which normally competes with levodopa for an active carrier mechanism). This increases the availability of levodopa in the brain. These agents are useful in patients with response fluctuation to levodopa.

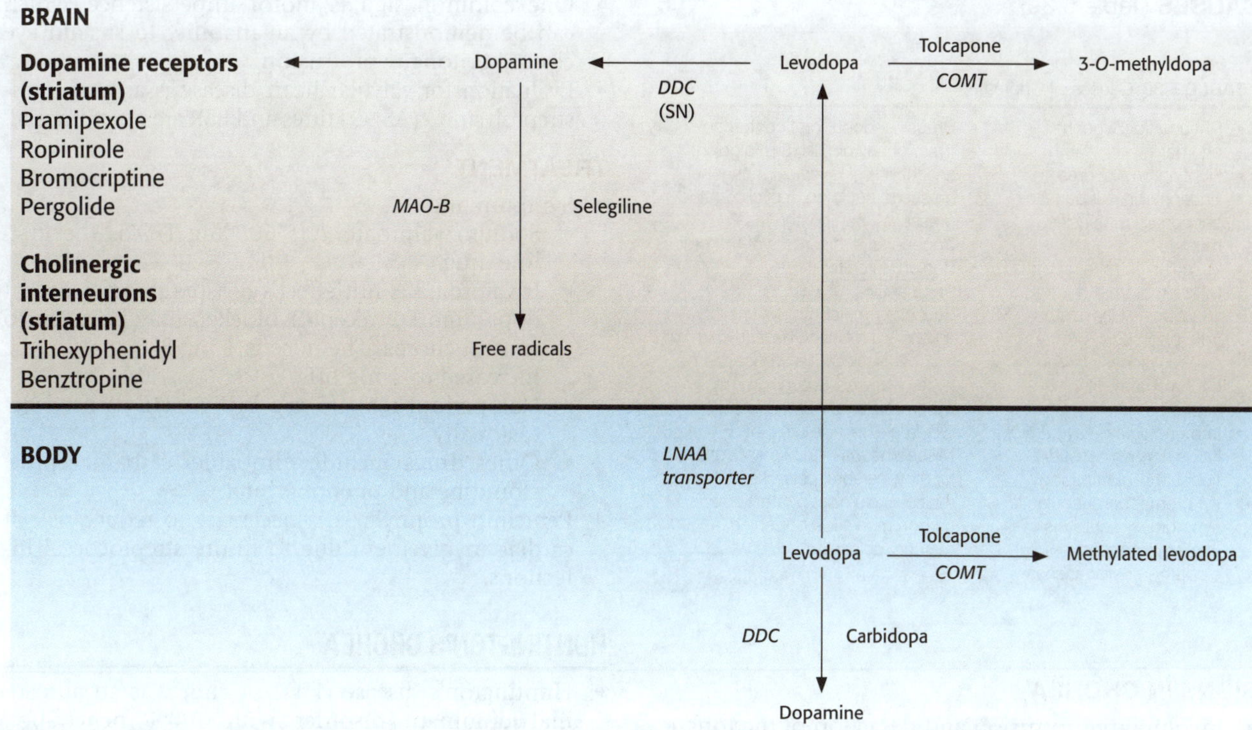

Flowchart 5.4 Sites of Action of Various Drugs Used in Parkinson's Disease. COMT, catechol-*O*-methyl transferase; DDC, dihydroxyphenylalanine decarboxylase; LNAA, large neutral amino acid; MAO-B, monoamine oxidase B; SN, substantia nigra.

Rivastigmine

- May be considered in patients with significant dementia.

MISCELLANEOUS DRUGS

- Istradefylline, an adenosine receptor A_{2A} antagonist, is useful to reduce wearing-off effect of levodopa.
- Pimavanserin, an atypical antipsychotic, is useful for the treatment of hallucinations and delusions.
- Botulinum toxin type A is useful to control tremors.

SUMMARY OF MEDICAL TREATMENT

- Flowchart 5.4 indicates sites of action of various drugs used in Parkinson's disease.

SURGERY

- Stereotactic thalamotomy (ventrolateral nucleus of thalamus) used to be performed in the past is largely given up due to excellent response to drugs.
- Deep brain stimulation (subthalamic nucleus and globus pallidus interna) has been used with success in severe disease.

Q. Discuss briefly the CNS disorders characterised by involuntary movements. (IM 19.2)

- A movement disorder indicates abnormal movement or paucity of movement either voluntary or automatic which is not attributable to weakness or spasticity or any other medical causes directly interfering with musculoskeletal system. It can be hyperkinetic or hypokinetic (bradykinesia in Parkinson's disease) (Table 5.38).

TABLE 5.38 Hyperkinetic Movement Disorders

Hyperkinetic Movement Disorders	Site of Lesion
• Parkinsonism (resting tremors)	Substantia nigra and corpus striatum
• Chorea	Caudate nucleus
• Athetosis	Putamen
• Hemiballismus	Subthalamic nucleus
• Dystonia	Not known
• Myoclonus	Several areas
• Tic	—
• Tremors	—
• Tardive dyskinesia	—

CHOREA

- Irregular, semipurposeful, abrupt, rapid, brief, jerky and unsustained movements that flow randomly from one part of the body to another. These movements disappear during sleep.
- When choreic movements are more severe, assuming a flinging, sometimes violent, character, they are called ballism.

CAUSES (Table 5.39)

TABLE 5.39 Causes of Chorea

• Rheumatic (Sydenham's chorea) • Huntington's chorea • Encephalitis—Japanese encephalitis, measles, mumps • Vascular—stroke, subdural haematoma • Infections—HIV-related (toxoplasmosis, progressive multifocal leukoencephalopathy, HIV encephalitis) • Immunological—systemic lupus erythematosus, antiphospholipid antibody syndrome, paraneoplastic syndromes, acute disseminated encephalomyelopathy, coeliac disease	• Drugs—L-dopa, oral contraceptives, phenytoin, lithium, digoxin, anticholinergics, calcium channel blockers, baclofen, tricyclic antidepressants, corticosteroids • Degenerative disorders of the brain • Benign hereditary • Pregnancy • Endocrine-metabolic dysfunction—adrenal insufficiency, hyperthyroidism, hypercalcaemia/hypocalcaemia, hyperglycaemia/hypoglycaemia, hypernatraemia, hyponatraemia, liver failure, renal failure • Miscellaneous—anoxic encephalopathy, cerebral palsy, kernicterus, multiple sclerosis, post-traumatic, carbon monoxide poisoning, mercury poisoning

SIGNS IN CHOREA

- Involuntary protrusion and retraction of the tongue.
- Respiratory irregularity.
- Inability to hold the hands above head with palms facing each other as it results in pronation of arms so that palms face outwards (pronator sign).
- Milking action of patient's fingers if asked to grasp the physician's fingers (milkmaid sign) due to fluctuating strength of the grip.
- Hung-up reflexes (sustained contractions and choreic movements of the leg after the knee-jerk reflex).
- 'Jack-in-the-box' tongue (or chameleon tongue—patient is unable to maintain tongue in a protruded state, and the tongue moves in and out).

SYDENHAM'S CHOREA (SAINT VITUS DANCE)

- It is the most common cause of chorea in children. It is a self-limiting, nonsuppurative complication of group A β-haemolytic streptococcal pharyngitis and it follows acute rheumatic fever by 4–6 months. Severity varies and disorder may continue for a few months.
- Based on the assumption of molecular mimicry between streptococcal and central nervous system antigens, it has been proposed that the bacterial infection in genetically predisposed subjects leads to formation of cross-reactive antibodies that disrupt the basal ganglia function. Inflammation has been seen in caudate nucleus.
- It is a neuropsychiatric disorder; the clinical features include both neurological abnormalities (chorea, weakness and hypotonia) and psychiatric disorders (such as emotional lability, hyperactivity, distractibility, obsessions and compulsions). These abnormalities lead to inability to perform normal ADL including eating, talking, dressing, writing, walking, learning and socialising, and thus impact negatively on the child's quality of life.
- One common sign is motor impersistence, which can be demonstrated by an inability to sustain eye closure or tongue protrusion.
- Evaluation for valvular heart disease is a must. Antistreptolysin-O (ASLO) titres and ESR are often normal.

TREATMENT

- Symptomatic.
  - Sodium valproate 200–600 mg TID is the first-line drug.
  - If valproate is not effective, risperidone, a potent dopamine D2 receptor blocker, may be given to control chorea. The dose is 1 mg BID that can be increased to 2 mg BID.
  - Haloperidol 0.5–1.5 mg BID or TID is used occasionally.
  - Other drugs include pimozide, carbamazepine, clonidine and phenobarbital.
- Penicillin prophylaxis is necessary to reduce risk of cardiac involvement due to future streptococcal infections.

HUNTINGTON'S CHOREA

- Huntington's disease (HD) or chorea is an autosomal dominant disorder with 100% penetrance, caused by an expansion of an unstable trinucleotide (CAG) repeat near the telomere of chromosome 4. The normal CAG repeat length in the gene is 35 or lower; expansions of 40 or more cause HD with complete penetrance. In successive generations, onset tends to develop earlier in life (correlating with longer repeat sizes—genetic anticipation).
- Age of onset is around 40 years. It progresses relentlessly over 15–17 years.
- Characterised by a triad of movement disorder, cognitive decline and behavioural changes.
- Main features are choreic movements and hypotonia. Rigidity may be seen in many cases.
- Personality and mood changes, psychosis and dementia are common.
- Oculomotor abnormalities occur in the form of slowing of saccades and increased response latency.
- No curative treatment is available. Symptomatic treatment is with dopamine-depleting agents such as reserpine, tetrabenazine or deutetrabenazine, and neuroleptics such as haloperidol. Other medications that may help suppress HD include amantadine, levetiracetam and clonazepam.
- Branaplam is being developed as a potential first orally administered disease-modifying therapy for HD.

ATHETOSIS

- Athetosis is slow, writhing, distal movements affecting fingers, hands, toes and feet (snake charmer's movement).
- Causes: Various causes of athetosis are listed in Box 5.48.
- Treatment:
  - Haloperidol, tetrabenazine.

BOX 5.48 Causes of Athetosis

- Kernicterus
- Degenerative brain disorders (involving basal ganglia)
- Cerebral palsy
- Encephalitis
- Thalamic stroke

BOX 5.49 Causes of Dystonia

- Drugs—prochlorperazine, metoclopramide, haloperidol, chloroquine, etc.
- Kernicterus
- Degenerative disorders
- Previous brain injury
- Familial

DYSTONIA

- Dystonia is a movement disorder characterised by sustained or intermittent muscle contractions causing abnormal, often repetitive, movements, postures or both. May be focal or generalised.
- Causes are listed in Box 5.49.
- Examples include cranial dystonia (blepharospasm or oromandibular or lingual dystonia), cervical dystonia (spasmodic torticollis), laryngeal dystonia (spasmodic dysphonia) and dystonic writer's cramp.
- Treatment:
  - Tetrabenazine, a dopamine-depleting drug.
  - High-dose anticholinergics (up to 24–30 mg of benzhexol per day; trihexyphenidyl up to 60–100 mg/day). Occasionally, L-dopa is useful in familial cases.
  - Sodium valproate (200–600 mg TID).
  - Botulinum toxin A and B for cervical dystonia, blepharospasm, oromandibular dystonia, laryngeal dystonia and writer's cramp.
  - Stereotactic thalamotomy or deep brain stimulation may be required if the disease is severe and distressing.
  - For drug-induced dystonia, benztropine, diphenhydramine, promethazine or diazepam can be used.

HEMIBALLISMUS

- It is violent flinging movements of the limbs. It is usually unilateral, and hence called hemiballismus.
- Cause:
  - Stroke affecting subthalamic nucleus (on contralateral side).
- Treatment:
  - Haloperidol 0.5–2.5 mg TID.
  - Tetrabenazine 25–50 mg TID.

MYOCLONUS

- Myoclonus is sudden, involuntary, brief, irregular, jerk-like contractions (positive myoclonus) or inhibition of contraction (negative myoclonus) of certain muscle groups. It may occur at two or more sites.
- Myoclonic muscle contractions are mostly accompanied by some movement of the affected body segment. In fasciculations or myokymia, twitches remain within affected body segment.
- Occasionally, myoclonus can be due to brief loss or inhibition of muscular tone, as in asterixis—for example in hepatic encephalopathy ('liver flap') or in uraemic encephalopathy. This is known as negative myoclonus.

CAUSES (Box 5.50)

BOX 5.50 Causes of Myoclonus

- Metabolic disturbances
  - Posthypoxic brain injury
  - Chronic renal failure
  - Chronic liver disease
  - Respiratory failure
  - Electrolyte imbalance
- Encephalitis
- Drug overdose
- Tricyclic antidepressants
- Lipid storage diseases
- Creutzfeldt–Jakob disease
- Myoclonic epilepsy

TREATMENT

- Correction of underlying disease.
- Sodium valproate (300–1200 mg/day).
- Clonazepam (0.5–10 mg/day).

TICS

- Abrupt, usually brief and often repetitive jerky and stereotyped movements, which vary in intensity and are repeated at irregular intervals.
- Patients usually have an inner urge that precedes the actual movement or a local feeling of discomfort in the region of the tic. These premonitory sensations are usually temporarily relieved by the occurrence of the tic.
- Tics are voluntarily suppressible for variable periods of time, but this usually occurs at the expense of mounting inner tension and an irresistible need to perform the tic, followed by a rebound burst of tics. Motor and phonic tics can persist during all stages of sleep.
- Many patients with childhood-onset tics have Tourette's syndrome, a genetic disorder typically manifested by a wide array of chronic, fluctuating, simple, and complex motor and phonic (vocal) tics. Associated comorbidities include attention-deficit disorder (with or without hyperactivity) and obsessive-compulsive disorder.
- Education and acceptance are often all that is required. Drug treatment includes clonidine, neuroleptic drugs (e.g. fluphenazine and risperidone), tetrabenazine (a monoamine-depleting drug), topiramate and clonazepam.

TARDIVE DYSKINESIA

- Tardive dyskinesia (TD) is a medication-induced hyperkinetic movement disorder associated with the use of dopamine receptor-blocking agents, including antipsychotic drugs (both first generation and second generation) and antiemetic agents, metoclopramide and prochlorperazine.

- It encompasses a wide range of abnormal, involuntary movements that often persist after discontinuation of the causative medication. It can be irreversible and lifelong.
- The involuntary movements and postures include chorea, athetosis, akathisia (motor restlessness resulting in repeated leg-crossing, weight-shifting, or stepping in place), stereotyped behaviours, dystonia, tics and respiratory dyskinesias (tachypnoea, irregular breathing rhythms and grunting noises).
- Oral, facial and lingual dyskinesia are the most common manifestations of TD. The movements may include protruding and twisting movements of the tongue, pouting, puckering, or smacking movements of the lips, chewing movements and blepharospasm.
- Tetrabenazine, valbenazine and deutetrabenazine are vesicular monoamine transporter-2 (VMAT2) inhibitors and have been found useful in managing patients with TD.

Q. Define tremors. How do you classify tremors? Describe them briefly.

- Tremor is rhythmic alternate movement at a joint due to synchronous or alternate contraction of antagonistic muscles.
- It is differentiated from other involuntary movement disorders, such as chorea, athetosis, ballism and myoclonus, by its repetitive, stereotyped movements of a regular amplitude and frequency.
- Tremor may be simple (when it occurs in a single plane) or compound (when it is multiplanar, e.g. pill-rolling tremor of Parkinson's disease).
- It may be physiological or pathological. Physiological tremor is a fine tremor occurring at a frequency of 8–12/second. Physiological tremor is barely visible to the unaided eye and is symptomatic only during activities that require extreme precision. It is accentuated during anxiety, fever, thyrotoxicosis and use of adrenergic drugs. Pathological tremor occurs in thyrotoxicosis, hypoglycaemia, hypocalcaemia, Cushing's syndrome, alcohol withdrawal, drug and toxin ingestion (Box 5.51) and several neurological conditions.
- Tremors may occur at rest (static) or on movement (kinesiogenic or action). Kinesiogenic tremor or action tremor is any tremor that emerges during voluntary contraction of muscles. It may be intentional (cerebellar) or postural action type.

BOX 5.51 Drugs/Toxins Causing Tremors

- Adrenergic agonists
- Valproic acid
- Lamotrigine
- Lithium
- Tricyclic antidepressants
- Antihistamines
- Thyroxine
- Nifedipine
- Neuroleptics
- Nicotine
- Theophylline
- Monoamine oxidase inhibitor
- Cyclosporin A
- Alcohol withdrawal
- Caffeine
- Corticosteroids

REST OR STATIC TREMOR

- Rest tremor (static tremor) is maximal at rest (with gravity eliminated) and becomes less prominent or disappears with activity.
- It is typically seen in parkinsonism where it may be of pill-rolling type. It is often associated with bradykinesia and rigidity.

ACTION TREMOR

- These occur while performing an action. It is of two types: postural tremor and intention (kinetic) tremor.

POSTURAL TREMOR

- Tremor is maximal when limb posture is actively maintained against gravity.
- It is reduced by rest and is not markedly enhanced during voluntary movements towards a target.
- It often occurs due to toxic and metabolic factors, or stress where the onset is relatively acute.
- Insidious onset of postural tremor indicates a benign or familial essential tremor. It affects hands in nearly all cases and frequently affects head, face/jaw, voice, tongue and lower limbs. Ethanol is surprisingly effective in reversing essential tremor temporarily.
- The two most often used drugs are nonselective β-blockers (e.g. propranolol) and primidone. Other drugs are topiramate, gabapentin and alprazolam. Intramuscular injections of botulinum toxin type A into intrinsic hand muscles can be considered in medically resistant cases. Lastly, deep brain stimulation in the ventral intermedius nucleus of thalamus is effective in more than 90% of patients.

INTENTION TREMOR

- Intention tremor is a cerebellar sign.
- Classic intention tremor is produced by lesions in the cerebellum or in the brachium conjunctivum pathway from deep cerebellar nuclei (dentate, globose and emboliform) to contralateral ventrolateral thalamus. Stroke, multiple sclerosis and tumour may affect the cerebellum and cerebellar pathways causing tremor. Drug toxicity (e.g. phenytoin, sodium valproate and amiodarone) is another important cause to exclude.
- It is brought on by voluntary movement and seen as rhythmic side-to-side oscillation as the limb reaches closer to the target, and stops on completion of the intended movement.
- Proximal limb muscles are usually involved more than distal ones.
- Clinically identified during finger–nose or heel–knee tests.

Q. What are the various signs in cerebellar diseases?

- **Dyssynergia:** Difficulty in carrying out complex movements resulting in breaking of an act into its components.
- **Dysdiadochokinesia:** Inability to perform alternating movements smoothly and rapidly (e.g. asking

the patient to tap the palm of one hand with the fingers of the other, and then rapidly turn over the fingers and tap the palm with the back of them, repeatedly, or asking the patient to supinate and pronate the hands rapidly).

- **Dysmetria:** Loss of ability to judge the distance, speed or power of movement. The act may be stopped before the target is reached or the patient overshoots the desired target (past-pointing during finger–nose test).
- **Intention tremor:** Discussed above.
- **Rebound phenomenon:** Inability to stop the movement of a body part when suddenly released after active resistance (e.g. when the patient is asked to flex his/her elbow against physician's resistance, and then the physician suddenly releases the patient's arm, the patient may strike his/her face with his/her hand).
- **Hypotonia:** The tone of muscles is reduced on the side of the lesion.
- **Pendular knee jerk:** The reflexes tend to be less brisk and rather slower in rise and fall producing pendular jerk at the knee (three or more swings at the knee when the knee reflex is elicited with patient in sitting position and the legs hanging from bedside).
- **Nystagmus:** Horizontal, coarse nystagmus, worse on looking to the side of lesion with fast component towards the affected side.
- **Titubation:** Rhythmic oscillation of head on the body or of the body itself. The patient may not sit or stand because of this and may fall backwards.
- **Gait ataxia:** Patient reels from side to side with a tendency to fall on the side of lesion. He/she cannot walk on a line (impaired tandem walking). If asked to walk around a chair, patient sways on the side of the lesion.
- **Speech disturbances:** Scanning (incoordination of tongue) or staccato speech (incoordination of the larynx) due to incoordination of the muscles of articulation. In staccato speech, each syllable is uttered separately. In scanning speech, syllables of words are separated by pauses.
- **Oculomotor abnormalities:** Irregular bursts of rapid eye movements which include opsoclonus, ocular flutter, up-beating nystagmus and down-beating nystagmus.

Q. Enumerate various gait disorders.

- Various gait disorders are described in Table 5.40. Fig. 5.10 depicts some of the abnormal gaits.

Q. Write a short note on cerebellar ataxias.

- Comprise a wide spectrum of neurological disorders with ataxia as the main symptom.
- Ataxia results from the involvement of cerebellar structures, or from a combination of cerebellar and extracerebellar lesions, especially due to brainstem involvement or sensory involvement.

CLASSIFICATION

- Causes of ataxias can be classified based on duration (Table 5.41) and based on whether they are hereditary or acquired (Table 5.42).

TABLE 5.40 Gait Disorders

Type of Gait	Features	Common Causes
Spastic gait		
• Unilateral	Circumduction of the affected leg during the swing phase of each step	Ischaemic stroke, intracerebral haemorrhage
• Bilateral	Scissoring due to increased tone in the adductor muscles so that the legs nearly touch with each step	Cerebral palsy, myelopathy, multiple sclerosis
Waddling gait	Weakness of gluteal medius muscles leads to drop of non-weight-bearing side resulting in excessive side-to-side trunk motion	Proximal muscle weakness (e.g. myopathy)
High steppage gait	Patient lifts the swinging leg higher to compensate for the toes' inability to clear the ground with each step; this leads to a slapping quality when foot lands on the ground	Weakness of ankle dorsiflexion (e.g. peripheral polyneuropathy, L5 radiculopathy, lead poisoning)
Shuffling gait	Shortened steps, reduced arm swing and forward flexed posture	Parkinsonism
Festinant gait	Steps become increasingly rapid and short so that gait takes on the appearance of running; tendency to fall	Advanced parkinsonism
Cerebellar ataxic gait	Wide-based, irregular, uncoordinated movements; step lengths are variable; turns are unsteady; side-to-side lurching is present	Cerebellar involvement
Sensory ataxic gait	Wide-based, shortened step, stomping gait (as the foot hits the ground); looks down while walks; worsens in dark	Peripheral neuropathy, posterior column involvement (e.g. vitamin B_{12} deficiency, syphilis)
Frontal gait	Impaired balance, reduced step length, wide gait, reduced step height; failure to initiate gait (feet may appear glued to the floor)	Frontal lobe diseases, normal pressure hydrocephalus

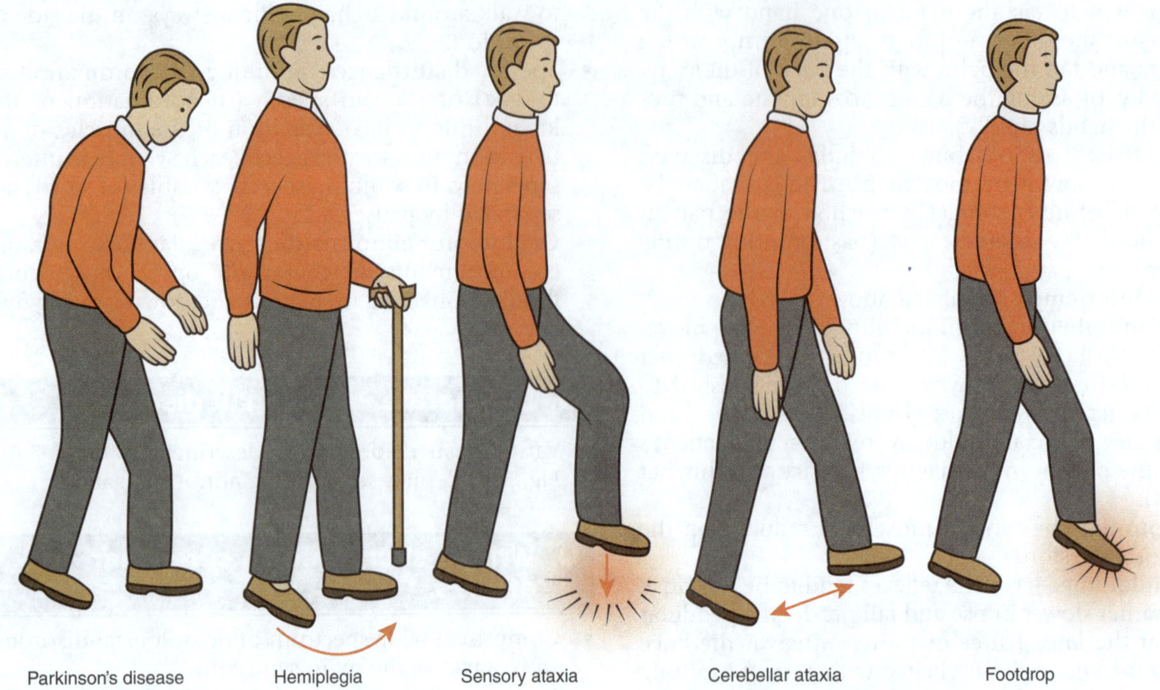

Fig. 5.10 Gait disorders.

TABLE 5.41 Causes of Ataxias Based on Duration

Acute ataxia	• Cerebellar haemorrhage • Cerebellar infarction • Alcohol • Drugs [antiepileptic agents, lithium, antineoplastics (cytarabine, 5-fluorouracil, capecitabine, vincristine), cyclosporin, metronidazole] • Toxins (heavy metals, carbon tetrachloride, phencyclidine, toluene) • Infections/postinfectious diseases (meningoencephalitis, cerebellar abscess, chickenpox, infectious mononucleosis)
• Subacute ataxia	• Infections (progressive multifocal leukoencephalopathy, prion disease) • Autoimmune diseases [acute disseminated encephalomyelitis, coeliac disease Hashimoto thyroiditis, Guillain–Barré syndrome (Miller Fisher variant), multiple sclerosis, vasculitis] • Primary or metastatic tumours • Paraneoplastic cerebellar degeneration • Wernicke encephalopathy • Vitamin B_{12} deficiency • Acquired hepatocerebral degeneration
• Chronic ataxia	• Spinocerebellar ataxias • Friedreich's ataxia • Ataxia telangiectasia • Xeroderma pigmentosum • Wilson's disease • Multiple system atrophy • Progressive supranuclear palsy

HEREDITARY CEREBELLAR ATAXIAS

- A heterogeneous group of neurological disorders, characterised by imbalance, progressive gait and limb incoordination, dysarthria and disturbances of eye movements. Additional neurological and systemic features are usually present in these patients.

TABLE 5.42 Hereditary or Acquired Causes of Ataxia

Acquired or sporadic ataxias:

- Multiple system atrophy (MSA)
- Progressive supranuclear palsy
- Stroke (infarction, haemorrhage)
- Wernicke's encephalopathy
- Toxin-induced ataxias
  - Ethanol
  - Drugs [antiepileptic agents, lithium, antineoplastics (cytarabine, 5-fluorouracil, capecitabine, vincristine), cyclosporin, metronidazole]
  - Toxins (heavy metals, carbon tetrachloride, phencyclidine, toluene)
- Immune-mediated
  - Multiple sclerosis
  - Miller Fisher syndrome
  - Systemic lupus erythematosus
  - Coeliac disease
  - Paraneoplastic syndrome (small-cell lung cancer, breast or ovarian cancer and lymphoma)
- Infectious/postinfectious diseases
  - Meningoencephalitis
  - Cerebellar abscess
  - Chickenpox, infectious mononucleosis
  - Progressive multifocal leukoencephalopathy
  - Creutzfeldt–Jakob disease
- Traumatic
- Neoplastic disorder
  - Cerebellar tumour
  - Metastatic disease
- Hypothyroidism
- Acquired hepatocerebral degeneration
- Chiari malformations

Hereditary ataxias:

- Autosomal dominant cerebellar ataxias
  - Spinocerebellar ataxias
  - Episodic ataxias
- Autosomal recessive cerebellar ataxias
  - Friedreich's ataxia
  - Abetalipoproteinaemia
  - Ataxia telangiectasia
  - Wilson's disease

SPINOCEREBELLAR ATAXIAS

- Autosomal dominant.
- Progressive disorders in which the cerebellum slowly degenerates, often accompanied by degenerative changes in brainstem and other parts of CNS, and less commonly the peripheral nervous system.
- Several types of spinocerebellar ataxias (SCAs); SCA1 is the most common type.
- Ataxia is usually of cerebellar type, but in some SCAs, predominant or a strong sensory ataxia.
- Patients with SCA1 suffer from a progressive cerebellar syndrome with ataxia of gait and stance, ataxia of limb movements, dysarthria and cerebellar oculomotor abnormalities.
- Additional noncerebellar signs in majority of patients.
- About half of the patients have supranuclear or nuclear gaze paresis and/or saccade slowing.
- Pyramidal tract signs with spasticity, extensor plantar responses, hyperreflexia, decreased vibration sense and dysphagia also common.

FRIEDREICH'S ATAXIA

- Autosomal recessive.
- Onset is early; typically present in children aged 8–15 years and almost always present before age 25 years.
- Progressive gait and limb ataxia, dysarthria, absent deep tendon reflexes, loss of joint position and vibration senses, and pyramidal weakness with extensor plantars.
- Ataxia is due to both posterior column involvement and spinocerebellar tract involvement.
- Hypertrophic cardiomyopathy in many patients.
- Axonal sensory neuropathy, distal wasting, scoliosis, sensorineural deafness, optic atrophy and diabetes are common features.

ATAXIA TELANGIECTASIA

- Autosomal recessive inheritance.
- Patients typically present in early childhood.
- The neurological presentation includes cerebellar ataxia, dysarthria, peripheral neuropathy and extrapyramidal features (dystonia, tremor and chorea).
- Patients have a characteristic eye movement disorder comprising oculomotor apraxia, slow saccades and nystagmus.
- Ocular telangiectasia appear by the age of 10 years; may also occur on the skin and pharyngeal wall.
- Immunodeficiency is common and patients develop recurrent infections, particularly respiratory tract infections, leading to bronchiectasis.
- Patients are predisposed to develop malignancy, particularly lymphoma and brain tumours, and diabetes mellitus.
- Serum alpha-foetoprotein is elevated.
- Death is due to infections or malignancy.

Q. Classify meningitis and enumerate its causes. (PA 35.1)

- Table 5.43 gives classification and causes of meningitis.
- Other noninfectious causes include the following:

TABLE 5.43 Classification and Causes of Meningitis

1. **Bacterial meningitis:**
• Common organisms
  • *Streptococcus pneumoniae* (30%–50%)
  • *Neisseria meningitidis* (10%–35%)
  • *Haemophilus influenzae* type B (1%–3%)
• Uncommon organisms
  • *Staphylococcus aureus*
  • *Staphylococcus epidermidis*
  • Group B streptococci
  • *Escherichia coli*
  • *Klebsiella*
  • *Proteus* spp.
  • *Citrobacter* spp.
  • *Pseudomonas* spp.
  • *Listeria monocytogenes*
2. **Tuberculous meningitis (TBM):**
• *Mycobacterium tuberculosis*
	3. **Viral meningitis (aseptic meningitis):**
	• Enteroviruses (*Coxsackie*, poliovirus)
	• Arboviruses
	• HIV
	• Herpes simplex-2
	• Mumps virus
	4. **Spirochaetal:**
	• Leptospirosis
	• Lyme disease
	• Syphilis
	5. **Rickettsial:**
	• Typhus fever
	6. **Protozoal:**
	• *Naegleria*
	7. **Fungal:**
	• *Cryptococcus*
	8. **Sarcoidosis**
	9. **Malignant disease:**
	• Leukaemic meningitis
	10. **Subarachnoid haemorrhage (SAH)** (causes meningismus)
	11. **Other noninfectious causes (see text)**

- Vasculitis:
  - Primary central nervous system vasculitis.
  - Eosinophilic granulomatosis with polyangiitis (Churg–Strauss syndrome).
  - Wegener granulomatosis.
- Connective tissue disease:
  - Systemic lupus erythematosus.
  - Rheumatoid arthritis.
  - Sjögren's syndrome.

Q. Discuss the aetiology, clinical features, investigations and treatment of pyogenic meningitis. Syn: acute bacterial meningitis (ABM). (MI 15.1)

AETIOLOGY

- Discussed in the Table 5.43.

INTRODUCTION

- ABM is an inflammation of the leptomeninges (arachnoid and pia), and fluid residing in the space that it encloses and also that in the ventricles of the brain. As the subarachnoid space is continuous around the brain, the spinal cord and the optic nerves, an infective agent gaining entry to any part of it may extend immediately to all of it, even its most remote recesses. Therefore, meningitis is always cerebrospinal. It also reaches the ventricles, either directly or by reflux through the basal foramina of Magendie and Luschka.
- Meningitis may be acute meningitis (with onset over hours to days) or chronic meningitis (syndrome persisting more than 4 weeks). Partially treated pyogenic meningitis may present with chronic meningitis.
- Inflammation of the meninges sometimes extends into the parenchyma with resultant symptoms and

BOX 5.52 Predisposing Factors for Pneumococcal Meningitis

- Acute otitis media
- Mastoiditis
- Pneumonia
- Diabetes mellitus
- Recent head injury
- Sickle cell disease
- Hodgkin's lymphoma
- Multiple myeloma
- Immunoglobulin deficiency
- Splenectomy
- Renal transplantation
- Bone marrow transplantation
- Chronic alcoholism

BOX 5.53 Predisposing Factors for *H. influenzae* Meningitis

- Anatomic defects like dermal sinus tract and old skull fracture
- Abnormality of immune defences
- Diabetes mellitus
- Alcoholism

signs of cerebral or spinal cord involvement, often termed meningoencephalitis or meningoencephalomyelitis.

- *Neisseria meningitidis* are Gram-negative, bean-shaped aerobic diplococci. Most infections are caused by organisms belonging to serogroups A, B, C, Y and W-135. Serogroups A and C predominate throughout Asia including India. The human naso-oropharyngeal mucosa is the only natural reservoir of *N. meningitidis*. Meningococci are transferred from one person to another by direct contact or via droplets.

PREDISPOSING FACTORS

- Predisposing factors for *N. meningitidis* meningitis are given in Box 5.52 while those for *H. influezae* meningitis are given in Box 5.53.

N. MENINGITIDIS MENINGITIS

- *N. meningitidis* meningitis occurs more often in patients with underlying immunodeficiency disorders and deficiency of any of the complement components.

LISTERIA MONOCYTOGENES MENINGITIS

- It has become an important pathogen, especially in elderly, debilitated and those who are immunosuppressed (transplantation, cancer therapy and connective tissue disorders). Alcoholism and high-dose steroids predispose to this. Infection is acquired by ingesting foods contaminated with this organism. Mortality rate is very high.

OTHERS

- Neurosurgical procedures are followed by *Staphylococcus aureus* meningitis. *Staphylococcus epidermidis* meningitis follows cerebral ventricular shunt infections.

PATHOGENESIS

- All three important organisms are normal inhabitants of nasopharynx. Antecedent viral infections of the upper respiratory tract or lungs predispose the colonised patient to bloodstream invasion, which is the usual route by which bacteria reach the meninges. Once blood-borne, pneumococcus, meningococcus and *Haemophilus influenzae* have a predilection for meninges. Transnasal spread through cribriform plate to subarachnoid space may also be important.
- Disruption of blood–CSF barrier by trauma, circulating endotoxin or an initial viral infection of the meninges also facilitates the entry of bacteria into subarachnoid space.
- A critical event after invasion is the inflammatory reaction produced by the invading bacteria. This results in production of several cytokines of which the most important are interleukin-1 and tumour necrosis factor. Many of the neurological manifestations and complications of bacterial meningitis are due to the immune response to the pathogens rather than from direct pathogen-induced tissue injury.

CLINICAL FEATURES

- Fever, headache and vomiting are the cardinal features.
- Seizures, impairment of consciousness, photophobia, stiff neck and stiff back.
- Three patterns of onset are documented:
  - Fulminant onset—patient becomes seriously ill within 24 hours, without antecedent respiratory tract infections (25%).
  - Meningitis developing over 1–7 days and associated with respiratory symptoms (50%).
  - Meningeal symptoms after 1–3 weeks of respiratory symptoms (20%).
- In elderly, immunocompromised and debilitated patients, the classic features of meningitis may be minimal, where low-grade fever and changes in mental status may occur without headache or neck rigidity.
- Meningococcal meningitis usually occurs as outbreaks. The evolution is extremely rapid and the onset is attended by petechial or purpuric skin eruptions and large ecchymoses. Circulatory collapse may occur.
- Pneumococcal meningitis is usually preceded by an infection in the lung, ear or sinuses. Heart valves may be affected.
- *H. influenzae* meningitis follows upper respiratory tract infections and ear infections in the young.

SIGNS OF MENINGEAL IRRITATION

- Neck stiffness (neck rigidity)—the examiner is unable to put the patient's chin on the chest by passive flexion of the neck (due to neck muscle spasm).
- Kernig's sign—with the patient's thigh flexed to 90° from the abdomen, try to extend the knee to more than 135° passively. The patient will resist leg extension owing to spasm of hamstrings or describe pain in the lower back or posterior thighs. This manoeuvre stretches roots of the sciatic nerve that are inflamed at their exits from the spinal theca.
- Brudzinski's neck sign—with the patient supine, the physician places one hand behind the patient's head and places the other hand on the patient's chest. The physician then raises the patient's head (with the hand behind the head) while the hand on the chest restrains the patient and prevents the patient from

BOX 5.54 CSF Analysis in Pyogenic Meningitis

- Appearance is turbid.
- Pressure is elevated above 180 mm H_2O.
- Cell count is raised, ranging from 5000 to 20,000/μL; neutrophil leucocytes predominate.
- Protein level is elevated (more than 45 mg/dL).
- Sugar level is decreased (less than 40 mg/dL or less than 40% of blood sugar).
- Gram stain of the sediment of CSF may show meningococci as Gram-negative, kidney-shaped, intracellular diplococci (inside neutrophils), and pneumococci as Gram-positive diplococci.
- Culture of CSF grows the pathogen in 70%–80% of cases.
- Measurement of bacterial antigen in the CSF (latex agglutination tests, immunochromatographic tests and PCR).

rising. Automatic flexion of both the legs at hip and knee is a positive sign.
- Brudzinski's leg sign—on passively flexing one lower limb, the other leg gets flexed automatically.
- Jolt accentuation manoeuvre—exacerbation of headache caused by rotation of the head horizontally two or three times per second.

INVESTIGATIONS

- Increased total leucocytes, polymorphonuclear leucocytosis and raised ESR.
- Lumbar puncture and cerebrospinal fluid studies (Box 5.54).
- Hyponatraemia due to syndrome of inappropriate antidiuretic hormone (SIADH).
- Blood culture may be positive for *H. influenzae*, meningococci or pneumococci.
- Culture of pus from middle ear or sinuses.
- Biopsy of skin lesions (if present) to demonstrate meningococci.
- Radiography:
  - Radiograph of chest for pneumonia and lung abscess.
  - Radiograph of skull for chronic osteomyelitis and fracture.
  - Radiograph of paranasal sinuses for sinusitis.
  - Radiograph of mastoids for mastoiditis.
- CT scan may detect evidences of cerebritis, vascular occlusion, encephalomalacia, hydrocephalus, brain abscess or subdural empyema. Commonest CT finding is increased contrast enhancement of meninges.

Note: A lumbar puncture is safe in patients with suspected meningitis who are conscious, and have no papilloedema or focal deficits. In such cases, lumbar puncture may be performed without a CT scan. Risk factors for elevated ICP include new-onset seizure, immunocompromised patient, decreased level of alertness, papilloedema or focal neurological signs. A CT should be done in these patients before performing a lumbar puncture. However, the patient must receive a dose of antibiotics and steroids before the CT scan.

TREATMENT

- Initial management includes airway protection and oxygenation, volume resuscitation, prevention of hypoglycaemia, control of seizures, reduction of hyperthermia and measures to reduce ICP. The latter measures include elevation of head, fluid restriction, mannitol and, in severe cases, hyperventilation for a short time.

ANTIBIOTICS

- Empirical antibiotics must be administered immediately in patients with suspected meningitis (Table 5.44). One should not wait for the results of lumbar puncture or CT scan of brain before administering antibiotics.
- The duration of treatment is: 7–10 days for *H. influenzae* or *N. meningitidis* meningitis, 10–14 days for *S. pneumoniae* meningitis and 21 days for *Listeria monocytogenes* meningitis.
- Ceftriaxone is the drug of choice in any patient with acute meningitis when empirical treatment is required or the aetiological agent has been found to be one of these three common pathogens. However, many of the penicillin-resistant pneumococci have reduced susceptibility to third-generation cephalosporins; therefore, empirical management of meningitis should include vancomycin plus cefotaxime or ceftriaxone.
- For children who are younger than 1 month, consider adding vancomycin to the usual antibiotic combination of a broad-spectrum cephalosporin and ampicillin.
- In patients with impaired cell-mediated immunity (such as HIV, lymphoma, corticosteroid use or cytotoxic chemotherapy), there is an increased risk for *L. monocytogenes* and Gram-negative bacilli. Ampicillin and cefepime (or meropenem) should be used to ensure coverage for these, in addition to vancomycin for *S. pneumoniae*.

STEROIDS

- Despite antibiotics, serious complications can occur in patients with meningitis. Corticosteroids have been found to reduce the incidence of hearing impairment in children with *H. influenzae* meningitis. They have also been found to be useful in adults with pneumococcal meningitis. Because it is often difficult to distinguish patients who have bacterial meningitis from those with viral meningitis in the emergency room and because data indicate that it is preferable to administer dexamethasone before initiation of antibiotic therapy, most patients with suspicion of meningitis should receive steroids in the emergency room itself.
- Dexamethasone is given in a dose of 0.15 mg/kg every 6 hours for 4 days.
- Adjunctive dexamethasone should not be used in patients who have already received antimicrobial therapy.

COMPLICATIONS

- Approximately 50% of adults with meningitis develop CNS complications including cerebrovascular involvement, cranial nerve palsies, focal neurological deficits, cerebral oedema and hydrocephalus.
- Pneumonia and otitis media are frequently seen in patients with meningitis.

TABLE 5.44 Empiric Antibiotic Therapy for Bacterial Meningitis

Age Group	Likely Organisms	Empirical Treatment (Dose/Day)
• Neonates	*E. coli*, *Streptococcus agalactiae*, *Listeria*	Ampicillin (100–150 mg/kg) plus cefotaxime (50 mg/kg) or ceftriaxone (50–100 mg/kg)
• Children (younger than 12 years)	*H. influenzae*, *N. meningitidis*, *S. pneumoniae*	Ceftriaxone (or cefotaxime) plus vancomycin (40 mg/kg)
• Adults	*N. meningitidis*, *S. pneumoniae*	Ceftriaxone (or cefotaxime) plus vancomycin
• Elderly	*S. pneumoniae*, *Listeria*, Gram-negative organisms	Ampicillin plus ceftriaxone or cefotaxime or ceftazidime plus vancomycin
• Immunocompromised	*S. pneumoniae*, *Listeria*, Gram-negative organisms, *Staphylococcus aureus*	Ampicillin plus vancomycin plus cefepime or meropenem

- Systemic complications include septic shock, acute respiratory distress syndrome and disseminated intravascular coagulation.

PROPHYLAXIS

N. MENINGITIDIS MENINGITIS

- Indications: Chemoprophylaxis is indicated in close contacts of patients with *N. meningitidis* meningitis. Administer it as soon as possible, preferably within 24 hours.
- Chemoprophylaxis regimens:
  - Rifampicin 10 mg/kg twice a day for 2 days. It is effective in about 95% of cases.
  - Ceftriaxone 125 mg intramuscularly if age is less than 15 years, otherwise 250 mg. It has 97% efficacy.
  - Ciprofloxacin 500 mg orally (single dose) is also effective.
- Vaccine:
  - The quadrivalent polysaccharide vaccine that provides protection against serogroups A, C, Y and W-135 and the bivalent polysaccharide vaccines (A and C) are available.
  - Vaccination, for both adults and children older than 2 years, is carried out by administering single 0.5-mL dose, subcutaneously.

H. INFLUENZAE MENINGITIS

- Indications: Prophylaxis for meningitis caused by *H. influenzae* type B is recommended for all household contacts when at least one contact is younger than 4 years.
- Chemoprophylaxis regimen:
  - Rifampicin is given for prophylaxis, though its efficacy is not clear.

Q. What is meant by Mollaret's meningitis?

- A syndrome of recurrent aseptic, self-limiting meningitis is characterised by large atypical monocytes (Mollaret cells) in the CSF.
- Most common aetiological agent is herpes simplex-2.
- Characterised by repeated self-limiting episodes of fever, meningismus and severe headache (usually of 2–5 days' duration) separated by symptom-free intervals.
- Diagnosis can be made by PCR testing for HSV DNA in CSF.

Q. Write a short note on aseptic meningitis.

- Aseptic meningitis is inflammation of the meninges with lymphocytic pleocytosis in CSF and no cause apparent after routine CSF stains and cultures. It does not typically cause notable parenchymal involvement of the brain (encephalitis) or spinal cord (myelitis). It has a more benign clinical course compared with bacterial meningitis, meningoencephalitis or encephalomyelitis.
- Viruses (e.g. herpes simplex virus, varicella zoster virus, HIV, enteroviruses, lymphocytic choriomeningitis virus, and occasionally Zika virus and SARS-CoV-2) are the most common cause. Other causes may be infectious (rickettsiae, spirochetes, parasites, etc.) and noninfectious (vaccine reactions—rabies, pertussis; drugs—azathioprine, carbamazepine, ciprofloxacin, isoniazid, naproxen, ibuprofen, etc.; malignancies—lymphoma, leukaemias; sarcoidosis; Behçet's disease, SLE, reaction to intrathecal drugs, etc.).
- Symptoms include fever, headache, vomiting and meningeal signs.
- Some may be asymptomatic but with CSF abnormalities.
- The CSF shows mildly or markedly elevated pressure and presence of 10 to >1000 lymphocytes/μL. Occasionally, a few neutrophils appear during the first few hours of viral meningitis. CSF glucose is normal and CSF protein is normal or mildly elevated. CSF may also be sent for viral culture and viral PCR and blood for virus-specific antibodies.
- Viral aseptic meningitis is usually self-limited.
- Treatment is symptomatic.

Q. Enumerate the causes of neck stiffness.

- A number of conditions can produce neck stiffness (Box 5.55).
- The term 'meningism' refers to symptoms that mimic those of meningitis but without inflammation of the meninges.

BOX 5.55 Conditions Producing Neck Stiffness

- Meningitis
- Meningism
- Leukaemic meningitis
- Subarachnoid haemorrhage
- Cervical spondylosis
- Neck trauma (fracture, dislocation of cervical spine, sprain, rupture of ligament, etc.)
- Tetanus
- Rupture of intracerebral abscess into subarachnoid space
- Elderly people

Q. Describe the causes, clinical features, investigations, differential diagnosis and sequelae of viral encephalitis. (MI 5.2)

- Encephalitis is defined as inflammation of the brain parenchyma associated with neurological dysfunction such as altered state of consciousness, seizures, personality changes, cranial nerve palsies, speech problems, and motor and sensory deficits.
- The inflammatory process can also involve the spinal cord (encephalomyelitis).

AETIOLOGY

- The most common cause of encephalitis is a viral infection (Box 5.56).
- The most common virus responsible for large-scale epidemics in India is Japanese B encephalitis virus. It is spread by the mosquito *Culex tritaeniorhynchus* that breeds extensively in rice ecosystem. The pigs act as the amplifying hosts. Humans are incidental to the transmission cycle.
- In immunocompetent adults, >90% of cases of herpes simplex encephalitis (HSE) result from infection with HSV-1, with the remainder due to HSV-2 infection. More than two-thirds of cases of encephalitis due to HSV-1 appear to result from reactivation of endogenous latent HSV-1 in individuals previously exposed to the virus.
- Influenza virus is an important cause of encephalitis, mostly seen in children.
- Besides viral causes, encephalitis can occur in scrub typhus, tuberculosis, bacterial meningitis, leptospirosis and others.
- Other causes of encephalitis include immune checkpoint inhibitors (PD-1, PD-L1 and CTLA) and autoimmune encephalitis.

BOX 5.56 Viruses Causing Encephalitis

- Enteroviruses
- Herpes simplex (usually type 1)
- Mumps virus
- Influenza virus
- Japanese encephalitis virus
- SARS-CoV-2
- Nipah virus
- Arboviruses
- Rabies virus
- HIV
- Lymphocytic choriomeningitis virus
- Dengue virus
- Chikungunya virus
- Zika virus

CLINICAL FEATURES

- Clinically characterised by association of encephalopathy, focal deficits, seizures and fever.
- Viral encephalitis is often preceded by nonspecific features (fever, myalgias and arthralgias).
- Onset is acute with fever and headache, similar to acute meningitis but with accompanying features of cerebral involvement. Cerebral features include variable degree of change in consciousness, confusion, disorientation, and mental changes such as delirium, agitation, hallucinations as well as focal signs such as hemiplegia, aphasia, cranial nerve deficits and involuntary movements. Seizures and raised ICP are common. Many show signs of meningeal irritation. Specific clinical signs may occur depending on particular virus, for example rabies virus predominantly affects brainstem and limbic system early in the course. Herpes simplex virus has affinity to involve temporal and frontal lobes.
- Associated myelitis may lead to flaccid, asymmetric paralysis of the limbs along with sensory changes and bladder involvement. This must be differentiated from acute epidural abscess.
- Additional features particularly seen in Japanese encephalitis include parkinsonian syndrome with mask-like facies, tremor, cogwheel rigidity and choreoathetoid movements.

HERPES SIMPLEX VIRAL ENCEPHALITIS (HSVE)

- It is important to suspect this condition as it is potentially treatable.
- Although there are no clinical features that are pathognomonic for HSVE, predilection of the virus for temporal and orbitofrontal lobes results in characteristic clinical picture that should alert the clinician to the condition. A 1-day to 4-day history of gradually increasing headache and fever is followed by alteration of consciousness, memory loss, personality changes, confusion, disorientation and olfactory hallucinations. Focal neurological signs such as hemiparesis, aphasia, focal or generalised seizures and signs of meningeal irritation may also be present.

INVESTIGATIONS

- CT scan is usually normal in encephalitis. In HSE, it may show low-attenuation areas, particularly in the temporal lobes with surrounding oedema (vs. Japanese encephalitis where lesions in thalamus are common).
- Cerebrospinal fluid:
  - Clear.
  - Increased pressure.
  - Protein levels are mildly elevated (70–700 mg/dL; values >800 mg/dL rarely seen).
  - Sugar is normal or mildly reduced.
  - Cell count is increased (usually 5–500/mm^3) and is lymphocytic. Red blood cells are common in HSE.
  - Antibodies to specific virus in increasing titres are seen if serial examinations are done. It is useless for immediate diagnosis. IgM antibodies are important for early diagnosis.

- PCR of CSF is the diagnostic method of choice for viral encephalitis including HSE and therapy should be instituted pending the results of PCR.
- EEG (spike and slow-wave or periodic sharp-wave patterns over the involved temporal lobe, or diffuse slowing) and MRI of brain (increased signal intensity in insular cortex and temporal lobe, usually on one side) are important in patients with suspected herpes encephalitis. In contrast, in JE, T2-weighted MRI images show increased signal over the thalamic region in most patients; similar lesions are less commonly found over the cortex, midbrain, cerebellum and spinal cord.
- Brain biopsy in select patients.

DIFFERENTIAL DIAGNOSIS

- Viral encephalitis should be differentiated from acute metabolic encephalopathies, postinfectious encephalomyelitis, bacterial or tubercular infections of the brain and stroke. This is possible from clinical examination, CT scan, CSF evaluation and blood biochemistry.

POSTINFECTIOUS ENCEPHALOMYELITIS

- It indicates encephalitis that follows a viral illness without actual viral invasion of CNS or following administration of some vaccines. It is thought to be due to autoimmune reaction to viral or vaccinal proteins which results in demyelination. An alternate explanation is increased vascular permeability and congestion in the CNS triggered by circulating immune complexes.
- Rabies vaccine (Semple vaccine, not used now) and measles infection are most common causes of postinfectious encephalitis.
- Two forms are described: acute disseminated encephalomyelitis (ADEM) and acute haemorrhagic leucoencephalitis (AHLE).

Acute Disseminated Encephalomyelitis

- The patient develops a multifocal inflammatory demyelinating process (ADEM) after 1–3 weeks following infection or vaccination. The preceding infection is typically a benign upper respiratory tract infection or a nonspecific febrile illness. Preceding infections consist mostly of various viral infections (measles, varicella and rubella), group A β-haemolytic streptococci and intracellular bacteria such as *Mycoplasma pneumoniae*.
- This process involves cranial nerves (e.g. optic nerve), cerebrum, brainstem and spinal cord.
- Characterised by acute onset (maximal neurological deficit reached within hours to days of onset) of focal neurological signs and encephalopathy (early evidence in the form of behavioural impairment, delirium and fluctuations of vigilance). Other features include fever and seizures.
- Key features that help in differentiating ADEM from encephalitis include a history of vaccination or a prodromal illness in the weeks preceding neurological signs and symptoms. In ADEM, demyelination involving the optic nerve or spinal cord can result in monocular visual loss, symptoms of spinal cord dysfunction (paraplegia or tetraplegia with deep tendon reflex abolition and acute urinary retention) or acute polyradiculoneuropathy, which are generally rare in acute encephalitis. Seizures are uncommon.
- MRI in ADEM typically shows multifocal lesions of same age with a predilection for the white matter in both hemispheres and infratentorial areas, whereas acute encephalitis usually produces lesions that involve both grey and white matters.
- CSF profiles are similar in ADEM and acute viral encephalitis. Oligoclonal bands should be sought in patients with a presumed diagnosis of ADEM as multiple sclerosis can present with similar features.
- Treatment is usually with high-dose intravenous corticosteroids alone or together with other immunomodulatory therapies, including intravenous immunoglobulin, plasma exchange or cyclophosphamide. Empiric treatment with acyclovir may also be initiated.

Acute Haemorrhagic Leucoencephalitis

- AHLE is considered a hyperacute variant of ADEM and has a fulminant course with haemorrhagic white matter lesions.
- In contrast to ADEM, which is more common in children and teenagers, AHLE mainly affects adult patients.
- Onset is acute, with fever, coma, seizures and focal neurological signs.
- CSF opening pressure is usually elevated and analysis shows a lymphocytic pleocytosis and up to 1000 red blood cells/mL with increased protein levels, ranging from 100 to 300 mg/dL.
- MRI shows widespread hyperintensities in white matter on both T1- and T2-weighted images.
- Treatment is similar to ADEM.

MANAGEMENT

- General measures to care for the unconscious patient should be started. Anticonvulsants are often necessary. Brain oedema is best controlled with dexamethasone 4 mg 6 hourly.
- HSE responds well to acyclovir (10 mg/kg IV 8 hourly for 14–21 days), if instituted early. As the drug is safe, it may be given to all patients with diagnosis of viral encephalitis as specific diagnosis is made only later or is impossible. It can produce renal insufficiency.
- Oseltamivir in influenza-associated encephalitis.

PROGNOSIS

- Highly variable. In large epidemics, high mortality is seen. Many may be left with residual deficit like dementia, focal deficits and epilepsy. Other sequelae include cerebellar and extrapyramidal signs, flexion deformities of the arms, hyperextension of the legs, language impairment, learning difficulties and behavioural problems. Many recover completely if the illness is mild.

Q. Describe the aetiology, clinical features, complications and treatment of herpes zoster.

AETIOLOGY

- Herpes zoster (shingles) is the result of reactivation of varicella zoster virus (VZV) lying dormant in the dorsal root ganglion following chicken pox in early life. This may occur spontaneously or with immunosuppression by other diseases, when it can be severe and widespread (e.g. use of steroids and HIV infection).

CLINICAL FEATURES

- Symptoms and signs are dermatomal in distribution. The dermatomes from T3 to L3 are most commonly involved, although cranial nerves may also be involved.
- First manifestation is pain in the involved dermatome.
- In 3 to 4 days, skin becomes red and vesicles appear (Fig. 5.11). Vesicles dry up in a week's time leaving scars.
- Pain, which is severe and burning in nature, persists as long as vesicles remain.
- Herpes over face usually involves the first division of the fifth nerve and occasionally seventh nerve (Ramsay Hunt syndrome).
- Some individuals may present only with prodromal symptoms, never developing the tell-tale rash. This phenomenon is known as 'zoster sine herpete'.
- Multidermatomal involvement or dissemination is seen in immunocompromised patients.

COMPLICATIONS

- Herpes zoster ophthalmicus is shingles involving the first division of the trigeminal nerve distribution with ocular involvement. Involvement of the nasociliary nerve is associated with cutaneous lesions on the tip of the nose (Hutchinson's sign) and predicts a high likelihood of ocular involvement (keratitis, uveitis, retinitis and choroiditis) (Fig. 5.12).
- Sometimes, pain persists for long time even after the vesicles have dried up. When pain persists even after 4–6 weeks, it is called postherpetic neuralgia. The risk for postherpetic neuralgia increases with age, and almost half of patients older than 60 years who experience herpes zoster will develop it, immunocompromised patients being more susceptible.

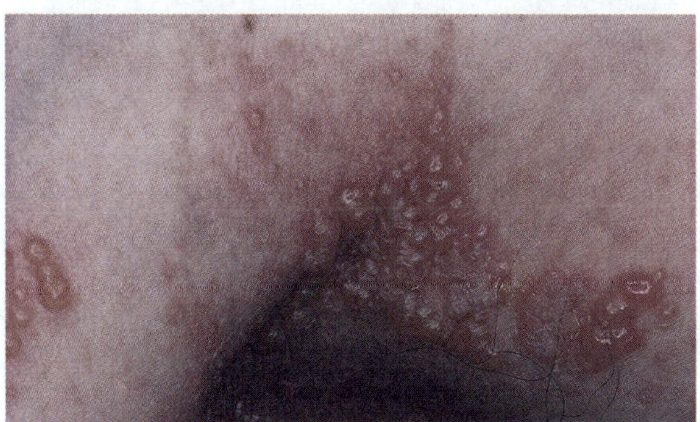

Fig. 5.11 Unilateral, dermatomal distribution of herpes zoster lesions.

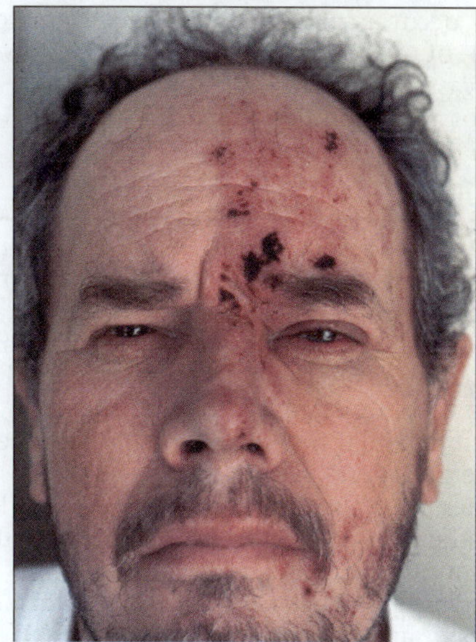

Fig. 5.12 Herpes zoster skin eruption with the classical involvement of the tip of the nose (Hutchinson's sign).

- Other potential complications include encephalitis, myelitis, meningitis and peripheral nerve palsies.

DIAGNOSIS

- The diagnosis is mainly clinical.
- Tzanck smear (from the base of the lesion) shows multinucleated giant cells.
- The polymerase chain reaction (PCR) technique is the most sensitive and specific diagnostic test, as it can detect VZV DNA in fluid from the vesicle. It can be used if diagnosis is not clear.

TREATMENT

- Idoxuridine 5% lotion over the skin or 0.1% solution for corneal instillation.
- Oral aciclovir (800 mg five times daily), famciclovir (500 mg three times daily) and valaciclovir (1 g three times daily) are useful in early stage of disease. They also reduce development of postherpetic neuralgia.
- Pain is controlled with analgesics.
- Calamine lotion is applied as a smoothening agent.
- Corticosteroid therapy along with antiviral drugs is recommended for special situations such as Ramsay Hunt syndrome and ocular complications.
- Postherpetic neuralgia may become very refractory but may respond to carbamazepine or amitriptyline or gabapentin or pregabalin. Topical capsaicin is also useful.

Q. Discuss the aetiopathogenesis, clinical features, complications and management of tuberculous meningitis.

AETIOPATHOGENESIS

- Tuberculous meningitis (TBM) is infection caused by *Mycobacterium tuberculosis*.

- It may occur as part of widespread haematogenous spread of mycobacteria in children. However, in most cases, it occurs by reactivation of a subpial focus of a dormant lesion (Rich's focus).

PATHOLOGY

- Subarachnoid space throughout CNS is involved. Basal cisterns and Sylvian fissure are maximally involved.
- Thick exudates cover the base of the brain and scattered tubercles are found in the meninges. This may lead to communicating hydrocephalus.
- Emerging cranial nerves are engulfed by these gelatin-like exudates.
- Exudates may also block foramina of Luschka and Magendie or any point of CSF pathway resulting in noncommunicating hydrocephalus.
- Blood vessels at base show inflammatory changes and may cause cerebral infarcts.
- Exudates can also surround lower part of spinal cord and cauda equine resulting in tuberculous radiculomyelopathy.

CLINICAL FEATURES

- It has a subacute or chronic course. Disease may occur at any age, but children are commonly affected.
- In children, early manifestations are lack of interest, malaise, fever, anorexia, urinary retention and constipation.
- Classical meningitis symptoms seen are fever, headache and vomiting appearing over a few days. Signs include neck rigidity and positive Kernig's and Brudzinski's signs.
- Further on, cranial nerve palsies (commonly blindness, diplopia due to ophthalmoplegia, facial palsy and deafness) with hemiparesis or paraplegia follow. These deficits may occur suddenly due to vascular involvement.
- Features of increased ICP due to hydrocephalus will result in change in intellect, altered consciousness, urinary incontinence and gait ataxia.
- Seizures are common.
- Movement disorders like chorea, hemiballismus, athetosis, generalised tremors, myoclonic jerks and ataxia may occur.
- SIADH secretion is a common complication leading to hyponatraemia.
- If left untreated, patient lapses into vegetative state and dies.
- Tuberculous spinal meningitis may manifest as an acute, subacute or chronic form. The dorsal cord seems to be affected most commonly, followed by the lumbar and the cervical regions:
  - The clinical picture in primary spinal meningitis is often characterised by myelopathy, with progressive ascending paralysis, eventually resulting in basal meningitis and associated sequelae.
  - In some cases with acute onset, acute paraplegia with sensory deficit and urinary retention may develop.
  - The subacute form is often dominated by myeloradiculopathy with radicular pain and progressive paraplegia or tetraplegia.
  - A less virulent chronic form might mimic a very slowly progressive spinal cord compression or a nonspecific arachnoiditis.

DIFFERENTIAL DIAGNOSIS (Box 5.57)

BOX 5.57 Differential Diagnosis of Tuberculous Meningitis

- Partially treated pyogenic meningitis
- Cryptococcal meningitis (particularly in HIV-positive patients)
- Syphilitic meningitis
- Other rare infections (e.g. *Brucella* and fungi)
- Neoplastic meningitis (leukaemia, lymphoma, metastasis)—CSF glucose is very low
- Miscellaneous (e.g. SLE, Behçet's disease and sarcoidosis)

INVESTIGATIONS

CT SCAN AND MRI

- Meningeal enhancement.
- Presence of exudates.
- Hydrocephalus.
- Cerebral infarcts.
- Gadolinium-enhanced MRI more sensitive than CT.

CEREBROSPINAL FLUID ANALYSIS (Box 5.58)

BOX 5.58 CSF Findings in Tuberculous Meningitis

- Pressure is increased
- Usually clear, but xanthochromia suggests block in the CSF flow in the spinal canal
- A fine clot or cobweb may form on allowing CSF to stand for some time
- Protein levels are elevated (100–800 mg/dL). Very high levels indicate block to CSF flow
- Sugar is lowered (to less than 40% of blood sugar)
- Cell counts are elevated and predominantly lymphocytic
- Ziehl–Neelsen staining or fluorescent staining of the coagulum may show mycobacteria
- Cultures are rarely positive and take 6 weeks
- Adenosine deaminase (ADA) levels are elevated; however, no cut-off has been defined to differentiate TBM from pyogenic meningitis
- Nucleic acid amplification tests (NAAT) on CSF—PCR tests to detect mycobacterial nucleic acids. The Xpert MTB/RIF assay uses real-time PCR

OTHER INVESTIGATIONS

- Chest radiograph—it may show evidence of pulmonary tuberculosis (old or active) in 50% of cases.

PARTIALLY TREATED PYOGENIC MENINGITIS VERSUS TUBERCULOUS MENINGITIS

- Features shown in Box 5.59 favour a diagnosis of TBM rather than partially treated pyogenic meningitis.

BOX 5.59 Features Favouring a Diagnosis of Tuberculous Meningitis

- Duration of illness >7 days
- Optic atrophy on fundus examination
- Focal neurological deficits
- Abnormal movements
- CSF findings
  - CSF white blood cell count <1000/μL
  - CSF lymphocyte count >90%
  - CSF protein content >200 mg/dL

MANAGEMENT

- Anti-TB chemotherapy should be started at the earliest. Early phase (first 2 months) involves intensive therapy combining rifampicin, INH, pyrazinamide and streptomycin or ethambutol. After a period of 2 months, rifampicin with INH is continued for another 7–10 months. Ethambutol and streptomycin do not penetrate blood–brain barrier effectively.
- All patients should receive prednisolone 40 mg a day to reduce meningeal adhesions and severity of arteritis. It is given for 3 weeks followed by tapering over next 3 weeks.
- For communicating hydrocephalus, acetazolamide or furosemide. For noncommunicating hydrocephalus, ventricular drainage or ventriculoperitoneal shunt.

PROGNOSIS

- If treatment is instituted early before neurological deficits appear, recovery may be complete. Presence of focal deficits and change in consciousness before therapy predict poor outcome. Residual deficits will include dementia, blindness, deafness, epilepsy, hemiparesis and paraparesis.

Q. How will you differentiate bacterial, viral and TBM on the basis of CSF examination?

- Differentiating features of bacterial, viral and TBM based on CSF examination are given in Table 5.45.

Q. What are the common causes of acute fever and altered sensorium (febrile encephalopathy)?

- Common causes of acute fever with altered sensorium are given in Box 5.60.

BOX 5.60 Common Causes of Fever With Altered Sensorium (Febrile Encephalopathy)

- Acute bacterial meningitis
- Tuberculous meningitis
- Viral encephalitis
- Acute disseminated encephalomyelitis
- Brain abscess
- Typhoid fever
- Cerebral malaria
- Leptospirosis
- Scrub typhus
- Sepsis-associated encephalopathy
- Cortical venous thrombosis
- Anticholinergic (e.g. dhatura) poisoning
- Sympathomimetic (e.g. cocaine, amphetamine) poisoning
- Heat stroke
- Neuroleptic malignant syndrome
- Serotonin syndrome
- Malignant hyperthermia

Q. Describe the clinical features and management of neurosyphilis.

- The organism (*Treponema pallidum*) invades nervous system within 3–18 months after primary infection.
- Initial event is asymptomatic meningitis. This may remain so and cause more damage later on.
- All forms of neurosyphilis have meningitis as a component, in variable severity.
- Vascular changes occur secondary to meningitis as endarteritis obliterans.

CLASSIFICATION

- Neurosyphilis is typically classified as early (within 1 to 2 years of infection) or late forms (more than 1 to 2 years after infection) (Flowchart 5.5).
  - Early stages include asymptomatic neurosyphilis, meningeal syphilis and meningovascular syphilis.
  - Late forms include general paresis of insane, tabes dorsalis and CNS gumma.

TABLE 5.45 CSF Findings in Bacterial Versus Viral Versus Tuberculous Meningitis

Characteristic	Bacterial Meningitis	Viral Meningitis	Tuberculous Meningitis
Opening pressure	Elevated; 20–50 cm H_2O	Normal to elevated; 6–30 cm H_2O	Elevated; 15–40 cm H_2O
Appearance	Turbid	Clear	Cobweb on standing
White cells	100–20,000 cells/μL (mean 800 cells/μL) >90% polymorphs	10–1000 cells/μL (mean 80 cells/μL) >90% lymphocytes (in some, majority cells are polymorphs in first 1 to 2 days)	10–2000 cells/μL (mean 200 cells/μL) >90% lymphocytes
Protein	>200 mg/dL	<60 mg/dL	100–4000 mg/dL
CSF:blood glucose ratio	<0.4	>0.6	<0.4
Gram stain	Positive in 60%–90%	No organisms	No organisms
Ziehl–Neelsen stain	Negative	Negative	Positive (in 35%–65% of cases)
Lactate	Elevated (usually >4 mmol/L)	Normal or mildly elevated	Elevated (usually >4 mmol/L)

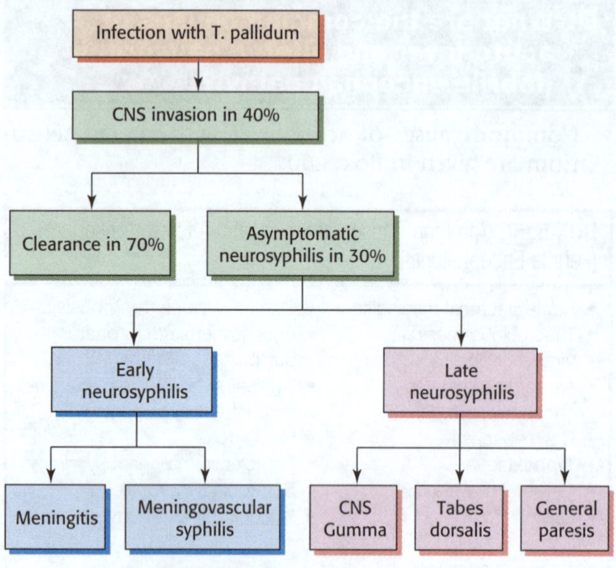

Flowchart 5.5 Natural History of Syphilis.

ASYMPTOMATIC NEUROSYPHILIS

- Asymptomatic invasion of CNS by *Treponema* is common within a few months of primary infection.
- Diagnosis is made by demonstrating CSF lymphocytosis with elevated protein and positive VDRL test.
- This is found in nearly 25% of cases with late latent form of syphilis. Many of these patients may go on to develop symptomatic neurosyphilis.
- These patients should be treated with penicillin.

SYMPTOMATIC NEUROSYPHILIS

- Although mixed features are common, the major categories are as follows:
  - Meningeal syphilis.
  - Meningovascular syphilis.
  - Parenchymatous syphilis that includes general paralysis of insane and tabes dorsalis.

MENINGEAL SYPHILIS

- Symptoms of meningitis may occur at any time after infection, but appear usually within 2 years.
- Symptoms consist of headache, stiff neck, cranial nerve palsies, convulsions and mental confusion.
- Papilloedema with symptoms of increased ICP may occur.
- Patient is afebrile. CSF is abnormal (Box 5.61).
- May have skin rash on palms and soles.

BOX 5.61 CSF Findings in Meningeal and Meningovascular Syphilis

- Pressure may be normal or raised
- Fluid is clear
- Protein is elevated (100–200 mg/dL)
- Sugar is normal
- Cell count is mildly elevated and is lymphocytic
- Gamma globulin levels are elevated
- VDRL and fluorescent treponemal antibody absorption (FTA-ABS) are positive

MENINGOVASCULAR SYPHILIS

- Meningovascular syphilis is a form of meningitis associated with vasculitis of small and medium size arteries in the central nervous system; it causes strokes and myelopathy.
- Presents usually 6 to 7 years after initial infection, but can be as early as 6 months to as late as 10–12 years.
- Should be suspected whenever a young patient presents with stroke resulting in hemiparesis, aphasia, visual loss, etc. Features of stroke are generally subacute in nature. Other features are headache, vertigo, insomnia and psychological abnormalities.
- The gold standard for diagnosis is VDRL from CSF, which is highly specific but only 30%–70% sensitive for neurosyphilis. CSF fluorescent treponemal antibody absorption (FTA-ABS) is more sensitive but not specific because false-positives are common.

GENERAL PARALYSIS OF INSANE

- It develops 20 years after primary infection.
- This is due to diffuse involvement of parenchyma producing a variety of manifestations which include personality changes, illusions, grandiose delusions, hallucinations, reduced memory, hyperactive reflexes and Argyll Robertson pupils.

TABES DORSALIS

- Tabes is the parenchymal form of neurosyphilis that involves posterior columns in the spinal cord.
- Usually develops 20–25 years after onset of infection.
- Symptoms are severe lightening pains in trunk and extremities, ataxia and urinary incontinence.
- Signs include variable patchy tactile sensory loss and severe impairment of proprioception with sensory ataxia (Romberg's sign—falling or stepping to one side when standing with feet together and eyes closed). Tendon jerks are absent. Muscular strength is normal. Trophic lesions, perforating ulcers of feet and Charcot joints are complications. Argyll Robertson pupils occur in tabes dorsalis also.
- The gait is characteristic and described as 'stamp and stick' sound—patient landing forcefully and flat footed on a wide base in order to detect the position of the feet and then striking a cane on the floor for stability.
- Visceral crisis consists of abrupt epigastric pain with vomiting lasting for hours. Barium studies show pylorospasm (gastric crisis). Similarly, intestinal crisis with diarrhoea, rectal crisis with tenesmus, genitourinary crisis with strangury, and pharyngeal–laryngeal crisis with gulping movements and dyspnoea may occur.
- CSF findings—as described previously.

TREATMENT OF NEUROSYPHILIS

- Treatment of neurosyphilis is given in Box 5.62.

BOX 5.62 Treatment of Neurosyphilis

RECOMMENDED REGIMENS:

- Crystalline penicillin 18–24 million units/day given in six divided doses for 10–14 days

Or

- Procaine penicillin G 1.8–2.4 million units IM once a day plus oral probenecid 500 mg four times daily, both for 10–14 days

IN PATIENTS WITH PENICILLIN ALLERGY:

- Ceftriaxone 2 g/day for 10–14 days

Or

- Doxycycline 200 mg 12 hourly for 28 days

FOLLOW-UP

- Patient should be re-examined every 3 months and CSF at 6-month interval. If CSF is normal and VDRL titres have come down, no further treatment is required. If CSF remains abnormal, another full course of penicillin should be given.

Q. Discuss briefly about Charcot joint.

- Charcot joint is the complication of chronic loss of proprioception and pain senses from lower extremities.
- Common causes include chronic severe sensory polyneuropathies (e.g. diabetes mellitus, leprosy and toxins), syringomyelia, tabes dorsalis, spina bifida, meningomyelocoele and cerebral palsy.
- Most frequently, hips, knees and ankles are affected. Occasionally, lumbar spine and upper limb joints are affected.
- Begins as osteoarthritis with repeated injuries to the insensitive joints, and progresses to destruction of articular surfaces.
- Often presents initially as a warm, swollen and erythematous joint (acute form).
- Frequent subluxation fractures with mild discomfort and minimal pain may occur. The initial treatment is immediate immobilisation and avoidance of weight bearing in early stages. Further mechanical injury should be prevented. Bisphosphonates, calcitonin and recombinant parathyroid hormone may help in the acute phase as they inhibit osteoclastic reabsorption, but evidence of their efficacy is lacking.

Q. What are the common demyelinating diseases?

- Demyelination is the loss or destruction of the nerve's myelin coating in the central or peripheral nervous system (brain, spinal cord, optic nerves and nerves) resulting in impairment or loss of function of neurons.
- Schwann cells supply the myelin for peripheral neurons, whereas oligodendrocytes myelinate the axons of CNS.
- Symptoms and signs will depend on the area that is involved.

COMMON CAUSES OF DEMYELINATION (Table 5.46)

TABLE 5.46 Common Causes of Demyelination

Demyelinating Diseases of CNS	Demyelinating Diseases of Peripheral Nervous System
• Multiple sclerosis • Neuromyelitis optica • Infectious or postinfectious—acute disseminated encephalomyelitis (ADEM), HIV encephalitis, progressive multifocal leucoencephalitis, subacute sclerosing panencephalitis, Creutzfeldt–Jakob encephalitis • Transverse myelitis • Nutritional—Wernicke's encephalopathy, subacute combined degeneration • Toxic—radiation, chemotherapeutic agents, toluene, mercury, methanol • Hypoxic/ischaemic—vasculitis, posterior reversible encephalopathy syndrome	• Dry beriberi • GB syndrome • Chronic inflammatory demyelinating polyneuropathy • Charcot–Marie–Tooth disease • Vitamin B_{12} deficiency • Organophosphate poisoning • Copper deficiency

Q. Describe the nerve supply of urinary bladder. Add a note on neurogenic bladder.

- Dysfunctions of bladder arising out of neurological disorders are termed neurogenic bladder.
- Bladder and its sphincters are innervated by sympathetic (from L1 and L2; via hypogastric nerve), parasympathetic (from detrusor nucleus at S2–S4 segments; via pelvic nerve) and somatic motor (from pudendal nucleus at S2–S4 segments; via pudendal nerve) fibres. Lumbosacral centres are under control from pontomesencephalic and cortical micturition centres.
- Sympathetic fibres are inhibitory to the detrusor and allow urine to collect. Parasympathetic fibres are facilitatory and aid in emptying the bladder by contraction of detrusor and relaxation of the internal sphincter of urethra (Fig. 5.13).
- Internal sphincter is in contracted state during rest and relaxes while micturating. External sphincter is under voluntary control. Cortical centre and its connection with frontal lobe control conscious aspects of micturition and have inhibitory influence over lower centre. Pontomesencephalic centre acts as a coordinator over entire afferent and efferent influences.
- During the storage phase of micturition, bladder filling activates afferent nerve fibres in the bladder wall. This afferent input results in stimulation of sympathetic efferent activity (via the hypogastric nerve), leading to contraction of smooth muscles in the bladder base and proximal urethra (via activation of α-adrenergic receptors) and relaxation of the detrusor (via activation of β-adrenergic receptors in the bladder body). Somatic efferent activity (via the pudendal nerve) also increases, resulting in increased tone of the striated external urethral sphincter. These

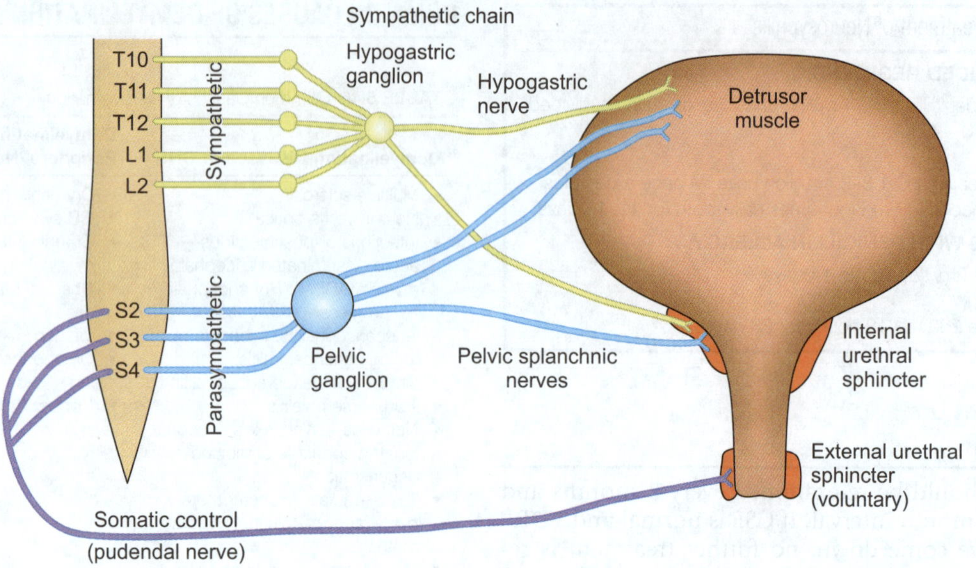

Fig. 5.13 Nerve supply to the bladder and sphincters.

responses promote continence. Parasympathetic system is largely inactive during urine storage.

- The voiding phase of micturition is initiated voluntarily by signals from cerebral cortex. Initial event is relaxation of striated external urethral sphincter caused by inhibition of somatic efferent activity. There is inhibition of sympathetic efferent activity with concomitant activation of parasympathetic outflow to the bladder and urethra.

NEUROGENIC BLADDER

- Neurogenic bladder dysfunctions are classified according to functional status of the bladder based on cystometry and urodynamic studies.
- Several patterns of bladder dysfunctions may arise. Basic principle involves consideration of detrusor (atonic or hypertonic) and sphincteric activity (coordinated or not with detrusor contraction) (Table 5.47).

TABLE 5.47 Types of Neurogenic Bladder

Type of Neurogenic Bladder	Features	Lesions
Uninhibited bladder	• Reduced awareness of bladder fullness • Low capacity of bladder due to reduction of inhibition of pontomesencephalic centre • Urge urinary incontinence with relatively low volumes of urine • Bladder pressure normal (due to normal function of detrusor and internal/external sphincters)	• Lesions above the pontomesencephalic centre (e.g. stroke, frontal tumours, parasagittal meningioma, hydrocephalus, head trauma)
Upper motor neuron bladder	• Bladder capacity is reduced due to high detrusor tone • Urine incontinence if detrusor pressure exceeds internal/external urinary sphincter pressure producing urgency, urge incontinence, incomplete voiding and increased residual urine • High bladder pressure due to simultaneous detrusor and external urinary sphincter contractions (individual will sense an overwhelming desire to urinate but only a small amount of urine may dribble out—detrusor-sphincter dyssynergia) leading to vesicoureteral reflux	• Lesions between the pontomesencephalic centre and sacral spinal cord (e.g. traumatic spinal cord injury, compressive myelopathy, multiple sclerosis)
Mixed, type A bladder	• Detrusor flaccid while the intact pudendal nucleus produces a hypertonic external urinary sphincter • Large bladder producing urinary retention which patient is unable to sense • Overflow incontinence may occur	• Sacral cord lesions which damage the detrusor nucleus but spare the pudendal nucleus
Mixed, type B bladder	• Flaccid external urinary sphincter due to the pudendal nucleus lesion while the bladder is spastic due to the disinhibited detrusor nucleus • Urinary incontinence • Low capacity of bladder but vesicular pressure is not elevated as there is little outflow resistance	• Sacral cord lesions that spare the detrusor nucleus but damage the pudendal nucleus
Lower motor neuron bladder	• Detrusor tone is low and internal urinary sphincter innervation is intact • Overflow urinary incontinence • Large bladder capacity and increased risk of urinary tract infections	• Sacral cord or sacral nerve root injuries, diabetes mellitus, tabes dorsalis

- Lesions of cerebral hemispheres, if located postcentrally, result in loss of awareness of bladder fullness and cause incontinence, whereas precentral lesions cause difficulty in initiating micturition. Residual urine is insignificant. More anteriorly located frontal lobe lesions cause loss of social inhibition resulting in unconcerned micturition at inappropriate places.
- Common causes include multiple sclerosis, parkinsonism, stroke, myelopathies, spinal cord injuries, spina bifida, diabetes mellitus with autonomic neuropathy, unintended sequelae following pelvic surgery and cauda equina.
- Neurogenic bladder predisposes to development of urinary infection and back pressure changes at upper urinary tract, and requires to be treated appropriately.
- Treatment requires correct assessment by urodynamic studies, followed by proper catheterisation techniques, use of pharmacological agents (anticholinergic drugs like oxybutynin or tolterodine for detrusor spasticity, α-adrenergic blockers like terazosin, if internal sphincter fails to relax) and surgery in certain cases. Botulinum toxin type A is useful in reducing episodes of urinary incontinence in patients with neurogenic detrusor overactivity.

Q. Tabulate spinal cord levels relative to vertebral levels.

- While examining and making a final diagnosis in a patient with myelopathy, it is important to write both the cord level and the vertebral level of the lesion. The relationship between spinal cord and vertebral levels is shown in Box 5.63.

BOX 5.63 Spinal Cord Level Relative to Vertebrae

Spinal Cord Level	Corresponding Vertebral Level
Upper cervical	Same as cord level
Lower cervical level	1 level higher
Upper thoracic	2 levels higher
Lower thoracic	2 to 3 levels higher
Lumbar	10th–12th thoracic vertebrae
Sacral	12th thoracic and 1st lumbar vertebrae

Q. Draw a diagram showing transverse section of spinal cord at upper cervical area.

- Transverse section of spinal cord at upper cervical area is shown in Fig. 5.14.

Q. Discuss causes and clinical features of various spinal cord syndromes.

- Various spinal cord syndromes are described in Table 5.48.

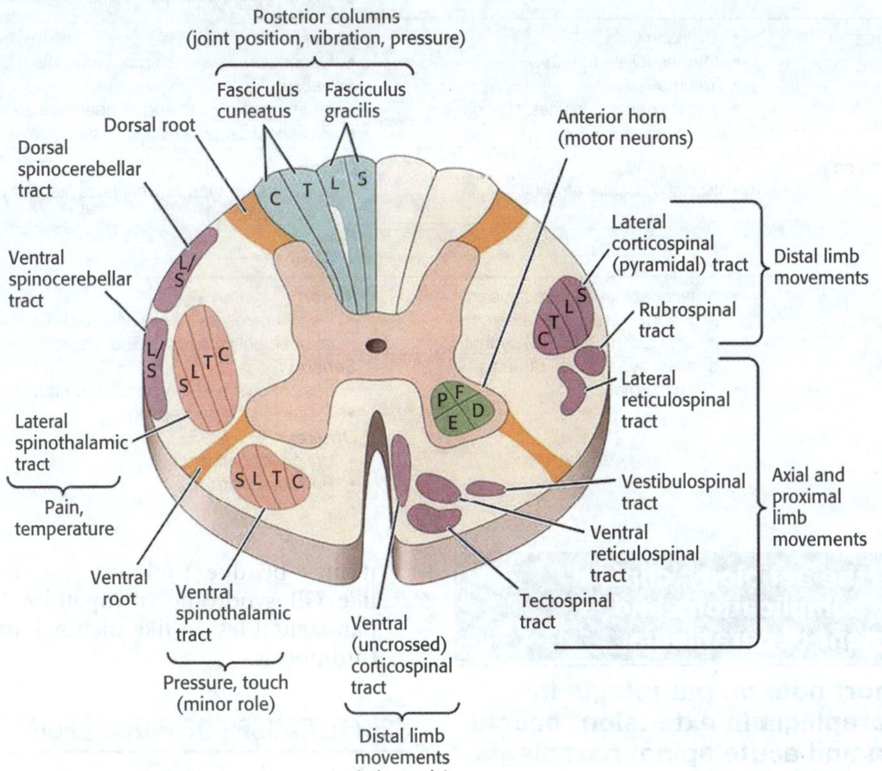

Fig. 5.14 Transverse section of spinal cord at upper cervical level. Left-sided tracts, ascending tracts; right-sided tracts, descending tracts; C, cervical; T, thoracic; L, lumbar; S, sacral.

TABLE 5.48 Spinal Cord Syndromes

Syndrome	Causes	Clinical Features
Complete transaction of spinal cord	• Trauma • Infarction • Metastatic malignancy • Multiple sclerosis • Spinal epidural haematoma or abscess • Transverse myelitis	***Motor:*** • Paraplegia due to corticospinal tract involvement • Initially spinal shock with flaccid paraplegia • Later, spastic paraplegia • Loss of abdominal and cremastric reflexes • May get lower motor type of paralysis at the level of lesion ***Sensory:*** • All sensations absent • Sensory level is generally two to three segments below the level of lesion • Segmental paraesthesias at the level of lesion ***Others:*** • Retention of urine • Constipation • Sexual dysfunction • Anhidrosis, trophic skin changes below the level of lesion
Brown-Sequard syndrome (occurs due to damage to one side of spinal cord)	• Extramedullary compressive myelopathy (e.g. abscess, tumour) • Penetrating injuries (e.g. gunshot) • Multiple sclerosis	***Motor:*** • Ipsilateral spastic weakness due to descending corticospinal tract involvement • Lower motor neuron signs at the level of lesion ***Sensory:*** • Ipsilateral loss of proprioception (vibration and position) due to involvement of posterior column • Contralateral loss of pain and temperature due to involvement of lateral spinothalamic tract
Posterior spinal cord syndrome	• Diabetes mellitus • Tabes dorsalis	***Motor:*** • None ***Sensory:*** • Impaired position and vibration sensation in lower limbs • Sensory ataxia • Positive Romberg's sign • Positive Lhermitte's sign ***Others:*** • Urinary incontinence • Absent knee and ankle jerks • Charcot's joint in late stages • Argyll-Robertson pupil (in syphilis)
Central cord syndrome	• Syringomyelia • Intramedullary tumours • Trauma • Hyperextension injuries of neck	***Motor:*** • Upper limb weakness more than lower limb weakness ***Sensory:*** • Impairment of pain and temperature sensation on both sides • Preserved proprioception (dissociative anaesthesia)
Anterior horn cell syndrome	• Poliomyelitis • Spinal muscular atrophy	***Motor:*** • Lower motor type of weakness (flaccidity, fasciculations, absent reflexes) ***Sensory:*** • None
Anterior spinal cord syndrome	• Anterior spinal artery occlusion (e.g. aortic dissection, atherosclerosis of aorta, SLE, HIV, syphilitic arteritis, hyperflexion of neck) • AV malformation	***Motor:*** • Flaccid paralysis initially and spastic paraparesis later due to involvement of corticospinal tracts ***Sensory:*** • Loss of pain and temperature on both sides • Preserved proprioception ***Others:*** • Urinary incontinence • Radicular pain

Q. Describe the aetiology, clinical features, complications and management of paraplegia.

Q. Write a short note on paraplegia in flexion, paraplegia in extension, flaccid paraplegia and acute spinal paraplegia.

- Paraplegia is dense paralysis of both lower limbs. It is usually due to disorders of spinal cord. Occasionally it may be due to lower motor neuron disorders like GB syndrome, myopathies or an intracranial parasagittal lesion like meningioma or sagittal sinus thrombosis.

SPINAL CAUSES OF PARAPLEGIA (Table 5.49)

- High cauda equina lesions (compressive) at L1 or L2 can cause paraplegia of lower motor neuron type.

TABLE 5.49 Spinal Causes of Paraplegia

• Acute	Trauma, transverse myelitis, multiple sclerosis, neuromyelitis optica, infarction of spinal cord (vasculitis, anterior spinal artery thrombosis), spinal epidural abscess
• Subacute or chronic	
• Spinal cord compression (extradural)	Spinal metastasis, tuberculosis of spine, primary bone tumours, disc prolapse or spondylosis at lower cervical region, ligamental hypertrophy in cervical region, extradural granulomas and neoplasms (usually lymphoma), extradural arteriovenous malformation
• Intraspinal tumours (intradural extramedullary)	Meningioma (including parasagittal meningioma of brain), neurofibroma
• Intramedullary tumours (intradural intramedullary)	Astrocytoma, ependymoma, syringomyelia
• Miscellaneous	Arachnoiditis, syringomyelia, radiation myelopathy, lathyrism, hereditary spastic paraplegia, tropical spastic paraplegia, subacute combined degeneration, fluorosis, HIV myelopathy, paraneoplastic, spinocerebellar ataxias, triorthocresyl phosphate (TOCP) poisoning, subacute myelopathic neuropathy (SMON), arsenic poisoning, radiation

CLINICAL FEATURES

- Acute-onset lesions result in flaccid, areflexic paralysis in both lower limbs and sensory loss till the level of lesion. Urinary retention is present. This phase of flaccid paralysis is due to spinal shock.
- Spinal shock gradually resolves and features of UMN lesion appear after 3 to 4 weeks.
- Spinal shock may persist for longer duration if infections occur or bed sores develop.
- Neurogenic shock may occur with cervical and high thoracic spine injury resulting in sudden loss of sympathetic tone. This leads to autonomic instability producing hypotension, bradyarrhythmia and temperature dysregulation (flushed warm skin). Treatment requires use of IV fluids, norepinephrine and atropine.
- Limbs may assume paraplegia in 'flexion' or 'extension' depending on the lesion.
  - When corticospinal tracts alone are affected, the extrapyramidal system takes the upper hand, resulting in increased tone of antigravity muscles (paraplegia in extension).
  - When the influence of extrapyramidal system is cut off, the spinal arc takes over and there is relative increase in the tone of flexors of legs (paraplegia in flexion).
- Subacute or chronic spinal paraplegias appear as 'spastic paraplegias'.
- Presence of sensory and bladder symptoms and signs depends on the underlying cause.

INVESTIGATIONS

- Plain radiograph of the spine to detect vertebral diseases, fractures, etc.
- CSF in evaluation of arachnoiditis.
- Appropriate diagnostic tests to determine the underlying cause. These include CT scan and MRI of spine.
- Brain MRI if paraparesis is associated with drowsiness, confusion, seizures or other hemispheric signs.
- Electrophysiologic studies if an underlying neuromuscular disorder is suspected.

COMPLICATIONS

- Complications of paraplegia may lead to death.
- Common complications of paraplegia are given in Box 5.64.

BOX 5.64 Complications of Paraplegia

- Pressure sore
- Urinary infection
- Renal calculi
- Faecal impaction with intestinal obstruction
- Contracture of limbs

MANAGEMENT

- Care of paraplegia is as important as treating the underlying cause.

SKIN

- Pressure sores have to be prevented as they occur due to loss of sensation and diminished blood supply.
- Patient should be turned every 2–4 hours to a position that avoids pressure over bony prominences.
- Skin must be kept dry and clean.
- If possible, patient should be nursed on a specially designed mattress like water or air-cushioned bed.
- If pressure sores develop, patient must not lie on the affected side. Aseptic care must be taken. Skin grafting may be necessary.

BLADDER

- Aseptic, intermittent catheterisation should be done.
- Indwelling catheter is not desirable as it predisposes to infection, reduces bladder capacity and promotes calculus formation.
- Occasionally, urinary diversion procedures may be necessary.
- Urinary infections should be treated promptly. Fluid intake should be adequate.

BOWEL

- Constipation is prevented by laxatives.
- If faecal matter becomes hard, manual evacuation is necessary.

PARALYSIS

- Spasticity can lead to contractures and flexor spasms.
- Regular passive movements of the limbs.
- Patient should be nursed in a posture that discourages flexion at joints.
- Drug treatment of spasticity is effective in many patients but it may reduce function as many patients use their spasticity as an aid to stand or walk.

Baclofen is the most effective drug for reducing spasticity. Diazepam and tizanidine also work well in most patients.
- In severe cases, intrathecal baclofen may be administered via a pump. If this is not effective, sectioning of the anterior roots (rhizotomy) may be done.

REHABILITATION

- Patient can be taught to use a calliper or wheelchair.
- With encouragement, patient can be made an active member of the society.

Q. Discuss the causes and differential diagnosis of spastic paraplegia.

- Spastic paraplegia denotes an upper motor neuron lesion causing paraplegia. It is invariably due to a lesion that appears subacutely or chronically. Acute lesions generally cause flaccid paralysis. Once spinal shock resolves in patients with acute causes of paraplegia (see 'Spinal Causes of Paraplegia'), paraplegia with spasticity develops.
- The term 'ataxic paraplegia' is used when ataxia is a predominant feature and is present with paraplegia (or paraparesis). Important causes include spinocerebellar degeneration and Friedreich's ataxia.

CAUSES OF SPASTIC PARAPLEGIA (Table 5.50)

- In elderly, motor neuron disease, spinal metastasis and cervical spondylosis are the common causes.
- In younger age group, hereditary spastic paraplegia, tuberculosis of spine, extradural granulomas and neurofibromas are the common causes.
- Hereditary spastic paraplegia has onset from early childhood to adulthood onwards, with insidious development of leg stiffness and/or abnormal wear of the shoes.
- Lathyrism and residual deficits from previous lesions occur in all age groups.
- Diagnosis may be arrived at by adequate history, physical signs, CT scan, MRI and CSF analysis. Arteriovenous malformations may require spinal angiography. Tumours and granulomas require surgery and biopsy for adequate diagnosis and further management.
- In some patients, antispasticity drugs such as baclofen and tizanidine can be helpful to reduce spasticity.

TABLE 5.50 Causes of Spastic Paraplegia

Group	Causes
• Pure motor syndromes (motor disturbance alone)	Any early cord compression, motor neuron disease, hereditary spastic paraplegia, Erb's spastic paraplegia (syphilitic), lathyrism, residual deficit from acute lesions (on partial recovery)
• With sensory and bladder involvement	See 'Spinal Causes of Paraplegia' (subacute or chronic)

TABLE 5.51 Causes of Acute Flaccid Paralysis

Acute neuropathy:
- Guillain–Barre syndrome
- Other acute neuropathies—vasculitis, porphyria, toxins (e.g. organophosphates, arsenic, thallium), infections (e.g. Lyme disease, diphtheria), critical illness neuropathy

Acute myopathy (no sensory loss, reflexes often preserved):
- Hypokalaemic periodic paralysis
- Hyperkalaemic periodic paralysis
- Hypophosphataemia
- Acute rhabdomyolysis
- Polymyositis (rare)

Anterior horn cell disease:
- Poliomyelitis

Acute neuromuscular junction disorders (tend to cause paralysis descending from the cranial nerves rather than ascending from the lower limbs):
- Myasthenic crisis
- Botulism
- Tick paralysis
- Neuroparalytic snake bite (krait and cobra)
- Organophosphate and carbamate poisoning
- Hypermagnesaemia
- Drug overdose (e.g. aminoglycosides, quinolones, polymyxin antibiotics, quinidine, procainamide, neuromuscular blockers)

Acute myelopathy (initially flaccid paralysis due to spinal shock)

Q. Enumerate causes of acute flaccid paralysis or weakness.

- Acute flaccid paralysis can be caused by several diseases including acute spinal cord diseases (refer Table 5.49). Various causes are mentioned in Table 5.51.

Q. What are the causes of episodic quadriparesis?

- Episodic quadriparesis can be caused by several diseases (Box 5.65).

BOX 5.65 Causes of Episodic Quadriparesis

Electrolyte disturbances	Hypokalaemia or hyperkalaemia Hypercalcaemia Hypophosphataemia Hypermagnesaemia
Muscle disorders	Channelopathies: periodic paralyses Metabolic defects of muscle: impaired carbohydrate or fatty acid utilisation; abnormal mitochondrial function
Neuromuscular junction disorders	Myasthenia gravis Lambert–Eaton myasthenic syndrome
Central nervous system disorders	Transient ischaemic attacks of the brainstem Transient global cerebral ischaemia Multiple sclerosis

Q. Describe briefly about transverse myelitis.

- Transverse myelitis (TM) is a heterogeneous group of inflammatory disorders characterised by acute or subacute motor, sensory and autonomic (bladder, bowel and sexual) spinal cord dysfunction. The term myelitis is a nonspecific term for inflammation of the spinal cord; transverse refers to involvement across one level of the spinal cord. The term 'myelopathy' is a broad, generic term which does not imply any particular aetiology; myelitis refers to an inflammatory disease process.

- TM occurs with optic neuritis in neuromyelitis optica (Devic's disease).

CAUSES (Box 5.66)

BOX 5.66 Causes of Transverse Myelitis

- Parainfectious (occurring at the time of and in association with an acute infection or an episode of infection)
  - Viral: Herpes simplex, herpes zoster, cytomegalovirus, Epstein–Barr virus, enteroviruses (poliomyelitis, Coxsackie virus, echovirus), human T-cell leukaemia virus-1 (HTLV-1), human immunodeficiency virus, influenza, rabies, chikungunya
  - Bacterial: *Mycoplasma*, Lyme borreliosis, syphilis, tuberculosis
- Postvaccinal (rabies)
- Systemic autoimmune disease
  - Systemic lupus erythematosus
  - Sjögren's syndrome
  - Behçet's disease
  - Antiphospholipid syndrome
- Sarcoidosis
- Multiple sclerosis
- Neuromyelitis optica
- Acute demyelinating encephalomyelitis
- Paraneoplastic syndrome
- Drugs and toxins
  - Tumour necrosis factor-alpha inhibitors
  - Sulphasalazine
  - Chemotherapeutic agents (cisplatin, gemcitabine)
  - Heroin abuse
- Vascular
  - Vasculitis secondary to heroin abuse
- Idiopathic

CLINICAL FEATURES

- TM symptoms develop rapidly over several hours to several days. Approximately 45% of patients worsen maximally within 24 hours. Incomplete deficit may or may not progress over several more days to a complete transverse sensorimotor myelopathy.
- Common presenting symptoms of TM include limb weakness, sensory disturbance, and bowel and bladder dysfunction.
- Neuropathic pain may occur in the midline (an aching, deep pain) or in a dermatomal distribution (radicular or lancinating pain or a sensation of burning or itching), with the latter pattern providing a clue to the anatomical level of the lesion.
- Almost all patients will develop leg weakness of varying degrees of severity. The arms are involved in a minority of cases and this is dependent on the level of spinal cord involvement.
- Acutely, limb tone and muscle stretch reflexes may be diminished and even absent (spinal shock syndrome) leading to possible diagnostic confusion with Guillain–Barre syndrome.
- Sensation is diminished below the level of spinal cord involvement (generally one to two segments below the level) in the majority of patients (sensory level).
- Some patients experience tingling or numbness in the legs.
- Pain and temperature sensation are diminished in the majority of patients.
- Appreciation of vibration and joint position sense may also be decreased or may be spared.
- Bladder and bowel sphincter control are disturbed in the majority of patients.
- Tonic spasms (recurrent short-lived episodes of involuntary painful flexor contractions lasting 30 seconds to a few minutes) are also seen in many patients.
- Demyelination is responsible for the presence of Lhermitte's sign (paraesthesias that radiate down the spine or limbs with neck flexion). It suggests an intrinsic cervical spinal cord lesion, typically affecting the dorsal columns. Another sign of demyelination is Uhthoff's phenomenon (transient worsening of neurologic symptoms from excessive heat).
- Recovery may be absent, partial or complete, and generally begins within 1–3 months.

DIAGNOSIS

- The first step is to exclude a mass-occupying lesion that might be compressing the spinal cord. This is important because early surgery to remove the compression may sometimes reverse neurological injury to the spinal cord.
- Diagnosis requires MRI and CSF analysis.
- MRI typically shows cord swelling and gadolinium-enhancing lesions (single or multiple). Lesions associated with multiple sclerosis usually span less than three vertebral segments. Longitudinally extensive TM ($\geq$3 vertebral segments) occurs in idiopathic TM, neuromyelitis optica, ADEM, cord infarction and myelitis associated with systemic diseases such as systemic lupus erythematosus. MRI also helps exclude other treatable causes of spinal cord dysfunction (e.g. spinal cord compression).
- CSF usually contains lymphocytes (<100/µL), protein content is slightly increased (100–120 mg/dL) and IgG index is elevated.
  - IgG index is a measure of intrathecal synthesis of immunoglobulin.
  - Calculated with the use of the following formula: ([CSF IgG]/[serum IgG])/([CSF albumin]/[serum albumin]) × 100. (IgG is in mg/dL, CSF albumin is in mg/dL while serum albumin is in g/dL.)
  - Normal <0.66.
- Tests to find out treatable causes of myelitis should include chest X-ray; tuberculin; serological tests for *Mycoplasma*, Lyme disease and HIV; vitamin B_{12} and folate levels; ESR; antinuclear antibodies; CSF

and blood for VDRL tests; and serum NMO-IgG antibody.

- Brain MRI as multiple sclerosis may present with TM.

DIAGNOSTIC CRITERIA (Box 5.67)

BOX 5.67 Diagnostic Criteria for Transverse Myelitis

- Bilateral (not necessarily symmetric) sensorimotor and autonomic spinal cord dysfunction
- Clearly defined sensory level
- Progression of clinical deficits to maximum between 4 hours and 21 days after symptom onset
- Demonstration of spinal cord inflammation
  - Cerebrospinal fluid pleocytosis
  - Elevated IgG index
  - MRI revealing a gadolinium-enhancing cord lesion
- Exclusion of compressive, postradiation, neoplastic and vascular causes

TREATMENT

- Despite the lack of randomised controlled studies, administration of high-dose IV corticosteroids (e.g. methylprednisolone 1 g daily for 5 days) should be started as early as possible in all patients. If it fails, plasma exchange should be tried. Some cases may respond to IVIg therapy.
- Treatment of the underlying cause.
- Otherwise, treatment is supportive (see 'paraplegia' on page 384).

Q. How do you differentiate between compressive and noncompressive myelopathy?

Q. How do you differentiate between extradural, intradural extramedullary and intramedullary myelopathies?

DIFFERENTIATION BETWEEN COMPRESSIVE AND NONCOMPRESSIVE MYELOPATHY (Table 5.52)

TABLE 5.52 Compressive Versus Noncompressive Myelopathy

Feature	Compressive Myelopathy	Noncompressive Myelopathy
Local deformity	±	-
Local pain	±	-
Girdle-like sensation	±	-
Radicular pain	±	-
Clear upper level of sensory level	+	Usually no
Onset and progression	Gradual	May be acute
Symmetry	Asymmetrical	Majority symmetrical
Flexor spasm	±	-
Bladder and bowel involvement	Late	Early or late
Examples	Pott's spine	Transverse myelitis, motor neuron disease

DIFFERENCES BETWEEN EXTRADURAL, INTRADURAL AND INTRAMEDULLARY MYELOPATHY (Table 5.53)

TABLE 5.53 Extradural Extramedullary Versus Intradural Extramedullary Versus Intramedullary Myelopathy

Feature	Extradural Extramedullary Myelopathy	Intradural Extramedullary Myelopathy	Intramedullary Myelopathy
• Onset	Asymmetrical	Asymmetrical	Often symmetrical
• Localised pain	Common and early	Uncommon	Rare
• Local deformity	May be present	Absent	Absent
• Root pains	Common	Less common compared to extradural	Uncommon
• Pyramidal signs	Late	Early onset producing spasticity	Late
• Lower motor nerve involvement	Localised to the site of involvement	Localised to the site of involvement	Spreads over many segments
• Bladder involvement	Late	Rare and late	Common and early
• Sacral sensory loss	Early	Early	Delayed ('sacral sparing')
• Dissociated sensory loss	Absent	Absent	May be present (e.g. syringomyelia)
• Examples	Pott's spine, intervertebral disc herniation, metastatic (breast, lung, prostate), multiple myeloma, primary vertebral column tumours, trauma, craniovertebral junction anomalies, fluorosis, epidural abscess or haematoma	Metastatic, neurofibroma, schwannoma, meningioma, epidermoid, dermoid, teratomas, arachnoiditis, sarcoidosis, AV malformation	Syringomyelia, ependymoma, astrocytoma, haemangioblastoma, haematomyelia, metastatic

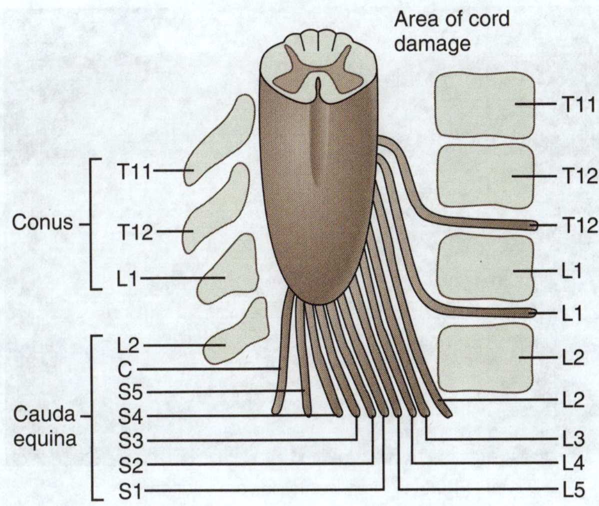

Fig. 5.15 Schematic representation of conus medullaris and cauda equina. C, coccygeal.

Q. How will you differentiate between conus medullaris lesions and cauda equina lesions?

- Spinal cord terminates at the level of intervertebral disc between the first and second lumbar vertebrae, forming the conus medullaris, below which is the filum terminale and a bundle of nerve roots.
- Cauda equina is formed by nerve roots caudal to the level of spinal cord termination (below L1 vertebral level) which give horsetail-like appearance (Fig. 5.15).
- Conus medullaris is the most distal bulbous part of the spinal cord. It consists of sacral spinal cord segments (Fig. 5.15).
- Cauda equina syndrome refers to a characteristic pattern of neuromuscular and urogenital symptoms resulting from simultaneous compression of multiple lumbosacral nerve roots below the level of conus medullaris. The nerves provide sensory innervation to saddle area, motor innervation to sphincters and parasympathetic innervation to bladder and lower bowel.
- Conus medullaris is in proximity to the nerve roots and any lesion of this area often results in a combination of upper motor neuron and lower motor neuron symptoms and signs in the dermatomes of the affected segments.
- Clinical features to differentiate cauda equina syndrome and conus medullaris syndrome are given in Table 5.54.

Q. Discuss briefly about neurocutaneous syndromes.

- Neurocutaneous syndromes are genetic disorders that lead to growth of tumours in various parts of the body. Involvement of skin and nervous system is typical of these disorders.

TABLE 5.54 Clinical Features Differentiating Cauda Equina Syndrome and Conus Medullaris Syndrome

Features	Cauda Equina	Conus Medullaris
• Onset	Asymmetrical and gradual	Symmetrical and acute
• Dissociated sensory loss	Absent	Present
• Root pain	Common	Rare
• Low backache	Common	Rare
• Fasciculations	Common	Rare
• Bladder and bowel involvement	Early or late (depends on root involvement)	Early
• Muscle tone	Decreased	Increased
• Knee and ankle reflexes	Both absent	Knee present but ankle absent
• Anal reflex	Absent or diminished	Normal
• Perianal (saddle) numbness	Yes (saddle anaesthesia)	No ('perianal' sparing)

NEUROFIBROMATOSIS

- Both types 1 and 2 neurofibromatoses have autosomal dominant inheritance.

NEUROFIBROMATOSIS TYPE 1 (VON RECKLINGHAUSEN'S DISEASE)

- Criteria to diagnose neurofibromatosis type 1 are given in Box 5.68.
- Selumetinib, a kinase inhibitor, is approved for the treatment of paediatric patients 2 years of age and older with neurofibromatosis type 1 who have symptomatic, inoperable plexiform neurofibromas.

NEUROFIBROMATOSIS TYPE 2

- Criteria to diagnose neurofibromatosis type 2 are given in Box 5.69.

TUBEROUS SCLEROSIS

- Features of tuberous sclerosis are described in Box 5.70.

BOX 5.68 Diagnostic Criteria of Neurofibromatosis Type 1

Two or more of the following:

1. Six or more café au lait spots, greater than 5 mm in diameter in prepubertal individuals and over 15 mm in diameter in postpubertal individuals
2. Two or more neurofibromas of any type or one plexiform neurofibroma
3. Axillary and/or inguinal freckling (Crowe's sign)
4. Optic nerve glioma
5. Two or more Lisch nodules (dome-shaped lesions around the iris on slit-lamp examination)
6. Osseous lesions such as dysplasia of the sphenoid wing, thinning of long bone cortex, with or without pseudoarthrosis
7. First-degree relative (parent, sibling or offspring) with NF type 1 according to above-mentioned criteria

BOX 5.69 Diagnostic Criteria of Neurofibromatosis Type 2

One of the following:

1. Bilateral vestibular schwannomas before age 70 years
2. Unilateral vestibular schwannoma before age 70 years PLUS first-degree relative with NF type 2
3. Any two of the following: Meningioma, nonvestibular schwannoma, neurofibroma, glioma, cerebral calcification, posterior subcapsular lens opacity; *PLUS*
   a. First-degree relative with NF2 *OR*
   b. Unilateral vestibular schwannoma
4. Multiple meningiomas *PLUS*
   a. Unilateral vestibular schwannoma *OR*
   b. Any two of the following: Nonvestibular schwannoma, glioma, neurofibroma cerebral calcification, posterior subcapsular lens opacity

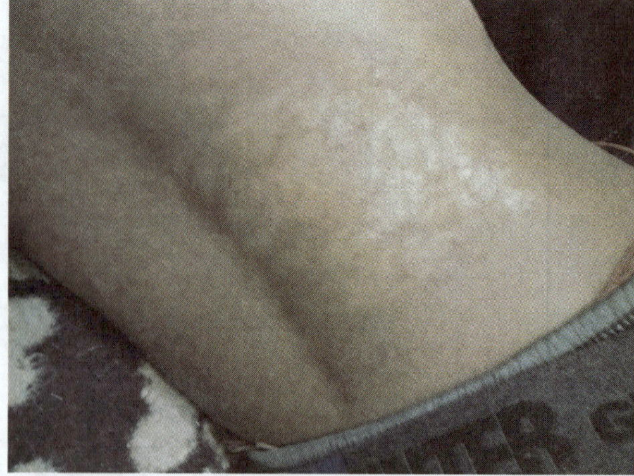

Fig. 5.17 Ash leaf hypopigmentation.

BOX 5.70 Tuberous Sclerosis

- Autosomal dominant
- Characterised by formation of hamartomas in multiple organ systems
- Clinically, characterised by seizures, cutaneous lesions and mental retardation
- Skin lesions:
  - Adenoma sebaceum—facial angiofibroma (Fig. 5.16)
  - Ash leaf hypopigmentation (Fig. 5.17)
  - Shagreen patch—an irregularly shaped, irregularly thickened, slightly elevated soft skin-coloured or yellowish patch over lumbosacral region or other areas (Fig. 5.18)
  - Calcified subependymal nodules
- Rhabdomyosarcomas of the myocardium
- Angiomyolipomas of the kidneys, liver, pancreas and adrenals
- Increased frequency of ependymomas and astrocytomas

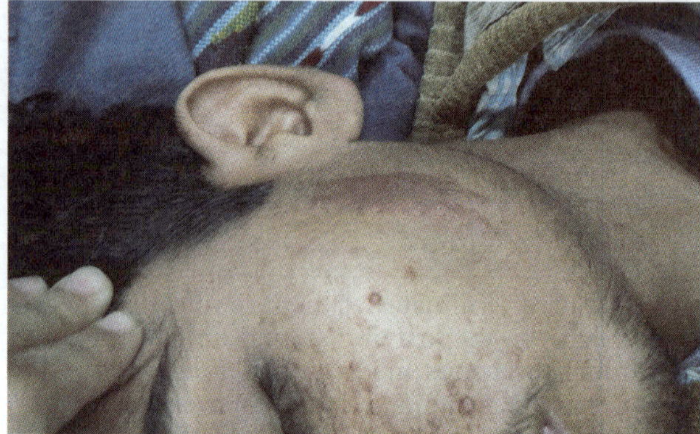

Fig. 5.18 Shagreen patch over face.

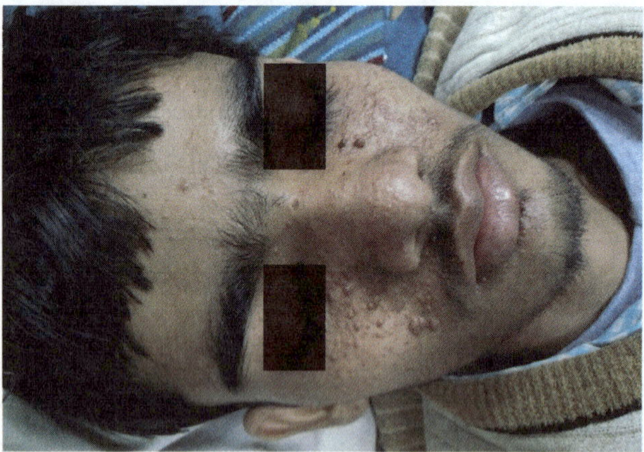

Fig. 5.16 Facial angiofibroma.

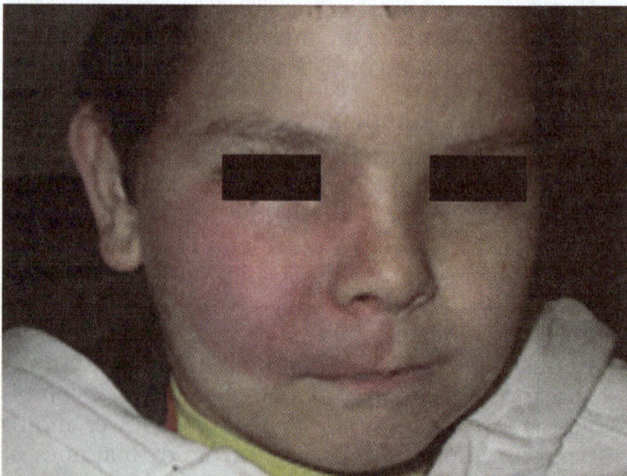

Fig. 5.19 Port wine stain in the distribution of maxillary branch of trigeminal nerve. Courtesy: Higueros,E, Roe E, Granell E, Baselga E. Sturge-Weber Syndrome: A Review. Actas Dermosifiliogr. 2017;108(5): 407–41.

STURGE–WEBER SYNDROME

- Sporadic disease.
- Characterised by vascular malformation with capillary venous angiomas that involve the face, choroid of the eye and leptomeninges.
- Facial angioma (port wine stain) has a predilection for the distribution of the first or second division of the trigeminal nerve (Fig. 5.19).
- Angiomatous meningeal malformation.
- Atrophy of the cerebral hemisphere often present.
- Usually unilateral.
- Focal seizures on contralateral side in most patients (80%).

- Mental retardation in more than 50% of patients.
- Glaucoma on the same side as the skin lesions.
- Radiographic hallmark on CT brain is 'tramline' or gyriform calcifications usually involving the occipital and parietal lobes.
- Everolimus is approved for the adjunctive treatment of patients aged 2 years and older with tuberous sclerosis-associated partial-onset seizures. Oral cannabidiol is also approved for control of seizures

VON HIPPEL–LINDAU SYNDROME

- Autosomal dominant.
- Retinal, cerebellar and spinal haemangioblastoma, CNS haemangioblastoma being the most commonly recognised manifestation (in 40% of patients).
- Renal cell carcinoma.
- Phaeochromocytomas.
- Cysts and tumours of kidney, pancreas and liver.

Q. Discuss the aetiology, clinical features, diagnosis and management of lumbago sciatica syndrome.

Q. Discuss the clinical manifestations, investigations and management of intervertebral disc prolapse (IVDP).

- Lumbago is acute low backache.
- Sciatica is the neuralgic pain that starts in the back and radiates along the posterior aspect of lower limb to heel.

CAUSES

- Combination of lumbago with sciatica is invariably due to acute intervertebral disc protrusion in the lumbar region (L3–L4; L4–L5; L5–S1).
- Other uncommon causes are the following:
  - Metastasis.
  - Tumours.
  - Tuberculosis of spine and epidural abscess.
  - Spinal canal stenosis.
  - Spondyloarthropathies.
  - Facet arthropathy.

CLINICAL FEATURES OF INTERVERTEBRAL DISC PROLAPSE

LUMBAGO

- Lumbago is localised low backache in the midline that increases on movements of spine or straining (like coughing, sneezing). There is associated paraspinal muscular spasm.
- Pain starts acutely, usually while attempting to lift weight in bent posture. Lumbago may or may not be associated with sciatica.

SCIATICA

- Also known as lumbar radicular pain.

TABLE 5.55 Neurologic Deficit in Sciatica

• **L4 root**	Weakness of invertors of foot, sensory impairment at L4 dermatome (inner aspect of leg) and depressed knee jerk
• **L5 root**	Weakness of extensor hallucis longus with sensory impairment at L5 dermatome (outer aspect of leg and dorsum of foot)
• **S1 root**	Weakness of plantar flexors of toes, foot and hamstrings with depressed ankle jerk and sensory impairment at S1 dermatome (outer aspect of foot)

- Occurs due to irritation of a spinal root compressed by the protruded disc close to the intervertebral foramen.
- Pain is shooting, burning or shock-like in character. It may be continuous or brought on by spinal movements and straining.
- Patient prefers to lie down on his/her sides with flexed lower limbs.
- Syndrome of pain may or may not be associated with symptoms of neurological deficit, which depends on the root involved (Table 5.55).
- Positive straight leg raising (SLR) test is present. A positive SLR test (also known as Lasegue's sign) results from gluteal or leg pain by passive straight leg flexion with the knee in extension.
- Large disc protrusions may cause bilateral, more extensive neurological deficit (cauda equina syndrome).

SPINAL CANAL STENOSIS

- Low back and leg pain are aggravated by walking and alleviated by bending forward. Often present with a wide-based gait and neurological weakness. These symptoms are referred to as intermittent neurogenic claudication.

INVESTIGATIONS

- Plain radiograph of lumbosacral spine:
  - Loss of lumbar lordosis.
  - Scoliosis.
  - Reduced intervertebral disc space.
  - On most occasions, radiograph is normal.
- CT scan shows the protruded disc. MRI is more sensitive and specific.

TREATMENT

- Conservative management is preferred when no neurological deficit is present.
- Bed rest for 1 week or so; however, presently, early return to daily activities is encouraged.
- Analgesics (NSAIDs) and muscle relaxants.
- Tramadol or duloxetine as second-line treatment.
- Gabapentin, pregabalin and antidepressants for neuropathic pain.
- The utility of lumbar epidural steroid injections is controversial.
- Surgery is recommended when neurological deficit is present.

Q. Discuss the aetiology, clinical features, investigations and management of syringomyelia.

Q. Give a brief account of dissociated suspended anaesthesia.

- Syringomyelia is a disorder where cavitation (syrinx) occurs within spinal cord along with dilated central canal. At times, syrinx can represent a focal dilation of the central canal.
- Syrinxes commonly develop in the lower cervical and high thoracic regions or in the high cervical region where they may extend proximally to the medulla or pons (syringobulbia).
- Many cases are associated with Chiari malformations (usually type I in which there is caudal herniation of the cerebellar tonsils exceeding 5 mm below the foramen magnum).

CAUSES

- Congenital development (or idiopathic).
- Associated with intramedullary tumours.
- Post-traumatic.
- Arachnoiditis.
- Postinflammatory (transverse myelitis and multiple sclerosis).

CLINICAL FEATURES OF IDIOPATHIC TYPE

- Disorder is chronic.
- Common in females.
- Age of onset is third to fourth decade of life.
- Numbness in upper limbs with frequent burns and injuries that are painless.
- Later, spastic weakness in lower limbs with urinary bladder involvement occurs.

SIGNS

- Physical findings suggest central cord syndrome or syringomyelic syndrome. They are the following:
  - Lower motor neuron (LMN) signs in upper limbs, usually at C_8-T_1 myotomes with wasting of muscles in the neck, shoulders, arms and hands with absent reflexes in the upper limb.
  - Dissociated suspended anaesthesia—there is loss of pain and temperature sensation bilaterally with intact touch and proprioception (dissociated) over dermatomes of upper limbs, and intact sensations above and below (suspended). This is due to lesion at anterior commissure of spinal cord. This disrupts crossing pain and temperature fibres at midline.
  - Pyramidal signs in lower limbs.
- At times, signs to suggest spinothalamic tract involvement may be seen on one side or bilaterally over trunk and lower limbs.
- Syringobulbia may produce dysphagia, nystagmus, pharyngeal and palatal weakness, asymmetric weakness and atrophy of the tongue, and sensory loss involving primarily pain and temperature senses in the distribution of the trigeminal nerve.
- Thoracic kyphoscoliosis is common.

INVESTIGATIONS

- Plain radiograph of cervical spine may show widened cervical spinal canal and associated bony craniovertebral anomalies like basilar invagination.
- CT scan shows the widened cord.
- MRI is the most sensitive method. It shows fluid-filled cavitation and dilated central canal. MRI of brain and entire spinal cord should be done.

TREATMENT

- Surgical removal of obstruction of CSF flow, if any, along with syringo-subarachnoid shunt.

Q. Discuss the clinical manifestations, investigations and management of cervical spondylosis/spondylitis. (OR 6.1)

- Spondylitis suggests inflammation of intervertebral joints. However, the term commonly refers to degenerative disorder of cervical spine, where intervertebral disc degenerates with changes in adjacent bones and ligaments, which eventually leads to formation of protruding bar-like structures at intervertebral areas. They may protrude and compromise spinal canal or intervertebral foramen. Maximum changes occur at C5–C6, C6–C7 and C4–C5 intervertebral disc spaces in that order.

CLINICAL FEATURES

- Bars or protrusions may just produce localised neck pain or cause neurological problems. Neurological problems present as one or both of the following:
  a. Radiculopathy
  b. Myelopathy

RADICULOPATHY

- Common roots affected are C5, C6 and C7. It results in root pain with neurological deficit (Table 5.56). Radiculopathy is a feature of dorsolateral protrusions. Onset is usually acute or may occasionally be chronic. Neck movements worsen pain.
- Spurling test: The patient's neck is turned to the side of the radicular pain and is then slightly extended. Downward pressure is applied to the top of the patient's head, which narrows the neural foramina on the affected side. If the pain is elicited or

TABLE 5.56 Neurologic Deficit in Cervical Radiculopathy

Root	Muscle	Sensory Loss	Reflex
• C5	Biceps, deltoid, spinatus	Upper lateral arm	Biceps
• C6	Brachioradialis	Radial aspect of lower arm extending to thumb	Supinator
• C7	Triceps	Middle finger	Triceps

worsened, it can be attributed to radiculopathy. The test may be repeated by turning the patient's head to the side opposite the pain; if the pain is worsened by this manoeuvre, a musculoskeletal cause is suggested.
- Shoulder-abduction test: This test is performed by placing the palm of the affected arm on top of the patient's head. If the pain is relieved, radiculopathy is the likely source of the pain.

MYELOPATHY

- Occurs when protrusions (bars) occur dorsomedially. It can also occur due to displacement of vertebral bodies (spondylolisthesis).
- Insidious onset with variable progression.
- Usually painless.
- Acute worsening may follow trauma.
- Pyramidal disturbance with impaired joint position sense (with positive Romberg's sign) is seen in lower limbs.
- Upper limbs get involved later in various combinations of upper and lower motor neuron lesions depending on the level of compression (C4, C5, C6 or C7). Multiple levels may be evident.
- Bladder gets involved later.

INVESTIGATIONS

- Plain radiograph of cervical spine shows reduced intervertebral spaces with bony protrusions (degenerative changes).
- CT scan or MRI can demonstrate the disordered (bony) anatomy and precise level of cord compression.

TREATMENT

- Conservative management is preferred when no neurological deficit is seen. It includes rest, analgesics, intermittent cervical traction and cervical collar followed by tonic neck exercises.
- Surgery is indicated when neurological deficit is present. Surgical procedures are laminectomy, foraminal decompression and discectomy from anterolateral approach.

PROGNOSIS

- Radiculopathy responds well to treatment.
- Myelopathy has variable prognosis, which may arrest or improve even without treatment.

Q. What are the causes and clinical manifestations of Brown-Sequard syndrome?

- Brown-Sequard syndrome refers to findings seen in hemisection of the spinal cord.
- In disease states, it is never seen in its pure form, except may be in stab injuries.

OTHER CAUSES (Box 5.71)

BOX 5.71 Causes of Brown-Sequard Syndrome Other Than Stab Injury

- Intradural tumours
- Infarction of spinal cord
- Radiation myelopathy
- Myelitis

} All produce incomplete or additional findings

CLINICAL MANIFESTATIONS (Table 5.57)

TABLE 5.57 Clinical Features of Brown-Sequard Syndrome

Features	Ipsilateral	Contralateral
• At level of lesion	• LMN signs (atrophy with depressed jerks) • All modalities of sensations are lost with or without hyperaesthesia	— —
• Below level of lesion	• UMN signs (hypertonia, exaggerated deep tendon reflexes and extensor plantar response) • Impaired joint position and vibration sense	• Impaired pain and temperature sense

Strictly unilateral lesions do not produce bladder problems. If lesion is large and extends across midline, bladder involvement is expected.

Q. What are the physical signs of posterior column lesion?

SENSATIONS CONVEYED BY POSTERIOR COLUMN

- Joint position sense.
- Vibration sense.
- Fine touch.
- Cortical sensations (form, shape, weight, location of tactile sensation).

PHYSICAL SIGNS OF POSTERIOR COLUMN LESION

- Sensory ataxia.
- Impaired joint position sense.
- Positive Romberg's sign.
- Impaired stereognosis, tactile localisation and discrimination.
- Impaired vibration sense.

ROMBERG'S SIGN

- Romberg's sign is seen in sensory ataxias.

Method of Eliciting

- Patient is asked to stand with his/her feet as close as possible (being steady) with eyes open. On closure of eyes, he/she tends to lose his/her balance if the sign is positive. When it is negative, closure of eyes makes no significant difference in maintaining steadiness.

Physiological Basis

- Necessary sensory information for maintaining equilibrium in upright posture comes from eyes, labyrinths, joints and muscles in lower limbs and trunk. Information is complementary to one another. In the absence or impairment of one, it is possible for CNS to compensate. In the presence of impaired proprioception, visual clues help CNS to maintain equilibrium. When such clues are removed, unsteadiness appears.

Q. What are the diseases affecting posterior column? Give the clinical features of any one of them.

Q. Discuss the aetiology, clinical features and management of subacute combined degeneration.

DISEASES AFFECTING POSTERIOR COLUMN (Box 5.72)

BOX 5.72 Diseases Affecting Posterior Columns of Spinal Cord

- Subacute combined degeneration
- Tabes dorsalis
- Posteriorly located compressive lesions
- AIDS myelopathy
- Cervical spondylosis with ligamentum flavum hypertrophy
- Any advanced cord compression
- Transverse myelitis
- Friedreich's ataxia

SUBACUTE COMBINED DEGENERATION

- It is a nutritional disorder of CNS due to vitamin B_{12} deficiency, including pernicious anaemia.
- Deficiency of vitamin B_{12} leads to lack of adenosylcobalamin that is required as a cofactor for the conversion of methylmalonyl-CoA to succinyl-CoA. This leads to accumulation of methylmalonyl-CoA, causing a decrease in normal myelin synthesis and incorporation of abnormal fatty acids into neuronal lipids.
- Condition is characterised by demyelination of corticospinal tracts and posterior column. It is usually associated with peripheral neuropathy, optic neuritis and mental changes.

CLINICAL FEATURES

- Subacute in onset (over weeks).
- Paraesthesia in lower limbs, associated with sensory ataxia.
- Examination shows impaired tactile sensation in glove and stocking distribution.
- Impaired joint position and vibration senses.
- Absent ankle jerks (due to associated peripheral neuropathy) with extensor plantar response and brisk knee jerks.
- Megaloblastic anaemia is usually present, but not necessarily.
- Associated optic neuritis and dementia may be seen.
- MR imaging of spinal cord shows abnormally increased T2-signal hyperintensity in posterior columns, and occasionally in lateral columns.

TREATMENT AND PROGNOSIS

- Injection hydroxocobalamin or cyanocobalamin 1 mg daily for 5 days followed by 1 mg once in 1–3 months. After improvement, injectable preparation may be changed to oral methylcobalamin.
- Anaemia responds very well to treatment.
- Ataxia and sensory signs improve well if treatment is initiated early.
- Dementia and spasticity often persist.

Q. Discuss the aetiology, clinical manifestations, management and prognosis of motor neuron disease.

AETIOLOGY

- Aetiology is unknown. There is loss of motor neurons and gliosis in motor cortex, motor nuclei of brainstem and anterior horn of spinal cord with degeneration of corticospinal tract in spinal cord.

CLASSIFICATION (Table 5.58)

TABLE 5.58 Motor Neuron Disease: Classification

Hereditary	Sporadic
• Werdnig–Hoffmann disease [infantile spinal muscular atrophy (infantile SMA)] • Kugelberg–Welander disease [adolescent spinal muscular atrophy (adolescent SMA)] • Others (including adult forms of spinal muscular atrophy)	• Amyotrophic lateral sclerosis (most common) • Progressive muscular atrophy (PMA) • Progressive bulbar palsy • Primary lateral sclerosis (PLS) • Multifocal motor neuropathy with conduction block

CLINICAL FEATURES

GENERAL

- Insidious onset and steadily progressive course.
- Combination of lesions of UMN and/or LMN is characteristic.
- Widespread fasciculations are common. There is no sensory or bladder involvement.
- Average age of onset is sixth decade.
- Four patterns are recognised in early stages that often merge with each other later.

PROGRESSIVE BULBAR PALSY

- Dysarthria, dysphagia and dysphonia.
- Impaired articulation occurs early with low volume of speech.
- Difficulty in swallowing and hoarseness occur later.
- Signs of true (nuclear or bulbar) as well as supranuclear (pseudobulbar) bulbar palsy often coexist.
- Wasting and fasciculations of tongue along with spasticity.

- Jaw jerk is exaggerated.
- Emotional lability with uncontrolled laughter and crying.

AMYOTROPHIC LATERAL SCLEROSIS

- Commonest mode of onset.
- 'Amyotrophic' means muscle atrophy and 'lateral sclerosis' refers to pathological changes in the spinal cord (and brainstem) that include degeneration of the lateral columns where the corticospinal tracts are located.
- Starts in the limbs in about two-thirds of patients (spinal form); bulbar onset in one-third of patients.
- Bulbar involvement can be UMN (pseudobulbar palsy) or LMN type (bulbar palsy):
  - Bulbar palsy is associated with upper and lower facial motor weakness and poverty of palatal movement with wasting and weakness, wasting and fasciculation of the tongue.
  - Pseudobulbar palsy is characterised by emotional lability (also known as pathological laughing or crying), brisk jaw jerk and dysarthria.
- In the extremities:
  - Generally, LMN signs in upper limbs and UMN signs in lower limbs.
- Cervical-onset amyotrophic lateral sclerosis (ALS) presents with upper limb symptoms, either bilateral or unilateral. Proximal weakness can present as difficulty with tasks associated with shoulder abduction (e.g. hair washing, combing), and distal weakness produces wasting of small muscles of hands that manifests with impairment of activities requiring pincer grip. Later, wasting and fasciculation spread to proximal arm muscles. In upper limbs, both UMN and LMN signs can occur. Thus, DTR in upper limbs becomes exaggerated (UMN involvement) in spite of atrophic muscles. Lower limbs would have UMN signs (spasticity of legs, extensor plantar response and exaggerated DTR in lower limbs).
- Lumbar onset implies degeneration of the anterior horn cells of the lumbar spinal area and is associated with LMN features in the legs, such as a tendency to trip (foot drop) or difficulty in climbing stairs (proximal weakness).
- Thoracic onset is generally diagnosed with paraspinal EMG.
- Fig. 5.20 depicts wasting seen in various muscle groups in a patient with ALS.

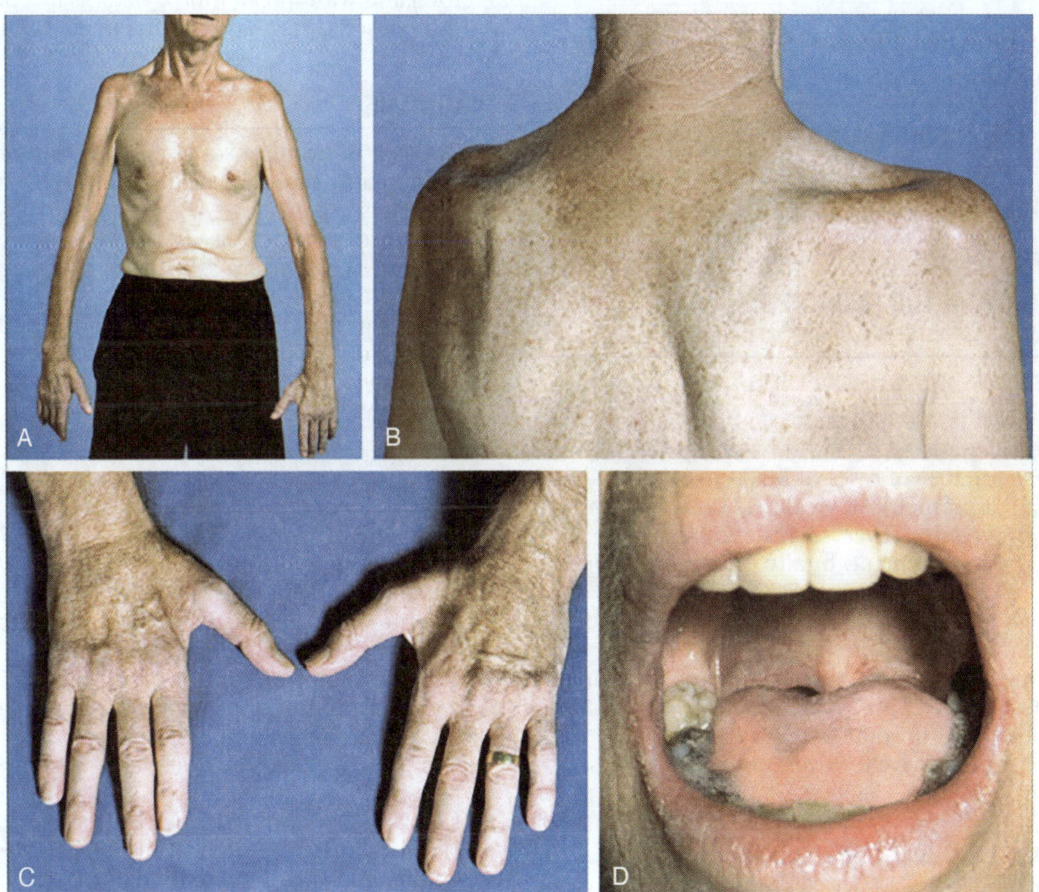

Fig. 5.20 Clinical features of muscle wasting in a patient with amyotrophic lateral sclerosis. (A) Proximal and symmetrical upper limb wasting. (B) Wasting of deltoid, supraspinatus and infraspinatus muscles. (C) Disproportionate wasting of the thenar muscles combined with the first dorsal interossei, the so-called 'split-hand'. (D) Substantial wasting of the tongue muscles in bulbar-onset ALS. Note the absence of palatal elevation present on vocalisation. *Courtesy*: Kiernan MC, Vucic S, Cheah BC, Turner MR, Eisen A, Hardiman O, Burrell JR, Zoing MC. Amyotrophic lateral sclerosis. Lancet. 2011 Mar 12;377(9769):942–55.

- Extraocular movements, sensation and bladder function are typically normal.
- Senses of hearing, sight, touch, smell and taste are intact.
- Depression is common in these patients.
- A definite diagnosis of ALS is made by confirming a progressive course of weakness, with both UMN and LMN findings in three out of four anatomically defined regions of the body: craniobulbar, cervical, thoracic and lumbosacral.

PROGRESSIVE MUSCULAR ATROPHY (PMA)

- PMA occurs when clinical disease is limited to the lower motor neuron, at least for an extended period of time at disease onset.
- Onset is asymmetrical with distal involvement more than proximal (in adult-onset spinal muscular atrophy, onset is symmetrical and weakness is more proximally than distally).
- Muscle weakness and wasting, first in hands and then in rest of lower body.
- Fasciculations are seen.
- By approximately 5 years after onset, 22% of patients will have upper motor neuron features of disease, and the disease is then considered ALS with lower motor neuron onset.

PRIMARY LATERAL SCLEROSIS (PLS)

- It is a rare form of MND.
- Typical onset around 50 years of age.
- Features are confined to upper motor neurons only.
- There is progressive tetraparesis starting in lower limbs, with terminal pseudobulbar palsy.

VARIANTS OF MOTOR NEURON DISEASE (Box 5.73)

MADRAS MOTOR NEURON DISEASE

- Age of onset is 20–30 years.
- Male:female ratio is 2:1.
- Accounts for 10% of cases of MND in South India.
- Gradual, asymmetrical weakness and wasting of limbs progressing over several years, along with pyramidal involvement, finally producing a picture of ALS.
- Weakness of facial and bulbar muscles (related to lower cranial nerves) present.
- Sensorineural deafness and optic atrophy in many patients.
- Cerebellar signs in some patients.
- Most patients survive for over 30 years after onset.

BOX 5.73 Variants of Motor Neuron Disease

- Madras motor neuron disease
- Monomelic amyotrophy
- Wasted leg syndrome
- Juvenile MND of North India
- Hemiplegic type of MND
- Crural ALS
- MND with dementia
- MND with parkinsonism

BOX 5.74 Differential Diagnosis of Motor Neuron Disease

- Parasagittal tumours
- Foramen magnum tumours
- Compressive spinal cord lesions
- Syringomyelia
- Polymyositis
- Chronic inflammatory demyelinating polyneuropathy
- Multiple motor neuropathy with conduction block
- Paraneoplastic
- HIV myelopathy
- Hyperthyroidism
- Hyperparathyroidism
- Myasthenia
- Subacute combined degeneration
- Toxins (lead, mercury, aluminium)
- Drugs (phenytoin)
- Radiation
- Poliomyelitis
- Multisystem atrophy

- Reduced serum citrate and increased serum pyruvate levels.

COURSE OF MOTOR NEURON DISEASE

- Variants are common. Pictures of different categories merge and final picture is of severe bulbar palsy + UMN + LMN signs in all four limbs. Final state consists of anarthria (severe dysarthria resulting in speechlessness), aphagia (complete inability to swallow) and widespread limb weakness in a person with full consciousness and normal intellectual abilities.

DIAGNOSIS

- Absence of overt sensory, sphincter and oculomotor dysfunction serves to distinguish MND from other disorders.
- Exclusion of other diseases (motor neuron disease mimics) is important as many of them are treatable. These are listed in Box 5.74.
- Investigations include spine radiography, EMG, nerve conduction velocity (to document LMN involvement), MRI of spine, thyroid function tests and occasionally lumbar puncture.

TREATMENT

- No curative medical treatment—walking aids, wheelchair and physiotherapy.
- Others include noninvasive ventilation.
- Symptomatic treatments include use of botulinum toxin and anticholinergic drugs (atropine, hyoscine, glycopyrrolate) to control drooling, gastrostomy to reduce aspiration, baclofen, tizanidine, gabapentin, benzodiazepines and levetiracetam for spasticity, and selective serotonin reuptake inhibitors for depression.
- Death occurs from pneumonia or respiratory failure.
- Usual duration of survival in bulbar palsy is about 2 years, ALS 4 to 5 years and PMA 8–10 years.
- There are two drugs which have some effect on survival: riluzole (a sodium-channel blocker that inhibits glutamate release) and edaravone (a novel neuroprotective agent). These agents slow down progression of ALS.

Q. Briefly discuss spinal muscular atrophy.

- Spinal muscular atrophy (SMA) are hereditary forms of motor neuron disease.
- SMA is caused by homozygous deletion or, less commonly, smaller mutations of SMN1, leading to deficiency of the ubiquitously expressed survival motor neuron (SMN) protein. This deficiency leads to muscle wasting and weakness, and feeding and respiratory difficulties.
- Disease severity is most often modified by the presence of a back-up gene, SMN2.
- Autosomal recessive inheritance in majority.
- SMA is divided into four types:
  - SMA type I or Werdnig–Hoffmann disease usually presents before 6 months of age. Infants are unable to sit unaided and death often occurs before 2 years without respiratory support.
  - Children with SMA type II (Dubowitz disease) become symptomatic before 18 months, can sit but not stand unaided, and survival is variable with 80% surviving to adulthood.
  - SMA type III (also known as Kugelberg–Welander disease) presents in adolescence. Patients can walk or run and survive to adulthood.
  - Type IV SMA denotes adult-onset cases.

TYPE IV SMA (ADULT-ONSET SMA)

- Male:female ratio is 5:1.
- Involvement of only LMN.
- Proximal muscles are usually more affected, or at least affected much sooner than the distal muscles. For example, the muscles of the thighs are weaker than the muscles of the lower legs and feet.
- The lower extremities are often more severely affected than the upper extremities.
- Deep tendon reflexes are diminished or absent.
- Most adults have normal life span.
- Nusinersen, an antisense oligonucleotide-based drug, can be used for all types of SMAs. It acts by modifying splicing of SMN2.
- Onasemnogene abeparvovec-xioi is the gene therapy approved to treat children less than 2 years of age with spinal muscular atrophy. It replaces the gene SMN1.
- The drug risdiplam, is also approved for the treatment of adults and children 2 months of age or older.

Q. Briefly outline classification, clinical features, investigations, diagnosis and treatment of multiple sclerosis.

- Multiple sclerosis (MS) is an autoimmune disease of white matter that occurs due to interaction of genetic factors with environmental factors. In some cases, deep cerebral cortex and cerebral nuclei may be involved. Some of the environmental factors which increase the risk of MS include smoking and vitamin D deficiency.
- Most frequently affects young and middle-aged people.
- Characterised by chronic inflammation, demyelination and axonal loss in many cases, with remissions and exacerbations of clinical symptoms and signs.

CLASSIFICATION (Fig. 5.21)

- Relapsing-remitting multiple sclerosis (RRMS)—85% of cases; symptoms and signs typically evolve over a period of several days, stabilise, and then often improve, spontaneously or in response to corticosteroids, within weeks. Patients are clinically stable between these episodes. Since not all relapses remit completely, disability develops over time with the stepwise accumulation of deficits.
- Primary progressive multiple sclerosis (PPMS)—10% of cases; characterised by gradual progression of disability without superimposed relapses.
- Secondary progressive multiple sclerosis (SPMS)—characterised by gradual progression of disability with or without superimposed relapses following initial RRMS.
- Progressive relapsing multiple sclerosis (PRMS)—5% of cases; characterised by gradual progression of disability from disease onset with relapses later in the course of disease.
- All MS types are further classified as either active or inactive (based on the prior 12 months). Additionally, SPMS and PPMS are further characterised as progressive or nonprogressive (based on the prior 12 months).

CLINICAL FEATURES

MOTOR FEATURES

- Predominantly upper motor neuron weakness of muscles (brisk deep tendon reflexes, Babinski's sign and loss of abdominal reflexes).
- Wasting of muscles of hands and spasticity in advanced cases.

SENSORY FEATURES

- Tingling and numbness common.
- Objective sensory loss, particularly posterior column features. Loss of pain and temperature sensation less common.

OTHER FEATURES

- Cerebellar signs common and include disequilibrium, truncal or limb ataxia, scanning speech and intention tremor.
- Optic neuritis usually occurs at the onset of disease.
  - Most often unilateral.
  - Pain with ocular movement is common (unlike ischaemic optic neuritis that is painless).
  - Patients may describe a dimming or bleaching of colour (colour desaturation).
  - Visual acuity may or may not be affected.
  - Visual field loss is often present. Central scotoma is common.
  - Optic disc often appears entirely normal because inflammation is predominately retrobulbar. Later, it becomes pale.

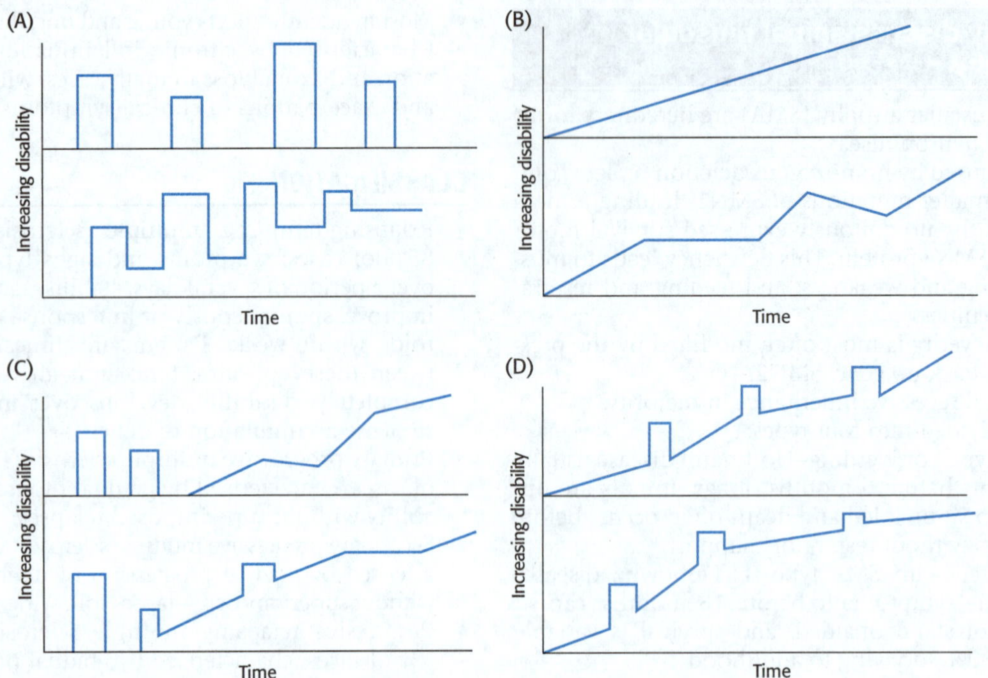

Fig. 5.21 Classification of multiple sclerosis. (A) **RRMS**. There may be residual deficit from an attack, but the baseline between attacks remains stable until the next attack. (B) **PPMS**. There are no acute attacks, but a gradual worsening over time. (C) **SPMS**. After an initial course of RRMS, the baseline deficit gradually worsens, with or without intervening acute attacks. (D) **PRMS**. Starts as primary progressive MS, but has subsequent acute attacks at some point after onset.

  - An afferent pupillary defect is typically present on the swinging flashlight test (Marcus Gunn pupil). The pupils will be equal in size before testing because of consensual light response. For swinging flashlight test, shining the light on normal pupil causes constriction of both pupils (direct and consensual reflex). The light is then swung to the opposite (affected) pupil. Both the pupils will dilate due to afferent defect.
  - Other ocular features include diplopia and nystagmus. Cranial nerve III palsy and internuclear ophthalmoplegia (usually bilateral) may occur.
  - Pulfrich effect may occur when conduction latencies between the eyes are unequal, resulting in a sense of disorientation in moving traffic.
- Bladder and bowel involvement.
- Uhthoff's phenomenon is worsening of symptoms on exposure to heat (hot water bath) or exercise, and occurs due to conduction block.

PAROXYSMAL FEATURES

- Trigeminal neuralgia.
- Facial weakness.
- Vertigo.
- Dysarthria.
- Epilepsy.
- Emotional changes and delusions.
- Lhermitte's sign or barber chair sign (shooting electric pain in the neck with radiation to the shoulders and back on flexing the neck and occurs due to posterior column involvement).

DIAGNOSIS

- Age of onset of MS between 10 and 50 years.
- The diagnosis of MS is based on finding clinical evidence of CNS lesions that are disseminated in time and space.
- An acute episode must last for at least 24 hours in the absence of fever or metabolic derangements.
- Dissemination in time means that there is more than one episode of CNS dysfunction. All events occurring within 30 days of an event are considered to be part of a single event.
- Dissemination in space indicates involvement of more than one area of the CNS.
- Both dissemination in time and space can be diagnosed by performing an MRI if only one episode or one site is obvious on history and examination. Dissemination in space can also be documented by evoked potentials that may indicate an involved area that is otherwise asymptomatic.
- Presence of prominent cortical signs like aphasia, apraxia, recurrent seizures, visual field loss (except central scotoma) and early dementia, or extrapyramidal signs such as chorea and rigidity generally exclude a diagnosis of MS.

INVESTIGATIONS

- Cerebrospinal fluid: Increased cells ($<75/\mu L$), raised protein (<1000 mg/dL) and increased IgG. Electrophoresis of CSF shows oligoclonal bands. CSF analysis is probably most useful for ruling out infectious or neoplastic conditions that mimic MS.

- Visual, auditory and somatosensory evoked potentials show prolongation, and help in diagnosing involvement of clinically silent lesions.
- MRI is very sensitive for detecting lesions that are typically periventricular in location. It can show lesions dispersed both in time [new and old lesions—simultaneous presence of gadolinium-enhancing (acute) and nonenhancing lesions (chronic)] and in space (at different locations—infratentorial, juxtacortical, cortical, periventricular and spinal cord). In patients with optic neuritis, gadolinium-enhanced T1 sequences reveal optic nerve enhancement in most patients.

DIAGNOSTIC CRITERIA (Table 5.59)

TABLE 5.59 2017 McDonald Criteria for Diagnosis of Relapsing-Remitting Multiple Sclerosis

Number of Clinical Attacks	Number of MRI Lesions	Additional Data Required for Diagnosis
≥2	≥2	None
≥2	1 (if clear-cut historical evidence of a previous attack involving a lesion in a different anatomical location)	None
≥2	1 (if clear-cut historical evidence of a previous attack involving a lesion in a different anatomical location is NOT present)	Dissemination in space demonstrated by an additional clinical attack implicating a different CNS site or by MRI
1	≥2	Dissemination in time demonstrated by additional clinical attack, MRI or CSF-specific oligoclonal bands
1	1	Dissemination in space demonstrated by an additional clinical attack implicating a different CNS site or by MRI AND dissemination in time demonstrated by additional clinical attack, MRI or CSF-specific oligoclonal bands

TREATMENT

ACUTE EXACERBATION

- Methylprednisolone 1 g IV daily for 3 days is the standard therapy to hasten recovery but does not alter extent of recovery. It is followed by oral prednisolone 60 mg for 5 days and then tapered off.
- Plasma exchange for those not responding to steroids.

DISEASE-MODIFYING DRUGS

- These include interferon β-1b, interferon β-1a, mitoxantrone, glatiramer acetate, cladribine and natalizumab. These are used to reduce disease progression and relapses. Others are fingolimod, siponimod, teriflunomide, ocrelizumab (anti-CD20 monoclonal antibody), alemtuzumab and dimethyl fumarate.
- May be used in RRMS and SPMS varieties.
- Mitoxantrone (a type II topoisomerase inhibitor) is the only medication approved for progressive disease. It can cause a dose-dependent cardiac toxicity in the form of heart failure.

SYMPTOMATIC TREATMENT

- Spasticity—baclofen (15–18 mg/day), tizanidine (2–8 mg/day) or diazepam (5–10 mg/day).
- Pain—carbamazepine (100–1200 mg/day), gabapentin (300–3600 mg/day) or phenytoin (300–400 mg/day).
- Fatigue—modafinil.
- Impaired ambulation—dalfampridine.
- Paroxysmal symptoms—carbamazepine, gabapentin or acetazolamide.
- Spastic bladder—anticholinergics like oxybutynin (5 mg TDS), tolterodine (1 to 2 mg BID) or propantheline (7.5–15 mg QID).

EXPERIMENTAL THERAPY

- Autologous haematopoietic stem cell transplantation

Q. Write a short note on neuromyelitis optica (Devic's disease).

- An idiopathic inflammatory, immune-mediated demyelinating disease which predominantly targets optic nerves and spinal cord and is distinct from MS.
- More common in females.
- Optic neuritis may be unilateral or bilateral. It is al most always acute, usually severe and may or may not be associated with retro-orbital pain. Visual loss is common.
- Neurological dysfunction due to myelitis is symmetrical. It worsens over several hours to days and involves motor, sensory and sphincter function. In contrast, myelitis in multiple sclerosis tends to be incomplete and asymmetric.
- Fatal autonomic disturbances may occur due to the involvement of autonomic outflow in thoracic myelitis.
- Lower brainstem involvement can occur from contiguous cervical myelitis, and produces nausea, intractable hiccups and respiratory failure. In some cases, hypothalamus and other areas of brain may be involved. Diencephalic involvement may manifest as hypersomnolence, narcolepsy, syndrome of inappropriate antidiuretic hormone secretion or menstrual irregularities.

- High frequency of coexisting autoimmune conditions including SLE, Sjögren's syndrome, juvenile rheumatoid arthritis, Graves' disease and autoimmune hepatitis.
- MRI of spinal cord helps in diagnosis. The spinal cord lesions are central, contiguous and longitudinally extensive (involving more than three spinal vertebral segments), often involving grey matter, and resemble those of complete acute TM. In contrast, in MS, spinal cord involvement is peripheral and restricted to one or two vertebral segmental levels.
- MRI brain abnormalities are present in many cases but are quite distinct from MS lesions. Cerebral lesions are usually linear, as opposed to oval lesions in MS.
- CSF oligoclonal bands are uncommon, whereas a neutrophilic pleocytosis (≥50 cells/mm^3 and ≥5 neutrophils/mm^3) occurs commonly during acute attacks.
- One or more autoantibodies, including antinuclear antibody, anti-double-stranded DNA antibody, extractable nuclear antigen and antithyroid antibodies, are commonly present at the time of diagnosis.
- Another autoantibody commonly present in serum is NMO IgG that is directed against water channel aquaporin-4 (aquaporins are membrane water channel proteins important in maintaining fluid homoeostasis in brain).

COURSE

- Optic neuritis and myelitis can occur simultaneously or in discrete attacks separated by weeks to years. Furthermore, NMO may have a monophasic course (10%) but has a relapsing course in nearly 90% of patients. Patients with a monophasic course have optic neuritis in both eyes and myelitis within a short interval and then have no recurrence.
- Patients with relapsing course have residual deficits following initial and subsequent attacks.
- Unlike in MS, a secondary progression course is uncommon in NMO.

TREATMENT

- Attacks of neuromyelitis optica are more severe, less often steroid responsive, and usually lead to significant morbidity and mortality from respiratory failure as a result of cervical myelopathy.
- Intravenous steroids for acute attack.
- Plasma exchange for those not responding to steroids.
- Immunosuppressives for prevention of relapses (oral steroids + azathioprine or mycophenolate mofetil; rituximab).
- Other drugs which are approved for treatment include eculizumab (a complement inhibitor), inebilizumab (an anti-CD19 agent) and satralizumab (an anti-interleukin-6 receptor).

Q. Enumerate the common neurological manifestations of vitamin deficiency.

NEUROLOGICAL MANIFESTATIONS OF VITAMIN DEFICIENCY (Table 5.60)

TABLE 5.60 Neurological Manifestations of Vitamin Deficiency

Vitamin	Deficiency State
• Vitamin A	• Night blindness
• Vitamin D	• Myopathy of osteomalacia
• Vitamin E	• Spinocerebellar syndrome (cerebellar ataxia, hyporeflexia, proprioceptive and vibratory loss, and an extensor plantar response), peripheral neuropathy, visual scotomas, muscle cramps
• Vitamin B complex	
• Thiamine (vitamin B_1)	• Sensorimotor, distal polyneuropathy (beriberi), Wernicke's encephalopathy, Korsakoff's psychosis
• Riboflavin (vitamin B_2)	• Polyneuropathy
• Niacin	• Dementia (pellagra includes diarrhoea, dermatitis and dementia), spasticity, myoclonus, peripheral neuropathy
• Pyridoxine (vitamin B_6)	• Polyneuropathy, convulsions in children (pure sensory neuropathy with vitamin B_6 intoxication)
• Cobalamin (vitamin B_{12})	• Subacute combined degeneration, optic neuritis, dementia, peripheral neuropathy

Q. What is peripheral neuropathy?

Q. What are the commonly encountered causes of polyneuropathies? Discuss the clinical presentation, investigations and management of polyneuropathies.

Q. What are the conditions associated with significant autonomic neuropathies?

DEFINITION

- Any disorder of the nervous system that lies outside the pia mater, that is in the peripheral nervous system, is considered peripheral neuropathy.
- Polyneuropathy is a definite clinical syndrome consisting of involvement of all peripheral neurons symmetrically to result in a characteristic clinical picture.
- Mononeuropathy is involvement of one nerve. Most cases are due to compression of a nerve (e.g. carpal tunnel syndrome). Commonly involved nerves are ulnar, median, radial and peroneal nerves. Diabetes mellitus is the most common cause of noncompressive mononeuropathy.
- Mononeuritis multiplex refers to simultaneous or sequential involvement of noncontiguous nerve trunks. Diabetes mellitus is the most common cause.

5

TABLE 5.61 Types of Peripheral Neuroaphies and Their Causes

Type	Site	Causes
• Monoradiculopathy	Spinal root	Trauma, tumour, disc protrusion
• Polyradiculopathy	Spinal roots	Arachnoiditis, GB syndrome
• Plexopathy		
• Brachial	Plexus	Trauma, tumours, neuralgia, radiotherapy
• Lumbosacral	Plexus	Tumours, trauma, idiopathic, radiotherapy
• Mononeuropathy	Single nerve trunk	Trauma, entrapment, leprosy, tumour (neurofibroma), infarction (see Table 5.62)
• Mononeuritis multiplex	Multiple nerve trunks	Leprosy, trauma, diabetes, PAN, familial pressure sensitive neuropathy (see Table 5.62)
• Polyneuropathy	Generalised	Separate list in Table 5.63.

TYPES OF PERIPHERAL NEUROPATHY AND THEIR CAUSES

- Various types of peripheral neuropathies and their causes are given in Tables 5.61 and 5.62.

TABLE 5.62 Causes of Mononeuropathy and Mononeuritis Multiplex

Focal Neuropathy (Mononeuropathy)	Mononeuritis Multiplex
• Leprosy	• Leprosy
• Entrapment	• Diabetes mellitus
• Myxoedema	• Vasculitis
• Rheumatoid arthritis	• Polyarteritis nodosa
• Amyloidosis	• Systemic lupus erythematosus
• Acromegaly	• Sjögren's syndrome
• Trauma	• Temporal arteritis
• Ischaemic lesions	• Sarcoidosis
• Diabetes mellitus	• HIV, hepatitis B or hepatitis C infection
• Vasculitis	• Paraneoplastic syndrome
• Sarcoidosis	• Lead poisoning
	• Polycythaemia
	• Cryoglobulinaemia

CLASSIFICATION AND CAUSES OF POLYNEUROPATHY (Table 5.63)

TABLE 5.63 Classification and Causes of Polyneuropathy

Cause	Nature (Clinical)	Nature (Pathological)
Acute		
• GB syndrome	Motor	Demyelinating
• Vasculitis (e.g. polyarteritis nodosa)	Sensory motor	Ischaemic
• Diphtheria	Motor	Demyelinating
• Dapsone	Sensory motor	Mixed
• Acute intermittent porphyria	Motor	Demyelinating
Subacute		
• Nutritional deficiency	Sensory motor	Axonal/mixed
• Toxins		
• Arsenic	Sensory	Axonal/mixed
• Lead	Motor	Demyelinating
• Drugs		
• Chloroquine	Sensory motor	Mixed
• Phenytoin	Sensory motor	Mixed
• Vincristine	Sensory motor	Mixed
• Industrial toxins		
• Carbon tetrachloride	Sensory	Axonal
• Acrylamide	Sensory	Axonal
• Aniline dyes	Sensory	Axonal

TABLE 5.63 Classification and Causes of Polyneuropathy—cont'd

Cause	Nature (Clinical)	Nature (Pathological)
Chronic		
• Diabetes	Sensory motor	Mixed
• HIV infection	Sensory	Axonal
• Carcinoma	Sensory motor	Demyelinating, axonal or mixed
• Chronic inflammatory demyelinating polyradiculoneuropathy (CIDP)	Sensory motor	Demyelinating
• Hypothyroidism	Sensory	Mixed
• Hereditary	Sensory or motor or mixed	Demyelinating, axonal or mixed
• POEMS syndrome	Sensory motor	Demyelinating, axonal or mixed

PROXIMAL AND DISTAL SYMMETRICAL NEUROPATHIES (Table 5.64)

TABLE 5.64 Causes of Proximal and Distal Symmetrical Neuropathies

Proximal Symmetrical Neuropathy (Mainly Motor)	Distal Symmetrical Sensorimotor Neuropathy
• GB syndrome	• Endocrine (diabetes mellitus, hypothyroidism)
• Chronic inflammatory demyelinating polyradiculoneuropathy (CIDP)	• Leprosy
• Diabetes mellitus	• Alcoholism
• Acute intermittent porphyria	• Vitamin B_{12} deficiency
• Diphtheria	• Thiamine deficiency
• HIV/AIDS	• Chronic kidney disease
• Hypothyroidism	• Critical illness polyneuropathy
	• Connective tissue diseases (vasculitic)
	• Rheumatoid arthritis
	• Polyarteritis nodosa
	• Systemic lupus erythematosus
	• Cryoglobulinaemia
	• HIV infection
	• Sarcoidosis
	• Cancer-associated (multiple myeloma, lymphoma, paraneoplastic)
	• Toxic neuropathy (acrylamide, carbon disulphide, organophosphorus compounds, arsenic and mercury intoxication)
	• Medications (vincristine, isoniazid, didanosine, dapsone, cisplatin)

CONDITIONS ASSOCIATED WITH SIGNIFICANT AUTONOMIC NEUROPATHIES (Table 5.65)

TABLE 5.65 Causes of Significant Autonomic Neuropathies

• GB syndrome • Diabetes • Amyloidosis	• Acute intermittent porphyria • Paraneoplastic • HIV infection • Certain specific genetically determined neuropathies

POLYNEUROPATHY

- Peripheral nerve fibres can be classified according to size, which correlates with the degree of myelination:
  - Large nerve fibres are heavily myelinated and include A-α fibres, which mediate motor strength, and A-β fibres, which mediate vibratory and touch sensation.
  - Medium-sized fibres, known as A-γ fibres, are also myelinated and carry information to muscle spindles.
  - Small fibres include myelinated A-δ fibres and unmyelinated C fibres, which include somatic (which mediate pain and thermal sensations) and autonomic fibres.
- When the cell body or its axon or myelin is the site of disease, neuron that is longest is affected earlier. Hence, early disturbance occurs at the distal-most point in the body.
- Depending on underlying cause and pathology, neuropathies may be purely motor, predominantly motor, pure sensory or sensorimotor, but most commonly mixed with equal degree of involvement.
- Electrophysiologically, it is possible to differentiate neuropathies into demyelinating, axonal or mixed that helps to narrow the diagnostic possibilities.

COMMON CAUSES OF SMALL FIBRE POLYNEUROPATHY (Box 5.75)

BOX 5.75 Common Causes of Small Fibre Polyneuropathy

• Diabetes mellitus (burning feet syndrome) • Alcoholism • Vitamin B_{12} deficiency • Amyloidosis • Pellagra • Arsenic intoxication • Connective tissue diseases	• Drug induced (antiretrovirals, cisplatin, isoniazid, metronidazole, nitrofurantoin, vincristine) • Infections (HIV, hepatitis C) • Paraneoplastic • POEMS syndrome • Hereditary (Fabry's disease, Wilson's disease)

CLINICAL FEATURES

- Onset may be acute (few hours to days), subacute (within 4 weeks) or chronic (over months and years) depending on underlying cause.
- Sensory symptoms may appear in two different ways. Positive sensory symptoms occur when aberrant sensation occurs in the absence of stimulation. Negative symptoms occur when adequate stimuli fail to produce a sensory response. Common features are distal paraesthesias (positive symptoms) initially at toes that ascend up to ankle and leg symmetrically on both sides. It is associated with disturbances of tactile and proprioceptive sensations (negative symptoms).
- Ankle jerk is lost very early (may not be lost in axonal neuropathies).
- Later, symptoms appear at fingers and ascend to wrist.
- Depending on nature of pathology, muscular weakness appears initially at toes, ankle, and fingers and wrist in that order. Muscle wasting develops over a period of time. Initial proximal weakness in neuropathies suggests a radicular (nerve roots) involvement or primary muscle involvement (myopathy).
- Fasciculations are rare; when present, suggest distal motor axonal involvement or more likely anterior horn cell disease.
- Autonomic involvement causes orthostatic hypotension, nocturnal diarrhoea, urinary retention, dry skin, dry mouth, heat intolerance and localised excessive sweating in unaffected areas.
- Other symptoms of autonomic dysfunction include bladder (atonic) dysfunction manifested by difficulty in voiding, sexual impotence, retrograde ejaculation, decreased tearing and pupillary abnormalities.
- Features of small fibre involvement include the following:
  - Burning pain, numbness and tingling in the feet that extends proximally in a 'glove and stocking' distribution.
  - Symptoms usually worse at night and often affect sleep.
  - Allodynia (perception of nonpainful stimuli as being painful), hyperalgesia (perception of painful stimuli as being more painful than expected), or reduced pinprick and thermal sensation in the affected area.
  - Vibratory sensation can be mildly reduced at the toes.
  - Motor strength, tendon reflexes and proprioception are preserved (because they are functions of large nerve fibres).
  - Autonomic features may be present.
- Chronic inflammatory demyelinating polyradiculoneuropathy (CIDP), an immune-mediated disorder, is characterised by progressive proximal, symmetrical limb weakness, areflexia and large fibre sensory loss (distal paraesthesias, poor balance and impaired proprioception). Peak of clinical features occurs at least 8 weeks after onset. It is associated with albuminocytological dissociation in the cerebrospinal fluid (increased albumin with near-normal cells). Treatment includes high-dose steroids and intravenous immunoglobulin (IVIg). Plasma exchange is an effective therapy for treatment-refractory cases of CIDP.
- Additional systemic findings are very important as they often give clues to underlying pathology:
  - Signs of nutritional deficiency.
  - Systemic signs of toxicity of drugs and toxins.
  - Presence of malignancy or connective tissue disorder.

- Presence of skeletal deformities (pes cavus, hammer toes and kyphoscoliosis), visual or auditory involvement in hereditary neuropathies.
- Thickened nerves (Box 5.76).

BOX 5.76 Causes of Thickened Nerves

- Leprosy
- Acromegaly
- Amyloidosis
- Neurofibromatosis
- Infiltration of nerves by lymphoma
- Chronic inflammatory demyelinating polyradiculoneuropathy
- Charcot–Marie–Tooth disease
- Refsum's disease

INVESTIGATIONS

- If no clinical clues are forthcoming, investigations are necessary (Box 5.77).
- Nerve conduction studies define distribution and extent of neuropathy and differentiate between axonal and demyelinating processes. In small fibre neuropathy, these tests are normal.
- Skin biopsy in suspected small fibre neuropathy.

BOX 5.77 Routing Investigations in Peripheral Neuropathy

- Blood biochemistry
  - Sugar
  - Renal function tests
  - Liver function tests
  - Thyroid function tests
  - Serum immunoglobulins
- Vitamin B_{12} level
- Serology
  - HBsAg
  - Antinuclear antibody
  - Rheumatoid factor
- Electrodiagnostic studies
- CSF evaluation
- Nerve biopsy

TREATMENT

- Curative treatment depends on the underlying cause.
- Corticosteroids, IVIg and plasma exchange are useful in CIDP.
- Symptomatic treatment includes the following:
  - Neuropathic pain and paraesthesias—gabapentin 300–900 mg/day, pregabalin 75–300 mg/day, amitriptyline 25–50 mg/day or duloxetine 30–120 mg/day.
  - Weakness—physiotherapy and occupational rehabilitation.
  - Autonomic disturbance—depends on end-organ involvement, for example bladder care, managing postural hypotension.

Q. How do you differentiate between large-fibre and small-fibre neuropathies?

- Features which help in differentiating small-fibre neuropathy from large-fibre neuropathy are given in Table 5.66.

TABLE 5.66 Small-Fibre Neuropathy Versus Large-Fibre Neuropathy

Feature	Small-Fibre Neuropathy	Large-Fibre Neuropathy
History	• Pain predominates • Allodynia	• Weakness, imbalance (sensory ataxia)
Examination	• Reduced sensation to pinprick and temperature • Reduced distal sweating pattern with increased sweating more proximally (autonomic dysfunction) • Preserved reflexes and motor strength	• Reduced proprioception and vibratory sensation • Reduced deep tendon reflexes • Motor weakness
Tests	• Skin biopsy for measurement of intraepidermal nerve fibre density • Quantitative sudomotor axon reflex test	• Abnormalities on nerve conduction testing

Q. How will you differentiate between axonal and demyelinating neuropathy?

- Differences between axonal and demyelinating neuropathy are given in Table 5.67.

Q. Write a brief note on Guillain–Barre syndrome (GB syndrome), postinfective polyneuropathy, acute inflammatory polyneuropathy or acute inflammatory demyelinating polyradiculoneuropathy (AIDP).

- GB syndrome (GBS) is the commonest acute demyelinating polyneuropathy that is presumed to be autoimmune in nature.
- It affects people at any age.
- It usually follows viral infection, rarely after surgery or immunisation. Zika virus infection may also produce it. Immune checkpoint inhibitors may also produce it.

PATHOGENESIS

- Exact pathogenesis is not known.
- GBS is a monophasic immunologically mediated inflammatory disorder of peripheral nerves. Multifocal demyelination with inflammation results in conduction block. Severe forms show secondary axonal degeneration.
- GBS commonly follows an infection. Antiganglioside antibodies are seen in at least one-third of GBS patients. These antibodies appear to cross-react with antigens in the lipopolysaccharides of some antecedent infective agents. These antibodies act against gangliosides, such as GM1, distributed throughout the myelin in the peripheral nervous system.
- Both cellular and humoral immune mechanisms probably play a role in its development.

TABLE 5.67 Demyelinating Neuropathy Versus Axonal Neuropathy

Features	Demyelinating Neuropathy	Axonal Neuropathy
• Onset	Acute or insidious	Insidious
• Pattern of sensory involvement	Minimal sensory loss; involvement of vibration and position sensation out of proportion to pain and temperature sensation	Glove and stocking distribution of loss of all sensations
• Reflexes	Loss of all deep tendon reflexes	Preservation of DTR except ankle reflex
• Motor involvement	Distal muscles are predominantly affected without significant wasting	Distal muscle weakness with wasting
• Recovery pattern	Rapid recovery (over few days to weeks)	Recovery over months to years (if occurs)
• Residual deficit	Less	Common
• Central involvement	Rare	Due to toxic agents
• CSF protein	Raised	Normal
• Nerve conduction	Very slow	Normal or slightly slow

- Since inflammation is important in its pathogenesis, the most common type of GBS is also known as AIDP.

CLINICAL FEATURES

- It is an acute disorder.
- It usually progresses for a few days and rarely up to 1 month.
- It is a predominant motor neuropathy.
- Sensory findings are minimum and consist of distal paraesthesias with mildly disturbed joint position sense.
- Motor paralysis is more striking and is symmetrical, involving proximal muscles more than distal. It begins in the legs, progressing over several days to involve arms, face and eyes (ascending paralysis).
- Reflexes are absent.
- Fifty per cent of patients show bifacial weakness.
- Some show bulbar muscular weakness.
- Respiratory paralysis occurs in a few.
- Autonomic disturbances occur in a few, resulting in sudden fluctuations in BP and heart rate.
- Bladder involvement is rare, and even when seen is mild and hardly lasts longer than 1 week.
- Clear sensory level, marked bladder involvement, persistent asymmetric weakness and prominent sensory symptoms without weakness are against the diagnosis of GBS.
- Box 5.78 summarises clinical features of GBS.

BOX 5.78 Summary of Clinical Features of GBS

- Acute onset
- Progressive monophasic illness up to 4 weeks
- Preceding infectious respiratory/gastrointestinal illness
- Symmetrical upper and lower extremity weakness
- Hypo/Areflexia
- Paraesthesias/numbness, pain (less common)
- Cranial neuropathies (bulbar, facial, extraocular muscles)
- Autonomic dysfunction (diarrhoea/constipation, hyponatraemia)

MILLER FISHER SYNDROME

- It is a variant of GBS and is characterised by areflexia, ataxia and ophthalmoplegia without significant limb weakness.
- Often preceded by *Campylobacter jejuni* infection (usually producing diarrhoea).

OTHER VARIANTS

- Acute motor axonal neuropathy:
  - Progresses more rapidly and has an earlier peak than demyelinating GBS.
  - Tendon reflexes are relatively preserved or even exaggerated.
  - Autonomic dysfunction is rare.
- Acute motor and sensory axonal neuropathy.

COURSE

- Muscle weakness gradually progresses over 1–3 weeks and then plateaus over next several days to weeks before gradual recovery. On recovery, nearly 15% of patients do not have any deficit while minor deficit and major deficits occur in nearly 70% and 5%–10% of cases, respectively.

INVESTIGATIONS

- CSF becomes abnormal after 1 week of illness and shows raised proteins (>45 mg/dL), and normal sugar and cell count (generally <10/mm^3; rarely cell count may go up to 50 cells/mm^3, but never above that). This is known as albuminocytological dissociation.
- Nerve conduction velocity studies show slowing of velocities and conduction block (demyelination pattern).
- Acute intermittent porphyria, postdiphtheritic neuritis and drug-induced acute polyneuropathies will need to be ruled out.

TREATMENT

- Immediate management of a patient with GBS consists of maintenance of airway, breathing and circulation. Ventilate if patient develops respiratory failure.

- Monitor pulse, blood pressure and cardiac activity using a cardiac monitor as these patients have autonomic instability.
- Steroids are of little value in these patients.
- Plasmapheresis (plasma exchange) and intravenous immunoglobulin (0.4 g/kg/day for 5 days or 2 g/day for 2 days) have been shown to accelerate recovery. Adverse effects of IVIg include headache, aseptic meningitis, nausea and hypocalcaemia. Rare but serious adverse effects include haemolytic anaemia, renal dysfunction and thrombotic events, such as deep vein thrombosis, pulmonary embolus, acute coronary syndrome and cerebral ischaemia. Plasma exchange combined with IVIg or corticosteroids does not provide better outcomes.

Q. Discuss the clinical features, investigations and management of myasthenia gravis.

Q. Briefly describe edrophonium test (Tensilon test).

- Myasthenia gravis (MG) is an autoimmune disorder where antibodies are produced against acetylcholine receptors located at motor end plates in myoneural junctions.
- Antibodies are produced by B-lymphocytes that are defectively regulated by T-lymphocytes. T-lymphocyte tolerance to self-antigens is established in the thymus, but in MG, this tolerance is lost that results in production of autoantibodies against acetylcholine receptors.
- Thymic hyperplasia is observed in about 65% of MG patients, and thymomas are present in about 10% of MG patients.

CLINICAL FEATURES

- Age of onset is 15–50 years.
- Females are more affected than males.
- Remissions and relapses are seen during the early course of illness.
- Characteristic feature is easy fatiguability associated with paresis of muscles.
- Repeated contractions worsen the weakness.
- Rest improves the muscular strength.
- Reflexes and sensations are normal.
- Diurnal variation is present.
- Ocular muscles are most commonly affected resulting in ptosis and diplopia. Pupils are not involved.
- Involvement of bulbar muscles results in dysphagia, nasal regurgitation and difficulty in speaking (nasal voice).
- Limb muscle involvement is of proximal group resulting in difficulty in raising the arm above shoulder, and problems in getting up from squatting or sitting positions.
- Involvement of respiratory muscles results in myasthenic crisis and can cause death.
- MG is termed ocular MG when weakness is exclusive to the eyelids and extraocular muscles, and generalised MG when weakness extends beyond these ocular muscles.

EXACERBATION OF WEAKNESS

- Patients being treated with anticholinesterase agents may present with exacerbation of weakness due to (i) myasthenic crisis or (ii) cholinergic crisis. Other causes of acute respiratory failure due to neuromuscular weakness include snake bite, botulism, organophosphate poisoning, GB syndrome and polymyositis.
  - Myasthenic crisis occurs in patients with MG who either are not on any treatment or are being undertreated due to low dosages or development of drug resistance. Other precipitating factors include exertion, extremes of temperature, infections, surgery, trauma and use of other drugs that can increase myasthenic weakness (Table 5.68). By definition, myasthenic crisis is characterised by severe weakness of the bulbar (innervated by cranial nerves) and/or respiratory muscles, enough to cause inability to maintain adequate ventilation, causing respiratory failure that requires artificial airway or ventilatory support. Edrophonium test is positive.
  - Cholinergic crisis occurs as a result of relative overdose of anticholinesterase drugs. Patients present with muscarinic features (excessive salivation, lacrimation, miosis, abdominal pain, diarrhoea, increased bronchial secretions and urinary incontinence) along with respiratory insufficiency. However, it may be difficult to differentiate this condition from myasthenic crisis on clinical grounds alone.

INVESTIGATIONS

TENSILON TEST (EDROPHONIUM TEST)

- Edrophonium is a rapidly acting acetylcholinesterase inhibitor. It has a short duration of action and reverses the muscular weakness dramatically in myasthenia. In adults, a 2-mg injection is given as a test dose (to check for tolerance) followed by another 8 mg that results in dramatic improvement in ptosis, diplopia, nasal voice, etc., within 30 seconds and persists up to 1 to 2 minutes. Positive test is highly suggestive of MG. Side effects like abdominal cramps can be relieved by atropine.

OTHERS

- Chest radiography and CT scan for thymoma.
- Thyroid function tests (10% may have associated hyperthyroidism).

TABLE 5.68 Drugs Which May Aggarvate Myasthenia Gravis

- Antibiotics—aminoglycosides (most important), polymyxins, colistin, tetracyclines, fluoroquinolones, macrolides, ritonavir
- Cardiovascular drugs—lidocaine, β-blockers, calcium channel blockers, quinidine, procainamide
- Others—chloroquine, penicillamine, interferons, statins, iodinated contrast agents, lithium, carbamazepine, phenytoin, muscle relaxants, curare-like neuromuscular blockers, magnesium, botulinum toxin, quinine, chloroquine, D-penicillamine

- Acetylcholine receptor antibody levels (present in >90% of patients with generalised myasthenia).
- Anti-muscle-specific protein (tyrosine) kinase (anti-MuSK) antibodies in many patients who are negative for ACh-receptor antibodies.
- Anti-low-density lipoprotein-related protein 4 (anti-LRP4) antibody in some patients who are negative for both anti-AChR and anti-MuSK antibodies.
- Electrodiagnostic studies (repetitive nerve stimulation producing decremental response, exercise testing and single-fibre electromyography).
- Ice test: In a patient with ptosis, a small cube of ice is placed over the eyelid for about 2 minutes. Improvement of the ptosis after this procedure suggests a disorder of neuromuscular transmission.

MANAGEMENT

- Anticholinesterases are effective in providing symptomatic relief. Neostigmine (15 mg) one to two tablets, three to six times a day or pyridostigmine 60–120 mg three to six times a day may be used. Dosage is titrated to the need of the patient. Cholinergic systemic side effects like abdominal cramps and increased salivation are managed with propantheline 15 mg two to three times a day. Pyridostigmine is generally better tolerated than neostigmine due to fewer gastrointestinal side effects. Treatment response with anticholinesterases is much less favourable in anti-MuSK MG, with a significantly increased risk of myasthenic crisis.
- Corticosteroids are useful in induction and maintenance of remission. However, in about 15% of patients, corticosteroids may worsen symptoms transiently during initial periods of treatment and may precipitate myasthenic crisis.
- Thymectomy can induce remission when the disease is generalised and has not been chronic. It is also recommended in patients with thymoma. Thymectomy may or may not reduce requirement of steroids.
- Immunosuppression with azathioprine, cyclophosphamide, cyclosporin, tacrolimus or mycophenolate mofetil is recommended when the dosage of steroid requirement is too high to maintain remission. Rituximab, eculizumab (a terminal complement inhibitor) and efgartigimod [an antibody fragment that binds to the neonatal Fc receptor (FcRn), preventing FcRn from recycling immunoglobulin G back into the blood] may be used in refractory cases.
- Plasma exchange and intravenous immunoglobulin are useful for inducing a short-term remission like prior to surgery or during myasthenic crisis.
- Supportive measures like ventilatory assistance and nasogastric tube feeding may be required in some cases.

DRUGS THAT MAY AGGRAVATE MYASTHENIA GRAVIS

- A number of drugs may aggravate MG and should be avoided (Table 5.68).

PROGNOSIS

- Prognosis is variable. Deaths are common if crisis occurs in the first 2 to 3 years. Deaths rarely occur after 5–7 years of illness.

Q. Explain muscular dystrophies or hereditary myopathies. (PY 3.13; PE 30.14)

- Group of hereditary disorders characterised by progressive muscle weakness and wasting with histopathological features of 'dystrophic' muscle (variation in muscle fibre size, muscle fibre degeneration and regeneration and replacement of muscle by fibrosis and fat).

CLASSIFICATION (Table 5.69)

TABLE 5.69 Classification of Muscular Dystrophies

- **X-linked muscular dystrophies:**
  - Duchenne muscular dystrophy
  - Becker muscular dystrophy
  - Emery–Dreifuss muscular dystrophy
- **Autosomal muscular dystrophies (can be dominant or recessive):**
  - Limb-girdle muscular dystrophy
  - Others
- **Autosomal dominant muscular dystrophies:**
  - Facioscapulohumeral muscular dystrophy
  - Ocular muscular dystrophy
  - Oculopharyngeal muscular dystrophy
  - Myotonic dystrophy
- **Sporadic:**
  - Congenital muscular dystrophy

DUCHENNE MUSCULAR DYSTROPHY

- X-linked recessive disorder, caused by absence of dystrophin due to mutation of Duchenne muscular dystrophy (DMD) (also known as dystrophin) gene.
- Onset between 3 and 5 years.
- Proximal muscles of lower limbs are affected first followed by proximal muscles of upper limbs. Boys fall frequently.
- On getting up from the floor, patient uses his/her hands to climb up himself/herself (Gower's sign) (Fig. 5.22).
- Later, neck muscles, extraocular muscles, diaphragm and facial muscles involved.
- Patient is bedridden by the age of 10 years.
- Pseudohypertrophy (muscles enlarged by the infiltration of fat) of calf muscles (Fig. 5.23) and occasionally deltoid muscles.
- Other features include contractures, macroglossia, absence of incisor teeth, mental retardation, skeletal atrophy and cardiac involvement (tachycardia, tall R-waves in right precordial leads, deep Q-waves in limb leads and left precordial leads, dilated cardiomyopathy).
- Serum creatine kinase elevated to at least 20 times the normal.
- EMG shows myopathic pattern (small, short-duration, and polyphasic muscle action potentials).

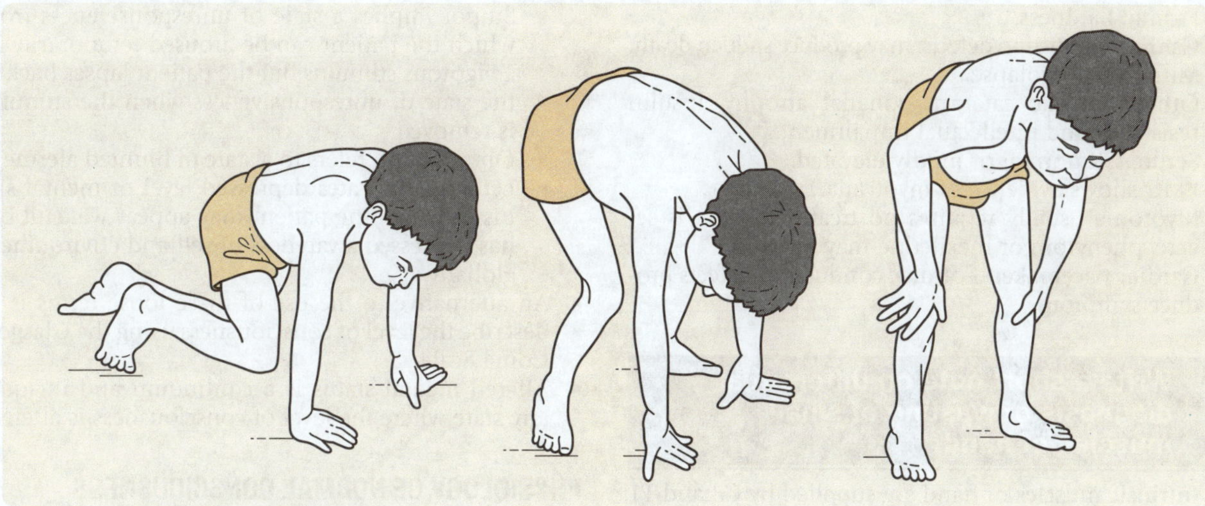

Fig. 5.22 Gower's sign.

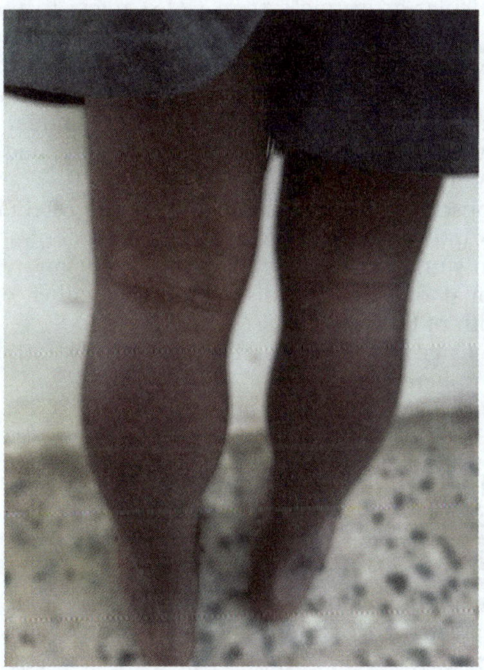

Fig. 5.23 Pseudohypertrophy of calf muscles in a patient of Duchenne muscular dystrophy.

- Muscle biopsy shows muscle fibres of varying size as well as small groups of necrosis and regenerating fibres. It also shows deficiency of dystrophin (a protein present on inner surface of sarcolemma) by Western blot test.
- Treatment with corticosteroids (prednisolone or deflazacort) may slow progression for up to 3 years.
- Novel therapy includes mutation-specific drug treatment such as casimersen, viltolarsen, golodirsen and eteplirsen.
- Others include physiotherapy, management of respiratory and cardiac complications and maintenance of nutrition.

BECKER MUSCULAR DYSTROPHY

- X-linked recessive disorder resulting from partial dystrophin deficiency.
- Onset between 5 and 25 years.
- Pelvic and pectoral muscles predominantly involved.
- Patient unable to walk after about 25 years of onset.
- Significant facial weakness is not common.
- Associated features include cardiac involvement, contractures and hypertrophy of muscles.
- Serum CK is raised.
- EMG shows myopathic pattern.

MYOTONIC DYSTROPHY

- Type 1 more common than type 2.
- Autosomal dominant.
- Onset during second decade of life.
- Typical 'hatchet-faced' appearance due to atrophy and weakness of temporalis, masseter and facial muscles.
- Neck flexors, sternocleidomastoid and distal limb muscles affected early.
- Dysarthria, nasal voice and swallowing difficulties due to palatal, pharyngeal and tongue involvement.
- Proximal muscles remain strong.
- Myotonia:
  - Percussion of thenar muscles or tongue produces contraction without immediate relaxation.
  - Slow relaxation of hand grip after a forced voluntary closure.
  - Causes of myotonia are listed in Box 5.79.

BOX 5.79 Causes of Myotonia

- Myotonic dystrophy
- Myotonia congenita
- Paramyotonia congenita
- Hypokalaemic periodic paralysis
- Hyperkalaemic periodic paralysis

- Frontal baldness.
- Cardiac conduction defects; may produce sudden death.
- Mitral valve prolapse.
- Others include cataract, gonadal atrophy, insulin resistance and intellectual impairment.
- Serum CK normal or mildly elevated.
- EMG shows evidence of myotonia.
- Myotonia usually requires no treatment. If it is severe, phenytoin or mexiletine may be used.
- Cardiac pacemaker if cardiac conduction defects produce symptoms.

Q. Write a short note on differential diagnosis of wasting of small muscles of hand.

- Intrinsic muscles of hand are supplied by C8 and T1 myotomes through median and ulnar nerves.

CAUSES (Table 5.70)

TABLE 5.70 Causes of Wasting of Small Muscles of Hand

Site	Causes
• Spinal cord lesions	Motor neuron disease, syringomyelia, intramedullary tumours, intradural tumours (rare)
• Plexus lesions	C8-T1 root lesions with Horner's syndrome (e.g. trauma, Pancoast's tumour), lower trunk and medial cord lesions (e.g. trauma, metastasis, thoracic outlet syndrome)
• Median nerve lesions	Trauma, carpal tunnel syndrome
• Ulnar nerve lesions	Trauma, leprosy, entrapment at ulnar groove or Guyon's tunnel
• Polyneuropathy	Causes—refer distal symmetrical sensorimotor polyneuropathy (Table 5.64)

Q. Outline the causes of coma. How do you proceed to investigate and manage a case of coma?

Q. Write a short note on Glasgow Coma Scale.

- Consciousness is a state of awareness of the self and the environment.
- Coma is a state where consciousness (wakeful state) is altered severely and is due to depressed brain function. It is defined as a state of altered consciousness from which a person cannot be aroused.

TERMS USED IN A PATIENT WITH ALTERED LEVEL OF CONSCIOUSNESS

- While assessing a patient with altered mental status, several terms are commonly used.
  - Coma is at one end of spectrum of decreased level of consciousness from which patient cannot be aroused.
  - Stupor implies a state of unresponsiveness from which the patient can be aroused temporarily by a vigorous stimulus but the patient lapses back to the state of unresponsiveness when the stimulus is removed.
  - Obtundation refers to a state of blunted alertness.
  - Lethargy indicates depressed level of mental status in which the patient may appear wakeful but has depressed awareness of self and environment globally.
- An alternative to the use of these loose terms is to describe the level of consciousness using the Glasgow Coma Scale.
- Altered mental status is a continuum and includes any state where the level of consciousness is altered.

PHYSIOLOGY OF NORMAL CONSCIOUSNESS

- Anatomic structures that maintain normal level of consciousness include brainstem reticular formation, ascending projectional system, thalamic nuclei, thalamocortical fibres and cerebral cortex; reticular activating system (RAS) refers to the first four structures.
- RAS mainly occupies the mid portion (tegmentum) of the pons and midbrain. Because of the compactness of RAS and its proximity to the cranial nerve nuclei, cranial nerve function is often impaired when RAS is damaged.
- Consciousness is maintained by active cerebral cortex under the influence of ascending RAS.
- Thus unconsciousness may be brought on by functional or structural disturbances of either one or both of the following:
  - Large areas of cerebral cortex (usually both hemispheres).
  - Upper brainstem structures.

PATHOPHYSIOLOGY OF ALTERED LEVEL OF CONSCIOUSNESS

METABOLIC DERANGEMENTS

- Metabolic derangements produce CNS dysfunction characterised by global depression of CNS activity resulting in *absence of focal deficits in most cases.*
- The pupillary reflexes are intact except in presence of certain toxins like anticholinergics and opiates.
- Occasionally, hypoglycaemia and hepatic failure can produce focal neurological deficits as the most sensitive neuron-groups are affected initially.
- If brain is deprived of its normal supply of oxygen due to impairment of systemic oxygen uptake or distribution for more than 10 seconds, loss of consciousness ensues.

STRUCTURAL DERANGEMENTS

- The level of consciousness is altered when a structural process disrupts either the RAS or both the cerebral hemispheres.
- Most often, these conditions produce *focal neurological deficits* and may also lead to *raised intracranial pressure (ICP).*

- Since rigid skull is nonexpandable, any increase in ICP is directly transmitted to the brain and vessels. Tentorium separates the cerebrum from cerebellum and brainstem. It has an opening in the centre (tentorial notch) through which passes the brainstem. Focal increases in the intracranial volume and ICP can lead to displacement and compression of brain resulting in herniation syndromes (see page 333).

CAUSES OF COMA

- Causes of coma include primary neurological disorders, various systemic disorders and toxins that can impair brain function (Table 5.71).

EVALUATION OF SEVERITY OF COMA

- One of the most commonly used score to evaluate severity of altered level of consciousness is Glasgow Coma Score (Table 5.72).

TABLE 5.72 Glasgow Coma Score

Eye Opening (E)	Score	Verbal Response (V)	Score
• Spontaneous	4	• Oriented	5
• To speech	3	• Confused conversation	4
• To pain	2		
• None	1	• Inappropriate words	3
		• Incomprehensible sounds	2
		• None	1
Best Motor Response (M)		**Coma Score**	**E + M + V**
• Obeys	6	• Fully conscious	15
• Localises	5	• Deeply comatose	3
• Withdraws	4		
• Abnormal flexion	3		
• Abnormal extension	2		
• None	1		

APPROACH TO PROBLEM OF COMA

INITIAL STABILISATION

- The first step is CABDE (Circulation, Airway, Breathing, Disability and Exposure). Make sure that there is no immediate danger to life by ensuring CAB (Circulation, Airway with cervical spine control, Breathing). Disability is assessed by abbreviated coma scale (AVPU—Alert, responds to Verbal commands, responds to Pain and Unconscious). The patient should be exposed completely for detailed examination taking care not to expose the patient to extremes of temperature.
- Attach a cardiac monitor and pulse oximeter and administer oxygen. Establish an intravenous access and withdraw blood for various investigations including bedside estimation of sugar, urea and electrolytes.

HISTORY

- After initial stabilisation, obtain a brief history from all the relatives and friends. Ask about the details of what happened, any trauma, use of medications, exposure to alcohol, history of seizures, diabetes, hypertension, cirrhosis, previous neurological diseases and associated symptoms like headache.

TABLE 5.71 Causes of Coma

Primary Neurological Disorders	Systemic Disorders Causing Coma
Cerebral hemispherical lesions:	**Metabolic encephalopathies:**
• Brain tumours	• Hypoglycaemia
• Abscess	• Hyponatraemia or hypernatraemia
• Cerebral infarcts (large)	• Hypocalcaemia or hypercalcaemia
• Cerebral haemorrhage	• Hyperglycaemia with or without ketosis
• Subarachnoid haemorrhage	• Severe hypoxia—severe heart failure, severe anaemia, severe lung disease
• Subdural haematoma	• Hypercapnia
• Sagittal sinus thrombosis	• Hyperpyrexia, heat stroke or hypothermia
• Hydrocephalus	• Hypoosmolar or hyperosmolar states
	• Hepatic and uraemic encephalopathy
	• Myxoedema
	• Severe peripheral circulatory failure
Brainstem lesions:	**Miscellaneous:**
• Infarct	• Toxic encephalopathies secondary to toxins (including alcohol intoxication)
• Pontine haemorrhage	• Systemic infections (including malaria, typhoid)
• Posterior fossa mass lesions	• Hypertensive encephalopathy
• Wernicke's encephalopathy	• Wernicke's encephalopathy
Combination of both (entire brain):	• Febrile encephalopathy (see page 379)
• Trauma	
• Meningitis, encephalitis	
• Anoxia (postcardiac arrest)	
• Severe shock states	
• Postictal state following a generalised fit	
• Cerebral depressant drugs (sedatives/hypnotics)	
• Raised ICP due to brain oedema from any cause, for example Reye's syndrome	

- Presence of empty pill bottle near the patient may suggest an overdose.
- Check the pockets of the patient for any clues about any medical diseases or drugs.
- History of mode of onset and evolution (or progression) gives clue to underlying mechanism (Table 5.73).
- Headache before onset of coma may suggest an intracranial haemorrhage; appearance of a focal deficit points to a structural lesion.
- High fever may indicate meningitis, encephalitis or cerebral malaria. Also, elicit a history of hypertension, diabetes, renal failure, liver disease, seizure disorder and cancer.
- Other important points include exposure to high temperature (heat stroke), alcohol bout, ear discharge (temporal abscess), toxemia of pregnancy (eclampsia) and recent delivery (cerebral vein thrombosis).

PHYSICAL EXAMINATION

- Assume cervical spine injury in all such patients until ruled out; therefore, immobilise the neck.
- Check the vital signs:
  - Presence of moderate to severe hypertension suggests the possibility of intracranial bleed or hypertensive encephalopathy. Do not presume hypertension to be due to raised intracranial pressure during the initial evaluation.
  - Hypotension may be due to occult blood loss, poisoning and septic or cardiogenic shock.
  - Consider tachypnoea a sign of inadequate oxygenation and not a sign of central nervous damage. It may be due to the presence of ketoacidosis, sepsis, poisoning due to salicylates or methanol, and herniation.
  - Bradypnoea on the other hand, may indicate poisoning due to opiates.
  - Check rectal temperature in all comatose patients to look for hypothermia or hyperthermia. Fever may indicate a systemic infection, meningitis, cerebral malaria, encephalitis, brain abscess, pontine haemorrhage, heat stroke or poisoning due to anticholinergics. Hypothermia may be due to sepsis or myxoedema.
  - Presence of hypertension and bradycardia may indicate raised ICP (Cushing's reflex).
- Look for evidence of trauma or previous surgeries:
  - Bruising and laceration of the scalp and face may indicate head injury.
  - Presence of haemotympanum, bilateral medial orbital ecchymosis (Raccoon eyes) or postauricular ecchymosis (Battle's sign) indicates basilar skull fracture.
  - Palpate scalp for craniotomy sites (which may indicate old surgery on brain and subsequent epileptic focus).
  - Palpate scalp for the reservoir of a ventricular shunt (which if noncompressible, may indicate blocked shunt and acute hydrocephalus).
  - A surgical scar on the neck may indicate a thyroid or parathyroid disease which may produce coma due to myxoedema or hypercalcaemia/hypocalcaemia.
- Examine the neck for asymmetries in the carotids or bruits over the vessels.
- The breath odour of the victim may be helpful in certain conditions like diabetic ketoacidosis (fruity smell), and ethanol and kerosene poisonings.
- Presence of petechiae may suggest meningococcemia or thrombotic thrombocytopenic purpura.
- A shunt in the forearm may indicate uraemia or electrolyte abnormalities as the cause of coma.
- Needle tracks on the skin suggest intravenous drug abuse.
- Evaluate cardiac system and look for arrhythmias (which can alter mental status due to reduced cardiac output), myocardial infarction and endocarditis.
- Examine abdomen to look for any organomegaly, pulsatile masses (e.g. aortic aneurysm), bruits and ascites.

NEUROLOGICAL EXAMINATION

- Assess the level of mental status using Glasgow coma scale. Reactions to verbal, painful and other stimuli are helpful in gauging the depth of coma. However, perform these manoeuvres cautiously as they may lead to increase in ICP. Use of pinprick or pinching may leave marks. A safe and more noxious stimulus is tickling of nasal cavity with cotton.
- Look for neck rigidity (meningitis or SAH). However, remember that in a comatose patient, it may not be apparent.
- Several respiratory patterns can occur in a comatose patient. However, their localising value is not absolute.
  - In Cheyne–Stokes breathing, the ventilatory effort varies in depth and rate leading to a crescendo-decrescendo type of respiration. In between, there is a phase of apnoea. It may occur with various metabolic abnormalities, congestive heart failure and bilateral cerebral hemispherical lesions.
  - Hyperventilation consists of continuous, rapid and deep respirations. It may be associated with hypoxia with patient making efforts to correct it, metabolic acidosis and partial midbrain damage.
  - Ataxic breathing is irregular in rhythm and depth and it frequently precedes respiratory arrest in patients with expanding posterior fossa lesions.

TABLE 5.73 Causes of Coma Based on Rapidity of Evolution

Abrupt (within seconds and minutes) / Acute (within a few hours)	Subacute (within several hours and a few days)
Abrupt (within seconds and minutes): • Cerebral haemorrhage • Subarachnoid haemorrhage • Massive cerebral infarct • Cardiac arrest • Epileptic fit • Trauma **Acute (within a few hours):** • Cerebral infarct or haemorrhage • Acute poisoning—alcohol, drugs • Hypoglycaemia in diabetics due to overdosage of insulin or oral antidiabetics	**Subacute (within several hours and a few days):** • Metabolic encephalopathies • Brain tumours, other mass lesions • Encephalitis and meningitis • Encephalopathies secondary to severe systemic infections

- Apneustic breathing has a prolonged inspiratory pause and it usually occurs with pontine damage near the fifth cranial nerve, and in some cases with hypoglycaemia and meningitis.
- Posture: A comatose patient may assume certain postures either spontaneously or in response to a painful stimulus.
  - A patient who is lying with legs crossed or folded up has an intact brainstem.
  - A decorticate posture indicates abnormal flexion of the upper limbs and extension of lower limbs. It may be associated with brain damage above the midbrain level.
  - A decerebrate posture indicates extension, adduction and internal rotation of all the four limbs. It is often associated with damage to diencephalon and midbrain with intact pons.
  - Lesions at other locations and sedative overdose can also produce these two postures.
- Examine carefully for subtle spontaneous movements including turning on bed, pulling up bed sheets, etc. Note any asymmetry in these movements.
- Presence of repetitive movements of any kind may indicate epileptic activity.
- Examine the motor system for muscle tone, asymmetry of movements and reflexes.
  - In acute lesions of brain, motor tone is reduced. This may be demonstrated by arm-drop or leg-drop tests.
  - For arm-drop test, hold the arms above the patient and then release. The hemiplegic arm will drop at right angle while the normal side will fall more slowly.
  - For leg-drop test, elevate the legs slightly, extend one leg and then the other, and then drop them in turn. A difference in tone may cause a difference in the rate of fall of the two legs.
  - Other manoeuvre includes opening the eyelids and releasing them simultaneously which results in slower closure of the eye on the hemiplegic side.
- The deep tendon reflexes and unilateral extensor plantar (Babinski's reflex) are useful in localising a structural brain lesion. Bilateral extensor plantars may be seen in any patient with coma; they may be absent in deep coma.
- Examine fundus for any evidence of raised ICP (papilloedema, absence of venous pulsations), SAH, diabetic retinopathy or hypertensive retinopathy. However, papilloedema is often not present in early stages of raised ICP.
- Pupils:
  - Check for the direct and consensual light pupillary reflexes. The reflex path for pupillary reflexes includes optic nerve, optic tracts, lateral geniculate bodies, portion of midbrain (Edinger–Westphal's nucleus), and intracranial course of cranial nerve III.
  - The pupillary pathways are relatively resistant to metabolic insults, and as a general rule, hemispheric disease has very little influence on pupillary function.
  - Patients with metabolic causes of coma usually have small to mid-sized pupils which are reactive to light.
  - A unilaterally dilated or sluggishly reacting pupil is a sign of an impending herniation. However, it may occur due to instillation of a cycloplegic agent in one eye and eye injury. A small degree of anisocoria (usually less than 1 mm) occurs in about 10% of normal population, but in the comatose patient, even minor pupillary asymmetry may reflect early III nerve compression.
  - Pinpoint, nonreactive pupils indicate a pontine lesion.
  - Toxins like opiates, cholinesterase inhibitors and barbiturates produce small pupils.
  - Destruction of midbrain produces midposition, fixed pupils because both cranial nerve III nuclei and pupillodilator sympathetic fibres are located together in this portion of brain.
- Extraocular movements:
  - These are controlled by cortex (anterior frontal lobe and posterior occipital lobe), pons, midbrain, III, IV and VI cranial nerves, and medial longitudinal fasciculus (MLF).
  - As these areas are located in proximity to the RAS, any lesion of the RAS will produce some alterations in the extraocular movements.
  - Examine the spontaneous position of the eyeballs carefully. Slight dysconjugate gaze is common in patients with coma.
  - Slow, conjugate movements of the eyes on both sides are often seen in a comatose patient. Full spontaneous horizontal movements of both the eyes indicate a relatively intact pons and midbrain.
  - In focal lesions of the cortex, the eyes may deviate conjugately to the side of lesion as the frontal lobe lateral gaze centres that deviate the eyes to the contralateral side are damaged.
  - During a focal seizure, the eyes frequently deviate conjugately away from the seizure focus.
  - Sustained conjugate downward eye deviation may occur with brainstem damage, SAH and in some metabolic encephalopathies.
  - A brainstem injury will result in dysconjugate eye movements.
  - A lesion of the VI nerve causes paralysis of abduction resulting in deviation of eye downwards and medially due to the unopposed action of III and IV nerves.
  - In III nerve palsy, the affected eye is turned outwards and downwards due to unopposed action of IV and VI nerves.
  - Lesions of MLF produce perfect eye alignment on straight gaze but paralysis of the adducting eye and nystagmus of the abducting eye during attempts to look towards contralateral side (internuclear ophthalmoplegia).
  - Uncommon spontaneous movements include ocular bobbing and ocular dipping.
    - Ocular bobbing indicates abrupt downwards movements of the eyes with slow return to

midposition. Previously, it was thought to be specific for intrapontine lesions but it has been reported in some cases of metabolic encephalopathies and cerebellar haemorrhage.
    - Ocular dipping is a cyclic downward conjugate movement of the eyes with a rapid upward movement. It is reported in hypoxic coma.
- Oculocephalic test:
    - Reflex eye movement on change of head position is called oculocephalic test.
    - Do not perform the oculocephalic test (also known as doll's eyes test) if any suspicion of cervical spine injury is present.
    - Normally, in an awake patient, as the head is turned to one side, the eyes turn to the opposite side due to intact cortex. For example, if the head is turned to left side, the eyes move to the right side. This is termed a positive response.
    - In a comatose patient with intact brainstem, cortical control is absent and brisk movements of the head from one side to other produce conjugate motion of the eyes in the direction opposite to that of the head.
    - It indicates integrity of vestibular and cervical proprioceptors, MLF, and III cranial nerves in the midbrain.
    - Patients with brainstem dysfunction will have an absent reflex (i.e. the eyes will remain fixed in the direction of head movement).
    - Patients with a variety of drug overdose particularly with phenytoin, antidepressant and barbiturate poisoning, may manifest sluggish or absent oculocephalic reflex despite intact brainstem.
- Oculovestibular or caloric test:
    - This test involves a stronger stimulus to the brainstem compared to the oculocephalic test. It is useful if oculocephalic reflex is absent or is contraindicated.
    - Before conducting this test, exclude tympanic membrane perforation.
    - Raise the head of the patient to 30° so as to stimulate the horizontal semicircular canal only.
    - Irrigate the ear with 50–100 mL of cold (~30°C) saline.
    - If the patient demonstrates turning of both eyes to the ipsilateral side and then the eyes rapidly jerk back to midline, that is nystagmus is away from the side of irrigation, he is not comatose but is awake, as it indicates intact cortex and brainstem.
    - The nystagmus component of the test depends upon the intact cortex so that in patients with cortical lesion but intact brainstem, both eyes deviate to the side of irrigation without showing any nystagmus.
    - If the patient has brainstem damage, no response occurs.
    - A few patients with large overdose of antidepressants and glutethimide may show absence of this response.
    - If the ipsilateral eye moves but the contralateral eye does not, an internuclear lesion involving MLF is present.
- Blinking response to corneal stimulation with cotton indicates intact V and VII nerves.
- The gag response indicates intactness of IX and X nerves.

INVESTIGATIONS

- The selection of laboratory and radiological tests is guided by the history and initial evaluation.
- During initial stabilisation, take blood for glucose, urea, sodium, calcium, bilirubin, haemoglobin, leucocyte count and arterial blood gas analysis. If facilities are available, take blood for toxicological screening.
- Specific tests like carboxyhaemoglobin levels are required if a diagnosis of carbon monoxide poisoning is suspected.
- Whenever trauma is suspected, get a cervical spine X-ray to rule out spine injury.
- Get a CT brain in patients in whom coma is suspected to be the result of a structural lesion of brain or if routine evaluation has failed to reveal the cause of coma.
- Analyse CSF if a nonfocal cause like meningitis is suspected.
- An ECG may be helpful in certain cases. Osborn J waves suggest hypothermia while widening of QRS complex suggests antidepressant poisoning. A prolonged QT interval may indicate hypocalcaemia, or antidepressant or phenothiazine toxicity.

DIFFERENTIAL DIAGNOSIS

- Coma vigil (akinetic mutism): This usually results from diffuse frontal lobe disease. The patient appears awake but is silent, and is extremely slow to respond to any stimuli. He may show visual tracking to sensory stimuli. He may not be aware of the environment.
- Minimally conscious state: A condition in which patient appears not only to be wakeful (like vegetative state patients) but also exhibits inconsistent (fluctuating) signs of awareness (unlike patients with vegetative state). The latter includes nonreflexive response to sensory stimulation, awareness of the self or the environment, or language comprehension or expression.
- Akinetic mutism: Akinetic mutism refers to a state in which the patient, although awake, remains entirely silent and motionless. The patient has sleep/wake cycles and can maintain vital functions, but does nothing voluntarily. This condition is often due to bilateral frontal lobe lesions, hydrocephalus and a mass in the region of third ventricle.
- Locked-in-state: The patient is aware and awake. However, due to severe impairment of motor function preventing communication, coma can be mistakenly diagnosed in these patients. This syndrome

is due to extensive transverse pontine and midbrain lesions. Patients' only form of communication may be through vertical eye movements and blinking.

- Vegetative state: In this state, the patient has no true cortical output. He can open the eyes and make some motor movements but information is not processed and therefore, he does not have any meaningful interaction with the environment, that is the patient is awake without being aware.
- Conversion reaction: Patients with conversion reaction (pseudocoma) have normal pupils, corneal reflexes and plantar reflexes. They may keep their eyes firmly shut and resist the opening of the eye by examiners. The eyes roll up when the lids are raised. Roving eye movements cannot be imitated and their presence indicates true coma. The presence of nystagmus during cold caloric testing suggests that coma is either feigned or hysterical.

APPROACH TO DIAGNOSIS OF COMA BASED ON COMBINED CLINICAL AND LABORATORY DATA (Table 5.74)

TABLE 5.74 Diagnosis of Cause of Coma Based on Clinical and Laboratory Data

Normal brainstem reflexes, no lateralising signs	
CT abnormal	**CT normal**
• Hydrocephalus • Bilateral subdural haematoma • Diffuse cerebral contusion or oedema • SAH • Brainstem haemorrhage • Cerebellar haemorrhage • Cerebellar infarct • Posterior fossa mass lesion • Large cerebral mass lesion with transtentorial herniation	• Drug induced (TS) • Metabolic encephalopathy (BB) • Shock, hypertensive encephalopathy • Meningitis, encephalitis (CSF) • Reye's syndrome (BB) • Brainstem infarction • Drug overdosage (TS) • Trauma, brain death
Normal brainstem reflexes with lateralising signs	
CT abnormal	**CT normal**
• Cerebral haemorrhage or infarct • Viral encephalitis • Subdural haematoma, tumours, abscess	• Early cerebral infarct • Metabolic encephalopathy with fleeting focal signs (BB) • Epileptic fit in postictal state

BB, blood biochemistry; CSF, CSF evaluation; TS, toxicology screening.

TREATMENT

- Maintain circulation, airway and breathing.
- Diagnose underlying cause at the earliest.
- Adopt appropriate specific treatment at the earliest.
- If patient is a diabetic, administer hypertonic glucose, without waiting for laboratory reports. However, it is best to get a bedside estimation of blood glucose and administer dextrose only if the blood glucose is below 80 mg/dL.
- If patient is an alcoholic, administer glucose and vitamin B_1 100 mg intravenously.

SUMMARY OF APPROACH TO A PATIENT WITH ALTERED LEVEL OF CONSCIOUSNESS (Flowchart 5.6)

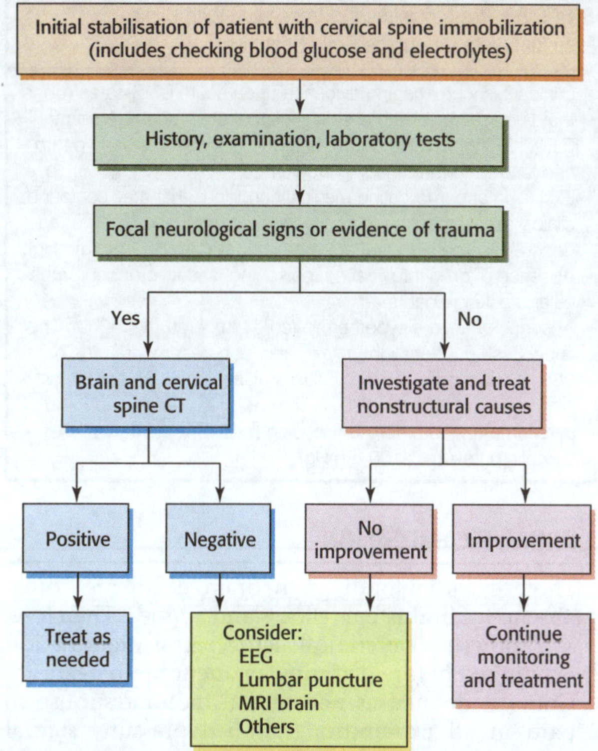

Flowchart 5.6 Approach to a Patient with Altered Level of Consciousness.

CARE OF UNCONSCIOUS PATIENT

- Maintain airway and clear off secretions—by frequent assisted clearance.
- Posture of the patient—prone or lateral position prevents aspiration of gastric contents.
- Nasogastric tube—to keep the stomach empty or to feed, depending on underlying situation.
- Bladder care—continuous indwelling catheter or clean intermittent catheterisation.
- Skin care—change of posture once in 2 to 3 hours, and skin should be kept clean and dry to prevent bedsores.
- Have a secure IV line.

Q. Write a short note on brain death.

- Defined as the irreversible loss of all functions of the brain, including the brainstem.
- Occurs when ICP exceeds CPP resulting in cessation of CBF and oxygen delivery.
- Concept of brain death is important as: (i) it allows withdrawal of costly life-saving equipment and drugs; and (ii) family can be offered opportunity for organ donation.
- Diagnosis of brain death is primarily clinical. Complete clinical examination including independent brain death determinations by two licensed physicians is conclusive.

PRE-REQUISITES FOR PROCEEDING WITH CLINICAL EXAMINATION TO DETERMINE BRAIN DEATH (Box 5.80)

BOX 5.80 Pre-requisites for Proceeding With Clinical Examination to Determine Brain Death

- Clinical or neuroimaging evidence of an acute CNS catastrophe that is compatible with the diagnosis of brain death. A normal CT scan should raise doubt as to the diagnosis of brain death and lead to further imaging studies.
- Exclusion of complicating medical conditions that may confound clinical assessment such as severe electrolyte, acid–base or endocrine disorders and refractory shock (systolic BP <90 mmHg).
- Absence of drug intoxication, poisoning, sedative or neuromuscular blocking agents.
- Absence of severe hypothermia (core temperature <32°C). This is because pupillary light reflex is lost at core temperatures of 28°C–32°C and brainstem reflexes disappear when core temperature drops below 28°C. A core body temperature of >36°C is recommended before proceeding to CNS examination.
- Systolic pressure >100 mmHg.

CLINICAL EXAMINATION

- Three essential findings in brain death are coma, absence of brainstem reflexes and apnoea. Therefore, a comprehensive clinical neurological examination is required before declaring a patient brain dead.
- Coma is defined as no cerebral motor response to pain in all extremities (nail-bed pressure, sternal pressure and supraorbital pressure).
- Absence of brainstem reflexes:
  - Pupils—round or oval pupils measuring 4–9 mm with no response to bright light.
  - Ocular movement—no oculocephalic movements on rapid turning of the head (performed only when no fracture or instability of cervical spine is present); no deviation of eyes to cold caloric stimulation, that is absent oculovestibular reflex (irrigate each ear with ice water after the head has been tilted 30° to check for eye deviation).
  - Facial sensation and facial motor response—no corneal reflex, no jaw reflex, no grimacing to deep pressure on nail bed, supraorbital ridge or temporomandibular joint.
  - Pharyngeal and tracheal reflexes—no response to stimulation of posterior pharynx with a tongue blade, no cough response to bronchial suctioning.
- Apnoea test:
  - Before performing apnoea test, the following conditions should be met:
    - Core temperature >36.5°C.
    - Euvolaemia.
    - Systolic pressure >90 mmHg.
    - Normal PCO_2.
  - Place on 100% oxygen for at least 10 minutes to maintain PaO_2 >200 mmHg.
  - After that, apnoea test is conducted as follows:
    - Connect a pulse oximeter and disconnect the ventilator.
    - Deliver 100% O_2 at 6–10 L/minute into trachea by placing a cannula at the level of carina.
    - Observe closely for any respiratory movements.
    - Must maintain SpO_2 >85%, mean arterial pressure >60 mmHg and systolic arterial pressure >90 mmHg (otherwise abort the test).
    - Measure arterial PO_2, PCO_2 and pH after approximately 8 minutes and reconnect the ventilator.
    - If respiratory movements are absent and arterial PCO_2 ≥60 mmHg, apnoea test result is positive (i.e. it supports the diagnosis of brain death).
    - If respiratory movements are observed, apnoea test result is negative.

CONFIRMATORY LABORATORY TESTS

- A confirmatory test is not mandatory, but is desirable in patients in whom specific components of clinical testing cannot be reliably performed.
  - Conventional angiography showing absence of intracerebral filling at the level of carotid bifurcation or circle of Willis.
  - EEG showing absence of electrical activity during at least 30 minutes of recording.
  - Transcranial Doppler ultrasonography showing small systolic peaks in early systole without diastolic flow, indicating very high vascular resistance associated with greatly increased ICP.
  - 99m-Technetium-labelled hexamethylpropyleneamine oxime cerebral blood flow scan showing absence of uptake of isotope in brain parenchyma.
  - Somatosensory evoked potentials showing absence of response with median nerve stimulation on both sides.

CLINICAL OBSERVATIONS COMPATIBLE WITH DIAGNOSIS OF BRAIN DEATH

- While observing a patient, a few findings may be seen that should not be misinterpreted as evidence for brainstem function. These are as follows:
  - Spontaneous limb movements other than pathological flexion or extension response.
  - Respiratory-like movements (shoulder elevation and adduction, back arching and intercostal expansion without significant tidal volumes).
  - Sweating.
  - Tachycardia.
  - Normal BP without pharmacological support.
  - Sudden increases in BP.
  - Absence of diabetes insipidus.
  - Presence of deep tendon reflexes or superficial abdominal reflexes.
  - Presence of extensor plantar reflex.
- Common physiological derangements after brain death:
  - Hypothermia.
  - Hypotension.
  - Cardiac arrhythmias.
  - Diabetes insipidus.
  - Disseminated intravascular coagulation.
  - Pulmonary oedema.

MCQs

IM17.1

1. A 65-year-old woman goes to see her GP complaining of 2 weeks of right-sided headache and a transient episode of right-sided blindness a day ago which has completely resolved. She notices that the pain on her head is exacerbated when she is combing her hair. On examination of her central and peripheral nervous systems, no abnormalities are found.
What is the most likely diagnosis?
A. Horner's syndrome
B. Giant cell arteritis
C. Malignant hypertension
D. Amaurosis fugax
E. Migraine

Ans: B. Giant cell arteritis

Headache is almost invariable in giant cell arteritis (GCA). Pain develops over inflamed superficial temporal and/or occipital arteries. Touching the skin over an inflamed vessel (e.g. combing hair) causes pain. Arterial pulsation is soon lost; the artery becomes hard, tortuous and thickened. The scalp over inflamed vessels may become red. Rarely, gangrenous patches appear. Urgent treatment with corticosteroids is needed to prevent permanent blindness.

(IM17.3)

2. A 24-year-old woman develops severe left-sided headache with nausea. Sounds and light make this headache worse. She notices that she is seeing zigzags in her vision. Clinical examination does not reveal any clinical or neurological abnormalities. What is the most likely cause of this presentation?
A. Cataract
B. Retinitis pigmentosa
C. Central retinal artery occlusion
D. Migraine
E. Acute glaucoma

Ans: D. Migraine

The classic symptoms of migraine are the premonitory aura, momentary loss of visual field and unilateral, severe headache and vomiting. The mechanisms are not well understood. Blood flow studies in patients during migraine attacks have shown changes in blood flow during the different phases but no consistent pattern.

3. A 60-year-old woman with a history of polymyalgia rheumatica presents with bilateral visual loss. What is the most likely diagnosis?
A. Closed angle glaucoma
B. Optic neuritis
C. Central retinal artery occlusion (CRAO)
D. Central retinal vein occlusion
E. Giant cell arteritis

Ans: E. Giant cell arteritis

Giant cell arteritis is vasculitis of large and medium arteries of the head. It is often associated with polymyalgia rheumatica. Inflammation of the temporal arteries can cause emboli to the central retinal artery causing visual loss.

4. A 55-year-old man presents with mild vertigo of onset over months. On examination, he has papilloedema, unilateral cerebellar signs and contralateral pyramidal signs. What is the most likely diagnosis from the list below?
A. Wernicke's encephalopathy
B. Ramsay Hunt syndrome
C. Posterior fossa tumour
D. Meniere's disease
E. Benign positional vertigo

Ans: C. Posterior fossa tumour

Tumours of the posterior fossa can lead to gradually increasing intracranial pressure due to progressive blockage of the flow of the spinal fluid. Examinations reveal bilateral papilloedema, ipsilateral absent corneal reflex, ipsilateral cerebellar symptoms and contralateral pyramidal signs.

5. A 34-year-old person, a chronic alcoholic, presents with confusion for one day. On examination, he has ophthalmoplegia, nystagmus and ataxia. What is the likely diagnosis?
A. Wernicke's encephalopathy
B. Delirium tremens
C. Posterior fossa tumour
D. Friedreich's ataxia,
E. Acute lead poisoning

Ans: A. Wernicke's encephalopathy

Wernicke's encephalopathy is an acute neurological condition characterised by a clinical triad of ophthalmoparesis with nystagmus, ataxia and confusion. This is a life-threatening illness caused by thiamine deficiency.

6. A 35-year-old man presents with one-sided facial weakness, vertigo and a painful rash in the ear canal. What is the most likely cause of this presentation from the list below?
A. Bell's palsy
B. Ramsay Hunt syndrome
C. Posterior fossa tumour
D. Acute stroke
E. Guillain-Barre syndrome

Ans: B. Ramsay Hunt syndrome

Ramsay Hunt syndrome is suggested by the presence of painful vesicles in the external auditory meatus. It is caused by reactivation of herpes zoster virus affecting cranial nerve VII, the facial nerve and may lead to ipsilateral facial palsy and associated hearing loss.

IM18.6

7. A 75-year-old man with prostate cancer presents with progressive weakness affecting both limbs and urinary retention on a background of increasing back pain. Examination reveals a spastic paraparesis and loss of anal tone. What is the most likely site of pathology?
A. Anterior horn cell

B. Corticospinal tract
C. Muscle
D. Neuromuscular junction
E. Peripheral nerve

Ans: B. Corticospinal tract

Spinal cord compression causes lower motor neurone signs at the level of the lesion and upper motor neurone symptoms below it. It is a neurosurgical emergency. Treatment involves steroids to reduce inflammation around tumour deposits, radiotherapy or surgical resection.

IM18.6

8. A 60-year-old man presents with chronic arm weakness that occurred after a childhood infection. On examination, there is wasting of the deltoid on the right with fasciculations in the muscle. There are no upper motor neuronal or sensory signs. What is the most likely site of pathology?
   A. Anterior horn cell
   B. Spinal portion of corticospinal tract
   C. Muscle
   D. Neuromuscular junction
   E. Peripheral nerve

Ans: Anterior horn cell

This is suggestive of polio-infection of the anterior horn cell causing lower motor neurone signs without sensory disturbance. Destruction of anterior horn cells causes muscle wasting and lower motor neurone signs.

IM17.1

9. A 46-year-old man presents with sudden-onset occipital headache associated with nausea and vomiting followed by the rapid onset of a left-sided flaccid hemiparesis. He has a past history of hypertension and was on amlodipine, ramipril and bisoprolol. What is the most likely diagnosis?
   A. Brain abscess
   B. Hemiplegic migraine
   C. Meningitis
   D. Subarachnoid haemorrhage
   E. Subdural haematoma

Ans: D. Subarachnoid haemorrhage

A sudden-onset, severe, occipital headache with vomiting is characteristic of a subarachnoid haemorrhage. Focal neurological signs may be present. An urgent CT scan and neurosurgical intervention may be required in these cases.

10. A 28-year-old woman who has previously had optic neuritis presents with worsening leg weakness. Examination reveals a spastic paraparesis. She is catheterised. What is the most likely diagnosis?
    A. Guillain-Barré syndrome
    B. Multiple sclerosis
    C. Motor neurone disease (MND)
    D. Brown-Sequard syndrome
    E. Spinal cord compression

Ans: B. Multiple sclerosis

Multiple sclerosis causes upper motor neurone disease. It follows a number of disease patterns but also causes bladder sphincter dysfunction. Optic neuritis may be the first presentation of multiple sclerosis.

11. A 50-year-old man presents with progressive weakness of both legs. He has noticed problems with swallowing and speech. Examination of his legs reveals spastic paraparesis with fasciculations in his upper limbs. Sensory examination is normal. What is the most likely diagnosis?
    A. Guillain-Barré syndrome
    B. Multiple sclerosis
    C. Motor neurone disease (MND)
    D. Brown-Sequard syndrome
    E. Spinal cord compression

Ans: C. Motor neurone disease (MND)

MND is a progressive condition with a combination of upper and lower motor neurone signs. The muscles of speech and swallowing are often involved and there is no sensory disturbance.

12. A 16-year-old girl presents with bilateral lower limb weakness of two days' onset. She had a preceding episode of diarrhoea 2 weeks previously. Examination reveals a bilateral lower motor neurone weakness of both legs. Sensory examination is normal. What is the most likely diagnosis?
    A. Guillain-Barré syndrome
    B. Multiple sclerosis
    C. Motor neurone disease (MND)
    D. Brown-Sequard syndrome
    E. Spinal cord compression

Ans: A. Guillain-Barré syndrome

This often follows a diarrhoea or flu-like illness and is usually self-limiting although recovery may be incomplete. There will be muscle weakness in the limbs and in severe cases bulbar and respiratory muscles may be involved. Less commonly, there may be autonomic nervous system involvement.

13. A 60-year-old man describes a gradual loss of hearing in his left ear occurring over a few months. He hears tinnitus and is troubled by mild intermittent vertigo unrelated to head position. What is the most likely diagnosis?
    A. Multiple sclerosis
    B. Benign paroxysmal positional vertigo (BPPV)
    C. Acoustic neuroma
    D. Meniere's disease

Ans: C. Acoustic neuroma

An acoustic neuroma is a benign, slow growing neoplasm of the Schwann cells of the eighth cranial nerve. Most patients present with unilateral, sensorineural deafness developing gradually over a period of months or years. A small percentage will have sudden hearing loss. Vertigo, which may be quite mild, and tinnitus are common.

IM6.12

14. A 62-year-old man presented with a 1-week history of progressive headache and intermittent weakness of his right arm. His wife said that he had not been himself in recent days and his behaviour had not seemed normal. He had been complaining of a painful rear tooth for some time and had generally poor dentition. On clinical examination, temperature was 37.0°C. He had a mild right arm upper motor neurone pattern weakness. Investigations: Haemoglobin 13.5 g/dL, White cell count 16,000/cmm. A noncontrast CT scan of brain showed a subtle abnormality in the left frontoparietal region. What is the next most appropriate diagnostic step?
 A. Lumbar puncture
 B. Blood culture
 C. Serum procalcitonin
 D. Magnetic resonance imaging
 E. Neurosurgical referral for biopsy

Ans: D. Magnetic resonance imaging

This patient is presenting with clinical features of a space-occupying lesion with focal neurological signs. Although he has no documented fever, that does not rule out an abscess as a possible cause of his symptoms. The noncontrast CT scan abnormality means that additional imaging is required to characterise the region of concern. A magnetic resonance imaging is likely to yield the most useful information in terms of a possible abscess and should be requested if available.

IM17.1

15. A 35-year-old woman complains of recurrent unilateral episodes of headaches that last up to 1 hour. During episodes of headaches, she also suffers from conjunctival injection, lacrimation and miosis. The headaches are retro-orbital. What is the most likely diagnosis?
 A. Giant cell arteritis
 B. Migraine
 C. Trigeminal neuralgia
 D. Cluster headaches
 E. Sinusitis

Ans: D. Cluster headaches

The pain is ipsilateral and related to ocular structures. There is the absence of aura (migraines) or a band-like headache (tension headache). Cluster headaches present with very intense pain localised around one eye that lasts for 15 minutes to 3 hours. There may be simultaneous lacrimation, miosis and nasal congestion. The episodes may occur in cluster several months apart.

16. A 28-year-old man has a sudden onset occipital headache and vomiting. On fundoscopy examination, the left eye has a subhyaloid haemorrhage. What is the most likely diagnosis?
 A. Giant cell arteritis
 B. Sagittal sinus thrombosis
 C. Meningitis
 D. Intracerebral haemorrhage
 E. Subarachnoid haemorrhage

Ans: E. Subarachnoid haemorrhage

Subhyaloid haemorrhages are seen in subarachnoid haemorrhages, traumatic vessel rupture and hypertension. A classic feature of subarachnoid haemorrhage is sudden-onset 'thunderclap' headaches in the occipital region.

IM17.1

17. A 47-year-old medical secretary visits her doctor with a 6-month history of headaches. The headaches occur across her forehead and tend to get worse throughout the day. She does not have any associated vomiting or visual disturbance. What is the most likely diagnosis?
 A. Giant cell arteritis
 B. Temporomandibular joint (TMJ) dysfunction
 C. Trigeminal neuralgia
 D. Migraine
 E. Tension headache

Ans: E. Tension headache

Tension headaches occur in a band across the forehead and get worse throughout the working day. There will be no aura or red flag features and they may disappear during annual leave.

IM19.2

18. A 68-year-old man has micrographia, a pill-rolling tremor and a stooped, stiff posture. What is the most likely gait present in this patient?
 A. Antalgic gait
 B. Festinating gait
 C. Cerebellar ataxic gait
 D. Circumduction gait
 E. Waddling gait

Ans: B. Festinating gait

A festinating gait is seen in Parkinsonism. It appears as a narrow-based, shuffling gait with a broken turn and reduced arm swing.

IM19.2

19. A 40-year-old woman presents with hypotonia, an intention tremor and slurred speech. What is the most likely gait present?
 A. Circumduction gait
 B. Festinating gait
 C. Cerebellar ataxic gait
 D. Antalgic gait
 E. Waddling gait

Ans: C. Cerebellar ataxic gait

Cerebellar signs include broad-based unstable gait, intention tremor, slurred speech, nystagmus, dysdiadochokinesis, past pointing and hypotonia.

IM19.2

20. A 35-year-old man presents with his partner who is worried as she feels that there are changes in his personality and cognition. He adds that he has worsening jerky, random movements, which he is unable to control. His father died at the age of 45 years. On examination, he has jerky, uncontrollable movements of hands. What is the most likely diagnosis?
 A. Wernicke's encephalopathy

B. Huntington's disease
C. Alzheimer's disease
D. Vascular dementia
E. Parkinson's disease

Ans: B. Huntington's disease

Huntington's disease is a progressive neurodegenerative autosomal dominant disorder. It results in abnormal involuntary writhing movements (chorea) followed by the development of cognitive and psychiatric symptoms.

IM17.1

21. A 30-year-old investment banker presents with frontal headaches that occur at work. He describes each episode of headache as a constant pressure especially behind the eyes. Physical examination is normal. What is the most likely diagnosis?
A. Cervical spondylosis
B. Giant cell arteritis
C. Trigeminal neuralgia
D. Temperomandibular joint (TMJ) dysfunction
E. Tension headache

Ans: E. Tension headache

Tight band sensations, pressure behind the eyes, throbbing and bursting sensations are common in tension headaches. It can be precipitated by stress, noise, eyestrain or hunger. Physical exam is usually normal. Treatment is with simple analgesia, addressing precipitating factors and reassurance.

IM24.15

22. A patient in hospital has a homonomous superior quadrantanopia. Where is the most likely lesion?
A. Parietal lobe
B. Temporal lobe
C. Occipital lobe
D. Frontal lobe
E. Optic chiasm

Ans: B. Temporal lobe

This is the most likely lesion site.

IM24.15

23. A patient presents to the emergency department with visual disturbance. On examination there is a homonomous inferior quadrantanopia with no other neurological deficit. Where is the most likely lesion?
A. Parietal lobe
B. Temporal lobe
C. Occipital lobe
D. Frontal lobe
E. Optic chiasm

Ans: A. Parietal lobe

This is the most likely lesion site as the optic radiations through the parietal lobe tend to account for visual field from inferior quadrants.

IM17.1

24. A 60-year-old woman presents with a 2-week history of gradually worsening occipital headache. The pain is made worse by coughing and tends to improve as the day goes on. Which of the following is the most likely cause of headache in this patient?
A. Temporal arteritis
B. Dental abscess
C. Trigeminal neuralgia
D. Tension headache
E. Raised intracranial pressure.

Ans: E. Raised intracranial pressure.

Headache due to raised intracranial pressure may be worse in the morning, or when coughing or straining; it may improve when standing up.

IM17.3

25. A 16-year-old girl presents with a 2-year history of episodic, unilateral throbbing headache associated with vomiting and photophobia. Which of the following is the most likely cause of headache in this patient?
A. Migraine
B. Temporal arteritis
C. Cervical disc protrusion at C5/6
D. Dental abscess
E. Raised intracranial pressure

Ans: A. Migraine

Classic migraine is unilateral and associated with photophobia; it affects young women more than any other patient group.

26. An 80-year-old woman presents with pain over her forehead, which was previously the site of an episode of shingles. Which of the following is the most likely cause of headache in this patient?
A. Acute bacterial meningitis
B. Cervical disc protrusion at C5/6
C. Dental abscess
D. Migraine
E. Postherpetic neuralgia

Ans: E. Postherpetic neuralgia

Postherpetic neuralgia is a common complication following herpes zoster infection, affecting 50% of patients over 60 years.

IM18.7

27. A patient who is unable to write and speak in an understandable manner but who can understand the questions asked and emit sounds most likely has an injury in the:
A. Left frontal lobe
B. Right frontal lobe
C. Left temporal lobe
D. Right temporal lobe
E. Left parietal lobe

Ans: A. Left frontal lobe

The Broca's area, which is essential for speech production, is located in the lower frontal circumvolution of the dominant hemisphere with respect to human language (in most cases, the left hemisphere). Damage to the Broca's area results in expressive aphasia. Patients with expressive aphasia have difficulty speaking and writing, although they can understand language relatively well.

IM19.2

28. A 36-year-old man is distressed by the development of jerky, random and uncontrollable movements, which originally started as restlessness and small, unintentionally initiated movements. His father developed similar symptoms at 40 years of age. What is the most likely diagnosis?
    A. Huntington's chorea
    B. Essential tremor
    C. Hemiballismus
    D. Parkinson's disease
    E. Wilson's disease

Ans: A. Huntington's chorea

An autosomal dominant mutation resulting in neurodegeneration. Acetylcholine and gamma-aminobutyric acid secretion from the corpus striatum is impaired with neuronal loss causing unintentional movements.

IM19.2

29. An 87-year-old man undergoes a postmortem. He had suffered from tremors, rigidity and akinesia for the last 10 years of his life. The pathologist reports that there are eosinophilic inclusion bodies present at the substantia nigra. What is the most likely diagnosis?
    A. Huntington's chorea
    B. Essential tremor
    C. Hemiballismus
    D. Parkinson's disease
    E. Wilson's disease

Ans: D. Parkinson's disease

Lewy bodies are described which cause loss of dopamine containing neurons in the substantia nigra resulting in tremor, rigidity, bradykinesia and postural instability.

IM18.2|IM24.9

30. An 84-year-old man presents to the Emergency Department with a 4-hour history of right-sided upper and lower limb weakness, right-sided facial droop and slurred speech. His past medical history includes atrial fibrillation. What is the most likely site of the lesion?
    A. Left anterior cerebral artery
    B. Left middle cerebral artery
    C. Left posterior cerebral artery
    D. Left superior cerebellar artery
    E. Left vertebral artery

Ans: B. Left middle cerebral artery

Occlusion of the MCA causes a contralateral paralysis that affects the arm, lower part of the face and leg, with contralateral sensory loss or inattention and a loss of language with dominant hemisphere involvement.

31. A 45-year-old woman presents with headache and an increase in her glove and shoe size. Her family have commented that her facial skin has become coarse and spaces between her lower teeth have appeared. You examine her visual fields. What is the most likely visual lesion you would expect?
    A. Central scotoma
    B. Bitemporal hemianopia
    C. Homonymous hemianopia
    D. Quadrantanopia
    E. Tunnel vision

Ans: B. Bitemporal hemianopia

She has features of acromegaly. A pituitary somatotroph adenoma can compress the optic chiasma and the afferents fibres from the nasal half of the retina from each eye as they cross in the chiasma causing visual loss.

IM17.11

32. A 30-year-old woman complains of a unilateral headache which appears to be initiated after eating chocolate or a glass of wine. The throbbing headache is preceded by flashing lights. The headaches last for 72 hours. Examination is unremarkable. What is the appropriate treatment of this patient's headache?
    A. Carbamazepine
    B. Sumatriptan
    C. Lithium
    D. Propranolol
    E. Tricyclic antidepressants

Ans: B. Sumatriptan

This patient has migraine.

IM17.11

33. A 40-year-old male smoker complains of recurrent headaches that occur daily for periods of 4 weeks at a time. Peri-orbit pain occurs on the left, and the eye is constantly watering. The GP examines him during an attack and notes that his left eye is injected, watering and the pupil is constricted. What is the appropriate treatment of this patient's facial pain?
    A. Carbamazepine
    B. Sumatriptan
    C. Lithium
    D. Propranolol
    E. Tricyclic antidepressants

Ans: B. Sumatriptan

This patient has cluster headache.

34. A 21-year-old girl presents to the emergency as she has been unsteady on her feet for a day, having had diarrhoea during the previous week. On examination, she is afebrile, has reduced muscle power and tone, and no tendon reflexes can be elicited in her lower limbs. Twelve hours later, she is unable to stand and the tendon reflexes in her upper limbs are now absent. She has no other medical problems and has been fully immunised. What is the most likely diagnosis?
    A. Guillain–Barré syndrome
    B. Myasthenia gravis
    C. Myotonic dystrophy
    D. Poliomyelitis
    E. Spinal muscular atrophy

Ans: A. Guillain–Barré syndrome

Guillain–Barré syndrome (postinfectious polyneuropathy). The classical presentation is with ascending weakness. It may follow Campylobacter gastroenteritis. She must be closely monitored, as a serious complication is respiratory failure. To monitor her respiratory function, you can ask her to cough (or sing) to assess diaphragmatic function and involvement of the nerves supplying the chest muscles

IM24.6

IM18.6

35. A 54-year-old woman has been referred to the neurologist with symptoms of nasal regurgitation of fluids and choking. She is otherwise fit and well and has no other past medical history. On examination, you find she has a fasciculating tongue and weakness of her palate. What condition is she suffering from?
   A. Acute cerebral vascular accident
   B. Myasthenia gravis
   C. Progressive bulbar palsy
   D. Progressive muscular atrophy
   E. Multiple sclerosis

Ans: C. Progressive bulbar palsy

Degeneration of motor neurons in the brain stem producing signs of lower motor neurone involvement producing lower cranial nerves involvement.

IM18.2

36. A 65-year-old woman presents to the Emergency Department with a 2-hour history of weakness in her left upper and lower limbs. Her past medical history shows that she suffers from atrial fibrillation, hypertension and type 2 diabetes. On neurological examination, she has no cranial nerve abnormalities and no focal motor or sensory abnormalities in the upper or lower limbs. What is the most likely diagnosis?
   A. Carotid artery dissection
   B. Transient ischaemic attack
   C. Transient global amnesia
   D. Dissecting aortic aneurysm
   E. Thromboembolic infarct

Ans: B. Transient ischaemic attack

Neurological symptoms disappearing in less than 24 hours and usually much briefer than this.

IM17.1

37. A 34-year-old man presents to the Emergency Department with a severe left-sided headache that woke him from his sleep. He is now complaining of a severe pain on the back of his left eye. He states that he has had this before and it typically lasts for about 30 minutes. He has suffered from these attacks for the past few nights. On this occasion, he denies any vomiting but he states that he has vomited with previous episodes. He is also complaining that his left nostril feels congested. On examination you find no abnormalities. What is your diagnosis?
   A. Cluster headache
   B. Migraine
   C. Tension headache
   D. Subarachnoid haemorrhage (SAH)
   E. Sinusitis

Ans: A. Cluster headache

A typical description of bouts of severe unilateral pain, often with nasal or eye symptoms.

IM19.2

38. A 55-year-old woman consults her doctor because she has noticed a problem with her hands shaking. She has had the tremors for 5 years and it is present in both hands. Tremors are worst when she is trying to perform a task and may subside when her hands are in her lap. She tells the doctor that they often improve with a glass of alcohol only to come back again. She has normal cranial nerve function including olfaction. She does not know whether she has a family history of any movement disorder. What is the most likely diagnosis?
   A. Dystonia
   B. Essential tremor
   C. Huntington's disease
   D. Idiopathic Parkinson's disease
   E. Vascular parkinsonism

Ans: B. Essential tremor

This is an often hereditary, alcohol sensitive, bilateral tremor without a rotational component.

39. A 25-year-old man with no significant past medical history presents with a 48-hour history of bilateral limb weakness initially affecting his feet but gradually ascending to involve his knees and hips. He has had some shooting pains and numbness in his feet over the same period. There is no associated autonomic dysfunction and no history of neck or back pain or injury. His sphincter function is intact. He describes a flu-like illness approximately 2 weeks previously. On examination, there is a bilateral, symmetrical pure lower motor neurone weakness of both lower limbs to the hip. What is the most appropriate next step?
   A. Measure vital capacity
   B. CT spine
   C. Measure peak expiratory flow rate
   D. Administer edrophonium
   E. Start immediate intravenous corticosteroids

Ans: A. Measure vital capacity

The most likely diagnosis is of Guillain–Barré syndrome—the main causes of death arise from respiratory failure.

6 Diseases of the Liver and Biliary System

Q. Enumerate important functions of liver. (PY 4.7)

- Important functions of liver are listed in Box 6.1.

BOX 6.1 Important Functions of Liver

- Carbohydrate metabolism including gluconeogenesis, glycogenolysis and glycogenesis
- Protein metabolism
- Lipid metabolism
- Bilirubin metabolism
- Bile acid formation and secretion
- Vitamin and mineral metabolism
- Hormone metabolism
- Drug and alcohol metabolism
- Cholesterol metabolism
- Synthesis of plasma proteins including clotting factors

Q. Discuss various liver function tests and their significance in jaundice. (PY 4.8)

BILIRUBIN IN THE BLOOD

- Normal serum bilirubin level is 0.3–1.0 mg/dL.
- Hyperbilirubinaemia may be of conjugated or unconjugated type.
    - Unconjugated hyperbilirubinaemia is characterised by a serum level less than 6 mg/dL and absence of bilirubinuria. The other tests of liver function are normal. Examples are haemolytic diseases, ineffective erythropoiesis and Gilbert's syndrome.
    - Conjugated hyperbilirubinaemia is generally characterised by higher levels of bilirubin and bilirubinuria. The other tests of liver function are often abnormal. Examples are parenchymal liver diseases and biliary tract obstructions.
    - Fluctuating hyperbilirubinaemia is seen in gallstones, carcinoma of ampulla of Vater, chronic hepatitis, haemolytic anaemias and Gilbert's syndrome.

BILIRUBIN IN THE URINE

- Normally, bilirubin cannot be detected in urine.
- In unconjugated hyperbilirubinaemia, there will be no bilirubin in the urine. Thus, absence of bilirubin in the urine in a jaundiced patient points to unconjugated hyperbilirubinaemia.
- In conjugated hyperbilirubinaemia, urine contains bilirubin. Thus, bilirubinuria in a jaundiced patient points to conjugated hyperbilirubinaemia (hepatobiliary disease).

URINE UROBILINOGEN

- Urinary urobilinogen is detected by Ehrlich's aldehyde test.
- No urobilinogen in urine in case of obstructive jaundice (bilirubinuria present).
- Increased urobilinogen in urine in viral hepatitis, cirrhosis, malignancy and heart failure (bilirubinuria present).
- Markedly increased urobilinogen in urine in case of haemolytic diseases (no bilirubinuria).

ENZYMES

AMINOTRANSFERASES

- Aspartate aminotransferase (AST, SGOT—serum glutamic oxaloacetic transaminase) and alanine aminotransferase (ALT, SGPT—serum glutamic pyruvic transaminase).
    - Normal value 5–40 IU/L.
    - Aminotransferase levels are useful to differentiate between hepatocellular jaundice and obstructive jaundice.
- Drugs such as erythromycin and furosemide may produce falsely elevated aminotransferase levels.

Alanine Aminotransferase

- Concentration of ALT is much higher in the liver than in other tissues (e.g. kidney, heart muscle). Hence, a raised ALT is a very sensitive index of hepatic damage.
    - 100–500 times rise occurs in paracetamol-induced liver damage.
    - 10–100 times rise occurs in:
        - Viral hepatitis (increase in ALT associated with hepatitis C infection tends to be more than that associated with hepatitis A or B).
        - Acute drug-induced hepatitis.
        - Acute circulatory failure (ischaemic liver injury).
        - Exacerbations of chronic hepatitis.
    - 2–10 times rise occurs in:
        - Infectious mononucleosis.
        - Cytomegalovirus infections.
    - Less than fivefold rise occurs in:
        - Alcoholic hepatitis (AST:ALT ratio >2).
        - Obstructive jaundice.
        - Cirrhosis of liver.
        - Nonalcoholic fatty liver.
        - Chronic hepatitis.
    - Pyridoxal 5´-phosphate is a coenzyme required for synthesis of transaminases, especially ALT. This enzyme is deficient in alcoholic patients; hence, AST:ALT ratio is more than 2 in patients with alcoholic liver disease.

Aspartate Aminotransferase

- AST exists as two different isoenzymes: mitochondrial and cytoplasmic form.
- AST is found in highest concentration in liver and heart compared with other tissues of the body such as skeletal muscle, kidney and brain.
- Elevated mitochondrial AST is seen in extensive tissue necrosis during myocardial infarction and also in acute and chronic liver diseases.
- About 80% of AST activity of liver is contributed by mitochondrial isoenzyme, whereas most of circulating AST activity in normal people is derived from cytosolic isoenzyme.
- A ratio of AST/ALT is >5, especially if ALT is normal or slightly elevated, is suggestive of injury to extrahepatic tissues, such as skeletal muscle in the case of rhabdomyolysis or strenuous exercise.

- ALT is present in highest concentration in periportal hepatocytes and in lowest concentration in hepatocytes surrounding the central vein. AST is present in hepatocytes at more constant levels.
- Hepatocytes around the central vein have the lowest oxygen concentration and thus are more prone to damage in the setting of acute hepatic ischaemia which results in AST value greater than ALT.
- After there is no further injury to hepatocytes, rate of decline of AST and ALT depends on their rate of clearance from the circulation. Plasma half-life of ALT is nearly three times that of AST. Hence, AST declines more rapidly than ALT, and ALT may be higher than AST in the recovery phase of injury.
- Falsely low serum AST (but not ALT) is seen in patients with renal failure or those taking isoniazid. In patients with renal failure, serum AST level increases significantly after haemodialysis.

ALKALINE PHOSPHATASE

- Serum contains alkaline phosphatase (ALP) activity derived from liver, bone, intestines, proximal tubules of kidneys and placenta. Normal serum level is 3–13 KA units (80–240 IU/L).
- In hepatocellular jaundice, only very small amount of ALP is liberated from the cells and the rise in ALP is less than 2.5-fold.
- In obstructive jaundice, due to obstruction of biliary tract at any level, new ALP is synthesised that escapes into blood. Hence, ALP levels are markedly raised in obstructive jaundice.
- If the source of ALP is not clear, determine the levels of two enzymes, γ-glutamyl transpeptidase (GGT) and 5′-nucleotidase. These are more specific for liver. The associated elevation of these two enzymes confirms the source of ALP as liver.
- Causes of raised ALP are given in the Box 6.2.
- Low levels of ALP can be present in patients with fulminant Wilson's disease, hypophosphatasia and haemolytic anaemia.

BOX 6.2 Causes of Elevated Serum Alkaline Phosphatase

- Choledocholithiasis
- Acute cholangitis
- Malignant bile duct obstruction—malignancies involving pancreas, gallbladder, ampulla of Vater, bile duct; metastasis to perihilar lymph nodes
- Biliary stricture
- Infections—AIDS cholangiopathy, roundworm, liver flukes
- Infiltrative disorders of liver (sarcoidosis, tuberculosis, lymphomas)
- Cholestasis—later phase of acute hepatitis, intrahepatic cholestasis of pregnancy, primary sclerosing cholangitis
- Primary biliary cholangitis
- Liver abscess
- Metastatic carcinoma to liver
- Metastatic bone tumours
- Paget's disease
- Adolescence
- Rickets and osteomalacia
- Sepsis
- Hyperparathyroidism
- Pregnancy
- Tumours of GI tract
- Drugs (antibiotics, antiepileptics and anabolic steroids)
- Total parenteral nutrition

γ-GLUTAMYL TRANSPEPTIDASE

- GGT is a microsomal enzyme present in hepatocytes and biliary epithelial cells, renal tubules, pancreas and intestine.
- Raised levels occur in biliary obstruction and parenchymal damage, but not in patients with bone disease.
- But more important is its rise in acute alcoholism. So, it is useful to detect and follow alcohol abuse in patients who deny it. Raised levels suggest prolonged intake of more than 60 g alcohol/day.
- Other causes of elevated GGT include nonalcoholic fatty liver, chronic obstructive lung disease, diabetes mellitus, hyperthyroidism, obesity and renal failure. It is also raised in patients taking barbiturates or phenytoin.

PLASMA PROTEINS

- Albumin is synthesised in liver. In chronic liver diseases like cirrhosis and chronic hepatitis, serum albumin is low. Fall indicates severe liver cell damage and bad prognosis. Normal serum albumin level is 4–5.5 g/dL.
- Globulins are synthesised by the reticuloendothelial system. The level rises in chronic liver diseases. Normal serum globulin level is 1.5–3.5 g/dL.
  - IgG is mainly raised in chronic hepatitis and cryptogenic cirrhosis.
  - IgA is mainly raised in alcoholic liver disease.
  - IgM is mainly raised in primary biliary cholangitis (previously called primary biliary cirrhosis.

COAGULATION FACTORS

- Liver synthesises all the coagulation factors, except factor VIII. Vitamin K is required to activate some factors. Prothrombin time depends on factors I, II, V, VII and X and it gets prolonged when the plasma concentration of any one of these falls below 30% of normal.
- Among vitamin K-dependent factors, factor VII is the most sensitive marker of liver injury due to shortest half-life time.
- Prothrombin time (normal value 11–12.5 seconds) is prolonged in:
  - Severe liver damage as in acute hepatitis, for example viral hepatitis.
  - Prolonged biliary obstruction that reduces vitamin K absorption.
  - Deficiency of vitamin K (including malabsorption, poor intake and antibiotic therapy which produces destruction of vitamin K-producing commensals).
  - Consumption coagulopathy.

CERULOPLASMIN

- Synthesised in liver and is an acute phase reactant.
- It binds with copper and serves as a major carrier for copper in the blood.

- Normal plasma level of ceruloplasmin is 20–60 mg/dL.
- Levels are elevated in infections, rheumatoid arthritis, pregnancy, liver diseases and obstructive jaundice.
- In Wilson's disease, ceruloplasmin level is depressed due to decreased rate of synthesis. Low levels may also be seen in neonates, Menkes' disease, kwashiorkor, marasmus, protein-losing enteropathy and copper deficiency.

BROMSULPHTHALEIN CLEARANCE

- Bromsulphthalein (BSP) clearance is delayed in Dubin–Johnson syndrome. Not done at present.

SUMMARY OF LIVER FUNCTION TESTS (Box 6.3)

BOX 6.3 Liver Function Tests—Summary

Test	Indicates
Bilirubin	Transport
Aminotransferases	Hepatocellular damage
Alkaline phosphatase (ALP)	Biliary tract obstruction
γ-glutamyl transpeptidase (GGT)	Enzyme induction
Proteins	Synthesis
Coagulation tests	Synthesis

Q. Write a short note on alpha-foetoprotein.

- α-Foetoprotein is mainly synthesised in foetal liver. Its production falls to low levels after birth.
- It acts as a transporter for several ligands, such as bilirubin, fatty acids, retinoids, steroids, heavy metals and possibly various drugs.
- Conditions associated with elevated levels of α-foetoprotein are given in Box 6.4.

Q. Briefly discuss the indications and significance of liver biopsy.

- Liver biopsy can be performed via three routes: percutaneous (most common), transjugular and laparoscopic.

BOX 6.4 Conditions Associated With Elevated α-Foetoprotein

- Hepatocellular carcinoma.
- Carcinomas of stomach, pancreas, gallbladder, bile ducts and lungs.
- Embryonic carcinomas.
- Viral hepatitis.
- Chronic hepatitis.
- Cirrhosis (markedly elevated level indicates development of hepatocellular carcinoma)
- Ataxia telangiectasia.

INDICATIONS (Box 6.5)

BOX 6.5 Indications of Liver Biopsy

- Suspected cirrhosis—clinical suspicion but not proved with other investigations; differentiating fatty liver without fibrosis from cirrhosis.
- Hepatic malignancy—primary (hepatoma) and secondaries
- Chronic hepatitis—for diagnosis, assessing the severity and stage of liver damage, assessing response to treatment
- Diagnosis of granulomatous diseases—tuberculosis, leprosy, sarcoidosis
- Storage and metabolic disorders—amyloidosis, glycogen storage disorders, haemochromatosis, Wilson's disease
- Pyrexia of unknown origin (when associated with hepatomegaly)—brucellosis, tuberculosis, lymphoproliferative malignancies
- Acute jaundice—if diagnosis not clear on routine investigations
- Staging of lymphoma
- After liver transplantation—to assess for rejection or presence of disease recurrence

COMPLICATIONS (Box 6.6)

BOX 6.6 Complications of Liver Biopsy

Pain	Bile peritonitis
Bleeding—intraperitoneal, haemobilia, intrahepatic or subcapsular haematoma	Haemothorax and pneumothorax
Sepsis	Malignant needle-track seeding

Q. Enumerate the contraindications of liver biopsy.

- Contraindications for liver biopsy are shown in Box 6.7.

Q. What is hepatic elastography? Explain briefly. (IM 5.13)

- Liver fibrosis is a response induced by chronic liver injury. It may lead to advanced liver cirrhosis and hepatocellular carcinoma.
- Conventional liver tests and imaging studies are not sensitive for hepatic fibrosis, which is an early stage of chronic liver disease and cirrhosis.

BOX 6.7 Contraindications of Liver Biopsy

Significant coagulopathy or thrombocytopenia	NSAID use in last 7 days
Severe jaundice	Haemangioma of liver
Ascites (gross)	Hydatid cyst
Hepatobiliary infections	Hepatocellular failure
Extrahepatic biliary obstruction	Uncooperative patient

- Hepatic elastography is a method for measurement of hepatic fibrosis in a noninvasive way.
- Can be accomplished by ultrasound or magnetic resonance, latter being more accurate.
- Useful to:
  - Estimate existing degree of liver damage.
  - Monitor disease progression or regression via serial measurements.
  - Guide prognosis and further management including treatment.

ULTRASOUND ELASTOGRAPHY

- Uses a mild amplitude, low frequency (50 Hz) vibration transmitted through the liver. It induces an elastic shear wave that is detected by pulse echo ultrasonography as the wave propagates through liver. The velocity of wave correlates with tissue stiffness; the wave travels faster through denser, fibrotic tissue.
- Can sample a much larger area than liver biopsy, providing a better understanding of the entire hepatic parenchyma. Moreover, it can be repeated without risk.
- Less effective in obese patients as adipose tissue attenuates the elastic wave.
- May overestimate degree of fibrosis some condition (Box 6.8).

Q. Explain endoscopic retrograde cholangiopancreatography. (IM 5.13)

- Endoscopic retrograde cholangiopancreatography (ERCP) is an endoscopic technique in which a specialised side-viewing endoscope is guided into the duodenum, allowing for instruments to be passed into the bile and pancreatic ducts.
- The facilities provided by endoscopic retrograde cholangiopancreatography (ERCP) include the following:
  - Direct visualisation and manipulation of the papilla of Vater.
  - Sphincterotomy and stone removal.
  - Manipulations within the common bile duct using balloon catheters, wire baskets and stents.
  - Tissue sampling for patients with pancreatic or biliary cancer.
  - Radiological imaging of biliary tree and pancreatic duct.
- Uses:
  - Biopsy of ampullary carcinoma.
  - Anatomical study of biliary tree and pancreatic duct in cholestasis of unknown cause.
  - Removal of stones from CBD.
  - Biliary drainage in malignant strictures.
  - Dilatation of benign strictures.
- Complications:
  - Pancreatitis (rectal administration of diclofenac or indomethacin just before ERCP reduces incidence of pancreatitis).
  - Cholangitis.
  - Bleeding.
  - Duodenal perforation.

BOX 6.8 Conditions in Which Ultrasound Elastography May Overestimate Fibrosis

- Liver inflammation (e.g. active hepatitis)
- Cholestasis (e.g. biliary obstruction)
- Mass lesions within the liver (e.g. tumour)
- Liver congestion (e.g. heart failure)

Q. Give a brief account of uses and complications of percutaneous transhepatic cholangiography (PTC).

- Procedure involves passing a Chiba needle into the liver under fluoroscopy or ultrasound guidance and injecting contrast material directly into an intrahepatic bile duct. This delineates the entire biliary tract.
- Usually, it is performed for evaluation of patients who are found to have biliary duct dilation on ultrasonography and who are not candidates for ERCP. Not commonly used at present.
- Uses:
  - Documentation and localisation of the site of obstruction of the biliary tract.
  - Preoperative planning of surgery.
  - Stent introduction in malignant strictures.
  - Dilation of benign biliary strictures.
  - Drainage of infected bile in the setting of cholangitis.
- Complications:
  - Bleeding.
  - Infection.
  - Biliary peritonitis.
  - Haemobilia.
- Percutaneous transhepatic biliary drainage (PTBD) is a minimally invasive procedure for drainage of the biliary system in obstructive jaundice when ERCP cannot be done.

Q. Write briefly on magnetic resonance cholangiopancreatography. (IM 5.13)

- It has largely replaced diagnostic ERCP.
- Magnetic resonance cholangiopancreatography (MRCP) is comparable to invasive ERCP for diagnosis of extrahepatic bile duct and pancreatic duct abnormalities such as choledocholithiasis, malignant obstruction of bile and pancreatic ducts, congenital anomalies and chronic pancreatitis.
- Other indications for MRCP usually include unsuccessful ERCP or a contraindication to ERCP.
- It is a little inferior to ERCP in diagnosis of sclerosing cholangitis.

Q. Write a short note on endoscopic ultrasound.

- Gradually replacing ERCP as a diagnostic modality:
  - Useful in imaging pancreatic and biliary diseases such as choledocholithiasis, pancreatic and biliary cancers and cystic lesions of the pancreas.

- In ampullary carcinoma, local tumour extension and regional lymph node metastasis can be evaluated by endoscopic ultrasound (EUS) and not by ERCP.
- Fine-needle aspiration can be performed from suspicious lesions under EUS guidance.
- Useful for other interventions also:
    - Injection of bupivacaine and alcohol into the coeliac ganglia to reduce pain in patients with unresectable pancreatic carcinoma.
    - Endoscopic management of pancreatic pseudocysts (drainage).
    - Localised therapy for pancreatic tumours.
    - Detection of small tumours (benign or malignant) in liver.
    - Liver elastography to detect fibrosis.
    - Guided treatment of gastric varices
    - Biopsy of mediastinal lymph nodes.
- Disadvantages:
    - High cost.
    - High degree of training required.
    - Possibility of missing small stones in the common bile duct.
    - Pigment stones may not produce any shadowing and may be missed.
    - Cannot differentiate benign from malignant tumours at the ampulla of Vater.

Q. What are the sources of bilirubin? Discuss the metabolism of bilirubin. (IM 5.1)

- Bilirubin metabolism can be discussed under the following headings:
    - Normal sources of bilirubin.
    - Transport of bilirubin.
    - Hepatic metabolism.
    - Intestinal phase of bilirubin metabolism.
    - Renal excretion of bilirubin.

NORMAL SOURCES OF BILIRUBIN

- 80%–85% of bilirubin is derived from the catabolism of the haemoglobin of senescent red blood cells (mostly in spleen and Kupffer cells of liver).
- 15%–20% is derived from bone marrow due to the destruction of maturing cells and from liver due to the turnover of haem and haem-containing precursors (cytochromes, myoglobin, catalase, etc.).
- Haem liberated from above sources is oxidised to biliverdin by the enzyme haem oxygenase.
- Biliverdin is then reduced to bilirubin by the enzyme biliverdin reductase present in mononuclear cells (Flowchart 6.1).

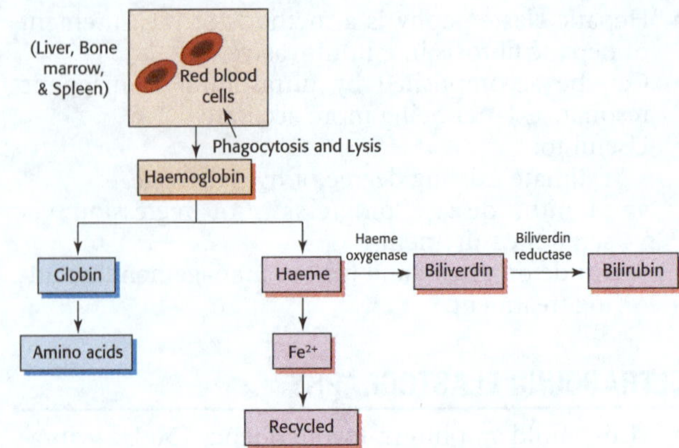

Flowchart 6.1 Formation of Bilirubin.

TRANSPORT OF BILIRUBIN

- Unconjugated bilirubin is liberated into plasma. This unconjugated bilirubin is tightly bound to albumin in a fully reversible manner. Thus, unconjugated bilirubin is transported in the plasma and bound to albumin. Unbound unconjugated bilirubin can cross blood–brain barrier and cause kernicterus in neonates with hyperbilirubinaemia.
- Conjugated bilirubin is also bound to albumin, but both in reversible and irreversible manner.

HEPATIC METABOLISM

- It has three distinct phases:
    - Hepatic uptake.
    - Conjugation.
    - Excretion into bile.

HEPATIC UPTAKE

- Unconjugated bilirubin-albumin complex is subjected to the liver cell, that is hepatocyte. Albumin dissociates and the unconjugated bilirubin enters the cell. In the cell, unconjugated bilirubin gets bound to several of the glutathione-S-transferases. This binding prevents the efflux of unconjugated bilirubin back into plasma.

CONJUGATION

- In the hepatocyte, the unconjugated bilirubin is conjugated by the enzyme bilirubin UDP-glucuronosyltransferase (UGT1A1). The co-substrate for bilirubin conjugation is UDP-glucuronic acid, a ubiquitous intracellular substance derived from glucose.
- Conjugation is a two-step reaction resulting first in the formation of bilirubin monoglucuronide and then bilirubin diglucuronide.
- Why conjugate? Unconjugated bilirubin is water-insoluble and so not excreted into bile. So, it must be converted to a water-soluble derivative (i.e. conjugated bilirubin or bilirubin glucuronide) in order to be excreted by the liver cell into bile.

EXCRETION OR SECRETION INTO BILE

- This is the rate limiting step of bilirubin metabolism. This step is the one that is most susceptible to impairment when liver cell is damaged.
- The secretion across the plasma membrane is by an ATP-dependent transport process mediated by a canalicular membrane protein called multidrug resistance-associated protein 2 (MRP2).

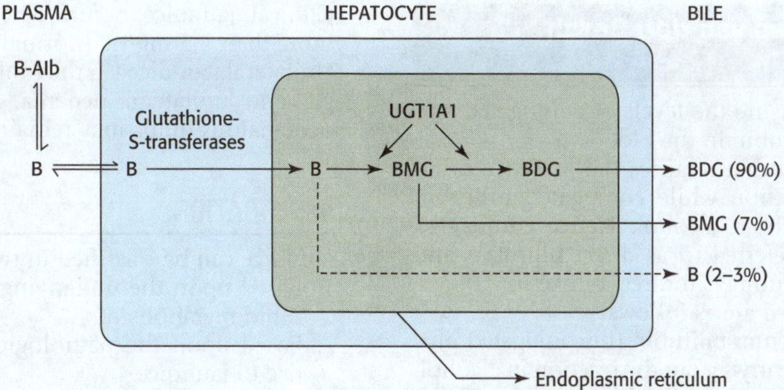

Fig. 6.1 Bilirubin metabolism. Alb, albumin endoplasmic reticulum; B, unconjugated bilirubin; BMG, bilirubin monoglucuronide; BDG, bilirubin diglucuronide; UGT1A1, UDP-glucuronosyltransferase.

- So conjugated bilirubin is secreted into bile. Normal bile contains 90% of bilirubin diglucuronide and 7% of bilirubin monoglucuronide with remaining 2%–3% as unconjugated bilirubin.
- When this step is compromised, two consequences occur:
  1. Decreased excretion of bilirubin into bile.
  2. Regurgitation or re-entry of conjugated bilirubin into the blood stream (conjugated hyperbilirubinaemia).
- Fig. 6.1 depicts bilirubin metabolism in the liver.

INTESTINAL PHASE OF BILIRUBIN METABOLISM

- Conjugated bilirubin (bilirubin diglucuronide and bilirubin monoglucuronide) reaches the intestinal lumen through bile. Conjugated bilirubin as such is not reabsorbed by the intestinal mucosa.
- This conjugated bilirubin has got two fates:
  1. Part of this conjugated bilirubin is excreted in the stool as such, that is bilirubin diglucuronide and bilirubin monoglucuronide.
  2. Rest of the conjugated bilirubin is metabolised in the lumen to urobilinogen by the action of intestinal bacteria. This urobilinogen has three fates:
     a. Part of this urobilinogen is reabsorbed from small intestine into the portal circulation, thus reaching liver (enterohepatic circulation). The liver re-excretes this urobilinogen into bile.
     b. Part of the urobilinogen is reabsorbed and excreted in the urine as urobilinogen (up to 4 mg/day).
        - So normal urine contains urobilinogen.
        - In obstructive jaundice or severe intrahepatic cholestasis, urobilinogen is absent in the urine.
        - In hepatocellular disease, haemolytic disease or intestinal bacterial overgrowth, urinary urobilinogen is increased markedly (more than 4 mg/day).
     c. Part of the urobilinogen in the intestine is excreted in the stool as stercobilinogen. Stercobilinogen gives the stool its normal colour. In obstructive jaundice, stercobilinogen is absent in the stool, and hence stools are pale or clay coloured.

RENAL EXCRETION OF BILIRUBIN

- In normal individuals, there is no bilirubin in urine since unconjugated bilirubin is tightly bound to albumin and hence not filtered by glomeruli.
- But with regard to conjugated bilirubin, a small fraction (5%) is less tightly bound to albumin and another small fraction is unbound. This unbound fraction is filtered and appears in the urine as bilirubin (bilirubinuria).
- So in contrast to unconjugated hyperbilirubinaemia, bilirubin appears in the urine in conjugated hyperbilirubinaemia (including obstructive jaundice).

BILIRUBIN METABOLISM—SUMMARY (Flowchart 6.2)

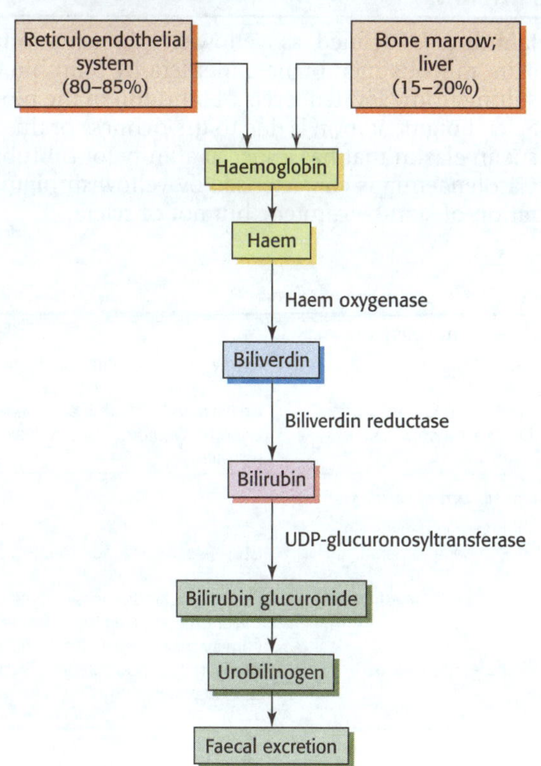

Flowchart 6.2 Summary of Bilirubin Metabolism.

Q. Briefly discuss van den Bergh reaction.

- It is meant to measure the levels of conjugated and unconjugated bilirubin in the blood.
- Unconjugated bilirubin requires the presence of alcohol for the reaction while conjugated bilirubin reacts directly without alcohol. Hence conjugated bilirubin is also referred to as direct bilirubin and unconjugated bilirubin as indirect bilirubin.
- Three steps involved are as follows:
  a. Measure total serum bilirubin (unconjugated plus conjugated) by carrying out the reaction in alcohol.
  b. Measure direct reacting bilirubin (conjugated) by carrying out the test without alcohol.
  c. Calculate indirect reacting bilirubin (unconjugated bilirubin) by finding the difference between total and conjugated bilirubin.
- Based on the van den Bergh reaction, the hyperbilirubinaemias can be classified into two types:
  a. Predominantly unconjugated hyperbilirubinaemia—where 80%–85% of total serum bilirubin is measured as indirect reacting (unconjugated).
  b. Predominantly conjugated hyperbilirubinaemia—where more than 50% of total serum bilirubin is of direct reacting type (conjugated).

Q. Enumerate the causes of jaundice. How will you arrive at the aetiology of jaundice? Give the points of differentiation in clinical features and investigations. (IM 5.1)

DEFINITION

- Jaundice is defined as yellowish pigmentation of skin, mucous membrane and sclera by bilirubin, resulting from elevated levels of bilirubin in the blood. Scleral pigmentation is due to the richness of this tissue in elastin that has a special affinity for bilirubin.
- Carotenaemia is characterised by yellowish pigmentation of skin by carotene but not of sclera.
- Clinical jaundice occurs when serum bilirubin is more than 2.5 mg/dL (normal is 0.3–1.0 mg/dL).
- Unilateral jaundice (in the limbs) is seen in hemiplegia and unilateral oedema. The hemiplegic and oedematous limbs may remain uncoloured.

CLASSIFICATION

- Jaundice can be classified in two ways:
  1. Based upon the underlying derangement of bilirubin metabolism.
  2. Based upon the pathological mechanism giving rise to jaundice.

CLASSIFICATION BASED ON THE UNDERLYING DERANGEMENT OF BILIRUBIN METABOLISM (Table 6.1)

- Predominantly unconjugated hyperbilirubinaemia.
- Predominantly conjugated hyperbilirubinaemia.

CLASSIFICATION OF JAUNDICE BASED ON THE PATHOLOGICAL MECHANISM GIVING RISE TO JAUNDICE (Box 6.9)

Haemolytic Jaundice

- Results from increased destruction of red blood cells or their precursors, resulting in increased production of unconjugated bilirubin. Various causes are given in Table 6.2.

Clinical Features

- Pallor due to anaemia.
- Jaundice is mild; no other signs of liver disease.
- Hepatosplenomegaly due to increased reticuloendothelial activity.
- Dark stools due to increased stercobilinogen.
- Urine turns dark yellow on standing due to increased urobilinogen in the urine getting converted to urobilin.

Investigations

- No bilirubin in urine.
- Urinary urobilinogen is increased (more than 4 mg/24 hours).

TABLE 6.1 Classification of Jaundice Based on Underlying Derangement of Bilirubin Metabolism

PREDOMINANTLY UNCONJUGATED	
• Overproduction	Extravascular or intravascular haemolysis, ineffective erythropoiesis, reabsorption of large haematoma, extravasation of blood in tissues
• Decreased hepatic uptake	Drugs (e.g. flavaspidic acid, atazanavir), sepsis, heart failure, portosystemic shunts
• Decreased conjugation	Gilbert's syndrome, Crigler–Najjar syndrome, neonatal jaundice, acquired transferase deficiency (e.g. cirrhosis, hepatitis)
PREDOMINANTLY CONJUGATED	
• Intrahepatic causes	
• Familial and hereditary	Dubin–Johnson syndrome, Rotor syndrome, recurrent benign intrahepatic cholestasis, cholestatic jaundice of pregnancy
• Acquired disorders	Hepatocellular diseases—acute viral hepatitis, alcoholic liver disease, nonalcoholic steatohepatitis, drug-induced liver injury, toxin-induced liver injury (e.g. amatoxin from mushrooms), autoimmune hepatitis, chronic hepatitis, cirrhosis, primary biliary cholangitis, ischaemic hepatitis, Wilson's disease, haemochromatosis, sepsis, total parenteral nutrition
• Extrahepatic causes	Stone in common bile duct, tumours and strictures of bile duct, primary sclerosing cholangitis, pancreatitis, periampullary carcinoma, carcinoma head of pancreas

Note: In hepatocellular disease (cirrhosis and hepatitis), there is usually interference in all three major steps of bilirubin metabolism—uptake, conjugation and excretion. However, excretion is the rate-limiting step, and is usually impaired to the greatest extent. As a result, conjugated hyperbilirubinaemia predominates.

BOX 6.9 Classification of Jaundice Based on Pathological Mechanism

- Congenital, nonhaemolytic jaundice (see page 430)
- Haemolytic jaundice
- Hepatocellular jaundice
- Cholestatic jaundice

TABLE 6.2 Causes of Haemolysis

• Intraerythrocytic defects	
• Hereditary	Spherocytosis, sickle cell disease, thalassaemia, G6PD deficiency
• Acquired	B_{12} and folate deficiency
• Extraerythrocytic defects	Antibodies (autoimmune and isoimmune haemolytic anaemias), malaria, prosthetic heart valves, drugs like sulphasalazine and dapsone, paroxysmal nocturnal haemoglobinuria, snake bite, copper sulphate poisoning

- Serum bilirubin is raised (less than 6 mg/dL).
- Predominantly unconjugated hyperbilirubinaemia.
- Other liver function tests are normal.
- Evidence of haemolytic anaemia.

Hepatocellular Jaundice

- Bilirubin transport across the hepatocyte may be impaired at any point between the uptake of unconjugated bilirubin into the cell and transport of conjugated bilirubin into biliary canaliculi.
- In addition, swelling of cells and oedema due to inflammation causes mechanical obstruction of intrahepatic biliary tree.
- Hence in hepatocellular jaundice, concentration of both unconjugated and conjugated bilirubin rises in the blood.
- Various causes of hepatocellular jaundice are given in Table 6.3.

Cholestatic Jaundice

- Cholestasis means failure of bile flow, and its cause may lie anywhere between hepatocyte and duodenum.
- Cholestatic jaundice is usually a 'surgical jaundice'.
- Cholestasis can be due to small duct obstruction (intrahepatic cholestasis) or large duct obstruction (extrahepatic cholestasis).

TABLE 6.3 Causes of Hepatocellular Jaundice

• Acute viral hepatitis	• Systemic causes:
• Alcoholic hepatitis	• Haemochromatosis
• Chronic hepatitis	• Wilson's disease
• Cirrhosis	• Budd–Chiari syndrome
• Drug-induced and toxin-induced hepatitis:	• Constrictive pericarditis
• Chlorpromazine, imipramine	• Acute ischaemia
• INH, rifampicin, erythromycin	• Right-sided heart failure
• Amitriptyline, halothane, methyldopa	• Veno-occlusive disease
• *Amanita phalloides* mushrooms	

TABLE 6.4 Causes of Cholestatic Jaundice

Small duct obstruction (intrahepatic cholestasis)	Large duct obstruction (extrahepatic cholestasis)
• Drugs, alcohol	• Gallstones in the CBD
• Viral hepatitis, cirrhosis	• Carcinoma head of pancreas
• Chronic hepatitis	• Carcinoma ampulla of Vater
• Primary biliary cholangitis	• Stricture of bile ducts
• Severe bacterial infections	• Sclerosing cholangitis
• Hodgkin's disease	• Helminths in the CBD
• Granulomas (tuberculosis, sarcoidosis)	• Carcinoma of bile ducts
	Inborn errors of bile secretion
• Widespread secondaries in liver	• Progressive familial intrahepatic cholestasis
• Ulcerative colitis	
• Hypotension	• Benign recurrent intrahepatic cholestasis
• Total parenteral nutrition	
• Pregnancy	

- The consequences are retention of bile acids and bilirubin in the liver and blood, and a deficiency of bile acids in the intestine.
- Causes of cholestatic jaundice are given in Table 6.4.

Clinical Features (*Table 6.5*)

TABLE 6.5 Clinical Features of Cholestatic Jaundice

Symptoms	Signs
• Jaundice (gradually progressive or fluctuating)	• Deep jaundice with a greenish hue
• Pruritus	• Scratch marks
• Pale or clay-coloured stools	• Xanthelasmas on eyelids (lipid deposit)
• Dark urine (increased conjugated bilirubin)	• Xanthomas over tendons (lipid deposit)
• Fever with chills and rigors (cholangitis)	• Palpable gallbladder (in carcinoma head of pancreas)
• Weight loss (malabsorption)	
• Haemorrhagic tendency (vitamin K deficiency)	• Large hard irregular liver (neoplasm)
• Bone pains (calcium and vitamin D deficiency)	• Secondary biliary cirrhosis (late)
• Abdominal pain	• Signs of liver cell failure (late)

Investigations

- Bilirubin present in urine.
- Urobilinogen absent in urine.
- Serum bilirubin markedly raised.
- Predominantly conjugated hyperbilirubinaemia.
- Serum ALP markedly raised (>3–4 times that of normal).
- Minimal biochemical changes of parenchymal damage.
- Ultrasonography (for underlying cause).
- Antimitochondrial antibody (primary biliary cholangitis).
- ERCP or MRCP.
- Percutaneous transhepatic cholangiography (PTC).
- Liver biopsy (only if there is evidence of liver cell disease with uncertain aetiology).

Q. How do you clinically differentiate haemolytic jaundice, hepatocellular jaundice and obstructive (cholestatic) jaundice?

- Clinical features which help in differentiating various types of jaundice are given in Table 6.6.

TABLE 6.6 Clinical Features of Various Types of Jaundice

Clinical Feature	Haemolytic	Hepatocellular	Obstructive
• Colour of jaundice	Lemon yellow	Orange yellow	Greenish yellow
• Depth of jaundice	Mild	Variable	Deep
• Pruritus	Absent	Variable	Present
• Bleeding tendency	Absent	Present	Present (late)
• Bradycardia	Absent	Absent	Present
• Anaemia	Present	Absent	Absent
• Splenomegaly	Present	Variable	Absent (late; after cirrhosis)
• Palpable gallbladder	Absent	Absent	May be present
• Features of hepatocellular failure	Absent	Present (early)	Present (late)

BOX 6.10 Congenital Nonhaemolytic Hyperbilirubinaemias

- Gilbert's syndrome
- Crigler–Najjar syndrome type I
- Crigler–Najjar syndrome type II
- Dubin–Johnson syndrome
- Rotor syndrome

Q. Discuss briefly the congenital nonhaemolytic hyperbilirubinaemias.

- Various congenital nonhaemolytic hyperbilirubinaemias are listed in Box 6.10.

GILBERT'S SYNDROME

- Also known as constitutional hepatic dysfunction and familial nonhaemolytic jaundice.
- Aetiology:
  - Mild deficiency of uridine diphosphate glucuronosyltransferase-1A1 (UGT1A1—reduced to 10%–35% of normal) enzyme resulting in unconjugated hyperbilirubinaemia.
  - Autosomal recessive inheritance.
- Clinical features:
  - More common in males; occurs in 5% of general population with onset during adolescence.
  - Usually asymptomatic and jaundice detected incidentally.
  - Rarely symptoms like anorexia, malaise and upper abdominal pain occur.
  - Depth of jaundice increases with infections, fatigue, exertion, fasting, dehydration and menstruation. During fasting, glucose is depleted that results in lower availability of UDP-glucuronic acid required for conjugation.
  - Increased incidence of adverse effects (mainly diarrhoea and neutropenia), if irinotecan is administered.
  - Physical examination is normal, except for mild jaundice.
- Investigations:
  - Unconjugated hyperbilirubinaemia (usually less than 3 mg/dL). Elevation of bilirubin levels during fasting is used as the most common diagnostic tool. Following reduced calorie intake of 400 kcal/day for 24–48 hours a significant increase in bilirubin blood levels is usually observed. Following intravenous nicotinic acid, a significant increase in bilirubin occurs within 3 hours.
  - Urobilinogen in the urine is increased.
  - No bilirubinuria.
  - Normal peripheral smear, reticulocyte count and serum haptoglobin.
  - Normal liver enzymes.
- Treatment:
  - Usually no treatment is necessary.
  - Glucuronosyltransferase activity may be increased by phenobarbital 60 mg BD.

CRIGLER–NAJJAR SYNDROME TYPE I

- Autosomal recessive inheritance.
- Complete absence of bilirubin-uridine-diphosphate–glucuronosyltransferase, and therefore bile is colourless.
- Pigment gallstones may occur in 40%–50% cases.
- Severe unconjugated hyperbilirubinaemia and kernicterus lead to death.
- Treatment includes daily phototherapy, plasma exchange and liver transplantation. Phenobarbital has no effect.

CRIGLER–NAJJAR SYNDROME TYPE II

- Autosomal recessive inheritance in most cases.
- Partial deficiency of UGT1A1 (<10% of normal).
- Jaundice is milder than type I (bilirubin 6–25 mg/dL); rarely causes kernicterus.
- Treatment includes ultraviolet light phototherapy, phenobarbital and in some cases, liver transplantation.

DUBIN–JOHNSON SYNDROME

- Autosomal recessive inheritance.
- Reduced ability to transport bilirubin diglucuronide into biliary canaliculi due to defective MRP2, which is required for secretion of conjugated bilirubin from the hepatocytes into canaliculi.
- Clinically presents with jaundice, generally after puberty. Pruritus is absent.

- Fifty per cent of bilirubin is conjugated with total bilirubin usually 2–5 mg/dL; bilirubinuria is present.
- The degree of hyperbilirubinaemia may be increased by intercurrent illness, oral contraceptives and pregnancy.
- Life expectancy is generally normal.
- Liver enzymes are normal.
- Gallbladder is usually not visualised on oral cholecystography.
- BSP retention test shows impaired clearance with reflux into blood at 90 minutes.
- Urinary total coproporphyrin is normal with coproporphyrin I more than 80%. In normal subjects, 75% of urinary coproporphyrin is coproporphyrin III.
- Factor VII levels are low.
- Liver biopsy shows dark pigment in lysosomes in the centrilobular hepatocytes. It is composed of polymers of epinephrine metabolites.
- No treatment is required in most cases.

ROTOR SYNDROME

- Autosomal recessive inheritance.
- Due to poor reuptake and storage of bilirubin by liver cells.
- Clinical presentation is with mild jaundice.
- Conjugated hyperbilirubinaemia and bilirubinuria.
- BSP retention test shows impaired clearance but there is no reflux back into blood.
- Gallbladder is visualised on oral cholecystography.
- Total coproporphyrin excretion in urine is elevated twofold to fivefold, with 65% constituting coproporphyrin I.
- Liver biopsy is normal and does not show dark pigment.

Q. Explain briefly about Charcot's triad.

- The presence of following triad in the presence of stones in bile ducts: (1) pain in the right hypochondrium; (2) intermittent or persistent jaundice; (3) fever with chills and rigors. It occurs due to acute cholangitis.
- Other causes of cholangitis include malignant lesion of common bile duct (CBD), benign stricture of CBD and sclerosing cholangitis. Rare causes include Mirizzi syndrome (mechanical pressure on the CBD due to stones in the gallbladder neck or cystic duct) and Lemmel syndrome (a diverticulum near the duodenal papilla compresses the opening of the CBD).

Q. Explain briefly Reynolds pentad.

- It is a combination of Charcot's triad (pain in the right hypochondrium, intermittent or persistent jaundice, fever with chills and rigors) with shock and altered mental status. It is again seen in acute cholangitis.

Q. Describe Courvoisier's law.

- In common bile duct obstruction with stone, the gallbladder as a rule is impalpable. Most patients with jaundice due to stones have a shrivelled, fibrotic, nondistensible gallbladder, and hence gallbladder will not be palpable.
- A jaundiced patient with malignant obstruction (e.g. carcinoma head of pancreas) will have distensible gallbladder, and hence gallbladder may be palpable.
- Courvoisier's law states that a painless, palpably enlarged gallbladder with jaundice is unlikely to be due to gallstones.

Q. Write a short note on drug- and toxin-induced liver injury. (IM 5.7)

- Two major types of chemical hepatotoxicity have been recognised: (1) direct toxic or predictable type and (2) idiosyncratic type.
- Direct toxic hepatitis is characterised by a predictable and dose-related toxicity, short latent period and absence of extrahepatic manifestations.
- Idiosyncratic drug reactions are characterised by unpredictable, most often dose-independent toxicity with variable latent period and presence of extrahepatic manifestations like fever, rashes, arthralgia and eosinophilia. However, for many drugs, idiosyncratic hepatotoxicity can be dose dependent. Drugs causing this type of reaction include halothane, isoniazid, chlorpromazine, amoxicillin/clavulanate, atorvastatin, nevirapine, carbamazepine and diclofenac.
- Based on clinical presentation, drug- and toxin-induced liver injury can be hepatotoxic injury, cholestatic injury or mixed injury. Some drugs produce autoimmune hepatitis.
  - The clinical pattern is defined as 'hepatocellular' when there is an ALT/ALP ratio ≥ 5 or an ALT $>$five times the normal limit.
  - Liver injury is called 'cholestatic' when there is an increase of 2 or more times the ALP alone or when ALT/ALP ratio <2.
  - When the ALT/ALP ratio is between 2 and 5, the clinical pattern is called 'mixed'.
- Based on histology, drug- and toxin-induced liver injury can be hepatitis, cholestatic, steatohepatitis, granulomatous, hepatic fibrosis/cirrhosis and chronic hepatitis.
- Severity may range from asymptomatic elevations of hepatic enzymes to fulminant hepatic failure to chronic liver disease.

COMMON HEPATOTOXIC DRUGS AND TOXINS WITH MORPHOLOGIC CHANGES (Table 6.7)

TABLE 6.7 Common Hepatotoxic Drugs and Toxins With Morphologic Changes

Cholestasis	Hepatitis
• Methyltestosterone • Methimazole • Erythromycin estolate • Chlorpropamide • Chlorpromazine • Anabolic steroids • Cyclosporin nimesulide • Amoxicillin/clavulanate • Herbal drugs	• Halothane • Phenytoin • Methyldopa • Isoniazid • Rifampicin • Ibuprofen • Ketoconazole • Fluconazole • Zidovudine • Chlorothiazide • Oxyphenisatin • Herbal drugs
Fatty liver	**Granulomas**
• Zidovudine • Amiodarone • Indinavir • Ritonavir • Methotrexate • Tetracyclines • Valproic acid • Tamoxifen	• Methyldopa • Sulphonamides • Allopurinol • Carbamazepine • Quinidine
Toxic (necrosis)	**Hepatic fibrosis/cirrhosis**
• Paracetamol • Carbon tetrachloride • Yellow phosphorus • Mushroom (*Amanita phalloides*)	• Methotrexate • Amiodarone • Valproic acid
	Chronic hepatitis
	• Phenytoin • Isoniazid • Valproic acid • Atorvastatin • Nitrofurantoin • Methyldopa

INVESTIGATIONS

- Acute viral hepatitis and autoimmune hepatitis should be excluded after stopping the drug.
- Abdominal imaging (ultrasound, computed tomography scan and MRI) should be performed in all instances of cholestatic jaundice to exclude biliary tract pathology and infiltrative processes.
- Liver biopsy if autoimmune hepatitis remains a competing aetiology.

TREATMENT

- Withdrawal of the suspected agent.
- Mainly supportive therapy as in viral hepatitis.
- N-acetylcysteine (NAC) for paracetamol toxicity.
- Corticosteroids for autoimmune-like drug-induced liver injury.
- Ursodeoxycholic acid may be tried to treat cholestatic drug-induced liver injury.
- Carnitine is used to treat valproate-related drug-induced liver injury.
- Liver transplantation in severe acute hepatic failure.

Q. Describe the aetiology, epidemiology, pathogenesis, clinical features and treatment of viral hepatitis. Add a note on the diagnosis and prevention. (IM 5.16, IM 5.17, IM 5.4)

Q. Give a brief account of aetiology and epidemiology of delta hepatitis.

Q. Briefly describe anicteric hepatitis.

TYPES OF VIRAL HEPATITIS

- Viral hepatitis can be caused by a number of viruses which are listed in Table 6.8.

HEPATITIS A

AETIOLOGY

- Caused by hepatitis A virus (HAV), an RNA virus belonging to the picornavirus group.
- HAV survives on human hands and fomites, and requires temperatures higher than 185°F (85°C) for inactivation. It is resistant to freezing, detergents and acids, but is inactivated by formalin and chlorine.

EPIDEMIOLOGY

- Incubation period is about 30 days (15–45 days).
- Source of the infection is a person incubating or suffering from the disease.
- HAV is transmitted almost exclusively by the faecal-oral route. Infected persons excrete the viruses in their faeces for 2 weeks before the onset and 5–7 days after the onset of the illness.
- Can rarely spread by blood transfusions and homosexual activity.
- Children are most commonly affected. Overcrowding and poor sanitation facilitate the spread.
- In outbreaks, water, milk and shell fish are all implicated.
- No carrier state has been identified.
- The single most important predictor of the clinical course of an acute hepatitis A infection is the age. Symptomatic infections are uncommon in young children. In adults 75%–90% of the infections are symptomatic, with jaundice in majority of cases.

TABLE 6.8 Causes of Viral Hepatitis

Hepatitis Caused by Common Viruses	Hepatitis Caused by Other Viruses
• Hepatitis A, caused by hepatitis A virus (HAV) • Hepatitis B, caused by hepatitis B virus (HBV) • Delta hepatitis, caused by hepatitis D virus (HDV) • Hepatitis C, caused by hepatitis C virus (HCV) • Hepatitis E, caused by hepatitis E virus (HEV)	• Cytomegalovirus • Epstein–Barr virus • Herpes simplex virus • Yellow fever virus • Hepatitis G virus • Dengue virus

PREVENTION

- At community level, prevention is attempted by improving social conditions, especially overcrowding and unhygienic situations.
- Immune serum globulin (0.1 mL/kg) can protect from infection for 2 months. It is used in those at particular risk, for example close contacts, those with other major diseases, pregnant females, immunocompromised persons and in outbreaks, for example, in a school or nursery. In household contacts, passive prophylaxis with immunoglobulin within 2 weeks of exposure reduces icteric disease by more than 80%, although the infection is not necessarily prevented. However, at present, active immunisation rather than passive immunisation is recommended to reduce chances of transmission.
- A vaccine is available for active immunisation. It is approved for use in persons above the age of 1 year. Two doses at 6 month interval are recommended. It seems to provide lifelong immunity. The exact role of this vaccine in Indian setup is not clear as most persons get infection with hepatitis A in early childhood when the disease has a mild course. It may be administered in high-risk groups (military personnel, food handlers). Patients with chronic hepatitis C or other chronic liver diseases may be at an increased risk of fulminant hepatitis or death with HAV superinfection. These patients may be administered HAV vaccine.

HEPATITIS B

AETIOLOGY

- Caused by hepatitis B virus (HBV), belonging to the group of hepadna viruses.
- HBV comprises a surface envelope (antigen expressed on it is called hepatitis B surface antigen [HBsAg]) and a nucleocapsid core containing DNA (antigen expressed on its surface is called hepatitis B core antigen [HBcAg], while another soluble antigen in the nucleocapsid is called hepatitis Be antigen [HBeAg]). Nucleocapsid core also has DNA polymerase enzyme.
- The corresponding antibodies are:
  - Anti-HBs.
  - Anti-HBc.
  - Anti-HBe.
- HBsAg-positive serum containing HBeAg is more likely to be highly infectious than HBeAg-negative or anti-HBe-positive serum.

EPIDEMIOLOGY

- Incubation period is about 90 days (50–150 days).
- Humans are the only source of infection, being individuals incubating or suffering from acute hepatitis, asymptomatic carriers or persons with chronic liver disease.
- Major route of transmission is parenteral but occasionally nonparenteral.
- Commonly follows transfusion of infected blood or blood products, injections with contaminated needles, intravenous drug use with needle sharing, tattooing and acupuncture. Albumin solutions and gammaglobulins are free of risk. At present, HBV accounts for only less than 10% cases of posttransfusion hepatitis.
- Nonparenteral means of transmission include spread through body fluids like saliva, urine, semen and vaginal secretions. However, this requires close personal contact, sexual intercourse and male homosexuality.
- Mother-to-child spread (perinatal transmission) is also common. It could be either transplacental transmission or transmission at or soon after birth.
- The groups with high-risk rates of HBV infection include spouses of acutely infected persons, sexually promiscuous males (homosexuals), health care workers exposed to blood, dentists, haemophiliacs and prisoners.
- Risk of transmission of hepatitis B through needlestick injury from an HBsAg positive person is about 30%.
- A chronic carrier state is described for HBV infection (1%–20%).
- Serum HBsAg is positive in 30% cases of Down's syndrome, lepromatous leprosy, leukaemia, Hodgkin's disease, polyarteritis nodosa, patients on chronic haemodialysis and needle-using drug addicts.
- The age at which a person is infected with the virus determines the disease outcome; 90% of those who acquire HBV perinatally or in early childhood will develop chronic hepatitis as their immune system cannot destroy and clear infected hepatocytes. In adults, 90% of infections are acute and only 5%–10% progress to chronic hepatitis.

PREVENTION

- For active immunisation, recombinant vaccines (containing HBsAg) are available which provide 95% efficacy against HBV infection. Since nonpercutaneous routes of transmission are quite prevalent in India, this vaccine is recommended in all children. It is also recommended in high-risk groups (health workers, haemodialysis patients, injection drug users, haemophiliacs and sexual contacts of HBsAg carriers). Injections are given at 0, 1 and 6 months for full immunity. Dose is 10 μg for children younger than 10 years and 20 μg in children older than 10 years. The duration of immunity provided is not known but protective levels of anti-HBs have been found for 5–10 years. Boosters are not recommended at present except in immunosuppressed. The vaccine is not effective in HBsAg carriers.
- Hyperimmune B immunoglobulin (HBIG) is prepared from blood containing anti-HBs. This can prevent or minimise hepatitis B infection. This should preferably be given within 24 hours or at most a week of exposure. Dose is 0.06 mL/kg. Indications are accidental needle puncture, gross personal contamination with infected blood, oral ingestion or contamination of mucous membranes and exposure to infected blood in the presence of cuts and grazes.
- Active-passive immunisation is vaccine being given together with hyperimmune globulin, and is recommended for postexposure prophylaxis in unvaccinated

persons. For perinatal exposure of infants born to HBsAg-positive mothers a single dose of 0.5 mL of HBIG in the thigh of newborn immediately after birth is followed by three doses of vaccine starting within 12 hours of birth.

DELTA HEPATITIS

AETIOLOGY

- Caused by hepatitis D virus (HDV), which is a defective RNA virus. The RNA genome is covered by an outer coat of HBsAg.
- It has no independent existence. It requires HBV for replication and expression.
- HDV can infect a person simultaneously with HBV (coinfection). HDV can superinfect a person who is already a chronic carrier of HBV (superinfection).

EPIDEMIOLOGY

- Two epidemiologic patterns exist: (i) Delta infection being endemic among those with hepatitis B, predominantly transmitted by nonparenteral route, especially close personal contact. (ii) In nonendemic areas, delta infection is confined to persons exposed frequently to blood and blood products, mainly intravenous drug addicts and haemophiliacs. Here, predominant transmission is by parenteral route.
- Coinfection gives rise to severe acute hepatitis that is limited by recovery from HBV infection.
- Superinfection causes rapidly progressive chronic hepatitis, with episodes of acute hepatitis.
- It can cause fulminant liver failure and rapid progression to cirrhosis (in 70% cases within 5–10 years) as well as an increased risk of liver cancer.

HEPATITIS C

AETIOLOGY

- It is a single-stranded RNA virus belonging to the family *Flaviviridae*.
- HCV has six genotypes. Chronic HCV 1 infection has poor response to therapy. In India, HCV 3 is most prevalent.
- HCV-RNA can be detected within a few days of infection, well before the appearance of antibodies to HCV (anti-HCV).

EPIDEMIOLOGY

- Incubation period is about 50 days (15–160 days).
- Major route of transmission is parenteral.
- More than 90% of cases of posttransfusion hepatitis are caused by HCV. It is also common in drug addicts.
- Common sources of infection are blood and blood products, particularly coagulation factor concentrates. Other modes include perinatal and sexual transmission.
- Transmission of hepatitis C through needle-stick injury from an infected person is 1%–3%.
- HCV is not transmitted by breastfeeding.
- Nearly 80% develop chronic hepatitis while only 20% are able to clear the virus.
- Prevention by vaccine, immunoglobulin or antiviral drugs is not possible.

HEPATITIS E

AETIOLOGY

- It is a single-stranded RNA virus with four genotypes.

EPIDEMIOLOGY

- Incubation period is about 40 days (15–60 days).
- The HEV genotypes 1 and 2 are common in Asia and Africa and are transmitted mainly by contaminated drinking water. On the contrary, HEV genotypes 3 and 4 are common in industrialised nations and are transmitted by consumption of raw meat products, fruits and blood transfusion.
- Accounts for epidemic, water-borne hepatitis; common in India.
- Commonly occurs after contamination of water supplies as after monsoon flooding.
- Can lead to chronic hepatitis especially in patients who are transplanted, have haematological malignancies requiring chemotherapy or have infection with HIV.

PREVENTION

- Similar to hepatitis A (no vaccine available).

CLINICAL FEATURES OF VIRAL HEPATITIS

- Prodromal symptoms usually last for a few days to 2 weeks before the onset of jaundice, characterised by fever, chills, headache, malaise and prominent gastrointestinal symptoms like anorexia and distaste for cigarettes. Nausea, vomiting and diarrhoea follow. Patients with HBV infection have polyarthralgia and occasionally a 'serum sickness syndrome' with skin rashes and polyarthritis.
- Steady upper abdominal pain, sometimes severe (due to stretching of liver capsule).
- Urine is dark with yellowish discolouration of sclera.
- With onset of clinical jaundice, constitutional symptoms diminish.
- Liver becomes palpable and tender.
- Enlarged cervical lymph nodes and splenomegaly in some cases.
- As obstruction to biliary canaliculi increases (cholestatic phase), jaundice deepens, stools become paler, urine becomes darker and liver becomes more palpable.
- Recovery phase—gradually appetite improves and gastrointestinal symptoms subside; jaundice decreases, stools and urine become normal, and liver size decreases. Over a period of 3–6 weeks, majority recover.
- Recovery phase is more prolonged in acute hepatitis B and hepatitis C.
- Complete clinical and biochemical recovery occurs in 1–2 months from the onset in cases of hepatitis A and E, and in 3–4 months from the onset in hepatitis B and C.
- Delta coinfection is indistinguishable from acute hepatitis B. But delta superinfection appears as a clinical exacerbation resembling acute viral hepatitis

in a person chronically infected with HBV. Chronic HDV superinfection is associated with a severe course of hepatitis that frequently leads to rapid fibrosis progression, hepatic decompensation and development of hepatocellular carcinoma.

- In hepatitis A infection, the likelihood of clinically apparent disease increases with age. In children ≤6 years of age, most infections (70%) are asymptomatic, and if illness does occur, it is usually anicteric. Among older children and adults, infection is usually symptomatic, with jaundice occurring in 70% of patients. In some cases, HAV can cause a second bout of jaundice (relapsing hepatitis) 6–12 weeks after primary infection. The symptoms during the relapse are usually less severe than the initial infection. There is no evidence of chronic liver disease or persistent infection following HAV infection. However, 15%–20% of the patients may have prolonged or relapsing disease lasting up to 6 months. Other atypical features include prolonged cholestasis and acute kidney injury.
- Acute HBV infection can range from a subclinical disease to an icteric hepatitis, the former being the most common presentation.
- HCV infection is infrequently diagnosed during the acute phase of infection. Most patients (60%–75%) are asymptomatic or have mild symptoms.
- In hepatitis B, D and E, fulminant hepatic failure can develop. It is uncommon with hepatitis C and rare in hepatitis A. With hepatitis E, fulminant hepatitis occurs in 1%–2% of cases but it occurs in nearly 20% cases in pregnant females.
- **Anicteric hepatitis** is a mild illness with an anicteric course (no clinical jaundice). Diagnosis is based on the history of contact with a definite case, vague gastrointestinal symptoms, malaise, bilirubinuria and aminotransferase elevation. Diagnosis of anicteric hepatitis needs a high index of suspicion.

COMPARISON OF HEPATITIS A, HEPATITIS B, HEPATITIS C AND HEPATITIS E (Table 6.9)

TABLE 6.9 Comparison of Hepatitis A, Hepatitis B, Hepatitis C and Hepatitis E

Features	Hepatitis A	Hepatitis B	Hepatitis C	Hepatitis E
• Incubation period	30 days (15–45)	90 days (50–150)	50 days (15–150)	40 days (15–60)
• Onset	Acute	Insidious	Insidious	Acute
• Age	Children, young	Any age	Adult, but of any age	Young adults
• Route of transmission				
• Faecal-oral	+++	–	Unknown	+++
• Other nonparenteral	+/–	++	++	+/–
• Parenteral	+	+++	+++	+/–
• Severity	Mild	Severe	Mild	Mild
• Prognosis	Good	Worse	Moderate	Good
• Chronicity	None	About 90% of infants infected; about 2%–6% of adult infected	50%–70%	Rare
• Prophylaxis	Immune serum globulin	Hyperimmune serum globulin and hepatitis B vaccine	None	None
• Carrier state	None	1%–30%	1%	None

INVESTIGATIONS

- Urine shows bilirubinuria (in early stages), slight microscopic haematuria and mild proteinuria.
- Total count is low with neutropenia, relative lymphocytosis and atypical lymphocytes.
- Aminotransferases (AST, ALT) are raised. Maximum levels are seen in the prodromal phase, varying from 400 to 4000 IU/L. They decline progressively during icteric and recovery phase.
- Bilirubin levels are variably raised. Both conjugated and unconjugated bilirubins are equally raised.
- ALP level may be raised but is usually less than two times the normal.
- Serum protein levels are normal.
- Prothrombin time—marked prolongation signifies extensive hepatocellular damage. This is one of the best indices of prognosis.
- Blood glucose level may be low.
- Antismooth muscle antibody, rheumatoid factor, antinuclear antibody and heterophil antibody may be present in low titres during prodromal phase.

IMMUNOLOGICAL TESTS FOR VIRAL HEPATITIS (Table 6.10)

TABLE 6.10 Immunological Tests for Viral Hepatitis

Hepatitis A

- Anti-HAV of the IgM type early in the course (diagnostic of recent infection)
- Anti-HAV of the IgG type later in the course that persists for years conferring immunity

Hepatitis B

- HBsAg—a reliable marker of infection and appears first before the appearance of symptoms; disappears over 3–6 months (persistence of HBsAg for longer than 6 months indicates an HBV carrier[a] or progression to chronic hepatitis B infection)
- Anti-HBs—appears after disappearance of HBsAg and persists lifelong; confers protection against subsequent infection[b]
- HBcAg—not found in the blood
- Anti-HBc—usually the first antibody to appear and persists lifelong; initially it is of IgM type and later IgG type
- HBeAg—detected transiently, early in the course; its persistence is correlated with continued viral replication, infectivity and progression to chronicity
- Anti-HBe—detected later during the course
- HBV-DNA—a marker of active viral replication and appears along with HBsAg

Delta hepatitis

- Delta antigen—occasionally detectable
- Anti-delta—initially of IgM type and later IgG type
- HDV-RNA—most reliable test

Hepatitis C

- Anti-HCV—appears 4–10 weeks after infection; disappears after recovery; persists in chronic hepatitis C
- HCV-RNA—after exposure, HCV-RNA becomes detectable in serum after 7–14 days, followed by aminotransferase elevation and later (after 4–10 weeks) by presence of antibodies; remains detectable in most, continuously or intermittently

Hepatitis E

- Anti-HEV—both IgM and IgG are present at onset

[a]It is not a truly 'inactive' disease phase and is now called hepatitis B 'e' antigen (HBeAg)-negative chronic infection in patients with previous HBV infection, or 'incidentally detected asymptomatic hepatitis B surface antigen (HBsAg)-positive subject' in patients who are incidentally detected during routine tests, without any previous or present symptoms of liver disease.

[b]Occasionally, appearance of anti-HBs may trail disappearance of HBsAg by several weeks to months. During this window period, both HBsAg and anti-HBs are negative; the sole markers of recent HBV infection during this time are antibodies against the HBV core antigen (IgM anti-HBc).

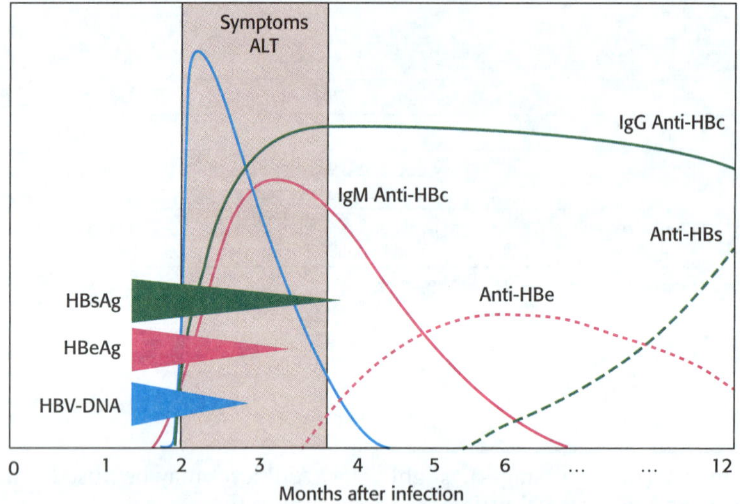

Fig. 6.2 Natural course of hepatitis B infection.

NATURAL COURSE OF HEPATITIS B INFECTION

- Fig. 6.2 gives the natural course of hepatitis B infection in terms of clinical symptoms, liver enzymes and antigens and antibodies.

COMPLICATIONS OF ACUTE VIRAL HEPATITIS

- Complications of viral hepatitis are listed in Box 6.11.

POOR PROGNOSTIC FEATURES

- Factors which indicate a poor prognosis in a patient with acute viral hepatitis are given in Box 6.12.

TREATMENT

- Rest:
  - During the acute symptomatic period, rest and thereafter gradual ambulation.

BOX 6.11 Complications of Acute Viral Hepatitis

• Fulminant hepatic failure	• Renal failure
• Relapsing hepatitis	• Henoch–Schonlein purpura
• Cholestatic hepatitis	• Chronic hepatitis
• Posthepatitis syndrome	• Cirrhosis
• Aplastic anaemia	• Hepatocellular carcinoma
• Polyarteritis nodosa	• Myocarditis
• Transverse myelitis	• Peripheral neuropathy

BOX 6.12 Poor Prognostic Factors in Acute Viral Hepatitis

• Marked increase in AST and ALT	• Recurring attacks of hypoglycaemia
• Bilirubin >20 mg/dL	• Renal failure
• Liver not enlarged	• Associated comorbid conditions
• Prolongation of prothrombin time by 5 seconds	• HBV, HCV or HDV infection

  - In high-risk patients (patients older than 50 years, pregnant and those with other major diseases), rest is continued till symptoms and signs have disappeared, and liver function tests have returned to near normal.
- Physical exertion, alcohol and hepatotoxic agents should be avoided.
- Diet:
  - Nutritious diet of 2000–3000 kcal/day. In the initial stage, when good diet is not tolerated, give a light diet, fruit drinks and glucose. There is no need to avoid fatty diets, but most patients cannot tolerate these diets.
  - Encourage good protein intake.
  - If vomiting is severe, intravenous fluids are given.
- Drugs:
  - Drugs should be avoided if possible (especially sedatives and hypnotics).
  - Alcohol to be avoided for next 6 months.
  - Oral contraceptives can be resumed after clinical and biochemical recovery.
- Antiviral drugs:
  - Some evidence suggests efficacy of interferon-α and direct-acting antiviral agents in patients with acute hepatitis C infection by reducing the rate of chronicity.
  - In acute hepatitis B, oral antiviral drugs (mainly lamivudine, entecavir or tenofovir) may be given in patients with severe hepatitis defined as presence of at least two of the following criteria: bilirubin >10 mg/dL, international normalised ratio (INR) >1.5 and hepatic encephalopathy.

Q. Write briefly on Australia antigen, HBsAg or hepatitis B surface antigen.

- HBsAg (Australia antigen, hepatitis B surface antigen) is located in the capsular material of the HBV.
- A negative test for HBsAg makes HBV infection very unlikely, but does not exclude it.
- HBsAg appears in blood late in the incubation period or prodromal phase of hepatitis B and usually lasts for 3–4 weeks or may persist up to 3 months.
- Persistence of HBsAg beyond 6 months may suggest a chronic hepatitis B infection. In such cases, anti-HBc remains positive while anti-HBs is mostly negative.

Q. Define fulminant (acute) hepatic failure. Discuss the causes, pathology, clinical features, investigations, complications and management of fulminant (acute) hepatic failure. (IM 5.2)

DEFINITION

- Fulminant or acute hepatic failure is a syndrome characterised by hepatic encephalopathy and coagulopathy (INR >1.5), resulting from sudden severe impairment of hepatic function, occurring within 4 weeks of onset of symptoms (jaundice) in the absence of any evidence of preexisting liver disease.
- Onset of encephalopathy within 7 days of onset of symptoms is known as hyperacute hepatic failure. It has better prognosis than acute hepatic failure.
- Onset of ascites between 4 weeks and 6 months of onset of symptoms is called subacute hepatic failure.

AETIOLOGY

- Various causes of acute liver failure are given in Box 6.13. In India, the most common cause of ALF is viral hepatitis followed by antitubercular drug-induced liver injury.

PATHOLOGY

- Extensive parenchymal necrosis.
- Less than 30% of the liver cells appear viable histologically.
- Severe fatty degeneration in tetracycline toxicity and pregnancy.

BOX 6.13 Causes of Acute Liver Failure

- Acute viral hepatitis (B, D and E and others)[a]
- Drugs (refer hepatotoxic drugs given on page 432)
- Pregnancy (acute fatty liver; HELLP[b]; eclampsia)
- Autoimmune hepatitis
- Hyperthermia/heat stroke
- Wilson's disease
- Budd–Chiari syndrome
- Shock
- Poisoning, for example *Amanita phalloides*, paracetamol
- Indeterminate (15%–20%)
- Reye's syndrome

[a]Fulminant hepatitis is uncommon with hepatitis C and not an uncommon complication of hepatitis A in India; the most common cause of ALF in pregnancy is HEV in India

[b]Coexistence of haemolysis, elevated liver enzymes and low platelets.

PATHOGENESIS

- Elevated ammonia in the blood apparently plays a role in the pathogenesis of hepatic encephalopathy.
- Other factors implicated include elevated levels of aromatic amino acids, reduced levels of branched-chain amino acids, short-chain fatty acids, mercaptans and false neurotransmitters (octopamine).
- Activation of the innate immune system responses causes large production of inflammatory mediators which produce systemic effects. Later circulating monocytes may become functionally impaired and less able to respond to infectious stimuli leading to sepsis and multiorgan failure.

CLINICAL FEATURES

- General features:
  - Weakness, nausea, vomiting.
  - Right hypochondrial pain and jaundice.
  - Liver may be enlarged initially, but later shrinks and becomes impalpable.
  - Liver dullness absent on percussion.
  - Ascites and oedema (later).
- Features of hepatic encephalopathy:
  - Reduced alertness, poor concentration, restlessness, manic episodes, drowsiness and coma.
  - Confusion, disorientation, inversion of sleep rhythm, yawning, slurred speech and convulsions.
  - Foetor hepaticus and flapping tremor (asterixis).
- Features of cerebral oedema:
  - Bradycardia, hypertension and irregular respiration (Cushing's triad).
  - Unequal or abnormally reacting pupils.
  - Fixed pupils.
  - Hyperventilation and profuse sweating.
  - Hyperreflexia and extensor plantars.
  - Myoclonus, focal fits and decerebration.
  - Papilloedema (late).
- Hepatic encephalopathy is graded into four grades (Table 6.11).
- Other features:
  - Coagulopathy resulting in bleeding from various sites including intracranial bleed.
  - Cardiac dysfunction and hypotension due to decreased systemic vascular resistance and cardiac involvement.
  - Hypotension due to adrenal involvement.

TABLE 6.11 Grading of Hepatic Encephalopathy

Grade	Features
• Grade 1	Trivial lack of awareness; euphoria or anxiety; shortened attention span; impaired addition or subtraction; incoordination, mild asterixis
• Grade 2	Lethargy or apathy; minimal disorientation for time or place; subtle personality change; inappropriate behaviour, asterixis
• Grade 3	Somnolence to semistupor, but responsive to verbal stimuli; confusion; gross disorientation; muscular rigidity, hyperreflexia, extensor plantars
• Grade 4	Coma (unresponsive to verbal or noxious stimuli); decerebration

INVESTIGATIONS

- Urine contains protein, bilirubin and urobilinogen.
- Leucocytosis, thrombocytopenia.
- Serum bilirubin is raised.
- Serum aminotransferase activity is initially raised but falls later.
- Hypoalbuminaemia.
- Prothrombin time is prolonged.
- Blood ammonia levels are elevated.
- Daily blood and urine cultures, and chest radiograph to exclude infection.
- EEG—characteristic of hepatic encephalopathy.
- Ultrasonography—shrunken liver.
- Intracranial pressure, as detected by intracranial pressure monitoring, is raised.
- Noninvasive assessment of intracranial pressure by optic nerve sheath diameter in all intubated patients. This should be done regularly.
- CSF is normal.
- Others include investigations relevant to find underlying aetiology.

COMPLICATIONS

- Complications of acute liver failure are given in Box 6.14.

MANAGEMENT

- Carries a high mortality (60%–80%).
- General measures:
  - Monitor vital signs, hourly urine output, central venous pressure, renal functions and electrolytes.
  - Monitor blood glucose every 2–3 hours as hypoglycaemia is common.
  - Fluid and electrolytes therapy. Patients are often volume depleted at presentation and require fluid resuscitation. In patients with normal intravascular volume, fluids may be restricted to two-third of maintenance requirement. Hypokalaemia should be corrected.
  - Calories are supplied as glucose (300 g/day) orally or by nasogastric tube or by infusion into a central vein.
  - Ventilatory support for respiratory failure.
  - Antibiotics (e.g. cefotaxime) and antifungals if there is any persistent hypotension or need for vasopressors, or if encephalopathy is worsening.
  - Omeprazole or pantoprazole to prevent gastrointestinal bleed.

BOX 6.14 Complications of Acute Liver Failure

• Encephalopathy	• Pancreatitis
• Cerebral oedema	• Acute kidney injury
• ARDS	• Hypothermia
• Bleeding	• Hypoglycaemia, hypokalaemia
• Hypotension	• Hypocalcaemia, hypomagnesaemia
• Infections	• Acid–base imbalance

- Renal failure is treated with renal replacement therapy (e.g. dialysis). Other indications for renal replacement therapy include refractory hyperammonaemia, progressive encephalopathy or evidence of intracranial hypertension.
- Treatment of encephalopathy:
  - Protein intake of at least 40 g/day is recommended.
  - Role of rifaximin, lactulose, bowel washes, etc. (refer hepatic encephalopathy on page 456) is controversial. Lactulose is catabolised by colonic bacterial flora to short-chain fatty acids (e.g. lactic acid and acetic acid) that lower the colonic pH. This reduction in pH favours the formation of the nonabsorbable ammonium ion from ammonia, trapping ammonia in the colon and thereby reducing plasma ammonia concentrations.
  - Avoid sedatives if possible.
  - Restlessness and excitement are treated with smallest possible dose of diazepam or midazolam intravenously.
- Treatment of cerebral oedema:
  - Head elevation at 30° and elective ventilation in patients with grade 3 or 4 encephalopathy. The head should be in the midline because neck rotation or flexion may compromise jugular venous drainage and increase intracranial pressure.
  - Mannitol 20% (1 g/kg body weight) intravenously over half an hour. Dose may be repeated every 6 hours with serum osmolarity kept below 310 mOsm/L.
  - 3% hypertonic saline to control cerebral oedema (sodium should be maintained between 145–150 mEq/L).
  - Controlled hyperventilation to maintain $PaCO_2$ between 30 and 35 mmHg (for short periods only).
  - Sodium thiopental can be used in controlling mannitol-resistant cerebral oedema.
- Other measures:
  - Consider corticosteroids in presence of persistent hypotension despite adequate volume resuscitation and the use of vasopressors (adrenal involvement can occur in ALF).
  - Administration of vitamin K for prolonged prothrombin time may be of some benefit in patients with malnutrition, but usually is ineffective. Fresh frozen plasma is reserved for clinical evidence of bleeding or before invasive procedures.
  - Coagulopathy is best assessed by thromboelastography (TEG). It can assess platelet function, clot strength and fibrinolysis. Based on findings on TEG, appropriate replacement therapy can be given to reverse coagulopathy.
  - N-acetylcysteine is recommended in all cases of acute liver failure with mild to moderate encephalopathy, particularly those with paracetamol toxicity.
  - Consider antiviral therapy for hepatitis B and herpes simplex virus-related failure; steroid therapy for autoimmune hepatitis-related failure; penicillin G or silibinin in *Amanita phalloides*-related failure; and emergent delivery for pregnancy-related acute liver failure.

BOX 6.15 Indications of Liver Transplantation in Non-Paracetamol-induced ALF

- INR > 6.5 regardless of grade of hepatic encephalopathy (HE)

  OR
- Any three of the following regardless of HE
  - Age < 10 or > 40 years
  - Aetiology indeterminate, drug-induced
  - Time interval from icterus to encephalopathy > 7 days
  - INR > 3.5
  - Bilirubin > 3.4 mg/dL

  - Exchange transfusion, plasmapheresis, charcoal haemoperfusion (molecular adsorbent recirculating system—MARS) and haemodialysis using special membranes have not been found to be helpful.
  - Liver transplantation in selected cases (Box 6.15).

Q. Give a brief account of subacute hepatic failure.

- Liver failure occurring between 4 and 26 weeks after onset of symptoms is called subacute liver failure. The diagnostic criteria for subacute liver failure are:
  - Persistent progressive jaundice for 4 weeks after its appearance in a patient with acute hepatitis.
  - Development of ascites 4 weeks after the appearance of jaundice.
  - Biochemical evidence of hepatocellular necrosis.
  - Submassive or bridging necrosis on liver biopsy.

CLINICAL FEATURES

- Ascites is common.
- Hepatic encephalopathy occurs in 20%–100% of the cases.
- Nausea, fever and abdominal pain.
- In contrast to acute liver failure, cerebral oedema is uncommon while spontaneous bacterial peritonitis (SBP) and renal failure are more common.
- Incidence of sepsis and gastrointestinal haemorrhage is similar in acute and subacute liver failure.
- Hepatomegaly can occur in about half of the patients in contrast to shrunken liver seen in patients with acute failure.

TREATMENT

- Stabilise airway, breathing and circulation of the patient and monitor blood glucose, electrolytes and renal functions.
- Role of glucose–insulin–potassium drip is controversial.
- The mortality ranges from 70% to 90% with renal failure accounting for about half of the deaths.
- Most of the survivors develop chronic liver disease.

Q. Describe Reye's syndrome.

- It is an acute encephalopathy with hepatic dysfunction due to mitochondrial damage.

- Usually in children and adolescents, rarely in adults.
- Follows an infectious illness like influenza or chickenpox.
- History of aspirin intake.
- Begins abruptly with vomiting and lethargy during the recovery period of a viral illness followed by acute encephalopathy and seizures with cerebral oedema.
- Severe fatty degeneration of the liver (causing elevations in ammonia levels and liver enzymes, but usually no jaundice).
- Treatment includes intensive supportive care, correction of metabolic abnormalities and control of intracranial pressure.
- Prognosis is generally good. However, encephalopathy can result in permanent neurologic sequelae.

Q. How do you classify chronic parenchymal liver diseases?

- Chronic parenchymal liver disease can be classified into two types: chronic hepatitis and cirrhosis (Flowchart 6.3).

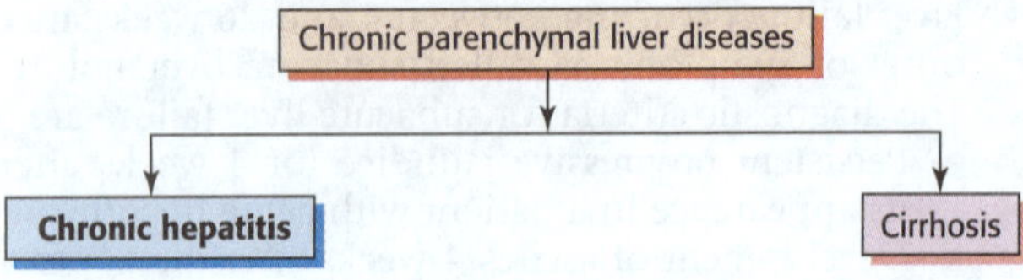

Flowchart 6.3 Classification of Chronic Parenchymal Diseases.

Q. Discuss the classification, aetiology, pathology, clinical features and management of chronic hepatitis.

Q. Write a short note on autoimmune hepatitis.

- Chronic hepatitis is diagnosed when liver disease is present on clinical or other grounds for more than 6 months.

CLASSIFICATION

- Based on combination of three factors:
  - Cause of chronic hepatitis.
  - Histologic activity or grade.
  - Degree of progression or stage.

CLASSIFICATION OF CHRONIC HEPATITIS BY CAUSE

- Causes of chronic live disease are given in Box 6.16.

BOX 6.16 Classification by Causes of Chronic Hepatitis

- Chronic hepatitis B
- Chronic hepatitis B plus hepatitis D
- Chronic hepatitis C
- Autoimmune hepatitis
- Drug-related chronic hepatitis (isoniazid, amiodarone, methotrexate, valproate, nitrofurantoin)
- Alcoholic hepatitis
- Nonalcoholic steatohepatitis
- Metabolic causes (primary biliary cholangitis, sclerosing cholangitis, Wilson's disease, haemochromatosis, α1-antitrypsin deficiency)
- Budd–Chiari syndrome
- Cryptogenic chronic hepatitis

CLASSIFICATION OF CHRONIC HEPATITIS BY GRADE

- Grade indicates severity of liver disease and is based on the histopathological evidence of inflammatory and necrotic findings. Based on the severity of following factors, a severity score (mild, moderate or severe) is assigned (Knodell–Ishak score or histologic activity index):
  - Periportal necrosis including piecemeal necrosis and/or bridging necrosis.
    - Piecemeal necrosis indicates swollen hepatocytes isolated in inflammatory cell infiltrate.
    - When piecemeal necrosis leads to septum formation linking portal tracts and central vein, it is known as bridging necrosis.
  - Intralobular necrosis.
  - Portal inflammation.
  - Fibrosis (a part of staging of chronic hepatitis).

CLASSIFICATION OF CHRONIC HEPATITIS BY STAGE

- Indicates level of progression of disease in term of fibrosis.
- Based on the degree of fibrosis:
  - Stage 0—no fibrosis.
  - Stage 1—mild fibrosis (portal fibrosis without septae).
  - Stage 2—moderate fibrosis (a few septae).
  - Stage 3—severe fibrosis (numerous septae without cirrhosis).
  - Stage 4—cirrhosis.

AUTOIMMUNE HEPATITIS (LUPOID HEPATITIS)

- It is a chronic immune-mediated liver disease of unknown aetiology. There are no features that are absolutely diagnostic and the existence of the condition can be established only by recognition of a constellation of compatible features and the exclusion of other diseases.

CLINICAL FEATURES

- Seen mainly in females during second or third decade.
- Fluctuating course is common.
- In majority, the onset is insidious with fatigue, anorexia and jaundice.
- In about 25% cases, the onset is acute like viral hepatitis but without the normal resolution.
- Fever, polyarthralgia, epistaxis and amenorrhoea.
- Jaundice (mild to moderate).
- Occasionally, maculopapular skin lesions, pleuritis, pericarditis and renal failure.
- Signs of chronic liver disease may be present—spider telangiectasia, hepatosplenomegaly, caput medusa, ascites, palmar erythema.
- Associated conditions are migrating polyarthritis of large joints, lymphadenopathy, thyrotoxicosis, Hashimoto's thyroiditis, myxoedema, vitiligo, Coombs' positive haemolytic anaemia, pleurisy, transient pulmonary

infiltrates, ulcerative colitis, glomerulonephritis and Sjogren's syndrome.
- Cholestasis is unusual and patients with pruritus, hyperpigmentation, xanthelasmas or disproportionately elevated serum alkaline phosphatase levels must be evaluated for other conditions.

INVESTIGATIONS

- Serum bilirubin is elevated by less than 6 mg%.
- Aminotransferases are elevated to more than 10 times during relapses.
- Hypoalbuminaemia and polyclonal hypergammaglobulinaemia with particular elevated level of serum IgG.
- Serum alkaline phosphatase is slightly raised.
- Prothrombin time is prolonged.
- Positive antinuclear antibodies (homogeneous pattern), antismooth muscle antibodies and antimitochondrial (type I autoimmune hepatitis) antibodies.
- Anti-LKM1 (anti–liver-kidney microsome type I—targeted against an antigen of the cytochrome P450 system) and anti-liver cytosol (LC)-1 antibodies are present in a subtype of autoimmune hepatitis (type II; seen more frequently in children).
- HBsAg is negative.
- Normal serum α1-antitrypsin and normal serum ceruloplasmin, iron and ferritin levels.
- Elastography may be used to assess the stage of hepatic fibrosis noninvasively.
- Liver biopsy shows aggressive hepatitis characterised by a chronic inflammatory cell infiltrate with or without cirrhosis.

PROGNOSIS

- Exacerbations and remissions are common.
- Progression to cirrhosis is limited in mild disease.
- Some may progress rapidly to hepatic failure and death.
- In about 30%, cirrhosis is present at the time of diagnosis.
- Hepatocellular carcinoma is uncommon.

TREATMENT

- Prednisolone 30–60 mg is given orally daily initially, then gradually tapered as the liver function improves. Maintenance therapy to be continued for at least 2 years after LFT has become normal. Budesonide (3 mg tid) can replace prednisolone unless patient has cirrhosis.
- Azathioprine 50–100 mg/day to be added if maintenance dose of prednisolone is more than 10 mg/day. In acute phase, prednisolone and azathioprine may be combined.
- Other immunosuppressive agents (mycophenolate mofetil, cyclosporin, tacrolimus, infliximab or rituximab) if no response.
- Liver transplantation is indicated for autoimmune hepatitis with decompensated cirrhosis or acute liver failure.

CHRONIC HEPATITIS B

- Chronic HBV infection affects 5% of the worldwide population and may lead to cirrhosis and hepatocellular carcinoma. HBV genotype C infection (prevalent in India) poses an increased risk for cirrhosis and hepatocellular carcinoma.
- HBV infection is considered as chronic when the surface antigen persists for more than 6 months.
- The risk of chronicity depends on the age at which the acute infection was contracted.
- If a child is infected at birth, acute infection is uncommon but chronic liver disease occurs in nearly 90% of cases.
- On the other hand, in immunocompetent adults, the incidence of acute hepatitis is high while chronic infection develops in only 2%–6% of cases.
- Other conditions where incidence of chronic hepatitis B infection is high are given in the Box 6.17.

PHASES OF CHRONIC HBV INFECTION

- Chronic HBV infection has four major phases: immune-tolerant, HBeAg-positive immunoactive, HBeAg-negative inactive disease (inactive chronic HBV or low replicative) and HBeAg-negative immunoreactive phases. Patients in the immunotolerance and HBeAg-negative inactive disease phases are asymptomatic while those in the HBeAg-positive immunoactive and HBeAg-negative immunoreactive disease phases can range from asymptomatic to liver failure. Very few patients with chronic HBV infection become HBsAg negative (resolution of chronic HBV infection).

Immune-tolerant Phase

- Characterised by active viral replication in liver but little or no evidence of disease activity.
- Immune system does not recognise the virus.
- Associated with high levels of HBV DNA (>20,000 IU/mL) in blood with normal or mildly elevated liver enzymes and without liver inflammation. HBsAg and HBeAg are positive.
- Lasts for 10–30 years in perinatally acquired HBV but is shorter in those infected as children or adults.
- No treatment is required.

HBeAg-positive Immune-active Disease (Chronic Hepatitis)

- Most patients will eventually progress from the immune-tolerant phase to the immune-active phase.
- Evidence of liver inflammation and elevated levels of liver enzymes.
- Elevated HBV DNA levels (though levels are lower than in the immunotolerant phase).
- HBsAg and HBeAg positive.
- Clinically, patients may range from asymptomatic to symptomatic liver failure with jaundice.
    - Intermittent deepening of jaundice with recurrence of malaise and anorexia (episodes resem-

BOX 6.17 Conditions Associated With Chronic Hepatitis B State

• Down's syndrome	• Polyarteritis nodosa
• Lepromatous leprosy	• Patients on chronic haemodialysis
• Leukaemias	• Needle using drug addicts
• Hodgkin's lymphoma	• HIV infection

bling acute hepatitis) may occur and may lead to progressive liver injury.
  - Mild hepatomegaly.
  - Complications of cirrhosis occur in end-stage liver disease.
  - Extrahepatic manifestations include arthralgias, arthritis, vasculitis, glomerulonephritis and polyarthritis nodosa.
  - Long-standing cases develop hepatocellular carcinoma.
- Treatment is indicated.

HBeAg-negative Inactive Disease (Low or Nonreplicative Phase or Inactive Carrier State)

- Immune response results in decline in HBV DNA levels (<2000 IU/mL) and HBeAg seroconversion (anti-HBe).
- Normal ALT.
- None to mild inflammation in liver histology.
- Individuals asymptomatic.
- No treatment is required.
- Outcome:
  - Majority (~60%) remain in this phase indefinitely (*inactive carrier state*).
  - About 25% will have recurrent episodes of immune-activation and intrahepatic inflammation (HBeAg-negative persistent immune-active disease) which requires treatment.
  - About 10% may become positive again for HBeAg (seroreversion).
  - About 10% will develop HBeAg-negative immune-active disease.

HBeAg-negative Immune-active Disease (Chronic Hepatitis)

- HBsAg and anti-HBe positive and HBeAg negative.
- ALT elevated.
- HBV DNA > 2000 IU/mL; may fluctuate.
- Moderate to severe necrosis and inflammation in liver histology.
- Clinically, patients may range from asymptomatic to symptomatic liver failure with jaundice.
- Treatment is required.

SUMMARY OF HBeAg-POSITIVE IMMUNE ACTIVE DISEASE AND INACTIVE CARRIER STATE (Box 6.18)

BOX 6.18 Criteria for HBeAg-positive Immune Active Disease and Inactive Carrier State

CRITERIA FOR HBeAg-POSITIVE IMMUNE ACTIVE DISEASE
- HBsAg positive >6 months
- Serum HBV DNA >20,000 IU/mL
- HBsAg- and HBeAg-positive
- Persistent or intermittent elevation in ALT/AST levels
- Liver biopsy showing chronic hepatitis with moderate or severe necroinflammation

CRITERIA FOR INACTIVE CARRIER STATE
- HBsAg-positive >6 months
- HBeAg-negative, anti-HBe-positive
- Serum HBV DNA <2000 IU/mL over 1 year
- Persistently normal ALT/AST levels over 1 year
- Liver biopsy confirms absence of significant hepatitis

INVESTIGATIONS

- Aminotransferase levels tend to be mildly elevated but may be as high as 1000 units. ALT (SGPT) tends to be more elevated as compared to AST (SGOT). Once cirrhosis develops AST exceeds ALT.
- The bilirubin level may be normal or elevated up to 10 mg/dL.
- Prolonged prothrombin time and hypoalbuminaemia occur in severe cases.
- Hyperglobulinaemia.
- Viral markers:
  - Positive HBsAg.
  - Positive IgG anti-HBc, negative IgM anti-HBc.
  - Positive HBe antigen or rarely, positive anti-HBe.
  - Positive HBV DNA.

TREATMENT

- Indications for treatment of chronic HBV infection are given in Box 6.19.
- In presence of cirrhosis (compensated or decompensated), oral drugs are recommended.

Drugs Used in Chronic HBV (Table 6.12)

Interferon α-2b

- Response to interferon α-2b (defined as loss of HBeAg and HBV DNA) occurs in 30%–40% of patients. Unfortunately, this therapy is associated with several

BOX 6.19 Criteria for Treating Chronic HBV

- HBV DNA >20,000 IU/mL and ALT greater than two times normal (regardless of liver histology)
- HBV DNA >2000 IU/mL and moderate fibrosis on fibroscan of liver
- HBV DNA >2000 IU/mL and at least moderate histological lesions (regardless of ALT)
- HBV DNA detectable and compensated or decompensated cirrhosis
- HBeAg-positive, HBV DNA >20,000 IU/mL and age >30 years (regardless of ALT and liver histology)
- HBV and HDV co-infected patients with HBV DNA persistently >2000 IU/mL
- HBV and HIV co-infection
- HBV and HCV co-infected patients receiving HCV direct-acting antivirals
- HBsAg-positive health care workers with HBV DNA >200 IU/mL (to reduce direct transmission to patients during exposure-prone procedures)
- HBsAg-positive patients under immunosuppression/chemotherapy

TABLE 6.12 Drugs Used in Chronic HBV

Interferons (IFN)	• IFNα-2a and IFNα-2b • Pegylated IFNα-2a
Nucleoside analogues	• Lamivudine (3TC) • Telbivudine (LdT) • Entecavir (ETV)
Nucleotide analogues	• Adefovir (ADV) • Tenofovir disoproxil (TDF) • Tenofovir alafenamide (TAF)

Note: The preferred IFN is PegIFNα-2a, and the preferred nucleoside/nucleotide analogues include ETV, TDF and TAF. Duration of treatment with oral drugs is at least 4–5 years but may be given lifelong.

side effects including flu-like symptoms, leucopenia, thrombocytopenia, depression, skin rash and others.

- Dose is 5 million units daily subcutaneously or 10 million units thrice a week for 48 weeks.
- Pegylated interferon-α-2a can be used once a week.

Lamivudine

- The results are similar to those achieved by interferon therapy but this drug is better tolerated and is given orally.
- Dose is 100 mg once a day until HBeAg becomes negative.
- However, development of resistance is high and therefore, tenofovir and entecavir are recommended as the first-line oral agents.

Entecavir

- A cyclopentyl guanosine analogue that is a potent inhibitor of HBV DNA polymerase.

Tenofovir

- It is a cytosine nucleoside analogue with antiviral activity against both HBV and HIV.

Adefovir Dipivoxil

- A nucleotide reverse transcriptase inhibitor and may be useful in patients who develop resistance to lamivudine.

Telbivudine

- An l-nucleoside that is structurally related to lamivudine; may cause elevation of CPK.

CHRONIC HEPATITIS C

- Chronicity is the hallmark of HCV infection. Approximately, 15%–30% of patients with acute hepatitis C infection recover spontaneously whereas the remaining 70%–85% patients develop chronic infection.
- Cirrhosis may develop in about 20% of cases after 20 years of exposure while hepatocellular carcinoma also develops in several patients (risk 1%–4% per year in patients with cirrhosis).
- A number of factors can accelerate progression to advanced liver disease, most notably alcohol consumption, coinfection with HIV or HBV, and older age at the time of infection.

CLINICAL FEATURES

- Clinical features are similar to those with chronic hepatitis B. Fatigue is the most common symptom. Jaundice is rare.
- Chronic cases have prominent extrahepatic features that are mostly in the form of autoimmune and lymphoproliferative states. These include essential mixed cryoglobulinaemia, membranoproliferative glomerulonephritis, uveitis, peripheral neuropathy, non-Hodgkin's lymphoma, lichen planus, sicca syndrome, hypothyroidism, insulin resistance and porphyria cutanea tarda.

INVESTIGATIONS

- Laboratory features are similar to those in patient with hepatitis B but aminotransferase levels tend to fluctuate more.
- Anti-HCV is positive in >95% cases.
- HCV-RNA is detectable in all patients, mostly continuously but occasionally intermittently.
- Cryoglobulins are present in nearly 50% cases.

TREATMENT

- As acute infection with hepatitis A or B in those with underlying chronic HCV infection can result in high morbidity, hepatitis A and B vaccination should be performed in those who are sero-negative for these viruses.
- Indications for antiviral treatment are:
  - Detectable HCV RNA with or without elevated ALT.
  - Findings of cirrhosis, fibrosis or moderate inflammation on biopsy (biopsy not mandatory); platelet count, FIB-4 score and fibroscan can be done.
    - Platelet count $<160,000/mm^3$ is suggestive of presence of cirrhosis.
    - FIB-4 (Fibrosis-4 score) = Age (years) × AST level (U/L)/platelet count (10^9/L) × $\sqrt{}$ALT (U/L). FIB-4 >3.25 quite accurately predict cirrhosis.

Interferon α

- Previously, untreated patients were given a combination of pegylated interferon α-2a (or pegylated interferon α-2b) and ribavirin. Pegylated interferon is given once a week. Sustained virological response occurs in about 50% of patients.
- Patients who have contraindications to ribavirin (pregnancy, end-stage renal failure, haemoglobinopathies, severe heart disease and uncontrolled hypertension) should be treated with interferon α-2a alone, preferably long-acting preparations of interferons, pegylated interferons. These long-acting preparations have been shown to be more effective as compared to the unmodified interferons.

Direct-acting Antivirals (DAAs)

- Standard of care at present is a combination of DAAs and can achieve cure rates above 95%.
- Safer and better-tolerated than the older therapies.
- Various DAAs which are in use to treat hepatitis C infection are given in Table 6.13.
- Commonly used combinations of DAAs are listed in Box 6.20.
- Liver transplant is the only available treatment option for patients with decompensated cirrhosis.

TABLE 6.13 Classification of DAAs Based on Mechanism of Action

Mechanism of Action	Drugs
NS3 protease inhibitors (*end with '-previr'*)	Paritaprevir, glecaprevir, grazoprevir, voxilaprevir
NS5A inhibitors (*end with '-asvir'*)	Ledipasvir, velpatasvir, pibrentasvir, ombitasvir, elbasvir, daclatasvir, glecaprvir
RNA-dependent RNA polymerase inhibitors (*end with '-buvir'*)	
Nucleoside/nucleotide analogues	Sofosbuvir
Nonnucleoside analogues	Dasabuvir

BOX 6.20 Commonly Used Combinations of DAAs

Sofosbuvir + velpatasvir (approved for all genotypes)
Sofosbuvir + velpatasvir + voxilaprevir
Sofosbuvir + simeprevir
Sofosbuvir + daclatasvir
Sofosbuvir + ledipasvir
Dasabuvir + ombitasvir
Glecaprevir + pibrentasvir (approved for all genotypes)
Elbasvir + grazoprevir

CHRONIC HEPATITIS D (PLUS HEPATITIS B)

- Chronic hepatitis D may follow acute coinfection with hepatitis B but development of chronicity is not higher than that seen with hepatitis B infection.
- When hepatitis D infects a person with chronic hepatitis B, there is worsening of liver disease. Cirrhosis incidence is three times higher with hepatitis D infection than with HBV mono-infection.
- LKM3 antibodies are present in chronic hepatitis D infection.
- Management is supportive. Only pegylated interferon-α has proven antiviral activity against HDV as it leads to HDV clearance in about 25% of patients.

Q. Briefly discuss alcoholic liver disease. (IM 5.5)

- Chronic and excessive ingestion of alcohol can cause liver disease:
  - Fatty liver.
  - Alcoholic steatohepatitis.
  - Alcoholic hepatitis.
  - Alcoholic cirrhosis (refer page 445).
- Threshold for developing alcoholic liver disease:
  - Intake of >60–80 g/day for 10 years in men.
  - Intake of >20–40 g/day for 10 years in women.

CONTENT OF ALCOHOL IN DIFFERENT ALCOHOLIC BEVERAGES

- Table 6.14 mentions the content of alcohol in various alcoholic beverages.

ALCOHOLIC FATTY LIVER (ALCOHOLIC STEATOSIS)

- Asymptomatic.
- Hepatomegaly.
- Occasionally, discomfort in right upper quadrant with tender hepatomegaly, nausea and jaundice.
- Progression to cirrhosis uncommon.
- Modest elevations of AST, ALT and GTP.
- Occasionally, elevated bilirubin.
- Elevated triglycerides, cholesterol.
- Ultrasound shows fatty liver.
- Biopsy if done shows accumulation of fat in perivenular hepatocytes and later in entire hepatic lobule.
- Cessation of alcohol results in normalisation of pathological changes.

ALCOHOLIC STEATOHEPATITIS

- With continued excessive alcohol ingestion, approximately 30% of patients with steatosis develop histological evidence of inflammation. This is termed alcoholic steatohepatitis.
- Presentation is similar to alcoholic steatosis.
- Many have significant fibrosis on biopsy.

ALCOHOLIC HEPATITIS

- Characterised by recent onset of jaundice with or without other signs of liver decompensation in patients with ongoing alcohol abuse. It is not uncommon for patients to have ceased alcohol consumption days or weeks before the onset of symptoms.
- Histopathology shows steatohepatitis.

Clinical Features

- Fever, rapid onset of jaundice, abdominal discomfort and proximal muscle wasting.
- Hepatomegaly.
- Features of chronic liver disease like spider angiomata, palmar erythema, chapped lips and gynaecomastia.
- In severe cases, portal hypertension, ascites, encephalopathy and variceal bleed can occur without cirrhosis.
- Nonhepatic manifestations of alcohol toxicity including polyneuropathy, cardiomyopathy and a history of chronic pancreatitis may be present.

Investigations

- AST and ALT elevated twofold to sevenfold, but usually <400 IU.
- AST:ALT ratio >2.
- Elevated bilirubin (>3 mg/dL).
- Mild increase in alkaline phosphatase.
- Reduced albumin.
- Prolonged prothrombin time.
- Leucocytosis (elevated neutrophils), elevated C-reactive protein.
- Neutrophil-to-lymphocyte ratio (NLR); patients with low (<5) or high (>8) NLR values do not appear to derive benefit from corticosteroid therapy.
- Infections are common and comprehensive investigations to exclude infections should be done.
- Biopsy shows ballooning degeneration of hepatocytes with leucocyte infiltration; Mallory bodies often present.
- Potentially reversible but many progress to cirrhosis.

TABLE 6.14 Content of Alcohol in Various Alcoholic Beverages

	Beer	Malt Liquor	Wine	Liqueur	Whisky/Tequila/Brandy
Alcohol percentage (weight/volume)	5%	7%	~12%	~24%	40%–45%
One drink equivalence (14 g of pure alcohol)	350 mL	~260 mL	~150 mL	~75 mL	45–50 mL

Prognosis

- High mortality in severe hepatitis.
- Poor prognostic factors include: Prothrombin time >5 seconds of control, anaemia, albumin <2.5 g/dL, bilirubin >8 mg/dL, renal failure, presence of ascites.
- Maddrey discriminant function (MDF) >32 carries poor prognosis:
  - 4.6 × (patient's prothrombin time – control prothrombin time) + serum bilirubin.
  - MDF score of >32 predict short-term mortality of 30% at 1 month and 40% within 6 months.

Treatment

- Complete abstinence from alcohol:
- Nutritional support (>3000 kcal/day; protein intake of 1.2–1.5 g/kg; multivitamins).
- Prednisolone may be tried for 4 weeks in severe cases (discriminant function >32).
- Pentoxifylline and N-acetylcysteine in severe cases although benefit is controversial.
- Liver transplantation in selected cases.

Q. Discuss the aetiology, pathology, pathogenesis, classification, clinical features, investigations, complications and treatment of cirrhosis. (IM 5.16, IM 5.6)

Q. Describe Laennec's cirrhosis and alcoholic cirrhosis.

Q. Enumerate the causes of gynaecomastia.

Q. Briefly explain Child–Pugh score or Child–Turcotte–Pugh score.

CAUSES

- Various causes of cirrhosis are given in Table 6.15.

PATHOLOGY AND PATHOGENESIS

- Cirrhotic changes affect the whole liver but not necessarily every lobule.
- Widespread necrosis of liver cells.
- Extensive fibrosis that distorts the hepatic architecture.
- Regenerative, nodular hyperplasia of the remaining surviving liver cells leads to regenerating nodules.
- Destruction and distortion of hepatic vasculature by fibrosis lead to obstruction of blood flow, which eventually leads to portal hypertension and its sequelae (gastroesophageal varices and splenomegaly).
- Ascites and hepatic encephalopathy result from both hepatocellular insufficiency and portal hypertension.
- Hepatocellular damage leads to jaundice, oedema, coagulopathy and a variety of metabolic abnormalities.
- Alcoholic cirrhosis:
  - Safe limits of alcohol are 200 g and 140 g of alcohol per week in males and females, respectively.
  - Occurrence of cirrhosis six times when alcohol intake is double the safety limit.
  - Ingestion of 180 g of alcohol/day for 25 years increases the risk of developing cirrhosis 25 times.
  - Hepatitis C infection is an important contributor for progression to cirrhosis.

TABLE 6.15 Aetiology of Cirrhosis

- Alcoholic cirrhosis
- Postnecrotic cirrhosis or postviral cirrhosis
  - Hepatitis B
  - Hepatitis C
  - Delta hepatitis (hepatitis D) + hepatitis B
  - Chronic autoimmune hepatitis
- Drug-induced cirrhosis
  - Methotrexate
  - Methyldopa, isoniazid
  - Sulphonamides
- Biliary cirrhosis
  - Primary
  - Secondary
- Nonalcoholic fatty liver disease (NAFLD) and nonalcoholic steatohepatitis (NASH)
- Cardiac cirrhosis
- Haemochromatosis
- Wilson's disease
- α1-antitrypsin deficiency
- Glycogen storage diseases
- Galactosaemia
- Intestinal bypass surgery
- Hepatic outflow tract obstruction
- Veno-occlusive disease
- Cryptogenic (Idiopathic) cirrhosis

CLASSIFICATION

- Micronodular cirrhosis (Laennec's cirrhosis):
  - Involvement of every lobule of whole liver.
  - Uniform, regular connective tissue septa.
  - Regenerating nodules of less than 3 mm diameter.
  - Most common cause is alcoholic cirrhosis.
- Macronodular cirrhosis:
  - Liver surface is grossly distorted.
  - Connective tissue septa vary in thickness.
  - Regenerating nodules show marked differences in size.
  - Coarse, irregular nodules growing up to several centimetres.
  - Most common cause is chronic viral hepatitis.
- Mixed cirrhosis:
  - Shows features of both micronodular and macronodular cirrhosis.

Note: This classification is rarely used at present as it is nonspecific for aetiology, morphologic appearance of the liver may change as the liver disease progresses, and serological markers available today are more specific than morphological appearance of the liver for determining the aetiology.

CLINICAL FEATURES

- Symptoms of cirrhosis are given in Box 6.21.

SIGNS

- Various signs of cirrhosis are given in Table 6.16.
- Jaundice:
  - In the initial stages, jaundice is fluctuating, but later the patient becomes chronically jaundiced.
  - Mechanisms of jaundice in cirrhosis are the following:
    - Failure of bilirubin metabolism (predominant mechanism).
    - Intrahepatic cholestasis.
    - Haemolysis.
- Diminished body hair:
  - Seen mainly in males, who slowly loose the male hair distribution.
  - Alopecia affects mainly the face, axilla and chest.

BOX 6.21 Symptoms of Cirrhosis

- Low-grade fever
- Weakness, fatigue and weight loss
- Anorexia, nausea, vomiting and upper abdominal discomfort
- Abdominal distension due to ascites
- Loss of libido
- Menstrual irregularities like amenorrhoea and irregular menses
- Haemorrhagic tendencies like easy bruising, purpura, epistaxis, menorrhagia and gastrointestinal bleeding[a]
- Symptoms of hepatic insufficiency (refer page 456)
- Symptoms of portal hypertension and its sequelae (refer page 450)

[a]Occur due to underproduction of coagulation factors by the liver and thrombocytopenia resulting from hypersplenism.

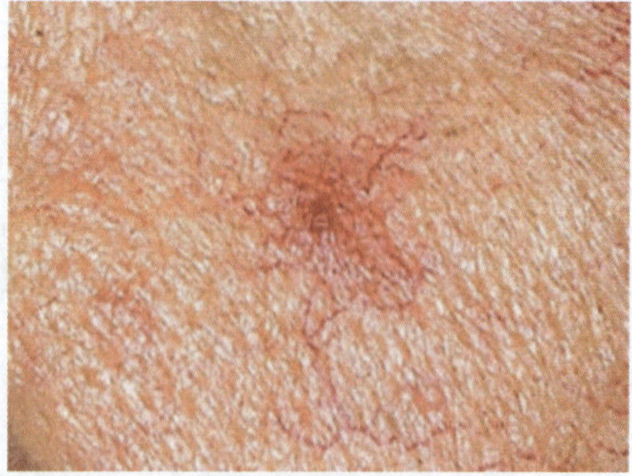

Fig. 6.3 Spider naevus.

BOX 6.22 Conditions Associated With Spiders

- 2% of healthy individuals (≤3 in number)
- Cirrhosis of liver
- Third trimester of pregnancy
- Viral hepatitis
- Alcoholic hepatitis
- Rheumatoid arthritis
- Thyrotoxicosis

TABLE 6.16 Signs in a Patient With Cirrhosis

Signs of hepatocellular failure

• Jaundice	• Palmar erythema	• Flapping tremors
• Parotid enlargement	• Dupuytren's contracture	• Gynaecomastia
• Diminished body hair	• Clubbing	• Testicular atrophy
• Spider naevi	• White nails	• Ascites

Features dominant in male cirrhosis

- Diminished body hair
- Gynaecomastia
- Testicular atrophy

Features dominant in alcoholic cirrhosis

- Parotid enlargement
- Gynaecomastia
- Spider naevi
- Dupuytren's contractures (related to alcoholism)
- Liver enlarged, normal or small in size

Features dominant in female cirrhotics

- Menstrual irregularities
- Signs of virilisation
- Breast atrophy

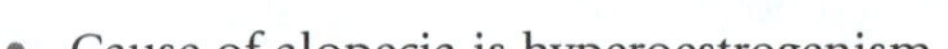

  - Cause of alopecia is hyperoestrogenism.
  - Hyperoestrogenism is due to increased peripheral formation of oestrogen resulting from diminished hepatic clearance of the precursor, androstenedione.
  - Hyperoestrogenism is responsible for alopecia, gynaecomastia and testicular atrophy.
- Spider naevi:
  - Syn: Spider telangiectasia; vascular spiders; spider angiomas; arterial spiders.
  - Thought to be due to arteriolar changes induced by hyperoestrogenism.
  - Seen in the territory drained by the superior vena cava (head and neck, upper limbs, front and back of upper chest).
  - Vary in size from 1–2 mm to 1–2 cm in diameter.
  - Seen as a central arteriole from which numerous small vessels radiate peripherally, resembling spider's legs (Fig. 6.3). Compression of the central arteriole with a pinhead makes the whole spider disappear. Releasing compression shows filling from centre to periphery.
  - Conditions associated with spiders are listed in Box 6.22.
- Palmar erythema (liver palm):
  - Palmar erythema is due to increased peripheral blood flow. In cirrhosis, circulatory changes occur in the form of increased peripheral blood flow and decreased visceral blood flow, especially to the kidneys.
  - Seen as erythema of palm, especially thenar and hypothenar eminences (Fig. 6.4).

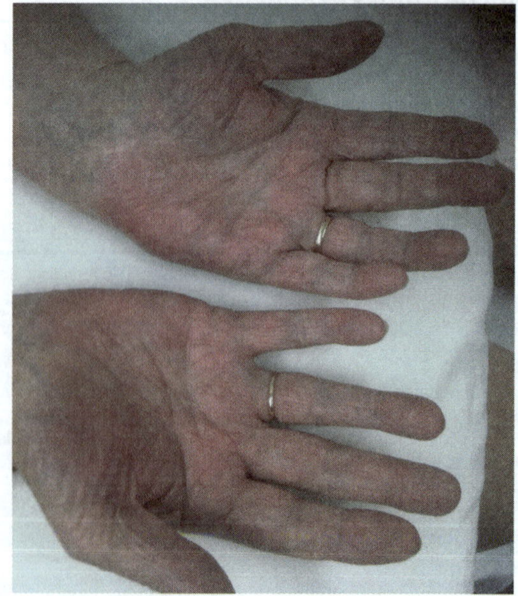

Fig. 6.4 Palmar eythema.

- May be seen on the sole; also seen in hyperdynamic circulatory states and in some normal people.
- Dupuytren's contracture:
  - Due to fibrosis of palmar aponeurosis.
  - Seen as a flexion contracture of the fingers, especially ring and little fingers, with loss of function (Fig. 6.5).
  - Probably caused by local microvessel ischaemia and platelet and fibroblast-derived growth factors that promote fibrosis.
  - Other causes include diabetes mellitus and manual labour. An autosomal dominance inherited form is also seen.
- Clubbing and central cyanosis:
  - Due to development of pulmonary arteriovenous shunts leading to hypoxaemia.
- Nail changes:
  - White (Terry's) nails (Fig. 6.6).
    - Due to hypoalbuminaemia.
    - Nails become chalky white and brittle.
  - Muehrcke's nails.
    - Pairs of transverse white lines that disappear on applying pressure.
    - Lines do not move with growth of nail.
- Flapping tremors:
  - Seen in hepatic precoma (for further details, refer hepatic encephalopathy).

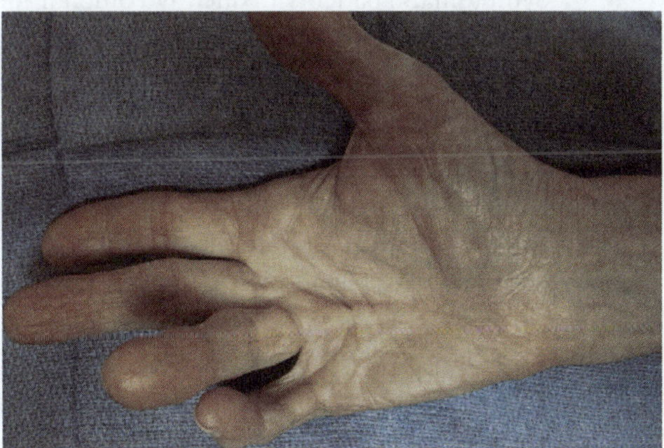

Fig. 6.5 Dupuytren's contracture.

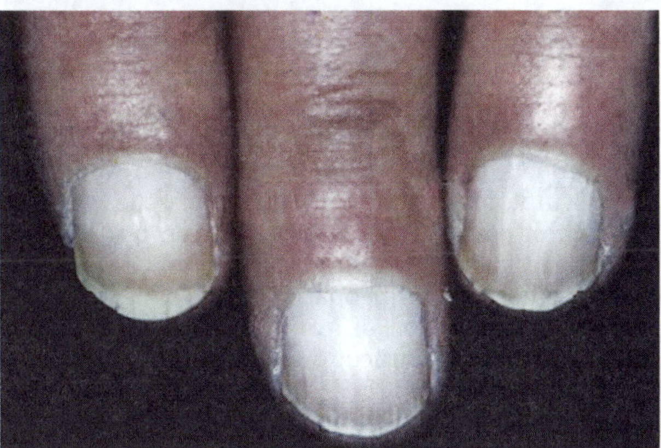

Fig. 6.6 Terry's nails.

- Foetor hepaticus:
  - A sweet and pungent smell in breath.
  - Caused by increased concentrations of dimethyl sulphide due to underlying severe portosystemic shunting.
- Gynaecomastia:
  - Seen in males (in females, there is atrophy of breasts).
  - Due to hyperoestrogenism.
  - Proliferation of male breast glandular tissue palpable as nodule (vs. pseudogynaecomastia—accumulation of subareolar fat tissue without palpable nodule).
  - Causes of gynaecomastia are given in Box 6.23.
- Testicular atrophy:
  - It is a consequence of hyperoestrogenic state.
  - Normal testicular volume in an adult is 15–25 mL. Measurement can be done by Prader orchidometer (Fig. 6.7).
- Ascites:
  - Results from both hepatocellular insufficiency and portal hypertension (refer ascites).
- Parotid and lacrimal gland enlargement:
  - Mechanism is not clear.
  - Seen more commonly in alcoholic cirrhosis.
- Skin pigmentation:
  - Generalised hyperpigmentation of skin occurs due to increased melanin deposition.
- Anaemia:
  - A number of factors can produce anaemia in cirrhosis (Box 6.24).

BOX 6.23 Causes of Gynaecomastia

• Physiological (infancy, puberty, ageing)	• Ketoconazole
• Cirrhosis of liver	• Oestrogens
• Spironolactone	• Other drugs (cyproterone acetate, flutamide, finasteride)
• Cimetidine	• Klinefelter's syndrome
• Digoxin	• Tumours of testes and lung
• Hyperthyroidism	• Hypogonadism

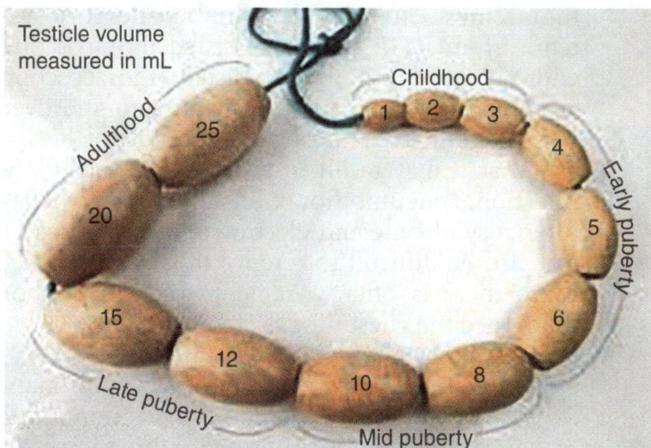

Fig. 6.7 Prader orchidometer.

BOX 6.24 Causes of Anaemia in Cirrhosis

- Acute and chronic blood loss from varices
- Nutritional deficiency of vitamin B_{12} and folate
- Hypersplenism
- Direct bone marrow suppression by alcohol
- Haemolysis due to the effect of hypercholesterolaemia on RBC membrane

- Hepatomegaly:
  - In early stages of cirrhosis due to any cause, liver is enlarged, firm to hard, irregular and nontender; more common in alcoholics.
  - In late stages, liver shrinks in size and becomes nonpalpable. This is due to progressive hepatocyte destruction and fibrosis.
  - Other causes of enlarged liver with cirrhosis include primary biliary cholangitis, primary sclerosing cholangitis, haemochromatosis and Wilson's disease.
- Portal hypertension, hepatic encephalopathy and renal failure:
  - These are major complications of cirrhosis.
  - Symptoms and signs of portal hypertension and its sequelae (refer page 450), hepatic encephalopathy (refer page 456) and renal failure (refer hepatorenal syndrome [HRS] page 460) often coexist with cirrhosis.
- Other extrahepatic consequences:
  - Pleural effusion (hepatic hydrothorax):
    - Defined as significant pleural effusion, usually greater than 500 mL, in a cirrhotic patient, without an underlying pulmonary or cardiac disease.
    - Most often develops on right side.
    - Ascites is also present in vast number of cases.
    - Proposed mechanisms include:
      - Hypoalbuminaemia—decreased colloid osmotic pressure.
      - Leakage of ascitic fluid via diaphragmatic defects.
      - Transdiaphragmatic migration of fluid via lymphatic channels.
    - Pleural fluid is transudative.
  - Treatment involves control of ascites, therapeutic thoracentesis, transjugular intrahepatic portosystemic shunt (TIPS), video-assisted thoracoscopy with pleurodesis, video-assisted thoracoscopy with repair of defects in the diaphragm and liver transplantation. A chest tube should not be inserted as it may result in protein loss, secondary infection, pneumothorax, haemothorax, hepatorenal syndrome and electrolyte disturbances. It can also be difficult to remove the chest tube because there is often a rapid reaccumulation of fluid once the chest tube is clamped.
  - Hepatopulmonary syndrome:
    - Results in hypoxaemia through pulmonary microvascular vasodilatation and intrapulmonary arteriovenous shunting resulting in ventilation-perfusion mismatch.

BOX 6.25 Diagnostic Triad for Hepatopulmonary Syndrome

- Presence of chronic liver disease
- Evidence of intrapulmonary vascular dilatation
- Partial oxygen pressure <80 mmHg or alveolar-arterial oxygen gradient >15 mmHg (or >20 mmHg for age > 65 years)

    - Triad of hepatopulmonary syndrome is given in Box 6.25.
    - Intrapulmonary capillary vasodilatation constitutes main anatomic disturbance leading to impaired arterial oxygenation through ventilation-perfusion mismatch. Intrapulmonary arteriovenous shunting constitutes another mechanism causing arterial hypoxia.
    - Nitric oxide overproduction and angiogenesis are hallmarks of this condition. Probably occur due to a defect in the synthesis and metabolism of pulmonary vasoactive substances by the impaired liver.
    - Vasodilatation and shunting predominates in middle and lower lung fields. Consequently, when a patient moves from a supine position to a standing position, blood flow to these fields increases and exacerbates the shunt and ensuing hypoxaemia (i.e. orthodeoxia).
    - Can occur even with mild liver disease.
    - Symptomatic patients frequently complain of insidious onset of progressive dyspnoea or orthodeoxia-platypnoea (platypnoea indicates dyspnoea accentuated by assumption of an upright position and relieved by assumption of a recumbent position).
    - Can also present with cyanosis and clubbing.
    - Chest radiograph may show a bibasilar interstitial pattern that reflects the predominantly basal vascular dilatations.
    - Diagnosis by contrast-enhanced (microbubble) echocardiography, perfusion lung scan and pulmonary angiography.
    - Treatment by oxygen inhalation, coil embolisation (in localised shunts) and in severe cases, lung transplantation.
- Portopulmonary hypertension characterised by an elevated mean pulmonary artery pressure (>25 mmHg), increased pulmonary vascular resistance (>240 dyn.s/cm^5) and normal wedge pressure (<15 mmHg) in a setting of underlying portal hypertension. The risk is independent of the severity of the liver disease. Dyspnoea on exertion is the most common symptom and other symptoms include orthopnoea, fatigue, syncope, chest pain and haemoptysis. It can lead to right heart failure.
- Cirrhotic cardiomyopathy:
  - Constellation of features indicative of abnormal heart structure and function in patients with cirrhosis.
  - Main clinical features include baseline increased cardiac output, attenuated systolic contraction or diastolic relaxation in response to

physiologic, pharmacologic and surgical stress and prolonged QT interval.
- Ultrasound and MRI are helpful to diagnose cirrhotic cardiomyopathy.

- Acquired hepatocerebral degeneration:
  - Refers to a neurological syndrome consisting of various movement disorders (parkinsonism and ataxia) and cognitive impairment in advanced cirrhosis or portosystemic shunt.
  - Characterised by a chronic, progressive and irreversible course.
- Hepatic osteodystrophy:
  - Osteoporosis and osteomalacia.

SEVERITY OF LIVER DISEASE

- The Child–Pugh (CP) scoring classification, originally devised to risk-stratify patients undergoing shunt surgery is useful to assess liver disease severity in patients with established cirrhosis (Table 6.17).

CLINICAL CATEGORIES OF CIRRHOSIS

Clinically, cirrhosis can be categorized into four categories (Box 6.26).

ACUTE-ON-CHRONIC LIVER FAILURE (ACLF)

- See page 458.

END STAGE CIRRHOSIS

- End stage of cirrhosis is characterised by:
  - Chronic jaundice.
  - Progressive, refractory ascites; worsening of signs of portal hypertension.
  - Progressive renal dysfunction.
  - Most of them die in hepatic encephalopathy.

TABLE 6.17 Child–Pugh Score or Child–Turcotte–Pugh Score

Parameter	Points		
	1	2	3
• Encephalopathy (grade)	None	1–2	3–4
• Ascites	None	Mild or controlled with diuretics	Moderate despite diuretics
• Prolongation of prothrombin time (seconds)	<4	4–6	>6
• Serum albumin (g/dL)	>3.5	2.8–3.5	<2.8
• Serum bilirubin (mg/dL)	<2	2–3	>3

Note: CP class A: Points 5–6; CP class B: 7–9; CP class C: >9 (range 5–15). These classes correlate with one- and two-year patient survival: class A: 100% and 85%; class B: 80% and 60%; and class C: 45% and 35%.

BOX 6.26 Clinical Categories of Cirrhosis

- Compensated cirrhosis—no overt manifestations of liver failure
- Decompensated cirrhosis—with overt manifestations of disease for example ascites, hepatic encephalopathy, infection or bleeding esophageal varices
- Acute-on-chronic liver failure—an acute deterioration of chronic liver disease often due to a precipitating event and resulting in associated extrahepatic organ failures and a high short-term mortality
- End stage cirrhosis

BOX 6.27 Complications of Cirrhosis

- Variceal haemorrhage
- Ascites
- Spontaneous bacterial peritonitis
- Hepatic encephalopathy
- Acute on chronic liver failure
- Hepatocellular carcinoma
- Hepatorenal syndrome
- Hepatopulmonary syndrome
- Hepatic hydrothorax
- Portopulmonary hypertension
- Cirrhotic cardiomyopathy
- Portal vein thrombosis
- Muscle wasting (sarcopaenia)

COMPLICATIONS

- Complications of cirrhosis are listed in Box 6.27.

INVESTIGATIONS

- Complete blood picture:
  - Anaemia.
  - Leucopenia and thrombocytopenia due to hypersplenism and bone marrow suppression by alcohol.
  - Acanthocytosis—spur-like projections on RBC.
    - The activity of serum lecithin cholesterol acyltransferase, an enzyme which converts free cholesterol into cholesterol ester, is decreased, and consequently, free cholesterol is elevated. This cholesterol accumulation increases erythrocyte surface area, altering its shape to acanthocytes (Fig. 6.8).
- Liver function tests:
  - Hyperbilirubinaemia of both conjugated and unconjugated types.
  - Serum proteins show A:G ratio reversal.
    - Hypoalbuminaemia due to impairment of hepatic protein synthesis.
    - Hyperglobulinaemia due to nonspecific stimulation of reticuloendothelial system.
  - Transaminases:
    - AST (SGOT) is raised.

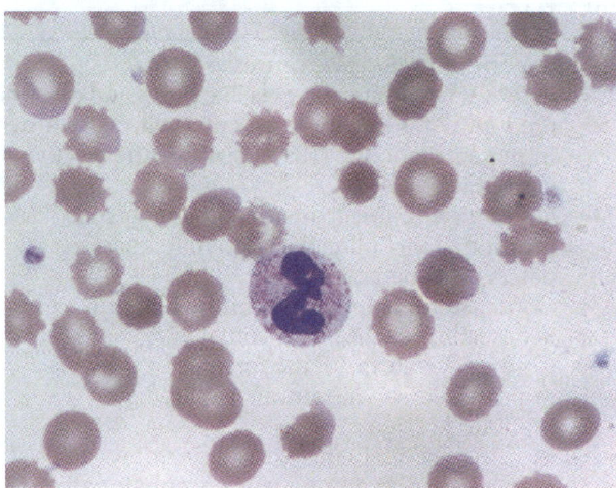

Fig. 6.8 Acanthocytes (spur cells).

- ALT (SGPT) is raised, but less than 300 units.
- AST:ALT ratio is more than 2 in alcoholic cirrhosis (in contrast to viral hepatitis-related cirrhosis where the ratio is less than 2).
- Alkaline phosphatase may be mildly raised.

- Prothrombin time:
  - Prolonged due to reduced synthesis of clotting proteins, especially the vitamin K-dependent factors.
- Hepatitis B and C markers.
- Blood ammonia estimation in cirrhosis is a reliable investigation, particularly in a situation where hepatic encephalopathy is suspected. The reasons for raised blood ammonia are:
  - Diminished hepatic clearance.
  - Shunting of portal venous blood around the liver to systemic circulation.
- Respiratory alkalosis:
  - Due to central hyperventilation.
- Metabolic abnormalities:
  - Glucose intolerance or hypoglycaemia.
  - Hyponatraemia.
  - Hypokalaemia.
  - Hypomagnesaemia.
  - Hypophosphataemia.
- Ultrasonographic examination:
  - Liver size small and coarse echotexture.
  - Macronodules.
  - Hypertrophied caudate lobe.
  - Splenic enlargement.
  - Portosystemic collaterals.
  - Ascites.
  - Ultrasound imaging every 6 months for hepatocellular carcinoma surveillance.
- Fibroscan to determine amount of fibrosis.
- Liver biopsy confirms the diagnosis of cirrhosis (not done routinely).
- Relevant investigations related to the specific aetiologies of cirrhosis in individual patients (serum α-foetoprotein, serum transferrin saturation level, serum ferritin, ceruloplasmin, α1-antitrypsin, antinuclear antibodies and antismooth muscle antibodies).
- Ascitic fluid examination, barium swallow for demonstration of varices, upper gastrointestinal endoscopy for delineation of varices.

TREATMENT

- Treatment of underlying causes:
  - Removal of causative agents like drugs and alcohol.
  - Oral antiviral therapy with entecavir or tenofovir in patients who are HBsAg positive irrespective of viral load.
  - Oral antiviral therapy with sofosbuvir plus NS5A inhibitors, including daclatasvir, ledipasvir or velpatasvir for hepatitis C.
  - Corticosteroids for autoimmune hepatitis.
  - Venesection for haemochromatosis.
  - Copper chelators or zinc for Wilson's disease.
- High-protein diet—minimum 1 g/kg/day.
- 2000–3000 kcal/day.
- Diets enriched in branched-chain amino acids, in patients predisposed to hepatic encephalopathy.
- Multivitamin supplementation daily.
- Thrombopoietin receptor agonists (avatrombopag and lusutrombopag) for correction of thrombocytopenia before an invasive procedure.
- Vaccination against hepatitis A and B viruses, influenza virus and pneumococcus as early as possible, because the antigenic response becomes weaker as cirrhosis progresses.
- Penicillamine inhibits the formation of cross-links in collagen; colchicine inhibits the assembly of collagen; however, none of them have shown any benefit.
- Specific treatment of complications—for example variceal bleeding, hepatic encephalopathy and ascites.

Q. Write a short note on anatomy of the portal venous system. How do you define and classify portal hypertension?

Q. Discuss the aetiology, pathogenesis, clinical features, investigations and complications of portal hypertension. (IM 5.16, IM 5.6)

ANATOMY OF PORTAL VENOUS SYSTEM

- Anatomy of portal venous system is shown in Fig. 6.9.

DEFINITION

- Portal hypertension is a condition characterised by prolonged elevation of portal venous pressure (more than 30 cm saline).
- Normal portal venous pressure is 10–15 cm saline or 7–10 mmHg.
- A better definition is hepatic venous pressure gradient (HVPG—difference in pressure between portal vein and hepatic vein) more than 5 mmHg. HVPG >10 mmHg defines significant portal hypertension.

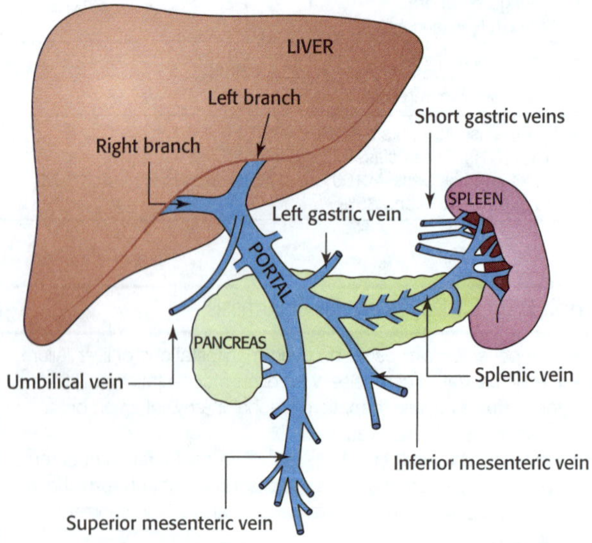

Fig. 6.9 Anatomy of the portal venous system.

CLASSIFICATION OF PORTAL HYPERTENSION (Table 6.18)

- In prehepatic portal hypertension, the obstruction is in the main portal vein.
- In presinusoidal intrahepatic portal hypertension, the obstruction is usually in the portal tracts.
- The causes of portal hypertension are represented diagrammatically in Fig. 6.10.

PATHOGENESIS

- Portal venous pressure is determined by:
  - Portal blood flow.
  - Portal vascular resistance.
- Increased portal vascular resistance is almost always the main factor producing portal hypertension, irrespective of its cause. Increased portal vascular resistance leads to:
  - Reduction in the flow of portal blood to the liver.
  - Development of collateral vessels allowing portal blood to bypass the liver and enter systemic circulation.

TABLE 6.18 Classification of Portal Hypertension

• Prehepatic	Portal vein thrombosis, splenic vein thrombosis, splenomegaly (e.g. lymphoma, Gaucher's disease)
• Intrahepatic	
• Presinusoidal	Noncirrhotic portal fibrosis, schistosomiasis, primary biliary cholangitis, primary sclerosing cholangitis, sarcoidosis, tuberculosis, Wilson's disease, haemochromatosis, adult polycystic liver disease,
• Sinusoidal	Liver cirrhosis, chronic viral hepatitis, alcoholic hepatitis, acute fatty liver of pregnancy, arsenic poisoning,
• Postsinusoidal	Veno-occlusion disease affecting central hepatic venules
• Extrahepatic	Hepatic vein thrombosis (Budd–Chiari disease), inferior vena caval occlusion, chronic right ventricular failure, chronic constrictive pericarditis, restrictive heart disease, tricuspid insufficiency

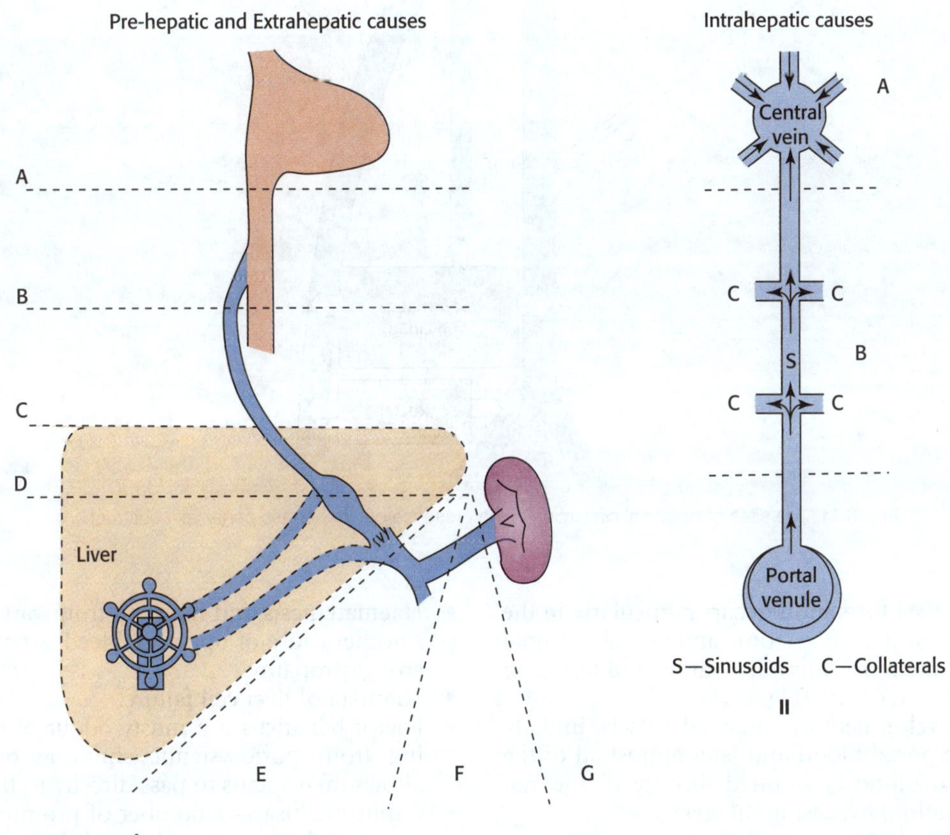

Fig. 6.10 Causes of portal hypertension.

I. **A. Heart:** Rise in atrial pressure, for example constrictive pericarditis. **B. Inferior vena cava:** Congenital webs, tumour invasion, thrombosis. **C. Large hepatic veins:** Thrombosis, webs, tumour invasion. **D. Small hepatic veins:** Veno-occlusive disease. **E. Portal vein:** Thrombosis, invasion or compression by tumours. **F. Splenic vein:** Thrombosis, invasion or compression by tumours. **G. Increased blood flow:** Idiopathic tropical splenomegaly, arteriovenous fistulae.

II. **A. Postsinusoidal causes:** Veno-occlusive disease, alcoholic central hyaline sclerosis. **B. Sinusoidal causes:** Cirrhosis, acute alcoholic hepatitis, cytotoxic drugs, vitamin A intoxication. **C. Presinusoidal causes:** Schistosomiasis, noncirrhotic portal fibrosis, congenital hepatic fibrosis, sarcoidosis, toxins (vinyl chloride, copper, arsenic), idiopathic portal hypertension.

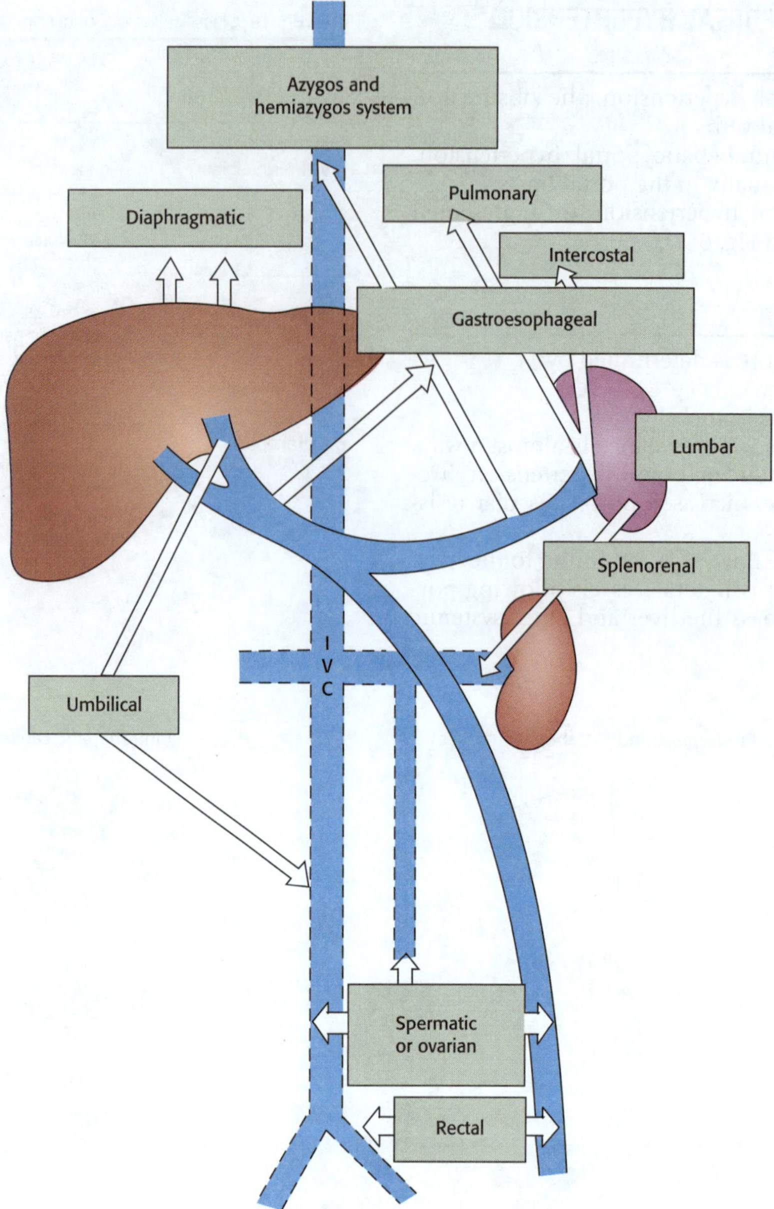

Fig. 6.11 The sites of collateral circulation in the presence of intrahepatic portal vein obstruction.

- Collateral vessel formation occurs particularly in the oesophagus, stomach, rectum, anterior abdominal wall and in the renal, lumbar, ovarian and testicular (spermatic) vasculature (Fig. 6.11).
- With the development of collateral vessels, initially most of the portal blood and later almost all of the entire portal blood is shunted directly to the systemic circulation, bypassing the liver.

CLINICAL FEATURES

- History and symptoms related to the aetiology of portal hypertension:
  - Alcoholism.
  - Past history of hepatitis.
  - Past history of abdominal inflammation (especially neonatal umbilical sepsis).
  - Prolonged use of oral contraceptives.
- Haematemesis and melaena from variceal bleeding. Another cause of upper GI bleed is portal hypertensive gastropathy.
- Stigmata of liver cell failure.
- Foetor hepaticus is a musty odour of breath, resulting from portosystemic shunting of blood that allows mercaptans to pass directly to the lungs.
- Caput medusae—a number of prominent collateral vessels radiating from the umbilicus. Typical caput medusae is rare. Usually only one or two veins are seen, especially in the epigastrium. The flow of blood is always away from the umbilicus.
- In postsinusoidal, extrahepatic portal hypertension, prominent dilated veins are seen in the left flank.
- A venous hum may be audible in the region of xiphoid process or umbilicus. This is due to the flow in collateral vessels. Very rarely, a thrill may

be palpable at the site of maximum intensity of venous hum.

- Cruveilhier–Baumgarten syndrome is the association of dilated abdominal wall veins and a loud venous hum at the umbilicus.
- Splenomegaly is the single most important diagnostic sign of portal hypertension. A diagnosis of portal hypertension is unlikely if splenomegaly cannot be documented clinically, radiographically or ultrasonography. Usually splenic size is less than 5 cm below costal margin. However, marked splenomegaly can occur in younger patients, those with macronodular cirrhosis and in presinusoidal intrahepatic portal hypertension. Hypersplenism is manifested as thrombocytopenia and leucopenia.
- Liver size may be enlarged or shrunken.
  - Small, contracted, fibrotic liver is associated with very high portal venous pressure.
  - Soft liver suggests extrahepatic portal vein obstruction.
  - Firm liver suggests cirrhosis and hence intrahepatic portal hypertension.
- Haemorrhoids may occur from dilation of rectal veins.
- Ascites occurs partly due to portal hypertension but is mainly due to liver cell failure. Portal hypertension determines the localisation of fluid to peritoneal cavity.
- Ascites and encephalopathy are uncommon in prehepatic and presinusoidal portal hypertension.

COMPLICATIONS OF PORTAL HYPERTENSION (Box 6.28)

BOX 6.28 Complications of Portal Hypertension

- Ascites
- Hepatic encephalopathy
- Variceal haemorrhage
- Spontaneous bacterial peritonitis
- Hepatorenal syndrome
- Hypersplenism
- Portal hypertensive gastropathy
- Hepatic hydrothorax
- Hepatopulmonary syndrome
- Portopulmonary hypertension
- Cirrhotic cardiomyopathy

INVESTIGATIONS

- Barium swallow usually shows varices as filling defects in the lower-third of oesophagus ('bag of worms appearance').
- Upper gastrointestinal endoscopy:
  - Most reliable method.
  - Oesophageal varices are seen as blue rounded projections under submucosa.
  - 'Cherry red spots' indicate impending rupture.
- Ultrasonography detects:
  - Size of liver and spleen.
  - Size and patency of portal vein and splenic vein.
  - Collaterals.
  - Ascites.
- Portal venography (splenoportal venogram) rarely done presently, can give information regarding the following:
  - Size and patency of portal vein and splenic vein.
  - Sites of collaterals.
  - Varices at unusual sites.
  - The intrahepatic pattern of splenoportal venogram in cirrhosis is called tree in winter appearance.
- Measurement of portal venous pressure by wedged hepatic venous pressure (WHVP) or transhepatic venous pressure:
  - Confirms portal hypertension.
  - Differentiates sinusoidal from presinusoidal forms.
- Proctoscopy and barium enema for rectal and colonic varices.
- Liver function tests for liver diseases.

TREATMENT

- Nonselective β-blockers (propranolol, carvedilol, timolol and nadolol) produce vasoconstriction of both splanchnic arterial bed and portal venous system along with reduced cardiac output. This reduces splanchnic blood flow. They also reduce recurrence of variceal bleed.
- Nitrates (nitroglycerine and isosorbide dinitrate) reduce venous return and postsinusoidal resistance and are useful in combination with β-blockers in reducing risk of variceal bleed.
- β-blockers with or without nitrates are used for primary prophylaxis of variceal bleed.
- Treatment of underlying disease.

Q. Discuss the diagnosis and management of variceal bleeding.
(IM 15.2, IM 5.16, IM 5.6)

- Commonest site of bleeding is oesophageal varices within 3–5 cm of the oesophagogastric junction.

PREDISPOSING FACTORS (Box 6.29)

BOX 6.29 Predisposing Factors for Variceal Bleeding

- Large varices
- High portal venous pressure
- Liver failure
- Salicylates and other nonsteroidal and anti-inflammatory drugs
- 'Cherry red spots' on endoscopy

CLINICAL FEATURES

- Painless, mild to massive haematemesis, with or without melaena.
- Associated signs vary from mild postural tachycardia to profound shock, depending on the extent of blood loss.
- Associated signs of liver cell failure, ascites and portal hypertension are usually present.

DIAGNOSIS

- Fibreoptic endoscopy done within 8 hours of bleed usually shows the bleeding site and varices. This is essential to exclude other causes of bleeding.
- Ultrasonography to confirm the patency of portal vein.

MANAGEMENT

- Management is considered under five headings, viz. general measures, reduction of portal pressure, local measures, prevention of recurrent bleeding and primary prophylaxis.

GENERAL MEASURES

- Immediate hospitalisation and intensive care management.
- Monitoring vital signs, intake, output, fluid and electrolyte balance.
- Cirrhotics to be graded on Child–Pugh score immediately.
- Emergency blood transfusion (if Hb is below 7 g/dL) has the first priority. The aim is to maintain Hb between 7 and 9 g/dL. Saline infusions must be avoided as far as possible.
- Deficiency of clotting factors is corrected by fresh blood or fresh frozen plasma. However, their role is still controversial unless guided by thromboelastography (TEG).
- Platelet transfusions to raise platelet counts above 50,000/mm^3.
- Injection of vitamin K intramuscularly.
- Nasogastric tube aspiration of blood which reduces nitrogen load in colon.
- H_2-receptor antagonists (like cimetidine, ranitidine or famotidine) or proton-pump inhibitors (like pantoprazole or omeprazole) to prevent stress ulcers although PPIs may increase risk of infection.
- Routine measures in cirrhotics to prevent hepatic encephalopathy (refer hepatic encephalopathy on page 456).
- Tense ascites is treated by careful paracentesis or spironolactone or amiloride.
- Antibiotic administration to prevent SBP, other infections and recurrence of bleed. Commonly used antibiotics include norfloxacin or ciprofloxacin or cefotaxime or ceftriaxone.

REDUCTION OF PORTAL VENOUS PRESSURE

- Vasopressin (Pitressin)
  - Constricts the splanchnic arterioles and reduces portal pressure and portal blood flow.
  - 20 units of vasopressin in 100 mL of 5% glucose is given intravenously over 10 minutes; repeated if necessary 3–4 times at hourly intervals. It can also be given as an infusion: 0.4 units/minute until bleeding stops or for 24 hours and then 0.2 units/minute for a further 24 hours.
  - Abdominal colic, evacuation of bowels and facial pallor indicate that vasopressin is active. Absence of these suggests an inert preparation.
  - Adverse effects of vasopressin are the following:
    - Angina.
    - Arrhythmias.
    - Myocardial infarction.
    - Mesenteric ischaemia.
  - Sublingual or intravenous nitroglycerine (0.4 mg) is given to combat these adverse effects.
- Terlipressin:
  - Terlipressin itself is not active, but vasopressin is released from it.
  - No systemic or cardiac side effects.
  - Given at a dose of 2 mg 6 hourly till bleeding stops and then 1 mg 6 hourly for a further 24 hours.
- Somatostatin and octreotide:
  - Somatostatin and its synthetic analogue octreotide stop variceal bleed in more than 80% of cases.
  - Equivalent to vasopressin and endoscopic therapy.
  - Dose of somatostatin is 250 μg as bolus followed by 250 μg/hour for 2–5 days.
  - Dose of octreotide is 50 μg as bolus followed by 50 μg/hour for 2–5 days.

LOCAL MEASURES

- Balloon tamponade:
  - Sengstaken tube with three lumens.
  - Minnesota tube with four lumens.
    - These tubes have two balloons, oesophageal and gastric balloons.
    - The tube is introduced into the stomach, preferably through the mouth. The gastric balloon is inflated and pulled back into the cardia of the stomach. If bleeding does not stop, oesophageal balloon is inflated for additional tamponade.
    - If oesophageal balloon is used, it should be deflated for about 10 minutes every 3 hours to avoid oesophageal mucosal damage.
    - One lumen allows the aspiration of oesophageal contents and the other lumen of gastric contents.
    - Complications of balloon tamponade include necrosis and ulcerations of oesophagus, obstruction to pharynx and asphyxia.
- Endoscopic procedures:
  - These include endoscopic sclerotherapy (stops bleeding in 80%–90% of cases) and endoscopic variceal band ligation (EVBL). EVBL is the treatment of choice.
  - In the absence of QT prolongation, infusion of erythromycin 250 mg as a prokinetic agent is useful to improve stomach clearance and thus facilitate endoscopy.
- Other procedures:
  - If the patient does not respond to these measures, transjugular intrahepatic portosystemic shunt (TIPS) is helpful in most patients. It involves transjugular insertion of an intrahepatic stent between a branch of the portal vein and a branch of the hepatic vein.
  - Surgical procedures should be considered for continued or recurrent haemorrhage. The options include portosystemic shunting (bypass the blood into the inferior vena cava by portacaval, mesocaval or proximal splenorenal shunts) and oesophageal staple transaction.

SUMMARY OF TREATMENT OF ACUTE VARICEAL BLEED

- Table 6.19 summarises treatment of acute variceal bleed. Flowchart 6.4 gives management of a patient with acute variceal bleed.

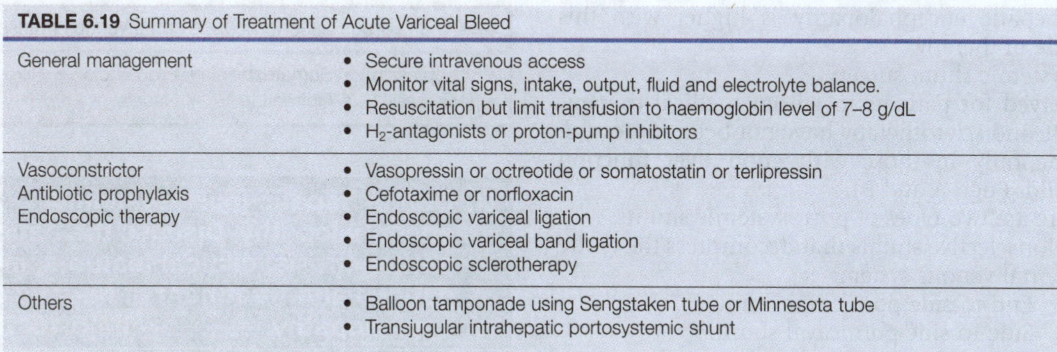

TABLE 6.19 Summary of Treatment of Acute Variceal Bleed

General management	• Secure intravenous access • Monitor vital signs, intake, output, fluid and electrolyte balance. • Resuscitation but limit transfusion to haemoglobin level of 7–8 g/dL • H_2-antagonists or proton-pump inhibitors
Vasoconstrictor Antibiotic prophylaxis Endoscopic therapy	• Vasopressin or octreotide or somatostatin or terlipressin • Cefotaxime or norfloxacin • Endoscopic variceal ligation • Endoscopic variceal band ligation • Endoscopic sclerotherapy
Others	• Balloon tamponade using Sengstaken tube or Minnesota tube • Transjugular intrahepatic portosystemic shunt

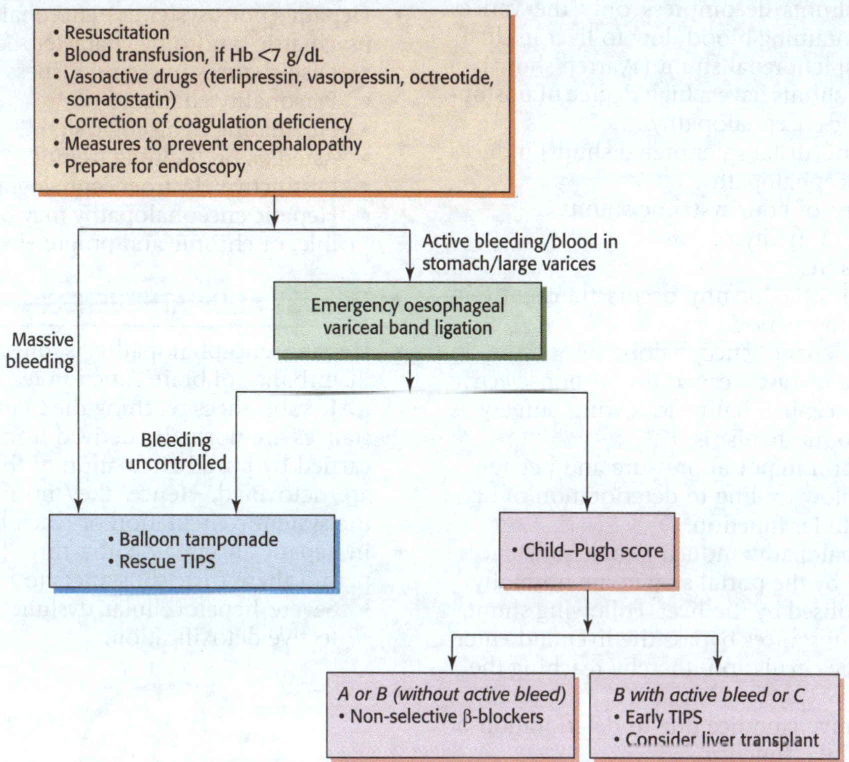

Flowchart 6.4 Management of Acute Variceal Bleed.

PREVENTION OF RECURRENT BLEEDING (SECONDARY PROPHYLAXIS)

- Bleeding reoccurs in approximately 65% of patients within 1 year after initial bleed.
- Medical treatment:
  - It consists of nonselective β-blockers (propranolol 80–160 mg/day) with or without nitrates.
- EVBL:
  - EVBL alone or in combination with β-blockers is the therapy of choice in these patients.
- Endoscopic sclerotherapy:
  - Endoscopic sclerotherapy may be considered if the patient cannot tolerate medical therapy and EVBL cannot be done.
  - Commonly used sclerosants are the following:
    - Ethanolamine oleate.
    - Sodium morrhuate.
    - Absolute alcohol.
    - Sodium tetradecyl sulphate.

BOX 6.30 Complications of Sclerotherapy

- 1% mortality
- Abdominal pain, fever and dysphagia
- Reappearance of varices
- Oesophageal ulceration and perforation
- Stricture formation
- Oesophageal reflux
- Pulmonary complications like chest pain, pleural effusion, mediastinitis and aspiration pneumonia
- Acute respiratory failure
- Spinal cord paralysis due to anterior spinal artery occlusion

  - Injections are repeated every 2 weeks thereafter until the varices are obliterated.
  - Complications of sclerotherapy are listed in Box 6.30.
- TIPS:
  - TIPS is more effective than EVBL for the prevention of recurrent variceal bleed but the incidence

of hepatic encephalopathy is higher with this mode of therapy.

- Portosystemic shunt surgery:
  - Reserved for patients in whom medical therapy, EVBL and sclerotherapy have not been successful.
  - Done only in those with good liver function (Child–Pugh A and B).
  - There are two types of portosystemic shunts:
    1. Nonselective shunts that decompress the entire portal venous system:
       - End-to-side portocaval shunt.
       - Side-to-side portocaval shunt.
       - Proximal splenorenal anastomosis.
       - Mesocaval shunt.
    2. Selective shunts decompress only the varices while maintaining blood flow to liver itself:
       - Distal splenorenal shunt (Warren shunt).
  - Nonselective shunts have a high degree of postoperative hepatic encephalopathy.
  - Selective shunt (distal splenorenal shunt) induces much less encephalopathy.
  - Complications of portosystemic shunts:
    - Operative mortality of 5%.
    - Shunt closure.
    - Hepatic encephalopathy occurs transiently in postoperative periods.
    - Chronic hepatic encephalopathy occurs in 20%–40% of cases, especially in nonselective shunts. Encephalopathy following surgery is due to two mechanisms:
      1. Reduction in portal pressure and hepatic blood flow leading to deterioration of hepatocellular function.
      2. Encephalopathy-inducing toxic substances carried by the portal system are normally metabolised by the liver. Following shunt, these substances bypass the liver and enter systemic circulation, thereby reaching the brain.
    - Postoperative jaundice due to deterioration of hepatocellular function.
    - Chronic ankle oedema.
    - Personality deterioration.

PRIMARY PROPHYLAXIS

- Nonselective β-blockers (e.g. propranolol, carvedilol, nadolol, timolol) in patients with medium to large or high-risk small varices (severe liver dysfunction as indicated by Child–Pugh class B or C, an alcoholic aetiology of liver disease and presence of 'red wale signs' on varices during an initial endoscopy).
- Nitrates may be added to nonselective β-blockers.
- EVBL if patients cannot tolerate β-blockers.
- Endoscopic sclerotherapy and shunt procedures not recommended for primary prophylaxis.

Q. Name the drugs that are used in the reduction of portal venous pressure.

- Drugs used to reduce portal venous pressure are listed in Box 6.31.

BOX 6.31 Drugs Used to Reduce Portal Venous Pressure

- Vasopressin
- Terlipressin
- Somatostatin
- Octreotide
- Propranolol
- Nadolol
- Nitroglycerine

Q. Define hepatic (portosystemic) encephalopathy. Discuss the aetiopathogenesis, clinical features, investigations and treatment of hepatic encephalopathy. (IM 5.16, IM 5.6)

DEFINITION

- Hepatic (portosystemic) encephalopathy is a neuropsychiatric syndrome characterised by the following:
  - Disturbances in consciousness and behaviour.
  - Personality changes.
  - Fluctuating neurologic signs.
  - Asterixis or 'flapping tremor'.
  - Distinctive electroencephalographic changes.
  - Hepatic encephalopathy may be acute and reversible, or chronic and progressive.

AETIOLOGY AND PATHOGENESIS

- Hepatic encephalopathy is due to a biochemical disturbance of brain function resulting from various toxic substances reaching the brain. These toxic substances are normally derived from the intestine and carried by portal circulation to the liver, where they are detoxified. Hence, they normally do not enter the systemic circulation or reach brain (Fig. 6.12).
- In hepatic encephalopathy, three factors operate that permit these toxic substances to reach brain.
  - Severe hepatocellular dysfunction leading to defective detoxification.

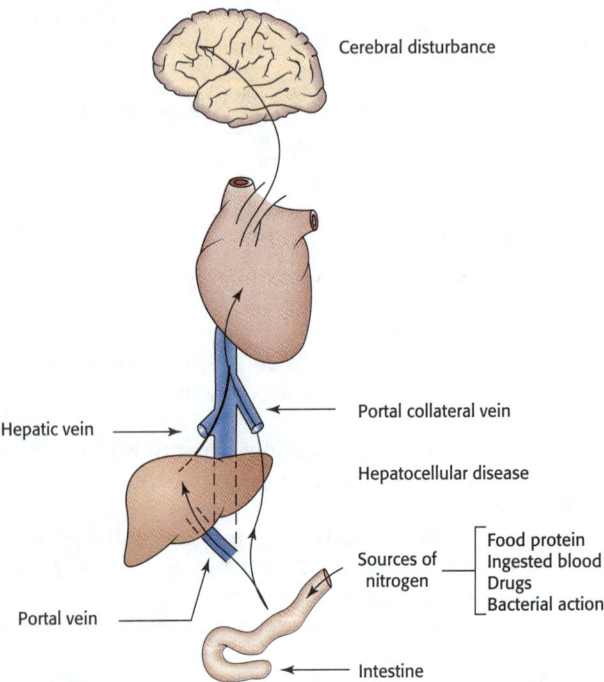

Fig. 6.12 The mechanism of portosystemic encephalopathy.

BOX 6.32 Toxic Substances in Hepatic Encephalopathy

- Ammonia—most important
- γ-Aminobutyric acid (GABA)
- Mercaptans derived from methionine
- Short-chain fatty acids
- Octopamine
- Amino acids
- Phenol

  - Intrahepatic and extrahepatic shunting (collaterals) of portal venous blood into systemic circulation, allowing toxins to enter the systemic circulation (Box 6.32). Here, the liver is 'bypassed'.
  - Increased permeability of the blood–brain barrier, allowing the toxins to enter the brain.
- Muscles are capable of temporarily detoxifying ammonia by converting ammonia into glutamine via glutamine synthetase. Impaired hepatic clearance of ammonia upregulates the gene coding for glutamine synthetase, and skeletal muscles become a significant site of ammonia metabolism for patients with cirrhosis. Therefore, sarcopaenia is a risk factor for hepatic encephalopathy and improving muscle mass is beneficial for its treatment.

PRECIPITATING FACTORS (Table 6.20)

- Gastrointestinal bleeding leads to an increase in the production of ammonia and other nitrogenous substances in the gut, which are absorbed and carried to brain.
- Increased dietary protein is acted upon by the intestinal bacteria to produce excess nitrogenous substances.
- Diuretics, paracentesis and vomiting precipitate hepatic encephalopathy by electrolyte imbalance, particularly hypokalaemic alkalosis.
- Mechanism of encephalopathy in surgical portosystemic shunts is discussed under 'shunt surgery'.
- Infections which can precipitate encephalopathy include SBP, urinary tract infections and *Clostridium difficile* colitis.

CLINICAL FEATURES

- Disturbances in consciousness and behaviour:
  - Hypersomnia is the earliest feature, which progresses to inversion of sleep rhythm with excessive daytime sleepiness.
  - Reduction of spontaneous movements, fixed stare, apathy, slowness and brevity of response.
  - Disorientation in time and space
  - Later, confusion, disorientation, drowsiness and eventually coma develop.
  - Convulsions occur rarely.
- Personality changes:
  - Childishness, irritability and loss of concern for family.
  - Slight impairment of organic mental function to gross confusion.
  - Defecating and micturating in inappropriate places.
- Fluctuating neurological signs:
  - Slurred speech.
  - Constructional apraxia.
  - Hypertonia.
  - Hyperreflexia.
  - Bilateral extensor plantar response.
  - Hyperventilation and hyperpyrexia.
- Asterixis or flapping tremor:
  - Most characteristic neurologic abnormality.
  - Due to impairment of flow of joint position sense and other afferent information to the brainstem reticular formation, resulting in lapses of postures (negative myoclonus).
  - It is best demonstrated by having the patient extend the arms and dorsiflex the hands. It is manifested as the rapid flexion extension movements at metacarpophalangeal and wrist joints, accompanied by lateral movement of digits.
  - Asterixis can also be demonstrated on head and trunk.
  - Other conditions associated with flapping tremor are the following:
    - Uraemia.
    - Respiratory failure.
    - Severe heart failure.

TABLE 6.20 Precipitating Factors for Hepatic Encephalopathy

Drugs and toxins • Sedatives • Alcohol	**Superimposed diseases** • Viral/alcoholic hepatitis • Hepatocellular carcinoma
Increased ammonia production, absorption or entry into the brain • Increased dietary protein • Gastrointestinal bleeding • Constipation • Hypokalaemia • Acute infections • Metabolic alkalosis	**Dehydration** • Vomiting and diarrhoea • Overzealous use of diuretics • Large volume paracentesis **Shunts** • Surgical shunts • TIPS **Miscellaneous** • Portal/hepatic vein thrombosis • Hyponatraemia

INVESTIGATIONS

- Blood ammonia levels are raised (upper limit of normal is 0.8–1 μg/mL)
- Electroencephalogram shows delta waves—the characteristic, symmetric, high voltage, slow wave (2–5 per second) waves.
- CT scan of head to exclude other causes of altered level of consciousness.
- Cerebrospinal fluid:
  - Normal proteins.
  - Increased glutamine.
  - Normal cell count.
- Visual evoked potential abnormalities may be present in incipient stages.
- Liver functions.

TREATMENT

- Treatment or removal of the precipitating causes.
- Maintain calories (glucose 300 g/day).
- Correct electrolyte imbalance.
- Avoid sedatives like benzodiazepines. Fentanyl may be used for sedation if required.

- Routine correction of coagulation test abnormalities is not indicated in patients without active bleeding or for minor procedures such as central line placement, thoracentesis or paracentesis.
- Restricting proteins in diet is not recommended at present. Administer 1.0–1.5 g/kg of proteins daily.
- In gastrointestinal bleeding, Ryle's tube aspiration and bowel washes are employed to remove the blood and blood products. This reduces the nitrogen production in the gut.
- Oral neomycin 0.5–1 g 6 hourly to sterilise the gut. This reduces the intestinal ammonia production by bacteria. Main side effects of neomycin are nephrotoxicity and ototoxicity. Therefore, at present, neomycin is not used commonly.
- Alternative includes rifaximin (a nonabsorbable derivative of rifampicin). Dose of rifaximin is 550 mg bid. The combination of lactulose and rifaximin seems to be more effective than either drug alone.
- Lactulose syrup 15–30 mL three times orally per day. Dose is increased gradually till there are two to three loose stools per day.
    - Metabolism of lactulose by colonic bacteria results in an acidic pH in the intestine, which favours conversion of ammonia to ammonium, which is poorly absorbed.
    - Lactulose diminishes ammonia production by its direct effect on bacterial metabolism.
    - Lactulose increases incorporation of ammonia by bacteria for synthesis of nitrogenous compounds.
    - Lactulose modifies the colonic flora, and displaces urease-producing bacteria with non-urease-producing *Lactobacillus*.
    - The cathartic effects of lactulose in the colon improves gastrointestinal transit, allowing less time for ammonia absorption with increased faecal nitrogen excretion.
- Lactitol has a similar action, more palatable and is a better option than lactulose.
- Lactulose and lactitol may also be given as enemas in patients who are unable to take them orally.
- Polyethylene glycol bowel irrigation can be used instead of lactulose or lactitol.
- Intravenous mannitol to reduce the spontaneous cerebral oedema (controversial).
- Role of levodopa, bromocriptine, keto-analogues of essential amino acids and branched chain amino acids (isoleucine, leucine and valine), L-ornithine-L-aspartate (stable salt of ornithine and aspartic acid) and L-carnitine is controversial.
- Faecal microbiota transplant (FMT) has also been studied and found useful in some patients. The microbiota in patients with liver cirrhosis have more urease-producing bacteria, associated with increased production of ammonia. Therefore, by manipulating the gut microbiome through FMT, there is potential to reverse intestinal dysbiosis.
- Haemoperfusion to remove toxic substances.
- Liver support systems include artificial liver support and bioartificial liver support. Artificial liver support removes circulating toxins via filtration, whereas bioartificial liver support uses filtration as well as liver cells to theoretically improve the detoxification process. Their use is still controversial.
- Hepatic transplantation is the ultimate cure.

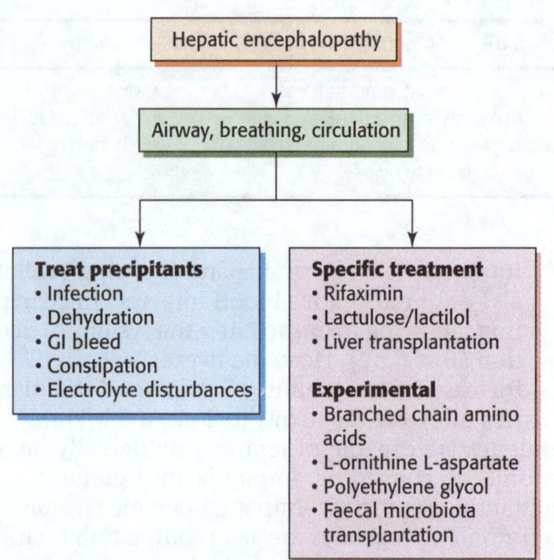

Flowchart 6.5 Summary of Management of Hepatic Encephalopathy.

SUMMARY OF MANAGEMENT OF HEPATIC ENCEPHALOPATHY

- Flowchart 6.5 summarises management of a patient with hepatic encephalopathy.

Q. Discuss acute-on-chronic liver failure (ACLF)

- Characterised by acute decompensation with organ failure.
- Carries a high short-term mortality.
- May occur either in compensated or in decompensated cirrhosis.

DEFINITIONS

EUROPEAN ASSOCIATION FOR THE STUDY OF THE LIVER—CHRONIC LIVER FAILURE CONSORTIUM

- The definition of ACLF is based on the existence of the failure of 1 of the 6 major organ systems. Organ failures include liver, renal, coagulation, cerebral, respiratory and circulatory.
- Triggered by hepatic (continuous alcohol consumption, hepatotropic viral infections including superinfection with HAV/HEV or reactivation, hepatotoxic drugs) or extra-hepatic factors (most common being infection).
- Organ failures are defined as shown in the Box 6.33.
- ACLF is divided into 3 grades of increasing severity (Table 6.21).

ASIAN PACIFIC ASSOCIATION FOR THE STUDY OF THE LIVER—ACLF RESEARCH CONSORTIUM

- The definition of ACLF is based on the presence of liver dysfunction. Extrahepatic organ failures may subsequently develop but are not included in the definition.

BOX 6.33 Definition of Organ Failure in ACLF

- Liver failure if the serum total bilirubin ≥12.0 mg/dL
- Kidney failure if the serum creatinine ≥ 2.0 mg/dL or the patient requires dialysis
- Encephalopathy (grade 3 or 4)
- Coagulation failure if the INR ≥2.5 or platelets ≤20,000/mm^3
- Circulatory failure if a vasopressor (dopamine, dobutamine, epinephrine or norepinephrine) or terlipressin is used
- Respiratory failure if the PaO/FiO$_2$ ratio ≤200

TABLE 6.21 Grades of ACLF

ACLF grade 1	• Patients with single kidney failure • Patients with single liver, coagulation, circulatory or lung failure that is associated with creatinine levels ranging from 1.5 mg/dL to 1.9 mg/dL or hepatic encephalopathy grade 1 or grade 2, or both • Patients with single brain failure with creatinine levels ranging from 1.5 mg/dL to 1.9 mg/dL
ACLF grade 2	• Patients with 2 organ failures
ACLF grade 3	• Patients with 3 organ failures or more

- Defined as acute hepatic insult manifesting as jaundice (total bilirubin levels ≥5 mg/dL) and coagulopathy (INR ≥1.5 or prothrombin activity <40%) complicated within 4 weeks by clinical ascites, encephalopathy, or both.

PATHOPHYSIOLOGY

- The pathophysiology of ACLF is unknown. Systemic inflammation may play a significant role as it correlates with the severity of ACLF. The greater the intensity of systemic inflammation, the larger the number of organ failures and the higher the short-term mortality. Bacterial infections and acute alcoholic hepatitis are two precipitants of systemic inflammation that are frequently associated with ACLF. Severe upper GI haemorrhage may cause ischaemic hepatitis which precipitates ACLS. In addition, gastrointestinal haemorrhage predisposes to infections via translocation of bacterial by-products from the intestinal lumen to the systemic circulation (Flowchart 6.6).

INVESTIGATIONS

- Leucocyte count, platelet count.
- Liver function tests.

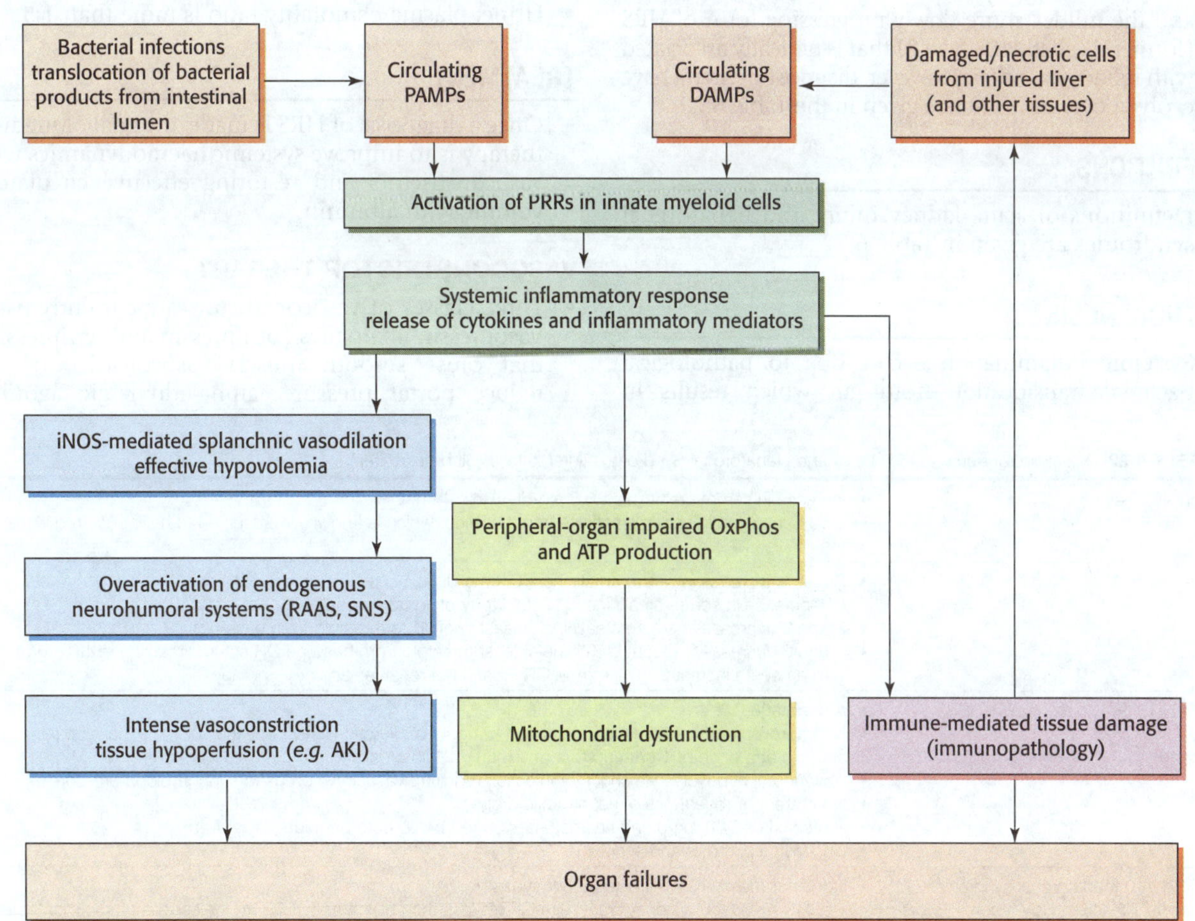

Flowchart 6.6 Pathophysiology of ACLF. PAMPs = Pathogen-associated molecular patterns; DAMPs = Damage-associated molecular patterns; PRRs = Pattern-recognition receptors; iNOS = Inducible nitric oxide synthase; OxPhos = Oxidative phosphorylation; RASS = Renin-angiotensin-aldosterone system; SNS = Sympathetic nervous system; AKI = Acute kidney injury.

- Prothrombin time and INR.
- Blood urea, creatinine, electrolytes.
- Cultures from possible sites of infection.

TREATMENT

- Treatment is supportive with control of infection with antibiotics, treatment of hepatitis viruses (e.g. tenofovir for hepatitis B, steroids for alcoholic hepatitis), renal replacement therapy, treatment of hepatic encephalopathy, ventilatory support, etc.
- Liver transplant.

Q. Write a short note on hepatorenal syndrome (HRS).

Q. Write a short note on acute kidney injury in cirrhotic patients.

- HRS is renal failure with normal tubular function in a patient with chronic liver disease in the absence of an identifiable cause of renal failure. It is a type of renal failure that can occur in patients with advanced cirrhosis and associated ascites.
- Previously, HRS was categorised into 2 major types: the severe and rapidly progressing form of HRS (formerly called HRS type 1) marked by cirrhosis with ascites, and the milder, more slowly progressing form of HRS (formerly called HRS type 2) that is typically associated with refractory ascites. However, diagnostic criteria have evolved over time and are given in the Table 6.22.

DEFINITIONS

- Definitions of acute kidney injury and hepatorenal syndromes are given in Table 6.22.

PATHOGENESIS

- Systemic inflammation occurs due to pathological bacterial translocation from gut which results in release of several pro-inflammatory cytokines resulting in splanchnic vasodilatation, microvascular dysfunction and cardiovascular dysfunction, all producing renal injury.
  - Splanchnic vasodilatation causes a reduction in effective arterial blood volume and a decrease in mean arterial pressure. Activation of sympathetic nervous system and renin–angiotensin–aldosterone system occurs which causes renal vasoconstriction.
  - Impairment of cardiac function can also be due to development of cirrhotic cardiomyopathy.

PRECIPITATING FACTORS

- Gastrointestinal bleeding.
- Sepsis including SBP.
- Diarrhoea.
- Diuretic therapy.
- Aggressive paracentesis.

INVESTIGATIONS

- Urinalysis is normal.
- Urea and creatinine levels are high. Serum sodium is less than 120 mEq/L.
- Urine sodium excretion is less than 10 mEq/day.
- Urine: plasma osmolality ratio is more than 1.5.

TREATMENT

- Once a diagnosis of HRS is made, the goal of medical therapy is to improve systemic haemodynamics with vasoconstrictors and restoring effective circulatory volume with albumin.

VASOCONSTRICTOR THERAPY

- Three classes of vasoconstrictors are currently used: Vasopressin analogues (ornipressin and terlipressin) that cause smooth muscle vasoconstriction and reduce portal pressure, alpha-adrenergic agonists

TABLE 6.22 Definitions of Acute Kidney Injury and Hepatorenal Syndromes (International Club of Ascites)

Acute kidney injury	• Increase in serum creatinine ≥0.3 mg/dL within 48 h, OR • ≥50% increase in serum creatinine from baseline, which is known or presumed to have occurred within the previous 7 days
Staging of AKI	• Stage 1: Increase in serum creatinine ≥0.3 mg/dL OR increase in serum creatinine ≥1.5-fold to twofold from baseline • Stage 2: Increase in serum creatinine at least twofold to threefold from baseline • Stage 3: Increase in serum creatinine at least threefold from baseline OR serum creatinine ≥4.0 mg/dL with an acute increase ≥0.3 mg/dL OR initiation of renal replacement therapy
AKI-HRS (Previously type 1 HRS)	• AKI ≥stage 2 • No improvement in serum creatinine after 48 hours of diuretic withdrawal and volume expansion with albumin at a dose of 1 g/kg up to a maximum of 100 g daily • Absence of hypovolaemic shock or infection requiring vasoactive drugs to support blood pressure • No current or recent use of nephrotoxic drugs • Proteinuria <500 mg/d and haematuria <50 red blood cells per high-power field • Underlying cirrhosis and ascites
HRS-NAKI (hepatorenal syndrome-non-AKI—previously type 2 HRS)	• Does not meet AKI-HRS criteria. Two types. • HRS-AKD (acute kidney disease): eGFR is less than 60 mL/min/1.73 m^2 for less than three months in absence of other potential causes of kidney disease • HRS-CKD (chronic kidney disease): eGFR is less than 60 mL/min/1.73 m^2 for more than three months in absence of other potential causes of kidney disease

TABLE 6.23 Vasoconstrictors Used in HRS

Drug	Dose	Route	Frequency	Adverse effects
Terlipressin	1 mg; titrate if no improvement (i.e. decrease in serum creatinine by 25% by day 3), increase up to maximum 12 mg/day	Intravenous	Every 4–6 hours	Diarrhea, abdominal pain, peripheral ischaemia, myocardial infarction, mesenteric ischaemia, pulmonary oedema
Norepinephrine	0.5–3 mg/h; titrate to achieve 10 mmHg increase in mean arterial pressure	Intravenous	Infusion	Nausea, vomiting, anxiety, cardiac dysrhythmias
Midodrine and octreotide	7.5–15 mg and 100–200 μg	Oral and subcutaneous	Three times a day	Bradyarrhythmias, paraesthesias, abdominal pain, diarrhoea, cholelithiasis, hyperglycaemia

(norepinephrine and midodrine) that lead to smooth muscle vasoconstriction and increase in systemic vascular resistance and octreotide (Table 6.23). Terlipressin is the agent of first choice for HRS-AKI. Midodrine is used along with octreotide.

ALBUMIN

- All vasoconstrictors should be combined with human albumin infusion given at a dose of 20–40 g/day.

RENAL REPLACEMENT THERAPY (RTT)

- RRT may be indicated for patients with AKI-HRS unresponsive to drug treatment and with volume overload, uraemia, or electrolyte derangements; however, RRT does not improve survival in hepatorenal syndrome, and it should be reserved for use as a bridge to transplantation.

LIVER TRANSPLANT

- Liver transplantation is the treatment of choice because it represents definitive treatment for HRS-AKI.

PREVENTION

- In patients with cirrhosis and ascites who do not yet have HRS-AKI, medical management to prevent HRS-AKI is focused on avoiding overuse of diuretics and nephrotoxic medications, preventing episodes of dehydration and monitoring patients closely following large-volume paracentesis. Infections should be identified early and treated promptly.

Q. Discuss the pathogenesis and management of ascites and refractory ascites in cirrhosis. (IM 5.16, IM 5.6)

- Ascites represents a state of total body sodium and water excess.

DEFINITIONS

- Ascites is graded into several categories (Table 6.24).

TABLE 6.24 Grades of Ascites

Grade 1 ascites	Ascites detectable only by ultrasound
Grade 2 ascites	Ascites causes symmetrical distension of the abdomen
Grade 3 ascites	Ascites causes marked abdominal distension (tense ascites)
Complicated ascites	Development of refractoriness, spontaneous bacterial peritonitis, hepato-renal syndrome
Recidivant ascites	Ascites occurs at least three times in 12 months despite optimisation of therapy
Diuretic-resistant ascites	Diuretic therapy failure due to unsatisfactory efficacy: intensive diuretic therapy for at least 1 week and salt-restricted diet with weight loss <0.8 kg over 4 days OR Reappearance of grade 2 or 3 ascites within 4 weeks of initial mobilisation
Diuretic-intractable ascites	Development of unacceptable side effects due to diuretic therapy which preclude the use of an effective diuretic dosage

PATHOGENESIS

- Ascites in cirrhosis results from a combination of the following:
  - Liver failure.
  - Portal hypertension.

MECHANISMS INVOLVED IN PATHOGENESIS (Flowchart. 6.7)

- Vasodilators:
  - Portal hypertension may cause release of vasodilators in the splanchnic circulation such as nitric oxide and carbon monoxide which can cause reduction in effective circulatory volume. This in turn causes activation of sympathetic nervous system, renin–angiotensin–aldosterone system and vasopressin release.
- Secondary hyperaldosteronism:
  - Decreased renal blood flow leads to increased release of renin, which stimulates the angiotensin system, which in turn leads to secondary hyperaldosteronism. The secondary hyperaldosteronism results in salt and water retention. Failure of liver to metabolise aldosterone intensifies secondary hyperaldosteronism.

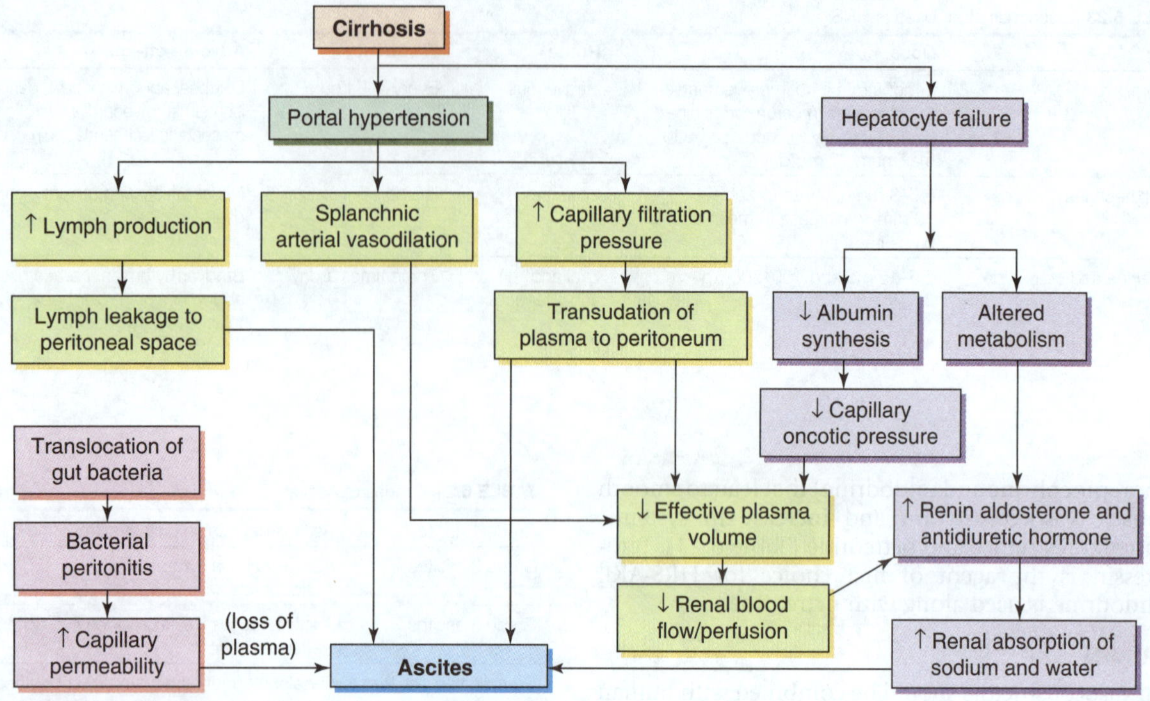

Flowchart 6.7 Pathogenesis of Ascites in Cirrhosis of Liver. (Courtesy: Aithal GP, Palaniyappan N, China L, Härmälä S, Macken L, Ryan JM, Wilkes EA, Moore K, Leithead JA, Hayes PC, O'Brien AJ, Verma S. Guidelines on the management of ascites in cirrhosis. Gut. 2021 Jan;70(1): 9-29).

- Vasopressin:
  - Failure of liver to metabolise vasopressin reduces renal water clearance that results in fluid retention.
- Increased capillary hydrostatic pressure:
  - Portal hypertension raises the hydrostatic pressure within the splanchnic capillary bed. This results in extravasation of fluid from plasma into the peritoneal cavity.
- Reduced plasma oncotic pressure:
  - Hypoalbuminaemia results in a reduction of plasma oncotic pressure. This again results in an extravasation of fluid (ascites and oedema).
- Hepatic lymph:
  - Hepatic lymph oozes freely from the surface of cirrhotic liver into the peritoneal cavity. This adds to the development of ascites.
  - So, portal hypertension and lymphatic ooze predispose to localisation of fluid within the peritoneal cavity.
- Translocation of bacteria:
  - Translocation of bacteria and bacterial products from gut to systemic circulation stimulate the release of pro-inflammatory cytokines leading to inflammation and further release of nitric oxide and carbon monoxide.

ASCITIC FLUID IN CIRRHOSIS (Table 6.25)

- Total ascitic fluid protein concentration <1.5 g/dL indicates an increased risk of SBP.

TABLE 6.25 Ascitic Fluid Analysis in Cirrhosis

• Appearance—clear, straw coloured or light green • Specific gravity—less than 1.016 • Protein—less than 2.5 g/dL • Total cell count—normal (<250/μL) • SAAG[a] ≥1.1 g/dL	• Differential cell count—majority of the cells are mesothelial cells and lymphocytes • Gram's stain—negative • Culture—negative • Malignant cells—absent

[a]SAAG—Serum-ascites albumin gradient, that is the difference between serum albumin and ascitic fluid albumin. It is a better test rather than simple estimation of protein in the ascitic fluid.

MANAGEMENT

- For grade 1 ascites, no specific measures are required to control it.
- The goal of the therapy is the loss of no more than 1.0 kg body weight daily if both ascites and peripheral oedema are present and no more than 0.5 kg body weight daily in patients with ascites alone. This is to avoid side effects such as renal impairment, hepatic encephalopathy, hyponatraemia, hypokalaemia, hypomagnesaemia and muscle cramps.
  - General measures:
    - Hospitalisation if ascites is massive.
    - Estimation of daily body weight.
    - Strict intake and output recording.
    - Estimation of abdominal girth daily.
    - Urinary electrolyte determination.
    - Estimation of serum electrolytes and renal function tests twice a week.

- Bed rest induces diuresis because renal blood flow increases in the horizontal position.
- Strict salt-free diet (2 g of salt/day) initially, but later allowing 4–6 g of salt (equivalent to a no added-salt diet with avoidance of preprepared meals).
- Fluid restriction to 1000–1500 mL/day, if there is hyponatraemia. Routine restriction of fluid intake not recommended.
- Diuretics.
  - Diuretics are introduced in a step-wise manner.
  - As there is secondary hyperaldosteronism, one of the aldosterone antagonists (potassium-sparing diuretics) is preferred— for example spironolactone, triamterene, amiloride.
  - Spironolactone is the drug of choice. It is started at a low dose of 25 mg QID and gradually stepped up every week to a maximum of 400 mg/day.
  - When a large dose of spironolactone has failed, add one of the potent diuretics (e.g. furosemide, torsemide, a thiazide, ethacrynic acid). Usual combination is spironolactone plus furosemide or torsemide.
  - Diuretic dosage is adjusted to achieve a rate of weight loss of no greater than 0.5 kg/day in patients without peripheral oedema and 1 kg/day in those with peripheral oedema (to prevent diuretic-induced renal failure and/or hyponatraemia).
  - Stop all diuretics if severe hyponatraemia (sodium <120 mEq/L), progressive renal failure or worsening hepatic encephalopathy develops.

TREATMENT OF REFRACTORY ASCITES

- Failure to respond to dietary and diuretic regime indicates refractory ascites. Such cases are managed on the following lines:
  1. Intravenous salt-poor albumin, 25 g in 3 hours.
  2. Large-volume paracentesis
     - Remove 5 L of fluid over 1–2 hours. Salt-free albumin (8 g per litre of ascitic fluid removed) should be infused to prevent paracentesis-induced circulatory dysfunction.
     - Can produce circulatory dysfunction due to a reduction of effective blood volume, a condition known as postparacentesis circulatory dysfunction.
  3. Vasoconstrictor like midodrine may ameliorate splanchnic vasodilatation and improve renal perfusion and filtration.
  4. Transjugular intrahepatic portosystemic shunt (TIPS) is applied in patients with refractory ascites who may require a transplant. Complications include hepatic encephalopathy and shunt thrombosis.
  5. LeVeen shunt. It is a peritoneovenous shunt that allows the peritoneal fluid to drain directly into the internal jugular vein. It should be considered in patients with refractory ascites who are not candidates for paracentesis, transplant or TIPS.
     - Common complications of LeVeen shunt are infection, superior vena caval thrombosis, pulmonary oedema, bleeding from oesophageal varices, disseminated intravascular coagulation.

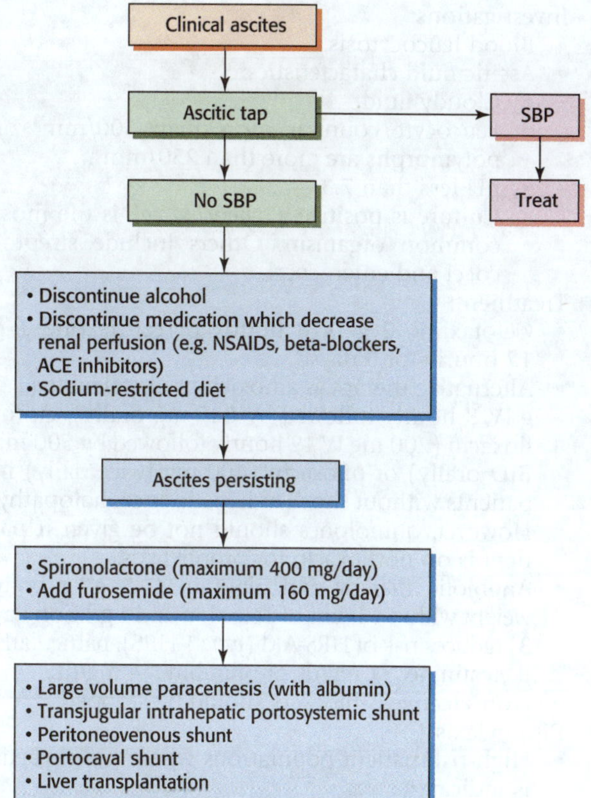

Flowchart 6.7(II) Summary of Management of Ascites in a Patient with Cirrhosis.

  6. A newer technique is drainage of peritoneal fluid into urinary bladder using a pump.
  7. Portocaval shunt.
  8. Liver transplantation.

SUMMARY OF MANAGEMENT OF ASCITES IN CIRRHOSIS

- Management of ascites in a patient with cirrhosis is summarised in Flowchart 6.7(II).

Q. Briefly explain spontaneous bacterial peritonitis. (IM 5.16, IM 5.6)

- Occurs due to translocation of bacteria from gut and reduced local and systemic immunity.
- Definition:
  - SBP is defined as infected ascitic fluid in the absence of a recognisable secondary cause of peritonitis.
- Clinical features:
  - May present as an abrupt deterioration or hepatic encephalopathy in a cirrhotic patient with ascites.
  - Usually, presentation is abrupt onset of fever with chills, abdominal pain and rebound abdominal tenderness.
  - A diagnostic paracentesis should be performed in patients with gastrointestinal bleeding, shock, fever, worsening liver and/or renal function and hepatic encephalopathy as incidence of SBP is high in these conditions.

- Investigations:
  - Blood leucocytosis.
  - Ascitic fluid characteristics:
    - Cloudy fluid.
    - Leucocyte count is more than $500/mm^3$ or polymorphs are more than $250/mm^3$.
    - pH less than 7.3.
    - Culture is positive. *Escherichia coli* is the most common organism. Others include streptococci and enterococci.
- Treatment:
  - Cefotaxime 2 g IV 8 hourly or ceftriaxone 1 g 12 hourly for 5 days.
  - Alternative therapy is amoxicillin/clavulanate (1.2 g IV 8 hourly followed by 625 mg orally), ciprofloxacin (200 mg IV 12 hourly followed by 500 mg BID orally) or ofloxacin (400 mg twice daily) in patients without shock or hepatic encephalopathy. However, quinolones should not be given if patient is on norfloxacin for prophylaxis.
  - Antibiotic therapy and albumin (1.5 g/kg body weight within 6 hours of detection and 1 g/kg on day 3) reduces risk of HRS-AKI (type 1 HRS), particularly if creatinine >1 mg/dL or bilirubin >4 mg/dL.
  - Nonselective β-blockers should be stopped.
- Prophylaxis:
  - High-risk patient populations where prophylaxis is indicated are:
    - Patients with acute gastrointestinal haemorrhage (primary prophylaxis; also decreases rate of rebleeding).
    - Patients with low total protein content <1.5 g/dL in ascitic fluid and advanced liver disease (Child–Pugh ≥9 and bilirubin ≥3 mg/dL or serum creatinine ≥1.2 mg/dL) (primary prophylaxis).
    - Patients with a previous history of SBP (secondary prophylaxis; recurrence in as many as 70% cases in first year).
  - In patients with upper GI haemorrhage, cefotaxime or ceftriaxone or norfloxacin (400 mg BID for 7 days).
  - In patients with low ascitic protein content or previous episode of SBP, long-term norfloxacin (400 mg/day) for prophylaxis. Alternative drugs include cotrimoxazole (800 mg sulphamethoxazole + 160 mg trimethoprim once a day) or ciprofloxacin (500 mg/day).

Q. Discuss the definition, mechanism, causes, clinical features and differential diagnosis of ascites.

Q. What is Puddle sign?

DEFINITION

- Ascites is defined as an accumulation of excess fluid within the peritoneal cavity.

MECHANISMS

- For mechanisms of ascites in cirrhosis and portal hypertension, refer 'ascites due to cirrhosis' on page 461.
- Inflammation of peritoneum leads to increased capillary permeability and exudation of fluid into the peritoneal cavity. The same mechanism is responsible for diminished reabsorption of fluid. Both these factors favour development of ascites in bacterial peritonitis and tuberculous peritonitis.
- Venous obstruction can lead to transudation of fluid into peritoneal cavity, for example inferior vena caval (IVC) obstruction.
- Lymphatic obstruction can lead to chylous ascites. Involvement of mesenteric lymph nodes, thoracic duct and abdominal lymphatic ducts can result in leakage of chyle into peritoneal cavity.
- Rupture of a viscus can result in outpouring of blood, cystic fluid or contaminated material, favouring ascites, for example pancreatitis.

CAUSES (Table 6.26)

TABLE 6.26 Causes of Ascites

Transudates	Exudates
• Cirrhosis and portal hypertension • Congestive cardiac failure • Nephrotic syndrome • Constrictive pericarditis • Beriberi • Hypoproteinaemia of any cause • IVC obstruction	• Tuberculous peritonitis • Malignant peritonitis • Bacterial peritonitis • Pancreatic ascites **Miscellaneous (exudative/ transudative)** • Meigs' syndrome • Chylous ascites • Budd–Chiari syndrome

CLINICAL FEATURES

SYMPTOMS

- Abdominal distension.
- Bloated feeling of abdomen.
- Dyspnoea and orthopnoea due to elevation of diaphragm.
- Indigestion and heart burns due to gastroesophageal reflux resulting from increased intraabdominal pressure.

SIGNS

- Abdominal distension and fullness of flanks.
- Skin over the abdominal wall may become stretched and shiny with striae albicans.
- Umbilicus may be flat or everted.
- Divarication of recti and herniae.
- Prominence of hypogastrium in the erect posture.
- Abdominal wall may show distended veins of two types. Veins radiating out from the umbilicus with flow away from the umbilicus represent collaterals due to portal hypertension (caput medusae). Prominent veins in the flanks with flow from below upwards represent the IVC collaterals, resulting from compression of IVC by severe ascites.
- In moderate ascites, the dullness is confined to only flanks. With larger amounts, the flanks and hypogastric areas are dull (horseshoe-shaped dullness). The epigastrium and umbilical regions remain resonant due to floating intestines. In massive ascites, the whole of the abdomen is dull except for a small area over the umbilical region.

- Shifting dullness elicitation requires a minimum of 1000 mL of fluid.
- Fluid thrill is elicitable in tense ascites.
- Paraumbilical zone of dullness is detected with smaller amounts of fluid. The patient is put in knee-elbow position and paraumbilical region percussed. Normally, the percussion note is tympanitic. Dullness indicates fluid.
- Puddle sign can detect even a volume as low as 120 mL. Patient lies prone for 5 minutes. The patient is then put in knee-elbow position. Apply the stethoscope on the most dependent part of the abdomen. Repeatedly flick one flank lightly. Diaphragm is moved gradually to the opposite flank. A marked change in the intensity and character of percussion note indicates fluid. However, since it is very uncomfortable to the patient, it is not advisable to do it.

SECONDARY EFFECTS

- Scrotal oedema.
- Pleural effusion, especially right sided. Pleural effusion develops due to defects in the diaphragm allowing the ascitic fluid to pass into the pleural space.
- Pedal oedema results from hypoproteinaemia and a functional block of IVC due to tense ascites.
- Cardiac apex is shifted upwards due to raised diaphragm.
- Neck veins may be distended secondary to an increase in right atrial pressure, which follows tense ascites and raised diaphragm.
- Meralgia paraesthetica can occur due to compression of lateral cutaneous nerve of thigh.

INVESTIGATIONS

- Ultrasonography is very sensitive in confirming ascites, detecting small amounts of fluid and in identifying the cause.
- Diagnostic paracentesis (Table 6.27).
- Laparoscopy and peritoneal biopsy.
- The ascitic fluid findings specific for individual aetiologies are discussed under the 'differential diagnosis of ascites'.

TABLE 6.27 Examination of Ascitic Fluid

Investigation	Interpretation
• Gross appearance	
• Clear, straw coloured or light green	Cirrhosis, congestive heart failure, nephrotic syndrome
• Haemorrhagic	Malignancy, tuberculosis, pancreatitis
• Cloudy, turbid	Bacterial peritonitis
• Deep green	Biliary leak
• Milky white (chylous)	Lymphatic obstruction
• Specific gravity	Less than 1.016 in transudates More than 1.016 in exudates
• Protein	Less than 2.5 g/dL in transudates More than 2.5 g/dL in exudates
• SAAG	*See below on the same page*
• Glucose	Low in malignancy, tuberculosis, peritonitis
• Amylase activity	More than 1000 units/L in pancreatitis
• Microscopy	
• Polymorphs	Less than 250/mm³ in cirrhosis More than 250/mm³ in bacterial peritonitis
• Lymphocytes	Tuberculosis, malignancy
• Gram's stain	Bacterial peritonitis
• Ziehl–Neelsen staining	Tuberculosis
• Cytological examination	Malignancy
• Culture	
• Pyogenic bacteria	Bacterial peritonitis
• Mycobacteria	Tuberculosis

DIFFERENCES BETWEEN TRANSUDATES AND EXUDATES (Table 6.28)

TABLE 6.28 Differences Between Transudates and Exudates

Feature	Transudate	Exudate
• Appearance	Clear, thin coloured	Turbid, haemorrhagic, straw
• Specific gravity	Less than 1.016	More than 1.016
• Protein	Less than 2.5 g/dL	More than 2.5 g/dL
• Total cell count	Considerably low (<250/μL)	Considerably high (>250/μL)
• Differential count	Mesothelial cells or lymphocytes	Polymorphs, lymphocytes or RBC

SERUM-ASCITES ALBUMIN GRADIENT

- A useful prognosticator of portal pressure.
- Calculated by subtracting the ascitic albumin concentration from the serum albumin concentration.
- Serum-ascites albumin gradient (SAAG) $\geq$1.1 g/dL indicates a high likelihood of portal hypertension.
- SAAG <1.1 g/dL indicates a high possibility of other causes.
- Ascitic fluid total protein level is typically used to define ascitic fluid as transudative (protein content <2.5 g/dL) or exudative (protein content $\geq$2.5 g/dL). However, many patients with SBP have a low rather than high ascitic fluid total protein level and many patients with portal hypertension secondary to heart failure have a high rather than the expected low ascitic fluid total protein level. SAAG is highly sensitive in these cases.

DIFFERENTIAL DIAGNOSIS OF ASCITES

CIRRHOSIS OF LIVER

- Clinical features and investigations are discussed under 'cirrhosis'.
- In cirrhosis, the ascitic fluid characteristics are:
  - Clear, straw coloured or light green.
  - Protein content less than 2.5 g/dL.
  - Polymorphonuclear leucocytes less than 250/mm³.

CONSTRICTIVE PERICARDITIS

- Common causes of constrictive pericarditis are:
  - Tuberculosis.

- Rheumatoid arthritis.
  - Haemopericardium.
  - Idiopathic.
- Because of constriction of the heart, the inflow to heart is reduced resulting in:
  - Decrease in cardiac output.
  - Increase in systemic venous pressure.
- Clinical features:
  - Raised JVP with a rapid γ descent.
  - Pulse is rapid and of low volume.
  - Pulsus paradoxus.
  - Kussmaul's sign (inspiratory augmentation of JVP).
  - Hepatomegaly.
  - Ascites and pedal oedema (late and minimal).
  - Pericardial knock.
- Chest radiograph might show a small-sized heart with calcification of pericardium.
- Ascitic fluid is a transudate (unless patient has associated tubercular involvement of peritoneum).
- Echocardiography confirms the diagnosis.
- Treatment includes medical management of the cause and pericardiectomy.

TUBERCULOUS PERITONITIS

- Tuberculous peritonitis results from one or more of the following:
  - Haematogenous seeding of peritoneum.
  - Lymphatics or mesenteric nodes.
  - Genitourinary source.
- Clinical features:
  - Evening rise of temperature, night sweets, weight loss and loss of appetite.
  - Malaise and gradual abdominal distension.
  - 'Doughy feel' of the abdomen.
  - Multiple palpable masses in the abdomen caused by matted omentum and loops of intestine.
- Ascitic fluid is usually straw coloured with a protein concentration more than 2.5 g/dL and lymphocytes more than 70%.
- Acid-fast bacilli may be demonstrated by Ziehl–Neelsen staining of ascitic fluid.
- Tubercle bacilli may be cultured from ascitic fluid.
- ADA levels are elevated.
- Diagnosis can be confirmed by the peritoneal biopsy of a granuloma under laparoscopy.
- Treatment is antituberculous chemotherapy.

MALIGNANT ASCITES

- Primaries of stomach, colon, ovary or other intraabdominal tumours may exude fluid into the peritoneal cavity.
- Any primary malignancy elsewhere may cause ascites by secondary deposits on peritoneal surface.
- Periumbilical subcutaneous tumour deposits are known as 'Sister Joseph's nodules'.
- Ascitic fluid characteristics are:
  - Exudate.
  - Haemorrhagic.
  - High in protein.
  - High in specific gravity.
  - Sediment contains malignant cells.
- Diagnosis can be confirmed by a laparoscopic biopsy of the peritoneum.
- Treatment is mainly palliative:
  - Repeated paracentesis.
  - Intraperitoneal instillation of methotrexate, nitrogen mustard or chloroquine may slow down the rate of reaccumulation of ascites.

PANCREATIC ASCITES

- Pancreatic ascites results from one of the following mechanisms:
  - Disruption of the main pancreatic duct, associated with internal fistula between the duct and peritoneal cavity.
  - Leaking from pancreatic pseudocyst in patients with chronic pancreatitis.
- Previous history suggestive of acute pancreatitis like severe abdominal pain radiating to the back and signs of acute abdomen followed by the development of ascites.
- Ascitic fluid characteristics are:
  - Exudate.
  - Haemorrhagic or turbid; protein more than 2.5 g/dL.
  - High levels of amylase (more than 1000 IU/L).
- Serum amylase is elevated.
- ERCP shows passage of contrast material from a major pancreatic duct or pseudocyst into the peritoneal cavity.
- Treatment:
  - Nasogastric suction and parenteral alimentation to reduce pancreatic secretions.
  - Ascitic tap to keep the peritoneal cavity free of fluid so as to hasten the sealing of leak. Octreotide (long-acting analogue of somatostatin) inhibits pancreatic secretion and is useful.
  - If there is no response over 2–3 weeks of medical treatment, surgical approach is required which includes stenting of disrupted main pancreatic duct or pancreatic resection.

BACTERIAL PERITONITIS

- Acute bacterial peritonitis.
- Chronic bacterial peritonitis.

Acute Bacterial Peritonitis

- Common causes are appendicitis, perforated viscus like peptic ulcer or typhoid ulcer, cholecystitis, ulcerative colitis, diverticulitis and gangrene of the small bowel.
- Symptoms and signs of acute bacterial peritonitis are:
  - Fever and severe abdominal pain.
  - Nausea and vomiting.
  - No flatus.
  - Thirst.
  - 'Hippocratic facies'.
  - Tachycardia, hypotension and shock.
  - Board-like rigidity.
  - Tenderness and rebound tenderness.
  - Absent peristaltic sounds.
- Plain radiograph of abdomen reveals dilated loops of intestine.
- Gas under the diaphragm in cases of perforation.
- Ascitic fluid characteristics are:
  - Exudate.
  - Turbid or purulent.
  - Presence of intestinal contents in the fluid.
  - Cell counts markedly raised.

- Polymorphs more than 250/mm^3.
- Gram staining for bacteria is positive.
- Culture grows the organism.
- Treatment:
  - Surgical emergency.
  - Correction of fluid and electrolyte disturbances.
  - Broad-spectrum antibiotic therapy.
  - Measures to combat shock.
  - Surgical measures.

Chronic Peritonitis

- Progressive ascites with intermittent subacute intestinal obstruction.
- Ascitic fluid is an exudate, high in protein and contains large number of chronic inflammatory cells.
- Treatment of the underlying cause relieves the condition.

MEIGS' SYNDROME

- Meigs' syndrome is a combination of:
  - Pleural effusion.
  - Ascites.
  - Nonmetastatic pelvic tumour (commonly fibroma of the ovary) in females.
- Pleural effusion is most commonly right sided, may be an exudate or transudate. It is thought to result from movement of ascitic fluid across the diaphragm.
- Both ascites and pleural effusion resolve dramatically following removal of the pelvic tumour.

CHYLOUS ASCITES

- Due to chyle (intestinal lymph) in the peritoneal cavity.
- Fluid is milky or creamy due to the presence of chylomicrons.
- Common causes of chylous ascites are:
  - Injuries (trauma) to the main lymph ducts in the abdomen.
  - Intestinal obstruction if associated with rupture of a major lymphatic channel.
  - Congenital lymphangiectasia.
  - Malignancy or tuberculosis obstructing the intestinal lymphatics, for example lymphoma.
  - Filariasis.
- Clinical manifestations are acute abdominal pain with signs of peritoneal irritation and leucocytosis. All these subside leaving the patient with a distended, nontender, fluid-filled abdomen (chylous ascites).
- Ascitic fluid characteristics are:
  - Milky or creamy.
  - High content of fat (triglycerides >200 mg/dL).
  - Sudan III staining demonstrates fat globules.
  - Cholesterol low (ascites/serum ratio <1).
- Treatment options include dietary measures (high-protein and low-fat diet with medium-chain triglycerides), use of pharmacological agents (e.g. orlistat which prevents conversion of dietary triglycerides into free fatty acids in the intestinal lumen) and surgical or percutaneous interventions in some select cases.

BUDD–CHIARI SYNDROME

- Refer page 472.

Q. What are various disorders associated with iron overload?

Q. Discuss the aetiology, pathology, clinical features, investigations and management of hereditary (primary) haemochromatosis ('bronzed diabetes').

DISORDERS CAUSING IRON OVERLOAD

- Various disorders causing iron overload are given in Table 6.29.
- In β-thalassaemia, sideroblastic anaemia and chronic haemolytic anaemias, there is increased iron absorption from GIT. Besides, these patients often require multiple blood transfusions.
- In secondary iron overload, iron accumulates in Kupffer cells rather than hepatocytes, as typically occurs in hereditary haemochromatosis. Features of haemosiderosis are similar to those of haemochromatosis with additional features of anaemia and underlying disease.
- Conditions that require blood transfusion also frequently exhibit ineffective erythropoiesis, and this also drives an increase in dietary iron absorption.

HEREDITARY HAEMOCHROMATOSIS

- In haemochromatosis, total body iron is increased to 20–60 g (normal is 4 g).
- High incidence of hepatocellular carcinoma.

AETIOLOGY

- Increased absorption of dietary iron over years. Patients with haemochromatosis absorb only a few milligrams of iron in excess of physiological need and thus clinical manifestations often occur at 40–60 years of age, when 20–40 g of excess iron have accumulated.
- Disease inherited as an autosomal recessive.
- The gene responsible for the disease in many cases is called *HFE* and is located on chromosome 6. This gene is responsible for regulating hepcidin, the primary iron regulatory hormone. Mutation leads to reduced hepcidin expression.
- About 90% of the patients are males. Females are protected by the iron loss in menstruation and pregnancy.

TABLE 6.29 Disorders Causing Iron Overload

Hereditary Haemochromatosis	Secondary Haemosiderosis

	• Chronic anaemias
	  • β-Thalassaemia
	  • Sideroblastic anaemia
	  • Chronic haemolytic anaemias
	• Exogenous iron overload
	• Multiple blood transfusions—haemolytic anaemias, myelodysplastic syndrome, aplastic anaemia
	• Repeated iron injections
	• Prolonged oral iron
	• Chronic liver diseases especially alcoholic liver disease, chronic hepatitis and nonalcoholic fatty liver disease

PATHOPHYSIOLOGY

- Pathophysiology of haemochromatosis is given in Flowchart 6.8.

PATHOLOGY

- Excess iron is deposited in various tissues resulting in damage to liver, pancreas, heart, pituitary gland and skin.

CLINICAL FEATURES

- Clinical features of haemochromatosis are given in Box 6.34.

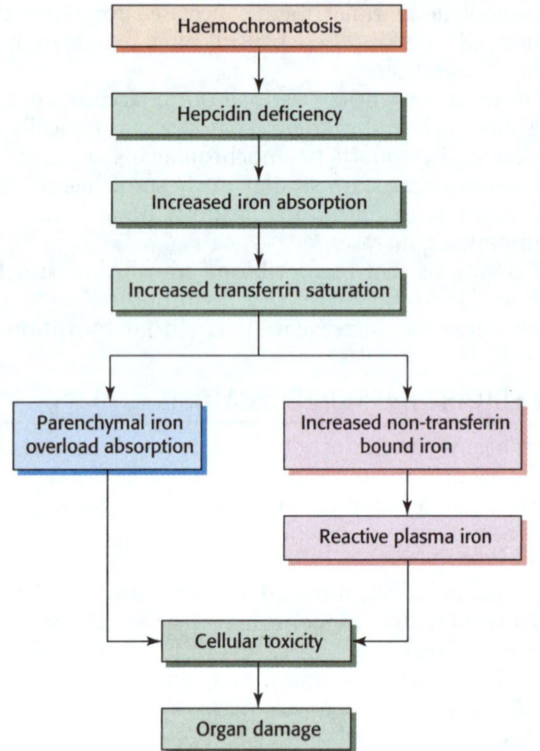

Flowchart 6.8 Pathophysiology of Haemochromatosis.

BOX 6.34 Haemochromatosis: Clinical Features

- Most often in males older than 40 years of age. In non-HFE-associated cases, onset in early adulthood
- Cirrhosis with hepatosplenomegaly, loss of libido, testicular atrophy, spiders, loss of body hair, jaundice and ascites; portal hypertension and live failure uncommon
- Diabetes mellitus in 30%–60% of cases
- Leaden-grey skin pigmentation due to excess melanin in exposed parts, axillae, groins and genitalia ('bronzed diabetes')
- Heart failure and cardiac arrhythmias
- Hypopituitarism
- Arthritis and chondrocalcinosis; arthritis particularly involves second and third metacarpophalangeal joints of the hands initially, but can progress to involve other joints including hips, wrists, ankles and knees
- Hypogonadism related to involvement of both pituitary gland and genitalia
- Hepatocellular carcinoma in 30% of patients with cirrhosis
- Many asymptomatic and identified by iron studies as part of screening studies and screening of family members of an affected individual

INVESTIGATIONS

- Plasma iron concentration is increased.
- Transferrin saturation is elevated (>45%–50%) which is highly sensitive for diagnosis.
- Serum ferritin levels are increased to more than 300 µg/L (also increased in alcoholic liver disease, hepatitis C infection, nonalcoholic steatohepatitis and also as acute phase reactant in other inflammatory and neoplastic conditions). Ferritin levels are less sensitive than transferrin saturation in screening tests for haemochromatosis.
- CT scan has poor sensitivity for iron deposits in liver.
- MRI is sensitive to detect increased hepatic iron content.
- Liver biopsy shows iron deposition and hepatic fibrosis leading on to cirrhosis. Due to availability of MRI, liver biopsy is often not performed.

MANAGEMENT

- Weekly venesection of 500 mL blood (which removes 250 mg of iron) until the serum iron is normal (may take 2 years or more). Thereafter, venesection is continued as required to keep serum ferritin normal. Blood removed can be used for routine transfusion.
- In rare cases, who cannot tolerate venesection (because of severe cardiac disease or anaemia), chelation therapy with desferrioxamine may be used in removing iron. Dose is 40–80 mg/kg/day subcutaneously. It removes 10–20 mg of iron/day. Oral iron chelators include deferiprone and deferasirox.
- Treatment of cirrhosis.
- Treatment of diabetes.
- Treatment of heart failure and cardiac arrhythmias.
- Alcohol consumption should be severely curtailed or eliminated because it increases the risk of cirrhosis nearly tenfold.
- Supplemental vitamin C must be avoided as pharmacological doses can accelerate iron mobilisation to a level that saturates circulating transferrin, resulting in an increase in pro-oxidant and free-radical activity.
- Raw shellfish should be avoided because of *Vibrio vulnificus*, a bacteria that can cause potentially fatal infection and that has been reported in patients with high iron levels.
- First-degree family members should be screened.

Q. Discuss the aetiology, pathology, clinical features, investigations and management of Wilson's disease (hepatolenticular degeneration).

Q. Explain in brief about Kayser–Fleischer ring.

AETIOLOGY

- Autosomal recessive inheritance.
- There is a failure of biliary copper excretion, causing its accumulation in the body.
- Wilson's disease is characterised by the following abnormalities:
  - Excessive accumulation of copper in the body.
  - Failure to synthesise ceruloplasmin.

CLINICAL FEATURES

- Presents between 5 and 30 years.
- Dominant features may be hepatic or neuropsychiatric:
  - In childhood and early adolescence, hepatic disease dominates.
  - In late adolescence, neuropsychiatric manifestations dominate.
- Liver involvement:
  - Asymptomatic hepatosplenomegaly.
  - Acute hepatitis.
  - Fulminant hepatic failure.
  - Chronic hepatitis.
  - Cirrhosis with portal hypertension.
- Brain involvement:
  - Characteristically produces neuropsychiatric manifestations.
  - Neurological manifestations.
    - Movement disorders, especially resting and intention tremors.
    - Less common manifestations include spasticity, rigidity, chorea, dysphagia and dysarthria.
  - Psychiatric manifestations.
    - Bizarre behavioural disturbances similar to schizophrenia, manic depressive psychosis and neurosis.
    - Others include irritability, personality change, impulsiveness, labile mood and declining school performance.
- Eye involvement:
  - Characteristic feature is Kayser–Fleischer rings, due to deposition of copper in the Descemet's membrane of cornea (Fig. 6.13).
    - Greenish-brown or golden-brown ring around the periphery of the cornea, appearing first at the upper periphery. It is best detected by slit-lamp examination.
    - Disappears with treatment.
    - Kayser–Fleischer rings may be associated with 'sunflower cataracts'.
    - May occasionally be seen in primary biliary cholangitis, primary sclerosing cholangitis.

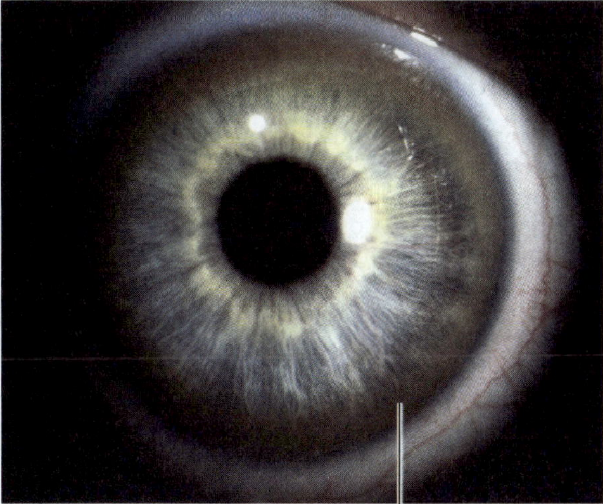

Fig. 6.13 Kayser–Fleischer ring.

- Other manifestations:
  - Kidney involvement resulting in renal tubular damage.
  - Skeletal involvement leading to osteoporosis.
  - Arthropathy.
  - Cardiomyopathy.
  - Haemolysis.

INVESTIGATIONS

- Slit-lamp examination of the eyes for Kayser–Fleischer ring.
- Low serum ceruloplasmin levels (less than 20 mg/dL). Levels can however, be normal in people with ongoing inflammation as it is an acute phase protein.
- Low total serum copper concentration.
- High urinary copper excretion (more than 100 μg/day).
- High hepatic copper content (more than 250 μg/g of dry tissue).
- Basal ganglia lesions on MRI.

MANAGEMENT

- Chelating drugs:
  - Penicillamine 1–4 g/day lifelong.
  - Alternative drug is trientine dihydrochloride 1.2–2.4 g/day. Adverse effects include aplastic and sideroblastic anaemias.
- Zinc acetate (equivalent to 150 mg zinc every day) for asymptomatic patients or after maximal improvement with penicillamine or trientine. It blocks absorption of copper from intestine. In addition, zinc increases levels of metallothionein in intestinal mucosal cells, which acts as an intracellular ligand that binds copper and holds it until it is excreted in the faeces with desquamated epithelial cells. However, zinc must not be administered with penicillamine or trientine since both the drugs chelate zinc.
- Patients with severe neurologic involvement, who do not improve with penicillamine or trientine, may be treated with intramuscular dimercaprol. Another agent is tetrathiomolybdate that acts by forming a tripartite complex with copper and protein, either in intestinal lumen where it prevents copper absorption or in circulation where it makes copper unavailable for cellular uptake.
- Liver transplantation in fulminant hepatic failure and advanced cirrhosis.
- All siblings of the patient should be screened for Wilson's disease and treated even if they are asymptomatic.

Q. Write a short note on an α_1-antitrypsin.

- It is an α-1-globulin produced by the liver. It comprises 90% of the α-1-globulin peak seen on serum electrophoresis.
- It is an acute phase reactant also and is released in response to acute inflammation.
- It is a protease inhibitor (Pi) that inhibits neutrophilic protease enzymes, particularly trypsin. This prevents breakdown of elastin and collagen by proteases.

- There are three forms of α-1-antitrypsin:
  - PiM (medium).
  - PiS (slow).
  - PiZ (very slow).
- PiMM is the normal phenotype, while the phenotype PiZZ gives low α-1-antitrypsin concentrations. Occasionally, PiZM may produce liver disease.
- α-1-antitrypsin deficiency is associated with liver disease (cirrhosis) and pulmonary disease (emphysema).
  - In neonates, α-1-AT deficiency produces cholestatic jaundice known as neonatal hepatitis syndrome.
  - In adults, the manifestations are:
    - Chronic hepatitis.
    - Cirrhosis.
    - Hepatocellular carcinoma and cholangiocarcinoma.
    - Chronic obstructive pulmonary disease.
    - Bronchiectasis.
    - Others: Panniculitis, vasculitis, pancreatitis and glomerulonephritis.
- Diagnosis:
  - Liver function tests and pulmonary function tests.
  - Serum protein electrophoresis shows absence of α-1-globulin peak.
  - Low plasma α-1-AT concentration (normal above 150 mg/dL).
  - α-1-AT containing globules can be demonstrated in the liver.
  - Genotyping for S and Z alleles.
- Treatment:
  - Abandon cigarette smoking and alcohol intake.
  - Supportive treatment for liver injury.
  - Management of COPD.
  - In adult patients (>18 years) with airway obstruction (FEV1 between 35% and 65% of predicted), who have severe deficiency and have stopped smoking, intravenous administration of exogenous α-1-AT derived from pooled human plasma has been shown to be of benefit. Not indicated for correcting liver disease.
  - Liver or lung transplantation.

Q. What is biliary cirrhosis?

Q. Discuss the aetiology, pathology, clinical features, investigations and management of primary biliary cholangitis (primary biliary cirrhosis).

- Biliary cirrhosis is the cirrhosis of the liver secondary to prolonged obstruction of biliary system, anywhere between the small interlobular bile ducts and the papilla of Vater. Obstruction results in progressive destruction of bile ducts.

PRIMARY BILIARY CHOLANGITIS (PRIMARY BILIARY CIRRHOSIS)

- Since many patients do not have cirrhosis, primary biliary cholangitis has replaced the previous term of primary biliary cirrhosis.

PATHOGENESIS

- It is a chronic autoimmune disease affecting interlobular bile ducts (cholangitis) leading to retention of bile salts into the liver (cholestasis) and secondary damage of hepatocytes.
- The disease is characterised by loss of immune tolerance to E2 component of the pyruvate dehydrogenase complex, a crucial enzyme of oxidative phosphorylation. This leads to interleukin-12 and IFN-γ driven immune-mediated lymphocytic cholangitis with consequent destructive chronic injury to the biliary epithelial cells.
- This loss of immune tolerance is precipitated by some environmental factors (chemical or infectious) which act through molecular mimicry.

PATHOLOGY

- Chronic granulomatous inflammation destroying the interlobular bile ducts, results in fibrosis and later cirrhosis of the liver and its complications.

CLINICAL FEATURES

- Occurs predominantly in females in the middle age (fifth or sixth decade).
- Asymptomatic patients are discovered on routine examination or investigations.
- Cardinal features are pruritus, hyperpigmentation and jaundice.
- Usually pruritus occurs months to years before jaundice. It is more at night.
- Liver involvement:
  - Intense pruritus, probably due to bile salts.
  - Progressive jaundice, later becoming intense.
  - Patient acquires a 'bottle green colour'.
  - Scratch marks and finger clubbing.
  - Hepatosplenomegaly.
  - Hepatocellular failure, portal hypertension and ascites.
- Hypercholesterolaemia:
  - Xanthelasmas around the eyes.
  - Xanthomas over joints, tendons, hand creases, elbows and knees.
  - Pain, tingling and numbness over feet and hands due to peripheral neuropathy resulting from lipid infiltration of peripheral nerves.
- Malabsorption:
  - Steatorrhoea and diarrhoea from malabsorption of fat.
  - Easy bruising and ecchymosis from vitamin K deficiency.
  - 'Hepatic osteodystrophy'—bone pains and fractures due to osteomalacia and osteoporosis resulting from malabsorption of vitamin D.
  - Night blindness due to vitamin A deficiency.
  - Dermatitis due to vitamin E deficiency.
- Associated diseases:
  - Sicca syndrome.
  - Thyroid diseases.
  - CRST syndrome (calcinosis, Raynaud's phenomenon, sclerodactyly and telangiectasia).
  - Scleroderma.

INVESTIGATIONS

- Hyperbilirubinaemia of the conjugated type.

- Mild elevation of transaminases.
- Twofold to fivefold rise of serum alkaline phosphatase which is persistent for >6 months.
- Marked rise of serum 5´-nucleotidase activity.
- Hyperlipidaemia (often no treatment is required unless other risk factors for CAD are present).
- Antimitochondrial antibodies in 85% cases; others are antinuclear antibodies (antiglycoprotein-210 or anti-sp100 antibodies).
- Elevated immunoglobulins especially IgM.
- Ultrasound to exclude biliary obstruction.
- MRCP shows normal biliary tree.
- Liver biopsy confirms the diagnosis but not required in many cases.

MANAGEMENT

- Ursodeoxycholic acid (10–15 mg/kg) improves bilirubin and aminotransferase values. UDCA appears to exert its beneficial effects by rendering bile composition less toxic for the injured biliary epithelium, reducing the retention of bile acids in hepatocytes and inhibiting bile-induced apoptosis of hepatocytes.
- Obeticholic acid, an analogue of chenodeoxycholic acid may be combined with UDCA if patient does not respond to it. It should be avoided in presence of advanced cirrhosis.
- Steroids (budesonide) may improve biochemical and histological disease but may lead to osteoporosis.
- Other therapies like azathioprine, colchicine, methotrexate and cyclosporin have shown little benefit.
- Steatorrhoea is treated by limiting fat intake and substituting long-chain triglycerides with medium-chain triglycerides in the diet.
- Monthly injections of vitamin K.
- Vitamin D (calciferol 1 mg/day) or alfacalcidol 1 μg/day.
- Calcium supplementation.
- Bisphosphonates (e.g. alendronate) to reduce osteoporosis.
- Liver transplantation.
- Management of pruritus:
  - Cholestyramine 4–16 g/day.
  - Rifampicin 150–600 mg/day is second-line agent.
  - Opiate antagonists (naloxone and naltrexone) have shown some benefit.
  - Sertraline 25–100 mg/day.
  - Antihistamines have no role.
- Sicca syndrome:
  - Artificial tears and saliva.
  - Pilocarpine or cevimeline in refractory cases.

Q. What is meant by secondary biliary cirrhosis?

- Secondary biliary cirrhosis results from prolonged obstruction to large biliary ducts by:
  - Stones.
  - Bile duct strictures.
  - Sclerosing cholangitis.
- Patients with malignant tumours of bile duct or pancreas rarely survive long enough to develop secondary biliary cirrhosis.
- Clinical features:
  - Recurrent abdominal pain in stones.
  - Fluctuating jaundice in stones.
  - Previous history of abdominal surgery in strictures.
  - Chronic cholestasis with episodes of ascending cholangitis and even liver abscess.
  - Right upper quadrant pain due to cholangitis or biliary colic.
  - Cirrhosis, ascites and portal hypertension are late features.
- Investigations:
  - Hyperbilirubinaemia of the conjugated type.
  - Markedly elevated serum alkaline phosphatase activity.
  - Ultrasound and CT of abdomen.
  - ERCP or MRCP.
  - Liver biopsy rarely required.
- Treatment:
  - Relief of obstruction to bile flow by ERCP or surgery.
  - Antibiotics in sclerosing cholangitis.

Q. What is cardiac cirrhosis?

- Prolonged severe right-sided congestive heart failure leads to cardiac cirrhosis. Common causes of right heart failure include severe mitral stenosis with tricuspid regurgitation, constrictive pericarditis, restrictive heart disease and cor pulmonale.
- In right heart failure, there is retrograde transmission of elevated venous pressure via the IVC and hepatic vein, into the liver. This leads to hepatic congestion. With prolonged passive venous congestion, liver becomes enlarged, tender and ultimately results in cirrhosis. Examination of liver shows a 'nutmeg liver' (alternating red-congested and pale-fibrotic areas).
- Clinical features:
  - Symptoms and signs of severe right heart failure (pulsatile liver initially, positive hepatojugular reflux—absent in Budd–Chiari syndrome).
  - Liver is enlarged, smooth and tender in initial stages.
  - More important is a chronic encephalopathy with a waxing and waning course.
- Diagnosis:
  - Firm enlarged liver with signs of chronic liver disease in a patient with valvular heart disease, constrictive pericarditis or cor pulmonale of long duration (more than 10 years).
  - Liver nonpulsatile despite presence of tricuspid regurgitation.
  - Liver biopsy confirms the diagnosis (not required in most cases).
- Treatment is that of the underlying cardiovascular disorder.

Q. Write a short note on noncirrhotic portal fibrosis or idiopathic noncirrhotic portal hypertension.

- Idiopathic noncirrhotic portal hypertension (INCPH) is characterised by presinusoidal increase in portal venous pressure in the absence of a known cause of liver disease and portal vein thrombosis.

- By definition, occlusion of the extrahepatic portal vein/hepatic veins, any disorder known to induce portal hypertension in the absence of cirrhosis (e.g. infiltrative diseases, vascular malignancies, schistosomiasis, congenital hepatic fibrosis, sarcoidosis) and any known cause of chronic liver disease must be excluded to make a diagnosis of INCPH.
- The term INCPH has replaced the previous terms like noncirrhotic portal fibrosis (NCPF) and hepatoportal sclerosis.
- INCPH (known as NCPF in India) is an idiopathic disease characterised by periportal fibrosis and involvement of small and medium branches of portal vein, resulting in development of portal hypertension and splenomegaly but without features of liver cell failure.

AETIOLOGY

- Postulated aetiologies include bacterial infections, exposure to toxins (particularly arsenic), immunological abnormalities and hypercoagulable states.

CLINICAL FEATURES

- The disease is characterised by upper GI bleed, massive splenomegaly with anaemia, preserved liver function and benign prognosis in a majority of patients.
- Development of ascites, jaundice and hepatic encephalopathy is uncommon and may be seen only after an episode of gastrointestinal haemorrhage.
- In late stages, the patient may develop some features of cirrhosis and ascites.

INVESTIGATIONS

- Liver function tests are usually normal. Pancytopenia may occur due to hypersplenism.
- Levels of vitamin B_{12} are low ($\leq$250 pg/mL), which may be helpful in distinguishing this condition from cirrhosis.
- On Doppler ultrasound, splenoportal axis and hepatic veins are patent. Thickened portal vein (>3 mm) with echogenic walls is characteristic. There is sudden narrowing or cut-off of intrahepatic second-degree and third-degree PV branches: so-called withered-tree appearance.
- MRI and CT show a nonnodular liver with enlarged caudate lobe, atrophic right lobe and preserved liver volume.
- Liver histology demonstrates maintained lobular architecture, portal fibrosis of variable degree, sclerosis and obliteration of small-sized portal vein radicals and subcapsular scarring with collapse of the underlying parenchyma.

TREATMENT

- Treatment is endoscopic sclerotherapy or banding to prevent variceal bleed and shunt surgery.
- TIPS (transjugular intrahepatic proto-systemic shunt) is an option if surgical shunt is not feasible.

Q. Discuss the aetiology, pathology, clinical features, investigations and management of hepatic venous outflow tract obstruction.

Q. Explain briefly about Budd–Chiari syndrome.

Q. Describe veno-occlusive disease or hepatic sinusoidal obstruction syndrome.

- Obstruction to the hepatic venous outflow (hepatic venous outflow tract [HVOT] obstruction) can occur at the following levels:
  - Central hepatic veins → Veno-occlusive disease.
  - Large hepatic veins → Budd–Chiari syndrome.
  - Suprahepatic portion of IVC → Budd–Chiari syndrome.

BUDD–CHIARI SYNDROME

DEFINITION

- Budd–Chiari syndrome is characterised by obstruction of hepatic venous outflow at any level from the small hepatic veins to the junction of the IVC with the right atrium. This term does not include cardiac or pericardial causes of hepatic outflow obstruction.
- Budd–Chiari syndrome comprises a triad of abdominal pain, ascites and hepatomegaly.

AETIOLOGY

- Causes of Budd–Chiari syndrome are given in Table 6.30 and depicted in Figure 6.14.

PATHOLOGY

- In the initial stages, liver shows centrilobular venous dilatation and congestion, with haemorrhage and central necrosis of hepatocytes.
- In the later stages, centrilobular fibrosis develops and the picture is that of cardiac cirrhosis.

TABLE 6.30 Aetiology of Budd–Chiari Syndrome

Hepatic Vein Obstruction	IVC Obstruction

• Venous thrombosis
  • Polycythaemia vera
  • Antiphospholipid syndrome
  • Pregnancy and postpartum period
  • Use of oral contraceptives
  • Sickle cell disease
  • Paroxysmal nocturnal haemoglobinuria
  • Other hypercoagulable diseases
• Compression (may also produce thrombosis)
  • Liver abscess
  • Hydatid cyst
• Radiation injury
• Webs (congenital)
	• Congenital
	  • Webs
	  • Diaphragms
	• Thrombosis
	  • Renal cell carcinoma
	  • Hepatoma
	  • Myeloproliferative syndrome
	  • Nephrotic syndrome
	• Vasculitis
	  • Behcet's syndrome
	  • Idiopathic

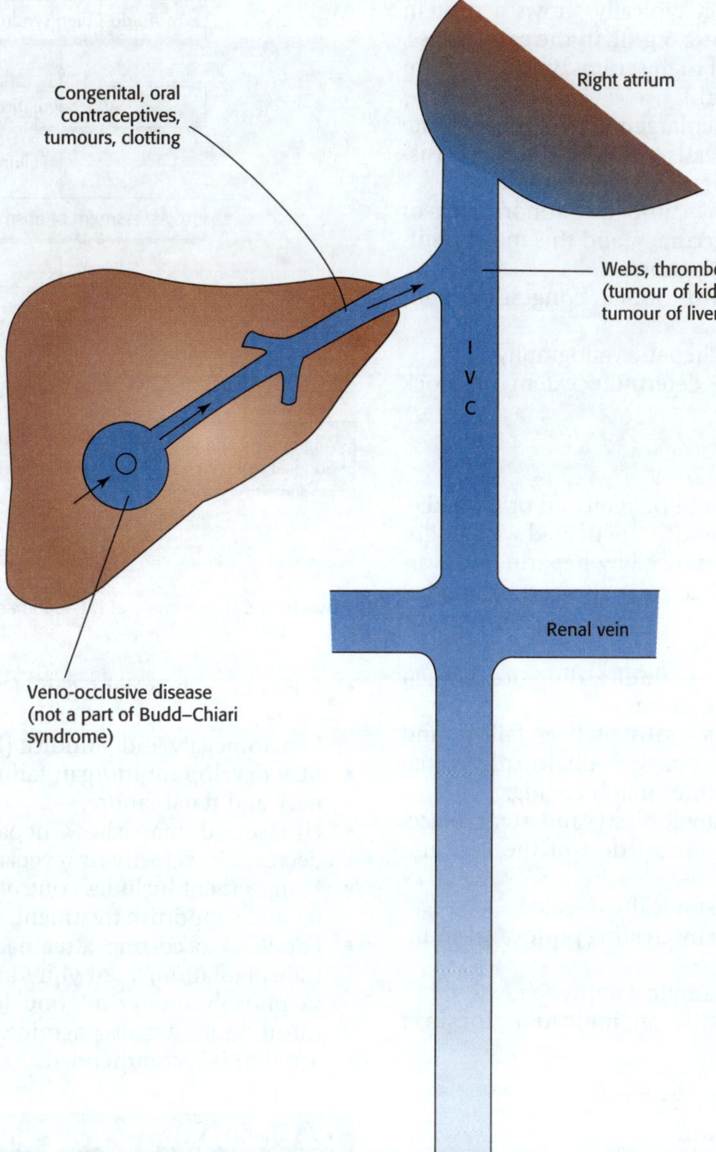

Fig. 6.14 Aetiological factors in Budd–Chiari syndrome.

CLINICAL FEATURES

- Fulminant form (fulminant Budd–Chiari syndrome)
  - Presents with fulminant hepatic failure due to liver necrosis. Ascites and renal failure are present.
- Acute form (acute Budd–Chiari)
  - Develops over a month or so and follows sudden venous occlusion (renal cell carcinoma, hepatoma and polycythaemia).
  - Presents with acute abdominal pain, vomiting, tender hepatomegaly, ascites and mild jaundice.
  - If venous occlusion is total, delirium, coma and hepatocellular failure develop.
- Subacute form (subacute Budd–Chiari)
  - Insidious onset.
  - Ascites and hepatic necrosis may be minimal, because the hepatic sinusoids have been decompressed by a portal and hepatic venous collateral circulation.
- Chronic form (chronic Budd–Chiari)
  - More usual presentation.
  - Manifests as cirrhosis and portal hypertension.
  - Pain in abdomen, tender hepatomegaly and ascites.
  - Icterus is mild or absent.
  - Negative hepatojugular reflux—that is pressure over the liver or other parts of abdomen fails to fill the jugular veins.
  - Gradual development of portal hypertension and splenomegaly.
  - Enlarged caudate lobe of the liver becomes palpable.
  - Obstruction in suprahepatic part of IVC manifests itself as bilateral pedal oedema and distended veins over abdomen, flanks and back.
  - Hepatocellular carcinoma may develop.

INVESTIGATIONS

- Liver function tests reveal mild hyperbilirubinaemia, raised alkaline phosphatase, low serum albumin and raised transaminases.

- Ascitic fluid examination typically shows a protein concentration more than 2.5 g/dL in the early stages, though later, ascites is of high serum-ascites albumin gradient (SAAG >1.1 g/dL).
- Ultrasound may show enlargement of the caudate lobe, intrahepatic collaterals, echogenic areas consistent with occlusion of hepatic veins and ascites.
- Doppler ultrasonography can detect abnormality of venous flow with high accuracy, and this may be sufficient to establish the diagnosis.
- Liver biopsy shows centrilobular congestion with fibrosis.
- Noninvasive CT or MRI hepatic venography.
- Hepatic venography to determine extent of block and caval pressures.

MANAGEMENT

- Predisposing causes should be removed or treated.
- Very early cases of thrombosis are treated with endovascular streptokinase followed by heparin and warfarin. Anticoagulation therapy is also recommended in most patients irrespective of whether thrombotic state is found.
- Ascites is treated with low-salt diet, diuretics, LeVeen shunt and portosystemic shunts.
- Management of complications of liver failure and portal hypertension, such as encephalopathy, renal insufficiency and gastrointestinal bleeding.
- Percutaneous balloon angioplasty and stent placement for membranous obstruction of the IVC and hepatic vein.
- Congenital web can be surgically resected.
- TIPS to decompress liver by creating portocaval shunt if above measures fail.
- Portosystemic shunt by surgical approach.
- Progressive liver failure is an indication for liver transplantation.

SUMMARY OF MANAGEMENT OF BUDD–CHIARI SYNDROME

- Flowchart 6.9 summarises management of a patient with Budd–Chiari syndrome.

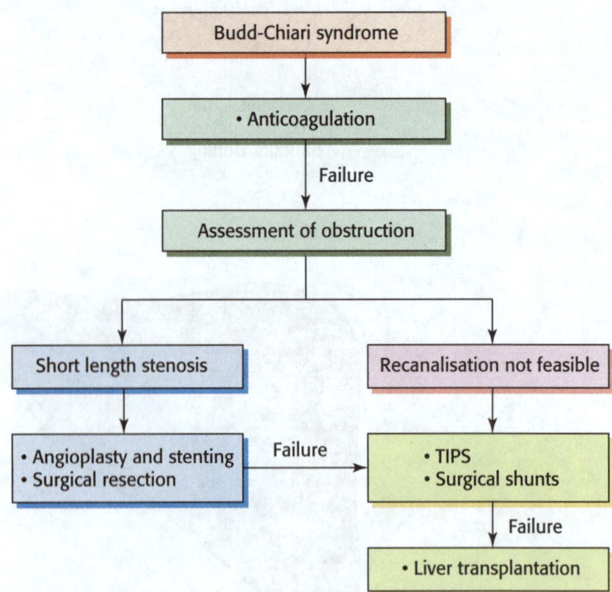

Flowchart 6.9 Summary of Management of Budd–Chiari Syndrome.

VENO-OCCLUSIVE DISEASE OR HEPATIC SINUSOIDAL OBSTRUCTION SYNDROME

- Veno-occlusive diseases (VOD), also known as hepatic sinusoidal obstruction syndrome, occurs most commonly as a complication of myeloablative regimens (particularly busulfan, cytarabine and cyclophosphamide) that are used to prepare patients for haematopoietic stem cell transplantation. Other causes include chemotherapeutic agents in conventional doses, chronic immunosuppression with azathioprine or 6-thioguanine, and ingestion of herbal teas made with pyrrolizidine alkaloids.
- Occurs due to circulatory obstruction at the level of central hepatic veins.
- Peak incidence of presentation is 12 days after haematopoietic cell transplantation and majority occur by 21 days.
- VOD due to ingestion of pyrrolizidine alkaloids can be acute or chronic in onset.
- Presents with weight gain (>5%) with or without ascites, right upper quadrant pain of liver origin, hepatomegaly and jaundice (bilirubin ≥2 mg/dL).
- May develop multiorgan failure, particularly pulmonary and renal failure.
- Ultrasound may show hepatomegaly, ascites and decrease in velocity or reversal of the portal flow.
- Management includes control of fluid overload, ascites and supportive treatment. TIPS is contraindicated.
- For VOD occurring after haematopoietic stem cell transplantation, methylprednisolone or defibrotide (a phosphodiester oligonucleotide with local antithrombotic, anti-ischaemic and anti-inflammatory activity) is recommended.

Q. Discuss fatty liver and its causes; non-alcoholic fatty liver disease; metabolic dysfunction-associated fatty liver disease; non-alcoholic steatohepatitis.

- Fatty liver indicates presence of excess fat in the liver.

CAUSES OF FATTY LIVER

- Causes of fatty liver are given in Table 6.31.

NON-ALCOHOLIC FATTY LIVER DISEASE (NAFLD) NON-ALCOHOLIC STEATOSIS AND NON-ALCOHOLIC STEATOHEPATITIS

- NAFLD (also called as metabolic dysfunction-associated fatty liver disease—MAFLD) is classified into two categories: simple fatty liver (non-alcoholic steatosis or non-alcoholic fatty liver) with a favourable clinical outcome and non-alcoholic steatohepatitis (NASH), which is intractable and progressive.
- Chronic liver disease such as viral hepatitis, Wilson's disease, haemochromatosis and autoimmune

TABLE 6.31 Causes of Fatty Liver

Alcohol

Nonalcoholic fatty liver disease (NAFLD) (nonalcoholic steatosis and nonalcoholic steatohepatitis [NASH])

1. **Drugs**
   - Glucocorticoids
   - Amiodarone
   - Aspirin
   - Tetracyclines
   - Methotrexate
   - Zidovudine
   - Didanosine
   - Tamoxifen
   - Amiodarone
2. **Nutritional**
   - Protein–calorie malnutrition
   - Total parenteral nutrition
   - Rapid weight loss/obesity
3. **Metabolic**
   - Lipodystrophy
   - Pregnancy (acute fatty liver)
   - Diabetes
4. **Miscellaneous**
   - Inflammatory bowel disease
   - HIV infection
   - Reye's syndrome
   - Toxic mushrooms (*Amanita phalloides*)
   - Obstructive sleep apnoea
   - Indian childhood cirrhosis
   - Chronic hepatitis C

TABLE 6.32 Risk Factors for Development of NAFLD

Main risk factors	Insulin resistance, obesity, sedentary lifestyle, type 2 diabetes mellitus, hypertension, dyslipidaemia
Drugs	Tamoxifen, corticosteroids amiodarone, methotrexate, oestrogens, valproic acid, antiretroviral medications
Miscellaneous	Total parenteral nutrition, rapid weight loss, obesity surgery (e.g. jejunoileal bypass), polycystic ovarian syndrome, hypothyroidism, obstructive sleep apnoea

hepatitis, starvation, lipodystrophy, coeliac disease, Cushing's disease and medications as mentioned in Table 6.31 should be excluded before labelling the disease as NAFLD.

RISK FACTORS FOR NAFLD

- There are several risk factors for development of NAFLD (Table 6.32).

PATHOGENESIS

- Hyperinsulinaemia and insulin resistance lead to increased adipocyte lipolysis and circulating free fatty acids which are taken up by hepatocytes initiating various complex metabolic pathways that lead to NAFLD (Flowchart 6.10).
- NASH is considered to be induced by two consecutive steps: excess fat accumulation and subsequent necroinflammation in the liver.

CLINICAL FEATURES

- Nonalcoholic fatty liver is a common cause for abnormal liver tests.
- Most patients have no symptoms at the time of diagnosis, although some have fatigue, malaise and a sensation of fullness in the upper abdomen. Other features may include daytime sleepiness and autonomic disturbances. Hepatomegaly is the only sign in most patients. Many patients are obese.

COURSE

- Patients with simple steatosis generally have a benign course whereas many with NASH show progression to cirrhosis and sometimes to hepatocellular carcinoma. Many patients with cryptogenic cirrhosis are likely to represent cases of previously unrecognised NASH, particularly because hepatic steatosis may disappear with the development of cirrhosis.
- Incidence of coronary artery disease and chronic kidney disease is increased in patients with NASH.

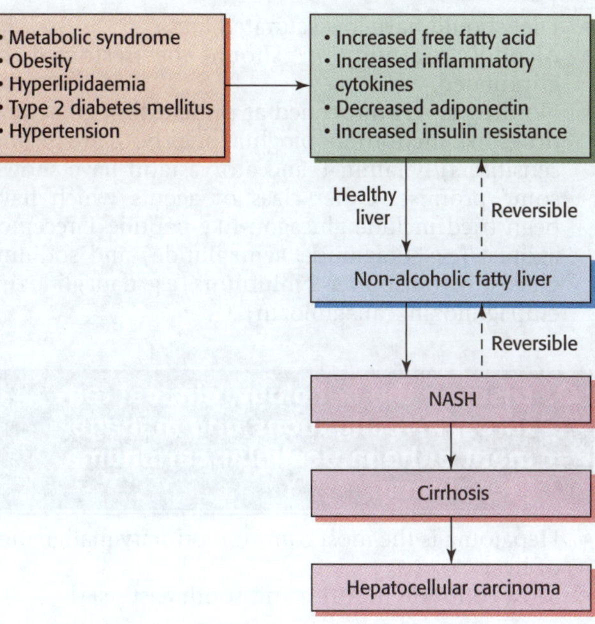

Flowchart 6.10 Pathogenesis of NAFLD.

INVESTIGATIONS

- Laboratory features include intermittent elevation in ALT and AST with AST:ALT <1. This ratio increases as fibrosis advances.
- Ferritin levels increased in 20%–50% of patients.
- Autoantibodies (e.g. antinuclear and antismooth muscle antibodies) identified in nearly 25% of patients and may be associated with more advanced fibrosis.
- Ultrasound shows diffuse increase in echogenicity as compared to the kidneys and spleen. On CT scan, fatty infiltration produces a low-density liver as compared to spleen. MRI is more sensitive.
- Ultrasound elastography and MRI elastography provide assessment of amount of liver fibrosis and may replace liver biopsy in many patients.
- Liver biopsy remains the best diagnostic tool for confirming fatty liver disease. It is also the most sensitive and specific mean of providing important prognostic information by distinguishing steatosis from NASH and by determining the stage of fibrosis.

TREATMENT

- Treatment includes control of weight, diabetes and hyperlipidaemia.
- Weight loss >5% of total body weight can decrease hepatic steatosis, weight loss >7% of total body weight can lead to resolution of NASH and weight loss >10% of total body weight can result in fibrosis regression or stability.
- Clinically significant weight loss generally requires a hypocaloric diet targeting 1200–1500 kcal/d or a reduction of 500–1000 kcal/d from baseline.

- Diet should have low saturated fats.
- Alcohol consumption should be restricted or eliminated.
- No drug is recommended at present though several drugs like metformin, pioglitazone (both are insulin sensitisers), vitamin E and atorvastatin have shown some promise. Other class of agents which have been tried include glucagon-like peptide-1 receptor agonist (e.g. liraglutide, semaglutide) and sodium-glucose cotransporter-2 inhibitors (e.g. dapagliflozin, empagliflozin, canagliflozin).

Q. Discuss the aetiology, clinical features, investigations and management of hepatocellular carcinoma (hepatoma).

- Hepatoma is the most common primary malignancy of liver.
- Most common in Africa and south-east Asia.

AETIOLOGY

- Table 6.33 gives a list of causes of hepatocellular carcinoma.

CLINICAL FEATURES

- Usually occurs in patients with underlying cirrhosis.
- Nonspecific symptoms like weakness, anorexia, weight loss and fever.
- Hepatomegaly with pain or tenderness is the most common presentation (more than 50%).
- Obstructive jaundice caused by invasion of the biliary tree or compression of intrahepatic ducts.
- Friction rub or bruit over the liver.
- Blood-tinged ascites.
- Metabolic disturbances (paraneoplastic features) include polycythaemia, hypoglycaemia, hypercholesterolaemia, acquired porphyria cutanea tarda, watery diarrhoea and hypercalcaemia.
- Intravascular invasion and growth into portal vein or IVC are common features.
- Features related to metastasis (bones, lungs, etc.).

INVESTIGATIONS

- Very high levels of serum alkaline phosphatase.
- A markedly increased (>500 μg/L) or rising levels of α-foetoprotein.
- Ultrasonography.
- CT scan of abdomen (triple-phase) or MRI abdomen.
- Liver scintigraphic scans.
- Hepatic artery angiography shows 'tumour blushes'.
- Liver aspiration or biopsy confirms the diagnosis.

TABLE 6.33 Causes of Hepatocellular Carcinoma

• Chronic HBV infection	• α-1-antitrypsin deficiency
• Chronic hepatitis C virus infection	• Wilson's disease
• Aflatoxin (a fungal toxin contaminating food)	• Thorotrast and arsenic exposure
• Alcoholic cirrhosis	• Oestrogens and androgens
• Primary biliary cholangitis	• Anabolic steroids
• Haemochromatosis	• Nonalcoholic steatohepatitis (NASH)
• Obesity	• Betel quid chewing

MANAGEMENT

- Curative intent (lesions one to three in number and <5 cm in size; no metastasis; compensated underlying liver disease with Child score A) possible in only 15% cases as most present with advanced disease.
  - Surgical removal (after successful resection, tumour recurs in the cirrhotic liver in about 70% of patients after 5 years).
  - Percutaneous ethanol injection (PEI) or percutaneous acetic acid injection (PAI).
  - Percutaneous radiofrequency thermal ablation.
- Palliative therapy:
  - PEI or acetic acid injection.
  - Transcatheter arterial chemoembolisation (TACE).
  - Transcatheter arterial embolisation.
  - Percutaneous radiofrequency thermal ablation.
  - Transarterial radioembolisation (TARE) with intra-arterial injection of yttrium-90 microspheres (^{90Y}).
  - Chemotherapy using sorafenib (a multikinase inhibitor).
  - Other agents approved for treatment include nivolumab (PD-1 receptor inhibitor), pembrolizumab (PD-1 receptor inhibitor) and atezolizumab (PD-L1 inhibitor) plus bevacizumab (VEGF inhibitor).
- Liver transplant is an option in presence of localised tumour and underlying advanced liver disease.

Q. Discuss the aetiology, clinical features, investigations and management of pyogenic liver abscess (bacterial liver abscess).

AETIOLOGY

- Bacteria reach the liver and cause abscess by one of the following five mechanisms:
  - Portal vein bacteraemia from appendicitis, diverticulitis and perforated bowel.
  - Systemic bacteraemia reaching liver via hepatic artery.
  - Ascending cholangitis.
  - Direct extension from a contiguous focus of infection like subphrenic abscess.
  - Penetrating trauma introducing the bacteria into liver or blunt trauma resulting in a hepatic haematoma that gets secondarily infected.
- Single abscesses are more common in the right lobe of the liver. Multiple abscesses are seen in elderly patients, usually due to ascending cholangitis.
- Common organisms are *E. coli*, *Klebsiella pneumoniae*, *Staphylococcus aureus*, anaerobic streptococci and *Bacteroides*.

CLINICAL FEATURES

- Most have a subacute onset.

- Fever with chills and rigors.
- Weight loss, anorexia, nausea and vomiting.
- Right upper quadrant pain radiating to right shoulder.
- Pleuritic chest pain.
- Tender hepatomegaly.
- Mild jaundice.
- Respiratory findings at the base of right lung (pleural effusion, crepitations).

INVESTIGATIONS

- Leucocytosis and raised ESR.
- Mildly elevated serum bilirubin and transaminases.
- Elevated serum alkaline phosphatase.
- Low serum albumin.
- Blood culture may be positive.
- Chest radiograph shows raised right dome of diaphragm, right basilar atelectasis and pneumonia or effusion.
- Ultrasonography confirms the diagnosis.
- CT scan of abdomen, if clinical suspicion is strong but ultrasound is normal.
- Needle aspiration of pus for culture sensitivity (both aerobic and anaerobic).

MANAGEMENT

- Percutaneous drainage with either catheter placement or needle aspiration followed by treatment with a combination of ampicillin plus gentamicin plus metronidazole, or ceftriaxone plus metronidazole, or piperacillin-tazobactam with or without metronidazole (to provide cover for amoebic liver abscess). Later, change the antibiotic according to the sensitivity reports. Duration is 4–8 weeks.
- Ultrasound-guided aspiration of the abscess. Indications include:
  - Abscess size is large (>6 cm).
  - Left lobe abscess.
  - Lack of response after 48–72 hours of medical therapy.
  - Ultrasonographic picture suggestive of large abscess with impending rupture.
- Surgical drainage for those who fail to respond or have multiloculated abscess, abscess with thick pus, multiple abscesses or left lobe abscess.

COMPLICATIONS

- Septic metastasis leading to endophthalmitis, septic pulmonary embolism, infection of the lungs and CNS.
- Rupture of abscess into peritoneal cavity.
- Rupture of abscess into pleural cavity, lung or pericardium producing pleural effusion, empyema, pneumonia, pericarditis or bronchopleural fistula.
- Multiorgan failure.

Q. Discuss the differential diagnosis of jaundice of 3 weeks' duration in an elderly person.

- Common causes of jaundice of 3 weeks' duration in an elderly person are listed in the Box 6.35.

BOX 6.35 Differential Diagnosis of Jaundice of 3 Weeks' Duration in an Elderly Person

- Viral hepatitis
- Drug-induced hepatitis
- Gallstone disease
- Hepatocellular carcinoma
- Alcoholic hepatitis
- Weil's disease
- Cirrhosis of liver
- Secondaries in liver
- Carcinoma of head of pancreas

Q. What are the common causes of hepatomegaly with tenderness (tender hepatomegaly)?

- Common causes of tender hepatomegaly are listed in Box 6.36.

BOX 6.36 Common Causes of Tender Hepatomegaly

- Hepatitis
  - Viral hepatitis
  - Drug-induced hepatitis
  - Alcoholic hepatitis
  - Chronic hepatitis
- Nonalcoholic fatty liver disease
- Congestive cardiac failure
- Amoebic liver abscess
- Pyogenic liver abscess
- Acute Budd–Chiari syndrome
- Hepatocellular carcinoma—late feature
- Secondaries—occasionally

Q. Enumerate the common causes of splenomegaly.

- Common causes of splenomegaly based on size of palpable spleen are given in the Table 6.34.

TABLE 6.34 Causes of Splenomegaly

Mild Enlargement (up to 5 cm)	Moderate Enlargement (5–8 cm)	Massive Splenomegaly (more than 8 cm)
• Malaria • Typhoid • Infective endocarditis • Disseminated tuberculosis • Viral hepatitis • Disseminated fungal infection • Septicaemia • Thalassaemia minor • Rheumatoid arthritis • Systemic lupus erythematosus • HIV infection • Congestive cardiac failure	• Cirrhosis of liver • Lymphomas • Leukaemias • Infectious mononucleosis • Haemolytic anaemias • Splenic abscess • Amyloidosis • Haemochromatosis • Polycythaemia vera	• Hyperreactive malarial syndrome (tropical splenomegaly) • Kala-azar • Chronic myeloid leukaemia • Extrahepatic portal vein obstruction • Thalassaemia major • Myelofibrosis • Myeloid metaplasia • Hairy cell leukaemia • Gaucher's disease • Niemann–Pick disease • Sarcoidosis • Splenic cysts

MCQs

1. A 45-year-old woman presents to the Gastroenterology Outpatient clinic with progressive jaundice, pruritis and chronic fatigue. Liver function tests: Bilirubin 5.15 mg/dL, alkaline phosphatase 540 IU/L (normal <147 IU/L), ALT 240 U/L. You suspect primary biliary cholangitis and arrange an autoimmune screen. Which autoantibody is associated with primary biliary cholangitis?
   A. Antimitochondrial antibodies (AMA)
   B. Anticentromere antibodies (ACA)
   C. Antineutrophil cytoplasmic antibody (ANCA)
   D. Antitransglutaminase (tTG)
   E. Anti-Scl-70 antibodies

Ans: A. Antimitochondrial antibodies (AMA)

IM5.14|IM5.12

2. In a patient with altered liver function tests, with predominance of alkaline phosphatase and gamma-glutamyl transferase (GGT) over ALT and AST, and excluding the most frequent liver diseases, the next diagnostic step would be:
   A. Evaluation of the bile duct with imaging test
   B. Liver biopsy
   C. Determination of antimitochondrial antibodies (AMA)
   D. Determination of p-ANCA
   E. Liver transplantation

Ans: A. Evaluation of the bile duct with imaging test

In the clinical situation described with predominance of cholestasis enzymes, priority is given to the evaluation of the bile duct by means of imaging tests: ultrasound, CT, MRI or cholangiography. If the bile duct is normal, autoantibodies would be ordered to support the diagnosis of primary biliary cholangitis or autoimmune cholangitis. If intrahepatic and extrahepatic short segmental biliary strictures appear alternating with normal ducts, it would support the existence of primary sclerosing cholangitis.

IM5.6|IM5.16

3. In patients with advanced liver cirrhosis, with variceal re-bleeding despite preventive pharmacological treatment and endoscopic band ligation, the therapeutic option of choice is:
   A. Transjugular intrahepatic portosystemic shunt (TIPS)
   B. Surgical portosystemic shunt
   C. Octreotide maintenance treatment
   D. Sclerosis of varicose veins
   E. Liver transplantation

Ans: Transjugular intrahepatic portosystemic shunt (TIPS)

In the above case, the therapeutic option of choice is the transjugular intrahepatic portosystemic shunt, whose perioperative mortality is lower, especially if a liver transplant is planned in the short term. Surgical portosystemic shunt would be the choice in liver cirrhosis with good liver function (Child's stage A).

IM5.6

4. In a patient with advanced hepatocellular carcinoma, ascites and portal hypertension, and a positive hepatitis C antibody test, who has gastrointestinal bleeding, the following statements are true, except:
   A. There is a defect in the synthesis of factors II, VII, IX, X
   B. Thrombocytopaenia may be related to hypersplenism
   C. Protein C, S and antithrombin levels are normal
   D. Fibrinolysis may be increased
   E. Prothrombin complex concentrates should not be used, or should be limited to very extreme situations

Ans: C. Protein C, S and antithrombin levels are normal

Coagulopathy in patients with liver disease is multifactorial. The above-mentioned proteins are the factors synthesised in the hepatocytes that suffer a decrease in production.

IM16.3

5. A patient with chronic alcoholism is diagnosed with chronic pancreatitis after an endoscopic retrograde cholangiopancreatography. The patient reports episodic, severe epigastric pain, radiating to the back, but with good response to nonopioid analgesics. For the last 5 months, he has lost 5 kg of weight. He has profuse, malodorous diarrhoea of up to six bowel movements a day. Which of the following is the most suitable action?
   A. Perform an abdominal ultrasound to rule out associated ileocaecal tuberculosis
   B. Assess for the presence of steatorrhoea by D-xylose test
   C. Start treatment with pancreatic enzymes
   D. Perform a colonoscopy with ileocaecal biopsy
   E. Recommend loperamide as it is probably an irritable bowel syndrome with predominant diarrhoea

Ans: C. Start treatment with pancreatic enzymes as his loose stools appear to be due to fat malabsorption caused by pancreatic exocrine deficiency.

IM5.6

6. A 45-year-old man presents with acute upper gastrointestinal bleeding. On further questioning, he admits to a 6-month history of lethargy, weight gain and pedal oedema. He has a past history of diabetes and impotence. Examination of his abdomen reveals moderate splenomegaly with a small amount of ascites. An upper gastrointestinal endoscopy shows multiple columns of oesophago-gastric varices that are treated with sclerotherapy. Which of the following is the most likely diagnosis?
   A. Haemochromatosis
   B. Nonalcoholic fatty liver
   C. Budd-Chiari syndrome
   D. Peritoneal mesothelioma
   E. Non-Hodgkin's lymphoma

Ans: A. Haemochromatosis

This causes liver cirrhosis with portal hypertension, diabetes and impotence as in this case and is treated with venesection and consideration of transplant.

IM5.6

7. A 55-year-old woman is found to have a raised alkaline phosphatase (ALP) through blood tests done during a medical examination for pruritus and jaundice. Which antibody is most likely to be present?
   A. Antivoltage gated Ca^{2+} antibodies
   B. Antiphospholipid antibodies
   C. Antimitochondrial antibodies
   D. Anticitrullinated protein antibody
   E. Anticentromere antibodies

Ans: C. Antimitochondrial antibodies

Primary biliary cholangitis is often characterised by the presence of antimitochondrial (M2 subtype) antibodies. Often asymptomatic and diagnosed after finding raised ALP on routine liver function tests. Lethargy and pruritus may occur and may precede jaundice.

IM5.6

8. A 28-year-old woman presents with sudden onset severe right upper quadrant pain, jaundice and abdominal distension. She has no other medical conditions and only takes the oral contraceptive pill. On examination, she is icteric, has a 3 cm palpable, tender liver and shifting dullness. What is the most likely diagnosis?
   A. Budd-Chiari syndrome
   B. Pancreatitis
   C. Acute cholecystitis
   D. Alcoholic liver disease
   E. Cardiac failure

Ans: A. Budd-Chiari syndrome

Budd-Chiari syndrome is hepatic vein thrombosis. It is associated with use of oral contraceptives and underlying thrombophilias. It presents with a triad of abdominal pain, hepatomegaly and ascites, and commonly sudden onset jaundice.

IM5.7

9. A 24-year-old woman develops deranged liver function tests and mild jaundice following a recent severe lower respiratory tract infection for which she received some treatment. What is the most likely drug causing the patient's hepatotoxicity?
   A. Codeine
   B. Chlorpheniramine
   C. Co-amoxiclav
   D. Dextromethorphan
   E. Paracetamol

Ans: C. Co-amoxiclav

Co-amoxiclav can cause a cholestatic picture on liver function tests. It is associated with liver parenchymal disruption, and hence impaired bile flow. It is likely that this patient received a course of co-amoxiclav for her respiratory tract infection, which then led to deranged liver function tests. This is usually transient and resolves after stopping the offensive drug.

IM16.1

10. A 36-year-old man presented with a 3-month history of loose stools five or six times a day. The stools were watery and occasionally pale in colour. There was occasional nocturnal diarrhoea. He had type 2 diabetes mellitus and was taking a sulphonylurea. He had had a cholecystectomy 2 years previously. There had been no weight loss, and the results of blood tests, including tissue transglutaminase were normal. Which of the following is the most likely cause of his diarrhoea?
    A. Bile acid diarrhoea
    B. Diverticular disease
    C. Drug-induced diarrhoea
    D. Helicobacter pylori infection
    E. Small intestinal bacterial overgrowth

Ans: A. Bile acid diarrhoea

Nocturnal diarrhoea with episodic pale stools raises the possibility of bile acid diarrhoea, especially post-cholecystectomy.

IM5.8

11. A 48-year-old woman presented with a 5-day history of colicky right upper abdominal pain and a 2-day history of jaundice and nausea. She had noticed that her stools had become pale and her urine was darker than usual. She was otherwise well and had no comorbidities. She had been taking regular paracetamol for pain relief. She had not lost any weight. On examination, she had a body mass index of 32 kg/m^2. She was jaundiced but afebrile and normotensive. She was tender in the right hypochondrium. Investigations: Haemoglobin 12.0 g/dL; White cell count $6400/mm^3$; Bilirubin 7.2 mg/dL; Alanine aminotransferase 160 U/L; Alkaline phosphatase 542 IU/L (normal 45–105); Albumin 3.6 g/dL; Globulin 3.2 g/dL; Gamm-glutamyl transferase 800 U/L (4–35); International normalised ratio 1.2. What is the most likely cause for the jaundice?
    A. Unintentional paracetamol overdose
    B. Pancreatic cancer
    C. Gallstone-related biliary obstruction
    D. Acute viral hepatitis
    E. Autoimmune hepatitis

Ans: C. Gallstone-related biliary obstruction

Gallstone-related biliary obstruction is the most likely cause in a patient with risk factors for developing gallstones who presents with symptoms of obstructive jaundice and pain.

Absence of weight loss make B less likely but important to exclude. The lack of significant hepatitis (disproportionately low alanine aminotransferase) and history make A and D unlikely, while normal globulin levels make E unlikely.

IM5.14

12. A 24-year-old man presented because his mother had noticed that he had been a bit yellow when he

returned after a night shift at the store where he had recently started as a shelf stocker. He said that he had lost his appetite since he had started working there. He felt otherwise well. He had no previous medical problems and did not regularly take any medications. He drank 60–90 mL of whiskey every night for the last 2 months. He had a new girlfriend. His mother had thyroid problems. Examination was normal with no evident jaundice. Investigations: Haemoglobin 15.9 g/dL; Mean corpuscular volume 91 fL; Reticulocyte count 1%; Sodium 139 mEq/L; Potassium 4.0 mEq/L; Urea 14 mg/dL; Creatinine 1.0 mg/dL; Bilirubin 2.57 mg/dL; Alanine aminotransferase 28 U/L; Aspartate aminotransferase 19 U/L; Alkaline phosphatase 88 U/L (normal 45–105); Albumin 4.2 g/dL; Gamma-glutamyl transferase 40 U/L (normal 4–35); International normalised ratio 1.0. Which of the following is the next most useful diagnostic test?
A. Conjugated and unconjugated bilirubin concentrations
B. Ultrasound scan
C. Urine urobilinogen
D. Peripheral smear for evidence of haemolysis
E. Liver biopsy

Ans: A.

Conjugated and unconjugated bilirubin is the most appropriate initial test for Gilbert's syndrome, which is the likely cause.

Normal alanine aminotransferase, alkaline phosphatase and γ-glutamyl transferase make parenchymal and/or biliary disease unlikely; hence ultrasound scan and liver biopsy would be unhelpful.

IM15.1

13. A 60-year-old man was admitted with vomiting of fresh blood. He also had an episode of melaena. He was otherwise well. He had been admitted with similar symptoms while on holiday 1 month previously. Investigations at that time were negative. He did not drink alcohol and was not taking nonsteroidal anti-inflammatory drugs. On examination, he was slightly pale, with a systolic blood pressure of 110 mmHg in supine position, falling to 100 mmHg on standing. His pulse was 100/minute. The remainder of the examination was normal. Investigations: Haemoglobin 12.5 g/dL on admission and 8.2 g/dL the following day (It had been 14.1 g/dL in the month prior to admission); Urea initially 60 mg/dL, falling to 40 mg/dL the following day; Creatinine 1.0 mg/dL. Upper gastrointestinal endoscopy within 24 hours was normal with good mucosal views. The patient responded well to intravenous fluid resuscitation. What is the most likely diagnosis?
A. Arteriovenous malformations
B. Gastric erosions
C. Mid-small bowel gastrointestinal stromal tumour
D. Dieulafoy's lesion
E. Mallory–Weiss tear

Ans: D. Dieulafoy's lesion

Arteriovenous malformations, gastric erosions and Mallory–Weiss tears would be seen on gastroscopy if they were responsible for the bleeding. Mid-small bowel lesions would not cause fresh haematemesis and would not be associated with a rise in urea concentration. The most appropriate answer is Dieulafoy's lesion.

IM15.2

14. A 45-year-old man was admitted as an emergency, vomiting copious amounts of fresh red blood and passing loose, tarry black stools, which continued in the emergency department. He was drinking around 150 mL of whiskey every day for the past 10 years and had been taking ibuprofen tablets for back pain for several months. On examination, he looked unwell, pale and clammy and was unable to sit up because of feeling light-headedness. His blood pressure was 85/40 mmHg, heart rate 170 bpm and temperature 36.0 °C. There were no definite clinical stigmata of chronic liver disease. What is the most important next step in management while waiting for blood test results to be available?
A. Rectal examination and erect and supine blood pressure measurements
B. Insert two wide-bore intravenous access needles and give intravenous saline
C. Insert two wide-bore intravenous access needles and give antibiotics and terlipressin
D. Telephone the on-call gastroenterology team immediately
E. Insert two wide-bore intravenous access needles and give fresh frozen plasma immediately

Ans: B. Insert two wide-bore intravenous access needles and give intravenous saline

Although rectal examination may be justified in some cases, this man is having a major gastrointestinal bleed with ongoing melaena and is therefore not a priority; the priorities are intravenous access and resuscitation. An erect blood pressure reading is unlikely to provide additional useful information as he already has low blood pressure and feels unwell in sitting position.

19. IM5.13

15. A 45-year-old woman presents to the Emergency Department with a history of recurrent abdominal pain in the right upper quadrant. She describes dark urine and pale stools. On examination she is tossing in bed due to pain. Abdominal examination elicits positive Murphy's sign. What is the most appropriate next step in the management?
A. Abdominal ultrasound
B. Endoscopy
C. CT abdomen
D. Emergency laparotomy
E. Erect chest and abdominal X-ray

Ans: A. Abdominal ultrasound

Ultrasound will provide the best imaging of the biliary system. X-ray will only detect 10% of all gallstones and will not provide information on biliary tract dilatation.

IM13.12

16. A 60-year-old man has a history of hepatitis B. He has presented with jaundice and weight loss. Ultrasound showed a mass lesion in the liver. Which of the following tumour markers would be the most appropriate to test in this patient?
    A. Alpha-fetoprotein (AFP)
    B. Calcitonin
    C. CA 125
    D. Carcinoembryonic antigen (CEA)
    E. Human chorionic gonadotropin (βHCG)

Ans: A. Alpha-fetoprotein (AFP)

Hepatocellular carcinoma is associated with HBV and causes raised AFP.

IM5.8

17. A 45-year-old woman presents to the Emergency Department with severe right upper quadrant abdominal pain and jaundice. She has a past history of cholecystectomy and had an endoscopic retrograde cholangiopancreatogram (ERCP) 3 days ago to remove retained common bile duct stones. You suspect ascending cholangitis.
    Which of the following is a classical feature of cholangitis?
    A. Ascites
    B. Encephalopathy
    C. Fever
    D. Purpura
    E. Hypoxia

Ans: C. Fever

Abdominal pain, jaundice and fever are the characteristic features of ascending cholangitis (Charcot's triad).

IM5.18

18. A normally fit and well 17-year-old woman is admitted feeling generally unwell. She is found to have markedly deranged liver function tests. After a week of admission, she becomes increasingly confused, and her INR increases to 6.8. You diagnose fulminant hepatic failure secondary to seronegative hepatitis. What is the most appropriate treatment?
    A. Mannitol
    B. Lactulose
    C. Haemofiltration
    D. Liver transplantation
    E. N-acetylcysteine

Ans: D. Liver transplantation

The patient has deteriorated rapidly and is unlikely to improve with supportive measures; therefore urgent liver transplantation is required. She also fulfills criteria for liver transplantation with INR >6.5.

IM16.15

19. A 25-year-old woman presents to the gastroenterology outpatient clinic with a 6-month history of weight loss and diarrhoea. Occasionally this diarrhoea is bloody, and she frequently passes large amounts of mucus. On examination she is very thin and has a tender mass in the right iliac fossa. You suspect a diagnosis of Crohn's disease.
    Which of the following is a common feature of Crohn's disease?
    A. Toxic megacolon
    B. Decreased incidence in smokers
    C. Shallow mucosal ulceration
    D. Fistulation is common
    E. Surgery is curative

Ans: D. Fistulation is common

Fistula formation is a common complication of Crohn's disease.

IM15.10

20. A 35-year-old smoker is admitted with sudden onset melaena and haematemesis. He is otherwise normally fit and well but admits to recently taking indomethacin for lower back pain. On admission his pulse rate is 110 beats/min, with a BP of 101/90 mmHg. Initial investigations show:
    Hb 6.0 g/dL
    Platelet 245,000/cmm
    Urea 48 mg/dL
    Creatinine 0.9 mg/dL
    Large calibre peripheral IV access is obtained, and fluid resuscitation is started. Despite aggressive crystalloid administration and 3 units of blood, he remains tachycardic and continues to pass large amounts of dark red blood per rectum. From the following options below, select the most appropriate investigation:
    A. Colonoscopy
    B. Mesenteric angiogram
    C. Flexible sigmoidoscopy
    D. Oesophagogastroduodenoscopy
    E. Barium swallow

Ans: D. Oesophagogastroduodenoscopy

This is the investigation of choice. An OGD in experienced hands can be both diagnostic and therapeutic. Obvious bleeding sites such as a duodenal ulcer can be managed via an endoscopic needle injection with adrenaline or endoscopic clips.

IM5.5

21. A 64-year-old labourer presents to the Emergency Department with haematemesis and melaena. Of note he has clubbing, several spider naevi and multiple small haemorrhages on his upper and lower limbs. His clotting results are shown below:
    Platelets: 105,000/cmm
    Activated partial thromboplastin time (aPTT) 56 seconds (normal 25–35 seconds), Prothrombin time (PT): 36 seconds
    Thrombin clotting time: 15 seconds (normal 12–14 seconds)
    What is the most likely cause of these results?
    A. Alcoholic liver disease
    B. Haemophilia A
    C. Heparin therapy
    D. Immune thrombocytopaenia
    E. Warfarin therapy

Ans: A. Alcoholic liver disease

All clotting tests are prolonged. This is most likely due to a liver problem (the site of clotting factor production). His low platelet count suggests portal hypertension and hypersplenism. He may also have vitamin K and folate deficiency due to poor nutrition.

IM15.14

22. A 55-year-old woman with known liver disease secondary to alcohol consumption presents with a large haematemesis probably related to oesophageal varices. Her blood pressure is 90/60 mmHg and she is alert. She is resuscitated initially with intravenous fluids and blood. What is the most appropriate next management step while waiting for the endoscopist to arrive?
    A. Insertion of a Sengstaken–Blakemore tube
    B. Propranolol infusion
    C. Terlipressin infusion
    D. Vasopressin infusion
    E. Pantoprazole infusion

Ans: C. Terlipressin infusion

Vasoconstrictor therapy is for emergency control of bleeding while waiting for endoscopy and in combination with endoscopic techniques. The aim of vasoconstrictor agents is to restrict portal inflow by splanchnic arterial constriction.

IM5.18

23. A 55-year-old woman has developed end-stage cirrhosis and asks about the possibility of liver transplantation. In which situation would this be an appropriate consideration?
    A. Alcohol intake cut down to 6 units of alcohol a day
    B. Chronic hepatitis B, high HBV DNA
    C. Associated cardiomyopathy with ejection fraction of 25%
    D. Autoimmune hepatitis not responding to treatment
    E. Primary biliary cholangitis with bilirubin 3.5 mg/dL

Ans: D. Autoimmune hepatitis not responding to treatment

In patients who have failed to respond to medical treatment or have major side effects of corticosteroid therapy, transplantation may be appropriate although the disease may recur.

IM5.6

24. A 56-year-old woman with chronic liver disease develops confusion, depressed consciousness, personality changes and intellectual impairment. A blood test is done which supports the diagnosis that the woman suffers from hepatic encephalopathy. Which of the following blood factors is the most likely cause of this condition?
    A. Ammonia
    B. Urea
    C. Arginine
    D. Citrulline
    E. Ornithine

Ans: A. Ammonia

Ammonia, generated by the amino acid deamination process, disappears almost completely from the blood and turns into urea. The synthesis of urea takes place in the liver. If the liver fails, ammonia builds up in the blood and is extremely toxic, severely affecting the brain.

7 Diseases of the Cardiovascular System

Q. Discuss the differential diagnosis of chest pain.

COMMON CAUSES OF CHEST PAIN

- Common causes of chest pain are shown in Box 7.1.
- Respiratory chest pain most commonly arises from parietal pleura (including the diaphragmatic pleura), chest wall and the mediastinal structures. Lung parenchyma and visceral pleura are insensitive to most painful stimuli. The peripheral part of the diaphragm and costal portion of parietal pleura are innervated by somatic intercostal nerves; thus pain felt in these areas is often localised to cutaneous distribution of involved neurons over the adjacent chest wall. Central portion of diaphragm is innervated by phrenic nerve; therefore central diaphragm irritation is referred to ipsilateral shoulder tip or even the neck.

BOX 7.1 Common Causes of Chest Pain

CARDIAC:
- Angina pectoris
- Myocardial infarction
- Mitral valve prolapse
- Pericarditis
- Hypertrophic cardiomyopathy
- Aortic stenosis/regurgitation
- Takotsubo cardiomyopathy

AORTIC:
- Dissecting aneurysm

LUNG AND PLEURA (RESPIRATORY):
- Pleurisy
- Pneumothorax
- Pulmonary embolism
- Lung malignancy

OESOPHAGEAL;
- Reflux oesophagitis
- Diffuse oesophageal spasm
- Oesophageal perforation
- Achalasia

HYPERADRENERGIC STATE:
- Cocaine intoxication

INTRAABDOMINAL CONDITIONS:
- Acute pancreatitis
- Acute cholecystitis
- Perforated peptic ulcer

MUSCULOSKELETAL

ANXIETY

MISCELLANEOUS CONDITIONS:
- Acute chest syndrome (sickle cell anaemia)
- Herpes zoster (including postherpetic neuralgia)

BOX 7.2 History to Be Elicited in a Patient With Chest Pain

- What is the character of pain?
- What were you doing when the pain started?
- What is the location of pain?
- Are there any precipitating or relieving factors?
- Does the pain radiate to any other site?
- Did you have associated sweating, palpitations, vomiting or shortness of breath?
- Any other associated symptoms like fever and cough?
- Did you lose consciousness?
- How long did the pain last?
- How often do you have the pain?
- Do you have any swelling or pain in leg?
- Are you on bed rest for some reason?
- Are there any skin lesions around the site of pain?
- Are you hypertensive or diabetic?
- Do you consume any illicit drugs?

BOX 7.3 Signs of Myocardial Ischaemia

• Rise in blood pressure and heart rate	• Dyskinetic segment around the apex
• Fourth heart sound	• Paradoxical splitting of second heart sound
• Murmur of mitral regurgitation due to papillary muscle dysfunction	• Relief of pain by carotid sinus massage (Levine test)

HISTORY

- Various points which need to be asked in the history are shown in Box 7.2.

ANGINA PECTORIS

- Pain is usually retrosternal in location and brought on by exertion. It is relieved by rest and sublingual nitrates. Pain seldom lasts more than 20 minutes. Character of the pain is squeezing, crushing or aching. Pain commonly radiates to left arm and less commonly to right arm, throat, back, chin and epigastrium. Often the pain comes on while walking uphill after a heavy meal on a cold winter day.
- Box 7.3 shows physical signs of 'myocardial ischaemia'. The presence of one or more of them during an attack of pain may be suggestive of ischaemia.
- Salient investigations include electrocardiography, echocardiography, exercise testing and coronary angiography.

MYOCARDIAL INFARCTION

- A history of previous episodes of anginal pain with recent worsening may be present. The pain of infarction is similar in character and distribution to anginal pain. But it is more severe, prolonged (lasts more than 20 minutes), persisting at rest and not responding to nitrates. There may be vomiting, anxiety, palpitations, breathlessness, sweating and a feeling of impending death.
- One or more of the physical signs of myocardial ischaemia may be present (mentioned in Box 7.3).
- Other common physical signs include pallor, sweating, cyanosis, hypotension, arrhythmias (most commonly ventricular ectopic beats), pericardial friction rub, signs of heart failure and cardiogenic shock.
- Salient investigations include serial electrocardiograms and cardiac injury enzymes.

MITRAL VALVE PROLAPSE

- History of nonspecific chest pain.
- Physical findings include a mid-systolic click and a late systolic murmur varying with posture and respiration.
- Echocardiography can confirm the diagnosis.

PERICARDITIS

- Pericardial pain is felt retrosternally to the left of the sternum or on the left or right shoulder. Pain is aggravated by deep breathing and rotating the trunk. It is worse in the lying down position and is relieved by sitting up and leaning forwards.
- Physical findings include the characteristic pericardial friction rub and evidence of pericardial effusion.

- Salient investigations include electrocardiography and echocardiography.

DISSECTING ANEURYSM OF AORTA

- Sudden onset of severe, sharp, stabbing or tearing pain over the anterior chest radiating to the back is the usual history. Dissection is more common in hypertensive males.
- Physical findings include asymmetry of brachial, carotid or femoral pulses, inappropriate bradycardia and an early diastolic murmur of aortic regurgitation. Neurological features (hemiparesis, paraparesis, etc.) may develop due to carotid artery or spinal artery involvement.
- Salient investigations include chest radiography, echocardiography, CT scanning and aortography.

PLEURISY

- Can occur due to inflammation, infection, neoplastic infiltration or trauma.
- Pleuritic pain is a well-localised pain that is cutting, stabbing or tearing in character. It is often aggravated by coughing, sneezing and deep inspiration. Commonest sites of pleuritic pain are axillae and beneath the breasts.
- Characteristic sign is a pleural friction rub.

PNEUMOTHORAX

- History of sudden-onset dyspnoea and chest pain following strenuous exertion or coughing. More common in tall, thin, young males.
- Depending on the size of pneumothorax, clinical features may include cyanosis, tachycardia, hypotension and distended neck veins. Respiratory system examination reveals shift of the mediastinum (trachea and apex beat) to the opposite side, with reduced chest movements, hyper-resonant percussion note, diminished vocal fremitus and vocal resonance, and markedly reduced to absent breath sounds on the involved side.
- Diagnosis is confirmed by chest radiography and ultrasound of chest.

ACUTE PULMONARY EMBOLISM

- Characteristic clinical setting may be obvious, for example prolonged immobilisation, recent surgery, previous history of thromboembolism, malignancy or intake of oral contraceptives.
- Clinical examination may reveal calf muscle tenderness, tachypnoea and tachycardia. Respiratory system examination may show a variety of physical signs like crepitations over the involved area, pleural rub or pleural effusion. Cardiovascular system examination may show evidence of acute right ventricular failure including increased intensity of the pulmonary component of second heart sound, a right-sided third heart sound and murmur of pulmonary regurgitation. However, examination may be entirely normal.
- Salient investigations include chest radiography, electrocardiogram, echocardiography, helical CT scan and radionuclide ventilation/perfusion scan.

REFLUX OESOPHAGITIS

- Characteristic history is 'heart burn', felt as a burning pain behind the sternum, radiating to the throat. It typically occurs after heavy meals and is brought on by bending, lifting or straining. Pain may occur on lying down in bed at night but relieved by sitting up. Other symptoms of gastro-oesophageal reflux are odynophagia and regurgitation of gastric contents into the mouth.
- Salient investigations include oesophagoscopy, barium studies and acid infusion studies. Often, a sliding hiatus hernia predisposes to reflux.

DIFFUSE OESOPHAGEAL SPASM

- Pain can mimic that of angina and is sometimes precipitated by exercise and relieved by nitrates. Usually the pain is related to food or drink intake. Dysphagia is often present.
- Salient investigations include oesophageal motility studies, barium studies and manometry.

MUSCULOSKELETAL PAIN

- Common causes of musculoskeletal pains are as follows:
  - Intercostal myalgia.
  - Costochondritis (Tietze's syndrome).
  - Fracture of the ribs (cough, trauma).
  - Secondaries (metastasis) in the ribs.
  - Intercostal neuralgias.
- Pain is usually well localised, variable in intensity and site, varying with posture and movement.
- Usually associated with severe local tenderness.

Q. Give a brief account of mechanism, causes, consequences and management of Cheyne–Stokes breathing.

DEFINITION

- This is a form of periodic breathing characterised by alternating periods of central apnoea (or hypopnoea) and hyperpnoea.
- The rate and depth of respiration increase to a maximum over a period of a few minutes, and then decrease until breathing virtually ceases. The patient lies motionless for 10–20 seconds (apnoea). Then the cycle is repeated (Fig. 7.1).

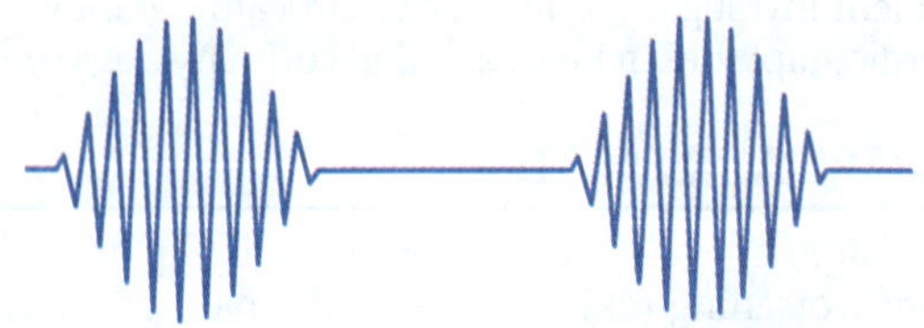

Fig. 7.1 Pattern of Cheyne–Stokes breathing.

MECHANISM

- Spontaneous rhythmic activity of breathing is abolished when there is anoxaemia. Consequent apnoea results in accumulation of carbon dioxide. This hypercapnia stimulates respiratory centres resulting in hyperventilation. The hyperventilation leads to carbon dioxide wash-out and results in depression of the respiratory centre leading to apnoea. The cycle is repeated.
- Delay between changes in ventilation and detection of the resulting $PaCO_2$ by the central chemoreceptors maintains a cyclic pattern of respiration. Factors which contribute to this delay include prolonged lung to brain circulation time, reduced tissue and lung CO_2 and O_2 stores, and increased ventilatory drive.
- Apnoeas are more severe when the patient is supine because pulmonary congestion worsens on lying flat, which activates afferent receptors present in lung ('J' receptors) and induces hyperventilation.
- In addition, in heart failure, the baseline arterial carbon dioxide tension is lower than normal which also leads to apnoea.
- Overnight polysomnogram is the gold standard diagnostic test.

CONDITIONS ASSOCIATED WITH CHEYNE–STOKES BREATHING (Box 7.4)

BOX 7.4 Conditions Associated With Cheyne–Stokes Breathing

• Severe heart failure	• Increased intracranial pressure
• Uraemia	• Severe pneumonia
• Chronic hypoxia	• Narcotic drug poisoning
• Cerebral trauma and haemorrhage	• Normal subjects living at high altitude
• Stroke	• During deep sleep

CONSEQUENCES

- Alternating cycles of hyperventilations and hypoventilations provoke oscillations in blood pressure, heart rate and tidal volume. This leads to a state of physiological instability in the already stressed cardiovascular system in patients with heart failure (HF).
- Poor sleep quality leads to daytime somnolence, fatigue, impaired quality of life and insomnia.

MANAGEMENT

- Treatment of underlying cause.
- In patients with HF, theophylline, acetazolamide or benzodiazepines have been used with varying success.
- Oxygen therapy.
- Continuous positive airway pressure ventilation during sleep.

Q. Discuss the approach to a patient with palpitations.

- Described as an uncomfortable awareness of one's own heartbeat.
- Occurrence of palpitations does not necessarily mean that an arrhythmia is present; conversely, an arrhythmia can occur without palpitations.

CAUSES OF PALPITATIONS (Table 7.1)

TABLE 7.1 Causes of Palpitations

Cardiac arrhythmias: • Paroxysmal atrial flutter/fibrillation • Paroxysmal supraventricular tachycardia • Premature atrial contractions • Sick sinus syndrome • Sinus tachycardia • Premature ventricular contractions • Ventricular tachycardia	**Drug-induced:** • Alcohol (use or withdrawal) • Amphetamines • Anticholinergic agents • Caffeine, nicotine • Cardiac glycosides • Cocaine • Adrenaline • Nitrates
High-cardiac-output states: • Anaemia • Arteriovenous fistula • Beriberi • Fever • Paget's disease • Pregnancy • Thyrotoxicosis	**Metabolic:** • Hyperthyroidism • Hypoglycaemia • Phaeochromocytoma **Psychiatric causes:** • Generalised anxiety • Hypochondriasis • Major depression • Panic disorder
Cardiac abnormalities: • Congenital heart disease (atrial septal defect, patent ductus arteriosus, ventricular septal defect) • Aortic or mitral regurgitation • Mitral valve prolapse • Pacemaker (function or failure) • Prosthetic heart valves • Atrial myxoma	**Miscellaneous:** • Emotional stress • Hyperventilation • Premenstrual syndrome • Scombroid fish poisoning • Strenuous physical activity

EVALUATION

- Primary goals are as follows:
  - To detect and identify presence and nature of any underlying arrhythmia.
  - To determine the presence of organic heart disease.
  - To determine the presence of precipitating causes.

HISTORY

Character of Palpitations

- Helpful to ask patients to tap out the rhythm of their palpitations to identify regularity and speed.
- A feeling of 'flip-flopping' in chest is usually secondary to a premature atrial or ventricular beat.
- A feeling of stoppage of heart is usually secondary to the pause that follows a premature beat.
- A feeling of pounding is usually due to a forceful beat caused by postextrasystolic potentiation after a premature beat.
- A feeling of rapid fluttering in chest is usually secondary to supraventricular or ventricular tachyarrhythmias.
- A feeling of neck pulsations may be due to atrioventricular (AV) nodal tachycardia caused by simultaneous contraction of atria and ventricles, causing reflux of

blood in superior vena cava. Associated 'shirt flapping' (visible movement of patient's clothes during the episode) can also be noted in AV node reentry tachycardia.
- An irregular heartbeat suggests atrial fibrillation.
- The association of polyuria and palpitations may indicate supraventricular tachycardia because increased atrial pressures stimulate production of natriuretic peptides.

Mode of Onset and Termination
- Palpitations that start and terminate abruptly usually indicate atrial or ventricular tachyarrhythmias.
- Palpitations that occur gradually usually indicate benign aetiologies, such as sinus tachycardia during exercise or anxiety.

Precipitating Factors
- A history of palpitations during strenuous activity is often normal, but palpitations during minimal stress suggest an underlying pathology, such as myocardial ischaemia, heart failure, atrial fibrillation, anaemia or thyrotoxicosis.
- Prolonged QT syndrome may present with palpitations during times of catecholamine excess and manifest itself as polymorphic ventricular tachycardia (VT) during these times.
- Use of drugs is another major precipitating cause of palpitations. Although patients may not be taking any prescribed medications, it is crucial to ask them if they have taken any over-the-counter remedies (e.g. sympathomimetic agents for allergies or colds), diet pills, illicit drugs (e.g. cocaine), alcohol, tobacco or even caffeinated beverages or chocolate.

Associated Symptoms
- Include syncope, anxiety, dizziness and chest pain.
- Syncope is a serious symptom in patients with palpitations and may represent VT or a very rapid supraventricular tachycardia.
- Palpitations associated with anxiety, a lump in the throat, dizziness and tingling in the hands and face suggest sinus tachycardia accompanying an anxiety state marked by hyperventilation.
- Palpitations associated with angina may suggest myocardial ischaemia precipitated by increased oxygen demand, secondary to a rapid heart rate.

Relief With Vagal Manoeuvres
- Termination of palpitations with carotid massage or other vagal manoeuvres (e.g. Valsalva's manoeuvre) may be effective in patients with supraventricular tachycardia.

Family History
- Family history of sudden cardiac death (e.g. arrhythmogenic right ventricular cardiomyopathy, hypertrophic cardiomyopathy, prolonged QT interval).

EXAMINATION
- Examination is often done during symptom-free period.
- Important signs to look for include features of anxiety (e.g. tremors), abnormal vital signs, pale skin, exophthalmos, goitre, jugular venous distension, carotid bruits, diminished carotid upstroke, heart murmurs, gallops and clicks, wheezes, crepitations, lower extremity oedema and calf tenderness.

Laboratory Studies
- Haemoglobin, serum glucose, electrolytes and thyroid function tests.
- Electrocardiogram—may show bundle branch block, short PR interval, delta waves, prolonged QT interval, ischaemia, chamber enlargement, prior myocardial infarction or other forms of organic heart disease.
- Holter monitoring.
- Exercise electrocardiography may be helpful in patients whose palpitations are precipitated by exercise and who have risk factors for ischaemic heart disease.
- Echocardiography to evaluate for any structural heart disease and assessment of left ventricular function.
- Electrophysiology study (an invasive test of electrical conduction system of heart) in selected patients.

Q. Discuss the differential diagnosis of syncope. (PY 5.11)

SYNCOPE (FAINTING)
- Comprises generalised weakness of muscles, loss of postural tone, inability to stand upright and brief loss of consciousness, with rapid and spontaneous recovery.

FAINTNESS (PRESYNCOPE)
- Refers to lack of strength with sensation of impending loss of consciousness.
- 'Faintness' reflects the prodromal phase of 'fainting' (syncope). The sequence of symptoms includes increasing light-headedness, blurring of vision proceeding to blackout, heaviness in the lower limbs progressing to swaying and loss of consciousness.

MECHANISM
- Fainting (syncope) is a sudden and brief loss of consciousness and postural tone secondary to hypoperfusion of the brain.
- Cerebral ischaemia may be due to sudden vasodilatation, a sudden fall in cardiac output or both simultaneously.

COMMON PRECIPITATING CAUSES OF SYNCOPE (Box 7.5)

BOX 7.5 Precipitating Causes of Syncope

• Warm environment, hot bath	• Rising after prolonged bed rest
• Postexercise	• Rapid postural change
• Prolonged motionless standing	• Valsalva
• Large meals (carbohydrate load)	• Alcohol
• Volume depletion	• Medications

CLASSIFICATION OF SYNCOPE (Table 7.2)

TABLE 7.2 Classification and Causes of Syncope

• Reflex syncope	• Vasovagal, situational (micturition, cough, postexercise), carotid sinus syndrome
• Syncope due to orthostatic hypotension	• Drug-induced, volume depletion, autonomic failure, postural tachycardia syndrome
• Cardiac syncope	• Arrhythmia (bradycardia or tachycardia), cardiac diseases, pulmonary embolism, acute aortic dissection, pulmonary hypertension

VASOVAGAL SYNCOPE

- Mechanisms include reflex slowing of heart mediated through vagus nerve, and marked fall in arterial pressure and peripheral vascular resistance.
- Causes include emotional stress, warm overcrowded room, sudden pain, mild blood loss, anaemia, fever, prolonged standing and fasting.
- Clinical features include a 'prodromal phase' characterised by nausea, sweating, yawning, epigastric distress, tachypnoea, weakness and confusion. This is followed by faintness, pallor, coldness of hand and feet, and eventually loss of consciousness. Physical examination reveals tachycardia during prodromal phase and bradycardia later with low blood pressure and weak pulse. Consciousness is regained rapidly without confusion, headache or focal neurological symptoms, though fatigue is frequent. Convulsions can result if recumbency is prevented.
- Vasovagal syncope is common in the young people.

CARDIAC SYNCOPE

- Cardiac syncope is due to a sudden reduction in cardiac output. This can occur when the heart is beating too fast or too slow or when it is not beating at all. It can also occur when there is obstruction to outflow of blood from the heart or cardiac contractility is reduced markedly.
- Common causes of cardiac syncope are given in Box 7.6.

BOX 7.6 Common Causes of Cardiac Syncope

- Complete heart block (Stokes–Adams–Morgagni syndrome)
- Paroxysmal tachycardias (supraventricular or ventricular)
- Sick sinus syndrome
- Acute massive myocardial infarction
- Aortic stenosis (exertional syncope)
- Aortic dissection
- Hypertrophic cardiomyopathy (exertional syncope)
- Primary pulmonary hypertension
- Pulmonary embolism
- Left atrial ball valve thrombus or myxoma
- Tetralogy of Fallot
- Long QT syndrome
- Brugada syndrome

BOX 7.7 Common Causes of Orthostatic Hypotension

• Drugs including antihypertensive drugs	• Physiological
• Volume loss (e.g. haemorrhage, gastroenteritis)	• Primary autonomic failure (e.g. pure autonomic failure, multiple system atrophy, Parkinson's disease, dementia with Lewy bodies)
• Diabetic neuropathy and tabes dorsalis	• Postural tachycardia syndrome
• Spinal cord injuries	• Idiopathic orthostatic hypotension

ORTHOSTATIC SYNCOPE (POSTURAL SYNCOPE)

- This occurs when the person suddenly gets up from a lying down position or stands still for a long time. Basic mechanism is postural hypotension resulting from loss of vasoconstrictor reflexes in the lower limb vessels.
- Orthostatic hypotension is defined as a sustained reduction of systolic BP ≥20 mmHg or diastolic BP ≥10 mmHg within 3 minutes of active standing or passive 60° head-up tilt using a tilt table.
- Common causes of orthostatic hypotension are given in Box 7.7.

DRUG-INDUCED SYNCOPE

- Common drugs which can produce syncope are listed in Table 7.3.

TABLE 7.3 Causes of Drug-Induced Syncope

Vasodilators/Volume Depletion	Arrhythmogenic and Vasodilators
• Angiotensin-converting enzyme inhibitors (ACE inhibitors) • β-Blockers • Calcium channel blockers • Diuretics	• Quinidine • Amiodarone • Tricyclic antidepressants • Antipsychotics • Opioids

SYNCOPE ASSOCIATED WITH CEREBROVASCULAR DISEASE

- Caused by occlusion in the large arteries in the neck.
- Physical activity can further reduce the blood flow (which is already compromised) to the brainstem resulting in loss of consciousness.

MISCELLANEOUS CAUSES OF SYNCOPE

- Carotid sinus syncope (hypersensitive carotid sinus) is common in elderly patients. It follows some form of compression on the carotid sinus as in turning the head to one side, tight collar or shaving over the region of carotid sinus.
- Vagal and glossopharyngeal neuralgia.
- Micturition syncope is seen in elderly patients during or after micturition, particularly after arising from the bed.

- Cough syncope follows paroxysms of cough in elderly patients with chronic bronchitis. During coughing, intrathoracic pressure is elevated, resulting in decreased venous return to the heart, in turn resulting in diminished cardiac output. Diaphragm contraction further impedes venous return by vena cava compression.
- Hyperventilation and hysterical fainting.

INVESTIGATIONS

- Haemoglobin and metabolic parameters, particularly blood sugar, sodium and urea.
- Electrocardiogram and cardiac monitoring.
- Echocardiography.
- Holter monitoring (ambulatory ECG).
- Carotid sinus massage in patients older than 40 years with syncope of unknown origin compatible with a reflex mechanism.
- Electroencephalogram.
- Tilt-table test and autonomic function tests.
- CT head.

MANAGEMENT

- Patients likely to have reflex or situational syncope, or syncope due to orthostatic hypotension may be discharged.
- Patients with orthostatic hypotension may be advised to discontinue medications which aggravate it. Use of stockings is helpful. Salt intake may be increased if possible. Drugs which are approved for postural hypotension include midodrine (an α1-adrenergic agonist), droxidopa (a synthetic norepinephrine precursor) and fludrocortisone (a synthetic mineralocorticoid).
- Patients likely to have a cardiac cause should be admitted and monitored, and treated based on underlying cause.

Q. Define cyanosis. Mention the causes and mechanisms of central and peripheral cyanosis. (PY 6.6)

Q. How will you differentiate central cyanosis from peripheral cyanosis?

Q. Explain in brief about differential cyanosis.

DEFINITION

- Cyanosis is defined as a bluish discolouration of the skin and mucous membranes, resulting from an increased amount of reduced haemoglobin (more than 5 g/dL), or of abnormal haemoglobin derivatives in the capillary blood, for example methaemoglobin and sulphmethaemoglobin (1.5 and 0.5 g/dL, respectively).
- Cyanosis is most marked in the lips, nail beds, ears and malar eminences.

TYPES OF CYANOSIS AND THEIR MECHANISMS

- Cyanosis can be subdivided into two: central cyanosis and peripheral cyanosis.
- Central cyanosis is due to decreased arterial oxygen saturation (most of the cases) or the presence of an abnormal haemoglobin derivative (rarely).
- Peripheral cyanosis is due to slowing of blood flow to an area, resulting in greater extraction of oxygen from normally saturated arterial blood. This results from vasoconstriction or diminished peripheral blood flow (reduced cardiac output).

CAUSES

- Various causes of cyanosis are given in Table 7.4. All causes of central cyanosis can also cause peripheral cyanosis.

DIFFERENTIATION BETWEEN CENTRAL AND PERIPHERAL CYANOSIS

- Differentiating features between central and peripheral cyanosis are given in Table 7.5.
- Cyanosis in HF is often of a mixed type due to both central and peripheral causes.
- 'Differential cyanosis' is cyanosis occurring in the lower limbs, but not in the upper limbs. This occurs in patients with patent ductus arteriosus with a reversal of shunt.
- Cyanosis of only upper limbs can occur in patients with patent ductus arteriosus with reversal of shunt in combination with transposition of great vessels.
- Cyanosis of left upper limb and both lower limbs (sparing right upper limb) can occur in patients with patent ductus arteriosus with reversal of shunt in combination with a preductal coarctation of aorta.
- Intermittent cyanosis in Ebstein's anomaly.

TABLE 7.4 Causes of Cyanosis

Central Cyanosis	Peripheral Cyanosis
• Due to decreased arterial oxygen saturation • Cardiac causes ◦ Fallot's tetralogy ◦ Eisenmenger's syndrome ◦ Heart failure • Pulmonary causes ◦ Chronic bronchitis ◦ Interstitial lung disease ◦ Pneumonia ◦ Pulmonary embolism ◦ Pulmonary arteriovenous fistula • High altitude • Hypoventilation (intracranial haemorrhage, tonic–clonic seizures, heroin overdose) • Cirrhosis of liver (hepatopulmonary syndrome) • Due to abnormal haemoglobin derivatives ◦ Methaemoglobinaemia ◦ Sulphaemoglobinaemia • Others ◦ Polycythaemia	• Due to diminished peripheral blood flow resulting from reduced cardiac output ◦ Mitral stenosis ◦ Heart failure ◦ Shock • Due to local vasoconstriction ◦ Cold exposure ◦ Raynaud's disease ◦ Peripheral vascular disease • Venous stasis or obstruction ◦ Deep vein thrombosis • Hyperviscosity ◦ Multiple myeloma ◦ Polycythaemia ◦ Waldenstrom's macroglobulinaemia

TABLE 7.5 Differentiation Between Central and Peripheral Cyanosis

Feature	Central Cyanosis	Peripheral Cyanosis
• Site	Both mucous membranes and skin are involved	Skin; sparing of mucous membranes of the oral cavity or those beneath the tongue
• Tongue	Affected	Unaffected
• Temperature of limb	Warm	Cold
• Clubbing	Present (shunts)	Absent
• Capillary refill time	Normal	Prolonged
• Polycythaemia	Present (shunts)	Absent
• Local warming	Cyanosis remains	Cyanosis may disappear
• Breathing pure oxygen for 10 minutes	Cyanosis may disappear	Cyanosis remains
• Arterial blood gas studies	Abnormal	Normal

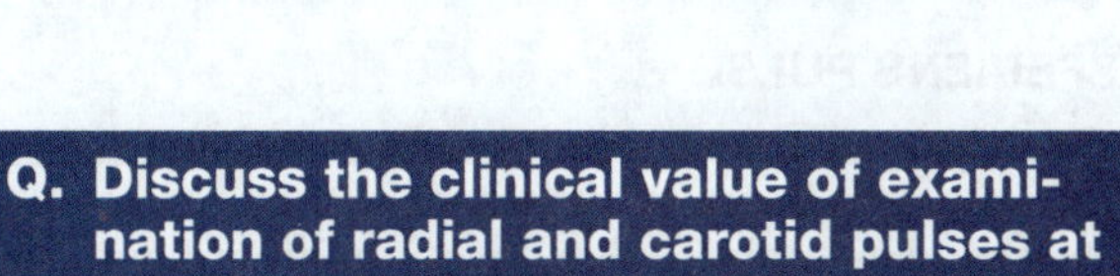

Q. Discuss the clinical value of examination of radial and carotid pulses at bedside.

- Study of peripheral arterial pulses includes the examination of radial, brachial, carotid, femoral, popliteal, posterior tibial and dorsalis pedis pulses.
- Examination should be performed under the heads given in Box 7.8.
- Rate and rhythm are assessed by palpating radial artery.
- Pulse volume is best assessed by palpating carotid artery.
- Pulse character is best assessed by palpating carotid artery except collapsing pulse that is better appreciated at radial artery.

NORMAL ARTERIAL PULSE TRACING

- Normal tracing of arterial pulse in relation to heart sounds and jugular venous pulse is shown in Fig. 7.2.

RATE

- Radial pulse is used to assess the rate.
    - Normal—resting pulse rate of 60–100 beats/minute.
    - Bradycardia—resting pulse rate less than 60 beats/minute (Table 7.6).
    - Tachycardia—resting pulse rate more than 100 beats/minute (Table 7.6).

BOX 7.8 Analysis of Pulse

• Rate	• Character or quality
• Rhythm	• Condition of vessel wall
• Volume	• Radiofemoral delay

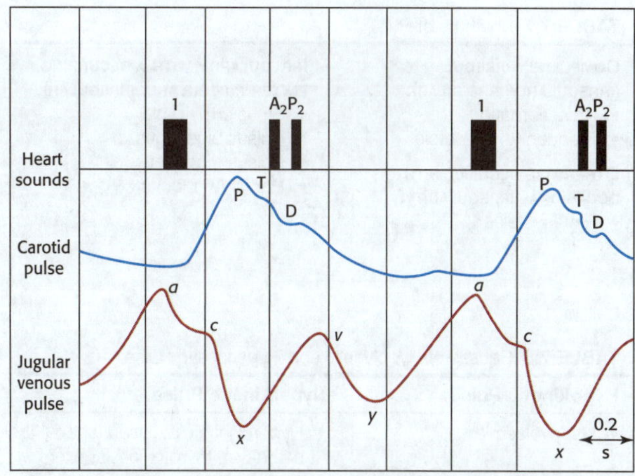

Fig. 7.2 Relationships between the heart sounds, arterial pulse and jugular venous pulse. 1, First heart sound; A_2, aortic component of the second heart sound; P_2, pulmonary component of the second heart sound; P, percussion wave; T, tidal wave; D, dicrotic notch; *a*, *c*, *x*, *v* and *y*, waves and troughs of the jugular venous pulse.

TABLE 7.6 Causes of Bradycardia and Tachycardia

Bradycardia (Less Than 60 Beats/Minute)	Tachycardia (More Than 100 Beats/Minute)
• Athletes	• Anxiety
• Hypothyroidism	• Fever
• Vasovagal syncope	• Pregnancy
• Drugs—β-blockers	• Hyperthyroidism
• Heart block	• Cardiac failure
• Sick sinus syndrome	• Tachyarrhythmias
• Hypothermia	• Drugs—salbutamol, terbutaline

- 'Pulse deficit' (apex-pulse deficit):
    - Definition—the difference between the heart rate counted by auscultation and pulse rate is called pulse deficit.
    - Significance—pulse deficit occurs in atrial fibrillation. Can also occur with multiple ventricular premature beats.
    - Mechanism—atrial fibrillation is characterised by cycles of varying lengths of diastole. This results in varying stroke volumes with some of the ventricular contractions too weak and unable to open the aortic valve, but at the same time many are good enough to close the mitral valve, thereby producing heart sounds. In multiple ventricular premature beats, ectopic beats may not be conducted to radial artery resulting in pulse deficit.

RHYTHM

- Radial pulse is used to assess the rhythm (Table 7.7).

VOLUME

- Carotid artery is used to assess the volume of pulse (Table 7.8).

TABLE 7.7 Rhythms of Pulse

Completely irregular (irregularly irregular):	Irregularity with a recurring pattern (regularly irregular):
• Atrial fibrillation • Frequent extrasystoles **Otherwise regular with occasional irregularity:** • Extrasystoles	• Sinus arrhythmia • Pulsus bigeminus • Pulsus trigeminus • Partial AV blocks

TABLE 7.8 Causes of Hypokinetic and Hyperkinetic Pulse

Hypokinetic Pulse	Hyperkinetic Pulse
• Hypovolaemia	• Hyperkinetic circulation (anaemia, fever, thyrotoxicosis, exercise, pregnancy)
• Shock	• Mitral regurgitation
• Heart failure	• Aortic regurgitation
• Acute myocardial infarction	• Patent ductus arteriosus
• Constrictive pericarditis	• Ventricular septal defect
• Mitral stenosis	• Peripheral arteriovenous fistulae
• Aortic stenosis	• Complete heart block

- Hypokinetic pulse (weak pulse; pulsus parvus) is seen in conditions associated with:
  - Decreased left ventricular stroke volume.
  - Narrow pulse pressure.
  - Increased peripheral vascular resistance.
- Hyperkinetic pulse (bounding pulse) is seen in conditions associated with:
  - Increased left ventricular stroke volume.
  - Wide pulse pressure.
  - Decreased peripheral vascular resistance.

CHARACTER OR QUALITY

- Carotid artery is generally used to assess the character of pulse, though sometimes radial artery gives better information.

PULSUS PARVUS

- A hypokinetic pulse, which is of low amplitude.
- Occurs as a result of a reduction in left ventricular stroke volume (e.g. heart failure) or a decrease in systemic arterial pressure.

PULSUS TARDUS

- A slow-rising pulse that peaks late in systole.
- Seen in aortic stenosis.

PULSUS PARVUS ET TARDUS

- Description—this is a small-volume ('parvus') pulse that rises slowly ('tardus') to a late systolic peak. There is an associated systolic thrill.
- Mechanism—this is the result of mechanical obstruction to left ventricular ejection.
- Significance—seen in aortic stenosis.

ANACROTIC PULSE

- Description—this is a variant of 'pulsus parvus et tardus', in which a notch is palpable on the upstroke of the pulse wave.
- Significance—occurs in severe aortic stenosis.

COLLAPSING (WATER HAMMER) PULSE

- Description—this is a pulse characterised by a rapid upstroke, a rapid downstroke and a high volume.
- Mechanism—the rapid upstroke is due to the markedly increased stroke volume. The rapid downstroke or the collapsing character is due to two factors:
  - The diastolic leak back into left ventricle.
  - Rapid run-off to the periphery because of low systemic vascular resistance.
- Significance—collapsing pulse is seen typically in aortic regurgitation. Various causes are listed in Box 7.9.
- Corrigan's pulse is largely used to describe abrupt distension and quick collapse of carotid pulse, whereas the term 'water hammer pulse' is used for the characteristic pulse seen in peripheral arteries like the radial artery.

BISFERIENS PULSE

- Description—this is a pulse with double peak (two peaks), both being felt in systole.
- Mechanism—this is due to a combination of the slow-rising pulse of aortic stenosis and collapsing pulse of aortic regurgitation:
  - Significance—bisferiens pulse is seen in the following conditions:
    - Combination of aortic stenosis and aortic regurgitation (regurgitation being dominant lesion).
    - Severe aortic regurgitation.
    - Hypertrophic cardiomyopathy.
    - Large patent ductus arteriosus.

DICROTIC PULSE

- Description—dicrotic pulse has two palpable waves, one in systole and other in diastole. Diastolic wave follows dicrotic notch.
- Mechanism—due to very low stroke volume.
- Significance—seen in the following conditions:
  - Dilated cardiomyopathy.
  - Extreme dehydration.
  - Advanced heart failure.
  - Cardiac tamponade.

PULSUS ALTERNANS

- Description—this is an alternation of large- and small-volume beats, with a normal rhythm. There is a difference of 10–40 mmHg in systolic pressure between beats.

BOX 7.9 Causes of Collapsing Pulse

- Aortic regurgitation (generally not seen in acute aortic regurgitation)
- Hyperkinetic circulatory states (anaemia, fever, thyrotoxicosis, exercise, pregnancy, Paget's disease, beriberi)
- Patent ductus arteriosus
- Ruptured sinus of Valsalva
- Large arteriovenous fistulae
- Truncus arteriosus
- Mitral regurgitation (occasional)
- Complete heart block (occasional)

- Mechanism—pulsus alternans is due to alternating left ventricular contractile force, that is the ventricle beats strongly, and then weakly, alternating with each other.
- Significance—seen in acute left ventricular failure. It may occur following paroxysmal tachycardia.

PULSUS BIGEMINUS

- Description—pulse with regular alteration of pressure pulse amplitude. This is clinically felt as two beats followed by a pause, thereby producing irregular rhythm (in contrast to pulsus alternans where rhythm is regular).
- Mechanism—it is caused by coupled ectopic beats, that is an ectopic beat following each regular beat.

PULSUS PARADOXUS

- Description—pulsus paradoxus is characterised by the following features:
  - A decrease in systolic blood pressure more than 10 mmHg during normal inspiration.
  - A radial pulse that gets smaller in volume (and may even disappear) with inspiration and larger in volume with expiration.
- It is important to note the following points in relation to pulsus paradoxus:
  - A decrease in systolic blood pressure by 3–10 mmHg and a small reduction in the volume of pulse during normal inspiration are physiological. Pulsus paradoxus is merely an exaggeration of this and NOT a reversal of this.
  - The 'paradox' in the pulse is that heart sounds are still audible at a time when no radial pulse is felt.
  - Mild cases of pulsus paradoxus may not alter the radial pulse volume, which may appear normal. But sphygmomanometric measurement of systolic pressure during slow respiration will detect a more than 10 mmHg fall during inspiration.

Mechanism of Pulsus Paradoxus

- In normal people, during inspiration, there is a reduction in intrathoracic pressure, resulting in the following:
  - Pooling of blood in pulmonary vasculature.
  - Pooling of blood in the right ventricle due to increased venous return.
- This generalised pooling of blood results in a reduction in the venous return to the left atrium and left ventricle. The net result is a reduction in cardiac output resulting in a drop of systolic blood pressure by 3–10 mmHg.
- In pulsus paradoxus, during inspiration, the increased right ventricular volume of blood results in a bulging of the interventricular septum into the left ventricular cavity. This results in a reduction in the left ventricular volume leading to a further reduction in cardiac output. This exaggerates the normal inspiratory reduction in blood pressure, allowing it to exceed 10 mmHg. In patients with severe asthma, obstructive airway disease or tension pneumothorax, the degree of negative pressure generated during inspiration is exaggerated. This results in enhanced pooling of blood, thereby causing pulsus paradoxus.

BOX 7.10 Causes of Pulsus Paradoxus

- Constrictive pericarditis
- Cardiac tamponade
- Pericardial effusion (rare)
- Restrictive cardiomyopathy
- Chronic obstructive airway disease (severe)
- Severe bronchial asthma
- Tension pneumothorax
- Pulmonary embolism (rare)
- Pregnancy (rare)

Conditions Associated With Pulsus Paradoxus

- Conditions which can produce pulsus paradoxus are listed in Box 7.10.

REVERSE PULSUS PARADOXUS

- Indicates inspiratory rise in arterial blood pressure.
- Seen in hypertrophic cardiomyopathy, intermittent positive-pressure ventilation and AV dissociation.

WAVE FORMS OF NORMAL AND ABNORMAL PULSES

- Waves forms of normal and abnormal pulses are depicted in Fig. 7.3.

RADIOFEMORAL DELAY

- Occurs in coarctation of aorta and sometimes in aortic dissection.
- Elicited by simultaneous palpation of right radial artery and one femoral artery.
- Features of radiofemoral delay are the following:
  - Femoral pulse is of small volume.
  - Femoral pulse occurs after radial pulse.
  - Lower limb blood pressures will be lower than upper limb blood pressures.

Q. Describe the normal wave patterns of jugular venous pulse and their variations.

Q. How will you differentiate jugular venous pulse from carotid pulse?

Q. Briefly describe hepatojugular reflux and abdominojugular reflux test.

Q. Give a brief account of Kussmaul's sign.

Q. How do you calculate central venous pressure from jugular venous pressure?

DEFINITION

- Jugular venous pulse (JVP) is the oscillating top of a height of venous blood in the internal jugular vein that faithfully reflects the pressure and haemodynamic changes in the right side of heart in all phases of the cardiac cycle.

SIGNIFICANCE

- Two main objectives of examining the JVP are the following:
  - Estimation of jugular venous pressure.
  - Studying the waveform.

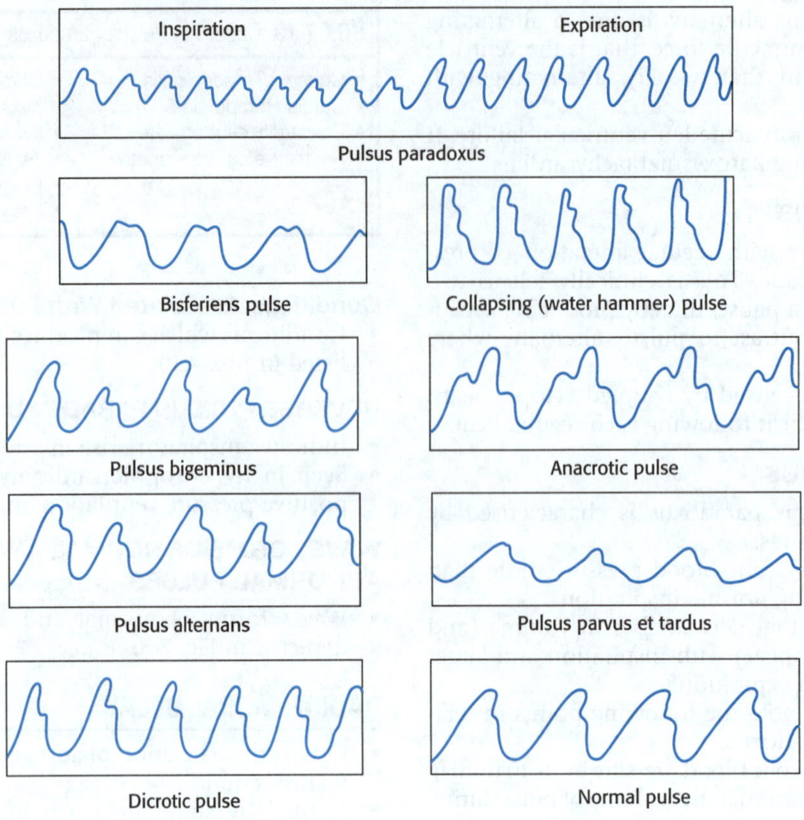

Fig. 7.3 Wave forms of various types of pulses.

JUGULAR VENOUS PRESSURE

- Examination of right jugular vein is preferred.
- Jugular venous pressure is expressed as the vertical distance in centimetres between the top of the venous column and the sternal angle, regardless of the body position. Normally, it is less than 3 cm. By convention, jugular venous pressure is measured from the sternal angle with the patient reclining at 45°.
- Central venous pressure can be accurately estimated from the jugular venous pressure. For this, the sternal angle is taken as the reference point. The centre of the right atrium lies 5 cm below the sternal angle, regardless of body position. The central venous pressure is calculated as 5 + jugular venous pressure in centimetres (e.g. if jugular venous pressure is 6 cm, the central venous pressure = 5 + 6 = 11 cm of water or blood).

NORMAL WAVE PATTERNS OF JUGULAR VENOUS PULSE

- The various waves on JVP reflect the phasic pressure changes in the right atrium.
- Normal JVP has three positive waves, namely, *a*, *c* and *v* waves, and two negative descents, namely, *x* descent and *y* descent.
- In normal persons, the *a* wave is more visible than the *v* wave, and the *x* descent is more prominent than the *y* descent. In fact, the *v* wave and *y* descent are often not visible in healthy adults owing to the very compliant normal right atrium (Fig. 7.4).

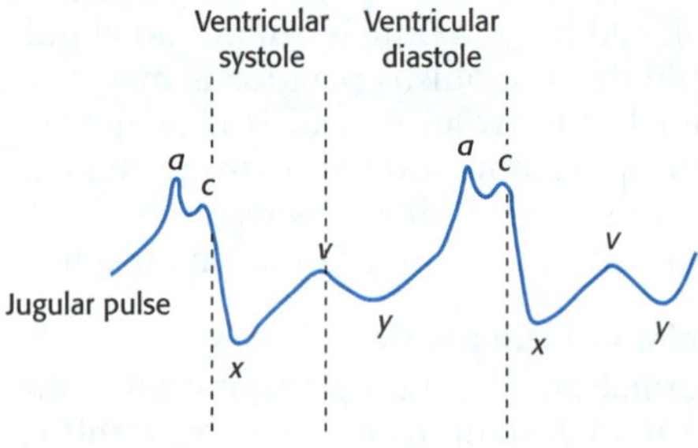

Fig. 7.4 Jugular venous pulse: normal wave patterns. *a*, Atrial contraction; *c*, onset of ventricular contraction; *v*, pressure peak immediately prior to opening of tricuspid valve; *c–x*, *x* descent; *v–y*, *y* descent.

MECHANISM

- The *a* wave is due to right atrial contraction. It occurs just before the first heart sound and before the onset of ventricular ejection (carotid pulse upstroke).
- The *c* wave is due to bulging of the tricuspid valve into the right atrium and impact of the adjacent carotid artery during ventricular systole.
- The *v* wave is due to passive right atrial filling during ventricular systole.
- The *x* descent ('systolic collapse') is due to atrial relaxation and downward displacement of tricuspid valve during systole. It occurs during systole and ends just prior to second heart sound.

- The *y* descent ('diastolic collapse') is due to opening of the tricuspid valve and the rapid flow of blood into the right ventricle. It occurs after second heart sound.

ABNORMALITIES IN JUGULAR VENOUS PRESSURE

CAUSES OF RAISED JUGULAR VENOUS PRESSURE

- Various causes of raised jugular venous pressure are given in Box 7.11.

ABNORMALITIES IN WAVEFORM

- Abnormalities in the jugular venous waveform can be in any of the waves as given in Table 7.9.

BOX 7.11 Causes of Raised Jugular Venous Pressure

• Right heart failure (commonest)	• Constrictive pericarditis
• Tricuspid regurgitation	• Cardiac tamponade
• Tricuspid stenosis	• Superior vena caval obstruction (nonpulsatile)
• Pulmonary embolism	• Acute nephritis
• Overuse of IV fluids	• Massive ascites or right-sided pleural effusion

TABLE 7.9 Abnormalities in Jugular Venous Waveforms

Abnormalities	Conditions
• Abnormalities of the *a* wave:	
• Large *a* waves	Tricuspid stenosis, pulmonary hypertension, pulmonary stenosis, right ventricular hypertrophy
• Regular 'cannon' *a* waves	Junctional rhythm
• Irregular 'cannon' *a* waves	Complete heart block, multiple ectopics
• Absent *a* waves	Atrial fibrillation
• Abnormalities of the *v* wave:	
• Large *v* waves	Tricuspid regurgitation, right ventricular failure
• Abnormalities of the *x* descent:	
• Increased prominence	Cardiac tamponade, constrictive pericarditis, atrial septal defect
• Decreased prominence	Tricuspid regurgitation (replaced by *c*–*v* wave), right ventricular failure, atrial fibrillation
• Abnormalities of the *y* descent:	
• Rapid *y* descent	Tricuspid regurgitation, restrictive heart disease including constrictive pericarditis, severe right heart failure
• Slow *y* descent	Tricuspid stenosis, right atrial myxoma, cardiac tamponade

TABLE 7.10 Differences Between Jugular Venous Pulse and Carotid Pulse

Jugular Venous Pulse	Carotid Pulse
• Definite upper level	• No definite upper level
• Upper level falls during inspiration	• No change with respiration
• On sitting up, appears lower in the neck	• On sitting up, appears higher in the neck
• Wavy column with two to three positive waves	• Jerky with only one wave
• Two descents (*x* and *y*)	• One descent
• Not palpable or palpable as a slight fluttering sensation	• Well palpable as a pulsation
• Obliterated by mild pressure at root of neck	• Not obliterated by pressure at root of neck
• Hepatojugular reflux present	• Hepatojugular reflux absent

DIFFERENTIATION OF JUGULAR VENOUS PULSE FROM CAROTID PULSE

- At times, it may become difficult to differentiate between carotid pulse and jugular venous wave in the neck. Table 7.10 gives some of the points which help in differentiating the two.

HEPATOJUGULAR REFLUX (ABDOMINOJUGULAR REFLUX TEST)

- Better term is abdominojugular reflux.
- Procedure—the palm of the hand is placed over the abdomen in periumbilical area and firm pressure is applied for a minimum period of 10 seconds, ensuring that the patient does not perform Valsalva's manoeuvre.
- Normal response—the upper level of jugular venous pulsation moves upwards by less than 3 cm and then falls down even when the pressure is continued.
- Positive abdominojugular reflux test—it is defined as an increase in JVP (more than 3 cm) during 10 seconds of firm mid-abdominal compression, remains high throughout the period of compression, followed by an abrupt drop in pressure of 4 cm of blood on release of compression.
- Clinical significance:
  - It is positive in early or incipient right HF.
  - Abdominojugular reflux test is positive in right HF, secondary to elevated left heart filling pressures.
  - The typical JVP of tricuspid regurgitation can be elicited even when the resting pulse wave is normal.
  - During abdominojugular reflux testing, the upper level of JVP does not move upward at all in inferior vena caval obstruction and Budd–Chiari syndrome (hepatic vein occlusion).

KUSSMAUL'S SIGN

- Normally, there is a decrease in the height of jugular venous pulsations and a drop in jugular venous pressure during inspiration.

BOX 7.12 Conditions in Which Kussmaul's Sign Is Present

• Constrictive pericarditis	• Acute severe asthma
• Restrictive cardiomyopathy	• Pulmonary embolism
• Severe right-sided heart failure	• Severe tricuspid regurgitation
• Right ventricular infarction	• Tricuspid stenosis

- Kussmaul's sign is an increase in the height of jugular venous pulsations and hence a rise in jugular venous pressure (central venous pressure) during inspiration.
- Kussmaul's sign is seen in the several conditions (Box 7.12).

Q. Discuss the clinical importance of apex beat.

DEFINITION

- Apex beat is the lowermost and outermost point of definite cardiac pulsation.
- Also known as 'point of maximum impulse'.

NORMAL APEX BEAT

- Left ventricle normally produces the apex beat.
- Site of the apex beat:
  - With the patient in supine or sitting posture, it is located 1 cm medial to the mid-clavicular line or 9 to 10 cm from the mid-sternal line, in the fifth left intercostal space.
  - With the patient lying on his/her left lateral side, the apex beat may move 1 to 2 cm laterally.
- Features of the normal apex beat:
  - It is palpable only during the first half of systole and lasts less than 30% of systole. On palpating the carotid artery simultaneously, the apical beat does not last longer than the carotid upstroke.
  - It gently raises the palpating finger.
  - It is detectable in only one intercostal space and is less than 3 cm in diameter.

ABNORMALITIES OF APICAL IMPULSE

- Abnormalities in character.
- Abnormalities in position.

ABNORMALITIES IN CHARACTER

- Hyperdynamic apex.
- Heaving apex.
- Tapping apex.
- Hypokinetic apex.
- Double apex.

Hyperdynamic Apex (Hyperkinetic Apex; Volume Overload Apex; Diffuse Apex; Forceful and Ill-Sustained Apex)

- Site of the apex beat:
  - Shifted downwards and laterally due to chamber enlargement resulting from volume overload.

TABLE 7.11 Causes of Hyperdynamic Apex Beat

Increased left ventricular stroke volume (volume overload):	Dilated cardiomyopathy Hyperdynamic circulatory states:
• Aortic regurgitation • Mitral regurgitation • Ventricular septal defect • Patent ductus arteriosus	• Exercise • Thyrotoxicosis • Severe anaemia

BOX 7.13 Causes of Heaving Apex Beat

• Aortic stenosis	• Coarctation of aorta
• Systemic hypertension	• Hypertrophic cardiomyopathy

- Features of the hyperdynamic apex beat:
  - The apical thrust is increased in amplitude.
  - It lifts the finger up, but the lift is not sustained.
  - It lasts more than 30% but less than 60% of systole.
  - It is detectable in more than one intercostal space and is more than 3 cm in diameter.
- Conditions associated with hyperdynamic apex beat are shown in Table 7.11.

Heaving Apex (Sustained Apex; Pressure Overload Apex; Forceful and Sustained Apex)

- Site of the apex beat:
  - Usually normal in position and results from left ventricular hypertrophy due to pressure overload.
- Features of the heaving apex beat are as follows:
  - The apical thrust is increased in amplitude and duration.
  - The duration of the thrust is prolonged and felt in the second half of systole also.
  - It lasts more than 60% of systole.
  - It lifts the finger up and the lift is sustained.
  - It is detectable in only one intercostal space and is less than 3 cm in diameter.
- Conditions associated with heaving apex beat (pressure overload of left ventricle) are shown in Box 7.13.

Tapping Apex

- It is due to palpable loud first heart sound.
- It imparts a tapping feeling to the palpating finger.
- Occurs in mitral stenosis.

Hypokinetic Apex or Absent Apical Impulse (Box 7.14).

BOX 7.14 Causes of Hypokinetic Apex Beat

• Obesity	• Pericardial effusion	• Shock
• Emphysema	• Constrictive pericarditis	• Myxoedema

Double Apex

- Occurs in hypertrophic cardiomyopathy and left ventricular aneurysm.

TABLE 7.12 Causes of Abnormalities in Position of Apical Beat

Cardiac Enlargement:	Cardiac Displacement:	Dextrocardia Pleural Diseases:
• Aortic regurgitation • Mitral regurgitation • Ventricular septal defect • Patent ductus arteriosus • Dilated cardiomyopathy	• Scoliosis, funnel chest **Pulmonary diseases:** • Pulmonary fibrosis • Collapse of lung • Large pulmonary masses	• Pleural effusion • Pneumothorax • Hydropneumothorax • Pleural fibrosis

Note: Pulmonary fibrosis, collapse of lung and pleural fibrosis cause shifting of apex to the side of abnormality while large pulmonary masses, pleural effusion and pneumothorax cause shift to the opposite side.

ABNORMALITIES IN POSITION

- Causes of abnormalities in position of apical beat are given in Table 7.12.

Q. Briefly discuss about left parasternal heave or left parasternal impulse.

- Indicates forward (anterior) movement of lower left parasternal area.
- Palpated with the base or ulnar aspect of hand.
- Three grades.
  - Grade 1: Visible but not palpable.
  - Grade 2: Visible and palpable but obliterable with pressure.
  - Grade 3: Visible and palpable but not obliterable with pressure.
- Seen in right ventricular enlargement (as in atrial septal defect, ventricular septal defect, pulmonic stenosis, pulmonary hypertension) and left atrial enlargement.

Q. What is the mechanism of first heart sound? Discuss the variations in first heart sound.

- The first heart sound (S_1) results from the closure of mitral and tricuspid valves. It has two components:
  - Mitral component (M_1) due to mitral valve closure.
  - Tricuspid component (T_1) due to tricuspid valve closure.
- The mitral component (M_1) is followed by the tricuspid component (T_1).
- Splitting of S_1 is usually not heard because the sound of tricuspid valve closure is too faint to hear.
- S_1 is best heard at the apex. It is best heard with the diaphragm of stethoscope.
- Intensity of S_1 is determined primarily by valve mobility, force of ventricular contraction and, most importantly, the velocity of valve closure and valve position at the onset of systole. S_1 is louder when onset of ventricular systole finds mitral leaflets still widely open such as in mitral stenosis with pliable leaflets, a short PR interval, tachycardias and increased diastolic flow rates. Alternatively, a soft S_1 occurs when the AV valves are partially closed at the onset of ventricular contraction, as with a long PR interval, acute aortic regurgitation and decreased flow rates (low cardiac output).
- Various causes of changes in intensity of first heart sound are given in Table 7.13.
- There can be abnormalities in splitting of first heart sound and the causes are listed in Table 7.14.

TABLE 7.13 Causes of Variations in the Intensity of First Heart Sound

Loud first heart sound:	Soft first heart sound:

• Mitral stenosis
• Short PR interval (preexcitation syndrome)
• Tachycardia
• Increased flow across mitral valve
  • Exercise
  • Anaemia
  • Fever
  • Thyrotoxicosis
  • Paget's disease
  • Pregnancy
  • Beriberi
  • Patent ductus arteriosus
  • Ventricular septal defect
• Increased flow across tricuspid valve:
  • Atrial septal defect
• Left atrial myxoma
• Tricuspid stenosis
• Thin chest wall
	• Mitral regurgitation
	• Calcified mitral valve
	• Long PR interval
	• Myocarditis
	• Left ventricular failure
	• Severe or acute aortic regurgitation
	• Left bundle branch block
	• Obesity
	• Emphysema
	• Pericardial effusion
	Varying intensity of first heart sound:
	• Atrial fibrillation
	• Premature beats
	• Complete AV block
	• Ventricular tachycardia
	• Severe cardiac tamponade (auscultatory alternans in which S_1 sounds are soft and loud with alternate beats)

TABLE 7.14 Abnormalities in Splitting of First Heart Sound

Wide Splitting of First Heart Sound	Reversed Splitting of First Heart Sound
• Ebstein's anomaly • Complete right bundle branch block • Ectopic beat from left ventricle • Right atrial myxoma	• Complete left bundle branch block • Severe mitral stenosis • Left atrial myxoma • Right ventricular pacing • Ectopic beat from right ventricle

Q. What is the mechanism of second heart sound? Discuss the variations in second heart sound.

- The second heart sound (S_2) is due to the closure of aortic and pulmonary valves. It has two components:
  - Aortic component (A_2) due to aortic valve closure.
  - Pulmonary component (P_2) due to pulmonary valve closure.
- The aortic component (A_2) is followed by the pulmonary component (P_2).
- Normally, during expiration, both valves close almost simultaneously, and, hence, second heart sound is single. During inspiration, the aortic valve closes early due to increased capacitance of pulmonary vascular bed while pulmonary valve closes late due to increase in right ventricular volume due to increased venous return. This results in a physiological inspiratory splitting of second heart sound.

TABLE 7.15 Variations in the Intensity of Second Heart Sound

Aortic Component (A_2)	Pulmonary Component (P_2)
• Increased intensity: • Essential hypertension • Syphilitic aortic regurgitation • Hyperdynamic circulatory states • Decreased intensity: • Aortic stenosis • Aortic regurgitation	• Increased intensity: • Pulmonary hypertension • Pulmonary artery dilatation • Decreased intensity: • Pulmonary stenosis • Tetralogy of Fallot • Pulmonary atresia

- Loudness of A_2 or P_2 is proportional to the respective pressures in aorta or pulmonary artery at the onset of diastole.

VARIATIONS IN THE INTENSITY OF SECOND HEART SOUND

- Causes of variations in intensity of second heart sound are given in Table 7.15.

ABNORMALITIES IN SPLITTING OF SECOND HEART SOUND

- Variations in splitting of second heart sound are listed in Table 7.16.

Q. Discuss the significance of third heart sound.

- Third heart sound (S_3) is produced in the ventricle due to abnormal filling pattern. It is a low-pitched sound heard at the end of rapid filling phase (early diastole). It occurs 0.14–0.22 second after the second heart sound.
- A third heart sound arising from the left ventricle is known as 'left-sided third heart sound' and the one arising from right ventricle as 'right-sided third heart sound'.
- S_3 is best heard with the bell of stethoscope.
- Left-sided S_3 is best heard during expiration with the patient in the left lateral position.
- Right-sided S_3 is best heard during inspiration.
- Left-sided S_3 may be physiological or pathological. Right-sided S_3 is always pathological.

CAUSES OF THIRD HEART SOUND

- Various causes of third heart sound are given in Table 7.17.

Q. Discuss the significance of fourth heart sound.

- Fourth heart sound (S_4) occurs as a result of forceful atrial contraction ('atrial kick'). It is a low-pitched

TABLE 7.16 Abnormalities in Splitting of Second Heart Sound

Wide Mobile Split	Reversed (Paradoxical) Splitting
• Delayed electrical activation of right ventricle	• Delayed electrical activation of left ventricle
• Right bundle branch block	• Left bundle branch block
• Ectopic from left ventricle	• Ectopic from right ventricle
• Prolonged right ventricular systole	• Prolonged left ventricular systole
• Pulmonary stenosis	• Hypertension
• Pulmonary hypertension	• Severe aortic stenosis
• Massive pulmonary embolism	• Hypertrophic cardiomyopathy
• Early aortic closure	• Patent ductus arteriosus
• Mitral regurgitation	• Severe left ventricular dysfunction
	• Early pulmonary valve closure • Tricuspid regurgitation
	• Early electrical activation of right ventricle • Wolff–Parkinson–White syndrome (type B)
Wide Fixed Splitting	**Single Second Heart Sound**
• Atrial septal defect	• Severe aortic stenosis (absent or markedly attenuated A_2)
• Severe pulmonary stenosis	• Severe pulmonary stenosis (absent or markedly attenuated P_2)
• Severe right ventricular failure	• Tetralogy of Fallot

TABLE 7.17 Causes of Third Heart Sound

Physiological S_3	Hyperdynamic States	Pathological Left-Sided S_3	Pathological Right-Sided S_3
• Children • Age less than 40 years • Athletes • Pregnancy	• Arterio-venous fistula • Thyrotoxicosis	• Left ventricular failure • Aortic regurgitation • Mitral regurgitation • Ischaemic heart disease • Cardiomyopathy	• Right ventricular failure

TABLE 7.18 Causes of Fourth Heart Sound

Left-Sided S_4	Right-Sided S_4

• Systemic hypertension
• Hypertrophic cardiomyopathy
• Ischaemic heart disease (especially acute myocardial infarction)
• Acute mitral regurgitation
• Anaemia, thyrotoxicosis and arterio-venous fistulae
	• Right ventricular hypertrophy due to:
	  • Pulmonary hypertension
	  • Pulmonary stenosis

sound heard in presystole (late diastole; before first heart sound). It is absent in atrial fibrillation.

- S_4 may be confused with spilt S_1. Firm pressure by the diaphragm of stethoscope eliminates S_4 but not split S_1.
- S_4 is always abnormal in younger persons.
- A fourth heart sound arising from the left side is known as 'left-sided fourth heart sound' and the one arising from right side as 'right-sided fourth heart sound'.
- Left-sided S_4 is best heard during expiration with the patient in the left lateral position.
- Right-sided S_4 is best heard during inspiration.

CAUSES OF FOURTH HEART SOUND

- Table 7.18 lists causes of fourth heart sound.

Q. What is summation gallop?

- It occurs when both S_3 and S_4 are present in a patient with tachycardia.
- Due to shortening of diastole, the two sounds (S_3 and S_4) merge to produce a single loud sound.

Q. Discuss other abnormal cardiac sounds on auscultation.

EJECTION CLICK

- Ejection click is a sharp, high-frequency sound audible immediately after S_1. It can occur with aortic valve stenosis, pulmonary valve stenosis as well as in dilation of ascending aorta and pulmonary artery.
- An aortic ejection click is audible over the entire precordium and varies little with respiration. A pulmonary click is most audible along the left upper sternal border, becoming louder during expiration and less audible or absent during inspiration.
- As the valves become stiff and calcified in aortic and pulmonary stenosis, ejection click disappears.

NONEJECTION CLICK

- Associated with mitral valve prolapse.
- High-frequency, sharp clicks occurring in mid-systole and heard over the apex or left-lower sternal border.
- May be an isolated finding or be followed by late systolic murmur.
- Manoeuvres such as squatting move a mid-systolic click towards S_2, whereas standing and performing Valsalva's manoeuvre move the click towards S_1.
- Mid-systolic click arises from sudden tension on the chordae tendineae or from sudden halt of prolapsing mitral valve leaflet during ventricular systole.

PROSTHETIC VALVE SOUNDS

- A ball-in-cage prosthesis (Starr–Edwards) has loud, clicking opening and closing sounds. In the case of aortic valve, opening sound has the same timing as an ejection sound (ES), and in the case of the mitral valve it occurs when an opening snap (OS) would occur. Closing sound corresponds to the component of the heart sounds contributed by that valve, that is mitral component of S_1 for mitral valve and aortic component of S_2 for an aortic valve.
- Disc valves produce distinct closing sounds but usually no audible opening sounds.
- Tissue valves do not normally produce additional sounds.

PERICARDIAL KNOCK

- In constrictive pericarditis, ventricular filling occurs mainly in early diastole which produces a sharp sound called pericardial knock.
- Its timing is earlier than a normal S_3 and typically occurs 0.10–0.12 seconds after S_2.

OTHERS

- OS, pericardial rub, tumour plop (in myxoma—early diastolic sound).

Q. Discuss the conduction system of the heart briefly.

- The rate and rhythm of the heart are controlled by the sinoatrial node (SA node) situated at the junction of superior vena cava and right atrium.
- The impulse from the SA node spreads through the atrial musculature and down to the AV node that is situated above the tricuspid valve.
- Passage through the AV node is relatively slow, accounting for the normal physiological delay in ventricular depolarisation.
- The impulse then travels downwards to the bundle of His and through its branches (right bundle branch and left bundle branch) to the Purkinje network of fibres that convey the impulse to the ventricular endocardium and then epicardium (Fig. 7.5).
- The SA node is the normal pacemaker of the heart as it has the fastest inherent discharge rate. However, potential pacemaking properties also exist in the cells of the AV node, bundle of His and Purkinje fibres.

Q. How do you analyse an electrocardiogram? (IM 1.18)

RATE

- The ECG is normally recorded at a speed of 25 mm/second so that each small square, that is 1 mm, represents 0.04 second.

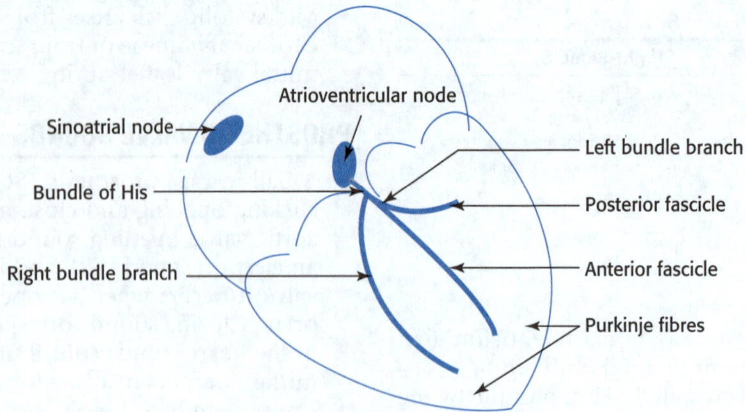

Fig. 7.5 Conduction system of the heart.

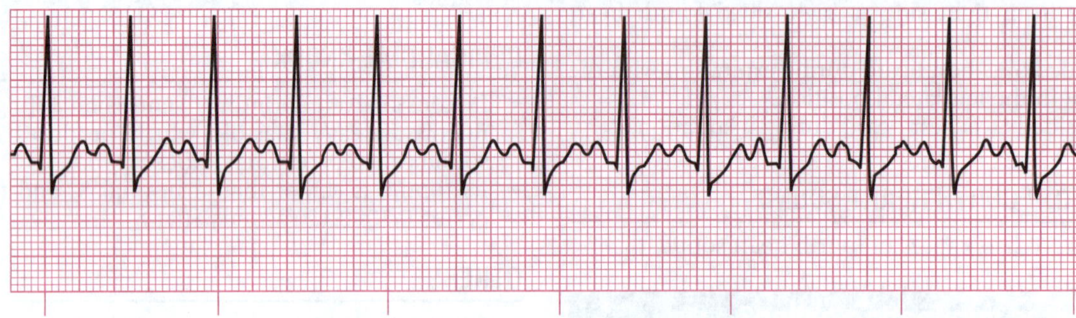

Fig. 7.6 Sinus tachycardia with a rate of 125/minute.

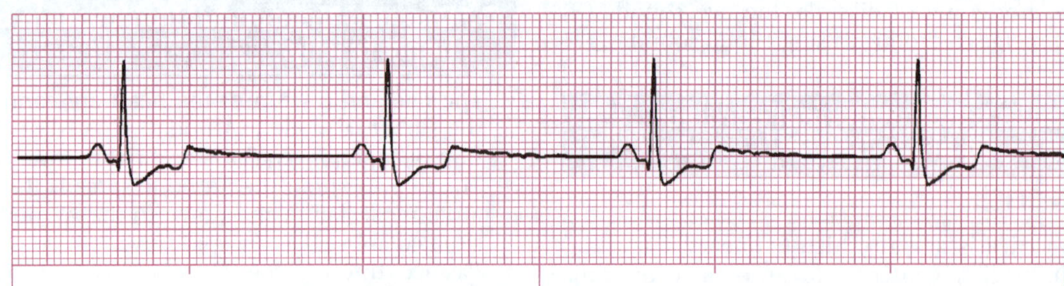

Fig. 7.7 Sinus bradycardia with a rate of 40/minute.

- The atrial and ventricular rates are calculated by counting the number of small squares between two consecutive P waves (PP interval) and R waves (RR interval), respectively. Dividing 1500 by PP and RR intervals gives the atrial and ventricular rates, respectively.
- Though normally both atrial and ventricular rates are equal, they should be calculated separately since they can be different in complete AV block and paroxysmal supraventricular tachycardia (PSVT) with 2° AV block.
- A heart rate >100/minute is tachycardia (Fig. 7.6) and <60/minute is bradycardia (Fig. 7.7).

RHYTHM

- See whether it is regular or irregular. If there is any doubt, use a piece of paper to map out three or four consecutive beats and see whether rate is same further along the ECG.
- Check for: P wave before each QRS complex, PR intervals (for AV blocks) and QRS interval (for bundle branch block).

REGULAR RHYTHM

- In sinus rhythm, P wave precedes every QRS complex with consistent PR interval.
- In nodal or junctional rhythm, no discernable P wave precedes each QRS complex; the QRS complexes are narrow and regular with constant RR interval.

IRREGULAR RHYTHM

- In atrial fibrillation, no discernable P waves precede each QRS complex; the QRS complexes are irregular with varying RR intervals (Fig. 7.8).

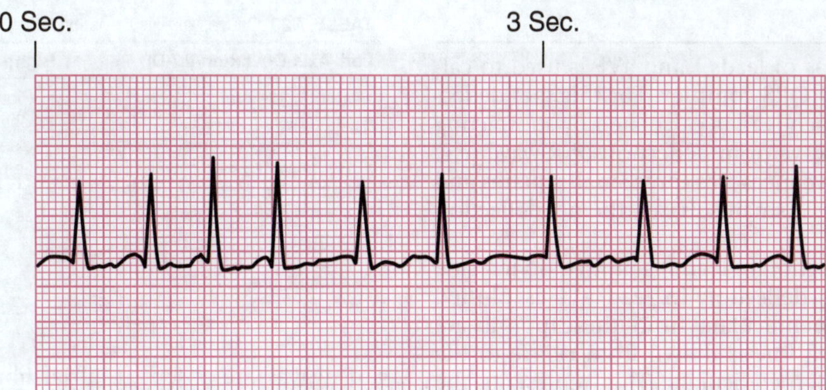

Fig. 7.8 Irregularly irregular rhythm in atrial fibrillation.

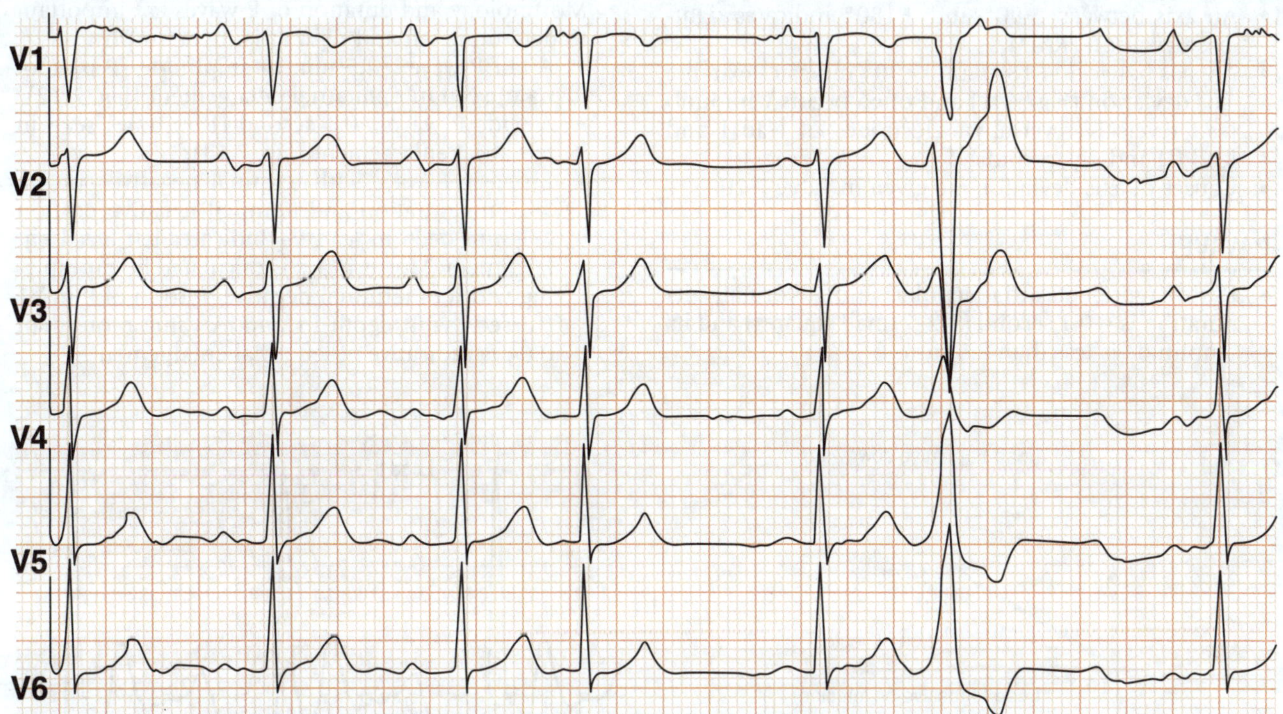

Fig. 7.9 ECG showing supraventricular ectopic (fourth beat—note incomplete compensatory pause) and ventricular ectopic (sixth beat—note complete compensatory pause).

- Irregular rhythm with P wave preceding each QRS with consistent PR interval is sinus arrhythmia.
- Premature beats—after a premature beat, the atria and the ventricles are in a refractory state, and hence, the next expected sinus impulse is blocked. This produces a pause that is known as compensatory pause. It is called complete when the duration of RR interval, including the premature beat, is twice that of the normal RR interval, and incomplete when it is less than twice the duration of the normal RR interval. Incomplete compensatory pause is a feature of supraventricular premature beats (Fig. 7.9), whereas complete compensatory pause is seen in ventricular premature beats (Fig. 7.9).

Causes of Irregular Rhythm (Table 7.19)

TABLE 7.19 Causes of Irregular Rhythm on ECG

Irregularly Irregular Rhythm	Regularly Irregular Rhythm

• Atrial fibrillation
• Multiple premature beats
  • Complete compensatory pause:
    • Ventricular premature beats
  • Incomplete compensatory pause:
    • Supraventricular premature beats
• Sinus arrhythmia
	• Complete compensatory pause:
	  • Ventricular premature beats
	• Incomplete compensatory pause:
	  • Supraventricular premature beats
	• 2° AV block of varying type
	• Atrial and ventricular bigeminy or trigeminy

AXIS

- Generally, the axis of leads I and aVF is used to calculate the axis of QRS complex. For this, net deflection of QRS in each lead is calculated by subtracting deflection of Q wave from deflection of R wave (e.g. if in lead I, Q wave measures three small squares and R-wave height is six small squares, the net deflection is +3).
- Net positive deflection in lead I is plotted on left side and net positive deflection in lead aVF is plotted downwards. Perpendiculars from these points are drawn and then a line is drawn from centre to the intersection of perpendiculars. This represents the axis of QRS complex (Fig. 7.10).
- The normal QRS axis is −30° to +90°.
- Left-axis deviation (LAD) is an axis between −30° and −90°.
- An axis between +90° and +180° indicates right-axis deviation (RAD).
- An axis between +180° and −90° indicates extreme axis deviation (Fig. 7.11) and often occurs with limb lead reversal (reversal of electrodes of lead I and lead II) and dextrocardia.
- Causes of axis deviation are given in Table 7.20.

P WAVE

- P wave represents atrial depolarisation. Normally, its duration is <0.1 second (<2.5 small squares) and its amplitude is less than 2.5 mm.

TABLE 7.20 Causes of Axis Deviation

Left-Axis Deviation (LAD)	Right-Axis Deviation
• Left bundle branch block • Left anterior hemiblock • Inferior wall myocardial infarction • Hypertrophic cardiomyopathy • Left ventricular hypertrophy • Wolff–Parkinson–White syndrome • Atrial septal defect (ostium primum type)	• Right ventricular hypertrophy • Chronic obstructive airway disease • Left posterior hemiblock • Atrial septal defect (ostium secundum type)

- P waves are absent in atrial fibrillation and before ventricular premature beats.
- Normally, all P waves are followed by QRS complexes. In third-degree AV block, P waves do not bear any relation to QRS complexes.
- Morphology and duration of P waves are important to determine left and right atrial hypertrophy.
  - A tall P wave >2.5 mm in amplitude (P pulmonale) seen in right atrial enlargement (Fig. 7.12).
  - A wide P wave >0.1 second (P mitrale) seen in left atrial enlargement (Fig. 7.13).
  - Biphasic P wave with terminal negative portion >40 ms duration and terminal negative portion >1 mm deep in lead V1 indicates left atrial enlargement. Morris index is calculated by multiplying width of terminal negative portion of P in V1 (in sec.) with depth in mm. A value more than 0.04 is indicative of left atrial enlargement.

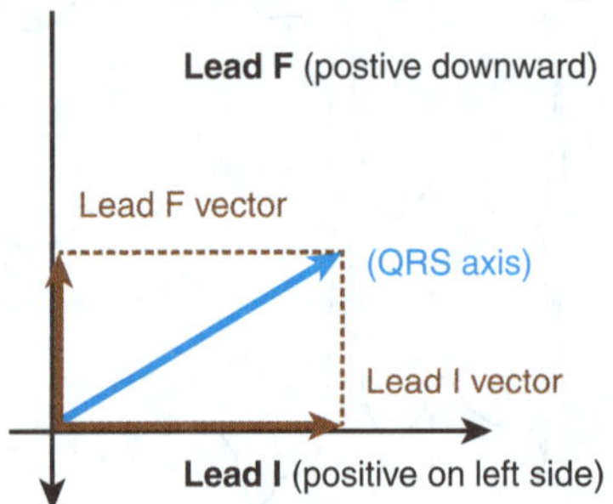

Fig. 7.10 Calculation of QRS axis.

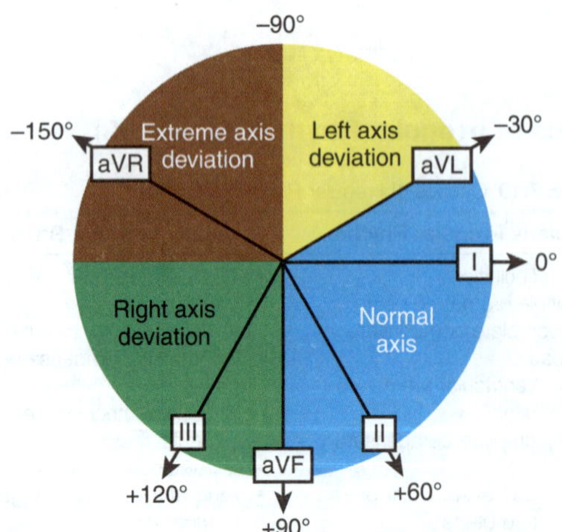

Fig. 7.11 Normal axis and extreme axis deviations.

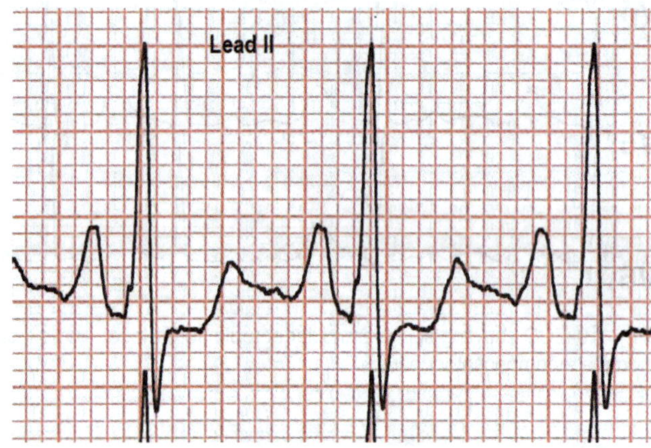

Fig. 7.12 P pulmonale.

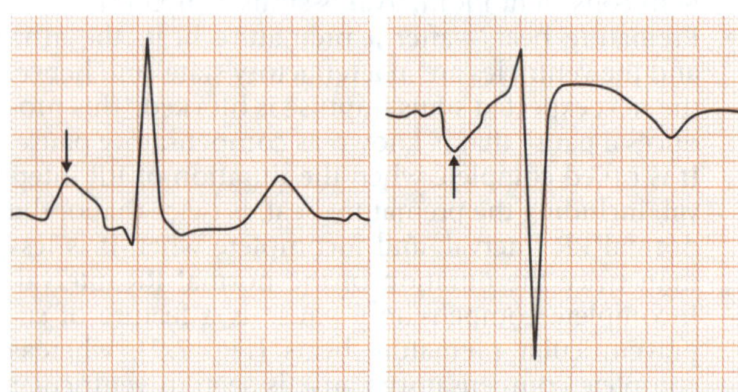

Fig. 7.13 P mitrale.

TABLE 7.21 Abnormalities in PR Interval

Prolongation of PR Interval (First-Degree AV Block)	Short PR Interval
• Rheumatic fever (carditis)	• Hypokalaemia
• Ischaemic heart disease	• Hypocalcaemia
• Digitalis effect	• Wolff–Parkinson–White syndrome
• Hyperkalaemia	• AV nodal rhythm
• Hypercalcaemia	• Supraventricular tachycardia
• Hypothermia	**Progressive Prolongation of PR Interval:**
	• Wenckebach's second-degree block

PR INTERVAL

- The PR interval (normally 0.12–0.20 seconds) reflects intraatrial, AV nodal and His–Purkinje conduction. It is the interval between the beginning of P wave and the beginning of QRS complex. Causes of abnormal PR interval are shown in Table 7.21.

QRS COMPLEX

- The QRS complex, representing ventricular depolarisation, has a normal duration of 0.04–0.10 seconds.
- Abnormal Q waves are present in myocardial infarction and hypertrophic cardiomyopathy.
- Wide QRS complexes are seen in right bundle branch block (RBBB) and left bundle branch block (LBBB).
  - In RBBB, QRS duration >0.12 seconds, rsR' pattern in lead V_1, and slurred and wide S waves in leads I, aVL and V_6 (Fig. 7.14).
  - In LBBB, QRS duration >0.12 seconds, dominant S wave in lead V_1, broad monophasic R wave in leads I, aVL, V_{5-6}, and absence of q waves in I, aVL and V_5-V_6 (Fig. 7.15).
- Wide and bizarre QRS complexes are seen in ventricular ectopics, ventricular tachycardia and supraventricular tachycardia with aberrant conduction.
- Increase in the height of QRS complexes may indicate right or left ventricular hypertrophy.
- Left ventricular hypertrophy:
  - Sum of S wave in lead V_1 and R wave in lead V_5 or V_6 >35 mm.
  - S wave in V_1 >25 mm or R wave in V_5 or V_6 >25 mm.
  - R wave in lead aVL >12 mm.
  - In systolic overload, q waves in leads I, aVL, V_5 and V_6 may disappear, ST become depressed and T wave becomes inverted.
  - In diastolic overload, q waves become deep in leads I, aVL, V_5 and V_6, and T waves become tall in V_5–V_6.
- Right ventricular hypertrophy:
  - Right-axis deviation.
  - Predominant R wave in V_1 and V_2 (R:S ratio >1) or R wave >5 mm in V_1.
  - Sum of R wave in V_1 or V_2 and S wave in V_5 or V_6 >10 mm.
- Box 7.15 lists causes of tall R waves in lead V_1.

ST-SEGMENT

- ST-segment elevation or depression is seen in ischaemic heart disease, cardiomyopathies, myocarditis and conduction blocks.
- Some drugs like digitalis can also produce ST-segment depression. Also seen with hypokalaemia and subarachnoid haemorrhage.
- ST-segment elevation in all leads (except aVR and V_1) in acute pericarditis.

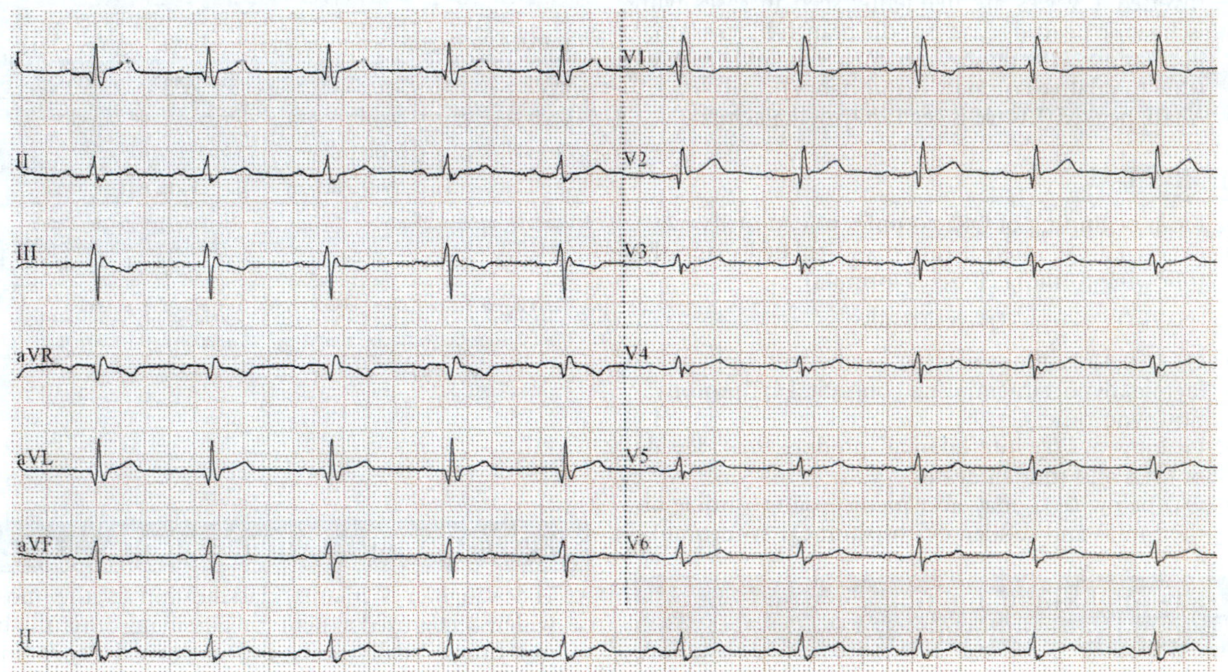

Fig. 7.14 Right bundle branch block (note prolonged PR interval).

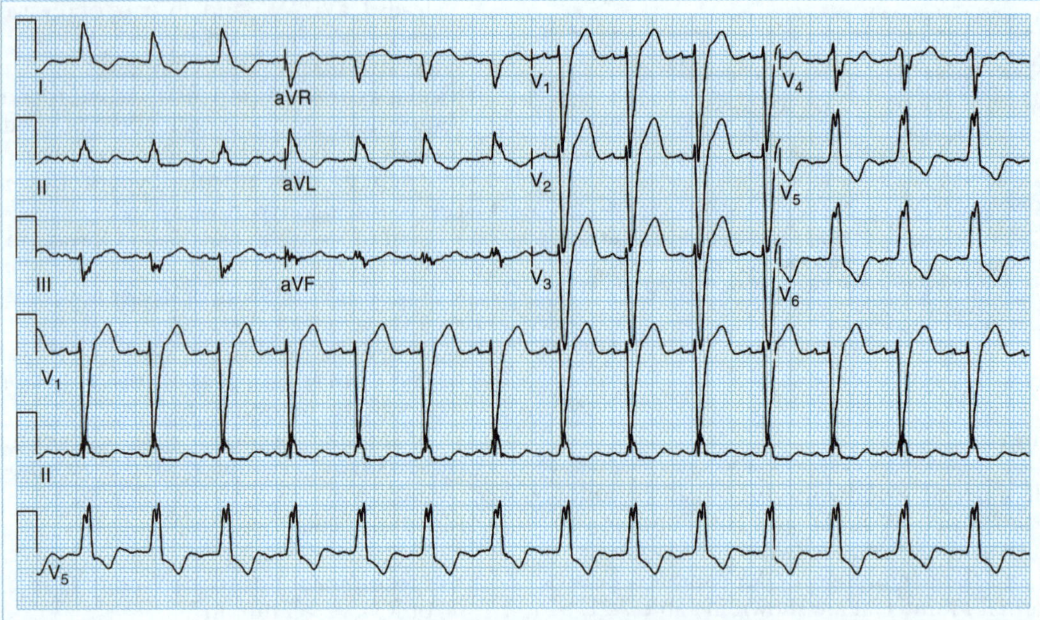

Fig. 7.15 Left bundle branch block.

BOX 7.15 Causes of Tall R Waves in V_1

- Right ventricular hypertrophy
- Dextrocardia
- Right bundle branch block
- Hypertrophic cardiomyopathy
- Wolff–Parkinson–White syndrome (type A)
- Posterior wall myocardial infarction

BOX 7.16 Usefulness of Electrocardiogram

- Myocardial ischaemia and infarction
- Cardiac arrhythmias
- Conduction defects
- Chamber (atrium or ventricle) hypertrophy
- Pericarditis
- Electrolyte abnormalities (hypokalaemia, hyperkalaemia, hypocalcaemia, hypercalcaemia)
- Effects of drugs (digitalis, tricyclic antidepressants)
- Hypothermia

T WAVES

- T waves represent ventricular repolarisation.
- Inverted T waves are frequently seen in cases with ischaemic heart disease, bundle branch blocks, atrial fibrillation with rapid ventricular rate and in PSVT (due to relative coronary insufficiency).
- A tall, peaked T wave is seen in hyperkalaemia.

QT INTERVAL

- From beginning of QRS complex to end of T wave.
- Corrected QT interval (QT_c) is calculated using the following formula (Bazett's formula):

$$QT_c = QT/\sqrt{RR}$$

- $QT_c > 0.45$ is abnormal that can be seen in hypokalaemia, hypocalcaemia and congenital QT prolongation syndrome.
- Prolonged QT_c interval may produce torsades de pointes and sudden death.
- QT_c below 0.32 may also predispose to cardiac arrhythmias and sudden death (short QT syndrome).

Q. Explain the usefulness of electrocardiogram.

- Electrocardiography is useful in diagnosing several conditions (Box 7.16).

TABLE 7.22 Classification of Antiarrhythmic Drugs

Class	Examples
Class Ia—sodium channel blockers	Procainamide, quinidine
Class Ib—sodium channel blockers	Mexiletine, lidocaine
Class Ic—sodium channel blockers	Flecainide, propafenone
Class II—beta blockers	Atenolol, bisoprolol, carvedilol, labetalol, metoprolol, propranolol, sotalol
Class III—potassium channel blockers	Amiodarone, sotalol
Class IV—calcium channel blockers	Verapamil, diltiazem
Class V—other agents	Adenosine, digoxin

Q. Classify antiarrhythmic agents.

- The Vaughan Williams classification is the most widely recognized system for classifying antiarrhythmic drugs. Medications are categorised depending on where they act within the cardiac action potential (Table 7.22).

TABLE 7.23 Classification of Cardiac Arrhythmias

Disturbances of Impulse Formation	Disturbances of Impulse Conduction

• Supraventricular arrhythmias (arrhythmias which originate in sinoatrial node, atrial myocardium or atrioventricular node)
• SA nodal:
  • Sinus tachycardia
  • Sinus bradycardia
  • Sinus arrhythmia
• Atrial:
  • Atrial premature contraction
  • Atrial fibrillation
  • Atrial flutter
  • Atrial tachycardia
  • Multifocal atrial tachycardia (MAT)
• AV nodal:
  • Paroxysmal supraventricular tachycardia (AV nodal reentrant tachycardia and AV reentrant tachycardia)
  • Junctional ectopics
  • Junctional rhythm
  • Junctional tachycardia
• Ventricular arrhythmias (arrhythmias which originate below atrioventricular node):
  • Ventricular ectopics
  • Idioventricular rhythm
  • Accelerated idioventricular rhythm
  • Ventricular tachycardia
  • Torsades de pointes
  • Ventricular fibrillation (VF)
	• Sinoatrial blocks
	• Tachycardia–bradycardia syndrome
	• AV nodal blocks:
	  • First-degree block
	  • Second-degree block
	    • Wenckebach's (Mobitz type I) block
	    • Mobitz type II block
	  • Complete or third-degree block
	• Bundle blocks:
	  • Right bundle branch block
	  • Left bundle branch block
	  • Left anterior hemiblock
	  • Left posterior hemiblock

Q. Define and classify cardiac arrhythmias. (IM 2.19)

- Any abnormal alteration in either rate or rhythm of heart is termed cardiac arrhythmia.

CLASSIFICATION

- Classification of cardiac arrhythmias is given in Table 7.23.

Q. Explain sinus arrhythmia.

- Definition—this is a phasic alteration in the heart rate in relation to breathing. The heart rate increases in inspiration and decreases in expiration (Fig. 7.16).
- P-wave morphology remains constant in individual leads [unlike multifocal atrial tachycardia (MAT)].
- Significance—this is the most common arrhythmia. It is a normal phenomenon and is a manifestation of normal autonomic nervous activity.

Q. What are ectopic beats (extrasystoles; premature beats)?

Q. Describe supraventricular ectopics (atrial ectopics; atrial premature beats).

Q. Explain briefly about ventricular ectopics (ventricular extrasystoles; ventricular premature beats, premature ventricular contractions—PVC).

ECTOPIC BEATS (EXTRASYSTOLES; PREMATURE BEATS)

- Definition—a heartbeat occurring as a result of an impulse originating in an area other than the SA node is known as an ectopic beat.
- Classification—ectopic beats are classified based on the origin of the impulse (ectopic focus).
  - Supraventricular:
    - Atrial (arising from atrium).
    - Junctional (arising from AV junction).
  - Ventricular.
- Haemodynamics—the normal sinus impulse (arising from SA node) following an ectopic impulse will find the ventricles refractory, and, hence, not conducted into the ventricles, resulting in a 'missed' or 'dropped' beat. This is responsible for the 'compensatory pause'. Compensatory pause allows more filling of the ventricles, and, hence, the subsequent beat is more forceful.
- Symptoms include extra beats, thumping beats or missed beats.
- Signs include irregularity in rhythm, missing of beats, postectopic bounding beat and cannon waves on JVP.

SUPRAVENTRICULAR ECTOPICS (ATRIAL ECTOPICS; ATRIAL PREMATURE BEATS)

- Causes are listed in Box 7.17.
- Electrocardiogram:
  - The ECG shows an abnormal P wave (P′ wave) that occurs early in the cardiac cycle. Sometimes, it may get buried in the preceding T wave. It may be inverted if the source of its origin is near the AV node.
  - Sum of RR interval preceding and following the ectopic beat is less than twice the basal RR interval,

BOX 7.17 Causes of Supraventricular Ectopics

- Idiopathic in healthy people
- Anxiety
- Excessive coffee, tea or tobacco
- Ischaemic heart disease
- Valvular heart diseases

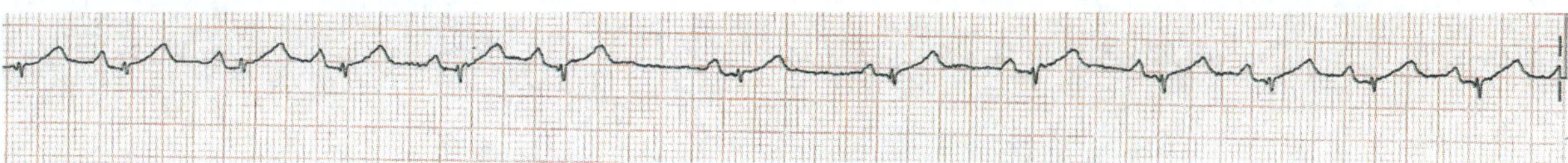

Fig. 7.16 Sinus arrhythmia.

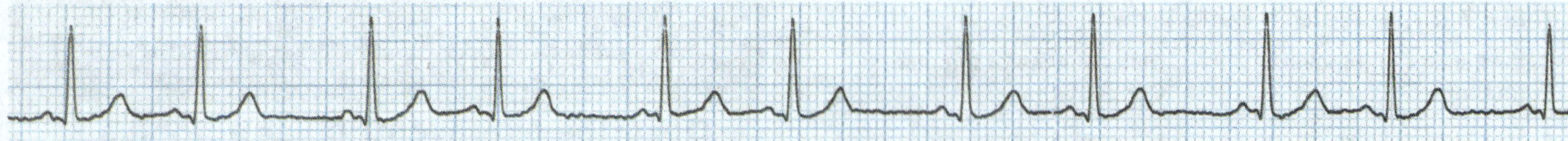

Fig. 7.17 Atrial bigeminy (regularly irregular).

that is the pause following the ectopic is not fully compensated.

- Most often, the QRS complex is narrow and identical to the sinus rhythm. However, occasionally, P′ is conducted aberrantly that results in a wide QRS complex. This must be distinguished from ventricular ectopic beat.
- Alternate supraventricular ectopics produce supraventricular bigeminy (Fig. 7.17).
- Supraventricular ectopics can sometimes precipitate atrial tachycardia, flutter and fibrillation.

- Treatment:
  - Treatment is that of the underlying cause.

VENTRICULAR ECTOPICS (VENTRICULAR EXTRASYSTOLES; VENTRICULAR PREMATURE BEATS)

- Causes of ventricular ectopics are listed in Box 7.18.
- Electrocardiogram:
  - A PVC is characterised on the ECG by a wide, bizarre QRS complex, more than 0.12 seconds in duration and usually without a preceding P wave.
  - Due to abnormal repolarisation, PVC is associated with secondary T-wave changes that include widening of T wave and deflection of T wave opposite to that of ectopic QRS complex.
  - The pause is fully compensated so that the sum of RR intervals preceding and following the ectopic QRS equals double the normal sinus RR interval.
  - When a PVC depolarises the ventricles at a similar time as a conducted atrial beat, a fusion beat is seen.
  - Ventricular bigeminy is present when a ventricular premature beat follows each sinus beat (Fig. 7.18).
  - Ventricular trigeminy is present when two sinus beats are followed by the ventricular premature beat. Thus every third beat is a ventricular premature beat.
- Treatment:
  - Treat the underlying cause.
  - In the absence of ischaemia, PVCs alone rarely require any specific pharmacological therapy.
  - In acute ischaemic heat disease, amiodarone may be required if the PVCs are multiform (varying morphology), couplets (two consecutive PVCs) are present, or R-on-T phenomenon (occurrence of PVC on the preceding T wave) is present.
  - Symptomatic healthy people can be treated with β-blockers, diltiazem, verapamil or amiodarone. If not controlled, radiofrequency ablation should be considered.

BOX 7.18 Causes of Ventricular Ectopics

- Idiopathic in healthy people
- Excessive tea, coffee and alcohol
- Beta-agonists, cocaine
- Acute myocardial infarction
- Myocardial ischaemia
- Myocarditis
- Digitalis toxicity
- Hypokalaemia
- Mitral valve prolapse

Q. Describe briefly about tachycardias.

Q. Write a brief note on narrow complex and wide complex tachycardias.

- Tachycardias are defined as a heart rate >100/minute.
- Tachycardias that utilise SA nodal, atrial or AV nodal tissue as part of their mechanism (i.e. arising above the bundle of His) are known as supraventricular tachycardia while those below as VT.
- Another way to classify tachycardias is narrow complex (QRS complex <0.12 seconds) and wide complex (QRS >0.12 seconds) tachycardias.
- In general, tachycardias that originate below the AV node produce wide QRS complexes while those originating from or above the AV node produce narrow QRS complexes.
- Common causes of wide complex tachycardias include:
  - Ventricular tachycardia.
  - Pacemaker-mediated tachycardia.
  - Some cases of supraventricular tachycardia.
  - Atrial fibrillation with Wolff–Parkinson–White syndrome.
  - Toxicity of certain medications (e.g. tricyclic antidepressants, diphenhydramine, cocaine).
  - Postresuscitation cardiac rhythm.
  - Hyperkalaemia (usually produces wide complexes with bradycardia).

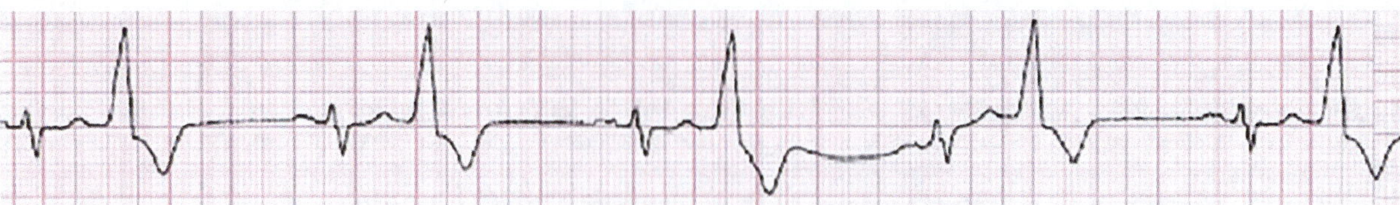

Fig. 7.18 Ventricular bigeminy.

- Sometimes, supraventricular tachycardias may produce widened QRS complexes due to:
  - Antegrade conduction from the atria to the ventricles via an accessory pathway (bundle of Kent and others).
  - Underlying preexisting bundle branch block (aberrant conduction).
  - Rate-related bundle branch block induced by the tachycardia itself (aberrant conduction).
- Wide complex tachycardia (QRS duration >0.12 seconds), thus, may be either supraventricular or ventricular in origin and differentiation between them is important from the therapeutic point of view.
- Look for any evidence of haemodynamic instability before attempting to differentiate these two types of tachycardias.
- In evaluating a patient with a regular wide complex tachycardia, the operating assumption must be that the tachycardia is of ventricular origin until proved to be otherwise.
- ECG criteria that suggest a VT are listed in Box 7.19.
- Capture beats are QRS complexes resulting from ventricular activation originating in supranodal tissue, using normal electrical conduction pathways. These are therefore narrow and are similar to a normal QRS complex.
- Fusion beats are hybrid QRS complexes and result from simultaneous activation of ventricles via normal conduction through AV node and through ventricular rhythm. They are therefore intermediate in morphology and width from either a capture or ventricular beat.
- Precordial concordance means that QRS direction on the ECG in all the precordial leads is monophasic, that is all are either completely positive or negative. Positive precordial concordance, however, may also occur during supraventricular tachycardia with aberrant conduction. Negative precordial concordance nearly always indicates VT.
- After termination of tachycardia, the ECG should be analysed during sinus rhythm for any evidence of QT prolongation, Brugada phenotype, ischaemic heart disease, preexcitation or an underlying cardiomyopathy; all of these features increase the probability of life-threatening arrhythmias.

BOX 7.19 ECG Criteria for Ventricular Tachycardia

- Precordial concordance (all QRS complexes in precordial leads are either completely positive or completely negative)
- Onset of QRS to nadir of S wave >0.1 second
- Presence of fusion beats
- Presence of AV dissociation
- Presence of capture beats
- QRS axis <–90° to ±180°
- QRS width >0.14 second if RBBB is present or >0.16 second if LBBB is present
- RBBB pattern with
  - Rsr′ or RS pattern in lead V_1
  - R/S <1 or QS pattern in V_6
- LBBB pattern with
  - Q in V_6
  - Notched downstroke S wave in V_1
  - R >0.03 second in V_1

ECG APPROACH TO TACHYCARDIAS

- Based on ECG, tachycardias can be classified as narrow-complex and wide-complex, regular or irregular (Flowchart 7.1).

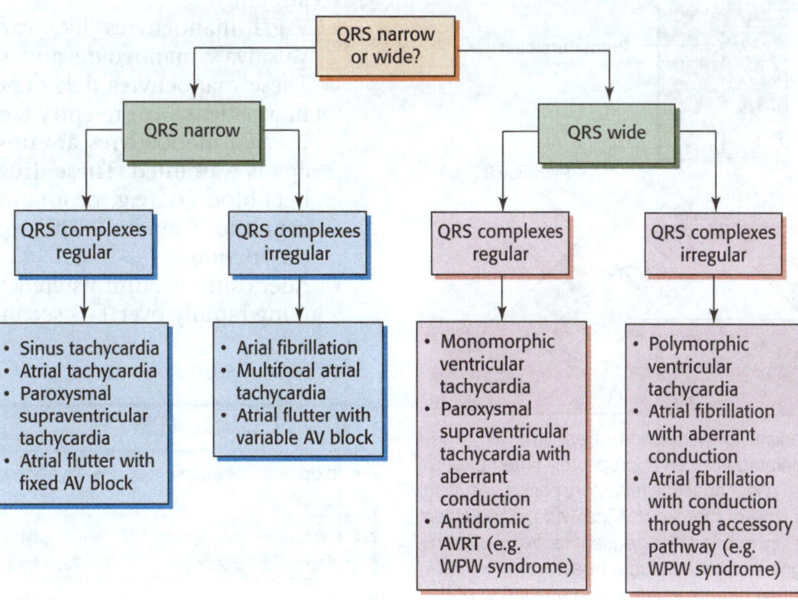

Flowchart 7.1 ECG Approach to Tachycardias.

Q. What do you understand by the term supraventricular tachycardias? Name various supraventricular tachycardias.

Q. What do you understand by the term 'reentry' arrhythmias?

- Supraventricular tachycardia refers to an arrhythmia having three or more complexes at rates exceeding 100 beats/minute and originating above the ventricle (i.e. in the SA node, atria or the AV junction).

BOX 7.20 Supraventricular Tachycardias

- Sinus tachycardia
- Atrial fibrillation
- Atrial flutter
- Multifocal atrial tachycardia
- Paroxysmal supraventricular tachycardia (PSVT)
- Wolff–Parkinson–White syndrome
- Junctional tachycardia

- Supraventricular tachycardia includes several conditions (Box 7.20).

RE-ENTRY

- The most common mechanism of arrhythmias is re-entry. This is particularly true for PSVT.
- Re-entry requires presence of two electrophysiologically distinct pathways around an insulated core (e.g. the AV valve annulus).
- In PSVT, re-entry occurs due to presence of an additional electrical connection between the atrium and ventricle (e.g. the bundle of Kent) or within the AV node itself.
- In re-entrant rhythms, electrical impulse can cycle and recycle repetitively (Fig. 7.19).

Q. Describe sinus tachycardia.

- It is characterised by a rate more than 100/minute and normal P waves, PR interval and QRS complexes.
- It is usually seen in patients with fever, anaemia, thyrotoxicosis, embolism, HF and shock.
- Treatment:
  - Identify underlying cause and correct it.
  - Use ivabradine alone or in combination with β-blockers if the fast rate produces myocardial ischaemia.

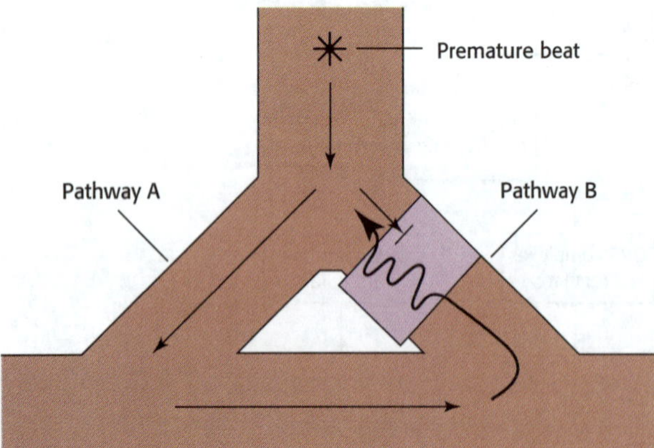

Fig. 7.19 Re-entry mechanism for generation of arrhythmias. In re-entry, electrical signals generated from an appropriately timed premature beat find pathway B still under absolute refractory period, resulting in conduction block in this limb of the circuit. Meanwhile, conduction down pathway A proceeds unimpeded. Subsequent recovery of pathway B allows electrical signals to be conducted backward (or retrograde), resulting in reactivation of pathway A and propagation of the re-entry circuit.

Q. Write a short note on paroxysmal supraventricular tachycardia.

- It is usually paroxysmal and recurrent, and has a rate of 140–220 beats/minute with 1:1 conduction.
- It usually results from re-entry of an atrial ectopic in the AV node (AV nodal re-entry tachycardia—AVNRT). PSVT can also result from re-entry in the accessory pathways (AV re-entry tachycardia—AVRT). Occasionally, it results from increased atrial automaticity.
- Usually, AVRT is orthodromic with activation transmitted from atria to ventricles via the AV node and back via the accessory pathway ('orthodromic' because the AV node is conducting in the 'correct direction'). Less commonly, the direction of activation is antidromic that leads to aberrant ventricular activation and broad QRS complexes.
- Causes of PSVT are given in Box 7.21.
- Clinical features:
  - The onset and termination of the arrhythmia are sudden.
  - Patients most commonly complain of palpitations, an odd feeling in the chest and, on occasion, light-headedness or syncope.
  - Those with significant heart disease may have additional symptoms during the arrhythmia such as dyspnoea and chest pain.
  - Some patients have polyuria and experience diuresis during or after PSVT.
- Electrocardiogram:
  - The P wave is usually buried in the QRS complex or occurs slightly before or after the QRS complex.
  - The QRS complexes occur at regular intervals (there is constant RR cycle length) and are similar to those seen during sinus rhythm (Fig. 7.20).
  - Significant ST-segment depression during tachycardia has been observed in 25%–50% of patients. Majority of these patients do not have underlying coronary artery disease.
- Treatment:
  - Vagal manoeuvres like carotid sinus massage, Valsalva's manoeuvre and gag reflex are useful. These manoeuvres delay conduction in AV node in a patient with re-entry tachycardia.
  - If vagal manoeuvres are unsuccessful, drug therapy is warranted. These drugs include adenosine, beta-blockers (e.g. propranolol, esmolol), diltiazem and verapamil. They prolong the AV refractory period.
  - Adenosine is administered as an initial bolus of 6 mg rapidly over 1–3 seconds followed immedi-

BOX 7.21 Causes of PSVT

• Idiopathic in healthy individuals	• Hyperthyroidism
• Excessive coffee, tea, alcohol or tobacco	• Organic heart disease (ischaemic, valvular or congenital)
• Anxiety	• Chronic lung disease

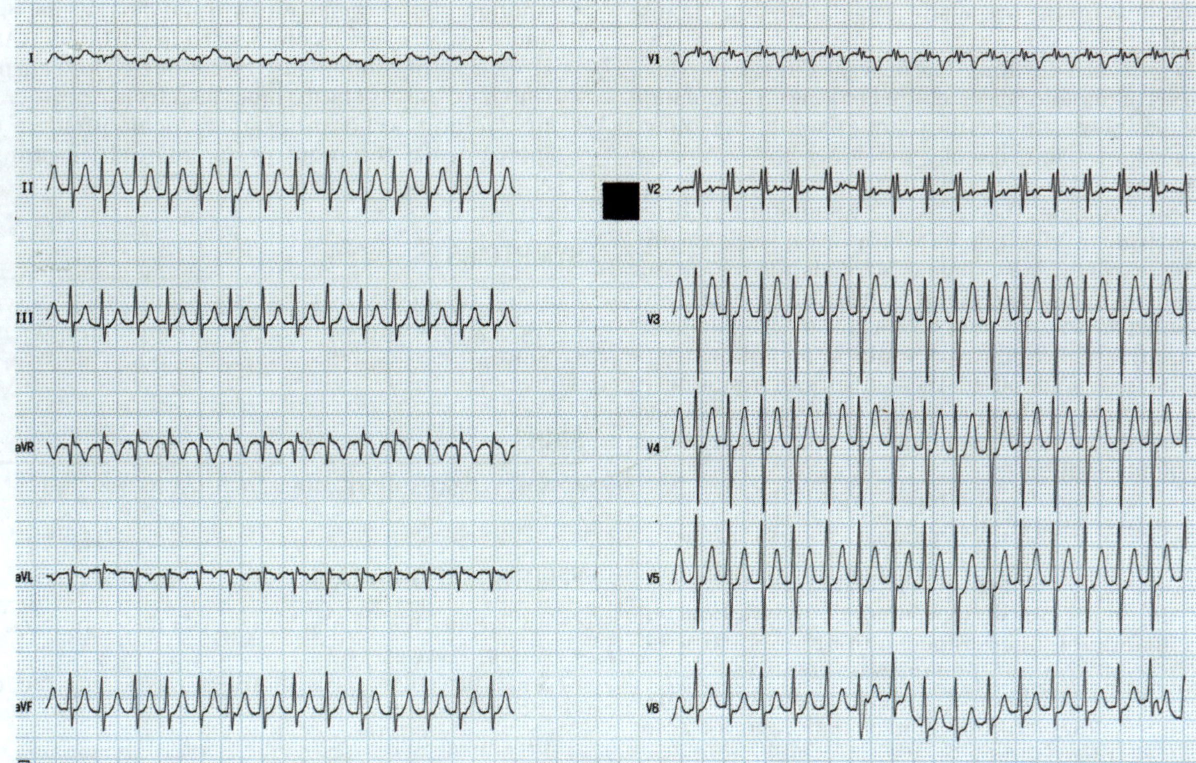

Fig. 7.20 Paroxysmal supraventricular tachycardia.

ately by 20 mL of saline. If required, a second and third dose of 12 mg is repeated in 1 to 2 minutes.

- Diltiazem is administered in a dose of 10 mg over 2 minutes; same dose may be repeated if conversion to sinus rhythm does not occur in 15 minutes. If required, an infusion can be started at 10 mg/hour.
- Synchronised cardioversion is performed if patient is haemodynamically compromised.
- Long-term control can be achieved by radiofrequency ablation of the reentrant pathway.

Q. Discuss the aetiology, pathophysiology, clinical features, complications and management of atrial fibrillation. (IM 1.8)

DEFINITION

- This is an arrhythmia where multiple atrial foci fire impulses at a rate of 350–600/minute. There is no atrial contraction but only fibrillation. The ventricles respond at irregular intervals, usually at a rate of 100–140/minute.
- Atrial fibrillation can be paroxysmal, persistent, long standing or permanent.
    - Paroxysmal atrial fibrillation means an episode which terminates spontaneously or with intervention within 7 days of onset.
    - Persistent atrial fibrillation means an episode which lasts longer than 7 days.
    - Long-standing persistent atrial fibrillation means that atrial fibrillation has lasted for more than 12 months.
    - Permanent atrial fibrillation means that the arrhythmia is persistent and a joint decision by the patient and clinician has been made to no longer pursue a rhythm control strategy.

AETIOLOGY (Box 7.22)

BOX 7.22 Causes of Atrial Fibrillation

- Rheumatic heart disease (especially mitral valvular disease)
- Ischaemic heart disease (especially acute myocardial infarction)
- Hypertension
- Thyrotoxicosis
- Congenital heart diseases (especially atrial septal defect)
- Cardiomyopathy
- Pericardial diseases
- Rare causes—alcohol, pulmonary embolism, exercise, sinoatrial disease, chronic lung diseases, electrocution

PATHOPHYSIOLOGY AND HAEMODYNAMICS

- Atria fire the impulses at a rate of 350–600/minute. Many of them reach the AV node in its refractory period and so are not conducted. However, a variable number (about 100–140/minute) of impulses are conducted to the ventricles at irregular intervals. This accounts for the irregularly irregular rhythm of pulse and heart.

- The irregular rhythm of heart results in varying durations of diastole (short, normal or long). The duration of diastole determines the volume of ventricular blood; the shorter the diastole, the lesser the ventricular volume, and the longer the diastole, the higher the ventricular volume. The ventricular volume in turn determines the cardiac output, which hence keeps varying. This varying cardiac output accounts for the varying volume of pulse and the pulse deficit (ventricular systoles that are so weak as to be not able to evoke a pulse).
- Lack of atrial contraction results in the following:
  - Stasis of blood in the left atrium resulting in thrombus formation and subsequent dislodgment of the thrombus resulting in systemic embolisation.
  - Disappearance of *a* waves from JVP (*a* waves are due to atrial contraction).
  - Disappearance of a fourth heart sound if it was already present (S_4 is due to atrial contraction).
  - In some cases, disappearance of presystolic accentuation of mid-diastolic murmur of mitral stenosis (atrial contraction may contribute to PSA).
  - Loss of 'atrial booster effect' (atrial contraction in presystole) resulting in precipitation or worsening of cardiac failure.
- Tachycardia-related cardiomyopathy in patients with poor rate control may further depress cardiac function. It usually occurs when the ventricular rate is persistently faster than 110/minute. It improves or completely reverses after adequate rate control or restoration of sinus rhythm.

RISK OF STROKE IN ATRIAL FIBRILLATION

- In patients with nonvalvular atrial fibrillation, the average annual risk for arterial thromboembolism including stroke is 5%, and the risk is higher in patients older than 75 years.
- A risk index (CHA_2DS_2-VASc) has been developed to determine the risk of stroke due to thromboembolism in patients with non-valvular atrial fibrillation (Table 7.24).
- CHA_2DS_2-VASc score of 9 predicts a stroke rate of 15.2% per year.
- Antithrombotic agents (warfarin and direct-acting oral anticoagulants) are recommended for CHA_2DS_2-VASc score ≥ 2. They should also be considered for patients who have one risk factor other than female sex.
- In addition, echocardiographic demonstration of intraauricular thrombus or an enlarged left atrium also indicates increased risk of emboli.

SYMPTOMS

- Usual symptoms include palpitations, fatigue, syncope, angina and symptoms of HF and thromboembolism.

SIGNS

- Signs of atrial fibrillation are listed in Box 7.23.

ELECTROCARDIOGRAM

- An irregularly irregular rhythm of QRS complexes.
- Absent P waves.
- Small, irregular waves (fibrillary waves) at a rate of 350–600/minute that are difficult to see on ECG (fine atrial fibrillation) (Fig. 7.21).
- At lower rates of 150–300, coarse fibrillary waves are seen (coarse atrial fibrillation).

Note: Patients with atrial fibrillation and digoxin toxicity may have regular RR intervals due to development of AV block and junctional rhythm; P waves are absent.

DIFFERENTIAL DIAGNOSIS

- Atrial flutter with variable block: Prominent sawtooth waves at lower rates of 250–350/minute are seen in the ECG.
- Atrial tachycardia with variable block: Atrial rate is approximately 150/minute that is regular but the conduction to the ventricles is not regular producing irregular pulse.
- Both multifocal atrial tachycardia and wandering atrial pacemaker can have irregular ventricular responses; P waves of differing morphology are present.

TABLE 7.24 CHA_2DS_2-VASc Score

Risk Factor	Score
• Congestive heart failure	1
• Hypertension	1
• Age ≥75 years	2
• Diabetes mellitus	1
• Stroke/transient ischaemic attack/thromboembolic event history	2
• Vascular disease (prior MI, peripheral artery disease)	1
• Age 65–74 years	1
• Sex category (female)	1

BOX 7.23 Signs in Atrial Fibrillation

• Irregularly irregular pulse	• Absence of '*a*' waves on JVP
• Varying volumes of pulse	• Disappearance of the PSA of the mid-diastolic murmur of mitral stenosis (MS) in some cases
• Pulse deficit (apex-pulse deficit)	• Disappearance of the fourth heart sound
• Varying intensity of the first heart sound	• Hypotension

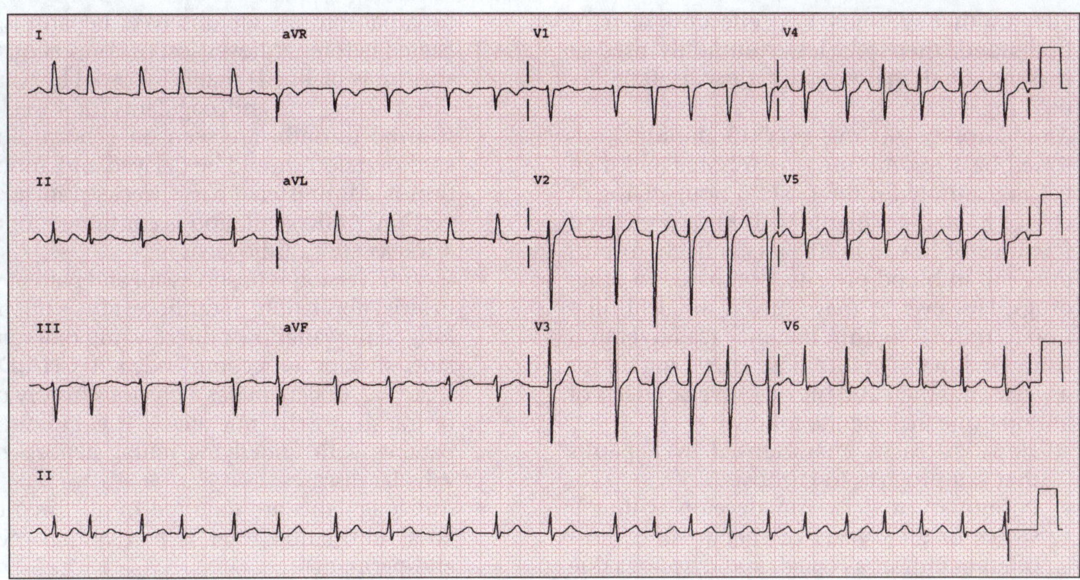

Fig. 7.21 Atrial fibrillation with fast ventricular rate.

COMPLICATIONS (Box 7.24)

BOX 7.24 Complications of Atrial Fibrillation

• Syncope	• Angina
• Thromboembolism	• Hypotension
• Precipitation/worsening of cardiac failure	• Precipitation of pulmonary oedema in mitral stenosis

TREATMENT

GOALS OF MANAGEMENT

- Haemodynamic stabilisation.
- Control of ventricular rate.
- Restoration of sinus rhythm.
- Prevention of embolic complications.
- Treatment of underlying cause.

1. If the patient's clinical status is severely compromised (presence of hypotension, angina, syncope, pulmonary oedema or altered sensorium), synchronised DC cardioversion starting at 100–200 J (using biphasic cardioverters) is the treatment of choice.
2. If the patient's clinical status is not severely compromised, treatment is in two steps:
   - ***Slowing the ventricular rate*** with verapamil, diltiazem, propranolol, esmolol or digoxin (Flowchart 7.2). In general, beta-blockers are initiated first. The goal is to achieve a resting ventricular rate of less than 110/minute. Controlling the ventricular rate increases cardiac output, decreases the metabolic demand of the heart and avoids the potentially dangerous side effects of rhythm control drugs. The doses of various drugs are as follows:
     - Diltiazem: 10 mg intravenously over 2 minutes; repeat same dose in 15 minutes if required; start an infusion at 10–15 mg/hour to maintain ventricular rate below 80/minute. Oral maintenance dose is 60–120 mg tid.
     - Verapamil: 5–10 mg intravenously over 2 minutes; repeat in 30 minutes if required. Oral maintenance dose is 40–240 mg bid.
     - Propranolol: 1 mg intravenously over 2 minutes; repeat every 5 minutes up to a maximum of 5 mg. Oral maintenance dose is 40–120 mg tid.
     - Metoprolol: 2.5–5.0 mg bolus; up to 4 doses. Oral maintenance dose is 25–100 mg bid.
     - Digoxin: 0.25–0.5 mg intravenously, and then 0.25 mg after 4–6 hours and another dose

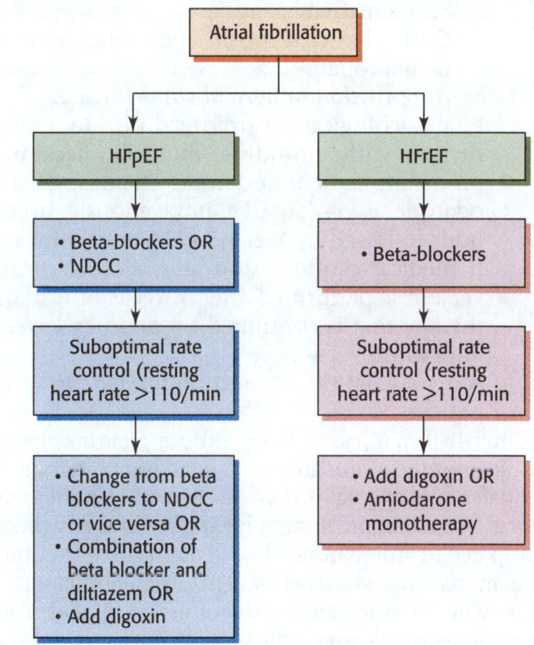

Flowchart 7.2 Rate Control in Atrial Fibrillation. NDCC, non-dihydropyridine calcium channel blockers (diltiazem and verapamil); HFpEF, heart failure with preserved ejection fraction; HFrEF, heart failure with reduced ejection fraction.

after another 12 hours. Peak effect not seen for hours and, therefore, less commonly used at present. Oral maintenance dose is 0.0625–0.25 mg od.

- Amiodarone: 150 mg over 10 minutes, followed by 1 mg/minute over 6 hours and then 0.5 mg/minute for the next 18 hours. Drug of choice in stable patients with known ejection fractions of less than 40%. Less likely to produce fall in blood pressure compared to other drugs. However, it may convert atrial fibrillation to normal rhythm that may lead to embolism. Oral maintenance dose is 200 mg tid for 4 weeks and then 200 mg od. Adverse effects of amiodarone include the following:
  - Hepatic toxicity characterised by hepatitis that can progress to cirrhosis.
  - Pulmonary toxicity can develop within 6 weeks or after years of therapy and most often manifests as cough and dyspnoea due to interstitial lung disease.
  - Thyroid dysfunction (hypothyroidism, hyperthyroidism).
  - Sun sensitivity.
  - Corneal microdeposits, light sensitivity, optic neuropathy.
- *Converting rhythm to normal sinus rhythm.*
  - Pharmacological cardioversion to sinus rhythm with quinidine, ibutilide, flecainide, propafenone or amiodarone. The dose of amiodarone is 5–7 mg/kg intravenously over 1 hour followed by 1.2–1.8 g/24-hour infusion.
  - If medical cardioversion fails, electric cardioversion is performed after 3 weeks of warfarin therapy that is continued for another 4 weeks after cardioversion.
  - Anticoagulation is recommended in such patients.

3. If sinus rhythm is restored by electric or pharmacological cardioversion, amiodarone, dronedarone, flecainide, propafenone or sotalol may be used to prevent recurrence. Dronedarone, though having better safety profile compared to amiodarone, should not be used to control rate in patients with permanent atrial fibrillation or those with HF as it increases risk of stroke, MI and death.
4. In patients in whom cardioversion is unsuccessful or in whom atrial fibrillation is likely to recur, treatment consists of the following:
   - Allow the patient to remain in atrial fibrillation but reduce the ventricular rate by diltiazem, verapamil, propranolol or digoxin. Goal is to achieve a resting heart rate of about 80/minute or <110/minute during moderate exercise. Resting rates <110/minute are also acceptable in most patients (lenient rate control strategy).
   - Chronic anticoagulation.
5. Antithrombotic (anticoagulant) therapy:
   - Early medical or electric cardioversion may be done without prior anticoagulation therapy when atrial fibrillation has been present for less than 48 hours.
   - If duration of atrial fibrillation exceeds 48 hours or is unknown, a transoesophageal echocardiography should be done to exclude an atrial thrombus. If no atrial thrombi are observed, heparin is administered before cardioversion (if conversion to sinus rhythm is planned) that is followed by warfarin or direct-acting oral anticoagulants for 4 weeks.
   - If atrial thrombi are seen on echocardiography, cardioversion should be delayed and anticoagulation is administered for 3 weeks prior to cardioversion. Anticoagulation is continued for another 4 weeks after cardioversion.
   - If cardioversion is unsuccessful and patient remains in atrial fibrillation, or cardioversion is not planned, long-term warfarin or direct-acting oral anticoagulants therapy is recommended if CHA_2DS_2-VASc score ≥2, or patient has a previous history of stroke or transient ischaemic attack. It is indicated in all patients with underlying mitral stenosis or other valvular diseases.
   - Anticoagulants are required in all three types of atrial fibrillation, that is paroxysmal, persistent and permanent.
   - Anticoagulants include warfarin and nonvitamin K antagonist oral anticoagulants (NOAC) like dabigatran (a direct thrombin inhibitor), rivaroxaban or apixaban (both are direct factor Xa inhibitors). NOACs are preferred over warfarin except in patients with moderate to severe mitral stenosis and prosthetic heart valves.
   - With warfarin, the INR should be maintained between 2.0 and 3.0 (between 2.5 and 3.5 if underlying valvular lesion is present).
6. Aspirin:
   - Aspirin (325 mg/day) plus clopidogrel (75 mg/day) does not provide adequate protection from stroke but can be used as an alternative to anticoagulants in the following situation:
     - Contraindication/allergy to anticoagulants.
7. Refractory cases are managed with catheter ablation therapy.

Note: Rate control strategies advocate medically slowing ventricular response to the fibrillating atrium and using anticoagulation to reduce stroke risk. On the other hand, rhythm control strategies involve medical or electrical conversion to sinus rhythm to improve haemodynamics and symptoms and, theoretically, reduce stroke risk. However, data available suggest no definite advantage of one approach over the other. Rate control along with chronic anticoagulation is possibly the best strategy for most patients with atrial fibrillation. In some select group patients (e.g. young patients or patients with left ventricular dysfunction producing symptoms), rhythm control may be tried, even though there are no data to support this line of action.

Q. Define atrial flutter. Discuss the causes, electrocardiographic features and management of atrial flutter.

- Definition:
  - Atrial flutter is characterised by a regular, rapid atrial rate of 250–350/minute, where ventricles respond to every second, third, fourth or fifth beat (2:1, 3:1, 4:1 or 5:1 AV block).

- Common causes:
  - Organic heart diseases (ischaemic, rheumatic, congenital).
  - Pericarditis.
  - Acute respiratory failure.
  - First week following open heart surgery.
- Electrocardiographic feature:
  - Characteristic flutter waves are seen as regular sawtooth waves ('F' waves) (Fig. 7.22).
- Management:
  - Immediate conversion to sinus rhythm can be accomplished by direct current cardioversion or atrial pacing.
  - Initial reduction of ventricular rate using digoxin, diltiazem, β-blockers or verapamil followed by conversion to sinus rhythm using quinidine, amiodarone, disopyramide or flecainide.
  - Prevention of recurrences can be accomplished by quinidine, amiodarone, disopyramide or flecainide.
  - The stroke risk is similar to that for atrial fibrillation and the management of anticoagulation is almost identical.

Q. Discuss briefly Wolff–Parkinson–White syndrome.

- Cause—presence of an abnormal band of atrial tissue connecting the atria and ventricles and bypassing the AV node which predispose the patient to various arrhythmias.
- During sinus rhythm, conduction takes place partly through the AV node and partly through the bypass tract. This results in a short PR interval (<0.12 seconds), a delta wave in the beginning of QRS complex due to activation of ventricles via the accessory pathway (preexcitation) and prolonged QRS complex (>0.12 seconds) due to fusion of excitation via two pathways (Fig. 7.23). The term Wolff–Parkinson–White (WPW) pattern indicates preexcitation on an ECG in the absence of symptomatic arrhythmias.
- This tract can act as a re-entry pathway and the patient may develop supraventricular tachycardia.
- The term WPW pattern is applied to the patient with preexcitation manifest on an ECG in the absence of symptomatic arrhythmias while the term WPW syndrome is applied to the patient with both preexcitation manifest on an ECG and symptomatic arrhythmias involving the accessory pathway.
- Clinical features:
  - Majority of patients with WPW pattern on ECG remain asymptomatic.
  - A small percentage of patients with the WPW pattern develop arrhythmias leading to palpitations, light-headedness, syncope, chest pain or cardiac arrest.
- Complications:
  - PSVT, atrial fibrillation, VT, ventricular fibrillation (VF) and death.
- Treatment:
  - Narrow complex tachycardia is treated in the same way as PSVT.
  - For broad complex tachycardia, procainamide and ibutilide are useful as these drugs increase the refractory period and reduce the conduction rate through the bypass tract.
  - Preferred treatment for patients with arrhythmias is radiofrequency ablation of the bypass tract.
  - In patients with WPW syndrome and atrial fibrillation, cardioversion is the treatment of choice. Caution should be employed when using digitalis, adenosine or verapamil in patients with WPW syndrome and atrial fibrillation because increase in AV nodal refractory period produces increased conduction through the accessory pathway which may precipitate VF.

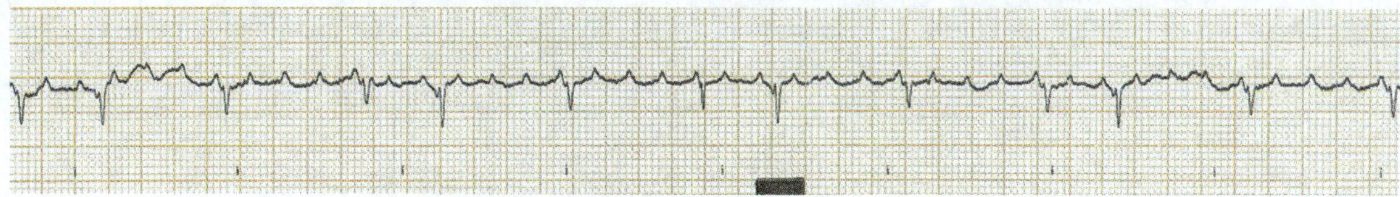

Fig. 7.22 Atrial flutter with variable block.

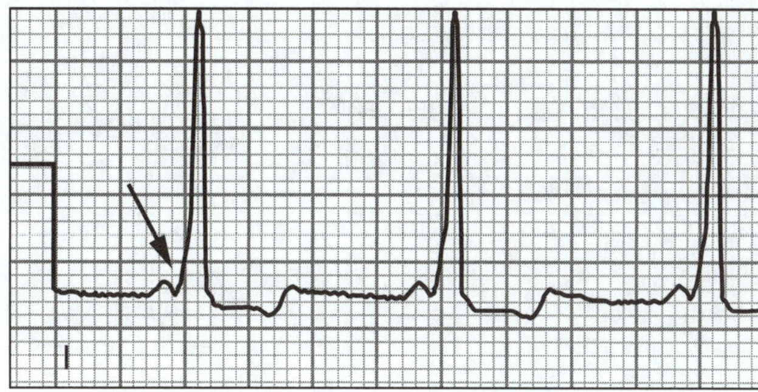

Fig. 7.23 Wolff–Parkinson–White pattern (note short PR interval and slurred QRS complex shown by arrow).

Q. Explain briefly about sick sinus syndrome or sinus node dysfunction.

- The term 'sick sinus syndrome' encompasses a number of abnormalities including sinus bradycardia, sinus arrest, combinations of sinoatrial and AV blocks, supraventricular tachycardias, particularly atrial fibrillation and flutter, and tachycardia–bradycardia.
- Defined by abnormal cardiac impulse formation and by abnormal propagation from the SA node which prevent it from performing its pacemaking function. It is characterised by sinus node dysfunction with an atrial rate inappropriate for physiological requirements.
- The abnormalities are usually due to ischaemia, fibrosis (often age-related and produced by dysfunction of ion channels within SA), drug-induced (beta-blockers, calcium channel blockers, digoxin, sympatholytic medications, antiarrhythmic medications, lithium), infiltrative disorders (haemochromatosis, sarcoidosis, connective tissue diseases) or autonomic dysfunction.
- Clinical features:
  - Many patients are asymptomatic.
  - In others, clinical features are related to cerebral hypoperfusion and reduced cardiac output. These can include syncope, palpitations and dizziness as well as symptoms caused by worsening of underlying conditions such as HF, angina pectoris and cerebrovascular accident.
  - Peripheral thromboembolism and stroke, which can occur in the presence of bradycardia–tachycardia syndrome (alternating bradyarrhythmias and tachyarrhythmias), may be related to dysrhythmia-induced emboli.
  - A slow heart rate in the presence of fever, left ventricular failure or pulmonary oedema may be suggestive of sick sinus syndrome.
- Treatment of recurrent symptomatic bradycardia or prolonged pauses requires implantation of a permanent pacemaker. Oral anticoagulation should be considered in patients with a history of intermittent tachycardias.

Q. Explain briefly about ventricular tachycardia.

- It is a wide complex tachycardia (rate >100/minute) with ≥3 consecutive complexes with regular rate and single QRS morphology (monomorphic VT) or varying QRS morphology (polymorphic VT).
- Nonsustained VT is a series of repetitive ventricular beats that have a duration of less than 30 seconds; sustained VT lasts for more than 30 seconds.
- Cause:
  - It usually occurs in the presence of some underlying heart disease and is rarely seen in normal hearts.
- Clinical features:
  - The patient may be asymptomatic or may present with palpitations or haemodynamic collapse.
  - The assumption that a haemodynamically stable patient cannot have VT is erroneous.
- Electrocardiogram (Fig. 7.24):
  - The width of the QRS complex is generally >0.16 seconds.

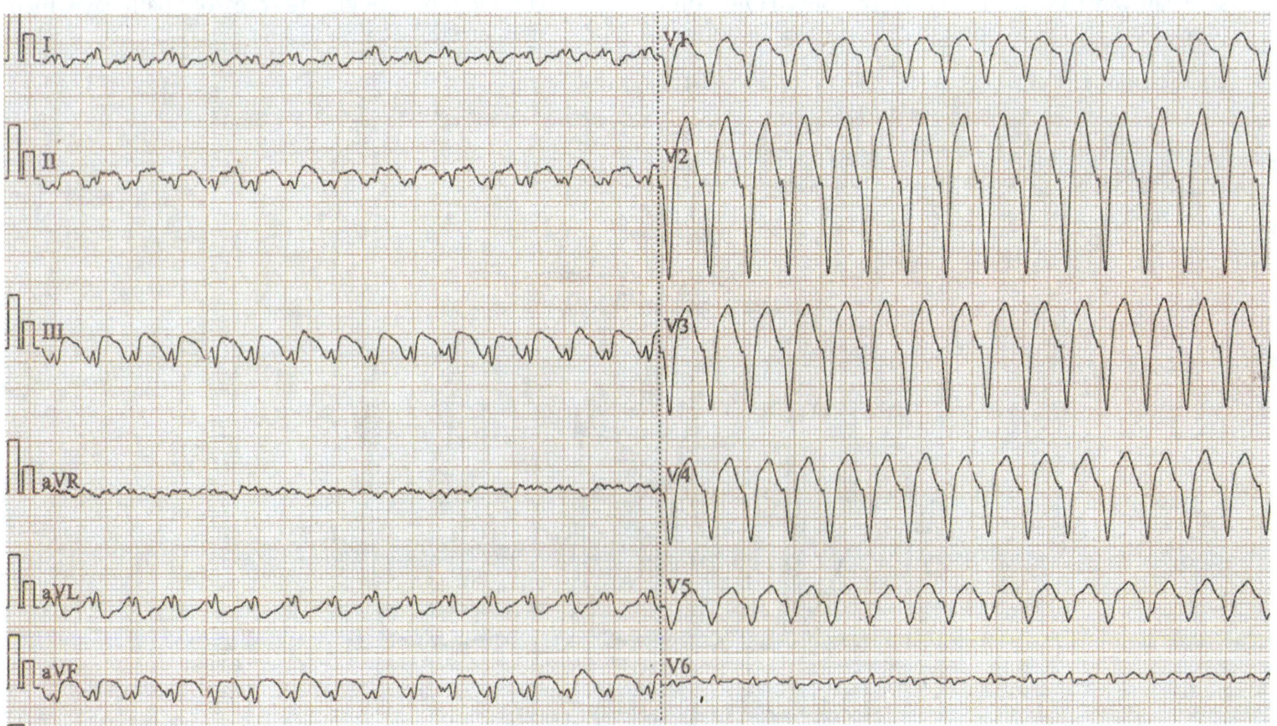

Fig. 7.24 Ventricular tachycardia.

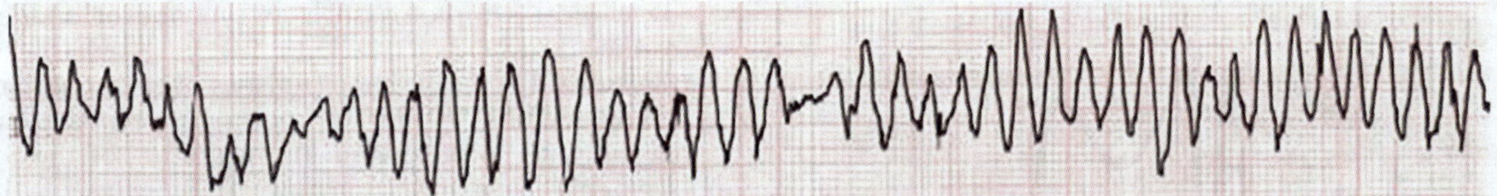

Fig. 7.25 Torsades de pointes.

- Positive or negative concordance of the QRS complex across the precordial leads (e.g. R waves or S waves only).
- A monophasic 'Rr' pattern in lead V_1 (termed rabbit ears) with a taller left ear.
- An indeterminate axis (between −90° and −180°).
- In severe underlying heart disease, the QRS morphology may be variable (polymorphic VT). The basal QT interval before onset of polymorphic VT is normal as compared to torsades de pointes.

- Treatment:
  - If the patient is haemodynamically unstable in the form of hypotension, angina, HF or altered sensorium, immediate cardioversion in synchronised mode is required.
  - If the patient is stable and has normal LV function, amiodarone, procainamide, sotalol and lidocaine are the drugs of choice. If the patient has LV dysfunction, amiodarone or lidocaine is preferred.
    - Amiodarone 150 mg intravenously over 10 minutes, then 1 mg/minute for 6 hours and then 0.5 mg/minute for next 18 hours.
    - Lidocaine 1–1.5 mg/kg IV over 1 minute followed by infusion at 1–4 mg/minute. A repeat bolus of 50 mg may be required during the first 30 minutes to avoid subtherapeutic blood levels.

Q. Write a short note on torsades de pointes.

- It is a special type of VT characterised by gradual changing of QRS axis so that it appears to twist around the isoelectric line (Fig. 7.25).
- The baseline ECG shows prolonged QT interval.
- Causes:
  - It can result from ingestion of certain drugs like quinidine, procainamide, antidepressants and phenothiazines, and electrolyte imbalances like hypokalaemia and hypocalcaemia.
  - Other causes are congenital long QT syndromes (Jervell and Lange-Nielsen syndrome—associated with deafness; and Romano-Ward syndrome—without deafness).
- Most of the episodes of torsades are self-limiting and do not produce haemodynamic compromise. However, these attacks may precipitate VF.
- Treatment:
  - Recurrence rates of torsades after spontaneous resolution are quite high. Therefore, treatment is primarily directed to prevent the recurrences rather than to terminate a given episode.
  - Magnesium in a dose of 2–4 g IV over a period of 30 minutes is quite effective in terminating an episode and preventing its recurrence.
  - Because the occurrence of torsades de pointes is dependent on relative bradycardia, isoproterenol and overdrive pacing are also usually effective.
  - Beta-blockers are useful in patients with congenital long QT syndrome.

Q. Give a brief outline of Brugada syndrome.

- It is characterised by coved-shaped ST-segment elevation (≥2 mm) in right precordial leads (V_1–V_3) followed by inverted T waves (Type 1—Fig. 7.26), incomplete or complete RBBB, and susceptibility to ventricular tachyarrhythmia (particularly polymorphic VT) and sudden cardiac death. Type 2 Brugada morphology is known as 'saddle-back type' and is characterised by a convex ST-segment elevation ≥0.5 mm in 1 or more right precordial leads (V_1–V_3) followed by a positive T-wave (Fig. 7.27).
- Syncope due to tachyarrhythmia usually occurs during sleep or at rest.
- Typically presents in third or fourth decade.
- Similar ECG patterns are seen in anterior wall infarction, arrhythmogenic right ventricular dysplasia, acute pericarditis, Duchenne muscular dystrophy, hypercalcaemia, hyperkalaemia and tricyclic antidepressant overdose.
- Genetically transmitted as an autosomal dominant syndrome with incomplete penetrance.

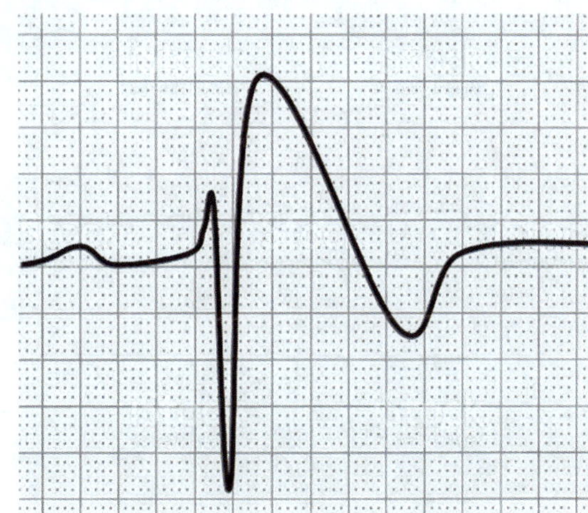

Fig. 7.26 Type 1 Brugada morphology.

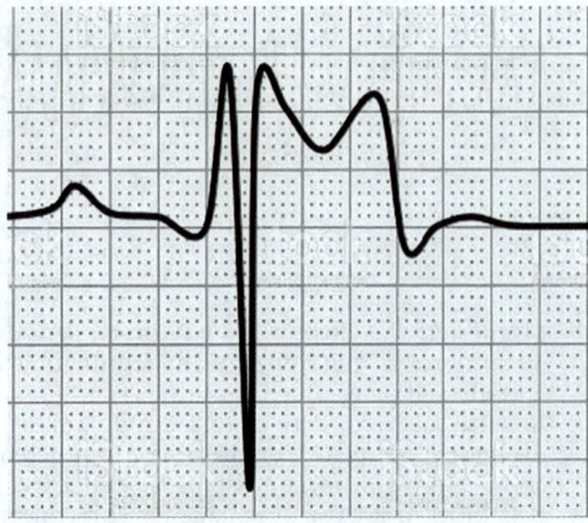

Fig. 7.27 Type 2 Brugada morphology.

- Treatment involves implantable cardioverter-defibrillator (ICD) in patients who have experienced at least one attack of cardiac arrest. Quinidine may be used if ICD implantation is not feasible. It can also be used along with ICD to reduce the number of shocks delivered by ICD.
- Radiofrequency catheter ablation, the use of ablation to suppress focal arrhythmogenic substrates, is another therapeutic option if standard therapy has failed.

Q. Describe briefly early repolarisation syndrome.

- The term early repolarisation syndrome is used when early repolarisation shown in ECG is accompanied by clinical symptoms such as syncope or sudden cardiac death.
- Electrocardiographic characteristics of early repolarisation include J-point (the point between the end of the QRS complex and the beginning of the ST-segment) elevation, notching or slurring of the terminal part of the QRS complex, and tall and symmetric T waves (Fig. 7.28).
- Previously, early repolarisation was considered a benign phenomenon which did not need further evaluation.
- However, it has been seen that early repolarisation in ECG, particularly in the inferior and lateral leads is associated with an increased risk of lethal ventricular arrhythmias and sudden cardiac death.
- Since an early repolarisation pattern is relatively frequent ECG-finding in the general population and the incidence of idiopathic VF or polymorphic VT is relatively low, the majority of individuals presenting an early repolarisation pattern on ECG will remain asymptomatic and the isolated presence of an early repolarisation pattern does not require further intervention.
- However, patients who survived sudden cardiac death will require insertion of an ICD.

Q. What is commotio cordis?

- Commotio cordis is occurrence of VF and sudden death triggered by a blunt, nonpenetrating and often innocent-appearing unintentional blow to the chest without damage to the ribs, sternum or heart (and in the absence of underlying cardiovascular disease).
- In Latin, it means agitation of the heart.
- Occurs primarily in children, adolescents and young adults.

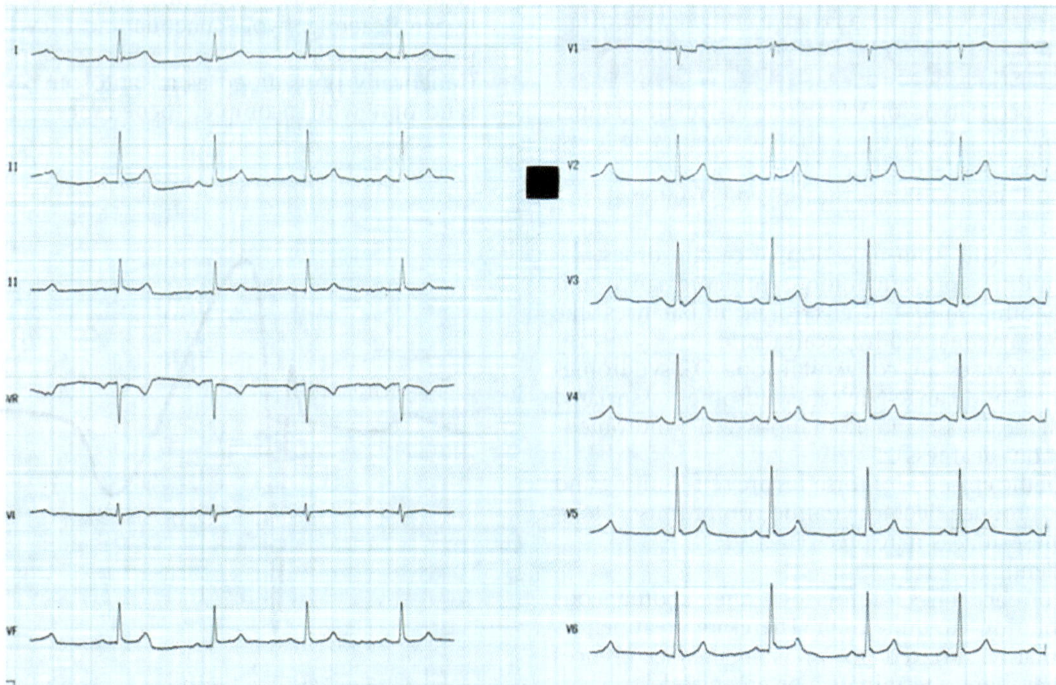

Fig. 7.28 Early repolarisation pattern.

Q. Write a short note on sudden cardiac death.

- Sudden cardiac death (SCD) is defined as an unexpected, nontraumatic death due to presumed cardiac causes occurring in a short time period (generally within 1 hour of symptom onset) in a person with known or unknown cardiac disease in whom no previously diagnosed fatal condition is apparent.
- The event is referred to as sudden cardiac arrest if there is restoration of circulation either spontaneously or by an intervention (e.g. defibrillation). However, the use of term SCD to describe both fatal and nonfatal cardiac arrest persists by convention.
- Nearly 85% of SCDs occur due to ventricular arrhythmias (either primary VF or brief VT degenerating to VF).

CAUSES

- Causes of SCD are shown in Box 7.25.

TREATMENT

- It involves primary prevention (preventing SCD in patients with high-risk conditions), secondary prevention (preventing SCD in patients revived from SCD) and cardiopulmonary resuscitation (CPR) in patients presenting cardiac arrest.
  - Traditional antiarrhythmic agents either have been ineffective in preventing/reducing sudden death or have increased sudden death and therefore are not recommended.
  - β-Blockers (bisoprolol, carvedilol or sustained-release metoprolol), ACE inhibitors (or angiotensin receptor blockers) and mineralocorticoid receptor antagonists (spironolactone or eplerenone) are recommended particularly in patients with HF and ejection fraction ≤40%.
  - Patients with sustained arrhythmias who survive SCD should be evaluated for ischaemic heart disease, and should be revascularised as appropriate.
  - ICD is the primary treatment modality in most patients.
  - Radiofrequency ablation for patients with AV bypass tracts, bundle branch block-associated VT, arrhythmogenic right ventricular dysplasia—conditions uncommonly seen.

BOX 7.25 Causes of Sudden Cardiac Death

- Coronary artery disease
- Ischaemic cardiomyopathy
- Nonischaemic cardiomyopathy
- Hypertrophic cardiomyopathy
- Aortic dissection
- Arrhythmogenic right ventricular dysplasia
- Arrhythmia from antiarrhythmic agents
- Cocaine
- Myocarditis
- Valvular heart disease (e.g. aortic stenosis)
- Congenital heart disease
- Long QT syndrome
- Brugada syndrome
- Wolff–Parkinson–White syndrome
- Early repolarisation syndrome
- Electrolyte abnormalities
- Sarcoidosis
- Amyloidosis
- Cardiac tumours

Q. Define cardiac arrest. What are the causes of cardiac arrest? How do you manage it?

Q. Explain about cardiopulmonary resuscitation. (IM 2.21, IM 2.22)

DEFINITION

- Cardiac arrest is defined as an abrupt loss of cardiac pump function which may be reversible by a prompt intervention, but will lead to death in its absence.
- Cardiac arrest may result from one of the following four mechanisms: (a) ventricular fibrillation (VF), (b) pulseless ventricular tachycardia (VT), (c) asystole and (d) pulseless electrical activity (PEA) (Box 7.26).

MANAGEMENT (CARDIOPULMONARY RESUSCITATION)

- CPR provides artificial ventilation and perfusion to the vital organs, particularly heart and brain, until spontaneous cardiopulmonary function is restored.
- It encompasses both basic life support (BLS) and advanced life support (ALS).
- Successful resuscitation following cardiac arrest requires an integrated set of coordinated actions represented by the links in the 'chain of survival' (Table 7.25).

BOX 7.26 Common Causes of Cardiac Arrest

VENTRICULAR FIBRILLATION:
- Myocardial ischaemia or infarction
- Electrocution
- Other structural heart diseases
- Hypokalaemia and hyperkalaemia
- Drugs

VENTRICULAR ASYSTOLE:
- Localised failure of conducting tissue
- Massive myocardial infarction

PULSELESS ELECTRICAL ACTIVITY (PEA):
- Cardiac rupture
- Massive pulmonary embolism

Note:
1. Initial rhythm of VT may degenerate into PEA or asystole with passage of time.
2. Reversible causes of refractory VT/VF, asystole and PEA are 5 Hs and 5 Ts, and have been listed later.

TABLE 7.25 Links in the Chain of Survival

Out-of-Hospital Cardiac Arrest	In-Hospital Cardiac Arrest
• Immediate recognition of cardiac arrest and activation of the emergency response system (ERS)	• Early recognition and prevention
• Early CPR with an emphasis on chest compressions (BLS)	• Activation of emergency response
• Rapid defibrillation	• Immediate high-quality CPR
• Basic and advanced emergency medical services during transport	• Rapid defibrillation
• Advanced life support (ALS) and postcardiac arrest care	• Postcardiac arrest care
• Recovery	• Recovery

BASIC LIFE SUPPORT

- BLS indicates manoeuvres which, without special equipment [except automated external defibrillator (AED) and a protective shield], either prevent circulatory and respiratory arrest or externally support the circulation and ventilation of a victim in arrest.
- The major goal of BLS is to provide adequate oxygen and perfusion to vital organs (brain and heart) until advanced cardiac life support is available.
- Most out-of-hospital cardiac arrests occur following a myocardial injury and present initially with VF or pulseless VT. The patient is therefore likely to be responsive to defibrillation that has become a part of BLS.
- Immediate recognition and activation of ERS (emergency response system), early CPR and rapid defibrillation (when appropriate) are the first three BLS links in the adult chain of survival.
- Scene safety is important before starting BLS.

IMMEDIATE RECOGNITION AND ACTIVATION OF EMERGENCY RESPONSE SYSTEM

- Early recognition that a cardiac arrest has occurred is the key to survival. For every minute a patient is in cardiac arrest, the chances of survival drop by roughly 10%. If a patient is unresponsive and is not breathing normally, he/she is presumed to be in cardiac arrest.
- If a lone rescuer finds an unresponsive adult, he/she should first ensure that the scene is safe.
- Rescuer should then check for a response by tapping the victim on the shoulder and shouting at the victim (Fig. 7.29).
- If the victim is unresponsive and has absent or abnormal breathing (i.e. only gasping), the rescuer should assume that the victim is in cardiac arrest. The trained or untrained lay person should activate the ERS.
    - If other rescuers are present, the first rescuer should direct them to activate the ERS and get the AED; the first rescuer should start CPR immediately (Fig. 7.30).
    - If a lone rescuer is present, he should activate the ERS first and then begin CPR.
    - If the rescuer is not trained in recognising abnormal breathing, the lay rescuer should phone the ERS once the rescuer finds that the victim is unresponsive; the dispatcher at ERS should be able to guide the lay rescuer to check for breathing and the steps of CPR.
    - The health-care provider can check for response and look for no breathing or no normal breathing (i.e. only gasping) before activating the ERS.
- After activation of the ERS, all rescuers should immediately begin CPR for adult victims who are unresponsive with no breathing or no normal breathing (only gasping). The rescuer should treat the victim who has occasional gasps as if he/she is not breathing.

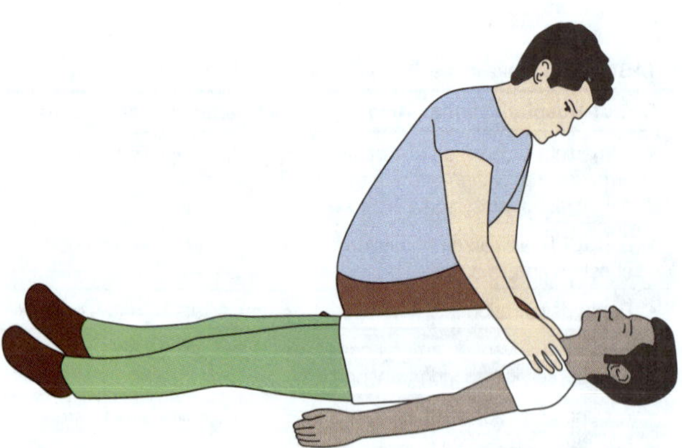

Fig. 7.29 Checking for response.

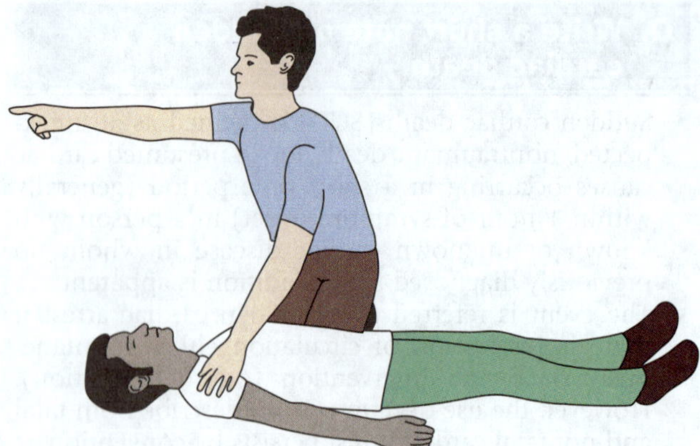

Fig. 7.30 Calling for help and asking other people to activate ERS.

PULSE CHECK

- Lay rescuer should not check for a pulse and should assume that cardiac arrest is present if an adult suddenly collapses or an unresponsive victim is not breathing normally.
- The health-care provider may palpate pulse (carotid artery) but should take no more than 10 seconds to check for a pulse.

EARLY CARDIOPULMONARY RESUSCITATION

- CPR includes four sequential steps: circulation, airway and breathing (CAB) and defibrillation.

Circulation

- Circulation is achieved by chest compressions.
- Chest compressions consist of forceful rhythmic applications of pressure over the lower half of the sternum. These compressions create blood flow by increasing intrathoracic pressure and directly compressing the heart. This generates blood flow and oxygen delivery to the myocardium and brain.
- Effective chest compressions are essential for providing blood flow during CPR. For this reason, all patients in cardiac arrest should receive chest compressions.
- For cardiac compression, the patient should be in a supine position on a firm surface.
- The rescuer should place the heel of one hand on the centre (middle) of the victim's chest in the lower half of the sternum and the heel of other hand on top of the first so that the hands are overlapped and parallel to each other. The arms should be held straight with shoulders of rescuer directly over the sternum of the victim (Fig. 7.31).

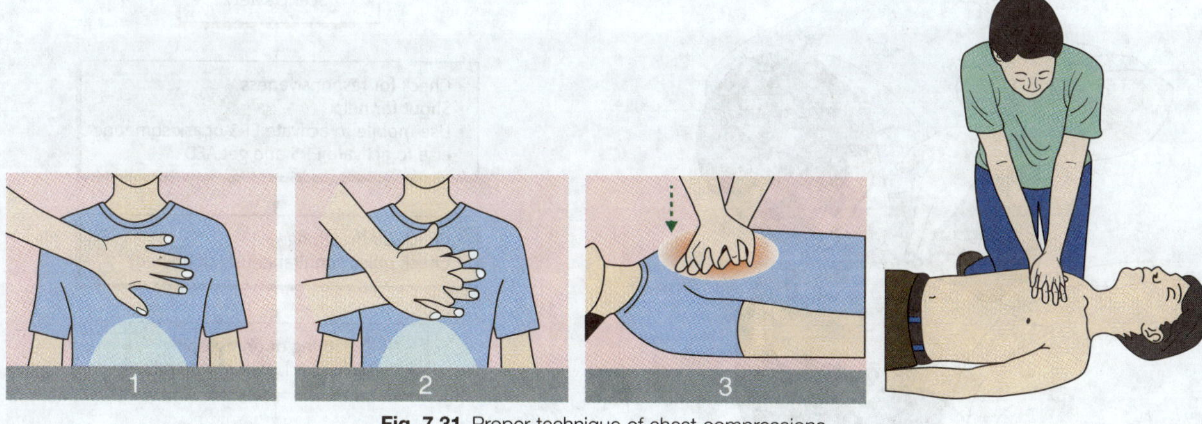

Fig. 7.31 Proper technique of chest compressions.

- Chest compression is performed at a rate of 100-120/minute with the compression phase occupying at least 50% of the whole cycle of compression–relaxation ('duty cycle'). The compression depth should be 2–2.4 inches (5–6 cm). Rescuers should allow complete recoil of the chest after each compression to allow the heart to fill completely before the next compression.
- In both single-rescuer and two-rescuer CPR, 30 compressions are delivered followed by 2 breaths. However, only 'hands-on' or 'compression-only' CPR is also recommended for a lay person who is reluctant to give mouth-to-mouth respiration or is not trained in that.
- The rescuer should interrupt chest compression as infrequently as possible and should limit interruptions to no more than 10 seconds at a time.
- When more than one rescuer is present, rescuers should change roles after every 2 minutes or five cycles of CPR. Every effort should be made to accomplish this switch in <5 seconds.

Airway

- The trained lay rescuer who feels confident that he/she can perform both compressions and ventilations should open the airway using a head tilt–chin lift manoeuvre.
- A health-care provider should use the head tilt–chin lift manoeuvre to open airway of a victim with no evidence of head or neck trauma.
- For victims with suspected spinal injury, rescuers should initially use manual spinal motion restriction (e.g. placing one hand on either side of victim's head to hold it still) while performing compressions. If a health-care provider suspects a cervical spine injury, he/she should open the airway using jaw thrust method. However, if he/she fails to open the airway using jaw thrust, head tilt–chin lift manoeuvre should be done.
  - In head tilt–chin lift method, the chin is moved forward with the index and middle fingers of one hand while the other hand is placed over the forehead so as to flex the neck in relation to the chest and extend the head in relation to the neck (Fig. 7.32).

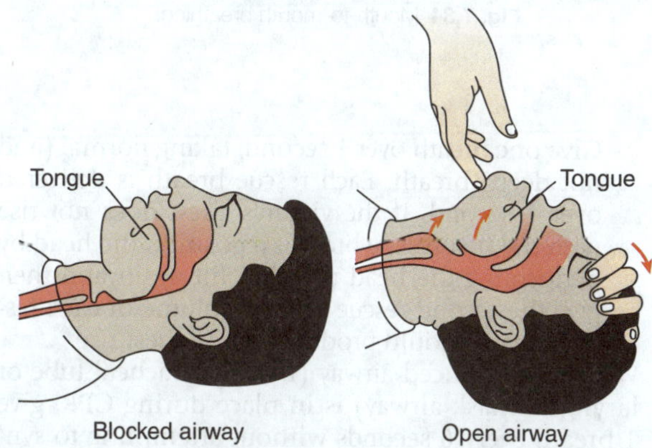

Fig. 7.32 Head-tilt chin-lift method.

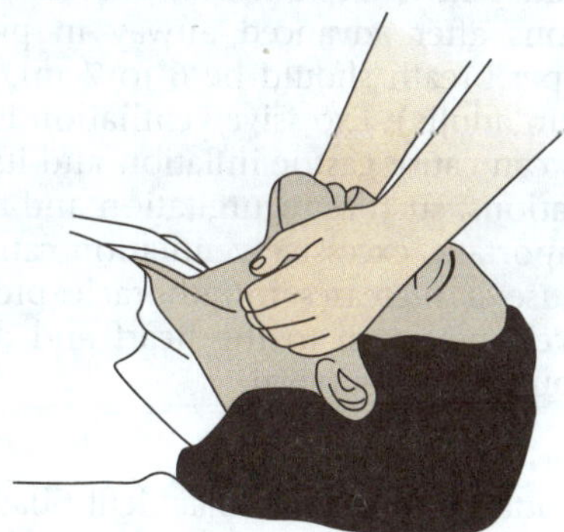

Fig. 7.33 Jaw thrust method.

  - In jaw-thrust method, the angles of mandible are grasped with both hands and the mandible is lifted forward (Fig. 7.33).

Breathing

- After opening the airway, mouth-to-mouth or mouth-to-nose or mouth-to-mask or bag-mask breathing is started with compression: ventilation ratio of 30:2.
  - To provide mouth-to-mouth rescue breaths, open the victim's airway, pinch the victim's nose and create an airtight mouth-to-mouth seal (Fig. 7.34).

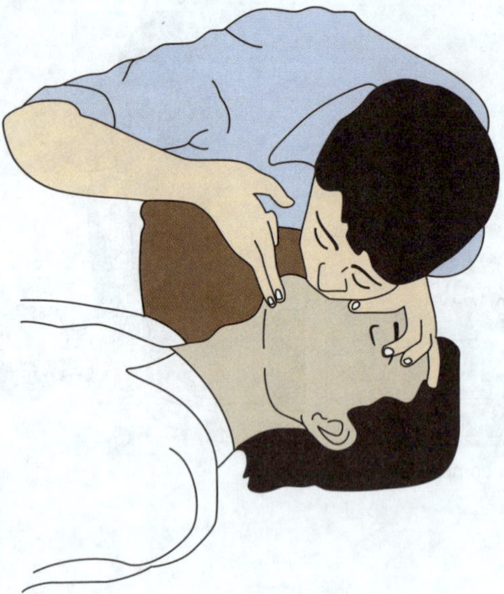

Fig. 7.34 Mouth-to-mouth breathing.

Give one breath over 1 second, taking normal (and not deep) breath. Each rescue breath is delivered over 1 second. If the victim's chest does not rise with the first rescue breath, reposition the head by performing the head tilt–chin lift again and then give the second rescue breath. Volume of each rescue breath should produce visible chest rise.

- When an advanced airway (i.e. endotracheal tube or laryngeal mask airway) is in place during CPR, give 1 breath every 6 seconds without attempting to synchronise breaths between compressions; this will result in delivery of 10 breaths/minute. There should be no pause in chest compressions for delivery of ventilations after advanced airway in place. Tidal volume per breath should be 6 to 7 mL/kg (about 600 mL in adults). Excessive ventilation is unnecessary and can cause gastric inflation and its resultant complications, such as regurgitation and aspiration. More important, excessive ventilation can be harmful because it increases intrathoracic pressure, decreases venous return to the heart and diminishes cardiac output and survival.

Early Defibrillation

- The importance of early cardiac defibrillation in patients of cardiac arrest has led to the development of AEDs. Since VF and pulseless VT are the major causes of cardiac arrest in adults, application of early defibrillation in field setting by the paramedics is important.
- Defibrillator should be used as soon as it is available.
- AEDs are capable of analysing cardiac rhythm and, if appropriate, advise/deliver an electric countershock. The operator merely places two self-adhesive electrode pads onto the patient and administers a shock when advised, standing clear when the AED is ready to discharge.
- CPR should be started immediately following 1 shock and continued for 5 cycles of 30:2 compression-to-ventilation ratio before rechecking the rhythm.

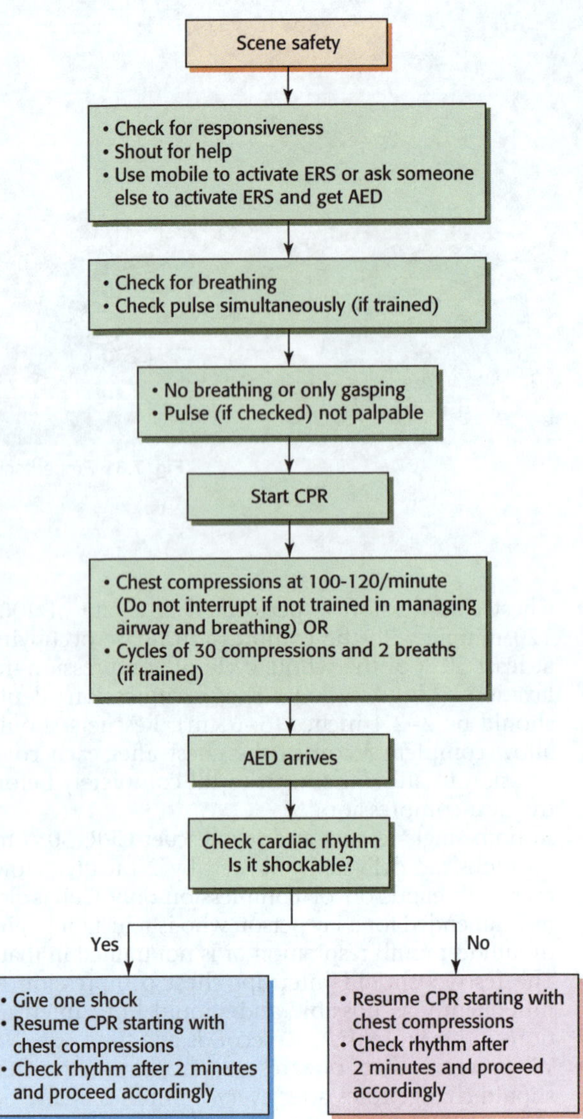

Flowchart 7.3 Adult Basic Life Support Algorithm.

SUMMARY OF BASIC LIFE SUPPORT

- Flowchart 7.3 summarises basic life support in adults.

ADVANCED LIFE SUPPORT

- ALS consists of BLS (CAB and early defibrillation) followed by use of special equipment and drugs for establishing and maintaining effective ventilation and circulation (ABCD, where *D* stands for defibrillation and for differential diagnoses which include treatable causes of cardiac arrest).

ADVANCED AIRWAY

- It includes the use of oral and nasal airways, bag mask, orotracheal and nasotracheal endotracheal tubes for intubations, laryngeal mask airway and surgical procedures like cricothyrotomy and tracheostomy.

ADVANCED BREATHING

- Confirmation of endotracheal tube placement using both clinical assessment (tube seen passing through

vocal cords; five-point auscultation—over epigastrium, left and right anterior chest, and left and right mid-axillary parts of chest; condensation of water vapour inside the tube) and use of a device (e.g. exhaled carbon dioxide detector, end-tidal CO_2 capnograph—$ETCO_2$ or oesophageal detector device). End-tidal carbon dioxide is the gold standard to confirm position of tube in trachea.
- Securing the endotracheal tube using tube holders (which are better than using tape or bandage to hold the tube).
- Ventilate at a tidal volume of 6 to 7 mL/kg and at a rate of 10 breaths/minute.
- Confirm effective ventilation and oxygenation by end-tidal CO_2 monitor and oxygen saturation monitor. If $ETCO_2$ is low or decreasing, reassess CPR quality.

High-Quality Cardiopulmonary Resuscitation (Box 7.27)

BOX 7.27 High Quality CPR

- Adequate rate (100–120/minute) and depth (2–2.4 inches or 5 to 6 cm) of compression.
- Allow chest wall to recoil back completely in between two compressions.
- Minimise interruptions during chest compressions.
- Rotate chest compressor every 2 minutes.
- Avoid excessive ventilation.
- 30:2 chest compression: ventilation ratio if advanced airway not in place.
- If end-tidal CO_2 <10 mmHg by quantitative waveform capnography, improve CPR quality.
- If intraarterial relaxation phase pressure <20 mmHg, improve CPR quality.

ADVANCED CIRCULATION

- It includes continuation of chest compression along with establishing an intravenous access, attaching a cardiac monitor/defibrillator and assessing the rhythm, defibrillation and administering drugs appropriate for rhythm and condition.
- With advanced airway in place, rescuers no longer provide cycles of compression with pauses for ventilation. The compression is done continuously at the rate of 100–120/minute and ventilation is provided at 10 breaths/minute (1 breath every 6 seconds).
- Basic rhythms commonly seen in patients with cardiac arrest include VF, pulseless VT, asystole and PEA. Of these, VT and fibrillation are the most common rhythm and are most amenable to therapy.
- Rhythm checks should be done only after 2 minutes of CPR and not immediately following a defibrillation attempt.
- Pulse check should be performed only after 2 minutes of CPR if the monitor shows a change in rhythm from previous one or it shows an organised rhythm.

Ventricular Fibrillation or Pulseless Ventricular Tachycardia (Shockable Rhythms)

- As soon as a defibrillator is available, it should be used for early conversion of the fibrillating heart to normally contracting heart. One shock at 360 J (monophasic defibrillators) or 150–200 J (biphasic defibrillators) is given that is followed by CPR immediately without checking the rhythm or the pulse.
- Continue CPR for 2 minutes, and then pause briefly to check the monitor for rhythm. If VT/VF persists:
  - Give second shock of same energy, resume CPR immediately and continue for 2 minutes, and repeat this cycle.
  - Immediately following second shock, give adrenaline (epinephrine) intravenously in a dose of 1 mg (10 mL of 1:10,000 solution) as an IV bolus followed by a rapid bolus of 20 mL of saline and elevating the arm up. If IV access is not available, intraosseous (IO) route should be accessed.
  - If VT/VF persists, continue giving shocks every 2 minutes.
  - Repeat adrenaline every 3–5 minutes if VT/VF persists.
  - If after two doses of adrenaline VT/VF persists, administer amiodarone 300 mg IV followed by 150 mg after 3–5 minutes if VT/VF persists; start amiodarone infusion (maximum cumulative dose: 2.2 g over 24 hours).
  - If amiodarone is not available or is not effective, give lidocaine. The initial dose of lidocaine is 1–1.5 mg/kg IV bolus. If VF or pulseless VT persists, additional doses of 0.5–0.75 mg/kg IV push may be administered at 5- to 10-minute intervals to a maximum dose of 3 mg/kg.
  - Look for reversible causes if VT/VF persists.
- If organised electrical activity is seen during brief pause in compressions every 2 minutes, check for pulse.
  - If a pulse is present, start postresuscitation care.
  - If a pulse is not present, continue CPR and switch to nonshockable rhythm sequence if VT or VF disappears.

Pulseless Electrical Activity and Asystole (Nonshockable Rhythms)

- PEA is defined as cardiac electrical activity in the absence of any palpable pulse. These patients often have some mechanical myocardial contractions but they are too weak to produce a detectable pulse. Asystole is commonly seen in patients of unwitnessed sudden cardiac arrest outside the hospital and in critically ill patients, and is nearly always fatal. Both are nonshockable rhythms.
- If the rhythm is PEA or asystole:
  - Continue CPR for 2 minutes before the rhythm check is repeated.
  - Give adrenaline 1 mg IV as soon as feasible.
  - Recheck rhythm after 2 minutes of CPR.
  - If PEA or asystole persists, continue CPR, recheck rhythm every 2 minutes and give adrenaline every 3–5 minutes. Atropine has no role in PEA or asystole.
  - If there is change in rhythm, check for pulse. If pulse is present, start postresuscitation care. If pulse is absent, continue CPR with rhythm check every 2 minutes and adrenaline every 3–5 minutes.
  - In case of asystole, check that the leads are connected properly and the gain on monitor is set at maximum.

- If at any time the rhythm develops into VF/VT, defibrillate the patient.
- Look for reversible causes (see section 'Differential Diagnoses' below) that can produce PEA or asystole.
- CPR can be stopped if:
  - VF:VT eliminated.
  - Advanced airway device placed and position confirmed.
  - Proper oxygenation and ventilation ensured using oxygen saturation monitor and end-tidal CO_2 monitor.
  - All rhythm-appropriate drugs administered.
  - All potentially reversible causes excluded.
  - CPR performed for 10 minutes after the rhythm confirmed to be PEA/asystole.

DIFFERENTIAL DIAGNOSES

- Try to search for reversible causes producing cardiac arrest rhythm and treat them. These causes have been listed as '5 Hs and 5 Ts' (Table 7.26).

RETURN OF SPONTANEOUS CIRCULATION

- Return of spontaneous circulation (ROSC) is indicated by appearance of pulse and blood pressure, abrupt and sustained increase in $ETCO_2$ (typically ≥40 mmHg), and spontaneous arterial pressure waves with intraarterial monitoring.

SUMMARY OF ADVANCED CARDIAC LIFE SUPPORT

- Flowchart 7.4 (given on next page) summarises the steps in advanced cardiac life support.

MISCELLANEOUS DRUGS/EQUIPMENT IN CARDIAC ARREST

- Sodium bicarbonate has no benefit when it is administered early during the CPR. In fact, bicarbonate may be detrimental to the patient. It may be used in patients with cardiac arrest related to hyperkalaemia or tricyclic antidepressant poisoning.
- Calcium is recommended only if there is some evidence to suggest hypocalcaemia, hyperkalaemia or calcium channel blocker overdose.
- Fibrinolytic therapy (e.g. streptokinase, tenecteplase) should not be routinely used in cardiac arrest. When pulmonary embolism is presumed or known to be the cause of cardiac arrest, empirical fibrinolytic therapy can be considered.

TABLE 7.26 Reversible Causes of Cardiac Arrest

5 Hs	5 Ts
• Hypoxia	• Tamponade, cardiac
• Hypovolaemia	• Tension pneumothorax
• Hypothermia	• Toxins/tablets
• Hydrogen ions (acidosis)	• Thrombosis, coronary (myocardial infarction)
• Hypokalaemia/hyperkalaemia	• Thrombosis, pulmonary (pulmonary embolism)

- Point-of-care ultrasound (POCUS) is useful in diagnosis of reversible causes of cardiac arrest, such as tamponade, pulmonary embolism, tension pneumothorax and hypovolaemia. It is also helpful in distinguishing a true asystole from a fine VF. POCUS is also helpful in intubating a patient and confirming its position in trachea.
- Extracorporeal cardiopulmonary resuscitation (ECPR) is the use of venoarterial extracorporeal membrane oxygenation to support systemic circulation and vital organ perfusion in patients in refractory cardiac arrest not responding to conventional CPR. It may be used in patients with witnessed cardiac arrest and good-quality CPR when a potentially reversible cause of arrest is present. It may be used to facilitate specific interventions (e.g. coronary angiography, pulmonary thrombectomy and rewarming after hypothermic cardiac arrest).

POSTRESUSCITATION CARE

- Ensure an adequate airway and support breathing. Hyperventilation should be avoided for routine care. Start at ventilation of 10–12/minute and ensure end-tidal CO_2 of 30–40 mmHg. Although 100% oxygen may have been used during initial resuscitation, titrate inspired oxygen to the lowest level required to achieve an arterial oxygen saturation of 94%, so as to avoid potential oxygen toxicity.
- Continuous cardiac monitoring.
- Use vasoactive medications and fluids to maintain mean arterial pressure above 65 mmHg. Drugs include noradrenaline and dobutamine.
  - Noradrenaline—0.1–0.5 μg/kg/minute.
  - Dobutamine—5–10 μg/kg/minute.
- Get an ECG done. If it shows ST-elevation myocardial infarction or if the patient has cardiogenic shock, immediate coronary angiography should be considered.
- Avoid hyperthermia.
- Targeted temperature management (TTM): Hypothermia (32°C–36°C) for at least 24 hours may be considered for any patient who is unable to follow verbal commands after resuscitation from cardiac arrest. One of the techniques recommended is to infuse 1 to 2 L of ice-cold isotonic saline or Ringer's lactate. Clinicians should continuously monitor the patient's core temperature using an oesophageal thermometer, bladder catheter in nonanuric patients or pulmonary artery catheter if one is placed for other indications. However, at present, maintaining normothermia instead of hypothermia after achieving ROSC is advised, particularly in out-of-hospital cardiac arrest patients..
- Avoid hyperglycaemia; maintain blood sugar <200 mg/dL.
- Overall the most common cause of cardiac arrest is cardiac ischaemia. Therefore, ECG should be obtained as soon as possible to detect ST elevation. If found, urgent primary percutaneous coronary intervention (PCI) should be done.
- Attention should be directed to treating the precipitating cause of cardiac arrest ('Hs' and 'Ts').

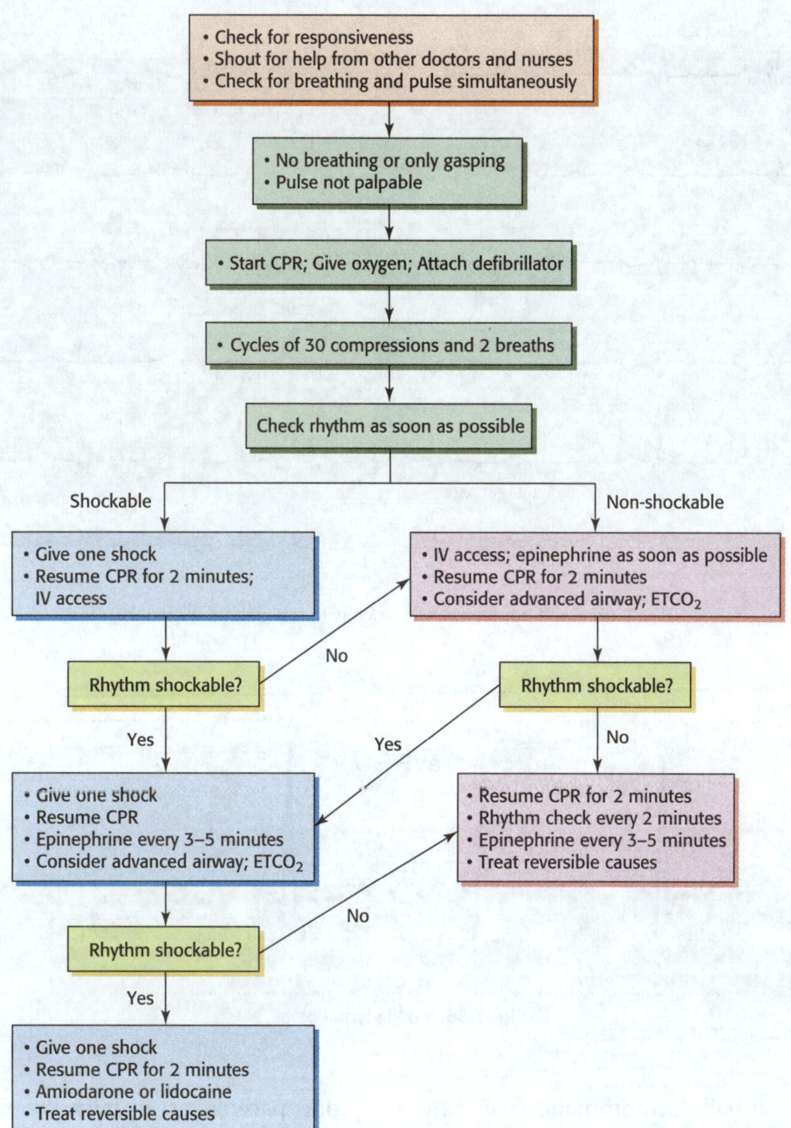

Flowchart 7.4 Adult Advanced Cardiac Life Support Algorithm.

Q. Discuss the causes, clinical features and management of atrioventricular blocks.

FIRST-DEGREE BLOCK

- First-degree AV block may be associated with electrolyte disturbances, use of digitalis, β-blockers or calcium channel blockers, myocarditis and acute myocardial infarction (usually inferior wall).
- It is usually asymptomatic.
- In the ECG, the PR interval is prolonged to more than 0.20 seconds. All the P waves are conducted and the QRS is normal as the delay is most often in the AV node (Fig. 7.35).
- Treatment includes correction of any electrolyte imbalance and removal of an offending agent. If it occurs as a result of acute MI, the patient should be observed to detect any progression to higher degrees of blocks.

SECOND-DEGREE BLOCK

- It can be subdivided into Mobitz type I and Mobitz type II blocks.
- Mobitz type I (Wenckebach) second-degree AV block:
  - It usually occurs in acute inferior wall myocardial infarction and use of digitalis, β-blockers or calcium channel blockers.
  - The block is usually transient and the patient is often asymptomatic.
  - It is characterised by progressive slowing of AV conduction until it is totally blocked. The ECG typically shows progressive prolongation of successive PR intervals until one P wave is not conducted. The PP interval remains unchanged. The QRS is usually normal (Fig. 7.36).
  - If the patient is symptomatic, atropine should be administered. Pacing is usually not required.
- Mobitz type II second-degree AV block:
  - This type of block usually occurs after anterior wall MI.

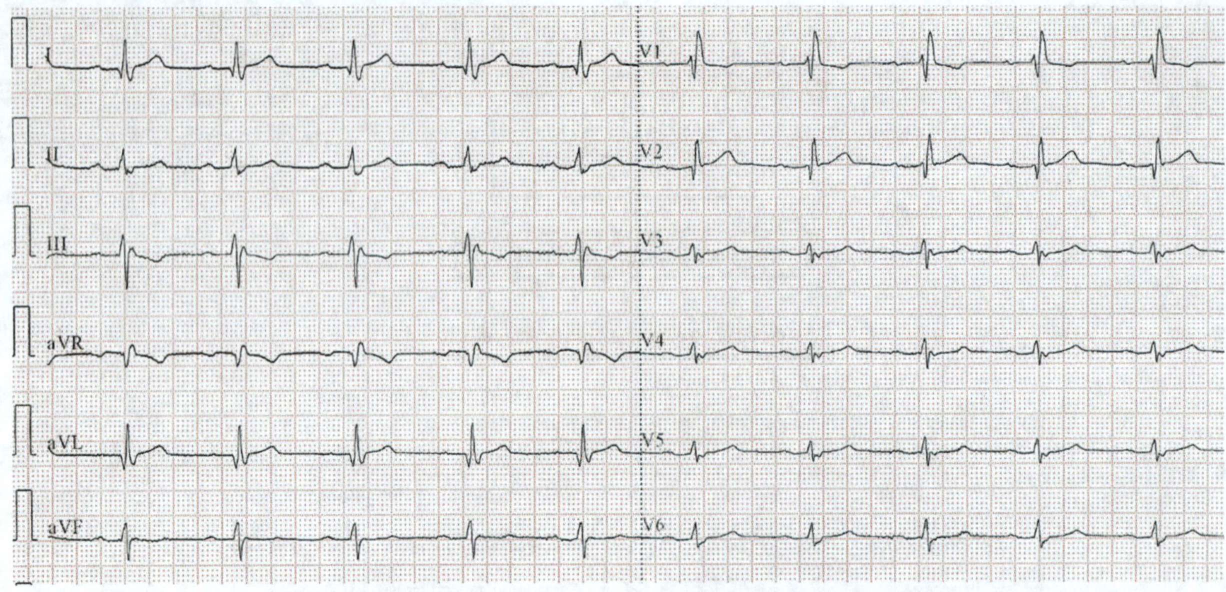

Fig. 7.35 Right bundle branch block with first degree AV block.

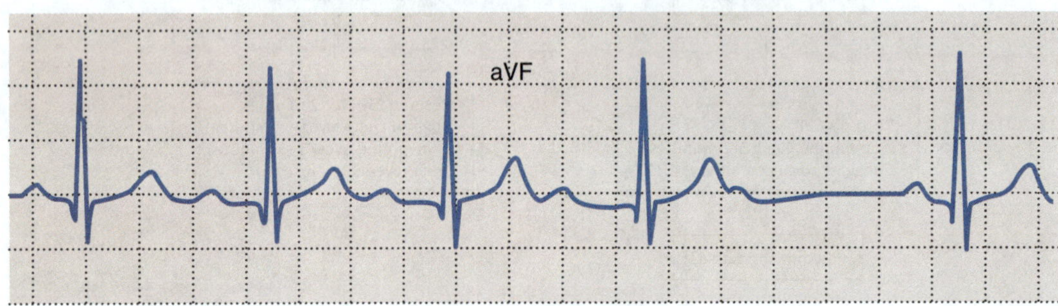

Fig. 7.36 Mobitz type I block.

- The patients are usually symptomatic (see complete heart block below) and there are high chances of its progression to third-degree AV block.
- The block is characterised by a constant PR interval with intermittent failure of atrial impulses to conduct to the ventricles. The block is defined by a ratio in which the first digit represents the total number of P waves and the second digit represents the number of P waves conducted, that is the number of QRS complexes. Thus, in a 3:1 block, of three P waves, one is conducted while two are blocked. In 2:1 block, of two P waves, one is conducted (Fig. 7.37).
- It occurs most often due to delay in conduction in the His-bundle and Purkinje system and, therefore, the QRS is often wide.
- Patients generally require a pacemaker. Atropine is of little use while response to isoproterenol is variable.

THIRD-DEGREE OR COMPLETE ATRIOVENTRICULAR BLOCK

- In complete heart block, none of the atrial impulses reach the ventricles. The atria are thus activated by one pacemaker, usually the sinus pacemaker. The ventricles are activated by another pacemaker situated in either the bundle of His or ventricles.

CAUSES OF COMPLETE HEART BLOCK (Table 7.27)

- Lenegre's disease is idiopathic sclerodegenerative disease of conducting system.
- Lev's disease is calcification and sclerosis of conducting system.

CLINICAL FEATURES (Box 7.28)

- The ECG shows constant PP and RR intervals but with complete AV dissociation, that is the atria and ventricles beat independently and there is no relation between the P waves and the QRS complexes (Fig. 7.38).

MANAGEMENT

- Complete heart block complicating acute inferior myocardial infarction usually does not require any treatment. If the patient deteriorates clinically, it may be treated with intravenous atropine (0.6 mg) that may be repeated every 3–5 minutes for a total of 3 mg. Doses of atropine <0.6 mg may paradoxically result in further slowing of the heart rate.

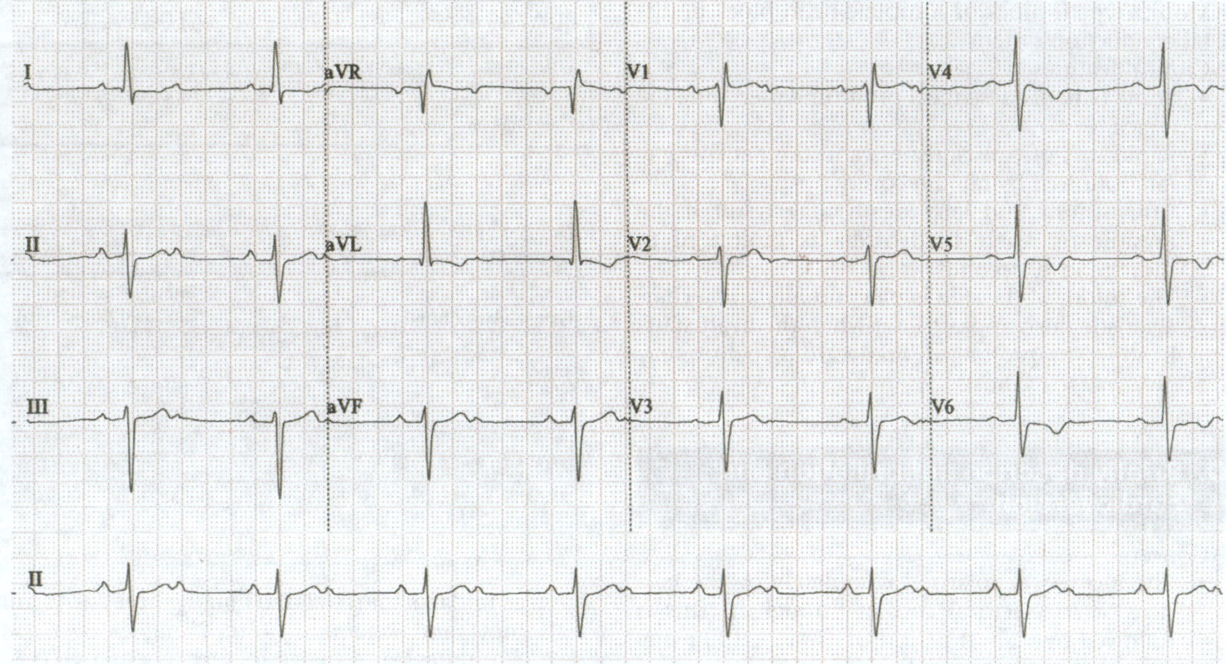

Fig. 7.37 Mobitz type II (2:1) block.

TABLE 7.27 Causes of Complete AV Block

Congenital	Acquired
• Autoimmune antibodies • Congenital heart disease • Idiopathic	• Lenegre's disease • Lev's disease • Myocardial ischaemia or infarction • Intracardiac surgery • Digitalis intoxication • Infective endocarditis • Tumours and infections involving the conducting system • Myocarditis • Acute rheumatic fever • Amyloidosis • Drugs (verapamil, diltiazem, beta-blockers, antiarrhythmics) • Sleep apnoea

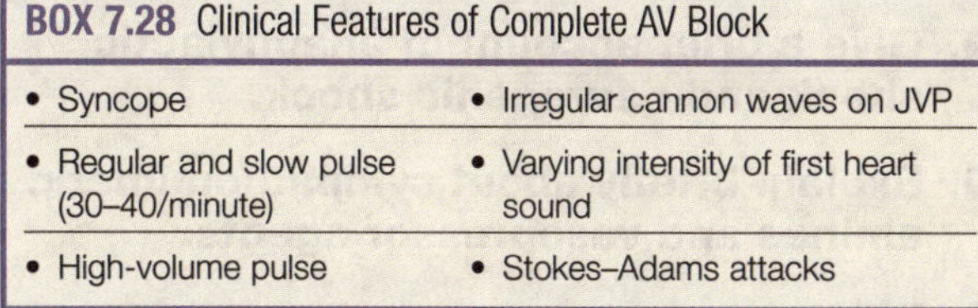

BOX 7.28 Clinical Features of Complete AV Block

• Syncope	• Irregular cannon waves on JVP
• Regular and slow pulse (30–40/minute)	• Varying intensity of first heart sound
• High-volume pulse	• Stokes–Adams attacks

- If bradycardia is unresponsive to atropine, intravenous infusion of β-adrenergic agonists with rate-accelerating effects (dopamine, adrenaline) or transcutaneous pacing can be effective while the patient is prepared for emergent transvenous temporary pacing.
- However, administration of atropine or other drugs should not delay implementation of external pacing for patients with poor perfusion (e.g. bradycardia causing shock, altered level of consciousness, acute HF or ischaemic chest pain).
- Complete heart block complicating acute anterior myocardial infarction should be treated by immediate insertion of temporary pacemaker.
- Chronic complete heart block should be treated by the implantation of a permanent pacemaker.

Q. What are Stokes–Adams attacks (Stokes–Adams–Morgagni attacks)? Write their clinical features.

- An episode of syncope caused by bradycardia related to AV block is called Stokes–Adams–Morgagni syndrome. These commonly occur due to an underlying

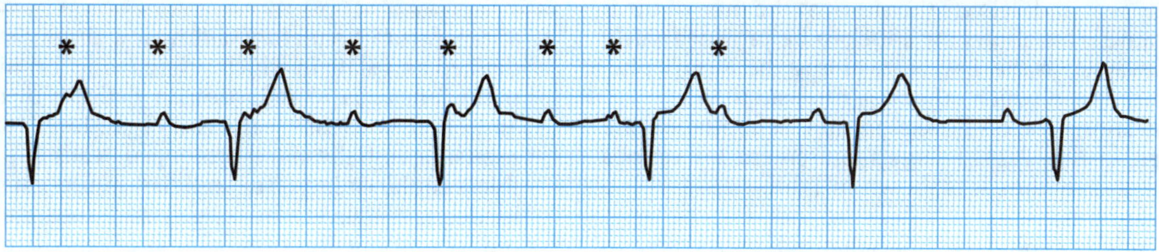

Fig. 7.38 Complete heart block (P-waves are marked by *).

Mobitz type II block or complete heart block in distal conduction system.

- Clinical features:
  - Some patients describe a prodrome preceding the attack.
  - Rapid loss of consciousness and the patient may fall, followed by rapid recovery.
  - Convulsions and later death may result if the asystole or severe bradycardia is prolonged to more than 10 seconds.
  - The colour of the skin is pale initially and a characteristic flush appears later when the heart starts beating. In prolonged bradycardia, pallor may give way to cyanosis.

Q. Briefly describe defibrillation and cardioversion.

- Concept:
  - The heart is depolarised completely by the passage of an electrical current through it. This is followed by a short period of asystole, following which normal sinus rhythm is resumed.
  - The equipment used for delivering energy may be monophasic or biphasic.
- Method:
  - Defibrillation is used to treat pulseless VT or VF. Defibrillators using direct current are used for this. An electric shock of high energy but short duration is delivered to the heart through the chest wall, using two electrodes. One electrode (or paddle) is applied over the sternum (or to the right of sternum) and the other over the left infrascapular area (or in the left axilla). When a patient is defibrillated, the energy is released through the electrodes (or paddles) immediately when the defibrillation buttons are pressed. The shock is delivered at whatever point the cardiac cycle happens to be in at that moment.
  - Cardioversion is done in a patient when pulse is still present but he/she is unstable. In it, the current is given in a synchronised way. To perform synchronised cardioversion, the defibrillator is placed into the 'synchronise' mode by pressing the appropriate button on the machine. This causes the monitor to track the R wave of each QRS complex. A synchronising marker will appear above each QRS complex, indicating that the synchronise feature is active. The appropriate energy level is then selected, and the shock button is pressed. The defibrillator does not release the shock immediately. Instead, it waits for the next R wave to appear and delivers the shock at the time of the R wave. This allows the shock to be provided safely away from the T wave, avoiding the R-on-T phenomenon which otherwise can lead to VF.
- Indications for cardioversion and defibrillation are given in Box 7.29. Energy requirement for various cardiac arrhythmias is shown in Table 7.28.
- Precautions:
  - Patient should be anaesthetised or sedated in elective cardioversion. Short acting sedatives such as midazolam (0.02–0.03 mg/kg over 2 to 3 minutes) and ketamine (1 to 2 mg/kg over 1 to 2 minutes), and analgesics such as fentanyl (0.5–1 µg/kg) can be administered before the procedure.
  - Digitalis therapy should be withdrawn at least 36 hours before cardioversion. If cardioversion is deemed necessary in a patient on digoxin, it should be carried out starting with a lower energy level and ensuring the correction of hypokalaemia.
  - Patients with long-standing atrial arrhythmias should be anticoagulated for at least 3 weeks before cardioversion.

BOX 7.29 Indications for Cardioversion and Defibrillation

- Ventricular fibrillation
- Ventricular tachycardia
- Atrial fibrillation
- Atrial flutter
- Supraventricular tachycardia

TABLE 7.28 Energy Requirements Commonly Used During Cardioversion and Defibrillation

Type of Arrhythmia	Energy Required in Biphasic Equipment
Atrial fibrillation	100–200 J
Atrial flutter	50–100 J
Paroxysmal supraventricular tachycardia	50–100 J
Ventricular tachycardia with pulse	100–200 J
Pulseless VT/ventricular fibrillation	150–200 J

Q. Define acute circulatory failure/shock.

Q. Give the classification, causes and management of shock. (SU 2.1)

Q. Give the causes and management of cardiogenic shock. (SU 2.2)

Q. Describe hypovolaemic shock, septic shock, SIRS and sepsis. (PY 5.11)

Q. Give a brief account of anaphylactic shock and neurogenic shock.

Q. Explain briefly about sympathomimetic amines and vasopressor agents.

Q. Write a note on adrenergic receptors.

DEFINITION

- Shock (acute circulatory failure; low-output state) is defined as a state in which severe reduction in tissue perfusion leads to reduction in delivery of oxygen and other nutrients at the end organ level. Shock is reversible initially, but if prolonged, leads to irreversible cellular injury. The cellular injury caused by inadequate delivery of oxygen and substrates also induces production of inflammatory mediators that further compromises perfusion.

- Cardiogenic shock is a clinical condition of inadequate tissue perfusion due to cardiac dysfunction. The definition of cardiogenic shock includes haemodynamic parameters: persistent hypotension (systolic blood pressure <90 mmHg or mean arterial pressure 30 mmHg lower than baseline) along with signs of impaired organ perfusion in the state of normovolaemia or hypervolaemia. Haemodynamic parameters for diagnosis include severe reduction in cardiac index (<1.8 L/minute/m^2 without support or <2.0 L/minute/m^2 with support) and adequate or elevated filling pressure (e.g. left ventricular end-diastolic pressure >18 mmHg or right ventricular end-diastolic pressure >10–15 mmHg).

CLASSIFICATION AND CAUSES

- Classified broadly into four types: distributive (characterised by severe peripheral vasodilatation and includes septic, anaphylactic and neurogenic shocks), cardiogenic, hypovolaemic and obstructive.
- The common types of shocks and their causes are given in Table 7.29.
- Various terms used in relation to conditions with systemic inflammation are shown in Table 7.30.

QUICK SEQUENTIAL ORGAN FAILURE ASSESSMENT SCORE (Box 7.30)

- Any patient having quick sequential organ failure assessment (qSOFA) score ≥2 is considered to have sepsis.

PATHOPHYSIOLOGY OF SHOCK

SYMPATHOADRENAL AND NEUROENDOCRINE RESPONSES

- Stimulation of baroreceptors and chemoreceptors by hypotension leads to increased sympathetic activity.

TABLE 7.29 Common Causes of Shock

Type of Shock	Causes
• Hypovolaemic shock	Haemorrhage, severe vomiting and diarrhoea, plasma loss in burns and acute pancreatitis, diabetic ketoacidosis
• Cardiogenic shock	Acute myocardial infarction (when more than 40% of myocardium is damaged), acute aortic regurgitation, acute mitral regurgitation, rupture of interventricular septum, rupture of papillary muscle, right ventricular infarction, myocarditis, cardiac arrhythmias, dilated cardiomyopathy, takotsubo cardiomyopathy, severe valvular stenosis
• Septic shock	Gram-positive and Gram-negative bacterial infections, other infections
• Anaphylactic shock	Drugs, insect stings
• Neurogenic shock	High cervical cord injury, severe head injury
• Obstructive shock	Acute massive pulmonary embolism, tension pneumothorax, cardiac tamponade, constrictive pericarditis, restrictive cardiomyopathy, atrial myxoma

TABLE 7.30 Terms Used in Relation to Conditions With Systemic Inflammation

Term	Definition
• Infection	An inflammatory response to microorganisms or invasion of normally sterile host tissue by microorganisms
• Bacteraemia	Presence of viable bacteria in the blood
• Systemic inflammatory response syndrome (SIRS)	Systemic inflammatory response to a variety of insults manifested by two or more of the following: • Temperature >38°C or <36°C • Heart rate >90 beats/minute • Respiratory rate >20/minute or $PaCO_2$ <32 mmHg • TLC count >12,000/mm^3 or <4000/mm^3 or >10% immature cells
• Sepsis	Previously defined as SIRS due to infection New definition: Life-threatening organ dysfunction caused by a dysregulated host response to infection (Sepsis 3.0 definition). Organ dysfunction can be identified as an acute change in qSOFA score ≥2 points due to the infection.
• Septic shock	A subset of sepsis in which underlying circulatory and cellular metabolism abnormalities are profound enough to substantially increase mortality. Diagnosed when patients with sepsis have persisting hypotension requiring vasopressors to maintain mean arterial pressure (MAP) ≥65 mmHg and having a serum lactate level >2 mmol/L despite adequate volume resuscitation.
• Multiple organ dysfunction syndrome (MODS)	Presence of altered multiple organ function in an acutely ill patient such that homeostasis cannot be maintained.
• Acute respiratory distress syndrome (ARDS)	See discussion on ARDS given on page 129).

BOX 7.30 Quick Sequential Organ Failure Assessment Score

- Respiratory rate ≥22/minute
- Altered mentation
- Systolic blood pressure ≤100 mmHg

- This is augmented by release of catecholamines from the adrenals.
- These changes produce increased myocardial contractility, tachycardia and vasoconstriction resulting in partial restoration of blood pressure.
- Reduction in blood flow to kidneys stimulates release of renin that ultimately results in enhanced production of aldosterone (via angiotensin I and II). This causes sodium and water retention.
- During shock, there is increased release of antidiuretic hormone and cortisol that helps in retaining fluid and sodium.
- All these effects try to restore blood pressure but at the expense of reduced perfusion to vital organs such as kidneys. If shock is not treated in the early stage, these responses can no longer maintain the blood pressure and a stage of irreversible shock develops.

INFLAMMATORY REACTION

- This occurs in patients with all types of shock but is more apparent in sepsis.
- There is activation of leucocytes and release of a variety of potentially damaging mediators.
- Endotoxin (a lipopolysaccharide) released by Gram-negative bacteria is a potent trigger of inflammatory response.
- There is a release of cytokines (important being tumour necrosis factor-α, interleukin-1 and interleukin-10), activation of complement components, release of platelet-activating factors, prostaglandins and leucotrienes. TNF-α and IL-6 have myocardial depressant action. TNF-α also induces coronary endothelial dysfunction, which may further diminish coronary flow in patients with cardiogenic shock.
- Endothelial cells also play a role in sepsis-induced shock as they produce increased amount of nitric oxide synthase. This enzyme increases the production of nitric oxide, a potent vasodilator that may contribute to prolonged shock and reduced reactivity to adrenergic agents.

CARDIOGENIC SHOCK

- Cardiogenic shock as a result of myocardial ischaemia/infarction has been described as a 'downward spiral'. Myocardial perfusion depends on the pressure gradient between the coronary arterial system and the left ventricle, and on the duration of diastole. When stroke volume decreases after an initial ischaemic insult, hypotension leads to a further decrease in myocardial perfusion. This decrease in perfusion leads to worsening ischaemia and progressive myocardial dysfunction. Ultimately, without intervention, this downward spiral leads to death (Flowchart 7.5).

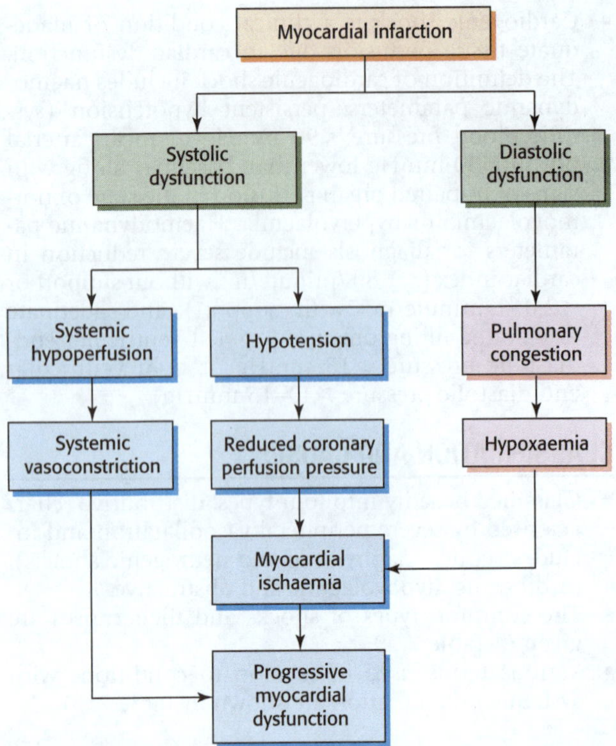

Flowchart 7.5 Pathophysiology of Cardiogenic Shock.

NEUROGENIC SHOCK

- Neurogenic shock is caused by the loss of sympathetic control of resistance vessels resulting in massive dilatation of arterioles and venules. Pooling of blood in venous system leads to reduced venous return to heart, which produces fall in stroke volume, cardiac output and blood pressure. Arteriolar dilatation reduces blood pressure further.

BOX 7.31 Cardinal Features of Shock

- Hypotension with a systolic blood pressure <90 mmHg
- Tachycardia (>100/minute) with thready pulse
- Cold, clammy skin
- Peripheral cyanosis often present
- Tachypnoea, Cheyne–Stokes breathing
- Altered mental status
- Urine output <30 mL/hour
- Hyperlactataemia indicating abnormal cellular oxygen metabolism (lactate >2 mmol/L)

Note:
- Some patients with septic shock may initially present with warm hyperperfused extremities ('warm shock') due to abnormal peripheral vasodilatation.
- Specific clinical manifestations of the underlying cause of shock are usually present.
- In neurogenic shock, the extremities are often warm due to arteriolar dilatation and patients have bradycardia.

CARDINAL FEATURES OF SHOCK

- Cardinal features of shock are given in Box 7.31.

PATHOPHYSIOLOGY AND CLINICAL MANIFESTATIONS OF SHOCK

- Flowchart 7.6 depicts pathophysiology and clinical manifestations of shock.

MANAGEMENT OF SHOCK

- Management of shock can be discussed under three headings:
  - Patient monitoring.
  - General measures.
  - Vasopressors and inotropes (sympathomimetic amines and vasopressin).
- Note that these measures are applicable to all shock syndromes. Special considerations in specific shock syndromes will be discussed later.

PATIENT MONITORING

- Clinical monitoring of pulse, blood pressure and respiration.
- Electrocardiographic monitoring for cardiac rate, rhythm and arrhythmias.
- Arterial blood gases and pH for correction of acidosis and hypoxia.

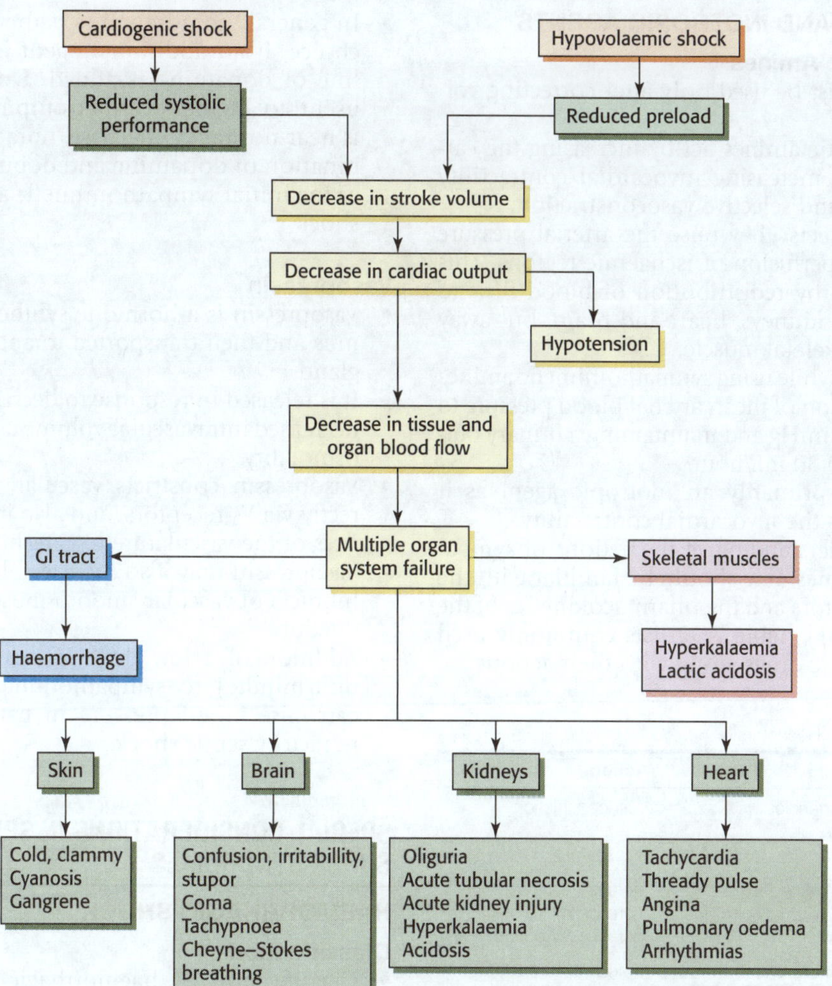

Flowchart 7.6 Pathophysiology and Clinical Manifestations of Shock.

- Central venous pressure monitoring or inferior vena cava (IVC) diameter (with respiratory variability) using an ultrasound for knowing the blood volume, and for guiding fluid replacement.
- Pulmonary capillary wedge pressure monitoring with a Swan–Ganz catheter in the management of cardiogenic shock.
- Urinary catheterisation to monitor hourly urinary output.
- Arterial catheterisation for monitoring arterial pressure (optional).

GENERAL MEASURES

- Care of the skin, airway, bowel and bladder, and nutrition.
- Pain and anxiety should be alleviated by reassurance.
- Patient should be put in a horizontal position with legs slightly elevated, unless this position is uncomfortable or causes shortness of breath. In that case, he/she should be allowed the most comfortable position.
- Correction of hypovolaemia:
  - Correction is based on the amount and nature of fluid lost, clinical state of the patient, and IVC diameter, central venous pressure or pulmonary artery wedge pressure (PAWP).
  - Hypovolaemia is corrected by blood, Ringer's lactate solution, isotonic saline solution, dextran, albumin or plasma depending on the situation.
- Prevention and treatment of renal complications:
  - In the initial stages of shock, there is renal vasoconstriction that if prolonged can lead to acute tubular necrosis and renal failure. Protection of the kidneys from vasoconstriction can be achieved by a rapid and adequate correction of hypovolaemia. There is no role of diuresis with furosemide or mannitol, and intravenous low-dose (2–4 μg/kg/minute) dopamine.
  - Once acute tubular necrosis and renal failure have set in, the patient should be managed as for acute kidney injury.
- Correction of hypoxia with oxygen by face masks or nasal prongs and, if necessary, by intubation and mechanical ventilation.
- Correction of acidosis with intravenous sodium bicarbonate (if acidosis is severe).
- Treatment of cardiac arrhythmias with drugs, electrical cardioversion or pacing.
- Treatment of sepsis with antibiotics and drainage of any abscesses.
- Low-dose corticosteroids in early stages of septic shock.

VASOPRESSORS AND INOTROPIC AGENTS

Sympathomimetic Amines

- These agents must be used only after correcting volume deficit.
- Sympathomimetic amines act by increasing the cardiac output (by increasing myocardial contractility and heart rate) and selective vasoconstriction.
- By these two effects, they raise the arterial pressure allowing better perfusion of ischaemic regions. This is accomplished by redistribution of blood flow to vital organs like kidneys, heart and brain, but away from skin and skeletal muscle.
- Main guidelines while using sympathomimetic amines should be elevation of mean arterial blood pressure to levels above 65 mmHg and maintaining a urinary output of more than 30 mL/hour.
- Dobutamine is primarily an inotropic agent as it mainly increases the myocardial contractility.
- For a better understanding of the actions of sympathomimetic amines, one should be familiar with the adrenergic receptors and the pharmacokinetics of the drugs (Table 7.31). Table 7.32 lists commonly used sympathomimetic drugs along with their actions.
- In general, noradrenaline is the first vasopressor of choice. If an additional agent is required, adrenaline or dopamine is added. Dobutamine alone is useful to augment cardiac output if arterial pressure is near-normal. Otherwise, noradrenaline or a combination of dopamine and dobutamine is preferred as the initial sympathomimetic agent in cardiogenic shock.

TABLE 7.31 Adrenergic Receptors

Receptors	Site	Action
α (Vascular)	Arterioles Venules Veins	Vasoconstriction
β-1 (Cardiac)	Myocardium Sinoatrial node AV node	Increase contraction Increase heart rate Increase AV conduction
β-2 (Vascular)	Arterioles Lungs	Vasodilatation Bronchial dilatation

Vasopressin

- Vasopressin is a hormone synthesised in hypothalamus and then transported to and stored in pituitary gland.
- It is released in response to decreased blood volume, decreased intravascular volume and increased plasma osmolality.
- Vasopressin constricts vascular smooth muscle directly via V_1 receptors, and also increases responsiveness of the vasculature to catecholamines.
- Vasopressin may also increase blood pressure by inhibition of vascular smooth muscle nitric oxide production.
- Addition of a low dose of vasopressin (0.01–0.04 unit/minute) to sympathomimetic catecholamines can raise blood pressure in patients with pressor-refractory septic shock.

SPECIAL CONSIDERATIONS IN SPECIFIC SHOCK SYNDROMES

HAEMORRHAGIC SHOCK

Classification

- Classification of haemorrhagic shock is given in Table 7.33.

TABLE 7.32 Commonly Used Sympathomimetic Amines

Amine (Dose)	Receptor Activated	Action
• Dopamine		
• 3 μg/kg/minute	Dopaminergic	Vasodilator action on renal, mesenteric, cerebral and coronary vessels
• 3–10 μg/kg/minute	β-1	Increased myocardial contractility, heart rate and cardiac output
• >10 μg/kg/minute	α	Vasoconstriction
• Dobutamine		
• 1–10 μg/kg/minute	β-1	Increase in myocardial contractility with minimal increase in heart rate and minimal vasodilatation of peripheral vessels
• Noradrenaline		
• 2–8 μg/minute	β-1	Increased myocardial contractility, heart rate and cardiac output
	α	Vasoconstriction in skin, muscle and splanchnic beds
	β-2	Coronary vasodilatation
• Adrenaline		
• 1–8 μg/minute	β-1	Increased myocardial contractility, heart rate and cardiac output
	α	Vasoconstriction in most vessels except skeletal muscles and coronaries
	β-2	Vasodilatation in skeletal muscles and coronaries
• Isoproterenol		
• 1–4 μg/minute	β-1	Increased myocardial contractility, heart rate and cardiac output
	β-2	Vasodilatation predominantly in skeletal muscles
• Phenylephrine		
• 20–200 μg/minute	α	Vasoconstriction

TABLE 7.33 Classification of Haemorrhagic Shock

Shock Class	Blood Loss in mL (%)	Heart Rate per Minute	Blood Pressure	Pulse Pressure	Respiratory Rate per Minute	Mental Status	Base Deficit (mEq/L)
I	750 (15%)	<100	Normal	Normal	14–20	Normal	0 to −2
II	750–1500 (15%–30%)	100–120	Normal	Narrowed	20–30	Anxious	−2 to −6
III	1500–2000 (30%–40%)	120–140	Reduced	Narrowed	30–40	Confused	−6 to −10
IV	>2000 (>40%)	>140	Reduced	Narrowed	>35	Lethargic	>−10

Treatment

- Rapid localisation and control of haemorrhage along with blood product resuscitation.
- Damage control resuscitation (particularly in traumatic shock):
  - Avoid or correct hypothermia.
  - Minimise crystalloid infusions (<3 L in the first 6 hours).
  - In trauma patients, use a massive transfusion protocol to ensure that sufficient blood products are rapidly available. Administer blood products in a ratio of 1:1:1 (plasma to platelets to red cells).
  - Obtain functional laboratory measures of coagulation (e.g. by means of thromboelastrography or rotational thromboelastometry) to guide targeted transfusion therapy.
  - Procoagulant haemostatic adjuncts (e.g. tranexamic acid) to promote clot formation may be considered.
  - Avoid delays in surgical, endoscopic or angiographic haemostasis.

CARDIOGENIC SHOCK

- Establish large-bore peripheral intravenous access.
- Correct any bradyarrhythmia (with atropine/temporary pacing) or tachyarrhythmia (with cardioversion), which may be contributing to hypotension.
- Insert a peripheral arterial line to monitor blood pressure and a urinary catheter.
- If clinical signs or haemodynamic monitoring indicates that the left ventricle is underfilled (PCWP <15 mmHg), infuse 100- to 200-mL boluses of intravenous fluid to optimise left ventricular filling pressures (aiming for PCWP of approximately 15 mmHg).
- If PCWP >18 mmHg, do not infuse intravenous fluid.
- Give diuretics in conjunction with inotropes (to prevent further hypotension).
- Commonly used vasopressor is noradrenaline. Dopamine, adrenaline or vasopressin as first-line agents are not recommended. Addition of an inotropic agent like dobutamine may help to improve stroke volume after haemodynamic stabilisation with a vasopressor. Levosimendan, a calcium sensitiser, and milrinone and enoximone, phosphodiesterase-3 (PDE-3) inhibitors, may also be used to improve cardiac contractility.
- Vasodilator therapy (in selected cases):
  - Venodilatation reduces central venous pressure and right ventricular output and slows the development of pulmonary oedema.
  - Arteriolar dilatation improves left ventricular function by reducing the afterload.
  - Commonly used agents are nitroglycerine and nitroprusside.
- Circulatory assist devices:
  - Circulatory assist devices may be beneficial in selected cases of cardiogenic shock. The various modalities include:
    - Intraaortic balloon counterpulsation (use of an IABP improves coronary and peripheral perfusion via diastolic balloon inflation and augments left ventricle performance via systolic balloon deflation with an acute decrease in afterload). Indicated in only those with mechanical complications of MI (e.g. papillary muscle rupture).
    - Partial cardiac bypass (left ventricular assist devices).
    - Extracorporeal membrane oxygenator (ECMO).
- PCI and thrombolytic therapy in selected cases of acute myocardial infarction (see pages 592–594). Thrombolytic therapy is less effective but is indicated when PCI is not possible or if a delay has occurred in transport for PCI, and when MI and cardiogenic shock onset is within 3 hours.
- Surgical therapy:
  - Role of surgical therapy in cardiogenic shock is mainly aimed at correction of underlying cause. It is indicated in selected cases of cardiogenic shock resulting from the following:
    - Ruptured papillary muscle and acute mitral regurgitation.
    - Rupture of the interventricular septum.
    - Selected cases of acute aortic regurgitation, aortic dissection and acute massive pulmonary embolism.
    - Myocardial infarction (where revascularisation is done by either PCI or coronary artery bypass surgery).

SEPTIC SHOCK (DISCUSSED IN SECTION 'DISEASES DUE TO INFECTIONS')

ANAPHYLACTIC SHOCK (DISCUSSED IN SECTION 'IMMUNOLOGICAL FACTORS IN DISEASE')

NEUROGENIC SHOCK

- Horizontal positioning of the patient.
- Maintain an adequate fluid balance. Large amount of fluids may be required.
- Noradrenaline may be required in some cases.

Q. Define pulmonary oedema. Enumerate the causes of pulmonary oedema.

Q. Discuss the aetiology, clinical presentation, investigations and management of cardiogenic pulmonary oedema. Add a note on the pathophysiology.

DEFINITION

- Acute pulmonary oedema is a condition characterised by accumulation of excess fluid in the interstitium and alveoli of the lung.

AETIOLOGY

- Various causes of acute pulmonary oedema are given in Table 7.34.
- Cardiogenic pulmonary oedema can also be classified as shown in Box 7.32.

PATHOPHYSIOLOGY OF CARDIOGENIC PULMONARY OEDEMA

- Cardiogenic pulmonary oedema is transudation of fluid, macromolecules and red blood cells from the pulmonary capillaries into initially the interstitium and later into alveoli and bronchioles.
- Normally pulmonary interstitium is efficiently drained by lymphatics. In pulmonary oedema, the rate of fluid accumulation in the interstitium exceeds the drainage capacity of lymphatics, which results in accumulation of fluid in the interstitium (Flowchart 7.7).
- Various factors that operate in the development of pulmonary oedema can be summarised as follows:
  - Elevated pulmonary capillary pressure favouring transudation of fluid.
  - Widening of the pulmonary capillary endothelial intercellular junctions, allowing passage of fluid, macromolecules and red blood cells into the interstitium (interstitial oedema).
  - Disruption of the intercellular junctions between the alveolar lining cells, allowing fluid, macromolecules and red blood cells to enter the alveoli (alveolar oedema).

TABLE 7.34 Aetiology of Pulmonary Oedema

- **Cardiogenic pulmonary oedema** (primary abnormality is elevated pulmonary capillary pressure)
  - Myocardial infarction
  - Hypertensive heart disease (including accelerated hypertension)
  - Mitral stenosis, mitral regurgitation
  - Aortic stenosis, aortic regurgitation
  - Congenital heart diseases
  - Myocarditis
  - Arrhythmias
- **Noncardiogenic pulmonary oedema** (primary abnormality is not elevated pulmonary capillary pressure)
  - Disruption of alveolar–capillary membranes, for example ARDS (for causes, refer ARDS on page 129)
  - Increased negativity of the interstitial pressure, for example rapid evacuation of a large pneumothorax or pleural effusion, and acute severe asthma
  - Impeding lymphatic drainage by lymphatic blockade, for example fibrotic and inflammatory diseases of lung and lymphangitis carcinomatosis
  - Precise mechanism is unknown, for example narcotic overdose (morphine, methadone, dextropropoxyphene), exposure to high altitude and neurogenic pulmonary oedema (postulated to be due to reduced PaO_2 causing pulmonary hypertension)

BOX 7.32 Classification of Cardiogenic Pulmonary Oedema

- Hypertensive pulmonary oedema presents with signs and symptoms of heart failure accompanied by high blood pressure (systolic >140 mmHg) and relatively preserved left ventricular function with a chest radiograph compatible with acute pulmonary oedema. These patients are often euvolaemic.
- Normotensive pulmonary oedema patients have normal blood pressure and volume overload with or without reduced left ventricular function.
- Hypotensive pulmonary oedema patients have cardiogenic shock with markedly depressed left ventricular function and pulmonary oedema.
- Sympathetic crashing acute pulmonary oedema (SCAPE) or flash pulmonary oedema.

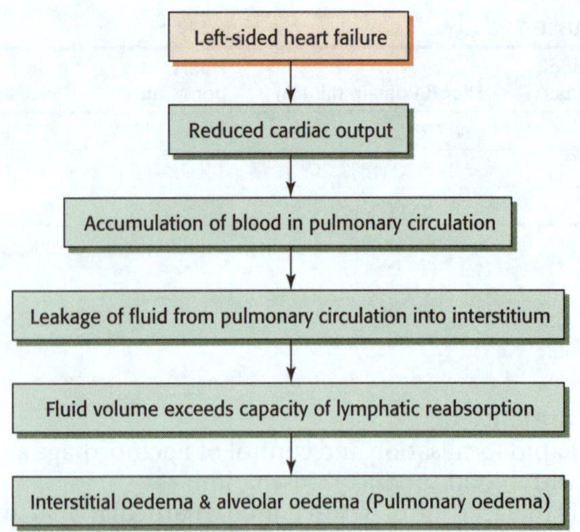

Flowchart 7.7 Pathogenesis of Cardiogenic Pulmonary Oedema.

SYMPATHETIC CRASHING ACUTE PULMONARY OEDEMA (SCAPE)

- Develops drastically within a few minutes to hours due to abrupt increase in sympathetic activity that causes a sudden increase in catecholamine release, subsequently increasing arterial tone and blood pressure, and precipitation of pulmonary oedema.
- Increased sympathetic tone also adversely affects the pulmonary circulation by increasing permeability.

STAGES IN DEVELOPMENT OF PULMONARY OEDEMA

- 'Interstitial oedema'—this is the early stage where oedema is confined to interstitium.
- 'Alveolar oedema'—this occurs later, with oedema fluid, macromolecules and red blood cells entering the alveoli.

CLINICAL FEATURES OF ACUTE CARDIOGENIC PULMONARY OEDEMA

- Clinical features of acute cardiogenic pulmonary oedema are given in Box 7.33.

BOX 7.33 Clinical Features of Acute Cardiogenic Pulmonary Oedema

- Severe dyspnoea and orthopnoea
- Cough initially dry, but later with copious, pinkish, frothy expectoration
- Anxiety, pallor, sweating, cyanosis
- Tachycardia, tachypnoea
- Cold, bluish extremities
- Bilateral scattered rhonchi
- Bilateral crepitations, predominantly basal
- Raised JVP
- Presence of S_3
- Signs of underlying heart disease
- Progressive hypoxia, hypercapnia and acidosis
- Eventually, respiratory arrest

TABLE 7.35 Radiological Features of Acute Cardiogenic Pulmonary Oedema

Radiological grading of pulmonary oedema	
• Grade 1	• Prominence of the upper lobe veins (reverse moustache sign; stag's antler sign) (Fig. 7.39)
• Grade 2 (interstitial oedema)	• Kerley A lines—thin nonbranching lines radiating from the hilum (Fig. 7.40) • Kerley B lines—transverse thin lines of 1–3 cm, seen at the lung bases, lying perpendicular to the pleura (Fig. 7.40) • Blurring of the outline of the central pulmonary vessels and hilum due to perivascular oedema • 'Endobronchial cuffing'—blurring seen around the end-on view of bronchi
• Grade 3 (alveolar oedema)	• Bilateral fluffy shadows in the lung fields • Confluencing of fluffy shadows around hilum giving the 'bat's wing' appearance (bilateral perihilar opacity dense at the hilum, fading towards periphery) (Fig. 7.41) • Pleural effusions at uncommon sites like lamellar effusion, interlobar effusion and subpulmonic effusion. Interlobar effucion might give the appearance of a tumour, but it disappears with treatment (hence called 'phantom', 'disappearing' or 'vanishing' tumour)

INVESTIGATIONS

- Arterial blood gas studies show hypoxia. Initially, the patient has hypocapnia but in late stages hypercapnia develops.
- Chest radiograph shows several features (Table 7.35).
- Ultrasound of lungs shows bilateral *B* lines (vertical artefacts which result from reverberation of sound waves off fluid-filled pulmonary interstitium) (Fig. 7.42).

TREATMENT OF ACUTE CARDIOGENIC PULMONARY OEDEMA

- Propped-up position or sitting position with legs hanging down along the side of the bed to reduce venous return.

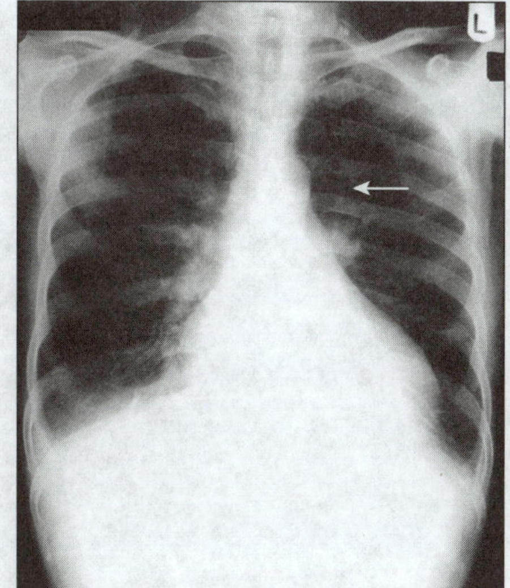

Fig. 7.39 Chest radiograph showing prominence of upper lobe veins (arrow).

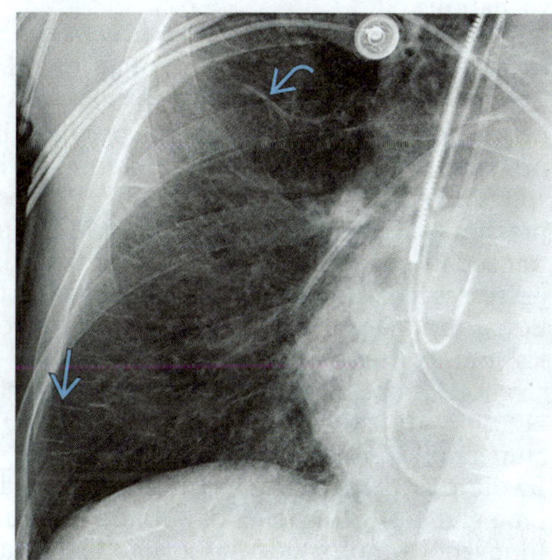

Fig. 7.40 Chest radiograph showing short thin (Kerley B) lines perpendicular to the lateral pleura and longer oblique (Kerley A) lines.

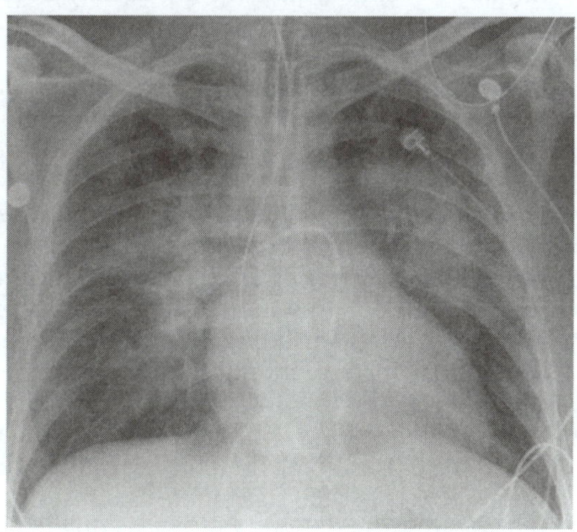

Fig. 7.41 Chest radiograph showing 'bat's wing' appearance in a patient with pulmonary oedema.

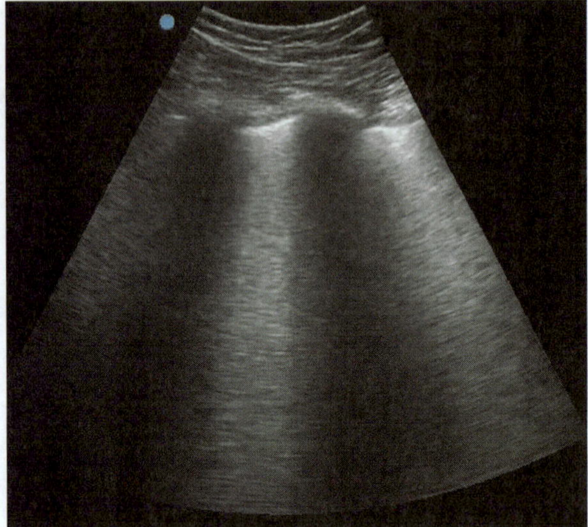

Fig. 7.42 Ultrasound of lung showing confluent 'B' lines in a patient with pulmonary oedema.

- Oxygenation:
  - One hundred per cent oxygen.
  - Noninvasive ventilation (NIV) may be tried if oxygen saturation remains below 90%. NIV can be provided by either continuous positive airway pressure (CPAP) or bilevel ventilation (both inspiratory and expiratory support, BiPAP). Positive pressure raises intraalveolar pressure reducing transudation of fluid. It augments cardiac output, decreases left ventricular afterload, increases functional residual capacity and respiratory mechanics, and reduces work of breathing.
- Intravenous loop diuretics, for example furosemide 40–100 mg (drug of choice), torsemide (10–20 mg) or bumetanide 1 mg:
  - By diuresis, they reduce the circulating blood volume and hasten the relief of pulmonary oedema.
  - Intravenous furosemide has a venodilator action by which it reduces venous return. This effect occurs within a few minutes while diuresis may take 30 minutes.
  - Diuretics should be avoided in hypertensive pulmonary oedema as patients are usually euvolaemic or even hypovolaemic.
- Morphine:
  - Morphine exerts vasodilatory effect which reduces preload and afterload to the heart and helps in reducing pulmonary oedema. It has anxiolytic effect as well.
  - However, it has several drawbacks including respiratory depression. It decreases both hypoxic and hypercapnic respiratory drive. It can produce vomiting with risk of aspiration. It reduces absorption of several drugs including clopidogrel. In addition, it may increase mortality.
- Vasodilators:
  - Preload reduction with nitrates sublingually (5–10 mg of isosorbide dinitrate) or nitroglycerine intravenously (5–100 μg/minute as infusion). Initial recommended dose of nitroglycerine is 10–20 μg/minute, and it is increased in increments of 5 μg/minute every 3–5 minutes as needed. Tachyphylaxis is common, necessitating incremental dosing. Major adverse effects of nitrates are hypotension, tachycardia and headache.
  - Afterload reduction with intravenous sodium nitroprusside 20–30 μg/minute in patients with systolic blood pressure more than 100 mmHg. Nitroprusside is particularly useful in settings in which acute afterload reduction is needed, including hypertensive emergency, acute aortic regurgitation, acute mitral regurgitation and acute ventricular septal defect. The major complication of nitroprusside therapy is hypotension and toxicity due to accumulation of cyanide or thiocyanate. This usually occurs only in patients who have been receiving high doses of nitroprusside for 24 hours or more, commonly in patients with renal failure.
  - Nesiritide, a recombinant form of human brain natriuretic peptide (BNP), is a venous and arterial vasodilator that may also potentiate the effect of diuretics. Hypotension and worsening of renal functions are important side effects.
- Inotropic agents: To increase the contractility of the myocardium, inotropic agents have been useful in hypotensive pulmonary oedema or cardiogenic shock. Intravenous dopamine or dobutamine are most often used for this purpose. Noradrenaline may be used if there is no response.
  - Dobutamine is useful in patients with pulmonary oedema with normal or low-normal blood pressure.
  - Noradrenaline and dopamine are preferred to dobutamine if shock is also present.
  - Intravenous digitalis has no role in pulmonary oedema; however, in presence of supraventricular tachycardia with fast ventricular rate, intravenous digoxin (0.5 mg) may be useful.
  - Milrinone increases the contractile state of the heart and reduces the systemic vascular resistance, both of which decrease the left ventricular afterload and filling pressures. However, it increases risk of life-threatening arrhythmias.
  - Levosimendan, a novel calcium sensitiser that improves cardiac contractility by binding to troponin-C in cardiomyocytes and has vasodilatory properties, has beneficial haemodynamic and clinical effects in patients with acute pulmonary oedema.
- Monitoring the intraarterial pressure and pulmonary vascular pressures through a Swan–Ganz catheter in selected cases.
- In refractory cases, rotating tourniquets may be applied to the limbs. Tourniquets with pressure just above the diastolic are applied to three of the four limbs and rotated every 15 minutes. However, their efficacy is unproven.
- Ultrafiltration (a method of fluid removal) may be useful in patients with renal dysfunction and expected diuretic resistance.
- Correction of precipitating causes like infection or arrhythmias.
- Treatment of underlying cause.

TREATMENT OF SYMPATHETIC CRASHING ACUTE PULMONARY OEDEMA

- Nitroglycerine in high doses of 400–800 μg as bolus over 2 minutes reduces both preload and afterload. This should be followed by a repeat dose if required or an infusion at 100–400 μg/minute which is rapidly tapered to 50–100 μg/minute once the patient is stable.
- Simultaneously, the patient should be started on NIV. Endotracheal intubation and mechanical ventilation may be avoided in a significant number of patients using high-dose nitroglycerine and NIV.

Q. Define orthopnoea, trepopnoea and platypnoea/orthodeoxia.

- Orthopnoea:
  - Dyspnoea that develops in recumbent position and is relieved by sitting up.
  - Occurs within a few minutes of assuming recumbent position.
  - Occurs in left heart failure.
- Platypnoea/orthodeoxia:
  - Platypnoea is dyspnoea that develops in upright position and gets relieved in supine position.
  - Orthodeoxia is deoxygenation when changing from a supine to an upright position.
  - Occurs in left atrial thrombus, left atrial myxoma, pulmonary arteriovenous fistula, liver cirrhosis and persistent foramen ovale.
- Trepopnoea:
  - Dyspnoea that occurs only in left or right lateral decubitus position.
  - May occur in patients with pathology of one lung and chronic HF.

Q. Define heart failure. Discuss the types, common causes, pathophysiology, clinical features, staging and management of heart failure. (IM 1.1, IM 1.24, IM 1.4, IM 1.5, IM 1.6, IM 1.7)

DEFINITION

- HF or cardiac failure is defined as a state in which the ventricles at normal filling pressures (i.e. adequate intravascular volume) cannot maintain an adequate cardiac output to meet the metabolic needs of peripheral tissues or can do so only with an elevated filling pressure. It results from any structural or functional impairment of ventricular filling or ejection of blood.
- The term HF is preferred over the older term congestive HF because not all patients with HF have volume overload.

PATHOPHYSIOLOGY

- To understand pathophysiology of HF, it is important to understand preload and afterload (Box 7.34).
- HF is characterised by a decrease in cardiac output (except in high-output failure). Cardiac output in turn is a function of preload, afterload and myocardial contractility. In HF, preload is increased, afterload is increased and myocardial contractility is decreased.
- In the initial stages of HF, reduction in cardiac output produces certain compensatory mechanisms. These compensatory mechanisms are initially beneficial, but later become counterproductive and account for most of the manifestations of HF. These compensatory mechanisms are mediated through renin–angiotensin system and autonomic nervous system. These mechanisms are discussed in the subsequent text and are shown in Flowchart 7.8.
  - Increased myocardial contractility: As the ventricle dilates (resulting in increased preload), the ventricular contractility increases, resulting in relatively increased volume of blood ejected (Frank–Starling law). However, there is a limit to which the myocardial cells can be stretched so as to enhance their contractility and beyond this limit, their contractility diminishes. The increased left ventricular filling pressures are transmitted to the pulmonary veins that result in alveolar transudation of fluid and pulmonary congestion. Finally, oxygen demand is enhanced due to increased contractility.
  - Myocardial hypertrophy occurs due to volume and pressure overload in the ventricle and helps in enhanced contractility and hence increased cardiac output. However, it produces increased oxygen demand and reduced compliance of the ventricle that results in increased preload that is again transmitted to the pulmonary vasculature.
  - Sympathetic stimulation results in peripheral vasoconstriction that in turn leads to salt and water retention due to direct and indirect effects on the renin–angiotensin system. Sympathetic stimulation also produces increased heart rate and enhances contractility. Increased afterload may be deleterious as it tends to reduce cardiac output and increases oxygen demand of the heart.
  - Myocardial remodelling: The fundamental mechanism that underlies the progressive nature of myocardial dysfunction has been termed remodelling. Important changes in structure and function of

BOX 7.34 Concept of Preload, Afterload and Myocardial Contractility

- Preload—refers to the pressure that fills the left ventricle during diastole. It is measured either directly as the left ventricular end-diastolic pressure or indirectly and more commonly as the PAWP. Main determinants of preload are left ventricular compliance and venous return.
- Afterload—refers to the pressure against which the left ventricle contracts and is measured as the mean aortic pressure. Main determinants of afterload are total peripheral resistance and left ventricle size.
- Myocardial contractility (inotropic state)—this mainly depends on the adrenergic nervous activity and the levels of circulating catecholamines.

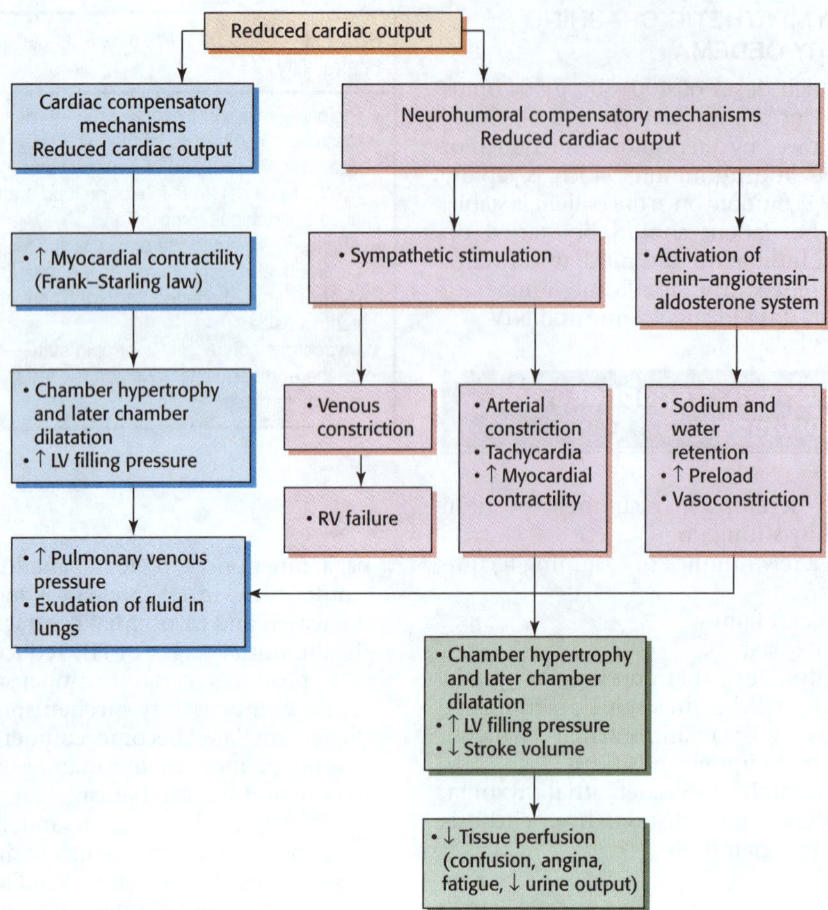

Flowchart 7.8 Pathophysiology of Heart Failure.

the myocardium include hypertrophy and apoptosis (programmed cell death) of myocytes, and alterations in the quantity and composition of extracellular matrix. Remodelling involves not only the ischaemic area but also the viable myocardium, resulting in gradual loss of contractility over a period of time.

TYPES OF HEART FAILURE

ACUTE AND CHRONIC HEART FAILURE

- Acute HF is rapid onset of new (de novo AHF) or worsening (acute decompensated HF) signs and symptoms of HF. The sudden reduction in cardiac output results in systemic hypotension without peripheral oedema. Best examples are acute myocardial infarction and rupture of a papillary muscle of mitral valve.
- Chronic HF develops gradually. Here systemic arterial pressure is well maintained, but oedema accumulates. Best examples are dilated cardiomyopathy and multivalvular disease.
- Compensated HF implies that the compensatory changes have prevented the development of overt HF. A minor insult like an infection may precipitate severe HF.

BASED ON LEFT VENTRICULAR EJECTION FRACTION

- HF with left ventricular ejection fraction (LVEF) ≥50%—HF with preserved ejection fraction (HFpEF).
- HF with LVEF ≤40%—HF with reduced ejection fraction (HFrEF).
- HF with LVEF between 40% and 50%—HF with mid-range ejection fraction (HFmrEF).
- For treatment considerations, HFpEF and HFmrEF are considered as one category.

LOW-OUTPUT AND HIGH-OUTPUT HEART FAILURE

- Low-output HF is associated with a low cardiac output. The heart fails to generate adequate output or can do so with high-filling pressures. Best examples are HF associated with ischaemic heart disease, hypertension, cardiomyopathy, valvular diseases and pericardial disease.
- In high-output HF, the heart fails to maintain sufficient circulation despite an increased cardiac output (defined as cardiac output >8 L/minute or a cardiac index >3.9 L/minute/m^2). Best examples are cardiac failure associated with hyperthyroidism, anaemia, pregnancy, arteriovenous fistulae, beriberi and Paget's disease. The underlying primary physiological problem in

high-output HF is of reduced systemic vascular resistance. This occurs due to either systemic arteriovenous shunting or peripheral vasodilatation. Both scenarios can lead to a fall in systemic arterial blood pressure, a feature of low-output HF. This can lead to sympathetic neural activation, a compensatory rise in cardiac output and neurohormonal activation. This process in turn can cause salt and water retention, and overt clinical HF. Thus, salt and water retention occurs in both low- and high-output HF due to a similar neurohormonal response to arterial hypotension. In the former it is due to low cardiac output and in the latter due to reduced systemic vascular resistance. In high-output HF, patients are likely to have warm rather than cold peripheries due to low systemic vascular resistance and peripheral vasodilatation. Right-sided HF is prominent in thiamine deficiency (wet beriberi).

LEFT-SIDED, RIGHT-SIDED AND BIVENTRICULAR HEART FAILURE

- 'Left side' is a term for the functional unit of left atrium, left ventricle, mitral valve and aortic valve.
- 'Right side' is a term for the functional unit of right atrium, right ventricle, tricuspid valve and pulmonary valve.

Left-Sided (Left Ventricular) Heart Failure

- Excess fluid accumulates upstream behind the failing left ventricle.
- There is reduction in left ventricular output, increase in left atrial pressure and increase in pulmonary venous pressure.
    - Acute increase in left atrial pressure causes pulmonary congestion and pulmonary oedema, for example myocardial infarction.
    - Gradual increase in left atrial pressure causes reflex pulmonary hypertension but no pulmonary oedema, for example aortic stenosis.

Right-Sided (Right Ventricular) Heart Failure

- Excess fluid accumulates upstream behind the failing right ventricle.
- There is reduction in right ventricular output that results in systemic venous congestion.
- Best examples are cor pulmonale, pulmonary valvular stenosis and multiple pulmonary emboli.

Biventricular Heart Failure

- There is failure of both left and right ventricles.
- Best examples are as follows:
    a. Disease processes affecting both ventricles like dilated cardiomyopathy and ischaemic heart disease.
    b. Diseases of left heart leading to chronic elevation of left atrial pressure, pulmonary hypertension and subsequent right ventricular failure.

FORWARD AND BACKWARD HEART FAILURE

- Forward HF is characterised by decreased cardiac output and inadequate perfusion of organs leading to poor tissue perfusion. Poor renal perfusion results in activation of renin–angiotensin–aldosterone system producing excessive absorption of sodium by renal tubules.
- Backward HF is characterised by a normal cardiac output, but marked salt and water retention, and pulmonary and systemic venous congestion.

SYSTOLIC AND DIASTOLIC HEART FAILURE

- Systolic HF is characterised by an abnormality of ventricular contraction. The ejection fraction is usually below 40%.
- Diastolic HF:
    - Characterised by an impaired ventricular relaxation and increased ventricular stiffness resulting in reduced filling (diastolic dysfunction).
    - Diagnosis of diastolic HF is based on three features—signs or symptoms of HF (usually dyspnoea), normal LV systolic function and diastolic LV dysfunction (using echocardiography or invasive pulmonary capillary wedge pressure).
    - Certain conditions such as ischaemia, left ventricular hypertrophy, hypertension and aortic stenosis predispose to diastolic dysfunction.
    - Survival similar to systolic HF.
    - ACE inhibitors, angiotensin receptor blockers (ARBs) and β-blockers do not offer significant benefit in outcome.
- The symptoms of HF may be identical whether failure is secondary to systolic or diastolic dysfunction.

COMMON CAUSES OF HEART FAILURE (Box 7.35)

- In practice, the most commonly encountered causes of HF are ischaemic heart disease, hypertensive heart disease, valvular heart diseases and cardiomyopathies.

PRECIPITATING AND AGGRAVATING CAUSES OF HEART FAILURE

- These are given in Box 7.36.

STAGES OF HEART FAILURE

- Various stages of heart failure are described in Table 7.36.

BOX 7.35 Common Causes of Heart Failure

PRESSURE OVERLOAD OF VENTRICLE:
- Systemic hypertension
- Pulmonary hypertension
- Aortic stenosis
- Pulmonary stenosis

VOLUME OVERLOAD OF VENTRICLE:
- Conditions associated with increased metabolic demand
- Mitral regurgitation
- Aortic regurgitation
- Ventricular septal defect
- Patent ductus arteriosus
- Atrial septal defect

INFLOW OBSTRUCTION OF VENTRICLE:
- Mitral stenosis
- Tricuspid stenosis
- Endomyocardial fibrosis

IMPAIRED VENTRICULAR FUNCTION:
- Diffuse myocardial disease
    - Myocarditis
    - Cardiomyopathy
- Segmental myocardial disease
- Myocardial infarction (ischaemic heart disease)

BOX 7.36 Precipitating Causes of Heart Failure

- Infections
- Anaemia, pregnancy, thyrotoxicosis
- Cardiac arrhythmias
- Supervening heart diseases like myocarditis, infective endocarditis, myocardial infarction
- Systemic hypertension
- Pulmonary embolism
- Drugs like β-blockers, corticosteroids and NSAIDs
- Excess salt intake
- Physical and emotional stress
- Poor compliance with therapy

TABLE 7.36 Stages of Heart Failure

Stage A	Patients have risk factors (e.g. hypertension, diabetes mellitus, hyperlipidaemia, coronary artery disease, thyroid disorders, alcohol use, tobacco use) for the development of HF but do not have structural or functional heart disease and are asymptomatic
Stage B	Patients who have already developed structural heart disease such as myocardial infarction, LV dysfunction or LV hypertrophy, but are asymptomatic
Stage C	Patients have structural heart disease with prior or current symptoms of HF
Stage D	Patients have advanced end-stage refractory HF and remain persistently symptomatic despite maximum pharmacological and device therapies

CLINICAL MANIFESTATIONS OF HEART FAILURE

DYSPNOEA

- Dyspnoea is initially exertional, but progressively worsens to a stage of breathlessness even at rest.
- The mechanisms underlying dyspnoea include:
  - Interstitial pulmonary oedema surrounding the pulmonary capillaries stimulates the juxtacapillary receptors (J receptors). This elicits a reflexly mediated, 'rapid and shallow breathing' of cardiac dyspnoea.
  - Respiratory muscle fatigue.
  - Bronchial mucosal oedema.
  - Increased bronchial mucus production.

ORTHOPNOEA

- Dyspnoea occurring soon after lying flat and relieved by sitting up is known as orthopnoea.
- Nocturnal cough has the same significance as orthopnoea.
- The mechanisms underlying orthopnoea include—in the lying down posture—the following:
  - Increased venous return from the lower limbs and abdomen to the lungs.
  - Elevation of the diaphragm.
  - Reabsorption of the peripheral oedema that had accumulated while ambulant.

PAROXYSMAL NOCTURNAL DYSPNOEA

- This is an attack of severe shortness of breath and coughing usually occurring at night, awakening the patient from sleep. Paroxysmal nocturnal dyspnoea (PND) persists even after sitting upright, whereas simple orthopnoea is relieved by sitting upright.
- Mechanisms underlying PND include:
  - Depression of the respiratory centre during sleep.
  - Reduced adrenergic stimulation of the myocardium at night resulting in further impairment of myocardial function.
  - In addition, mechanisms causing orthopnoea also contribute to PND.

CARDIAC ASTHMA

- This is closely related to PND and nocturnal cough. It is characterised by wheezing secondary to bronchospasm, most prominent at night. Acute pulmonary oedema is a severe form of cardiac asthma.
- The classic explanation for wheezing in HF is that it is caused by pulmonary oedema and accompanying bronchial wall oedema. However, it may also be due to bronchial hyper-reactivity.

ACUTE PULMONARY OEDEMA

- It is a severe form of cardiac asthma resulting from marked elevation of pulmonary capillary pressure leading to alveolar oedema.
- Clinically, it is characterised by severe breathlessness, cough with copious, pinkish frothy expectoration and bilateral crepitations.

CHEYNE–STOKES RESPIRATION

- A type of periodic breathing with alternate periods of apnoea and hyperventilation seen in advanced HF.
- Mechanisms underlying Cheyne–Stokes respiration include:
  - Diminished sensitivity of the respiratory centre to arterial PCO_2 is the main mechanism.
  - Prolongation of the circulation time from lungs to brain that occurs in HF.

NOCTURIA

- A feature of early HF.
- Underlying mechanism is a better renal perfusion and diuresis at night when the patient is supine.

CEREBRAL SYMPTOMS

- Confusion, difficulty in concentration, memory impairment, headache, insomnia and anxiety.
- Underlying mechanisms include:
  - Arterial hypoxaemia.
  - Reduced cerebral perfusion.

NONSPECIFIC SYMPTOMS

- Fatigue and weakness from reduced perfusion of skeletal muscles.
- Low-grade fever from reduction of cutaneous flow.
- Anorexia, nausea, abdominal pain and fullness from congestion of liver and portal venous system.

CARDIAC OEDEMA

- Due to gravity, cardiac oedema accumulates over dependent parts. In ambulant patients, it occurs symmetrically in the legs, particularly in the pretibial region and around the ankles. It is less in the morning and more towards the evening. Oedema is sacral in bedridden patients.

- In advanced stages, there is anasarca with oedema fluid accumulating throughout the body. Face and arms are typically spared until the terminal stages.

CYANOSIS

- Mainly affects lips and nail beds.
- Extremities are cold and pale due to reduced blood flow, and also cyanosed.

PULSE

- Sinus tachycardia.
- Pulsus alternans is a sign of severe HF.

BLOOD PRESSURE

- Diminished pulse pressure due to reduced stroke volume.
- Diastolic blood pressure may be slightly raised occasionally due to generalised vasoconstriction.

JUGULAR VENOUS PRESSURE

- Jugular venous pressure is raised as a consequence of elevated systemic venous pressure.
- In the early stages, jugular venous pressure may not be raised at rest. But it becomes raised:
  - During and immediately after exercise.
  - With sustained pressure on the abdomen (positive hepatojugular or abdominojugular reflux). A positive abdominojugular reflux suggests reduced right ventricular compliance so that right ventricle cannot accommodate an increase in venous return.

THIRD HEART SOUND AND FOURTH HEART SOUND

- The presence of a third heart sound in an adult is highly suggestive of HF.
- The presence of either of the two (S_3 or S_4) is known as triple rhythm ($S_1 + S_2 + S_3$ or $S_1 + S_2 + S_4$).
- The presence of both of them (S_3 and S_4) is known as quadruple rhythm ($S_1 + S_2 + S_3 + S_4$).
- In some cases, S_3 and S_4 merge to become a single sound that sounds like a triple rhythm, but known as summation gallop.
- The timing of S_1, S_2 and either of S_3 or S_4 in association with an increased heart rate results in a characteristic cadence of a 'gallop', when it is known as gallop rhythm (S_3 gallop or S_4 gallop).

RESPIRATORY SYSTEM

- Inspiratory fine crepitations over lung bases.
- In patients with pulmonary oedema, crepitations are coarse and heard widely over both lung fields associated with expiratory rhonchi.

LIVER (CONGESTIVE HEPATOMEGALY)

- Right upper quadrant pain from stretching of the capsule of the liver.
- Liver is enlarged and tender due to systemic venous hypertension.
- Cardiac cirrhosis occurs in prolonged HF which results in atrophy and centrilobular necrosis of liver cells, leading later to extensive fibrosis.
- Hypoglycaemia can occur in long-standing cases due to depletion of liver glycogen stores and increased production of lactic acid from glucose, induced by hypoxia.
- With prolonged hepatomegaly, spleen may also become enlarged.
- Jaundice is a late feature characterised by hyperbilirubinaemia of both conjugated and unconjugated types. In acute hepatic congestion, jaundice is severe and enzymes are markedly elevated.

PLEURAL EFFUSION, ASCITES AND PERICARDIAL EFFUSION

- Pleural effusion is more common on the right side and results from elevation of pleural capillary pressure and transudation of fluid into pleural space.
- Ascites results from transudation secondary to elevated pressures in hepatic veins, portal veins and veins draining the peritoneum.
- Pericardial effusion can occur rarely.

KIDNEY

- Oliguria.
- Urinary sodium is low; specific gravity is high and contains proteins (less than 1 g/day).
- Prerenal azotaemia is common. Blood urea is typically elevated out of proportion to serum creatinine.

CARDIAC CACHEXIA

- Advanced HF is associated with severe anorexia, weight loss and malnutrition.

HAEMATOLOGICAL FEATURES

- Anaemia in HF is common and develops due to a complex interaction of iron deficiency, kidney disease, reduced erythropoietin production and cytokine production. Blood loss may contribute.

COMMON DIAGNOSTIC STUDIES

- Chest radiograph may show cardiomegaly, prominence of upper lobe veins, Kerley A and B lines, and other features of pulmonary oedema.
  - Prominence of upper lobe veins.
  - Kerley B lines—engorged peripheral lymphatics seen in lower lobe.
  - Phantom tumour—fluid in horizontal or oblique fissures of lungs; disappears with diuretics.
  - 'Bat's wing'—increased bronchovascular markings (also known as inverted moustache signs) in perihilar area.
  - Pleural effusion (bilateral or unilateral).
  - Cardiomegaly.
- Electrocardiography (may show presence of ventricular hypertrophy, atrial abnormality, arrhythmias, electrical alternans—Figure 7.43, conduction abnormalities, previous MI and active ischaemia).
- BNP.
  - Serum levels of BNP and NT-proBNP are elevated in HF. These tests are highly sensitive for diagnosis of HF as the cause of dyspnoea and are often used to differentiate cardiac from respiratory cause of acute dyspnoea in emergency departments. These markers are also used as independent mortality predictors in patients with HF.

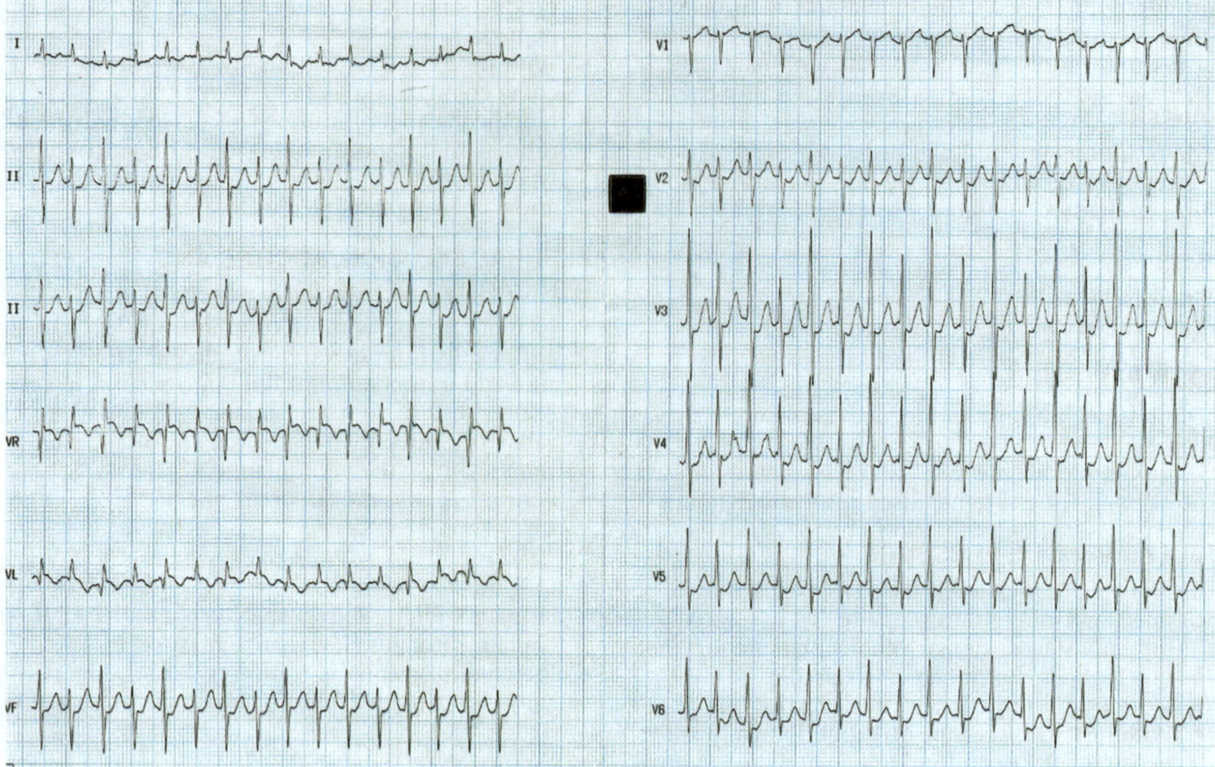

Fig. 7.43 Electrical alternans with PSVT.

- Assessment of ejection fraction, valvular functions and chamber size and shape by echocardiography. It can also differentiate between systolic and diastolic HF.
- Assessment of ejection fraction by radionuclide ventriculography.
- Exercise stress testing and cardiac catheterisation, if indicated.
- Ambulatory Holter monitoring if arrhythmias are suspected.
- Renal and liver functions as baseline.
- Thyroid function tests to exclude occult thyroid disease.

MANAGEMENT OF HEART FAILURE

- Physical and emotional rest:
  - Absolute bed rest is rarely required.
  - Small doses of tranquillisers may be used.
  - Correction of obesity by restriction of caloric intake.
- Salt-restricted diet and avoidance of salt-retaining medicines (e.g. NSAIDs):
  - In mild HF, mild sodium restriction.
  - In more severe HF, more rigid control of sodium intake (1 to 2 g/day).
  - In severe HF, sodium chloride intake should be less than 0.5–1 g/day.
  - Restriction of water intake is advised only in most severe cases.

  Note: Normal diet contains 6–10 g of sodium chloride.
- ACE inhibitors and ARBs—recommended for all patients with HF, whether symptoms are mild, moderate or severe, unless not tolerated or contraindicated.
- Sacubitril/valsartan combines a neprilysin inhibitor with an ARB and is categorised as an angiotensin receptor–neprilysin inhibitor (ARNI). Neprilysin inhibition prevents degradation of BNP and other compensatory peptides (e.g. bradykinin, adrenomedullin), thus increasing plasma levels of these peptides and enhancing their beneficial effects, which include vasodilation, natriuresis, diuresis and inhibition of pathogenic growth and fibrosis. Valsartan counterbalances the increase of angiotensin II that also results from neprilysin inhibition, while simultaneously exerting the beneficial effects of ARBs. ARNI is the first choice in the treatment of HFrEF. Patients with chronic, symptomatic HF (NYHA class II or III symptoms) may be switched from ACE inhibitors or ARBs to the ARNI to further

TABLE 7.37 Indications for ARNI, Ivabradine and SGLT-2 Inhibitor Use

Indications for use of an ARNI (sacubitril/valsartan): • HFrEF (EF ≤40%) • NYHA class II–IV HF • Administered in place of an ACE inhibitor or ARB
Indications for use of ivabradine: • HFrEF (EF ≤35%) • On maximum tolerated dose of beta-blocker • Sinus rhythm with a resting heart rate ≥70/minute • NYHA class II or III HF
Indications for use of an SGLT-2 inhibitor: • HFrEF (EF ≤40%) with or without diabetes • NYHA class II–IV HF • Administered in conjunction with an ARNI

reduce morbidity and mortality (Table 7.37). Low dose is 24 mg sacubitril + 26 valsartan while the target dose is 97 md sacubitril + 103 mg valsartan. It should be avoided if an ACE inhibitor or ARB is taken within last 36 hours.

- β-Blockers (carvedilol, metoprolol succinate and bisoprolol)—recommended for all patients with HF (except very severe cases) who remain symptomatic despite appropriate doses of ACE inhibitors.
- Diuretics—used if patient has volume overload.
- Digoxin—for details regarding digoxin therapy, refer page 544.
- Mineralocorticoid receptor blocker (previously called aldosterone receptor blocker)—spironolactone or eplerenone—recommended for patients who remain symptomatic despite appropriate doses of ACE inhibitors and diuretics. Aldosterone promotes fibrosis in the heart and contributes to diastolic stiffness. Spironolactone and eplerenone reduce mortality related to HF.
- Vasodilators—for details regarding vasodilator therapy, refer page 546.
- Sympathomimetic amines—improve myocardial contractility in HF. They are dopamine, dobutamine, adrenaline and isoproterenol (isoprenaline). Of these drugs, dopamine and dobutamine are used in acute or refractory HF.
  - Dopamine is useful in HF associated with hypotension.
  - Dobutamine (continuous intravenous infusion of 2.5–10 μg/kg/minute) is useful in acute HF without hypotension.
- Inotropic agents (including milrinone and amrinone) can be used short term to stabilise cardiogenic shock and to allow for other therapies, including revascularisation, valve repair or initiation of more traditional therapies. In addition, inotropic agents can be used to bridge a patient to cardiac transplantation or insertion of a left ventricular assist device. Finally, inotropic agents can be used as palliation when HF becomes refractory and the patient is not a candidate for either cardiac transplantation or a ventricular assist device.
- Mechanical removal of fluid by thoracentesis, paracentesis and dialysis are measures used in severe cases.
- Miscellaneous:
  - Anticoagulation therapy is indicated in patients with HF who are at risk for thromboembolism (patients with atrial fibrillation, valvular heart disease, documented left ventricular thrombus or a history of embolic stroke). It may also be given in patients with a very low ejection fraction.
  - Ivabradine (an inhibitor of the hyperpolarisation-activated cyclic nucleotide-gated channel responsible for diastolic depolarisation of pacemaker cells in the SA node) is purely a heart rate-reducing agent. It may be used only in patients with normal sinus rhythm and discontinued if patients develop atrial fibrillation. (Table 7.37). It is contraindicated in patients with HFpEF.
  - Sodium-glucose cotransporter-2 (SGLT-2) inhibitors (dapagliflozin and empagliflozin) exhibit a beneficial class effect in patients with HFrEF (Table 7.37). They may also be useful in patients with HFpEF.
    - SGLT-2 inhibitors also reduce cardiovascular events and heart failure in patients with type 2 diabetes mellitus.
    - Exact mechanisms of beneficial effects are not known. Postulated mechanisms include improved glycaemic control in diabetic patients, diuresis, weight reduction and reduction in blood pressure.
    - Other potential mechanisms include improved cardiomyocyte calcium handling, enhanced myocardial energetics, induced autophagy and reduced epicardial fat.
- Treatment of iron-deficiency anaemia with intravenous iron.
- Routine use of anticoagulation in people with HF who remain in sinus rhythm is not recommended.
- Omega-3 polyunsaturated fatty acid (PUFA) supplementation is reasonable to use as adjunctive therapy in patients with NYHA class II–IV symptoms to reduce mortality and cardiovascular hospitalisations.
- Biventricular pacing and ICD in select group of patients.
  - Consider placement of an ICD to monitor heart rate and rhythm and to correct arrhythmia in patients with left ventricular dysfunction and an ejection fraction less than 30%.
  - Cardiac resynchronisation therapy (biventricular pacing) in patients with an ejection fraction <35%, a QRS interval >150 milliseconds or QRS >120 milliseconds with LBBB and symptoms despite maximum medical therapy.
- Surgical treatment options include left ventricular aneurysmectomy, left ventricular assist devices and cardiac transplantation.

SUMMARY OF MANAGEMENT OF HEART FAILURE

- The overall management of HF is summarised in Flowchart 7.9.
- Steps in managing patients with chronic HF based on New York Heart Association classification are shown in Table 7.38.

Q. Write a note on acute heart failure.

- Acute HF is rapid onset of new (de novo AHF) or worsening (acute decompensated HF) signs and symptoms of HF. The sudden reduction in cardiac output results in systemic hypotension without peripheral oedema.

CLINICAL CLASSIFICATION

- Clinically, classification is based on evidence of hypoperfusion and congestion (Table 7.39).
- Based on evidence of pulmonary congestion and hypoperfusion, AHF is classified into four types (Table 7.40).

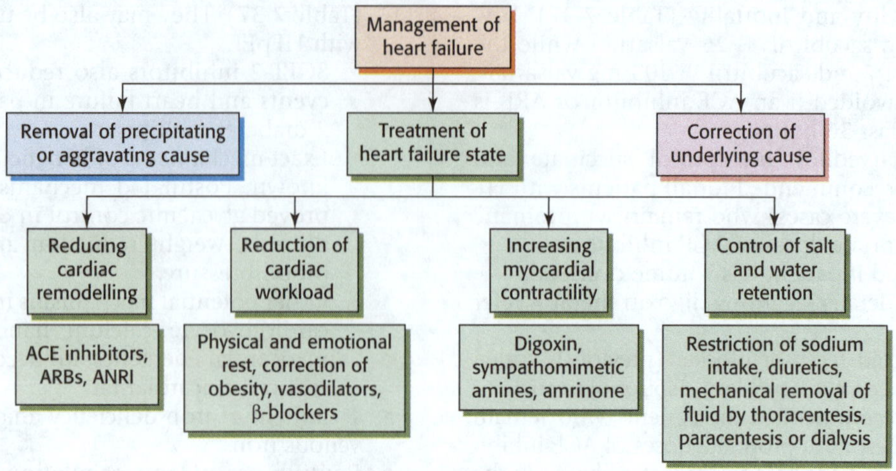

Flowchart 7.9 Management of Heart Failure.

TABLE 7.38 Steps in the Management of Chronic Heart Failure

Functional Class I	Functional Class II	Functional Class III	Functional Class IV
• Angiotensin receptor-neprilysin inhibitor (ARNI) • ACE inhibitors or angiotensin receptor blockers (if ARNI not possible to give) • β-Blockers	• Mild restriction of activity • Mild sodium restriction • ARNI • ACE inhibitors or angiotensin receptor blockers (if ARNI is not possible to give) • β-Blockers • Mineralocorticoid receptor antagonist (e.g. spironolactone) • SGLT-2 inhibitor (e.g. dapagliflozin and empagliflozin) • Diuretics (for volume overload) • Digoxin (if symptoms persist in presence of atrial fibrillation)	• Moderate restriction of activity • Moderate sodium restriction • As in class II patients • Ivabradine • Direct vasodilators (hydralazine plus nitrates)	• Severe restriction of activity • Severe sodium restriction • As in class III patients • Intravenous dopamine/dobutamine and amrinone (if required) • Cardiac resynchronisation therapy (if QRS >150 ms with LBBB in ECG) • Cardiac transplantation

TABLE 7.39 Evidences for Hypoperfusion and Congestion

Evidence of hypoperfusion	Narrow pulse pressure, symptomatic hypotension, cool extremities, impaired mental status
Evidence of pulmonary congestion	Orthopnoea/paroxysmal nocturnal dyspnoea, peripheral oedema, distended jugular veins, crepitations, hepatojugular reflux, ascites

TABLE 7.40 Classification of Acute Heart Failure

	Pulmonary Congestion Absent	Pulmonary Congestion Present
Hypoperfusion absent	Warm-dry	Warm-wet
Hypoperfusion present	Cold-dry	Cold-wet

TREATMENT

- Oxygen therapy and/or ventilatory support (NIV or mechanical ventilation).
- Correction of precipitating cause.
- Intravenous loop diuretics are key for symptomatic treatment in AHF patients with signs of significant fluid overload and congestion. De novo AHF or diuretic naïve patients should receive initial intravenous furosemide bolus of 20–40 mg, while patients on chronic oral diuretic therapy should be administered intravenous bolus of at least equal to their oral dose.
- Vasodilators should be used if systolic blood pressure >90 mmHg.
- Treatment of AHF is given in Table 7.41.

Q. Discuss the pathogenesis of ascites in heart failure.

- Increase in hepatic venous pressure and portal venous pressure results in transudation of fluid into the peritoneal cavity.
- Decrease in renal perfusion leads to activation of renin–angiotensin–aldosterone system, which in turn is responsible for salt and water retention (contributing to ascites and oedema).
- Congestion of gastrointestinal tract results in diminished appetite and protein intake, leading to hypoproteinaemia (contributing to ascites and oedema).
- Chronic congestive HF results in cardiac cirrhosis leading to ascites.

TABLE 7.41 Treatment of Acute Heart Failure

Warm-Dry	Cold-Dry	Warm-Wet		Cold-Wet	
		Predominant Congestion	**Predominant Hypertension**	**Systolic Blood Pressure <90 mmHg**	**Systolic Blood Pressure ≥90 mmHg**
Adjust oral therapy	• Fluid challenge • Consider inotropic agent if hypoperfusion persists	• Diuretic • Vasodilator • Consider ultrafiltration if resistant to diuretics	• Vasodilator • Diuretics	• Inotropic agents • Vasopressor in refractory cases • Consider mechanical circulatory support	• Vasodilator • Diuretic • Consider inotropic agents in refractory cases

Q. What are the features of left ventricular failure (left-sided failure; left heart failure)?

- Features of left ventricular failure are listed in Box 7.37.

Q. What are the features of right ventricular failure (right-sided failure; right heart failure)?

- Features of right ventricular failure are listed in Box 7.38.

Q. What is refractory or advanced heart failure? How will you manage a case of refractory heart failure?

- When the response to maximum therapy is inadequate, HF is considered to be refractory or advanced.

MANAGEMENT

- Look for and correct an underlying cause or precipitating cause of HF that was overlooked.
- Look for and correct the complications of overly vigorous therapy, for example digitalis toxicity, hypovolaemia or electrolyte imbalance.
- Overzealous treatment with diuretics is managed by temporary cessation of diuretic and salt restriction.
- Hyponatraemia is treated with temporary cessation of diuretic therapy and restriction of oral water intake.
- Intravenous vasodilator (sodium nitroprusside) along with dopamine or dobutamine may be useful in refractory cases.
- Intravenous nesiritide, a recombinant form of BNP, is beneficial. It is a potent vasodilator that provides both early and sustained reduction in filling pressures.
- Intravenous amrinone with an angiotensin-converting enzyme inhibitor (ACE inhibitor) in refractory cases.
- Cardiac transplantation to be considered if all the above-mentioned measures fail.

BOX 7.37 Features of Left Ventricular Failure

• Dyspnoea, orthopnoea	• Pulsus alternans
• Paroxysmal nocturnal dyspnoea (PND)	• Narrow pulse pressure
• Nocturia	• S_3 gallop of left ventricular origin
• Acute pulmonary oedema	• S_4 gallop
• Tachypnoea, pallor, sweating	• Basal crepitations

BOX 7.38 Features of Right Ventricular Failure

• Anorexia, nausea, vomiting	• Raised JVP, hepatojugular reflux
• Right hypochondrial pain	• Enlarged tender liver
• Peripheral oedema and cyanosis	• Ascites and pleural effusion

Q. Give a brief account of brain natriuretic peptide.

PATHOPHYSIOLOGY

- Cardiac myocardium secretes several natriuretic peptides to maintain stable blood pressure and plasma volume and to prevent excess salt and water retention.
- Atrial natriuretic peptide (ANP) is secreted by the atrial myocardium.
- BNP was initially isolated in porcine brains.
- In humans, BNP is primarily secreted by the ventricles in the heart as a response to left ventricular stretching or wall tension. It is activated only after a prolonged period of volume overload.
- Cardiac myocytes secrete a BNP precursor—proBNP, which consists of 108 amino acids. After it is secreted into the ventricles, proBNP is cleaved into the biologically active C-terminal portion (BNP) and the biologically inactive N-terminal (NT-proBNP) portion.
- Natriuretic peptides have several actions:
  - Downregulating the sympathetic nervous system.
  - Downregulating the renin–angiotensin system.
  - Facilitating natriuresis and diuresis through the afferent and efferent haemodynamic mechanisms of the kidney and distal tubules.
  - Decreasing peripheral vascular resistance.
  - Increasing smooth muscle relaxation.

UTILITY

- BNP levels are used in the diagnosis of HF. It can be useful in patients presenting in the emergency room when the clinical diagnosis of HF is uncertain.
- Elevated BNP levels also have been associated with renal failure (because of reduced clearance), pulmonary

embolism, pulmonary hypertension, chronic hypoxia, atrial fibrillation, acute myocardial infarction, obese patients and sepsis.

- Elevated BNP levels in patients with HF may be associated with an increased risk of death or cardiovascular events.
- BNP measurement is a potential tool for monitoring treatment response in patients with HF.

Q. Give a brief account of digoxin. (IM 1.24)

Q. What are the manifestations of digoxin toxicity? How will you manage a case of digoxin toxicity?

- Digoxin is a purified glycoside from the plant *Digitalis lanata*.

ACTION

- Increases myocardial contractility.
- Prolongs the refractory period of AV node, thereby slowing ventricular rate.
- Reflex vasodilatation from withdrawal of sympathetic constrictor activity in patients with HF.

PHARMACOKINETICS

- Bioavailability of digoxin tablet is 60%–80%.
- Plasma contains only 1% of the body stores of digoxin; the rest is tissue bound. Hence, digoxin is not effectively removed from body by dialysis.
- Concentration of digoxin in the heart is 30 times than that in the plasma.
- Half-life of digoxin is 1.6 days, and the effects may persist for 24–36 hours after the last dose.
- Eighty-five per cent of digoxin is excreted by the kidneys and the remaining 15% in the stool through biliary excretion.

INDICATIONS

- Cardiac arrhythmias, particularly supraventricular tachycardia and atrial fibrillation with a fast ventricular rate.
- Severe HF in sinus rhythm; most effective in those with impaired ventricular contractility. It has an impact on symptoms and hospitalisation rates but not on mortality in patients with HF.
- HF accompanied by atrial fibrillation or flutter with a rapid ventricular rate (often used in combination with β-blockers).

DOSAGE AND ROUTE OF ADMINISTRATION

- Digoxin loading is done by giving 0.25–0.5 mg orally or intravenously initially, followed by 0.25 mg 6 hourly to a total dose of 1–1.5 mg.
- Maintenance therapy is by a daily oral dose of 0.125–0.375 mg (0.5–1.5 tablets). Maintenance dose should be reduced in those with renal impairment.

TABLE 7.42 Digoxin Toxicity and Its Management

Cardiac Manifestations	Extracardiac Manifestations	Management of Toxicity
• Bradycardia • Multiple ventricular ectopics • Ventricular bigeminy • Paroxysmal atrial tachycardia with block • Ventricular tachycardia (VT) • Bidirectional VT • Ventricular fibrillation • Conduction defects	• Anorexia, nausea, vomiting, diarrhoea • Altered colour vision • Hyperkalaemia	• Stop digoxin, check urea, electrolytes and plasma digoxin concentration • Correct hypokalaemia and dehydration; avoid calcium for treating hyperkalaemia • Correct bradycardia using atropine or pacing • Treat atrial tachycardia with β-blockers • Treat VT with lignocaine or amiodarone • Antidigoxin antibodies in severe cases

DIGOXIN TOXICITY AND ITS MANAGEMENT

- Manifestations of digoxin toxicity and its management are described in Table 7.42.

Q. Discuss the role of diuretic therapy in the management of heart failure. (IM 1.24)

- Diuretics should be used if necessary to achieve euvolaemia in fluid-overloaded patients. In patients with systolic left ventricular dysfunction, use of diuretics as monotherapy should be avoided. They should always be combined with an ARNI or ACE inhibitor to maintain euvolaemia.
- The site of action, dosage, route of administration and individual side effects of the commonly used diuretics are summarised in Box 7.39.

RELATIVE POTENCY OF DIURETICS

- Low potency—acetazolamide and potassium-sparing diuretics.
- Medium potency—thiazides.
- High potency—loop diuretics.

THIAZIDES

- Mechanism of action:
  - Inhibit reabsorption of sodium and chloride mainly in the distal tubule and also in the proximal tubule to a lesser degree.
- Side effects:
  - Main side effects are hypokalaemia and metabolic alkalosis.
  - Other side effects—hyperuricaemia, hyperglycaemia, hyperlipidaemia, hyponatraemia, hypersensitivity.
- Notes:
  - Thiazides are ineffective when the glomerular filtration rate is less than 30 mL/minute.

7

BOX 7.39 Diuretics in Common Use

Group/Name	Site of Action	Dose/Day, Route	Individual Side Effects
• **Thiazides**			
• Chlorothiazide	Distal tubule	250–1000 mg PO, IV	Electrolyte disturbances
• Hydrochlorothiazide	Distal tubule	25–100 mg PO	Electrolyte disturbances
• Chlorthalidone	Distal tubule	25–100 mg PO	
• Indapamide	Distal tubule	2.5–5 mg PO	
• Metolazone	Proximal and distal tubules	2.5–20 mg PO	Hyperuricaemia, glucose intolerance
• **Carbonic anhydrase inhibitors**			
• Acetazolamide	Proximal tubule	250–500 mg PO	Hypokalaemia, acidosis, hypersensitivity
• **Loop diuretics**			
• Furosemide	Loop of Henle	20–60 mg PO, IV, IM	Ototoxicity
• Bumetanide	Loop of Henle	0.5–2 mg PO, IV, IM	Myalgia
• Ethacrynic acid	Loop of Henle	25–100 mg PO, IV	Ototoxicity
• Torasemide	Loop of Henle	5–100 mg PO, IV	Acid–base disturbances
• **Potassium-sparing diuretics**			
• Spironolactone	Distal tubule and collecting duct	50–200 mg PO	Gynaecomastia, hyperkalaemia, acidosis
• Triamterene	Distal tubule and collecting duct	100–200 mg PO	Hyperkalaemia, acidosis, renal stones
• Amiloride	Distal tubule and collecting duct	5–10 mg PO	Hyperkalaemia, acidosis

- Hypokalaemia induced by thiazides is prevented by either oral potassium chloride supplementation or combining with a potassium-sparing diuretic.
- Thiazides are useful in the initial management of chronic HF of mild to moderate severity.

CARBONIC ANHYDRASE INHIBITORS

- Acetazolamide is the only drug currently used.
- Mechanism of action:
  - Inhibits the reabsorption of sodium bicarbonate mainly in the proximal tubule, and to a lesser degree in the distal tubule.
- Side effects:
  - For side effects, refer to Box 7.39.
- Note:
  - Rarely used at present. May be useful in patients with high serum bicarbonate levels (e.g. cor pulmonale, metabolic alkalosis). Used in prophylaxis of acute mountain sickness.

LOOP DIURETICS

- Mechanism of action:
  - Inhibit reabsorption of sodium, chloride and potassium, mainly in the thick-ascending limb of loop of Henle and to a lesser degree in the proximal tubule.
  - Increase renal blood flow by cortical vasodilatation.
- Side effects:
  - Main side effects are hypokalaemia and metabolic alkalosis.
  - Other side effects are postural hypotension, hypomagnesaemia, hyperuricaemia, hyperglycaemia and hypersensitivity.
- Notes:
  - Loop diuretics are of particular value in three situations:
    - Acute pulmonary oedema.
    - Severe refractory HF.
    - When renal function is impaired.
  - All nonsteroidal antiinflammatory drugs including aspirin blunt the response of loop diuretics.
  - Hypokalaemia induced by loop diuretics is prevented by oral potassium chloride supplementation or combining it with a potassium-sparing diuretic.
  - In acute HF or worsening of chronic HF, intravenous loop diuretics are often used. When compared with intermittent bolus dosing, a loading dose followed by continuous infusion has been shown to have a larger diuretic and natriuretic effect.
  - Torasemide has been shown to have a greater bioavailability and more consistent rate of absorption in patients with HF than furosemide or bumetanide.

POTASSIUM-SPARING DIURETICS

- Mechanism of action:
  - Spironolactone and eplerenone are aldosterone antagonists and act on the distal tubule and collecting duct by competitive inhibition of aldosterone. These are called mineralocorticoid receptor inhibitors.
  - Amiloride and triamterene block sodium reabsorption and secondarily inhibit potassium secretion in the distal tubules.
- Side effects:
  - For individual side effects of the three drugs, refer Box 7.39.

- Notes:
  - Therapeutic efficacy of potassium-sparing diuretics is low when used alone. They are more effective in combination with thiazides or loop diuretics.
  - Potassium-sparing diuretics should not be administered alone to patients with hyperkalaemia, renal failure or hyponatraemia.

CHOICE OF DIURETIC

- Combined use of diuretics is indicated for three reasons:
  - To avoid electrolyte disturbances that occur with the isolated use of a powerful agent like a loop diuretic.
  - For increasing salt and water excretion in refractory oedema.
  - To avoid the ototoxicity from large doses of loop diuretics.
- Oral thiazides are useful for chronic cardiac oedema of mild to moderate degree.
- A loop diuretic given alone or in combination with a potassium-sparing diuretic is the agent of choice in severe HF refractory to other diuretics.
- A combination of a loop diuretic plus a thiazide plus a potassium-sparing diuretic is used in very severe HF.
- In severe HF, metolazone may be added with frequent measurement of creatinine and electrolytes.
- In patients who are unable to tolerate even low doses of spironolactone due to hyperkalaemia and renal dysfunction, amiloride or triamterene may be used.
- Diuretics should never be used alone to treat HF because they do not prevent the progression of disease or maintain clinical stability over time.

SPIRONOLACTONE AND EPLERENONE (MINERALOCORTICOID BLOCKERS; ALDOSTERONE ANTAGONISTS)

- These are very effective in patients with HF and severe secondary hyperaldosteronism and lower mortality and morbidity in patients with systolic dysfunction who have class III or IV symptoms despite use of other drugs and ejection fraction ≤35%. Since hyperkalaemia is a common adverse effect, spironolactone or eplerenone may be combined with other diuretics. The combination of ACE inhibitors, angiotensin receptor blockers and spironolactone (or eplerenone) should be used carefully because of a significantly increased risk for hyperkalaemia.

Q. Discuss the role of vasodilator therapy in heart failure. (IM 1.24)

Q. Briefly explain about afterload reduction therapy.

- HF is associated with:
  - Increase in left ventricular afterload from peripheral vasoconstriction.
  - Increase in preload from an elevated ventricular end-diastolic volume.
- Vasodilator therapy in HF is designed to reduce the preload or afterload or both of a failing ventricle. This is accomplished by relaxation of vascular smooth muscle in the periphery (vasodilatation).
- Vasodilators should not be used in patients with hypotension.

CLASSIFICATION

VENOUS DILATORS

- Act by relaxing the vascular smooth muscle of the systemic venous bed.
- They reduce the preload by pooling of blood in the venous bed and hence reducing the venous return, which results in a reduction in ventricular end-diastolic volume.

ARTERIOLAR DILATORS

- Act by relaxing the vascular smooth muscle of the arterial bed.
- They reduce the left ventricular afterload and hence increase the stroke volume.

BALANCED VASODILATORS

- Act by a generalised relaxing effect on the vascular smooth muscle of both venous and arterial beds.
- They reduce both preload and afterload.

VASODILATORS USED IN THE TREATMENT OF HEART FAILURE (Table 7.43)

- Angiotensin receptor-neprilysin inhibitors (ARNIs), angiotensin converting enzyme inhibitors (ACE inhibitors) or angiotensin receptor blockers (ARBs) are the drugs of choice in the treatment of HF and are superior to other vasodilators. An example of ARNI is sacubitril/valsartan.
- If the patient cannot tolerate ARNI or ACE inhibitors or has contraindications to their use, other vasodilators may be used. One of the recommended combinations is the use of hydralazine and long-acting nitrates. This combination improves clinical outcome and decreases mortality in patients with HF and depressed ejection fraction.

TABLE 7.43 Vasodilators Used in the Treatment of Heart Failure

Venous Dilators (Preload Reduction)	Arteriolar Dilators (Afterload Reduction)	Balanced Dilators (Preload and Afterload Reduction)
• Nitroglycerine • 10–200 µg/minute IV • 0.5–1 inch TID TD • 0.3–0.6 mg/dose SL • Isosorbide dinitrate • 10–60 mg TID PO	• Hydralazine • 25–100 mg TID PO	• Sodium nitroprusside • 10–300 µg/minute IV • Prazosin • 1–10 mg TID PO • Angiotensin receptor-neprilysin inhibitor • ACE inhibitors • Angiotensin receptor blockers

TD, transdermal; SL, sublingual; PO, per oral

- Intravenous vasodilators are used in acute HF.
- Nesiritide (synthetic form of BNP) is useful in acute left ventricular failure. Besides its vasodilatory effect, it also attenuates neurohormonal activity. It decreases sympathetic tone as well as inhibits production of renin, aldosterone and endothelin. Additionally, it promotes natriuresis and diuresis at the level of the kidney while maintaining glomerular filtration rate and renal blood flow. A concern with its use is a possibility of worsening of renal function, particularly in patients with systolic blood pressure <90 mmHg.

Q. What is the role of angiotensin-converting enzyme inhibitors in the management of heart failure? (IM 1.24)

Q. Explain the role of angiotensin-converting enzyme inhibitors in hypertension.

- ACE inhibitor therapy should be considered a priority in all patients with HF.
- Asymptomatic patients with a documented left ventricular systolic dysfunction should also be treated with an ACE inhibitor to delay or prevent the development of HF. ACE inhibitors also reduce the risk of myocardial infarction and sudden death in this setting.
- For a proper understanding of the ACE inhibitors, one should be familiar with the renin–angiotensin–aldosterone system. The renin–angiotensin–aldosterone system is summarised in Flowchart 7.10.
- ACE inhibitors inhibit the conversion of angiotensin I to angiotensin II. Hence, the ACE inhibitors counteract the actions of angiotensin II.
- They act in HF by the following:
  - The vasodilator effect that will reduce preload and afterload and so improves cardiac function.
  - Diuresis with elimination of sodium and water. Plasma potassium levels are preserved.
  - An important effect of ACE inhibitors is to reduce the cardiac remodelling that otherwise has a deleterious effect and is responsible for progression of HF, particularly in patients with ischaemic heart disease.
- They act in hypertension by:
  - Inhibiting the generation of angiotensin II that is a potent vasoconstrictor.
  - Inhibiting the degradation of bradykinin that is a potent vasodilator.
  - Altering prostaglandin production.
  - Blocking the angiotensin-mediated increase in sympathetic activity.

PRECAUTIONS WITH ANGIOTENSIN-CONVERTING ENZYME INHIBITORS

- Can cause profound hypotension with postural symptoms.
- Can cause deterioration in renal function, especially in patients with bilateral renal artery stenosis or pre-existing renal disease. So renal functions should be monitored.
- Severe hypotension can occur with the first dose, especially with captopril if given in the presence of hypovolaemia or hyponatraemia.
- Withhold diuretics for at least 24 hours before the initiation of therapy.
- Start the drug only with a small dose (e.g. 6.25 mg of captopril) while the patient is supine and under observation.

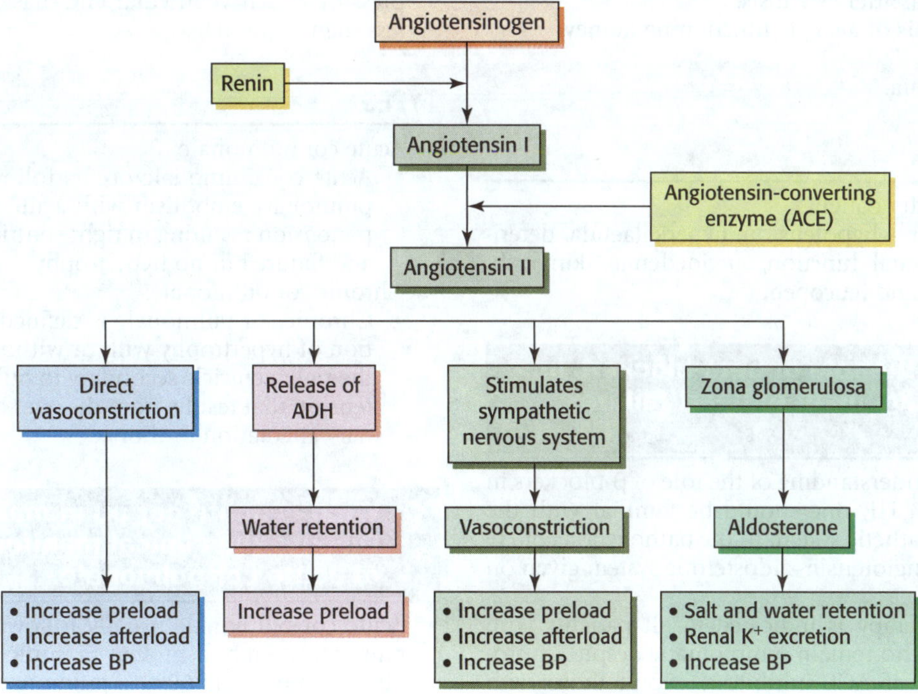

Flowchart 7.10 Renin–Angiotensin–Aldosterone System.

- Risk of hyperkalaemia with simultaneous administration of potassium supplements or potassium-sparing diuretics should be kept in mind.

COMMONLY USED ANGIOTENSIN-CONVERTING ENZYME INHIBITORS (Table 7.44)

TABLE 7.44 ACE Inhibitors

Drug	Initial Dose	Target Dose
• Captopril	6.25 mg TID	12.5–50 mg TID
• Enalapril	2.5 mg/day	10 mg BID
• Lisinopril	2.5 mg/day	20 mg/day
• Ramipril	1.25 mg/day	5 mg BID
• Perindopril	2 mg/day	8–16 mg OD

Note: Every effort should be made to uptitrate to the highest-tolerated dose of ACE inhibitor in patients with HF. The end point for blood pressure can be as low as 90 mmHg systolic blood pressure as long as the patient is asymptomatic. If this is not possible, a lower dose is preferable to none at all.

INDICATIONS

- Mild to severe forms of HF, particularly with systolic dysfunction.
- Hypertension (particularly with high plasma renin activity), renal or renovascular hypertension, accelerated hypertension and malignant hypertension.

Note: Angiotensin receptor antagonists (e.g. candesartan, valsartan, losartan) may be used as an alternative to ACE inhibitors for patients who are ACE intolerant.

CONTRAINDICATIONS

- Bilateral renal artery stenosis.
- Artery stenosis of a single functioning kidney.
- Pregnancy.
- Hyperkalaemia.

SIDE EFFECTS

- Common—dry cough.
- Less common—hypotension, hyperkalaemia, deterioration in renal function, angioedema, skin rash, altered taste and leucopenia.

Q. What is the role of beta-blockers in the management of heart failure? (IM 1.24)

- For proper understanding of the role of β-blockers in patients with HF, one should be familiar with the role of sympathetic system in the pathogenesis of HF (see renin–angiotensin–aldosterone system given on page 547).
- β-Blocker therapy is indicated in all patients with systolic HF who remain symptomatic despite appropriate doses of ACE inhibitors, except those with dyspnoea at rest, those who are volume overloaded, those who are haemodynamically unstable or those with contraindications to their use (bradycardia, bronchospasm, heart block). Those with asymptomatic systolic failure also benefit from the use of these agents.
- Commonly used β-blockers include carvedilol, metoprolol succinate (long acting) and bisoprolol (Table 7.45).
- The starting dose should be low which is doubled every 3 to 4 weeks until the patient is unable to tolerate it (due to bradycardia, hypotension or side effects) or the target dose is reached.

TABLE 7.45 Commonly Used Beta-Blockers in Heart Failure

Drug	Initial Dose	Target Dose
• Carvedilol	3.125 mg/day	12.5–25 mg/day
• Bisoprolol	1.25 mg/day	10 mg/day
• Metoprolol	25 mg/day	100–200 mg/day

Q. Define cor pulmonale. What are the types of cor pulmonale?

- Cor pulmonale is the dilatation and/or hypertrophy of right ventricle due to an increase in its afterload, which results from diseases of lung, pulmonary circulation or thorax, but without left-sided heart disease. The right heart dysfunction results from pulmonary hypertension.
- The presence of overt right HF is not essential to make the diagnosis of cor pulmonale but right HF is a common consequence.
- Pulmonary hypertension in cor pulmonale is defined as pulmonary arterial pressure above 25 mmHg with a pulmonary capillary wedge pressure, left atrial pressure or left ventricular end-diastolic pressure of less than 15 mmHg.

TYPES

- Acute cor pulmonale:
  - Acute cor pulmonale occurs following a massive pulmonary embolism with acute pulmonary hypertension resulting in right ventricular dilatation and failure but no hypertrophy.
- Chronic cor pulmonale:
  - Chronic cor pulmonale is defined as a combination of hypertrophy with or without dilatation of the right ventricle secondary to pulmonary hypertension that results from diseases of lung, pulmonary circulation or thorax.

Q. What is acute cor pulmonale? Discuss the clinical manifestations of acute cor pulmonale.

- Acute cor pulmonale usually follows acute massive pulmonary embolism that is sufficient enough to obstruct more than 60% of pulmonary circulation. It leads to acute pulmonary hypertension, acute right ventricular dilatation and failure. It can also occur due to ARDS.

CLINICAL FEATURES (Box 7.40)

BOX 7.40 Clinical Features of Acute Cor Pulmonale

Sign Related to Pulmonary Embolism	Signs of Acute Right Ventricular Failure
• Signs of deep venous thrombosis • Acute dyspnoea, haemoptysis • Syncope or cardiac arrest • Tachypnoea, tachycardia, hypotension • Chest pain	• Raised jugular venous pressure • Parasternal heave • Right ventricular third heart sound and gallop

Q. Discuss the aetiology, pathogenesis, clinical features, investigations and management of chronic cor pulmonale.

- Chronic cor pulmonale is defined as hypertrophy with or without dilatation of the right ventricle secondary to pulmonary hypertension, which results from diseases of lung, pulmonary circulation or thorax.

AETIOLOGY (Box 7.41)

- Chronic obstructive pulmonary disease (COPD—including chronic bronchitis and emphysema) causes more than 50% of cases of chronic cor pulmonale.
  - Patients with chronic bronchitis develop erythrocytosis, oedema and early onset of cor pulmonale (blue bloaters).
  - Patients with emphysema develop cor pulmonale later (pink puffers).
  - Chronic bronchial asthma rarely leads to chronic cor pulmonale.

BOX 7.41 Aetiology of Chronic Cor Pulmonale

Diseases of Lung:	Diseases of Pulmonary Circulation:
• Chronic obstructive pulmonary disease (COPD) • Chronic bronchial asthma (uncommon) • Pulmonary tuberculosis • Interstitial lung disease • Diffuse bronchiectasis • High-altitude dwelling • Cystic fibrosis • Pleural fibrosis	• Recurrent pulmonary thromboembolism • Primary pulmonary hypertension • Collagen vascular diseases • Chronic liver disease **Diseases of Thorax:** • Kyphoscoliosis • Neuromuscular diseases • Obesity • Sleep apnoea syndrome

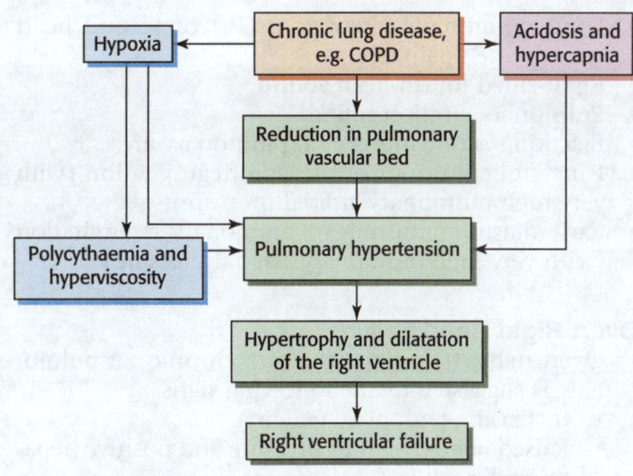

Flowchart 7.11 Pathogenesis of Chronic Cor Pulmonale.

PATHOGENESIS (Flowchart 7.11)

- Increased pulmonary vascular resistance and pulmonary hypertension are the central mechanisms in all cases of chronic cor pulmonale.
- Hypoxaemia not only promotes vasoconstriction but also contributes to the process of vascular remodelling by stimulating smooth muscle proliferation.
- Hypoxaemia produces polycythaemia and hyperviscosity which produce pulmonary hypertension.
- Other possible mechanisms include action of inflammatory mediators on pulmonary vasculature and endothelial dysfunction (disturbance in balanced release of mediators with vasodilatory properties such as nitric oxide or prostacyclin, and mediators with vasoconstrictive properties such as endothelin-1 or angiotensin).

CLINICAL FEATURES

SYMPTOMS

- There is no symptom that is specific for chronic cor pulmonale. There is overlap between symptoms of cor pulmonale and those due to underlying COPD.
  - Dyspnoea not relieved by sitting up, due to pulmonary hypertension.
  - Exertional dyspnoea not fully explained by the degree of underlying disease.
  - Rapid decline of arterial oxygenation on exercise.
  - Dry cough.
  - Fatigue.
  - Atypical anterior chest pain due to dilatation of the root of pulmonary artery.
  - Exercise-induced peripheral cyanosis and excessive daytime somnolence.
  - Swelling on feet.

SIGNS

- Tachypnoea, even on mild exertion.
- Pedal oedema.
- Prominent *a* waves on JVP.
- Right ventricular heave in the left parasternal region and epigastrium.

- Loud pulmonary component (P_2) of second heart sound, often palpable.
- Right-sided fourth heart sound.
- Pulmonary ejection sound.
- Ejection systolic murmur at pulmonary area.
- Pansystolic murmur of tricuspid regurgitation (with very high pulmonary arterial pressure).
- Early diastolic murmur of pulmonary regurgitation (with very high pulmonary arterial pressure).

Overt Right Heart Failure

- Overt right HF in a patient with chronic cor pulmonale is suggested by the following signs:
  - Increasing peripheral oedema.
  - Raised jugular venous pressure and positive hepatojugular reflux.
  - Tender hepatomegaly.
  - Cardiac enlargement.
  - Right ventricular third heart sound and a gallop rhythm.
- However, symptoms and signs of right HF as peripheral oedema, distended jugular veins and palpable liver can be observed in patients with COPD and cor pulmonale without right HF.

ADDITIONAL CLINICAL FEATURES IN CHRONIC BRONCHITIS (BLUE BLOATERS)

- Chronic cough with sputum production.
- Frequent mucopurulent exacerbations.
- Secondary erythrocytosis.
- Repeated episodes of right HF and respiratory failure.

ADDITIONAL CLINICAL FEATURES IN EMPHYSEMA (PINK PUFFERS)

- Severe exertional dyspnoea.
- Cough and sputum production are considerably less prominent.
- Erythrocytosis is uncommon.
- Right HF and respiratory failure usually occur late as a terminal event.

INVESTIGATIONS

- Chest radiography (cardiac enlargement due to dilatation of right ventricle, enlarged main and hilar pulmonary arterial shadows with peripheral vascular pruning).
- Electrocardiogram (features of right atrial enlargement and right ventricular hypertrophy).
- Arterial blood gas studies (hypoxia, hypercapnia).
- BNP (may be a useful biomarker for pulmonary hypertension in patients with COPD).
- Echocardiography (chamber hypertrophy and enlargement, elevated pulmonary systolic pressure by Doppler echocardiography).
- Ventilation–perfusion scan (for pulmonary embolism).
- CT pulmonary angiography (for acute pulmonary embolism).
- Right heart catheterisation (rarely required).

MANAGEMENT OF CHRONIC COR PULMONALE

- General measures.
- Additional measures in COPD-induced cor pulmonale.
- Surgical treatment.

GENERAL MEASURES

- Treatment to decrease pulmonary hypertension.
- Treatment of right HF.

Treatment to Decrease Pulmonary Hypertension

- Treatment of underlying disease.
- Oxygen therapy is the most important treatment in reducing pulmonary hypertension. In fact, long-term oxygen therapy is the only treatment shown to retard the progression of pulmonary hypertension.
  - Chronic oxygen therapy is initiated if the arterial oxygen tension is 55 mmHg or less.
  - Oxygen should be administered in a controlled manner. The inspired oxygen concentration is adjusted to produce PaO_2 of 60 mmHg or more.
  - Oxygen should be administered for a minimum period of 12–15 hours/day.

Treatment of Right Heart Failure

- Salt restriction.
- Digoxin (if associated with atrial fibrillation or left ventricular failure).
- Diuretics.
- Phlebotomy when haematocrit is more than 60%.
- Vasodilator therapy to reduce afterload with hydralazine and nifedipine appears to be beneficial if given for a short period. These are, however, not recommended because of their potential detrimental effects on gas exchange produced by inhibition of hypoxic pulmonary vasoconstriction and their lack of effectiveness after long-term treatment.
- Prostacycline analogues (epoprostenol and treprostinil) may be useful in some patients, although they have not been studied systematically in cor pulmonale secondary to lung diseases.
- Sildenafil, a phosphodiesterase-4 inhibitor, has also been used in the treatment of pulmonary hypertension with variable results.
- Bosentan, an endothelin-1 receptor blocker, has some role in idiopathic pulmonary hypertension.

ADDITIONAL MEASURES IN COPD-INDUCED COR PULMONALE

- Avoidance of airway irritants like tobacco smoke.
- Bronchial toilet for removal of secretions.
- Treatment of respiratory infections with antibiotics.
- Bronchodilators are useful.
- Corticosteroids may be beneficial in patients with bronchospasm.
- Tranquillisers, sedatives and narcotics are preferably avoided.

SURGICAL TREATMENT

- Pulmonary embolectomy in unresolved pulmonary emboli.
- Heart–lung transplantation in patients with primary pulmonary hypertension.

- Unilateral lung transplantation in patients with interstitial lung disease.

Q. Define rheumatic fever. Discuss the aetiology, pathogenesis, clinical features, investigations and management of rheumatic fever. Add a note on rheumatic fever prophylaxis.
(IM 1.27, IM 1.3, IM 1.9)

DEFINITION

- Rheumatic fever is an inflammatory disease occurring as a delayed sequel to pharyngeal infection with group A streptococci. It primarily involves the heart, joints, central nervous system, skin and subcutaneous tissues.

AETIOLOGY

- Rheumatic fever follows an antecedent pharyngeal infection with group A β-haemolytic *Streptococcus*. The latent period between the pharyngeal infection and the onset of rheumatic fever ranges from 1 to 5 weeks, the average duration being 19 days.
- Cutaneous streptococcal infection that commonly causes acute poststreptococcal glomerulonephritis has not been shown to cause rheumatic fever.
- The various serotypes of group A streptococci vary in their rheumatogenic potential. M-protein is one of the best-defined determinants of bacterial virulence. The highly prevalent M-type 12 usually does not produce rheumatic fever. M-type 5 commonly causes rheumatic fever. The other rheumatogenic serotypes include 1, 3, 6, 14, 18, 19 and 24.
- Fewer than 2% to 3% of previously healthy persons develop rheumatic fever following group A β-haemolytic streptococcal pharyngitis.

PATHOGENESIS

- Precise pathogenetic mechanisms of rheumatic fever have not been defined.

MOLECULAR MIMICRY

- *Streptococcus*-induced autoimmunity is believed to be the mechanism resulting in rheumatic process. Several streptococcal antigens have demonstrated cross-reactivity with cardiac and other tissues ('molecular mimicry').

STREPTOCOCCAL SUPERANTIGENS

- Superantigens are a unique group of glycoproteins synthesised by bacteria and viruses that can bridge class II major histocompatibility complex molecules to specific T-cell receptors, stimulating antigen binding. The T cells are activated to release cytokines or become cytotoxic, and these can become autoreactive.
- Some of the superantigens on streptococci include M-protein fragments and pyrogenic exotoxin that may have a role in the pathogenesis of rheumatic fever.
- Superantigens may also stimulate B lymphocytes. Streptococcal erythrogenic toxin may behave like a superantigen for B cell leading to production of autoreactive antibodies.

HOST FACTORS

- There is strong evidence that an autoimmune response to streptococcal antigens mediates the development of rheumatic fever only in a susceptible host (only 0.3%–3% of individuals with acute streptococcal pharyngitis go on to develop rheumatic fever).
- In India, HLA-DR3 is present more frequently in rheumatic fever patients. Also, Indians with rheumatic fever have low frequency of HLA-DR2.

EPIDEMIOLOGY

- Rheumatic fever is a worldwide disease. It is a major cause of death and disability in children and adolescents in socio-economically deprived areas.
- It is most prevalent in areas of poor economic conditions, overcrowding and substandard housing. All of these factors in general reflect the frequency and severity of streptococcal pharyngitis.
- It is common to see multiple cases among the siblings and others in the same family.
- In India, the annual incidence of rheumatic fever has been estimated to be between 0.18 and 0.3 per 1000 school children.
- The peak incidence is between 5 and 15 years. It is relatively rare in infants and young children younger than 5 years.
- No clear-cut sex predilection exists though certain clinical manifestations, such as mitral stenosis and Sydenham's chorea, have a female preponderance after puberty.

PATHOLOGY

- Acute rheumatic fever is characterised by exudative and proliferative inflammatory lesions of the connective tissues. It mainly involves the heart, joints and subcutaneous tissues.

HEART

- In the heart, all three layers (endocardium, myocardium and pericardium) are involved resulting in rheumatic pancarditis.
- Myocardium:
  - Myocardium shows the pathognomonic myocardial Aschoff body. Aschoff bodies are small granulomas with a central zone of fibrinoid degeneration surrounded by lymphocytes, plasma cells and large basophilic giant cells (Aschoff giant cells) and fibroblasts.
  - Aschoff bodies may persist for many years in chronic rheumatic inflammation, especially in those who develop severe mitral stenosis.
  - Eventually, the Aschoff body is converted into a spindle-shaped or triangular scar.
- Endocardium:
  - Rheumatic endocarditis produces verrucous valvulitis. It may later lead to healing with fibrous

thickening and adhesions of valve commissures, leaflets and chordae tendineae. End result of this is varying degrees of stenosis and regurgitation of valves.
  - Mitral valve is the most commonly involved, aortic valve next, tricuspid valve rarely and pulmonary valve almost never.
- Pericardium:
  - Pericarditis produces pericardial effusion and a thick serous exudate that gives the 'bread and butter' appearance macroscopically.

EXTRACARDIAC LESIONS

- Joint involvement with an effusion later healing without any residual deformity.
- Subcutaneous nodules showing many histological features similar to those of Aschoff body.
- Pleural lesions (fibrinous pleurisy).
- Pulmonary lesions (rheumatic pneumonitis).
- Nonspecific findings in the brain of patients with chorea.

CLINICAL MANIFESTATIONS

SORE THROAT

- Only two-thirds of patients remember having any upper respiratory symptoms in the past 1–5 weeks.

POLYARTHRITIS

- Arthritis is the most common major manifestation of rheumatic fever and is present in nearly 75% of cases.
- Classical presentation is acute migratory polyarthritis with features of a febrile illness.
- Most commonly involved joints are large joints of the extremities.
- Hips and small joints of hands and feet are affected occasionally.
- Involvement of spine, sternoclavicular and temporomandibular joints is rare.
- Affected joints show signs of inflammation with or without effusion.
- 'Migratory involvement' or 'flitting' nature is characteristic. As pain and swelling subside in one joint, others tend to get involved.
- Over a period of time, involved joints heal without any residual deformity. Jaccoud's arthritis is a rare deformity of the metacarpophalangeal joints following repeated attacks of rheumatic fever.
- To be acceptable as a major criterion for diagnosis:
  - Polyarthritis should involve two or more joints.
  - Should be associated with at least two minor manifestations.
  - Should be associated with a high titre of one of the streptococcal antibodies.

Post-streptococcal Reactive Arthritis

- Development of arthritis after an episode of group A streptococcal pharyngitis without other major criteria of acute rheumatic fever.
- Occurs 10 days after pharyngitis and does not respond readily to acetylsalicylic acid. Arthritis of rheumatic fever occurs 14–21 days after an episode of group A streptococcal pharyngitis and responds rapidly to acetylsalicylic acid.
- Arthritis of poststreptococcal reactive arthritis (PSRA) is cumulative and persistent, and can involve large joints, small joints or axial skeleton. On the other hand, arthritis of rheumatic fever is migratory and transient, and usually involves only the large joints.
- A small proportion of patients with PSRA may subsequently develop valvular heart disease; therefore, patients should be observed carefully for several months for evidence of carditis.

CARDITIS

- Features of carditis develop early (within 3 weeks of onset) and occur in 40%–50% of cases.
- It is more common in younger children, and may be asymptomatic and picked up on echocardiography only.
- Rheumatic fever may involve endocardium, myocardium and pericardium resulting in pancarditis.
- Involvement of myocardium alone without pericardial and endocardial involvement does not constitute major criterion.
- Usual sequence of events in carditis is given in Flowchart 7.12.

Manifestations of Carditis (Box 7.42)

- Myocarditis:
  - Tachycardia disproportionate to fever and persisting in sleep.
  - Dropped beats.
  - Third heart sound (S_3), fourth heart sound (S_4) or a summation gallop.
  - Foetal or 'tic-tac' quality of heart sounds.

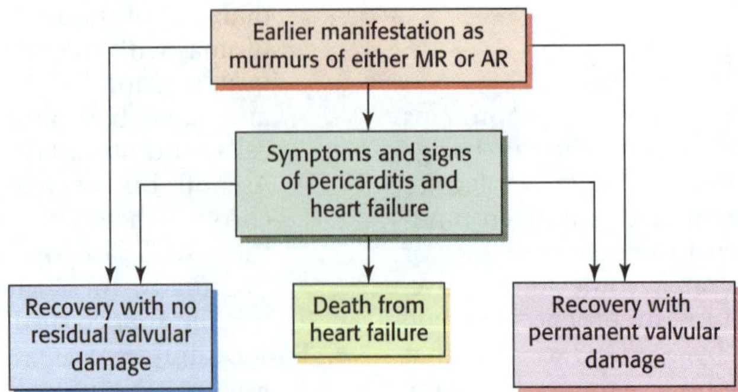

Flowchart 7.12 Usual Sequence of Events in Carditis.

BOX 7.42 Cardinal Features of Acute Rheumatic Carditis

- Murmurs
  - Apical systolic murmur
  - Apical mid-diastolic murmur (Carey–Coombs murmur)
  - Basal diastolic murmur
- Pericarditis
- Cardiomegaly
- Heart failure

  - Arrhythmias of which prolongation of PR interval is the commonest.
  - Features of HF.
- Endocarditis:
  - Apical systolic murmur of mitral regurgitation.
  - Apical mid-diastolic murmur (Carey Coombs' murmur) due to nodules on the mitral valve leaflets.
  - Basal early diastolic murmur of aortic regurgitation.
  - In an individual with previous RHD
    - A definite change in character of murmurs.
    - Appearance of a new significant murmur.
- Pericarditis:
  - Pericardial pain.
  - Pericardial friction rub.
  - Pericardial effusion (uncommon and always small).

Diagnosis of Carditis

- Requires the presence of one or more of the following:
  - Appearance of or change in the character of organic murmurs.
  - Cardiomegaly.
  - Pericarditis or pericardial effusion.
  - HF.

SUBCUTANEOUS NODULES

- Subcutaneous nodules are usually associated with severe carditis and tend to occur several weeks after its onset.
- Description—small, pea-sized, painless nodules over bony prominences.
- Common sites—extensor tendons of hands and feet, elbows, margins of patellae, scalp, occiput, over scapulae and over spinous processes of vertebrae.
- Easily missed as skin over them is not inflamed.
- They usually persist for 1 to 2 weeks.

ERYTHEMA MARGINATUM

- Occurs in nearly 10% of cases of acute rheumatic fever.
- Characterised by erythematous pink rashes with a clear centre and round or serpiginous margins (Fig. 7.44). These rashes are transient, migrating from place to place, nonpruritic, not indurated and blanch on pressure. They are brought on by application of heat.
- They are most commonly seen on the trunk and proximal parts of extremities, but never on face.

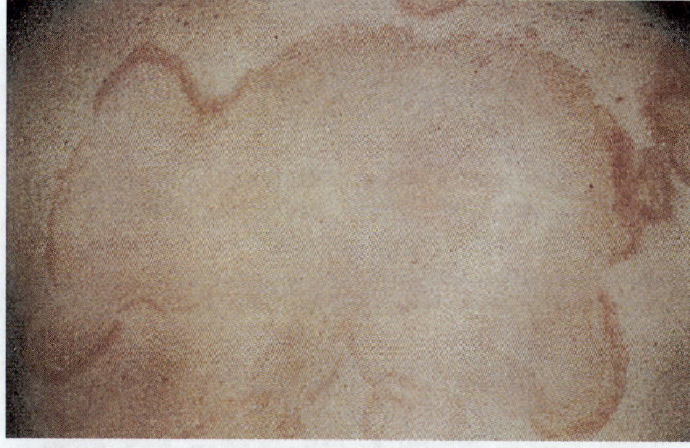

Fig. 7.44 Erythema marginatum (note serpiginous margins with clear centre).

CHOREA (SYDENHAM'S CHOREA; CHOREA MINOR; SAINT VITUS' DANCE)

- For a detailed description and management of chorea, refer page 365 and also to page 556.
- Chorea usually appears after a long latent period (up to 6 months) after the initial streptococcal infection.
- It occurs in nearly 15% of first attacks of acute rheumatic fever and is most common between the ages of 7 and 14 years. It is rare after puberty.
- Chorea is characterised by sudden, aimless, irregular movements associated with muscle weakness, emotional instability, obsessions and compulsions, tics and psychotic features.
- Pure chorea is the term used when no previous rheumatic manifestations are noted.

OTHER CLINICAL MANIFESTATIONS OF RHEUMATIC FEVER

- Other clinical manifestations include fever, arthralgia, abdominal pain and epistaxis.

DURATION OF ATTACK

- The average duration of an untreated attack of acute rheumatic fever is approximately 3 months.
- Chronic rheumatic fever, generally defined as disease persisting for longer than 6 months, occurs in less than 5% of cases and is a cause of persisting HF.

LABORATORY FEATURES

ISOLATION OF GROUP A STREPTOCOCCI

- Group A streptococci may be isolated by throat culture only in a minority of cases. Hence, serological tests are preferred.

STREPTOCOCCAL ANTIBODY TESTS (SEROLOGICAL TESTS)

- These tests confirm a recent streptococcal infection.
- Streptococcal antibody levels are raised in the early stages of acute rheumatic fever. However, their levels may be low or declining in two situations:
  - When the interval between the streptococcal pharyngeal infection and detection of rheumatic fever is more than 2 months (e.g. chorea).
  - In those patients whose only major manifestation is rheumatic carditis.
- Common serological tests done are as follows:
  - Antistreptolysin O (ASO).
  - Anti-DNase B.
  - Antihyaluronidase (AH).
  - Antistreptozyme (ASTZ).

- Single titres of ASO more than 250 Todd units in adults and 333 Todd units in children older than 5 years are taken as positive. However, a rising titre is even more significant. ASO test is positive in 80% of cases.
- ASTZ test is a very sensitive indicator of recent streptococcal infection. Titres more than 200 units/mL are considered positive. The real value of ASTZ test is in ruling out rheumatic fever.
- These four tests when combined together give an accuracy rate of more than 95%.

ACUTE-PHASE REACTANTS

- These tests confirm the presence of an inflammatory process, but are nonspecific.
  - Erythrocyte sedimentation rate (ESR) is raised.
  - C-reactive protein (CRP) is raised.
- These two are often normal in chorea.

OTHER TESTS CONFIRMING AN INFLAMMATORY REACTION

- Polymorphonuclear leucocytosis.
- Increase in serum complements.
- Increase in serum mucoproteins, α_2 and γ globulin levels.
- Anaemia due to suppression of erythropoiesis.

ELECTROCARDIOGRAM

- The most consistent abnormality is a prolongation of the PR interval.
- Less common findings are second-degree AV block and some other nonspecific changes.

CHEST RADIOGRAPHY

- Chest radiography may show evidence of cardiac failure.
  - Cardiomegaly.
  - Pulmonary congestion.

ECHOCARDIOGRAPHY

- Echocardiography can detect:
  - Myocardial dysfunction.
  - Valvular dysfunction.
  - Pericardial effusion.

DIAGNOSIS OF ACUTE RHEUMATIC FEVER

- For diagnosis, modified T. Duckett Jones criteria (revised Jones criteria) or WHO criteria are applied.

REVISED JONES CRITERIA (1992)

- Revised Jones criteria (1992) are for diagnosis of first episode of acute rheumatic fever (Table 7.46).
- Two major manifestations or one major and two minor manifestations indicate a high probability, with one supporting evidence of preceding streptococcal infection, for example:
  - Recent scarlet fever.
  - Positive throat culture for group A *Streptococcus.*
  - Increased streptococcal antibodies.

TABLE 7.46 Revised Jones' Criteria to Diagnose First Episode of Rheumatic Fever (1992)

Major Manifestations	Minor Manifestations
• Carditis • Polyarthritis • Chorea • Erythema marginatum • Subcutaneous nodules	• Fever • Arthralgia • Previous rheumatic fever or rheumatic heart disease • Raised ESR • Positive CRP • Prolonged PR interval

BOX 7.43 WHO Criteria for Diagnosis of Rheumatic Fever

- First episode—as per Jones' criteria (1992)
- Recurrent episode:
  - In a patient without established RHD: as per first episode
  - In a patient with established RHD: requires only two minor manifestations plus evidence of antecedent group A *Streptococcus* infection as per Jones' criteria
- Chorea and indolent carditis do not require evidence of antecedent group A *Streptococcus* infection or other major criteria

WHO CRITERIA

- WHO criteria can be used for both first episode and recurrent episodes of acute rheumatic fever (Box 7.43). Supporting evidence of preceding streptococcal infection also includes positive rapid antigen test for group A streptococci on throat swab.

REVISED JONES' CRITERIA (2015)

- In the revised 2015 Jones criteria, a low- and medium-to-high-risk population was identified (Table 7.47). India comes under high-risk category.
- A low-risk population is one in which cases of acute RF occur in ≤2/100,000 school-age children or rheumatic heart disease is diagnosed in ≤1/1000 patients at any age during 1 year. Diagnosis of first episode of RF

TABLE 7.47 Revised Jones' Criteria (2015) for First and Subsequent Attacks of Rheumatic Fever

Major Criteria	
Low-Risk Population	**High-Risk Population**
• Carditis (clinical or by echocardiography) • Arthritis—only polyarthritis • Chorea • Erythema marginatum • Subcutaneous nodules	• Carditis (clinical or by echocardiography) • Arthritis—monoarthritis or polyarthritis • Polyarthralgia • Chorea • Erythema marginatum • Subcutaneous nodules
Minor Criteria	
Low-Risk Population	**High-Risk Population**
• Polyarthralgia • Fever (≥38.5°C) • ESR ≥60 mm/hour and/or CRP ≥3.0 mg/dL • Prolonged PR interval (if there is no carditis as a major criterion)	• Monoarthralgia • Fever (≥38.0°C) • ESR ≥30 mm/hour and/or CRP ≥3.0 mg/dL • Prolonged PR interval (if there is no carditis as a major criterion)

requires evidence of antecedent group A beta-haemolytic streptococcal infection along with two major criteria or one major and two minor criteria.
- Diagnosis of subsequent episodes of RF requires a confirmation of two major criteria or one major and two minor criteria or three minor criteria (plus evidence of preceding group A streptococcal infection).

MANAGEMENT OF ACUTE RHEUMATIC FEVER

BED REST

- Patients who have not had carditis should be advised bed rest until temperature and ESR are normal.
- Patients who have had carditis should continue to have bed rest for 2–6 weeks after the ESR and temperature have returned to normal.

ANTISTREPTOCOCCAL THERAPY

- A course of antibiotic should be given to eradicate the streptococci, even if the throat culture is negative. One of the following regimens may be used:
  - Single injection of benzathine penicillin 1.2 million units intramuscularly.
  - Daily injection of procaine penicillin 600,000 units intramuscularly for 10 days.
  - Oral erythromycin 20–40 mg/kg/day in three divided doses or azithromycin in a dose of 500 mg once a day for 5 days in patients who are sensitive to penicillin.

SALICYLATES

- Aspirin is effective in providing symptomatic relief.
- Aspirin is started at doses of 60 mg/kg/day in six divided doses. Dose is increased gradually until the drug produces either a clinical improvement or systemic toxicity (tinnitus, headache or hyperpnoea). This dose might go up to 120 mg/kg/day or a maximum of 8 g/day.
- Aspirin at this dose should be continued until the ESR is normal and then gradually tapered over 4–6 weeks.

CORTICOSTEROIDS

- Indications:
  - Patients who have severe carditis manifested by HF not responding to aspirin.
  - Patients with severe arthritis whose symptoms and signs are not adequately suppressed by aspirin.
- Prednisolone is given orally at a dose of 60–120 mg/day in four divided doses until the ESR is normal. It is then gradually tailed off over a period of 4–6 weeks.
- To prevent a 'poststeroid rebound', an 'overlap' course of aspirin may be added when the steroid is being tapered off. Aspirin is then continued for an additional 2 to 3 weeks.
- Monitoring the corticosteroid or aspirin therapy during acute phase as well as while being tapered should be based on indices of healing process:
  - ESR
  - CRP

SUPPORTIVE THERAPY

- Includes treatment of HF, valvular lesions, heart blocks and chorea.

PREVENTION OF RHEUMATIC FEVER

- Prevention of rheumatic fever includes:
  - 'Primary prevention'—prevention of initial rheumatic attacks.
  - 'Secondary prevention'—prevention of recurrence of rheumatic fever.

PRIMARY PREVENTION

- Primary prevention can be summarised as 'accurate diagnosis and treatment of group A streptococcal pharyngeal infection'.
- An outbreak of rheumatic fever in a closed population is best treated by mass penicillin prophylaxis.
- Established streptococcal pharyngitis can be treated by procaine penicillin, benzathine penicillin or oral penicillin, or erythromycin or azithromycin.
- In communities where rheumatic fever is endemic, sore throat in children (3–15 years) should be regarded as streptococcal infection and be treated as such unless any one of the following clinical characteristics is present: ulceration, hoarseness, watery nasal secretion or conjunctivitis.

SECONDARY PREVENTION (RHEUMATIC FEVER PROPHYLAXIS)

- Rheumatic fever prophylaxis should be given to all patients who have experienced a documented attack of rheumatic fever.
- Duration of prophylaxis is controversial. Broad outlines are as follows:
  - No carditis: For 5 years or until 18 years of age (whichever is longer).
  - Resolved carditis: For 10 years or until 25 years of age (whichever is longer).
  - Severe RHD or if surgery is required: Lifelong or at least till the age of 40 years.
- Decision to continue prophylaxis beyond 5 or 10 years (in first or second group mentioned above) depends on many variables like age of the patient, relative risk of acquiring infection and socioeconomic state.
- Regimens: One of the following regimens may be used:
  - Intramuscular injection of 1.2 million units of benzathine penicillin every 3 weeks (most efficient regimen).
  - Oral penicillin V 500 mg twice a day (less effective than benzathine penicillin).
  - Sulphadiazine 1 g/day orally as a single dose (in those allergic to penicillins).
  - Erythromycin 250 mg twice a day orally or azithromycin 500 mg once a day (in those allergic to penicillins and sulpha).

Q. Discuss the aetiology, clinical features and management of rheumatic chorea (Sydenham's chorea; chorea minor; Saint Vitus' dance).

DEFINITION

- Rheumatic chorea is a syndrome characterised by choreic movements, muscle weakness and emotional instability (also refer page 365).

AETIOLOGY

- Pharyngeal infection by group A streptococci.
- Chorea is a delayed manifestation of rheumatic fever. Often, there is a long latent period of up to 6 months.
- When no previous rheumatic manifestations are noted, the term pure chorea is used.
- Chorea is more common in females in the age group 5–15 years.

CLINICAL FEATURES

- Mild forms will appear like increased fidgetiness and may be difficult to diagnose. Following three signs are helpful in mild cases:
  - 'Milkmaid's grip'—it is due to inability to maintain muscular contraction. When the patient is asked to squeeze the examiner's fingers, a squeezing and relaxing motion (like milking a cow) occurs, which is described as milkmaid's grip.
  - 'Bag-of-worms appearance'—this is asynchronous contraction of the lingual muscles.
  - 'Jack-in-the-box sign'—when the patient is asked to keep the tongue protruded out, it retracts involuntarily.
- Well-established cases are easy to diagnose. There are intermittent or continuous, fast, jerky, involuntary movements of the extremities that interfere with normal activity. Movements may be more on one side (hemichorea). Facial chorea results in frequent grimacing, blinking and slurring of speech. These movements subside in sleep and get worsened with emotional disturbances, and during voluntary movements.
- In severe cases, the person is unable to get up or sit and has violent continuous jerks that may cause physical injury.

ADDITIONAL FEATURES

- Hypotonia.
- Pendular knee jerks.
- Generalised muscular weakness (mild).
- Emotional instability.

MANAGEMENT

- Complete mental and physical rest.
- Keep the patient in a quiet room.
- Padded sideboards for beds to prevent injury.
- Haloperidol or sodium valproate with diazepam.
- Rheumatic fever prophylaxis.

Q. Discuss the aetiology, pathophysiology, clinical features, investigations and complications of mitral stenosis.

Q. How do you grade the severity of mitral stenosis based on mitral valve orifice size?

Q. Explain briefly about juvenile mitral stenosis and paediatric mitral stenosis.

ANATOMY OF NORMAL MITRAL VALVE

- The mitral valve apparatus is a funnel-shaped structure with its apex in the left ventricle.
- Normal mitral valve orifice is about 4–6 cm^2 (average 5 cm^2).
- The mitral valve apparatus has a mitral annulus and two leaflets, namely anterior mitral leaflet (AML) and posterior mitral leaflet (PML). The two leaflets are attached by about 120 chordae tendineae to 2 papillary muscles.

ALTERED ANATOMY IN RHEUMATIC MITRAL STENOSIS

PRIMARY PATHOLOGICAL FEATURES

- Thickened mitral cusps with or without calcification.
- Fusion of valve commissures (major cause of obstruction).
- Shortening and fusion of chordae tendineae.

SECONDARY PATHOLOGICAL FEATURES

- Left atrial hypertrophy and dilatation.
- Left atrial thrombi.
- Changes of venous and arterial hypertension in pulmonary vasculature.
- Right ventricular hypertrophy.

AETIOLOGY OF MITRAL STENOSIS

- Mitral stenosis can be caused by several diseases, most common being rheumatic fever (Box 7.44).

BOX 7.44 Mitral Stenosis: Aetiology

• Rheumatic fever	• Malignant carcinoid
• Congenital mitral stenosis	• Gout
• Coxsackie B virus carditis	• Mitral annular calcification
• Systemic lupus erythematosus	• Mucopolysaccharidosis
• Atrial myxoma (behaves like mitral stenosis)	• Infective endocarditis (extremely rare)
• Methysergide treatment	• Rheumatoid arthritis (extremely rare)

- Rheumatic fever is the most common cause of mitral stenosis. But only about one-half of the patients with mitral stenosis will give a history of rheumatic fever or chorea.
- Two-thirds of all patients with mitral stenosis are females.
- In India, the latent period from the first attack of rheumatic fever to the onset of symptoms of mitral stenosis is much shorter than in the West (where it is average 20 years). This period may be as short as 1 to 2 years. This is due to repeated attacks of severe carditis in India.
- Juvenile mitral stenosis is common in India. The clinical manifestations occur below the age of 19 years.
- Paediatric mitral stenosis indicates development of clinical manifestations below the age of 12 years.

SEVERITY OF STENOSIS ACCORDING TO MITRAL VALVE SIZE

- Severity of mitral stenosis can be graded according to mitral valve size as shown in Table 7.48.

PATHOPHYSIOLOGY AND HAEMODYNAMICS

- In mitral stenosis, the obstruction to the flow of blood from left atrium to left ventricle leads to elevation in left atrial pressure (up to 25 mmHg in severe cases). This rise in left atrial pressure occurs only during exercise in the initial stages, but later it remains elevated even at rest.
- The elevated left atrial pressure is reflected back in the pulmonary veins resulting in pulmonary venous hypertension.
- Subsequently, pulmonary arterial hypertension develops. Symptoms and signs of pulmonary venous hypertension abate when pulmonary arterial hypertension sets in.
- Pulmonary arterial hypertension (pulmonary hypertension) results from the following:
  - 'Passive pulmonary hypertension'—passive backward transmission of elevated left atrial pressure.
  - 'Reactive pulmonary hypertension'—reflex spasm of pulmonary arterioles in response to elevated pulmonary venous and left atrial pressure.
  - Organic obliterative changes in the pulmonary vascular bed.
- This chronic pulmonary hypertension results in the following consequences:
  - Right ventricular hypertrophy and later dilatation, ultimately resulting in right ventricular failure.
  - Functional tricuspid regurgitation from tricuspid valve ring dilatation secondary to right ventricular dilatation.
  - Pulmonary incompetence (regurgitation) due to pulmonary valve ring dilatation.
- The elevated left atrial pressure results in left atrial dilatation. This enlarged left atrium is prone to:
  - Atrial fibrillation.
  - Stasis of blood with thrombus formation.
  - Detachment of the thrombus resulting in systemic embolism.
- Ejection fraction of left ventricle reduced in approximately one-third of patients due to:
  - Decreased preload from impaired filling.
  - Increased afterload secondary to reflex vasoconstriction (secondary to reduced cardiac output).
- Patients with severe mitral stenosis easily decompensate with tachycardia (due to shortened diastolic period during which flow from left atrium to left ventricle occurs) or high flow.
- Atrial contraction helps to maintain flow across the stenotic mitral valve; atrial fibrillation, which is associated with tachycardia, irregular RR interval and lack of atrial contraction, is often an important precipitating factor for symptoms of dyspnoea.
- Flowchart 7.13 summarises pathophysiology of mitral stenosis.

TABLE 7.48 Severity of Mitral Stenosis as Per Mitral Valve Size

Severity/Stage	Mitral Valve Orifice
• Minimal	More than 2.5 cm^2
• Mild	1.4–2.5 cm^2
• Moderate	1.0–1.4 cm^2
• Severe (critical, tight)	Less than 1.0 cm^2
	(Normal mitral valve orifice is 4–6 cm^2)

CLINICAL FEATURES

SYMPTOMS

- Mild to moderate mitral stenosis may remain asymptomatic. Lymphatic hyperfunction in such patients may help prevent pulmonary congestion and its attendant symptoms.
- The natural history of mitral stenosis is such that once the patient becomes symptomatic, there is gradual and steady deterioration. Persistent inflammatory valve damage and haemodynamic injury contribute to gradual progression. Death occurs in 2–5 years unless the stenosis is corrected.

Dyspnoea

- Dyspnoea is initially exertional, but gradually progresses to a state of breathlessness even at rest.
- Dyspnoea results from pulmonary venous congestion occurring as a result of pulmonary venous hypertension. The fluid is driven out of the pulmonary capillaries into the interstitium, which leads to a decrease in the compliance of the lungs, and consequently increases the work of breathing. This results in dyspnoea.
- Severe exertion, excitement, fever, anaemia, sexual intercourse, pregnancy, thyrotoxicosis and atrial fibrillation can all precipitate or aggravate dyspnoea by elevation of pulmonary capillary pressure.

Orthopnoea and Paroxysmal Nocturnal Dyspnoea

- In the supine position, there is increased venous return to the heart, which will increase pulmonary venous pressure, resulting in orthopnoea and PND.

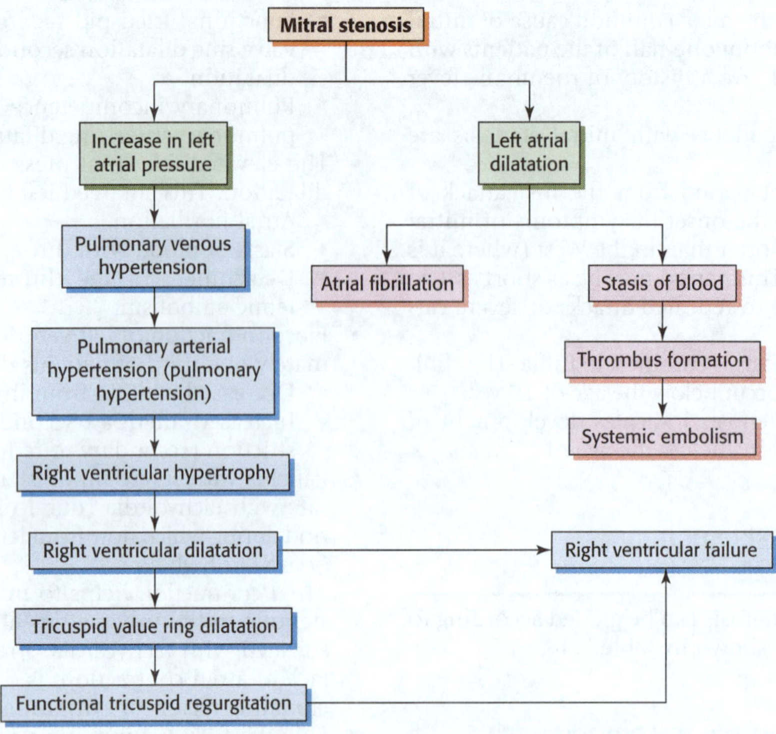

Flowchart 7.13 Pathophysiology of Mitral Stenosis.

Pulmonary Oedema

- Pulmonary oedema develops when pulmonary capillary pressure exceeds 25 mmHg and the resulting transudate cannot be cleared by lymphatics.
- Common precipitating factors of pulmonary oedema are the same as those for dyspnoea.
- Pulmonary oedema can develop in two forms, either suddenly or gradually, preceded by orthopnoea and PND.

Haemoptysis

- Causes of haemoptysis in mitral stenosis are listed in Box 7.45.
- Haemoptysis subsides as pulmonary arterial hypertension develops.

Winter Bronchitis

- Patients with mitral stenosis are prone to recurrent attacks of bronchitis, particularly in the winter season.

Other Symptoms

- Palpitation.
- Fatigue, loss of appetite and chest pain due to pulmonary hypertension and HF.

BOX 7.45 Causes of Haemoptysis is Mitral Stenosis

- Rupture of pulmonary–bronchial venous connections secondary to pulmonary venous hypertension
- Pink frothy sputum of pulmonary oedema
- Blood-streaked sputum of recurrent bronchitis
- Pulmonary infarction due to pulmonary embolism

- Symptoms of right ventricular failure like peripheral oedema and right hypochondrial pain.
- Symptoms related to complications may be present (vide infra).

PHYSICAL SIGNS

General Examination

- Peripheral and facial cyanosis occurs in extremely severe cases.
- Mitral facies is seen in severe cases with low cardiac output and peripheral vasoconstriction. The lips and face are cyanotic. Despite this cyanosis, there may be a 'malar flush' or 'florid countenance' (florid appearance) due to dilated veins in the cheek.
- Peripheral oedema in HF.

Pulse

- Low volume in severe mitral stenosis.
- Irregularly irregular rhythm and varying volume in atrial fibrillation.

Blood Pressure

- May be slightly reduced.

Jugular Veins

- Jugular venous pressure is elevated in HF.
- Jugular venous pulse.
  - Prominent *a* waves with pulmonary hypertension.
  - Absent *a* waves in atrial fibrillation.
  - Prominent *v* waves (*c–v* waves) and rapid *y* descent in functional tricuspid regurgitation.

Inspection and Palpation

- Precordial bulge in long-standing cases with onset of illness early in life.

- Apex beat is normal in position in isolated mitral stenosis, whereas it may be shifted with the development of right ventricular hypertrophy.
- Apex beat is tapping in character due to the loud palpable first heart sound.
- Diastolic thrill at the apex, which is best felt with the patient in left lateral position with breath held in expiration.
- Exercise accentuates the thrill.
- Visible and palpable pulsations in the second left intercostal space from the underlying dilated pulmonary artery in pulmonary hypertension.
- Palpable pulmonary component of the second heart sound (P_2) in the pulmonary area due to pulmonary hypertension.
- Visible and palpable left parasternal heave and epigastric pulsation due to right ventricular hypertrophy.

Auscultation

Loud First Heart Sound

- This is an important finding in mitral stenosis. It is due to closure of the diseased mitral valve with rapid apposition of the leaflets.
- In associated atrial fibrillation, the first heart sound varies in intensity.
- A low intensity of the first heart sound may occur in some conditions (Box 7.46).

Loud Second Heart Sound

- This is an important sign of pulmonary hypertension.
- The second heart sound is closely split and the pulmonary component of the second heart sound (P_2) is accentuated.

Mitral Opening Snap

- OS is a sharp, snappy sound occurring in early diastole, following aortic valve closure (A_2).
- It is best heard during expiration, at or just medial to the cardiac apex (sometimes, it is widely heard).
- OS occurs due to abrupt halt in leaflet motion in early diastole after rapid initial rapid opening, due to fusion at the leaflet tips.
- Significance:
  - A_2–OS interval signifies severity of mitral stenosis, being close with tighter stenosis. It varies from 0.04 to 0.12 seconds.
  - The OS may become dull (soft) or even absent in severe mitral stenosis if there is calcification or severe fibrosis of the mitral valve. It may also be absent in severe mitral stenosis due to extreme clockwise rotation of heart.

BOX 7.46 Causes of Reduced Intensity of First Heart Sound in Mitral Stenosis

- Dominant associated aortic regurgitation
- Dominant associated mitral regurgitation
- Calcification and/or fibrosis of the mitral valve

Ejection Click

- A pulmonary systolic ejection click may be heard in severe pulmonary hypertension with marked dilatation of pulmonary artery.

Murmur of Mitral Stenosis

- This is a diastolic murmur well localised to the mitral area. It is low pitched, rough and rumbling in character, best heard at the apex with the bell of the stethoscope, with the patient in left lateral position and during expiration. Murmur is accentuated by exercise carried out just before auscultation.
- In early stages of mitral stenosis, the murmur is confined to mid-diastole or presystole. Still later, the murmur becomes longer and extends to the first heart sound (S_1), often with a presystolic accentuation.
- In patients with sinus rhythm, the murmur is accentuated during atrial systole ('presystolic accentuation') as the atrial contraction increases the rate of flow across the stenosed mitral valve.
- The presystolic accentuation of the murmur is present:
  - With regular sinus rhythm.
  - During long RR interval in atrial fibrillation.
- The presystolic accentuation of the murmur is absent (even with significant mitral stenosis) in:
  - Rigid or calcified mitral valve.
  - Very low cardiac output.
  - Atrial fibrillation (although rarely it may be present during long RR interval).
- Duration of the murmur is variable. In general, the duration of the murmur correlates with the severity of stenosis (the longer the murmur, the more severe the stenosis).
- The classical diastolic murmur of severe mitral stenosis (mitral valve orifice less than 1 cm^2) starts immediately after the OS, is characteristically long and loud, and is present throughout the rest of the diastole with a presystolic accentuation, ending in a loud first heart sound.

Murmur of Tricuspid Regurgitation

- This is a loud pansystolic murmur heard at the lower left sternal border. It is accentuated during inspiration (De-Carvallo's sign). This murmur should be differentiated from an organic mitral regurgitation murmur, which could be an associated lesion.

Murmur of Pulmonary Regurgitation (Graham Steell's Murmur)

- This is a high-pitched early diastolic decrescendo murmur along the left sternal border. Pulmonary regurgitation results from dilatation of the pulmonary valve ring that occurs with severe pulmonary hypertension. This murmur should be differentiated from the more common mild aortic regurgitation murmur, which could be an associated lesion.

Other Findings

- Tender hepatomegaly, peripheral oedema, ascites and right-sided pleural effusion may occur with severe right ventricular failure.

SIGNS INDICATING SEVERITY OF MITRAL STENOSIS (Box 7.47)

BOX 7.47 Indicators of Severity of Mitral Stenosis	
• Narrow A_2–OS interval	• Long diastolic murmur
• Signs of pulmonary arterial hypertension	• Signs of right ventricular overload

INVESTIGATIONS IN MITRAL STENOSIS

- Electrocardiogram can confirm:
  - Left atrial enlargement ('P' mitrale)
  - Right ventricular hypertrophy.
  - Atrial fibrillation.

RADIOLOGICAL FEATURES OF MITRAL STENOSIS (Box 7.48)

- Echocardiogram can reveal:
  - Mitral stenosis and the valve orifice size.
  - Anatomy of the mitral valve apparatus.
  - Size of cardiac chambers.
  - Pulmonary artery pressure.
  - Calcification of mitral valve.
  - Other associated valvular lesions.
- Transoesophageal echocardiography can reveal:
  - An improved image of mitral valve anatomy including presence of calcification.
  - A clot in the left atrium or in the left atrial appendage.

BOX 7.48 Radiological Features of Mitral Stenosis

DUE TO LEFT ATRIAL ENLARGEMENT:
- Straightening of left heart margin (mitralisation) due to enlargement of left atrial appendage (Fig. 7.45)
- Double right heart margin (shadow through shadow or double bubble) (Fig. 7.45)
- Widening of carinal angle and elevation of left main bronchus (Fig. 7.45)
- Indentation of oesophagus on barium swallow

DUE TO PULMONARY VENOUS HYPERTENSION:
- Prominence of upper lobe veins (stag's antler sign or reverse moustache sign)
- Kerley A (straight lines up to 4 cm long, running towards hilum) and Kerley B (short, horizontal lines near costophrenic angles) lines
- Endobronchial cuffing
- Bilateral perihilar opacity dense at the hilum, fading towards periphery (bat's wing sign)

DUE TO PULMONARY ARTERIAL HYPERTENSION:
- Prominent pulmonary conus
- Prominence of pulmonary arteries and their main branches
- Peripheral pruning of the small pulmonary arteries
- Right ventricular enlargement

DUE TO CHANGES IN THE MITRAL VALVE:
- Calcification of the mitral valve, best seen on fluoroscopy

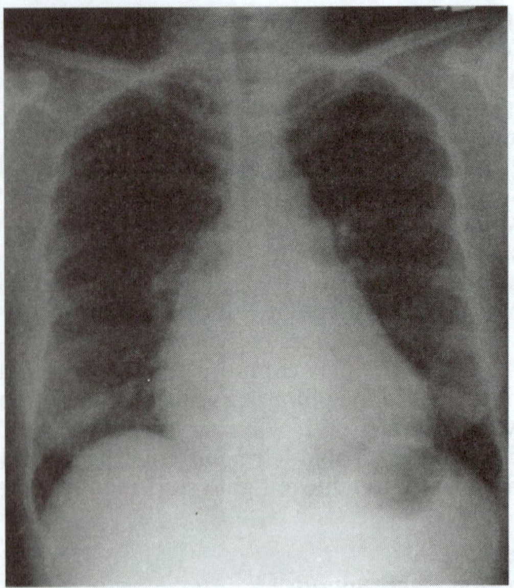

Fig. 7.45 Chest radiograph demonstrating straightening of the left heart border by the enlarged left atrium, double density noted along the right heart border due to enlarged left atrium and elevation of left mainstem bronchus due to enlarged left atrium.

- Cardiac catheterisation:
  - Rarely needed as imaging methods discussed above are accurate.
  - Occasionally used to assess discrepancies between symptoms and echocardiography findings.
  - Occasionally used to image coronary arteries in elderly patients.

COMPLICATIONS OF MITRAL STENOSIS (Box 7.49)

ATRIAL FIBRILLATION IN MITRAL STENOSIS

- Most common complication of mitral stenosis, occurs in up to 40% of patients.
- Atrial fibrillation can occur as a transient episode or a sustained arrhythmia.
- Loss of atrial contraction with the development of atrial fibrillation decreases the cardiac output by 15%–20%. Since cardiac output is related to heart rate, atrial fibrillation with a rapid ventricular rate decreases the diastolic filling time and further compromises cardiac output.
- Atrial fibrillation predisposes to systemic embolism.
- The incidence of atrial fibrillation in mitral stenosis is related to:
  - Size of the left atrium (the larger the size, the more frequent).

BOX 7.49 Complications of Mitral Stenosis	
• Atrial fibrillation	• Winter bronchitis
• Pulmonary hypertension	• Dysphagia due to oesophageal compression by the left atrium
• Right ventricular failure	• Ortner's syndrome
• Systemic thromboembolism	• Infective endocarditis (very rare)
• Haemoptysis	

- Age of the patient (the older the patient, the more frequent).
- Residual rheumatic inflammation.
- Left atrial fibrosis.

SYSTEMIC EMBOLISM IN MITRAL STENOSIS

- Systemic embolism occurs from the clots formed in the left atrium.
- Usually, it is the freshly formed clots that get dislodged, rather than the old ones.
- Embolisation commonly occurs in brain (60%–70%), kidneys, spleen and extremities.
- Embolism is more frequent in the following situations:
  - Atrial fibrillation.
  - Older patients (older than 35 years).
  - Those with reduced cardiac output.
  - Those who already had one or more embolic episodes.
  - Those having a large left atrial appendage.

INFECTIVE ENDOCARDITIS

- Occurs infrequently in patients with isolated mitral stenosis.
- In patients with mitral stenosis alone, it occurs more frequently in mild mitral stenosis with pliable valves and less frequently in severe stenosis with rigid, calcified valves.

ORTNER'S SYNDROME

- This is a very rare complication of severe pulmonary hypertension secondary to mitral stenosis. There is hoarseness of voice due to paralysis of left recurrent laryngeal nerve. There is compression of the nerve between the enlarged tense pulmonary artery and the aorta, at ligamentum arteriosum.

MANAGEMENT OF MITRAL STENOSIS

MEDICAL MANAGEMENT

- Treatment of atrial fibrillation with anticoagulants, verapamil, diltiazem, β-blockers, digoxin and cardioversion.
- Treatment of right ventricular failure with salt restriction, diuretics, digoxin, etc.
- Infective endocarditis prophylaxis is not recommended in patients with mitral stenosis unless mitral valve replacement or mitral valve repair using prosthetic material has been done or patient had previous endocarditis.
- Rheumatic fever prophylaxis.

SURGICAL MANAGEMENT

- Indicated in patients with class III or IV symptoms. Other considerations include valve anatomy and onset of complications even in absence of symptoms (e.g. atrial fibrillation, pulmonary arterial hypertension and embolic events).
- Balloon mitral valvotomy (BMV), also known as percutaneous balloon valvuloplasty (PBV), in young patients without extensive valvular calcification or thickening, no atrial thrombus and no or mild mitral regurgitation. Also a procedure of choice in pregnant females.
- Closed surgical mitral commissurotomy (closed mitral valvotomy) is rarely performed as BMV is superior to it.
- Open mitral commissurotomy (open mitral valvotomy).
- Mitral valve replacement is performed if significant mitral regurgitation is present, if leaflets are immobile, heavily calcified or if there is severe subvalvular scarring.
  - Mechanical prosthetic valves: Require lifelong anticoagulation.
    - Types:
      - Caged-ball valve (Starr–Edwards prosthesis).
      - Tilting-disc valve (Bjork–Shiley valve).
    - Tilting-disc valve is preferred as compared to caged-ball valve because:
      - It occupies less space and hence can be used in patients with small left ventricle.
      - Incidence of haemolysis is lower.
      - Incidence of strut (ring on which valve is attached) fracture is lower.
  - Bioprosthetic valves: Low incidence of thrombosis.
    - Types:
      - Porcine bioprosthetic valve.
      - Pericardial xenograft prosthetic valve.
    - Useful in pregnancy when oral anticoagulants are contraindicated.
    - Because of rapid deterioration of valve, it is not used in patients younger than 35 years.

Q. How will you clinically differentiate between mitral opening snap and split second heart sound?

- Particularly when the OS is heard at the pulmonary area, it has to be differentiated from a split second sound. The question is whether the second component is P_2 or OS. The differentiation is based on the character and behaviour of the second component as well as the split (Table 7.49).

TABLE 7.49 Differentiation Between Opening Snap and Split Second Sound

Mitral Opening Snap (OS)	Split Second Sound (Split S_2)
• OS is high pitched and loud	• P_2 is soft, unless accentuated
• OS best heard medial to apex	• P_2 best heard at pulmonary area
• Split widens on standing (A_2–OS interval increases)	• Split narrows on standing (A_2–P_2 interval decreases)
• Split narrows on inspiration	• Split widens on inspiration
• OS is louder during expiration	• P_2 is louder during inspiration
• Intensity of OS is unchanged on leg raising	• Intensity of P_2 is louder on leg raising
• Loud S_1 and other evidence of MS	• S_1 may or may not be loud

TABLE 7.50 Differentiation Between Opening Snap and Third Heart Sound

Mitral Opening Snap (OS)	Left-Sided Third Heart Sound (S_3)
• High-pitched, sharp, snappy sound	• Low-pitched thud or boom
• Best heard medial to the apex	• Best heard at the apex
• May be heard extensively along the left sternal edge or at the base of the heart	• Well localised to the apex
• Best heard with the diaphragm of the stethoscope	• Best heard with the bell piece of the stethoscope, with the patient in the left lateral position
• Less widely separated from S_2 (A_2–OS interval is 0.04–0.12 second)	• More widely separated from S_2 (A_2–S_3 interval is 0.14–0.16 second)
• Separates further from A_2 on standing (A_2–OS interval increases)	• Does not move on standing (A_2–S_3 interval is unchanged)
• Louder during expiration	• Decreases during inspiration
• Intensity unchanged with leg raising and sustained hand grip	• Intensity increases with leg raising and sustained hand grip
• Usually associated with a loud S_1 and other evidence of MS	• May or may not be associated with a loud S_1

Q. How will you differentiate between the mitral opening snap and left ventricular third heart sound?

- The mitral OS and third heart sound (S_3) occur in early diastole. At times, it becomes difficult to differentiate between the two (Table 7.50).

Q. Discuss the aetiology, pathophysiology, clinical features, investigations, complications and management of chronic mitral regurgitation. How do you clinically assess the severity of mitral regurgitation?

Q. Discuss briefly about acute mitral regurgitation.

AETIOLOGY

CHRONIC MITRAL REGURGITATION

- Causes of chronic mitral regurgitation (MR) are given in Table 7.51.
- In myocardial ischaemia or infarction, regional wall motion abnormality may distort the mitral valve apparatus resulting in inadequate leaflet closure.

TABLE 7.51 Causes of Chronic Mitral Regurgitation

Common Causes	Less Common Causes
• Rheumatic heart disease (40%) • Rupture of chordae tendineae (20%) • Degenerative mitral valve disease, for example mitral valve prolapse (15%) • Ischaemic papillary muscle dysfunction (10%) • Infective endocarditis (5%)	• Congenital mitral regurgitation • Ischaemia or infarction of myocardium • Marked LV enlargement of any cause • Cardiomyopathies (dilated and hypertrophic) • Mitral annulus calcification • Systemic lupus erythematosus, rheumatoid arthritis, ankylosing spondylitis • Marfan's syndrome • Drug-related (ergotamine, methysergide, pergolide, anorexiant medications)

ACUTE MITRAL REGURGITATION

- Infective endocarditis.
- Acute myocardial infarction with rupture of a papillary muscle or one of its heads.
- Chest trauma.
- Cardiac surgery.
- Acute rheumatic fever with carditis.
- Prosthetic valve dysfunction.
- Atrial myxoma.

RHEUMATIC MITRAL REGURGITATION

- Commonest cause of chronic MR in India.
- Pure or predominant MR is more common in males.
- Rheumatic involvement of mitral valve causes marked fibrosis, thickening, calcification and shortening of both mitral leaflets and chordae tendineae. These result in improper closure of valve cusps during systole resulting in MR.

PRIMARY (OR ORGANIC) VERSUS SECONDARY (OR FUNCTIONAL) MITRAL REGURGITATION

- Primary MR is caused by structural abnormalities of valve leaflets and subvalvular apparatus, including stretching or rupture of chordae tendineae.
- Secondary MR is caused by both ischaemic (coronary artery disease) and nonischaemic (e.g. dilated cardiomyopathy) heart diseases via multiple mechanisms including impaired left ventricular wall motion, left ventricular dilatation, and papillary muscle displacement and dysfunction. Here the valve is normal.

PATHOPHYSIOLOGY OF ACUTE MITRAL REGURGITATION

- With sudden onset of MR, the regurgitant blood flows into small, noncompliant left atrium causing acute elevation of left atrial pressure and pulmonary arterial pressure.
- Left ventricle is unable to effectively increase cardiac output.
- Both these factors lead to acute pulmonary oedema and cardiogenic shock.

PATHOPHYSIOLOGY OF SEVERE CHRONIC MITRAL REGURGITATION (Flowchart 7.14)

- In chronic MR, atrium is more compliant, and therefore mechanical energy generated by left ventricle

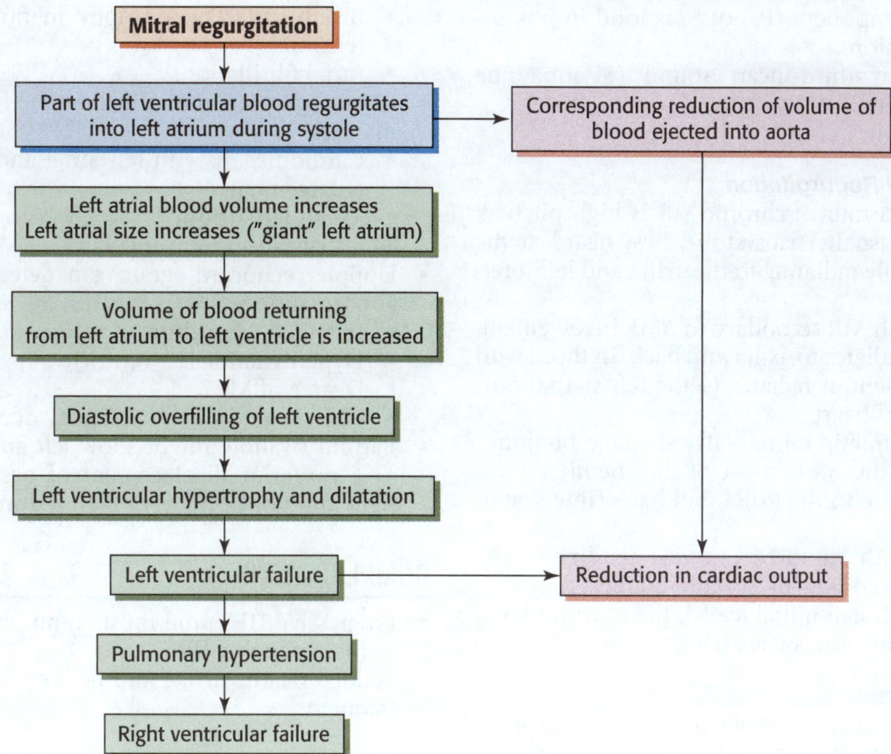

Flowchart 7.14 Pathophysiology of Severe Chronic Mitral Regurgitation.

causes volume overload and atrial enlargement rather than an increase in intraatrial pressure.

- Patients with chronic MR often remain asymptomatic for many years. Over time, the left ventricle dilates to accommodate increased volume load and maintains cardiac output. Chronic left ventricular volume overload leads to contractile dysfunction, heart failure and increased risk of sudden death.

CLINICAL FEATURES

SYMPTOMS

- Patients with chronic MR may remain asymptomatic for several years.
- Palpitation is the most common symptom.
- Symptoms of reduced cardiac output like fatigability, weakness, exhaustion, weight loss and cachexia are common.
- Symptoms of left ventricular failure like exertional breathlessness, orthopnoea and PND occur late in the course of MR.
- Features of right-sided HF like tender hepatomegaly, peripheral oedema, raised jugular venous pressure, ascites and functional tricuspid regurgitation are uncommon, and occur very late in the course of MR. They are seen in patients with pulmonary hypertension.
- In acute MR, the symptoms are due to acute pulmonary oedema.
- In severe MR, sudden death may occur with rupture of chordae tendineae which causes about 25% of deaths of patients on medical treatment.

SIGNS

- Pulse:
  - High volume that in severe MR may become collapsing.
  - Irregular rhythm and varying volume in atrial fibrillation associated with long-standing MR.
- Jugular veins:
  - JVP is normal in uncomplicated MR.
  - With atrial fibrillation, *a* waves disappear. With pulmonary hypertension, *a* waves are more prominent.
  - With right ventricular failure and functional tricuspid regurgitation, jugular venous pressure is raised and *v* waves become very prominent.
- Blood pressure:
  - Wide pulse pressure in severe MR.

Inspection and Palpation

- 'Rocking motion of the precordium' with each cardiac cycle due to a combination of retraction of the left ventricle and expansion of the left atrium during systole.
- Apex beat is shifted downwards and laterally, and is hyperdynamic (forceful but ill-sustained) in character.
- Systolic thrill at the apex.
- Sustained left parasternal heave and palpable pulmonary component of second heart sound (P_2) in pulmonary hypertension.

Auscultation

- First heart sound (S_1) is usually soft.
- In severe MR, the second heart sound (S_2) is widely split due to aortic valve closure (A_1) occurring early.

- Pulmonary component (P_2) of S_2 is loud in pulmonary hypertension.
- Left ventricular third heart sound (S_3) may be present in severe MR.
- Pulmonary ES in pulmonary hypertension.

Murmur of Mitral Regurgitation

- The typical murmur of chronic MR is high pitched, blowing and usually pansystolic, best heard at the apex, commonly radiating to the axilla and left interscapular area.
- In patients with MR secondary to AML involvement, the murmur radiates to axilla and back. In those with PML involvement, it radiates to the left sternal border and base of heart.
- Since the rheumatic mitral valve damage predominantly affects the AML, most of the rheumatic MR murmurs radiate to the axilla and back (interscapular area).
- In patients with ruptured chordae tendineae, the murmur has a 'cooing' or 'seagull' quality.
- In patients with flail mitral leaflet, the murmur has a 'musical' quality and is late systolic.

Mitral Flow Murmur

- A short, rumbling mid-diastolic murmur may be audible at the apex in severe cases due to an increased flow across the mitral valve.

Other Murmurs

- Ejection systolic murmur at pulmonary area due to pulmonary hypertension.
- Pansystolic murmur at lower left sternal border due to functional tricuspid regurgitation.

SIGNS INDICATING SEVERITY OF MITRAL REGURGITATION (Box 7.50)

BOX 7.50 Signs of Severe Mitral Regurgitation

• High-volume pulse	• Wide mobile split of second heart sound (S_2)
• Cardiomegaly with hyperdynamic apex	• Loud pansystolic murmur
• Left ventricular third heart sound (S_3)	• Mid-diastolic flow murmur at apex

SIGNS IN ACUTE MITRAL REGURGITATION

- Normal apical impulse as ventricle is not yet dilated.
- Third heart sound and/or fourth heart sound.
- An early systolic or pansystolic murmur (may be absent).

INVESTIGATIONS

- Electrocardiogram can detect the following abnormalities:
  - Left atrial enlargement.
  - Left ventricular hypertrophy.
  - Biventricular hypertrophy in pulmonary hypertension.
  - Atrial fibrillation.
- Chest radiography might show the following abnormalities:
  - Cardiomegaly with left atrial and left ventricular enlargement.
  - 'Giant left atrium'.
  - Calcification of mitral valve.
- Doppler echocardiogram can detect the following abnormalities:
  - Enlarged left atrium.
  - Hyperdynamic left ventricle.
  - Degree of MR.
  - Clues regarding the aetiology of MR.
- Barium swallow might show left atrial enlargement as a posterior displacement of oesophagus in the right anterior oblique view (not done routinely).

COMPLICATIONS

- Progressive HF is the most common cause of death in these patients (Box 7.51).
- Sudden death, stroke and fatal endocarditis are less frequent.

MANAGEMENT

MEDICAL MANAGEMENT

- Infective endocarditis prophylaxis is not indicated in patients with MR. However, it is mandatory for patients after mitral valve repair or after mitral valve replacement (MVR).
- Rheumatic fever prophylaxis.
- Restriction of physical activity.
- Evaluation and modification of coronary artery disease risk factors to prevent its development.
- Follow up asymptomatic patients with echocardiography in order to assess left ventricular dilatation and systolic dysfunction.
- Treatment of HF with salt restriction, diuretics, ACE inhibitors, β-blockers, mineralocorticoid antagonists, digoxin and vasodilators.
- Treatment of atrial fibrillation with verapamil, diltiazem, β-blockers, digoxin, anticoagulation and cardioversion.
- In acute MR, nitrates and diuretics to reduce filling pressures.

SURGICAL MANAGEMENT

- Reconstruction of mitral valve apparatus by mitral valvuloplasty or mitral annuloplasty. Preferred to mitral valve replacement (MVR) whenever feasible.

BOX 7.51 Complications of Mitral Regurgitation

• Atrial fibrillation	• Pulmonary hypertension (late)
• Infective endocarditis	• Right ventricular failure (very late)
• Left ventricular failure	• Systemic embolism (rare)

- MVR with a prosthesis.
- Indications for surgery.
  - Acute MR.
  - Chronic severe MR and NYHA functional class II, III or IV symptoms in the presence of severe left ventricular dysfunction (defined as ejection fraction <30% and/or left ventricular end-systolic dimension >55 mm).
  - Asymptomatic or symptomatic patients with mild (EF ≤60% and left ventricular end-systolic diameter 40–50 mm) or moderate (EF 30%–50% and left ventricular end-systolic diameter 50–55 mm) left ventricular dysfunction.
  - Asymptomatic severe MR with normal left ventricular size and function (ejection fraction >60% and left ventricular end-systolic dimension <40 mm), only if likelihood of successful mitral valve repair is high.
  - If EF ≤30%, mitral valve repair only if high likelihood of success.

Q. In the presence of combined mitral stenosis and mitral regurgitation, how will you clinically assess the dominance of lesions?

- Features suggesting predominant mitral regurgitation versus mitral stenosis are given in Box 7.52.

Q. Discuss the aetiology, clinical features, complications and management of mitral valve prolapse or Barlow's syndrome.

- Mitral valve prolapse (MVP) is an abnormal systolic valve movement of one or both of the mitral leaflets towards the left atrium (≥2 mm beyond annular plane). Thus, in MVP, mitral leaflets bulge into the left atrium during ventricular systole, with or without MR.

BOX 7.52 Predominant Mitral Regurgitation Versus Predominant Mitral Stenosis

Signs of Predominant Mitral Regurgitation	Signs of Predominant Mitral Stenosis
• High-volume pulse	• Low-volume pulse
• Left ventricular enlargement	• Evidence of right ventricular hypertrophy
• Hyperdynamic apex	• Evidence of pulmonary hypertension
• Soft first heart sound	• Loud first heart sound
• Wide splitting of second heart sound	• Narrow splitting of second heart sound
• Left ventricular third heart sound	• Distinct OS with a narrow A_2–OS interval
• Short mid-diastolic flow murmur	• Long mid-diastolic murmur with presystolic accentuation

AETIOLOGIC CONSIDERATIONS

- More common in females aged between 15 and 30 years; however, severe MR caused by prolapse is more frequent in older males than in young females.
- Redundant mitral leaflet tissue and chordae tendineae.
- Structural abnormalities causing mitral prolapse include diffuse myxomatous degeneration of mitral valve and primary flail leaflet with ruptured chords. These conditions predominantly affect the posterior mitral leaflet.
- Familial type associated with an autosomal dominant mode of inheritance.
- Commonly associated with Marfan's syndrome and cystic medial necrosis.
- MVP may be associated with the following conditions:
  - Congenital heart diseases, especially atrial septal defect.
  - Acute rheumatic fever, chronic rheumatic heart disease.
  - Ischaemic heart disease, cardiomyopathies.

CLINICAL FEATURES (Box 7.53 and Box 7.54)

- Mid or late systolic click results from a sudden tensing of mitral valve apparatus as the leaflets prolapse into left atrium.
- When end-diastolic volume is decreased (as with standing), click–murmur complex occurs shortly after S_1. Manoeuvres that increase end-diastolic volume (such as squatting) cause click–murmur complex to move towards S_2.

BOX 7.53 Symptoms of MVP

- Asymptomatic
- Atypical chest pain (precordial, stabbing)
- Palpitation (due to ventricular ectopics, supraventricular tachycardia, ventricular tachycardia)
- Syncope or presyncope (light-headedness, dizziness)
- Orthostatic phenomena (orthostatic tachycardia, hypotension and arrhythmias)
- Fatigue
- Rarely, symptoms of left ventricular failure like exertional dyspnoea, orthopnoea and paroxysmal nocturnal dyspnoea in patients with severe mitral regurgitation
- Rarely, sudden death
- Rarely, transient ischaemic attacks

BOX 7.54 Signs of MVP

- Abnormalities of chest wall and thoracic spine (scoliosis, narrow anteroposterior chest diameter, straight back or pectus excavatum).
- Bifid apical impulse.
- Mid or late systolic click(s)—occur ≥0.14 second after S_1 (non-ejection click).
- Mid-systolic or late systolic apical murmur (rarely 'whooping' or 'honking') may or may not be present.
- The systolic murmur of mitral valve prolapse increases during standing and Valsalva manoeuvre, but decreases during squatting and isometric exercise.

INVESTIGATIONS

- Electrocardiogram usually shows nonspecific ST–T changes in leads II, III and aVF.
- Echocardiography (transthoracic and transoesophageal) can confirm the diagnosis. Serial echocardiography is usually not necessary unless MR is present.
- Colour Doppler to assess MR.
- Cardiovascular magnetic resonance (CMR) for the assessment of LV volumes, function and MR severity, especially when echo does not address these issues satisfactorily.

COMPLICATIONS (Box 7.55)

BOX 7.55 Complications of MVP

• Arrhythmias	• Transient cerebral ischaemic attacks and embolic episodes (rare)
• Infective endocarditis	• Acute severe mitral regurgitation (rare)
• Progressive mitral regurgitation	• Sudden death (rare)

MANAGEMENT

- Reassurance in asymptomatic patients.
- Infective endocarditis prophylaxis is not recommended.
- β-Blockers in atypical chest pain.
- Antiarrhythmic drugs in significant arrhythmias.
- Aspirin or anticoagulants in transient ischaemic attacks (not required to prevent first attack).
- Mitral valve repair or replacement in severe MR (defined as symptomatic patient or EF <60% with left ventricular end systolic diameter >45 mm).

Q. Classify aortic stenosis.

Q. Discuss the aetiology, clinical features, investigations and management of valvular aortic stenosis.

CLASSIFICATION

- Valvular aortic stenosis.
- Subvalvular aortic stenosis.
- Supravalvular aortic stenosis.

AORTIC VALVE

- The normal aortic valve area averages 3 to 4 cm^2, and there should normally be minimal gradient across it (<10 mmHg).
- A valve area of less than 0.8 cm^2 or a gradient of more than 50 mmHg represents critical stenosis.

AETIOLOGY OF AORTIC STENOSIS (Table 7.52)

TABLE 7.52 Aetiology of Aortic Stenosis

Valvular aortic stenosis:
• Acquired
  • Rheumatic heart disease
  • Fibrocalcific deformity of a bicuspid valve
  • Fibrocalcific deformity of three cusped valve or calcific stenosis of a trileaflet aortic valve (aortic sclerosis)
  • Systemic lupus erythematosus (SLE)
  • Fabry's disease
  • Type II hyperlipoproteinaemia
  • Infective endocarditis
  • Radiation exposure
• Congenital
  • Unicuspid unicommissural valve
  • Three cusped valve with fusion of commissures
  • Hypoplastic annulus
	Subvalvular aortic stenosis:
	• Membranous diaphragm
	• Tunnel deformity
	• Hypertrophic cardiomyopathy
	Supravalvular aortic stenosis:
	• Hourglass constriction of aorta
	• Hypoplasia of aorta
	• Fibromembranous lesion of aorta

CLINICAL FEATURES

SYMPTOMS

- Natural history characterised by years of asymptomatic progression.
- Decreased exercise tolerance is usually the first symptom and occurs due to angina in the compensated phase (average survival 4 years).
- Exertional dizziness and syncope (average survival 3 years).
- Exertional breathlessness, orthopnoea and PND due to HF which occurs in the decompensated phase (average survival 2 years).
- Haematemesis and melaena from AV malformations of right colon, small intestine and stomach (Heyde's syndrome).

SIGNS

- Pulsus tardus is a slow-rising arterial pulse best felt in carotids (delayed carotid upstroke) due to prolongation of ejection phase. The classic anacrotic pulse is seen in severe aortic stenosis. Another type of pulse seen in severe aortic stenosis is pulsus parvus et tardus (slow rising with delayed peak).
- Low systolic blood pressure (<100 mmHg).
- In congenital supravalvular aortic stenosis, systolic blood pressure is usually higher by approximately 30 mmHg in right arm than in left arm.
- Normal JVP; however, prominent *a* waves may be present due to reduced right ventricular compliance produced by hypertrophy of interventricular septum.
- Systolic thrill in carotids.
- Systolic thrill at aortic area radiating to carotids, lower left sternal border and even mitral area (cross-belt area).
- Heaving (forceful and sustained) apical impulse.
- No cardiomegaly in the initial stages of concentric hypertrophy. Cardiomegaly develops later, with left ventricular dilatation and failure.

Auscultation

- The aortic component of second heart sound (A_2) is delayed, resulting in a narrow splitting of second heart sound in mild to moderate aortic stenosis, and a paradoxical splitting of second heart sound in severe aortic stenosis.
- Intensity of A_2 component is decreased and may even be inaudible, when the second heart sound appears single (single S_2). In congenital valvular aortic stenosis, A_2 is usually heard as the valve remains flexible.
- Ejection click of valvular origin in young patients where the valve is not immobilised by calcification. It does not vary with respiration.
- Left ventricular third heart sound (LVS_3) in left ventricular failure.
- Fourth heart sound due to vigorous atrial contraction.
- The murmur of aortic stenosis is an ejection systolic murmur (ESM) best heard at aortic area, conducted to carotids. It is best heard with the patient sitting up, leaning forwards and breath held in expiration.
  - Soft, short ESM with early peaking suggests mild stenosis.
  - Harsh, loud, long ESM with late peaking suggests severe stenosis.
  - At times, as one moves downwards from aortic area to mitral area, the murmur initially becomes softer and then again increases in intensity. This phenomenon is known as 'hourglass conduction'.
  - In calcific aortic stenosis, the murmur is loud and harsh in the aortic area, but it has a musical quality along the left sternal border and at apex. This difference in quality of the same murmur at two different sites is referred to as 'Gallavardin phenomenon'. It may be confused with murmur of mitral regurgitation. However, the murmur of aortic stenosis at apex is musical and high pitched while that of MR is harsh holosystolic murmur.
- In congenital subvalvular stenosis, aortic regurgitation may develop producing a diastolic murmur.

SUPRAVALVULAR AORTIC STENOSIS

- Narrowing of ascending aorta that can occur as a discreet hourglass deformity or as a diffuse hypoplasia originating at the superior margin of the sinuses of Valsalva just above the level of the coronary arteries.
- Narrowing of several other arteries often present. This includes narrowing of peripheral pulmonary arteries (peripheral pulmonary artery stenosis) and narrowing of other arteries like coronary, renal, carotid, innominate and mesenteric arteries. Coarctation of aorta may also be present.
- Sporadic or familial; in latter form, it is transmitted as an autosomal dominant trait with incomplete penetrance and variable expressivity.
- Asymptomatic or presentation with dyspnoea, chest pain due to aortic stenosis, myocardial infarction due to coronary abnormalities, stroke or even sudden death occurring during exercise. Infants may present with features of HF.

Examination

- Systolic thrill and murmur, best at the first right intercostal space.
- No election click (in contrast to aortic valve stenosis).
- Continuous murmur if peripheral pulmonary artery stenosis is present.
- Disparity of pulse and blood pressure between the arms due to selective streaming of blood into innominate artery (blood pressure in right arm may exceed the pressure in the left one by 20 mmHg or more).
- Femoral pulse reduced if coarctation of aorta also present.
- Hoarse voice, hernias, lax skin and stiffness of joints due to deficient elastin.

WILLIAMS' SYNDROME

- Comprises several features:
  - Supravalvular aortic stenosis.
  - Elfin facies (prominent forehead, widely spaced eyes, upturned nose, underdeveloped mandible, dental hypoplasia, patulous lips).
  - Mental retardation.
  - Hypercalcaemia.

INVESTIGATIONS

- Chest radiography:
  - Normal heart size (due to concentric hypertrophy of left ventricle in initial stages).
  - Poststenotic dilatation of aorta.
  - Calcification of aortic valve (best appreciated in lateral X-ray).
- ECG shows left ventricular hypertrophy with or without strain, first-degree AV block or bundle branch block.
- Echocardiography:
  - Accurate assessment of aortic valve area.
  - Number of aortic valve cusps.
  - Pattern of thickening of aortic cusps.
  - Transvalvular gradient.
  - Left ventricular hypertrophy and ejection fraction.
- Exercise stress testing and serum BNP level may help determine the appropriateness of valve replacement in asymptomatic patients with severe aortic stenosis.
- Cardiac catheterisation with coronary angiography before aortic valve surgery.

TREATMENT

- No strenuous physical work.
- Avoid hot baths, steam rooms and saunas so as to avoid hypotension that may result from peripheral vasodilation.
- Infective endocarditis prophylaxis in patients who have undergone aortic valve replacement. It is not recommended for patients with aortic stenosis or other acquired valve diseases. Absolute risk of endocarditis is sufficiently low (well under 1% per year) and, therefore, the benefit of antibiotic prophylaxis before any invasive procedure does not outweigh the risk.
- Rheumatic fever prophylaxis in aortic stenosis of rheumatic aetiology.
- Treatment of angina, atrial fibrillation and left ventricular failure.

- Treatment of systemic hypertension with ACE inhibitors. Nitrates should be used with caution in patients with angina as this may lead to orthostatic hypotension and syncope. β-Blockers are avoided in severe aortic stenosis because the patient may be critically sensitive to a small fall in contractility.
- Though previously thought to be detrimental, arterial vasodilators in low doses may be tried in patients with severe AS and HF.
- For asymptomatic patients with preserved LV ejection fraction, follow-up echocardiographs to monitor the gradient and LV systolic function every 3–5 years for mild aortic stenosis and every 6–12 months for severe aortic stenosis.
- Surgery:
  - Surgery is advised when the patient has moderately severe aortic stenosis with symptoms or signs of left ventricular failure. It is also recommended in severe aortic stenosis with ejection fraction <50%, patients with transvalvular pressure gradient ≥40 mmHg or peak velocity across aortic valve ≥4 m/second, patients with moderate or severe aortic stenosis undergoing other cardiac surgery, and presence of dilated aortic root.
  - Open commissurotomy or valvuloplasty for noncalcific stenosis.
  - Aortic valve replacement (open or transcatheter aortic valve replacement—TAVR) for calcific aortic stenosis.
- Percutaneous balloon valvotomy generally not useful:
  - High risk for stroke, aortic regurgitation, and other complications.
  - High risk for restenosis.

Q. What is the mechanism of angina in aortic stenosis?

- Increase in left ventricular muscle mass leads to increased oxygen demand.
- Left ventricular systolic hypertension leads to increase in myocardial oxygen need and impedance in systolic coronary flow.
- Prolongation of systole leads to increased myocardial oxygen consumption.
- Limiting the duration of diastole leads to reduced coronary filling.
- Coronary atherosclerosis.

Q. How will you clinically assess the severity of aortic stenosis?

- Severe aortic stenosis is characterised by one or more of the features shown in Box 7.56.

BOX 7.56 Features of Severe Aortic Stenosis

• Low systolic blood pressure	• Paradoxical splitting of S_2
• Heaving apical impulse	• Harsh, loud, long ejection systolic murmur with late peaking
• Soft A_2 or single S_2	• Orthopnoea, paroxysmal nocturnal dyspnoea, cardiomegaly and S_3

Q. Discuss briefly about aortic sclerosis.

- Defined as thickening and calcification of a tricuspid (three cusps) aortic valve without any obstruction to left ventricular outflow.
- Fairly common in elderly people affecting 21%–26% of adults older than 65 years.
- Patients asymptomatic.
- Examination may show a soft mid-systolic murmur at the aortic area, a normal split of second heart sound and a normal-volume carotid pulse.
- Risks:
  - Progression to aortic stenosis (calcific aortic valve disease): Risk factors like hypercholesterolaemia, raised lipoprotein Lp(a), smoking, hypertension and diabetes increase the rate of progression to calcific aortic stenosis. These factors are also associated with a higher frequency of aortic sclerosis without aortic stenosis in a given population.
  - Aortic sclerosis may be accompanied by mitral annulus calcification (up to 50%).
  - Increased cardiovascular morbidity and mortality possibly due to increased rate of atherosclerosis.
  - Patients without presence of atherosclerosis risk factors still have an increased frequency of cardiovascular events and mortality.
  - Development of aortic regurgitation is rare.
- Diagnosed by echocardiography that shows leaflet thickening, stiffness, increased echogenicity, and normal excursion of leaflets with peak Doppler velocities across the valve <2 m/second. The commissures are not fused.
- Quantification of aortic valve calcification by electron beam tomography; using this technique, valve calcification can be sequentially monitored.
- Treatment:
  - Reducing risk factors by appropriate therapy, although effect on aortic sclerosis is unproven.
  - Careful follow-up to detect severe aortic stenosis.
  - Endocarditis prophylaxis is not recommended in patients with aortic valve sclerosis.

Q. Write a short note on bicuspid aortic valve disease.

- Most common congenital cardiac defect.
- Male to female ratio of 3:1.
- Often associated with other congenital cardiac lesions, most frequent being dilatation of proximal ascending aorta secondary to abnormalities of the aortic media. Others include coarctation of aorta, hypoplastic left heart syndrome, ventricular septal defect (VSD) and atrial septal defect.
- Symptoms often develop in adulthood, although the patient may remain asymptomatic throughout his/her life.
- Complications include aortic valve stenosis, aortic regurgitation, endocarditis, aortic aneurysm formation and aortic dissection.

- Auscultatory findings include an ejection sound best heard at the apex, often accompanied by a brief ejection systolic murmur. There may be associated murmurs of aortic stenosis or aortic regurgitation.
- Despite potential complications, life expectancy is usually not shortened in asymptomatic persons.
- Diagnosis by echocardiography. Calcification is common in adults with bicuspid aortic valve.
- Cardiac MRI augments the diagnostic process as it enables views of the valve without interference from calcification. It also allows for excellent assessment of the aorta.
- Follow-up echocardiography to detect complications.
- Medical management includes control of hypertension and use of β-blockers. Endocarditis prophylaxis is not indicated.
- Surgical treatment includes aortic valve replacement. Many will also need aortic root surgery.

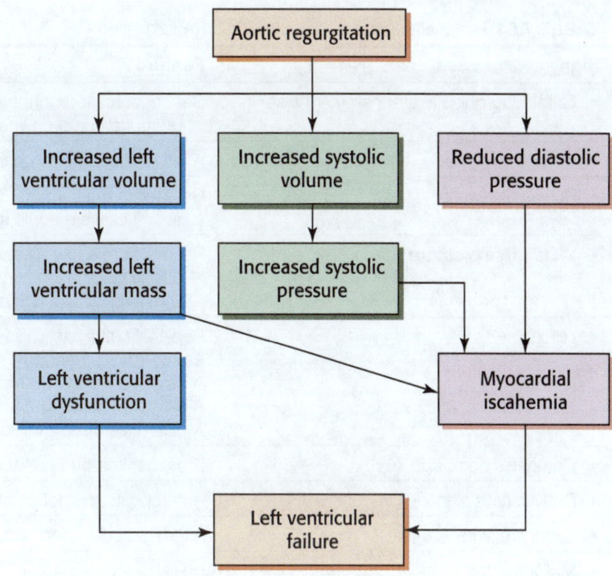

Flowchart 7.15 Pathophysiology of Chronic Aortic Regurgitation.

Q. Discuss the aetiology, clinical features, complications, investigations and treatment of aortic regurgitation.

Q. What are the peripheral signs of aortic regurgitation?

- Aortic regurgitation (AR) can be acute or chronic.

AETIOLOGY

- Various causes of acute and chronic aortic regurgitation are listed in Table 7.53.

PATHOPHYSIOLOGY (Flowchart 7.15)

- In chronic aortic regurgitation (AR), left ventricle enlarges, producing a greater total stroke volume, which is ejected into aorta. With progression, there is decline in left ventricular (LV) function that causes left ventricle to dilate, leading to increase in LV end-diastolic volume without further elevation of the regurgitant volume. Ultimately, ejection fraction and forward stroke volume decline during rest and ventricular emptying is impaired. In advanced stages, left atrium pressure, pulmonary artery wedge pressure, pulmonary artery pressure and right atrium pressure rise and cardiac output falls.
- In cases of acute AR, left ventricle does not have time to adapt to increased diastolic volume. Thus, the patient develops acute LV failure without typical high-cardiac-output state.

TABLE 7.53 Causes of Aortic Regurgitation

Acute Aortic Regurgitation	Chronic Aortic Regurgitation	
	Common causes	**Uncommon causes**
• Trauma	• Rheumatic (two-thirds of cases)	• Infective endocarditis
• Rheumatic fever	• Syphilis	• Ventricular septal defect (VSD)
• Infective endocarditis	• Bicuspid aortic valve	• Marfan's syndrome
• Dissecting aneurysm	• Atherosclerotic aortic valve (aortic sclerosis)	• Rheumatoid arthritis
• Post-aortic balloon valvuloplasty		• Ehlers–Danlos syndrome
• Acute aortic prosthetic valve dysfunction		• Systemic lupus erythematosus
		• Ankylosing spondylitis
		• Reiter's syndrome
		• Takayasu's disease
		• Aneurysm of aorta
		• Severe hypertension

CLINICAL FEATURES

SYMPTOMS

- Remain asymptomatic for years or decades, but once decompensated, they deteriorate rapidly.
- Palpitations, forceful pulsations in the neck.
- Angina.
- Exertional breathlessness, orthopnoea and paroxysmal nocturnal dyspnoea.
- Syncope.
- Symptoms of right ventricular failure (late).

SIGNS

- Peripheral signs of chronic aortic regurgitation are listed in Table 7.54.

Inspection and Palpation

- Prominent neck pulsations.
- Thrill in the carotids.
- Hyperdynamic precordium.
- Hyperdynamic apex that is shifted down and out.
- Suprasternal pulsations.

Auscultation

- First heart sound (S_1) may be soft.
- A_2 component of second heart sound (S_2) is soft in rheumatic AR but loud and 'tambour' like in syphilitic AR.
- Narrowly split, single or paradoxically split second heart sound.
- Third heart sound (S_3) in patients with LV failure.
- Fourth heart sound (S_4) in prominent LV hypertrophy.

TABLE 7.54 Peripheral Signs of Chronic Aortic Regurgitation

Sign	Feature
• Collapsing pulse (water hammer pulse)	Best appreciated on the radial artery when the arm is elevated. This is characterised by a rapid upstroke, rapid downstroke and a high volume
• Corrigan's pulse	A jerky carotid pulse characterised by full expansion followed by quick collapse
• Pulsus bisferiens	Best felt in the carotids. This is a pulse with double peak (two peaks), both being felt in systole. It is seen in severe aortic regurgitation (AR)
• Wide pulse pressure	Results from a low diastolic pressure from aortic run-off and high systolic pressure from increased stroke volume (on auscultation, Korotkoff sounds may disappear at a low point, may be even 0 mmHg; phase IV may be taken as indicative of diastolic pressure)
• Hill's sign	Popliteal cuff systolic pressure exceeding brachial cuff systolic pressure by more than 20 mmHg (measured manually) A difference of 20–39 mmHg indicates mild AR A difference of 40–59 mmHg indicates moderate AR A difference of 60 mmHg or more indicates severe AR
• Corrigan's neck sign	Prominent carotid pulsations visible in the neck
• De-Musset's sign	Anteroposterior motion of the head (head nodding) synchronous with cardiac cycle
• Landolfi's sign	Alternating dilatation and constriction of pupil synchronous with cardiac cycle
• Muller's sign	Pulsations of the uvula
• Lighthouse sign	Capillary pulsations on the forehead and face resulting in alternate blanching and flushing
• Quincke's sign	Alternate paling and flushing of lightly compressed nail bed or mucous membrane of mouth
• Rosenbach's sign	Pulsations of the liver
• Gerhardt's sign	Pulsations of an enlarged spleen
• Pistol-shot femorals	Booming sound synchronous with systole heard over the femoral arteries
• Traube's sign	Booming systolic and diastolic sounds heard over the femoral artery
• Duroziez's sign	A systolic murmur heard over the femoral artery when it is compressed proximally and a diastolic murmur when it is compressed distally
• Mayne's sign	More than a 15-mmHg decrease in diastolic blood pressure with arm elevation from the value obtained with the arm in the standard position
• Becker's sign	Accentuated retinal artery pulsations

- Early diastolic murmur (EDM) of AR—a high-pitched, early diastolic, decrescendo murmur best heard at Erb's point, also known as neo-aortic area (left third intercostal space near sternum) in rheumatic AR and at aortic area in syphilitic AR. The murmur is best heard with the diaphragm of the stethoscope, with the patient sitting up and leaning forwards, breath held in deep expiration and hands clenched. Rheumatic AR murmur is soft blowing in character. The character of syphilitic AR murmur is described as 'cooing dove' or 'seagull'. A similar character is seen also in AR of infective endocarditis and trauma.
- Ejection systolic murmur—an ejection systolic murmur is heard at aortic area or Erb's point, which might even be conducted to carotids. This is a flow murmur due to increased flow across the aortic valve, and not due to organic aortic stenosis. This murmur may be quite loud. It is often higher-pitched, shorter and less grating in quality than the ejection systolic murmur of aortic stenosis.
- Mid-diastolic murmur (Austin Flint murmur)—a mid-diastolic rumbling murmur is heard at the apex in severe AR. It is a functional murmur and does not represent mitral stenosis.
- A blowing, pansystolic murmur, often radiating to the axilla may be heard at the apex. It is due to marked dilatation of left ventricle and functional mitral regurgitation.

Duroziez's Sign

- Elicited by compression of femoral artery with cephalad and caudad tilting of the stethoscope.
- Produces systolic and diastolic murmurs, respectively.
- Systolic portion of the murmur caused by increased forward flow into the lower extremity.
- Diastolic murmur caused by AR (backward flow).

ACUTE AORTIC REGURGITATION

- Onset is sudden with patient presenting with acute LV failure.
- Pulse pressure is normal with near-normal systolic and diastolic pressures.
- Apical impulse is usually not hyperdynamic.
- S_1 is soft or absent.
- P_2 is normal or increased.
- S_3 is commonly heard.
- EDM is short, while functional systolic murmur across aortic valve is less loud.
- Austin Flint murmur is usually absent.
- ECG and chest radiograph generally do not show evidence of LV enlargement.

TABLE 7.55 Acute Versus Chronic Aortic Regurgitation

Feature	Acute AR	Chronic AR
Pulse pressure	• Normal or reduced	• Increased
Blood pressure	• Normal or near-normal	• Elevated systolic and diminished diastolic
Apex	• Normal in position and character	• Shifted down and out, hyperdynamic
S_1	• Soft	• Normal or diminished
S_2	• Normal or loud P_2	• Narrow split
S_3	• Present	• Present in late stages
Murmurs	• Soft, early diastolic • Functional systolic murmur soft	• Decrescendo or holodiastolic • Functional systolic murmur loud
ECG	• No left ventricular hypertrophy	• Left ventricular hypertrophy
Chest X-ray	• Normal cardiac shadow • Pulmonary venous hypertension	• Enlarged cardiac shadow due to left ventricular dilatation • Pulmonary venous hypertension uncommon

- Pulmonary venous hypertension in the form of redistribution of upper lobe vessels seen on chest radiograph.
- Differentiating acute from chronic AR is shown in Table 7.55.

INVESTIGATIONS

- VDRL and *Treponema pallidum* hemagglutination (TPHA) tests to rule out syphilitic aetiology.
- Rheumatoid factor, ANA, ESR and CRP to exclude connective tissue disorders.
- ECG shows diastolic overload pattern of left ventricle (LV hypertrophy with ST depression and T inversion in I, aVL, V_5 and V_6).
- Chest radiograph shows gross cardiomegaly of LV type (cor bovinum) and evidence of pulmonary oedema later. In bicuspid aortic valve or rheumatic cause of aortic regurgitation, calcification of aortic valve may be seen. In syphilitic AR, calcification of ascending aorta may occur.
- Echocardiography—for diagnosis, severity, possible cause and LV function.
- Cardiac catheterisation.
- Coronary angiography.

TREATMENT

- Treatment of the underlying cause.
- Infective endocarditis prophylaxis is not indicated.
- Rheumatic fever prophylaxis.
- Medical treatment of cardiac failure with digoxin, diuretics, salt restriction and fluid restriction.
- Afterload reduction therapy:
  - Isosorbide dinitrate 20–40 mg 6 hourly (mainly causes preload reduction).
  - Hydralazine 50 mg 6 hourly.
  - Angiotensin-converting enzyme inhibitors or angiotensin receptor blockers.
  - Dihydropyridine calcium channel blockers (e.g. nifedipine).
- Asymptomatic patients with normal LV size and systolic function do not require surgery but should be monitored carefully for development of symptoms, LV dysfunction or progressive LV dilatation.
- Surgical therapy is required in symptomatic patients or those with LV ejection fraction <50% or end-systolic LV diameter >50 mm (even if asymptomatic). It involves aortic valve replacement (open or TAVR).
- Prompt surgical intervention is indicated for acute severe AR resulting from aortic dissection, infective endocarditis and trauma especially when haemodynamically unstable. While waiting for surgery, medical therapy is often necessary to augment forward flow and achieve haemodynamic stability. Inotropes and/or vasodilators should be carefully chosen based on arterial pressures.

Q. Explain the clinical assessment of severity of aortic regurgitation.

- The presence of one or more of the points listed in Box 7.57 suggests that AR is severe.

Q. Describe angina in aortic regurgitation.

Q. What is nocturnal angina?

- Angina is a common symptom in AR, particularly of syphilitic aetiology.
- 'Nocturnal angina' is an unusual form of angina occurring in aortic regurgitation. It is characterised by paroxysmal, nocturnal anginal pains associated with nightmares, dyspnoea, palpitations, skin flushing, profuse sweating and wide pulse pressure. It does not respond to sublingual nitroglycerine.

BOX 7.57 Indicators of Severe Aortic Regurgitation

• Presence of peripheral signs	• Hyperdynamic apex, shifted down and out
• Pulsus bisferiens	• Early diastolic murmur (EDM) lasting more than two-thirds of diastole
• Hill's sign more than 60 mmHg	• Presence of Austin Flint murmur

MECHANISMS OF ANGINA IN AORTIC REGURGITATION

- Associated coronary artery disease.
- Low aortic diastolic pressure leading to decreased myocardial perfusion (since coronary flow occurs mainly in diastole).
- Increased myocardial oxygen demand due to myocardial hypertrophy.
- During sleep, bradycardia develops which leads to increased diastolic time, thereby further reducing diastolic blood pressure and coronary blood flow.

Q. How do you differentiate between aortic regurgitation of rheumatic and syphilitic aetiology?

- Table 7.56 shows features which help in differentiating rheumatic AR from syphilitic AR.

Q. How will you clinically differentiate the early diastolic murmur of aortic regurgitation from that of pulmonary regurgitation?

- Table 7.57 shows features which help in differentiating early diastolic murmur of AR from that of pulmonary regurgitation.

TABLE 7.56 Rheumatic AR Versus Syphilitic AR

Rheumatic AR	Syphilitic AR
• Younger age group (10–40)	• Older age group (more than 40)
• Anginal pains less common	• Anginal pains more common (due to associated coronary artery involvement)
• Decompensation relatively late	• Decompensation relatively early
• Soft A_2 component	• Loud and tambour like A_2
• EDM best heard at Erb's area	• EDM best heard at aortic area
• Soft, blowing character of EDM	• Cooing dove or seagull character of EDM

TABLE 7.57 Early Diastolic Murmur of AR Versus Early Diastolic Murmur of PR

Aortic Regurgitation Murmur	Pulmonary Regurgitation Murmur
• Best heard at Erb's area or aortic area	• Best heard at pulmonary area
• Better heard during expiration	• Better heard during inspiration
• Begins just after A_2	• Begins just after P_2
• Decreases with amyl nitrite inhalation	• No effect
• Increases with hand grip and IV phenylephrine	• No effect

Q. What is meant by Austin Flint murmur (AFM)?

- Mid-diastolic, low-pitched, rumbling murmur heard at the apex in severe AR.
- Resembles mitral stenotic murmur.
- Best heard at apex using diaphragm of stethoscope with patient in left lateral position.

POSSIBLE MECHANISMS

- Diastolic mitral regurgitation.
- Relative mitral stenosis due to aortic regurgitant jet pushing the anterior mitral leaflet upwards, thus impeding the flow of blood from left atrium.
- Low-pitched vibrations of the AR murmur itself being heard at the apex due to acoustical filtering properties of chest.
- Turbulence generated by the mixing of antegrade mitral flow stream with retrograde aortic flow within the left ventricular cavity.

Q. How will you clinically differentiate Austin Flint murmur from the murmur of mitral stenosis (MS)?

- Table 7.58 shows features which help in differentiating Austin Flint murmur (AFM) from the murmur of mitral stenosis (MS).

Q. Discuss the aetiology, clinical features and management of tricuspid stenosis (TS).

- Aetiology:
  - Rheumatic (usually associated with mitral and aortic valve disease).
  - Carcinoid syndrome.
  - Right atrial myxoma (can obstruct flow through the tricuspid valve).

TABLE 7.58 Austin Flint Murmur Versus Mitral Stenosis Murmur

Feature	AFM	MS
• Diastolic thrill	–	+
• Loud first heart sound (S_1)	–	+
• Third heart sound (S_3)	+	–
• Opening snap (OS)	–	+
• Evidence of pulmonary hypertension	–	+
• Evidence of RV enlargement and/or hypertrophy	–	+
• Evidence of LV enlargement and/or hypertrophy	+	–
• Presystolic accentuation	±	+
• Murmur decreases with amyl nitrite	+	–
• Atrial fibrillation	–	+

- Infective endocarditis.
- Fibrosis of tricuspid valve apparatus associated with endocardial pacemaker lead.
- Congenital.
- Clinical features:
  - Clinical manifestations of associated mitral stenosis may dominate.
  - Little or no dyspnoea.
  - Fatigue is common.
  - Refractory oedema, ascites and marked hepatomegaly with presystolic pulsation.
  - JVP is raised with prominent *a* waves (giant *a* waves) and slow *y* descent.
  - At lower left sternal border, loud first heart sound, a tricuspid opening snap (OS) and a mid-diastolic murmur with presystolic accentuation are heard.
  - Tricuspid murmur increases during inspiration (De-Carvallo's sign), leg raising and squatting.
- Treatment:
  - Salt and fluid restriction.
  - Diuretics.
  - Surgical relief of TS (balloon valvotomy, valve repair or valve replacement).

Q. Discuss the aetiology, clinical features and management of tricuspid regurgitation.

Q. What is De-Carvallo's sign?

- Aetiology:
  - Functional tricuspid regurgitation (most common)—rheumatic or congenital heart diseases with severe pulmonary hypertension, inferior wall infarction, cardiomyopathy and cor pulmonale.
  - Organic tricuspid regurgitation—rheumatic, Ebstein's anomaly, tricuspid valve prolapse, carcinoid syndrome, infective endocarditis, endomyocardial fibrosis, radiation therapy and trauma (e.g. endomyocardial biopsies, pacemaker lead placement).
- Clinical features:
  - Symptoms of right ventricular failure become intensified.
  - Oedema, ascites and pleural effusion.
  - Hepatomegaly with systolic pulsations.
  - JVP is raised with prominent *v* waves and rapid *y* descent.
  - A blowing pansystolic murmur at the lower left sternal border, which is intensified during inspiration (De-Carvallo's sign).
- Treatment:
  - Treatment of underlying heart disease reduces functional tricuspid regurgitation.
  - Surgical treatment of tricuspid regurgitation consists of tricuspid valve replacement or repair of the annulus.
  - In those undergoing left-sided valve surgery, tricuspid valve repair is universally recommended in the presence of severe coexistent TR.

Q. Discuss the clinical manifestations, investigations and management of pulmonary stenosis (PS).

- Majority are congenital and may be associated with maternal rubella syndrome (cataract, deafness, microcephaly, pulmonary artery stenosis or pulmonary valvular stenosis).
- May be an isolated lesion or associated with Fallot's tetralogy.
- Acquired pulmonic stenosis is most often due to carcinoid syndrome.
- Rheumatic aetiology very uncommon.
- May be supravalvular, valvular or infundibular.
- Symptoms:
  - Dyspnoea, fatigue.
  - Central cyanosis, if right-to-left shunt develops (increased right ventricular pressure in congenital pulmonic stenosis may force open foramen ovale).
  - Angina or syncope indicates severe stenosis and occurs due to an inability to augment pulmonary blood flow during exertion.
- Physical findings:
  - Prominent *a* waves on JVP.
  - Increased right ventricular thrust in the form of left parasternal heave and epigastric pulsation.
  - Systolic thrill, best felt with patient sitting up, leaning forwards and during inspiration.
  - Wide splitting of second heart sound.
  - A right-sided fourth heart sound.
  - Ejection click in valvular pulmonic stenosis. It is the only right-sided sound that is best heard during expiration and not accentuated with inspiration.
  - Ejection systolic murmur, best heard to the left of upper sternum, radiating to left shoulder and increasing with inspiration. The murmur duration increases with increasing degrees of stenosis and its peak intensity occurs later in systole.
  - Murmurs of tricuspid regurgitation and pulmonary regurgitation may be detected.
- Investigations:
  - ECG shows right ventricular hypertrophy and in severe cases, right atrial enlargement.
  - Chest radiography shows poststenotic dilatation of pulmonary artery, characteristically extending into the left pulmonary artery branch.
  - Doppler echocardiographic study.
  - Cardiac catheterisation.
- Treatment:
  - Mild to moderate stenosis requires no treatment except periodic evaluations.
  - Severe stenosis is treated by percutaneous pulmonary balloon valvotomy, surgical valvuloplasty or valve replacement.

Q. Discuss the manoeuvres useful in differentiating murmurs due to various cardiac diseases.

- Table 7.59 shows various manoeuvres that are useful in differentiating murmurs due to various cardiac diseases.

TABLE 7.59 Effect of Various Manoeuvres on Cardiac Murmurs

Manoeuvre	Effect
• **Valsalva**	During active strain phase against closed glottis, most murmurs reduce in intensity, except (a) murmur of hypertrophic cardiomyopathy (HCM) that gets louder and (b) murmur of mitral valve prolapse (MVP) that gets longer and louder
• **Respiration**	Right-sided sounds and murmurs get louder with inspiration except pulmonary ejection click
• **Handgrip**	By increasing afterload, handgrip augments murmur of mitral regurgitation (MR), aortic regurgitation (AR); does not affect murmur of aortic stenosis (AS) and decreases murmur of HCM and MVP
• **Squatting**	Causes a rapid increase in venous return and peripheral resistance, thereby increases left ventricular volume. Murmurs of MR and AR get louder while that of HCM gets softer
• **Post-extrasystolic beat**	Both HCM and AS murmurs get louder because of increased post-extrasystolic contractility while MR murmur is unaffected

Q. Discuss the aetiology, pathology, clinical features, investigations, treatment and prophylaxis of infective endocarditis. (IM 1.21)

Q. Explain in brief about postoperative endocarditis.

- Infective endocarditis is due to microbial infection of the heart valve or the lining of cardiac chamber (endothelium).
- The causative organism could be bacterium, fungus or *Rickettsia*.
- Streptococci and staphylococci account for the vast majority of cases.

TYPES OF INFECTIVE ENDOCARDITIS

- Subacute endocarditis and acute endocarditis.
- Native valve endocarditis and prosthetic valve or postoperative endocarditis.
- Left-sided endocarditis and right-sided endocarditis.

Note: Most physicians do not differentiate between subacute and acute infective endocarditis, and simply state them as infective endocarditis.

- Another classification of infective endocarditis is left-sided infective endocarditis, left-sided prosthetic infective endocarditis, right-sided infective endocarditis and device-related (permanent pacemaker, implantable cardioverter-defibrillator) infective endocarditis.

SUBACUTE ENDOCARDITIS

- Caused by organisms of relatively low virulence.
- Occurs on the damaged valves or at sites where the endothelium is damaged by a high-pressure jet of blood (VSD, PDA, MR, AS, AR).
- Characterised by formation of vegetations, embolic episodes, mycotic aneurysms, valve regurgitation, splenic and renal infarcts, and immune glomerulonephritis.
- Common sources of infection are procedures in the presence of periodontal infections (dental treatment), gastrointestinal tract infections and urinary tract infections.

ACUTE ENDOCARDITIS

- A source of infection or portal of entry is often evident.
- Caused by highly virulent and invasive organisms.
- Can affect damaged valves as well as normal hearts.
- Has a fulminant course, vegetations are more florid, valve destruction is greater and abscess (local and metastatic) formation is common.

POSTOPERATIVE ENDOCARDITIS OR PROSTHETIC VALVE ENDOCARDITIS

- Follows cardiac surgery using prosthetic valves and other prosthetic materials.
- May occurs early (within 60 days of surgery) due to intraoperative or hospital-acquired infections or late (after 1 year) due to infection with community-acquired organisms. Those occurring between 60 days and 1 year are a mixture of hospital-acquired episodes caused by less virulent organisms and community-acquired episodes.
- Aortic prosthetic valve more prone than mitral prosthetic valve.
- During the first 3 months, after surgery, mechanical heart valves are at higher risk for infection than are bio-prosthetic ones but the rates of infection for the two valve types congregate later on and are comparable at 5 years.
- In early prosthetic valve endocarditis, *Staphylococcus aureus* predominates followed by coagulase-negative staphylococci and fungi. After 2 months, additional organisms include *viridans* streptococci and enterococci. In late endocarditis, offending agents are the same which cause native valve endocarditis.

RIGHT-SIDED ENDOCARDITIS

- Occurs in intravenous drug users.
- Caused predominantly by organisms found on the skin (e.g. *S. aureus, Candida*).
- Affects right-sided valves, particularly tricuspid valve.
- May present with acute endocarditis.

PREDISPOSING FACTORS

- A variety of factors predispose to infective endocarditis. However, antibiotic prophylaxis is recommended only for a patient with a high risk of severe adverse outcome, should the patient develop endocarditis (Box 7.58).
- Prophylaxis is not recommended for MVP, rheumatic heart disease, ASD, VSD, calcific aortic sclerosis and bicuspid aortic valve.
- Procedures that are associated with high risk of endocarditis are shown in Table 7.60.

BOX 7.58 Cardiac Conditions Associated With the Highest Risk of Adverse Outcome From Endocarditis (Require Antibiotic Prophylaxis Before High-Risk Procedures)

- Prosthetic cardiac valve or prosthetic material used for cardiac valve repair
- Previous infective endocarditis
- Congenital heart disease (CHD)
  - Unrepaired cyanotic CHD including palliative shunts and conduits
  - Completely repaired congenital heart defect with prosthetic material or device whether placed by surgery or by catheter intervention, during the first 6 months after procedure
  - Repaired CHD with residual defects at the site or adjacent to the site of a prosthetic patch or prosthetic device (which inhibit endothelialisation)
- Cardiac transplantation recipients who develop cardiac valvulopathy

TABLE 7.60 Procedures Associated With High Risk of Endocarditis

Procedures	Procedures
Procedures on Respiratory Tract • Tonsillectomy and/or adenoidectomy • Surgical operations (incision or biopsy) that involve respiratory mucosa • An invasive respiratory tract procedure to treat an established infection (e.g. drainage of an abscess or empyema) **Procedures in Oral Cavity** • All dental procedures that involve manipulation of gingival tissue or the periapical region of teeth or perforation of the oral mucosa (e.g. dental extractions, suture removal, placement of orthodontic band, root canal treatment, dental procedures with intraligamentous anaesthesia and re-implantation of avulsed tooth)	**Procedures on Gastrointestinal Tract** • None unless procedure is done during an established infection **Procedures on Genitourinary Tract** • None unless procedure is done during an established infection (e.g. cystoscopy during known enterococcal UTI) **Procedures on Skin and Musculoskeletal System** • None unless procedure involves infected tissue

Note: Prophylaxis is not needed for routine anaesthetic injections through noninfected tissue, dental radiographs, placement of removable prosthodontic or orthodontic appliances, adjustment of orthodontic appliances, placement of orthodontic brackets, shedding of deciduous teeth, bleeding from trauma to the lips or oral mucosa, vaginal delivery, hysterectomy or tattooing. It is also not recommended for bronchoscopy, laryngoscopy, endotracheal intubation, cystoscopy, colonoscopy or skin suturing.

TABLE 7.61 Common Organisms Producing Endocarditis

Subacute Endocarditis	Acute Endocarditis	Postoperative Endocarditis

• *Viridans* streptococci
  ◦ *Streptococcus sanguis*
  ◦ *Streptococcus mitis*
• *Streptococcus milleri*
• *Streptococcus bovis*
• *Enteroccocus faecalis*
• *S. aureus*
• HACEK group[a]
	• *Staphylococcus aureus*
	• *Pseudomonas*
	• *Candida*
	• *Streptococcus pneumoniae*
	• *Neisseria gonorrhoeae*
		• All organisms causing acute and subacute endocarditis
		• *Staphylococcus albus*
		• *Candida*
		• *Aspergillus*

[a]*Haemophilus, Aggregatibacter* (formerly *Actinobacillus*), *Cardiobacterium, Eikenella* and *Kingella*.

COMMON ORGANISMS (Table 7.61)

- The commonest organism causing subacute endocarditis is *Streptococcus sanguis*. It is an α-haemolytic streptococcus belonging to *Streptococcus viridans* group. It is a normal inhabitant of oropharynx and gastrointestinal tract. *S. sanguis* is highly sensitive to penicillin.

PATHOLOGY AND PATHOGENESIS (Flowchart 7.16)

ENDOCARDIAL INJURY AND VEGETATION FORMATION

- The first step is endocardial injury which may occur by many mechanisms. The most common mechanism is

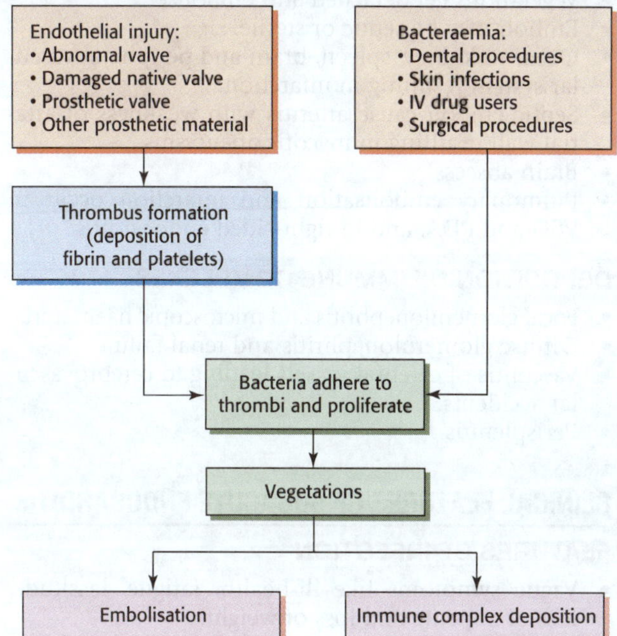

Flowchart 7.16 Pathogenesis of Infective Endocarditis.

injury by turbulent blood flow from an acquired or congenital intracardiac abnormality. Alternatively, an intravascular catheter or another device may directly abrade endocardium. In injection drug users, direct injection of contaminating debris may damage tricuspid valve surface.
- The endothelial damage triggers sterile thrombus formation, which occurs by deposition of fibrin and platelets.
- Once a sterile thrombus is present, transient bacteraemia can seed the thrombus.
- Once bacteria have attached to the endocardium, additional deposition of fibrin and bacterial proliferation lead to mature vegetation formation.

VEGETATIONS

- Vegetations are fibrin–platelet bacteria complexes.
- Vegetations have three layers, an inner layer of RBC, WBC and platelets, a middle layer of bacteria and an outer layer of fibrin.

BOX 7.59 Location of Vegetations

- Mitral valve—atrial surface and line of apposition of valve cusps.
- VSD—on the right ventricular endocardium and around the defect.
- Aortic valve—on the ventricular surface.
- PDA—on the pulmonary artery and ductus.
- Chordae tendineae and papillary muscles may have vegetations and lead to rupture.

- Vegetations are located differently on various valves (Box 7.59).

EMBOLISATION

- Vegetations get detached and embolise.
- Emboli may be septic or sterile.
- Occur to kidney, spleen, brain and peripheral vascular system resulting in infarction.
- Septic emboli cause arteritis with weakness of arterial wall resulting in mycotic aneurysms.
- Brain abscess.
- Pulmonary embolisation and infarction occur in VSD and PDA, and in right-sided endocarditis.

DEPOSITION OF IMMUNE COMPLEXES

- Focal glomerulonephritis and microscopic haematuria.
- Diffuse glomerulonephritis and renal failure.
- Vasculitis of cerebral vessels leading to cerebrovascular accidents.
- Perisplenitis.

CLINICAL FEATURES OF SUBACUTE ENDOCARDITIS

FEATURES OF INFECTION

- Vague symptoms like ill-health, fatigue, lassitude, loss of appetite and loss of weight.
- Low-grade or high-grade, intermittent or continuous fever with chills and rigors.
- Clubbing.
- Splenomegaly.
- Brownish pigmentation of face and limbs called cafe au lait pigmentation.

FEATURES OF HAEMODYNAMIC CHANGES

- Appearance of new murmurs, particularly a diastolic murmur.
- Change in the character of an existing murmur.
- Development of MR and TR due to rupture of papillary muscles or chordae tendineae.
- Worsening of cardiac failure.
- Acute left ventricular failure and pulmonary oedema due to rupture of valve cusps.

FEATURES OF EMBOLISM

- Cutaneous embolism—Janeway lesions on palms and soles.
- Nails—splinter haemorrhages (Fig. 7.46).
- Spleen—painful splenomegaly.
- Peripheral arteries—claudication, absence of peripheral pulses and gangrene.

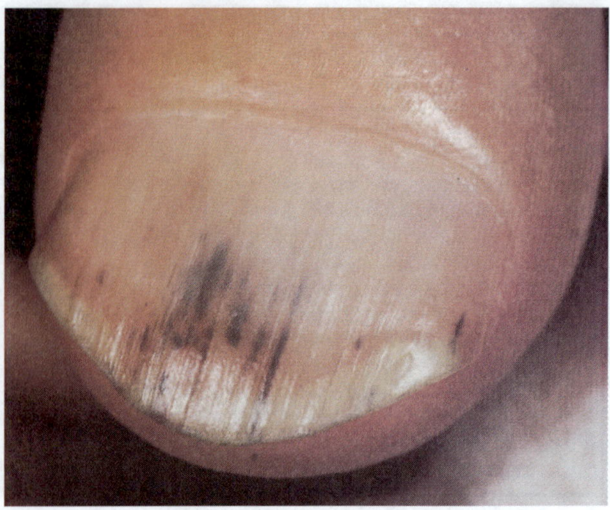

Fig. 7.46 Splinter haemorrhages.

- Central nervous system—convulsions, haemiplegia, aphasia, loss of vision and cerebellar disturbances.
- Kidneys—loin pain, haematuria and renal failure.
- Lungs—pulmonary infarction, pleurisy and pleural effusion (right-sided endocarditis).

FEATURES OF IMMUNOLOGICAL DISTURBANCES

- Osler's nodes—painful, tender, swollen nodules in pulps of fingers.
- Roth spots—circular retinal haemorrhages with white central spots.
- Glomerulonephritis and haematuria.

CLINICAL FEATURES OF ACUTE ENDOCARDITIS

- Severe, abrupt onset of febrile illness.
- Prominent and changing heart murmurs.
- Embolic episodes more common.
- Rapid development of renal and cardiac failure.

CLINICAL FEATURES OF POSTOPERATIVE ENDOCARDITIS

- Presents as an unexplained fever in a patient who has had cardiac valve surgery.
- Course depends on the virulence of the organism—prominent and changing heart murmurs, frequent embolic episodes and rapid development of renal and cardiac failure.

CLINICAL FEATURES OF RIGHT-SIDED ENDOCARDITIS

- Pulmonary infarction, pleurisy and pleural effusion due to vegetation embolism.
- Generally has a favourable prognosis.

INVESTIGATIONS

- Normocytic normochromic anaemia.
- Leucocytosis.

- Microscopic haematuria and albuminuria.
- Raised ESR and CRP.
- Blood culture—three specimens of 10 mL blood each are taken at least at an interval of 1 hour from one another. Both aerobic and anaerobic cultures are done, rarely fungal culture also.

NEGATIVE BLOOD CULTURES IN ENDOCARDITIS

- Defined as endocarditis without aetiology following inoculation of at least three independent blood samples in a standard blood culture system with negative cultures after 7 days of incubation and subculturing.
- Various causes are shown in Box 7.60.

OTHER INVESTIGATIONS

- Serological tests for *Bartonella*, *Coxiella burnetii* and *Brucella* in patients with negative blood cultures who have risk factors for these infections.
- Hyperglobulinaemia, positive rheumatoid factor, reduction in the complement levels and presence of circulating immune complexes.
- Echocardiography can detect the vegetations and identify the valve lesion, chamber dilatation and new prosthetic dehiscence. Transthoracic echocardiography has a sensitivity of about 75% for the diagnosis of vegetations. Transoesophageal echocardiography is mandatory in cases of doubtful transthoracic examination, in prosthetic and pacemaker endocarditis or when an abscess is suspected.
- High-resolution multislice cardiac CT for diagnosing paravalvular complications such as abscess.
- ^{18}F-fluorodeoxyglucose PET–CT to look for active foci and is useful particularly if endocarditis is related to a prosthetic valve or cardiac device.

MODIFIED DUKE CRITERIA FOR INFECTIVE ENDOCARDITIS (Table 7.62)

- Has a mean sensitivity of 80% for diagnosing infective endocarditis (IE).
- Diagnosis of IE is definite in the presence of:
  - Pathological criteria.
  - Two major criteria.
  - One major and two minor criteria.
  - Five minor criteria.
- Diagnosis of IE is possible in the presence of one major and one minor criteria, or three minor criteria.

BOX 7.60 Causes of Negative Blood Cultures in Endocarditis

- Prior antibiotic treatment (most common cause)
- Inadequate quantity of blood taken for culture
- Right-sided endocarditis
- Anaerobic infection
- Infection with fastidious organisms (e.g. *Haemophilus parainfluenzae, Brucella*)
- Fungal infections (*Candida, Histoplasma*)
- Non-infective endocarditis

TABLE 7.62 Modified Duke Criteria for Infective Endocarditis

MAJOR CRITERIA

- Blood cultures positive
  - Typical microorganisms consistent with infective endocarditis from two blood cultures:
    - *Viridans* streptococci, *Streptococcus bovis*, HACEK group (*Heamophilus*, *Actinobacillus*, *Cardiobacterium*, *Eikenella*, *Kingella*)
    - Community-acquired *Staphylococcus aureus* or enterococci in the absence of a primary focus

    OR
  - Other microorganisms consistent with IE from persistently positive blood cultures defined as:
    - Two positive cultures of blood samples drawn >12 hours apart
    - All of three or a majority of four separate cultures of blood (with first and last samples drawn 1 hour apart)

    OR
  - Single positive blood culture for *Coxiella burnetii* or positive serology for Q fever, *Bartonella* species and *Chlamydia psittaci*
- Evidence of endocardial involvement
  - Echocardiogram positive for IE
    - Oscillating intracardiac mass without alternative explanation
    - Abscess
    - New partial dehiscence of prosthetic valve
    - New valvular regurgitation (worsening or changing of preexisting murmur not sufficient)

MINOR CRITERIA

- Predisposition to infective endocarditis: Predisposing heart condition, injection drug use, previous infective endocarditis, or prosthetic valve or material
- Fever, temperature >38°C
- Vascular phenomena: Major arterial emboli, septic pulmonary infarcts, mycotic aneurysm, intracranial haemorrhages, subconjunctival petechiae, Janeway lesions
- Immunological phenomena: Glomerulonephritis, Osler's nodes, Roth spots, positive rheumatoid factor
- Microbiological evidence: Positive blood culture but does not meet a major criterion or serological evidence of active infection with organisms consistent with infective endocarditis

PATHOLOGICAL CRITERIA

- Positive microbiology or histology of pathological tissue material attained at surgery or autopsy (vegetations, valve tissue, embolic fragments or tissue/pus from intracardiac abscesses)

MEDICAL TREATMENT (Table 7.63)

- In right-sided endocarditis due to *S. aureus* with pulmonary abscesses, daptomycin can be used.
- In case of infection of prosthetic valve, the treatment should be continued for at least 6 weeks.

SURGICAL TREATMENT—INDICATIONS

- Progressive cardiac failure from valve damage.
- Endocarditis of prosthetic valve.
- Large vegetation (>10 mm) on a left-sided valve with an episode of embolisation, or very large (>15 mm) and mobile vegetation (high risk of embolism).
- Active infection persisting in spite of adequate treatment (when fever and bacteraemia are evident for more than 7–10 days despite adequate antibiotic treatment).
- Abscess formation, perivalvular involvement and fungal endocarditis are also considered indications for early surgery.

TABLE 7.63 Medical Treatment of Infective Endocarditis

Organism	Treatment
• Infective endocarditis awaiting culture report or culture negative	Benzylpenicillin 2–3 million units IV 4 hourly plus gentamicin 3 mg/kg once a day for 4–6 weeks OR Ceftriaxone 2 g once a day for 4–6 weeks OR Amoxillin/clavulanate 12 g/day in four divided doses plus gentamicin 1.5 mg/kg twice a day for 4–6 weeks Vancomycin in penicillin-allergic patients
• Suspected staphylococcal endocarditis	Vancomycin 30 mg/kg/day in two divided doses (not to exceed 2 g/day) for 6 weeks and gentamicin 1 mg/kg three times a day for 1–2 weeks. Add rifampicin 20 mg/kg/day in two divided doses in prosthetic valve endocarditis
• Streptococci highly sensitive to penicillin	Benzylpenicillin 2–3 million units IV 4 hourly for 4 weeks OR Ceftriaxone 2 g IV once a day for 4 weeks OR Benzylpenicillin or ceftriaxone for 2 weeks plus gentamicin 3 mg/kg once a day for 2 weeks Vancomycin 30 mg/kg/day in two divided doses (not to exceed 2 g/day) for 4 weeks in penicillin-sensitive patients
• Streptococci less sensitive to penicillin	Benzylpenicillin (24 million units/day in six divided doses) or ceftriaxone for 4–6 weeks and gentamicin 3 mg/kg/day (as single infusion) for at least 2 weeks
• Anaerobic streptococci	Benzylpenicillin, metronidazole
• Staphylococcal endocarditis (methicillin-sensitive)	Cloxacillin 2 g 4 hourly or cefazolin 2 g 8 hourly for 6 weeks plus gentamicin 1.5 mg/kg twice a day for 3–5 days
• Staphylococcal endocarditis (methicillin resistant)	Vancomycin for 6 weeks OR Daptomycin 10 mg/kg/day for 6 weeks
• Enterococcal endocarditis	Ampicillin 2 g 4 hourly or vancomycin plus gentamicin 1.5 mg/kg two times a day for 6 weeks OR Ampicillin plus ceftriaoxone for 4 weeks OR Vancomycin plus gentamicin for 6 weeks
• *Candida*	Amphotericin

TABLE 7.64 Infective Endocarditis Prophylaxis for Oral Procedures

Patient Group	Antibiotic	Dose (Single 30–60 Minutes Before Procedure)
• Able to take oral medicine	Amoxicillin	2 g
• Unable to take oral medicine	Ampicillin or Cefazolin or Ceftriaxone	2 g IM/IV 1 g IM/IV 1 g IM/IV
• Allergic to penicillins or ampicillin and able to take oral medication	Cephalexin or Clindamycin or Azithromycin/clarithromycin	2 g 600 mg 500 mg
• Allergic to penicillins or ampicillin and unable to take oral medication	Cefazolin or Ceftriaxone or Clindamycin or Vancomycin	1 g 1 g 600 mg 15 mg/kg (not to exceed 1 g)

Note: Cephalosporins should not be given to a patient who has a history of anaphylaxis, angio-oedema or urticaria with penicillins or ampicillin.

PROPHYLAXIS

INFECTIVE ENDOCARDITIS PROPHYLAXIS FOR ORAL PROCEDURES

- Prophylaxis for infective endocarditis in oral procedures is given in Table 7.64.

INFECTIVE ENDOCARDITIS PROPHYLAXIS FOR RESPIRATORY TRACT PROCEDURES

- As per Table 7.64 for oral procedures.
- For patients who undergo an invasive respiratory tract procedure to treat an established infection (e.g. drainage of an abscess or empyema), antibiotic regimen should contain an agent active against *viridans* streptococci. If such infection is known to be caused by *S. aureus*, the regimen should contain an antistaphylococcal penicillin or cephalosporin, or vancomycin (in patients allergic to β-lactams). Vancomycin should also be administered if the infection is known or suspected to be caused by a methicillin-resistant strain of *S. aureus*.

INFECTIVE ENDOCARDITIS PROPHYLAXIS FOR GENITOURINARY AND GASTROINTESTINAL TRACT PROCEDURES

- Not recommended for patients who undergo genitourinary or gastrointestinal tract procedures including diagnostic oesophagogastroduodenoscopy or colonoscopy.
- For patients who have an established gastrointestinal or genitourinary tract infection or for those who receive antibiotic therapy to prevent wound infection or sepsis associated with a GI or GU tract procedure, it may be reasonable that the antibiotic regimen includes an agent active against enterococci, such as penicillin, ampicillin, piperacillin or vancomycin.

INFECTIVE ENDOCARDITIS PROPHYLAXIS FOR SKIN AND SOFT TISSUE SURGERIES

- No prophylaxis indicated for routine surgeries.
- If a surgical procedure involves infected skin or musculoskeletal tissue, the therapeutic regimen should

contain an agent active against staphylococci and β-haemolytic streptococci, such as an antistaphylococcal penicillin or a cephalosporin. In case of allergy or suspected infection by methicillin-resistant strain of *Staphylococcus*, vancomycin or clindamycin should be administered.

Q. Write a brief note on Osler's nodes.

- Box 7.61 gives a brief account of Osler's nodes.

Q. Give a brief account of Janeway lesions.

- Box 7.62 gives a brief account of Janeway lesions.

Q. Enumerate the important features of Roth spots.

- Features of Roth spots are given in Box 7.63.

Q. Briefly explain non-infective endocarditis.

Q. Write a short note on marantic endocarditis.

Q. Write a short note on Libman-Sacks endocarditis.

- Refers to formation of sterile platelet and fibrin thrombi on cardiac valves and adjacent endocardium

BOX 7.61 Osler's Nodes

- Result from vasculitis
- Small, raised, painful, tender nodules of 0.5–1.5 cm diameter
- Seen on the pulps of fingers and toes, thenar and hypothenar eminences (Fig. 7.47)
- Last for 1–5 days
- Seen in infective endocarditis, SLE, gonococcal and typhoid infections

BOX 7.62 Janeway Lesions

- Subepithelial microabscesses.
- Bacteria can be identified near but not in the lesion.
- Seen in infective endocarditis.
- Small, red, raised, painless lesions over the palms and soles (Fig. 7.48).

BOX 7.63 Important Features of Roth Spots

- Seen in infective endocarditis
- Due to immune complex deposition
- Elliptical or circular-shaped haemorrhagic areas with central white spots (Fig. 7.49)
- Seen on the retina by fundoscopy
- May also be seen in anaemia, thrombocytopenia, leukaemia, hypertensive retinopathy, preeclampsia, HIV infection, anoxia

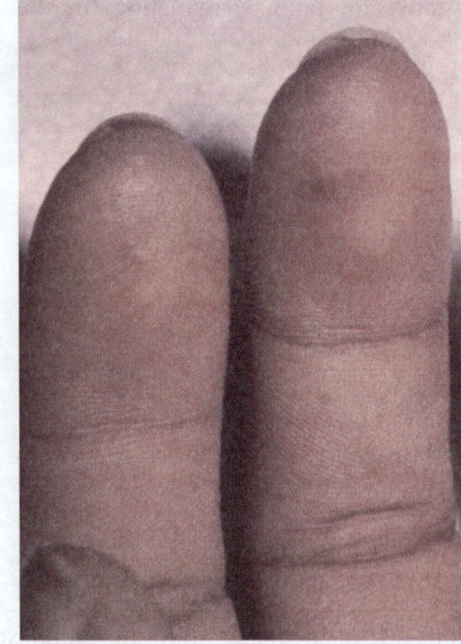

Fig. 7.47 Osler's nodes on pulp of fingers.

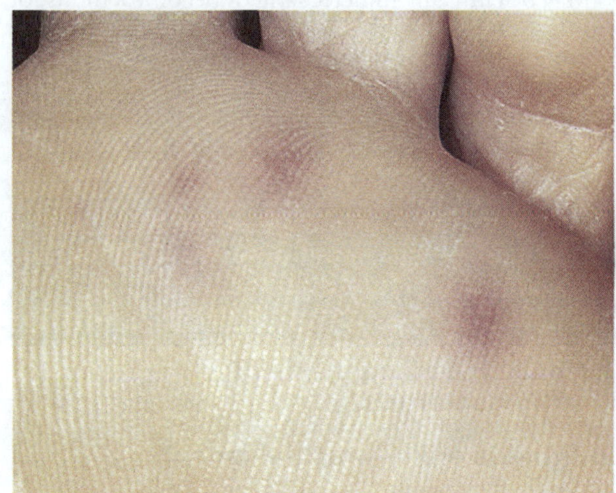

Fig. 7.48 Janeway lesions on sole.

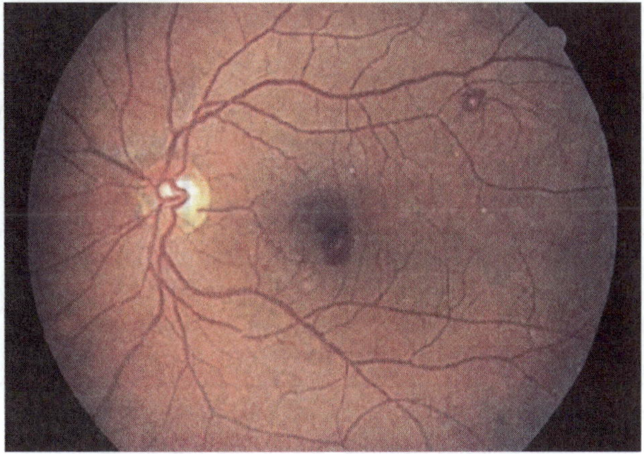

Fig. 7.49 Roth spots (white-centered haemorrhages).

in response to trauma, circulating immune complexes, vasculitis or a hypercoagulable state.
- Symptoms are those of systemic arterial embolism.
- Diagnosis by echocardiography and negative blood cultures.
- Treatment consists of anticoagulants and treatment of underlying cause.
- Prognosis is generally poor, more because of the seriousness of predisposing disorders than the cardiac lesion.

MARANTIC ENDOCARDITIS

- Also known as non-bacterial thrombotic endocarditis.
- Thrombotic vegetations.
- Vegetations tend to form on congenitally abnormal cardiac valves or those damaged by rheumatic fever.
- Occurs in malignancy and wasting disorders.

LIBMAN–SACKS ENDOCARDITIS

- Develops due to circulating immune complexes.
- Vegetations 3–4 mm in size.
- Vegetations composed of degenerating valve tissue.
- Most common on ventricular surface of mitral valve; aortic valve is rarely involved.
- May be clinically undetectable or become a nidus for infection (leading to infective endocarditis), produce emboli or impair valvular function.
- Seen in systemic lupus erythematosus.
- Medical treatment is not well established. Treatment of underlying disease should be initiated.

Q. Discuss the aetiology and risk factors of ischaemic heart disease (IHD) or coronary artery disease. (IM 2.1, IM 2.2)

Q. Discuss pathogenesis of atherosclerosis.

Q. What is ankle–brachial index?

- Ischaemic heart disease (IHD) is a condition in which there is an imbalance between myocardial blood supply and its oxygen demand.
- The term coronary artery disease indicates IHD due to diseases of coronary arteries.

AETIOLOGY

- Most IHD are due to atheroma and its complications (coronary artery disease).
- Uncommon causes include severe aortic stenosis, congenital abnormalities of coronary arteries (aberrant origin of coronary arteries, myocardial bridging, etc.) and arteritis due to connective tissue disorders.

PATHOGENESIS OF ATHEROSCLEROSIS

- Initial lesions of atherosclerosis are fatty streaks.
  - Lipoprotein particles accumulate within intima.
  - Lipoprotein particles undergo oxidative modifications within fatty streaks.
  - Inflammatory cells infiltrate the early lesions of atherosclerosis. These cells include monocyte-derived macrophages and lymphocytes. Macrophages digest oxidised low-density lipoprotein transforming into foam cells and causing the formation of fatty streaks.
  - The activated macrophages release chemoattractants and cytokines that perpetuate the process by recruiting additional macrophages and vascular smooth muscle cells (which synthesise extracellular matrix components) at the site of the plaque.
- Not all fatty streaks progress to atheromas. Circulating monocytes may remove lipids from intima. High-density lipoprotein also mediates lipid removal from fatty streaks and atheroma. This reverse cholesterol transport by HDL explains its antiatherogenic action. In addition, HDL maintains endothelial function and protects against thrombosis.
- Some lipid-laden foam cells die due to apoptosis (programmed cell death) which results in a lipid-rich, necrotic core.
- Fibrous tissue is formed around the lipid-laden macrophages. Smooth muscle cells synthesise fibrous tissue around the lipid core resulting in formation of a fibrous plaque. There is also proliferation of smooth muscle cells in plaques.
- Endothelial dysfunction has been shown to be a major factor in initiation of atherosclerosis. It is associated with hypercholesterolaemia, diabetes, hypertension, cigarette smoking, etc. Endothelial dysfunction may result in diminished vasodilatation or even vasoconstriction in response to various stimuli, including exercise.
- Pathogenesis of atherosclerosis is shown in Flowchart 7.17.
- As plaques advance, they also accumulate calcium (calcification of plaque).
- Some plaques bulge into the lumen of the coronary artery and narrow it. This may lead to flow limitation, particularly during increased myocardial demand leading to ischaemic symptoms.
- Sometimes haemorrhage occurs in a plaque, or its fibrous cap becomes cracked or partially detached. This flap may further narrow coronary lumen. The exposed thrombogenic material within the plaque may precipitate thrombosis, thus completely blocking the vessel lumen acutely and precipitating acute coronary syndromes.
- Characteristics of high-risk or vulnerable plaques include a large lipid core, thin fibrous caps, a high density of macrophages and T lymphocytes, a relative paucity of smooth muscle cells, increase in plaque neovascularity and intraplaque haemorrhage.

RISK FACTORS

MODIFIABLE (MODIFIABLE BY LIFESTYLE AND/OR PHARMACOTHERAPY)

- Smoking:
  - There is a dose-linked relationship between smoking and IHD.

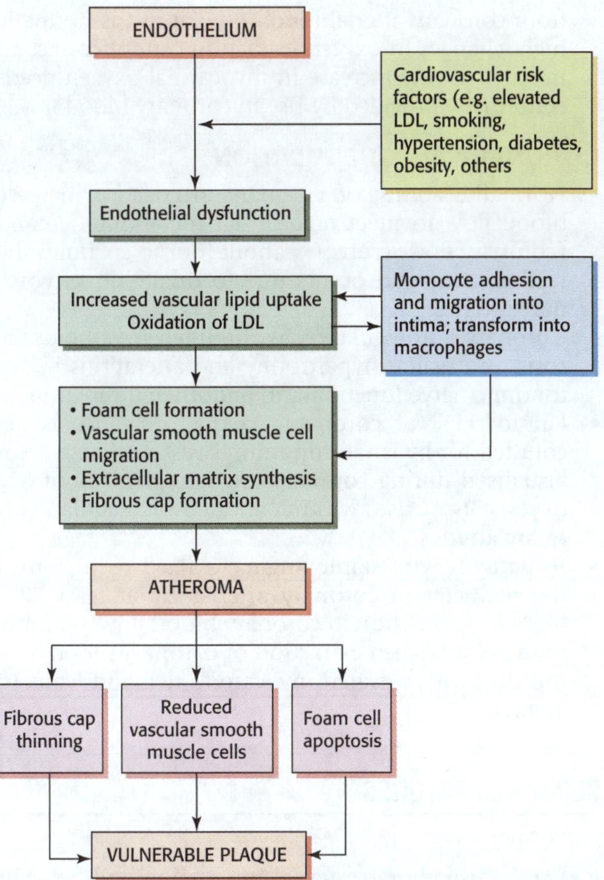

Flowchart 7.17 Pathogenesis of Atherosclerosis.

- The relative risk of death from IHD for smokers compared to that for nonsmokers is highest in the young and less in older people.
- Cholesterol:
  - Hypercholesterolaemia (elevated LDL) predisposes to IHD. Lowering the high cholesterol concentration by diet or drugs reduces the risk of cardiac events.
  - Low HDL cholesterol (<40 mg/dL).

Note: HDL ≥60 mg/dL is a 'negative' risk factor, that is it protects a person from IHD. Blood levels of HDL vary inversely with those of triglycerides. Independent role of triglycerides in IHD is controversial.

- Arterial hypertension:
  - Blood pressure ≥140/90 mmHg or on antihypertensive medications.
  - Even mild arterial hypertension is a risk factor for IHD.
- Diabetes mellitus:
  - Associated with diffuse coronary atheroma and IHD.
  - Insulin resistance (metabolic syndrome) may be associated with lipoprotein abnormalities (diabetic dyslipidaemia) that include small, dense LDL particles, low HDL and elevated triglycerides, all of which may increase IHD risk.
- Physical inactivity.
- Dietary factors:
  - Diets deficient in polyunsaturated fatty acids (PUFA).
  - Low vitamin C and vitamin E.
- Coagulation factors:
  - Fibrinogen and factor VII are associated with an increased risk of myocardial infarction.
- Obesity:
  - Obesity (BMI ≥30 kg/m^2) predisposes to IHD.
- Stress factors:
  - Occupations and events of stressful nature are risk factors for IHD.

NON-MODIFIABLE

- Geographical influences:
  - In some countries the incidence of IHD is increasing, whereas in other countries it is declining.
- Family history of premature CAD:
  - At the age of <55 years in males.
  - At the age of <65 years in females.
- Age:
  - Men ≥45 years.
  - Females ≥55 years (postmenopausal).
- Genetic factors:
  - Forty per cent of the risk of developing IHD is controlled by genetic factors.
  - Genetic factors operate in hyperlipidaemia, plasma fibrinogen concentration and other coagulation factors, some of which can be modified using lifestyle changes.

EMERGING RISK FACTORS (REMAIN CONTROVERSIAL)

- Apolipoprotein B
- Lipoprotein(a) [Lp(a)]
- C-reactive protein (high sensitivity)
- Hyperhomocysteinaemia
- Infection
- Small and dense LDL particles
- Impaired fasting glucose

SUMMARY OF RISK FACTORS

- The risk factors are summarised in Box 7.64.

BOX 7.64 Risk Factors for Atherosclerosis

MODIFIABLE RISK FACTORS (MAJOR)
- Smoking
- Hypercholesterolaemia (elevated LDL)
- Hypertension
- Diabetes mellitus

MODIFIABLE ADDITIONAL RISK FACTORS
- Physical inactivity
- Dietary factors
- Obesity
- Stress factors

NON-MODIFIABLE FACTORS
- Age (≥45 years in males and ≥55 years in females)
- Male gender
- Geographical factors
- Family history of premature CAD
- Genetic factors
- Others:
  - Elevated procoagulant levels
  - Elevated CRP levels
  - Hyperhomocysteinaemia
  - Small and dense LDL particles
  - Apolipoprotein B
  - Lipoprotein(a) [Lp(a)]

ANKLE–BRACHIAL INDEX

- Ratio of systolic blood pressure at the ankle to systolic blood pressure at the brachial artery.
- One of the most widely available markers of atherosclerosis and least expensive to perform.
- In the primary care setting, effectively used to assess cardiovascular risk and diagnose peripheral artery disease (PAD).
- An ABI ≤0.9 is the threshold for confirming lower-extremity PAD.
- An ABI ≤0.9 or ≥1.4 indicates increased risk of cardiovascular events and mortality regardless of presence of PAD symptoms or other cardiovascular risk factors.

Q. Discuss the clinical manifestations, investigations and management of angina pectoris.

Q. Write a short note on angina decubitus, nocturnal angina, Prinzmetal's angina (variant angina) and microvascular angina.

ANGINA PECTORIS

- A clinical syndrome of discomfort which occurs due to transient myocardial ischaemia.
- Transient myocardial ischaemia is due to the following:
  - Obstruction of coronary flow by atheroma.
  - Coronary arterial spasm.
  - Microvascular coronary dysfunction.
- Angina is worsened by factors that increase myocardial oxygen requirement or reduce supply (Box 7.65).

PATHOPHYSIOLOGY

MYOCARDIAL ENERGY (OXYGEN) BALANCE

- Myocardial ischaemia results from an imbalance between myocardial energy supply (oxygen and energy substrates like glucose and free fatty acids) and myocardial oxygen demand. Besides substrate supply, utilisation and enzymatic activities involved in metabolism may also play a role in the pathogenesis of myocardial ischaemia.
- Major determinants of myocardial oxygen demand are heart rate, blood pressure and myocardial wall tension (which is influenced by preload, afterload and contractility). Since myocardial oxygen extraction from coronary arterial blood flow at rest is normally high, changes in oxygen extraction cannot correct an imbalance. Any increase in myocardial oxygen needs is normally provided by rise in coronary blood flow.

BOX 7.65 Factors Which Increase Myocardial Oxygen Demand

• Exercise	• Hyperthyroidism
• Anaemia	• Aortic stenosis
• Tachycardia	• Aortic regurgitation
• Hypertension	• Arrhythmias
• Emotional stress (anger, fright, stress)	• Cold wind

CORONARY AUTOREGULATION

- Normally, ability of coronary arteries to increase blood flow to meet myocardial metabolic demand (coronary flow reserve) is about four to six times the resting value and occurs due to dilatation of coronary arteries.
- Coronary autoregulation is modified by atherosclerosis, ventricular hypertrophy and alterations in autonomic nerve function and endothelial function.
- Up to 95% of coronary arterial resistance is accounted for by small intramural vessels that are not visualised during coronary angiography. About 5% of resistance arises within conductive epicardial coronary arteries.
- In patients with stable angina, a fixed reduction in the diameter of coronary arteries by at least 70% leads to a reduction in coronary blood flow. Inability to increase oxygen extraction or coronary blood flow together with elevated myocardial demand leads to angina.

CLINICAL FEATURES

HISTORY

- Pain is usually retrosternal in location and brought on by exertion. It is relieved by rest and sublingual nitrates. Pain seldom lasts more than 20 minutes. Character of the pain is squeezing, crushing, tightening, heaviness or aching. Pain commonly radiates to left arm, or less commonly to right arm, throat, back, chin and epigastrium. Often, the pain comes on while walking uphill after a heavy meal on a cold winter day. This defines chronic stable angina.
- Precipitating circumstances remain similar between episodes; thresholds may be predicted by patients and relief patterns become known.
  - Angina severity is classified by New York Heart Association Classification into classes I–IV.
  - Many patients with angina also have silent episodes of angina, that is without any symptoms.
- Angina decubitus is pain while lying flat that raises end-diastolic left ventricular volume, myocardial wall tension and hence oxygen demand.
- Nocturnal angina is an unusual form of angina occurring in aortic regurgitation. It is characterised by paroxysmal, nocturnal anginal pains associated with nightmares, dyspnoea, palpitations, skin flushing, profuse sweating and wide pulse pressure. It does not respond to sublingual nitroglycerine. Nocturnal angina may also occur without associated aortic regurgitation and is due to respiratory pattern changes, episodic tachycardia and hypoxia due to respiratory changes or recumbency.
- Prinzmetal's angina or variant angina or vasospastic angina is pain that comes capriciously due to coronary arterial spasm and is accompanied by transient ST-segment elevation (sometimes depression) on

ECG. It occurs at night, at rest or with exertion. Exercise capacity is preserved. Attacks can be precipitated by hyperventilation. Provocation tests using ergonovine, acetylcholine or hyperventilation during angiography may reveal coronary vasospasm. Smoking and migraine are the most important predisposing risk factors. Prognosis is generally better than those with fixed, significant obstructive lesions, although response to treatment may be poor to β-blockers. Calcium channel blockers with or without long-acting nitrates are the main drugs used in this type of angina. β-blockers alone should not be used. Sublingual nitrates are useful in acute attacks.

- 'Microvascular' angina or cardiac syndrome X or ischaemia with no obstructive coronary arteries indicates angina-like pain, normal coronary angiograms and positive exercise tests. It is more common in women. Response to nitrates is less reliable. β-Blockers are more effective. Hormonal abnormalities, changes in pain perception with exaggerated sensitivity, insulin resistance and psychological overlays may be factors related to this type of angina. Pathogenesis includes endothelial dysfunction, release of vasoactive substances, autonomic dysfunction, vascular smooth muscle dysfunction and loss of oestrogen. About 1% of patients die and 0.6% suffer a stroke within 1 year after their first hospital admission.
- Angina equivalents mean symptoms of myocardial ischaemia other than pain. These include dyspnoea, faintness, fatigue and eructations precipitated by exertion and relieved with rest. At times, there may be no symptoms (silent angina). Angina equivalents and silent angina are more common in women, elderly and diabetics.

PHYSICAL EXAMINATION

- Usually negative, but may find tendon xanthomas, thickening of Achilles tendons, arcus lipoidosis in a young patient, aortic valve disease, diabetes, peripheral vascular disease, thyroid disease or obesity.
- Physical signs shown in Box 7.66 are those of 'myocardial ischaemia'. The presence of one or more of them during an attack of pain may be suggestive.

INVESTIGATIONS

- Electrocardiography—ECG is normal in most patients at rest and in between attacks. Most convincing evidence is demonstration of reversible ST-segment depression or elevation, with or without T wave inversion during an attack of pain. Patient may require exercise testing, for example treadmill testing or bicycle ergometry.
- Stress myocardial perfusion scanning using radioactive thallium (^{201}thallium) or technetium (^{99m}technetium-sestamibi). If a patient cannot perform exercise, pharmacological challenge is performed using dipyridamole, adenosine or dobutamine. Dipyridamole and adenosine raise blood flow in healthy coronary arteries, stealing blood from myocardium served by obstructed vessels. Dobutamine raises myocardial oxygen demand and is useful in patients who cannot raise their heart rates adequately during exercise.
- Echocardiography (including stress echocardiography) and radionuclide blood-pool scanning provide information about ventricular function.
- Coronary angiography (arteriography) provides detailed information about the extent and site of coronary artery stenosis. Indications for coronary angiography are given in Box 7.67.
- Newer modalities for diagnosing coronary artery disease include intravascular ultrasound, multiple-slice spiral computed tomographic coronary angiography (CTCA), magnetic resonance coronary angiography (MRCA) and positron emission tomography (which assesses myocardial viability using glucose metabolism).

BOX 7.66 Phsyical Signs Which May Occur During Anginal Pain

• Rise in blood pressure and heart rate	• Dyskinetic segment around the apex
• Fourth heart sound	• Paradoxical splitting of second heart sound
• Murmur of mitral regurgitation due to papillary muscle dysfunction	• Relief of pain by carotid sinus massage (Levine test)

MANAGEMENT

- The management of angina pectoris can be discussed under three headings:
  - General measures.
  - Drug treatment.
  - Surgical treatment.

GENERAL MEASURES

- Proper explanation about the disease.
- Avoid walking after meals particularly in cold, against a wind.
- Avoid unaccustomed strenuous exercises, stop smoking and reduce weight.
- Hyperlipidaemia treated with diet and drugs (with the goal of reducing LDL <70 mg/dL).

BOX 7.67 Indications for Coronary Angiography in a Patient With Angina

• Markedly positive stress test	• Prior re-vascularisation procedure
• Strong indication for left main coronary artery or three-vessel disease	• Indeterminate stress tests but clinical features of IHD
• Non-atherosclerotic cause of ischaemia (e.g. coronary arterial anomaly)	• Presence of heart failure
• Frequent readmissions for chest pain	• Unable to perform noninvasive tests
• Resistance to medical therapy	• Occupation demands a definitive diagnosis

- Control of hypertension and diabetes (ACE inhibitors are useful in these patients).
- Correction of precipitating conditions such as anaemia, valvular disease and arrhythmias.

DRUG TREATMENT

- Following groups of drugs are used in the management of angina pectoris:
  - Nitrates.
  - β-adrenergic receptor antagonists (β-blockers).
  - Calcium antagonists.
  - Platelet inhibitors.
  - Miscellaneous (ranolazine, trimetazidine, nicorandil and ivabradine).

Nitrates

- Glyceryl trinitrate (GTN) acts by venous and arteriolar dilatation, which lowers blood pressure, reduces venous return to heart and dilates coronary vessels. By producing venodilation, end-diastolic volume and pressure is reduced, leading to increased subendocardial perfusion.
- Fresh glyceryl trinitrate (500 μg) sublingually relieves pain in 2–3 minutes and produces mild headache. Patient is instructed to spit out or swallow the tablet once pain is relieved.
- Best use of GTN is prophylactically before exercise known to produce pain.
- Not more than two tablets per hour should be used. Use of GTN should be encouraged because physical activity promotes the formation of collateral vessels. GTN can be given sublingually, percutaneously as paste or patch, and slow-release buccal tablet. It is virtually ineffective when swallowed. It deteriorates on exposure to air, light and moisture.
- Isosorbide dinitrate has prolonged action (10–20 mg two to three times a day) and is given orally. It can also be given sublingually. Headache is a common side effect. Tolerance develops and dose needs to be increased. It is important to have a 10- to 12-hour nitrate-free period to avoid tolerance. Hence, doses are given in the morning and afternoon. Patients using patches must remember to remove them at night to avoid development of tolerance.
- Isosorbide mononitrate needs to be given once or twice a day.
- Long-acting nitrates are often used if symptoms are not controlled with β-blockers and/or calcium channel blockers. Although there is no evidence that nitrates improve patient prognosis, long-acting nitrates reduce the frequency and severity of angina attacks in patients with stable angina.
- Phosphodiesterase inhibitors (type 5 or PDE5), such as sildenafil, tadalafil and vardenafil, must not be used with nitrates within the same 24 hour period because of risk of severe hypotension.
- Other contraindications to nitrate use include hypertrophic cardiomyopathy, severe aortic stenosis, constrictive pericarditis, mitral stenosis and closed-angle glaucoma.

Beta-blockers

- They reduce myocardial oxygen demand by reducing heart rate for a given level of exercise, reducing heart rate response to anxiety and reducing myocardial contractility. In addition, because of their negative chronotropic effect, β-blockers prolong diastole, raising coronary artery blood flow and myocardial perfusion.
- Propranolol is started in a small initial dose (20 mg thrice daily) and gradually increased to 80–120 mg thrice daily.
- Cardioselective β-blockers have fewer peripheral side effects. These include metoprolol (50–200 mg/day) and atenolol (50–200 mg/day).
- Carvedilol (3.125–25 mg twice a day) has additional unique effects that include its antiarrhythmic effects, antioxidant and antiproliferative properties that inhibit apoptosis.
- β-Blockers should not be withdrawn abruptly as there is a risk of dangerous arrhythmias and myocardial infarction. This occurs due to upregulation of β-adrenergic receptors when patients are treated with β-blockers.
- Absolute contraindications to β-blockers are severe bradycardia, conduction system disease (sinus node dysfunction and/or high-grade AV block), asthma, peripheral vascular disease, depression and pulmonary oedema.
- Prinzmetal's angina may worsen with β-blockers due to an unopposed α-adrenergic effect.
- Patients with cocaine-induced coronary vasoconstriction may develop severe hypertension when given β-blockers.

Calcium Channel Blockers

- They inhibit the slow inward current caused by the entry of extracellular calcium through cell membrane of excited cells, particularly arteriolar smooth muscle and cardiac atrial cells. In arterioles, it results in vasodilatation and hence reduces blood pressure. In cardiac muscle, it reduces inotropy and conductivity. Dilatation of peripheral arteries reduces blood pressure (afterload), thereby reducing myocardial wall tension and hence myocardial oxygen consumption.
- Dihydropyridine calcium channel blockers (amlodipine, nifedipine, felodipine and nicardipine) produce coronary and peripheral arterial dilatation and negative inotropy while nondihydropyridine calcium channel blockers (verapamil, diltiazem) in addition reduce conductivity.
- Nifedipine is a powerful coronary and systemic arteriolar dilator. This can provoke reflex tachycardia. Only long-acting preparations are recommended at present, usually along with a β-blocker. Short-acting nifedipine can increase mortality due to myocardial infarction.
- Verapamil is given at a dose of 40–80 mg thrice daily. Common side effect is constipation. It has a negative inotropic effect and should be avoided in patients with impaired ventricular function.
- Both verapamil and diltiazem are contraindicated in patients with uncompensated heart failure because of their negative inotropic effects.
- Since β-blockers have been shown to reduce mortality after myocardial infarction, it is reasonable to

start a β-blocker and then add a calcium channel blocker if required. However, β-blockers should not be combined with verapamil as both have synergistic effect on rate and myocardial contractility.

- Calcium blockers are indicated in the following situations:
  - Response to β-blockers inadequate.
  - History of asthma, chronic obstructive airway disease or peripheral vascular disease where β-blockers should be avoided.
  - Sick sinus syndrome or significant atrioventricular blocks.
  - Prinzmetal's angina.
  - Adverse effects to β-blockers.

Antiplatelet Agents

Aspirin

- The antianginal drugs discussed above have been shown to ameliorate symptoms only; they may not reduce mortality.
- Aspirin (and lipid-lowering agents) have been shown to improve survival.
- Inhibits the synthesis of prostaglandins, notably thromboxane A_2, a potent vasoconstrictor and platelet activator.
- Dose is 75–150 mg/day.

$P2Y_{12}$ Antagonists

- Clopidogrel is a platelet inhibitor that is useful in patients who cannot tolerate aspirin.
- It may have a synergistic effect when combined with aspirin in patients following acute coronary syndrome or implantation of a drug-eluting stent; benefit of combination has not been shown in chronic stable angina.
- Prasugrel and ticagrelor are other $P2Y_{12}$ antagonists that achieve greater platelet inhibition compared to clopidogrel.

Miscellaneous Drugs

Angiotensin-Converting Enzyme Inhibitors

- These agents reduce total mortality, MI, stroke and heart failure among specific subgroups of patients, including those with heart failure, chronic kidney disease, hypertension and diabetes.

Ranolazine

- Ranolazine is a late sodium ion channel inhibitor. By preventing intracellular sodium overload, calcium accumulation is thwarted, diastolic muscle relaxation is normalised and myocardial oxygen balance and myocardial blood perfusion are preserved.
- It exerts its antianginal effect without affecting heart rate and blood pressure, making it an ideal drug of choice in bradycardic and hypotensive patients.
- Can be combined with other medications.
- Dose is 500–1000 mg twice a day.

Nicorandil

- It increases potassium ion conductance by opening ATP-sensitive potassium channels. It also produces smooth muscle relaxation causing vasodilatation.
- Useful for protection of myocardium during ischaemia and prevention of intracellular calcium toxicity.
- Dose is 10–40 mg twice a day.

Ivabradine

- Selectively inhibits inward sodium–potassium current, an important pacemaking current in SA node cells. This slows the rate of diastolic depolarisation and lowers heart rate ('bradycardic' drug).
- Does not affect contractility, AV nodal conduction or haemodynamics.
- Can be combined with other agents.
- An important side effect is brightness in visual fields because the drug also blocks the retinal current. This side effect is often transient.

Trimetazidine

- A metabolic modulator that improves myocardial energetics at several levels, partially inhibiting oxidation of fats by decreasing activity of mitochondrial enzyme 3-ketoacyl coenzyme A thiolase (3-KAT). It increases myocardial glucose utilisation, prevents decrease in ATP levels in response to hypoxia or ischaemia, minimises free radical production and protects against intracellular calcium overload.
- It raises coronary flow reserve, lowers frequency of anginal episodes, improves exercise performance and spares the use of nitrates without changes in heart rate, negative inotropic or vasodilator actions.
- May be added to other drugs.

SURGICAL TREATMENT

- Percutaneous coronary interventions (PCI)—percutaneous transluminal coronary angioplasty (PTCA) is the dilatation of coronary artery stenosis by a small balloon introduced percutaneously via an arterial catheter. Ideal for single-vessel coronary disease. Dilatation can be repeated if there is recurrence of symptoms.
  - Angioplasty is often combined with placement of a stent at the site of block that reduces the risk of re-occlusion. These stents are of two types: bare metal stents and drug-eluting stents. The latter stents are coated with drugs (e.g. sirolimus and paclitaxel) which may reduce the risk of re-occlusion.
  - Indications for PCI are:
    - Double-vessel or triple-vessel disease without significant proximal left anterior descending arterial (LAD) lesions, with anatomy enabling catheter-based therapy and normal left ventricular ejection fraction.
    - Single-vessel or double-vessel disease without significant proximal LAD lesions, with high risk on noninvasive testing and a large area of viable myocardium.
    - Prior PCI with either recurrence of stenosis or high risk on noninvasive testing.
    - Failure of optimum medical therapy and with acceptable risk for PCI.

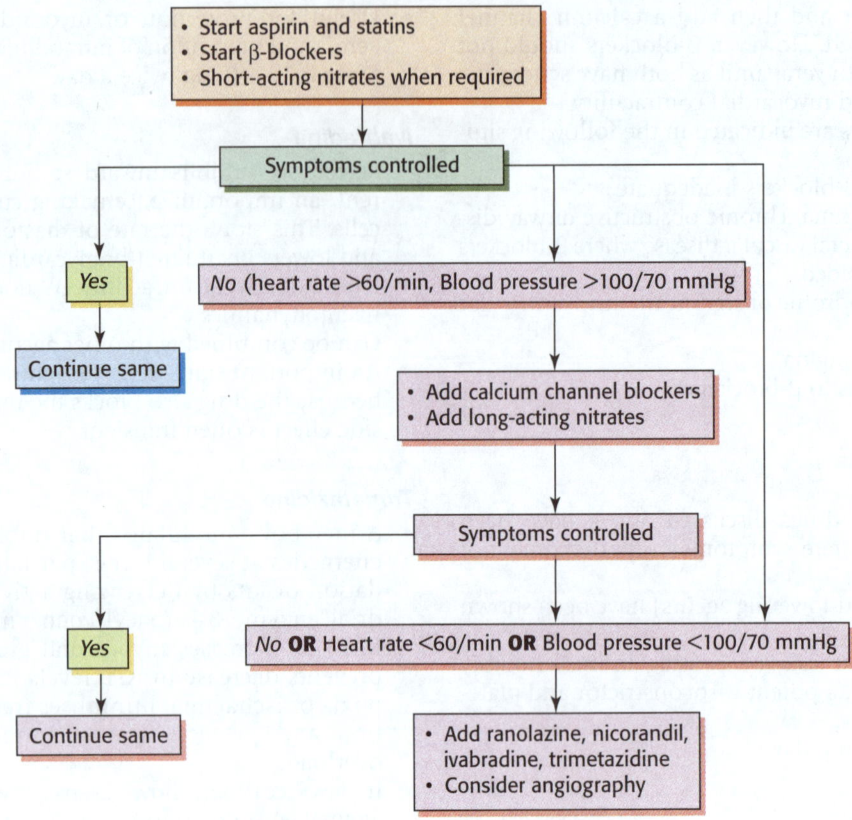

Note: 1. Avoid combination of beta-blockers and verapamil
2. Monitor blood pressure when nitrates are combined with dihydropyridine calcium-channel blocker

Flowchart 7.18 Summary of Management of Stable Angina.

- Coronary artery bypass grafting (CABG)—patient's saphenous vein is anastomosed to the aorta at one end and to a coronary vessel distal to a stenosis at the other. Ideal for left main coronary artery stenosis and significant stenosis in all three major coronary vessels. Alternatively, internal mammary artery can be used for grafting. Important indications of CABG are:
  - Significant left main coronary disease >50%.
  - Triple-vessel disease (particularly if left ventricular ejection fraction <50%).
  - Double-vessel disease with significant proximal left anterior descending artery disease and either LVEF <50% or demonstrable ischaemia on non-invasive testing.
  - Failure of optimum medical therapy and with acceptable risk for CABG.

MISCELLANEOUS THERAPIES

- Enhanced external counterpulsation. It stimulates opening or formation of collaterals.
- Transmyocardial laser re-vascularisation. Laser is used to make tiny channels through the heart muscle of left ventricle. When oxygen-rich blood enters the left ventricle, some of that blood can flow through the tiny channels and carry much-needed oxygen to the heart muscle.

SUMMARY OF MANAGEMENT OF STABLE ANGINA (Flowchart 7.18)

Q. What are acute coronary syndromes? (IM 2.5)

- Acute coronary syndrome refers to the constellation of symptoms manifesting as a result of acute myocardial ischaemia and occurring due to sudden, reduced blood flow to the heart.
- It includes the following conditions:
  - ST-elevation myocardial infarction (STEMI).
  - Unstable angina includes patients with acute coronary syndrome with normal ECG and without positive cardiac injury markers in the blood.
  - Non-ST-segment elevation myocardial infarction (NSTEMI) is diagnosed when cardiac markers are elevated but there is no ST elevation in the ECG.
  - Since management of unstable angina and NSTEMI is similar, they are grouped as non-ST-elevation acute coronary syndrome and are discussed together.
- Acute coronary syndromes as well as stable angina form parts of the spectrum of IHD, the most common cause being coronary artery disease (CAD).

Q. Discuss the clinical features, complications, investigations and management of acute myocardial infarction (ST-elevation myocardial infarction—STEMI). (IM 2.14, IM 2.15, IM 2.16, IM 2.17, IM 2.19, IM 2.20, IM 2.23)

Q. Describe thrombolytic therapy in acute myocardial infarction. (IM 2.16)

ACUTE MYOCARDIAL INFARCTION

- Myocardial infarction is myocardial necrosis occurring as a result of a critical imbalance between coronary blood supply and myocardial demand. It is usually due to the formation of an occlusive thrombus at the site of rupture of an atheromatous plaque in a coronary artery.
- In young patients, a hypercoagulable state may result in acute myocardial infarction.
- Another important cause of myocardial infarction is the use of cocaine. Cocaine use results in acute MI by various mechanisms including coronary vasospasm and hypercoagulability in the background of heightened sympathetic activity. Long-term cocaine use also results in hastened atherosclerosis.
- Silent infarct is characterised by no symptoms but only ECG changes.

CLINICAL FEATURES

SYMPTOMS

- Cardinal symptom is chest pain, but breathlessness, syncope, vomiting and extreme tiredness are common. Pain is at the same site as for angina but is more severe and prolonged. It is severe, with pallor and a peculiar facial expression. Pain is described as tightness, heaviness or constriction.
- Pain may be absent in patients with prior heart failure, prior stroke, age >75 years and diabetes mellitus. Painless MI also more common in females compared to in males.

SIGNS

- Many patients with acute myocardial infarction do not show any abnormalities on physical examination.
- Others may show one or more of the signs as shown in Box 7.68.

BOX 7.68 Possible Signs in Acute MI

• Mild fever	• Diffuse apical impulse
• Pallor, sweating	• Soft first heart sound
• Tachycardia or bradycardia	• Third heart sound
• Arrhythmias	• Pericardial friction rub
• Narrow pulse pressure	• Systolic murmur due to mitral regurgitation or uncommonly due to VSD
• Raised JVP	• Basal crepitations

Note: A small proportion of patients with acute MI or unstable angina have their pain partially or fully reproduced on chest wall palpation. Hence, local chest wall tenderness should not be used as a criterion to exclude acute coronary syndrome.

COMPLICATIONS

ARRHYTHMIAS

- Commonly encountered arrhythmias in acute myocardial infarction are listed in Box 7.69.

BOX 7.69 Arrhythmias Which May Occur in Acute Myocardial Infarction

- Sinus bradycardia
- Sinus tachycardia
- Ventricular ectopic beats
- Ventricular tachycardia
- Accelerated idioventricular rhythm
- Atrial tachycardia
- Atrial fibrillation
- Ventricular fibrillation
- Heart blocks

CARDIOGENIC SHOCK

- May be caused by an arrhythmia; its correction would bring about dramatic relief.
- Hypovolaemia due to excessive diuretic therapy or recurrent vomiting is another cause.
- If none of these is responsible, cardiogenic shock usually reflects extensive myocardial damage and indicates a bad prognosis.
- Risk factors for development of cardiogenic shock include older age, anterior MI, hypertension, diabetes mellitus, multivessel coronary artery disease, prior MI or angina, prior diagnosis of heart failure, STEMI and left bundle branch block.

OTHER COMPLICATIONS

- Cardiac failure, most commonly manifesting as pulmonary oedema.
  - Killip classification is used to classify heart failure in acute MI (Table 7.65).
- Infarction of the mitral papillary muscle leading to mitral regurgitation and pulmonary oedema.
- Rupture of interventricular septum leading to a murmur of VSD and severe hypotension.
- Cardiac tamponade due to rupture of ventricle into pericardial sac.
- Cerebral and peripheral embolism resulting from the detachment of a ventricular mural thrombus.

TABLE 7.65 Killip Classification for Heart Failure During Acute MI

Class	Description
I	No evidence of heart failure
II	Findings consistent with mild to moderate heart failure (e.g. S_3 gallop, basal lung crepitations or jugular venous distension)
III	Frank pulmonary oedema
IV	Cardiogenic shock

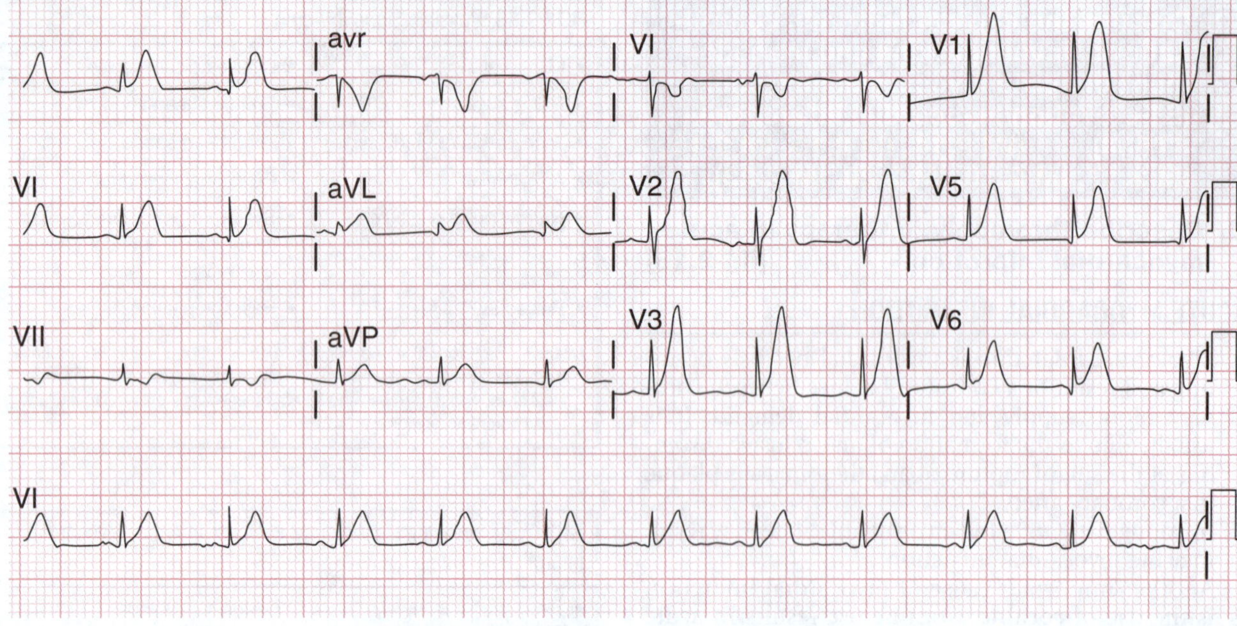

Fig. 7.50 Hyperacute T waves in V_2–V_6 suggesting anterior wall MI.

- Deep vein thrombosis and pulmonary embolism in patients on prolonged bed rest.
- Ventricular aneurysm and dyskinetic or akinetic segments.
- Dressler's syndrome, otherwise known as postmyocardial infarction syndrome, is an autoimmune reaction to necrotic muscle. Syndrome is characterised by fever, pericarditis and pleurisy. Occurs a few weeks or even months after the infarction. Treatment is with aspirin or other non-steroidal anti-inflammatory drugs (NSAIDs) or corticosteroids.

INVESTIGATIONS

ELECTROCARDIOGRAM

- Should be done and interpreted within 10 minutes of arrival.
- ECG is useful in confirming the diagnosis. The typical changes are seen in leads facing the infarcted area (e.g. anteroseptal, anterolateral, strict anterior, inferior, posterior wall as well as right ventricular infarction). These changes include:
  - ST-segment elevation (with reciprocal depression in the opposite leads) in two contiguous leads ≥0.1 mV in all leads other than leads V_2–V_3.
  - For leads V_2–V_3, ST-segment elevation ≥2 mm in men ≥40 years, ≥2.5 mm in men younger than 40 years or ≥1.5 mm in women regardless of age.
  - A bundle branch block, particularly left bundle branch block, with typical history suggesting acute MI also indicates acute infarction and qualifies for re-perfusion therapy.
  - Appearance of pathological Q waves, that is initial negative deflections of 0.04 second or more in leads other than aVR and V_1.
  - In very early MI, the T waves may become tall and peaked (hyperacute myocardial infarction). These are transient and last for a few hours only (Fig. 7.50).
  - ST depression in ≥2 precordial leads (V_1–V_4) may indicate STEMI of posterior wall.
  - Multilead ST depression with coexistent ST elevation in lead aVR indicates left main or proximal left anterior descending artery occlusion.

ECG and Location of MI

- Inferior wall MI—changes in leads II, II and aVF (Fig. 7.51)
- Anterior wall MI—changes in leads V_1–V_6, I and aVL (Fig. 7.52)
- Anteroseptal MI—changes in leads V_1–V_3 (Fig. 7.53)
- Anterolateral MI—changes in leads V_4–V_6, I and aVL (Fig. 7.54)
- Posterior wall MI—tall R and ST depression in leads V_1 and V_2 (Fig. 7.55)
- Right ventricular infarction—ST elevation in in V_4R

PLASMA ENZYMES (CARDIAC INJURY ENZYMES)

1. Creatine kinase (CK)
2. Aspartate aminotransferase (AST)
3. Lactate dehydrogenase (LDH)
4. Myoglobin
5. Troponins (troponin I and troponin T)

- Serial tests are done over 6–12 hours to show rise/fall in cardiac enzyme levels.
- CK starts to rise at 4–6 hours, peaks by about 12 hours and falls to normal in 48–72 hours. Measurement of the myocardial isoenzymes of CK (CK-MB) is more specific for myocardial infarction. Total CK is also elevated in skeletal muscle diseases (e.g. polymyositis and muscular dystrophies), cardioversion, skeletal muscle damage, hypothyroidism and stroke.

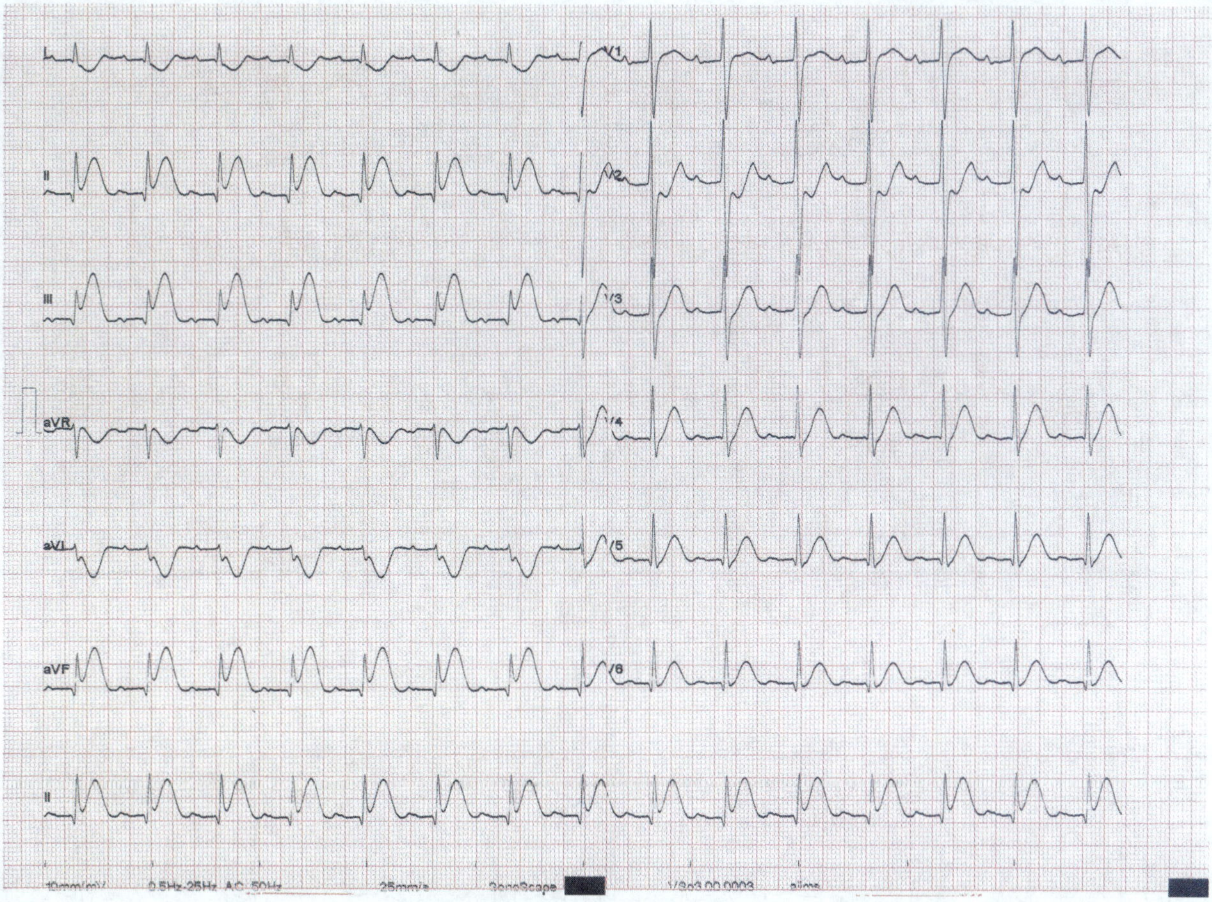

Fig. 7.51 Inferior wall ST elevation MI.

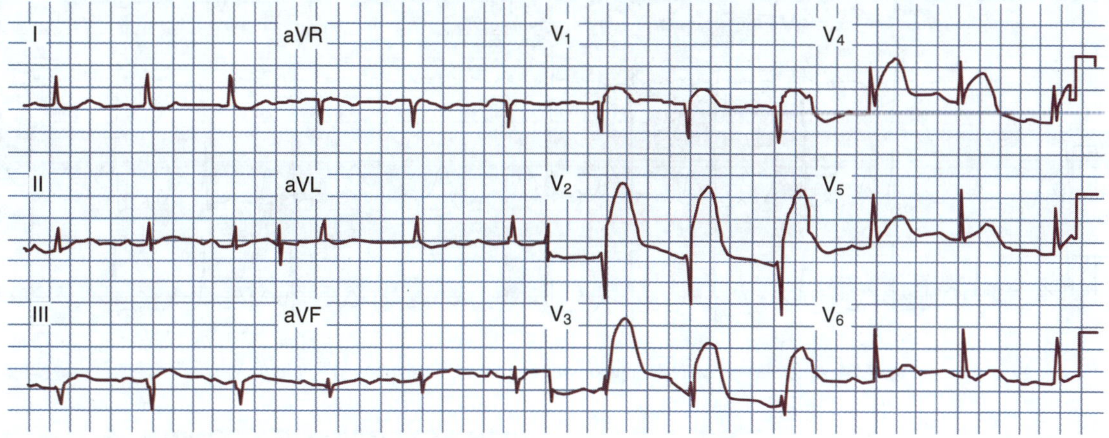

Fig. 7.52 Anterior wall MI (ST elevation in V_1–V_5).

- AST starts to rise by about 12 hours and reaches a peak on the first or second day.
- LDH starts to rise after 12 hours, reaches a peak after 2–3 days and may remain elevated for a week. A rise in the level of LDH_1 (an isoenzyme of LDH) is a more sensitive indicator of myocardial infarction than total LDH.
- Myoglobin is increased within 2–6 hours of onset of symptoms and remains elevated for 7–12 hours.
- Cardiac troponins include cardiac troponin T (cTnT) and cardiac troponin I (cTnI). The sensitivity of troponins is similar to that of CK-MB. However, cTn remains elevated for 100–200 hours after

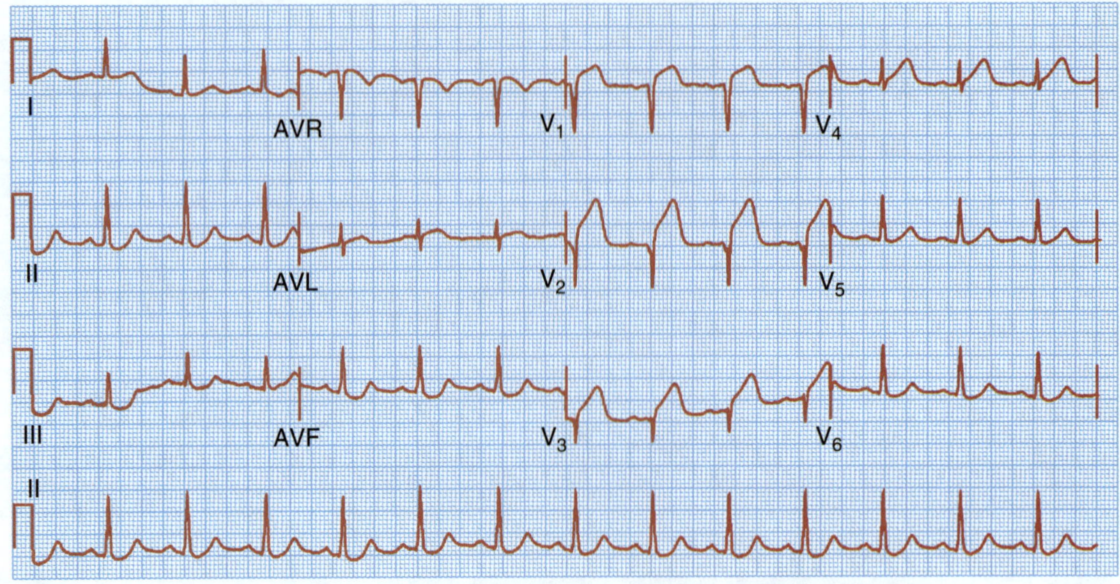

Fig. 7.53 Anteroseptal MI (ST elevation in V_1–V_3).

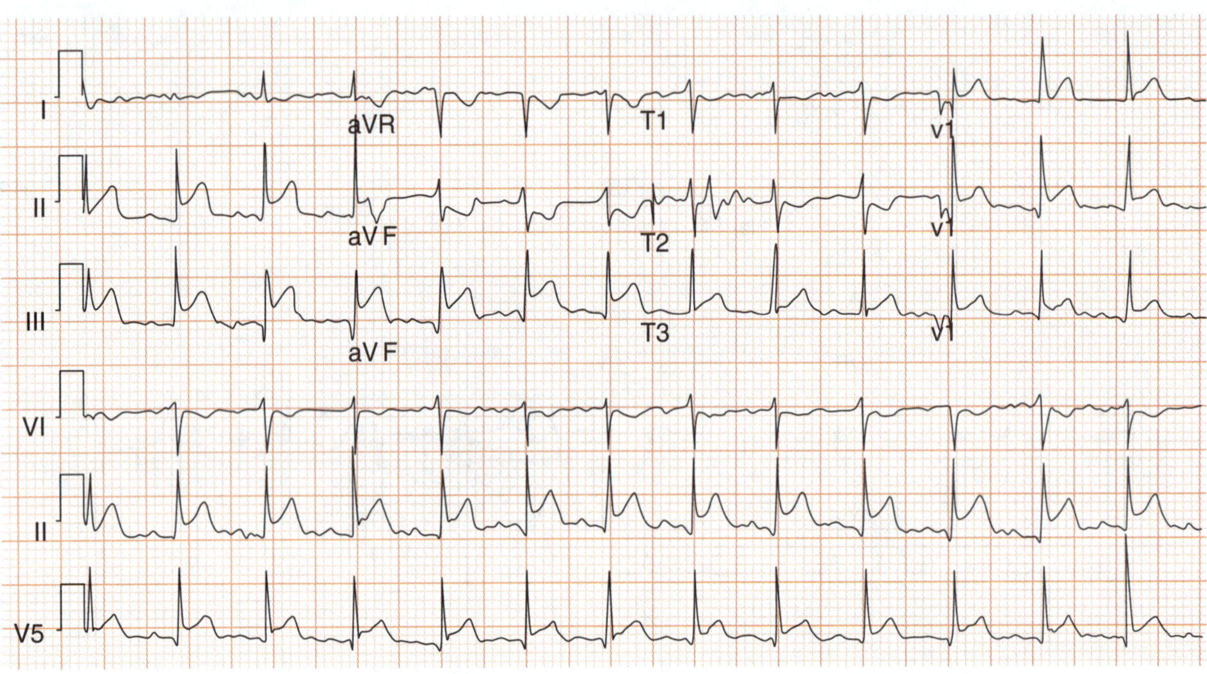

Fig. 7.54 Anterolateral MI (with inferior wall MI; note ST elevation in II, II, aVF, V_4–V_6).

acute MI and, therefore, this assay may have particular utility in the evaluation of patients who present sufficiently long after their episode of chest pain.

- Other conditions that may produce elevation of troponins include sepsis, hypotension, atrial fibrillation, intracranial haemorrhage, cardiac contusion, cardioversion, myocarditis, pulmonary embolism and chronic renal failure.

- Changes in plasma enzyme concentrations after myocardial infarction are shown in Fig. 7.56.

HIGH-SENSITIVITY TROPONIN

- It means that the laboratory is capable of detecting the presence of traditional cardiac biomarkers (troponin I and troponin T) at much lower concentrations than previously achievable with standard assays. The characteristics of assay are:
  - The assay must be sufficiently sensitive to detect the presence of circulating troponin in at least 50% of healthy, asymptomatic individuals.
  - The upper limit of normal value of hs-Tn is defined by the 99th percentile, which is the value that is not exceeded in 99% of healthy individuals.

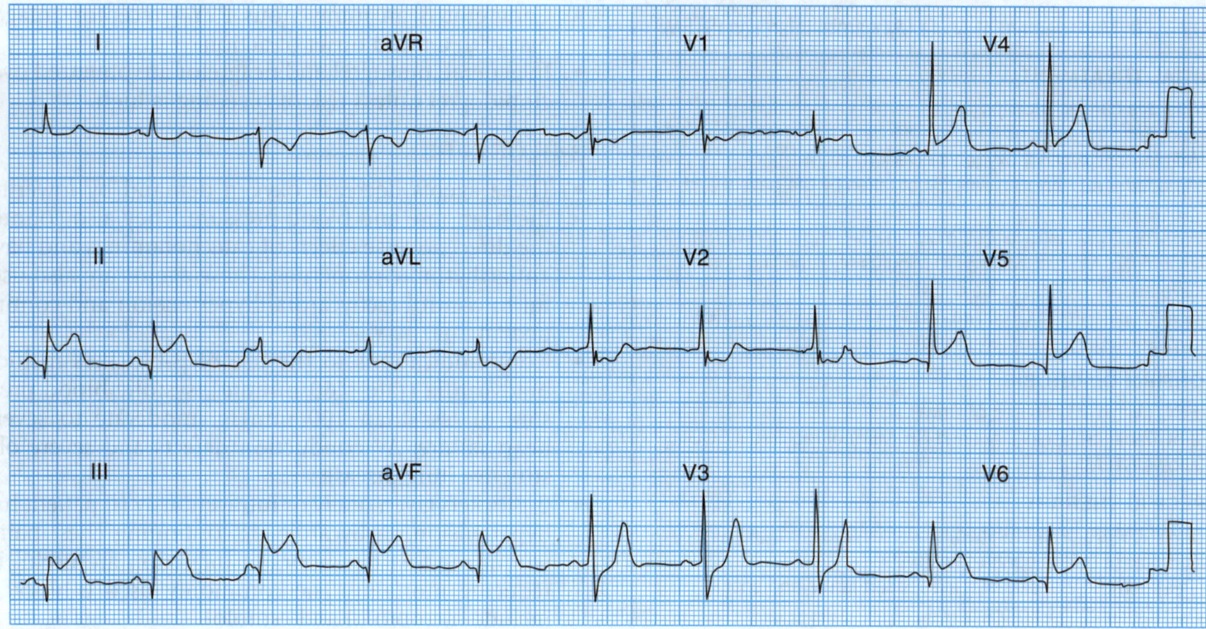

Fig. 7.55 Inferolateral and posterior wall MI (ST elevation in II, II, aVF, V_5, V_6; prominent 'R' and Sr depression in V_1 and V_2).

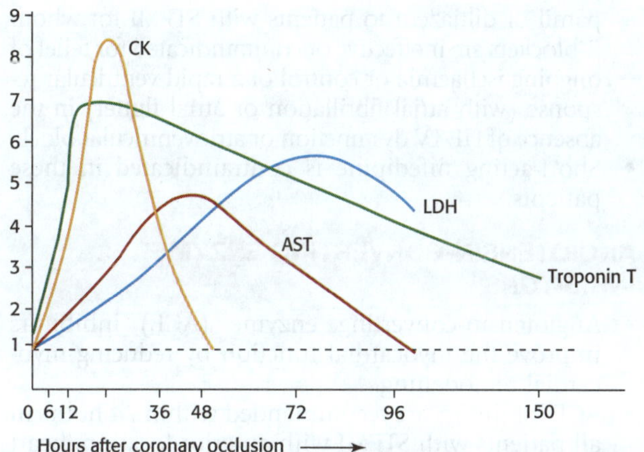

Note: CK and troponins are the first to rise, followed by AST and then LDH.

Fig. 7.56 Changes in plasma concentration of cardiac enzymes after MI.

- The assay must be precise with a coefficient in variation of <10%.
- May be used to 'rule out' MI (both STEMI and non-STEMI) when hsTn is below the upper reference limit at presentation and 1 hour ('0h/1h') in low-risk patients or when change in hsTn level between '0' and '3' hours is less than 50%.

OTHER INVESTIGATIONS

- Leucocytosis with a peak on the first day.
- Raised ESR that may remain so for days.
- Elevated C-reactive protein.
- Chest radiography:
  - Heart size is usually normal. Enlargement of cardiac shadow may indicate previous myocardial damage or pericardial effusion.
  - Evidence of pulmonary oedema.
- Radionuclide scanning shows the site of necrosis and the extent of impairment of ventricular function.
- Echocardiography for regional wall motion abnormality and ejection fraction.

MANAGEMENT (BOX 7.70)

- In the first 24–48 hours when the risk of fatal arrhythmia is highest, the patients are best treated in an intensive coronary care unit.

OXYGEN

- Hypoxaemia in patients with uncomplicated MI is usually caused by ventilation–perfusion abnormalities and may be exacerbated by HF. Therefore, oxygen is administered to patients suspected of having an acute ischaemic syndrome and oxygen saturation <90%.

NITRATES

- Nitrates reduce oxygen demand and myocardial wall stress by reducing both preload and afterload.
- If patient is stable, sublingual nitrate should be given.
- Intravenous nitroglycerine is recommended in patients with pulmonary oedema, accelerated hypertension and continuing chest pain.

CONTROL OF PAIN

- Morphine in a dose of 3–5 mg is administered intravenously every 10–15 minutes along with an antiemetic.
- The beneficial effects of morphine are mainly due to sedation and analgesia produced by it which result in reduction of myocardial oxygen demand. It also reduces preload to some extent which may be beneficial

BOX 7.70 Management of Acute Myocardial Infarction (STEMI)

INITIAL TREATMENT

- Attach a cardiac monitor.
- Secure an intravenous line.
- Administer oxygen if oxygen saturation <90%.
- Administer sublingual nitrate (if not taken by the patient and pain is present).
- If no relief, give intravenous morphine 3–5 mg along with an antiemetic. May repeat it 5–10 minutes after the first dose.
- Give aspirin 150 mg to be chewed.
- Give clopidogrel 300–600 mg orally (unless coronary artery bypass surgery is contemplated).

CONFIRM DIAGNOSIS

- ECG (within 10 minutes of arrival).
- If available, troponin T or I and CK-MB (not required if ECG shows STEMI).

SPECIFIC THERAPY

- Thrombolysis or percutaneous coronary interventions.
- β-Blockers unless contraindicated.
- Treat complications (arrhythmias, heart failure and shock).
- Admit in intensive coronary unit.

in patients with MI. β-Blockers, nitroglycerine and thrombolysis may also help in relieving pain.

- However, studies have shown that use of morphine may increase mortality and complications of MI as it delays platelet-inhibiting activity of antiplatelet drugs. Hence, use of morphine is not recommended if pain is relieved with nitrates.

ANTIPLATELET AGENTS

- Early administration of aspirin to patients with acute MI has been shown to be of significant benefit in AMI. The patient is asked to chew 150 mg non-enteric-coated aspirin.
- Administer clopidogrel ($P2Y_{12}$ receptor antagonist) to all patients unless the need for coronary artery bypass surgery is likely.
  - If percutaneous coronary intervention (PCI) is planned, loading dose is 600 mg.
  - If fibrinolysis is planned, loading dose is 300 mg if age <75 years; patients older than 75 years should receive 75 mg/day without loading dose.
  - It should be continued for at least 14 days, although it is reasonable to continue for 1 year particularly after stent placement.
- Prasugrel is another orally administered $P2Y_{12}$ receptor antagonist that is more potent, has more rapid action and is more consistent in its inhibition of platelet aggregation than are currently approved doses of clopidogrel. However, there is increased risk of bleeding in patients with a history of transient ischaemic attack or stroke; those older than 75 years or those who weigh <60 kg do not benefit from it. It is given in a loading dose of 60 mg followed by 10 mg/day.
- Third $P2Y_{12}$ receptor antagonist is ticagrelor which is a reversible inhibitor and is given in a loading dose of 180 mg followed by 90 mg twice a day.
- Cangrelor is an intravenous $P2Y_{12}$ receptor antagonist with a rapid onset of action.
- In general, prasugrel and ticagrelor are preferred over clopidogrel unless risk of bleeding is high.

β-BLOCKERS

- These agents decrease oxygen demand by lowering the heart rate and blood pressure. They also counter the direct adverse effects of catecholamines and have antiarrhythmic properties. These agents are also useful to control tachycardia, hypertension and continued angina.
- Contraindications to the use of β-blockers include bradycardia (rate <60/minute), systolic blood pressure of less than 100 mmHg, moderate to severe heart failure, AV conduction defects and severe obstructive lung disease.
- β-Blockers given orally or intravenously (if patient has hypertension, tachycardia or continuing chest pain) within the first few hours of infarction are useful in reducing mortality. The commonly used β-blockers include metoprolol and esmolol.

CALCIUM CHANNEL BLOCKERS

- These agents are not recommended in the management of AMI. However, it is reasonable to give verapamil or diltiazem to patients with STEMI for whom β-blockers are ineffective or contraindicated for relief of ongoing ischaemia or control of a rapid ventricular response (with atrial fibrillation or atrial flutter) in the absence of HF, LV dysfunction or atrioventricular block.
- Short-acting nifedipine is contraindicated in these patients.

ANGIOTENSIN-CONVERTING ENZYME INHIBITORS

- Angiotensin-converting enzyme (ACE) inhibitors improve the myocardial function by reducing myocardial remodelling.
- ACE inhibitors are recommended within 24 hours in all patients with STEMI with anterior location, heart failure or ejection fraction ≤40%. Initiate the treatment with short-acting ACE inhibitor, captopril, in a dose of 12.5 mg. If the systolic pressure remains above 100 mmHg, increase the dose to 25 mg 8 hourly with a constant watch on blood pressure. If patient is intolerant to ACE inhibitors, angiotensin receptor blocking agents may be given.

STATINS

- Intensive statin treatment (e.g. atorvastatin 40–80 mg) should be considered as early as possible but within 24 hours after hospital admission.
- Besides lowering cholesterol, beneficial effects are also related to direct effects on endothelial function, oxidative stress, inflammation, thrombosis as well as plaque stabilisation.

THROMBOLYTIC (OR FIBRINOLYTIC) THERAPY

- The goal is to initiate fibrinolytic therapy within 30 minutes (door-to-needle time or first medical contact [FMC]-to-needle time).

- Thrombolytic agents: These include streptokinase (STK), urokinase (UK), recombinant plasminogen activator (rt-PA, alteplase), reteplase, tenecteplase, anisoylated plasminogen streptokinase activator complex (APSAC and anistreplase) and single-chain urokinase plasminogen activator (scu-PA). All these agents act as direct or indirect plasminogen activators leading to generation of plasmin that lyses the clot. rt-PA, reteplase, tenecteplase and scu-PA do this only at the site of clot (fibrin-specific fibrinolytics), whereas others generate plasmin in the systemic circulation leading to a systemic lytic state that leads to a reduction in blood viscosity and exerts strong anticoagulant and antiplatelet effects.
- Fibrin-specific fibrinolytic agents have been shown to reduce mortality compared to STK.
- Fibrin-specific fibrinolytics also lack the significant acute side effects of hypotension and allergy caused by STK.
- STK may be associated with a lower incidence of intracranial haemorrhage, particularly in older people, but the overall mortality is still lower with the use of fibrin-specific fibrinolytic agents.
- Thrombolytic therapy is not recommended for patients with NSTEMI and unstable angina.

Indications for Thrombolysis in Acute Myocardial Infarction

- Various indications are given in Box 7.71.
- STK is used in a dose of 1.5 million units intravenously as an infusion over a period of 1 hour.
- In patients >65 kg, rt-PA (alteplase) is given in a dose of 15 mg bolus followed by 50 mg over 30 minutes and 35 mg over the next 60 minutes. For patients <65 kg, dose is 15 mg bolus, and then 0.75 mg/kg over 30 minutes and 0.5 mg/kg over the next 60 minutes.
- Signs of re-perfusion:
  - Sudden relief of chest pain.
  - Reduction by 50% of the initial ST-segment elevation within 60–90 minutes of fibrinolytic therapy.
  - Onset of re-perfusion arrhythmias (mainly accelerated idioventricular rhythm and frequent ventricular ectopics).
  - Early peaking of CK-MB enzyme.

BOX 7.71 Indications of Thrombolysis in Acute Myocardial Infarction

THROMBOLYSIS SHOWN TO BE OF DEFINITE VALUE

- ST-segment elevation MI with time to therapy 12 hours or less
- Bundle branch block (obscuring ST-segment analysis) and history suggestive of acute MI for less than 12 hours

THROMBOLYSIS MAY BE OF SOME BENEFIT

- ST-segment elevation with time to therapy 12–24 hours if there is clinical and/or ECG evidence of ongoing ischaemia or haemodynamic instability provided PCI is not available (controversial indication)

THROMBOLYSIS NOT INDICATED/MAY BE HARMFUL

- ST-segment depression only (unless leads V_1–V_4 show ST depression related to posterior wall MI)
- Time to therapy >24 hours

- Complications:
  - The major complication of thrombolytic therapy is haemorrhage that occurs in about 30% of cases.
  - The most common sites of haemorrhage are puncture sites and genitourinary system.
  - Intracranial haemorrhage occurs in about 0.5% of cases.
  - Use of STK and APSAC may be associated with allergic reactions.
  - Hypotension may occur if STK is infused rapidly.

Contraindications to Thrombolytic Therapy (Table 7.66)

TABLE 7.66 Contraindications of Thrombolytic Therapy

Major Contraindications	Other Contraindications
• Active bleeding (except menses) • Severe uncontrolled hypertension • History of haemorrhagic stroke • Ischaemic stroke within 3 months (except for acute ischaemic stroke within 3–4.5 hours) • Suspected aortic dissection • Known intracranial aneurysm or AV malformation • Known intracranial neoplasm (primary or metastatic) • Intracranial/spinal surgery within past 3 months • Significant cranial/spinal trauma in past 3 months	• History of poorly controlled severe hypertension • History of ischaemic stroke more than 3 months previously • Significant trauma within past 6 weeks • Traumatic or prolonged (>10 minutes) cardiopulmonary resuscitation • For streptokinase (STK), previous exposure (>5 days previously) or previous allergic reaction to STK • Major surgery within past 6 weeks • GI bleed within past 6 weeks • Pregnancy • Acute pericarditis

ANTITHROMBIN THERAPY

- Antithrombin therapy in the form of heparin is required before the completion of infusion of rt-PA or tenecteplase. It is also recommended in patients receiving STK.
- Unfractionated heparin should be given as an initial bolus dose of 60 IU/kg (with a maximum dose of 4000 units) followed by an initial infusion of 12 IU/kg/hour (maximum 1000 units/hour), adjusted to attain the activated partial thromboplastin time at 1.5–2 times control.
- Low-molecular-weight heparin (LMWH) as an adjunct to thrombolytics may result in higher re-perfusion rate and lower re-occlusion rate compared to unfractionated heparin.
- Direct thrombin inhibitors (hirudin and bivalirudin) can be used as an alternative to heparin and GP IIb/IIIa inhibitors in patients undergoing PCI.
- Another option is the use of fondaparinux unless PCI is planned when it should not be used as sole agent.
- These agents should be continued for at least 48 hours and preferably for 8 days after fibrinolysis or till PCI is performed.

PROPHYLACTIC ANTICOAGULANTS

- Use of low-dose heparin, that is 5000 units, twice a day subcutaneously to prevent deep vein thrombosis and pulmonary embolism is indicated in those who do not receive fibrinolytic agents.

PERCUTANEOUS CORONARY INTERVENTIONS

- These interventions include angioplasty (percutaneous transluminal coronary angioplasty—PTCA) or stent placement in the coronary artery. The goal is to achieve door-to device time of less than 90 minutes if the patient has reached a PCI-capable centre, or 120 minutes from first medical contact (FMC) to device if patient is transferred from a centre which is not PCI-capable.
- Stents may be bare metallic or drug-eluting, the latter containing sirolimus or paclitaxel. Though drug-eluting stents are considered to have lower risk of re-stenosis (by inhibiting intimal hyperplasia), recent data suggest both types of stents to be equally effective over long-term follow-up.
- Manual aspiration thrombectomy is reasonable for patients undergoing primary PCI before placing stents.
- PCI may be used solely in acute MI (primary PCI) or in combination with thrombolytic therapy when thrombolysis fails (rescue PCI).
- Glycoprotein IIb/IIIa inhibitors (abciximab and tirofiban) may be administered in some high risk patients undergoing percutaneous interventions.

Thrombolysis Versus Percutaneous Coronary Interventions

- In general, PCI is the treatment of choice provided it can be performed promptly by a qualified interventional cardiologist in an appropriate facility.
- The maximum acceptable delay from presentation to balloon inflation or device is:
  - Ninety minutes if a patient presents to a PCI-enabled hospital (door-to-device time).
  - One hundred and twenty minutes if a patient is referred from another hospital (FMC to device time) with door-in to door-out time in the first hospital <30 minutes.
- Fibrinolysis should be considered early when anticipated FMC-to-device time at a PCI-capable hospital exceeds 120 minutes because of unavoidable delays. It should be performed within 30 minutes of arrival (door-to-needle time).
- Re-perfusion is not routinely recommended in patients who present more than 12 hours after symptom of onset.
- Beyond 12 hours, PCI may be of benefit in patients who continue to be symptomatic or develop cardiogenic shock or heart failure.

Rescue PCI

- Rescue PCI is defined as PCI after failed fibrinolysis for patients with continuing or recurrent myocardial ischaemia.
- Indicated for patients with STEMI (younger than 75 years) who have received fibrinolytic therapy and continue to have persistent ischaemic symptoms or have cardiogenic shock, severe HF (Killip class III) or haemodynamically compromising ventricular arrhythmias.

Facilitated PCI

- Facilitated PCI refers to a strategy of planned immediate PCI after administration of an initial pharmacological regimen aimed at improving patency of coronary arteries before PCI. Such regimens may include GP IIb/IIIa inhibitors, full dose or reduced dose of fibrinolytic therapy and combination of a GP IIb/IIIa inhibitor and a reduced-dose fibrinolytic agent.
- However, facilitated PCI is usually not recommended in most patients with STEMI.

Pharmacoinvasive PCI

- This is routine PCI within 3–24 hours after successful primary PCI.
- Some studies have shown better outcomes after this strategy. However, it may not be feasible in most hospitals.

Re-Perfusion Options for STEMI

- Box 7.72 summarises reperfusion options for STEMI patients.

GLYCOPROTEIN IIB/IIIA INHIBITORS

- It is reasonable to use intravenous GP IIb/IIIa receptor antagonist such as abciximab, tirofiban or eptifibatide at the time of primary PCI in selected patients with STEMI who are receiving unfractionated heparin. These are contraindicated in patients receiving fibrinolytics.

CORONARY ARTERY BYPASS GRAFTING

- It is probably of little use in the setting of uncomplicated acute myocardial infarction. It offers benefit in patients with acute myocardial infarction with persistent pain or deteriorating haemodynamic status, and patients who develop coronary occlusion during coronary angiography and PTCA.

MANAGEMENT OF RIGHT VENTRICULAR INFARCTION

- In this type of infarction, there is reduced right ventricular stroke volume producing impaired left

BOX 7.72 Re-Perfusion Options for STEMI

FIBRINOLYSIS IS GENERALLY PREFERRED

- Early presentation (≤3 hours from symptom onset), although PCI also equally effective
- Primary PCI is not an option for the following reasons:
  - Catheterisation laboratory occupied/unavailable
  - Vascular access difficulties
  - Lack of access to a skilled PCI laboratory
- Delay to primary PCI
  - Door-to-device time minus door-to-needle time is >60 minutes.
- Door-to-device time is >90 minutes.

PRIMARY PCI IS GENERALLY PREFERRED

- Skilled PCI laboratory available with surgical backup
  - Door-to-device time is ≤90 minutes.
  - Door-to-device time minus door-to-needle time is ≤60 minutes.
- High risk from STEMI irrespective of time delay
  - Cardiogenic shock
  - Killip class HF ≥III
- Contraindications to fibrinolysis (including increased risk of bleeding and ICH) irrespective of time delay
- Late presentation (>3 hours after symptom of onset)

ventricular filling. This results in hypotension, raised JVP and clear lungs on auscultation.

- Volume expansion is the initial treatment of choice for haemodynamically significant right ventricular infarction.
- Patients with right ventricular infarction are treated in a manner similar to those with acute ST-elevation MI. This includes the early use of dual oral antiplatelets, statin therapy and re-perfusion therapy.
- Avoid opioids, diuretics, ACE inhibitors and nitrates.
- Inotropics (dobutamine) and vasopressors (norepinephrine and dopamine) may also be required especially when a significant component of associated left ventricular dysfunction is also present.
- These patients should be routinely considered for reperfusion therapy (fibrinolysis or PCI).

MANAGEMENT OF COMPLICATIONS

ARRHYTHMIAS

- Pain relief, reassurance, rest and correction of hypokalaemia play a major role in prevention of arrhythmias.
- Manage heart failure.
- Amiodarone is given after resuscitation from ventricular fibrillation, and for treatment of ventricular tachycardia with a rapid rate, multiple ectopic beats and R-on-T ectopics. Lidocaine, mexiletine or an intravenous β-blocker (atenolol or sotalol) may be used alternatively.
- Defibrillation is the treatment of ventricular fibrillation.
- Verapamil, diltiazem, esmolol or digoxin is used to treat atrial tachycardia, flutter or fibrillation with a fast ventricular rate.
- Atropine is used to treat symptomatic sinus bradycardia and heart block.
- Temporary pacemaker in heart block complicating inferior wall infarction and anterior wall infarction.
- Cardiopulmonary resuscitation to treat asystole.

CARDIOGENIC SHOCK

- Management is discussed on page 531.
- Cardiogenic shock is not a contraindication to fibrinolysis, but PCI is preferred if the patient is at a facility with PCI capabilities. PCI is reasonable in those who develop shock within 36 hours of symptom of onset.
- Intraaortic balloon counterpulsation (IABP) works synergistically with fibrinolytic agents or PCI in this setting.

AFTERCARE AND REHABILITATION

- Restrict physical activities for 4–6 weeks since infarct takes 4–6 weeks to become replaced with fibrous tissue.
- Gradual mobilisation and return to work over 6 weeks.
- When there are complications, the regimen has to be modified accordingly.
- Exercise within the limits set by angina and tiredness will do no harm but much good. Same limits apply to sexual activity.
- Control of obesity, regular exercises, cessation of smoking, adoption of a less hectic way of life and control of plasma lipids by diets and drugs.

MEDICATIONS

- Aspirin, 75–150 mg daily unless contraindicated.
- Clopidogrel, 75 mg daily for up to 12 months, in particular after stent implantation. May also be prescribed as an alternative when aspirin is contraindicated, or in addition to aspirin, particularly in patients with unstable angina or recurrent cardiac events.
- β-Blockers, unless contraindicated, are continued indefinitely. Carvedilol, bisoprolol or metoprolol (extended release) should be used in patients with heart failure.
- ACE inhibitor given early after an acute coronary syndrome.
- Statin therapy initiated in hospital for all patients with coronary heart disease.
- Warfarin after myocardial infarction for those at high risk of systemic thromboembolism because of atrial fibrillation, mural thrombus, heart failure or previous embolisation.
- Nitrates, short-acting for chest pain. Long-acting nitrates for symptom relief if β-blocker treatment alone is unsuccessful or is contraindicated.
- Mineralocorticoid antagonist (e.g. spironolactone and eplerenone) considered early after myocardial infarction in those who have LVEF ≤40% despite optimum doses of ACE inhibitors and β-blockers, and have either HF or diabetes.

Q. Briefly discuss unstable angina and non-ST-elevation myocardial infarction. (IM 2.14, IM 2.15, IM 2.17, IM 2.19, IM 2.20, IM 2.23)

- Unstable angina (UA) and non-ST-elevation myocardial infarction (NSTEMI) are part of acute coronary syndrome in which the patient presents with chest pain or its anginal equivalent (e.g. dyspnoea, jaw or arm pain) due to reduced coronary blood flow. They are also known as 'non-ST-segment elevation acute coronary syndrome' (NSTEACS).
- These are caused by coronary artery spasm and progression of the underlying CAD or haemorrhage into a nonoccluding plaque with subsequent thrombosis producing coronary obstruction over a period of few hours. An additional mechanism is complete occlusion in presence of collaterals.

NON-ST-ELEVATION MI

- It is often characterised by ST depression and T inversion along with elevation in cardiac enzymes. In some cases, ECG may be normal and the only abnormality is elevated cardiac enzymes.
- The myocardial function as shown by ejection fraction is less deranged as compared to STEMI. However, early as well as late re-infarction rates are higher in the NSTEMI as compared to in the latter.

UNSTABLE ANGINA

- UA angina includes:
  - Exertional angina of recent onset (within 6 weeks) with ≥class III severity.

TABLE 7.67 Risk Categories of NSTEMI/UA

Very High-Risk Criteria	High-Risk Criteria	Intermediate-Risk Criteria	Low-Risk Criteria
• Haemodynamic instability or cardiogenic shock • Recurrent or ongoing chest pain refractory to medical treatment • Life-threatening arrhythmias or cardiac arrest • Mechanical complications of MI • Acute heart failure • Recurrent dynamic ST–T wave changes, particularly with intermittent ST elevation	• Rise or fall in cardiac troponin compatible with MI • Dynamic ST wave or T wave changes (symptomatic or silent) • GRACE score >140	• Diabetes mellitus • Renal insufficiency (eGFR <60 mL/min/1.73 m^2) • LVEF <40% or heart failure • Early postinfarction angina • Prior PCI • Prior CABG • GRACE risk score >109 or <140	• Absence of any criteria mentioned under other three groups

Note: GRACE score is Global Registry of Acute Coronary Events Score.

- Angina at rest or minimal exertion, generally lasting for >20 minutes.
- Angina of worsening severity as shown by increasing duration or severity of pain, pain occurring on exerting less as compared to previous episodes and increasing requirement of nitrates.

- The ECG is usually normal but may show ischaemic ST–T changes. Cardiac enzymes are normal.
- UA and NSTEMI differ primarily in whether the ischaemia is severe enough to cause sufficient myocardial damage to release detectable quantities of cardiac enzymes.
- Patients with UA are at a high risk of developing MI or sudden death as compared to patients with stable angina and therefore require aggressive treatment in the hospital.

BOX 7.73 TIMI Score (One Point Score for Every Parameter)

- Age greater than or equal to 65 years
- More than three coronary risk factors (early family history, as defined by infarction or sudden cardiac death in first-degree male relatives age <55 years or in first-degree female relatives age <65 years, diabetes mellitus, hypertension, hyperlipidaemia or current smoking status)
- More than two angina events within 24 hours
- Use of aspirin within 7 days
- Prior angiographic coronary obstruction (≥50%)
- Elevated levels of cardiac biomarkers
- ST-segment deviation (≥0.5 mm)

RISK CATEGORIES IN NSTEMI/UA

- Define short-term risk of adverse effects in patients presenting with features suggestive of acute coronary syndrome and ECG showing no evidence of STEMI.
- One of the risk criteria is given in Table 7.67.
- Another classification for prognosis is the use of Thrombolytics in Myocardial Infarction (TIMI) risk score that uses a 7-point score (Box 7.73). A score ≥3 predicts a high risk for death, non-fatal MI or severe ischaemia requiring urgent re-vascularisation at 14 days after presentation and therefore warrants early requirement of invasive management.

MANAGEMENT

- Management of both NSTEMI and UA is similar. Patient should be hospitalised. Goals are to provide relief of ischaemia and to prevent recurrence of adverse ischaemic events.
- Risk stratify all patients with NSTEMI and UA to direct management decisions.
- Administer aspirin, oxygen (if saturation <90%), nitroglycerine (NTG), morphine, β-blockers, statins, P2PY$_{12}$ agents and others as in patients with STEMI. However, as per recent guidelines, routine administration of P2Y$_{12}$ inhibitors is not recommended in patients in whom coronary artery anatomy is not known and an early invasive management is planned.
- *NTG:* Patients with ongoing ischaemic discomfort should be given sublingual NTG every 5 minutes for a total of three doses, If pain persists or patient develops heart failure or remains hypertensive, administration of intravenous NTG should be initiated (initial rate of 5–10 μg/minute with increases of 10 μg/minute every 3–5 minutes until symptoms are relieved or if systolic blood pressure falls below 100 mmHg). Nitrates should not be administered to patients with systolic blood pressure less than 90 or ≥30 mmHg below baseline, severe bradycardia (<50 beats/minute), tachycardia (>100 beats/minute) without heart failure or right ventricular infarction.
- *Calcium channel blockers:* Routine use is not recommended. Diltiazem or verapamil may be administered as initial therapy for patients with ongoing ischaemia when β-blockers are contraindicated and there is no heart failure or left ventricular dysfunction.
- *ACE inhibitors:* Recommended for patients with hypertension despite treatment with NTG and a β-blocker, and with LV systolic dysfunction or HF. Also recommended in presence of diabetes.
- *P2Y$_{12}$* agents: These agents should be avoided if patient is likely to require emergency coronary bypass

surgery (those with severe widespread ST-segment depression or haemodynamic instability).

- *Anticoagulation:* Add intravenous unfractionated heparin (60 units/kg as bolus and then 12 units/kg/hour infusion) with monitoring of activated partial thromboplastin time (aPTT); goal is to maintain aPTT between 1.5 and 2.0 times the control. An alternative is subcutaneous LMWH (e.g. enoxaparin). Enoxaparin is slightly better than unfractionated heparin in terms of reducing mortality and recurrence of infarction particularly if conservative treatment is planned. Other options include bivalirudin (in patients selected for an early invasive strategy) and fondaparinux (particularly for patients who are selected for a conservative treatment strategy and who are at an increased risk of bleeding). These drugs should be continued for at least 48 hours after presentation.
- *Platelet GP IIb/IIIa receptor antagonist* is recommended in high-risk patients in whom an invasive strategy is planned. Administration should start as soon as a high-risk feature is identified. These drugs include eptifibatide, tirofiban and abciximab. Abciximab should not be administered if PCI is not being planned. Risk of bleeding increases with concomitant use of aspirin and heparin.
- Thrombolytic agents are contraindicated.

VERY HIGH-RISK GROUP OR TIMI SCORE >4

- Early coronary angiography (within 2 hours) and revascularisation is recommended.

HIGH-RISK OR TIMI SCORE 3–4

- Medical treatment as above.
- Consider an early invasive approach (<24 hours).

INTERMEDIATE AND LOW-RISK GROUP OR TIMI SCORE 0–2

- After an appropriate period of observation and assessment, these patients may be discharged on medical therapy for outpatient follow-up. The medications include aspirin, a $P2Y_{12}$ receptor antagonist (particularly ticagrelor), a β-blocker, an ACE inhibitor and a statin.
- Another option for intermediate-risk and low-risk patients is to perform an early noninvasive testing (e.g. stress echocardiography). The goals of noninvasive testing are to determine whether ischaemia is present in patients with low or intermediate risk categories and to estimate prognosis. It can be performed in patients who have been free of ischaemia at rest (or with low-level activity) and free of heart failure for a minimum of 12–24 hours. It can be performed during hospital stay or early after discharge in stable patients.

SUMMARY OF TREATMENT OF STEMI AND NON-STEMI (Flowchart 7.19)

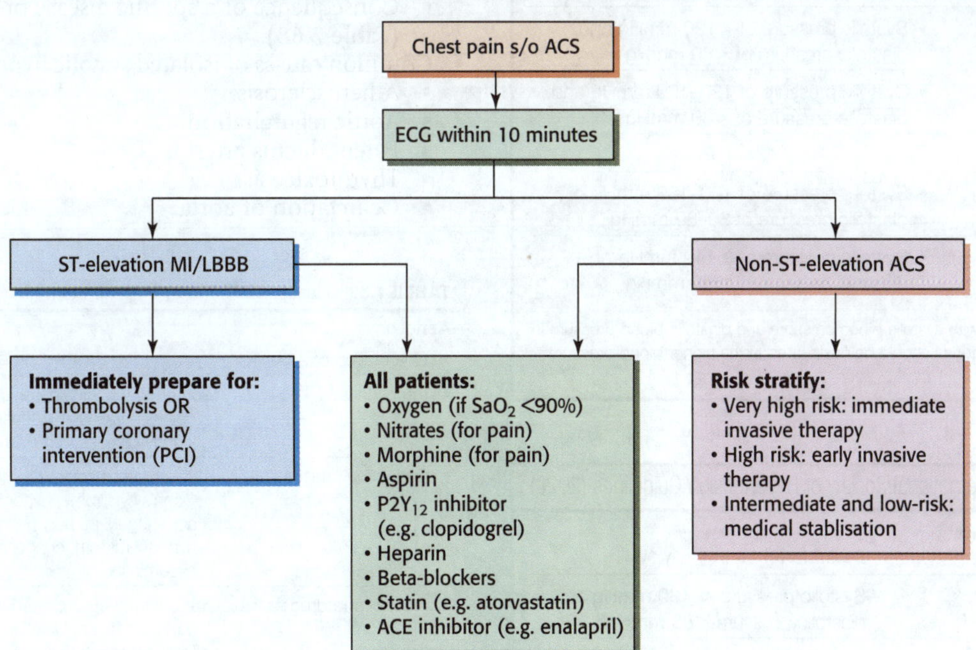

Flowchart 7.19 Summary of Management of Acute Coronary Syndrome.

Q. Classify hypertension. Discuss the pathophysiology, clinical features, complications and management of essential hypertension. (IM 8.14, IM 8.2, IM 8.4, IM 8.8)

Q. Discuss the causes and investigations of secondary hypertension. (IM 8.1, IM 8.12)

Q. Explain briefly about malignant hypertension.

- Fifteen per cent of the general population can be regarded as hypertensive.
- As per the latest guidelines, hypertension is defined as shown in Boxes 7.74 and 7.75.
- Ambulatory blood pressure monitoring is the standard for measuring blood pressure.
- White coat hypertension:
  - A transient increase in blood pressure in normal individuals when blood pressure is recorded in a hospital or in a physician's clinic.
  - Consider either carefully obtained home values using an appropriately calibrated BP monitor or obtaining 24 hour ambulatory BP measurements.

BOX 7.74 American College of Cardiology–American Heart Association Guidelines for Hypertension (2017)

Blood Pressure Category	Definition
Normal	• Systolic pressure of <120 mmHg and diastolic pressure of <80 mmHg
Elevated	• Systolic pressure of 120–129 mmHg and diastolic pressure of <80 mmHg
Hypertension:	
Stage 1	• Systolic pressure of 130–139 mmHg or diastolic pressure of 80–89 mmHg
Stage 2	• Systolic pressure of ≥140 mmHg or diastolic pressure of ≥90 mmHg

Note: Persons with systolic blood pressure and diastolic blood pressure in different categories should be designated in the higher blood pressure category.

BOX 7.75 International Society of Hypertension Guidelines (2020)

Blood Pressure Category	Definition
Normal	Systolic pressure < 130 mmHg and diastolic pressure <85 mmHg
High-normal	Systolic pressure 130–139 mmHg and/or diastolic pressure 85–89 mmHg
Grade 1 hypertension	Systolic pressure 140–159 mmHg and/or diastolic pressure 90–99 mmHg
Grade 2 hypertension	Systolic pressure ≥160 mmHg and/or diastolic pressure ≥100 mmHg

- Isolated ambulatory or masked hypertension
  - It is reverse phenomenon of 'white coat hypertension' in which individuals with normal clinic blood pressure (<140/90 mmHg) may have elevated ambulatory or home blood pressure values.
  - Such individuals have been shown to have greater than normal prevalence of organ damage and an increased prevalence of metabolic risk factors compared to subjects with a truly normal blood pressure.
- Paradoxical hypertension
  - Patients on antihypertensive agents paradoxically show increase in blood pressure.
    - Patients with diabetes and hypertension on β-blockers develop paradoxical rise in blood pressure if they develop hypoglycaemia. This occurs due to sympathetic stimulation following hypoglycaemia.
    - Patients with bilateral renal artery stenosis who are given angiotensin-converting enzyme (ACE) inhibitors.
    - Administration of pure β-blockers to patients with phaeochromocytoma.

CLASSIFICATION

- Primary or essential hypertension:
  - Accounts for 85% of the cases.
  - Not possible to define a specific underlying cause.
  - Seventy per cent of them have a positive family history.
- Secondary hypertension:
  - Accounts for 15% of the cases.
  - Consequence of a specific disease or abnormality (Table 7.68).
- Common causes of isolated systolic hypertension are:
  - Atherosclerosis.
  - Aortic regurgitation.
  - Patent ductus arteriosus.
  - Thyrotoxicosis.
  - Coarctation of aorta.

TABLE 7.68 Causes of Secondary Hypertension

Aetiology	
• Coarctation of aorta	
• Renal causes	Glomerulonephritis, chronic pyelonephritis, collagen vascular diseases, polycystic kidney disease, renal artery stenosis
• Endocrine causes	Phaeochromocytoma, Cushing's syndrome, Conn's syndrome, hyperparathyroidism, acromegaly, primary hypothyroidism, hyperthyroidism, congenital adrenal hyperplasia
• Alcohol and drugs	Oral contraceptives, anabolic steroids, corticosteroids, NSAIDs, COX-2 inhibitors, carbenoxolone, sympathomimetics, cyclosporin, tacrolimus, sibutramine, bromocriptine, erythropoietin, bevacizumab
• Preeclamptic toxaemia	
• Miscellaneous	Obstructive sleep apnoea, cocaine, phencyclidine

MEASUREMENT OF BLOOD PRESSURE

- BP must be measured twice—first with the patient supine or seated, and then after the patient has been standing for ≥2 minutes on three separate days. The average of these measurements is used for diagnosis. Blood pressure in standing is required to exclude significant postural drop that may get accentuated with medications.
- Ideally patient should be sitting comfortably in a chair with back supported and both feet flat on the floor, no intake of caffeine or use of tobacco for at least 30–45 minutes before measurement and resting with the arm supported at heart level for 5–10 minutes.
- BP is measured in both arms; if BP in one arm is much higher, the higher value is used. A difference of more than 10 mmHg between two arms suggests obstructive lesions of aorta, innominate artery or subclavian artery.
- An appropriately sized cuff covers two-thirds of the biceps; the bladder is long enough to encircle >80% of the arm, and bladder width equals at least 40% of the arm's circumference.
- The pressure at which the first heartbeat is heard as the pressure falls is systolic BP (phase I of Korotkoff sounds). Disappearance of the sound (phase V of Korotkoff sounds) marks diastolic BP.
- Auscultatory gap.
  - Occasionally, after initial appearance of Korotkoff sounds at systolic pressure, the sounds disappear for sometimes, re-appear again and finally disappear at the diastolic pressure. This is auscultatory gap.
  - Seen in some patients with hypertension.
  - Overestimates diastolic pressure and underestimates systolic pressure depending on which phase is auscultated. To avoid errors due to auscultatory gap, palpatory method of estimating systolic pressure should precede the auscultatory method.

PATHOPHYSIOLOGY

- Blood pressure is determined by several factors including blood volume, arterial tone and cardiac output. These in turn are affected by various genetic, environmental and neurohumoral mechanisms.

GENETIC FACTORS

- Multiple genes are involved in primary hypertension which may produce hypertension by interacting with environmental and neurohumoral mechanisms.

ENVIRONMENTAL FACTORS

- Several environmental factors interact with genetic predisposition to produce hypertension. These include high sodium intake, mental stress, poor sleep quality, excess alcohol intake, etc.

NEUROHUMORAL FACTORS

- Neurohumoral system includes renin–angiotensin–aldosterone system (RAAS), natriuretic peptides, endothelium and sympathetic nervous system.

RAAS

- RAAS has several effects including sodium retention, sodium diuresis, vasoconstriction, endothelial dysfunction and vascular injury.
- Angiotensin II, formed by the action of ACE on angiotensin I, enhances sodium reabsorption in the proximal tubule. It also increases aldosterone synthesis and release which again produces sodium retention. Both aldosterone and angiotensin II produce endothelial dysfunction.

Sodium Homeostatic Mechanisms

- When a normotensive person takes excessive salt, the body tries to reduce its harmful effects by reducing vascular resistance and increasing production of nitric oxide, a vasodilator from endothelial cells.
- In presence of endothelial dysfunction (due to genetic factors), release of nitric oxide is impaired which results in hypertension. These persons are 'salt-sensitive' which is defined as elevation in systolic blood pressure ≥10 mmHg within a few hours of ingestion of ≥5 g sodium.
- Chronic high salt ingestion (environmental factor) can result in endothelial dysfunction even in individuals who are not salt-sensitive.

Natriuretic Peptides

- Atrial natriuretic peptide (ANP) and brain natriuretic peptide (BNP) display natriuretic and vasodilator properties which help in maintaining sodium balance and lowering blood pressure.
- Deficiency of natriuretic peptides may lead to hypertension.

Endothelium

- Endothelial cells produce nitric oxide, a vasodilator as well as other factors like endothelin-1 which is a vasoconstrictor.
- Endothelium dysfunction can lead to reduced production of NO and increased levels or sensitivity to endothelin-1, both of which can produce hypertension.

Sympathetic Nervous System

- Baroreceptors situated in various arteries, particularly in the internal carotid artery, respond to stretch and modulate sympathetic outflow from brain.
- Sympathetic activity is generally more in persons with hypertension than in normotensive individuals.
- Besides producing direct vasoconstriction, increased sympathetic activity also increases renal sodium reabsorption. It also causes endothelium dysfunction.

SUMMARY OF PATHOGENESIS OF HYPERTENSION

- Pathogenesis of hypertension is summarised in Fig. 7.57.

CLINICAL FEATURES

- There are three objectives of clinical examination:
  - Identify any underlying cause.
  - Recognise risk factors for the development of complications.
  - Detect any complications already present.

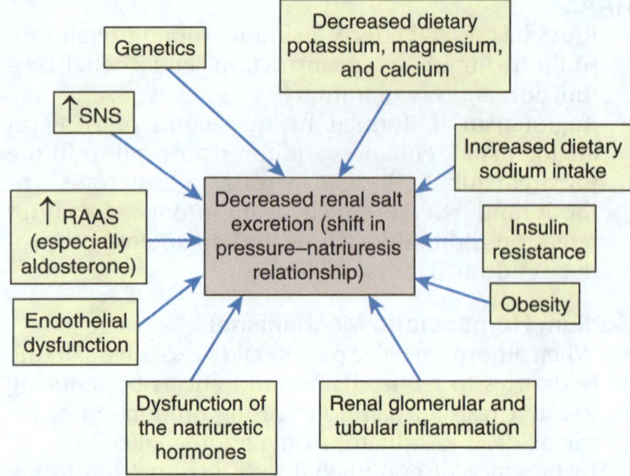

Fig. 7.57 Pathogenesis of hypertension (renal salt excretion leads to hypertension). SNS, sympathetic nervous system; RAAS, renin–angiotensin–aldosterone system.

- Risk factors are smoking, obesity, hyperlipidaemia, diabetes mellitus, physical inactivity, high salt intake and family history of premature CAD, all of which interact with hypertension, especially in the genesis of ischaemic heart disease.
- Clinical features of hypertension are due to hypertension per se and the underlying cause of hypertension.

CLINICAL FEATURES DUE TO HYPERTENSION PER SE

- Majority are asymptomatic and hypertension is detected on routine examination.
- Acute hypertension causes transient headache and polyuria.
- Long-standing hypertension leads to left ventricular hypertrophy and heaving apical impulse.
- Left atrial hypertrophy and fourth heart sound.
- Aortic component (A_2) of second heart sound is accentuated.
- Very short early diastolic murmur.
- Fundal changes (refer section heading 'Complications of Hypertension' below).

CLINICAL FEATURES DUE TO CAUSES OF HYPERTENSION

- History of intake of alcohol or drugs like oral contraceptives, corticosteroids, NSAIDs, carbenoxolone or sympathomimetic agents.
- Radiofemoral delay, upper limb hypertension, collaterals around scapulae and systolic murmur over spine suggest coarctation of aorta.
- Panic attacks, paroxysmal headache and palpitations suggest phaeochromocytoma. Skin stigmata of neurofibromatosis may also suggest phaeochromocytoma.
- Recurrent back pain, undiagnosed fever and recurrent urinary infections suggest chronic pyelonephritis.
- Enlarged palpable kidneys in polycystic kidney disease.
- Bruit over the abdomen in the lumbar region suggests renal artery stenosis.
- Characteristic facies and habitus in Cushing's syndrome.

COMPLICATIONS OF HYPERTENSION

CENTRAL NERVOUS SYSTEM COMPLICATIONS

- Transient ischaemic attacks.
- Cerebrovascular accidents (strokes) due to cerebral ischaemia, thrombosis or haemorrhage.
- Subarachnoid haemorrhage.
- Hypertensive encephalopathy.
- Multiinfarct dementia.

OPHTHALMIC COMPLICATIONS

- Hypertensive retinopathy is characterised by thickening of the walls of the retinal arterioles, diffuse or segmental narrowing of blood columns, varying width of the light reflex from vessel walls, arteriovenous nipping, retinal haemorrhages, soft and hard exudates and papilloedema (Table 7.69 and Fig. 7.58A and B). Severe retinopathy can cause visual field defects and blindness.

CARDIOVASCULAR COMPLICATIONS

- Coronary artery disease (angina and myocardial infarction).
- Diastolic dysfunction.
- Heart failure with preserved ejection fraction.
- Left ventricular hypertrophy.
- Heart failure with reduced ejection fraction.
- Aortic aneurysm.
- Aortic dissection.
- Atherosclerotic occlusive disease with limb or organ ischaemia.

RENAL COMPLICATIONS

- Proteinuria.
- Progressive renal failure.

MALIGNANT HYPERTENSION

- It was initially described as a clinical syndrome of markedly high blood pressure with retinal haemorrhages, exudates and papilloedema.
- However, now it is defined as a syndrome of markedly high blood pressure with multiorgan damage, particularly kidney, heart and brain. It characterises the condition of severe hypertension with concomitant retinopathy, microangiopathy, disseminated intravascular coagulation, encephalopathy, acute heart failure, or acute deterioration in renal function. The patient often presents with confusion, headache, vomiting, visual disturbances, dyspnoea and deterioration in renal functions.

TABLE 7.69 Grading of Hypertensive Retinopathy

Grade	Features
• Grade I	Arteriolar narrowing and increase in light reflex over the arterioles
• Grade II	Marked arteriolar narrowing and arteriovenous nipping
• Grade III	Grade II plus flame-shaped haemorrhages and soft exudates
• Grade IV	Grade III plus papilloedema

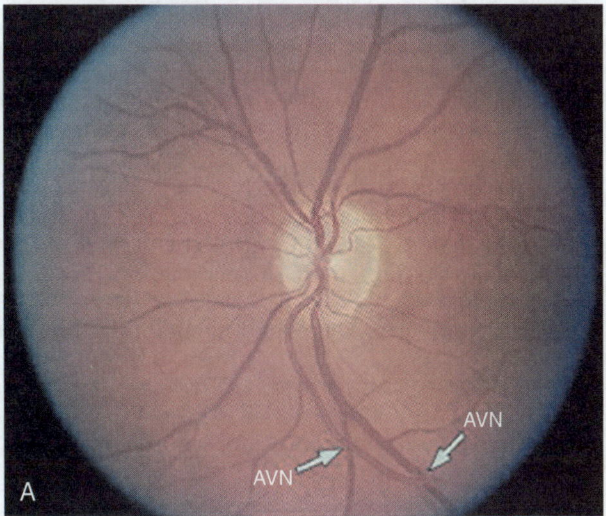

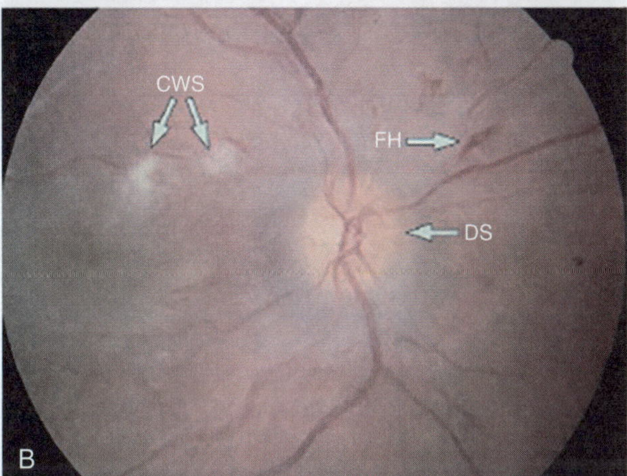

Fig. 7.58 A: Signs of mild hypertensive retinopathy in an eye with ischaemic optic neuropathy. B: Signs of severe hypertensive retinopathy. AVN, arteriovenous nipping; CWS, cotton-wool spots; FH, flame-shaped retina haemorrhage; DS, swelling of the optic disc. Courtesy: Wong TY, Mitchell P. The eye in hypertension. Lancet. 2007 Feb 3;369(9559):425 35.

BOX 7.76 When to Suspect a Secondary Cause in a Hypertensive Patient?

- Poor response to therapy (resistant hypertension)
- Worsening of control in previously stable patient
- Systolic pressure >180 mmHg or diastolic pressure >110 mmHg
- Onset of hypertension in persons younger than 20 years or older than 50 years
- Significant hypertensive target organ damage
- Lack of family history of hypertension
- Findings on history, physical examination or routine investigations that suggest a secondary cause

REASONS TO SUSPECT A SECONDARY CAUSE OF HYPERTENSION

- Box 7.76 gives reasons to suspect a secondary cause of hypertension.

INVESTIGATIONS

BASIC STUDIES

- Urine analysis for protein, blood and glucose, and microscopic examination for casts or pus cells.
- Blood urea and creatinine (to assess renal function).
- Serum electrolytes (for hypokalaemia and alkalosis in hyperaldosteronism).
- Fasting and postprandial blood glucose (for hyperglycaemia).
- Serum cholesterol and triglycerides.
- Serum calcium and uric acid.
- Electrocardiogram (for left ventricular hypertrophy).
- Chest radiograph (for cardiac size, evidence of cardiac failure and aortic dilatation).

STUDIES TO FIND A SECONDARY CAUSE

- Table 7.70 lists the studies required to find a secondary cause of hypertension.

TREATMENT

- For patients with stage 1 hypertension with no diabetes, chronic kidney disease or cardiovascular disease, the guideline recommends calculation of the estimated 10-year risk of cardiovascular disease. If this risk is <10%, lifestyle modifications alone should be implemented for a period of 3–6 months before initiating antihypertensive drug to lower blood pressure below 130/80 mmHg.
- For those with stage 2 hypertension or stage 1 hypertension with preexisting cardiovascular disease, diabetes mellitus, chronic kidney disease or a 10-year risk of cardiovascular disease of ≥10%, both lifestyle modifications and antihypertensives should be initiated. Re-evaluation is done after 1 month.

TABLE 7.70 Studies to Detect Secondary Causes of Hypertension

Underlying Disease	Investigations
Phaeochromocytoma	• 24-Hour urinary catecholamine, metanephrines and VMA levels, ^{123}I-labelled metaiodobenzylguanidine scanning
Cushing's syndrome	• Plasma cortisol levels, 24-hour urinary cortisol and dexamethasone suppression test
Renal artery stenosis	• Captopril-enhanced radionuclide scan (99m-technetium diethylenetriamine-penta acetic acid—DTPA scan), Doppler ultrasound, CT angiogram, MRI angiogram and renal arteriogram
Polycystic renal disease	• Ultrasonography
Primary aldosteronism	• Hypokalaemia, high aldosterone levels and low plasma renin activity, tests after oral or intravenous sodium loading, fludrocortisone suppression or captopril test, adrenal CT scan, adrenal vein sampling
Acromegaly	• GH levels and radiograph of the skull
Primary hypothyroidism	• T3, T4 and TSH levels
Coarctation of aorta	• Chest radiography for rib notching and catheterisation

- For all patients with hypertension, a blood pressure target of <130/80 mmHg is recommended.
- Treatment of hypertension can be discussed under three headings:
  - General measures.
  - Antihypertensive drug therapy.
  - Treatment of underlying cause (in secondary hypertension).

GENERAL MEASURES

- Lifestyle modifications are recommended for all patients with hypertension. A reduction in systolic blood pressure of 5 mmHg has been associated with about 10% reduction in mortality caused by stroke and heart disease.
  - Reassurance.
  - Control of obesity.
  - Low-sodium diet (<100 mEq sodium or <6 g salt)
  - Other dietary recommendations—diet rich in fruit, vegetables, potassium and low-fat dairy products, with low total and saturated fat (Dietary Approaches to Stop Hypertension or DASH eating plan).
  - Smoking to be abandoned.
  - Alcohol consumption to be moderated (males no more than two alcoholic drinks of 30 mL/day and females no more than one per day).
  - Regular aerobic exercises.
  - Relaxation classes, meditation and biofeedback.

ANTIHYPERTENSIVE DRUG THERAPY (Table 7.71)

- Required if target blood pressure is not achieved with general measures.

TABLE 7.71 Antihypertensive Drugs

Class	Drugs	Dose
• Diuretics		
• Thiazide diuretics	Chlorthalidone	12.5–25 mg OD
	Chlorothiazide	125–500 mg OD
	Hydrochlorothiazide	12.5–25 mg OD
	Metolazone	2.5–5.0 mg OD
	Indapamide[a]	1.25–2.5 mg OD
• Loop diuretics	Furosemide	10–40 mg BID (not used)
	Bumetanide	0.5–1.0 mg BID
	Torasemide or torsemide	2.5–10 mg OD
• Potassium-sparing diuretics	Amiloride	5–10 mg OD
	Triamterene	25–100 mg OD
• Mineralocorticoid receptor antagonists	Spironolactone	25–100 mg OD
	Eplerenone	50–100 mg OD
• β-Blockers	Propranolol	20–80 mg BID or TID
	Metoprolol	25–100 mg BID
	Atenolol	25–100 mg OD
	Bisoprolol	2.5–10 mg OD
	Nebivolol	5–10 mg OD
	Carvedilol	6.25–25 mg BID
• Combined α- and β-blockers	Labetalol	100–900 mg BID
• Angiotensin-converting enzyme (ACE) inhibitors	Captopril	12.5–50 mg TID
	Enalapril	2.5–20 mg OD or BID
	Lisinopril	2.5–40 mg OD
	Ramipril	2.5–20 mg OD
	Perindopril	2–8 mg OD
	Quinapril	10–80 mg OD
• Angiotensin II receptor antagonists (ARBs)	Losartan	25–50 mg BID
	Candesartan	8–32 mg OD
	Irbesartan	75–300 mg OD
	Valsartan	80–320 mg
	Telmisartan	20–80 mg OD
	Olmesartan	20–40 mg OD
	Azilsartan	40–80 mg OD
• Direct rennin inhibitors	Aliskiren	75–300 mg OD
• Calcium channel blockers	Nifedipine (SR)	30–60 mg OD
	Verapamil	40–160 mg BID
	Diltiazem	40–160 mg BID
	Diltiazem (SR)	90–360 mg OD
	Amlodipine	2.5–20 mg OD
	Felodipine	2.5–20 mg OD
	Nicardipine (SR)	60–120 mg BID
	Cilnidipine	5–20 mg OD
	Azelnidipine	8–16 mg OD

TABLE 7.71 Antihypertensive Drugs—cont'd

Class	Drugs	Dose
• α-Blockers	Prazosin Terazosin Doxazosin	2.5–5.0 mg OD or BID 1–20 mg OD 1–16 mg OD
• Direct vasodilators	Hydralazine Minoxidil	12.5–50 mg BID 1.25–40 mg BID
• Central α_2-blockers and other centrally acting drugs	Clonidine α-Methyldopa Reserpine Moxonidine	0.05–0.3 mg BID 250–1000 mg QID 0.05–0.25 mg OD 0.2–0.3 mg OD or BID

[a]Indapamide has mild diuretic and vasodilator action.

Diuretics

Thiazide Diuretics

- Mechanism of action—thiazide diuretics have an influence on carbonic anhydrase and so they inhibit the reabsorption of sodium bicarbonate in proximal tubules. They depress the sodium and chloride reabsorption in the early distal convoluted tubules. Potassium depletion results from reduced H^+ secretion and increased delivery of sodium and water to the distal tubules.
- Adverse effects—impotence, postural hypotension, allergic rashes, marrow depression, hyperuricaemia, hypercalcaemia and diabetes.
- If blood pressure cannot be controlled with a thiazide diuretic, ACE inhibitors, angiotensin receptor blockers or calcium channel blockers may be added.

Loop Diuretics

- Furosemide or others are used if there is renal impairment or when greater sodium excretion is needed.

β-Adrenoreceptor Antagonists (β-Blockers)

Uses of β-Blockers

- Various uses of beta-blockers are given in Box 7.77.

Contraindications of β-Blockers

- Contraindications to the use of beta-blockers are given in Box 7.78.

BOX 7.77 Uses of Beta-Blockers

- Angina pectoris
- Acute myocardial infarction and postmyocardial infarction period (to prevent re-infarction)
- Chronic open-angle glaucoma
- Cardiac arrhythmias
- Hypertension
- Thyrotoxicosis
- Hypertrophic cardiomyopathy
- Fallot's tetralogy (cyanotic spells)
- Phaeochromocytoma (after α-blocker)
- Anxiety with somatic symptoms
- Portal hypertension
- Migraine prophylaxis
- Essential tremor

BOX 7.78 Contraindications of Beta-Blockers

- Chronic obstructive pulmonary disease and asthma
- Severe heart failure
- Heart block
- Peripheral vascular disease
- Diabetes mellitus (masks sympathetic signs of hypoglycaemia)

Various Beta-blockers

Propranolol

- Mechanism of action includes sympatholytic effect, antihypertensive effect and relief of anxiety, palpitation and angina.
- A large portion of the drug is destroyed in its first passage through liver.
- Treatment is started with 40 mg twice a day and gradually increased to 160 mg 6 hourly. Slow-release forms are given as a single daily dose.
- Side effects—gastric disturbances, bradycardia, cardiac failure, bronchospasm, tiredness, bad dreams, hallucinations, cold hands and muscle weakness.

Metoprolol and Atenolol

- Cardioselective β-1 antagonists with mechanism of action similar to that of propranolol. They have a greater effect on the cardiac β-1 receptors than on the β-2 receptors (β-2 receptors subserve bronchodilatation and vasodilatation).
- Dose—metoprolol 50 mg twice daily to 100 mg thrice daily and atenolol 50–100 mg once daily. Sustained-release preparations of metoprolol are given in a dose of 12.5–100 mg OD.
- They may be used in hypertensive patients who have mild airway obstruction (COPD and asthma), peripheral vascular disease and type 1 diabetes; however, caution is required.
- Other indications—ischaemic heart disease and supraventricular tachycardia.
- Side effects—same as for propranolol but additionally cause hyperkalaemia.

Labetalol

- It has a combined α and β adrenoreceptor antagonistic action. Dose—100 to 200 mg twice daily. Side effects—same as of propranolol.

Angiotensin-Converting Enzyme Inhibitors (Captopril, Enalapril, Lisinopril, Ramipril and Perindopril)

- For a detailed account of ACE inhibitors, refer page 547.
- Indicated as vasodilator therapy in hypertension and chronic cardiac failure.
- Mechanism of action includes powerful arteriolar and venous dilatation, and inhibition of formation of angiotensin II, thereby reducing aldosterone release.
- Contraindicated in patients with impaired renal function (creatinine >3 mg/dL) and bilateral renal artery stenosis.

- Dose—start with a small dose (captopril 6.25 mg and enalapril 2.5 mg) and then gradually increase.
- Side effects—cough, angio-oedema, postural hypotension, rashes, blood dyscrasias, neuropathy and diarrhoea.

Angiotensin Receptor Blockers

Mechanism of Action

- The RAAS plays a pivotal role in the homeostatic regulation of blood pressure.
- Renin catalyses cleavage of angiotensinogen producing angiotensin I.
- Angiotensin II is produced from angiotensin I by the action of ACE. It is the most active hormone of the renin–angiotensin system.
- In humans, two angiotensin II receptors have been identified: AT_1 and AT_2. In adults, most effects of angiotensin II are mediated by the AT_1 receptor; the function of the AT_2 is not established.
- Binding of angiotensin II to its AT_1 receptors, besides mediating its main biological effects (including vasoconstriction, cell proliferation, hypertrophy and aldosterone secretion), provides feedback inhibition of further renin release by the kidney.
- Angiotensin receptor blockers block the action of angiotensin II by blocking AT_1 receptors.

Angiotensin Receptor Blockers

- Losartan.
- Irbesartan.
- Candesartan.
- Valsartan.
- Telmisartan.
- Olmesartan.
- Azilsartan.

Side Effects

- Better tolerated compared to ACE inhibitors.
- Side effects include hypotension, drowsiness and dizziness.
- Cough is rare.

Uses

- These agents are useful in the treatment of hypertension, myocardial infarction (to reduce myocardial remodelling) and diabetic nephropathy (to slow its progression).

Peripheral Vasodilators

- Act by producing peripheral arteriolar and venous vasodilatation by acting on arteriolar smooth muscles or smooth muscles of venules.
- Drugs in this category include hydralazine, prazosin, diazoxide, sodium nitroprusside and minoxidil.

Calcium Channel Blockers (Calcium Antagonists)

Uses of Calcium Channel Blockers

- Various indications of calcium channel blockers are given in Box 7.79.

BOX 7.79 Uses of Calcium Channel Blockers

• Angina pectoris/Prinzmetal's angina	• Achalasia cardia
• Hypertension	• Biliary dyskinesia
• Antiarrhythmic agent	• Pulmonary hypertension
• Peripheral vasospastic conditions, e.g. Raynaud's disease	• Cor pulmonale (chronic bronchitis with pulmonary hypertension) – possible role
• Migraine	• Heart failure
• Subarachnoid haemorrhage (to prevent vasospasm)	• Valvular diseases—MR and AR

Nifedipine and Verapamil

- Mechanism of action—they act on cell membrane selectively to block the access of calcium and exert negative inotropic action. They increase myocardial oxygen supply, prevent coronary artery spasm, increase coronary blood flow and reduce peripheral vascular resistance.
- Dose—nifedipine (sustained-release) 10–40 mg once or twice a day and verapamil 180–360 mg/day in divided doses.
- Short-acting nifedipine should be avoided.

Centrally Acting Drugs

Reserpine

- Mild antihypertensive with central and peripheral action. Dose—0.1 to 0.5 mg daily. Side effects—nasal congestion, depression and parkinsonism.

α-Methyldopa

- Mechanism of action—both central and peripheral. Dose—250 to 500 mg twice or thrice daily. Side effects—dryness of mouth, sedation, extrapyramidal features, fever, hepatitis and haemolytic anaemia.

Clonidine

- Mechanism of action—central only. Dose—0.1 to 1.0 mg daily. Side effects—dryness of mouth, drowsiness and rebound hypertension on sudden withdrawal.

BROAD GUIDELINES ON SELECTION OF DRUGS

- In the general nonblack population including those with diabetes, initial antihypertensive treatment should include a thiazide-type diuretic, dihydropyridine calcium channel blocker, ACE inhibitor or angiotensin receptor blocker.
- In the general black population including those with diabetes, initial antihypertensive treatment should include a thiazide-type diuretic or dihydropyridine calcium channel blocker.
- In the patient with chronic kidney disease and hypertension (irrespective of race and diabetic status), initial antihypertensive treatment should include an ACE inhibitor or aldosterone receptor blocking agent so as to improve kidney outcomes.
- Beta-blockers are first-line agents in patients with heart failure with reduced left ventricular ejection fraction or postmyocardial infarction.
- Combination of ACE inhibitors and angiotensin receptor blockers adds little blood pressure-lowering effects while increasing the risk of renal dysfunction and hyperkalaemia.

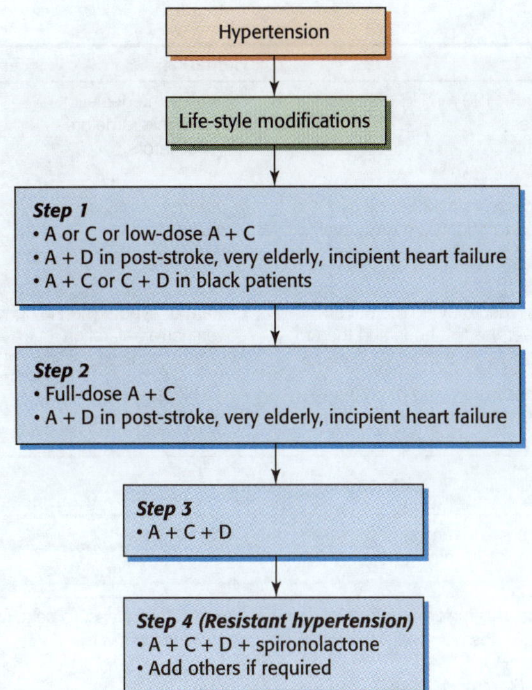

Flowchart 7.20 Summary of Management of Hypertension. A = ACE-inhibitor or Angiotensin receptor blocker; C = Calcium channel blocker; D = Thiazide-like diuretic.

- If goal BP is not reached within a month of treatment, increase the dose of the initial drug or add a second drug from one of the other classes.
- Flowchart 7.20 summarises management of hypertension.

RESISTANT HYPERTENSION

- Defined as a seated blood pressure of at least 140 mmHg systolic or 90 mmHg diastolic despite treatment with the maximally tolerated dose of three or more antihypertensive agents, one of which must be a diuretic.
- It is important to distinguish pseudoresistant or apparent hypertension from true resistant hypertension. Aetiologies of apparent resistant hypertension include measurement error and medication nonadherence. It can also be due to use of medications which interfere with actions of antihypertensive drugs.
- Renal denervation is an option to manage resistant hypertension.

Q. Discuss the clinical presentation and management of hypertensive encephalopathy.

- Hypertensive encephalopathy is characterised by a very high blood pressure and neurological disturbances including transient abnormalities in speech or vision, paraesthesia, disorientation, seizures, loss of consciousness and papilloedema.
- Neurological deficit is fully reversible if the hypertension is properly controlled.

TREATMENT

- The initial aim of treatment is to lower the blood pressure by 10%–20% in the first hour with more gradual lowering by about 25% over the next 6 hours. Too rapid fall in blood pressure might cause cerebral ischaemia, blindness, myocardial infarction or renal insufficiency.
- Intravenous sodium nitroprusside (0.3–1.0 μg/kg/minute) is the most effective drug. It has to be used very carefully in an intensive care setup.
- Alternatively, parenteral labetalol (20 mg/minute to a maximum of 200 mg), hydralazine (5–10 mg every 30 minutes to a maximum of 300 mg) or nitroglycerine (5–100 μg/minute as infusion) may be used.
- Do not use sublingual nifedipine as it can produce precipitous fall in blood pressure leading to acute myocardial ischaemia or stroke.

Q. Discuss briefly about hypertensive emergencies. (IM 8.15, IM 8.6)

- A hypertensive emergency involves an elevated blood pressure (usually >180 mmHg systolic) in association with signs and/or symptoms of acute target organ damage. The resultant vascular compromise of the affected organ may include hypertensive encephalopathy, acute heart failure with pulmonary oedema, dissecting aortic aneurysm, acute renal failure, unstable angina or myocardial infarction, intracranial bleed, acute ischaemic stroke or subarachnoid haemorrhage.
- The term hypertensive urgency indicates severe increase in blood pressure without associated end-organ damage. The blood pressure does not require urgent reduction but instead can be reduced over the course of days.

MANAGEMENT OF HYPERTENSIVE EMERGENCIES

- Management of hypertensive emergencies is given in Table 7.72.

DRUGS USED IN HYPERTENSIVE EMERGENCIES

- Drugs which are used to manage hypertensive emergencies are given in Table 7.73.

Q. Discuss the aetiology, pathophysiology, clinical features and investigations of pulmonary hypertension.

Q. Briefly explain about Graham Steell murmur.

DEFINITION

- Pulmonary hypertension (PH) is an elevation in pulmonary vascular pressure that can be caused by an isolated increase in pulmonary arterial pressure or by increases in both pulmonary arterial and pulmonary venous pressures.

TABLE 7.72 Management of Hypertensive Emergencies

Diagnosis	Suggested Drugs	Targets	Remarks
Acute aortic dissection	Labetalol IV Esmolol bolus and then infusion Nitroprusside infusion (after β-blockade)	Systolic pressure <120 mmHg within 20–30 minutes Pulse <60/minute	Avoid volume depletion Use β-blockers before vasodilators
Acute pulmonary oedema	Nitroglycerine infusion Enalaprilat IV Nitroprusside infusion Furosemide IV	Reduce blood pressure by 20–30% over the first hour, then to 160/100 mmHg over the next 2–6 hours	Hypotension may occur with enalaprilat
Acute coronary syndrome	Nitroglycerine infusion β-Blockers (metoprolol or labetalol)	Reduce blood pressure by no more than 20%–30% over the first hour, and then to 160/100 mmHg over the next 2–6 hours	Beware of hypotension in right ventricular infarction Avoid hypotension
Acute renal failure	Labetalol IV Nicardipine infusion Dialysis	Reduce blood pressure by no more than 20%–30% over the first hour, and then to 160/100 mmHg over the next 2–6 hours	Avoid nitroprusside Avoid ACE inhibitors
Hypertensive encephalopathy	See above on 605 page		
Subarachnoid haemorrhage	Labetalol bolus and infusion Esmolol bolus and infusion Nicardipine infusion	Systolic pressure <160 mmHg or mean arterial pressure <130 mmHg (to reduce recurrence)	Control of pain
Intracerebral haemorrhage	Labetalol bolus and infusion Esmolol bolus and infusion Nicardipine infusion	Systolic pressure 140 mmHg within 1 hour if initially, it is below 220 mmHg. If above 220 mmHg, reduce it to 160 mmHg	Avoid systolic pressure below 120 mmHg
Acute ischaemic stroke	Labetalol bolus and infusion Nitroglycerine infusion	If fibrinolytic therapy planned, treat if >185/110 mmHg Otherwise treat if >220/120 mmHg on the third measurement done 15 minutes apart	Avoid lowering blood pressure by more than 10%–15% in 24 hours
Phaeochromocytoma	Nicardipine, phentolamine	Systolic pressure <120 mmHg within 20–30 minutes	Avoid use of beta-blockers as sole agents
Eclampsia	Hydralazine, labetalol, nicardipine	Reduce systolic pressure below 140 mmHg within 20–30 minutes	Avoid ACE inhibitors, ARBs and nitroprusside

TABLE 7.73 Dosages of Drugs Used in Hypertensive Emergencies

Drug	Dose
Labetalol	Bolus: 20 mg IV every 2 minutes or 40–80 mg every 10–20 minutes to a total of 300 mg, OR Infusion: 2 mg/minute to a total of 300 mg
Esmolol	250–500 μg/kg over 1–3 minutes, followed by 50 μg/minute; may be increased by 50 μg/minute every 4 minutes till response or till 200 μg/minute is reached. Every 4 minutes, additional loading doses can also be given
Nicardipine	5 mg/hour; increase by 2.5 mg/hour every 15 minutes till response or 15 mg/hour is reached
Nitroglycerine	Start at 5 μg/minute and increase by 5–10 μg/minute every 3–5 minutes till 200 μg/minute is reached
Nitroprusside	0.3–0.5 μg/kg/minute; increase by 0.3–0.5 μg/kg/minute every 3–5 minutes to the desired effect. Rates >2 μg/kg/minute may produce cyanide toxicity
Enalaprilat	1.25 mg over 5 minutes IV every 4–6 hours

- It is defined as a resting mean pulmonary artery pressure greater than 20 mmHg (previous definition was greater than 25 mmHg).
- Pulmonary arterial wedge pressure (PAWP) and pulmonary vascular resistance (PVR) are important in classifying PH. Therefore, stress is given on the need for right heart catheterisation with measurement of cardiac output, PVR and PAWP.

AETIOLOGY AND CLASSIFICATION OF PULMONARY HYPERTENSION

- Classification and causes of pulmonary hypertension are given in Table 7.74.
- PH can occur in patients with portal hypertension with or without underlying liver disease.

PATHOPHYSIOLOGY

- Normal pulmonary artery systolic pressure at rest is less than 20 mmHg, with a mean of 12–16 mmHg. This low pressure is due to the large cross-sectional area of the pulmonary circulation which results in low resistance.
- PH results from one or both of the following:
  - Increase in pulmonary vascular resistance.
  - Increase in pulmonary blood flow.
- Pathophysiology of PH is summarised in Flowchart 7.21.

CLINICAL FEATURES

SYMPTOMS OF PULMONARY HYPERTENSION AND ITS CONSEQUENCES

- Fatigue, dyspnoea, syncope and angina due to reduced cardiac output.

TABLE 7.74 Aetiology and Classification (Updated 6th World Symposium on Pulmonary Hypertension Classification 2018)

1. Pulmonary arterial hypertension (PAH)— PAWP ≤ 15 mmHg, PVR ≥ 3 Wood units
   - Idiopathic PAH
   - Heritable PAH
   - Drug and toxin induced (fenfluramine, aminorex, toxic rape seed oil, amphetamines, dasatinib)
   - Associated with:
     - Connective tissue diseases (e.g. CREST syndrome, scleroderma, SLE, Sjogren's syndrome, polymyositis)
     - HIV infection
     - Portal hypertension
     - Congenital heart diseases
     - Schistosomiasis
   - PAH long-term responders to calcium channel blockers
   - PAH with overt features of venous/capillaries involvement (pulmonary veno-occlusive disease)/capillaries involvement (pulmonary capillary haemangiomatosis)
   - Persistent PH of the newborn syndrome
2. PH due to left heart disease— PAWP >15 mmHg
   - PH due to heart failure with preserved LVEF
   - PH due to heart failure with reduced LVEF
   - Valvular heart disease
   - Congenital/acquired cardiovascular conditions leading to postcapillary PH
3. PH due to lung diseases and/or hypoxia— PAWP ≤15 mmHg, PVR ≥3 Wood units
   - Obstructive lung disease
   - Restrictive lung disease
   - Other lung disease with mixed restrictive/obstructive pattern
   - Hypoxia without lung disease (e.g. sleep-disordered breathing, alveolar hypoventilation disorders, chronic exposure to high altitude)
   - Developmental lung disorders
4. PH due to pulmonary artery obstructions— PAWP ≤15 mmHg, PVR ≥3 Wood units
   - Chronic thromboembolic PH
   - Other pulmonary artery obstructions
5. PH with unclear and/or multifactorial mechanisms—variable PAWP and PVR
   - Haematological disorders (e.g. myeloproliferative disorders, chronic haemolytic anaemia, splenoctomy)
   - Systemic and metabolic disorders (e.g. sarcoidosis, pulmonary Langerhans cell histiocytosis, lymphangioleiomyomatosis, neurofibromatosis, vasculitis, glycogen storage disease, Gaucher disease)
   - Others (e.g. tumoural obstruction, fibrosing mediastinitis, chronic renal failure)
   - Complex congenital heart disease

(*Source: Eur Respir J:* Simonneau G, Montani D, Celermajer DS, et al. Haemodynamic definitions and updated clinical classification of pulmonary hypertension, Table 2, page 6, 2019; 53: 1801913)

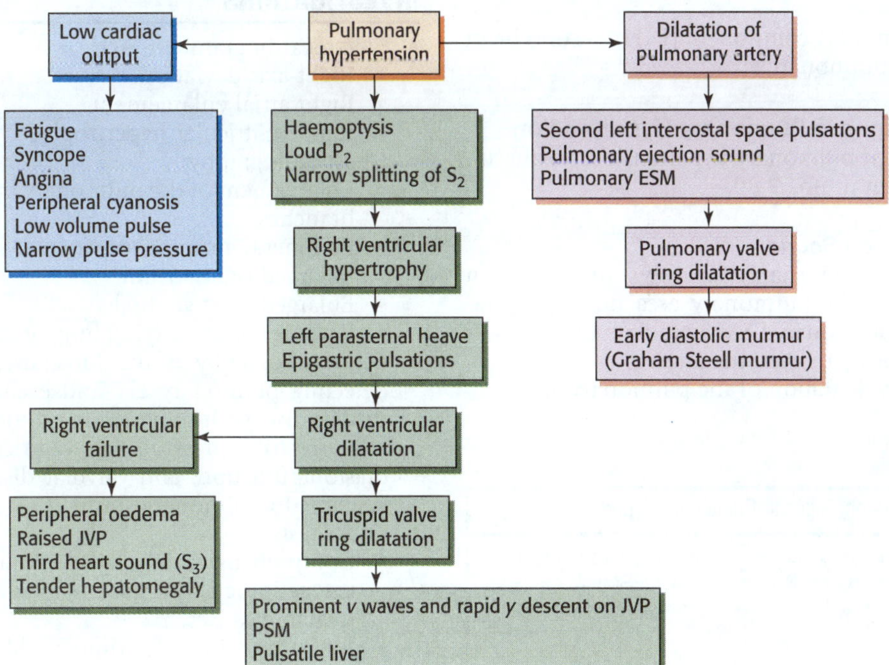

Flowchart 7.21 Pathophysiology of Pulmonary Hypertension.

- Haemoptysis is uncommon and occurs due to rupture of distended pulmonary vessels.
- Peripheral oedema, tender hepatomegaly and raised jugular venous pressure due to right ventricular failure.
- Raynaud's phenomenon occurs in approximately 2% of patients with idiopathic PH but is more common in patients with PH related to connective tissue disease.

SIGNS OF PULMONARY HYPERTENSION

Cyanosis

- Peripheral cyanosis due to reduced cardiac output and skin blood flow.
- Central cyanosis occurs only when a patent foramen ovale permits right-to-left shunt.

Pulse

- Low-volume pulse due to reduced cardiac output and left ventricular stroke volume.

Blood Pressure

- Narrow pulse pressure due to reduced cardiac output and left ventricular stroke volume.

Jugular Veins

- Prominent *a* waves.
- Jugular venous pressure is elevated with right ventricular failure.
- Prominent *v* waves and rapid *y* descent with functional tricuspid regurgitation.

Inspection and Palpation

- Apical impulse may be shifted outwards indicating right ventricular hypertrophy and dilatation.
- Visible and palpable left parasternal heave and epigastric pulsations indicating right ventricular hypertrophy.
- Visible and palpable pulsations in the second left intercostal space from an underlying dilated pulmonary artery.
- Palpable pulmonary component (P_2) of second heart sound in the pulmonary area.

Auscultatory Signs in Pulmonary Hypertension

- Various signs of pulmonary hypertension on auscultation are given in Box 7.80.

Pulmonary Ejection Sound

- It is a high-pitched, sharp, clicking sound heard in systole, best in the pulmonary area during expiration. A loud pulmonary ES may radiate to the lower left sternal border or even the apex.
- It results from dilatation of the pulmonary artery.

BOX 7.80 Auscultatory Signs in Pulmonary Hypertension

- Pulmonary ejection sound (ES)
- Loud second heart sound (S_2)
- Right atrial fourth heart sound (S_4)
- Right ventricular third heart sound (S_3)
- Pulmonary ejection systolic murmur (ESM)
- Pulmonary early diastolic murmur (EDM)
- Tricuspid pansystolic murmur (PSM)

Abnormal Second Heart Sound (S_2)

- Loud pulmonary component (P_2) of the second heart sound.
- Wide splitting of the second heart sound; in presence of severe right ventricular failure, split becomes fixed.

Right Atrial Fourth Heart Sound (S_4)

- It is best heard at the lower left sternal border and becomes louder during inspiration.

Right Ventricular Third Heart Sound (S_3)

- It is a low-frequency sound, best heard at the lower left sternal border and becomes louder during inspiration.
- This is a sign of right ventricular failure.

Pulmonary Ejection Systolic Murmur

- This is an ESM best heard at the pulmonary area.
- It results from the ejection of blood into a dilated pulmonary artery.

Pulmonary Early Diastolic Murmur (Graham Steell Murmur)

- This is a high-pitched, soft, blowing, decrescendo, early diastolic murmur which begins with or immediately after a loud P_2. It is usually confined to the second and third left intercostal spaces and close to the sternum.
- The murmur results from pulmonary regurgitation secondary to pulmonary valve ring dilatation.

Tricuspid Pansystolic Murmur

- This is a high-pitched PSM best heard at the lower left sternal border. The murmur increases in intensity during active inspiration ('inspiratory augmentation' or De-Carvallo's sign).
- The murmur results from functional tricuspid regurgitation secondary to the dilatation of tricuspid valve ring in right ventricular dilatation.

INVESTIGATIONS

- Electrocardiogram:
  - Right-axis deviation.
  - Right atrial enlargement.
  - Right ventricular hypertrophy.
- Chest radiography:
  - Enlargement of the pulmonary trunk and its main branches.
  - Peripheral 'pruning' of vascular shadows.
  - Enlarged right atrium.
  - Enlarged right ventricle.
  - Findings of underlying lung or cardiac pathology.
- Echocardiography is the most useful modality for detecting pulmonary HT and excluding underlying cardiac disease. It provides an estimate of pulmonary artery systolic pressure, left ventricular systolic and diastolic function, and valvular disease, and detects systemic-to-pulmonary shunt.
- Other tests:
  - Comprehensive laboratory evaluation to clarify the aetiology. The goal is to identify or exclude treatable causes.
  - Initial tests include complete blood counts, prothrombin time, partial thromboplastin time and liver profile.

- Autoantibodies if a collagen vascular disease is suspected.
- HIV ELISA if the patient has risk factors.
- Arterial blood gas to exclude hypoxia and acidosis as contributors to PH.
- Sleep studies if sleep apnoea suspected.
- Pulmonary function tests to establish airflow obstruction or restrictive lung disease.
- High-resolution computed tomography of chest to exclude occult interstitial lung disease.
- Helical CT to detect pulmonary thromboembolism.
- Ventilation–perfusion scanning to differentiate chronic thromboembolism from primary PH.
- Right heart catheterisation in patients with unexplained PH. It is also required to diagnose PH, assess the severity of haemodynamic deterioration and analyse vasoreactivity of pulmonary circulation so as to identify patients who may benefit from treatment with calcium channel blockers.

TREATMENT

- Treatment is directed at early recognition and treatment of the underlying cause.
- Pulmonary endarterectomy is the current mainstay of therapy for chronic thromboembolic PH.
- Since hypoxia is a potent pulmonary vasoconstrictor, it is critical to identify and reverse hypoxaemia. Low-flow supplemental oxygen therapy prolongs life in such patients.
- Vaccination against influenza and pneumococcal pneumonia is recommended.
- Women in reproductive age group are strongly counselled to use contraceptive measures.
- Excessive diuretics should be avoided as this may reduce the cardiac output further.
- Digoxin improves right ventricular contractility and cardiac output. However, no data support its long-term use in PH.
- Oral anticoagulants may benefit some patients particularly those with idiopathic PH and heritable PH.
- Calcium channel blockers (nifedipine, diltiazem, amlodipine) in those who demonstrate a favourable response to acute vasodilator testing (vasoreactive).
- Targeted pharmacotherapy: Currently approved drugs for treatment in patients with or without vasoreactivity include:
  - Prostanoids (epoprostenol, iloprost, treprostinil and selexipag) stimulate cAMP.
  - Endothelin receptor antagonists (bosentan, ambrisentan, macitentan) block endothelin signalling.
  - Phosphodiesterase-5 inhibitors (sildenafil and tadalafil) stimulate nitric oxide–cyclic GMP system. Cyclic GMP causes smooth muscle cell relaxation, decreases proliferation of pulmonary artery smooth muscle cells (PASMCs) and increases apoptosis of PASMCs.
  - Riociguat directly activates soluble guanylate cyclase to generate cyclic GMP.
- Combination therapy can be used if tolerated by the patient.
- These drug therapies are of little benefit in PH due to primary lung pathology like COPD and ILD.
- Lung transplantation.
- Creation of an interatrial right-to-left shunt can decompress the right heart chambers and increase LV preload and cardiac output.
- For treatment of idiopathic or primary pulmonary hypertension, please see the next section.

Q. What is primary pulmonary arterial hypertension? Discuss the clinical manifestations and management of primary pulmonary hypertension (PPH).

Q. Discuss about idiopathic pulmonary arterial hypertension.

- Primary pulmonary hypertension is the term used to describe pulmonary arterial hypertension (PAH) that occurs without a demonstrable cause, and may occur sporadically (idiopathic PAH) or as an inherited condition (heritable PAH).
- It is an intrinsic, idiopathic, obstructive disease of the small pulmonary arteries and arterioles.
- The aetiology is unknown. However, pregnancy, oral contraceptives and familial occurrence are noteworthy.
- Primary pulmonary hypertension is more common in females (female to male ratio is 5:1). The mean patient age is 20–30 years. Death commonly occurs within 5 years of the onset of symptoms.
- Clinically dyspnoea, weakness, fatigue, exercise-induced syncope and chest pain in an otherwise healthy, young, acyanotic female with no history of heart disease or cardiac murmurs suggest primary pulmonary hypertension. Sudden death may occur.
- Physical signs are the same as those for pulmonary hypertension.
- As many as 40% of patients with idiopathic PAH have serological abnormalities, usually an antinuclear antibody in a low titre and nonspecific pattern.
- Other investigations have been described above under pulmonary hypertension.

MANAGEMENT

- Restrict physical activities. Encourage cautious, graduated physical activity. Heavy physical activity can precipitate exertional syncope.
- Hot baths are discouraged because the resultant peripheral vasodilatation can produce systemic hypotension and syncope.
- Avoid excessive sodium intake.
- Careful use of diuretics in patients with right ventricular failure and functional tricuspid regurgitation.
- Supplemental oxygen if oxygen saturation falls below 90%.
- Calcium channel blockers (nifedipine) may alleviate pulmonary vasoconstriction and prolong life in about 20% of cases. They should be given only to those who show response on cardiac catheterisation. Verapamil should be avoided because of its negative inotropic effect.
- Epoprostenol (a prostacyclin) is a potent short-acting vasodilator. Continuous intravenous infusion

of this agent has been shown to prolong life. Iloprost, another prostacyclin, has also been used intravenously or via nasal route.

- Endothelin-I receptor antagonists (e.g. bosentan) and selective phosphodiesterase-5 inhibitors (e.g. sildenafil) are useful in some patients.
- Chronic anticoagulation with warfarin is recommended to prevent thrombosis in patients with primary pulmonary hypertension. Maintaining an International Normalised Ratio (INR) of 1.5–2.5 is recommended.
- Atrial septostomy—creation of a right-to-left interatrial shunt to decompress the failing pressure- and volume-overloaded right heart—may be used as a palliative procedure or as a stabilising bridge to lung transplantation.
- Ultimate answer is lung transplantation (with or without heart transplantation).

Q. Discuss the risk factors, clinical features, investigations and treatment of venous thrombosis (deep venous thrombosis—DVT).

Q. Discuss the prophylaxis of venous thrombosis (deep venous thrombosis—DVT).

Q. Explain about Wells probability score.

- Venous thrombosis implies thrombus formation in the systemic or right side of the heart.
- Deep venous thrombosis (DVT) means thrombus formation in the deep venous system, especially of the lower extremities and pelvis.

SIGNIFICANCE

- Venous thrombi can embolise to lung resulting in pulmonary embolism (pulmonary thromboembolism—PTE) and cause pulmonary infarction.
- It is during the first few days (7–10 days) after the formation of the thrombus that embolic risk is the highest.

SITES OF VENOUS THROMBOSIS

- Common sites of venous thrombosis are given in Box 7.81.

BOX 7.81 Common Sites of Venous Thrombosis

- Deep venous system of lower extremities (95% of pulmonary emboli arise from here)
- Other systemic veins, especially pelvic veins
- Left atrium, especially in patients with atrial fibrillation and cardiac failure
- Right ventricle
- Right atrium, especially in patients with right-sided pacemaker leads, ventricular or atrial septal closure devices and indwelling central venous lines

TABLE 7.75 Risk Factors for Venous Thrombosis

Biochemical	
• Disorders with hypercoagulable states (e.g. antithrombin deficiency, protein C deficiency, protein S deficiency, antiphospholipid syndrome)	
Clinical	
• Low cardiac output	• Long surgical procedures under GA
• Obesity, advancing age	• Fractures or injuries of lower limbs
• Prolonged bed rest	• Left and right ventricular failure
• Dehydration	• Carcinoma
• Polycythaemia	• Use of oestrogens
• Post-partum period	

PATHOGENESIS

- The three factors which promote DVT are defined by Virchow:
  - Stasis of blood.
  - Abnormalities of vessel wall.
  - Hypercoagulable state.

RISK FACTORS OF VENOUS THROMBOSIS

- A number of factors predispose to venous thrombosis (Table 7.75).

CLINICAL FEATURES OF DEEP VENOUS THROMBOSIS

- Clinical detection is difficult as DVT is silent in 50% of cases.
- Low-grade fever.
- Pain, tenderness, warmth and swelling of calf muscles.
- 'Homan's sign' is pain in the calf on forceful dorsiflexion of foot.
- Later, there is cyanosis, oedema and venous gangrene of the affected limb.

WELLS CLINICAL PREDICTION GUIDE FOR DIAGNOSIS OF DVT

- Quantifies probability of DVT.
- Stratifies patients into high-, moderate- or low-risk categories for having DVT (Table 7.76).

COMPLICATIONS

- Venous gangrene.
- Pulmonary embolism.
- Postthrombotic syndrome (oedema, nocturnal cramping, venous claudication, skin pigmentation, dermatitis, ulceration and lifelong limb pain).

INVESTIGATIONS

- D-dimer is elevated (>500 ng/mL) in most patients but is not specific. Also elevated in trauma, recent surgery, haemorrhage, cancer, elderly, pregnancy and

TABLE 7.76 Wells Probability Score for Deep Venous Thrombosis

Clinical Parameter	Score
• Active cancer (treatment ongoing or within 6 months or palliative)	+1
• Paralysis or recent plaster immobilisation of the lower extremities	+1
• Recently bedridden for >3 days or major surgery <4 weeks	+1
• Localised tenderness along the distribution of the deep venous system	+1
• Entire leg swollen	+1
• Calf swelling >3 cm compared to the asymptomatic leg	+1
• Pitting oedema (greater in the symptomatic leg)	+1
• Previous DVT documented	+1
• Collateral superficial veins (nonvaricose)	+1
• Alternative diagnosis (at least as likely as DVT)	−2

Low probability, score ≤0; moderate probability, score 1 or 2; high probability, score ≥3.

sepsis. In DVT, it remains elevated for 7 days. D-dimer results should be used as follows:

- A negative D-dimer assay rules out DVT in patients with Wells score ≤1.
- All patients with a positive D-dimer assay and all patients with a moderate to high risk of DVT (Wells score ≥2) require a diagnostic study (Doppler ultrasonography).

- Doppler (duplex) ultrasonography is useful but highly operator dependent. The major criterion for detecting venous thrombosis is failure to compress the vascular lumen. At times, thrombus may be seen inside the vein. Absence of normal phasic Doppler signals arising from the changes in venous flow provides indirect evidence of venous occlusion.
- Ascending contrast venography (phlebography) is the best method but is rarely performed presently due to availability of Doppler ultrasound.
- Impedance plethysmography (IPG) accurately detects above-knee thrombi. However, it cannot distinguish between thrombotic occlusion and extravascular compression of the vein.
- Radiofibrinogen method is very accurate in calf vein and lower thigh thrombi. However, results can be obtained only after several hours of injecting radiofibrinogen.

ALGORITHM FOR DIAGNOSING DVT

- Flowchart 7.22 gives algorithm to diagnose deep venous thrombosis.

TREATMENT OF DEEP VENOUS THROMBOSIS

- Bed rest with legs elevated to 15 degrees.
- Physiotherapy to legs.
- Graduated elastic stockings (compression stockings) should be used routinely to prevent postthrombotic syndrome, beginning within 1 month of diagnosis of proximal DVT and continuing for a minimum of 1 year after diagnosis.
- Start treatment with heparin (as in pulmonary embolism) as well as warfarin and continue with warfarin. No loading dose of warfarin is recommended at present. Anticoagulation with warfarin should be maintained for 3–6 months for DVT secondary to transient risk factors, and for more than 12 months for recurrent DVT (with INR between 2.0 and 3.0). In

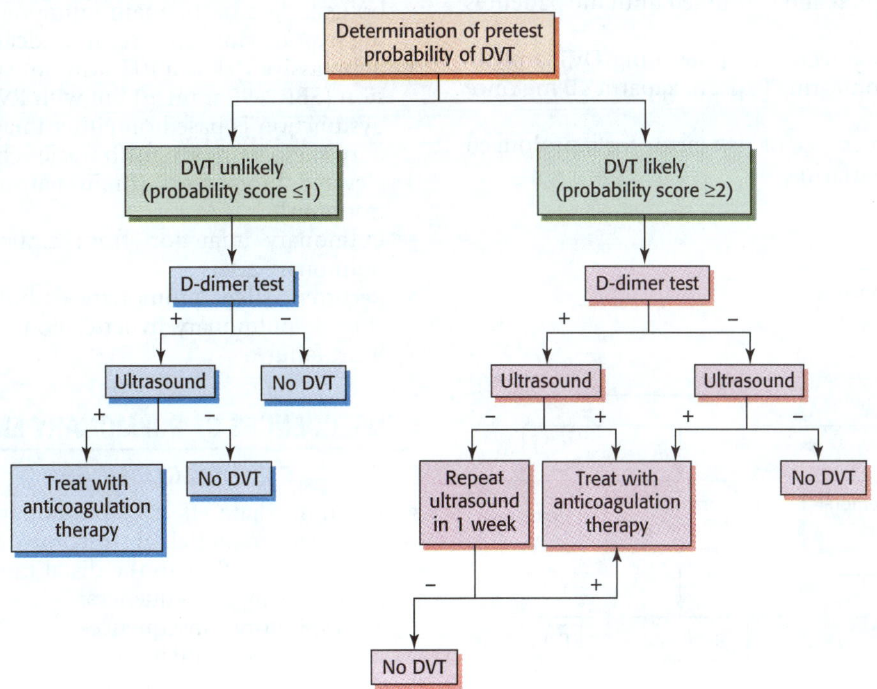

Flowchart 7.22 Algorithm for Diagnosing Deep Venous Thrombosis.

place of warfarin, direct-acting oral anticoagulants may be used. For idiopathic DVT, anticoagulation should be continued for at least 6 months, though extended-duration therapy may be more beneficial.

- LMWHs may be used in place of conventional heparin in the initial period. Consistent evidence demonstrates that LMWH is superior to unfractionated heparin for the initial treatment of DVT. Outpatient treatment of DVT with LMWH is safe and cost-effective for selected patients.
- Thrombolysis with streptokinase has little role in DVT as its efficacy in preventing embolism may not be better than heparin. One area where thrombolytic therapy is increasingly useful is when using catheter-guided lytic therapy to re-canalise the vein in massive DVT involving common femoral or iliac system.
- Thrombectomy (rarely).
- Inferior vena cava filters in patients with acute proximal DVT of the leg and contraindication to anticoagulation.
- Early ambulation is recommended over initial bed rest unless patient has severe pain or oedema.
- Treatment is summarised in Flowchart 7.23.

PROPHYLAXIS

- Prophylaxis is indicated in patients at high risk for DVT and pulmonary embolism (Box 7.82).
- Measures useful in the prophylaxis of DVT include the following:
  - Graduated elastic stockings.
  - Physiotherapy with active leg exercises.
  - Devices that compress the calf intermittently (usually once a minute)—intermittent pneumatic compression.
  - Low-dose subcutaneous heparin—5000 units 12 hourly, beginning before operation or on admission to hospital and continued until the patient is ambulatory.
  - LMWHs are effective in preventing DVT and require no monitoring (e.g. enoxaparin 40 mg once a day).
  - In case of presence of risk factor for a prolonged time, add warfarin.

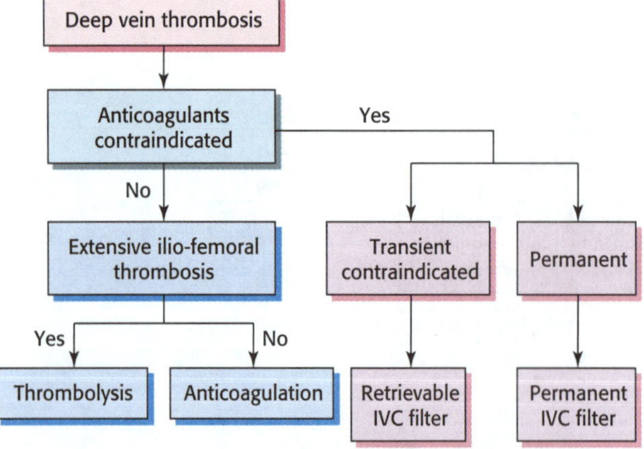

Flowchart 7.23 Summary of Treatment of Deep Vein Thrombosis.

BOX 7.82 Indications for Prophylaxis for Deep Venous Thrombosis

- Fractures of pelvis or extremities
- Those undergoing major abdominal, thoracic or gynaecological surgery
- Major medical diseases in admitted patients
  - Acute coronary syndrome
  - Acute heart failure (NYHA classes III, IV)
  - Active cancer requiring therapy
  - Sepsis
  - Acute respiratory diseases (respiratory failure with or without mechanical ventilation)
  - Chronic respiratory disease (e.g. chronic obstructive pulmonary disease)
  - Inflammatory bowel disease
  - Acute arthritis of lower extremities
  - Stroke
  - Paraplegia
  - Obesity

Q. Discuss the aetiology, clinical features, investigations and management of pulmonary embolism and pulmonary infarction.

- Occlusion of the pulmonary artery or its branches by emboli constitutes pulmonary embolism (pulmonary thromboembolism—PTE).
- Pulmonary infarction is ischaemic necrosis of lung tissue following embolic occlusion. It occurs in only less than 10% of cases of pulmonary embolism.

TYPES

- Acute massive pulmonary embolism where the embolus lodges in the main pulmonary artery producing hypotension (may result in death).
- Submassive PTE is a PTE without systemic hypotension (SBP >90 mmHg) but with RV dysfunction. RV dysfunction is based on either imaging (CT pulmonary angiogram or transthoracic echocardiogram) or elevated biomarkers (brain natriuretic peptide or troponin).
- Pulmonary infarction from embolism to smaller pulmonary artery.
- Recurrent silent pulmonary embolism resulting in chronic pulmonary hypertension and chronic right heart failure.

CONSEQUENCES OF PULMONARY EMBOLISM

IMMEDIATE CONSEQUENCES

- The immediate effect of pulmonary embolism is a complete or partial obstruction of the pulmonary arterial blood flow to the distal lung. This results in the following consequences:
  a. Respiratory consequences
     - 'Wasted ventilation' resulting from embolic occlusion producing a zone of lung that is ventilated but not perfused.

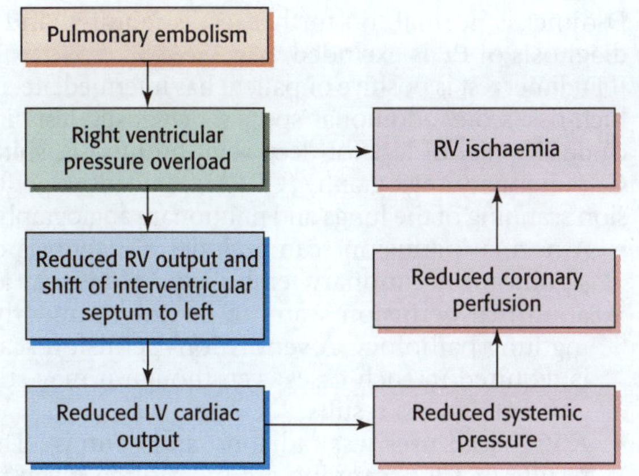

Flowchart 7.24 Haemodynamic Changes in Pulmonary Embolism.

- Loss of alveolar surfactant resulting in alveolar collapse and frank atelectasis.
- Arterial hypoxaemia.

b. Haemodynamic consequences (Flowchart 7.24)
- Acute pulmonary hypertension.
- Acute right ventricular failure and right ventricular ischaemia.
- Pulmonary infarction.
- Shock in massive embolism.
- Reduced preload to left ventricle
- Reduced LV cardiac output
- Reduced coronary perfusion

Note: The severity of haemodynamic consequences depends on the extent of embolic obstruction. At least 50% of vascular area must be obstructed for significant elevation of pulmonary arterial pressure.

LATE CONSEQUENCES

- Vast majority of pulmonary emboli resolve while few do not.
- Recurrent 'silent' small pulmonary emboli present only with late consequences like pulmonary hypertension and chronic right heart failure.

CAUSES AND RISK FACTORS

- Pulmonary embolism usually results from dislodgement of venous thrombi of the deep veins of lower limbs and pelvis. Rarely, emboli can arise from right atrium or right ventricle.
- Causes of pulmonary embolism are the same as those for venous thrombosis (refer page 610).
- Risk factors (predisposing factors) of pulmonary embolism are the same as those for venous thrombosis (refer Table 7.75).
- Additional risk factors include atrial fibrillation, COPD and sickle cell anaemia.
- 'Economy class syndrome' (or traveller's thrombosis) is a rare condition. The incidence through various studies appears to be in the range of 0.25/100,000 passengers in economic-class flights longer than 8 hours. An increased risk of thrombosis has not yet been confirmed in flights of less than 4 hours.

CLINICAL FEATURES OF PULMONARY EMBOLISM AND PULMONARY INFARCTION

- Sudden onset of unexplained breathlessness.
- Retrosternal discomfort from right ventricular ischaemia.
- Syncope.
- Haemoptysis.
- Pleuritic chest pain and haemoptysis in pulmonary infarction.
- Supraventricular tachyarrhythmias.
- Sudden onset or worsening of heart failure.
- Sudden deterioration in a patient with chronic obstructive lung disease.
- Sudden cardiac arrest.
- Paradoxical embolism (through patent foramen ovale or intrapulmonary shunts) resulting in stroke, myocardial infarction, etc.

PHYSICAL FINDINGS

- There may be no abnormal physical findings.
- A low-grade fever may occur with infarction.
- Central cyanosis in massive pulmonary infarction.
- Pleural friction rub and a small pleural effusion may be seen with pulmonary infarction.
- Tachycardia is the most consistent and most important physical sign.
- The possibility of pulmonary embolism should be considered if a patient has pleuritic chest pain, syncope, haemoptysis or dyspnoea out of proportion to the size of pleural effusion.
- In a massive pulmonary embolism, the following signs may be present:
  - Raised JVP with prominent *a* waves.
  - Left parasternal (right ventricular) lift.
  - Loud pulmonary component (P_2) of second heart sound.
  - Wide splitting of second heart sound indicating severe pulmonary hypertension and right ventricular failure.
  - Right ventricular third heart sound (RVS_3 or RV gallop).
  - Ejection systolic murmur at pulmonary area.
  - Clinical evidence of DVT may be present (refer page 610).

WELLS SCORING SYSTEM

- To determine probability of pulmonary embolism, Wells scoring system is used (Table 7.77).

PULMONARY EMBOLISM RULE-OUT CRITERIA

- Another criteria which is used in low-risk patients (when clinical risk of pulmonary embolism is less than 15%) is Pulmonary Embolism Rule-Out Criteria (PERC) (Box 7.83).

DIAGNOSIS

- Polymorphonuclear leucocytosis and raised erythrocyte sedimentation rate (ESR) with pulmonary infarction.
- Electrocardiogram may show tachycardia, changes of acute pulmonary hypertension and right ventricular enlargement with strain (R>S in lead V_1 with

TABLE 7.77 Wells Score for Pulmonary Embolism

Parameter	Score
• Symptoms of DVT	3
• PE most likely diagnosis	3
• Heart rate >100/minute	1.5
• Immobilised in past 4 weeks	1.5
• Previous PE or DVT	1.5
• Haemoptysis	1
• Malignancy	1

Clinical probability of PE: high if score >6; intermediate if score 2–6; low if score <2.

BOX 7.83 Pulmonary Embolism Rule-Out Criteria

- Age ≥50 years
- Heart rate ≥100/minute
- Oxygen saturation <95%
- Haemoptysis
- Oestrogen use
- Prior DVT or PE
- Unilateral leg swelling
- Surgery/trauma within the previous 4 weeks

Pulmonary embolism can be ruled out in low-risk patients if none of the above-mentioned criteria are present.

inverted T wave). Other abnormalities include atrial fibrillation or flutter; an S wave in lead I, a Q in lead III and an inverted T in lead III (S_1, Q_3 and T_3 pattern) (Fig. 7.59).

- Arterial blood gas studies may reveal hypoxaemia, hypocapnia and respiratory alkalosis.
- In large pulmonary embolism, echocardiogram may show large right ventricle and right atrium with flattening of interventricular septum indicating acute pulmonary hypertension ('D' sign).
- Based on Wells score, patients with low probability should undergo D-dimer estimation. If age-adjusted D-dimer is normal, no further test is required and a diagnosis of PE is excluded.
- If D-dimer test is positive or patient has intermediate- or high-risk score, additional specific diagnostic tests include Doppler of legs for deep vein thrombosis, spiral CT pulmonary angiography (CT-PA), ventilation–perfusion scanning of the lungs and pulmonary angiography.
  - A normal perfusion scan excludes a diagnosis of significant pulmonary embolism. However, an abnormal perfusion scan can be due to underlying lung pathology. A ventilation–perfusion scan is required in such cases even though it may still give ambiguous results.
  - A V/Q scan uses less radiation and contrast. The results of V/Q scanning are most often given as high, intermediate or low probability.

RADIOLOGICAL FEATURES

- Radiological features of pulmonary embolism are given in Box 7.84.

ALGORITHM FOR DIAGNOSIS OF PULMONARY EMBOLISM

- Diagnosis of pulmonary embolism is summarised in Flowchart 7.25.

MANAGEMENT

SUPPORTIVE MEASURES

- Bed rest in acute stage.
- Oxygen and analgesics.
- Intravenous saline and/or noradrenaline may be necessary to maintain venous pressure in massive embolism.

ANTICOAGULATION

- Unfractionated heparin is given at an initial dose of 80 units/kg intravenously followed by maintenance.
- For maintenance, any one of the following three regimens may be used:
  - Continuous intravenous.
  - Intermittent intravenous.
  - Intermittent subcutaneous.

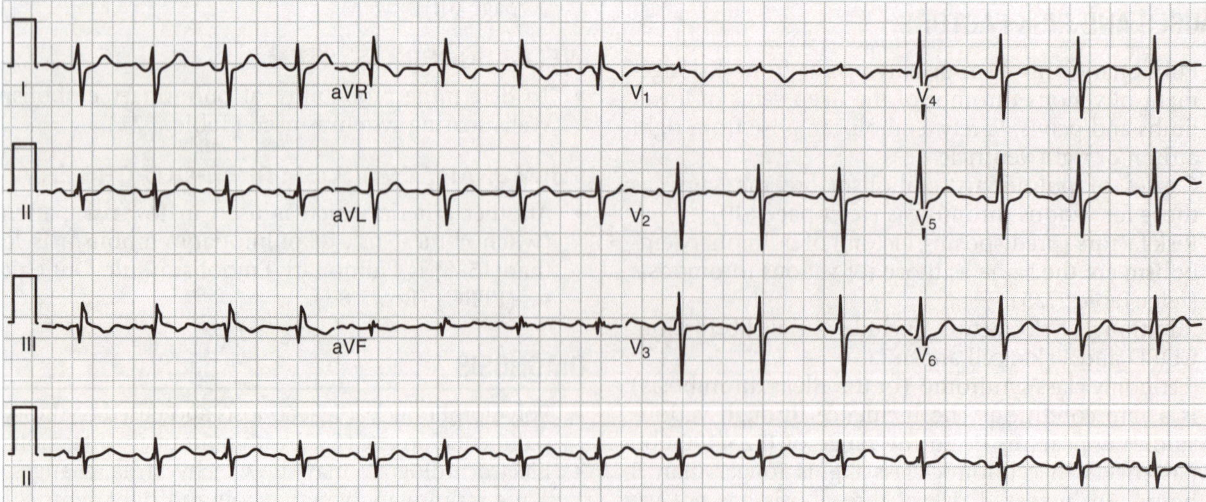

Fig. 7.59 $S_1Q_3T_3$ pattern in a patient with pulmonary embolism.

BOX 7.84 Radiological Features of Pulmonary Embolism

PULMONARY EMBOLISM

- Normal
- Increased radiolucency in lung zones due to diminished or absent blood flow (Westermark sign) (Fig. 7.60)
- Small infiltrative shadows due to atelectasis
- Elevation of the haemidiaphragm
- Difference in the diameter of pulmonary arteries and their main branches on either side; prominent descending pulmonary artery on one side is known as Palla sign (Fig. 7.60)
- Abrupt 'cut-off' of a vessel

PULMONARY INFARCTION

- May be normal, especially in early stages
- Parenchymal, wedge-shaped, infiltrative shadow abutting against the pleura (usually appears 12–36 hours later) (Hampton hump) (Fig. 7.61)
- Small pleural effusion

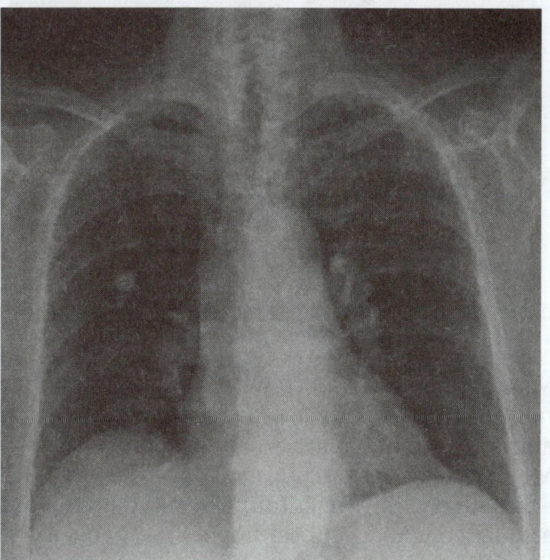

Fig. 7.60 Chest radiograph showing Westermark sign (reduced vascularity on right side) and Palla sign (dilated right inferior pulmonary artery).

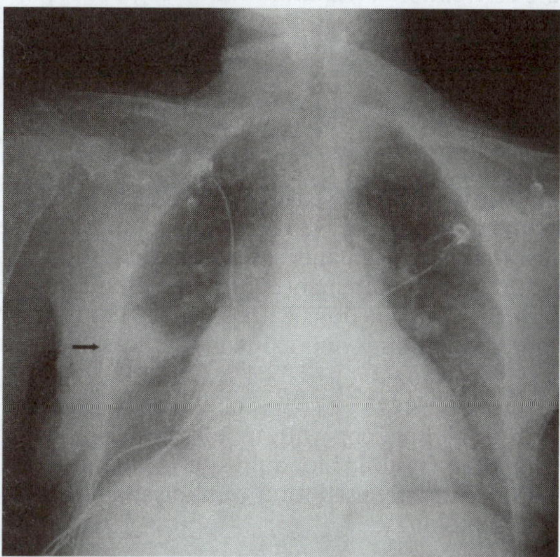

Fig. 7.61 Chest radiograph showing a wedge-shaped lesions abutting pleura (Hampton hump).

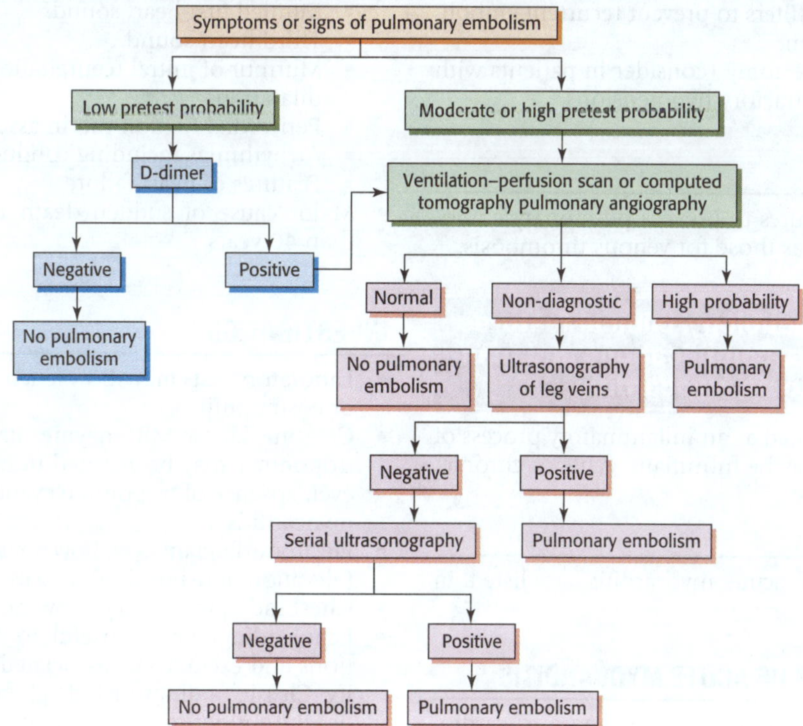

Flowchart 7.25 Algorithm for Diagnosis of Pulmonary Embolism.

- 'Continuous intravenous maintenance' is the most popular. Here, heparin is administered using an infusion pump at a rate of 18 units/kg/hour.
- Heparin therapy is monitored with activated partial thromboplastin time (aPTT) which is maintained at 1.5–2 times the control value.
- Intravenous heparin therapy should be continued for 5–7 days.
- Heparin prevents additional thrombus formation and permits the endogenous fibrinolytic system to lyse the clot in the pulmonary arteries.
- LMWHs (enoxaparin, dalteparin, tinzaparin) have been shown to be more efficacious as compared to the conventional heparin. Monitoring of the patient by performing repeated aPTT is also not required. Enoxaparin may be used in a dose of 1 mg/kg twice a day subcutaneously.
- An alternative to LMWH is fondaparinux.
- Along with heparin, oral warfarin should be started with the intention of keeping the INR at 2.5–3.0. This may take 4–5 days after which heparin is stopped. Instead of warfarin, nonvitamin K antagonist oral anticoagulants can be given in fixed doses without the requirement for routine monitoring and have fewer interactions with other medications.
- Anticoagulation is maintained for at least 6 months.

THROMBOLYTIC THERAPY

- It is used in patients with major embolism with hypotension (systolic blood pressure <90 mmHg).
- Agents currently used for thrombolysis are:
  - Streptokinase.
  - Tenecteplase.
  - Tissue plasminogen activator (tPA).

SURGICAL THERAPY

- Inferior vena cava filters to prevent recurrent emboli.
- Venous interruption.
- Pulmonary embolectomy (consider in patients with cardiac arrest or refractory hypotension).

PROPHYLAXIS

- Prophylactic measures to prevent pulmonary embolism are the same as those for venous thrombosis.

Q. Discuss the aetiology, clinical features, investigations, complications and management of acute myocarditis.

- Myocarditis is defined as an inflammatory process of myocardium. It may be fulminant, acute or chronic.

AETIOLOGY

- Various causes of acute myocarditis are listed in Table 7.78.

TABLE 7.78 Aetiology of Acute Myocarditis

• Infections	Viral (Coxsackie A and B, adenoviruses, influenza, HIV, dengue virus, parvovirus B19, SARS-CoV-2, zika, hepatitis C, Epstein–Barr virus), bacterial (diphtheria, *S. aureus*, *Mycoplasma pneumoniae*), protozoal (malaria, trypanosomiasis, toxoplasmosis), spirochaetal (Lyme disease), fungal
• Collagen vascular diseases	Scleroderma, systemic lupus erythematosus, polyarteritis nodosa
• Hypersensitivity reactions	Drugs: Azithromycin, benzodiazepines, clozapine, cephalosporins, dapsone, gefitinib, lithium, loop diuretics, methyldopa, NSAIDs, penicillins, phenobarbital, smallpox vaccination, streptomycin, sulphonamides, tetanus toxoid, tetracycline, thiazide diuretics, tricyclic antidepressants Others: Bee venom, wasp venom, scorpion venom, snake venom
• Miscellaneous	Acute rheumatic fever, drugs (anthracyclines), toxins (cocaine, alcohol, arsenic), chemical agents, radiation, sarcoidosis, Kawasaki disease, thyrotoxicosis, coeliac disease, immune checkpoint inhibitors (CTLA-4-blockers, PD-1 blockers and PD-L1 blockers)

CLINICAL FEATURES OF ACUTE MYOCARDITIS

- Range from asymptomatic ECG changes to cardiogenic shock.
- May have a viral prodrome of fever, myalgias, respiratory symptoms or gastroenteritis followed by an abrupt onset of haemodynamic collapse.
- May present with acute chest pain. Chest pain in acute myocarditis may mimic typical angina and be associated with electrocardiographic changes, including ST-segment elevation.
- Physical examination may be normal.
- Other findings include:
  - Inappropriate tachycardia.
  - Muffled first heart sound.
  - Third heart sound.
  - Murmur of mitral regurgitation due to ventricular dilatation.
  - Pericardial friction rub in associated pericarditis.
  - Arrhythmias including conduction blocks.
  - Features of heart failure.
- Major cause of sudden death in patients younger than 40 years.

INVESTIGATIONS

- Laboratory tests may show leucocytosis, elevated ESR or eosinophilia.
- Creatine kinase-MB enzyme, BNP/NT-ProBNP and troponin T may be elevated in many patients. However, absence of troponin elevation does not exclude myocarditis.
- Electrocardiogram may show nonspecific ST–T changes (elevation or depression), blocks or arrhythmias.
- Chest radiography may show cardiomegaly.
- Echocardiography is useful to assess cardiac functions and exclude any associated valvular abnormality. Classic findings include global hypokinesia with or without pericardial effusion.
- Routine viral serology testing is not recommended.

- Contrast-enhanced MRI and indium-111-labelled antimyosin scintigraphy are noninvasive tests to identify myocardial inflammation. MRI can also differentiate myocarditis from myocardial infarction.
- Endomyocardial biopsy can confirm the diagnosis. PCR helps to diagnose specific viral pathogens in the myocardium. However, its utility is limited because of sampling error from patchy inflammatory infiltrates and variability in observer interpretation. Indications of biopsy include:
  - Patients with new-onset heart failure (<2 weeks) associated with a normal or dilated left ventricle with haemodynamic compromise.
  - Patients with new-onset heart failure of 2 weeks' to 3 months' duration with a dilated left ventricle, ventricular arrhythmia or high-degree atrioventricular blockade.
  - Patients whose condition fails to respond to treatment in 1–2 weeks.

COMPLICATIONS

- Arrhythmias and heart block.
- Heart failure.
- Acute pericarditis.
- Progression to chronic myocarditis.
- Progression to chronic dilated cardiomyopathy.

NATURAL HISTORY

- Variable course.
- Patients with fulminant myocarditis (rapid onset of symptoms and severe haemodynamic compromise at presentation) have a good long-term survival rate if they survive the initial phase.
- Patients with acute myocarditis in whom development of symptoms is more protracted and the clinical picture less dramatic often have a worse long-term outcome.
- Patients who present with mildly compromised ventricular function (left ventricular ejection fraction of 40%–50%) typically improve within weeks to months.
- Among those presenting with more advanced left ventricular dysfunction (LVEF ≤35%), 50% will develop chronic ventricular dysfunction.

MANAGEMENT

- Prolonged bed rest in severe cases and restriction of physical activities in less severe cases (till ECG is normal).
- Treatment of heart failure (using ACE inhibitors, β-blockers and diuretics).
- Antiarrhythmic therapy should not be given for asymptomatic atrial and ventricular premature beats or for asymptomatic nonsustained arrhythmias. For other tachyarrthythmias, amiodarone and β-blockers can be given. Temporary pacemaker is required for heart blocks.
- Mineralocorticoid receptor antagonists (eplerenone or spironolactone) in patients not responding to above treatment.
- In severe heart failure, intravenous nitroglycerine or sodium nitroprusside may be required to reduce high filling pressures. If forward flow is a problem, inotropic agents (milrinone and dobutamine) may be used.
- Digoxin should be used with caution and at low doses only.
- Anticoagulation in the setting of concomitant atrial fibrillation or arterial or venous thromboembolism.
- NSAIDs are not effective and may actually increase mortality.
- Immunosuppressives (including steroids and azathioprine) should not be used in the routine treatment of patients with myocarditis. However, these agents are very useful in the treatment of patients with cardiac involvement due to a systemic autoimmune disease, sarcoidosis or hypersensitivity reaction. They are also useful in giant-cell myocarditis and chronic inflammatory dilated cardiomyopathy where symptoms last for more than 6 months. Interferons have been used in many patients with variable results. Other immunosuppressants include mycophenolate mofetil, cyclosporine and rituximab. Immunoadsorption using IVIg has also been successful in some cases.
- Ventricular assist devices and intraaortic balloon pump in refractory patients that may provide a bridge to transplant or to recovery.
- Extracorporeal membrane oxygenation (ECMO) as a short-term bridge to transplant or recovery, but usually in patients with sustained ventricular arrhythmias.

VIRAL MYOCARDITIS

- A brief about viral myocarditis is mentioned in Box 7.85.

BOX 7.85 Viral Myocarditis

- Commonest myocarditis, Coxsackie B virus being the most common virus
- Preceding upper respiratory illness
- Virus may be isolated from stools, pharyngeal washings or other body fluids
- Rising titres of specific antibodies in the blood
- Treatment—as above
- Usually a self-limited disease, but may progress to a chronic form

Q. Define cardiomyopathy. How do you classify cardiomyopathies? (PA 27.9)

DEFINITION

- Cardiomyopathies are diseases that involve the myocardium primarily and are NOT as a result of hypertension, congenital heart diseases, valvular heart diseases, coronary heart disease, pericardial diseases or pulmonary diseases.
- The term 'ischaemic cardiomyopathy' is frequently used, but it is not a cardiomyopathy as the primary involvement is that of coronary arteries and not the myocardium.

TABLE 7.79 Features of Cardiomyopathies

Type	Structural Abnormality	Functional Abnormality	Dysfunction
• **Dilated/Congestive**	Enlargement of ventricle	Poor ventricular contraction	Systolic dysfunction
• **Restrictive/Obliterative**	Small ventricle with 'stiff wall'	Impairment of ventricular filling	Diastolic dysfunction
• **Hypertrophic**	Hypertrophy of left ventricle which may be generalised, but usually involving the upper portion of interventricular septum predominantly	Impairment of ventricular filling; impairment of left ventricular ejection due to outflow tract obstruction (in 25%)	Predominantly diastolic dysfunction

CLASSIFICATION

- Cardiomyopathies are classified into three major groups based on the abnormalities of structure and function. These are dilated, restrictive and hypertrophic cardiomyopathies. Other cardiomyopathies are arrhythmogenic right ventricular cardiomyopathy and unclassified cardiomyopathies (e.g. takotsubo cardiomyopathy, tachycardia-induced cardiomyopathy and others).
- The salient features of the three major groups are summarised in Table 7.79.

Q. What are the causes, clinical features, salient investigations and treatment of dilated cardiomyopathy (congestive cardiomyopathy)?

FEATURES

- In dilated cardiomyopathy, there is enlargement of the ventricle and impairment of ventricular contraction, often affecting both ventricles.

COMMON CAUSES OF DILATED CARDIOMYOPATHY

- Causes of dilated cardiomyopathy are listed in Table 7.80.

TABLE 7.80 Common Causes of Dilated Cardiomyopathy

Inflammatory • Postinfective • Autoimmune diseases (SLE, systemic sclerosis, dermatomyositis) **Nutritional** • Thiamine deficiency • Selenium deficiency **Endocrine** • Diabetes mellitus • Thyrotoxicosis • Hypothyroidism **Haematological** • Sickle cell anaemia **Peripartum** **Tachycardia-Mediated Cardiomyopathy**	**Toxic** • Alcohol • Cocaine • Adriamycin • Trastuzumab • Cyclophosphamide **Infiltrative** • Haemochromatosis **Neuromuscular** • Muscular dystrophies • Friedreich's ataxia • Myotonic dystrophy **Metabolic** • Glycogen storage disease **Idiopathic (50%)**

Note: Some diseases can produce combined types of cardiomyopathies.

CLINICAL FEATURES

SYMPTOMS

- Symptoms of progressive left-sided and later right-sided heart failure.
- Sudden death is common (due to arrhythmia).
- Symptoms of systemic embolisation of left ventricular mural thrombi or pulmonary embolism due to embolism of right ventricular thrombi.

SIGNS

- Narrow pulse pressure and raised jugular venous pressure.
- Cardiomegaly.
- Signs of heart failure.
- Third and fourth heart sounds.
- Mitral and/or tricuspid regurgitation (functional).
- Arrhythmias are common.

INVESTIGATIONS

- Chest radiography:
  - Left ventricular enlargement or biventricular cardiomegaly.
  - Evidence of pulmonary venous hypertension and interstitial or alveolar oedema.
- Electrocardiogram:
  - Nonspecific ST–T wave changes.
  - Sinus tachycardia, atrial fibrillation or other arrhythmias.
  - Atrial and ventricular enlargement.
- Echocardiography can confirm the diagnosis. It reveals dilatation of left and/or right ventricle with poor global contraction function.
- Circulating levels of BNP are elevated.
- Angiography should be performed in older patients to exclude CAD.

TREATMENT

- Avoid strenuous exertion.
- Treatment of heart failure (diuretics, angiotensin receptor neprilysin inhibitor, ACE inhibitors and β-blockers).
- Additional vasodilators include nitrates, amlodipine and hydralazine.
- Use of mineralocorticoid receptor antagonists (spironolactone and eplerenone).
- Inotropes (digoxin, dopamine and dobutamine) in severe cases not responding to other medicines.
- Anticoagulation to prevent embolism.

- Prevention and treatment of arrhythmias (antiarrhythmic drugs, permanent pacemaker, implantable cardioverter-defibrillator).
- Cardiac resynchronisation therapy in patients who have evidence of dyssynchrony and who have NYHA class III or IV heart failure and continued symptoms despite maximal medical therapy.
- Left ventricular assist devices.
- Cardiac transplantation.

ALCOHOLIC CARDIOMYOPATHY

- Develops in individuals who consume large quantities (>90 g/day) of alcohol over several years.
- Presentation and treatment similar to those for idiopathic DCM.
- Another form of alcoholic cardiotoxicity (not cardiomyopathy) is 'holiday heart syndrome' that appears after a drinking binge. The name is derived from the fact that episodes are initially observed more frequently after weekends or public holidays, though in many patients, there is no such relation. Presentation is with recurrent supraventricular (particularly atrial fibrillation) and occasionally ventricular arrhythmias.
  - Given the generally transient nature of alcohol-induced atrial fibrillation in the structurally normal heart, rate control and supportive care for alcohol intoxication is generally adequate.

PERIPARTUM CARDIOMYOPATHY

- Usually occurs in multiparous females after the age of 30 years. Other risk factors include hypertension, preeclampsia and multiple (twins or triplets) gestations.
- Defined as:
  - Features of dilated cardiomyopathy during the last month of pregnancy or within 6 months of delivery.
  - Absence of a demonstrable cause for the cardiac failure.
  - Absence of demonstrable heart disease before the last month of pregnancy.
  - Documented systolic dysfunction.
- Management is similar to that of patients with dilated cardiomyopathy. Pregnancy must be avoided as the condition may recur.

Q. Discuss the causes, clinical features, investigations and treatment of restrictive cardiomyopathy (obliterative cardiomyopathy).

FEATURES

- Ventricular walls are excessively stiff, resulting in impairment of ventricular filling in diastole (abnormal diastolic function). This leads to high atrial pressures with atrial hypertrophy, dilatation and later atrial fibrillation.

TABLE 7.81 Common Causes of Restrictive Heart Disease

Primary	Infiltrative
• Endomyocardial fibrosis	• Amyloidosis
• Eosinophilic endomyocardial disease	• Sarcoidosis
• Idiopathic	• Neoplasm
	• Haemochromatosis
Metabolic	**Mediastinal Radiation**
• Glycogen storage disease	
• Fabry's disease	

COMMON CAUSES OF RESTRICTIVE HEART DISEASE

- Restrictive heart disease or restrictive cardiomyopathy can be due to several causes (Table 7.81).

CLINICAL FEATURES

- Clinical features are similar to those of constrictive pericarditis (see page 625).
- Exercise intolerance and dyspnoea are the most common symptoms.
- Systemic embolism occurs in nearly 25% of cases.
- Jugular venous pressure may be elevated with diastolic collapse (rapid *y* descent) and positive Kussmaul's sign.
- Peripheral oedema, ascites and enlarged, tender liver.
- In most patients, there is mild cardiac enlargement, the cardiac apex is easily palpable and a mitral regurgitation murmur may be heard (these features are not seen with constrictive pericarditis).
- Heart sounds are soft.
- Third and fourth heart sounds may be heard.

INVESTIGATIONS

- Electrocardiogram:
  - Nonspecific ST–T wave changes.
  - Low voltage.
  - Arrhythmias.
- Chest radiography shows mild cardiomegaly without any pericardial calcification.
- Echocardiography can confirm the diagnosis. It shows symmetrically thickened left ventricular walls.
- Cardiac MRI and CT typically show symmetrically thickened left ventricle wall, and normal or slightly reduced ventricular volumes and systolic function. These help in excluding constrictive pericarditis by showing normal pericardium (in constrictive pericarditis, CT or MRI may show thickened pericardium with or without calcification).
- Cardiac catheterisation shows increased ventricular filling pressures with typical dip-and-plateau (square-root) pattern in some cases. In contrast to equalisation of left- and right-sided diastolic pressures in constrictive pericarditis, left and right ventricular diastolic pressures are separable by more than 5 mmHg in restrictive cardiomyopathy due to unequal involvement and compliance of two ventricles.

TREATMENT

- Mainly symptomatic (careful use of diuretics).
- Chronic anticoagulation.
- Excision of fibrotic endocardium (in endomyocardial fibrosis).
- Cardiac transplantation.

Q. Discuss the clinical features, investigations and treatment of hypertrophic cardiomyopathy (HCM).

Q. Briefly outline hypertrophic obstructive cardiomyopathy (HOCM) and idiopathic hypertrophic subaortic stenosis (IHSS).

- Hypertrophic cardiomyopathy (previously called idiopathic subaortic stenosis) is characterised by presence of increased left ventricular wall thickness that is not explained by abnormal loading conditions such as hypertension or valvular disease.

FEATURES

- There is left ventricular hypertrophy that may be generalised but usually involving the interventricular septum predominantly. The upper portion of the interventricular septum is more hypertrophied (asymmetrical septal hypertrophy—ASH) and may result in left ventricular outflow tract obstruction (in 50%–75%).
- Cases with outflow tract obstruction were referred to as HOCM and those without obstruction as HCM. However, since obstruction is dynamic, the term HOCM is not used nowadays.
- The overall annual death rate in patients with HCM is estimated at ~1% per year, whereas that in patients with obstruction is ~2% per year.
- In most cases, the disease is familial and transmitted as an autosomal dominant trait. Nongenetic causes include amyloidosis, neonate of diabetic mother and drug-induced (tacrolimus, steroid).

CLINICAL FEATURES

- Many patients are asymptomatic.
- Family history of sudden death may be positive.
- Dyspnoea, fatigue, angina (due to ventricular hypertrophy which increases myocardial oxygen demand particularly during exertion), syncope or near syncope.
- Sudden death during or after physical exertion.
- Arrhythmias are common.
- Rapidly rising carotid pulse ('jerky').
- Bisferiens pulse (two systolic peaks). This results from sudden deceleration of blood due to development of midsystolic obstruction to blood flow and partial closure of aortic valve.
- Double apical impulse, due to atrial and ventricular systole.
- Second sound is normally split; however, the split may be paradoxic if there is severe left ventricular outflow tract obstruction.
- Loud fourth heart sound.
- Harsh ejection systolic murmur best heard at the lower left sternal border as well as at the apex due to left ventricular outflow tract obstruction. This murmur increases during standing and Valsalva manoeuvre (which reduce ventricular preload) but decreases during squatting and sustained hand grip (which increase afterload), and also by leg raising (which increases preload). This situation is in contrast to a murmur of aortic stenosis in which these manoeuvres decrease the intensity of the murmur.
- Pansystolic murmur at mitral area due to mitral regurgitation.

INVESTIGATIONS

- Electrocardiogram shows left ventricular hypertrophy and widespread deep and broad Q waves ('dagger-like' Q-waves), particularly in inferior and lateral precordial leads.
- Chest radiograph is normal or shows mild to moderate cardiac enlargement.
- Echocardiography is diagnostic. It may also show systolic anterior motion of anterior leaflet of mitral valve which is a major contributor to left ventricular outflow tract obstruction and the accompanying mitral regurgitation.
- Cardiovascular magnetic resonance most reliably assesses LV morphology.
- Ambulatory Holter electrocardiographic monitoring should be performed in the initial evaluation and as part of periodic follow-up (every 1 to 2 years) to identify patients who are at risk for sudden cardiac death and guide management of arrhythmias.

TREATMENT

- β-Blockers in angina and syncope. Treatment with β-blockers improves ventricular relaxation, increases diastolic filling time and reduces susceptibility to ventricular and supraventricular arrhythmias.
- Amiodarone for controlling arrhythmias.
- Calcium channel blockers like verapamil and diltiazem that do not have significant vasodilatory action are also beneficial because of their negative inotropic and chronotropic effects. They should not be used in presence of left ventricular outflow tract obstruction.
- If β-blockers alone are not sufficient, disopyramide (which also has a negative inotropic effect) along with β-blockers is helpful to reduce outflow tract obstruction.
- Patients with persistent or paroxysmal atrial fibrillation have a sufficiently increased risk of stroke; therefore, oral anticoagulation should be considered independent of the CHA_2DS_2VASc score.
- Surgical myotomy or myectomy of the hypertrophied septum.
- Digoxin, diuretics, nifedipine, nitrates and β-agonists should be avoided since they increase outflow tract obstruction.
- Implantable cardioverter-defibrillator in high-risk patients (cardiac arrest survivors, spontaneous sustained

or nonsustained ventricular tachycardia, family history of premature sudden death, unexplained syncope, left ventricular thickness ≥30 mm and abnormal blood pressure during exercise).
- Septal alcohol ablation is being increasingly used.
- Evaluation of first-degree family members.

Q. Write a short note on takotsubo cardiomyopathy.

- Takotsubo cardiomyopathy is an acute cardiomyopathy that mimics an acute coronary syndrome with left ventricular systolic dysfunction without obstructive coronary artery disease.
- Also known as stress cardiomyopathy, broken heart syndrome and transient apical ballooning.
- The term takotsubo originated from the Japanese word for an octopus trap because of the characteristic wall motion abnormalities of the left ventricle, including hypokinesia of the left ventricular apex (apical ballooning) with hyperkinetic function of the basal segments of the left ventricle resembling the shape of a Japanese octopus trap.
- It is commonly observed in postmenopausal women, although also reported in men, young women, and children.

TRIGGERING FACTORS

- Trigger can be physical, emotional or combined. Physical triggers include surgery, pneumonia, acute asthma, stroke, epilepsy, head injury and others. Emotional triggers include death of loved one, a relationship ending, financial problems, domestic abuse, gambling losses, anxiety and distress regarding public speaking).

CLINICAL FEATURES

- Most of the patients present with acute chest pain.
- Dyspnoea is the second common clinical manifestation.
- Other features include syncope (due to arrhythmias), cardiogenic shock (hypotension, abnormal mental status, cold extremities, oliguria or respiratory distress) and sudden death.
- Thromboembolic events (from apical thrombus) may occur in some patients.

INVESTIGATIONS

ELECTROCARDIOGRAM

- ST segment elevation, most commonly in anterior precordial leads is frequent.
- ST depression is a less common finding.
- Other findings include QT interval prolongation, T wave inversion and abnormal Q waves.

CARDIAC ENZYMES

- Cardiac troponin and natriuretic peptide levels are elevated while creatine kinase is usually normal.

ECHOCARDIOGRAPHY

- More than 80% patients demonstrate systolic apical ballooning of the left ventricle with hyperkinesia of the basal segments of left ventricle. In 15%, hypokinesia may be limited to mid-ventricle while in small number of patients, it may be limited to basal part of left ventricle (inverted takotsubo).

CORONARY ANGIOGRAPHY

- Coronary angiography characteristically demonstrates either normal vessels or no significant coronary atherosclerosis. Obstructive coronary artery disease (CAD) can be seen in some patients; however, the localisation and extent of the CAD are not responsible for the regional wall motion abnormalities.

DIAGNOSIS

- The diagnosis should be suspected when a patient, particularly a postmenopausal woman presents with features of acute coronary syndrome when the clinical manifestations and ECG abnormalities are out of proportion to the degree of elevation in cardiac biomarkers. A physical or emotional trigger is often but not always present.
- Mayo Clinic diagnostic criteria are used to make a diagnosis. All the four criterias need to be present.
  1. Transient left ventricular systolic (LV) dysfunction (hypokinesis, akinesis or dyskinesis). The wall motion abnormalities are typically regional and extend beyond a single epicardial coronary distribution; rare exceptions are the focal (within one coronary distribution) and the global type.
  2. Absence of obstructive coronary disease or angiographic evidence of acute plaque rupture. If coronary disease is found, the diagnosis of stress cardiomyopathy can still be made if the wall motion abnormalities are not in the distribution of the coronary disease. This exception is made since some patients with stress cardiomyopathy have concurrent coronary disease.
  3. New electrocardiographic abnormalities (either ST-segment elevation and/or T wave inversion) or modest elevation in cardiac troponin.
  4. Absence of phaeochromocytoma or myocarditis.

MANAGEMENT

- Patients presenting with ST elevation who are in centres where primary percutaneous coronary intervention can be done should undergo it in the usual manner. If the patient has stress cardiomyopathy, angiographic findings will suggest the diagnosis by typically showing no critical culprit coronary stenosis and the presence of apical ballooning on left ventricular angiography.
- Patients with ST elevation meeting criteria for reperfusion therapy presenting in a setting without availability of urgent angiography and PCI may be treated with thrombolytic therapy.
- Otherwise, the management is of the acute coronary syndrome, heart failure and cardiogenic shock.

PROGNOSIS

- Although acute heart failure is reversible, cardiogenic shock, life-threatening arrhythmias, or thromboembolic complications may contribute to the mortality rate, which is around 1%–5%.

Q. Discuss the aetiology, clinical features, investigations and management of acute pericarditis. (PA 27.7)

- Acute pericarditis is defined as an acute inflammatory disease of pericardium.

AETIOLOGY

- Various causes of acute pericarditis are mentioned in Table 7.82.

CLASSIFICATION OF PERICARDITIS

- Depending on the underlying cause, the inflammatory response in pericarditis may produce serous fluid, pus or dense fibrinous material.
- Pericarditis may be classified as acute (<6 weeks), subacute (6 weeks to 6 months) or chronic (>6 months) depending on the duration.

CLINICAL FEATURES

- Pericardial pain, pericardial friction rub and pericardial effusion with or without cardiac tamponade and pulsus paradoxus (paradoxical pulse) are the cardinal clinical manifestations of acute pericarditis.
- Nonspecific prodrome of fever, malaise and chest pain occurs in viral or idiopathic pericarditis.
- Myocarditis may be associated with pericarditis. Features of myocarditis have been discussed previously on page 616.
- Recurrence in about 30% of cases.

PERICARDIAL PAIN

- It is characteristically retrosternal in location, radiating to shoulders and neck. Radiation to one or both trapezius muscle ridges is suggestive of pericardial pain.
- Pain may be steady and constrictive or worsened by inspiration, coughing and change of body position ('pleuritic').
- It may be relieved by sitting up and leaning forward.
- Chest pain may be absent in patients with uraemic pericarditis, pericarditis associated with a rheumatic disorder, and neoplastic and post-irradiation pericarditis.

PERICARDIAL FRICTION RUB

- Pericardial friction rub is a superficial scratching sound, best heard to the left of sternum, often better heard (louder) by applying firm pressure with the diaphragm.
- It is usually better heard with the patient sitting upright and leaning forward.
- Pericardial friction rub has a to-and-fro, leathery character. It is often transitory, disappearing and re-appearing repeatedly.
- Classic pericardial rub has three phases that correspond to movement of heart during three phases of cardiac cycle: (a) atrial systole, (b) ventricular systole and (c) rapid ventricular filling during early diastole. However, some rubs are present in only one (monophasic) or two (biphasic) components of cardiac cycle.

PERICARDIAL EFFUSION AND CARDIAC TAMPONADE

- A detailed account of the clinical manifestations of pericardial effusion and cardiac tamponade is given later.

PULSUS PARADOXUS

- Pulsus paradoxus (paradoxical pulse) is characterised by weakness or disappearance of arterial pulse during inspiration.

TABLE 7.82 Aetiology of Acute Pericarditis

Common Causes	Less Common Causes
• Tuberculosis • Viral—Coxsackie B virus, mumps, varicella, rubella • Post-myocardial infarction syndrome (Dressler's syndrome) • Connective tissue diseases—SLE, rheumatoid arthritis, systemic sclerosis • Acute myocardial infarction • Idiopathic (majority)	• Rheumatic fever • Uraemia • Malignant disease • Hypothyroidism • Secondary to bacterial infections (including pneumonia) • Trauma and postsurgical • Radiation therapy • Drugs—hydralazine, procainamide, cytotoxics, phenytoin, penicillin, anticoagulants, methysergide • Ovarian hyperstimulation syndrome

INVESTIGATIONS

- Nonspecific elevation in total leucocyte count, CRP and ESR.
- Normal cardiac enzymes (CPK-MB and troponin T) unless associated myocarditis present.
- Autoantibodies if connective tissue diseases are suspected clinically.

ELECTROCARDIOGRAM

- Widespread ST-segment elevation in multiple leads (particularly leads I, II, aVL, aVF and V_1–V_3), with concavity upwards ('smiling face'); ST depressed in aVR and sometimes in V_1; depression of PR segment (Stage 1—occurs during the first hours to days) (Fig. 7.62).
- Subsequently, ST segments normalise with flattening of T waves (Stage 2—1 to 3 weeks).
- T waves become inverted later when ST segments become normal (Stage 3—3 to several weeks).
- In the final stage, ECG becomes normal (Stage 4—several weeks onwards).
- QRS voltage is reduced with pericardial effusion.
- Electrical alternans in large pericardial effusion.

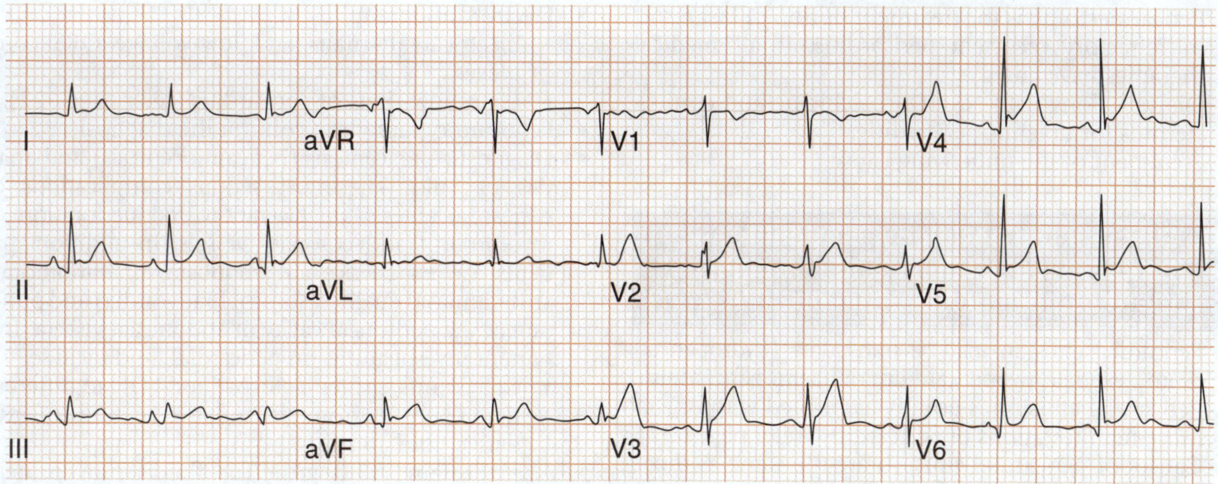

Fig. 7.62 ECG in acute pericarditis showing PR segment depression (prominent in leads II and III) and ST elevation in multiple leads with concavity upwards.

Comparison of ECG Changes in Acute Pericarditis and Acute ST-Elevation Myocardial Infarction

- ECG changes seen in acute pericarditis can be confused with those seen in ST-elevation MI. However, there are certain features which help in differentiating the two conditions (Table 7.83).

OTHER INVESTIGATIONS

- Chest radiography:
  - Without an effusion, chest radiograph is normal.
  - Rapid increase in the size of the cardiac shadow occurs in pericardial effusion or due to associated myocarditis.
  - 'Pear-shaped' or 'water-bottle' appearance of heart in pericardial effusion.
- Echocardiography can confirm the pericardial effusion.
- Cardiac MRI may be done to look for pericardial inflammation and also involvement of myocardium.
- Diagnostic paracentesis in pericardial effusion (refer page 624). It is indicated when the patient has tamponade or a large or symptomatic effusion despite medical therapy, and in cases in which tuberculous, purulent or neoplastic pericarditis is highly suspected.

TABLE 7.83 ECG Changes in Acute Pericarditis and Acute ST-Elevation Myocardial Infarction

ECG Finding	Acute Pericarditis	Acute ST-Elevation MI
• ST-segment shape	• Concave upward	• Convex upward
• Reciprocal ST-segment changes	• Absent	• Present
• Location of ST-segment changes	• Diffuse (except aVR and V_1)	• Depends on coronary artery involved
• Q waves	• Absent	• Present
• PR-segment depression	• Present	• Absent
• Concomitant presence of ST and T changes	• Absent (T wave inversion occurs after ST segments have normalised)	• Present

TREATMENT

- Rest and avoidance of physical activity.
- Hospitalisation if high-risk features (i.e. presence of specific, nonidiopathic, nonviral aetiology or high likelihood of complications) present:
  - Fever (temperature >38°C).
  - Leucocytosis.
  - Large pericardial effusion (echo-free space >20 mm).
  - Cardiac tamponade.
  - Acute trauma.
  - Immunosuppressed state.
  - Concurrent oral anticoagulation.
  - Elevated troponin levels.
  - Recurrent pericarditis.
  - Lack of response to NSAIDs after 1 week of therapy.
- Aspirin 600 mg 4 hourly or ibuprofen 300–800 mg 8 hourly for relief of pain and reduction in inflammation in idiopathic or viral pericarditis. Can be continued till pain and pericardial effusion disappear and ESR and CRP normalise (usually 7–10 days), followed by tapering over the next few weeks.
- Colchicine (0.5 mg twice a day) in addition to NSAIDs is more effective for initial attack and prevention of recurrences than aspirin alone.
- Corticosteroids (10–30 mg/day for 2–4 weeks) in selected cases (pericarditis associated with uraemia and connective tissue diseases) or those who do not respond to NSAIDs or where NSAIDs are contraindicated. This is followed by tapering over the next few months. However, use of corticosteroids in viral aetiology is associated with an increased risk of pericarditis recurrence.
- For patients with corticosteroid-dependent pericarditis and colchicine-resistant pericarditis, alternatives include azathioprine, intravenous immunoglobulins and anakinra (a nonselective interleukin-1 receptor antagonist).

- Pericardiectomy is the treatment option of last resort in refractory recurrent pericarditis, if all medical therapies have failed.
- Dialysis along with NSAIDs, colchicine and corticosteroids for uraemic pericarditis.
- Treatment of the underlying cause.

Q. Discuss the aetiology, clinical features, investigations and management of pericardial effusion. (PA 27.7)

- Pericardial effusion may be transudate (hydropericardium), exudate, pyopericardium or haemopericardium.
- Pericardial effusion is usually associated with one or more manifestations of pericarditis (refer page 622).
- Causes of pericardial effusion are the same as those for pericarditis (refer page 622).
- Effusion that develops slowly can be remarkably asymptomatic. If it develops over a short period, it may lead to cardiac tamponade.

CLINICAL SIGNS

- Apical impulse may not be palpable but sometimes it may be palpable well medial to the left border of cardiac dullness.
- Increase in cardiac dullness on percussion.
- Heart sounds are faint or muffled. A pericardial friction rub may or may not be audible.
- In a large effusion, there may be an area of dullness and tubular breathing at the lower angle of left scapula resulting from compression of lung (Ewart's sign).

INVESTIGATIONS

- Chest radiography:
  - Enlarged cardiac silhouette.
  - 'Water-bottle' appearance of heart shadow (Fig. 7.63).
  - Lucent pericardial fat lines.
- Fluoroscopy shows diminished ventricular pulsations.

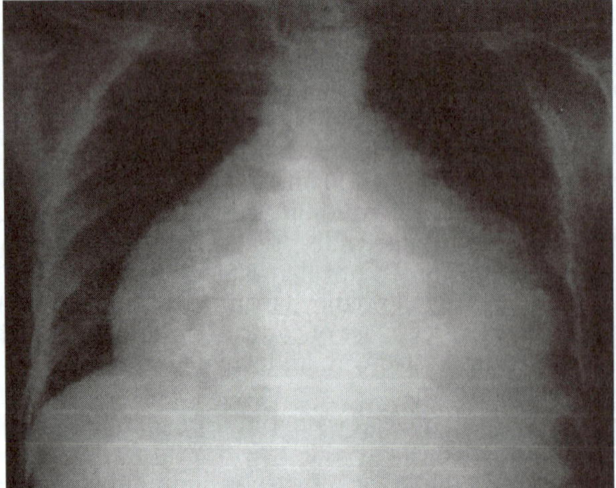

Fig. 7.63 Massive pericardial effusion producing 'water-bottle' appearance of heart.

- Electrocardiogram:
  - Electrical alternans and low-voltage QRS complexes.
  - May show signs of pericarditis (refer page 622).
- Echocardiography can confirm the diagnosis.
- Diagnostic paracentesis (pericardiocentesis) and analysis of fluid. The most serious complications of pericardiocentesis are laceration and perforation of myocardium and coronary vessels. In addition, patients can experience air embolism, pneumothorax, arrhythmias (usually vasovagal bradycardia) and puncture of the peritoneal cavity or abdominal viscera. Important investigations on pericardial fluid include:
  - Cell counts, protein, glucose and LDH to differentiate exudates from transudates. Features of exudative fluid are:
    - Protein >3.0 g/dL (or fluid:serum protein ratio >0.5).
    - LDH >200 mg/dL (or fluid:serum LDH ratio >0.6).
    - Glucose <two-thirds serum glucose in exudates.
    - White cell count is high in inflammatory diseases (bacterial and rheumatologic) and low in myxoedema.
  - Cholesterol is high (>100 mg/dL) in bacterial and malignant pericardial fluids.
  - Gram's stains and AFB stain.
  - Cytology for malignant cells.
  - Adenosine deaminase (ADA) and interferon-γ in tuberculosis.
  - *Mycobacterium* culture or radiometric growth detection (e.g. BACTEC).
  - PCR analyses for tuberculosis and viruses.
  - Tumour markers (carcinoembryonic antigen and cytokeratin 19 fragment).
- Thoracic and abdominal CT to rule out presence of lymphadenopathies and masses.

TREATMENT

- Therapeutic paracentesis with aspiration of effusion in selected cases. May be done using a pigtail catheter insertion under echocardiogram.
- Antiinflammatory drugs like aspirin or indomethacin.
- Treatment of underlying cause.
- In neoplastic conditions causing recurrent effusion, intrapericardial instillation of chemotherapeutic agents may be done.

Q. Give a brief account of tuberculous pericarditis.

- Usually secondary to pulmonary tuberculosis.
- Insidious onset and slow progression with weight loss, fever and fatigue.
- Clinical examination reveals a pericardial effusion (refer above).
- Associated pleural effusion is common.
- Natural history of tuberculous pericarditis is that of a chronic pericardial effusion with eventual thickening of pericardium, later leading to constrictive pericarditis.

INVESTIGATIONS

- Chest radiograph shows a 'water-bottle' configuration of heart.
- Echocardiography is important to confirm pericardial effusion. It may show cardiac tamponade, calcification of pericardium or features of constrictive pericarditis.
- Diagnosis is confirmed by aspiration of the fluid (which is an exudate with low sugar and elevated ADA), direct examination and culture for tubercle bacilli, and PCR for *Mycobacterium. tuberculosis*.
- Other investigations include chest radiograph for pulmonary tuberculosis and tuberculin skin test.
- Pericardial biopsy is rarely needed for confirmation of diagnosis.

TREATMENT

- Antituberculous chemotherapy for 6–9 months.
- Corticosteroids will reduce the incidence of constrictive pericarditis.
- Therapeutic aspiration (rarely) to relieve symptoms.
- Balloon pericardiotomy or pericardiectomy may be required at a later stage if constrictive pericarditis develops.

Q. Discuss the causes, clinical features, investigations and treatment of cardiac tamponade.

- Cardiac tamponade results from the accumulation of fluid in the pericardium in an amount sufficient to cause compression of the heart and impairment of diastolic filling.
- The minimum amount of fluid required for tamponade depends on the speed of accumulation (about 250 mL in rapidly developing effusions and more than 2000 mL in slowly developing effusions).
- Clinical features result from fall in cardiac output and systemic venous congestion.

AETIOLOGY

- Pericardial effusion (refer pages 622 and 624).
- Haemopericardium (anticoagulants, thrombolytics, recent cardiac surgery, indwelling catheters and blunt trauma chest).

CLINICAL FEATURES

- Dyspnoea and orthopnoea.
- Substernal chest discomfort radiating to neck and jaw.
- Right upper quadrant pain and pedal oedema in slowly developing cardiac tamponade (subacute tamponade).
- Tachycardia.
- Pulsus paradoxus or paradoxical pulse is the hallmark of tamponade.
- Hypotension.
- Raised jugular venous pressure with prominent x descent but absence or attenuation of y descent.
- Increase in cardiac dullness to percussion.
- Faint heart sounds; pericardial rub uncommon.
- Raised JVP, hypotension and muffled heart sounds constitute Beck's triad.
- Normal respiratory sounds.
- Tender hepatomegaly.
- Kussmaul's sign (rise in jugular venous pressure with inspiration) uncommon (see constrictive pericarditis below).

INVESTIGATIONS

- Chest radiography shows clear lung fields and normal or enlarged cardiac silhouette depending on rate of accumulation of pericardial fluid. Rapid accumulation of small amount of pericardial fluid is sufficient to produce features of tamponade (acute tamponade) but without cardiac enlargement on chest radiograph.
- Diminished cardiac pulsations on fluoroscopy.
- Electrocardiogram may show sinus tachycardia, reduction in QRS voltage, nonspecific ST–T changes and electrical alternans (alteration of QRS complex amplitude or axis between beats).
- Echocardiography can confirm the diagnosis by showing characteristic swinging motion of the heart, or systolic collapse of right atrium and diastolic collapse of right ventricle and dilated inferior vena cava without any respiratory variability.

MANAGEMENT

- Emergency pericardiocentesis.
- In a hypotensive patient, volume expansion with saline can be used as a temporary measure.
- Positive-pressure mechanical ventilation should be avoided in acute tamponade because it further reduces cardiac filling.
- Treatment of underlying cause.

Q. Describe chronic pericarditis.

- Chronic (>6 months) pericarditis includes effusive (inflammatory or hydropericardium in heart failure), adhesive and constrictive forms.
- Important causes include tuberculosis, histoplasmosis, toxoplasmosis, myxoedema, autoimmune diseases and systemic diseases.
- Symptoms are usually mild (chest pain, palpitations and fatigue) and are related to degree of cardiac compression and pericardial inflammation.
- Treatment includes management of underlying cause and pericardiocentesis. For frequent and symptomatic recurrences, balloon pericardiotomy or pericardiectomy may be done.

Q. Discuss the aetiology, clinical features, investigations and management of chronic constrictive pericarditis.

Q. Describe in brief about Kussmaul's sign.

- The pericardium becomes gradually fibrosed, thickened and inelastic. It acts as a rigid case, encasing the heart. It interferes with the diastolic relaxation of heart and hence ventricular filling. Hence, the inflow to the heart is reduced that is more during inspiration. The net result is a reduction in cardiac output and elevation of systemic venous pressure during inspiration.

AETIOLOGY

- Tuberculosis (commonest).
- Haemopericardium and cardiac surgery.
- Mediastinal irradiation.
- Rheumatoid arthritis and systemic lupus erythematosus.
- Uraemia.
- Asbestosis.
- Acute pericarditis (rare).
- Malignancy (rare).

CLINICAL FEATURES

- Clinical features result from reduced cardiac output and elevated systemic venous pressure.
- Weakness, fatigue, weight loss and anorexia.
- Patient appears emaciated with a protuberant abdomen due to ascites.
- Pulse is of low volume and rarely pulsus paradoxus may be present.
- Neck veins are distended (engorged) with a sharp *y* descent, a deep *y* trough and rapid ascent to baseline. A rapid *x* descent may also be seen in some cases.
- 'Kussmaul's sign' may be positive. This is an increase in the height of jugular venous pulsations (and hence a rise in jugular venous pressure) during inspiration.
- Atrial fibrillation may be present.
- Apical impulse may not be palpable (easily palpable in patients with restrictive heart disease).
- Heart sounds may be muffled.
- An early diastolic sound, 'pericardial knock' may be audible (occurs 0.09–0.12 seconds after A_2).
- Mitral regurgitation murmur is not heard (may be heard in patients with restrictive heart diseases).
- Congestive hepatomegaly.
- Ascites is more common, early and more severe than peripheral oedema.
- Protein-losing enteropathy may develop producing hypoalbuminaemia.

INVESTIGATIONS

- Chest radiography:
  - Heart size is normal or reduced (enlarged in patients with restrictive heart diseases).
  - Pericardial calcification (absent in patients with restrictive heart diseases), best seen in a lateral view and located over right ventricle and diaphragmatic surface of heart (Fig. 7.64).
- Fluoroscopy shows reduced cardiac pulsations.
- Electrocardiogram may show low-voltage QRS complexes and nonspecific T wave changes. Bundle branch block, ventricular hypertrophy, pathological Q waves and impaired atrioventricular conduction are rarely seen; presence of these features strongly favours restrictive cardiomyopathy.
- Echocardiography can confirm pericardial thickening and calcification.
- Magnetic resonance imaging can confirm pericardial thickening.
- Cardiac catheterisation in selected patients.
  - Elevation and near equalisation of diastolic pressures in right atrium, right ventricle and pulmonary wedge pressure which corresponds to left heart diastolic pressure.
  - Rapid *y* descent in jugular venous pressure and plateau during right heart catheterisation (dip and plateau sign or square-root sign).
  - Respiratory variation in filling of left and right ventricles (not present in patients with restrictive cardiomyopathy).

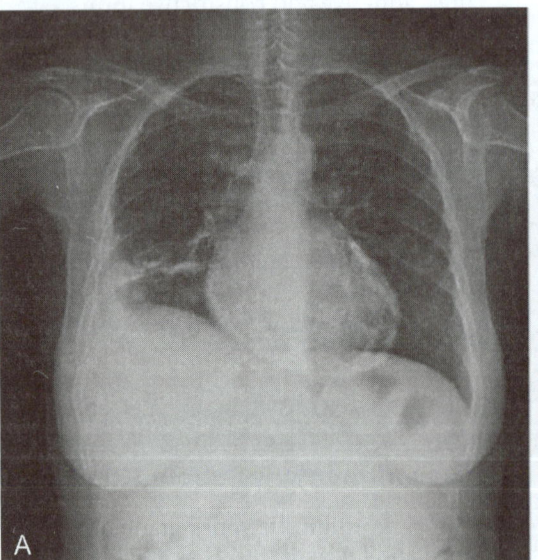

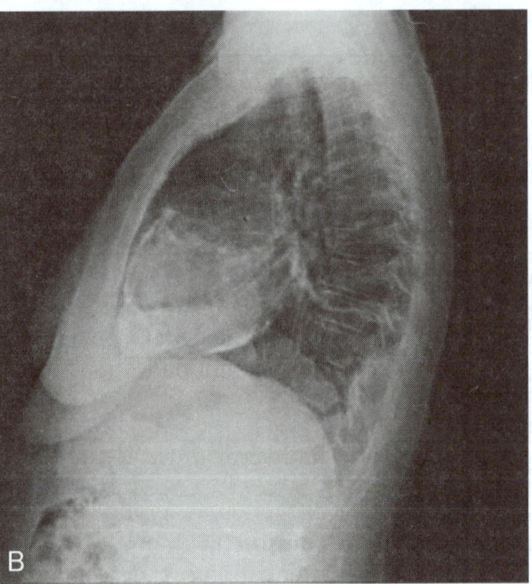

Fig. 7.64 Chest radiograph (PA and lateral) showing extensive pericardial calcification.

TREATMENT

- Pericardiectomy (resection of the pericardium) is the only definitive treatment.

Q. How will you differentiate between constrictive pericarditis and restrictive heart disease?

- Table 7.84 gives differences between constrictive pericarditis and restrictive heart disease.

Q. Enumerate the common congenital heart diseases seen in adults. (IM 1.28)

Acyanotic Congenital Heart Diseases	Cyanotic Congenital Heart Diseases
• Ventricular septal defect • Atrial septal defect • Patent ductus arteriosus • Pulmonary stenosis • Aortic stenosis • Coarctation of aorta	• Tetralogy of Fallot • Transposition of great arteries

Q. Discuss the clinical features, investigations, complications and management of coarctation of aorta (COA). (IM 1.29)

Q. Explain briefly about Suzman's sign and radiofemoral delay.

- Coarctation of the aorta (COA) is a narrowing of the lumen of aorta. It can occur anywhere from distal part of arch of aorta to bifurcation of abdominal aorta, but it is commonly located immediately below the origin of the left subclavian artery (Fig. 7.65). It is typically located at the insertion of the ductus arteriosus (juxta-ductal) but can be located distal to the ductus (post-ductal) or proximal to the ductus (preductal).
- Shone syndrome is a constellation of left-sided obstructive defects, including supramitral ring, parachute mitral valve, subaortic stenosis, along with aortic coarctation, which suggests a common developmental origin.

CLINICAL FEATURES

- More common in males.
- Commonly associated with bicuspid aortic valve (in 70%), berry aneurysms in the circle of Willis (10%) and Turner's syndrome. Other associated lesions include ventricular septal defect and patent ductus arteriosus.
- Commonly diagnosed during workup for hypertension in adults.
- Minor symptoms include headache and epistaxis (due to hypertension) and leg fatigue or claudication (from decreased circulation in the lower part of body).
- Major symptoms are related to four major complications:
  - Heart failure.
  - Infective endocarditis.
  - Cerebral haemorrhage due to rupture of berry aneurysm.
  - Rupture or dissection of aorta.
- Recurrent episodes of haematemesis and melaena are harbingers of impending rupture.
- Most patients with significant coarctation who do not undergo surgery die before the age of 40 years due to complications.

TABLE 7.84 Differences Between Constrictive Pericarditis and Restrictive Heart Disease

Features	Constrictive Pericarditis	Restrictive Heart Disease
Prior history	Pericarditis, trauma, cardiac surgery or a systemic disease that affects the pericardium (e.g. tuberculosis, connective tissue disease, malignancy)	An infiltrative disease that may involve the heart muscle (e.g. amyloidosis, sarcoidosis)
Ascites	Prominent	Less prominent
Pulsus paradoxus	Uncommon	Absent
Apical impulse	Not palpable	Easily palpable
Kussmaul's sign	More common	Less common
Third heart sound	Absent	Often present
Pericardial knock	Often present	Absent
Murmur of mitral regurgitation	Absent	May be present
BNP levels	Usually normal	Usually elevated
Bundle branch block, ventricular hypertrophy, pathologic Q waves in ECG	Uncommon	Common
Cardiomegaly on chest X-ray	Absent	Often present
Calcification of pericardium on Chest X-ray	Often present	Absent
Echo	Pericardial thickness > 4 mm	Pericardium not thickened
Cardiac catheterisation	Near equalisation of left and right ventricular diastolic pressures	Left and right ventricular diastolic pressures are separable by more than 5 mmHg

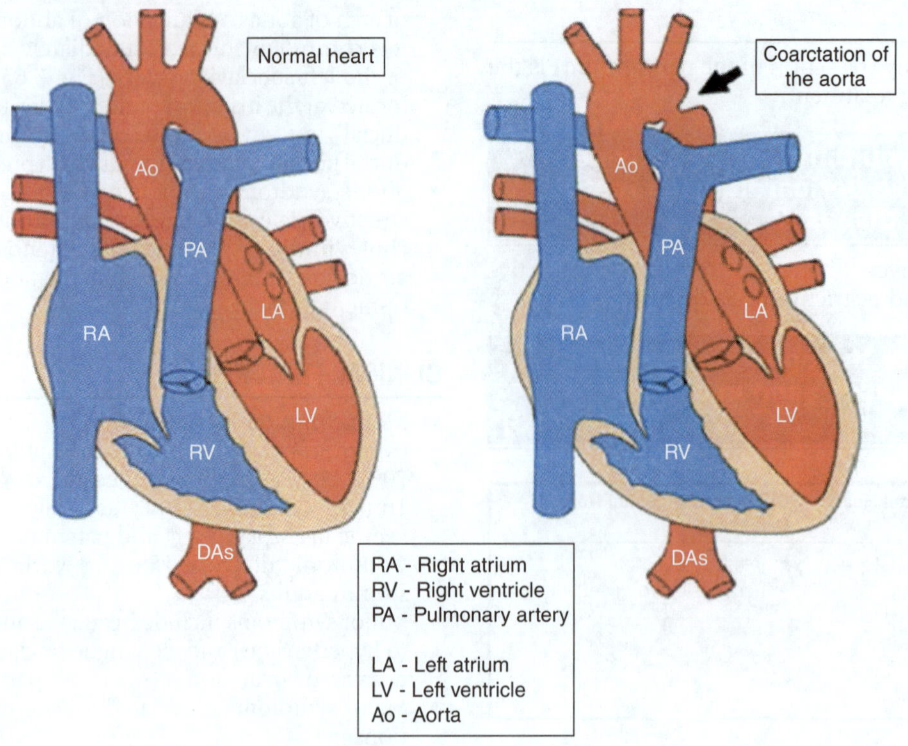

Fig. 7.65 Coarctation of aorta.

SIGNS

- Lower segment of the body may be underdeveloped.
- Hypertension in the upper limbs with low or normal pressure in lower limbs (difference >20 mmHg).
- Weak and delayed femoral pulses (radiofemoral delay).
- Prominent pulsations in the neck.
- 'Suzman's sign' is dilated, tortuous, pulsatile, collateral arteries seen around the scapulae and intercostal regions in the back. It is better seen with the patient bent forwards and hands hanging down.
- 'Corkscrew'-shaped retinal arteries.
- Heaving apical impulse.
- Load A_2.
- Aortic ejection sound if associated with bicuspid aortic valve.

Murmurs in Coarctation of Aorta

- In coarctation of aorta, several murmurs may be heard (Box 7.86).

BOX 7.86 Murmurs in Coarctation of Aorta

- Ejection systolic murmur (ESM) over the spine from coarctation itself
- Systolic or continuous murmurs over lateral thoracic wall, arising from collaterals
- Ejection systolic murmur (from the associated bicuspid aortic valve) or early diastolic murmur (from aortic regurgitation) in the aortic area

INVESTIGATIONS

- Electrocardiography (showing LVH), echocardiography (may show coarctation as well as associated cardiac lesions), radiological studies and angiography can confirm the diagnosis.

RADIOLOGICAL FEATURES OF COARCTATION OF AORTA

- Coarcatation of aorta may produce several signs on radiological investigations (Box 7.87).
- CT and MRI to look for aortic aneurysm and coarctation.

BOX 7.87 Radiological Features of Coarctation of Aorta

- 'Rib notching' or 'Dock's sign' is the notching of the undersurfaces of posterior ribs, extending from third to ninth ribs. It may be unilateral or bilateral and is seen only after the age of 6 years. Occurs due to dilated collaterals pressing on the lower part of ribs (Fig. 7.66).
- 'Post-stenotic dilatation' is the dilatation of the aorta distal to coarctation.
- '3 sign' is a combination of dilated prestenotic aorta and left subclavian artery above, stenosed, coarcted segment in the middle and dilated poststenotic aorta below (Fig. 7.66).
- 'E sign' is seen on the lateral view on a barium swallow. This results from the dilated prestenotic aorta and left subclavian artery and dilated poststenotic aorta indenting the barium-filled oesophagus.

- Cardiac catheterisation to assess associated cardiac lesions.

COMPLICATIONS

- Hypertension.
- Left ventricular failure.

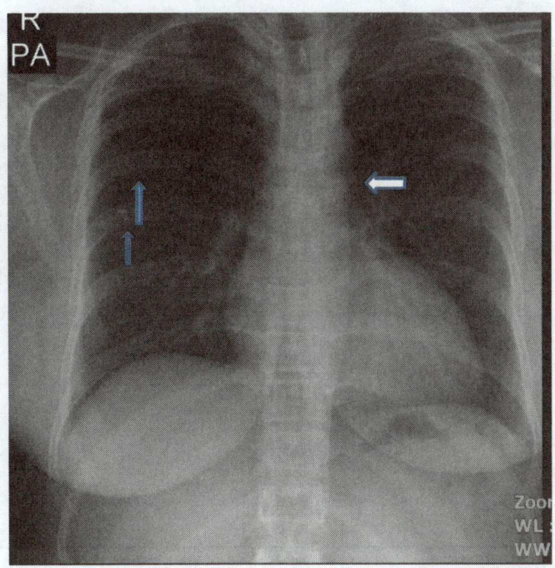

Fig. 7.66 Chest radiograph showing rib notching (blue arrows) and '3 sign' (white arrow).

- Cerebral aneurysm and haemorrhage.
- Aortic dissection and rupture of aorta.
- Infective endocarditis at the site of coarctation, bicuspid aortic valve or collateral channels.
- Persistent renal damage if surgery is delayed.

TREATMENT

- Treatment of hypertension and heart failure. Avoid ACE inhibitors and angiotensin II receptor antagonists as they may result in inadequate lower-body perfusion and may precipitate renal failure.
- Surgical correction (hypertension persists in many patients even after surgery).
- Endovascular stenting for isolated CoA (without other cardiac lesions).

Q. Discuss briefly the haemodynamics, clinical features, investigations, complications and management of persistent ductus arteriosus (patent ductus arteriosus—PDA). (IM 1.29)

Q. Give a brief account of differential cyanosis.

- Ductus arteriosus is a vessel leading from the bifurcation of the pulmonary artery to the aorta just distal and opposite to the origin of left subclavian artery (Fig. 7.67).
- This is functional in foetus and diverts desaturated blood from main pulmonary artery into the descending aorta and placenta for oxygenation. It closes by birth due to postnatal drop in circulating prostaglandin E2 levels as well as rise in systemic oxygen tension. In premature infants, the ductus arteriosus does not close rapidly and may require pharmacological or surgical closure.

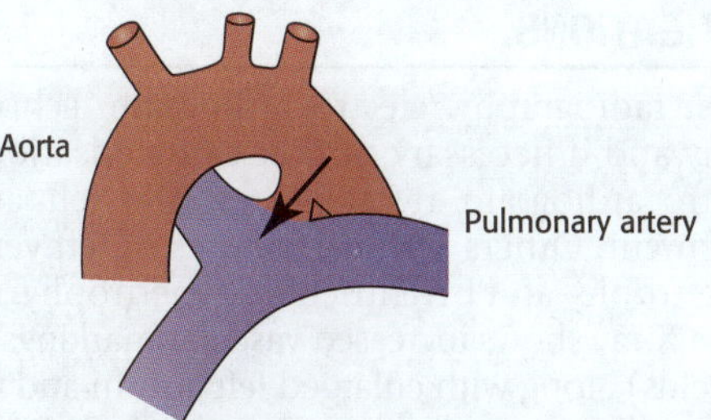

Fig. 7.67 Persistent ductus arteriosus (PDA).

- Persistence of the patency of this is known as patent ductus arteriosus (PDA).
- Higher incidence in premature newborns and those born at high altitude.
- Maternal rubella in the first trimester predisposes to persistent ductus arteriosus.

HAEMODYNAMICS

- Since the pressure in the aorta is higher than in the pulmonary artery (during both systole and diastole), there will be a continuous flow of blood from aorta to pulmonary artery (L → R shunt) in both systole and diastole.
- When pulmonary hypertension develops, this blood flow diminishes initially in diastole.
- Later, with the development of Eisenmenger's syndrome (see page 633), the blood flow is reversed (R → L shunt). Now, the blood flows from pulmonary artery to aorta (i.e. reversal of the shunt).

CLINICAL FEATURES

- More common in females.
- Retardation of growth and development in children.
- Dyspnoea.
- Collapsing pulse.
- Apex beat is shifted down and out and hyperdynamic in character.
- Continuous thrill at the upper left sternal edge.
- First heart sound is loud (due to loud mitral component).
- Continuous 'machinery murmur' with late systolic accentuation at the upper left sternal edge. Multiple ejection clicks are heard within this murmur. It should be distinguished from 'to-and-fro' murmur that is a combination of an ejection systolic murmur and an early diastolic decrescendo murmur (e.g. aortic stenosis and insufficiency). There is a definite gap between the end of the ejection murmur and the second heart sound in 'to-and-fro' murmur.
- Left ventricular third heart sound and a mid-diastolic flow murmur at the apex with large L → R shunt.
- With the development of pulmonary hypertension, signs of pulmonary hypertension develop.
- With the development of Eisenmenger's syndrome, shunt reverses (R → L), and central cyanosis and clubbing develop. Cyanosis and clubbing develop only in lower limbs but not in the upper limbs (differential cyanosis). The continuous murmur becomes quieter, confined to systole and later disappears.

INVESTIGATIONS

- Chest radiography, electrocardiogram, echocardiography and if necessary cardiac catheterisation.
- Electrocardiogram frequently shows left atrial enlargement. Others include features of left ventricular hypertrophy and biventricular hypertrophy.
- Chest X-ray shows increased vascular markings (plethoric fields) along with enlarged left atrium and ventricle.
- Echocardiogram and colour Doppler show PDA as well as amount of blood flow through the ductus arteriosus.

COMPLICATIONS

- Heart failure.
- Infective endocarditis.
- Paradoxical embolism.
- Pulmonary hypertension and Eisenmenger's syndrome.
- Rupture of the ductus.

MANAGEMENT

- Surgical ligation or division of the ductus (ideal treatment).
- Transcatheter occluding devices (e.g. coils, buttons and umbrellas) are increasingly used.
- Video-assisted thoracoscopic clip closure.
- In premature babies, a 'medical closure' of the ductus may be attempted using indomethacin (it inhibits prostaglandin synthesis). However, it may produce necrotising enterocolitis and renal insufficiency. Use of ibuprofen has been found to be as effective as indomethacin with lower incidence of adverse effects. These are rarely effective in full-term babies.

Q. What is reversed differential cyanosis?

- Cyanosis of upper limbs exceeds that of the lower limbs.
- Seen in transposition of great arteries (blood from right ventricle ejected into the aorta reaches the upper limbs and head, blood from left ventricle is ejected into pulmonary artery and reaches the lower limbs via PDA).

Q. Discuss briefly the haemodynamics, clinical features, investigations, complications and management of atrial septal defect (ASD). (IM 1.29)

Q. What is Lutembacher's syndrome.

Q. Explain briefly about patent foramen ovale?

TYPES

- Atrial septal defect (ASD) is a defect in the interatrial septum. Based on the location of the defect, it can be classified into three types:
  - Ostium secundum type (commonest) that involves the fossa ovalis in the mid-septal region. Twenty per cent of these cases are associated with mitral valve prolapse. This should not be confused with patent foramen ovale that is a normal variant and not a true septal defect.
  - Ostium primum type (rare)—it occurs when the septum does not fuse with the endocardial cushions leaving a defect at the base of the interatrial septum. The AV valves may also be deformed (AV septal defects or AV canal defects or endocardial cushion defects).
  - Sinus venosus type (rare)—it occurs high in the atrial septum near the entry of superior vena cava and is almost always associated with partial anomalous pulmonary venous return (to SVC or right atrium).
- Lutembacher's syndrome is a rare combination of ASD and rheumatic (or congenital) mitral stenosis.

PATENT FORAMEN OVALE

- Patent foramen ovale may be seen in >25% of adult population and is haemodynamically insignificant.
- During foetal development, a PFO is required for oxygenated blood to flow from the right to the left atrium.
- Usually asymptomatic but is associated with paradoxical emboli and increased incidence of embolic stroke (cryptogenic stroke).
- Other complications include migraine, decompression syndrome and air embolism, orthodeoxia–platypnoea syndrome (dyspnoea and arterial desaturation induced by upright posture and relieved by recumbence) and peripheral embolism.
- Transoesophageal echocardiography with contrast at rest, with cough, and following Valsalva is generally considered the most definitive diagnostic test.
- An incidentally detected patent foramen ovale generally requires no follow-up or treatment. If an embolic stroke has occurred and is likely caused by patent foramen ovale, medical therapy with antiplatelet agents or anticoagulation, and surgical or percutaneous closure of the defect are the options. Indications for surgical closure after a cryptogenic stroke are given in Box 7.88.

HAEMODYNAMICS

- In ASD, blood is shunted from left atrium to right atrium and then to right ventricle. The right ventricular output and hence pulmonary blood flow is markedly increased. This leads to progressive enlargement of

BOX 7.88 General Indications of PFO Closure for Secondary Prevention of Stroke (Should Fulfill All)

- Age ≤60 years
- No large vessel disease
- No lacunar infarction
- No cardioembolic source
- No other identifiable cause
- No autoimmune disease
- No hypercoagulability
- Controlled hypertension, diabetes
- Life expectancy >1 year

right atrium, right ventricle and pulmonary arteries. Eventually, pulmonary hypertension appears with reversal of the shunt (R → L shunt).

CLINICAL FEATURES

- Commonest congenital heart disease seen in adults. More common in females.
- Many asymptomatic and diagnosed on routine examination.
- Palpitations and fatigue.
- Recurrent respiratory infections.
- Retarded growth and development.
- Dyspnoea, cardiac failure and arrhythmias like atrial fibrillation occur late in the course of illness.
- Occasionally, a paradoxical embolism.

SIGNS

- Hyperdynamic precordium.
- Visible and palpable pulmonary artery pulsations in the second left intercostal space.
- Left parasternal heave.
- Systolic thrill over the pulmonary area (uncommon).
- S_1 is loud (due to accentuated tricuspid component of first sound).
- Second heart sound is widely split and fixed in relation to respiration.
  - 'Widely split' because the pulmonary valve closure is delayed by the larger volume of blood to be ejected by the right ventricle.
  - 'Fixed split' since the volume of blood ejected across the pulmonary valve is the same in inspiration and expiration.
- Ejection systolic murmur over the pulmonary area due to increased flow across the pulmonary valve.
- Mid-diastolic rumbling murmur (flow murmur) over the tricuspid area due to increased flow across the tricuspid valve.
- A pansystolic murmur of tricuspid regurgitation produced by dilatation of right ventricle.
- A pansystolic murmur of mitral regurgitation is characteristic of primum ASD.
- No audible murmur occurs secondary to flow across ASD.
- With the onset of pulmonary hypertension, signs of pulmonary hypertension develop.
- With the development of Eisenmenger's syndrome, central cyanosis and digital clubbing develop. Both pulmonary and tricuspid murmurs decrease in intensity and later disappear. Development of pulmonary hypertension and reversal of the shunt (Eisenmenger's syndrome) are late events in ASD (usually by third and fourth decades of life).

INVESTIGATIONS

- Chest radiography, electrocardiogram, echocardiography and if necessary cardiac catheterisation.
- Chest radiography reveals a prominent pulmonary artery and increased pulmonary vascular markings or pulmonary plethora (seen in all L to R shunts). Cardiomegaly may occur due to right ventricular enlargement. A small aortic knuckle is characteristic, which occurs due to chronically low systemic cardiac output.
- The electrocardiogram shows right atrial enlargement (*P* pulmonale), mild right ventricular hypertrophy, right-axis deviation and rSR′ pattern (right bundle branch block) in the right chest leads in ostium secundum ASD. In ostium primum ASD, ECG shows prolonged PR interval and left-axis deviation with right bundle branch block. In sinus venosus type of ASD, inverted P waves are seen in inferior leads.
- Echocardiogram reveals enlarged right ventricle with paradoxical septal motion, particularly well demonstrable on M-mode echocardiogram. By two-dimensional echocardiogram, the defect can be clearly visualised.
- Cardiac MRI may be useful and may give the same type of information that echocardiography can provide. It provides assessment of right ventricular size and function.
- Cardiac catheterisation is rarely required; most catheterisations are done with the intention to close the defect percutaneously. In selected patients, angiography is done to delineate associated anomalies not shown by noninvasive imaging. When catheterisation is performed, step-up in oxygen saturation is seen at the right atrial level.

COMPLICATIONS

- Heart failure (in neonates).
- Recurrent respiratory infections
- Paradoxical embolism (with right-to-left shunt).
- Atrial fibrillation.
- Pulmonary hypertension (late).
- Eisenmenger's syndrome (very late).
- Infective endocarditis (extremely rare).

MANAGEMENT

- Prompt treatment of respiratory infections.
- Surgical closure of the defect in patients older than 3 years, provided there are no signs of pulmonary hypertension, have right ventricular volume overloading (dilatation of right atrium and right ventricle with flat or paradoxical interventricular septal motion) and the pulmonary flow is 50% more than the systemic blood flow (Qp:Qs >1.5/1).
- A percutaneous transcatheter septal occluder may be used as an alternative to surgical closure for patients with ostium secundum—type ASD.
- Uncorrected ASD does not require antibiotic prophylaxis for endocarditis (see 'infective endocarditis' on page 574).

Q. Discuss briefly the haemodynamics, clinical features, investigations, complications and management of congenital ventricular septal defect (VSD). (IM 1.29)

Q. What is maladie de Roger?

- The interventricular septum has a membranous and a muscular portion. VSD implies a defect in the interventricular septum. Most of the VSDs are 'peri-

membranous', that is at the junction of membranous and muscular portions. Muscular defect is uncommon.
- May be associated with ASD, PDA or pulmonic stenosis.
- Maladie de Roger—small VSDs in muscular portion, presenting in older children as a loud pansystolic murmur without other haemodynamic changes. Such defects usually close spontaneously.

HAEMODYNAMICS

- The blood flows from the left ventricle to the right ventricle and then to the pulmonary artery. This ultimately results in a volume overload of the ventricles if the shunt is large. Pulmonary hypertension and reversal of shunt occur at a later stage.

CLINICAL FEATURES

- Commonest congenital heart disease in paediatric age group. Detected due to presence of a murmur on routine examination.
- Clinical features depend on the size of the defect and magnitude of the shunt.
- Recurrent respiratory infections.
- Failure to thrive.
- Heart failure.
- Hyperdynamic precordium.
- Apex beat is shifted down and out and is hyperdynamic in character.
- Systolic thrill at the third or fourth left intercostal space.
- Pulmonary component of second sound normal or increased depending on the degree of elevation of pulmonary artery pressure.
- Harsh pansystolic murmur, best heard at the third or fourth left intercostal space, but radiating all over precordium. No consistent relationship of intensity of murmur with the size of the defect. If the defect is muscular, murmur may stop well before S_2 because the defect decreases in size or obliterates in the later part of systole.
- Left ventricular third heart sound and a mid-diastolic rumbling murmur (flow murmur) at the apex due to increased flow across the mitral valve. Indicates pulmonary:systemic (Qp:Qs) blood flow ratio >2:1.
- Incidence of ventricular arrhythmias increased in VSD.
- With the development of pulmonary hypertension, signs of pulmonary hypertension appear. Later, with reversal of the shunt (Eisenmenger's syndrome), the murmur of VSD disappears, and central cyanosis and clubbing appear.

INVESTIGATIONS

- Chest radiography, electrocardiography, echocardiography and, if necessary, cardiac catheterisation.
- Chest X-ray shows cardiomegaly and increased pulmonary vascular markings if the shunt is large. Left atrial enlargement may also be noted.
- Electrocardiogram may be normal in small defects or may show evidence of left ventricular hypertrophy in small to moderate defects while it may show biventricular or right ventricular hypertrophy in moderate to large defects. Features of left atrial enlargement may also be seen. Another common finding is presence of intraventricular conduction defect or right bundle branch block.
- Echocardiography to assess location and size of VSD as well as blood flow across it. It can also define associated cardiac lesions.
- Cardiac catheterisation to assess pulmonary vascular resistance in complicated VSD.

COMPLICATIONS

- Heart failure.
- Recurrent chest infections.
- Arrhythmias.
- Pulmonary hypertension.
- Eisenmenger's syndrome.
- Right ventricular outflow tract obstruction.
- Aortic regurgitation.
- Infective endocarditis (rare).

NATURAL HISTORY

- Spontaneous closure in approximately 40% of cases.
- Additional 25%–30% of defects may become small enough not to require surgical intervention.
- Majority of defects close by age 2 years; most close by age 5–7 years.
- Pulmonary vascular obstructive disease may develop in 10%.
- Infundibular stenosis (Gasul's transformation) may occur in 8% of the defects. Though patient will require surgery, it prevents development of pulmonary vascular obstructive disease.
- Aortic insufficiency develops in approximately 5% of patients. This may be related to either prolapse of an aortic valve cusp into VSD or lack of support to the aortic root. This complication appears to occur more with advancing age.

MANAGEMENT

- Small VSDs with small shunts require no treatment as they are likely to close spontaneously.
- Heart failure is treated with diuretics and afterload reduction by ACE inhibitors.
- Operative correction is indicated in moderate to large defects with significant left-to-right shunt (pulmonary-to-systemic blood flow ratio >1.5:1.0). Also indicated after an episode of infective endocarditis irrespective of degree of shunting.
- Large VSDs with severe elevation of pulmonary resistance (irreversible pulmonary vascular obstructive disease) are not candidates for surgery. Symptomatic treatment and venesection for symptoms of polycythaemia should be undertaken. These patients may eventually become candidates for lung transplantation.

Q. What is Eisenmenger's syndrome? Discuss the clinical presentation of Eisenmenger's syndrome.

- Eisenmenger's syndrome is the consequence of the reversal of a left-to-right shunt to a right-to-left shunt. It occurs in patients with congenital heart diseases, especially PDA, VSD and ASD.
- Basically (before the reversal of the shunt), in patients with L → R shunt (ASD, VSD and PDA), the oxygenated blood from the left side of the heart gets mixed with the deoxygenated blood of the right side of the heart. Over a period of time, pulmonary vascular disease sets in and pulmonary vascular resistance goes up, ultimately resulting in pulmonary hypertension.
- When pulmonary arterial pressure goes up (pulmonary hypertension), the pressure in the pulmonary circuit exceeds the pressure of systemic side. This results in an obligatory reversal of shunt, now from right side to left side (R → L shunt). This is termed Eisenmenger's syndrome.

CLINICAL FEATURES

- Dyspnoea, cyanosis, fatigue, dizziness and syncope.
- Central cyanosis and clubbing occur from mixing of deoxygenated blood with oxygenated blood. It is generalised in ASD and VSD reversal, while it is differential (only lower limbs) in PDA with reversal.
- Conditions that cause systemic vasodilatation (e.g. fever, exertion and hot weather) may exaggerate shunt from right to left, resulting in systemic desaturation.
- Signs of pulmonary hypertension and its sequelae (refer 'pulmonary hypertension' on page 605).
- S_2 is loud with palpable P_2:
  - S_2 fixed but narrowly split in ASD with reversal.
  - S_2 single in VSD with reversal.
  - S_2 mobile but narrowly split in PDA with reversal.
- Eventually, patient dies of right heart failure. Other causes of death include pulmonary infections, infective endocarditis, severe haemoptysis, secondary erythrocytosis, pulmonary thrombosis with infarction, brain abscess, cerebral stroke and ventricular arrhythmias. These complications are uncommon in idiopathic pulmonary arterial hypertension.
- Survival is better in Eisenmenger's syndrome as compared to in idiopathic pulmonary arterial hypertension.
- The characteristic murmurs of the underlying defect (ASD, VSD and PDA) decrease in intensity and duration, and finally disappear with the development of Eisenmenger's syndrome.

TREATMENT

- Surgery with correction of an underlying defect in early phase where pulmonary hypertension is due to increased volume load and not due to increased pulmonary vascular resistance.
- Vasodilator therapy using calcium channel blockers may be detrimental as systemic vasodilatation may further increase right-to-left shunt.
- Long-term oxygen inhalation may improve symptoms.
- Diuretics and digoxin may be helpful in a few patients.
- Phlebotomy in patients with hyperviscosity syndrome due to erythrocytosis with haematocrit >65%. Fluid replacement (750–1000 mL) of isotonic saline while removing 400–500 mL of blood should be undertaken.
- Avoid iron deficiency.
- To prevent paradoxical air embolism, air bubbles in intravenous tubing should be carefully removed.
- Oral anticoagulation is recommended in patients with intrapulmonary thrombi, confirmed paradoxic embolism and in the presence of atrial flutter or fibrillation.
- Prostanoids (e.g. epoprostenol, iloprost and treprostinil), endothelin receptor antagonists (e.g. ambrisentan and bosentan) and phosphodiesterase-5 inhibitors (e.g. sildenafil and tadalafil) may improve symptoms.
- The only curative treatment is heart–lung transplantation.

Q. Describe Fallot's tetralogy or tetralogy of Fallot (TOF).

- It is the most common congenital cyanotic heart disease in adults. It consists of four features (Fig. 7.68):
  - VSD (almost always large).
  - Right ventricular hypertrophy.
  - Pulmonary stenosis, most commonly subvalvular or infundibular.
  - Overriding aorta (biventricular connection of the aortic root).
- Presence of ASD along with TOF is known as pentalogy of Fallot.

CLINICAL FEATURES

- Children at birth and early neonatal period are generally asymptomatic except for presence of cyanosis.

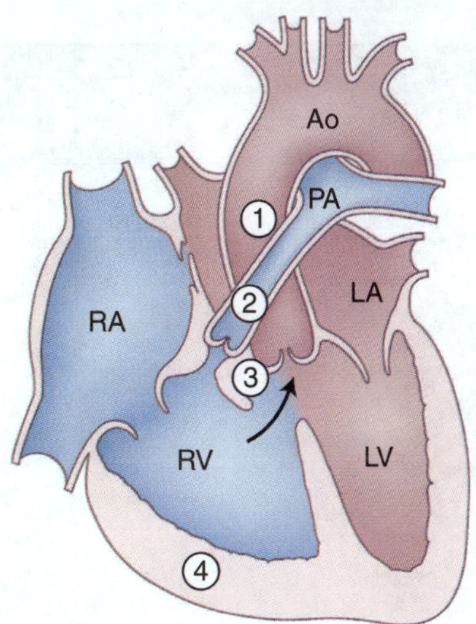

Fig. 7.68 Components of tetralogy of Fallot. 1=overriding of aorta; 2=pulmonary infundibular stenosis; 3=ventricular septal defect; 4=right ventricular hypertrophy.

- Within a few weeks to months of birth, children with TOF often develop dyspnoea, fatigue and hypoxic (cyanotic) spells on exertion (deepening of cyanosis with possible syncope).
- Cyanotic spells (tet spells) occur during feeding, crying, fever or exercise due to systemic vasodilatation producing increased right-to-left shunting across VSD. These factors also increase right ventricular obstruction. With progression of spell, metabolic acidosis develops that further reduces systemic resistance and increases pulmonary vascular resistance. This can result in sudden death. Squatting is common as it increases peripheral resistance, thereby reducing right-to-left shunting, and increases systemic venous return.
- Adults tend to have growth retardation, fatigue and dyspnoea on exertion but cyanotic spells are not the usual features. Polycythaemia secondary to chronic hypoxia is common and can lead to thrombotic strokes.
- Examination shows clubbing, central cyanosis, parasternal heave, systolic thrill, single loud second heart sound (pulmonary component is too soft to be heard) and ejection systolic murmur in the second and third left intercostal spaces (due to pulmonary outflow obstruction). Intensity and duration of murmur is inversely proportional to severity of right ventricular outflow tract obstruction. Since VSD is large, its murmur is not heard.

INVESTIGATIONS

- Low arterial oxygen which does not increase with oxygen therapy.
- Chest radiography shows a large right ventricle and a small pulmonary artery ('Coeur en Sabot' or 'boot-shaped' heart—'boot' by enlarged right ventricle, and concavity by underdeveloped right ventricular outflow tract and main pulmonary artery). The lung fields are oligaemic (Fig. 7.69).

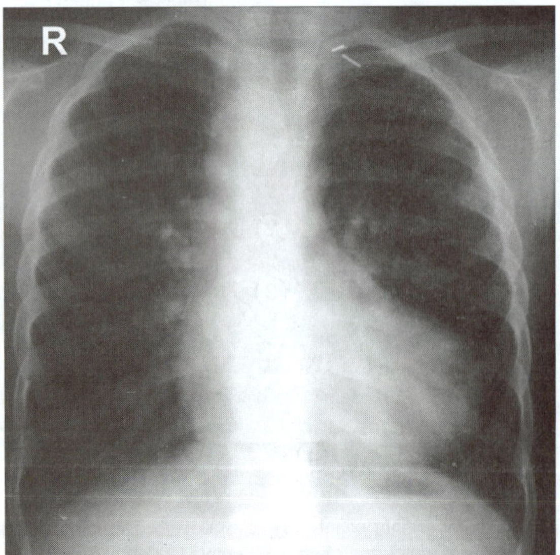

Fig. 7.69 Chest radiograph showing 'boot-shaped' heart.

- Right ventricular hypertrophy and right atrial enlargement in the electrocardiogram.
- Echocardiography.
- Cardiac catheterisation is rarely needed as echocardiography is highly sensitive.

COMPLICATIONS

- Intravascular thrombosis due to polycythaemia resulting in cerebrovascular accidents and embolism.
- Brain abscess.
- Higher incidence of pulmonary tuberculosis.
- Infective endocarditis.

TREATMENT

- Complete correction in infants and children.
- Blalock–Taussig shunt (a shunt between a subclavian artery and a pulmonary artery on the same side) in very young infants and premature babies in order to increase the blood supply to the lungs.
- Cyanotic spells:
  - The management goals for cyanotic spells are to increase pulmonary blood flow by increasing preload, provide pulmonary vasodilatation and increase afterload in order to reverse right-to-left shunting and promote pulmonary blood flow (Box 7.89).
- Antibiotic prophylaxis for endocarditis.
- Pneumococcal and influenza vaccination.

Q. Explain briefly about Raynaud's phenomenon. (DR 16.2)

Q. Discuss the clinical presentation and management of Raynaud's disease.

- Classified into primary (idiopathic) and secondary Raynaud's phenomenon.

BOX 7.89 Management of Cyanotic Spells

- Asking the patient to squat ('knee-to-chest' position) in order to increase venous return to the heart and increase systemic vascular resistance to mitigate right-to-left shunting.
- Administering oxygen.
- Administering intravenous fluids (5–10 mL/kg) to increase venous return.
- Administering morphine at a dose of 0.1 mg/kg intravenously to reduce release of catecholamines. This will increase period of right ventricular filling by decreasing heart rate and promote relaxation of infundibular spasm.
- Administering propranolol at a dose of 0.01 mg/kg intravenously followed by oral dose of 3–5 mg/kg/day in divided doses. It relaxes right ventricular outflow obstruction. However, β-blockers can produce hypotension.
- Administering sodium bicarbonate 2 mEq/kg intravenously to treat acidosis and promote pulmonary vasodilatation.
- Administering ketamine (1–3 mg/kg IV) which can also increase systemic vascular resistance and provide sedation.
- Administering phenylephrine 2–10 μg/kg/min to increase systemic vascular resistance.

AETIOLOGY OF RAYNAUD'S PHENOMENON

- Raynaud's phenomenon can be produced by several causes (Box 7.90).

CLINICAL FEATURES

- More common in females.
- Raynaud's phenomenon—on exposure to cold, fingers and less commonly toes become initially very pale (due to vasospasm of digital arteries and concomitant reduction in blood flow) (Fig. 7.70), then cyanosed (due to pooling of deoxygenated blood caused by vasoconstriction of the postcapillary venules) and then red and painful (due to refilling of vasospastic vessels with oxygenated blood). Approximately 60% of patients will exhibit all three colour changes. Pallor is the most specific sign and redness is the least specific. Some patients will exhibit only one or two of these changes. These changes are associated with throbbing pain. Thumb may be relatively spared in some patients.
- Raynaud's phenomenon can also result from emotional stress which is a common precipitant in Raynaud's disease.
- As the digital arteries become more constricted, other outward changes including chronic paronychia, nail pitting, hair loss, scarring, fissures and ulcerations of fingers become apparent.
- It can eventually lead to tissue necrosis and gangrene.
- Patients have been documented to have decreases in myocardial perfusion during cold challenge and there is a higher incidence of angina in patients with Raynaud's phenomenon.
- It should not be confused with acrocyanosis—a disorder primarily affecting young women in which digits turn blue whenever exposed to cold but there is no pain or any of the other outward physical changes associated with Raynaud's phenomenon.

BOX 7.90 Aetiology of Raynaud's Phenomenon

• Idiopathic (Raynaud's disease)	• Vaso-occlusive disease: cryoglobulinaemia, cold agglutinin disease, paraproteinaemia
• β-Blockers and ergot	• Systemic sclerosis
• Other drugs: bleomycin, cisplatin, cyclosporin, methysergide	• CREST syndrome
• Pneumatic drill usage	• SLE, rheumatoid arthritis, Sjogren's syndrome, mixed connective tissue disease
• Occupational exposure to cold	• Diabetes mellitus
• Peripheral vascular disease	• Large vessel: compressive (e.g. cervical rib), neurogenic (thoracic outlet obstruction), thromboangiitis obliterans, atherosclerosis

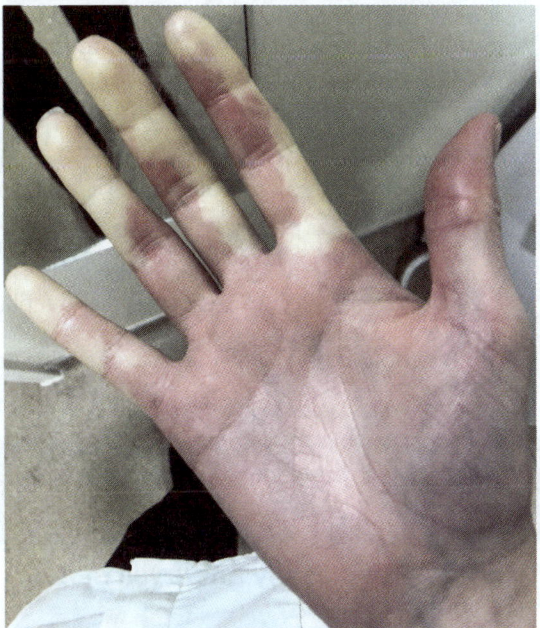

Fig. 7.70 Blanching phase of Raynaud's phenomenon. Note relative sparing of thumb. Courtesy: Herrick AL, Wigley FM. Raynaud's phenomenon. Best Pract Res Clin Rheumatol. 2020 Feb;34(1).

NAIL CAPILLARY MICROSCOPY

- Enlarged or distorted capillary loops and a relative paucity of loops suggest an underlying connective tissue disease, particularly systemic sclerosis.

RAYNAUD'S DISEASE

- Also known as idiopathic Raynaud's phenomenon.
- Age of onset between 15 and 30 years.
- More common in females.
- Symmetric episodic attacks without any evidence of peripheral vascular disease, tissue gangrene, digital pitting, negative nail fold capillary examination, normal ESR and negative antinuclear antibody test.

TREATMENT

- Stop smoking and withdraw offending drugs.
- Avoid exposure to cold.
- Treatment of underlying cause.
- Analgesics.
- Nifedipine 10 mg thrice daily which may be increased to higher doses if required. If patient is unable to tolerate it, amlodipine may be tried.
- If calcium channel blockers fail, other options are prostaglandins (e.g. iloprost), phosphodiesterase-5 inhibitors (sildenafil, tadalafil and vardenafil) and endothelin receptor antagonists (e.g. bosentan).
- Other drugs include ACE inhibitors or angiotensin receptor blockers, α-blockers (prazosin), selective serotonin reuptake inhibitors, and topical nitroglycerine.
- In severe cases, digital sympathectomy and botulinum toxin can be tried.
- Amputation is rarely needed.

Q. What are acute aortic syndromes?

Q. Classify aortic aneurysms. What are the common causes of aortic aneurysms?

ACUTE AORTIC SYNDROMES

- Acute aortic syndromes are a constellation of life-threatening medical conditions involving aorta. These include:
  - Acute aortic dissection.
  - Intramural haematoma.
  - Penetrating atherosclerotic aortic ulcer.

TYPES OF AORTIC ANEURYSMS

- Fusiform aneurysm.
- Saccular aneurysm.

SITES OF AORTIC ANEURYSMS

- Thoracic part of aorta.
  - Ascending aorta.
  - Arch of aorta.
  - Descending aorta.
- Abdominal aorta.
  - Any part of abdominal aorta, but commonest site being infrarenal portion.

AETIOLOGY OF AORTIC ANEURYSMS

- Aortic aneurysm has several aetiologies (Box 7.91).

Q. Discuss the clinical manifestations, complications, investigations and management of abdominal aortic aneurysms (AAA).

- An aneurysm is a permanent focal, full-thickness dilatation of an artery to 1.5 times its normal diameter. Normal infrarenal aortic diameters in patients older than 50 years are 1.5 cm in females and 1.7 cm in males. By convention, an infrarenal aorta 3 cm in diameter or larger is considered aneurysmal. In contrast, pseudoaneurysm represents a collection of blood and connective tissue outside the aortic wall.
- The most common cause of AAA is atherosclerosis. Smoking is an important risk factor for AAA.
- Common in males older than 60 years.
- Most common location is between the renal arteries and the iliac arteries.
- Clinical features of AAAs:
  - Most cases are asymptomatic.
  - Typically, aneurysms are noted on studies performed for other reasons as opposed to during physical examination.
  - Symptoms are back pain, abdominal pain and claudication.
  - Physical sign is a pulsatile, nontender mass in the abdomen. It imparts an expansile pulsation.
  - Classic presentation of a ruptured aneurysm includes the triad of hypotension, abdominal, flank or back pain and a pulsatile abdominal mass. However, pulsatile mass is often absent after rupture. Other common symptoms include urinary retention, constipation, urge to defaecate and haematuria. Flank or periumbilical ecchymosis (Grey Turner or Cullen signs, respectively) may be seen.
- Complications of AAAs:
  - 'Leaking aneurysm' is characterised by severe abdominal pain and tenderness.
  - 'Ruptured aneurysm' is characterised by acute severe abdominal pain and hypotension.
- Investigations in AAAs:
  - Abdominal radiograph may show the calcified outline of the aneurysm.
  - Ultrasonography (unreliable after rupture but should be performed while resuscitating patient).
  - CT angiography (gold standard for diagnosing rupture if patient is haemodynamically stable) and MRI.
  - Angiography confirms the diagnosis.
- Screening sonography above the age of 66 years advisable in those with:
  - Chronic obstructive pulmonary disease (COPD)
  - Coronary, cerebrovascular or peripheral arterial disease
  - Family history of AAA
  - Hyperlipidaemia
  - Hypertension
  - History of smoking
- Management of AAAs:
  - Rupture—emergency surgery preceded by volume resuscitation using fluids and blood to maintain a systolic blood pressure around 80–90 mmHg (permissive hypotension). Overresuscitation should be avoided because it can lead to clot disruption.
  - Asymptomatic.
    - Aneurysms of more than 5.5 cm diameter—surgery or endovascular aneurysm repair (EVAR).
    - Aneurysm more than 4.0 cm diameter and has grown by more than 1 cm in 1 year—surgery or EVAR.
    - Aneurysms of less than 5.5 cm diameter—serial follow-up with ultrasound.
  - Surgical treatment of AAA is excision and replacement with a graft.
  - Another option is EVAR using an expandable graft system.

BOX 7.91 Aetiology of Aortic Aneurysms

- Atherosclerosis (commonest cause)
- Smoking
- Cystic medial necrosis
- Syphilis (aneurysm of ascending aorta)
- Rheumatic aortitis
- Trauma
- Takayasu arteritis

Q. Discuss the clinical features, investigations and management of aneurysm of thoracic aorta.

Q. How do you classify aneurysms of thoracic aorta?

CLASSIFICATION

- Aneurysm of ascending aorta.
- Aneurysm of arch of aorta.

- Aneurysm of descending thoracic aorta.

CLINICAL FEATURES

- Clinical features of aneurysms of thoracic aorta may be discussed under four major headings.

GENERAL FEATURES

- These are features common to aneurysms of ascending, arch and descending thoracic aorta.
- Pain due to compression or erosion of adjacent musculoskeletal structures.
- Visible and pulsatile (expansile) mass over anterior chest in the corresponding area.
- Rupture is characterised by excruciating pain (may rupture into bronchus, pleura, oesophagus, mediastinum, pulmonary artery or pericardium).

CLINICAL FEATURES OF ANEURYSM OF ASCENDING AORTA

- Commonest cause of aneurysm of ascending aorta is cystic medial necrosis—syphilis was the most common cause a few decades ago.
- Pulsations in the second and third right intercostal spaces.
- Right parasternal dullness on percussion.
- Aortic regurgitation from aortic valve ring dilatation.
- Aortic ejection systolic murmur and a 'tambour'-like A_2.
- Superior vena caval syndrome from pressure on superior vena cava.
- Dry cough and recurrent pneumonias from compression of right main bronchus.
- Compression of pulmonary artery.

CLINICAL FEATURES OF ANEURYSM OF ARCH OF AORTA

- Suprasternal pulsations and pulsations over manubrium sterni.
- Dullness on percussion over the upper part of sternum.
- Right and left radial pulse difference.
- Tracheal tug is a tugging sensation felt when the neck is extended and larynx is held up.
- Cough, dyspnoea, stridor and recurrent pneumonias from tracheobronchial compression.
- Dysphagia from oesophageal compression.
- Hoarseness of voice from recurrent laryngeal nerve compression.
- Horner's syndrome from sympathetic nerve compression.
- Hiccups and diaphragmatic paralysis from phrenic nerve compression.
- Vertebral pain from vertebral compression.

CLINICAL FEATURES OF ANEURYSM OF DESCENDING THORACIC AORTA

- Compression of lung.
- Erosion of vertebrae and ribs.
- Compression of nerve roots.

INVESTIGATIONS

- Commonly done investigations include chest radiography, electrocardiogram, ultrasonogram, CT scan, MRI and angiogram.

TREATMENT

- Only definitive treatment is surgical or thoracic endovascular aortic repair (TEVAR).

Q. Discuss the predisposing factors, classification, clinical features, investigations and management of aortic dissection.

- Aortic dissection is caused by a tear of the intima with subsequent penetration of blood, which splits the aortic wall layers. This creates a cavity within the medial layer, the so-called false lumen which is separated from the native true lumen by dissection membrane. A second tear in dissection membrane allows blood to re-enter the true lumen.
- The dissection usually propagates distally but may also propagate proximally. The dissection usually produces aortic dilatation resulting in dissecting aneurysm of aorta.
- Afflicts males more than females in their fifth and sixth decades.

PREDISPOSING FACTORS

- Predisposing factors for aortic dissection are given in Box 7.92.

CLASSIFICATION

- There are two main classifications for aortic dissections (Table 7.85 and Fig. 7.71).

CLINICAL FEATURES

- Sudden-onset pain in the front or back of chest, often in the interscapular area. The pain is described as 'severe, ripping or tearing'.
- Syncope, dyspnoea and weakness.
- Hypertension or hypotension.
- Asymmetry of pulses and blood pressure in upper limbs (in 30% of cases only).

BOX 7.92 Predisposing Factors for Aortic Dissection

- Systemic hypertension (70%)
- Cystic medial necrosis, Marfan's syndrome
- Bicuspid aortic valve (BAV)
- Coarctation of aorta (COA)
- Third trimester of pregnancy
- Giant cell arteritis
- Behcet's disease
- Syphilis
- Trauma

TABLE 7.85 Classification of Aortic Dissection

Stanford Classification	DeBakey Classification
• Type A—dissection involving the ascending aorta independent of site of tear and distal extension • Type B—dissection limited to descending aorta	• Type I—involves ascending to descending aorta • Type II—limited to ascending aorta • Type III—involves descending aorta only

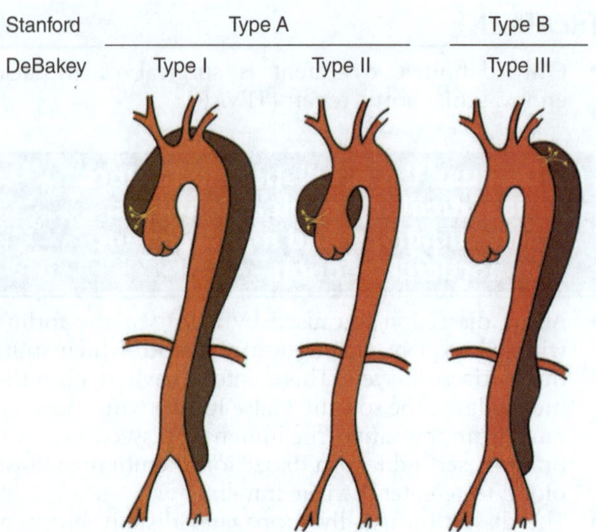

Fig. 7.71 Aortic dissections—Stanford and DeBakey classification.

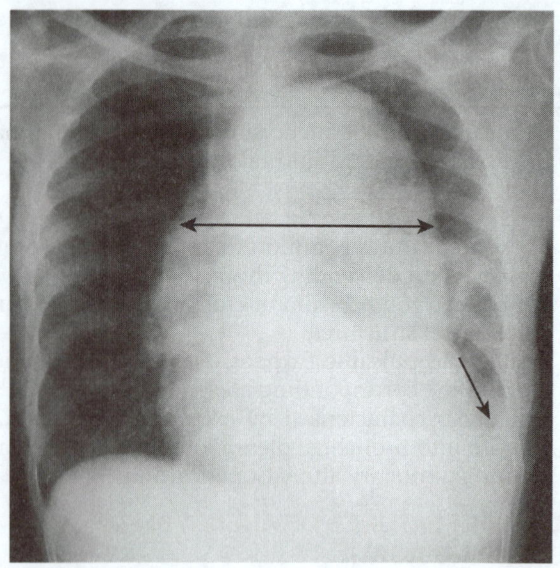

Fig. 7.72 Chest radiograph showing widening of mediastinum (double black arrow) and a left pleural effusion (single black arrow).

- Dissection can occlude orifices of branches of aorta resulting in ischaemia of brain, heart, bowel, kidney, spinal cord (paraplegia) and extremities (leg pain and paraesthesias).
- Aortic regurgitation, haemopericardium and cardiac tamponade can occur in type A dissection with retrograde propagation.
- Pulmonary oedema and cardiogenic shock due to acute AR.
- In the event of development of a 'dissecting aneurysm', symptoms resulting from compression of superior vena cava, superior cervical ganglion, bronchus and oesophagus can manifest.
- Bicuspid aortic valve is commonly associated with dissection and can produce a systolic murmur.
- Table 7.86 describes Aortic Dissection Detection risk score. Presence of any high-risk condition, high-risk pain feature and high-risk examination feature is given one point.

TABLE 7.86 Aortic Dissection Detection Risk Score

High-Risk Conditions	High-Risk Pain Features	High-Risk Examination Features

• Marfan syndrome
• Family history of aortic disease
• Known aortic valve disease
• Recent aortic manipulation
• Known thoracic aortic aneurysm
	• Chest, back or abdominal pain described as any one of the following:
	  • Abrupt onset
	  • Severe intensity
	  • Ripping or tearing
		• Evidence of perfusion deficit:
		  • Pulse deficit
		  • Systolic blood pressure differential
		  • Focal neurological deficit (in conjunction with pain)
		• Murmur of aortic regurgitation (new and with pain)
		• Hypotension or shock state

A score ≤1 with BNP <500 ng/mL or normal chest X-ray indicates a very low probability of aortic dissection.

INVESTIGATIONS

- D-dimer is elevated in majority of patients.
- Chest radiography:
  - Dissection involving ascending aorta presents as widening of superior mediastinum and a small pleural effusion, usually left sided (Fig. 7.72).
  - Dissection involving descending thoracic aorta presents as widening of mediastinum. Descending aorta may appear wider than ascending aorta.
- Electrocardiogram to differentiate from acute myocardial infarction. It shows nonspecific ST–T wave changes.
- Echocardiography—limited value for evaluation of the descending thoracic aorta for dissection but is highly useful in identifying proximal aortic dissection.
- Spiral CT scan is the modality of choice for diagnosis.
- Magnetic resonance imaging is useful in some patients.
- Aortography confirms the diagnosis but is rarely done presently.

TREATMENT

- Type A dissection is preferably treated by emergency surgical correction, pending which medical treatment as given in the subsequent text is started.
- Type B dissection that is stable and uncomplicated is preferably treated by medical measures (in selected cases, surgical treatment is indicated).
  - Medical therapy is aimed at reducing cardiac contractility and systemic arterial pressure to 100–120 mmHg systolic.
    - Parenteral administration of a β-blocker (esmolol or metoprolol). Target is to achieve a systolic blood pressure of 100–120 mmHg and a pulse of around 60/minute.
    - If β-blockers are contraindicated, parenteral calcium channel blockers may be used.

- If β-blockers alone do not control blood pressure, vasodilators (e.g. sodium nitroprusside or nitroglycerine) may be given.
- Direct vasodilators (diazoxide and hydralazine) as monotherapy are contraindicated because they increase the force of left ventricular ejection.
- Surgical therapy involves reconstruction of the aorta. Another option for type B dissection is thoracic endovascular aortic repair (TEVAR).

Q. Discuss the clinical spectrum of cardiovascular syphilis.

- Manifestations of cardiovascular syphilis are seen in the tertiary stage and are given in Box 7.93.
- Aortitis—commonly involves ascending aorta. Most are asymptomatic. Clinical features include burning retrosternal chest pain, dilatation of aorta, aortic ejection systolic murmur and a loud 'tambour'-like second heart sound.
- Aortic regurgitation—results from annular dilatation with normal valve cusps. For a detailed account of syphilitic aortic regurgitation, refer aortic regurgitation on pages 569–571.
- Aneurysms of aorta—clinical manifestations of aortic aneurysms are discussed under aortic aneurysm on page 636.
- Coronary ostial stenosis—manifests as angina (nocturnal angina), sudden death or arrhythmias. Myocardial infarction is rare.
- Myocardial gumma—clinical diagnosis is extremely difficult. May manifest as bundle branch block, AV block or rarely ECG pattern simulating myocardial infarction.
- Diagnosis of cardiovascular syphilis is based on syphilitic serological tests (positive TPHA and VDRL).
- Treatment of cardiovascular syphilis is with parenteral penicillin for 2 weeks with surgical correction.

Q. Mention the common causes of left ventricular hypertrophy.

- Box 7.94 gives common causes of left ventricular hypertrophy.

Q. Mention the common causes of left ventricular dilatation.

- Common causes of left ventricular dilatation are given in Box 7.95.

BOX 7.93 Manifestations of Cardiovascular Syphilis

• Aortitis	• Coronary ostial stenosis
• Aortic regurgitation	• Myocardial gumma
• Aneurysm of aorta	• Endarteritis

BOX 7.94 Common Causes of Left Ventricular Hypertrophy

• Systemic hypertension	• Coarctation of aorta (COA)
• Aortic stenosis (AS)	• Hypertrophic cardiomyopathy (HCM)

BOX 7.95 Common Causes of Left Ventricular Dilatation

• Aortic regurgitation (AR) • Mitral regurgitation (MR) • Ventricular septal defect (VSD) • Persistent ductus arteriosus (PDA)	• Dilated cardiomyopathy • Ischaemic heart disease (IHD) • Hyperkinetic circulatory states like anaemia, thyrotoxicosis and beriberi

Q. Discuss the differential diagnosis of ejection systolic murmurs (ESMs). (IM 1.16)

Q. Discuss in brief about straight back syndrome (SBS).

Q. Give a brief outline of idiopathic dilatation of pulmonary artery (IDPA).

- Ejection systolic murmur (ESM), also known as midsystolic murmur, starts shortly after the first heart sound (S_1) and ends before the second heart sound. It is a crescendo–decrescendo or diamond-shaped murmur (Fig. 7.73).
- ESMs are usually produced at aortic or pulmonary valves.

CAUSES

- Causes of ejection systolic murmur are given in Table 7.87.

DIFFERENTIAL DIAGNOSIS

- Diagnosis is based on the behaviour of the murmur and associated features.

AORTIC STENOSIS

Murmur

- Loud, harsh ESM best heard in the second right intercostal space (aortic area), radiating to carotid arteries. It diminishes with sustained hand grip.

Associated Features

- Pulsus tardus and low systolic blood pressure (less than 100 mmHg).

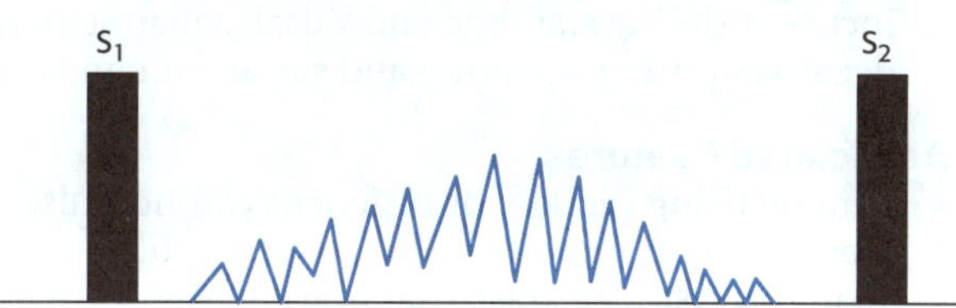

Fig. 7.73 Ejection systolic murmur (ESM).

TABLE 7.87 Causes of Ejection Systolic Murmurs

Organic valvular diseases	Flow murmur from intracardiac causes
• Aortic stenosis (AS) • Pulmonary stenosis (PS) • Hypertrophic cardiomyopathy (HCM) • Sclerotic aortic valve • Bicuspid aortic valve (BAV) • Tetralogy of Fallot (TOF)	• Atrial septal defect (ASD) • Aortic regurgitation (AR) • Mitral regurgitation (MR) **Miscellaneous** • Coarctation of aorta (COA) • Thin chest wall • Pectus excavatum • Straight back syndrome (SBS) • Idiopathic dilatation of pulmonary artery • Aneurysm of ascending aorta • Innocent murmur
Flow murmur from extracardiac causes • Exercise, pregnancy • Thyrotoxicosis • Severe anaemia • Systemic arteriovenous fistulae	

Note: 1. Flow ejection murmurs occur due to increased flow across semilunar (aortic or pulmonary) valves.
2. Mitral valve prolapse produces late systolic murmur.

- Left ventricular hypertrophy and heaving apical impulse.
- Systolic thrill at the second right intercostal space radiating to lower left sternal border and carotids ('cross-belt' area).
- Intensity of A_2 is decreased or A_2 may even be absent.
- Second heart sound may be single or narrowly split or rarely paradoxically split.
- Aortic ejection sound in second right intercostal space in valvular AS.

PULMONARY STENOSIS

Murmur

- Loud, harsh ESM best heard at the second left intercostal space (pulmonary area) radiating towards left shoulder. The murmur increases with inspiration and decreases with expiration.

Associated Features

- Prominent *a* waves on JVP.
- Left parasternal heave and epigastric pulsations due to right ventricular hypertrophy.
- Systolic thrill at the second left intercostal space (pulmonary area).
- Wide splitting of second heart sound due to delay in right ventricular ejection and hence delayed P_2.
- Pulmonary component (P_2) of second heart sound is soft or may even be absent.
- Murmur is often preceded by a pulmonary ejection sound.

HYPERTROPHIC CARDIOMYOPATHY

Murmur

- Harsh ESM best heard at the lower left sternal border as well as at the apex with no radiation. The murmur increases during standing and Valsalva manoeuvre. It decreases during squatting and sustained handgrip.

Associated Features

- Rapidly rising ('jerky') or bisferiens carotid pulse.
- Double apical impulse (bifid apical impulse).
- Giant presystolic parasternal heave.
- Loud fourth heart sound.
- Pansystolic murmur at the apex due to associated mitral regurgitation (MR).

SCLEROTIC AORTIC VALVE

- About 50% of the people older than 50 years have an aortic ESM from a sclerotic aortic valve without valve stenosis. It is benign, nonstenotic (nonobstructive) deformity of the aortic valve of old age.

Murmur

- Rough ESM of short duration (but less harsh and less intense than AS murmur), best heard in the second right intercostal space (aortic area), commonly radiating to apex and may even be maximal at the apex.

Associated Features

- Thrill is rare.
- Arterial pulse, JVP, apical impulse and heart sounds are normal.
- No extra sounds are audible.
- No other murmurs of other valvular lesions are audible.

BICUSPID AORTIC VALVE

- Common cause of isolated AS.
- Increased risk of infective endocarditis.

Murmur

- Soft ESM in the second right intercostal space (aortic area).

Associated Features

- Arterial pulse, JVP, apical impulse and heart sounds are normal.
- The murmur is usually preceded by an aortic ejection sound.
- Associated aortic regurgitation may be present.
- Associated AS, coarctation of aorta (COA) or dissection of aorta may be present.

TETRALOGY OF FALLOT

Murmur

- Loud, harsh ESM best heard at the second and third left intercostal spaces due to PS.

Associated Features

- Cyanotic spells ('Fallot spells' or 'tet spells').
- Squatting.
- Central cyanosis, finger clubbing and polycythaemia.
- Prominent *a* waves on JVP if PS is severe.
- Systolic thrill may be felt in the second or third left intercostal space.
- Second heart sound is single due to absent pulmonary component (P_2).

ATRIAL SEPTAL DEFECT

Murmur

- ESM at the second left intercostal space (pulmonary area) due to increased flow of blood across the pulmonary valve.

Associated Features

- Hyperdynamic precordium.
- Pulsations in the second left intercostal space from dilated pulmonary artery.

- Systolic thrill over second left intercostal space (pulmonary area).
- Wide and fixed splitting of second heart sound in relation to respiration.
- Rumbling mid-diastolic flow murmur at tricuspid area.

COARCTATION OF AORTA

Murmur

- ESM over the spine posteriorly from the coarctation itself.

Associated Features

- Underdeveloped lower segment of the body.
- Hypertension in the upper limbs.
- Radiofemoral delay.
- 'Suzman's sign'—pulsatile collaterals around scapulae and intercostal regions in the back.
- 'Corkscrew'-shaped retinal arteries.
- Heaving apical impulse.
- Aortic ejection sound in associated BAV.
- Systolic or continuous murmurs over lateral thoracic wall arising from collaterals.
- ESM and/or early diastolic murmur over the second right intercostal space (aortic area) from the associated BAV.

THIN CHEST WALL

- Increased transmission of sound through the thin chest wall can cause an ESM over precordium in otherwise normal people.

PECTUS EXCAVATUM

- The murmur is the result of distortion of the underlying structures by the deformity.
- Soft ESM, best heard at the base of the heart.
- No evidence of chamber enlargement or abnormal heart sounds.

STRAIGHT BACK SYNDROME

- In SBS, the normal thoracic kyphosis of the spine is lost and thoracic spine becomes 'straight'. This results in a reduction of anteroposterior diameter of the thorax, and the heart is compressed between the sternum anteriorly and the spine posteriorly. The murmur results from the distortion of the outflow tract and great vessels.
- ESM is best heard at the second left intercostal space (pulmonary area). It is probably caused by compression of right ventricular outflow tract by sternum which reduces with deep inspiration.
- Examination of the spine reveals absence of the normal thoracic kyphosis.
- No evidence of chamber enlargement or abnormal heart sounds.
- ECG often shows right bundle branch block.
- If the loss of thoracic inlet space is severe enough, tracheal compression may ensue and lead to dyspnoea. An additional cause of tracheal compression can be the brachiocephalic artery as it crosses the trachea in a narrowed space.
- Many patients have associated mitral valve prolapse.

IDIOPATHIC DILATATION OF PULMONARY ARTERY

- Dilatation of main pulmonary artery with or without dilatation of right and left pulmonary arteries.
- Majority are asymptomatic. Some may present with exertional dyspnoea, palpitation, fatigue and chest pain.
- ESM best heard at the second left intercostal space (pulmonary area). The murmur increases during inspiration. Compared to murmur of pulmonic stenosis, it is not transmitted to subclavicular or interscapular area.
- Pulsations in the second left intercostal space from the underlying dilated pulmonary artery.
- No signs of right ventricular hypertrophy.
- Ejection click at the pulmonary area.
- Pulmonary component (P_2) of the second heart sound may be loud. Split is generally fixed.
- No cardiac or extracardiac shunts.
- No chronic pulmonary disease.

Q. Discuss the differential diagnosis of pansystolic (holosystolic) murmurs (PSMs) over precordium. (IM 1.16)

- PSM starts immediately with the first heart sound and continues through to the second heart sound. Typically, it has a uniform intensity throughout (Fig. 7.74).

CAUSES

- Causes of pansystolic murmurs are given in Box 7.96.

DIFFERENTIAL DIAGNOSIS

- Diagnosis is based on the behaviour of the murmur and associated features.

MITRAL REGURGITATION

Murmur

- High-pitched, blowing, PSM best heard at the apex. It commonly radiates to axilla and back (left interscapular area) when the anterior mitral leaflet is predominantly involved. With predominant posterior mitral leaflet involvement, the murmur radiates to left sternal border and base of heart.
- It increases during expiration, sustained handgrip and transient exercise. The murmur is unchanged or decreases during inspiration.

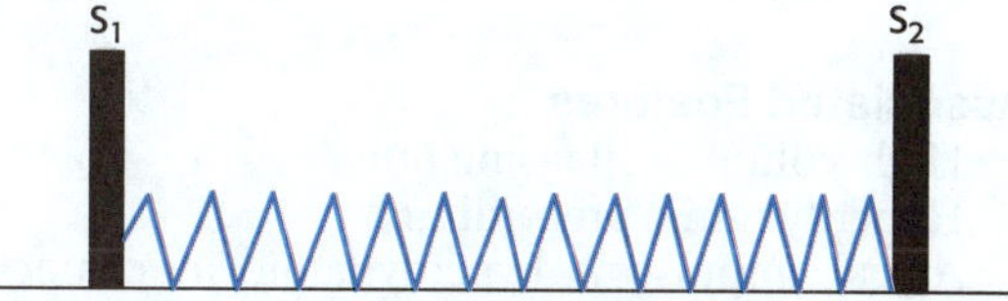

Fig. 7.74 Pansystolic murmur (PSM).

BOX 7.96 Causes of Pansystolic Murmur

• Mitral regurgitation (MR)	• Ventricular septal defect (VSD)
• Tricuspid regurgitation (TR)	• Aortopulmonary shunts (rare)

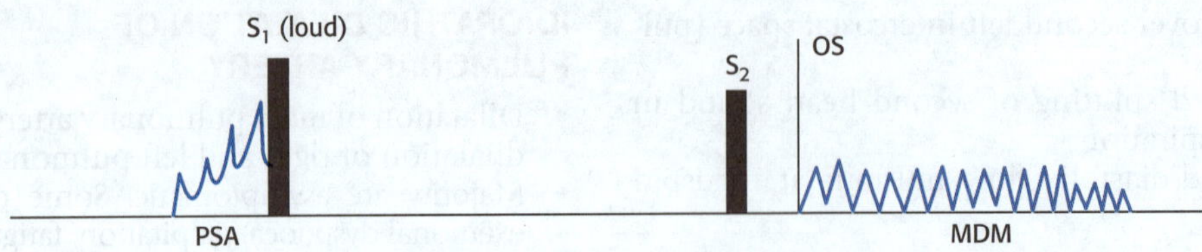

Fig. 7.75 Mid-diastolic murmur of mitral stenosis.

Associated Features

- High-volume collapsing pulse and wide pulse pressure.
- 'Rocking motion' of the precordium.
- Apical impulse is hyperdynamic in character and shifted down and out.
- Systolic thrill at the apex.
- First heart sound is soft.
- Second heart sound is widely split but mobile.
- Left ventricular third heart sound is common.
- Rumbling, mid-diastolic flow murmur at the apex in pure severe MR.

TRICUSPID REGURGITATION

Murmur

- Blowing PSM best heard at the lower left sternal border (tricuspid area), radiating to lower right sternal border or pulmonary area. It may be heard up to the apex but never beyond it. The murmur is intensified during inspiration and decreases during expiration (De-Carvallo's sign).

Associated Features

- JVP shows prominent *v* waves and rapid *y* descent.
- Hepatomegaly with systolic pulsations.
- Signs of pulmonary hypertension including functional TR.
- Rarely systolic thrill at lower left sternal border.
- Right ventricular third heart sound may be heard.
- Rumbling mid-diastolic flow murmur at lower left sternal border in pure severe TR.

VENTRICULAR SEPTAL DEFECT

Murmur

- Harsh PSM best heard at the third or fourth left intercostal space but radiating all over precordium. The murmur increases during transient exercise but is unchanged by respiration.

Associated Features

- High-volume collapsing pulse.
- Hyperdynamic precordium.
- Apical impulse is hyperdynamic in character and shifted down and out.
- Systolic thrill at the third or fourth left intercostal space.
- Second heart sound is widely split but mobile.
- Left ventricular third heart sound is common.
- Rumbling mid-diastolic flow murmur at the apex in large shunts.

Q. Discuss the differential diagnosis of mid-diastolic murmurs (MDMs). (IM 1.16)

Q. Briefly outline left atrial myxoma, Carey–Coombs murmur and Austin Flint murmur.

- Mid-diastolic murmur (MDM) is characterised by a short gap after the second heart sound, before the beginning of the murmur.
- MDM usually arises from the atrioventricular valves (mitral valve and tricuspid valve). It results from a disproportion between valve orifice size and flow rate. The classical MDM of mitral stenosis (MS) is shown in Figure 7.75.

CAUSES

- Causes of mid-diastolic murmur are given in Table 7.88.

DIFFERENTIAL DIAGNOSIS

- Diagnosis is based on the behaviour of the murmur and associated features.

MITRAL STENOSIS

Murmur

- MDM, often with a presystolic accentuation, well localised to the apex. It is low-pitched, rough and rumbling in character, best heard at the apex with the bell of the stethoscope with the patient in left

TABLE 7.88 Causes of Mid-Diastolic Murmur

At the Apex	At the Tricuspid Area

• **Organic**
  • Mitral stenosis (MS)
  • Rheumatic carditis (Carey–Coombs murmur)
  • Left atrial myxoma
  • Left atrial valve thrombus
• **Functional** (due to increased flow)
  • Aortic regurgitation (Austin Flint murmur)
  • Mitral regurgitation (MR)
  • Ventricular septal defect (VSD)
  • Persistent ductus arteriosus (PDA)
	• **Organic**
	  • Tricuspid stenosis (TS)
	• **Functional** (due to increased flow)
	  • Atrial septal defect (ASD)
	  • Severe tricuspid regurgitation (TR)

lateral position and during expiration. Murmur is accentuated by exercise carried out just before auscultation.

Associated Features

- Mitral facies.
- Tapping apical impulse with a diastolic thrill.
- Evidence of atrial fibrillation.
- Evidence of pulmonary hypertension.
- Loud first heart sound.
- Opening snap (OS).
- Loud pulmonary component (P_2) of second heart sound in pulmonary hypertension.
- Pansystolic murmur of tricuspid regurgitation (TR) in advanced cases with right ventricular dilatation.
- Early diastolic murmur of pulmonary regurgitation in advanced pulmonary hypertension.

CAREY–COOMBS MURMUR OF RHEUMATIC CARDITIS

Murmur

- Soft MDM, well localised to the apex without presystolic accentuation.

Associated Features

- Fever.
- Migratory polyarthritis.
- Subcutaneous nodules.
- Erythema marginatum.
- Chorea.
- S_1 normal.
- Evidence of myocarditis like tachycardia, third and fourth heart sounds, summation gallop, 'tic-tac' quality of heart sounds, arrhythmias and heart failure.
- Evidence of endocarditis like apical pansystolic murmur of mitral regurgitation (MR) and basal early diastolic murmur of aortic regurgitation (AR).
- Evidence of pericarditis like pericardial pain and pericardial friction rub.

LEFT ATRIAL MYXOMA

- Left atrial myxoma is a pedunculated, polypoidal, benign tumour arising from left atrium. It obstructs the mitral valve resulting in murmurs of stenosis or regurgitation. Diagnosis is by echocardiography and cardiac MRI. Surgical excision is required because of complications including sudden death.

Murmur

- MDM, often with a presystolic accentuation, best heard at the apex. The character and duration of the murmur vary from time to time or with a change in the position of the patient.

Associated Features

- Higher incidence in females.
- Systemic features like fever, fatigue, anaemia and weight loss are very common (in 90%).
- Systemic embolisation of tumour fragments or surface clots is common.
- Pulmonary hypertension and right heart failure can occur.
- First heart sound is loud.
- Pulmonary component (P_2) of the second heart sound is usually loud.
- 'Tumour plop' is an early diastolic sound.
- Apical systolic murmur from associated MR.
- Anaemia and increase in ESR, CRP and globulin levels.
- Features which differentiate atrial myxoma from mitral stenosis are shown in Box 7.97.

> **BOX 7.97** Differentiating Features Between Atrial Myxoma and Mitral Stenosis
>
> - Presence of constitutional symptoms, persistence of sinus rhythm, shorter duration of illness and changing character of murmur with posture and time differentiate left atrial myxoma from rheumatic mitral stenosis.

AUSTIN FLINT MURMUR OF AORTIC REGURGITATION

Murmur

- Rumbling MDM without a presystolic accentuation even in the presence of sinus rhythm. It is best heard at the apex. It is separate from early diastolic murmur of AR.

Associated Features

- Peripheral signs of AR
- Hyperdynamic precordium.
- Hyperdynamic apical impulse that is shifted down and out.
- Left ventricular third heart sound.
- Early diastolic murmur of AR in the Erb's area (third intercostal space on the left sternal border) or aortic area.
- Aortic ejection systolic murmur due to increased flow.

MITRAL REGURGITATION, VENTRICULAR SEPTAL DEFECT AND PERSISTENT DUCTUS ARTERIOSUS

- These conditions are associated with an increased flow of blood across the mitral valve, resulting in a MDM.

Murmur

- Rumbling MDM, best heard at the apex.

Associated Features

- All these conditions result in a hyperdynamic apex that is shifted down and out, and left ventricular third heart sound.
- MR
  - Systolic thrill at apex.
  - Soft first heart sound.
  - Pansystolic murmur at apex radiating to axilla and back.
- VSD
  - Systolic thrill at third or fourth left intercostal space.
  - Widely split, but mobile second heart sound.
  - Pansystolic murmur maximal at third or fourth left intercostal space and radiating all over precordium.

- PDA
  - Continuous thrill at the upper left sternal edge.
  - Continuous 'machinery murmur' with late systolic accentuation at the upper left sternal edge.

TRICUSPID STENOSIS

Murmur

- MDM, often with a presystolic accentuation, best heard at the lower left sternal border (tricuspid area). The murmur increases during inspiration (De-Carvallo's sign).

Associated Features

- Refractory oedema and ascites.
- Hepatomegaly with presystolic pulsations.
- Raised jugular venous pressure with prominent *a* waves (giant *a* waves) and slow *x* descent.
- Loud first heart sound and tricuspid OS

ATRIAL SEPTAL DEFECT AND TRICUSPID REGURGITATION

- These conditions are associated with an increased flow of blood across the tricuspid valve, resulting in MDM.

Murmur

- Rumbling MDM, best heard at the lower left sternal border (tricuspid area).

Associated Features

- ASD:
  - Hyperdynamic precordium.
  - Pulsations in the second left intercostal space.
  - Wide and fixed splitting of second heart sound.
  - Ejection systolic murmur at the second left intercostal space (pulmonary area).
- TR:
  - Hepatomegaly with systolic pulsations.
  - Raised jugular pressure with prominent *v* waves and rapid *y* descent.
  - Blowing pansystolic murmur at the lower left sternal border which is intensified during inspiration.

Q. Enumerate the common causes of continuous murmurs. (IM 1.16)

- Continuous murmurs begin in systole, peak near second heart sound and continue into diastole (Fig. 7.76).

BOX 7.98 Causes of Continuous Murmur

CONTINUOUS MURMURS

- Patent ductus arteriosus (upper left sternal edge)
- Surgically produced shunts in tetralogy of Fallot (right or left or upper sternum)
- Systemic arteriovenous fistula (directly over the fistula)
- Coarctation of aorta (posteriorly over the spine and lateral chest wall)
- Pulmonary arteriovenous fistula (over lower lobe or right middle lobe of lung)
- Coronary arteriovenous fistula (apicosternal region)
- Anomalous origin of the left coronary artery from the pulmonary artery
- Rupture of aneurysm of sinus of Valsalva (fourth left intercostal space)
- Jugular venous hum (medial aspect of the right supraclavicular fossa)
- Mammary souffle (right or left sternal border, from second to fourth intercostal spaces)

CAUSES

- Causes of continuous murmur are given in Box 7.98.

Q. Write a brief note on innocent murmurs.

Q. Describe briefly about venous hum (jugular venous hum; cervical venous hum).

Q. Explain mammary souffle.

- Innocent murmurs are those not due to recognisable lesions of the heart or blood vessels. They are most common in children and adolescents.

WHAT NOT IS AN INNOCENT MURMUR?

- There are some murmurs or associated features which should not be considered innocent (Box 7.99).

TYPES OF INNOCENT MURMURS

- Pulmonary ejection murmur:
  - Originates in the right ventricular outflow area to the pulmonary arteries.
  - It is high pitched and is best heard with diaphragm of stethoscope in the second left intercostal space

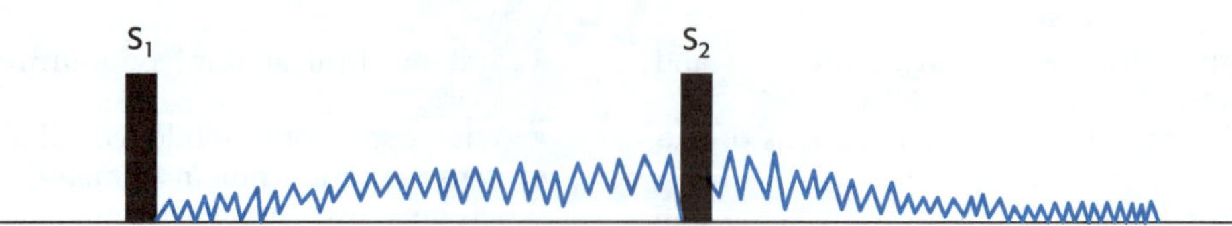

Fig. 7.76 Continuous murmur.

BOX 7.99 Features Suggesting a Murmur to Be Not an Innocent Murmur

- Diastolic murmurs
- Loud murmurs, grade IV or above
- Regurgitant (pansystolic) murmurs
- Murmurs associated with a click
- Murmurs associated with other signs or symptoms (e.g. cyanosis)
- Abnormal second heart sound (fixed split or single)

(pulmonary area) with radiation to lower left sternal border and apex.
  - The murmur is usually ejection systolic and is heard at the beginning of systole or mid-systole. It is louder on lying down and held expiration. It is heard more clearly in situations of increased cardiac output such as fever, anxiety, acute disease and postexercise; it decreases with the Valsalva manoeuvre and standing position.
  - In contrast to pulmonary valvular stenosis, there is no ejection click or thrill.
  - Most common in children and adolescents aged between 8 and 14 years, particularly those with pectus excavatum or kyphoscoliosis.
- Vibratory murmur or Still's murmur:
  - Found in many school-age children.
  - Best heard at the lower left sternal border or apex with wide radiation.
  - The murmur is usually ejection systolic or early systolic with a musical or twanging quality. It increases with the patient lying down and decreases in the erect posture. The murmur might disappear on extension of the neck.
  - It results from changes in flow produced by passage from the left ventricle to the aorta. However, exact pathogenesis is not clear.
- Supraclavicular arterial bruit:
  - Best heard on the right side of the neck and louder above the clavicle than below it.
  - The murmur is usually ejection systolic or early systolic. It increases with slight compression of subclavian artery and decreases or disappears with marked compression of the subclavian artery and hyperextension of shoulder.
  - This murmur is mostly found in adolescents and young adults and is low-pitched and of low intensity, sometimes associated with slight neck thrill.
- Venous hum (jugular venous hum; cervical venous hum):
  - Best heard with the bell at the root of the neck over the medial part of supraclavicular fossa (just lateral to sternocleidomastoid) with the head turned in the opposite direction. It is more common on the right side.
  - The murmur is continuous murmur that increases on sitting up. It decreases on lying down and is obliterated by compression of internal jugular vein, and by turning neck towards the side of murmur.
  - It originates where jugular, subclavian and brachiocephalic veins join the superior vena cava.
  - Mainly detected in children aged between 3 and 8 years.
- Mammary souffle:
  - Best heard at the right or left sternal border, extending from second to fourth intercostal spaces.
  - The murmur is a continuous murmur with systolic accentuation. It occurs in late pregnancy and during lactation. The murmur is obliterated by firm pressure with the stethoscope. It is due to increased blood flow to breast tissue and disappears after lactation.

Q. How do you differentiate bronchial asthma from cardiac asthma?

- Cardiac asthma has been defined as wheezing, coughing and orthopnoea due to congestive heart failure. It should be differentiated from bronchial asthma (Table 7.89).

TABLE 7.89 Features Differentiating Between Bronchial Asthma and Cardiac Asthma

Bronchial Asthma	Cardiac Asthma
• Longer duration of breathlessness	• Shorter duration of breathlessness
• Usually occurs in early morning hours	• Usually occurs 2–3 hours after sleep
• Scanty whitish sputum	• Copious pink frothy sputum
• No cardiomegaly	• Cardiomegaly may be present
• No third heart sound	• Third heart sound is heard
• Evidence of pulmonary disease	• Evidence of cardiac disease
• Predominantly rhonchi	• Starts with fine basal crepitations
• Usually relieved by bronchodilators	• Usually relieved by sitting up or diuretics
• Chest X-ray shows hyperinflation and normal heart size	• Chest X-ray shows cardiomegaly and other evidence of pulmonary oedema
• Electrocardiogram is usually normal	• Electrocardiogram is usually abnormal

MCQs

IM2.4

1. A 56-year-old man with a history of a throbbing sensation in the abdomen suffered severe abdominal and lumbar pain and collapsed. He was transferred to the emergency room where his death was certified. A rupture of an abdominal aortic aneurysm and multiple atherosclerotic plaques along the thoracic and abdominal aorta was observed during the necropsy. Which of the following cells played an important role in the genesis of this abdominal aortic aneurysm?
   A. Smooth muscle cells
   B. Macrophages
   C. Foam cells
   D. Platelets

E. All of the previous options

Ans: E. All of the previous options

The pathogenesis of atherosclerosis involves a chronic inflammatory response to endothelial cell injury. This results in endothelial dysfunction resulting in increased expression of leucocyte adhesion molecules. Circulating monocytes adhere to the altered endothelium, followed by migration to the intima where they become macrophages. Macrophages (B response) pick up and oxidise the filtered LDL. Macrophages charged with lipids become foam cells (C response) forming part of the atheroma. Activated macrophages secrete growth factors and inflammatory cytokines that promote the proliferation of other cell types within the atherosclerotic lesion. Platelets (D response) adhere to the damaged endothelium. Activated platelets release PDGF, which stimulates smooth muscle cells (A response) to migrate to the intima, where they proliferate and synthesise extracellular matrix.

IM2.4

2. A 60-year-old man with a history of elevated serum LDL and C-reactive protein suffers an acute myocardial infarction and dies before the ambulance sent arrives. Which of the following cells has contributed most to the pathogenesis of the vascular disease that led to his myocardial infarction?
   A. B lymphocytes
   B. Plasma cells
   C. Macrophages
   D. Mast cells
   E. Eosinophils

Ans: C. Macrophages

The pathogenesis of atherosclerosis that has led to the patient's myocardial infarction entails a chronic inflammatory response to the injury. The focal endothelial lesion is the first event that causes the recruitment of monocytes in the altered endothelium, followed by their migration to the tunica intima, where they become macrophages. Macrophages pick up and oxidise filtered LDL. Macrophages charged with lipids become foamy cells that form part of the atheroma. Activated macrophages secrete growth factors and inflammatory cytokines that promote the proliferation of other cell types within the atherosclerotic lesion. Option A is incorrect. B lymphocytes are not known to be involved in the pathogenesis of atherosclerotic inflammation. Option B is incorrect. Plasma cells are B lymphocytes secreting antibodies, which play no role in the pathogenesis of atherosclerosis. Option D is incorrect. Mast cells are important actors in the pathogenesis of type I hypersensitivity reactions. They are not known to contribute to atherogenesis. Option E is incorrect. Like mast cells, eosinophils play an important role in the pathogenesis of type I hypersensitivity reactions. They are also involved in the death of helminths. They are not known to contribute to atherogenesis.

IM1.15

3. A 58-year-old patient presents with a history of a heart murmur. He has had a history of palpitations and progressive dyspnoea for the last 3 years. On examination: blood pressure 140/40 mmHg, heart rate 102 bpm, apex shifted to the left and down. An early decrescendo diastolic murmur is heard in the aortic area. What entity will we suspect?
   A. Pulmonary regurgitation
   B. Mitral stenosis secondary to rheumatic fever
   D. Aortic stenosis
   C. Aortic insufficiency
   E. Dilated cardiomyopathy

Ans: C. Aortic insufficiency

4. Following statement is true regarding a 76-year-old hypertensive patient with persistent atrial fibrillation:
   A. Must be anticoagulated with oral anticoagulants
   B. Must be anticoagulated with oral anticoagulants only if heart rate is above 110/minute
   C. Must receive antiplatelet agents
   D. The patient should only be anticoagulated if he/she has had a history of embolism
   E. The patient should not receive antiplatelet or anticoagulant treatment because of increased risk of bleeding in elderly patients

Ans: A. Must be anticoagulated with oral anticoagulants

As per CHA_2DS_2-VASc score, age ≥75 years is an embolic risk factor in patients with atrial fibrillation. Arterial hypertension is also a second factor. So the indication for chronic anticoagulation treatment is clear in this patient.

IM2.17

IM1.25

5. A 55-year-old patient, after suffering an extensive previous infarction with severe secondary systolic dysfunction, presents minimal effort dyspnoea despite maximum medical treatment and no possibility of revascularisation. What other therapeutic possibilities could you offer him?
   A. Pacemaker implantation
   B. Cardiac transplantation
   C. Coranary artery bypass graft
   D. Valve replacements
   E. None of the above

Ans: B. Cardiac transplantation

In patients with refractory heart failure despite correct medical treatment and no possibility of aetiological treatment, heart transplantation is the only treatment that has been shown to strongly modify the prognosis.

IM1.24

6. A heart failure (HF) patient with minimal effort dyspnoea has just started beta-blocker therapy. He comes to your clinic due to a worsening of his usual dyspnoea since he started treatment. Which of the following therapeutic options do you think is the most appropriate for this patient?
   A. Increasing the dose of diuretics
   B. Suspending the beta-blocker treatment as it is contraindicated in this patient with advanced HF
   C. Switching from beta-blocker treatment to digoxin
   D. Increasing the dose of beta-blocker
   E. They are all correct

Ans: A. Increasing the dose of diuretics

When starting the beta-blocker treatment in these patients, an initial clinical worsening is common; it should be controlled by increasing the diuretic dose.

IM8.8

7. A 78-year-old patient was hospitalised for heart failure for the first time. Chest X-ray shows interstitial oedema and absence of cardiomegaly. The blood pressure is 160/95 mmHg. Cardiovascular system examination does not reveal any murmurs. The electrocardiogram shows left ventricular hypertrophy. What do you think is the causal aetiology of heart failure?
   A. Ischaemic heart disease
   B. Senile aortic stenosis
   C. Hypertrophic cardiomyopathy
   D. Arterial hypertension
   E. Atrial septal defect

Ans: D. Arterial hypertension

The most frequently observed aetiology in elderly patients hospitalised for heart failure is high blood pressure. The presence of hypertrophy in the electrocardiogram, absence of cardiomegaly and high blood pressure support this aetiology. The absence of murmurs and ischaemic changes on ECG rules out other pathologies.

IM1.1

8. A 56-year-old man presents with breathlessness. On examination, his pulse is irregularly irregular at 110 beats/minute. Blood pressure is 150/67 mmHg. Auscultation of his heart reveals a pansystolic murmur loudest at the apex which radiates to the axilla. What is the most likely diagnosis?
   A. Mitral regurgitation
   B. Mitral valve prolapse
   C. Atrial septal defect
   D. Aortic regurgitation
   E. Severe aortic stenosis

Ans: A. Mitral regurgitation

A pansystolic murmur loudest at the apex, which radiates to the axilla, is classical of mitral regurgitation. Chronic mitral regurgitation is usually due to rheumatic heart disease or due to left ventricular dilatation such as in hypertensive heart disease or ischaemia.

IM1.1

9. A 32-year-old woman attends a cardiology clinic for routine review. Auscultation of her heart reveals a mid to late systolic murmur with an initial click. The murmur increases in intensity with Valsalva manoeuvre. There are no signs of heart failure. What is the most likely diagnosis?
   A. Mitral regurgitation
   B. Mitral valve prolapse
   C. Atrial septal defect
   D. Aortic regurgitation
   E. Severe aortic stenosis

Ans: B. Mitral valve prolapse

Mitral valve prolapse is a relatively common condition, particularly in tall people and can be associated with conditions such as polycystic kidney disease. A mid to late systolic murmur with an initial mid-systolic click will be heard.

IM2.11

10. A 45-year-old woman has been admitted after an episode of chest pain lasting for 20 minutes that resolved with sublingual nitrate. Her three ECGs are normal. At what time interval will the troponin peak?
    A. 3–6 hours
    B. 6–9 hours
    C. 9–12 hours
    D. 12–18 hours
    E. 18–36 hours

Ans: E. 18–36 hours

IM2.23

11. A 55-year-old man presents with sudden onset central chest pain for 30 minutes. He is treated with oxygen, aspirin 300 mg and sublingual nitrate. His pain settled in 5 minutes and is admitted for observation. He has no ECG changes. After about an hour, he again developed chest pain. His repeat ECG remains unchanged. What is the most appropriate next step?
    A. Morphine 2.5 mg IV
    B. Streptokinase
    C. Nitroglycerine infusion
    D. Further aspirin 75 mg
    E. Metoprolol 5 mg IV

Ans: C. Nitroglycerine infusion

IV nitroglycerine is an effective treatment for the pain of coronary ischaemia.

IM2.16

12. A 65-year-old man presents to his local teaching hospital with a 2-hour history of chest pain and breathlessness. On examination, he is diaphoretic and tachycardic at 110 beats/minute. His blood pressure is 100/60 mmHg. Auscultation of his chest reveals basal crepitations and his SpO_2 on room air is 93%. His 12-lead ECG is shown below. What is the most appropriate step?

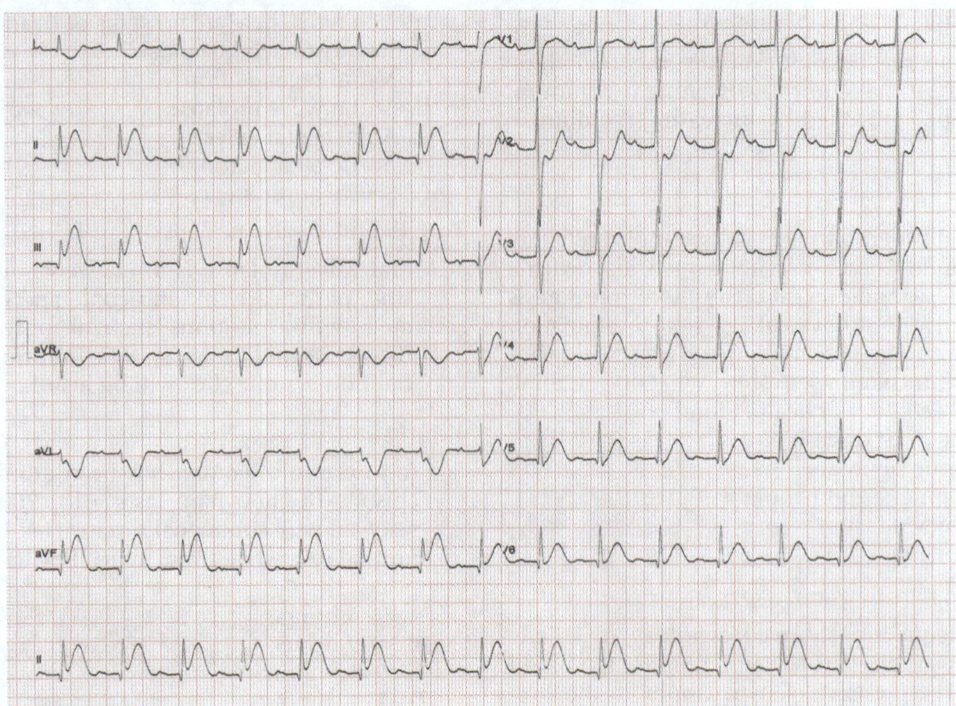

A. Furosemide 40 mg IV
B. Nitroglycerine infusion
C. Alteplase
D. Primary percutaneous coronary intervention
E. Dobutamine

Ans: D. Primary percutaneous coronary intervention

Urgent PCI with stenting or angioplasty to the lesion is indicated.

IM2.13

13. A 16-year-old man presents with a 2-day history of sharp central pain relieved by sitting forward. An ECG shows widespread ST segment elevation except in aVR and V_1. Which is the most appropriate next investigation?
    A. Echocardiogram
    B. Stress test
    C. Troponin
    D. Chest X-ray
    E. CT chest

Ans: A. Echocardiogram

Pericarditis is the most likely diagnosis here. An echocardiogram will help elucidate the presence of an associated pericardial effusion. Most cases are viral and require supportive treatment only.

14. A 28-year-old girl on the oral contraceptive presents with sudden-onset breathlessness and central chest pain. On examination, she is tachycardic with SpO_2 of 89% on room air and blood pressure of 100/60 mmHg. Which is the most appropriate next investigation?
    A. Echocardiogram
    B. D-Dimer
    C. Troponin
    D. Chest X-ray
    E. CT pulmonary angiography

Ans: E. CT pulmonary angiography

D-dimer testing may be useful in low to moderate risk patients to exclude pulmonary embolism. Where the risk is high, clinicians should move directly onto imaging.

IM2.11

15. A 55-year-old woman with a history of dyslipidaemia and hypertension presents with a 2-hour history of chest heaviness which was relieved with sublingual nitrate. Serial ECGs are normal. Which is the most appropriate next investigation?
    A. Echocardiogram
    B. D-Dimer
    C. Troponin
    D. Chest X-ray
    E. CT chest

Ans: C. Troponin

This is suggestive of cardiac ischaemia. Troponins are sensitive markers of myocardial damage.

16. A 66-year-old woman presents with syncope while climbing the stairs. There was no aura or prodrome. Examination reveals an ejection systolic murmur at the left sternal edge. Which is the most appropriate next investigation?
    A. Echocardiogram
    B. ECG
    C. Lying and standing blood pressure
    D. Electroencephalogram
    E. Tilt testing

Ans: A. Echocardiogram

The likely diagnosis is aortic stenosis and an echocardiogram is required to investigate this. Syncope is an indication for valve replacement.

IM2.4

17. A 60-year-old man complains of sudden-onset palpitations while an inpatient in the coronary care unit 2 days after an acute myocardial infarction. His pulse is 145 and regular and his blood pressure is 110/70 mmHg. ECG shows a broad-complex tachycardia. What is the most likely diagnosis?
    A. Supraventricular tachycardia
    B. Atrial flutter
    C. Complete heart block
    D. Ventricular tachycardia
    E. Sinus tachycardia

Ans: D. Ventricular tachycardia

Ventricular tachycardia (VT) is a serious broad-complex tachycardia. It may occur during cardiac arrest and is a shockable rhythm. A VT with pulse may also occur, commonly after damage to the heart or ischaemia, for example after an acute myocardial infarction. A VT with pulse may be treated with amiodarone.

18. A 26-year-old primigravida 36 weeks into her first pregnancy presents to the Emergency Department complaining of sudden onset breathlessness and chest pain. On arrival, she is in extremis: her pulse is 140 beats/minute, blood pressure 70/40 mmHg and SpO_2 88% on high flow oxygen. Auscultation of her chest reveals normal air entry in all lung fields with no additional sounds. Portable chest X-ray is normal. What is the most useful immediate investigation?
    A. D-dimer testing
    B. CT pulmonary angiography
    C. Transthoracic echocardiogram
    D. Full blood count
    E. Ventilation/perfusion scanning

Ans: C. Transthoracic echocardiogram

The main differential in this situation is an acute pulmonary embolism. This patient is clearly unstable and not in a position to be moved to radiology. An echo may demonstrate right heart dysfunction and add weight to the diagnosis. Based on echo findings, patient may be thombolysed.

IM1.24

19. A 65-year-old woman has been admitted for the third time in 3 months with decompensated cardiac failure. She has a past history of atrial fibrillation and hypertension. She is on furosemide 40 mg daily. Her pulse is 65 beats/minute and blood pressure 148/95 mmHg. Her echo shows an ejection fraction of 35%. Blood tests show Na^+ 142 mmol/L, K^+ 4.1 mmol/L, urea 32 mg/dL and creatinine 1.0 mg/dL. What medication should be added next?
    A. Beta-blocker
    B. Angiotensin receptor-neprilysin inhibitor
    C. ACE-inhibitor
    D. Angiotensin receptor blocker
    E. Calcium channel blocker

Ans: B. Angiotensin receptor-neprilysin inhibitor

ARNI is the first choice in the treatment of heart failure with reduced ejection fraction.

20. A 65-year-old gentleman is admitted for an open oesophagectomy. The anaesthetist places a central line into his right internal jugular vein. Immediately following the procedure, he develops tachycardia and tachypnoea. A chest X-ray is normal. Heart sounds are inaudible. He worsens and suffers a cardiac arrest with a nonshockable rhythm. What is the most appropriate next intervention?
    A. Pericardiocentesis
    B. Bilateral needle thoracentesis
    C. External pacing
    D. Lidocaine
    E. Amiodarone

Ans: A. Pericardiocentesis

Risks from central venous cannulation include pneumothorax, cardiac tamponade and dysrhythmias due to mechanical irritation by the wire. Since this patient had inaudible heart sounds, likely diagnosis is cardiac tamponade.

21. A 30-year-old woman is admitted with sudden onset of palpitations. On arrival in the Emergency Department, she is tachycardic with a pulse of 150 beats/minute. Her blood pressure is 130/65 mmHg. An ECG shows supraventricular tachycardia. What is the most appropriate initial drug treatment?
    A. Digoxin
    B. Propranolol
    C. Overdrive pacing
    D. Amiodarone
    E. Adenosine

Ans: E. Adenosine

IM1.24

22. A 35-year-old man presents with a history of erectile dysfunction for the last 3 months. He was diagnosed with hypertension 6 months ago for which he takes some medication. What is the most likely diagnosis for his erectile dysfunction?
    A. Psychogenic
    B. Beta-blocker medication
    C. Injury to penile nerve supply
    D. Peripheral vascular disease
    E. Varicocele

Ans: B. Beta-blocker medication

One of the adverse drug effects of β-blockers is that they can cause erectile dysfunction.

23. A 74-year-old man presented with a 6-month history of exertional chest pain radiating down his left arm. He described dull aches when pushing himself up at a fast pace once or twice a month. His past medical history included hypertension, benign prostate hyperplasia and osteoarthritis. He was taking losartan, tamsulosin and paracetamol. Clinical examination was unremarkable. What is the next most appropriate management of this patient?
    A. Arrange an exercise treadmill test and start him on a statin and aspirin
    B. Start patient on aspirin, statin, arrange an outpatient myocardial perfusion scan, stress

echocardiogram or stress cardiac MRI and reassess in a few weeks' time
C. Reassure him that this is atypical chest pain and discharge him from care
D. Arrange urgent outpatient coronary angiography and start him on a statin
E. Start him on aspirin, a statin and antianginal medication and reassess him in few weeks

Ans: E. Start him on aspirin, a statin and antianginal medication and reassess him in few weeks

This patient is presenting with a history suggestive of typical angina on effort, having been stable for several months and not treated with any antianginal or secondary prevention medication.

IM2.19|PA27.5

24. A 58-year-old woman presented with collapse and chest discomfort. She had been having an argument with a colleague and had felt unwell before losing consciousness which lasted for 5 minutes. On clinical examination, her heart rate was 100 beats/minute, and blood pressure was 100/60 mmHg. Investigations: ECG demonstrated ST elevation in anterior leads. Troponin was moderately elevated. An emergency coronary angiography was pefoshowed unobstructed coronary arteries. Left ventriculogram demonstrated regional wall motion abnormalities in the left ventricle primarily affecting the apex with hyperdynamic wall motion near the valves. What is the most likely diagnosis?
A. Coronary dissection
B. Coronary vasospasm
C. Takotsubo's cardiomyopathy
D. Thrombotic embolisation
E. ST elevation myocardial infarction with spontaneous recanalisation

Ans: C. Takotsubo's cardiomyopathy

This patient presented with changes of ST elevation myocardial infarction associated with chest pains and collapse after an emotional encounter. Unobstructed coronaries and the left ventriculogram changes are pathognomonic of Takotsubo's cardiomyopathy, which is commoner in women. ST elevation and increased troponin levels will be seen, and in the acute phase, there is a drop in cardiac output with clinical consequences of low blood pressure and possibly heart failure. ECGs, troponin levels and heart failure gradually return to normal with supportive management as the myocardium invariably recovers.

IM2.19

25. A 48-year-old man developed acute central chest pain 6 hours after admission to a medical ward. He had been admitted with a 2-week history of feeling feverish and unwell. He had a history of aortic valve replacement. On clinical examination, his temperature was 38.8°C, heart rate 120 beats/minute, and blood pressure was 134/88 mmHg. There was a diastolic murmur to the right of the sternum. The ECG demonstrated an anterior ST elevation myocardial infarction. What is the likely cause of the acute coronary syndrome?
A. Coronary dissection
B. Coronary vasospasm
C. Coronary embolisation
D. Plaque rupture
E. Plaque shift

Ans: C. Coronary embolisation

Infective endocarditis should be considered in any patient with a fever and a prosthetic valve. Embolisation occurs in many sites, including down a coronary artery. This would manifest as acute coronary syndrome and ST elevation myocardial infarction. Embolic phenomena in endocarditis carries a high risk and should prompt urgent cardiothoracic surgical referral.

26. A 65-year-old man presented with recurrent episodes of palpitations. He had no previous significant medical history. On clinical examination, his heart rate was 165 beats/minute and regular. Blood pressure was 148/90 mmHg. ECG confirmed SVT and adenosine reverts him to sinus rhythm. What is the most appropriate first-line therapy to consider?
A. Pacemaker
B. Flecainide
C. Ablation therapy
D. Anticoagulation
E. Digoxin

Ans: C. Ablation therapy

While there are many possible therapies for SVT, in general, all causes are amenable to ablation with a high chance of success and a low risk of complication.

IM1.1

27. A 73-year-old man presented with a 3-month history of increasing shortness of breath on exertion. He had a myocardial infarction 5 years previously. On clinical examination, there was moderate ankle oedema. Heart rate was 105 beats/minute and irregular, jugular venous pressure was raised 7 cm and blood pressure was 108/72 mmHg. Heart sounds were normal, but a grade 2/6 pansystolic murmur was audible in the mitral area. Which of the following hormonal abnormalities are likely in this situation?
A. Low plasma aldosterone
B. Low plasma angiotensin ll
C. Low plasma antidiuretic hormone
D. High plasma natriuretic peptide
E. High plasma tumour necrosis factor-α

Ans: D. High plasma natriuretic peptide

Natriuretic peptides are elevated in HF, unless the syndrome is very mild and the patient is on optimal therapy.

IM1.24

28. A 78-year-old woman presented with a 3-hour history of swollen lips and face but no wheeze. She

had recently been found to have severe nonischaemic cardiomyopathy. She had been advised to take furosemide, digoxin, ramipril, eplerenone and carvedilol. On clinical examination, she had swollen lips and face. Heart rate was 84 beats/min and blood pressure was 134/90 mmHg. There was no other abnormality. Which drug is the most likely cause of her presentation?

A. Carvedilol
B. Digoxin
C. Eplerenone
D. Furosemide
E. Ramipril

Ans: E. Ramipril

This is angioedema (as opposed to anaphylaxis, in which case the patient would appear much sicker and the onset would be more rapid), and ACE inhibitors are a well-recognised cause of this.

IM1.15

29. A 14-year-old child presented with persistent headaches. On clinical examination, his blood pressure (right arm) was 140/96 mmHg. There was a soft ejection systolic murmur heard between the scapulae. The femoral pulses were much weaker than the radial pulses. Oxygen saturations were 100%. What is the most likely diagnosis?
   A. Tetralogy of Fallot
   B. Ventricular septal defect
   C. Aortic stenosis
   D. Patent ductus arteriosus
   E. Coarctation of the aorta

Ans: E. Coarctation of the aorta

There is upper body hypertension with weak distal pulses resulting from coarctation of the aorta. None of the other diagnoses would present with weak femoral pulses compared to the radial pulses.

IM2.19

30. A 56-year-old man developed acute severe central chest pain and was attended by ambulance paramedics. On clinical examination, his heart rate was 96 beats/minute, and blood pressure was 148/88 mmHg. A 12-lead ECG showed ST segment elevation in V1-V4. A diagnosis of acute ST elevation myocardial infarction was made and it was decided to transport the patient to the nearest interventional cardiac centre. A cannula was placed in a peripheral vein before transport, and the patient's heart was monitored en route via defibrillator electrodes. When the ambulance was 5 km away from the hospital, the patient developed ventricular fibrillation, losing consciousness. The driver stopped the vehicle at the request of the paramedic. What is the best course of action?
   A. Commence chest compressions at a rate of 100/minute with asynchronous ventilation (10/minute)
   B. Defibrillate immediately
   C. Give two rescue breaths and then commence chest compressions
   D. Perform a precordial thump
   E. Turn on the sirens and blue lights and proceed to the hospital as quickly as possible

Ans: B. Defibrillate immediately

This is a patient who had a cardiac arrest witnessed by a highly trained healthcare professional and already had a defibrillator attached. Ventricular fibrillation occurring in the early stages of myocardial infarction is readily reversible by defibrillation. The priority is to defibrillate as soon as possible.

IM2.19

31. A 26-year-old woman presented to the Emergency Department following an intentional overdose of unknown quantities of some drug around 3 hours earlier. A resting ECG showed a heart rate of 64 bpm, with a QT interval of 498 msec. What action is likely to be required as a result of this finding?
   A. Insertion of a pacing wire
   B. Intravenous administration of magnesium
   C. Oral administration of activated charcoal
   D. Intravenous administration of sodium bicarbonate
   E. Intravenous administration of calcium gluconate

Ans: B. Intravenous administration of magnesium

The QT interval is prolonged and indicates that the patient is at risk of torsades de pointes arrhythmia. Treatment should include correction of any electrolyte imbalance, consideration of intravenous magnesium and monitoring for arrhythmia.

IM2.18|BI4.1

32. A 56-year-old woman presented with an abnormal fasting lipid profile on a routine health check. She was asymptomatic and clinical examination was normal. Investigations Serum total cholesterol 270 mg/dL, LDL 190 mg/dL, triglycerides 278 mg/dL. After excluding possible secondary causes, what is the best initial lipid-modulating therapy?
   A. A fibrate
   B. A statin
   C. A statin and a fibrate
   D. A bile acid sequestrant
   E. Hormone replacement therapy

Ans: B. A statin

This woman has a mixed dyslipidaemia as both total cholesterol and triglycerides are elevated. A statin would initially be best. Triglyceride concentrations can be expected to fall to some degree when cholesterol is reduced.

IM14.11|BI4.1

33. A 34-year old man presents concerns about his HDL-C. He has been informed previously 'that it is low' and wants to know how to improve it. Which of the following is known to increase HDL-C?
   A. A fibrate
   B. A statin
   C. Increased physical activity level
   D. β-adrenoceptor blockers

E. A bile acid sequestrant

Ans: C. Increased physical activity level

Increased physical activity, cessation of smoking, optimum diabetic control help to increase HDL cholesterol.

34. A 65-year-old man was admitted following a collapse. He reported at least half a dozen previous collapses with no warning. All had been in the standing position except two, which had occurred while he was reversing his car into a parking space. Two others had occurred while crossing the road. An eyewitness account described him 'just going down' with a quick recovery. His wife was extremely concerned about his risk of serious injury because of these collapses. His past medical history consisted of type 2 diabetes mellitus and he was taking metformin. He was otherwise well. Clinical examination was normal. There was no drop in blood pressure after standing. On investigation, a 12-lead ECG was normal. What is the most likely diagnosis?
   A. Carotid sinus hypersensitivity
   B. Cardiac arrhythmia
   C. Transient ischaemic attacks
   D. Epilepsy
   E. Vasovagal syncope

Ans: A. Carotid sinus hypersensitivity

Although a classic history of head-turning is rare, it is present here.

IM1.1

35. You are examining a 66-year-old woman with a past history of hypertension and dyslipidaemia. She is due for an abdominal hysterectomy. She describes a 12- month history of exertional breathlessness and one episode of syncope. On auscultation of his heart, you note the presence of an ejection systolic murmur at the left sternal edge. What is the most likely diagnosis?
   A. Mitral stenosis
   B. Mitral regurgitation
   C. Aortic stenosis
   D. Aortic regurgitation
   E. Atrial septal defect

Ans: C. Aortic stenosis

IM1.15

36. A 66-year-old hypertensive patient presents with sudden-onset sharp chest pain radiating to the back. Auscultation of his heart reveals an early diastolic murmur. What is the most likely diagnosis?
   A. Ventricular septal defect
   B. Pericarditis
   C. Thoracic aortic dissection
   D. Myocardial infarction
   E. Aortic stenosis

Ans: C. Thoracic aortic dissection

There is evidence of aortic incompetence but this is likely to be acute secondary to an aortic dissection. This requires emergency surgery and has a high mortality.

IM1.28

37. A 50-year-old woman presents with dyspnoea and fainting on exertion. On examination, she has blue fingertips and lips, jugular venous distension, oedema of the lower limbs. On auscultation of the heart, a harsh mid-systolic murmur is present. Chest X-ray shows a prominent pulmonary artery. Which of the following conditions is most likely present in this patient?
   A. Patent ductus arteriosus
   B. Tetralogy of Fallot
   C. Pulmonary stenosis
   D. Hypertrophic cardiomyopathy
   E. Patent foramen ovale

Ans: C. Pulmonary stenosis

Usually congenital or secondary to rheumatic fever. Associated with right heart failure (jugular venous distension, enlarged liver, peripheral oedema). Harsh mid-systolic ejection murmur heard in right, second intercostal space.

IM1.24

38. An 80-year-old woman is brought to the Emergency Department by a concerned neighbour after she is found wandering about her yard at 6 o' clock in the morning. Her comorbidities include heart failure, hypertension, osteoarthritis and type 2 diabetes, which is well-controlled. Her medications are gliclazide, metformin, digoxin, atenolol, frusemide and paracetamol. In the Emergency Department, she vomited several times and passed stools six times. Her pulse rate is 40 beats/minute and regular. Her blood pressure is 150/90 mmHg and blood glucose is 90 mg/dL. She also complains of blurred vision and seeing a yellow haze. Toxicity of which of her medications would explain her acute presentation?
   A. Gliclazide
   B. Atenolol
   C. Metformin
   D. Paracetamol
   E. Digoxin

Ans: E. Digoxin

This woman has overdosed on digoxin, most probably due to her declining cognitive function. Digoxin is a cardiac glycoside with negative chronotropic effects. This would explain the bradycardia. Digoxin overdose also results in nausea, vomiting, diarrhoea and disturbances of colour vision. The 'yellow haze' is typical but not always present.

IM1.15

39. A 24-year-old IV drug user presents to the Emergency Department with a fever for 7 days, lethargy and shortness of breath. Inflammatory markers are raised and a cardiac murmur is heard. Which murmur is most likely to have on auscultation?
   A. Ejection systolic murmur radiating to the neck
   B. Mid-diastolic murmur louder on inspiration
   C. Late-systolic murmur with mid-systolic click

D. Pansystolic murmur increasing on inspiration and loudest at left sternal edge
E. Systolic murmur loudest over apex and radiating to the axilla

Ans: D. Pansystolic murmur increasing on inspiration and loudest at left sternal edge

40. A 20-year-old man presents to the Emergency Department with a sprained ankle. An incidental ECG shows a right bundle branch block pattern with 'coved' ST elevation in V1-V3. What is the inferred ECG diagnosis in this case?
A. Bartter's syndrome
B. Brugada syndrome
C. Hypertrophic cardiomyopathy
D. Arrhythmogenic right ventricular cardiomyopathy
E. Wellens syndrome

Ans: B. Brugada syndrome

This inheritable condition accounts for part of a group of patients with idiopathic ventricular fibrillation who have no evidence of causative structural cardiac disease. It is more common in young male adults and in South East Asia. The diagnosis is made by identifying the classic ECG changes that may be present spontaneously or be provoked by the administration of a class I antiarrhythmic (flecainide or ajmaline): right bundle branch block with coved ST elevation in leads V1-V3. In 20% of cases, it is a monogenic inheritable condition associated with loss of sodium channel function due to a mutation in the SCN5A gene. Other mutations in the glycerol-3-phosphate dehydrogenase-1-like gene (GPD1LL-type) and genes related to calcium channel subunits (CACNA1C and CACNB2) have also been implicated in the genesis of this syndrome. It can present with sudden death during sleep, resuscitated cardiac arrest and syncope, or the patient may be asymptomatic and diagnosed incidentally or during familial assessment. There is a high risk of sudden death, particularly in the symptomatic patient or those with spontaneous ECG changes. The only successful treatment is an ICD. Beta-blockade is not helpful and may be harmful in this syndrome.

8 Diseases of the Gastrointestinal System

Q. What are the common causes of loss of appetite (anorexia)?

- Common causes of anorexia are given in Table 8.1.

Q. What are the common causes of persistent vomiting?

- Common causes of persistent vomiting are listed in Table 8.2.

Q. What are the causes of hiccough (or singultus) in an elderly male? Give the symptomatic treatment of hiccough.

- Hiccough is a phenomenon resulting from sudden spasmodic involuntary contraction of the diaphragm with the glottis remaining closed.

TABLE 8.1 Common Causes of Anorexia

Infections	Viral fever and pulmonary tuberculosis
Endocrine causes	Hypothyroidism, Addison's disease, hyperparathyroidism and panhypopituitarism
Liver diseases	Hepatitis and cirrhosis
Renal disease	Chronic renal disease
Malignancies	Carcinoma stomach, pancreas or any other malignancy; leukaemias, lymphomas
Psychiatric	Depression and anorexia nervosa
Miscellaneous	Heart failure

- Classified based on duration: hiccough bouts (up to 48 hours), persistent hiccoughs (48 hours to 1 month) and intractable hiccoughs (more than 1 month).
- Intractable hiccoughs can lead to malnutrition, weight loss, fatigue, dehydration, insomnia, psychological stress and decreased quality of life.
- Table 8.3 lists causes of hiccough.

TABLE 8.2 Common Causes of Persistent Vomiting

Acute abdominal emergencies	Acute appendicitis, acute pancreatitis, acute cholecystitis, intestinal obstruction, acute peritonitis
Gastro-oesophageal diseases	Gastro-oesophageal reflux, gastroparesis
Acute infections	Hepatitis, viral, bacterial and parasitic infestations of intestine
Central nervous system disorders	Raised intracranial tension, cerebral tumours, meningitis, encephalitis
Disorders of labyrinth or its connections	Acute migraine, acute labyrinthitis, Meniere's disease
Endocrine disorders	Diabetic ketoacidosis, adrenal crisis
Cardiac diseases	Congestive cardiac failure, acute myocardial infarction
Miscellaneous	Psychogenic vomiting, morning sickness of early pregnancy

TABLE 8.3 Causes of Hiccough

Habit of food ingestion	Hasty ingestion of food and fluids
Gastro-intestinal diseases	Gastro-oesophageal reflux, hiatus hernia, peptic ulcer disease
Irritation of the phrenic nerve	Tumours, pericarditis, mediastinitis, aortic aneurysm, surgery of thorax and abdomen
CNS disorders	Cerebrovascular accidents, encephalitis, brain tumours, multiple sclerosis
Local irritation of the diaphragm	Gaseous distension of stomach and intestines, subphrenic abscess, peritonitis, acute myocardial infarction
Electrolyte and metabolic disturbances	Hyponatraemia, hypokalaemia, hypocalcaemia, hypocapnia
Miscellaneous	Renal failure, hepatic failure, diabetic ketoacidosis, respiratory failure
Obscure	

SYMPTOMATIC TREATMENT

- Drinking cold water.
- Pressure over the eyeballs.
- Holding breath, Valsalva manoeuvre (produce hypercarbia).
- Pull on the tongue.
- Leaning forward, pulling knees to chest (both decrease diaphragmatic irritation).
- Local infiltration of phrenic nerve with procaine.
- Drug therapy:
  - Chlorpromazine 25–50 mg orally or intramuscularly.
  - Domperidone 10 mg thrice daily.
  - Metoclopramide 10 mg thrice daily.
  - Pantoprazole, omeprazole, lansoprazole, rabeprazole.
  - Xylocaine viscus 15 mL thrice a day.
  - Others—baclofen, gabapentin.

Q. Define constipation. What are the common causes of constipation? Discuss briefly about its management.

- Constipation—patients having bowel movements less frequently than three times a week. If stool is hard and difficult to pass, patient is constipated whatever be the frequency.

ROME IV CRITERIA FOR DEFINING CHRONIC, FUNCTIONAL CONSTIPATION (Box 8.1)

Box 8.1 ROME IV Criteria for Defining Chronic Functional Constipation

Following criteria for at least 12 weeks with onset ≥6 months:

- Presence of ≥2 of the following criteria:
  - Straining during ≥25% of defecations
  - Lumpy or hard stools in at least 25% of defecations
  - Sensation of incomplete evacuation for at least 25% of defecations
  - Sensation of anorectal obstruction or blockade for at least 25% of defecations
  - Digital evacuation to facilitate ≥25% of defecations
  - Fewer than three defecations per week
- Loose stools are rarely present without the use of laxatives.
- Insufficient criteria for irritable bowel syndrome.

CAUSES OF CHRONIC CONSTIPATION (Table 8.4)

TABLE 8.4 Causes of Chronic Constipation

Acute (<1 week)

Dehydration

Acute intestinal obstruction

Acute appendicitis

Chronic (>12 weeks)

I. Functional
   A. Rectal stasis
      - Faulty habits
      - Impaired consciousness
      - Painful anal area (anal fissure)
   B. Colonic stasis
      - Decreased food intake
      - Decreased fibre residue
   C. Irritable bowel syndrome (constipation-predominant)

II. Organic
   A. Endocrine and metabolic diseases
      - Myxoedema
      - Diabetes mellitus
      - Hypercalcaemia
      - Hyperparathyroidism
      - Hypokalaemia
   B. Myopathic diseases
      - Amyloidosis
      - Systemic sclerosis
      - Myotonic dystrophy
   C. Neurological diseases
      - Autonomic neuropathy
      - Cerebrovascular disease
      - Hirschsprung's disease
      - Multiple sclerosis
      - Parkinson's disease
      - Spinal cord diseases
   D. Structural diseases
      - Anal fissure
      - Haemorrhoids
      - Megacolon
      - Diverticulitis
   E. Psychological conditions
      - Depression
   F. Medications (antacids, anticholinergics, antidepressants, antihistamines, calcium, calcium channel blockers, clonidine, diuretics, iron, opioids)
   G. Others
      - Pressure on rectum from tumours or gravid uterus

INVESTIGATIONS

- Complete blood count, serum glucose, thyroid-stimulating hormone, calcium and creatinine levels.
- Stool examination including occult blood.

- Sigmoidoscopy or colonoscopy to exclude colon cancer in:
  - Patients older than 50 years.
  - Patients with concomitant rectal bleeding or weight loss.
  - Patients with haem-positive stools or iron-deficiency anaemia.
  - Family history of colonic cancer.
- Others—colonic transit time, anorectal manometry, balloon expulsion test and barium and magnetic resonance defaecography.

TREATMENT

- Eliminate offending medication.
- Treat underlying medical condition causing constipation.
- If no secondary cause of constipation identified, empirical treatment for functional constipation:
  - Nonpharmacological methods to improve bowel regularity.
  - Laxatives.

NON-PHARMACOLOGICAL TREATMENT

- Maintain a diary for stool frequency, consistency, size and degree of straining. Many patients incorrectly believe that they need to have a bowel movement every day.
- Patients should be educated on recognising and responding to the urge to defecate.
- Patients should be encouraged to attempt defecation first thing in the morning when the bowel is more active, and 30 minutes after meals to take advantage of the gastrocolic reflex.
- Patients should be encouraged to increase their intake of fibre-rich foods such as bran, fruits, vegetables and nuts.
- Adequate hydration.
- Patients should be encouraged to be as physically active as possible.

LAXATIVES

- Bulk laxatives:
  - Contain soluble (ispaghula or psyllium, pectin or guar) or insoluble (methyl cellulose) products.
  - Absorb water from intestinal lumen to increase stool mass and soften stool consistency.
  - Generally well tolerated.
  - Bloating and excessive gas production may be the adverse effects.
- Emollient laxatives (stool softeners):
  - Include docusate sodium and docusate calcium.
  - Act by lowering surface tension, allowing water to enter the bowel more readily.
  - Generally well tolerated.
  - Useful for patients with anal fissures or haemorrhoids that cause painful defecation.
- Mineral oil is not recommended because of potential to deplete fat-soluble vitamins and the risk of aspiration.
- Osmotic laxatives:
  - Hyperosmolar agents that cause secretion of water into the intestinal lumen by osmotic activity.
  - They include:
    - Magnesium hydroxide (milk of magnesia), magnesium citrate and sodium biphosphate, which are relatively safe, but may precipitate hypokalaemia, fluid and salt overload and diarrhoea. These are avoided in patients with congestive heart failure and chronic renal failure.
    - Sorbitol and lactulose that are metabolised by bacteria into hydrogen and organic acids. Poor absorption of these agents may lead to flatulence and abdominal distension.
    - Polyethylene glycol is a safe and effective laxative.
- Stimulant laxatives:
  - Include senna, castor oil, sodium picosulphate and bisacodyl (also available as suppository).
  - Increase intestinal motility and secretion of water and electrolytes into the bowel.
  - Continuous daily ingestion may produce hypokalaemia and protein-losing enteropathy.
- Serotonergic agents increase intestinal motility by acting on 5-HT4 receptors.
  - Prucalopride.
- Prosecretory agents:
  - Act by increasing fluid secretion into the intestinal lumen through direct action on intestinal epithelial cells.
  - Include linaclotide, lubiprostone and plecanatide.
  - Linaclotide is a minimally absorbed peptide agonist of the guanylate cyclase-C (GC-C) receptor that stimulates intestinal fluid secretion and transit. It reduces activation of colonic sensory neurons, thereby reducing pain, and activates colonic motor neurons, thereby increasing smooth muscle contraction and promoting bowel movements.
  - Lubiprostone activates chloride channels on the intestinal epithelial cells, thus secreting chloride and water into gut lumen. May be used in constipation-predominant irritable bowel syndrome (IBS).

OPIOID-INDUCED CONSTIPATION

- Peripherally acting μ-opioid receptor antagonists (PAMORAs) constitute a class of drugs which reverse opioid-induced constipation.
- They have very limited ability to cross the blood–brain barrier and thus they are able to antagonise peripheral but not central μ-opioid receptors. Therefore, they do not diminish the analgesic effect of opioid therapy.
- These include methyltrexone, naldemedine and naloxegol.

Q. Enumerate the common causes of acute diarrhoea in the tropics. (IM 16.1)

- Diarrhoea is described as three or more loose or watery stools a day.
- Acute diarrhoea is defined as an episode lasting less than 2 weeks.

CAUSES (Table 8.5)

TABLE 8.5 Causes of Acute Diarrhoea

Toxin-Induced Gastroenteritis	Gastroenteritis due to Changes in Mucosa

• Preformed toxins
  • *Staphylococcus aureus*
  • *Bacillus cereus*
  • Ciguatera fish poisoning[a]
  • Food borne botulism[a]
• Enterotoxins produced in the intestine
  • *Vibrio cholerae*
  • *Escherichia coli* (enterotoxigenic)
  • *Clostridium perfringens*
• *Clostridioides* (formerly *Clostridium*) *difficile* (antibiotic-associated diarrhoea)
	• Mucosal alteration without invasion
	  • Rotavirus
	  • Norovirus
	  • Adenovirus
	• Invasion of mucosa with destruction
	  • *Shigella*
	  • *E. coli* (enteroinvasive)
	  • *E. coli* (Enterohaemorrhagic or shiga toxin-producing E. coli—STEC)
	  • *Campylobacter*
	  • *Yersinia enterocolitica*
	  • *Salmonella*
	  • *Entamoeba histolytica*
	• Other causes
	  • Heavy metals (arsenic)
	  • Monosodium glutamate
	  • Mushrooms

[a]May present with predominant neurologic features with minimal GI features

Q. Enumerate the intestinal causes of chronic diarrhoea. (IM 16.1)

- Chronic diarrhoea is defined as one lasting longer than 2 weeks.

CAUSES (Table 8.6)

TABLE 8.6 Causes of Chronic Diarrhoea

1. Chronic enteric infections
  • *Salmonella*
  • *Streptococcus*
  • Fungi
  • Viruses
2. Parasitic causes
  • Amoebic colitis
  • Giardiasis
  • *Strongyloides stercoralis*
  • Trichuriasis
  • *Cryptosporidium*
  • *Microsporidium* (common in patients with AIDS)
  • *Isospora*
	3. Malabsorption syndrome
	4. Postoperative—enterocolostomy, gastrectomy
	5. Intestinal, biliary and gastric fistulae
	6. Pellagra
	7. Inflammatory bowel diseases
	  • Ulcerative colitis
	  • Crohn's disease
	8. Intestinal tuberculosis
	9. Diverticulitis
	10. Colonic neoplasms
	11. Colitis due to toxins—mercury, arsenic
	12. Laxative abuse
	13. Miscellaneous—hyperthyroidism, radiation injury, carcinoid, vipoma, HIV infection

Q. What is food poisoning?

- A foodborne disease outbreak where a cluster of two or more individuals develop similar symptoms following the ingestion of a common food.
- The most common form of food poisoning is gastroenteritis following consumption of food containing preformed toxin or organisms that produce toxin in the gut.
- Common causes have been listed above under 'common causes of acute diarrhoea' in Table 8.5.
- In case of ingestion of contaminated food having preformed toxin, the symptoms of acute upper gastrointestinal (UGI) upset (nausea and vomiting) start within 6 hours of ingestion. If the food contains organisms that produce toxin in the gut, the main feature is diarrhoea that usually develops within 6–72 hours of exposure.
- Botulism is also a type of food poisoning that does not produce symptoms of gastroenteritis.

Q. How will you evaluate and manage a patient with acute diarrhoea? (IM 16.11; IM 16.14; IM 16.2)

- Acute diarrhoea is defined as stool with increased water content, volume (at least 200 g/day) or frequency (at least thrice per day) that lasts <2 weeks.

EVALUATION OF A PATIENT WITH ACUTE DIARRHOEA

- Assess for:
  - Severity of dehydration.
  - Requirement for any diagnostic tests.
  - Any evident specific cause.
  - Requirement for any treatment.

HISTORY (Box 8.2)

BOX 8.2 Points to Be Asked in History in a Patient With Acute Diarrhoea

• Duration of diarrhoea • Stool volume • Frequency of loose stools • Appearance of stools (e.g. rice water) • Associated blood or mucus in the stools • Associated pain abdomen, fever • Associated with vomiting	• Urine output • Any change in the level of consciousness • Any other family member or close associate affected • History of having food outside in the recent past • Whether the patient is taking any antibiotics • Occupation of the patient

EXAMINATION

- Assess pulse, blood pressure (including postural change), skin turgor, dryness of mucous membranes, mental status and any acidotic breathing.
- Assess muscle strength and muscle reflexes as these may be reduced in hypokalaemia.
- Examine abdomen to exclude any surgical cause including intestinal obstruction.

LABORATORY INVESTIGATIONS

- Laboratory studies, in general, are usually not helpful in the acute management of a patient with diarrhoea as most cases are self-limiting.
- Specific diagnostic investigation may be required for patients with severe dehydration, persistent fever, bloody stool or immunosuppression, and for cases of suspected nosocomial infection or outbreak.

- A high leucocyte count with shift to the left suggests an invasive bacterial infection but may not always be present.
- Lactoferrin—a marker for leucocytes which is released by damaged cells and increases in the setting of bacterial infections.
- In patients with severe dehydration, check electrolytes and acid–base status. Severe diarrhoea produces metabolic acidosis.
- Obtain blood cultures when bacteraemia or a systemic infection is suspected.
- In severe cases, examine stool for the presence of leucocytes, red cells and cysts or trophozoites. Also look for the characteristic darting motility of *Vibrio cholerae* organisms.
- Stool culture if patient has grossly bloody stool, severe dehydration, signs of inflammatory disease, symptoms lasting more than 3–7 days or immunosuppression.
- *Clostridium difficile* toxins A and B for patients who develop unexplained diarrhoea after hospitalisation or during or after antibiotic use.

SEVERITY OF DEHYDRATION (Table 8.7)

TABLE 8.7 Severity of Dehydration

Features	Mild Dehydration	Moderate Dehydration	Severe Dehydration
• Urine output	Normal	Reduced	Markedly reduced
• Level of consciousness	Normal	Normal	Depressed
• Oral mucosa	Dry	Markedly dry	Parched
• Skin	Normal	Cool	Cool, mottled
• Skin turgor	Normal	Reduced	Markedly reduced
• Eyes	Normal	Sunken	Markedly sunken
• Pulse rate	Normal or mild increase	Tachycardia	Marked tachycardia
• Blood pressure	Normal	Postural drop or reduced	Shock
• Respiration	Normal	Normal	Acidotic
• Mental status	Normal or irritable	Lethargic	Comatose
• Urine specific gravity	<1.020	>1.020	>1.035
• Blood urea	Normal	Normal to raised	High

DIAGNOSIS

- Incubation period in a patient with toxigenic diarrhoea (usually associated with vomiting) is shorter (2–12 hours) as compared to that in inflammatory diarrhoea.
- Sudden onset in toxic diarrhoea while it is subacute in inflammatory diarrhoea.
- Presence of fever, severe abdominal tenderness or tenesmus suggests inflammatory colitis.
- Vomiting developing suddenly along with diarrhoea indicates toxin-mediated event. However, if other associated features like headache and fever are present, infection is likely.
- Diarrhoea with blood suggests *Shigella*, *Escherichia coli* or *Entemoeba histolytica* infection.
- If patient is previously on an antibiotic, consider *C. difficile* infection.
- Outbreaks indicate toxigenic cause.
- If stool does not have leucocytes, consider toxin-induced causes. If leucocytes are present or the illness continues, consider inflammatory causes (*Shigella*, *Salmonella*, *Campylobacter*, *E. coli*, *Entamoeba* and *C. difficile*).

SMALL BOWEL VERSUS LARGE BOWEL DIARRHOEA (Table 8.8)

TABLE 8.8 Small Bowel Versus Large Bowel Diarrhoea

Features	Small Bowel Diarrhoea	Large Bowel Diarrhoea
Volume of stools	• Large	• Frequent, small volume
Character of stools	• Watery without mucous; may have melaena; haematochezia absent	• Mucus often present; melaena absent; may be grossly bloody
Excessive flatulence	• Yes	• No

TABLE 8.8 Small Bowel Versus Large Bowel Diarrhoea—cont'd

Features	Small Bowel Diarrhoea	Large Bowel Diarrhoea
Associated abdominal features	• Cramping, bloating and gas formation	• Gripping pain in lower abdomen
Tenesmus	• No	• Often present
Urgency	• No	• Often present
Fever	• Uncommon	• Often present
Microscopy of stools	• Absence of inflammatory cells	• Red blood cells and inflammatory cells

MANAGEMENT

- Most cases are self-limiting and require fluid therapy only.

REHYDRATION

- Toxin-induced diarrhoea produces stools that are nearly isotonic. Sodium and chloride concentrations are slightly less than those in plasma while bicarbonate concentration is double that of plasma. The stools also contain significant amount of potassium.
- In inflammatory diarrhoea, the electrolyte loss is of less magnitude compared to toxigenic diarrhoea.
- Oral rehydration solution (ORS):
  - Exploits absorption of glucose-coupled sodium which remains intact even in severe diarrhoea.
  - Traditionally, ORS was prepared by adding 3.5 g of sodium chloride (three-fourth teaspoon of salt), 2.5 g of sodium bicarbonate (one teaspoon of baking soda) or 2.9 g of sodium citrate, 1.5 g of potassium chloride (one cup of orange juice or two bananas) and 20 g of glucose (four teaspoons of sugar) to 1 L of boiled water. Final solution contains 90 mmol of sodium, 20 mmol of potassium, 80 mmol of chloride, 30 mmol of bicarbonate and 111 mmol of glucose/L (osmolarity 331 mOsm/L).
  - Presently, ORS of lower osmolarity is used as it reduces stool output and vomiting, and also the need for intravenous rehydration as compared to standard ORS (Table 8.9). The final concentrations are sodium 75 mmol/L, chloride 65 mmol/L, potassium 20 mEq/L, glucose 75 mmol/L and citrate 10 mmol/L with an osmolarity of 245 mOsm/L.
- Intravenous fluids:
  - For moderate to severe dehydration.
  - Normal saline not ideal as it has no potassium and bicarbonate.
  - Ringer's lactate is usually administered.
  - In severe cases, fluids at a rate of 20 mL/kg/hour for the first 2–3 hours are administered. If the patient improves, reduce the rate to 10 mL/kg/hour for the next 2–4 hours.
  - Start concurrent oral rehydration therapy.

TABLE 8.9 Composition of ORS

Sodium chloride	2.6 g
Potassium chloride	1.5 g
Sodium citrate	2.9 g
Glucose	13.5 g

EARLY FEEDING

- Early refeeding decreases intestinal permeability caused by infections, reduces illness duration and improves outcomes.
- Many patients develop secondary lactose malabsorption; therefore, temporary avoidance of dairy products (except curd) is reasonable.

ADSORBENTS

- Kaolin may be useful in some patients as it adsorbs the toxin.
- Does not influence the course of the disease.

ANTIMOTILITY DRUGS

- Consider these agents for symptomatic treatment of toxin-induced diarrhoea in adults only.
- Can be given in inflammatory, nonbloody diarrhoea along with antibiotics.
- Should not be used in young children and elderly.
- Various agents are as follows:
  - Opiates (e.g. morphine and codeine). May produce respiratory depression.
  - Diphenoxylate/atropine combination. May produce respiratory depression and anticholinergic side effects.
  - Loperamide has the fewest side effects of all antimotility agents. Dose is two tablets of 4 mg each initially, and then 2 mg after each unformed stool, not to exceed 16 mg/day for ≤2 days.
  - Bismuth subsalicylate acts as an antisecretory agent and can provide effective clinical relief without significant side effects. Dose is one tablet every 30 minutes for a total of eight doses or 60 mL every 6 hourly.

ANTISECRETORY AGENTS

- Racecadotril:
  - Decreases hypersecretion of water and electrolytes into the intestinal lumen.
  - Inhibits enkephalinase, an enzyme that degrades enkephalins.
  - Dose is 100 mg TID.
  - Should be used in patients with acute and watery diarrhoea only.
  - Contraindicated in renal insufficiency, pregnancy and breastfeeding.

ANTISPASMODICS

- Mild antispasmodics (dicyclomine and hyoscine) in patients with significant abdominal cramps.

ANTIBIOTICS

- Antibiotics may be used in the following situations:
  - Symptomatic patients with inflammatory diarrhoea (high fever, toxicity and abdominal pain).
  - Patients presenting with an acute febrile dysentery illness.
  - Diarrhoea due to *Campylobacter jejuni*, where early use of azithromycin limits the duration of illness.
  - Severe disease (fever, more than six stools per day, volume depletion warranting hospitalisation)
- If clinical presentation suggests a possibility of Shiga toxin-producing *E. coli* (e.g. bloody diarrhoea without fever), antibiotics should be avoided because they may increase the risk of haemolytic uraemic syndrome.
- Commonly used antibiotics are quinolones (norfloxacin 400 mg and ciprofloxacin 500 mg, both given twice daily, or levofloxacin 500 mg given once a day) or azithromycin (500 mg once a day) for 3–5 days.
- In patients with suspected cholera, administer doxycycline in a dose of 300 mg as a single dose. Alternatives include azithromycin (1 g single dose) and ciprofloxacin (1 g single dose). Most strains are resistant to trimethoprim-sulphamethoxazole and furazolidone.

PROBIOTICS

- Probiotics are commonly recommended by physicians to limit the duration of diarrhoea. These agents are used along with ORS when antibiotics are not indicated.

ZINC

- In children older than 6 months, zinc supplementation helps in treating and preventing acute diarrhoea.

MISCELLANEOUS

- Somatostatin and analogues (octreotide, lanreotide and pasireotide) effective in postgastrectomy patients.
- Enterocyte apical membrane chloride channel inhibitor (crofelemer) for diarrhoea associated with HIV.

Q. What are the causes of chronic blood and mucus in the stools? Mention the investigations done in such cases. Stress the importance of stool examination in such a case.

CAUSES (Box 8.3)

BOX 8.3 Causes of Chronic Blood and Mucus in Stools

- Amoebic dysentery
- Bacillary dysentery
- Ulcerative colitis
- Crohn's disease
- Intestinal tuberculosis
- Carcinoma of the lower large bowel—rectum, sigmoid and colon
- Diverticulitis
- Necrotising enterocolitis
- Mesenteric vascular disease

BOX 8.4 Microscopic Examination of Stools in Patients With Chronic Blood and Mucus

- Ova
- Cysts
- Trophozoites
- Bacteria
- Pus cells
- Red blood cells
- Macrophages

INVESTIGATIONS

- Stool:
  - Macroscopy:
    - Fresh blood? Altered blood? Sticky? Foul smelling? Bulky? Floats in water? Mucus?
  - Microscopy (Box 8.4).
  - Culture and sensitivity—grows the organism.
- Proctoscopy—detects ulcers and tumours of rectum, haemorrhoids, masses.
- Sigmoidoscopy—visualises sigmoid colon, detects ulcers and tumours.
- Colonoscopy—visualisation of colon.
- Barium enema—detects growths or filling defects, strictures, ulcers and diverticula.
- Biopsy—of an ulcer or growth can be done using sigmoidoscope or colonoscope.

Q. Write a short note on occult blood in the stool.

- Patients with gastroduodenal bleeding of up to 60–100 mL/day may have normal-appearing stools (i.e. no melaena).
- Faecal blood loss in normal individuals varies from 0.5 to 1.5 mL/day; most faecal occult blood tests begin to become positive at a level of around 2 mL of blood loss per day.
- Occult blood in stools is detected by guaiac test—should be performed for several successive days because bleeding from the gastrointestinal tract is often intermittent. Unlike previous belief, this test is negative in a person on iron or bismuth. Conditions in which occult blood is positive in stools are given in Table 8.10.
- Other tests include faecal immunochemical tests for blood and haeme-porphyrin test. Faecal immunohistochemical testing detects only globin and therefore does not detect upper GI bleeding since the globin is digested in transit.

TABLE 8.10 Conditions Where Occult Blood Is Positive

- Upper gastrointestinal bleeding—peptic ulcer, malignancy, gastritis, oesophagitis, varices, portal hypertensive gastropathy, gastric antral vascular ectasias (GAVE)
- Lower gastrointestinal bleeding—malignancy, haemorrhoids, diverticulitis, inflammatory bowel disease, coeliac sprue, angiodysplasia, tuberculosis
- Hookworm disease, strongyloidiasis, ascariasis
- Some patients on aspirin or steroids[a]
- Mesenteric vascular disease

[a]A positive test in a patient on aspirin or steroids should not be assumed to be due to these agents but should be investigated.

INVESTIGATIONS

- Investigations which may be required in a patient with positive stool occult blood are listed in Box 8.5.

BOX 8.5 Investigations in a Patient With Stool Occult Blood Positive

Investigations include colonoscopy, oesophagogastroduodenoscopy, enteroscopy, video capsule endoscopy, enteroclysis, CT abdomen, angiography and radionuclide studies using technetium Tc-99m–labelled red blood cells

Q. What are the causes of haematemesis? Discuss the management of a patient with UGI bleeding. (IM 15.1; IM 15.10)

- UGI bleeding indicates bleeding proximal to the duodenojejunal junction (ligament of Treitz).
- Presents with haematemesis, melaena or both.

AETIOLOGY (Table 8.11)

- Erosive gastritis:
  - Can occur after ingestion of nonsteroidal antiinflammatory drugs (NSAIDs) and alcohol.
  - Can occur due to stress like trauma, burns, sepsis and shock.
- Variceal bleeding usually occurs from the lower 5 cm of oesophagus.
- Mallory–Weiss syndrome is an uncommon cause of UGI bleeding. It results from a linear tear in the distal oesophagus and proximal stomach. An episode of forceful retching precedes the onset of bleeding in most cases.
- Selective serotonin reuptake inhibitors decrease platelet serotonin resulting in defective platelet aggregation and impaired haemostasis.

CLINICAL FEATURES

- The patient most often presents with haematemesis and/or melaena.
- Colour of the vomitus depends on how long the blood has been in the stomach; bright red blood suggests a rapid and sizeable haemorrhage, while 'coffee ground' colour is consistent with a small bleed.

TABLE 8.11 Aetiology of Upper Gastrointestinal Bleed

Oesophageal causes	• Oesophageal varices, oesophagitis, oesophageal carcinoma, Mallory–Weiss syndrome
Gastroduodenal causes	• Erosive gastritis or duodenitis, stress ulcers, peptic ulcer (gastric and duodenal), gastric carcinoma, portal hypertensive gastropathy, gastric antral vascular ectasia (GAVE)
Miscellaneous causes	• Rupture of aortic aneurysm, coagulation defects, angiodysplasia or vascular malformations, selective serotonin reuptake inhibitors

- Melaena indicates black, tarry stools. It occurs when more than 60 mL blood is lost into the UGI tract. The stool has an offensive smell and is often difficult to flush away.
- Passage of frank blood per rectum (haematochezia) in massive bleed.
- Occasionally presentation is with symptoms of acute blood loss only. These include dizziness, extreme pallor, shock, angina or syncope.

FEATURES SUGGESTING SEVERE BLEEDING (Box 8.6)

BOX 8.6 Features Suggestive of Severe Bleeding

- Presence of clots in the vomitus
- Fresh blood in the nasogastric aspirate
- Haematochezia
- Hypotension and tachycardia
- A fall in systolic blood pressure >10 mmHg and a rise in pulse rate of >20 beats/minute on change of posture from lying to sitting position

DIAGNOSIS

- History of alcohol or drug (NSAIDs) ingestion, trauma, burns or sepsis suggests bleeding from gastric erosions.
- History of use of other drugs like antiplatelet agents (aspirin, clopidogrel) and anticoagulants indicates coagulation defect.
- A history suggestive of peptic ulcer (even though many patients with peptic ulcer may not give such history).
- History of jaundice, pedal oedema, abdominal distension and presence of splenomegaly, ascites, dilated abdominal veins or other features of liver cell failure (spider naevi, palmar erythema, jaundice and gynaecomastia) suggest variceal bleed.
- Haematemesis preceded by retching and a blood-free vomitus suggests a Mallory–Weiss tear.
- History of dysphagia and weight loss prior to bleed suggests a malignant cause.

INVESTIGATIONS

- Type and cross-match of blood, haemoglobin and haematocrit, blood urea and creatinine, coagulation profile, platelet count and liver function tests. An elevation of blood urea is associated with upper GI bleed. In the absence of renal failure, a blood urea to creatinine ratio of more than 72 indicates upper GI bleed rather than a lower GI bleed.
- ECG if suspicion of acute coronary syndrome.
- Nasogastric aspirate.
- Upper GI endoscopy.
- Angiography.

MANAGEMENT

- In case of massive bleeding, insert two wide-bore intravenous lines and resuscitate and replenish

intravascular volume with fluids and blood before any diagnostic measures and other therapeutic measures. Aim is to maintain haemoglobin above 7–8 g/dL.
  - Harmful effects of blood transfusion are due to impaired haemostasis, adverse effects on coagulation and increased splanchnic blood flow and pressure that might impair clot formation and stability.
- Assess the pulse, blood pressure, postural hypotension, urine output and level of consciousness.

GASTRIC LAVAGE

- Perform a gastric lavage by instilling 500 mL of tap water or saline (both are equally effective) every 30–60 minutes. However, in nonvariceal bleed, there are no guidelines which indicate benefit of a lavage.
- Do not apply vigorous suction for aspiration as it may produce further mucosal damage that may interfere with interpretation of endoscopic findings.
- Addition of noradrenaline in the lavage fluid does not give additional benefit over tap water.
- Lavage leads to at least temporary cessation of bleeding in 80%–90% of patients.
- Nasogastric tube should be kept for 24 hours after cessation of bleed to facilitate detection of rebleed.
- Gastric aspiration helps to:
  - Assess the rate of bleeding.
  - Clear the stomach prior to endoscopy.
  - Remove blood, thereby reducing the risk of encephalopathy in patients with liver disease.
  - Dilute acid pepsin in stomach, thereby reducing bleeding from erosions.

ENDOSCOPY

- Upper GI endoscopy as soon as the patient is haemodynamically stable. If bleeding has stopped, it can be postponed by a few hours. It helps in:
  - Early diagnosis.
  - Identifying patients who may rebleed.
  - Treatment of underlying condition (e.g. sclerotherapy or banding in oesophageal variceal bleed).
- Features indicating a high risk of rebleed from varices:
  - Large-sized varices.
  - Presence of daughter varices.
  - Presence of cherry red spots over the varices.
- Features indicating a high risk of rebleed from peptic ulcer:
  - Presence of a sentinel clot over the ulcer.
  - Presence of exposed blood vessel (nonbleeding blood vessels) at the base of the ulcer.

OTHER INVESTIGATIONS

- Angiography or radionuclide scan to delineate the anatomical site of bleeding if endoscopy fails.

OTHER MANAGEMENT STRATEGIES

Proton-Pump Inhibitors

- Omeprazole 40–80 mg intravenously followed by 8 mg/hour infusion or pantoprazole 40 mg intravenously followed by 8 mg/hour infusion.

Fresh Frozen Plasma and Platelets

- Fresh frozen plasma in patients with active bleeding and coagulopathy.
- Prothrombin complex concentrate in patients with active bleed who are on warfarin.
- Platelet transfusion in patients with active bleeding and thrombocytopenia.

Prokinetics

- Intravenous erythromycin before endoscopy is beneficial in terms of improved mucosal visualisation during endoscopy and reduction in blood transfused.

Balloon Tamponade, Vasopressin, Octreotide

- Discussed under 'variceal bleed' on page 454, Chapter 6.

Endoscopic Therapeutic Measures

- Thermal measures:
  - These include use of lasers, argon plasma coagulation, electrocoagulation and heater probe thermocoagulation.
- Nonthermal measures:
  - Endoscopic band ligation of bleeding vein and application of an arterial clip.
  - Endoscopic sclerotherapy (EST).
  - Injection of dilute (1:10,000) adrenaline in 1-mL aliquots around bleeding points along with fibrin glue.
  - Mechanical (clipping) therapy and application of topical haemostatic powders.

Antifibrinolytic Drug

- Tranexamic acid may be used in selected patients.

Radiological Measures

- Embolisation of the bleeding artery using autologous clot, gel foam or metallic coil may be effective in some patients in whom angiography is able to localise the site of bleed.

Surgical Measures

- If variceal bleed cannot be controlled with medical measures, emergency surgery is required. This includes shunt surgery or transaction–devascularisation of oesophageal varices.
- In patients with bleeding ulcer, surgery is contemplated if bleeding cannot be controlled with medical measures or if patient rebleeds after initial control.
- In patients with gastric erosions, total gastrectomy or vagotomy with drainage is required if medical measures fail.

SUMMARY OF MANAGEMENT (Flowchart 8.1)

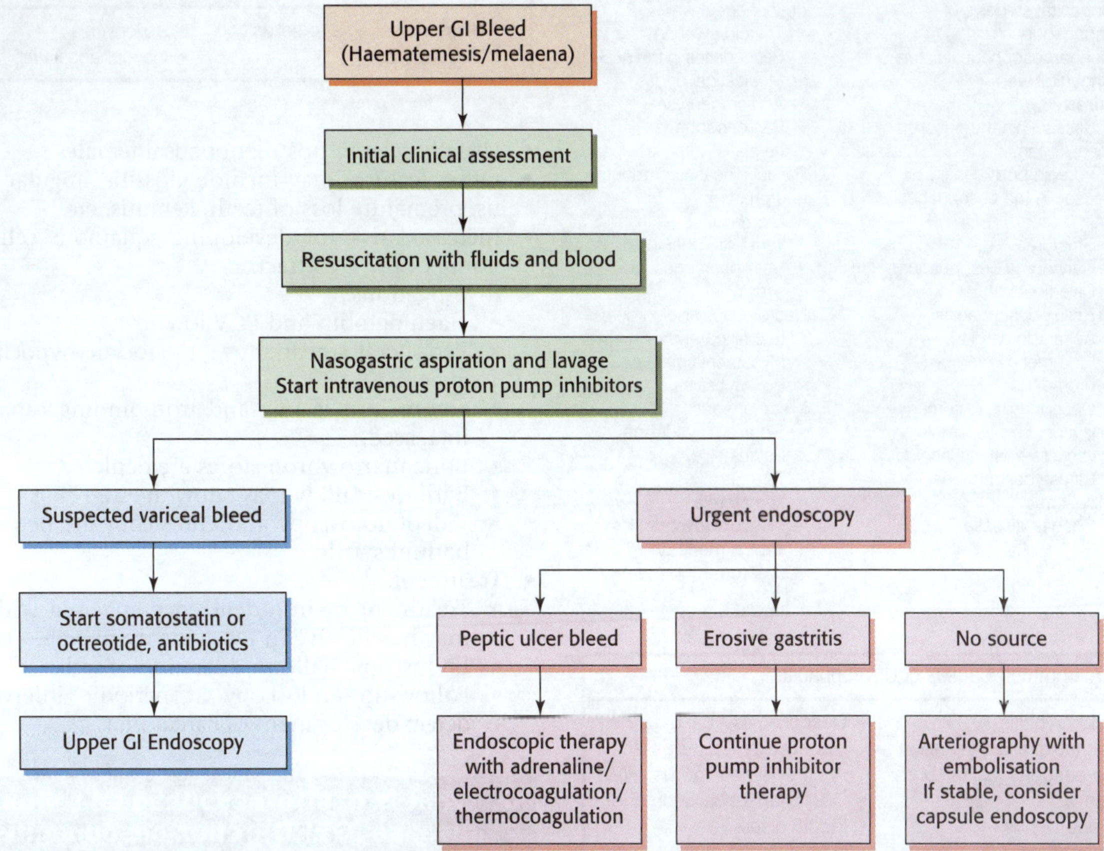

Flowchart 8.1 Summary of Management of Upper GI Bleed.

Q. List down the common causes of weight loss.

- Weight loss is defined as loss of more than 5% of usual body weight over 6 months.

CAUSES OF WEIGHT LOSS

- Causes of weight loss are given in Table 8.12.

TABLE 8.12 Causes of Weight Loss

- Diabetes mellitus
- Endocrine diseases—hyperthyroidism, pheochromocytoma, panhypopituitarism, adrenal insufficiency
- Gastrointestinal causes—tropical sprue, chronic pancreatitis, chronic diarrhoea due to ulcerative colitis and Crohn's disease, parasitic infestations, malabsorption
- Infections—tuberculosis, fungal infections, amoebiasis, bacterial endocarditis, HIV, giardiasis
- Malignancy—any occult malignancy (including cancer of stomach, pancreas, liver), lymphoma, leukaemia
- Psychiatric—anorexia nervosa, depression, schizophrenia
- Renal disease—chronic renal failure
- Drugs and toxins—anticonvulsants, antidepressants, levodopa, digoxin, metformin, exenatide, liraglutide, theophylline, alcohol, cocaine, amphetamines
- Miscellaneous—chronic obstructive pulmonary disease (pulmonary cachexia), chronic cardiac failure (cardiac cachexia), dementia, Parkinson's disease, motor neuron disease, stroke

Q. What are the causes of glossitis?

- Glossitis is inflammation of the tongue and denotes soreness and redness of the tongue.

CAUSES

- B-complex deficiency, megaloblastic anaemia, cirrhosis, pernicious anaemia, iron-deficiency anaemia, pellagra, scarlet fever, syphilis, gonorrhoea and tuberculosis
- Medications: ACE inhibitors, salbutamol, sulphonamides, oral contraceptive pills, lithium

Q. What are the causes of dysphagia? How will you investigate a case of dysphagia?

- Dysphagia is defined as a subjective sensation of difficulty or abnormality of swallowing.
- Odynophagia is defined as pain while swallowing.
- Causes of dysphagia are shown in Table 8.13.
- In general, mechanical causes commonly lead to dysphagia for solid foods initially, whereas patients with motility disorders tend to complain of progressive or nonprogressive dysphagia for both liquids and solids from the onset.
- Common causes of odynophagia are listed in Box 8.7.

TABLE 8.13 Common Causes of Dysphagia

I. **Congenital** • Congenital stenosis of oesophagus • Tracheo-oesophageal fistula • Congenital web II. **Acquired** A. Causes within the oesophageal lumen • Foreign body B. Causes in the oesophageal wall • Strictures • Carcinoma oesophagus • Diverticulum • Reflux oesophagitis • Achalasia cardia • Plummer–Vinson syndrome • Oesophagitis (cytomegalovirus, herpes simplex, varicella-zoster, *Candida*) • Diffuse oesophageal spasm • Chagas disease	C. Causes outside the oesophageal wall • Thyroid swelling • Secondaries in the neck • Mediastinal nodes • Aortic aneurysm • Paraoesophageal hernia D. Painful diseases of mouth and pharynx • Stomatitis • Tonsillitis, pharyngitis • Retropharyngeal abscess E. Neuromuscular disorders • Bulbar paralysis • Myasthenia gravis • Polymyositis F. Miscellaneous • Sjogren's syndrome • Rabies • Tetanus • Xerostomia • Muscular dystrophies • Lateral medullary syndrome

BOX 8.7 Common Causes of Odynophagia

- Acute pharyngitis
- Caustic (acid. alkali) ingestion
- Gastro-oesophageal reflux disease
- Injury due to pills—bisphosphonates, NSAIDs, iron, potassium chloride, zidovudine
- Oesophagitis—candida, herpes simplex, Epstein–Barr virus, cytomegalovirus, HIV
- Oesophageal carcinoma
- Mouth ulcers

INVESTIGATIONS

- Haemoglobin and peripheral smear for anaemia.
- Chest radiograph detects retrosternal goitre, mediastinal lymph nodes, aortic aneurysms and primary and secondary malignancies of lungs.
- Barium swallow detects tumours as filling defects or strictures (rat-tail appearance).
- Videofluoroscopic swallowing study (modified barium swallow).
- Oesophagoscopy allows removal of foreign body, visualisation and biopsy of tumours, ulcers, strictures, etc.
- CT scan of thorax.
- Biopsy from the growth, ulcer or inflamed mucosa.
- Oesophageal motility studies (oesophageal manometry).

Q. Briefly describe about Plummer–Vinson syndrome (Patterson–Kelly syndrome).

Q. Write a short note on sideropenic dysphagia.

- A syndrome characterised by features shown in Box 8.8.
- Dysphagia is due to a thin web in the postcricoid area. The web is formed of degenerated epithelial cells.

BOX 8.8 Features of Plummer–Vinson Syndrome/Sideropenic Dysphagia/Patterson–Kelly Syndrome

- Painless dysphagia to solids
- Iron deficiency
- Koilonychia
- Oesophageal web

- Usually seen in postmenopausal females.
- Other features may include glossitis, angular cheilitis, premature loss of teeth, keratitis, etc.
- Increased risk for developing squamous cell carcinoma of the UGI tract.
- Investigations:
  - Haemoglobin and PCV low.
  - Peripheral smear shows microcytic hypochromic anaemia.
  - Serum iron is low and iron-binding capacity is increased.
  - Bone marrow iron stores are depleted.
  - Barium swallow may show the web (Fig. 8.1).
  - Videofluoroscopy and endoscopy are better than barium swallow.
- Treatment:
  - Treatment of iron-deficiency anaemia with iron may be effective in resolving dysphagia.
  - Endoscopic balloon dilatation of web.
  - Follow-up endoscopy at periodic intervals to detect development of carcinoma.

Q. What is gastro-oesophageal reflux disease (GERD; reflux oesophagitis)?

Q. What are the normal mechanisms preventing reflux?

Q. Give the causes, clinical features, investigations, complications and treatment of reflux oesophagitis.

- GERD is defined as heartburn symptoms or complications resulting from the reflux of gastric contents into the oesophagus, up to the oral cavity and lungs.

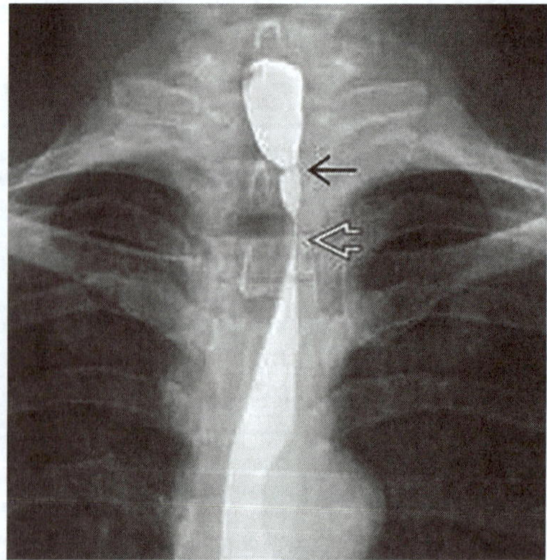

Fig. 8.1 Barium swallow in a patient with Plummer–Vinson syndrome shows oesophageal web and stricture.

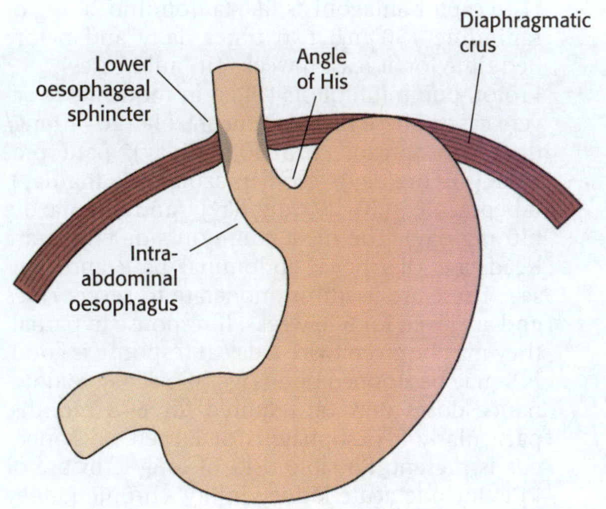

Fig. 8.2 Anatomy of normal antireflux barrier at the lower oesophagus. Courtesy: Mullassery D, Jones MO. Gastro-oesophageal reflux in children: surgical management. Paediatric Surgery 2019;37(4):204-207, 2019.

- Reflux oesophagitis occurs when the mucosal defences are unable to counteract the damage produced by refluxed acid, pepsin and bile.
- In long-standing oesophagitis, the lower oesophageal mucosa may change from squamous to columnar type (Barrett's mucosa). Barrett's mucosa is susceptible to ulcers, strictures and malignant changes (adenocarcinoma of oesophagus).

MECHANISMS PREVENTING REFLUX AND REFLUX OESOPHAGITIS (Fig. 8.2)

- Lower oesophageal sphincter (LES) is located at the lower end of oesophagus below the diaphragm. It is a 3- to 4-cm segment of tonically contracted circular smooth muscle at the distal end of the oesophagus.
- Striated muscles of the diaphragmatic crura.
- Anatomical flap valve at oesophagogastric junction. It keeps the distal part of LES in the abdominal cavity and maintains the angle of His.
- Intraabdominal pressure reinforces the LES tone.
- Oblique entry of oesophagus into the stomach (angle of His).
- Secondary peristaltic waves in the oesophagus clear the refluxed material.
- Swallowed saliva neutralises the refluxed acid.

AETIOPATHOGENESIS

- Sliding hiatus hernia—in this type of hernia, the oesophagogastric junction slides up through the diaphragm. This results in:
  a. Loss of the obliquity of entry of oesophagus into stomach.
  b. Loss of the reinforcing effect of intraabdominal pressure on the LES (refer above).
    - These two factors facilitate gastro-oesophageal reflux.
    - So hiatus hernia facilitates gastro-oesophageal reflux but does not directly cause it.
- Cardiomyotomy and vagotomy reduce the efficiency of the LES.
- Pregnancy, obesity, ascites, weightlifting and straining act by increasing the intraabdominal pressure.
- Cigarette smoking, alcohol, fatty foods and caffeine act by reducing the LES tone.
- Impaired gastric emptying due to gastric outlet obstruction, anticholinergic drugs and fatty food act by increasing the gastric content available for reflux.
- Large-volume meals act by the above mechanism.
- Systemic sclerosis causing reduced peristalsis of oesophagus and an incompetent LES.
- Drugs (aminophylline, β-agonists, nitrates, calcium channel blockers) that reduce the tone of LES.
- Acid pocket—in postprandial period, a layer of unbuffered acidic gastric juice sits on top of the meal close to the cardia; this is known as acid pocket. A more proximal location of acid pocket is seen in patients with GERD.
- Hypersensitivity to acid reflux.

HELICOBACTER PYLORI

- *H. pylori*, a spiral-shaped bacterium located in the mucous layer of the stomach, may inhibit or exacerbate acid reflux depending on how the infection affects the stomach.
- Distal gastritis increases the production of gastric acid. In this condition, the eradication of *H. pylori* reduces not only the risk of peptic ulceration but also the risk of acid reflux.
- Conversely, generalised atrophic gastritis decreases the production of gastric acid; as a result, *H. pylori* eradication may increase the severity of reflux.
- Since chronic *H. pylori* infection is associated with an increased risk of peptic ulceration and gastric cancer, *H. pylori* eradication is recommended even though *H. pylori* does not have an important role in pathogenesis of GERD.

CLINICAL FEATURES

- Heartburn (pyrosis) is deeply placed burning pain behind the sternum radiating to the throat. It occurs after meals, brought on by bending, lifting weight and straining. Heartburn occurs on lying down in bed at night and is then relieved by sitting up.
- Regurgitation of gastric contents into the mouth (acid eructation) without associated nausea or retching.
- Tracheal aspiration with coughing or laryngismus or aspiration pneumonia results from the regurgitated gastric contents in the mouth.
- Odynophagia—painful swallowing.
- Transient dysphagia to solids due to oesophageal spasm.
- Persistent dysphagia to solids due to strictures or development of oesophageal carcinoma.
- Iron-deficiency anaemia due to blood loss.
- Extra-oesophageal symptoms include hoarseness, sore throat, sinusitis, otitis media, chronic cough, laryngitis, non-atopic asthma, recurrent aspiration and pulmonary fibrosis.

COMPLICATIONS (Box 8.9)

BOX 8.9 Complication of GERD

- Oesophagitis
- Oesophageal ulcers
- Barrett's oesophagus
- Carcinoma oesophagus
- Strictures
- Aspiration pneumonia
- Iron-deficiency anaemia
- Dental erosions

ALARMING SYMPTOMS (Box 8.10)

BOX 8.10 Alarming Symptoms of GERD

- Weight loss
- GI bleeding
- Nausea and vomiting
- Dysphagia
- Odynophagia
- Family history of cancer

DIFFERENTIAL DIAGNOSIS

- Coronary artery disease
- Gastrointestinal malignancy
- Peptic ulcer disease
- Biliary tract disease
- Oesophagitis
- Achalasia.

INVESTIGATIONS

- Endoscopy:
  - Oesophagitis can be visualised and confirmed by biopsy.
  - Strictures can be visualised.
  - Barrett's mucosa can be confirmed by biopsy.
- Barium swallow and meal can reveal a hiatus hernia.
- Ambulatory 24-hour oesophageal pH metry may reveal a sudden decrease in intra-oesophageal pH from above to below 4.0. Wireless capsule is also available for oesophageal pH recording.
- Resting ECG and stress ECG to rule out ischaemic heart disease.
- Oesophageal manometry (primarily done before surgical intervention to exclude achalasia and other motility disorders and not for diagnosis of GERD).

TREATMENT

- General measures:
  - Weight reduction and cessation of smoking.
  - Small-volume, frequent feeds.
  - Avoid alcohol, fatty food, spicy food, caffeine, mint, orange juice and some medications. Avoid late-night meals.
  - Avoid weightlifting, stooping and bending at waist. Head end of the bed should be elevated to 15°.
- Medical treatment:
  - Liquid antacid 10–15 mL, 1 and 3 hours after meal, relieves heartburn (in mild cases). Treatment with alginate–antacid preparations abolishes acid pocket and helps in reducing GERD.
  - H_2-receptor antagonists like famotidine 20 mg or ranitidine 150 mg, two times daily and before bed time for at least 6 weeks (in mild cases).
  - Proton-pump inhibitors (PPIs) in moderate to severe cases: These include omeprazole (20–40 mg/day), lansoprazole (15–30 mg/day), pantoprazole (40 mg/day), esomeprazole (40 mg/day), rabeprazole (10–20 mg/day) and ilaprazole (10 mg/day). The most common side effects are headache, diarrhoea, abdominal pain and nausea. These are useful in moderate to severe cases and are given for 6–8 weeks. If response in partial, they may be given twice a day. If response is good, PPI may be stopped or dosage is lowered. Maintenance doses may be required for 6–8 months, particularly if oesophagitis or Barrett's oesophagus is present. Possible risks of long-term use of PPIs include acute kidney injury, chronic kidney disease, osteoporosis and *C. difficile* infection.
  - Metoclopramide or domperidone 10 mg thrice daily increases the LES tone and promotes gastric emptying. Other prokinetics include mosapride, itopride and levosulpiride. However, none of them have been shown to be useful in GERD patients. In addition, they have their own safety issues.
  - Patients who show resistance to PPIs may be treated with vonoprazan which belongs to a new class of acid suppressant medications, the potassium-competitive acid blocker.
  - Therapy for *H. pylori* if infection is evident on serology or urea breath test. It improves histological signs of gastric inflammation but does not improve symptoms or rates of recurrence of GERD.
  - Oesophageal stricture is treated by repeated dilatations.
  - Oral iron or blood transfusion for anaemia.
- Surgical treatment:
  - Surgical resection of strictures.
  - Surgical return of LES to the abdomen and construction of an additional valve mechanism (fundoplication) for sliding hiatus hernia.

Q. Give a brief account of hiatus hernia.

- A hiatal hernia is herniation of part of stomach into the thoracic cavity through the diaphragmatic hiatus.
  - In sliding hiatus hernia, gastro-oesophageal junction and the fundus of stomach slide upward (Fig. 8.3A).
  - In paraoesophageal hiatus hernia, gastro-oesophageal junction remains below the diaphragm while stomach herniates through diaphragm (Fig. 8.3B).
- Aetiology:
  - Unknown.
  - Obesity, pregnancy and ascites may be aetiological factors.
  - Occurs in 33% of normal adults and 50% of elderly.
- Clinical features:
  - Majority are asymptomatic.
  - Hiatus hernia predisposes to gastro-oesophageal reflux and hence symptoms of reflux may be present.

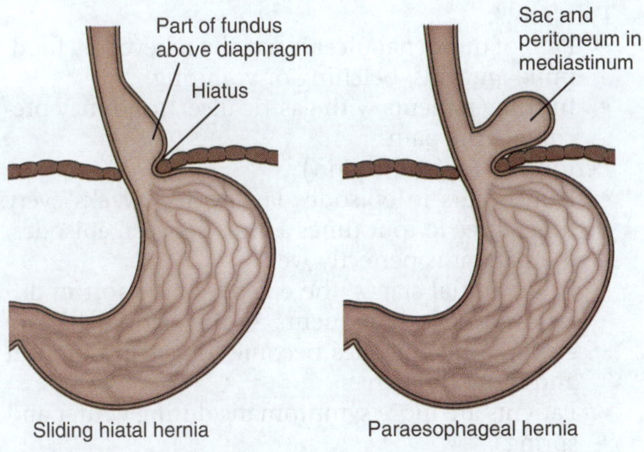

Fig. 8.3 A and B Sliding and paraoesophageal hiatal hernias.

- Complications include volvulus of stomach, bleeding from gastric ulcer, gastritis or gastric erosions and respiratory complications from mechanical compression of the lung by a large hernia.
- Investigations:
  - Chest X-ray may show fundal air–fluid level in chest. Chest X-ray after inserting a nasogastric tube will show its end in the chest.
  - Barium swallow will demonstrate the presence of gastro-oesophageal junction in the thorax in sliding hiatus hernia. It will demonstrate stomach in thorax in paraoesophageal hiatus hernia
  - Endoscopy.
- Management:
  - Asymptomatic hiatus hernias do not require any treatment.
  - If gastro-oesophageal reflux is present, surgical repair (either open laparotomy or laparoscopic approaches) of hernia is done in selected cases. Surgery involves repair of the diaphragmatic defect and fixing the stomach in the abdominal cavity (fundoplication) combined with an antireflux procedure.

Q. Discuss the aetiopathogenesis, clinical features and management of acid peptic disease or peptic ulcer disease. (IM 15.15; IM 15.16)

Q. Briefly describe about *Helicobacter pylori*. (IM 15.15)

- Peptic ulcer refers to an ulcer in the lower oesophagus, stomach or duodenum, in the jejunum after surgical anastomosis to stomach, and in the ileum adjacent to a Meckel's diverticulum.
- Incidence—10% of all adult males.
- Approximately 90% of peptic ulcers are caused by *H. pylori* infection or NSAID use.

AETIOPATHOGENESIS

- Heredity:
  - Strong family history with gastric ulcers but less strong family history with duodenal ulcers.
- Acid pepsin versus mucosal resistance:
  - Cause of peptic ulceration is digestion of the mucosa with acid and pepsin of gastric juice. Normal stomach is capable of resisting this digestion. So the concept of peptic ulceration is acid plus pepsin versus mucosal resistance. Factors that tilt this balance produce ulcers.
  - Gastric hypersecretion:
    - Ulcers occur only in the presence of acid and pepsin. Severe ulceration occurs in Zollinger–Ellison syndrome which is characterised by very high acid secretion. Acid secretion is more important in the aetiology of duodenal ulcer than in gastric ulcer.
  - Mucosal resistance:
    - Several mechanisms protect gastric mucosa from the acid.
      - Surface epithelial cells secrete bicarbonate under the influence of mucosal prostaglandins and this bicarbonate neutralises the acid.
      - The surface cells also secrete mucus that impedes the diffusion of ions and molecules such as pepsin.
      - The tight intercellular junctions and the surface lipoprotein layer provide a mechanical barrier.
      - Normal turnover of epithelial cells has a protective function. In addition, migration of epithelial cells bordering site of injury restores a damaged region.
      - The submucosal area provides adequate micronutrients and oxygen while removing toxic metabolic by-products of gastric epithelial cells.
  - Collectively, these mechanisms can be described as the 'gastric mucosal barrier'.
  - Prostaglandins play a central role in mucosal resistance. They regulate the release of mucosal bicarbonate and mucus, inhibit parietal cell secretion and are important in maintaining mucosal blood flow. This explains the ulcerogenic properties of NSAIDs.
  - Factors reducing mucosal resistance:
    - Several drugs, particularly those used in rheumatoid arthritis.
    - Aspirin is an important aetiological factor in gastric ulcer. It damages the membrane and tight junctions. It also inhibits prostaglandin synthesis, thus reducing bicarbonate secretion.
    - The organism *H. pylori.*
    - Reflux of bile and intestinal contents into stomach.
- Other risk factors include smoking and alcohol consumption.

H. PYLORI

- Majority of gastric and duodenal ulcers can be attributed to NSAIDs and *H. pylori.*
- *H. pylori* also plays a role in the development of gastritis, mucosal-associated lymphoid tissue (MALT) lymphoma, gastric adenocarcinoma and dyspepsia.
- *H. pylori* is a Gram-negative bacillus that produces mucosal damage.

- In a developing country, nearly 80% of persons are colonised with it by the age of 20 years. Other risk factors for acquiring *H. pylori* infection include poor socioeconomic conditions and family overcrowding.
- Transmission occurs following oral–oral or faeco-oral route.
- Postulated mechanisms for ulcer development:
  - Key factor secreted by the bacillus is urease which converts urea into ammonia, thus alkalinising the surrounding acidic medium for its survival but simultaneously producing ammonia-induced mucosal damage. Production of ammonia by bacteria prevents D cells in the antral glands from sensing the true level of acidity leading to inappropriate release of somatostatin and an increase in gastrin, and consequently excess acid secretion.
  - Neural pathways are also affected by *H. pylori* which results in downregulation of acid production.
  - *H. pylori* causes an inflammatory response in gastric mucosa with induction of epithelium-derived cytokines (interleukin-8 and interleukin-1 β). Influx of neutrophils and macrophages into the gastric mucosa with release of lysosomal enzymes, leucotrienes and reactive oxygen species impairs mucosal defence.
  - Inflammatory response also results in release of additional factors with ulcerogenic potential including platelet-activating factor and complement factors.

AETIOLOGY OF ACUTE AND STRESS ULCERS

- Aspirin.
- Head injury, burns, severe sepsis, surgery and trauma lead to peptic ulceration known as stress ulcers.
  - Head injury causes ulcers by gastric hypersecretion (Cushing's ulcer).
  - Burns and shock produce ulcers by reflux of duodenal contents and mucosal ischaemia.

CLINICAL FEATURES

- Peptic ulcer is a chronic condition with a natural history of spontaneous relapses and remissions lasting for decades or even life.
- The most common presentation is that of recurrent abdominal pain that has three notable characters:
  - Localisation to the epigastrium.
  - Relationship to food.
  - Periodicity.
- Epigastric pain:
  - Pain is referred to epigastrium and is so sharply localised that the patient will localise the site with one finger (pointing sign). It is usually burning in character.
- Pain:
  - Duodenal ulcer pain occurs on empty stomach (hunger pain) and is relieved by food or antacids. By contrast, patients with gastric ulcers have postprandial abdominal pain, nausea, vomiting and weight loss.
- Night pain:
  - Typically, the pain in duodenal ulcer wakes the patient from sleep around 3 a.m. and is relieved by food, milk or antacids.
- Pain relief:
  - Pain of duodenal ulcer is usually relieved by food, milk, antacids, belching or vomiting.
  - In some patients with gastric ulcer, food may precipitate the pain.
- Periodicity (episodic pain):
  - Pain occurs in episodes lasting 1–3 weeks every time, three to four times a year. Between episodes, the patient is perfectly well.
  - In the initial stages, the episodes are short in duration and less frequent. As the natural history evolves, the episodes become longer in duration and more frequent.
  - Patients are more symptomatic during winter and spring.
  - Relapses are more common in smokers than in nonsmokers.
- Other symptoms:
  - Water brash (excessive salivation), heartburn, loss of appetite and vomiting.
  - Anorexia, nausea, fullness, bloating and dyspepsia.
  - Occasionally, the patient may present for the first time with anaemia of chronic blood loss, abrupt haematemesis and acute perforation or gastric outlet obstruction.

DIFFERENCES BETWEEN GASTRIC ULCER AND DUODENAL ULCER (Table 8.14)

TABLE 8.14 Gastric Ulcer Versus Duodenal Ulcer

Factors	Gastric Ulcer	Duodenal Ulcer
• Age	More than 40 years	20–50 years
• Sex	Equal in both sexes	More in males
• Course of the illness	Less remittent	More remittent
• Episodes of pain	Relatively longer in duration	Relatively shorter in duration
• Antacids	Relief of pain not consistent	Relief of pain prompt
• Food	Provokes the pain	Relieves the pain
• Heartburn	Less common	More common
• Night pains	Less common	More common
• Anorexia and nausea	More common	Less common

ALARMING SYMPTOMS

- Symptoms in peptic ulcer disease which may suggest underlying gastric malignancy are given in Box 8.11.

BOX 8.11 Alarming Symptoms in Peptic Ulcer Disease

- Symptom onset after 55 years of age
- Progressive dysphagia
- Persistent or recurrent vomiting
- Severe abdominal pain
- Weight loss and/or anorexia
- Family history of gastric malignancy
- Blood in stool, melaena, haematemesis and/or anaemia

COMPLICATIONS

- Upper gastrointestinal bleed.
- Perforation.
- Gastric outlet obstruction (with fluid and electrolyte imbalance).
- Gastric malignancy.
- Pancreatitis (due to posterior penetration of ulcer).

INVESTIGATIONS

- Double-contrast barium meal may show the ulcer as a crater or as a deformed duodenal cap.
- Endoscopy can visualise the ulcer. Typical location is duodenal bulb and lesser curvature of stomach. A biopsy can be taken from a gastric ulcer to rule out malignancy (10% of gastric ulcers are malignant) and *H. pylori* infection.
- Tests for *H. pylori*.
- Serum gastrin and gastric acid analysis in patients suspected to have Zollinger–Ellison syndrome.

TESTS FOR *H. PYLORI* (Box 8.12)

BOX 8.12 Tests for *Helicobacter pylori* Infection

On Endoscopic Biopsy Material
- Rapid urease test (false-negative with recent use of proton-pump inhibitors, antibiotics)
- Histology (sensitivity reduced with use of proton-pump inhibitors, antibiotics and bismuth-containing compounds)
- Molecular tests like polymerase chain reaction
- Culture (technically demanding)

Non-invasive
- Serology for immunoglobulin G (positive results may persist for months after eradication)
- Urea breath test via release of exhaled labelled CO_2 (false-negative with recent use of proton-pump inhibitors, antibiotics)
- *H. pylori* stool antigen test (test for cure 7 days after therapy is accurate; sensitivity is reduced with use of proton-pump inhibitors, antibiotics and bismuth-containing compounds)

TREATMENT

- Short-term management.
- Long-term management:
  - Intermittent treatment.
  - Maintenance treatment.
  - Surgical treatment.

SHORT-TERM MANAGEMENT

GENERAL MEASURES

- Avoid smoking.
- Avoid aspirin and NSAIDs.
- Alcohol to be moderated.
- No special dietary advice, though patients should avoid any foods that precipitate symptoms.

ANTACIDS

- Mainly prescribed for symptomatic relief only.
- Act by neutralising acidity.
- Minor pain is treated with tablet preparations and severe pain with liquid preparations.
- Dose is 15–30 mL liquid antacid 1 and 3 hours after food and at bedtime for 4–6 weeks. Rarely used at present.
- Commonly used antacids are a combination of aluminium and magnesium compounds, sodium bicarbonate and calcium carbonate.

Side Effects

- Aluminium compounds cause constipation and phosphate depletion, and block the absorption of digoxin and tetracycline.
- Magnesium compounds cause diarrhoea, hypercalcaemia and hypermagnesaemia.
- Calcium compounds cause constipation, hypercalcaemia and milk-alkali syndrome (hypercalcaemia, alkalosis and renal impairment).
- Bicarbonate preparations cause alkalosis.
- All antacids contain significant sodium which will lead to water retention and hence exacerbation of cardiac failure and ascites.

HISTAMINE H_2-RECEPTOR ANTAGONISTS

- Include cimetidine, ranitidine, famotidine and nizatidine. Tablets of ranitidine have been found to be contaminated with human carcinogen N-nitrosodimethylamine, and all brands of ranitidine are banned in USA and European countries.
- All the four drugs are equally effective. Their doses and side effects are given in Table 8.15.
- The mechanism of action is inhibition of acid and pepsin secretion by blocking H_2-receptors.
- Can be prescribed as twice-daily doses or as a single large dose at bedtime.
- Symptomatic relief occurs within days and ulcer healing within weeks.
- Duration of treatment of duodenal ulcer patients is 4 weeks. In smokers and in patients who have had recent major complications (haematemesis and perforation), treatment should be prolonged to 6–8 weeks.
- Gastric ulcer patients are treated for 6 weeks followed by endoscopy and further treatment if necessary. A gastric ulcer that has not healed by

TABLE 8.15 H_2-Receptor Antagonists Used in Peptic Ulcer Disease

H_2-receptor Antagonist	Dose	Side Effects
• Cimetidine	• 400 mg BD or 800 mg at night	• Gynaecomastia in males, confusion in elderly, oligospermia, delay in elimination of warfarin, phenytoin and theophylline
• Ranitidine	• 150 mg BD or 300 mg at night	• Confusion, liver dysfunction
• Famotidine	• 20 mg BD or 40 mg at night	• Headache, dizziness, dry mouth
• Nizatidine	• 150 mg BD or 300 mg at night	• Sweating, urticaria, somnolence

12 weeks should be treated with one of the PPIs or surgery.

PROTON-PUMP INHIBITORS

- These are substituted benzimidazoles and include omeprazole, lansoprazole, pantoprazole, esomeprazole, rabeprazole and ilaprazole.
- Omeprazole, lansoprazole and esomeprazole should be taken 30 minutes before a meal.
- Rabeprazole and pantoprazole may be taken without regard to meals.

Mechanism of Action

- PPIs cross the parietal cell membrane and enter the acidic parietal cell canaliculus.
- In the acidic environment, the PPI becomes protonated, producing the activated form of the drug which binds covalently with the H^+/K^+-ATPase enzyme that results in irreversible inhibition of acid secretion by the proton pump.
- The parietal cell must then produce new proton pumps or activate resting pumps to resume its acid secretion.

Efficacy in Peptic Ulcer Disease

- PPIs have superior healing rates, shorter healing time and faster symptom relief compared to H_2-blockers.
- All PPIs appear to have similar efficacy in the treatment of various acid peptic disorders.

Side Effects

- The most common side effects are headache, diarrhoea (including pseudomembranous colitis produced by *C. difficile*), abdominal pain and nausea.
- Other possible effects include B_{12}, iron and calcium malabsorption, osteoporosis and related fractures and interaction with some drugs. Some evidence suggests occurrence of acute kidney injury and chronic kidney disease in patients on long-term therapy with PPIs.
- Omeprazole and esomeprazole reduce effectiveness of clopidogrel by interfering with its metabolism to active metabolite.

Drug Interactions (Table 8.16)

Dosage

- Omeprazole: 20 mg daily for 4–8 weeks.
- Lansoprazole: 15–30 mg daily for 4–8 weeks.
- Esomeprazole: 20–40 mg daily for 4–8 weeks.
- Pantoprazole: 40 mg daily for 4–8 weeks.
- Rabeprazole: 20 mg daily for 4–8 weeks.
- Ilaprazole: 10 mg daily for 4–8 weeks.

Indications

- Reflux oesophagitis and GERD.
- Peptic ulcer unresponsive to other medical measures.
- As an adjunct to anti-*H. pylori* treatment.
- Zollinger–Ellison syndrome.

PROSTAGLANDIN ANALOGUES

- Misoprostol 200 μg four times daily. Useful in preventing NSAID-induced mucosal injury.
- It inhibits acid secretion and stimulates bicarbonate and mucus secretion.
- Side effects are diarrhoea, uterine bleeding, uterine contractions and abortifacient activity.

COLLOIDAL BISMUTH COMPOUNDS

- Bismuth subsalicylate and colloidal bismuth subcitrate.
- Mechanisms of action are two:
  1. These precipitate in acid conditions, binding with proteins in the ulcer base to form a coat that protects against further acid pepsin digestion.
  2. Powerful antimicrobial effect against *H. pylori*.
- Side effects include blackening of tongue, teeth and face, and bismuth toxicity (neurotoxicity).
- At present, bismuth compounds are mostly used as a combination therapy for eradication of *H. pylori*.

SUCRALPHATE (SUCRALFATE)

- Dose is 2 g BID.
- Forms a protective coating over the ulcers.
- Side effects are reduction in the absorption of warfarin, phenytoin, tetracycline and digoxin.

TREATMENT FOR *H. PYLORI*

- Many clinicians administer drugs against *H. pylori* to all patients with peptic ulcer disease even without documenting the presence of bacteria.

TABLE 8.16 Drug Interactions of Various PPIs

Drug	Omeprazole	Lansoprazole	Pantoprazole	Rabeprazole
• Carbamazepine	↓ Metabolism	Unknown	None	Unknown
• Diazepam	↓ Metabolism	None	None	None
• Digoxin	↑ Absorption	Unknown	↑ Absorption	↑ Absorption
• Ketoconazole	↓ Absorption	↓ Absorption	Unknown	↓ Absorption
• Oral contraceptives	None	None	None	None
• Phenytoin	↓ Metabolism	None	None	None
• Warfarin	↓ Metabolism	None	None	None
• Theophylline	None	↑ Metabolism	None	None

TABLE 8.17 Treatment of *Helicobacter pylori*

- Triple therapy
  - PPI[a] + clarithromycin (500 mg BID) + metronidazole (500 mg BID) for 14 days
  - PPI[a] + clarithromycin (500 mg BID) + amoxicillin (1 g BID) for 14 days
  - PPI[a] + tinidazole (500 mg BID) + amoxicillin (750 mg BID) for 14 days
- Quadruple therapy
  - PPI[b] + bismuth subsalicylate (525 mg QID) + metronidazole (250 mg QID) + tetracycline (500 mg QID) for 14 days
  - PPI[b] + clarithromycin (500 mg BID) + metronidazole (500 mg BID) + amoxicillin (1 g BID) for 14 days

[a]Standard or double dose (omeprazole 40 mg, lansoprazole 60 mg, rabeprazole 40 mg, esomeprazole 40 mg) BID.
[b]Standard dose (omeprazole 20 mg, lansoprazole 30 mg, rabeprazole 20 mg, esomeprazole 20 mg) BID.

- It reduces the risk of recurrence of ulcer formation.
- Triple or quadruple therapy is recommended (Table 8.17).

LONG-TERM MANAGEMENT

INTERMITTENT TREATMENT

- For symptomatic relapses less than four times a year.
- Four-week course of one of the ulcer healing agents.

MAINTENANCE TREATMENT

- Indicated in:
  - Symptomatic relapses more than four times per year.
  - History of life-threatening complications like repeated bleeding or perforation.
- Long-term maintenance is with H_2-receptor antagonists (cimetidine 400 mg at night, ranitidine 150 mg at night, famotidine 20 mg at night or nizatidine 150 mg at night).

SURGICAL TREATMENT

- For disease refractory to medical therapy, suspicion of malignancy, bleeding ulcer, gastric outlet obstruction and perforated ulcer.
- For gastric ulcer, the procedure of choice is partial gastrectomy with a Billroth I anastomosis (stomach is anastomosed directly to the duodenum).
- Duodenal ulcer treatment includes:
  - Truncal vagotomy plus pyloroplasty or gastroenterostomy.
  - Selective vagotomy with pyloroplasty.
  - Highly selective vagotomy.

Q. Write a short note on dumping syndrome.

- Dumping syndrome refers to symptoms and signs that occur when food reaches the small bowel too rapidly; usually follows surgery for peptic ulcer disease.
- It usually occurs after a sweet food.
- Two phases of dumping may occur: early and late dumping.
  - Early dumping syndrome occurs 15–30 minutes after meals and consists of crampy abdominal pain, nausea, diarrhoea, borborygmi, bloating, sweating, tachycardia, palpitations, desire to lie down, light-headedness and occasionally syncope. It occurs due to rapid emptying of hyperosmolar gastric contents into the small intestine resulting in fluid shift from blood into the lumen of the gut. This causes intravascular volume contraction and intestinal distension. Mechanical stretching of the intestinal wall also results in vasomotor activation with compensatory activation of the renin-angiotensin system and hypersecretion of intestinal peptide hormones.
  - Late dumping occurs 2–3 hours after meals. The patient gets sweating, light-headedness, palpitations, tachycardia and occasionally syncope. Due to the lack of predigestion, relatively large amounts of rapidly absorbable carbohydrates enter the small intestine, initially leading to hyperglycaemia and followed by excessive insulin secretion with consecutive hypoglycaemia.
- Provocative test for assessing dumping syndrome:
  - A solution of 50–75 g glucose given orally after an overnight fast.
  - Immediately before and up to 180 minutes after ingestion of glucose solution, blood glucose, haematocrit, pulse rate and blood pressure are measured at 30-minute intervals.
  - Test considered positive if an early (30-minute) increase in pulse rate (>10/minute) or haematocrit >3% occurs, or if late (120- to 180-minute) hypoglycaemia occurs.
- Treatment:
  - Patient should be asked to avoid simple carbohydrate food and also to take meals in small amounts at frequent intervals with liquids withheld until 30 minutes after a meal as this accelerates food passage and increases the feeling of satiety.
  - Ingesting up to 15 g of guar gum or pectin that increases viscosity of food, thereby slowing down gastric emptying.
  - α-Glycosidase inhibitors (e.g. acarbose) for late dumping. Acarbose reduces rapid absorption of glucose by prevention of enzymatic cleaving of polysaccharides into smaller molecules.
  - Octreotide given subcutaneously before the meal may be used in refractory cases.

Q. Discuss the aetiology, clinical features, salient investigations and management of Zollinger–Ellison syndrome.

- It defines severe peptic ulcer disease secondary to unregulated gastrin release from a non-β-cell neuroendocrine tumour (gastrinoma).
- Aetiology:
  - More than 80% of gastrinomas are localised in the triangle of the gastrinoma—the convergence of cystic duct and common bile duct superiorly, the junction of second and third portion of

duodenum inferiorly, and the junction of head and body of pancreas medially.
- Most gastrinomas arise from the duodenum (about 75%), whereas they are localised in the pancreas in 25% of cases. Other sites include stomach, bones, ovaries, liver and others.
- Although more than 60% of these tumours are malignant, they grow slowly in about 70% of cases. Metastases occur in local lymph nodes, liver and bones.
- Besides gastrin, these tumours may secrete pancreatic peptide, somatostatin, adrenocorticotropic hormone (ACTH) and vasoactive intestinal peptide (VIP).
- Gastrinoma may be a part of multiple endocrine neoplasia type I (MEN-I).
  - An autosomal dominant syndrome.
  - Characterised by hyperplasia and/or multiple tumours in the parathyroid, pancreas, duodenum, anterior pituitary, foregut-derived neuroendocrine tissue and adrenocortical glands.

- Pathophysiology:
  - Excess gastrin stimulates the parietal cells of stomach to produce excess acid.
  - Excess acid leads to severe peptic ulceration.
  - Excess acid reaches the upper small intestine where it reduces the luminal pH to less than 2. At this low pH, pancreatic lipase is inactivated and bile acids are precipitated. This leads to steatorrhoea and diarrhoea.
- Clinical features:
  - Most commonly presents between 30 and 50 years of age.
  - Manifestations of peptic ulcerations but of shorter duration. Ulcers are severe, multiple and occur at unusual sites like jejunum or oesophagus.
  - Bleeding and perforation are common. May present as intractable recurrent ulceration, following surgery for peptic ulcer.
  - Diarrhoea occurs in nearly 50% of cases.
  - Triad of abdominal pain, weight loss and diarrhoea in the presence of ulcer disease suggests gastrinoma.
  - About one-third of the patients have MEN-I.
- Investigations:
  - Barium meal shows abnormally coarse gastric mucosal folds and ulcers.
  - Endoscopy reveals multiple ulcers at atypical sites.
  - Fasting gastrin level in blood is markedly raised (other causes of elevated gastrin level include achlorhydria, *H. pylori* infection, pyloric obstruction, renal failure and patients on H_2-blockers or PPIs). A serum gastrin value greater than 10 times the upper limit of normal in the presence of a gastric pH below 2 is diagnostic.
  - Gastrin provocating tests (secretin stimulation test, calcium infusion test and a standard meal test).
  - Elevated serum chromogranin A level (may be falsely elevated with proton pump inhibitor use).
  - Tumour localisation done by ultrasound, endoscopic ultrasound (EUS) and CT abdomen. The most important study for localisation is somatostatin receptor scintigraphy using ^{111}In-pentetreotide with single-photon emission tomography (SPECT) scanning (octreoscan).
  - Investigations for MEN-I.
- Treatment:
  - Surgical removal of the tumour whenever possible.
  - Omeprazole can heal the ulcers but in a higher dose (60 mg/day) and longer duration of treatment. Other PPIs include esomeprazole, pantoprazole, rabeprazole and lansoprazole.
  - Somatostatin and its analogues (octreotide, lanreotide) reduce gastric acid and serum gastrin levels in these patients. They can also reduce progression of tumour in some patients.
  - Unresponsive patients are treated by total gastrectomy.

BOX 8.13 Symptoms of Dyspepsia

- Upper abdominal pain, related or unrelated to food
- Gastro-oesophageal reflux and heartburn
- Anorexia, nausea and vomiting
- Early repletion or satiety after meals
- Feeling of abdominal distension or bloating
- Flatulence (burping, belching) and aerography

Q. Briefly discuss the causes and differential diagnosis of dyspepsia.

- Dyspepsia is a collective description of a variety of gastrointestinal symptoms (Box 8.13).
- Organic dyspepsia means that clinical and laboratory investigations indicate an underlying organic disease that is likely to be the cause of the symptoms. Ulcer dyspepsia is one form of organic dyspepsia where dyspeptic symptoms are associated with peptic ulcer.
- Nonulcer dyspepsia (functional dyspepsia) is dyspepsia for which no cause can be found.
- Flatulent dyspepsia is usually due to a functional disorder where dyspeptic symptoms like early satiety, flatulence, bloating and belching predominate.

CAUSES (Table 8.18)

- Causes of dyspepsia are given in Table 8.18.

TABLE 8.18 Causes of Dyspepsia

- Functional dyspepsia
- Dyspepsia associated with organic diseases of upper gastrointestinal tract
  - Peptic ulcer
  - Peptic oesophagitis and gastro-oesophageal reflux disease (GERD)
  - Gastric carcinoma
  - Lactose intolerance
- Dyspepsia associated with other conditions
  - Pancreatic diseases
  - Crohn's disease
  - Colon malignancy
  - Cardiac, renal, hepatic failure
  - Carcinoma lung
- Drugs
- Alcohol
- Pregnancy
- Depression
- Anxiety neurosis

8

COMMON DRUGS CAUSING DYSPEPSIA (Box 8.14)

BOX 8.14 Common Drugs Causing Dyspepsia

- Acarbose
- Bisphosphonates (e.g. alendronate)
- Antibiotics (e.g. erythromycin)
- Codeine
- Corticosteroids
- Iron
- Metformin
- Miglitol
- Nonsteroidal antiinflammatory drugs
- Orlistat
- Theophylline

DIFFERENTIAL DIAGNOSIS

- GERD:
  - Predominant heartburn, heartburn relieved by an antacid and heartburn exacerbated by stooping or lying flat.
  - Regurgitation.
- Peptic ulcer disease:
  - Predominant epigastric pain or discomfort.
  - Periodic symptoms (present for some months of the year and absent for other months).
  - Pain or discomfort relieved with food or causes nocturnal waking.
- Gastric malignancy:
  - Progressive dysphagia, weight loss, gastrointestinal bleeding, anaemia or persistent vomiting.
  - A history of pernicious anaemia or partial gastrectomy (increased incidence of gastric malignancy).

Q. Discuss the aetiology, clinical features, investigations and management of non-ulcer dyspepsia (functional dyspepsia; nervous dyspepsia; nonorganic dyspepsia).

AETIOLOGY

- Even on detailed investigation, no cause can be found.
- Symptoms are believed to be generated by disturbances in the motor function of the gastrointestinal tract.
- The motor dysfunction is analogous to that occurring in the IBS and indeed both IBS and nonulcer dyspepsia often exist together in the same individual.
- *H. pylori* may be responsible in some cases.
- Besides psychological factors, neurological and gut peptide factors are also implicated in the genesis.

CLINICAL FEATURES

- Usually in young females (younger than 40 years of age).
- All the dyspeptic symptoms are present in varying degrees.
- Abdominal pain, nausea and bloating after meals.
- Pain and nausea on waking in the morning is characteristic.
- Symptoms of IBS such as pellet-like stools and feeling of incomplete evacuation after defecation.
- History of stress factors like worries, concern about finance, employment and family affairs.
- Examination reveals inappropriate abdominal tenderness.
- All the organic causes of dyspepsia like drug intake, depression, pregnancy and alcohol abuse have to be excluded before making a diagnosis of nonulcer dyspepsia.
- Alarming features that merit thorough investigations include weight loss, anorexia, dysphagia and haematemesis or melaena.

INVESTIGATIONS

- Blood count, ESR and occult blood in stools to exclude organic disorders.
- Liver function tests to exclude alcoholism.
- Pregnancy tests to exclude pregnancy.
- Barium meal to exclude organic diseases.
- Endoscopy to exclude organic diseases. Required before a trial of H_2-blockers or PPIs in presence of any of the following:
  - Age >55 years.
  - Dysphagia.
  - Protracted vomiting.
  - Anorexia or unexplained weight loss.
  - Melaena or anaemia.
  - Palpable mass.
  - Previous peptic ulcer disease.
  - Jaundice.
  - Family history of gastric malignancy.
- Noninvasive tests for *H. pylori* if above-mentioned risk factors are absent.

DIAGNOSTIC CRITERIA (Table 8.19)

- Rome IV criteria divide functional dyspepsia into two types: Epigastric pain syndrome (EPS) and postprandial distress syndrome (PDS). Any one of first

TABLE 8.19 Rome IV Criteria for Functional Dyspepsia

A. At least 3 months with onset at least 6 months previously, of one or more of the following four:	
1. Bothersome postprandial fullness 2. Early satiation	Severe enough to impact on regular activities or finishing a regular-size meal for at least 3 days per week
3. Bothersome epigastric pain 4. Bothersome epigastric burning	For at least 1 day per week
AND	
B. No evidence of structural disease (including at upper endoscopy) that is likely to explain the symptoms	

two criteria under *point A* in Table 8.19 is for PDS while any one of last two criteria is for EPS.

MANAGEMENT

- Proper explanation and reassurance.
- Stress factors tackled by counselling.
- Avoid cigarette smoking and alcohol abuse.
- Small and frequent low-fat food.
- If endoscopy is noncontributory, initiate empirical treatment.
- *H. pylori* eradication if test is positive; may provide long-term benefit.
- H_2-receptor antagonists or PPIs for 4–6 weeks for EPS type of dyspepsia.
- Centrally active neuromodulators like tricyclic antidepressants.
- Prokinetic agents useful in PDS type of dyspepsia. These include metoclopramide 10 mg TID (for not more than 12 weeks), domperidone 10 mg TID, cinitapride 1 mg TID, and itopride 50 mg TID. These are to be used only after failure of *H. pylori* eradication and PPIs.
- Another category of drugs for PDS is fundus-relaxing drugs. These include acotiamide 100 mg TID and buspirone 7.5–15 mg BID.

SUMMARY OF MANAGEMENT (Flowchart 8.2)

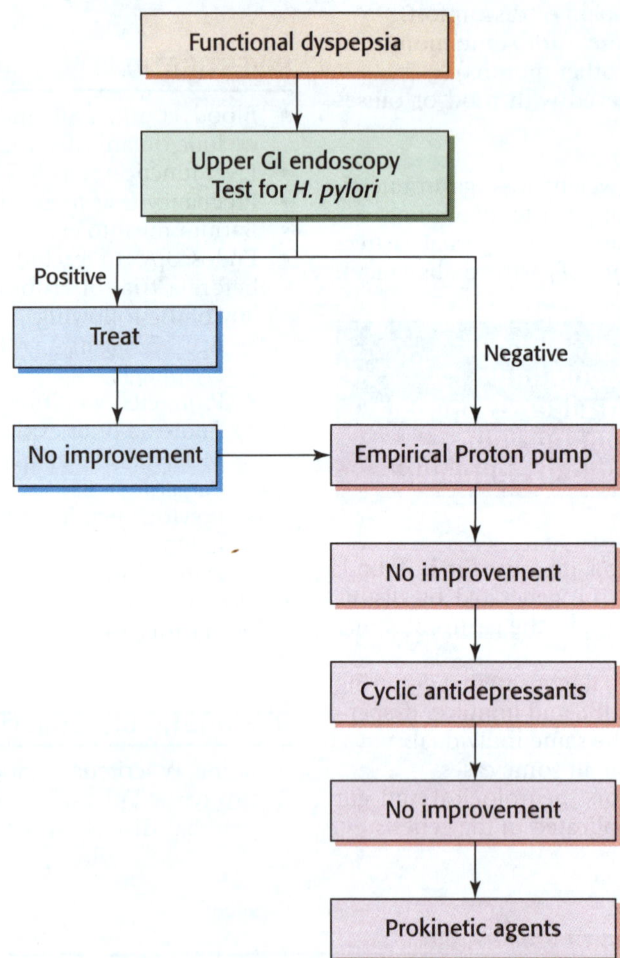

Flowchart 8.2 Summary of Management of Functional Dyspepsia.

DISTINGUISHING FEATURES (Table 8.20)

TABLE 8.20 Nonulcer Dyspepsia Versus Ulcer Dyspepsia

Nonulcer Dyspepsia	Ulcer Dyspepsia
• Pain not episodic	• Pain episodic (periodicity)
• Pain present throughout the day	• Pain occurs only on empty stomach
• Unaffected by antacids	• Relieved by antacids
• Pain provoked by food	• Pain relieved by food
• Diffuse abdominal pain referred to more than one site	• Localised abdominal pain referred to epigastrium
• Pain at night, waking the patient from sleep is rare	• Pain at night, waking the patient from sleep is common
• Pain not relieved by vomiting and patient cannot eat afterwards	• Pain relieved by vomiting and patient can eat immediately

Q. Discuss the classification, aetiology, clinical features, investigations and management of malabsorption syndrome. (IM 16.3)

- The term 'maldigestion' indicates impaired breakdown of nutrients (carbohydrates, proteins and fats) to absorbable split products (monosaccharides, disaccharides or oligosaccharides, amino acids, oligopeptides, fatty acids, monoglycerides). On the other hand, the term malabsorption strictly means defective mucosal uptake and transport of adequately digested nutrients including vitamins and trace elements.
- However, in practice, malabsorption is defined as impairment of digestion and/or absorption from gastrointestinal tract.

CLASSIFICATION AND AETIOLOGY OF MALABSORPTION SYNDROME

- Classification and aetiology of malabsorption syndrome is given in Table 8.21.

TABLE 8.21 Classification and Aetiology of Malabsorption Syndrome

Disorders of intraluminal digestion	
A. Defect in substrate hydrolysis • Enzyme deficiency • Enzyme inactivation • Rapid transit of food through gut	• Chronic pancreatitis • Cystic fibrosis • Pancreatic carcinoma • Zollinger–Ellison syndrome • Gastro-enterostomy • Partial gastrectomy
B. Defect in fat solubilisation • Reduced bile salt synthesis • Reduced bile secretion • Bile salt deconjugation and precipitation in gut • Increased bile salt loss in faeces	• Parenchymal liver diseases • Cholestatic jaundice • Zollinger–Ellison syndrome • Stagnant loop syndrome or blind loop syndrome (colonisation of small bowel by bacteria) • Terminal ileal disease (e.g. Crohn's disease, tuberculosis) • Terminal ileal resection
C. Defect in luminal availability of factors • Lack of intrinsic factor • Increased vitamin B_{12} consumption in gut	• Pernicious anaemia
Disorders of transport in the intestinal mucosal cell	
A. Defect in brush-border hydrolysis (mucosa normal histologically)	• Lactase deficiency
B. Defect in epithelial transport (mucosa often abnormal histologically)	• Coeliac disease • Tropical sprue • Lymphoma • Whipple's disease • Giardiasis • Radiation enteritis • AIDS
Disorders of transport from mucosal cell	
A. Lymphatic obstruction	• Abdominal lymphoma • Tuberculosis • Lymphangiectasia
B. Defect in epithelial processing	• Abetalipoproteinaemia
Drugs and systemic diseases causing malabsorption (see Tables 8.22 and 8.23)	

DRUGS CAUSING MALABSORPTION (Table 8.22)

TABLE 8.22 Drugs Causing Malabsorption

Drug	Mechanisms
• Colchicine	• Inhibits crypt cell division and lactase
• Neomycin	• Precipitation of bile salts in gut; inhibition of lactase
• Methotrexate	• Folic acid antagonist causing inhibition of crypt cell division
• Cholestyramine	• Binding bile salts
• Laxatives	• Multiple mechanisms

SYSTEMIC DISEASES ASSOCIATED WITH MALABSORPTION (Table 8.23)

TABLE 8.23 Systemic Diseases Associated With Malabsorption

Disease	Mechanisms
• Addison's disease	• Not clear
• Thyrotoxicosis	• Rapid transit through gut
• Hypothyroidism	• Villous atrophy; pancreatic insufficiency
• Diabetes mellitus	• Autonomic insufficiency; bacterial overgrowth; pancreatic insufficiency (causing diabetes)
• Collagen vascular diseases	• Villous atrophy; bacterial overgrowth; amyloidosis

CLINICAL FEATURES

- Insidious onset and gradual progression.
- General features:
  - Include diarrhoea, abdominal pain, distension, loss of weight, anaemia and vague ill health.
- Specific features:
  - Due to defective absorption of different constituents (Table 8.24).
- Bile acid malabsorption:
  - Failure of absorption of bile acids (e.g. chenodeoxycholic and deoxycholic acids) by distal ileum results in spillover of bile acids into colon where they induce secretion of sodium and water producing loose and watery stools.

INVESTIGATIONS

- Barium meal follow-through:
  - Shows nonspecific features such as dilated loops with flocculation and segmentation of barium.
  - Specific structural abnormalities in Crohn's disease, diverticula and strictures.
- Tests for fat absorption:
  - Sudan III staining of stool for fat globules.
  - Stool fat excretion in 1 day is more than 7 g (normal is less than 7 g/day on 100 g/day of fat diet). Generally stools are collected over a period of 72 hours. It does not differentiate between small intestinal, hepatobiliary and pancreatic causes.
  - Measurement of fat-soluble vitamin (A, D, E, K) levels in the blood; prothrombin time.
  - Plasma vitamin A level after 2–3 days of oral retinol will be lower than normal.
  - Near-infrared reflectance analysis.
  - ^{14}C-triolein breath test involves measurement of breath carbon dioxide after ingestion of radiolabelled triglyceride triolein.
- Tests for carbohydrate absorption:
  - Glucose tolerance test shows absence of rise in blood glucose levels.
  - d-Xylose absorption test measures urinary excretion of d-xylose over 5 hours after ingestion of a 25-g oral dose; less than 4 g is abnormal. It indicates enteric malabsorption instead of pancreatic cause.
  - Lactose tolerance test (LTT) is abnormal—after 50 g lactose is given orally, blood samples are taken every 20 minutes for 2 hours. Normally blood glucose shows a rise of more than 20 mg/dL.
  - Hydrogen breath test to diagnose lactase deficiency—50 g lactose is given orally and breath hydrogen measured every hour for 4 hours. A rise in hydrogen concentration of 20 ppm over baseline is considered diagnostic of lactose malabsorption.
- Tests for protein absorption:
  - Serum albumin level will be low.
  - Measurement of nitrogen in the 24-hour stool will be more than 2.5 g.

TABLE 8.24 Specific Features due to Malabsorption of Different Food Constituents

• **Protein**	Progressive emaciation, pitting pedal oedema
• **Fat**	Loss of weight, diarrhoea and loose, pale, bulky, offensive stool that float on water and are difficult to flush away (steatorrhoea)
• **Carbohydrate**	Abdominal distension, belching, bloating feeling in abdomen
• **Vitamins**	
• Vitamin A	Follicular keratosis, night blindness, xerophthalmia, keratomalacia
• Vitamin D	Muscular irritability, tetany, features of osteomalacia
• Vitamin K	Haemorrhagic tendencies
• Vitamins B_1 and B_2	Angular stomatitis, cheilosis, glossitis, neuropathy
• Folic acid	Macrocytic anaemia, glossitis
• **Minerals and electrolytes**	
• Sodium	Muscle cramps, weakness, hypotension
• Potassium	Weakness, areflexia, intestinal distension, cardiac arrhythmias
• Calcium	Muscular irritability, tetany, features of rickets, features of osteomalacia
• Magnesium	Weakness, tingling sensation, tetany
• Zinc	Anorexia, weakness, tingling, impaired taste
• Iron	Hypochromic microcytic anaemia, glossitis, koilonychia
• Water	Dehydration, low blood volume

- Labelling serum proteins with radioactive chromium and measuring radioactivity in stool is a test for protein-losing enteropathy.
- α_1-Anti-trypsin content in a 3-day collection of stools (normally no antitrypsin in stool).
- Test for bile acid malabsorption.
  - Selenium homocholic acid taurine (SeHCAT) test in which Se-labelled bile acid is administered orally and total body retention is measured with a gamma camera after 7 days. Retention value of less than 10% is considered abnormal.
- Tests for absorption of other substances:
  - Serum B_{12} level will be low.
  - Serum levels of iron, folate and calcium will be low.
  - Macrocytic anaemia in B_{12} and folic acid deficiency.
  - Prolonged prothrombin time.
  - Low serum sodium and potassium.
  - Low serum magnesium and zinc levels.
- Tests for pancreatic exocrine function:
  - Faecal elastase-1.
  - Faecal chymotrypsin.
  - Serum trypsinogen.
  - Secretin stimulation test.
- Tests for bacterial overgrowth:
  - $^{14}CO_2$ in breath after ingestion of cholyl-^{14}C-glycine.
  - Quantitative measurement of bacterial counts from aspirated intestinal fluid.
- Wireless capsule endoscopy:
  - Allows for visualisation of entire small bowel and allows for much more detailed evaluation of small bowel mucosal disease than barium studies.
- Small intestinal biopsy (duodenal or jejunal).

TREATMENT

- Gluten-free diet in coeliac disease:
- Pancreatic supplements in pancreatic insufficiency.
- Low-fat diet and cholestyramine for bile acid deficiency.
- Replacement therapy for anaemia, bone disease and coagulation defects.
- Oral folic acid, oral iron and intramuscular B_{12}.
- Vitamin D and calcium supplements.
- Vitamin B complex.
- Cholestyramine (bile acid binder) for bile acid malabsorption.
- Treat dehydration and electrolyte deficiency by intravenous infusion.

Q. Discuss the aetiology, pathology, clinical features, complications, investigations and treatment of coeliac disease (nontropical sprue; gluten-induced enteropathy).

DEFINITION

- A chronic immune-mediated intestinal disease producing malabsorption and caused in genetically susceptible individuals by ingestion of gluten.
- Clinical and histological improvement after withdrawal of dietary gluten.

AETIOLOGY

- Immunological damage of the mucosa due to gluten protein of wheat. Gluten is also present in barley and rye. The toxic component in gluten is gliadin.
- High association with HLA DQ2 and DQ8.

PATHOPHYSIOLOGY

- Gluten is the water-insoluble seed storage protein in wheat, rye and barley. Gliadin is the alcohol-soluble component of gluten.
- α-Gliadin and other related peptides bind with tissue transglutaminase (tTG) in enterocytes.
- α-Gliadin is rich in glutamine; transglutaminase deaminates glutamine residues forming glutamic acid. Deamidation enhances immunogenicity of α-Gliadin.
- These altered gliadin peptides are then presented to local intestinal T cells and recognised as foreign, thereby stimulating an immune response.
- Subsequently, CD4+T lymphocytes infiltrate in lamina propria and CD8+in intestinal epithelium.
- Recognition of HLA-bound gluten peptides by T cells leads to their activation and clonal expansion of B cells that produce antibodies.
- Antibodies produced by plasma cells are directed against a variety of antigens including transglutaminase, endomysium, gliadin and reticulin. This leads to intense local inflammatory reaction in the intestines producing villous fattening. This in turn leads to carbohydrate, protein and fat malabsorption.
- Osmotic and secretory diarrhoea occur due to undigested nutrients.
- Pathophysiology is summarised in Flowchart 8.3.

PATHOLOGY

- Mucosa of duodenojejunal flexure shows the abnormalities.
- Characteristic features are partial villous atrophy or subtotal villous atrophy.
- Lamina propria demonstrates cellular infiltrates consisting of plasma cells and lymphocytes.

CLINICAL FEATURES

- Seen in both children and adults but more common in children.
- Diagnosed typically in early childhood around the age of 2 years. A second peak is found around the age of 40 years.
- Features in adults:
  - Range from mild anaemia to florid malabsorptive state.
  - The most common cause of anaemia is iron deficiency; less commonly, it is due to folate and/or vitamin B_{12} deficiency.
  - Diarrhoea and weight loss.
  - Peripheral neuropathy (B_1 and B_{12} deficiency), hypoproteinaemia, oedema, bone pain and tetany.

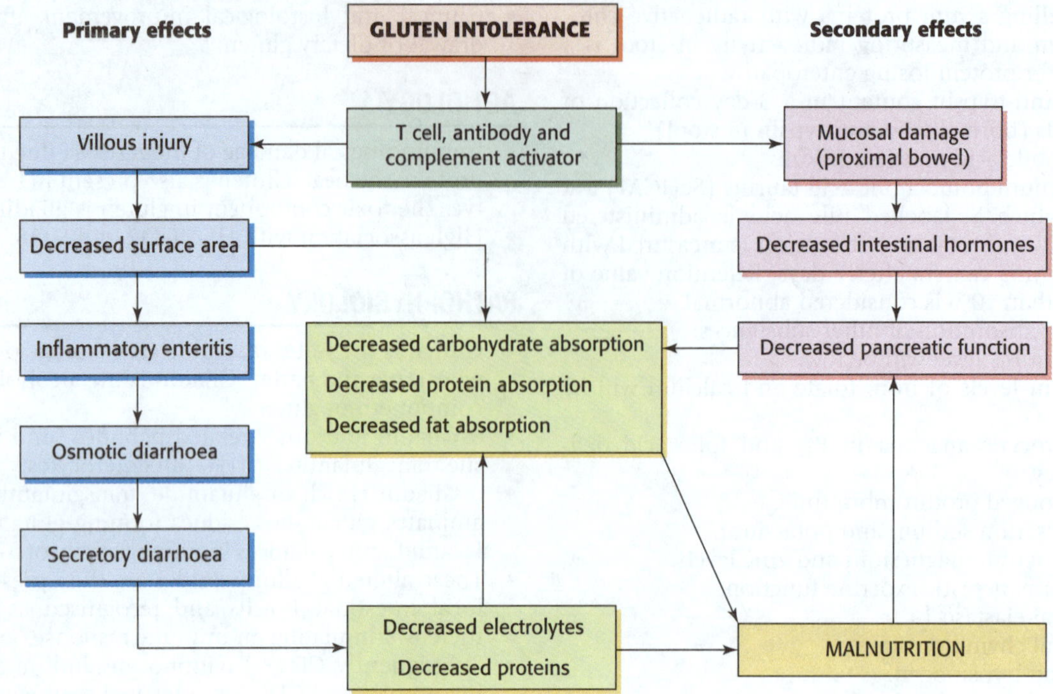

Flowchart 8.3 Pathophysiology of Coeliac Disease.

- Vitamin deficiency features.
- Clubbing (20%), glossitis, angular stomatitis and skin pigmentation.
- Amenorrhoea and infertility.
- Fingerprints show epidermal ridge atrophy in 90%.
- A number of other autoimmune syndromes have been associated with coeliac disease. These include type 1 diabetes, autoimmune thyroid disease, rheumatoid arthritis, systemic lupus erythematosus, Addison's disease and others.
- Other uncommon extraintestinal features include idiopathic pulmonary haemosiderosis, IgA nephropathy, elevated liver enzymes and liver failure, myocarditis and arthritis.

COMPLICATIONS

- Complications of coeliac disease are listed in Box 8.15.

DERMATITIS HERPETIFORMIS

- Chronic pruritic disease characterised by presence of intensely pruritic, symmetrical papulovesicular rash that evolves to crusting lesions broadly distributed over the body but especially on the forearms, knees (Fig. 8.4), buttocks, wrists and scalp.

BOX 8.15 Complications of Coeliac Disease

- Dermatitis herpetiformis
- Malignancies, particularly intestinal lymphoma mainly involving jejunum
- Pneumococcal infections
- Psoriasis
- Osteomalacia, osteoporosis
- Peripheral neuropathy, epilepsy, migraine and ataxia
- Amyloidosis
- Microscopic colitis
- Pericarditis, myocarditis

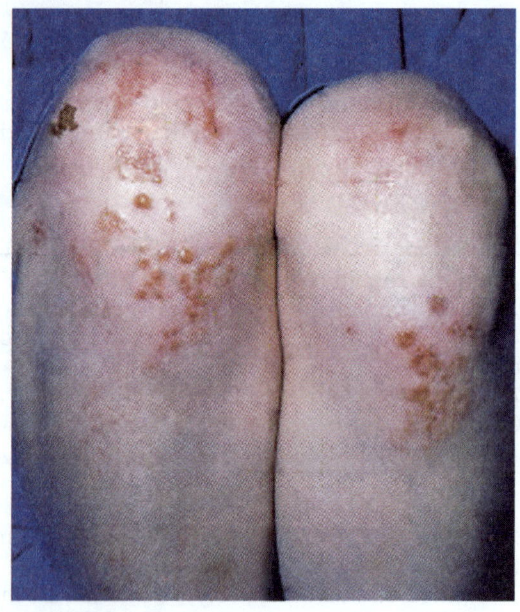

Fig. 8.4 Dermatitis herpetiformis. From James WD et al: Andrews' diseases of the skin, ed 12, Philadelphia, 2016, Elsevier.

- Mucous membranes are uncommonly involved.
- On biopsy, papillary dermal neutrophilic microabscesses are characteristically seen.
- On direct immunofluorescence, granular deposition of immunoglobulin A is detected.
- Direct immunofluorescence confirms the diagnosis.
- Also have IgA antibodies directed against epidermal transglutaminase which is homologous to tTG antibody.
- Gluten-free diet is the treatment of choice.
- If not responsive, dapsone may be tried.

INVESTIGATIONS

- Serological tests:
  - IgA antiendomysial antibodies (EMA; 85%–100% sensitive and 95%–100% specific).
  - IgA anti-tTG antibodies.
  - IgG and IgA antigliadin antibodies (not routinely recommended for diagnosing coeliac disease).
  - IgG deamidated gliadin peptide antibodies better than antigliadin antibodies.
  - Patients should not restrict their diet before testing for antibodies.
  - Sensitivity and specificity of various serological tests in coeliac disease are given in Table 8.25.
- Abnormal jejunal biopsy:
  - A biopsy may be omitted if patient has high antibody titres (tTG >10 times upper limit of normal and positive EMA) and an appropriate HLA type.
  - Biopsy is indicated for diagnosis in cases of IgA deficiency
- Tests indicating malabsorption of proteins, carbohydrate, fat and vitamins.
- Bone densitometry either at the time of diagnosis or 1 year after starting treatment because of high frequency of osteoporosis.

TREATMENT

- Strict gluten-free diet indefinitely. Avoid wheat and wheat products (e.g. *maida, dalia, sooji*, noodles, pastas), rye and barley.
- Rice, corn, soybean, potato, pulses, gram flour (*besan*), millets (*bajra*), milk, eggs, meat and fruits are safe. Pure oat in moderate quantities is also safe.
- Beer must be completely avoided, even from alcohol-free brands, as its manufacture involves the fermentation of various gluten-containing cereals. The same is true for all kinds of whisky obtained from malt distillation procedures.
- Corticosteroids (e.g. budesonide) are required rarely. Useful in critically ill patients who present with acute coeliac crisis manifested by severe diarrhoea, dehydration, weight loss, acidosis, hypocalcaemia and hypoproteinaemia. Also required for the rare patients who present with gliadin shock after a gluten challenge.
- Vitamin and mineral supplementation including iron administration.
- Dairy products are avoided in beginning as secondary lactase deficiency is often associated with coeliac disease.

TABLE 8.25 Sensitivity and Specificity of Various Serological Tests for Coeliac Diseases

Assay	Sensitivity (%)	Specificity (%)
• IgA antiendomysial antibody	85–98	96–100
• IgA antitissue transglutaminase antibody	90–98	94–97
• IgA antigliadin antibody	80–90	85–95
• IgG antigliadin antibody	75–85	75–90

Q. Discuss the aetiology, pathology, clinical features, investigations and treatment of tropical sprue (idiopathic tropical malabsorption syndrome).

DEFINITION

- Malabsorption occurring in patients of tropics in the absence of other intestinal diseases or parasites.

AETIOLOGY

- It is unknown, but some infective organism is suspected as antibiotics are very useful in the treatment of this disease.
- Some of the implicated bacteria include *E. coli, Klebsiella* and *Enterobacter*.
- Folic acid deficiency is another postulation.

PATHOLOGY

- Jejunal biopsy shows partial villous atrophy. This results in a decrease in total absorptive surface area.
- A normal jejunal biopsy rules out tropical sprue but an abnormal biopsy does not diagnose it since similar abnormalities are seen in some normal tropical subjects and also in some other conditions.

CLINICAL FEATURES

- Three phases:
  - Initial phase of active diarrhoea (common in India).
  - Intermediate phase.
  - Last phase (frank malabsorption).
- Spontaneous remissions and relapses may occur.
- Diarrhoea, abdominal distension, anorexia, weight loss and fatigue.
- Megaloblastic anaemia, oedema, glossitis and stomatitis.

INVESTIGATIONS

- Stool examination to exclude *Giardia, E. histolytica, Yersinia, Cryptosporidium* and other pathogens.
- Megaloblastic anaemia.
- Hypoalbuminaemia.
- Barium study will show thickening of mucosal folds.
- Abnormal tests for fat absorption.
- d-Xylose test abnormal.
- Vitamin B_{12} malabsorption.
- tTG and endomysial antibodies negative.
- Partial villous atrophy on jejunal biopsy.

TREATMENT

- Tetracycline or oxytetracycline 1 g daily in four divided doses for 6 months.
- Folic acid 5 mg daily (along with tetracycline).
- Correction of deficiencies of fluids, electrolytes, vitamins and iron.
- Symptomatic treatment for diarrhoea.

Q. Discuss the aetiology, clinical features, investigations and management of lactose intolerance.

AETIOLOGY

- The term lactose intolerance indicates that lactose malabsorption causes gastrointestinal symptoms. It occurs due to deficiency of lactase, an enzyme occurring in the brush border membrane of the intestinal mucosa that hydrolyses lactose to its components galactose and glucose.
- Lactose (primary carbohydrate in milk) cannot be hydrolysed and hence it goes to colon where it is fermented by bacteria to produce methane, hydrogen and carbon dioxide which can lead to gastrointestinal symptoms.
- Primary lactase deficiency is inherited and characterised by normal intestinal biopsy. Lactase activity begins to decrease after weaning usually after 2 years of age.
- Secondary lactase deficiency can be the consequence of any condition that damages the small intestinal mucosa brush border or significantly increases the gastrointestinal transit time. It is often associated with abnormal intestinal biopsy. Seen in coeliac disease, tropical sprue, Crohn's disease, giardiasis and viral gastroenteritis.

CLINICAL FEATURES

- Low lactase levels per se do not result in symptoms. Whether and to what extent symptoms occur depend on several factors such as amount of lactose consumed, individual sensitivity and rate of gastric emptying.
- Abdominal colic, abdominal distension, increased flatus and diarrhoea after ingesting milk or milk products. Symptoms generally appear 1 hour after ingesting milk and resolve after 5–7 days of avoidance of lactose-containing foods.
- Headache, light-headedness, loss of concentration, fatigue, cardiac dysrhythmias and mouth ulcers may be associated with lactose malabsorption.
- Improvement of symptoms on withdrawal of milk or milk products.

INVESTIGATIONS

- Hydrogen breath test:
  - Undigested lactose is fermented by the colonic microflora with production of hydrogen detectable in expired air.
  - It involves ingestion of 25–50 g of lactose and the measurement of hydrogen every 15 min for 3–6 hours. An increase in breath hydrogen concentration greater than 20 parts per million over baseline suggests lactase deficiency.
- Measurement of lactase activity in a jejunal biopsy specimen.

TREATMENT

- Lactose-free or lactose-restricted diet (avoidance of milk and dairy products). However, it may produce serious nutritional deficiencies, particularly calcium and protein deficiency. Most people with lactose intolerance can tolerate some amount of lactose in their diet.
- Gradually introducing small amounts of milk or milk products may help some people adapt to them with fewer symptoms. Often, people can better tolerate milk or milk products by taking them with meals.
- Exogenous β-galactosidase:
  - Enzyme replacement therapy with microbial exogenous lactase (obtained from yeasts or fungi) seems to be effective without any significant side effects.
  - Given together with milk and dairy products.
- Other therapeutic modalities include use of yoghurt and probiotics as source of β-galactosidase. Yoghurt delays gastric emptying and intestinal transit causing slower delivery of lactose to the intestine, thus optimising the action of residual β-galactosidase in the small bowel and decreasing the osmotic load of lactose. It also contains microorganisms that produce lactase.
- Increase calcium and vitamin D consumption.

Q. Briefly discuss the aetiology, clinical features, investigations and treatment of giardiasis.

AETIOLOGY

- Organism is *Giardia lamblia.*
- Infection occurs by ingestion of cysts through contaminated water or by faecal–oral route.
- Trophozoites attach to the mucosa of duodenum and jejunum causing alteration in small bowel functions. Most often, there is no local destruction or invasion.
  - The trophozoite is pear-shaped and measures 12–20 μm in length and 5–10 μm in width.
  - It has two symmetric nuclei and four pairs of flagella.
  - Trophozoites replicate by binary fission.
  - Detached trophozoites pass down the small intestine into the colon and encyst. Cysts are excreted in the faeces.
- Malabsorption that occurs in many patients is due to loss of brush border enzyme activities while in some cases there is flattening of villi.
- Patients with hypogammaglobulinaemia suffer from prolonged and severe infection that may be unresponsive to standard treatment.

CLINICAL FEATURES

- Incubation period is 1–3 weeks (median 7–10 days).
- Starts as diarrhoea, nausea, vomiting, anorexia, weakness and abdominal pain. Fever, tenesmus and blood in stool are rare.
- Symptoms may persist from a few days to weeks or months to years.
- Secondary lactase deficiency is common.
- Many patients are asymptomatic.
- Individuals with chronic giardiasis may present with or without having experienced antecedent acute

symptoms. Diarrhoea may not be a prominent symptom in these patients who often have increased flatus, loose stools, malabsorption, weight loss and growth retardation.

INVESTIGATIONS

- Repeated examination of stool for trophozoites and cysts.
- Detection of *Giardia* antigen in stool using immunoassays or PCR.
- Duodenal or jejunal fluid microscopy will demonstrate the organism.
- Jejunal biopsy shows the *Giardia* on the mucosa.
- Long-standing cases show steatorrhoea, malabsorption of xylose, vitamin B_{12} and lactose intolerance.

TREATMENT

- Maintain optimal hydration and electrolyte balance.
- Tinidazole 2 g or ornidazole 2 g as a single dose, repeated after 1 week.
- Metronidazole 2 g daily for 3 days or metronidazole 200 mg thrice daily for 7 days.
- Ornidazole 500 mg twice a day for 2–3 days.
- Nitazoxanide 500 mg twice a day for 3 days.
- Metronidazole 800 mg TID for 3 weeks in refractory cases.
- Albendazole 400 mg once a day for 5–10 days.
- Other drugs include paromomycin, furazolidone and quinacrine.
- Treatment of asymptomatic carriers is generally not recommended except in special instances like outbreak control (e.g. in day-care centres, prevention of household transmission by toddlers to pregnant women and susceptible individuals such as those with hypogammaglobulinaemia or cystic fibrosis, and food handlers).
- Avoid lactose-containing foods for at least 1 month after therapy.

Q. What is traveller's diarrhoea? Briefly explain.

- Travellers' diarrhoea is generally defined as the passage of ≥3 unformed stools per 24 hours plus at least one additional symptom (such as nausea, vomiting, abdominal cramps, fever, blood/mucus in the stools, or faecal urgency) that develop while abroad or within 10 days of returning from any resource-limited destinations.
  - Mild diarrhoea is tolerable, not distressing and does not interfere with planned activities.
  - Moderate diarrhoea is distressing or interferes with planned activities.
  - Severe diarrhoea is incapacitating or completely prevents planned activities. All dysentery is considered severe.
- Food and water contaminated with faecal matter are the main reservoirs for the pathogens that cause traveller's diarrhoea.

BOX 8.16 Aetiology of Traveller's Diarrhoea

- *Escherichia coli* (enterotoxigenic—ETEC and enteroaggregative)
- *Vibrio parahaemolyticus*
- *Vibrio cholerae*—El Tor biotype
- *Shigella*
- *Salmonella* (nontyphoid)
- *Campylobacter*
- *Giardia lamblia*
- *Entamoeba histolytica*
- Rotavirus
- Norovirus
- Commonly, no organism is identified

AETIOLOGY (Box 8.16)

- *E. coli*, especially enterotoxigenic E. coli (ETEC) is the most common pathogen worldwide.

CLINICAL FEATURES

- Usually affects intercontinental travellers.
- Abrupt onset, watery diarrhoea lasting 2–5 days.
- Abdominal cramps, nausea, vomiting, anorexia and fever.
- Diffuse tenderness over abdomen.

INVESTIGATIONS

- Laboratory evaluation is generally unnecessary.
- If the patient appears toxic, has high fever, is hospitalised, develops bloody or rice-water diarrhoea, has severe abdominal cramps, is immunocompromised, has a significant underlying medical condition or has persistent diarrhoea not responding to empiric therapy, stool should be examined for ova, cyst and parasites.

TREATMENT

- Usually self-limited and no treatment is required.
- Correction of dehydration by oral rehydration supplements.
- Antidiarrhoeal agents and antibiotics are required rarely. Loperamide may be used for short term if stools do not contain blood and patient is afebrile. It should not be given to children below the age of 2 years because of the potential risk of central nervous system depression. If patient has fever or has bloody diarrhoea with fever, norfloxacin or ciprofloxacin may be used. Azithromycin is used if patient is allergic to quinolones or is pregnant.
- Rifaximin, a poorly absorbed rifampicin derivative, is highly effective against noninvasive bacterial pathogens. Dose is 200 mg thrice a day for 3 days. It is less effective for the treatment of invasive pathogens and should not be used for the treatment of dysentery.
- For moderate diarrhoea without fever, ciprofloxacin or rifaximin can be given for 3 days or azithromycin 1000 mg once only. Trimethoprim–sulphamethoxazole and doxycycline are no longer recommended because of the development of widespread resistance.
- Loperamide may be used along with an antibiotic to reduce symptoms.

RECOMMENDATIONS ON TREATMENT (Table 8.26)

TABLE 8.26 Recommendations on Treatment by International Society of Travel Medicine

Mild traveller's diarrhoea	Oral rehydration Loperamide if required No antibiotics
Moderate traveller's diarrhoea	Oral rehydration Loperamide Azithromycin or a fluoroquinolone or rifaximin
Severe traveller's diarrhoea	Oral rehydration Azithromycin or a fluoroquinolone Loperamide (in absence of fever and dysentery)

PREVENTION

- Personal hygiene.
- Chemoprophylaxis should not be routinely used because of potential of alteration of gut flora, development of adverse events, development of antimicrobial resistance and possible drug interactions. If required, one of the following may be used:
  - Bismuth subsalicylate is given 60 mL four times a day. Avoid if allergic to aspirin, pregnant or on anticoagulants. Also avoid if taking doxycycline (e.g. for malaria prophylaxis).
  - Rifaximin once a day.
  - Doxycycline 100 mg/day for a few weeks.
- Probiotics may be useful.

Q. Briefly describe carcinoid tumours and carcinoid syndrome.

Q. Briefly describe gastrointestinal neuroendocrinal tumours.

- Carcinoid tumours are neoplasms of neuroendocrine cells (e.g. enterochromaffin cells). These are now categorised as well-differentiated neuroendocrine tumours (NET).
- Classified on the basis of their embryologic origin:
  - Foregut (lungs, bronchi and stomach).
  - Midgut (small intestine, appendix and proximal large bowel).
  - Hindgut (distal large bowel, rectum).
- Common sites of NET in the gastrointestinal tract are ileum, appendix and rectum. Other includes pancreas.
- Carcinoid syndrome refers to the systemic symptoms produced when the secretory products of these tumours are released into the systemic circulation.
  - This syndrome usually occurs after hepatic metastasis of midgut carcinoids as normally liver is able to deactivate these secretory products.
  - In contrast, patients with foregut (bronchial and extraintestinal) carcinoids can present with carcinoid syndrome without hepatic metastases since their secretory products normally bypass liver and enter systemic circulation directly.
  - Hindgut tumours seldom produce this syndrome since they do not secrete these products.

BOX 8.17 Secretory Products of Carcinoids

- Serotonin
- Histamine
- Tachykinins
- Motilin
- Bradykinins
- Adrenocorticotropic hormone
- Corticotropin-releasing factor
- Prostaglandins

- Intestinal carcinoids show a high tendency for hepatic metastases.
- Secretory products are listed in Box 8.17.

CLINICAL FEATURES

CLINICAL FEATURES DUE TO CARCINOID SYNDROME

- Cutaneous flushing involving head and neck (blush area) associated with lacrimation, periorbital oedema, tachycardia and hypotension. This may last for a few minutes to hours. Flushing may be precipitated by cheese, nuts, eggs, fish, chicken, turkey, red meat and wine.
- Diarrhoea with borborygmi cramps and malabsorption. Flushing and diarrhoea are precipitated by food, alcohol or exercise.
- Facial telangiectasia is purple telangiectasia most marked over malar area.
- Right heart valve lesions, especially tricuspid regurgitation and pulmonary stenosis. The left side is usually spared due to the inactivation of humoral substances by the lung.
- Wheeze occurs due to bronchoconstriction.
- Pellagra-like lesions are due to conversion of tryptophan to serotonin. Normally, niacin is produced from tryptophan. This leads to niacin deficiency. Symptoms of pellagra include rough scaly skin, angular stomatitis, glossitis, diarrhoea and encephalopathy.
- A carcinoid crisis is a potentially life-threatening complication of carcinoid syndrome caused by sudden release of vasoactive peptides which is precipitated by tumour manipulation during surgery, percutaneous needle biopsy or even anaesthesia. It manifests as hypotension or hypertension, diarrhoea, bronchoconstriction, flushing and acidosis.

CLINICAL FEATURES DUE TO CARCINOID TUMOURS

- General features include hepatomegaly due to hepatic metastases, intestinal obstruction and bleeding, and tumour-associated myasthenia.
- Occasionally local symptoms such as obstruction, bleeding or ischaemia caused by the tumour.

DIAGNOSIS

- Increased urinary excretion of 5-hydroxyindoleacetic acid (5-HIAA) in 24-hour collection (more than 9 mg).
- Elevated plasma levels of chromogranin A.
- Serotonin level in blood and platelets is high.

- CT, MRI and somatostatin receptor scintigraphy, positron emission tomography (PET) with radiolabelled 5-hydroxytryptophan, indium-111 pentetreotide or 68-gallium Dotatate, and occasionally laparotomy for localisation.
- Measurement of increased concentration of serotonin in tumour tissue.

TREATMENT

- Avoidance of conditions and diets precipitating flushing and diarrhoea.
- Supplementation of food with niacin.
- Bronchodilators for wheeze.
- Loperamide for diarrhoea.
- Serotonin receptor antagonists (cyproheptadine, methysergide and ondansetron) to control diarrhoea. These agents may also control flushing in some cases.
- Analogues of somatostatin (e.g. octreotide and lanreotide) are useful to control flushing.
- Telotristat (a tryptophan hydroxylase inhibitor which is the rate-limiting enzyme in serotonin synthesis) along with somatostatin analogues useful in patients with diarrhoea.
- Treatment of valvular disease and heart failure.
- Surgical resection of the tumour.
- Excision of hepatic metastases or hepatic artery embolisation with or without chemotherapy.

Q. Discuss the aetiology, clinical features, investigations and management of ischaemic colitis.

BLOOD SUPPLY

- Superior mesenteric artery supplies caecum, ascending colon and proximal two-thirds of transverse colon.
- Inferior mesenteric artery supplies distal transverse colon, descending colon, sigmoid colon and proximal aspect of rectum.
- Internal iliac artery supplies mid and distal rectum via rectal arteries.
- Marginal artery of Drummond extends along the periphery of colonic mesentery, giving rise to vasa recta and linking inferior mesenteric artery to superior mesenteric artery. Collateral vessels help to ensure adequate perfusion if one of the main branches becomes occluded.
- Splenic flexure (Griffiths' point) and sigmoid colon (Sudeck's point) are the most sensitive areas to decreased blood flow. These 'watershed' areas are where circulation from superior mesenteric artery and inferior mesenteric artery, and inferior mesenteric artery and rectal arteries, respectively meet. These areas rely on marginal artery of Drummond to provide collateral flow.
- Thus, left colon and splenic flexure are involved in 75% of ischaemic colitis.
- Severity of ischaemia will determine whether transmural necrosis (gangrenous colitis) occurs or only mucosa and/or submucosa is involved (nongangrenous colitis).

AETIOLOGY

- Systemic hypoperfusion.
- Occlusion of the inferior mesenteric artery leading to ischaemia of left colon (thrombosis and embolism).
- Occasionally it can develop due to vasculitis or ingestion of oral contraceptives.
- Drugs (e.g. alosetron, antihypertensive drugs, digoxin, cocaine).
- Sickle cell disease.
- IBS and COPD (two to four times more prone to develop ischaemic colitis).

CLINICAL FEATURES

- Most patients are older than 60 years.
- Colonic ischaemia can present acutely or chronically.

ACUTE ISCHAEMIC COLITIS

- Patients with acute colonic ischaemia usually present with rapid onset of mild cramping abdominal pain, often associated with urge to defecate, nausea and vomiting.
- Mild-to-moderate amounts of rectal bleeding (bright or maroon blood) or bloody diarrhoea usually develops within 24 hours of the onset of abdominal pain, though bleeding without prior abdominal pain also occurs frequently.
- Tenderness and guarding over left lower abdomen, especially left iliac fossa.
- Needs to be differentiated from acute mesenteric ischaemia (most patients with mesenteric ischaemia present with sudden onset of severe abdominal pain out of proportion to tenderness; they appear profoundly ill and they do not have bloody stools until the late stages).
- Transmural necrosis as a consequence of severe hypoperfusion presents as colon perforation with localised or generalised peritonitis.

CHRONIC ISCHAEMIC COLITIS

- Presents with recurrent abdominal pain, persistent bleeding, weight loss or symptomatic colonic strictures.

INVESTIGATIONS

- Leucocytosis and elevated lactate.
- Plain radiograph of abdomen shows 'thumb printing' of involved colon (Fig. 8.5).
- Double-contrast barium enema demonstrates involvement of splenic flexure and descending colon. Mucosal abnormalities are thumb printing and ulceration.
- CT abdomen shows oedema and thickening of the bowel wall in a segmental pattern (thumbprinting).
- Colonoscopy has replaced barium studies as it is more sensitive. Sigmoidoscopy shows normal rectal

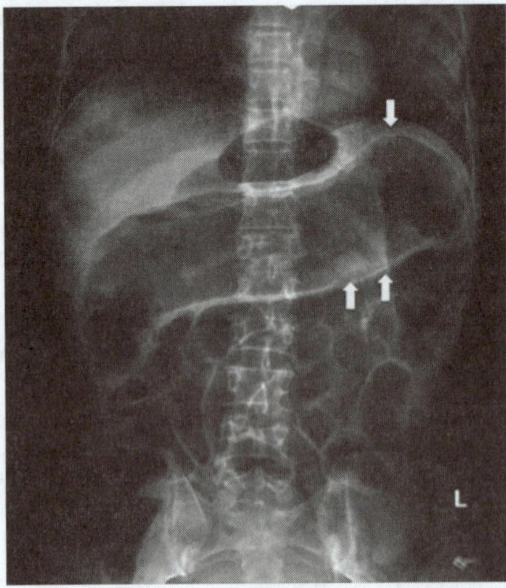

Fig. 8.5 Dilated transverse colon with 'thumb printing' seen on the left half (arrows).

mucosa and bleeding from above. It can also show stricture formation.

- Arteriography confirms the diagnosis in patients with obstructive lesions only.

TREATMENT

- Conservative management with intravenous fluids, haemodynamic stabilisation, discontinuation or avoidance of vasoconstrictive agents, bowel rest and empirical antibiotics.
- Anticoagulant therapy is indicated for patients who develop colonic ischaemia due to mesenteric venous thrombosis or related to mesenteric thromboembolism.
- Surgical treatment for peritonitis and strictures.

Q. What are the causes of lower gastrointestinal bleeding? (IM 15.1)

- Lower gastrointestinal bleeding is bleeding below the ligament of Treitz.
- Various causes of lower gastrointestinal bleeding are given in Box 8.18.

BOX 8.18 Causes of Lower Gastrointestinal Bleed

- Haemorrhoids, polyps
- Infective colitis (amoebic, bacillary)
- Carcinoma colon and rectum
- Diverticular disease
- Angiodysplasia
- Ulcerative colitis
- Ischaemic colitis
- AV malformations
- Meckel's diverticulum

Q. Discuss the aetiology, clinical features, investigations and treatment of pseudomembranous colitis (antibiotic-associated colitis).

AETIOLOGY

- Diarrhoea occurs due to a toxin produced by *Clostridioides difficile* (formerly known as *Clostridium difficile)* when the normal bacterial flora is altered or suppressed by antibiotics.
- Commonly implicated agents are as follows:
  - Tetracycline.
  - Ampicillin.
  - Lincomycin.
  - Clindamycin.
  - Others—diphenoxylate, quinolones, other antibiotics, proton pump inhibitors.
- Other risk factors include prolonged hospital stay and elderly patients.

PATHOGENESIS

- Two prerequisites for developing *C. difficile*–associated diarrhoea:
  - Disruption of normal gastrointestinal flora causing diminished colonisation resistance favouring *C. difficile.*
  - Acquisition of *C. difficile* from an exogenous source.
- Toxins required to cause diarrhoea:
  - Toxin A disrupts colonic mucosal cell adherence to colonic basement membrane and damages villous tips.
  - Toxin B enters the cell by endocytosis and induces apoptosis.
  - Another toxin produced by some strains is binary toxin or *C. difficile* transferase. Infection with such strains produces higher mortality.
- These toxins stimulate monocytes and macrophages which in turn release interleukin-8, resulting in tissue infiltration with neutrophils.

PATHOLOGY

- Rectum and colon show a yellowish membrane adherent to the eroded mucosa (pseudomembrane).
- Membrane is made up of fibrin and polymorphs.

CLINICAL FEATURES

- It usually occurs in adults.
- Patient is usually on antibiotics or would have received antibiotics within the past 8 weeks.
- Profuse watery diarrhoea (three or more unformed stools per 24 hours) with abdominal cramps.
- Blood in the stools may occur but is uncommon.
- Severe cases may present with fever and leucocytosis.
- Complications include dehydration, electrolyte disturbances, hypoalbuminaemia, toxic megacolon, bowel perforation, hypotension, renal failure, sepsis and death. Diarrhoea may be absent if patient develops paralytic ileus or fulminant colitis.

INVESTIGATIONS

- Sigmoidoscopy or colonoscopy shows yellowish membrane (pseudomembrane) (Fig. 8.6).

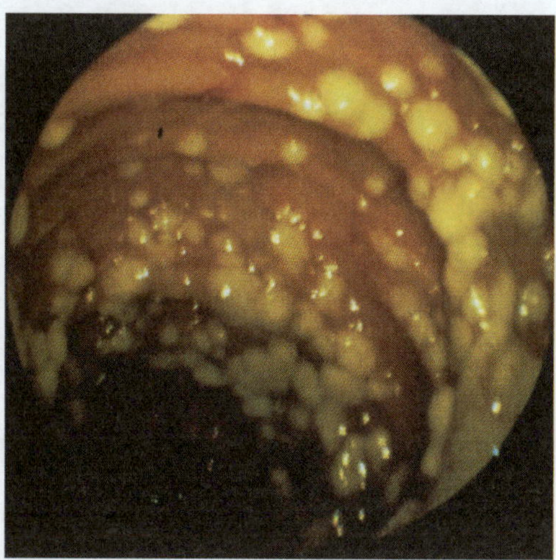

Fig. 8.6 *Clostridium difficile*-associated pseudomembranous colitis showing patchy, creamy plaques with intervening erythematous colonic mucosa.

- Histological features of pseudomembrane (polymorphs and fibrin).
- Stool contains toxin produced by *C. difficile* (should be done only on diarrhoeal stools unless paralytic ileus is suspected).
- Glutamate dehydrogenase detection in stool by enzyme immunoassay (present in both toxigenic and nontoxigenic strains of *C. difficile*). Helpful in ruling out disease.
- Stool culture.
- Nucleic acid amplification tests (e.g. PCR) for detecting genes of toxin A and B.

TREATMENT

- Withdraw the offending drug.
- Oral or intravenous rehydration.
- Oral metronidazole 500 mg thrice daily for 10–14 days in mild to moderate cases.
- Oral vancomycin 125–500 mg 6 hourly for 14 days in severe cases.
- Oral vancomycin plus intravenous metronidazole in refractory cases.
- Intravenous vancomycin not effective.
- Oral probiotic therapy (use of live nonpathogenic bacteria to restabilise the gut flora and provide colonisation resistance against *C. difficile*) often used in resistant or relapsed cases. Probiotics use organisms resistant to gastric acid. *Lactobacillus acidophilus* and *Saccharomyces boulardii* produce proteases that digest *C. difficile* toxins. However, clinical benefits not shown; may rarely produce sepsis.
- Fidaxomicin selectively eradicates *C. difficile* with a minimum effect on the intestinal microbiota.
- Bezlotoxumab, a human monoclonal antibody directed against *C. difficile* toxin B for prevention of recurrent disease.
- Antimotility drugs (loperamide or diphenoxylate) should not be given as they can precipitate toxic megacolon.
- Faecal microbiota transplantation for patients with refractory disease. It involves infusion of stool from an uninfected donor into the intestinal tract of the involved recipient. This will reconstitute intestinal microbiota in the recipient.
- Colectomy in severely ill, refractory patients.
- Management is summarised in Flowchart 8.4.

PREVENTION

- Hand washing, glove use, isolation of patients in a single room, barrier precautions and cleaning of the physical environment throughout the duration of symptomatic disease.
- Healthcare workers should wash their hands with soap and water rather than with alcohol-based hand-sanitising agents because alcohol is ineffective in killing *C. difficile* spores.

Q. Briefly explain Gardner's syndrome.

- Features of Gardner's syndrome are mentioned in Box 8.19.

Q. Give a brief account of Peutz–Jeghers syndrome.

- Features of Peutz–Jeghers syndrome are presented in Box 8.20.

Q. Discuss briefly the psychosomatic disorders of the gastrointestinal tract.

Q. Describe the aetiology, clinical features, investigations and management of irritable bowel syndrome.

DEFINITION

- A functional disorder of the gastrointestinal tract is one for which no structural, infective or biochemical cause can be found. A classification of the functional disorders of gastrointestinal tract is given in Box 8.21.

GLOBUS HYSTERICUS

- Persistent or intermittent, nonpainful sensation of a lump or foreign body in throat.
- Occurrence of the sensation between meals (i.e. sensation is independent of swallowing).
- Absence of dysphagia or odynophagia.
- Absence of evidence that gastro-oesophageal reflux is the cause of the symptom.
- Absence of histopathology-based oesophageal motility disorders.

FUNCTIONAL OR PSYCHOGENIC VOMITING

- May occur in anxiety neurosis.
- Usually occurs on awakening or immediately after breakfast.
- In the young, it may be due to school phobia.

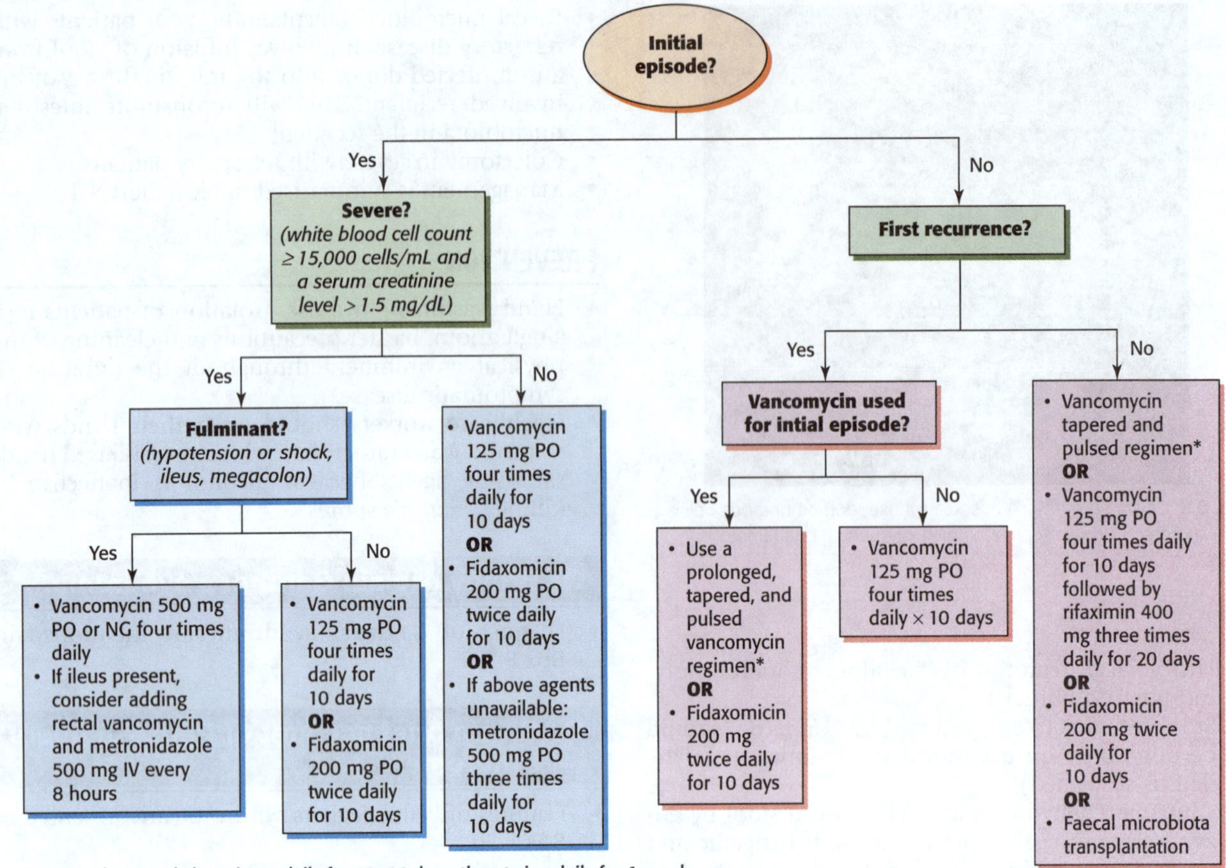

*125 mg by mouth four times daily for 10–14 days, then twice daily for 1 week, then once daily for 1 week, then every 2–3 days for 2–8 weeks.

Flowchart 8.4 *Clostridium difficile* Infection Treatment. (Source: Pharmacologic Approach to Management of *Clostridium difficile* Infection: Lukas T. Martin, Shelbi Vincent, Sarah Gillian, et al. Crit Care Nurs Q, Vol. 42, No. 1, pp. 2–11, 2019, Wolters Kluwer Health, Inc.)

BOX 8.19 Gardner's Syndrome

- Autosomal dominant disorder
- Numerous adenomatous polyps in colon
- Few gastric and duodenal polyps
- Hypertrophy of retinal pigment epithelium
- Benign soft-tissue tumours like lipomas, fibromas and sebaceous cysts
- Dental abnormalities—impacted or unerupted teeth, tooth ankylosis, congenitally missing teeth, supernumerary teeth
- Osteomas particularly involving jaw and skull
- Treatment is prophylactic total colectomy for fear of carcinoma colon

BOX 8.20 Peutz–Jeghers Syndrome

- Autosomal dominant disorder
- Multiple hamartomatous polyps of the entire GIT but mainly in small intestine
- Pigmentation of skin, lips and buccal mucosa (Fig. 8.7)
- Polyps may cause anaemia, rectal bleeding, abdominal pain, intestinal obstruction, intussusception
- Tumours of ovary, breast, pancreas, lung and endometrium in some cases
- Malignant potential of polyps
- Diagnosis and treatment by intraoperative enteroscopy (IOE) and double balloon enteroscopy (DBE) to remove all small intestinal polyps
- Follow-up surveillance for various cancers by periodic colonoscopy, upper endoscopy, capsule endoscopy, CT, MRI or ultrasound of the pancreas, chest X-ray, mammography and pelvic examination with ultrasound in women, testicular examination in men, carbohydrate antigen 19-9 (CA 19-9) and cancer antigen (CA-125)

- Characterised by retching alone or vomiting of gastric secretions or food.
- Little or no weight loss.
- Exclude pregnancy, alcohol abuse, depression, CNS disorders, metabolic causes and chronic cannabis use.
- Treatment is basically of the underlying psychological disturbances, tranquillisers and antiemetics.

IRRITABLE BOWEL SYNDROME

- IBS is a benign, chronic symptom complex of altered bowel habits and abdominal pain.

AETIOLOGY

- No organic cause can be found.
- Altered GI motility occurs in the form of exaggerated gastrocolic reflex, altered gastric emptying, increased small bowel contractions and increased small intestinal transit.

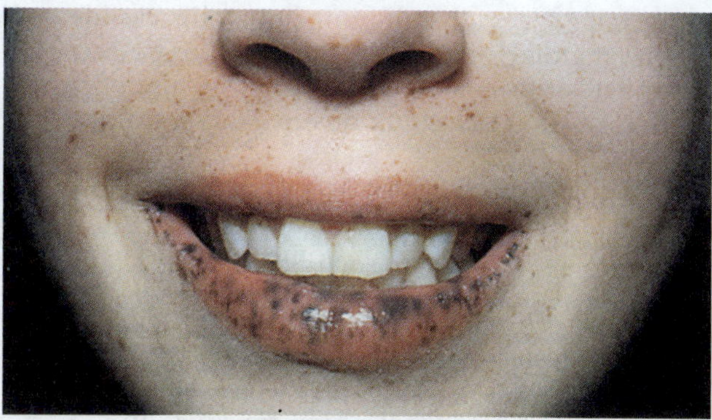

Fig. 8.7 Peutz–Jeghers Syndrome. Note the pigmentary changes.

BOX 8.21 Classification of Functional Disorders of Gastrointestinal Tract

- Bad taste (cacogeusia) or foul smell of breath (halitosis)
- Functional heartburn
- Noncardiac chest pain due to oesophageal dysmotility
- Functional dyspepsia
- Functional bloating
- Globus hystericus
- Aerophagia and unspecified excessive belching
- Functional vomiting and cyclic vomiting syndrome
- Irritable bowel syndrome
- Functional diarrhoea and functional constipation

- Neurotransmitters such as serotonin may be an important factor. It stimulates intestinal secretion and peristalsis in addition to visceral pain receptors via 5-HT_3 and 5-HT_4 pathways. Serotonin signalling is terminated by a specific serotonin reuptake transporter (SERT) located on enterocytes within the intestinal mucosa. A decrease in SERT leads to increased serotonin concentrations at the receptors.
- Psychological disturbances like anxiety, tension and excessive worry are all aetiologically significant.
- Certain foods may precipitate an attack.
- Although some studies show that patients with IBS have a different gastrointestinal microbiome to that of healthy controls, the role of the microbiota is still questioned, particularly because what constitutes a healthy microbiome is unclear.

CLINICAL FEATURES

- Three clinical variants:
  - Those with spastic colitis having primarily chronic abdominal pain and constipation (IBS with constipation or constipation-predominant IBS—at least 25% of stools are hard and fewer than 25% are loose or watery).
  - Those with chronic intermittent, watery diarrhoea often without pain (IBS with diarrhoea or diarrhoea-predominant IBS—at least 25% of stools are loose or watery and fewer than 25% are hard).
  - Those with both features and alternating diarrhoea and constipation (mixed IBS—at least 25% of stools are loose or watery and at least 25% are hard).
- More common in females of the age group 20–40 years.
- Abdominal pain is the most common symptom. Pain is referred to left or right iliac fossa or hypogastrium.
- Pain often provoked by food and relieved by defecation.
- Diarrhoea is often painless, occurs in the morning but never at night.
- In constipation-predominant IBS, stools are described as pellet-like, ribbon-like or pencil-like.
- Mucus may or may not be present.
- Postprandial tenesmus is common, due to an exaggerated gastrocolic reflex.
- Other symptoms are abdominal distension, feeling of incomplete evacuation of rectum, excessive flatus, dyspepsia and heartburns.
- Extraintestinal symptoms frequent and include headache, back pain, fatigue, myalgia, dyspareunia and urinary frequency.
- Physical examination is usually negative except for a tender sigmoid full of faeces and empty rectal ampulla.

INVESTIGATIONS

- Prime aim of investigations is to exclude organic bowel diseases.
  - Stool examination for leucocytes, parasites, ova and occult blood.
  - Routine testing for coeliac disease is advisable.
  - Sigmoidoscopy:
    - Usually normal or might show a prominent vascular pattern.
    - Large amounts of mucus may be seen.
    - Bowel shows marked motor activity.
    - Difficulty in negotiating rectosigmoid curve due to spasm.
  - Barium enema.
    - Usually normal.
    - Spasticity of sigmoid, accentuated haustral markings and a tubular appearance of the descending colon may be seen.
  - Exclude lactase deficiency, hyperthyroidism and alcohol abuse.
  - Measurement of the faecal calprotectin level which is a cytosol protein released by neutrophils, is useful as it can discriminate between IBS and inflammatory bowel disease with good accuracy.

DIAGNOSTIC CRITERIA (Box 8.22)

BOX 8.22 Rome IV Criteria for Diagnosis of Irritable Bowel Syndrome

Recurrent abdominal pain at least 1 day per week in the past 3 months (with symptom onset at least 6 months prior to diagnosis) associated with two or more of the following:

- Related to defecation (may be increased or unchanged by defecation)
- Associated with a change in stool frequency
- Associated with a change in stool form or appearance

Other symptoms that are not essential but support the diagnosis of IBS:

- Abnormal stool frequency (>3 bowel movements/day or <3 bowel movements/week)
- Abnormal stool form (lumpy/hard or loose/watery stool)
- Abnormal stool passage (straining, urgency or feeling of incomplete bowel movement)
- Passage of mucus
- Bloating or feeling of abdominal distension

BOX 8.23 Alarming Features Warranting Further Investigations

- Age >50 years
- Unexplained weight loss
- Presence of rectal bleeding
- Presence of iron-deficiency anaemia
- Family history of colorectal cancer, inflammatory bowel disease or coeliac disease
- Presence of obstructive symptoms (e.g. excessive straining, sense of incomplete rectal evacuation or digitation of the anus to facilitate defecation)
- Recent change in bowel habit

ALARMING FEATURES

- Presence of certain features necessitates investigations to exclude serious underlying causes of symptoms. These features are listed in Box 8.23.

TREATMENT

- Reassurance of the patient and explanation for the symptoms.
- Low FODMAP (fermentable oligosaccharides, disaccharides and monosaccharides and polyols) diet may be useful in some patients. FODMAPs are present in stone fruits, legumes, lactose-containing foods and artificial sweeteners.

Constipation-Predominant IBS

- Increase the roughage content of the diet and add a bulk laxative (methylcellulose, ispaghula husk, psyllium and corn fibre).
- Prokinetic agents like mosapride and levosulpiride are not useful in most patients.
- Tegaserod and prucalopride, 5-HT_4 agonists and prokinetic drugs, stimulate intestinal secretion of water and chloride and decrease the nociceptive response to rectal distension. However, use of tegaserod is restricted to women younger than 55 years with no cardiovascular morbidity, who are severely distressed due to symptoms (including pain) and who are educated about possible side effects, particularly severe diarrhoea and ischaemic cardiovascular events.
- Osmotic agents like polyethylene glycol, lactulose and milk of magnesia may be tried if fibre supplementation fails.
- Secretagogues (i.e. lubiprostone, linaclotide and plecanatide) increase intestinal chloride secretion by activating channels on the apical enterocyte surface causing net efflux of ions and water into the intestine.
    - Lubiprostone, which acts on apical type 2 chloride channel to increase water secretion into the faeces, can be used in women.
    - Linaclotide and plecanatide are agonists of GC-C. They activate GC-C receptors on intestinal enterocytes causing chloride channel activation.
- Tenapanor is a sodium-hydrogen exchange inhibitor and may be used for IBS with constipation.
- If abdominal pain is not adequately relieved, give a short-term trial of an anticholinergic agent (dicyclomine 10 mg TID) or an antispasmodic (mebeverine 135 mg TID).
- Psychotropic agents like amitriptyline (10–25 mg initially) may be useful in patients with abdominal pain.

Diarrhoea-Predominant IBS

- Give loperamide (2–4 mg up to four times a day).
- Cholestyramine (4 g four to six times a day), a bile acid–sequestrating agent, is a second-line agent. This is because bile acids stimulate colonic secretion and motility.
- 5-HT_3 receptor antagonists inhibit GI motility and benefit abdominal pain by reducing visceral sensitivity. Ondansetron, granisetron, alosetron and cilansetron are all selective 5-HT_3. Alosetron can produce severe ischaemic colitis and is approved for women with severe symptoms not responding to other treatment. It is contraindicated in patients with constipation.
- Rifaximin (550 mg TID) may be helpful in the treatment for bloating and may relieve global symptoms.
- Probiotics may be useful in some patients.
- Anticholinergics for pain control.
- Eluxadoline is a μ-opioid receptor agonist and δ-opioid receptor antagonist that decreases bowel contractions, inhibits colonic transit and reduces fluid/ion secretion. Useful if no response to other therapies. Can cause pancreatitis particularly in those without a gallbladder.

SUMMARY OF MANAGEMENT (Flowchart 8.5)

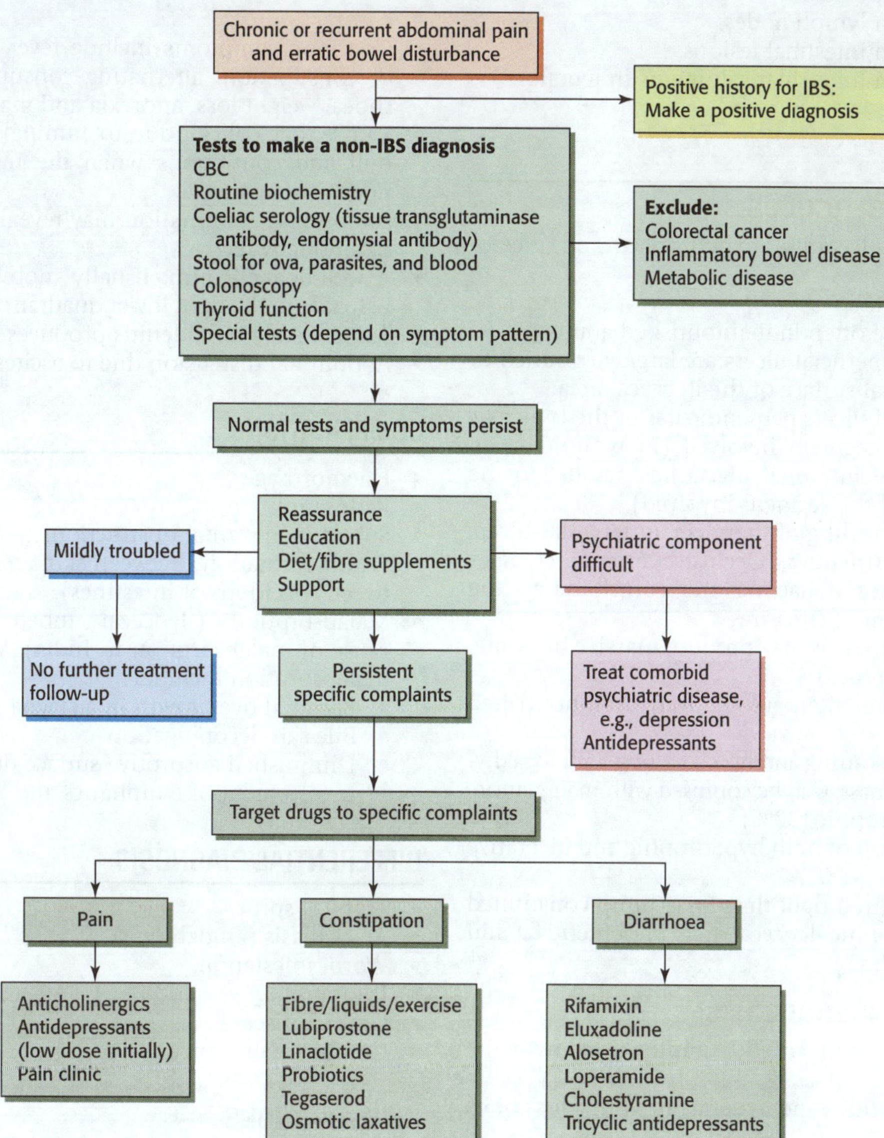

Flowchart 8.5 Summary of Management of Irritable Bowel Syndrome.

Q. Describe the aetiology, pathology, clinical features, complications, differential diagnosis, investigations and treatment of abdominal tuberculosis.

- Abdominal tuberculosis indicates tubercular involvement of gut, abdominal lymph nodes and peritoneum either individually or in various combinations.
- Intestinal tuberculosis commonly affects ileocecal region in 70% of patients. This is possibly related to:
  - Increased physiological stasis.
  - Increased rate of fluid and electrolyte absorption.
  - Minimal digestive activity.
  - Abundance of lymphoid tissue.
- Other areas that can get affected include ascending colon, jejunum, sigmoid colon, rectum, duodenum, stomach and oesophagus.

AETIOLOGY

- *Mycobacterium tuberculosis.*

ROUTES OF SPREAD

- Intestinal tuberculosis:
  - Haematogenous spread from the primary lung focus in childhood with reactivation later.
  - Ingestion of bacilli in sputum from active pulmonary focus.

  - Direct spread from adjacent organs.
  - Through lymph channels from infected nodes.
- Peritoneal tuberculosis:
  - Spread from lymph nodes.
  - Spread from intestinal lesions.
  - Spread from tubercular salpingitis in females.

PATHOLOGY

INTESTINAL TUBERCULOSIS

- Three types (ulcerative, hypertrophic and ulcero-hypertrophic).
- Ulcerative (60%):
  - Found more often in malnourished adults.
  - Multiple superficial ulcers are largely confined to the epithelial surface of the ileocecal area.
  - Long axis of ulcers perpendicular to the long axis of the gut segment involved (in typhoid fever, long axis of intestinal ulcers lies parallel to the long axis of the segment involved).
  - Cicatricial healing of these circumferential ulcers results in strictures. Occlusive arterial changes may produce ischaemia and contribute to the development of strictures.
  - Rarely endarteritis may produce massive bleeding.
- Hypertrophic (10%):
  - Found more often in relatively well-nourished adults.
  - Consists of scarring and fibrosis along with local hypertrophic mass. Can be confused with malignancy.
- Ulcero-hypertrophic (30%):
  - Combination of both hypertrophic and ulcerative forms.
  - Presents with a right iliac fossa lump constituted by hypertrophic ileocecal area, mesenteric fat and lymph nodes.

PERITONEAL TUBERCULOSIS

- Peritoneum is studded with multiple yellow-white tubercles.
- Peritoneum is thick and hyperaemic with a loss of its shiny lustre.
- The omentum is also thickened.
- Occurs in three forms:
  - Wet type presents with ascites.
  - Encysted (loculated) type presents with a localised abdominal swelling.
  - Fibrotic type presents with abdominal masses composed of mesenteric and omental thickening with matted bowel loops felt as lumps in the abdomen. Adhesions may involve the bowel loops producing subacute intestinal obstruction.
  - A combination of these types is also common.

LYMPH NODAL TUBERCULOSIS

- Involvement of mesenteric, omental, periportal and peripancreatic lymph nodes.
- Nodes may become palpable as rounded masses (tabes mesenterica).
- Usually seen in young adults.
- May be confused with lymphoma.

CLINICAL FEATURES

- Predominantly seen in young adults.
- Clinical presentation is acute, chronic or acute on chronic.
- Common symptoms include fever, pain, diarrhoea or constipation, alternating constipation and diarrhoea, weight loss, anorexia and malaise.
- Pain either colicky due to luminal compromise or dull and continuous when the mesenteric lymph nodes are involved.
- Abdominal examination may reveal no abnormality or a doughy feel.
- A well-defined, firm, usually mobile mass is often palpable in the right lower quadrant of the abdomen.
- Associated lymphadenitis produces mass.
- Abdominal distension due to ascites.

COMPLICATIONS

- Haemorrhage.
- Perforation.
- Subacute intestinal obstruction.
- Fistula formation (between skin and intestine or between two loops of intestines).
- Malabsorption (ileocecal tuberculosis common cause of malabsorption in India). Various causes of malabsorption include:
  - Bacterial overgrowth in a stagnant loop.
  - Bile salt deconjugation.
  - Diminished absorptive surface due to ulceration.
  - Involvement of lymphatics and lymph nodes.

DIFFERENTIAL DIAGNOSIS

- Tropical sprue.
- Amoebiasis (amoeboma).
- Worm infestation.
- Lymphoma.
- Crohn's disease.
- Colonic malignancy.

INVESTIGATIONS

- Raised ESR, anaemia and hypoalbuminaemia.
- Chest X-ray.
  - May show evidence of active or old tubercular lesion.
- Plain X-ray of abdomen.
  - Calcified lymph nodes.
  - Dilated bowel loops with multiple air–fluid levels due to obstruction.
  - Air under diaphragm and dilated loops due to perforation.
- Barium meal:
  - May show hypermotility (accelerated intestinal transit).
  - Hypersegmentation of the barium column ('chicken intestine').
  - Precipitation, flocculation and dilution of the barium.
  - Luminal stenosis with smooth but stiff contours ('hourglass stenosis').

- Multiple strictures with segmental dilatation of bowel loops.
- Stierlin's sign—repeated emptying of the caecum seen radiographically as barium remaining in the terminal part of ileum and in transverse colon. This occurs due to irritation of the cecum caused by bacteria.
- String sign—a thin stream of barium seen in the terminal ileum.

Note: Both Stierlin's and String's signs can also be seen in Crohn's disease, and, hence, are not specific for tuberculosis.

- Barium enema:
  - Wide gaping of ileocecal valve with narrowing of the terminal ileum ('Fleischner' or 'inverted umbrella sign').
  - Fold thickening and contour irregularity of terminal ileum shrunken in size ('conical caecum').
  - Pulled-up caecum due to contraction and fibrosis of the mesocolon.
  - Loss of normal ileocecal angle and dilated terminal ileum, appearing suspended from a retracted, fibrosed caecum ('goose-neck deformity').
  - Localised stenosis opposite the ileocecal valve with a rounded-off smooth caecum and a dilated terminal ileum ('purse-string stenosis').
- Abdominal ultrasound:
  - Intraabdominal fluid (free or loculated; with or without debris and septae).
  - Localised fluid between radially oriented bowel loops due to local exudation from the inflamed bowel (interloop ascites; 'club sandwich' or 'sliced bread' sign).
  - Lymphadenopathy, discrete or matted with heterogenous echotexture due to caseation; useful for taking biopsy or fine-needle aspiration of lymph node.
  - Uniform and concentric bowel wall thickening in the ileocecal region (vs. eccentric thickening at the mesenteric border found in Crohn's disease and variegated appearance of malignancy).
- Contrast-enhanced CT scan:
  - Symmetric circumferential thickening of caecum and terminal ileum.
  - Regional lymph nodes.
  - Mesenteric thickening.
  - Ulceration or nodularity within the terminal ileum, along with narrowing and proximal dilatation.
  - Ascitic fluid of high attenuation value.
  - Thickened peritoneum and enhancing peritoneal nodules.
  - Omental thickening seen as an omental cake appearance.
  - Caseating lymph nodes with hypodense centres and peripheral rim enhancement.
  - Retroperitoneal nodes (periaortic and pericaval) almost never seen in isolation, unlike lymphoma.
- Ascitic fluid examination:
  - See 'ascites' on page 464, Chapter 6.
- Biopsy of peritoneum:
  - Punch.
  - Laparoscopic.
- Colonoscopy:
  - Mucosal nodules and ulcers in colon.
  - Biopsy from the edge of ulcers. Perform PCR for *M. tuberculosis* and histopathology on biopsy specimen.

TREATMENT

- Antitubercular treatment similar to treatment of pulmonary tuberculosis.
- Surgery:
  - Strictureplasty for strictures that reduce the lumen by 50% or more and that cause proximal dilation.
  - Resection of segment having multiple strictures.
  - Treatment of perforation.

Q. Enumerate the conditions causing ulcers in intestine.

- Conditions producing intestinal ulceration are listed in Box 8.24.

Q. What are the inflammatory bowel diseases?

Q. Give the aetiology, pathology, clinical features, investigations and treatment of ulcerative colitis. (IM 16.16; IM 16.17)

- Inflammatory bowel diseases are chronic inflammatory disorders of gastrointestinal tract characterised by a relapsing and remitting course.
- Inflammatory bowel diseases include several conditions, most common being:
  - Ulcerative colitis.
  - Crohn's disease.
- Other uncommon inflammatory bowel diseases include:
  - Microscopic ulcerative colitis.
  - Microscopic lymphocytic colitis.
  - Microscopic collagenous colitis.

ULCERATIVE COLITIS

DEFINITION

- Ulcerative colitis is an inflammatory disease affecting mainly the large intestine, characterised clinically by recurrent attacks of bloody diarrhoea and pathologically by diffuse inflammation of colonic mucosa.

BOX 8.24 Common Conditions Causing Ulcers in Intestines

• Enteric fever	• Gram-negative bacillary dysentery
• Tuberculosis	• Zollinger–Ellison syndrome
• Amoebiasis	• Malignant ulcers
• Ulcerative colitis	• Mesenteric artery occlusion
• Crohn's disease	• Ischaemic colitis

- Disease extent can be broadly divided into distal and more extensive disease.
  - Distal disease refers to colitis confined to the rectum (proctitis) or rectum and sigmoid colon (proctosigmoiditis).
  - More extensive disease includes 'left-sided colitis' (up to the splenic flexure), 'extensive colitis' (up to the hepatic flexure) and pancolitis (affecting the whole colon).

AETIOLOGY

- Exact aetiology is not known.
- Familial or genetic:
  - Strong family history.
  - Occurrence in monozygotic twins.
- Infectious:
  - Possible pathogens include:
    - *Mycobacterium* (*M. avium paratuberculosis*).
    - Measles virus.
    - *Listeria monocytogenes.*
    - Yeast.
    - Endogenous bacteria.
      - *Bacteroides.*
      - *E. coli.*
- Dietary factors:
  - Deficiency or excess of certain nutrients (butyric acid, sulphides, l-arginine and glutamine).
- Smoking:
  - Patients with Crohn's disease are more likely to be smokers and smoking can exacerbate it.
  - There is an increased risk of ulcerative colitis in nonsmokers.
- Psychological:
  - Characteristic personality and major psychological stresses are related to flare-ups and precipitation of symptoms.
- Defective immune regulation:
  - Many immunological abnormalities have been described that include stimulation of macrophages leading to excessive production of cytokines (interleukin-1, interleukin-6 and tumour necrosis factor-α). There is also activation of other cells (eosinophils, mast cells and fibroblasts).
  - Immune complexes may be responsible for extraintestinal manifestations.

PATHOLOGY

- Primarily involves the colonic mucosa.
- Mucosal involvement is uniform and continuous with no intervening areas of normal mucosa.
- Rectum is involved in 95% of cases (proctitis).
- From the rectum, the disease extends proximally into the colon in a continuous fashion.
- Back wash ileitis is involvement of a few centimetres of ileum when the entire colon is involved.
- Macroscopically, the mucosa appears hyperaemic, haemorrhagic or ulcerated. Ulcers do not usually extend deeper beyond the submucosa.
- 'Pseudopolyps' are regenerating islands of mucosa surrounded by areas of ulceration and denuded mucosa. They protrude into the lumen of colon like polyps.
- Microscopically, the lamina propria is infiltrated with lymphocytes and plasma cells. There is loss of goblet cells also.
- Crypt abscesses are characteristic with infiltration of crypts with neutrophils.
- In toxic megacolon, transverse colon is dilated, walls are thin, mucosa denuded and inflammation extends to serosa. It may rupture later.
- In the chronic variety, there is fibrosis and shortening of the colon with loss of normal haustral pattern. The surface epithelium may show features of dysplasia.
- Strictures, anal fissures and anal abscesses are uncommon.

CLINICAL FEATURES

General

- Severity of symptoms reflects the extent of colonic involvement and the intensity of inflammation.
  - Exacerbations and remissions are characteristic; exacerbations are associated with emotional stress, intercurrent infections and use of antibiotics.
  - Bloody diarrhoea with mucus and pus.
  - Abdominal pain, especially lower abdominal.
  - Fever, weight loss and loss of appetite.
  - Symptoms and signs of dehydration and anaemia.
  - Extraintestinal manifestations in one-third of patients (may be present even when the disease is inactive).
  - Tenderness on palpation over the colon especially in the left iliac fossa.
  - Incidence of carcinoma of colon is high especially in cases of total colitis, duration more than 10 years and early age of onset.

Acute Variety

- Disease usually involves the entire colon.
- Severe systemic symptoms like fever, weight loss and loss of appetite.
- Exhausting diarrhoea and dehydration.
- Tachycardia and postural hypotension.
- Tenesmus, lower abdominal pain and left iliac fossa tenderness due to serosal involvement.
- Toxic megacolon and rupture may occur.

Chronic Variety

- Bowel permanently damaged by fibrosis; colon behaves as a rigid tube incapable of absorbing fluids and acting like a faecal reservoir.
- No systemic manifestations or toxaemia.
- Patient lives in chronic ill health with chronic diarrhoea.

Disease Confined to Rectum (Proctitis)

- Systemic symptoms are trivial or absent.
- Loose motions and blood streaking of stools.
- Severe tenesmus and frequent, small, loose stools.
- Bleeding and mucus per rectum.

Distal Colitis

- Constipation rather than diarrhoea.
- Retention of faeces in the proximal colon and small, hard stools.

SEVERITY OF ULCERATIVE COLITIS (Table 8.27)

TABLE 8.27 Montreal Classification of Ulcerative Colitis Based on the Severity of Disease

S0	Clinical remission	No symptoms
S1	Mild UC	Four or less stools per day (with or without blood), absence of systemic symptoms, normal inflammatory markers
S2	Moderate UC	More than four stools per day, minimal signs of systemic toxicity
S3	Severe UC	Six or more bloody stools per day, pulse rate of ≥90/min, Temp ≥37.5°C, haemoglobin <10.5 g/dL, ESR ≥30 mm/h

INVESTIGATIONS

General

- Anaemia, raised ESR and CRP, leucocytosis.
- Electrolyte abnormalities (hypokalaemia, hyponatraemia, etc.).
- Hypoproteinaemia.
- Abnormal liver function tests.
- Blood culture in sepsis.
- Stool examination and culture to exclude infective pathology.
- Stool for *C. difficile* toxin.
- Elevated faecal calprotectin (released from neutrophils) and lactoferrin levels.

Plain Radiograph of Abdomen

- To exclude toxic dilatation of colon (Fig. 8.8).
- May help assess disease extent in ulcerative colitis.

Barium Enema

- Earliest features are irritability and incomplete filling.
- Ulcerations.
- Pseudopolyps and strictures.

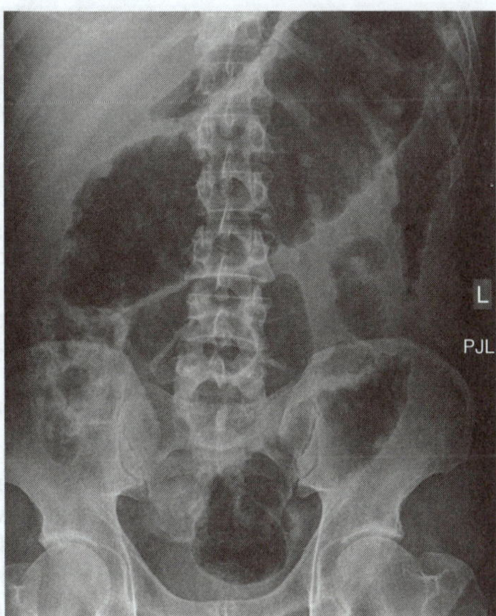

Fig. 8.8 Severe dilatation of the transverse colon with diffuse pseudopolyps along the colonic walls, consistent with ulcerative colitis and toxic megacolon.

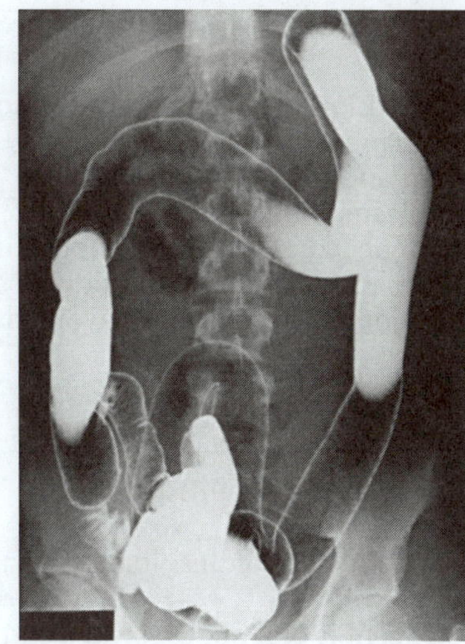

Fig. 8.9 A double-contrast barium enema in a patient with long-standing ulcerative colitis demonstrates a marked loss of haustration. The terminal ileum is normal.

- Chronic stage of the disease is characterised by shortening of the bowel, depression of flexures, narrowing of bowel lumen and rigidity. The bowel has asymmetric, ahaustral and tubular (pipe stem) appearance (Fig. 8.9).

Sigmoidoscopy

- Uniform, continuous involvement of the mucosa.
- Loss of mucosal vascularity.
- Diffuse hyperaemia or erythema.
- Exudate of mucus, pus and blood.
- Mucosal friability—gentle rubbing of the mucosa with a cotton swab shows the appearance of diffuse, small bleeding points.
- Shallow but small or confluent ulcers.
- Pseudopolyps.

Colonoscopy

- For mild to moderate disease, colonoscopy is preferable to flexible sigmoidoscopy because the extent of disease can be assessed. In moderate to severe disease, there is a higher risk of bowel perforation and flexible sigmoidoscopy is safer.

Rectal Biopsy

- Mucosal inflammation.

Serological Markers (Table 8.28)

TABLE 8.28 Serological Markers

Type of Antibodies	Positivity in Ulcerative Colitis (%)	Positivity in Crohn's Disease (%)
• Perinuclear antineutrophilic cytoplasmic antibody (p-ANCA)	60–75	5–10
• Anti-*Saccharomyces cerevisiae* antibodies (ASCA)	10–15	60–70
• Anti-goblet cell autoantibodies	30–40	30–40
• Anti-glycan antibodies (e.g. antilaminaribioside carbohydrate antibody)	<10	30–40

TREATMENT

General Measures

- Parenteral nutrition through a central venous line in seriously ill patients.
- High-protein and low-residue diet.
- Blood and plasma infusions.
- Correction of dehydration and electrolyte imbalance.
- Parenteral broad-spectrum antibiotics in sepsis.
- Loperamide for mild diarrhoea (avoided in severe disease).

Corticosteroids

- For inducing remission in moderate to severe cases.
- No role in maintaining remissions.
- Local treatment:
  - Hydrocortisone or prednisolone enemas, suppositories or foam.
  - Another agent is oral budesonide, a corticosteroid with minimal absorption and, therefore, minimal systemic exposure.
  - Choice of topical formulation is determined by proximal extent of the inflammation (suppositories for disease of the rectosigmoid junction; foam or liquid enemas for more proximal disease).
  - Duration of treatment is 3–6 weeks.
  - Proctitis is treated with corticosteroid suppositories twice daily.
  - Distal colitis with mild symptoms is treated with corticosteroid enema once or twice daily.
  - Topical steroids are less effective than topical 5-aminosalicylic acid (5-ASA).
- Systemic treatment:
  - Prednisolone 40–60 mg orally daily for 3–6 weeks.
  - Intravenous hydrocortisone 100–200 mg 6 hourly in severe cases.
  - Steroids once started are gradually tapered and withdrawn.

Aminosalicylates

- Useful in controlling acute exacerbation as well as to prevent relapses. Maintenance therapy may reduce the risk of colorectal cancer by up to 75%.
- Available as oral tablets, sachets, liquid or foam enemas.
- Act on epithelial cells by a variety of mechanisms to moderate the release of lipid mediators, cytokines and reactive oxygen species.
- Include 5-ASA or mesalazine alone, or combination of 5-ASA with a carrier which releases 5-ASA after splitting by bacteria in colon (sulphasalazine, olsalazine and balsalazide).
- Sulphasalazine, the most frequently used agent, is a combination of:
  - 5-ASA (active agent).
  - Sulphapyridine (acting as a 'carrier').
  - The compound is broken down in colon by bacterial action liberating 5-ASA that acts locally.
  - Side effects include nausea, headache, rashes, sterility in males, haemolytic anaemia, Stevens–Johnson syndrome and agranulocytosis. Dose is 2–4 g/day in mild to moderate attack and 0.5 g QID to prevent relapses, as a maintenance.
- Mesalazine uses 5-ASA with an enteric coating.
- Azodisalicylate joins two molecules of 5-ASA by an azo bond that is split by bacteria in the colon. An example is olsalazine. A side effect unique to olsalazine is diarrhoea resulting from excessive production of fluid in the intestines (secretory diarrhoea).
- In disease limited to rectosigmoid, topical (as enema or foam) 5-ASA (1 g/day) may be tried before resorting to topical steroids.

Note: 5-ASA in free form is absorbed in the small intestine and may produce renal toxicity.

Immunosuppressive Agents

- Both azathioprine and 6-mercaptopurine are useful in maintaining remission and have steroid-sparing properties. Long-term treatment is required to prevent relapse.
  - Useful in patients who require two or more corticosteroid courses within a calendar year, and those whose disease relapses as the dose of prednisolone is reduced below 15 mg, or relapse within 6 weeks of stopping steroid.
- Methotrexate useful in patients who do not respond to azathioprine.
- Cyclosporin, an inhibitor of calcineurin, prevents clonal expansion of T-cell subsets. Intravenous cyclosporin is effective in severe ulcerative colitis refractory to steroids. After response, azathioprine or 6-mercaptopurine is required to maintain remission.
- Tacrolimus has shown efficacy in refractory or extensive disease.
- In patients resistant to immunosuppressives, anti-TNF-α antibodies (e.g. infliximab, adalimumab and certolizumab) have been shown to be effective.
- Vedolizumab and ustekinumab, newer biological therapies in those who are intolerant to or who have lost response to the anti-TNF drugs.
- Other agents are tofacitinib (an oral, pan-JAK inhibitor) and ozanimod (a sphingosine 1 phosphate receptors modulator).
- Adsorptive cytapheresis (selective depletion of myeloid lineage cells like neutrophils and monocytes) to maintain remission in moderate to severe cases.

SUMMARY OF TREATMENT OF ULCERATIVE COLITIS (Flowchart 8.6)

SURGICAL MANAGEMENT (Table 8.29)

- Emergency surgical procedure is colectomy with ileostomy with the rectum and distal colon removed at a later stage.
- Elective surgical procedure is total proctocolectomy with ileostomy or ileorectal anastomosis or ileoanal anastomosis.

MISCELLANEOUS

- Colonoscopy with multiple biopsies is recommended every 3 years in patients with extensive colitis of more than 10 years' duration to assess for any dysplastic or malignant changes. In those with disease for more than 20 years, colonoscopy is recommended every 2 years and after that every year. Four random biopsies every 10 cm from the entire colon are best taken with additional samples of suspicious

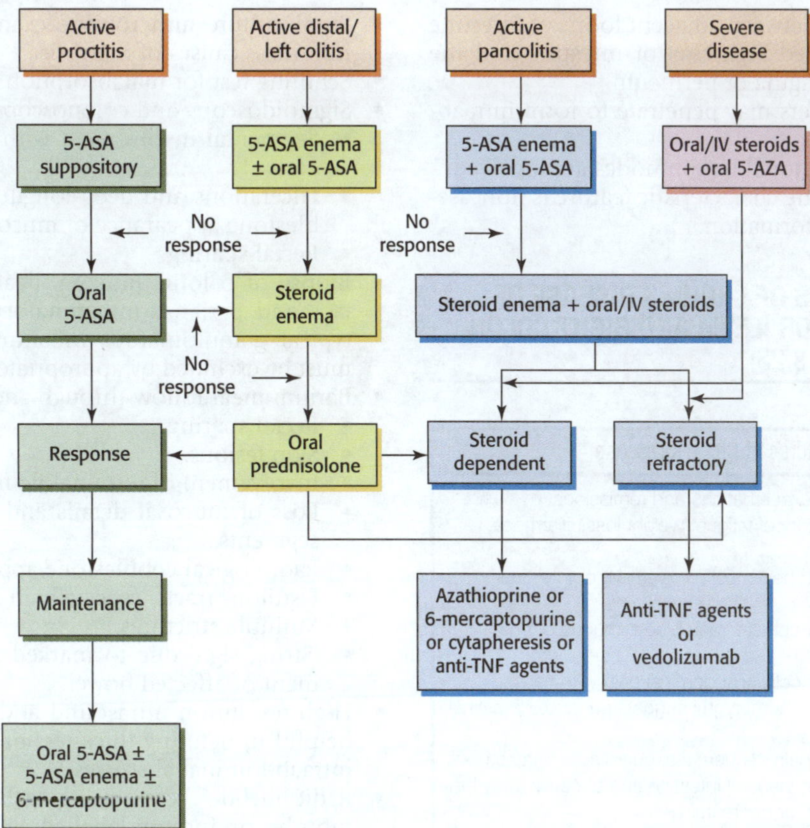

Flowchart 8.6 Treatment of Active Ulcerative Colitis.

TABLE 8.29 Ulcerative Colitis: Surgical Management

Indications of Emergency Surgery	Indications of Elective Surgery
• Severe forms of the disease	• Acute disease that fails to respond to medical treatment
• Toxic dilatation of colon	• Frequent relapses in spite of adequate treatment
• Perforation	• Chronic disease with permanently damaged bowel; strictures
• Severe haemorrhage	• Total bowel involvement with activity extending over >10 years

areas. If the biopsy shows high-grade dysplasia, total colectomy may be done.

- Newer methods for targeted biopsies include chromoendoscopy, narrow band imaging or confocal endomicroscopy.

Q. Discuss the aetiology, pathology, clinical features, investigations and management of Crohn's disease. (IM 16.16)

DEFINITION

- Crohn's disease is characterised by patchy and transmural inflammation, which may affect any part of the gastrointestinal tract.
- It may be defined by location (terminal ileal, colonic and ileocolic, UGI) or by pattern of disease (inflammatory, fistulating or stricturing).

AETIOLOGY

- Factors listed under section heading Ulcerative Colitis.

PATHOLOGY

- Affects small and large bowels but more common in small bowel. Can affect any part of the gastrointestinal tract from mouth to anus.
- Commonly involved sites in the order of frequency are the following:
    - Terminal ileum and right side of colon.
    - Colon alone.
    - Terminal ileum alone.
    - Ileum and jejunum.
- Inflammation extends through all the layers of the intestinal wall.
- Characteristically, the involvement is discontinuous. Involved segments of intestine are separated from each other by intervening segments of normal bowel.
- Bowel wall is greatly thickened and leathery with the lumen narrowed (stenosis).
- Mucosa has a nodular, cobblestoned look.
- Mucosal involvement is characteristically patchy. The inflammatory process is interrupted by islands of normal mucosa. A small area separated from a major area of involvement is known as a 'skip lesion'.

- Fistulae develop between adjacent loops of intestine or between affected segments of intestine and the bladder, uterus, vagina or perineum.
- The intestinal ulcers may penetrate to form intraabdominal abscesses.
- Mesentery and regional lymph nodes are involved.
- Microscopically, the characteristic feature is noncaseating granuloma formation.

CLINICAL FEATURES OF CROHN'S DISEASE OF SMALL INTESTINE OR ILEUM AND RIGHT COLON (ILEOCOLITIS) (Box 8.25)

BOX 8.25 Clinical Features of Crohn's Disease

- Chronic disease with exacerbations and remissions
- Young adults with history of fatigue, weight loss, diarrhoea, fever and pallor
- Abdominal pain due to peritoneal involvement or intestinal obstruction
- Stool usually does not contain frank blood, mucus or pus unless colon is involved
- Recurrent episodes of colicky abdominal pain with nausea, vomiting and excessive borborygmi suggest subacute intestinal obstruction
- Right lower quadrant pain, tenderness, guarding and mass
- Mass reflects adherent loops of intestine and abscess (may be palpable per abdomen or per rectal)
- Anal lesions such as oedematous skin tags, fistulae, fissures, perianal and perirectal abscesses are characteristic of the disease
- Features of malabsorption, e.g. weight loss and anaemia (iron, folic acid and B_{12} malabsorption)
- Sodium, potassium, water, magnesium and zinc deficiency due to chronic diarrhoea

COMPLICATIONS

- Intrabdominal complications are listed in the Box 8.26.

INVESTIGATIONS

- Normochromic normocytic or macrocytic (due to vitamin B_{12} malabsorption) or hypochromic anaemia.
- Raised ESR and leucocytosis.
- Abnormal liver function tests.
- Hypoproteinaemia.

BOX 8.26 Intrabdominal Complications of Crohn's Disease

- Intestinal obstruction
- Fistula formation
    - Ileovesical fistula leads to recurrent urinary infection, cystitis and pneumaturia
    - Fistulae between contiguous segments of intestines
    - Cutaneous fistulae
- Abscesses
- Free perforation
- Rectal fissures
- High incidence of carcinoma of intestine
- Gastric outlet obstruction or duodenal obstruction
- Gallstones and urinary oxalate stones
- Secondary amyloidosis in long-standing cases (hepatosplenomegaly with proteinuria)

- Stool culture and routine examination to exclude infectious causes of diarrhoea.
- Schilling test for malabsorption of vitamin B_{12}.
- Sigmoidoscopy and colonoscopy:
    - Segmental involvement with intervening normal area.
    - Ulcerations and deep longitudinal fissures. Cobblestone appearance of mucosa.
    - Rectal sparing.
- Biopsy of colonic mucosa, ileal mucosa, anal skin tags and perianal inflammatory lesions will show typical granulomatous inflammation. Tuberculosis must be excluded by appropriate histological tissues.
- Barium meal follow-through and barium enema:
    - Rectal sparing.
    - Skip lesions.
    - Involvement of terminal ileum.
    - Loss of mucosal details and rigidity of involved segments.
    - Radiological cobblestone appearance of mucosa.
    - Fistulous tracts, especially in ileocecal area.
    - Multiple strictures.
    - 'String sign' due to marked narrowing of a segment of affected bowel.
- High-resolution ultrasound and spiral CT scanning helpful in defining thickness of the bowel wall and intraabdominal abscesses.
- Radionuclide scan using gallium-labelled polymorphs or indium-labelled leucocytes to identify intestinal and colonic disease and localise extraintestinal abscesses.
- Serological markers:
    - See under section heading Ulcerative Colitis on page 693.

TREATMENT

- Diet and nutrition:
    - High-protein and high-energy diet.
    - Enteral feeding by nasogastric tube. Total parenteral nutrition in very ill patients.
    - Plasma or blood transfusion.
    - Low-residue diet in colic and subacute obstruction.
    - Low-fat diet and low linoleic acid in diet.
    - Milk-free diet in lactose intolerance.
    - Antibiotics (metronidazole and ciprofloxacin) for bacterial colonisation of gut and fistula.
    - Supplementation of iron, folic acid, calcium, zinc, vitamins D, B_{12} and electrolytes.
- Drug treatment:
    - Loperamide or codeine for diarrhoea.
    - In long-standing cases, diarrhoea may be due to bile salt malabsorption. Cholestyramine should be tried in such cases.
    - 5-ASA (e.g. mesalazine 4 g daily or sulphasalazine 2 g twice daily) as maintenance in mild to moderate ileocolonic disease. It reduces disease activity but its benefits in maintaining remission are not proven.
    - Prednisolone 40–60 mg daily initially which is gradually tapered and withdrawn (for inducing remission).

- The use of immunosuppressive agents (azathioprine, 6-mercaptopurine, methotrexate and cyclosporin) and anti-TNF agents (infliximab) has been discussed under section heading Ulcerative Colitis on page 694.
- Natalizumab, a monoclonal antibody directed against α4 integrins, is effective for induction and maintenance of remission in patients with moderate to severe Crohn's disease when therapy with TNF-α blocker has failed. It can produce progressive multifocal leucoencephalopathy.

SUMMARY OF TREATMENT OF CROHN'S DISEASE (Flowchart 8.7)

SURGICAL TREATMENT

- Indicated in repeated episodes of subacute obstruction, abscess, perforation, extensive and severe involvement of colon.
- Minimal resections for strictures and fistulae.

Q. Give a brief account of toxic dilatation of colon (toxic megacolon).

- Toxic dilatation of colon occurs most commonly in ulcerative colitis and occasionally in Crohn's disease. In fact, it is a severe form of ulcerative colitis with an additional feature of colonic dilatation. It is thought that neuromuscular tone of bowel is affected resulting in dilatation. Drugs like codeine, diphenoxylate, loperamide and anticholinergics used in the treatment of diarrhoea can precipitate this complication. Barium enema is another precipitating factor.
- Other causes include infectious colitis (including *C. difficile* infection), ischaemic colitis, volvulus, diverticulitis and obstructive colon cancer.

CLINICAL FEATURES

- Clinical features of severe colitis.
- High fever, tachycardia, dehydration, electrolyte imbalance and abdominal pain.
- Patient is toxic and ill.
- Examination reveals colonic dilatation and severe abdominal tenderness.
- Wall of the colon is thin and may rupture.
- Transverse colon is most commonly involved.
- Plain radiograph of abdomen may show colonic dilatation with transverse colonic diameter more than 5.5 cm (Fig. 8.10). Air may be seen in the wall of the colon.

TREATMENT

- Medical therapy for IBD-related toxic megacolon includes fluid and electrolyte therapy, nasogastric aspiration, discontinuation of all antimotility drugs (e.g. loperamide, anticholinergics), broad-spectrum antibiotics, intravenous hydrocortisone, deep vein thrombosis and gastric ulcer prophylaxis, and repeated abdominal radiographs.

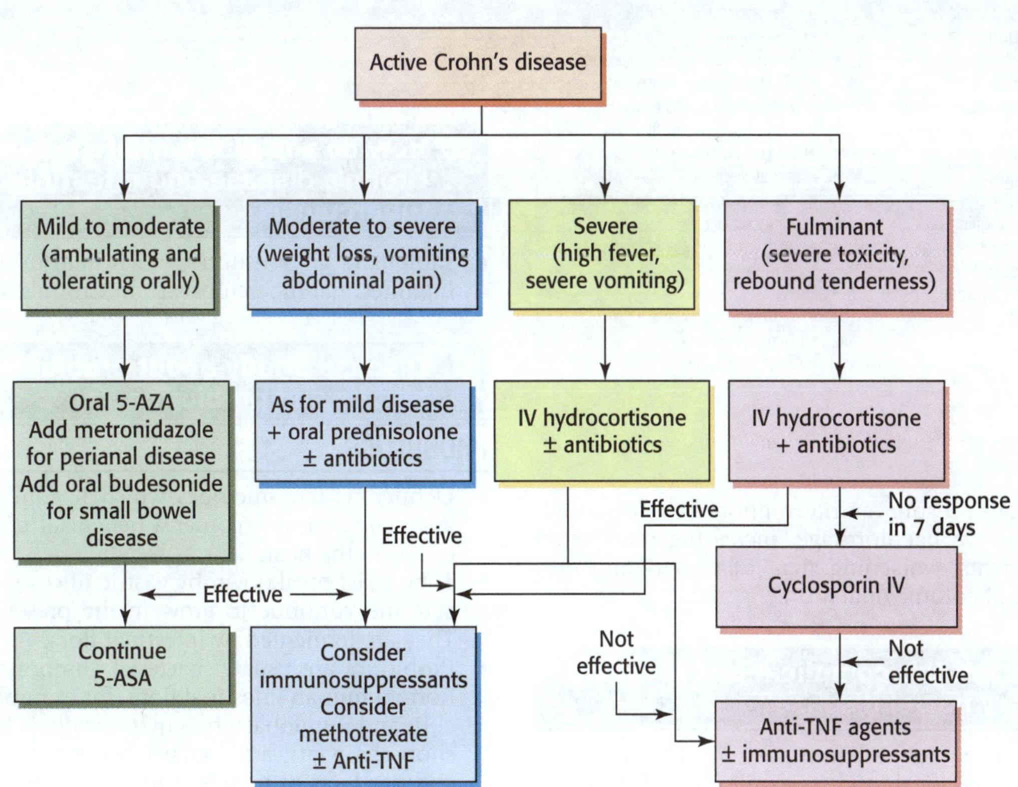

Flowchart 8.7 Treatment of Crohn's Disease.

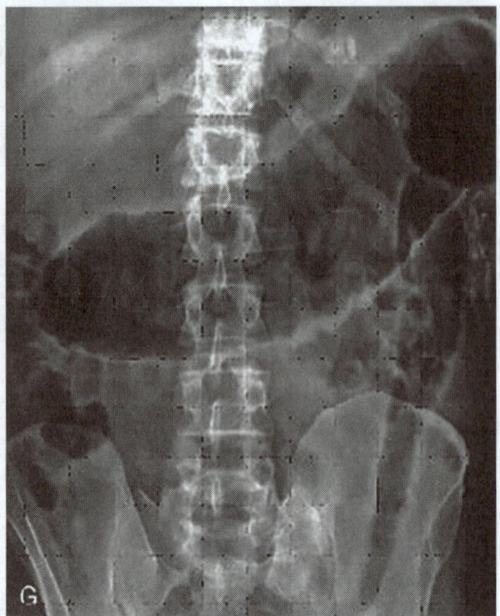

Fig. 8.10 Toxic megacolon.

TABLE 8.30 Complications of Inflammatory Bowel Disease

Local complications

- Fistulae, abscess and strictures
- Perforation
- Toxic dilatation (toxic megacolon)
- Carcinoma (cumulative risk is 5% after 20 years and 12% after 25 years in ulcerative colitis)

Systemic (extraintestinal) complications

- Nutritional and metabolic
  - Weight loss and anaemia
  - Electrolyte imbalance
  - Hypoalbuminaemia
- Eyes
  - Iritis and uveitis
  - Episcleritis and conjunctivitis
- Hepatobiliary
  - Fatty liver
  - Gallstones
  - Pericholangitis
  - Sclerosing cholangitis
  - Bile duct carcinoma
  - Chronic hepatitis
  - Cirrhosis
- Amyloidosis
- Musculoskeletal
  - Ankylosing spondylitis
  - Seronegative arthritis
  - Sacroiliitis
- Skin and mucous membranes
  - Erythema nodosum
  - Pyoderma gangrenosum
  - Aphthous stomatitis
  - Finger clubbing
- Haematological
  - Venous thrombosis; thromboembolism
  - Autoimmune haemolytic anaemia
- Renal
  - Calculous disease
  - Amyloidosis
  - Pyelonephritis

- Indications for surgical intervention include perforation, massive haemorrhage, increasing transfusion requirements, worsening signs of toxicity and progression of colonic dilatation.

Q. What are the complications of inflammatory bowel disease?

- Complications of inflammatory bowel disease are classified as local and systemic (extraintestinal) (Table 8.30).

Q. Differentiate between ulcerative colitis and Crohn's disease of the colon. (IM 16.15)

- Differences between ulcerative colitis and Crohn's disease of the colon are given in Table 8.31.

TABLE 8.31 Ulcerative Colitis Versus Crohn's Disease of Colon

Ulcerative Colitis	Crohn's Disease
Pathological Features	
• Continuous involvement	• Segmental involvement
• Inflammation is mucosal and submucosal	• Inflammation is transmucosal
• Granulomas are absent	• Granulomas are common
• Crypt abscesses are common	• Crypt abscesses are uncommon
• Loss of goblet cells	• No loss of goblet cells
• Strictures, fissures and fistulae uncommon	• Strictures, fissures and fistulae are common
• No mesenteric and lymph nodal involvement	• Mesenteric and lymph nodal involvement are common
Clinical Features	
• Rectal bleeding common	• Rectal bleeding is uncommon
• Abdominal pain is less common	• Abdominal pain is more common
• Weight loss infrequent	• Weight loss common
• No palpable abdominal masses	• Palpable abdominal masses
• Fistulae, fissures and perianal involvement are uncommon	• Fistulae, fissures and perianal involvement are characteristic
• Small bowel involvement is uncommon	• Small bowel involvement is common
• Rectal and colonic involvement is common	• Rectal and colonic involvement is rare
• Toxic dilatation is relatively common	• Toxic dilatation is uncommon

Q. How do you differentiate between Crohn's disease and intestinal tuberculosis?

- Table 8.32 gives features which help in differentiating intestinal tuberculosis from Crohn's disease.

Q. Discuss briefly about probiotics, postbiotics and prebiotics.

PROBIOTICS

- Defined as live microbes which if administered in adequate amounts confer a beneficial physiological effect on the host.
- They resist breakdown by gastric juices in the stomach and continue to grow in the presence of bile. They are fermented by intestinal flora.
- Probiotics are usually bacterial components of the normal human intestinal flora, for example, lactobacilli and bifidobacteria, that produce lactate and short-chain fatty acids such as acetate and butyrate as end products of metabolism. *S. boulardii*, a yeast, is also an important probiotic.

TABLE 8.32 Differentiating Features Between Intestinal Tuberculosis and Crohn's Disease

Feature	Intestinal Tuberculosis	Crohn's Disease
Clinical		
Duration of symptoms	Relatively shorter	Long-standing
Fever	Common	Less common
Diarrhoea	Less common	More common
Rectal bleeding	Less common	More common
Perianal fistulae	Less common	More common
Radiological		
Involvement of ileocaecal area	Caecal involvement more common	Ileal involvement more common
Involvement of multiple sites	Uncommon	Common
Length of intestine involved	Short segment	Long segment
Skip lesions	Very uncommon	Common
Intestinal fistula	Uncommon	Common
Intra-abdominal abscess	Uncommon	Common
Stricture	Concentric	Eccentric
Increased mesenteric vascularity	Uncommon	Common
Mesenteric lymph nodes	Necrotic	Homogeneous
Ascites	Often seen	Uncommon
Endoscopy		
Ulcer	Transverse	Longitudinal
Skip lesions	Uncommon	Common
'Cobblestone' mucosa	Uncommon	Common
Patulous ileocaecal valve	Common	Uncommon
Histology		
Disproportionate submucosal inflammation	Common	Rare
Granuloma	Caseation necrosis	No caseation necrosis
Acid-fast bacilli	Positive	Negative

- A commonly used probiotic is yoghurt in which milk is fermented by bacteria that convert lactose into lactic acid.
- Probiotics are also available as freeze dried bacteria in capsule, tablet or powder form. Their composition is variable but most contain *L. acidophilus*, often with *Bifidobacterium*.
- Exact mechanism of action of probiotics in various conditions is not clear. Postulated mechanisms are:
    - Suppression of growth or epithelial binding/invasion by pathogenic bacteria
    - Improvement of intestinal barrier function
    - Modulation of the immune system
    - Modulation of pain perception

POSTBIOTICS

- Nonviable bacterial products or metabolic by-products from probiotic microorganisms that confer a health benefit on the host.
- General postbiotics include bacterial metabolic by-products such as bacteriocins, organic acids, ethanol, diacetyl, acetaldehydes and hydrogen peroxide.
- Resistance to hydrolysis by GIT enzymes.
- They have a broad inhibitory property towards pathogenic microbes.

PREBIOTICS

- A selectively fermented ingredient that results in specific changes in the composition and/or activity of the gastrointestinal microbiota, thus conferring benefit upon host health.
- Prebiotics are selected as being nondigestible by the host and not metabolised by nonprobiotic gut flora such as *Bacteroides* spp. and *E. coli*.
- Prebiotics can be obtained naturally from sources like vegetables, fruits and grains.
- Synthetic prebiotics are oligosaccharides based on fructose or galactose known as fructose–oligosaccharides (FOS) and galactose–oligosaccharides (GOS), respectively. Lactulose is also a prebiotic.
- Can be added to foods or combined with a probiotic to make a synbiotic.

POTENTIAL USES

- Probiotics helpful in normalising the nutritional status of malnourished children. Use of yoghurt is suggested by the World Health Organization for nutritional recovery. Probiotic species that show a positive effect include *L. acidophilus*, yoghurt organisms

(*L. delbrueckii* var. *bulgaricus and Streptococcus salivarius* var. *thermophilus*), *L. plantarum* and *Bifidobacterium lactis.*
- Lactose intolerance where yoghurt is preferred source of probiotics.
- Pouchitis.
- Prebiotic like lactulose is useful in hepatic encephalopathy.
- Investigative role in preventing osteoporosis as prebiotics may increase calcium absorption.
- Chronic constipation and IBS.
- Ulcerative colitis.
- Antibiotic-associated diarrhoea—probiotics containing *S. boulardii* (a yeast) may be effective to some extent in the prevention and treatment of antibiotic-associated diarrhoea.
- Rotavirus-induced diarrhoea.
- Possible role in improving immunity.
- Necrotising enterocolitis in neonates.
- Reducing development of colonic cancer.
- Obesity management.

SAFETY

- The safety record of probiotics is remarkable. Nevertheless, there have been a few reports of bacteraemia.

Q. Discuss acute pancreatitis.

AETIOLOGY

- Various causes of acute pancreatitis are given in Table 8.33.

TABLE 8.33 Aetiology of Acute Pancreatitis

• Alcohol ingestion (acute and chronic)
• Biliary calculus
• Postoperative (abdominal and non-abdominal)
• Post-ERCP[a]
• Trauma to abdomen
• Metabolic conditions
  • Renal failure
  • Postrenal transplantation
  • Hypertriglyceridaemia
  • Hypercalcaemia
  • Acute fatty liver of pregnancy
• Penetrating peptic ulcer
• Connective tissue diseases
  • Systemic lupus erythematosus
  • Polyarteritis nodosa
• Infections
  • Viral hepatitis
  • Mumps
  • Roundworm
  • *Mycoplasma*
  • *Toxoplasma*
	• Drugs
	  • Sulphonamides
	  • Tetracyclines
	  • All-*trans*-retinoic acid
	  • Oestrogens
	  • Tamoxifen
	  • l-Asparaginase
	  • Azathioprine
	  • Thiazides
	  • Frusemide
	  • Didanosine
	  • Pentamidine
	  • Valproic acid
	  • Corticosteroids
	  • ACE inhibitors
	• Hereditary pancreatitis
	• Organophosphate poisoning
	• Thrombotic thrombocytopenic purpura
	• Scorpion sting

[a]Endoscopic retrograde cholangiopancreatography.

PATHOLOGY

- Oedematous pancreatitis (diffuse enlargement of pancreas with lack of pancreatic parenchymal necrosis or peripancreatic necrosis evident on imaging).
- Necrotising pancreatitis (presence of tissue necrosis of either pancreatic parenchyma or peripancreatic tissues; may be infected or sterile).
- Haemorrhagic pancreatitis.

PATHOPHYSIOLOGY

- Pathophysiology of acute pancreatitis is summarised in Flowchart 8.8.

CLINICAL FEATURES

SYMPTOMS

- The cardinal symptom of acute pancreatitis is pain.
  - Mild to severe intensity.
  - Dull, boring and steady.
  - Sudden pain in onset and gradually increases in severity.
  - Usually located in the epigastric region, though may be perceived more on the left or right side depending on which portion of the pancreas is involved.
  - Radiates directly through the abdomen to the back.
  - Partial relief if patient sits up and leans forwards.
  - Lasts for more than 1 day.
- Nausea and vomiting.
- Anorexia.

SIGNS

- Fever (low-grade).
- Tachycardia.
- Tachypnoea (secondary to inflammation of lungs, atelectasis and pleural effusion).
- Hypotension (secondary to exudation of plasma in peritoneal cavity, kinin-induced vasodilatation, systemic effects of proteolytic and lipolytic enzymes released into circulation).
- Jaundice.
- Abdominal tenderness, muscular guarding and distension.
- Bowel sounds often hypoactive.
- Lungs:
  - Cyanosis.
  - Basal crepitations.
  - Pleural effusion.
- Skin:
  - Erythematous skin nodules due to focal subcutaneous fat necrosis.
  - Bluish discolouration around the umbilicus (Cullen's sign). Also seen with ruptured ectopic pregnancy, ruptured aortic aneurysm, ruptured spleen and hepatocellular carcinoma.
  - Bluish or green-brown discolouration in the flanks (Turner's sign) due to haemoperitoneum. Other causes include blunt abdominal trauma, ruptured abdominal aortic aneurysm, ruptured ectopic pregnancy and spontaneous bleeding secondary to coagulopathy.
  - Cullen's sign and Turner's sign indicate severe necrotising pancreatitis.
- Others:
  - Haematemesis or melaena.

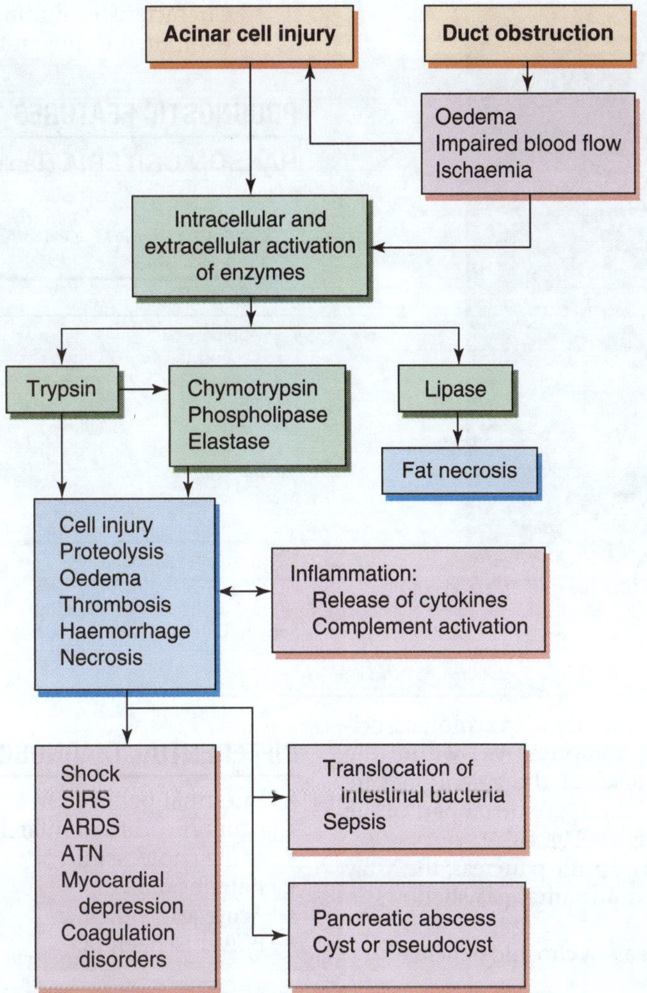

Flowchart 8.8 Pathophysiology of Acute Pancreatitis. ARDS = acute respiratory distress syndrome; ATN = acute tubular necrosis; SIRS = systemic inflammatory response syndrome.

- Ischaemic injury to retina is seen on fundus examination (Purtscher's retinopathy).

INVESTIGATIONS

- Serum amylase:
  - Levels increase for initial 24 hours and then decline to normal in 3–5 days.
  - Remains elevated in pancreatic abscess or pseudotumour formation.
  - Hypertriglyceridaemia occurs in 15%–20% of patients with acute pancreatitis and serum amylase levels are often spuriously normal in such cases.
  - A number of causes can produce elevated serum amylase level (Box 8.27).
- Serum lipase:
  - Preferable for diagnosis as its elevation is more specific than that of amylase.
  - Lipase takes longer time to clear from the blood, so it is a more useful indicator of pancreatitis than amylase.
  - Marked elevation in pleural or peritoneal fluid (>5000 IU/dL) suggests pancreatitis.

BOX 8.27 Causes of Elevated Serum Amylase

• Acute pancreatitis	• Mumps
• Small intestinal obstruction	• Diabetic ketoacidosis
• Perforation of peptic ulcer	• Burns
• Mesenteric ischaemia	• Ectopic pregnancy
• Tubo-ovarian disease	• Pancreatic carcinoma
• Renal insufficiency	• Macroamylasaemia

- Other investigations:
  - Blood glucose, total leucocyte count, platelet count, blood urea, serum calcium and other electrolytes, triglycerides.
  - Blood gases.
  - Urinary trypsinogen activation peptide is more useful than amylase in severe pancreatitis.
- Plain X-ray abdomen and chest:
  - To exclude other causes of acute abdominal pain (e.g. perforation).
  - A gas-filled duodenum (sentinel loop) secondary to localised ileus may be seen.

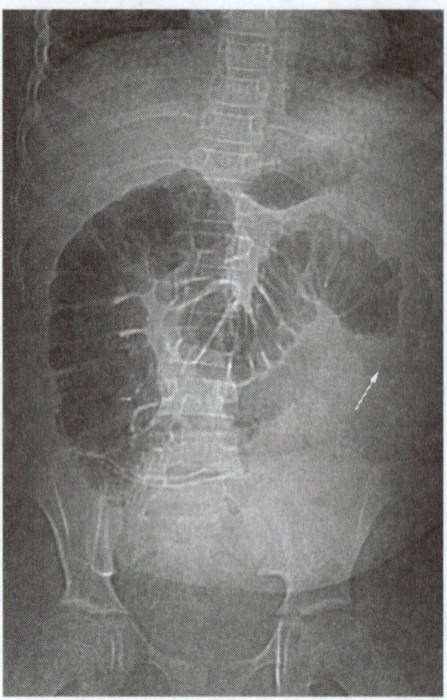

Fig. 8.11 Abdominal radiograph shows the classic 'colon cut-off sign' (arrow).

- Gaseous distension in the proximal colon associated with abrupt termination of gas within the colon usually at the level of the splenic flexure and decompression of the more distal part of the colon (colon cut-off sign) (Fig. 8.11).
- If abscess forms in the necrotic pancreas, the X-ray may show multiple extraluminal gas shadows in the pancreatic area.
- Calcification in pancreas in chronic pancreatitis.
- Ultrasound of abdomen:
  - To evaluate gallbladder and biliary tree.
  - It can detect acute pancreatitis in more than 60% of cases. However, pancreatic evaluation may be obscured by bowel gas.
- CT scan of abdomen:
  - May show solid mass of swollen pancreas (phlegmon), pseudocyst or pancreatic abscess.
- MRI abdomen:
  - Greater sensitivity for detecting mild acute pancreatitis as compared to CT scan.
  - Highly effective at identifying fluid collections and pancreatic necrosis.
  - Magnetic resonance cholangiopancreatography (MRCP) can be performed at the same time and stones within common bile duct can be readily identified if biliary pancreatitis is suspected.
- Endoscopic ultrasound (EUS):
  - Can be used to evaluate common bile duct for the presence of stones.
  - If stones are seen, ERCP can be performed at the same time to remove them.

DIAGNOSIS

- Presence of at least two of the following criteria:
  - Abdominal pain characteristic of acute pancreatitis.
  - Serum amylase and/or lipase ≥3 times the upper limit of normal.
  - Characteristic findings of acute pancreatitis on computed tomography scan.

PROGNOSTIC FEATURES

RANSON CRITERIA (Table 8.34)

TABLE 8.34 Ranson Criteria to Assess Severity of Acute Pancreatitis

At Admission	During Initial 48 Hours
• Age 55 years • Leucocytosis >6000/mm^3 • Blood sugar >200 mg/dL • Serum LDH >400 IU/L • Serum AST >250 IU/L	• Fall in haematocrit >10% of baseline • Fluid sequestration >4000 mL • Hypocalcaemia <8 mg/dL • Hypoxaemia with paO_2 <60 mmHg • Rise in blood urea >10 mg/dL after IV fluids • Hypoalbuminaemia <3.2 g/dL

0–2 Criteria—Mortality 2%
3–4 Criteria—Mortality 15%
5–6 Criteria—Mortality 40%
>6 Criteria—Mortality 100%

DIFFERENTIAL DIAGNOSIS

- Intestinal perforation.
- Acute myocardial infarction.
- Acute cholecystitis.
- Pneumonia.
- Acute appendicitis.
- Bowel ischaemia.

COMPLICATIONS (Table 8.35)

TABLE 8.35 Complications of Acute Pancreatitis

Local	Systemic
• Necrosis (sterile or infected) • Pseudocyst • Pancreatic abscess • Pancreatic ascites • Intraperitoneal haemorrhage • Obstructive jaundice • Intestinal obstruction • Splenic vein thrombosis	• Hypovolaemic shock • Acute respiratory distress syndrome • Multiple organ failure • Renal failure • Disseminated intravascular coagulation • Gastrointestinal haemorrhage • Fat necrosis • Hypocalcaemia • Pleural effusion

TREATMENT

- Nil orally initially with gradual return to oral intake as abdominal pain recedes and hunger returns. Enteral feeding should be restarted within 2–3 days even in severe cases. This can be done by oral intake or use of nasogastric or nasojejunal tube.
- Intravenous fluids to maintain intravascular volume in the first few days.
- Pain control with analgesics.

- Nasogastric aspiration if pain continues, patient has protracted vomiting or obstruction is seen on plain X-ray abdomen.
- Monitor pulse, blood pressure, abdominal girth, urine output, blood glucose and calcium and blood gases. Severe cases should be monitored in intensive care units.
- Prophylactic antibiotics, carbapenems (imipenem or meropenem) or ceftazidime in severe cases, though efficacy is not clear if infection is not suspected.
- Other drugs include PPIs, glucagon, octreotide and aprotinin (protease inhibitor).
- Surgery is indicated for:
  - Infected pancreatic necrosis.
  - Diagnostic uncertainty.
  - Complications.
- ERCP within first 36–48 hours in patients with gallstone pancreatitis who have evidence of cholangitis.
- Cholecystectomy during initial hospitalisation in patients with acute biliary pancreatitis.
- Most acute peripancreatic fluid collections and/or pseudocysts do not require interventions unless they become infected or cause significant extrinsic compression of other organs.

Q. Discuss briefly about chronic pancreatitis.

- Chronic inflammation and fibrosis of pancreas presenting as recurrent pain, endocrine deficiency (diabetes mellitus), exocrine deficiency (malabsorption) or a combination of two or all three features.

AETIOLOGY (Box 8.28)

BOX 8.28 Aetiology of Chronic Pancreatitis

- Chronic alcohol ingestion
- Cholelithiasis
- Cigarette smoke
- Drugs: valproate, thiazide, oestrogens, azathioprine
- Stenosis of sphincter of Oddi
- Autoimmune pancreatitis
- Associated with autoimmune diseases (Sjogren's syndrome, primary biliary cholangitis)
- Chronic kidney disease
- Cystic fibrosis
- Hypercalcaemia
- Hyperlipidaemia
- HIV infection
- Familial
- Idiopathic—tropical or fibrocalculous

CLINICAL FEATURES

- Pain, acute or recurrent, continuous or intermittent. May be referred to chest or back.
- Pain is often increased by alcohol or heavy meals.
- Features of local complications (e.g. pseudocyst, obstruction of adjacent organs or vascular thrombosis).
- Features of malabsorption—diarrhoea, steatorrhoea, weight loss, features of fat-soluble vitamin deficiency and vitamin B_{12} deficiency (exocrine failure).
- Diabetes mellitus (endocrine failure).
- In late stages, mechanical obstruction of common bile duct can occur.
- The risk of developing pancreatic carcinoma is high.

INVESTIGATIONS

- Serum amylase and lipase are usually normal.
- Hyperlipidaemia or hypercalcaemia (if cause of chronic pancreatitis is elevated calcium).
- Plain X-ray of abdomen:
  - Calcification in pancreatic area (in 30%).
  - Sensitivity for picking calcification increases when both anteroposterior and oblique views are taken.
- Ultrasound abdomen and CT scan of abdomen:
  - Pancreatic atrophy.
  - Calcifications.
  - Dilatation of bile duct.
  - Stricture of bile duct.
- ERCP is the gold standard for diagnosis as it most accurately demonstrates pancreatic ducts.
- MRCP may replace ERCP.
- EUS to evaluate pancreas.
- Pancreatic function tests:
  - Secretin/cholecystokinin (CCK) stimulation test (reduction in bicarbonate and enzyme secretion).
  - Faecal chymotrypsin or elastase concentration.
  - Twenty-four-hour faecal fat.
  - Oral glucose tolerance test.

TREATMENT

- Abstinence of alcohol.
- Diet rich in medium-chain triglycerides that do not require lipase for digestion.
- Pancreatic enzymes, particularly lipase, 20,000–75,000 units should be taken before each meal to reduce faecal fat excretion.
- PPIs or H_2-blockers to prevent inactivation of pancreatic enzymes by gastric acid.
- Treatment of pain by opioids or NSAIDs. Co-analgesics such as antidepressants and anticonvulsants (e.g. gabapentin, pregabalin) are also effective and can reduce the need for opioids. In intractable pain, coeliac ganglion blockade may be tried.
- Steroids in autoimmune pancreatitis.
- Treatment of diabetes.
- Endoscopic therapy with or without stents in painful chronic pancreatitis to allow pancreatic duct drainage in patients with obstructed ducts and treatment of complications such as pseudocysts and bile duct obstruction with jaundice.
- Surgery for unremitting pain; includes pancreatectomy along with islet cell auto-transplantation, and pancreato-jejunostomy.

Q. Describe the features of tropical pancreatitis or fibrocalculous pancreatic diabetes.

- Tropical pancreatitis is a juvenile form of chronic calcific pancreatitis that is not related to alcohol intake. When patients with tropical pancreatitis

develop diabetes, they are referred to as fibrocalculous pancreatic diabetes.
- Seen almost exclusively in tropical countries.
- In India, it is more common in southern states (Kerala and Tamil Nadu).

AETIOLOGY

- Various postulated aetiologies are as follows:
  - Malnutrition.
  - Diet rich in cassava that contains cyanogenic glycosides.
  - Oxidant stress.
  - Infections (Coxsackie and viral hepatitis).
  - Familial.

PATHOLOGY

- The gross appearance of the pancreas varies with the stage of the disease. In the initial stages, the size can be normal while it may shrink to a small size in the later stages.
- Cut sections show varying degrees of fibrosis and calcification with the presence of large intraductal calculi of varying size and shape.

CLINICAL FEATURES

- Affects young people, generally males.
- Pursues a relatively accelerated course.
- Presents with recurrent abdominal pain, typically in epigastric area with radiation to back. Pain gets precipitated by heavy meals.
- Associated features include malnutrition, enlarged parotid glands, abdominal distension and a peculiar cyanotic hue of the lips.
- Pancreatic exocrine deficiency presents with steatorrhoea and malabsorption.
- Diabetes mellitus is common. Even without insulin treatment, ketosis is uncommon. Patients have sufficient insulin reserve to prevent lipolysis and subsequent ketone body formation. They are also deficient in glucagon, a counterregulatory hormone that plays a pivotal role in ketogenesis. Episodes of hypoglycaemia with insulin are frequent.

INVESTIGATIONS

- Plain X-ray and ultrasound of abdomen show multiple and large intraductal calculi.

TREATMENT

- As with chronic pancreatitis.
- High doses of insulin are often required with careful watch over hypoglycaemia.

Q. How will you differentiate tropical pancreatitis from alcoholic pancreatitis?

- Table 8.36 gives differentiating features between alcoholic pancreatitis and tropical pancreatitis.

TABLE 8.36 Alcoholic Pancreatitis Versus Tropical Pancreatitis

Features	Alcoholic Pancreatitis	Tropical Pancreatitis
Age	• 35–45 years	• 20–40 years
Sex	• Males	• Males > females
Diabetes	• Less common (50%)	• More common (70%)
Steatorrhoea	• More common	• Less common
Intraductal calculi	• Less common; small	• Frequent; large
Pancreatic malignancy	• Less common	• More common

Q. Discuss the differential diagnosis of sudden upper abdominal pain in a 40-year-old male.

- Sudden upper abdominal pain in a 40-year-old patient can be due to several causes (Box 8.29).

PEPTIC ULCER PERFORATION

- History of recurrent epigastric pain with relation to food and periodicity.
- Perforation results initially in severe epigastric pain, but it soon becomes generalised.
- Shoulder pain due to irritation of diaphragm.
- Abdominal examination reveals board-like rigidity, absent peristaltic sounds and reduction or absence of liver dullness.
- Features of generalised peritonitis follow the initial phase of peritoneal irritation.
- Plain radiograph of abdomen in the erect posture may show gas under the diaphragm.

ACUTE PANCREATITIS

- History of precipitating factors like alcohol, gallstones and pancreatic stones.
- Acute severe pain in the epigastrium, usually 12–24 hours following heavy meal or alcohol.
- Pain may radiate to the back.
- Severe vomiting.
- Examination reveals hypotension, tachycardia and epigastric tenderness.
- Features of peritonitis.
- Cullen's sign and Grey Turner's sign (uncommon).
- High serum amylase and lipase activity.
- Plain radiograph of abdomen shows paralytic ileus or obstruction.
- Chest radiograph might show left pleural effusion, collapse or consolidation of lung.
- Ultrasonography and CT scan show swollen, oedematous pancreas, stones and ascites.

BOX 8.29 Common Causes of Sudden Upper Abdominal Pain

- Peptic ulcer perforation
- Acute pancreatitis
- Acute mesenteric artery occlusion
- Aortic dissection or rupture
- Acute myocardial infarction
- Acute cholecystitis

MESENTERIC ARTERY OCCLUSION

- Previous history of recurrent abdominal pain after food (postprandial angina).
- Occlusion causes sudden onset of severe pain in the epigastrium and umbilical region.
- History of passing black stools.
- Clinical examination reveals signs of acute abdomen like guarding, rigidity, tenderness and paralytic ileus.
- Mesenteric arteriography confirms the diagnosis.

AORTIC DISSECTION

- Sudden tearing pain radiating to the back.
- Evidence of associated diseases may be present.
  - Hypertension.
  - Diabetes mellitus.
  - Atherosclerosis.
  - Aortic regurgitation.
  - Marfan's syndrome.
- Urine output may be decreased if there is renal artery occlusion.
- Aortogram clinches the diagnosis.

ACUTE MYOCARDIAL INFARCTION

- Previous history of ischaemic heart disease (angina), hypertension, diabetes and other risk factors.
- Sudden onset of pain in the epigastrium, squeezing in type, associated with restlessness, pallor and profuse sweating.
- Clinical examination of cardiovascular system is usually normal.
- Occasionally, third heart sound and fourth heart sound are heard.
- A systolic murmur may be heard at the apex.
- ECG shows evidence of infarction.
- Cardiac injury enzymes (CK, troponin, AST and LDH) may be raised.

ACUTE CHOLECYSTITIS

- Pain in the right upper quadrant, epigastrium, right shoulder tip or interscapular region.
- Restlessness, pallor, sweating and vomiting.
- Clinical examination shows fever.
- Tenderness in the right hypochondrium and rigidity, worse on inspiration (Murphy's sign).
- Gallbladder may be palpable.
- Leucocytosis, jaundice and minor elevations of transaminases.
- Plain radiograph of abdomen may show gallstones (rare).
- Ultrasonography detects gall stones and gallbladder thickening.
- Cholescintigraphy shows cystic duct obstruction.

9 Diseases of the Connective Tissues and Joints

Q. How do you classify polyarthritis? What are the causes of polyarthritis? (IM 7.3, IM 7.8)

- Classification and causes of polyarthritis are given in Table 9.1.

Q. Discuss the clinical manifestations, diagnosis and management of rheumatoid arthritis (RA). (IM 7.19, IM 7.22, IM 7.23)

- RA is a chronic inflammatory joint disease with multisystem involvement.
- Females are affected three times more often than males (3:1).
- Onset is usually during fourth and fifth decades of life.
- Factors producing RA include infectious trigger, genetic predisposition and autoimmune response.
  - The role of genetic influences in the aetiology of RA is marked by association with HLA-DR4 in 70% of patients.
  - Autoimmune factors include activated T cells, auto-reactive B cells, macrophages and inflammatory cytokines like interleukin-1 and tumour necrosis factor-α.

CLINICAL FEATURES

ONSET

- Insidious onset with fatigue, anorexia, weakness and vague musculoskeletal symptoms.

TABLE 9.1 Classification and Causes of Polyarthritis

Category	Causes
• Inflammatory	
• Infections	Acute bacterial arthritis, sepsis, gonococcal arthritis, tuberculous arthritis, mycotic arthritis, syphilitic arthritis, viral arthritis, bacterial endocarditis, Lyme disease
• Immunological	Rheumatoid arthritis (RA), rheumatic fever, seronegative spondyloarthritides, systemic lupus erythematosus (SLE), polymyositis, systemic vasculitis, systemic sclerosis, adult-onset Still's disease, sarcoidosis
• Crystal induced	Gout, pseudogout (calcium pyrophosphate dihydrate deposition disease [CPPD]), calcium hydroxyapatite deposition disease
• Reactive	Reactive arthritis, Behcet's syndrome, sexually acquired reactive arthritis (SARA)
• Mechanical	Degenerative joint disease—osteoarthrosis
• Metabolic	Hypothyroidism, acromegaly, hyperparathyroidism, Cushing's disease, ochronosis, haemochromatosis, amyloidosis, Wilson's disease, hyperlipidaemia
• Neoplastic	Paraneoplastic arthropathies, carcinomatous arthropathy or neuromyopathy, hypertrophic osteoarthropathy (in some cases)
• Drug-induced	Thiazides causing gout, drug-induced lupus, corticosteroids
• Miscellaneous	Intestinal bypass arthritis, Whipple's disease

- Acute onset with rapid development of polyarthritis accompanied by constitutional symptoms including fever, lymphadenopathy and splenomegaly.
- Palindromic onset where recurrent acute episodes of joint pain and stiffness occur in individual joints lasting only a few hours or days. The joints look and feel normal between attacks, and the attacks do not cause any lasting damage to the joints.

ARTICULAR MANIFESTATIONS

- Joint involvement is usually symmetric. It is characterised by pain, swelling, tenderness and painful limitation of movements. The metacarpophalangeal and proximal interphalangeal joints of the hands, wrists, knees, and the metatarsophalangeal and proximal interphalangeal joints of the feet are the most common joints involved.
- Generalised stiffness may occur but 'morning stiffness' lasting more than 1 hour is a characteristic feature. The intensity and duration of morning stiffness is a measure of disease activity.

Hand and Wrist

- Swelling of the proximal but not the distal interphalangeal joints results in 'spindling' of the fingers.
- Hyperextension of the proximal interphalangeal joints with flexion of the distal interphalangeal joints results in 'swan-neck' deformity (Fig. 9.1A).
- Flexion of the proximal interphalangeal joints and extension of the distal interphalangeal joints result in 'boutonniere' or buttonhole deformity (Fig. 9.1B).
- Hyperextension of the first interphalangeal joint and flexion of the first metacarpophalangeal joint with a consequent loss of thumb mobility and pinch can occur.
- Extensor tendon rheumatoid granulomata and tendon rupture result in 'dropped finger'.
- Radial deviation of the wrist with ulnar deviation of the digits often with palmar subluxation of the proximal phalanges results in the 'Z' deformity (Fig. 9.2).
- Wrist synovitis with median nerve entrapment can result in carpal tunnel syndrome.
- Whole of hand may be swollen in very acute cases with pitting oedema over dorsum giving rise to the 'boxing glove' appearance.

Foot and Ankle

- Swelling of the metatarsophalangeal joints results in 'broadening' of the forefoot.
- Lateral deviation and dorsal subluxation of the toes.
- Plantar subluxation of the metatarsal heads.
- Eversion at the hindfoot (subtalar joint).
- Hallux valgus deformity.

Other Joints

- Flexion contractures of elbows, wrists, knees and hips.
- Shoulder joint involvement can occur as glenohumeral arthritis, rotator cuff fraying and rupture.
- Cervical spine involvement can result in atlanto-axial subluxation with progressive spastic quadriparesis.

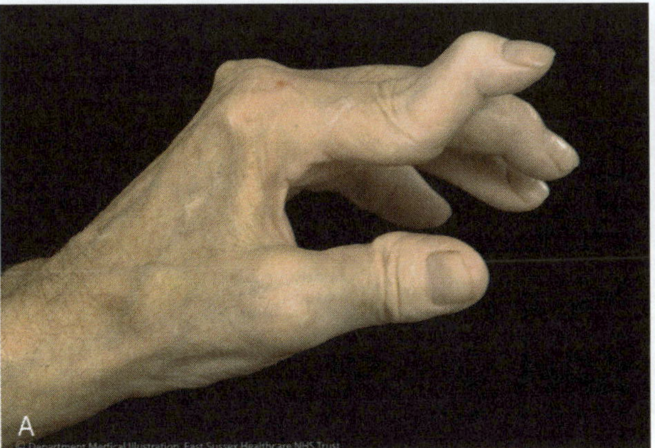

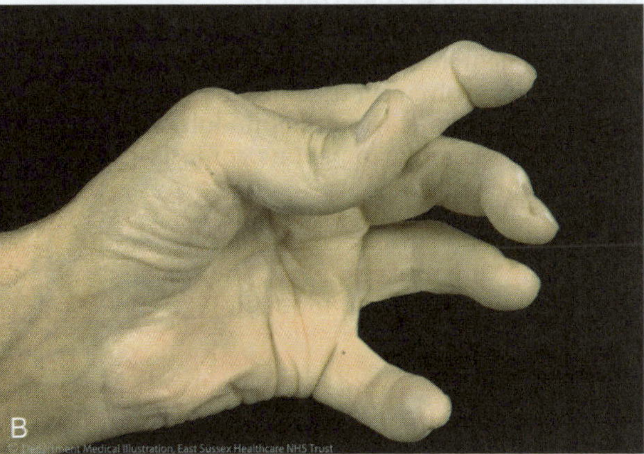

Fig. 9.1 (A) Swan-neck deformity of index finger, (B) Boutonniere deformity of thumb.

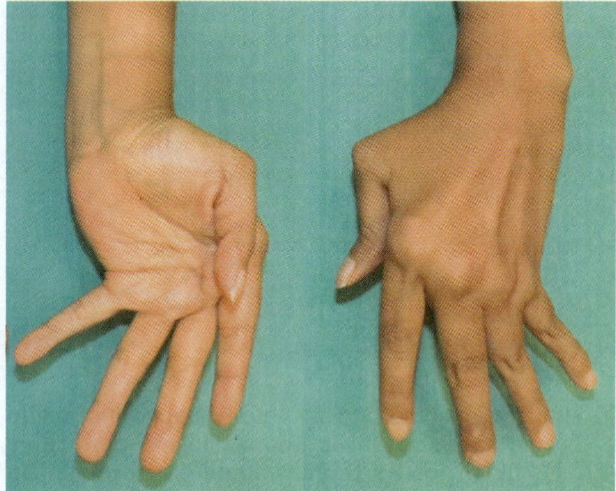

Fig. 9.2 'Z'-deformity.

- Cricoarytenoid joint involvement results in hoarseness of voice and stridor.
- Pain and swelling behind the knee can result from extension of inflamed synovium into the popliteal space (popliteal cyst or Baker's cyst).

EXTRA-ARTICULAR MANIFESTATIONS

Rheumatoid Nodules

- These develop in 25% of persons with RA. They are firm, round masses felt in the subcutaneous tissues, for example olecranon bursa, proximal ulna, Achilles tendon and occiput. Visceral structures like heart, lungs and pleura may also be involved.
- Rheumatoid nodules are clinical predictors of more severe arthritis, seropositivity, joint erosions and rheumatoid vasculitis.

Rheumatoid Vasculitis

- These manifestations are seen in patients with a high titre of circulating rheumatoid factor. Vasculitis results in the following manifestations:
- Polyneuropathy and mononeuritis multiplex.
- Cutaneous ulcerations, palpable purpurae and distal gangrene.
- Visceral infarction resulting in stroke, acute myocardial infarction and mesenteric ischaemia.

Pleuropulmonary Manifestations

- Pleural involvement results in effusion with low levels of pleural fluid glucose (less than 10 mg/dL).
- Pulmonary involvement resulting in interstitial fibrosis.
- Caplan's syndrome—multiple nodules and interstitial lung disease due to pneumoconiosis.

Cardiovascular Manifestations

- Pericarditis and chronic constrictive pericarditis.
- Premature atherosclerosis (an important cause of increased morbidity and mortality).
- Valvular involvement.
- Conduction defects.

Neurological Manifestations

- Nerve entrapment syndromes, for example carpal and tarsal tunnel syndromes.
- Spinal compression due to atlanto-axial subluxation.
- Peripheral neuropathies.

Ophthalmological Manifestations

- Scleritis, episcleritis and scleromalacia perforans.
- Sicca complex comprising keratoconjunctivitis sicca, xerostomia and salivary gland enlargement.
- Glaucoma.

Felty's Syndrome

- This is the association of splenomegaly and neutropenia with RA.

Osteoporosis

- Osteoporosis secondary to rheumatoid involvement is very common. It may be aggravated by corticosteroid therapy and immobilisation.

Haematological Manifestations

- Normocytic normochromic anaemia.
- Thrombocytosis.
- Eosinophilia and mild leucocytosis.

SUMMARY OF EXTRA-ARTICULAR COMPLICATIONS OF RHEUMATOID ARTHRITIS

- Table 9.2 summarises extra-articular complications of rheumatoid arthritis.

DIAGNOSIS

- Diagnosis of RA should be considered in patients with bilateral, symmetric, inflammatory polyarthritis involving small and large joints with sparing of the axial skeleton except the cervical spine.
- The criteria for diagnosis are shown in Table 9.3.

INVESTIGATIONS

- Markers of acute inflammation—raised ESR, anaemia, thrombocytosis, increased levels of acute-phase proteins (e.g. C-reactive protein [CRP]) and increased plasma viscosity.
- Rheumatoid factor.
- Anticitrullinated protein antibodies (ACPA), usually detected by anticyclic citrullinated peptide (CCP) antibodies.

TABLE 9.2 Extra-Articular Complications of Rheumatoid Arthritis

Pleuropulmonary	Pleuritis, pleural effusion, rheumatoid lung nodules, interstitial lung disease
Cardiovascular	Atherosclerosis, myocardial infarction, pericarditis, arrhythmias, valvular heart disease
Neurological	Entrapment neuropathy, mononeuritis multiplex, cervical subluxation producing cervical myelopathy, rheumatoid meningitis
Renal	Glomerulonephritis, secondary amyloidosis
Haematological	Felty's syndrome, anaemia, thrombocytosis
Vascular	Vasculitis
Ocular	Scleritis, episcleritis, keratoconjunctivitis sicca
Cutaneous	Rheumatoid nodules, ulcers

TABLE 9.3 American College of Rheumatology/European League Against Rheumatism Classification Criteria for Rheumatoid Arthritis (2010)

Features	Score
A. Joint involvement[a]	
1 large joint[b]	0
2–10 large joints	1
1–3 small joints[c] (with or without involvement of large joints)	2
4–10 small joints (with or without involvement of large joints)	3
>10 joints (at least one small joint)[d]	5
B. Serology (at least one test result is needed for classification)	
Negative RF and negative anticitrullinated protein antibodies (ACPA)	0
Low-positive RF *or* low-positive ACPA	2
High-positive RF *or* high-positive ACPA	3
C. Acute-phase reactants (at least one test result is needed for classification)	
Normal CRP *and* normal ESR	0
Abnormal CRP *or* abnormal ESR	1
D. Duration of symptoms	
<6 weeks	0
≥6 weeks	1

Add score of categories A–D; a score of ≥6/10 is needed for classification of a patient as having definite RA. Patients with a score of <6/10 are not classifiable as having RA, but their status can be re-assessed over time.
[a]Joint involvement: any swollen or tender joint on examination, which may be confirmed by imaging evidence of synovitis. Distal interphalangeal joints, first carpometacarpal joints and first metatarsophalangeal joints are excluded from assessment.
[b]Large joints: shoulders, elbows, hips, knees and ankles.
[c]Small joints: metacarpophalangeal joints, proximal interphalangeal joints, second to fifth metatarsophalangeal joints, thumb interphalangeal joints and wrists.
[d]Includes other joints not specifically listed (e.g. temporomandibular, acromioclavicular, sternoclavicular).
(*Source:* Adapted from *Arthritis & Rheumatism*. 2010 Rheumatoid Arthritis Classification: Daniel Aletaha, Tuhina Neogi, Alan J. Silman, et. al. Vol. 62, No. 9, pp 2569–2581, Table 2, September 2010, American College of Rheumatology. Links: http://www.arthritisrheum.org/ and http://www.interscience.wiley.com/)

- Radiographs of the affected joints may be useful. The characteristic radiological changes are symmetrical pattern of involvement, juxta-articular osteoporosis, soft-tissue swelling, bone erosions and joint space narrowing.
- Ultrasonography and MRI have greater sensitivity than plain radiographs for the detection of soft-tissue synovitis before joint damage occurs.
- Rarely, synovial fluid analysis, synovial biopsy and arthroscopy are required. The synovial fluid contains 2000–50,000 leucocytes/μL with no crystals or organism.

MANAGEMENT

- Rest and splinting of the joints should be instituted in the acute stage of illness.
- Active and passive physiotherapy helps in mobilisation and prevention of contractures.

ANALGESICS

- Nonsteroidal antiinflammatory drugs (NSAIDs) are the first-line drugs used in the management of RA. They act by suppression of inflammation. None of the NSAIDs has been shown to be more effective than aspirin in the treatment of RA.

DISEASE-MODIFYING ANTIRHEUMATIC DRUGS

- DMARDs are indicated in most cases. The conventional DMARDs are:
  - Hydroxychloroquine.
  - Oral gold (auranofin)—rarely used.
  - Parenteral (intramuscular) gold—rarely used.
  - d-Penicillamine—rarely used.
  - Sulphasalazine.
  - Methotrexate.
  - Leflunomide.
- Most patients should be started on a combination of DMARDs and analgesics in the early course of disease.
- DMARDs reduce inflammation and prevent damage to joints, bones and ligaments.
- These agents take 3–4 months before their full effect.
- Biologicals are also DMARDs but are discussed below separately.

Methotrexate

- Currently, methotrexate is the drug of choice for RA. It may be given alone or in combination with hydroxychloroquine (hydroxychloroquine alone may not be effective in halting the progression of disease).
- The usual starting dose is 7.5–10 mg/week orally. If a positive response does not occur within 4–8 weeks and there has been no toxicity, the dose should be increased by 2.5–5 mg/week each month to 20–25 mg/week before considering the treatment a failure.
- To improve the efficacy of MTX at dosages of 20–25 mg weekly, a change to subcutaneous administration should be considered.
- Folic acid is given in a dose of 5 mg once a week, on the day following methotrexate dose. It reduces some adverse events (gastrointestinal intolerance, stomatitis, hepatotoxicity, hyperhomocysteinaemia and alopecia) associated with methotrexate.

- Regular monitoring of liver enzymes and blood counts required as it can produce liver toxicity and can suppress bone marrow.
- Can also produce pulmonary toxicity (hypersensitivity pneumonitis, organising pneumonia, fibrosis).

Other DMARDs

- If the patient does not respond to methotrexate, the options include gold or D-penicillamine, sulphasalazine or leflunomide.
- A combination of methotrexate and leflunomide may be more effective than either drug alone.
- Leflunomide is a pyrimidine antagonist that blocks the enzyme dihydroorotate dehydrogenase, thereby blocking the synthesis of DNA. It has an efficacy similar to that of methotrexate. It can be used either alone or in combination with methotrexate. Dose is 10–20 mg/day.

Targeted DMARDs

- A novel subgroup of DMARDs recognised as JAK inhibitors inhibit the JAK or Janus kinase, which is involved in immune response of the body. These agents inhibit inflammation and prevent joint damage refractory to biologics and DMARDs.
- Tofacitinib is a JAK kinase inhibitor that is administered orally. It inhibits enzymes involved in joint inflammatory process. Others include baricitinib and upadacitinib.

BIOLOGICAL RESPONSE MODIFIERS (OR BIOLOGICALS)

- Biological response modifiers are the agents that block specific immune factors leading to RA.
- These agents include tumour necrosis factor-α blockers, interleukin-1 receptor antagonists and anti-CD20 B-cell agents.
- Anti-TNF-α inhibitors include monoclonal antibodies (infliximab, adalimumab, golimumab and certolizumab) and a soluble receptor fusion protein (etanercept).
- Other biologicals include rituximab (anti-CD20 antibody that blocks CD20 present on B cells), tocilizumab (a monoclonal antibody that binds to IL-6 receptors), abatacept (T-cell receptor CTLA4 that downregulates T cells) and anakinra (IL-1 receptor blocker).
- Usually given along with methotrexate or other conventional DMARDs.
- Infliximab:
    - A chimeric IgG1 monoclonal antibody (a chimera of human constant and mouse variable regions).
    - Binds to TNF-α and TNF-β and lyses TNF-producing cells to neutralise their activity.
    - Initial dose 3 mg/kg is given intravenously over 2 hours.
    - Same dose repeated at 2 and 6 weeks and then every 8 weeks.
    - Dose can be increased to 10 mg/kg or infusion interval can be shortened if an adequate response is not attained.
    - Patient monitored for any side effects during and 1 hour after infusion.
    - Side effects include pruritus, influenza-like symptoms, headache and hypotension. Occasionally, serum sickness can develop 1–2 weeks after infusion.
    - Reactivation of tuberculosis can occur. Other important side effects include soft-tissue and joint infections, fungal infections and demyelination.
- Etanercept:
    - A soluble dimeric fusion protein consisting of soluble human p75-TNF receptor and Fc portion of human IgG1.
    - It blocks the TNF receptor.
    - Dose is 25 mg subcutaneously twice a week.
    - Injection site reactions in the form of redness and swelling can occur.
- Adalimumab:
    - A humanised IgG1 monoclonal antibody (fully human constant and variable regions).

Summary of Disease-Modifying Antirheumatic Drugs (Table 9.4)

TABLE 9.4 Disease-Modifying Antirheumatic Drugs

Synthetic DMARDs	
Conventional DMARDs	Methotrexate Sulphasalazine Leflunomide Hydroxychloroquine Corticosteroids
Targeted DMARDs	Janus kinase inhibitors—tofacitinib, baricitinib, upadacitinib
Biological DMARDs	
Tumour necrosis factor-α antagonists	Adalimumab Golimumab Certolizumab Infliximab Etanercept
IL-1 receptor antagonist	Anakinra
IL-6 receptor antagonist	Tocilizumab Sarilumab
Anti-CD20 monoclonal antibody	Rituximab
CTLA-4-Ig fusion protein	Abatacept

CORTICOSTEROIDS

- Oral corticosteroid (e.g. prednisolone) is often combined with DMARDs in the early part of treatment and then tapered off in a few months.
- Parenteral corticosteroids used in the presence of incapacitating constitutional symptoms such as fever and weight loss, neuropathy and rheumatoid vasculitis.
- Intraarticular corticosteroid injections useful in the acute stage.

IMMUNOSUPPRESSANTS

- Immunosuppressants are used as third-line drugs for disease that recurs or does not respond to second-line agents. They inhibit the immune system and have potentially serious side effects. These include cyclophosphamide and azathioprine. However, in acute vasculitis causing serious organ involvement, intravenous cyclophosphamide may be lifesaving.

SURGICAL THERAPY

- Surgical therapy is useful in maintenance of joint function and prevention and correction of deformities. Various modalities include reconstructive hand surgery, arthroplasties, total joint replacements, tenosynovectomy and open or close synovectomy.

POOR PROGNOSTIC FACTORS

- Poor prognostic factors in patients with rheumatoid arthritis are listed in Box 9.1.

SUMMARY OF TREATMENT OF RHEUMATOID ARTHRITIS

- Flowchart 9.1 summarises treatment of rheumatoid arthritis.

BOX 9.1 Poor Prognostic Factors in Rheumatoid Arthritis

- Persistently moderate or high disease activity despite conventional DMARD therapy
- High acute phase reactant levels
- High swollen joint count
- Presence of rheumatoid factor and/or anticitrullinated protein antibodies at high levels
- Presence of early joint erosions
- Failure of two or more conventional DMARDs

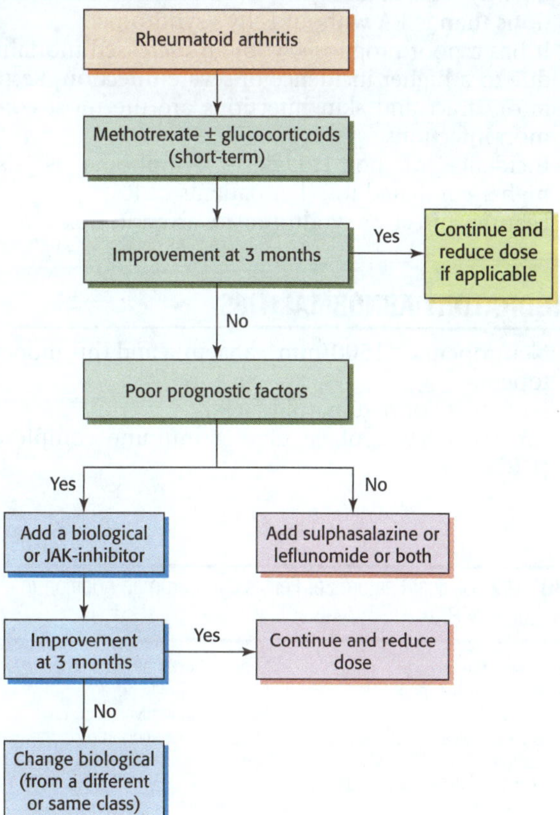

Flowchart 9.1 Treatment of Rheumatoid Arthritis.

TABLE 9.5 Conditions Associated With a Positive Rheumatoid Factor

Rheumatic Conditions (Prevalence)	Other Conditions
• Rheumatoid arthritis (80%)	• Age >60 years
• Sjögren's syndrome (75%–95%)	• Infections (endocarditis, tuberculosis, syphilis, mumps)
• Systemic lupus erythematosus (SLE) (15%–30%)	• Chronic liver disease
• Systemic sclerosis (20%–30%)	• Sarcoidosis
• Cryoglobulinaemia (40%–90%)	• Interstitial lung disease
• Mixed connective tissue disease (CTD) (50%–60%)	• Primary biliary cholangitis

Q. Explain rheumatoid factor. (IM 7.15)

- Rheumatoid factors (RFs) are IgM and IgG autoantibodies against the Fc portion of IgG. In clinical practice, IgM RF is widely used.
- RF is present in about 80% of patients with RA. It can also be present in a number of other conditions (Table 9.5).
- RF testing is appropriate in patients suspected of having RA. If clinical suspicion is low, RF testing is unlikely to be helpful. RF is also a good screening tool when Sjögren's syndrome or cryoglobulinaemia is suspected.
- In patients with RA, RF titres generally correlate with extra-articular manifestations and disease severity. However, RF titres are not useful in following disease progression. Hence, if a patient is RF-positive, there is no need to repeat it later.

Q. What are anticitrullinated protein antibodies? Explain. (IM 7.15)

Q. Write a short note on anticyclic citrullinated peptide (anti-CCP) antibody. (IM 7.15)

- Autoantibodies seen in patients with RA.
- Anticitrullinated protein antibodies (ACPA) recognise citrulline-containing peptides/proteins as common antigenic entity.
- Citrulline is a nonstandard amino acid generated by posttranslational modification of arginine during a variety of biological processes which include inflammation. Some of the citrullinated proteins include filaggrin, fibrin, fibrinogen, vimentin, types I and II collagens and modified cyclic citrullinated peptides (CCPs).
- IgG CCP antibody is a type of ACPA where antibody is directed against the antikeratin epitope that contains citrulline.
- Citrullinated extracellular fibrin is found within the synovium of patients with RA.
- Highly specific (97%) but less sensitive (50%) for diagnosis of RA. Positive results can occur in other

diseases, including SLE, systemic sclerosis, tuberculosis and sometimes chronic lung disease.
- It is more likely to be present early in the course of the disease and may be helpful in confirming the serological diagnosis in patients with a negative or equivocal rheumatoid factor.
- Presence of anti-CCP antibody may be a marker for the development of more severe erosive disease. Thus, anti-CCP-positive patients may require aggressive treatment.

Q. Discuss COX enzymes and COX-2 inhibitors. (IM 7.20)

- NSAIDs exert their antiinflammatory effects through the inhibition of prostaglandin synthesis from arachidonic acid by blocking cyclooxygenase (COX) enzyme.
- There are two isoforms of COX: COX-1 and COX-2.
  - COX-1 enzyme is constitutively expressed in gastrointestinal tract, kidneys and platelets. It is responsible for the production of thromboxane A_2 and prostaglandins. Under the influence of COX-1, prostaglandins maintain integrity of the gastric mucosa, mediate platelet function and regulate renal blood flow. Thromboxane A_2 is a vasoconstrictor and potent stimulator of platelet aggregation.
  - COX-2 is primarily induced at the site of inflammation, producing prostaglandins that mediate inflammation and pain. Prostaglandin I_2, a potent vasodilator and inhibitor of platelet function, is predominantly regulated by the COX-2 isoform.
- Conventional NSAIDs inhibit both the isoforms of COX in varying degrees.
- Inhibition of COX-1 is necessary for antiinflammatory and analgesic effects but may account for adverse effects associated with traditional NSAIDs.
- COX-2 inhibitors are NSAIDs that play a major role in the management of inflammation and pain caused by arthritis. These agents selectively inhibit the COX-2 enzyme and have minimal antiplatelet effects because they do not affect the thromboxane A2 pathway.
- With respect to their analgesic and antiinflammatory properties, there is no significant difference among traditional NSAIDs and COX-2 inhibitors.
- COX-2 inhibitors have relatively lesser gastrointestinal side effects (including lower incidence of peptic ulcer) compared to the conventional and nonselective NSAIDs.
- These agents do not have significant effect on platelets.
- Selective COX-2 inhibitors appear to have little risk of precipitating bronchospasm in patients with aspirin-induced asthma.
- Like traditional NSAIDs, COX-2 inhibitors can produce significant changes in renal functions and, hence, should be cautiously used in patients with diabetes, dehydration and congestive heart failure.
- This class of drugs includes celecoxib, rofecoxib, valdecoxib, etoricoxib and etodolac.
- Unfortunately, trials indicated a higher risk of myocardial infarction, heart failure and stroke (thromboembolic complications) in patients using COX-2 inhibitors compared to those taking other NSAIDs. Hence, two COX-2 inhibitors (rofecoxib and valdecoxib) were withdrawn. Celecoxib, etodolac and etoricoxib are available for clinical use.
- A possible explanation for a prothrombotic state induced with these agents is that they inhibit the vasodilating effects of endothelial prostaglandin I2 without affecting thromboxane A2 (a product of platelet COX-1 activity) resulting in an unbalanced prothrombotic state in patients at risk.

Q. What is Felty's syndrome? Enumerate the clinical manifestations and laboratory abnormalities of Felty's syndrome.

- Felty's syndrome refers to the constellation of neutropenia, splenomegaly and RA. It is considered an extra-articular manifestation of RA.
- It is seen in patients with long-standing (generally >10 years), chronic, seropositive RA. Most often, rheumatoid arthritis is present for several years before neutropenia and splenomegaly become apparent.
- RA in patients with Felty's syndrome is typically severe, with erosions and deformities and is more frequently associated with extra-articular manifestations than is RA without Felty's syndrome.
- It has a poor prognosis, with an increased mortality due to a higher incidence of severe infection. Respiratory tract and skin infections are the most common infections.
- Incidence of non-Hodgkin's lymphoma is also higher compared to other patients of RA.
- Features of Felty's syndrome are given in Box 9.2.

LABORATORY ABNORMALITIES

- Neutropenia <1500/mm^3, anaemia and thrombocytopenia.
- High titres of rheumatoid factor.
- Increased levels of circulating immune complexes (CIC).

BOX 9.2 Clinical Features of Felty's Syndrome (in Addition to Features of RA)

- Splenomegaly
- Skin pigmentation
- Weight loss
- Subcutaneous rheumatoid nodules
- Recurrent infections and chronic leg ulcers
- Lymphadenopathy
- Carpal tunnel syndrome
- Keratoconjunctivitis sicca
- Vasculitis resulting in mononeuritis multiplex and necrotising skin lesions
- Greater risk of developing non-Hodgkin's lymphoma

TREATMENT

- Treatment of underlying RA.
- Immunosuppressive agents, particularly methotrexate and azathioprine, are beneficial. Tumour necrosis factor inhibitors are avoided.
- In patients with life-threatening or refractory bacterial infection, G-CSF may be given to rapidly reverse neutropenia.
- Splenectomy is indicated in:
  - Recurrent or serious infections.
  - Severe leg ulcers.
  - Severe and persistent granulocytopenia (<500 mm^3), despite DMARD therapy for rheumatoid arthritis.
  - Severe anaemia due to hypersplenism.
  - Thrombocytopenia and haemorrhage due to hypersplenism.

Q. What is Still's disease?

- Still's disease, currently known as systemic juvenile idiopathic arthritis (sJIA) is systemic-onset, seronegative RA (JIA) occurring in children. Children with this illness comprise between 10% and 20% of all cases of JIA.
- Characteristically, the disease presents with high fever, arthralgia and arthritis, myalgia and also hepatosplenomegaly, lymphadenopathy, evanescent skin rashes, anaemia, leucocytosis and thrombocytosis. Pleurisy and pericarditis may occur.
- Fever is typically quotidian type, that is there is one spike of fever a day with normal temperature during the rest of the 24-hour period. Affected children are characteristically ill appearing when febrile but seem to improve dramatically when their temperature is normal.
- An evanescent, macular, salmon-pink rash is frequently present. The rash often fades as the temperature returns to normal, only to reappear with the next fever spike. The rash also may appear following stroking of the skin or other minor trauma—Koebner phenomenon.
- Approximately 10% of children develop overt clinical features of macrophage activation syndrome, a life-threatening condition characterised by fever, organomegaly, cytopenia, hyperferritinaemia, hypertriglyceridaemia, hypofibrinogenaemia and coagulopathy, The diagnostic hallmark is the presence on bone marrow examination of numerous, well-differentiated macrophages that are engaged actively in the phagocytosis of haematopoietic elements. Unlike Still's disease, these patients may have leucopenia, thrombocytopenia and very high levels of serum triglyceride.
- Tests for rheumatoid factor and antinuclear antibodies are negative but there is neutrophilia, thrombocytosis and elevated ESR.
- A work-up for fever of unknown origin is recommended prior to treatment to exclude infection, malignancy and other conditions.
- The disease has a good prognosis and most of the patients with mild to moderate disease respond to NSAIDs, steroids or DMARDs (particularly methotrexate). Biologicals like IL-1 and IL-6 inhibitors alone or with NSAIDs may be required for moderate to severe disease. Steroids may be added to biologicals for severe disease.

Q. Describe adult-onset Still's disease.

- It is a form of Still's disease that occurs in adults (older than 16 years) and is characterised by a triad of high spiking fever, a characteristic evanescent skin rash and arthritis/arthralgias.
- Fever is transient, lasting typically under 4 hours and is most commonly quotidian (once a day) or double quotidian (twice a day) in pattern.
- Rash is maculopapular, nonpruritic and predominantly found on the proximal limbs and trunk. It tends to occur during episodes of fever and disappear after fever subsides.
- Joints affected most frequently are the knees, wrists and ankles. Initially, arthritis may be mild, transient and oligoarticular. Some patients may develop severe and destructive polyarthritis.
- Other manifestations include lymphadenopathy, hepatomegaly, splenomegaly, pleuritis and pericarditis.
- Macrophage activation syndrome can occur in some patients.
- Investigations show anaemia, neutrophilic leucocytosis, thrombocytosis, raised ESR and CRP, and elevated liver enzymes.
- Ferritin levels are usually higher than those found in patients with other autoimmune or inflammatory diseases. A more useful marker is reduced level (<20%) of glycosylated fraction of ferritin.
- Course:
  - Self-limited or monocyclic pattern characterised by remission within 1 year from the onset.
  - Intermittent or polycyclic pattern with recurrent flares, with or without articular symptomatology.
  - Chronic articular pattern with dominant articular manifestations that can lead to joint destruction.
- Treatment is with NSAIDs and steroids. DMARDs (biological and nonbiological) may be used in refractory or severe cases or when prednisolone dose cannot be tapered to below 10 mg/day.

Q. Discuss briefly juvenile idiopathic arthritis or juvenile rheumatoid arthritis or juvenile chronic arthritis and its treatment.

- Criteria for diagnosis of juvenile idiopathic arthritis (JIA) include age of onset less than 16 years, disease duration greater than 6 weeks, arthritis and exclusion of other forms of juvenile arthritis.
- The terms juvenile rheumatoid arthritis (JRA) and juvenile chronic arthritis (JCA) are not used at present.
- JIA is subdivided into the following types:
  - Polyarticular JIA affects more than four joints during the first 6 months of disease and is more

common in young females than in young males. Symptoms include swelling or pain in five or more joints. The small joints of the hands are affected as well as the weight-bearing joints such as the knees, hips, ankles, feet and neck. In addition, the child may have low-grade fever and nodules over bony prominence. Based on the presence or absence of rheumatoid factor, it is termed polyarticular JIA, RF^+ or polyarticular JIA, RF^-.

- Oligoarticular or pauciarticular JIA affects fewer than five joints during the first 6 months of disease. Symptoms include pain, stiffness or swelling of affected joints. Knee and wrist joints are the most commonly affected. Eye involvement in the form of iridocyclitis can occur. These patients are more often antinuclear antibody (ANA)-positive compared to other categories. Oligoarticular or pauciarticular JIA is divided into persistent and extended based on whether the arthritis remains localised to <5 joints or not during the course of disease.
- Still's disease or systemic JIA presents with evanescent skin rash and fever in addition to arthritis. It may involve internal organs (e.g. splenomegaly, hepatomegaly, pericarditis, pleural effusion).
- Enthesitis-related JIA presents with asymmetric joint involvement of lower limbs with enthesitis (tenderness at the insertion of a tendon, ligament, joint capsule or fascia to the bone). Sacroiliitis with pain is often present. Eye involvement can occur. HLA-B27 is positive in majority. History of ankylosing spondylitis, enthesitis-related arthritis, sacroiliitis with inflammatory bowel disease or acute anterior uveitis in a first-degree relative often present.
- Psoriatic JIA presents with symmetrical or asymmetrical arthritis and psoriasis along with dactylitis, nail pitting, onycholysis or psoriasis in a first-degree relative.
- Undifferentiated arthritis presents with features that do not match any of the above-mentioned criteria to be included in a single subset of patients.

TREATMENT

- For oligoarticular JIA, intraarticular injections of steroids and appropriate use of NSAIDs (naproxen, meloxicam, celecoxib and ibuprofen) are the mainstay of treatment. Disease-modifying antirheumatic drugs (DMARDs) are generally not recommended for this group, although, occasionally, methotrexate may be used in difficult-to-control uveitis or when damage to a critical joint threatens function (e.g. shoulder, wrist and hip). Sulphasalazine and leflunomide are alternate DMARDs available if the child has contraindications or intolerance to methotrexate.
- For polyarticular JIA, treatment is similar to that for RA.
- For systemic JIA, NSAIDs and corticosteroids are indicated. Methotrexate and TNF inhibitors are not very effective. Biological agents which inhibit IL-1 (anakinra, canakinumab) or IL-6 (tocilizumab, sarilumab) are recommended as glucocorticoid-sparing therapies.

Q. What are the pleuropulmonary manifestations of rheumatoid arthritis?

- Pleuropulmonary manifestations of rheumatoid arthritis are the extra-articular features. These include the following entities:
  - Pleural effusion with a characteristically low pleural fluid glucose level (<10 mg/dL).
  - Interstitial lung disease—fibrosing alveolitis.
  - Rheumatoid nodules manifesting as solitary pulmonary nodules.
  - Cavitated rheumatoid nodules.
  - Bronchiolitis obliterans organising pneumonia (also known as cryptogenic organising pneumonia).
  - Granulomatous pneumonitis.
  - Pulmonary arteritis (vasculitis) resulting in infarction.
  - Caplan's syndrome—coexistence of seropositive RA and rounded, fibrotic, peripherally located pulmonary nodules of 0.5–5 cm diameter in patients with coal worker's pneumoconiosis (CWP).

Q. Discuss the classification, clinical manifestations, diagnosis and management of Sjögren's syndrome.

Q. Describe keratoconjunctivitis sicca.

- Sjögren's syndrome is an immunological disorder characterised by progressive destruction of exocrine glands leading to mucosal and conjunctival dryness. A diagnosis of Sjögren's syndrome is made when there is a triad of keratoconjunctivitis sicca, xerostomia and mononuclear cell infiltration of salivary gland.

CLASSIFICATION

- Classification and types of Sjogren's syndrome are given in Table 9.6.

TABLE 9.6 Classification and Types of Sjögren's Syndrome

• Primary (sicca syndrome)	The disease occurs by itself in the absence of any connective tissue disorder or in association with organ-specific autoimmune diseases such as thyroiditis, primary biliary cirrhosis or cholangitis
• Secondary	The disease is accompanied by a variety of systemic autoimmune disorders. These include RA, SLE, progressive systemic sclerosis or polymyositis
• Glandular type	The only clinical manifestations are within the exocrine system
• Extraglandular type	Other tissues are also involved

INCIDENCE

- The disease occurs in third to fourth decades and predominantly affects females.
- The two main mechanisms of tissue destruction in Sjögren's syndrome are lymphocytic infiltration and immune-complex deposition.

CLINICAL FEATURES

- Xerophthalmia encompasses itching and grittiness and may be associated with soreness, photosensitivity, ocular fatigue and reduced visual acuity. Diminished tear secretion may lead to chronic irritation and destruction of conjunctival epithelia (keratoconjunctivitis sicca). Complications include corneal ulceration and infection of the eyelids.
- Xerostomia is dryness of mouth resulting from lack of salivary secretion. This leads to increased local bacterial and fungal infections and dental caries.
- Xerosis (dryness of skin).
- Enlargement of the parotid or other major salivary glands occur in 65% of patients with primary Sjögren's syndrome but is uncommon in secondary Sjögren's syndrome.
- Mikulicz syndrome is characterised by prominent parotid and lacrimal glandular enlargement. It may result from Sjogren syndrome as well as other conditions
- Fatigue is common and seen in 70% cases.
- Renal involvement occurs in the form of interstitial nephritis or glomerulonephritis. Interstitial nephritis may lead to renal tubular acidosis (both type 1 and 2).
- Arthralgias are commonly seen while nonerosive arthritis is less frequent.
- Cutaneous and systemic vasculitis.
- Nasal crusting, epistaxis, recurrent sinusitis, dry cough and dyspnoea occur due to dry nose, dry trachea, small airway obstruction and/or interstitial lung disease.
- Polyneuropathies or mononeuritis multiplex.
- Approximately 10% of these patients develop a lymphoproliferative process that may go on to develop a non-Hodgkin's lymphoma. Salivary glands are the most common site of involvement. Persistent parotid gland enlargement, lymphadenopathy, lymphopenia and cryoglobulinaemia are manifestations suggesting the development of lymphoma.
- Hashimoto's thyroiditis is a common accompaniment of Sjögren's syndrome.

LABORATORY INVESTIGATIONS

- Common laboratory abnormalities are raised ESR, leucopenia, thrombocytosis, elevated levels of circulating immune complexes and autoantibodies (antibodies to Ro/SSA or La/SSB, ANA or RF). Anti-Ro (SSA) is the most specific antibody.
- Schirmer's test is positive. A folded test strip of sterile filter paper is placed over the margin of each lower eyelid at the junction of the middle and lateral thirds. The extent of wetting is measured over 5 minutes with the patient's eyes gently closed. Wetting <5 mm without anaesthesia is indicative of aqueous tear deficiency.
- Rose Bengal test evaluates damage to corneal epithelium.
- Measurement of salivary flow by salivary sialometry.
- Salivary gland involvement by salivary scintigraphy.
- High-frequency ultrasound and MRI can be used to define characteristic changes in the salivary gland parenchyma.
- Histopathology of minor (labial) salivary glands.

TREATMENT

- Ocular and mucosal lubricants like artificial tears, ophthalmological lubricating ointments, lubricating agents for dryness of mouth, nasal sprays of normal saline and moisturising skin lotions.
- Cyclosporin emulsion useful in ocular dryness.
- Muscarinic agonists (pilocarpine and cevimeline) approved for the treatment of the sicca symptoms. These agents stimulate the M1 and M3 receptors present on salivary glands and tear glands leading to increased secretory function.
- Hydroxychloroquine is helpful for arthralgias.
- Corticosteroids are useful particularly in the management of glomerulonephritis and interstitial lung disease. Immunosuppressives (cyclophosphamide and mycophenolate mofetil) may be added for treatment of ILD.
- Immunosuppressive therapy (cyclosporin A, azathioprine, methotrexate and mycophenolic acid) is indicated for systemic vasculitis.
- Few studies are available on the use of biological agents in the treatment of Sjögren's syndrome.

Q. What are spondyloarthropathies? (IM 7.6)

Q. What are seronegative spondyloarthropathies (SSA)?

- Also known as spondyloarthritides.
- Diverse group of inflammatory arthritides that share genetic predisposing factors and clinical features (inflammatory back pain due to sacroiliitis and spondylitis, peripheral arthritis, enthesitis—inflammation at sites where tendons, ligaments or joint capsules attach to bone, dactylitis and acute anterior uveitis).
- Associated with HLA-B27.
- Rheumatoid factor negative, therefore known as 'seronegative'.

CLINICAL CRITERIA FOR INFLAMMATORY BACK PAIN

- Clinical criteria for inflammatory back pain are given in Box 9.3.

BOX 9.3 Clinical Criteria for Inflammatory Back Pain

- Onset before age of 45 years
- Insidious onset
- Improvement with exercise
- No improvement with rest
- Morning stiffness >30 minutes
- Persistence (for at least 3 months)
- Awaking from pain, especially during second half of night, with improvement on arising
- Alternating buttock pain

Note: Coexistence of four or more criteria allows the definition of inflammatory back pain.

DIFFERENTIATING INFLAMMATORY FROM MECHANICAL BACK PAIN

- Table 9.7 gives differentiating features between inflammatory and mechanical back pain.

CLASSIFICATION OF SPONDYLOARTHROPATHIES

- Spondyloarthropathies can be divided into two subgroups: axial and peripheral (asymmetrical arthritis, generally in the lower limbs) according to the predominant location of arthritis; however, both may occur.
- Classification of spondyloarthropathies is given in Box 9.4.

FEATURES

- Features of spondyloarthropathies are given in Box 9.5.

DIAGNOSIS

- No specific diagnostic tests:
  - Raised ESR, CRP and anaemia.
  - Sacroiliitis or spondylitis on radiographs.
  - Ultrasound for enthesitis.
  - MRI more sensitive in diagnosing early sacroiliitis.

BOX 9.4 Classification of Spondyloarthropathies

- Radiographic axial spondyloarthropathy (ankylosing spondylitis)
- Nonradiographic axial spondyloarthropathy
- Reactive arthritis (infection-associated arthritis)
- Psoriatic spondyloarthritis—predominantly peripheral or predominantly axial
- Enteropathic spondyloarthritis (associated with inflammatory bowel disease)—predominantly peripheral or predominantly axial
- Juvenile-onset spondyloarthritis (enthesitis-related juvenile idiopathic arthritis)
- Peripheral spondyloarthropathy (lower limb, asymmetrical arthritis, dactylitis, enthesitis)
- Undifferentiated spondyloarthritis

BOX 9.5 Features of Seronegative Spondyloarthropathies

- Inflammatory spinal pain or synovitis predominantly involving lower limbs in an asymmetric fashion with one or more of the following:
  - Radiographic sacroiliitis with or without accompanying spondylitis
  - Enthesitis and dactylitis
  - Association with chronic inflammatory bowel disease
  - Association with psoriasis and other mucocutaneous lesions
  - Urethritis or cervicitis or acute diarrhoea occurring within 1 month before arthritis
  - Tendency for anterior ocular inflammation
  - Increased familial incidence
  - Occasional aortitis and heart block
  - No association with rheumatoid factor
  - Strong association with HLA-B27

Q. Explain ankylosing spondylitis, rheumatoid spondylitis or Marie–Strumpell disease.

- Ankylosing spondylitis is a seronegative chronic inflammatory arthritis that primarily affects the axial skeleton with a predilection for lumbar spine and sacroiliac joints.
- Ninety per cent of the affected people carry the histocompatibility antigen HLA-B27.
- It is also associated with inflammatory bowel disease.

TABLE 9.7 Features Differentiating Inflammatory From Mechanical Back Pain

Feature	Inflammatory Back Pain	Mechanical Back Pain
Usual age of onset	<45 years	Any but most often >45 years
Onset	Insidious	Acute to insidious
Chronicity	>3 months	Variable
Awakening during night due to pain	Yes	May or may not occur
Morning stiffness	Yes, >30 minutes	None to mild
Effect of physical activity	Improves	Worsens
Location and characteristics of pain	Low back pain common but may affect any area of the spine; may cause alternating buttock pain; does not radiate into legs; does not cause numbness, burning or tingling	Anywhere in spine; may radiate into legs; may cause numbness, burning or tingling
ESR and CRP	Elevated	Normal
Response to NSAIDs	Good	Variable

- The disease usually occurs in the second and third decades with a male to female ratio of 3:1.

CLINICAL FEATURES

- Involvement of the lumbar spine results in low back pain with nocturnal exacerbations. Characteristically, this is associated with low-back morning stiffness that improves with activity. Low-back stiffness may be precipitated by inactivity. Early physical signs include failure to obliterate the lumbar lordosis on forward flexion and restriction of the movements of lumbar spine in all directions. The limitation of forward flexion of lumbar spine can be measured by the Schober's test:
  - Mark points on the spine 5 cm below and 10 cm above the posterior superior iliac spines.
  - Ask the patient to bend forward maximally.
  - The distance between the two marks should increase by 5 cm or more in normal persons. An increase of less than 5 cm suggests decreased range of motion of the lumbar spine.
- Involvement of the sacroiliac joints causes low back pain. Pain in the sacroiliac joints may be elicited either by direct pressure or by manoeuvres that stress the joint, for example 'Figure of 4 test' (Patrick's test) (Fig. 9.3).
  - One limb is guided into 'Figure of 4' position with the ipsilateral ankle resting across the contralateral thigh.
  - The ipsilateral knee is then pressed downwards with one hand, while providing counterpressure with the other hand on the contralateral anterior superior iliac spine.
  - This manoeuvre tends to stress the sacroiliac joint on the side being tested.
- Enthesitis is common. Inflammation at the Achilles tendon and plantar fascia calcaneal insertions is particularly common and manifests as heel pain. Like arthritis, enthesitis typically is aggravated by rest and improved with activity. Other areas of enthesitis include superior and inferior aspects of patella, metatarsal heads and spinal ligament insertions on vertebral bodies.
- Involvement of the thoracic spine, costovertebral joints and costosternal joints results in chest pain, diminished chest expansion (<5 cm) and thoracic kyphosis.

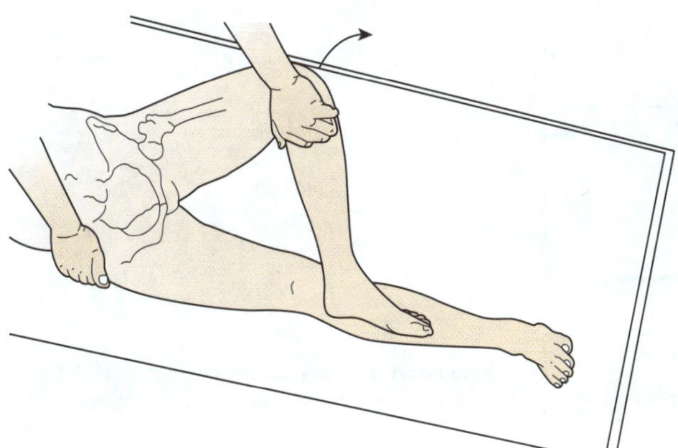

Fig. 9.3 Figure of 4 test (Patrick's test).

- Involvement of the cervical spine results in neck pain and a forward stoop of the neck.
- Peripheral arthritis is usually late and asymmetric. Involvement of hips and shoulders results in pain and limitation of movement. Hip involvement may lead to flexion contractures, compensated by flexion at knees.

EXTRA-ARTICULAR MANIFESTATIONS

- Extra-articular manifestations of ankylosing spondylitis are given in Box 9.6.

INVESTIGATIONS

- Erythrocyte sedimentation rate (ESR) is raised. Tests for rheumatoid factor (RF) are negative.
- HLA-B27 is present in >90% cases.
- MRI and bone scan can pick up early sacroiliitis.
- Ultrasonography can be useful in detecting enthesitis.

RADIOLOGICAL MANIFESTATIONS (Box 9.7)

DIAGNOSTIC CRITERIA

- Ankylosing spondylitis can be diagnosed based on the criteria given in Box 9.8 or shown in Flowchart 9.2.

MANAGEMENT

- Regular exercises, active and passive physiotherapy.
- Symptomatic relief can be obtained with NSAIDs. Indomethacin is the most effective drug. It may be given up to a maximum daily dose of 100 mg.
- Sulphasalazine and methotrexate are useful to control peripheral joint symptoms but not for axial symptoms.

BOX 9.6 Extra-Articular Manifestations of Ankylosing Spondylitis

- Acute anterior uveitis
- Iritis
- Aortic regurgitation and heart failure
- Cardiac conduction defects
- Apical pulmonary fibrosis and cavitation
- Osteoporosis
- Myelopathy secondary to atlanto-axial subluxation and spinal fracture
- Cauda equina syndrome
- Amyloidosis

BOX 9.7 Radiological Manifestations of Ankylosing Spondylitis

- Blurring of sacroiliac joint margins followed by erosions and sclerosis
- Erosion and sclerosis at the anterior corners of vertebrae
- Syndesmophyte (ossification of annulus fibrosus) formation, marginal
- 'Squaring' of lumbar vertebrae (due to enthesitis involving spine)
- Bamboo spine (multiple syndesmophytes bridging the intervertebral spaces) (Fig. 9.4)
- Diffuse osteoporosis of spine
- Atlanto-axial subluxation and vertebral fractures
- Erosive changes in symphysis pubis, ischial tuberosities and peripheral joints

BOX 9.8 Modified New York Criteria (1984)

RADIOLOGICAL CRITERIA

- Sacroiliitis, grade ≥2 bilaterally

Or

- Sacroiliitis, from grades 3 to 4 unilaterally

CLINICAL CRITERIA (TWO OF THE FOLLOWING THREE)

- Low back pain and stiffness for more than 3 months that improves with exercise but is not relieved by rest
- Limitation of motion of the lumbar spine in both the sagittal and frontal planes
- Limitation of chest expansion relative to normal values correlated for age and sex

Grade 2, sclerosis with some erosions; Grade 3, severe erosions, partial ankylosis; Grade 4, complete ankylosis.

- Local corticosteroid injections into peripheral joints, sacroiliac joints or entheses could provide immediate symptom; rarely systemic corticosteroids may be necessary.

ANTI-TNF-α AGENTS

- Infliximab, etanercept, golimumab, adalimumab and certolizumab are options for the treatment of patients with active ankylosing spondylitis who are not satisfactorily responding to NSAIDs. Duration of treatment is 2–3 years. These agents are useful for axial joint involvement not responding to adequate doses of NSAIDs given for 3 months. Also useful in peripheral arthritis not responding to sulphasalazine for 4 months.
  - Infliximab—5 mg/kg intravenously every 6–8 weeks.
  - Etanercept—25 mg subcutaneously twice a week initially.
  - Both these agents are also approved for RA, psoriasis, psoriatic arthritis and JIA.
  - In addition, infliximab also approved for Crohn's disease.
  - Contraindicated in pregnant patients, patients with active infection, SLE or multiple sclerosis.
  - Monitor patient for development of tuberculosis.

ANTI-INTERLEUKIN-17 AGENT

- Secukinumab.

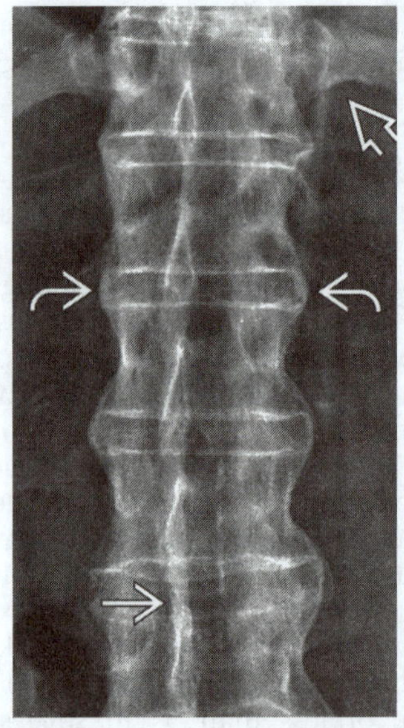

Fig. 9.4 AP radiograph shows the bamboo spine typical of advanced ankylosing spondylitis (AS), where ossification of the outer fibres of the annulus fibrosus mimics the joints of the bamboo plant.

OTHERS

- Rituximab and tofacitinib (a JAK-inhibitor) if anti-TNF-α agents are not effective.
- Reconstructive surgery including spinal corrective osteotomy, hip replacement.
- Control of uveitis by local steroid drugs.

Q. Write a short note on Reiter's syndrome.

Q. Discuss the clinical features, diagnosis and management of reactive arthritis.

- Classical Reiter's syndrome is a triad of nonspecific urethritis in males or cervicitis in females, conjunctivitis and arthritis 2–4 weeks following enteric or urogenital infections. However, this term is not used at present and is replaced by the term 'reactive arthritis'.

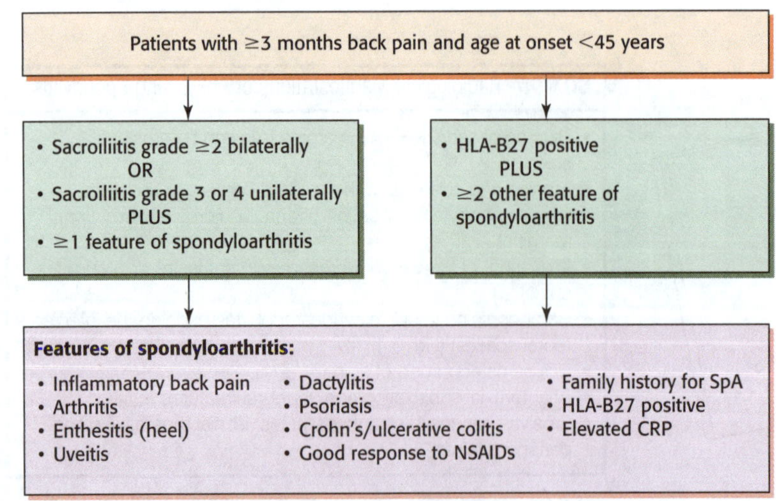

Flowchart 9.2 Assessment of Spondyloarthritis International Society (ASAS) Criteria. (*Source:* The Assessment of Spondyloarthritis international Society (ASAS) handbook: a guide to assess spondyloarthritis: J Sieper, M Rudwaleit, X Baraliakos, et al. *Ann Rheum Dis* 2009; 68 (Suppl II): Box4, ii3.)

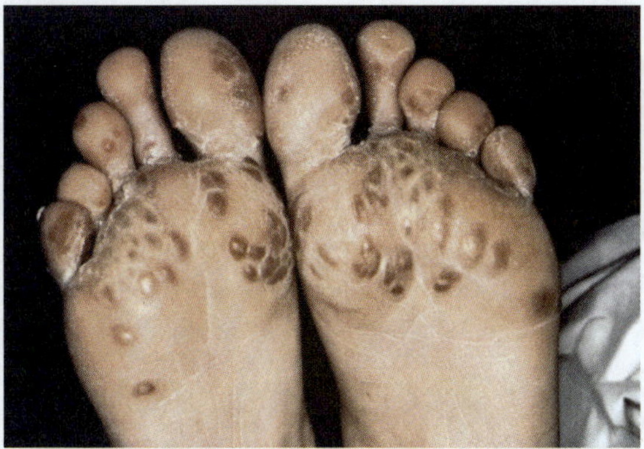

Fig. 9.5 Keratoderma blennorrhagica. (Courtesy of Dr. M.F. Rein and Centers for Disease Control and Prevention Public Health Image Library, 1976. Image #6950.)

- The term 'reactive arthritis' includes a case of spondyloarthropathy which arises following an infection, although the pathogens cannot be cultured from the affected joints.
- Poncet's disease is a reactive arthritis to tuberculous infection. Resolution of arthritis on starting of adequate antituberculous therapy is mostly within a few weeks. Chronic arthritis does not occur.
- More than 75% of the patients have the histocompatibility antigen HLA-B27.
- Common enteric pathogens triggering the disease are *Shigella*, *Salmonella*, *Yersinia* and *Campylobacter* species, and *Clostridioides* (formerly *Clostridium*) *difficile*.
- Common urogenital pathogens are *Chlamydia trachomatis*, *Neisseria gonorrhoeae* and *Streptococcus pyogenes*.
- However, a similar spectrum of clinical manifestations can occur after infection with other organisms at other sites also.

CLINICAL FEATURES

- The clinical symptoms of reactive arthritis usually develop with a delay of 1–3 weeks after onset of infection.
- Onset of arthritis is typically acute, particularly affecting joints of lower limbs in an asymmetrical fashion. Arthritis is generally oligoarticular with involvement of <5 joints.
- Enthesitis and dactylitis (inflammation of entire digit including joints, tendons and surrounding connective tissue) are very common.
- Keratoderma blennorrhagica—hyperkeratotic lesions on the palms of the hands or the soles of the feet—may be seen (Fig. 9.5).
- Circinate balanitis—a painless erythematous lesion of the glans penis.
- Usually a self-limiting course of 3–12 months.
- Up to 50% of patients have recurrent bouts of arthritis and 15%–30% develop chronic arthritis or sacroiliitis.
- Clinical features of reactive arthritis are given in Table 9.8.

TABLE 9.8 Clinical Features of Reactive Arthritis

• Constitutional	Fatigue, malaise, fever, weight loss
• Musculoskeletal	Arthritis (particularly affecting joints of the lower limbs), sacroiliitis, dactylitis or 'sausage digit' (diffuse swelling of a finger), Achilles tendonitis, plantar fasciitis
• Urogenital	Urethritis, acute haemorrhagic cystitis, prostatitis, cervicitis, salpingitis
• Ocular	Conjunctivitis, anterior uveitis, acute iritis
• Mucocutaneous	Keratoderma blennorrhagica, circinate balanitis, nail dystrophy, heaped-up hyperkeratosis
• Others	Aortic regurgitation, conduction defects, central or peripheral nervous system involvement, pericarditis, pleurisy

INVESTIGATIONS

- Raised erythrocyte sedimentation rate (ESR).
- Anaemia and polymorphonuclear leucocytosis.
- Characteristic synovial fluid findings (more than 2000 white blood cells/mL with a predominance of neutrophils).
- HLA-B27 is positive in more than 75% of cases.
- Serum tests for rheumatoid factor and antinuclear antibodies are negative.

RADIOLOGICAL FEATURES

- Juxta-articular osteoporosis.
- Erosive changes and reduction in joint space.
- Periostitis with reactive new bone formation due to enthesitis.
- Spurs at the insertion of the plantar fascia.
- Sacroiliitis (less common than ankylosing spondylitis).
- Discontinuous spondylitis with nonmarginal syndesmophytes.

MANAGEMENT

- Rest and NSAIDs (naproxen, indomethacin, diclofenac).
- Intraarticular or local steroid injections and rarely systemic steroids.
- Nonspecific urethritis is treated with a short course of tetracycline or ciprofloxacin. In patients with acute *Chlamydia*, induced reactive arthritis, a prolonged course of antibiotics (from 4 to 12 weeks), either tetracycline or ciprofloxacin, should be given.
- No role of antibiotics in reactive spondyloarthropathy secondary to enteric infections.
- Sulphasalazine, azathioprine and methotrexate may be useful in patients with persistent symptoms.
- Biologicals like infliximab, etanercept and adalimumab in refractory cases.

Q. What are the types of psoriatic arthritis? Discuss briefly the clinical manifestations, diagnosis and management of psoriatic arthritis.

- Psoriatic arthritis is a seronegative arthritis found in patients with psoriasis, a past or family history of psoriasis or characteristic nail changes.
- Occurs in about 20% of patients with psoriasis.
- Arthritis appears after the onset of skin lesions in the majority of patients. However, it can precede the skin disease in approximately 15% of patients while in another 15%, both skin lesions and arthritis occur at the same time.

BOX 9.9 Types of Psoriatic Arthritis

- Symmetric psoriatic arthritis
- Asymmetric psoriatic arthritis
- Arthritis mutilans
- Psoriatic spondyloarthritis
- Predominant distal interphalangeal arthritis

TYPES

- Various types of psoriatic arthritis are given in Box 9.9.

CLINICAL FEATURES

- The most common form (asymmetric arthritis) is characterised by frequent involvement of proximal and distal interphalangeal joints with characteristic 'sausage-shaped' digits (dactylitis—inflammatory involvement of tendons and tendon sheaths leading to swelling of affected fingers or toes). Usually, less than four joints are involved.
- Symmetric arthritis affects joints on both sides simultaneously and presents like rheumatoid arthritis (RA).
- Spondylitis form is characterised by stiffness of the lower spine or cervical spine. Joints of hands and feet can also be affected. Sacroiliitis, often asymmetrical, occurs in about 40% of patients.
- Distal interphalangeal psoriatic arthritis is characterised by inflammation and stiffness of distal interphalangeal joints of hands and feet. Nail changes are often marked in this type of arthritis.
- Arthritis mutilans is a severe, deforming and destructive arthritis that can progress over months or years causing severe joint damage.
- Enthesitis is common.
- Characteristic skin lesions of psoriasis may be present. These are widespread scaling silvery lesions, seen typically over extensor surfaces, scalp, ears and perineum. In the majority of cases, skin manifestations precede joint involvement, although the reverse occurs in 15%–20% of cases.
- Characteristic nail changes of psoriasis are pitting, onycholysis, subungual hyperkeratosis and horizontal ridging. These are present in nearly 80% of patients with arthritis.
- Uveitis, unilateral or bilateral and generally chronic.

DIAGNOSIS

- Raised ESR and negative tests for rheumatoid factor and antinuclear antibodies.
- Radiological findings are similar to those of RA but osteoporosis is relatively less common. Radiographs of distal interphalangeal joints may show 'pencil-in-cup' changes because of marked resorption of bone (Fig. 9.6). Other findings include enthesitis with periosteal reaction, sacroiliitis and spondylitis.

PSORIATIC ARTHRITIS VERSUS RHEUMATOID ARTHRITIS

- Clinical features are important to differentiate seronegative (rheumatoid factor-negative) RA with coincidental psoriasis from patients with peripheral psoriatic arthritis. Important features favouring diagnosis of psoriatic arthritis include the following:
  - Presence of nail psoriasis.
  - Absence of features characteristic of RA (e.g. rheumatoid nodules, extra-articular involvement and high titres of rheumatoid factor).
  - Involved joints are usually less tender and swollen and less symmetric in distribution than in RA.
  - Dactylitis, enthesitis and distal interphalangeal joint involvement are common.
  - Sacroiliitis and spondylitis common.

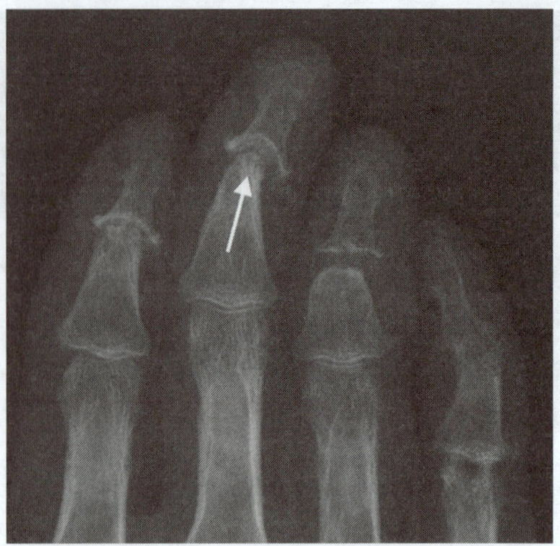

Fig. 9.6 Radiograph showing 'Pencil-in-cup' deformity.

MANAGEMENT

- Majority of the patients respond to NSAIDs.
- Other modalities of treatment include sulphasalazine, methotrexate, cyclosporin, photochemotherapy and intraarticular steroid injections.
- Anti-TNF-α agents (infliximab, etanercept, adalimumab, golimumab and certolizumab) and IL-17 inhibitor (secukinumab) in severe cases. JAK inhibitor, tofacitinib, is also approved.

Q. Discuss briefly about spondyloarthropathy associated with inflammatory bowel disease.

- Also known as enteropathic spondyloarthropathy.
- Occurs in about 20% of patients who have inflammatory bowel disease (IBD).
- Occurs more often in patients with Crohn's disease than in those with ulcerative colitis.
- May manifest before clinically apparent bowel disease.

CLINICAL FEATURES

PERIPHERAL ARTHRITIS

- Type 1 involves less than five joints and is clinically characterised by acute self-limiting attacks of less than 10-week duration, often paralleling intestinal inflammatory activity. Moreover, it is strongly associated with other extraintestinal manifestations of IBD such as erythema nodosum.

- Type 2 is polyarticular, involving five or more joints with symptoms that persist for months and years running independently from IBD flares. Metacarpophalangeal joints are most often involved. Approximately one-half of the patients have migratory arthritis. This type is associated with uveitis but not with other extraintestinal manifestations.
- At present, both are considered to be peripheral arthritis without any further differentiation.
- Both types are usually nonerosive and nondeforming but may become chronic and erosive in 10% of patients.
- No significant association between peripheral arthropathies and HLA-B27 in IBD.

INFLAMMATORY BACK PAIN

- Insidious in onset, frequently unilateral and intermittent at onset, more intense at rest, associated with stiffness but relieved by movement, exacerbated by cough or sneezing and accompanied by fatigue.
- May manifest as spondylitis indistinguishable from ankylosing spondylitis.
- Axial disease (spondylitis disease) is generally independent of IBD activity.
- May be associated with peripheral arthritis.
- Strongly associated with HLA-B27.

OTHERS

- Enthesitis.
- Dactylitis.
- Uveitis.
- Extra-articular manifestations of IBD.

TREATMENT

- NSAIDs to be used cautiously because they can exacerbate IBD. However, they still form the first-line treatment for IBD-associated spondyloarthropathy.
- Local joint injections of glucocorticoids for oligoarticular involvement.
- Sulphasalazine effective in the treatment of IBD and arthritis.
- Azathioprine and methotrexate may also be useful.
- Anti-TNF-α inhibitors beneficial in axial involvement. Also required in patients with peripheral joint involvement resistant to sulphasalazine and methotrexate.

Q. Describe undifferentiated spondyloarthropathy.

- This entity indicates involvement of spine and joints producing typical features of spondyloarthropathy but without any criteria for any of the well-defined spondyloarthropathies (discussed above).
- Over time, a small proportion of these patients develop a well-defined spondyloarthropathy.
- Clinical features include inflammatory back pain, unilateral or alternating buttock pain, enthesitis, dactylitis and occasionally extra-articular manifestations.
- Generally good prognosis with good response to NSAIDs.

Q. How will you differentiate various spondyloarthropathies?

- Differentiating points among various types of spondyloarthropathies are given in Table 9.9.

TABLE 9.9 Differentiation Among Various Types of Spondyloarthropathies

Feature	Ankylosing Spondylitis	Reactive Arthritis	Psoriatic Arthritis	IBD-associated Spondyloarthropathies
• Age at onset	Late teens to early adulthood	Late teens to early adulthood	35–45 years	Any age
• Male to female ratio	3:1	3:1	1:1	2:1
• HLA-B27 positive	90%	80%	40%	30%
• Frequency of sacroiliitis	100%	40%–60%	40%	20%
• Distribution of sacroiliitis	Symmetrical	Asymmetrical	Asymmetrical	Symmetrical
• Syndesmophytes	Marginal	Nonmarginal	Nonmarginal	Marginal
• Enthesitis	Common	Very common	Very common	Occasional
• Dactylitis	Uncommon	Common	Common	Uncommon
• Skin changes	None	Circinate balanitis, keratoderma blennorrhagica	Psoriatic lesions	Erythema nodosum, pyoderma gangrenosum
• Nail changes	None	Onycholysis	Pitting, onycholysis	Clubbing
• Uveitis	Acute	Acute	Chronic	Chronic
• Pulmonary involvement	Upper lobe fibrosis	None	None	None
• GI involvement	None	Diarrhoea	None	Features of associated Crohn's disease or ulcerative colitis
• Genitourinary involvement	None	Urethritis, cervicitis	None	None
• Cardiac involvement	Aortic regurgitation, conduction defects	Aortic regurgitation, conduction defects	Aortic regurgitation, conduction defects	Aortic regurgitation

Q. Discuss briefly symptoms, diagnosis and treatment of Behcet's disease.

- Behcet's disease is characterised by recurrent oral and genital ulcerations, uveitis and arthritis.
- This is an autoimmune disease with circulating autoantibodies to human oral mucous membrane and immune complexes seen in 50% of the cases.

CRITERIA FOR DIAGNOSIS

- Diagnostic criteria for Behcet's disease are given in Box 9.10.

CLINICAL FEATURES

MUCOCUTANEOUS LESIONS

- Painful oral ulcers on tongue, pharynx, buccal and labial mucosal membranes. Typical lesion is round with a sharp, erythematous and elevated border, mostly 2–30 mm in diameter.
- Genital ulcers occur in 60%–65% of cases and are painful. In men, they are localised on the scrotum, less frequently on the penis or in the urethra and in women on the vulva and vagina.
- Ulcers can also occur in the oesophagus, stomach and small intestine and can lead to perforation.
- Erythema nodosum.
- Behcet's pustulosis is a vasculitis characterised by a dome-shaped sterile pustule on an erythematous-oedematous base. Seen mostly on lower limbs and pubic area.

OCULAR INVOLVEMENT

- Often bilateral.
- Anterior uveitis, cataract, glaucoma, posterior uveitis, retinitis, venous or arterial occlusion.

VASCULAR MANIFESTATIONS

- Vasculitis.
- Venous thrombophlebitis.
- Arterial thrombosis.

ARTICULAR MANIFESTATIONS

- Nondeforming arthralgia and/or arthritis occur in 45% of cases.
- Knees and ankles are most involved, although smaller joints may also be affected.
- X-ray is generally normal.

NEUROLOGICAL MANIFESTATIONS

- Cerebral venous thrombosis or arterial aneurysm.
- Meningitis or meningoencephalitis, seizures, haemiplegia and cranial nerve palsies.

BOX 9.10 Diagnostic Criteria for Behcet's Disease

IN THE ABSENCE OF OTHER CLINICAL EXPLANATIONS, PATIENTS MUST HAVE:

1. Recurrent oral ulceration (aphthous or herpetiform) observed by the physician or patient recurring at least three times in a 12-month period

AND TWO OF THE FOLLOWING:

1. Recurrent painful genital ulceration
2. Eye lesions: anterior uveitis, posterior uveitis, cells in the vitreous by slit lamp examination or retinal vasculitis observed by an ophthalmologist
3. Skin lesions: erythema nodosum, papulopustular lesions (Behcet's pustulosis)
4. Pathergy, read by a physician at 24–48 hours

DIAGNOSIS

- Based on clinical features.
- Pathergy test:
  - A hypersensitivity phenomenon of skin to trauma.
  - The forearm is pricked with a small and sterile needle.
  - Occurrence of a small erythematous nodule or pustule at the site of needle insertion 1–2 days after the test indicates a positive test.
  - Although a positive pathergy test is helpful in the diagnosis of Behcet's disease, only about 50% of Behcet's patients demonstrate the pathergy phenomenon.

TREATMENT

- For mucocutaneous manifestations, local steroids and oral colchicine are used. If not effective, levamisole, dapsone or thalidomide can be tried.
- Apremilast, an oral phosphodiesterase-4 inhibitor is second-line agent for oral ulcers
- For joint manifestations, NSAIDs are sufficient. If no response occurs, methotrexate, sulphasalazine and low-dose prednisolone may be given.
- Aspirin is given for thrombophlebitis. Glucocorticoids and immunosuppressive agents (azathioprine, cyclophosphamide or cyclosporine A) are recommended for the management of acute deep venous thrombosis.
- Systemic steroids along with cytotoxic drugs (methotrexate, azathioprine, chlorambucil, cyclosporin A or cyclophosphamide) for uveitis.
- Same combination for central nervous system involvement except that cyclosporin is contraindicated. Cyclophosphamide pulses are recommended as first-line treatment for CNS vasculitis.
- Biologics such as infliximab and adalimumab in refractory cases.

Q. What is Henoch–Schönlein purpura?

Q. Explain anaphylactoid purpura or immunoglobulin A vasculitis.

- Current term for Henoch–Schönlein purpura and anaphylactoid purpura is immunoglobulin A vasculitis (IgA vasculitis).
- Most common form of systemic small vessel vasculitis usually seen in children which most often is self-limiting.

FEATURES

- The characteristic features are vasculitic purpura, abdominal pain, haematuria and acute arthritis.

- The purpuric lesions (nonthrombocytopenic purpura; palpable purpura) are palpable and found typically over buttocks and lower legs. These are almost always present on lateral malleolus.
- Recurrent colicky abdominal pain is common. In some cases, this results from intussusception. This may be associated with nausea, vomiting, diarrhoea and passage of blood and mucus per rectum.
- Arthralgia or arthritis commonly affects the knees and ankles but resolves without permanent damage to joints.
- Glomerulonephritis results in haematuria and red cell casts in urine. The proportion of those progressing to renal failure or end-stage renal disease is 1%–7%.

- With increasing age, hypertension, nephrotic syndrome and renal failure may develop.
- Diagnosis can be confirmed by direct immunofluorescence of the skin biopsy sample which demonstrates leucocytoclastic vasculitis with perivascular IgA, C3 and fibrin deposits. Kidney biopsy changes range from isolated mesangial proliferation to severe crescentic glomerulonephritis.

DIAGNOSTIC CRITERIA

- Diagnostic criteria for Henoch–Schönlein purpura are given in Box 9.11

TREATMENT

- Most patients respond to bed rest, paracetamol and NSAIDs.
- Corticosteroids are indicated in severe systemic disease including severe pain.
- Use of corticosteroids at the initial presentation does not prevent development of nephritis.
- Immunosuppressive therapy, generally methylprednisolone, should be considered only in patients who present with marked proteinuria (>1 g/day) and/or impaired kidney function during the acute episode.

Q. What are Clutton's joints?

Q. Describe the articular manifestations of syphilis.

- Articular disease can occur in congenital, secondary and tertiary syphilis.
  - Soon after birth, the infant may present with 'parrot's pseudoparalysis'. This is a painful limitation of joints resulting from osteochondritis.
  - At puberty, typically painless bilateral effusions may occur in knees and elbows (Clutton's joints).
  - Secondary syphilis may be associated with a migrating polyarthralgia.
  - Charcot's (neuropathic) joints are painless, deformed joints seen in neurosyphilis.

BOX 9.11 Diagnostic Criteria for Henoch–Schönlein Purpura

PALPABLE PURPURA (ESSENTIAL) IN THE PRESENCE OF ONE OF THE FOLLOWING:

- Diffuse abdominal pain
- Any biopsy showing predominant IgA (skin or kidney)
- Acute arthritis/arthralgia
- Renal involvement defined as proteinuria >0.3 g/24 and/or haematuria with red blood cell >5 per high-power field or ≥2+ on dipstick or red blood cell casts in the urinary sediment

Q. Discuss the clinical manifestations, diagnosis and management of systemic lupus erythematosus (SLE). (IM 7.19, IM 7.22)

Q. List down the various autoantibodies in systemic lupus erythematosus (SLE).

- SLE is a multisystem CTD characterised by the presence of numerous autoantibodies, circulatory immune complexes and widespread immune-mediated tissue damage.
- The onset is most commonly in the second and third decades with a female/male ratio of 9:1.

CLINICAL FEATURES (Table 9.10)

CONSTITUTIONAL SYMPTOMS

- These include fatigue, malaise, nausea, weight loss and fever.
- Though not life threatening, they have a significant impact on quality of life.

RENAL DISEASE (LUPUS NEPHRITIS)

- Affects about 30% of patients with SLE.
- Often asymptomatic, particularly initially; hence, regular urinalysis and blood pressure monitoring crucial.
- Characterised by proteinuria (>0.5 g/24 hours) and/or red cell casts.
- Histologically, lupus nephritis is classified as shown in Box 9.12.

NEUROPSYCHIATRIC FEATURES

- Seen in about 20% of cases.
- Clinical features include central nervous system involvement causing headache and seizures, psychiatric features including depression and psychosis and pe-

TABLE 9.10 Clinical Features of SLE

• Systemic	Fatigue, malaise, fever, anorexia, nausea, weight loss
• Musculoskeletal	Arthralgias, myalgias, nonerosive polyarthritis, myopathy
• Mucocutaneous	Malar rash ('butterfly' rash), discoid rash, other rashes, photosensitivity, oral ulcers, alopecia
• Haematological	Anaemia, leucopenia, lymphopenia, thrombocytopenia, splenomegaly, lymphadenopathy
• Neurological	Organic brain syndromes, psychosis, seizures, peripheral neuropathy
• Cardiopulmonary	Pleurisy, pericarditis, myocarditis, endocarditis (Libman–Sacks), pleural effusions
• Renal	Nephrotic syndrome, renal failure, proteinuria, cellular casts
• Gastrointestinal	Nonspecific symptoms, bleeding or perforation, abnormal liver enzymes
• Ocular	Retinal vasculitis, conjunctivitis, episcleritis, sicca syndrome

BOX 9.12 Histological Classification of Lupus Nephritis

- Class I—minimal mesangial lupus nephritis
- Class II—mesangial proliferative lupus nephritis
- Class III—focal lupus nephritis
- Class IV—diffuse lupus nephritis
- Class V—membranous lupus nephritis
- Class VI—advanced sclerosing lupus nephritis (≥90% globally sclerosed glomeruli without residual activity)

ripheral nervous system involvement causing neuropathy. Seizures and psychosis occur in the absence of offending drugs or known metabolic derangements.

MUSCULOSKELETAL FEATURES

- Arthralgia and myalgia in most patients.
- Nonerosive arthritis involving two or more peripheral joints
- The classical 'Jaccoud's arthropathy' can result in significant deformity and functional impairment. It is a nonerosive, deforming arthropathy of the metacarpophalangeal (MCP) and proximal interphalangeal joints, which presents with ulnar deviation and subluxation of the MCP. It occurs due to ligament laxity and muscle imbalance rather than the loss of bone and joint instability.

MUCOCUTANEOUS FEATURES

- Classic malar rash (fixed erythema, flat or raised, over the malar eminences and tending to spare the nasolabial folds) (Fig. 9.7).
- Discoid rash (erythematous, raised patches with adherent keratotic scaling and follicular plugging).
  - Presence of only discoid rash without any systemic features occurs in discoid lupus erythematosus. The rash is primarily on the face but can occur on any part of the body. In a small percentage of patients of discoid LE, SLE may ultimately develop.
  - Only 5% of people with DLE have SLE but, conversely, among individuals with SLE, 20% will have DLE.
- Generalised photosensitivity (skin rash on exposure to sunlight).
- Alopecia.
  - Scarring, when associated with discoid lesions.
  - Diffused, often fluctuating with disease activity.
- Recurrent crops of painless mouth ulcers, generally observed by physician.

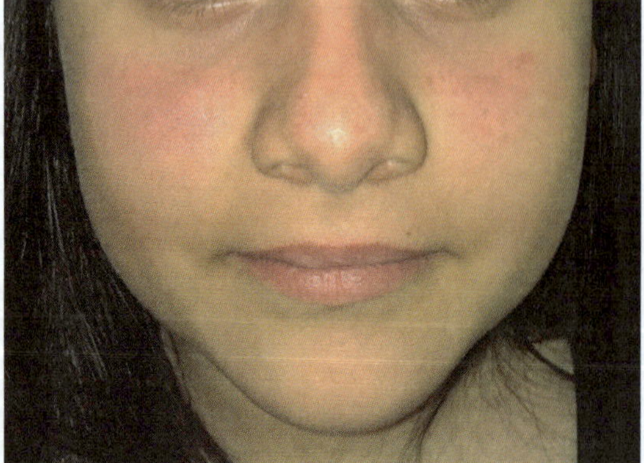

Fig. 9.7 Malar rash in a SLE patient. Note sparing of nasolabial folds.

- Cutaneous vasculitis presenting as palpable purpura and erythematous punctate lesions on the fingertips and palms.
- Other oral manifestations include dryness as a result of secondary Sjögren's syndrome.

HAEMATOLOGICAL FEATURES

- Normocytic normochromic anaemia.
- Coombs' positive haemolytic anaemia.
- Thrombocytopenia.
- Leucopenia.

CARDIOVASCULAR FEATURES

- Myocarditis and pericarditis.
- Pericardial effusion
- Endocarditis (Libman–Sacks endocarditis).
- A higher risk of coronary artery disease compared to in general population due to increased risk of atherosclerosis and vasculitis.

PULMONARY FEATURES

- Pleurisy.
- Pleural effusion, exudative with low C3 and positive ANA test in the fluid. Can also develop due to pulmonary embolism.
- Pneumonitis (infection must be excluded before ascribing a lung lesion to SLE).
- Vanishing or shrinking lung syndrome (progressive dyspnoea, usually accompanied by pleuritic chest pain, diaphragmatic elevation, lung volume reduction with no parenchymal abnormalities and a restrictive ventilatory defect in pulmonary function tests).
- Diffuse pulmonary haemorrhage.
- Pulmonary artery hypertension.

GASTROINTESTINAL FEATURES

- Nonspecific abdominal pain and dyspepsia.
- Hepatosplenomegaly.
- Mesenteric vasculitis.

OTHERS

- An increased risk of haematological cancer (particularly non-Hodgkin's lymphoma) and possibly lung and hepatobiliary cancers.

SUMMARY OF CLINICAL FEATURES

- Clinical features are summarised in Figure 9.8.

CAUSES OF DEATH

- Infections and renal failure are the leading causes of death in the first decade of disease, whereas thromboembolic events are frequently the cause of death in the second and later decades.
- Atherosclerosis occurs prematurely in patients with SLE and is an independent risk factor for cardiovascular causes of death.

INVESTIGATIONS

IMMUNOLOGICAL ABNORMALITIES

- The immunological abnormalities found in SLE are listed in Box 9.13.
- ANA is the best screening test. More than 90% of the patients have a positive test. A positive test is not specific

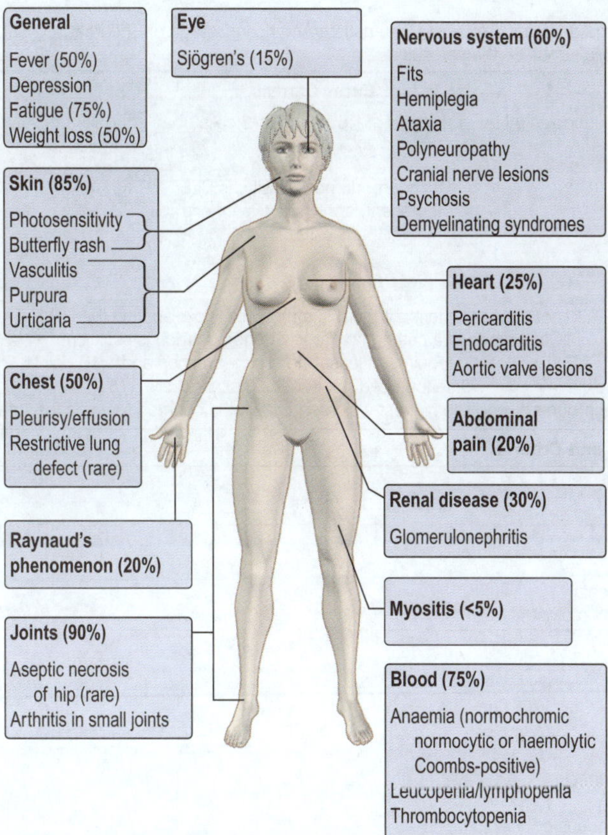

Fig. 9.8 Clinical features of SLE.

BOX 9.13 Autoantibodies in Patients With SLE

• Antinuclear antibodies (ANA)	• Anti-Ro (SSA)	• Antierythrocyte
• Anti-DNA (anti-dsDNA and anti-ssDNA)	• Anti-La (SSB)	• Antiplatelet
• Anti-Smith (Anti-Sm)	• Antihistone	• Antilymphocyte
• Anti-RNP	• Anticardiolipin (aCL)	• Antineuronal

for SLE as it can occur in a variety of other situations like in some normal people (especially elderly), other autoimmune diseases, acute viral infections, chronic inflammatory processes and with certain drugs.

- Anti-double-stranded DNA (anti-dsDNA) and anti-Sm are relatively specific for SLE.
- Rising levels of anti-dsDNA and low levels of complement (C3 and C4) usually reflect disease activity.

OTHER ABNORMALITIES

- The ESR is raised in some patients.
- The CRP, unlike the ESR, does not usually rise with disease activity unless there is arthritis or serositis. Infection should be excluded if a raised CRP is found in a patient with SLE.
- Anaemia (normocytic normochromic and Coombs' positive), leucopenia, lymphopenia and thrombocytopenia may be present.
- Low C3 and C4.
- With active nephritis, urinalysis shows proteinuria, haematuria and cellular or granular casts. Blood urea and serum creatinine may be elevated. Renal biopsy confirms renal involvement.
- Prolonged partial thromboplastin time in patients with lupus anticoagulant (LA).
- Other nonspecific abnormalities include false-positive tests for syphilis and positive tests for rheumatoid factor.
- Central nervous system disease usually warrants magnetic resonance imaging (MRI) of brain or spinal cord and examination of the cerebrospinal fluid where appropriate.

DIAGNOSTIC CRITERIA

- Diagnostic criteria of SLE are given in Table 9.11.

MANAGEMENT

- Patients with mild features (arthralgias, arthritis, myalgias, fever and mild serositis) should be managed with NSAIDs. Hydroxychloroquine may be added if required.
- Skin lesions also respond to hydroxychloroquine.
    - Side effects of hydroxychloroquine include ocular toxicity (retinopathy), prolongation of QT interval and hyperpigmentation of skin.
- Photosensitive skin lesions require application of sunscreen lotions.

TABLE 9.11 European League Against Rheumatism/American College of Rheumatology Classification Criteria for Systemic Lupus Erythematosus

ENTRY CRITERIA

Antinuclear antibodies (ANA) at a titre of ≥1:80 on HEp-2 cells or an equivalent positive test (ever)

↓

If absent, do not classify as SLE
If present, apply additive criteria

↓

ADDITIVE CRITERIA

Do not count a criterion if there is a more likely explanation than SLE
Occurrence of a criterion on at least one occasion is sufficient
SLE classification requires at least one clinical criterion and ≥10 points
Criterion need not occur simultaneously
Within each domain, only the highest weighted criterion is counted towards the total score

Clinical Domain and Criteria	Weight (Points)
Constitutional:	
Fever	2
Haematologic:	
Leucopenia	3
Thrombocytopenia	4
Autoimmune haemolysis	4
Neuropsychiatric:	
Delirium	2
Psychosis	3
Seizure	5
Mucocutaneous:	
Nonscarring alopecia	2
Oral ulcers	2
Subacute cutaneous or discoid lupus	4
Acute cutaneous lupus	6
Serosal:	
Pleural or pericardial effusion	5
Acute pericarditis	6
Musculoskeletal:	
Joint involvement	6
Renal:	
Proteinuria >0.5 g per 24 hours	4
Renal biopsy class II or V lupus nephritis	8
Renal biopsy class III or IV lupus nephritis	10
Immunologic Domains and Criteria	**Weight (Points)**
Antiphospholipid antibodies:	
Anticardiolipin antibodies OR anti-beta-2 glycoprotein 1 antibodies OR lupus anticoagulant	2
Complement proteins:	
Low C3 OR low C4	3
Low C3 AND low C4	4
SLE-specific antibodies:	
Anti-dsDNA OR anti-Sm antibodies	6

A total score of ≥10 and ≥1 clinical criterion is required to classify SLE.

- Patients with severe symptoms or life-threatening features should receive corticosteroids.
- Acutely ill patients and patients with proliferative glomerulonephritis may be treated with 'pulses' of methylprednisolone for 3 days (1 g/day) followed by oral steroids. Hydroxychloroquine is added to oral steroids. Belimumab (a BLyS-specific inhibitor) and voclosporin (a calcineurin inhibitor) are also approved for use in lupus nephritis.
- Immunosuppressants like azathioprine, methotrexate, cyclophosphamide and mycophenolate mofetil are also useful in controlling severe disease. These agents are particularly useful in patients with renal involvement. In this regard, a combination of intravenous cyclophosphamide and 'pulses' of steroids is the most effective regimen. Following induction, oral mycophenolate mofetil or azathioprine along with low-dose prednisolone are given to maintain remission.
- Belimumab, a monoclonal human antibody that inactivates B-lymphocyte stimulator, may be used for the treatment of patients with active disease who are refractory to standard treatment.

Q. Explain briefly drug-induced lupus.

- Caused by several medications, including anti-TNF blockers (e.g. infliximab), chlorpromazine, hydralazine, isoniazid, methyldopa, minocycline, procainamide and quinidine.
- Symptoms generally resolve after termination of drug.
- Significant differences between drug-induced lupus and SLE:
  - Males and females almost equally affected.
  - Renal and CNS involvement uncommon.
  - Antinuclear antibodies positive; antihistone antibodies positive; autoantibodies to DNA absent.
  - C_3 levels normal.

Q. What are antinuclear antibodies?

- Antinuclear antibodies (ANA) are antibodies that bind to various nuclear antigens. These are generally detected using indirect immunofluorescence. Most laboratories employ a HEp-2 cell line (a line of human epithelial cells).
- Higher titres of ANA (>1:160) are more likely to be true-positive than low titres.
- ANA is positive in several conditions. In SLE and drug-induced lupus, its sensitivity is more than 95% while the specificity for SLE is more than 90%.
- A negative ANA test does not exclude SLE. Rarely, patients with anti-Ro (anti-SSA) antibodies have a negative ANA.
- Titres of ANA do not correlate with disease activity and should not be used to monitor the course of SLE or other diseases.

CONDITIONS ASSOCIATED WITH A POSITIVE ANA TEST (Box 9.14)

- The nuclear pattern of a positive ANA is also important. This pattern reflects the intranuclear target of ANA. Various patterns are:
  - Homogeneous pattern—reflects antibodies directed against histone proteins and DNA and is highly suggestive of SLE; may also be seen in Sjögren's syndrome, scleroderma and rheumatoid arthritis.
  - Rim pattern—highly suggestive of SLE. Also seen with systemic sclerosis.
  - Speckled pattern—may be due to antibodies against U1-ribonucleoprotein (RNP), Smith (Sm), and Ro and La antigens; common with SLE, Sjögren's syndrome, polymyositis and mixed CTD.
  - Nucleolar pattern—signifies antibodies against RNA polymerase; common in systemic sclerosis. May also be seen with SLE, polymyositis.
  - Centromeric pattern—typically is found in patients with CREST syndrome.

BOX 9.14 Conditions Associated With a Positive ANA Test

- SLE
- Drug-induced lupus
- Systemic sclerosis
- Sjögren's syndrome
- Mixed CTD
- Polymyositis/dermatomyositis
- Rheumatoid arthritis
- Bacterial endocarditis
- Autoimmune hepatitis
- Primary biliary cholangitis
- Hashimoto's thyroiditis
- Interstitial lung disease
- Malignancies
- Elderly individuals

Q. Describe extractable nuclear antibodies.

- Extractable nuclear antibodies are directed against small ribonuclear proteins (RNA).
- Include anti-Sm, anti-uracil-rich 1 ribonucleoprotein (U1RNP), anti-SSA/Ro, anti-SSB/La, anti-tRNA synthetases (found in polymyositis/dermatomyositis), anti-topoisomerase-1 antibodies and anticentromere antibodies.
- Have a high specificity and should be ordered only in ANA-positive patients with clinical features suggestive of a particular CTD and in ANA-negative patients with known or suspected CTD.
- Do not correlate with disease activity and, therefore, may be found in patients without active disease.

Q. Discuss briefly about various antibodies seen in patients with connective tissue diseases. (IM 7.15)

- Autoantibodies see in patients with connective tissue diseases are discussed in Table 9.12.

Q. Describe antiphospholipid antibody syndrome and antiphospholipid antibodies.

- Antiphospholipid antibody (APLA) syndrome or antiphospholipid syndrome (APS) is characterised by the presence of APLAs and a syndrome of hypercoagulability.

CLASSIFICATION

- Based on presence or absence of underlying disease:
  - Primary APS occurs in patients without clinical evidence of another autoimmune disease.
  - Secondary APS occurs in association with other autoimmune diseases like SLE.
- Based on type of clinical manifestation:
  - Thrombotic—venous or arterial thrombosis
  - Obstetric—foetal death after 10 weeks of gestation, premature birth due to severe preeclampsia or placental insufficiency, or multiple embryonic losses before 10 weeks gestation.
  - Combined thrombotic and obstetric.
  - Catastrophic—life-threatening, multiorgan involvement due to thrombosis.

CLINICAL FEATURES

- Clinical features of APLA are given in Table 9.13.

TABLE 9.12 Autoantibodies in Various Connective Tissue Diseases (CTDs)

Autoantibodies	Importance
• Rheumatoid factor	• Discussed separately
• Anticyclic citrullinated peptide	• Discussed separately
• Antinuclear antibodies	• Discussed above
• Anti-double-stranded DNA (anti-dsDNA)	• Highly specific for SLE • Positive in only about 60% cases of SLE • Low titres also seen in Sjögren's syndrome, RA • Levels often correlate with disease activity • Presence correlates with lupus nephritis • Usually absent in drug-induced SLE
• Antihistone	• Sensitive for drug-induced lupus but not specific • Useful in patients with a positive ANA and a history of exposure to medications that can produce lupus
• Anti-Smith (anti-Sm)	• Highly specific for SLE but present in only 20%–30% cases
• Anti-U1 ribonucleoproteins (RNP)	• Present in 20%–30% cases of SLE • High titres in syndromes with features of polymyositis, lupus, scleroderma and mixed CTD • In anti-DNA-negative SLE, indicates low risk of nephritis
• Anti-Ro (anti-SSA)	• Common in Sjögren's syndrome with extraglandular features • Positive in 40% cases of SLE and is associated with photosensitive rash and pulmonary disease • May be positive in ANA-negative lupus • Indicates higher risk of lupus nephritis • May be positive in neonatal lupus or congenital heart block due to maternal antibodies
• Anti-La (anti-SS-B)	• Present in 10%–15% cases of SLE • Presence indicates low risk of nephritis • Associated with Sjögren's syndrome
• Antiphospholipid	• Present in nearly 50% cases of SLE • Three types: lupus anticoagulant (LA), anticardiolipin (aCL) and false-positive for syphilis • LA and IgG aCL associated with APLA syndrome
• Anticentromere	• Found in 20%–35% cases of systemic sclerosis • Associated with CREST syndrome (calcinosis, Raynaud's phenomenon, oesophageal dysfunction, sclerodactyly and telangiectasia) • Also present in primary biliary cirrhosis
• Antitopoisomerase I (anti-scl-70)	• Highly specific for systemic sclerosis • Found in 20%–40% cases of systemic sclerosis • Associated with diffuse cutaneous, pulmonary and cardiac involvements
• Anti-Jo-1	• Present in 30% cases with polymyositis or dermatomyositis • Associated with Raynaud's phenomenon
• Antineutrophil cytoplasmic antibodies (ANCA)	• Discussed separately

TABLE 9.13 Clinical Features of Antiphospholipid Antibody (APLA) Syndrome

Organ/System	Manifestations
• Arterial/venous	Thrombosis in any artery or vein
• Cardiac	Angina, myocardial infarction, valvular vegetations
• Haematological	Thrombocytopenia (in 40%–50% of patients), haemolytic anaemia, disseminated intravascular coagulation
• Neurological	Transient ischaemic attack, stroke, headache, mononeuritis multiplex
• Obstetrical	Pregnancy loss, intrauterine growth retardation
• Ophthalmological	Retinal artery/vein thrombosis
• Renal	Thrombosis of renal artery/vein, renal infarction, acute renal failure, haematuria
• Gastrointestinal	Budd–Chiari syndrome, hepatic infarction, intestinal infarction, splenic infarction, pancreatitis
• Cutaneous	Ulcers and infarcts in the skin, gangrene, livedo reticularis
• Pulmonary	Pulmonary embolism, pulmonary hypertension

INVESTIGATIONS

ANTIPHOSPHOLIPID ANTIBODIES

- These are a heterogeneous group of autoantibodies directed against phospholipid-binding proteins.
- These are LA, aCL antibodies and anti-β_2-glycoprotein I antibodies.
- LA antibodies:
  - Identified by coagulation assays in which they prolong the clotting times.
  - Failure of the prolonged clotting time to correct after a 1:1 mix with normal platelet-free plasma and correction of the clotting time after addition of excess phospholipids confirms the presence of LA.
  - For LA screening, two or more phospholipid-dependent coagulation tests including the activated partial thromboplastin time, dilute Russell viper venom time and kaolin clotting time required.
- aCL antibodies target cardiolipin (a bovine cardiac protein) and are detected by immunoassays.
- Anti-β_2-glycoprotein I antibodies are directed against β_2-glycoprotein I and may be causal in APLA syndrome.

TABLE 9.14 Criteria for Diagnosis of APLA

Clinical Features	Laboratory Features

• Vascular thrombosis (arterial, venous or small vessel)
• Complications of pregnancy:
  • One of more unexplained deaths of morphologically normal foetuses at birth or after 10 weeks of gestation with normal foetal morphology documented by ultrasound or direct examination of the foetus
Or
  • One or more premature births of morphologically normal neonates at or before 34th week of gestation because of eclampsia, pre-eclampsia or placental insufficiency
Or
  • Three or more unexplained consecutive spontaneous abortions before the 10th week of gestation
	• aCL antibodies (on two or more occasions at least 12 weeks apart)
	• LA antibodies (on two or more occasions at least 12 weeks apart)
	• Anti-β_2-glycoprotein I (IgG and/or IgM) on two or more occasions at least 12 weeks apart

- LA antibodies are more specific while aCL antibodies are more sensitive for APS. IgG aCL antibodies are more specific compared to IgM type.
- APLAs may be found in 10% of normal population and 30%–50% of patients with SLE.
- These antibodies are also found in patients with infections such as human immunodeficiency virus and may develop during therapy with medications such as chlorpromazine.

OTHER TESTS

- Mild thrombocytopenia
- Prolongation of activated partial thromboplastin time.
- False positive serologic test for syphilis.

DIAGNOSIS

- Table 9.14 gives diagnostic criteria for APLA.
- A diagnosis of definite APS is made if the patient has one clinical and one laboratory criteria.

TREATMENT

TREATMENT OF VENOUS OR ARTERIAL THROMBOSIS

- Anticoagulation with heparin and oral warfarin followed by oral warfarin to maintain international normalised ratio (INR) between 2 and 3. Duration of treatment is probably lifelong.
- Steroids are often added to this treatment.
- In severe cases of generalised thrombosis, plasmapheresis or intravenous immunoglobulin may be tried.

PREVENTION OF RECURRENCE OF ARTERIAL OR VENOUS THROMBOSIS

- Aspirin 325 mg/day (for arterial thrombosis) plus warfarin with INR between 1.4 and 2.8.

PROPHYLAXIS OF ANY THROMBOTIC EPISODE

- Aspirin may be useful in preventing thrombosis in females with previous pregnancy loss.
- In the presence of underlying SLE with APLAs positive, aspirin along with hydroxychloroquine should be started.
- Modification of other risk factors like hypercholesterolemia and smoking.

MANAGEMENT OF PREGNANCY IN PATIENTS WITH ANTIPHOSPHOLIPID SYNDROME

- Females with APLAs and a history of two or more early pregnancy losses, or one or more late pregnancy losses that have no prior history of thrombosis should receive combination of aspirin and heparin (unfractionated or low molecular weight) during pregnancy.
- Aspirin should be started with attempted conception.
- Heparin (5000–10,000 units every 12 hours) or low-molecular-weight heparin in prophylactic doses (enoxaparin 1 mg/kg; dalteparin 5000 units once a day) should be started, when a viable intrauterine pregnancy is documented on ultrasound and continued until late in the third trimester.

CATASTROPHIC ANTIPHOSPHOLIPID SYNDROME

- Can occur at onset or later after diagnosis.
- Presents with rapidly progressive multiorgan involvement with histopathological evidence of small vessel occlusions.
- Common clinical features include intraabdominal features (involvement of kidney, liver, gastrointestinal tract and spleen), ARDS, cerebral manifestations (multiple microinfarctions, seizures), cardiac involvement (cardiac failure, infarction) and skin complications (livedo reticularis, skin necrosis).
- Thrombocytopenia, haemolysis, schistocytes and activation of coagulation system are common laboratory findings.
- High ferritin is common.
- Diagnosis of catastrophic antiphospholipid syndrome requires involvement of three or more organs (or systems or tissues), manifestations that have developed within one week, histopathology of small vessel occlusion and confirmation of antiphospholipid antibodies
- Despite treatment, mortality is nearly 50%.
- The mainstay of treatment is intravenous heparin along with high-dose corticosteroids. Early addition of plasma exchange and/or intravenous immunoglobulin should be considered in patients who do not respond promptly to heparin and corticosteroids.

Q. Write a short note on scleroderma.

Q. Describe CREST syndrome.

Q. Discuss the clinical manifestations, diagnosis and management of systemic sclerosis.

- Systemic sclerosis is a multisystem disorder affecting skin (scleroderma—thickened, hardened skin), gastrointestinal tract, musculoskeletal system, lungs, heart and kidneys. The disease can also occur in a localised form without systemic involvement (localised scleroderma).

- Two subsets of the systemic form of the disease have been identified. They are diffuse cutaneous systemic sclerosis and limited cutaneous systemic sclerosis.
- Two subsets of the localised scleroderma are morphoea and linear scleroderma.
- Systemic sclerosis sine scleroderma (ssSSc) is a very rare subset characterised by absence of skin thickening, presence of Raynaud's phenomenon, pulmonary hypertension and involvement of internal organ involvement along with serological abnormalities.

CLINICAL MANIFESTATIONS

- Raynaud's phenomenon is usually the first manifestation. It may precede other features by months or years.
- Diffuse cutaneous scleroderma is characterised by rapid development of symmetrical skin thickening of proximal and distal extremities, face and trunk. These patients also have a high risk of developing kidney disease, interstitial lung disease, cardiac involvement and other systemic involvement.
- Limited cutaneous scleroderma is associated with skin thickening limited to distal extremities (distal to knees and elbows) and face. These patients generally have prominent vascular manifestations, including severe Raynaud's phenomenon and mucocutaneous telangiectasia. A few patients may develop interstitial lung disease, pulmonary arterial hypertension (due to fibrosis of pulmonary artery) or biliary cirrhosis after several years. This subset may also have features of CREST syndrome (i.e. calcinosis, Raynaud's phenomenon, oesophageal dysfunction, sclerodactyly and telangiectasia).

SKIN MANIFESTATIONS

- In the early stages (oedematous phase), there is non-pitting oedema and induration of the skin.
- As the disease advances (indurative phase), the skin becomes firm, thickened and eventually tightly bound to underlying subcutaneous tissue.
- After many years of disease, the skin may become thin and atrophic.
- Skin shows hyperpigmentation and depigmentation ('salt and pepper')
- Facial skin changes result in taut skin, 'mask-like' face, 'beaking' of the nose and microstomia (Fig. 9.9).
- Other skin manifestations are flexion contractures, ulcers over fingertips and bony prominences, pigmentation, telangiectasia, calcinosis cutis and dry, coarse skin (Fig. 9.10).

MUSCULOSKELETAL MANIFESTATIONS

- Muscle weakness occurs due to disuse atrophy, myopathy and myositis.
- Arthralgia of fingers and knees, symmetric polyarthritis, 'leathery' crepitations over joints (especially knees), joint contractures and resorption of terminal phalanges.

GASTROINTESTINAL MANIFESTATIONS

- Oesophageal involvement can manifest as dysphagia, reflux oesophagitis, sliding hiatus hernia, peptic oesophagitis, strictures, dilatation and atony of lower oesophagus.
- Gastric involvement results in dilatation, atony and delayed gastric emptying. Vascular ectasia (angiodysplasia) in the antrum of the stomach ('watermelon stomach') is frequent and may be a cause of chronic unexplained gastrointestinal bleeding and anaemia.

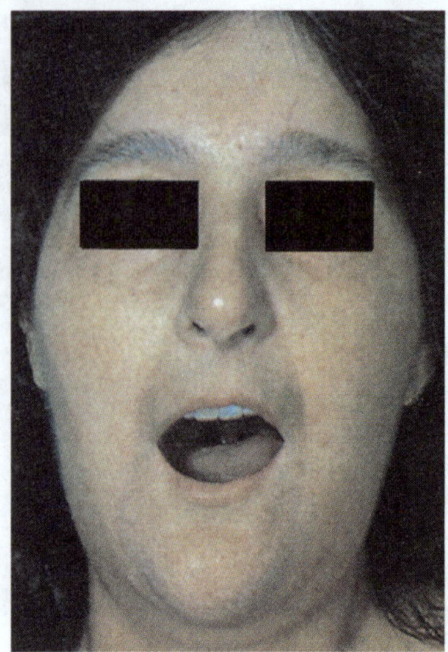

Fig. 9.9 Microstomia (limited mouth opening).

- Small and large bowel involvements result in abdominal distension, abdominal pain, constipation, intestinal obstruction, malabsorption and steatorrhoea.

PULMONARY INVOLVEMENT

- Pulmonary fibrosis manifests as exertional breathlessness, bilateral basal crepitations and 'honeycomb' lung on chest radiograph.
- Other pulmonary manifestations are aspiration pneumonia, pulmonary hypertension with right-heart failure and alveolar cell and bronchial carcinoma.

OTHER MANIFESTATIONS

- Cardiac involvement can manifest as pericarditis with or without effusion, heart failure, heart blocks, arrhythmias and cardiomyopathy.
- Renal involvement can manifest as progressive renal failure. It can also present as renal crisis manifesting as acute renal failure with malignant hypertension, hypertensive encephalopathy and left ventricular failure. Urine examination shows mild proteinuria with few cells or casts. Microangiopathic haemolysis anaemia and thrombocytopenia may also occur.
- Rare manifestations are dryness of mouth and eyes, hypothyroidism, cranial and peripheral nerve involvement and impotence in males.

SUMMARY

- Fig. 9.11 summarises manifestations of systemic sclerosis.

DIFFUSE VERSUS LIMITED CUTANEOUS SYSTEMIC SCLEROSIS

- Differences between diffuse and limited cutaneous systemic sclerosis are given in Table 9.15.

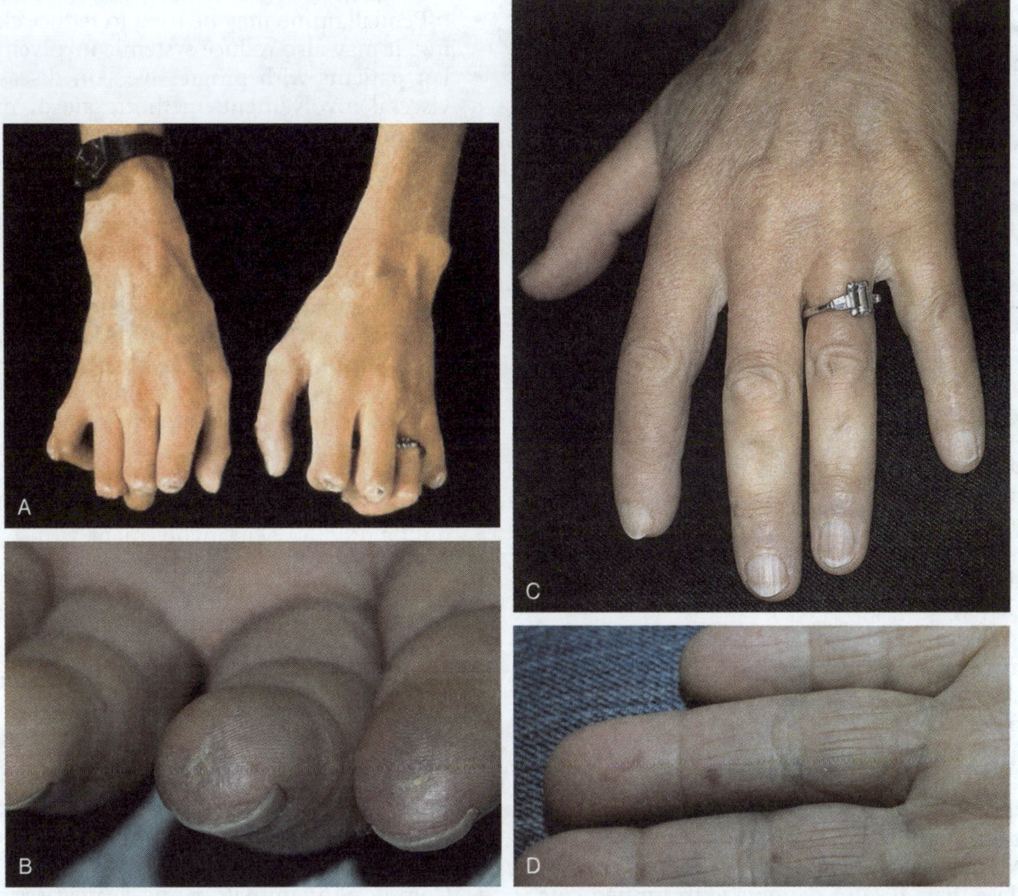

Fig. 9.10 Acral signs of systemic sclerosis: (A) Sclerodactyly, tethered smooth skin, calcinosis, ulceration and fixed flexion deformities of the fingers, (B) scarring secondary to digital pulp infarcts, (C) oedematous phase of systemic sclerosis, (D) telangieactasias.

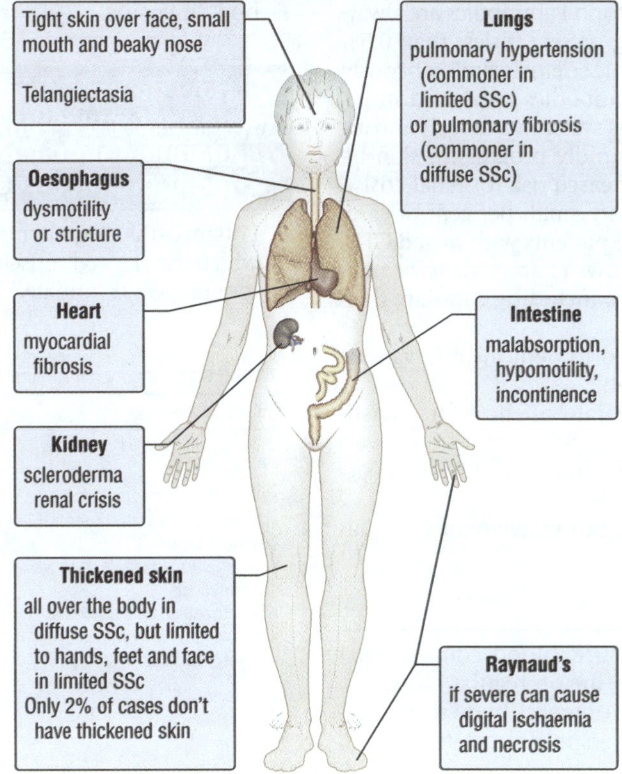

Fig. 9.11 Summary of clinical manifestations of systemic sclerosis.

TABLE 9.15 Differentiating Diffuse Versus Limited Cutaneous Systemic Sclerosis

Diffuse Cutaneous Systemic Sclerosis	Limited Cutaneous Systemic Sclerosis
• Proximal limb or trunk involvement with skin sclerosis	• Distal skin sclerosis
• Short history of Raynaud's phenomenon	• Long history of Raynaud's phenomenon
• Increased risk of renal crisis and cardiac involvement	• Late-stage complications frequent
• High frequency of severe lung fibrosis	• Pulmonary arterial hypertension and severe gut disease frequent

INVESTIGATIONS

- Elevated ESR.
- Anaemia related to:
  - Chronic disease.
  - Iron deficiency due to gastrointestinal bleed.
  - Blind loop syndrome producing folate and B_{12} deficiency.
  - Microangiopathic haemolytic anaemia due to renal involvement.
- Antinuclear antibodies in 90% cases and rheumatoid factor in 25% cases.
- Antinuclear antibodies which are highly specific for systemic sclerosis include antitopoisomerase I (antitopo I; previously called anti-Scl-70) and anticentromere.
  - Antitopo I antibodies are found in about 40% of patients with diffuse cutaneous systemic sclerosis and less than 10% of patients with limited cutaneous systemic sclerosis.
  - Anticentromere antibodies are seen in 30%–40% of patients with limited cutaneous involvement.
  - Anticentromere and antitopo I antibodies are always mutually exclusive, being present in less than 0.5% of all patients with systemic sclerosis simultaneously.
- Anti-RNA polymerase III antibodies are found in patients with diffuse cutaneous systemic sclerosis and are generally associated with rapidly progressive skin involvement as well as an increased risk for renal crisis.
- Anti-U1 RNP is found in very small per cent of cases but is present in virtually all patients with mixed CTD.
- Nailfold capillaroscopy shows characteristic of nailfold capillary abnormalities including capillary dilatation and loop dropout.
- Barium swallow test is used to demonstrate various abnormalities in oesophagus.
- X-ray and computed tomogram of chest for interstitial lung disease.
- Pulmonary function tests including diffusion capacity for interstitial lung disease.
- Echocardiography for cardiac involvement and pulmonary hypertension.

TREATMENT

- Monitoring of blood pressure, blood counts, renal functions and analysis of urine on regular basis.
- Control of Raynaud's phenomenon by oral nifedipine and phosphodiesterase-5 inhibitors (sildenafil, tadalafil, vardenafil).
- Management of gastro-oesophageal reflux.
- D-Penicillamine may be used to reduce skin thickening. It may also reduce systemic involvement.
- For patients with progressive skin diseases without visceral involvement, methotrexate or mycophenolate mofetil may be used.
- Cyclophosphamide remains the treatment of choice for lung disease and severe skin disease.
- For lung disease, mycophenolate mofetil is preferred as initial therapy over cyclophosphamide due to its better safety profile and comparable efficacy. Azathioprine is an alternative which may be considered for patients with contraindications or intolerance to cyclophosphamide and mycophenolate. Other drug which can be used is tocilizumab.
- Methotrexate is the treatment of choice for scleroderma overlap syndromes.
- Steroids are indicated in patients with myositis, pericarditis or pulmonary fibrosis. However, they should not be used for skin involvement.
- Antihypertensives in renal crisis (most important drugs are ACE inhibitors).
- Treatment of pulmonary hypertension includes endothelin receptor antagonists, epoprostenol analogues and phosphodiesterase-5 inhibitors.

Q. What are inflammatory muscle diseases?

- A heterogenous group of muscle diseases characterised by inflammation.
- Common inflammatory muscle diseases are given in Table 9.16.
- Three major forms of autoimmune muscle diseases are: polymyositis, dermatomyositis and inclusion body myositis.

Q. How do you classify polymyositis and dermatomyositis? Discuss the clinical manifestations, diagnosis and management of polymyositis–dermatomyositis.

- Polymyositis and dermatomyositis are conditions in which the skeletal muscle is damaged by an inflammatory process dominated by lymphocytic infiltration.

TABLE 9.16 Common Inflammatory Muscle Diseases

Infective Forms	Autoimmune (Idiopathic)
• Viral (coxsackie B, influenza A and B, HIV) • Bacterial (*Streptococcus*, *Staphylococcus*, clostridial, mycobacterial) • Fungal (candidiasis, coccidioidomycosis) • Protozoal (toxoplasmosis) • Helminthic (trichinosis, cysticercosis)	A. Generalised • Dermatomyositis • Polymyositis • Inclusion body myositis • Overlap syndromes • Necrotising myopathy (paraneoplastic, drugs, toxins) • Eosinophilic myositis • Granulomatous myositis B. Focal forms • Monomelic myositis • Eosinophilic myositis • Macrophagic myofasciitis • Orbital myositis

TABLE 9.17 Classification of Idiopathic Inflammatory Myositis

• Group I	Primary idiopathic polymyositis
• Group II	Primary idiopathic dermatomyositis
• Group III	Dermatomyositis (or polymyositis) associated with neoplasia
• Group IV	Juvenile dermatomyositis (or polymyositis) associated with vasculitis
• Group V	Polymyositis (or dermatomyositis) with associated collagen vascular disease
• Group VI	Inclusion body myositis
• Group VII	Miscellaneous

BOX 9.15 Another Classification of Inflammatory Myositis

- Dermatomyositis
- Overlap myositis (including antisynthetase syndrome)
- Immune-mediated necrotising myopathy
- Inclusion body myositis
- Polymyositis

- The term polymyositis is applied when the condition spares the skin and the term dermatomyositis when polymyositis is associated with a characteristic skin rash.
- Classification of idiopathic inflammatory myositis is given in Table 9.17. Another classification is given in Box 9.15.

CLINICAL MANIFESTATIONS

PRIMARY IDIOPATHIC POLYMYOSITIS

- Weakness of the proximal muscles of the lower limbs (hips and thighs) results in difficulty in arising from the squatting or kneeling position and in climbing or descending stairs.
- Weakness of the proximal muscles of the upper limbs (shoulder girdle muscles) results in difficulty in placing an object on a high shelf or combing hair. Various causes of proximal muscle weakness are given in Table 9.18.
- Weakness of the trunk muscles and flexor muscles of the neck may be present.
- Pain and tenderness of the involved muscles of buttocks, thighs and calves may be present.
- The distal muscles are spared in most of the patients.
- Involvement of facial and ocular muscles is uncommon.
- Other features are dysphagia (due to weakness of oropharyngeal muscles and striated muscle of upper third of oesophagus), respiratory impairment, myocarditis resulting in ECG abnormalities, heart failure, arrhythmias, arthralgia and interstitial lung disease.
- Muscle biopsy shows single fibre muscle necrosis and infiltration with CD^{8+} lymphocytes.

PRIMARY IDIOPATHIC DERMATOMYOSITIS

- This term is used when polymyositis is associated with characteristic skin changes.

TABLE 9.18 Causes of Proximal Muscle Weakness

• Endocrine	Diabetic neuropathy, hyperthyroidism/hypothyroidism, acromegaly, Cushing's syndrome
• Drug-induced myopathies	Steroids, statins, clofibrate, D-penicillamine, chloroquine, zidovudine, amiodarone
• Inherited myopathies	Muscular dystrophies (Becker/Duchenne, facioscapulohumeral, limb girdle), myotonia congenita
• Neurological	Spinal muscular atrophies, amyotrophic lateral sclerosis, Guillain–Barré syndrome, chronic inflammatory demyelinating polyneuropathy, myasthenia gravis, Eaton–Lambert syndrome
• Metabolic	Glycogen storage disease, hypokalaemia, hypercalcaemia/hypocalcaemia, vitamin D deficiency, uraemia, alcoholism, acute intermittent porphyria
• Infections	Influenza, hepatitis B, rickettsia, pyomyositis, trichinella
• Autoimmune myositis	List given in Table 9.17
• Others	Periodic paralysis, acute rhabdomyolysis, sarcoidosis

- The skin changes may precede or follow the muscle syndrome and include a localised or diffuse erythema, maculopapular eruption or scaling eczematoid dermatitis.
- The classic lilac-coloured (heliotrope) rash is seen on the upper eyelids. Periorbital oedema is frequent (Fig. 9.12).
- Other pathognomonic cutaneous manifestations include:
  - Gottron's papules are violaceous papules overlying the dorsal interphalangeal or metacarpophalangeal areas (Fig. 9.13). When fully formed, these papules become slightly depressed at the centre which can assume a white, atrophic appearance. Associated telangiectasia can be present.
  - Gottron's sign is symmetrical, erythematous or violaceous, often atrophic macules or plaques overlying dorsal aspect of interphalangeal and metacarpophalangeal joints, olecranon processes, patellae (Fig. 9.14) and medial malleoli.
  - Periungual telangiectasias.
  - Shawl sign is the occurrence of erythematous macules distributed in a 'shawl' pattern over the shoulders and back (Fig. 9.15). The V sign is occurrence

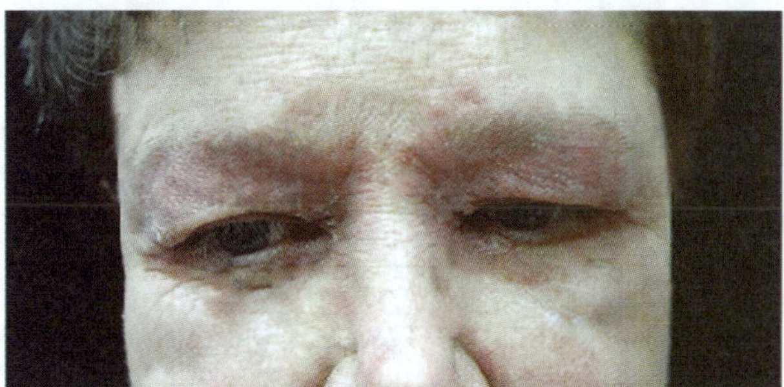

Fig. 9.12 Heliotrope rash and eyelid oedema (From: Callen JP, Jorisso JL, Bolognia JL, Piette WW, Zone JZ. Dermatological signs of internal disease, 4th edn. Elsevier; 2009).

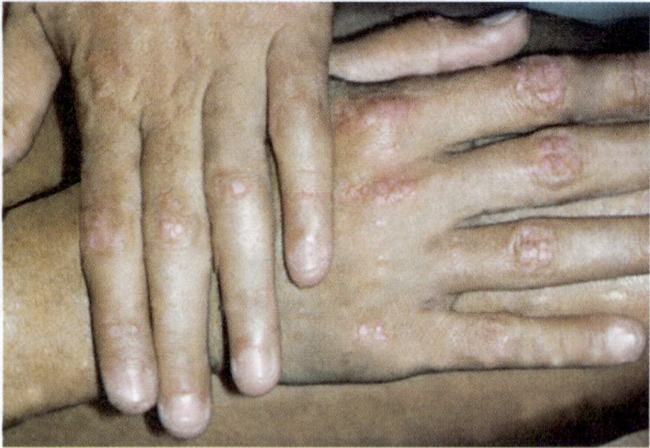

Fig. 9.13 Gottron's papules.

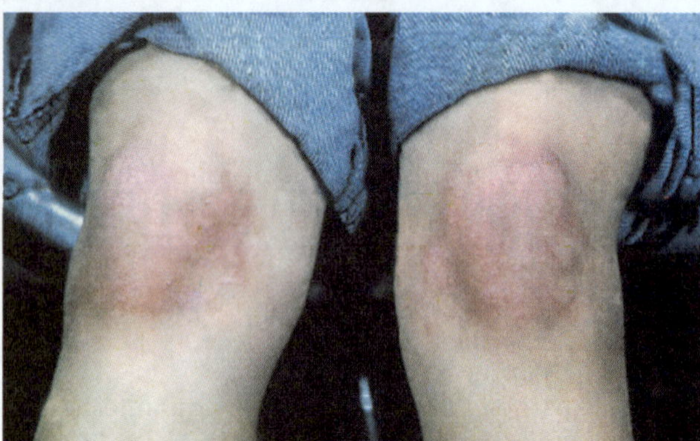

Fig. 9.14 Gottron's sign.

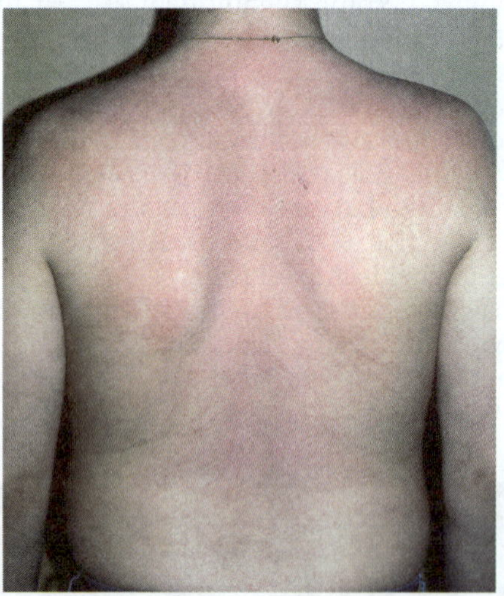

Fig. 9.15 Shawl sign. Courtesy: Steven Binnick, MD.

of erythematous lesions over the upper chest and neck.
  - The hands may be fissured, scaly and hyperkeratotic (mechanic's hand).
- Calcium deposition (calcinosis cutis) may occur on the buttocks, elbows, knees or traumatised areas and is more common in children.
- Muscle biopsy shows muscle necrosis (single fibres or in groups), perifasicular atrophy and infiltration with B cells and CD^{4+} lymphocytes.
- Pathognomonic skin lesion without muscle involvement is known as amyopathic dermatomyositis or dermatomyositis sine myositis.
- A few patients older than 50 years with dermatomyositis have an underlying malignancy. The most commonly reported malignancies are ovarian and gastric carcinoma, small cell lung cancer and lymphoma. Malignancies (non-Hodgkin lymphoma, lung and bladder cancers) can also rarely develop in patients with polymyositis.

DIAGNOSIS

- ESR and CRP are usually raised.
- Elevated serum levels of the muscle enzymes such as creatine kinase (CK), aldolase, serum glutamic oxaloacetic transaminase (SGOT), lactic dehydrogenase (LDH) and serum glutamic pyruvate transaminase (SGPT).
- Antinuclear antibodies are frequently raised.
- There are no known specific autoantibodies associated with the subgroup of polymyositis.
- Autoantibodies associated with dermatomyositis are subdivided into myositis specific autoantibodies (MSA) and myositis associated autoantibodies (MAA). MSAs are found in approximately 50%–60% of patients while MAAs are found in other autoimmune diseases also.
- Myositis-specific antibodies also help to define the phenotype of dermatomyositis and are separated in three groups, namely antisynthetase antibodies, which is the most common followed by antisignal recognition particle (SRP) antibodies and anti-Mi2 antibodies.
  - The most common antisynthetase antibody is anti-Jo-1; positivity to it is referred to as antisynthetase syndrome and is characterised by the Raynaud's syndrome, interstitial lung disease, mechanic's hands, fever and arthritis.
  - Those with anti-SRP antibodies have severe, acute resistant dermatomyositis with cardiac involvement, acute necrotising myopathy and rare cutaneous features.
  - Anti-Mi2 antibody positivity is highly specific for dermatomyositis, and these patients have classic cutaneous features, lower risk of myopathy and good response to treatment.
- The presence of myositis associated antibodies such as anti-PM/Scl, anti-Ro, anti-U1RNP, anti-Ku and anti-La may help to detect the presence of an overlapping connective tissue disorder.
- Characteristic EMG findings (myopathic pattern—increased insertional activity and spontaneous fibrillations and low-amplitude, short-duration polyphasic motor unit potential) may be present.
- Muscle biopsy shows the typical pathological changes of myositis.
- MRI aids in choosing sites of maximal inflammation for biopsy and to monitor treatment response.

MANAGEMENT

- The treatment of choice is prednisolone at a dose of 1 mg/kg daily till patient shows significant improvement. Then the dose is tapered to 10–15 mg/day over several weeks.
- If no improvement occurs with prednisolone, azathioprine (2–3 mg/kg/day) may be added. It also has some steroid-sparing effect.
- Other useful drugs include methotrexate, mycophenolate mofetil, cyclosporin and tacrolimus. Because 50% of anti-Jo-1-positive patients either have or will develop interstitial lung disease, methotrexate should be avoided in such patients.
- Patients with mainly skin involvement can be treated with hydroxychloroquine.
- In severe cases, intravenous immunoglobulins or rituximab.

Q. Define mixed connective tissue disease (MCTD).

- Defined as a generalised connective tissue disorder characterised by the presence of high-titre anti-U1 ribonucleoprotein (RNP) antibodies in combination with clinical features commonly seen in systemic lupus erythematosus, systemic sclerosis and polymyositis/dermatomyositis.
- Overlapping features tend to occur sequentially rather than concurrently.
- Early clinical features are nonspecific and may consist of general malaise, arthralgias, myalgias and low-grade fever.
- A key feature in suspecting a diagnosis of MCTD is the presence of unexplained Raynaud's phenomenon.
- Other features include swollen hands or puffy fingers, absence of severe renal and central nervous system disease, severe arthritis and insidious onset of pulmonary hypertension (not related to lung fibrosis). These features differentiate MCTD from pure SLE or systemic sclerosis.
- The therapy is directed by clinical manifestations and organ involvement.
  - Arthritis and arthralgia usually respond to NSAIDs and hydroxychloroquine. For refractory synovitis, corticosteroids and methotrexate can be used.
  - Pleuritis, pericarditis, myositis, myocarditis and aseptic meningitis usually respond to steroids. Steroid-sparing agents (methotrexate, cyclosporine, azathioprine and mycophenolate mofetil) are commonly used as a second-line agent.

Q. Write a brief note on polymyalgia rheumatica.

- This is a descriptive term for an aching syndrome usually seen in the elderly patients with an elevated ESR that cannot be attributed to more defined rheumatic, infectious or neoplastic disorders.
- Women are two to three times more likely than men to be affected by it.

CLINICAL FEATURES

- Proximal myalgias are characteristic. There is chronic, symmetric, proximal muscle aching and morning stiffness (lasting for >45 minutes but generally several hours), usually involving shoulder, hip, pelvic girdle and neck. Patients often report being unable to stand up from a chair, get out of bed without assistance, or lift their arms to comb their hair.
- On physical examination, active range of motion is restricted due to pain, without actual weakness, while passive range of motion may be normal. Muscles may be tender on palpation.
- Constitutional symptoms like malaise, fatigue, anorexia, weight loss, fever and night sweats may be present.
- Neuropsychiatric manifestations are frequent, particularly depression.
- A considerable number of patients (15%–30%) may have peripheral arthritis mainly involving knee and wrist, pitting oedema and carpal tunnel syndrome.
- Ten to thirty per cent of these patients have associated temporal arteritis.

INVESTIGATIONS

- Elevated ESR (more than 50 mm/hour), CRP and normocytic–normochromic anaemia.
- Tests for rheumatoid factor, anticitrullinated peptide antibody and antinuclear antibodies are usually negative.
- Liver enzyme, particularly alkaline phosphatase may be elevated.
- Temporal artery biopsy may show evidence of giant cell arteritis.
- Muscle enzymes are characteristically normal.
- Ultrasound may show bursitis or tenosynovitis.

TREATMENT

- Prednisolone given at dose of 15–20 mg/day is rapidly effective (Flowchart 9.3). A prompt and dramatic clinical response is considered by some to be an absolute criterion for diagnosis. Symptoms resolve in 48–72 hours in majority and the ESR normalises after 7–10 days. Dose is tapered very gradually with duration of therapy of 2–3 years.
- NSAIDs are useful to suppress rheumatic symptoms.

Q. Explain temporal arteritis, cranial arteritis or giant cell arteritis.

- This is a disease of the elderly occurring almost exclusively in people older than 55 years. Nearly half of patients have evidence of polymyalgia rheumatica.
- It is a chronic granulomatous vasculitis affecting the aorta and its branches.
- Arteritis can occur in any large and medium artery, although it has a predilection for the extracranial carotid artery and its branches such as the superficial temporal, occipital, ophthalmic, posterior ciliary arteries and vertebral arteries.

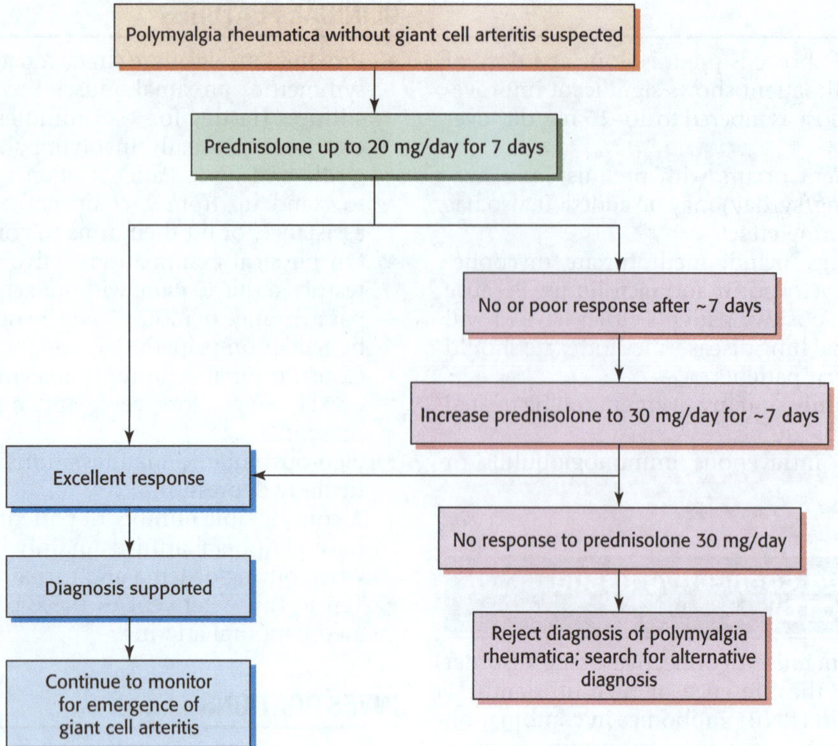

Flowchart 9.3 Algorithm for Diagnosing and Treating Polymyalgia Rheumatica. (From: Firestein GS et. al: Kelly's textbook of rheumatology, ed 9, Philadelphia, 2013, Saunders).

- The disease is characterised by the classic complex of fever, anaemia, high ESR and CRP and headache (usually temporal) in an elderly patient.
- The temporal artery may become tender, thickened and cord-like or nodular.
- Scalp pain and claudication of tongue and jaw are frequent.
- Visual symptoms including diplopia and even sudden blindness may result from ischaemic optic neuritis. The contralateral eye is often affected within 1–2 weeks, making prompt recognition and treatment critical.
- Involvement can extend to the aorta, its primary and secondary branches including subclavian and axillary arteries which leads to upper extremity ischaemia, absent or asymmetrical pulses and blood pressure readings.
- Neurological manifestations occur in about 30% of patients and include mononeuropathies, peripheral polyneuropathies of upper or lower extremities and, occasionally, transient ischaemic attacks and strokes.
- Thoracic aortic aneurysm or dissection is typically a late complication.
- The diagnosis is confirmed by biopsy of the temporal artery.
- Duplex ultrasonography can detect the characteristic appearance of a hypoechoic 'halo', occlusions and stenosis of temporal artery.
- CT angiography or MR angiography.
- FDG-PET imaging is useful for detection of vessel wall inflammation and diagnosis.
- This condition is exquisitely sensitive to corticosteroid therapy. Prednisolone is given at a dose of 40–60 mg/day. Dramatic response to a trial of prednisolone can confirm the diagnosis other than a temporal artery biopsy.
- Tocilizumab (IL-6 inhibitor) is approved as an alternative as steroid-sparing agent after initial control with prednisolone.

Q. Discuss the clinical features, diagnosis and management of classic polyarteritis nodosa (PAN).

- PAN is a multisystem, necrotising vasculitis of small- and medium-sized muscular arteries. The organ systems commonly involved are kidneys, heart, liver and gastrointestinal tract. PAN does not involve pulmonary arteries.
- Most cases of PAN are idiopathic, although hepatitis B or C virus infection and hairy cell leukaemia are important in the pathogenesis of some cases. Minocycline has also been implicated in some cases of PAN. Rarely, PAN can occur due to deficiency of adenosine deaminase-2.

CLINICAL FEATURES

- PAN predominantly affects males (M:F = 2.5:1).
- Common clinical manifestations are constitutional symptoms (fatigue, weight loss, weakness, fever), skin involvement, hypertension, renal failure, polyarthritis, myalgia, peripheral neuropathy and mononeuritis multiplex (Table 9.19).
  - Skin manifestations include tender erythematous nodules, palpable purpura and ulcers.

TABLE 9.19 Clinical Features of Polyarteritis Nodosa

• Systemic symptoms	Fever, malaise, weight loss
• Neuropathy	Mononeuritis multiplex, polyneuropathy
• Musculoskeletal	Arthralgias, myalgias, arthritis
• Skin	Palpable purpura, ulcers, erythematous nodules
• Kidneys	Hypertension, elevated creatinine, haematuria, glomerulonephritis
• Gastrointestinal symptoms	Diarrhoea, abdominal pain, rectal bleeding, intestinal ischaemia
• Central nervous system disease	Stroke
• Others	Peripheral vascular disease, cardiac ischaemia, pericarditis, myocarditis, testicular pain

- Renal involvement leads to renal ischaemia, infarcts, hypertension and renal insufficiency.
- Less commonly, clinical features result from involvement of gastrointestinal system, heart, genitourinary system and central nervous system.

DIAGNOSIS

- Anaemia, raised ESR and neutrophil leucocytosis.
- Thirty per cent of these patients are positive for hepatitis B surface antigen (HBsAg).
- p-ANCA is present in only about 20% of cases.
- Arteriograms usually reveal microaneurysms in the kidneys and abdominal viscera. Typically, they are saccular or fusiform, and 1–5 mm in diameter. CT and MR angiography are alternative to conventional angiography though they may not pick up smaller aneurysms.
- Characteristic finding of necrotising vasculitis on biopsy material of involved organ confirms the diagnosis.

TREATMENT

- Mild cases are treated with oral glucocorticoids (e.g. prednisolone 1 mg/kg daily).
- Various treatment modalities for severe cases include corticosteroids, cyclophosphamide and plasma exchange (see Microscopic Polyangiitis).
- For hepatitis-B associated PAN, combination of plasma exchange (to clear immune complexes) and antiviral agents (such as interferon α or lamivudine) is the standard treatment. Steroids should be used for short periods in critically ill patients.
- Tumour necrosis factor inhibitors are the treatment of choice for PAN associated with adenosine deaminase-2 deficiency.

Q. Describe microscopic polyangiitis.

- It is the most common antineutrophil cytoplasmic autoantibody (ANCA)-associated, necrotising, small vessel vasculitis and is characterised by absence of immune deposits in the involved vessels. Other ANCA-associated, necrotising small vessel vasculitis include granulomatosis with polyangiitis (GPA) and eosinophilic granulomatosis with polyangiitis (EGPA).

CLINICAL FEATURES

- The most common age of onset is 40–60 years. It is more common in males compared to in females.
- Upper and lower respiratory tracts, and the kidneys are most commonly affected.
- Presentation is by variable combinations of renal involvement, malaise, low-grade fever, weight loss, palpable purpura, abdominal pain, cough and haemoptysis.
- Kidney involvement is present in nearly 90% cases. It manifests in the form of microscopic haematuria with cellular casts in combination with proteinuria and rapidly progressive glomerulonephritis.
- Pulmonary haemorrhage (diffuse alveolar haemorrhage) is a very serious condition particularly in those patients who also have rapidly progressive glomerulonephritis (pulmonary-renal syndrome).
- Others: mononeuritis multiplex, sensorineural hearing loss, sinusitis, otitis media, purulent/bloody nasal discharge, skin purpura.

DIAGNOSIS

- Most patients have positive p-ANCA, although c-ANCA may also be present in 40% of cases.
- Urine for proteinuria and casts.
- Chest radiograph and computed tomography to look for lung involvement.
- Histological confirmation by skin biopsy, kidney biopsy (ranging from mild focal and segmental glomerulonephritis to diffuse necrotising and crescentic glomerulonephritis with few or no immune deposits) and occasionally, lung or nasal biopsy.

TREATMENT

- Combined treatment with cyclophosphamide and corticosteroids has reduced mortality and morbidity significantly.
- In severe cases, high-dose (500–1000 mg) intravenous methylprednisolone for 3 days combined with intravenous cyclophosphamide (500–1000 mg/m^2 body surface area) is recommended to induce remission. The regimen is repeated once every 4 weeks, though pulses of steroids can be repeated after 1 week.
- In severe cases (e.g. renal failure or diffuse alveolar haemorrhage), additional use of plasma exchange is beneficial. It may not be of value in patients with eosinophilic granulomatosis with polyangiitis (Churg–Strauss syndrome) and PAN.
- Maintenance is with tapering doses of steroids along with oral cyclophosphamide for 12–18 months. Methotrexate, azathioprine or rituximab can replace cyclophosphamide after initial remission of disease to complete 18 months of treatment.

Q. Discuss eosinophilic granulomatosis with polyangiitis.

Q. Describe Churg–Strauss syndrome.

- Eosinophilic granulomatosis with polyangiitis (EGPA), previously called Churg–Strauss syndrome (CSS) or allergic granulomatous angiitis, is a rare syndrome that affects small- and medium-sized arteries and veins.
- It is a systemic disorder characterised by asthma, transient pulmonary infiltrates, hypereosinophilia and a systemic vasculitis.

CLINICAL FEATURES

- The patient has a history of asthma and allergic rhinitis that is followed by small vessel vasculitis and granulomatous inflammation.
- Unlike in classical bronchial asthma, in CSS, asthma does not show the typical seasonal exacerbations.
- Almost 40% of patients present with pulmonary opacities, asthma and peripheral eosinophilia prior to the development of systemic vasculitis (polyangiitis).
- The vasculitic phase usually develops within 8–10 years of onset of asthma.
- Vasculitis, granuloma and eosinophilia may involve any organ system including lung, CNS, kidney, lymph nodes, muscle and skin. Common features are listed in Box 9.16.
- EGPA is typically suspected in patients whose asthma is poorly controlled on moderate doses of inhaled glucocorticoids.

INVESTIGATIONS

- Eosinophils >10% in peripheral blood.
- Elevated ESR and CRP.
- Urine showing RBC casts and proteinuria.
- Increased IgE levels.
- Positive antinuclear cytoplasmic antibodies against myeloperoxidase (p-ANCA) in 30%–60% of cases.
- Chest X-ray and CT chest may show infiltrates, miliary opacities, bilateral nodular disease without cavitation, and pleural effusion.

BOX 9.16 Clinical Features of Eosinophilic Granulomatosis With Polyangiitis

- Arthralgias and arthritis
- Purpura, tender subcutaneous nodules on the extensor surfaces of elbows, hands and legs
- Peripheral, patchy, migratory infiltrates in the lungs
- Serous otitis media, nasal obstruction, recurrent sinusitis, nasal polyposis
- Heart failure, pericarditis, myocardial infarction
- Abdominal pain, diarrhoea, GI bleed
- Mononeuritis multiplex
- Deep vein thrombosis, pulmonary embolism
- Isolated urinary abnormalities (microscopic haematuria, proteinuria), rapidly progressive glomerulonephritis
- Stroke
- Coronary arteritis, myocarditis (principal causes of morbidity and mortality)

BOX 9.17 Diagnostic Criteria[a] for Eosinophilic Granulomatosis With Polyangiitis

- Asthma
- Eosinophilia greater than 10% on a differential WBC count
- Mononeuropathy or polyneuropathy
- Nonfixed pulmonary infiltrates
- Paranasal sinus abnormalities
- Biopsy containing a blood vessel with extravascular granulomas

Note: To be used in patients with documented vasculitis.
[a]The finding of four of the six criteria has a sensitivity of 85% and a specificity of >99%.

- Histopathology of involved tissues (e.g. skin, nerves) showing necrotising vasculitis.

DIAGNOSTIC CRITERIA

- Box 9.17 gives the diagnostic criteria for eosinophilic granulomatosis with polyangiitis.

TREATMENT

- Most patients respond to high-dose steroids, though some cases may require addition of cytotoxic drugs like cyclophosphamide. Moderately severe cases may require addition of methotrexate or azathioprine to steroids.
- If response to steroids is not good, mepolizumab (anti-IL-5) may be added.
- In severe cases, anti-TNF-α agents like infliximab and etanercept may be used.

Q. Write briefly on clinical features, diagnosis and treatment of Wegener's granulomatosis or granulomatosis with polyangiitis.

- Granulomatosis with polyangiitis (formerly called Wegener's granulomatosis) is an idiopathic vasculitis of medium and small arteries characterised by granulomatous vasculitis of upper and lower respiratory tracts together with glomerulonephritis.

CLINICAL FEATURES

- Constitutional symptoms including fever, migratory arthralgias, malaise, anorexia and weight loss.
- Paranasal sinus pain and discharge, nasal mucosal ulcerations, saddle nose deformity and hearing loss.
- Pulmonary involvement may produce hoarseness, cough, haemoptysis, wheezing and dyspnoea.
- Renal involvement occurs in the form of glomerulonephritis resulting in proteinuria, haematuria and red blood cell casts in the urine. Rapidly progressive glomerulonephritis and acute renal failure may occur.
- Other manifestations are palpable purpurae, conjunctivitis, episcleritis, scleritis, cranial neuritis and mononeuritis multiplex.

DIAGNOSIS

- The ESR is markedly elevated.
- Other nonspecific abnormalities include mild anaemia, leucocytosis and mild hypergammaglobulinaemia.

- Chest radiograph may reveal patchy or diffuse pulmonary opacities, fleeting pulmonary infiltrates and nodules that may cavitate.
- A CT scan of chest may reveal many cavitating nodules not visible on plain chest X-ray.
- A CT scan of the sinuses may reveal mucosal thickening, bone destruction and infiltration of the orbits.
- Serum antiproteinase 3 (c-ANCA) is positive in nearly 95% of cases.
- The diagnosis can be confirmed by lung biopsy which will show the characteristic necrotising granulomatous vasculitis. Renal biopsy shows a segmental necrotising crescentic glomerulonephritis with no immunoglobulin deposition ('pauci-immune').

TREATMENT

- Treatment is similar to that for microscopic polyangiitis.

Q. Define and classify vasculitis.

- Vasculitis is a clinicopathological process characterised by inflammation of blood vessel walls and the surrounding interstitium.
- May affect large-, medium- or small-sized arteries, arterioles, venules or veins.
  - The large vessels include the aorta and its largest branches (clinically affecting the extremities and head/neck).
  - The medium-sized vessels refer to the main visceral arteries (e.g. renal, hepatic, coronary, mesenteric).
  - The small vessels refer to the capillaries, venules and arterioles.
- Small-vessel vasculitis may be associated with autoantibodies.

CLASSIFICATION (Table 9.20 and Fig. 9.16)

- Leucocytoclastic vasculitis is a histopathological diagnosis given to cutaneous, small vessel vasculitis.
- Most often idiopathic but can be seen with infections, neoplasms, inflammatory disorders and drugs.
- Key clinical features include palpable purpura with lower extremity location.
- Extracutaneous involvement (low-grade fevers, malaise, weight loss, myalgias and arthralgias) seen in approximately 30% of patients.
- Most are self-limiting.

CLINICAL FEATURES

- Clinical features of various vasculitides are given in Table 9.21.

TABLE 9.21 Clinical Features of Various Vasculitides

Large Vessel Vasculitis	Medium Vessel Vasculitis	Small Vessel Vasculitis
Asymmetric	Skin nodules and ulcers	Purpura
Hypertension	Livedo reticularis	Glomerulonephritis
Absence of pulses	Digital gangrene	Alveolar haemorrhage
Presence of bruits	Renovascular hypertension	Necrotising granuloma
Aortic dilatation	Haematuria	Peripheral neuropathy
Jaw claudication	Mononeuritis multiplex	Mononeuritis multiplex
Visual loss	Microaneurysms	

Q. Discuss briefly the clinical features associated with small vessel vasculitis. What are the laboratory investigations in a case with vasculitis? How do you treat it?

- Small vessel vasculitis is defined as vasculitis that affects vessels smaller than arteries (i.e. arterioles, venules and capillaries).

TABLE 9.20 Classification of Vasculitis

Large Vessel Vasculitis	Small Vessel Vasculitis	
• Takayasu's disease • Giant cell arteritis (temporal arteritis) **Medium Vessel Vasculitis** • Polyarteritis nodosa (PAN) • Kawasaki's disease • Primary CNS vasculitis • Buerger disease	***ANCA-associated*** • Granulomatosis with polyangiitis (Wegener's granulomatosis) • Microscopic polyangiitis • Eosinophilic granulomatosis with polyangiitis (Churg–Strauss syndrome) • Drug-induced vasculitis (cefotaxime, minocycline, carbimazole, methimazole, propylthiouracil, adalimumab, etanercept, infliximab, clozapine, thioridazine, allopurinol, D-penicillamine, hydralazine, levamisole, phenytoin and sulphasalazine)	***Non-ANCA-associated*** *Immune complex deposition (hypersensitivity vasculitis or leucocytoclastic vasculitis)* • Henoch–Schönlein purpura • SLE • RA • Mixed cryoglobulinaemia • Goodpasture's syndrome • Behcet's disease *Others (can also cause leucocytoclastic vasculitis)* • Drug-induced vasculitis • Infection-induced vasculitis • Inflammatory bowel disease

ANCA, antineutrophil cytoplasmic antibodies.

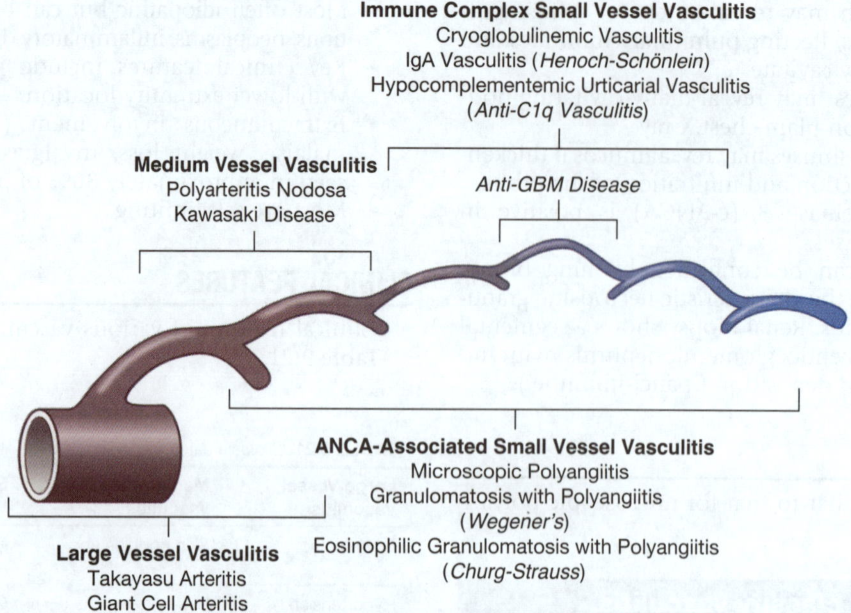

Fig. 9.16 The updated 2012 Chapel Hill Consensus Conference Classification of Vasculitis (From: Jennette JC, Falk RJ, Bacon PA, et al: 2012 revised International Chapel Hill Consensus Conference Nomenclature of Vasculitides. Arthritis Rheum 2013;65:1-11).

TABLE 9.22 Clinical Features of Small Vessel Vasculitis

• Constitutional features	Fever, anorexia, malaise, weight loss
• Musculoskeletal features	Myalgias, arthralgias, arthritis
• Skin	Palpable purpura, urticaria
• Kidneys	Haematuria, proteinuria, renal failure, necrotising glomerulonephritis (in ANCA-positive cases)
• Nervous system	Peripheral neuropathy, cranial nerve involvement, mononeuritis multiplex
• Cardiovascular system	Hypertension
• Respiratory system	Cough, haemoptysis, dyspnoea, lung infiltrates, diffuse alveolar haemorrhage

CLINICAL FEATURES

- Clinical features of small vessel vasculitis are given in Table 9.22.

LABORATORY INVESTIGATIONS

- Haemoglobin, total and differential leucocyte count, platelet count and ESR.
- Routine chemistry profile.
- Urinalysis.
- Chest radiograph and paranasal sinus radiograph.
- Antinuclear antibodies, rheumatoid factor, ANCA and cryoglobulins.
- Antibody to hepatitis B and C.
- ELISA for human immunodeficiency virus.
- Other tests depend on clinical circumstances and include nerve conduction velocity, nerve biopsy, angiography, skin biopsy and kidney biopsy.

MANAGEMENT

- It depends on the underlying cause of vasculitis.
- Most commonly used drugs include corticosteroids, azathioprine, cyclophosphamide and other immunosuppressants.

Q. What are antineutrophil cytoplasmic antibodies (ANCA)? Discuss their significance.

- ANCA are specific antibodies against antigens in cytoplasmic granules of neutrophils and lysosomes of monocytes.
- Two major patterns of staining are seen:
  - Cytoplasmic ANCA (c-ANCA) are mainly antibodies to proteinase 3.
  - Perinuclear ANCA (p-ANCA) are antibodies to myeloperoxidase.
- For their significance in small vessel vasculitis, ANCA should be assayed with indirect immunofluorescence (screening test) and then with direct ELISA for proteinase-3 or myeloperoxidase.
- Significance:
  - A number of conditions are associated with ANCA positivity (see above).
  - ANCA is present in majority of patients with microscopic polyangiitis, granulomatosis with polyangiitis (Wegener's granulomatosis) and eosinophilic granulomatosis with polyangiitis (Churg–Strauss syndrome). However, a negative ANCA does not exclude these diagnoses. Similarly, a positive ANCA assay is not solely diagnostic of ANCA-associated diseases.
  - ANCA detected by indirect immunofluorescence may be seen in RA, Felty's syndrome, SLE, ulcerative colitis, chronic hepatitis, primary sclerosing

cholangitis, HIV infection, active tuberculosis and subacute bacterial endocarditis.

Q. Discuss the aetiology, clinical manifestations, diagnosis and management of gout.

Q. Give a brief account of the various causes, clinical manifestations, investigations and management of hyperuricaemia. (IM 7.21)

AETIOLOGY OF GOUT AND HYPERURICAEMIA

- Various causes of hyperuricaemia and gout are given in Table 9.23.

CLINICAL FEATURES

- The full natural history of gout comprises four stages:
  1. Asymptomatic hyperuricaemia.
  2. Acute gouty arthritis.
  3. Intercritical period.
  4. Chronic tophaceous gout (tophi and chronic gouty arthritis).
- The onset may be insidious or explosively sudden. Most often, onset to peak intensity of pain is less than 12 hours. Triggers for gout flares include meals high in purine, alcohol intake, joint trauma and acute illness.
- The metatarsophalangeal joint of the great toe is the site of the first attack of acute gouty arthritis (podagra) in 70% of patients.
- Other joints that can get affected include tarsal joints, ankles, knees and wrists. Central joints such as hips, shoulders and spine are seldom affected, possibly because higher temperatures in these joints are not conducive to crystallisation.
- The affected joint is hot, red and swollen with shiny overlying skin and dilated veins. The joint is excruciatingly painful and tender. These joint manifestations may be associated with anorexia, nausea, fever, leucocytosis and raised ESR.

TABLE 9.23 Aetiology of Gout and Hyperuricaemia

Increased Production of Uric Acid	Decreased Renal Excretion of Uric Acid
• Increased purine synthesis de novo • Hypoxanthine-guanine phosphoribosyl transferase (HGPRT) deficiency • Phosphoribosyl pyrophosphate (PRPP) synthetase overactivity • Glucose-6-phosphatase deficiency • Idiopathic • Increased turnover of purines • Myeloproliferative disorders • Lymphoproliferative disorders • Cancer chemotherapy • Haemolysis	• Renal failure • Lead poisoning • Alcohol • Drugs—diuretics, low-dose aspirin, pyrazinamide, cyclosporin, levodopa • Lactic acidosis • Hyperparathyroidism • Myxoedema • Down's syndrome • Unidentified inherited defects

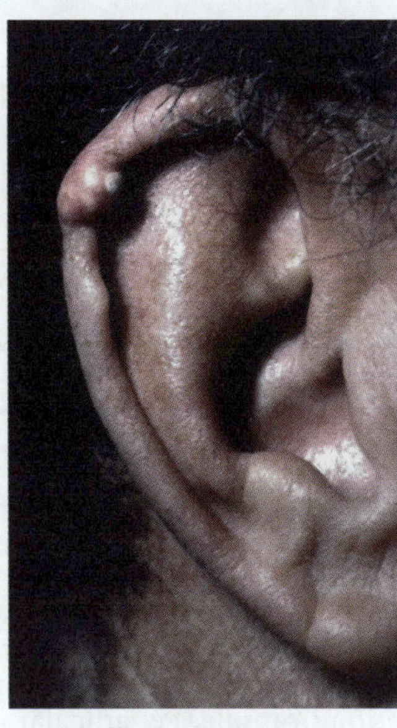

Fig. 9.17 Tophus.

- The joint manifestations may last only 1 or 2 days, or up to several weeks but characteristically subside spontaneously.
- Gout can also cause bursitis and tenosynovitis.
- This is followed by an asymptomatic phase (intercritical period) that is diagnostically important.
- In chronic tophaceous gouty arthritis, crystal deposits appear in cartilage, synovial membranes, tendons and soft tissues. The classic location of a tophus is the helix and antihelix of the ear (Fig. 9.17).

NEPHROPATHY

- Nephropathy is seen in 90% of subjects with gouty arthritis. Two types of parenchymal renal damage have been described:
  - Urate nephropathy results from deposition of urate crystals in the interstitial tissue, leading to albuminuria, isosthenuria or renal failure.
  - Obstructive uropathy (nephrolithiasis) results from the formation of uric acid crystals in the collecting tubules, renal pelvis or ureter with blockage of urine flow. The formation of urate calculi is favoured by hyperuricosuria, purine overproduction, excessive purine ingestion, uricosuric drugs and acidic urine.

OTHER FEATURES

- Gout may be associated with increased incidence of hypertension and cardiovascular disorders.
- On the other hand, hypertension is also a risk factor for development of gout.

DIAGNOSIS (Box 9.18)

- Serum uric acid levels are elevated. However, during an acute attack, serum uric acid may be normal in 50% cases.
- Synovial fluid examination done by compensated polarised microscopy can demonstrate urate crystals. They are seen as slender, needle-shaped and negatively birefringent structures.

BOX 9.18 Cardinal Features of Gout

- Increase in serum uric acid concentration (>7.0 mg/dL in males and >6.0 mg/dL in females)
- Recurrent attacks of a characteristic acute arthritis in which crystals of monosodium urate monohydrate are demonstrable in leucocytes of synovial fluid
- Aggregated deposits of monosodium urate monohydrate (tophi) in and around the joints
- Renal disease involving interstitial tissue and blood vessels
- Uric acid nephrolithiasis

- Plain radiographs are helpful to differentiate chronic tophaceous gout from RA.
    - Erosions in gout are characteristically punched out with overhanging sclerotic margins and are situated away from joint margins, sometimes outside the joint capsule. Periarticular osteopenia is absent and joint space is preserved in gout.
    - RA causes marginal erosions, always within the limits of the joint capsule.

MANAGEMENT

TREATMENT OF ACUTE ATTACK

- NSAIDs are the agents of choice. All NSAIDs are equally effective. Commonly used NSAIDs are indomethacin (50 mg 6 hourly), naproxen and fenoprofen.
- Colchicine is the second choice of drug. It is highly effective at a dose of 1.0 mg stat followed by 0.5 mg hourly till symptoms subside or GI side effects (vomiting and diarrhoea) occur or a total of 4 mg of colchicine has been given. To avoid toxic effects, another regimen is 1 mg stat followed by 0.5 mg two to three times a day.
- If patient does not tolerate NSAIDs or colchicine, intraarticular corticosteroids may be tried if a medium or large joint is involved.
- In patients with polyarticular involvement not responding to NSAIDs or colchicine, prednisolone 20–30 mg/day with tapering over 7–10 days is effective.
- Drug therapy for lowering uric acid may be started during an acute attack if effective antiinflammatory management has been instituted.

PROPHYLAXIS

- Avoidance of alcohol.
- Avoidance of meat and seafood. However, consumption of oatmeal and purine-rich vegetables (e.g. peas, beans, lentils, spinach, mushrooms and cauliflower) does not produce increased risk of gout.
- Controlled weight reduction in obese patients.
- Avoiding use of thiazides or loop diuretics, calcineurin inhibitors and niacin.

Drugs for Prophylaxis

- Sixty-two per cent of patients experience a second episode within 1 year and 78% within 2 years, while 7% have no further episode for 10 years even without antihyperuricaemic drugs.
- Antihyperuricaemic drugs are therefore appropriate under the following circumstances:
    - Two or more flares per year.
    - Chronic tophaceous gout.
    - Radiological erosions.
    - Urate calculi.
    - Asymptomatic patients with urinary urate excretion >1100 mg/24 hours (there is a 50% chance of developing renal calculi in these patients).
    - Persistently raised serum urate (>13 mg/dL in males and >10 mg/dL in females) as there is high risk of urate nephropathy.
- Goal of prophylactic therapy is to lower uric acid to below 6 mg/dL.
- Allopurinol reduces uric acid production through competitive inhibition of xanthine oxidase, which converts xanthine and hypoxanthine to uric acid. Its dose is 300–900 mg daily.
    - Allopurinol is generally well tolerated, but a rash requiring cessation of therapy occurs in 1%–2% of patients. In addition, it can rarely cause potentially life-threatening allopurinol hypersensitivity syndrome, characterised by severe cutaneous reactions (Stevens-Johnson syndrome or toxic epidermal necrolysis), acute kidney injury, hepatitis and eosinophilia.
- Febuxostat is a nonpurine selective inhibitor of xanthine oxidase. Dose is 40–120 mg/day. However, an increased risk of cardiovascular and all-cause mortality has been found with compared to allopurinol, although a study conducted later did not find these results.
- Uricosuric agents like probenecid and sulphinpyrazone are indicated in selected cases (when uric acid excretion in the urine is below 600 mg/day). Uricosuric drugs are risky if urinary urate excretion is already >800 mg/24 hours. These are contraindicated in those with urate calculi. Uricosurics are ineffective in renal impairment (creatinine clearance <50 mL/minute).
- Uricase is an enzyme which converts uric acid into soluble allantoin. Pegloticase, a polyethylene-glycolated modified porcine recombinant uricase, may be used in chronic gout refractory to conventional treatments. It is given intravenously every 15 days. Rasburicase, another uricase, is approved for use in preventing tumour lysis syndrome.

Q. Describe pseudogout, calcium pyrophosphate dihydrate (CPPD) deposition disease or pyrophosphate arthropathy.

- In this disease, CPPD crystal deposition occurs in fibrous and articular cartilage. Release of CPPD crystals into the joint space provokes an acute attack of synovitis—'pseudogout'.
- Conditions associated with CPPD include primary hyperparathyroidism, haemochromatosis, chronic tophaceous gout and others.
- Mostly asymptomatic; identified as an incidental finding on radiographs.
- The knee is the most frequently affected joint. Other sites include wrist, shoulder, ankle, elbow and hands. Acute attacks of pseudogout may be precipitated by trauma, joint surgery, sprain or even a long walk.

- Chronic pyrophosphate arthropathy resembles osteoarthritis involving knees, wrists, metacarpophalangeal joints (particularly second and third), shoulders and hips.

DIAGNOSIS

- Radiographs of joints may show chondrocalcinosis (calcification of articular fibrocartilage or hyaline cartilage) that occurs due to CPPD deposition.
- Ultrasound may be more sensitive than plain radiography of joints in picking up CPPD deposition.
- CPPD crystals can be demonstrated in synovial fluid or articular tissue by polarising microscopy. They are seen as rod- or rhomboid-shaped weakly positive birefringent crystals.

TREATMENT

- Various treatment modalities are joint aspiration, NSAIDs, intraarticular corticosteroids and colchicine.

10 Acute Poisoning and Environmental Emergencies

Q. Describe briefly the management of a patient who has ingested a poison. (IM21.1)

Q. What are antidotes? (IM21.1)

- Kerosene oil and pesticides are the most common poisons in childhood poisoning, while in adults, pesticides, particularly insecticides (organophosphates and carbamates), are most often involved in poisoning.
- Management requires several complementary steps. Besides the first two steps, other steps are followed concurrently and not sequentially. These are given in Box 10.1.

RESUSCITATION AND INITIAL STABILISATION

- The initial priorities are the maintenance of airway, breathing and circulation.
- Airway should be secured early in case of caustic ingestion. In case of altered level of consciousness, cervical spine should be immobilised while opening the airway.
- Breathing may require assistance in presence of hypoventilation or acute respiratory distress syndrome (ARDS).
- Hypotension should be treated first with crystalloids as it is most often due to loss of fluids or toxin-induced vasodilatation. Be careful in patients who have ingested beta-blockers or calcium channel blockers as these agents have negative inotropic effect on myocardium and infusing lot of fluids may precipitate heart failure. Cardiac arrhythmias should be first treated by correcting associated electrolyte and metabolic disturbances, and administration of an antidote. For cardiovascular complications due to prolonged QRS interval, sodium bicarbonate should be administered, while for prolonged QT interval, magnesium sulphate should be administered.
- Before infusing fluids, blood should be collected for investigations including sugar, urea, electrolytes and acid–base status, and toxicological investigations.
- Blood glucose should be checked by a bedside method in all patients with altered level of consciousness. Hypertonic dextrose (50%) should be infused only if the blood glucose is below 80 mg/dL.
- Toxin-induced seizures are best treated with benzodiazepines (diazepam, lorazepam and midazolam). Second-line agents include phenobarbitone and propofol. For isoniazid-induced seizures, pyridoxine in high doses should be given. Phenytoin has no role in toxin-induced seizures.
- If the patient is in altered sensorium and has miosis or respiratory depression, naloxone (an opioid antagonist) should be given empirically. In view of

BOX 10.1 Steps in Managing a Patient With Acute Poisoning

- Remove the patient from the site of external exposure (e.g. exposure to gas) and decontaminate after removing clothes (avoiding self-contamination).
- Resuscitation and initial stabilisation.
- Diagnosis of type of poison by history, examination and laboratory investigations.
- Nonspecific therapy to reduce the levels of toxin in the body.
- Specific therapy to reduce the toxic effects on the body (use of antidotes).
- Supportive care to support the functions of vital organs.

possibility of precipitating withdrawal reaction, naloxone is generally given in a dose of 0.1 mg initially unless the patient has respiratory severe depression when a loading dose of 2 mg is justified. If there is no response to 0.1 mg and there is no feature of opioid withdrawal, the dose is increased to 0.4–2 mg that is given every 2–3 minutes for a total of 10 mg.
- Thiamine can be used in patients with altered sensorium if the patient is malnourished or an alcoholic.
- Flumazenil, a benzodiazepine antagonist, is not recommended for empiric use in patients with altered level of consciousness.
- Rectal temperature should be obtained in all patients with altered sensorium to exclude hypothermia or hyperthermia.

DIAGNOSIS OF TYPE OF TOXIN

- This is based on history, examination and simple laboratory investigations.

TOXIDROMES

- Based on history and examination findings, it may be possible to define a syndrome associated with certain poisons. This is known as toxidrome. Various toxidromes are listed in Table 10.1, and Table 10.2 compares clinical features among various toxidromes.

SIMPLE LABORATORY TESTS

- Colour of urine: A pinkish colour of urine occurs in phenothiazine intoxication as well as in myoglobinuria and haemoglobinuria.
- Colour of blood: Chocolate-coloured blood is indicative of methaemoglobinaemia.
- Crystals in urine (in ethylene glycol poisoning).
- Ketonuria (in salicylate poisoning).
- Anion gap (normal 10–14 mmol/L):
  - Mnemonic for increased anion gap is MUDPILES (Table 10.3).
  - Low anion gap is seen in lithium and bromide poisoning, hypoalbuminaemia and multiple myeloma.

TABLE 10.1 Toxidromes

Toxidrome	Clinical Features	Examples
• Cholinergic	Muscarinic features (DUMBELS): Diarrhoea; urinary incontinence; miosis; bradycardia, bronchorrhoea and bronchospasm; emesis; lacrimation, low blood pressure; salivation and sweating Nicotinic features: Abdominal cramps, hypertension, fasciculations, muscle weakness, respiratory muscle weakness CNS features: Confusion, coma, seizures	Carbamates and organophosphates, nicotine, nerve agents (sarin, soman, tabun, VX)
• Anticholinergic	Dry, flushed skin, dry mucous membranes, urine retention, reduced bowel sounds, abnormal movements, picking at objects, mydriasis (nonreactive pupils), hypertension, tachycardia, hyperthermia, hallucinations, delirium, seizures	Datura, antidepressants, antihistamines, phenothiazines
• Narcotic	Miosis, CNS depression, coma, bradycardia, hypothermia, respiratory depression	Opioids
• Sympathomimetic	Sweating, tremors, tachycardia, hypertension, hyperthermia, mydriasis (reactive pupils), tachypnoea, agitation, hyperalert, seizures	Amphetamines, cocaine, ephedrine, theophylline, caffeine
• Sedative-hypnotic	CNS depression, confusion, stupor, coma, bradycardia, hypotension, hypopnoea, miosis, hyporeflexia	Barbiturates, benzodiazepines
• Hallucinogenic	Hallucinations, depersonalisation, agitation, hyperthermia, tachycardia, hypertension, nystagmus, mydriasis	Phencyclidine, lysergic acid diethylamide (LSD)

TABLE 10.2 Comparison of Clinical Features in Various Toxidromes

Toxidrome	Pulse	Blood Pressure	Respiratory Rate	Temperature	Pupils	Skin	Mental Status
Cholinergic	↓ or ↑	↓, N or ↑	↑	N or ↓	Miosis	Wet	Depressed, confused, seizures
Anticholinergic	↑	↑	N	↑	Mydriasis (nonreactive)	Dry	Confusion, delirium, seizures
Narcotic	↓	↓	↓	↓ or N	Miosis	N	Depressed, coma
Sympathomimetic	↑	↑	N or ↑	↑	Mydriasis (reactive)	Wet	Agitated, seizures
Sedative-hypnotic	N or ↓	N or ↓	N or ↓	N or ↓	N or miosis	N	Depressed, coma
Hallucinogenic	↑	↑	N or ↑	N or ↑	N or mydriasis	N or wet	Confused, hallucinations

N = normal

TABLE 10.3 Causes of Increased Anion Gap

• M	**M**ethanol, **M**etformin and **M**assive ingestions
• U	**U**raemia
• D	**D**iabetic, alcoholic and starvation ketosis
• P	**P**aracetamol
• I	**I**soniazid and **I**ron
• L	**L**actic acidosis
• E	**E**thylene glycol
• S	**S**alicylate poisoning

- Osmolal gap is the difference between the measured osmolality and calculated osmolality and is normally <10 mOsm/kg. Osmolal gap is elevated in patients with ethanol, methanol, ethylene glycol and isopropanol poisoning. Calculated osmolality is derived as follows:

  Calculated osmolality = 2 × Na^+ + serum glucose (mg/dL)/18 + blood urea nitrogen (mg/dL)/2.8

NONSPECIFIC TREATMENT

- It includes removal of unabsorbed poison from the gut (gut decontamination) and increasing the excretion of absorbed poison from the body.
- Gut decontamination includes induction of emesis, gastric lavage, use of activated charcoal and cathartics and whole bowel irrigation.
- Gastric emptying includes induction of emesis and gastric lavage.

REMOVING UNABSORBED POISON FROM GUT (GASTROINTESTINAL DECONTAMINATION)

- It is recommended that gut decontamination should not be performed unless a patient has ingested a potentially lethal amount of a toxin within the last 60 minutes. However, many physicians perform it up to 2 hours after ingestion.
- Before performing a procedure for gut decontamination, consider three factors:
  - Whether the ingestion is potentially dangerous.
  - Can the procedure remove a significant amount of toxin?
  - Whether the benefits of a procedure outweigh its risks.
- If the patient has ingested a nontoxic agent or nontoxic dose of a toxic agent, or if he/she is free of symptoms despite passage of time during which the toxin is known to produce features of toxicity, do not perform a gut decontamination procedure.
- Gut decontamination is also not indicated if the patient had prior repeated vomiting, the toxin is absorbed rapidly or the patient presents late after ingestion.
- If the risks of a procedure outweigh the possible benefits, gastric emptying should be avoided (e.g. ingestion of volatile hydrocarbons where risk of aspiration is present and caustics where risk of perforation is high).
- If the patient has ingested a high-risk toxin (cyanide and paracetamol), gastric emptying is indicated even if he/she is asymptomatic.

INDUCTION OF EMESIS

- Syrup of ipecac is used to induce emesis with the intention to remove the poison from the stomach. Vomiting occurs within 30 minutes of ingestion of ipecac.
- At present, it is not indicated in any patient due to several limitations.
- It is contraindicated in:
  - Comatose patients.
  - Patients with seizures.
  - Patients likely to deteriorate rapidly.
  - Patients who have ingested hydrocarbons or corrosives.

GASTRIC LAVAGE

- For orogastric lavage, the patient should be in a left lateral position with the head lower than the feet so as to avoid aspiration. If a patient is unconscious, intubate the patient before passing a lavage tube.
- Gastric lavage may be considered in a patient who has ingested a potentially life-threatening amount of a toxic agent within the past 60 minutes. It may also be used within 2–4 hours of ingestion of chemical poisons but its utility in such situations has not been proven.
- Lavage is contraindicated following ingestion of strong caustics, nontoxic agents and volatile hydrocarbons unless they contain a toxic agent.

CATHARTICS

- Commonly used cathartics are magnesium sulphate, sorbitol and magnesium citrate.
- Repetitive doses of these agents should be avoided.
- There are no data to support their efficacy and their use is not recommended at present.

ACTIVATED CHARCOAL

- Activated charcoal has enormous surface area and can adsorb large amounts of chemicals.
- The usual dose is 1 g/kg body weight or 10 parts of charcoal for every 1 part of toxin, whichever is greater.
- Activated charcoal is contraindicated in patients with unprotected airway and caustic ingestion.
- Activated charcoal is not effective in adsorbing lithium, iron, DDT, methanol, ethanol, metals and hydrocarbons.

WHOLE BOWEL IRRIGATION

- For whole bowel irrigation, isotonic solution of polyethylene glycol electrolytes in a dose of 2 L/hour is used orally for 4–6 hours or till the rectal effluent is clear.
- The components of this solution are not absorbed through the intestines; instead, it flushes the gut mechanically.
- At present, there are no established indications for the use of whole bowel irrigation.
- It is an option for potentially toxic ingestions of sustained-release drugs, enteric-coated drugs, iron, lead and drug packets (body packer syndrome).
- It is contraindicated in patients with bowel obstruction, perforation and ileus, and in patients with haemodynamic instability or compromised unprotected airways.

ENHANCEMENT OF EXCRETION OF TOXIN

- Important methods for enhancing excretion are forced diuresis, alteration in urinary pH, multiple doses of charcoal, peritoneal and haemodialysis, haemoperfusion, haemofiltration and exchange transfusion.

Forced Diuresis

- Infusing large amount of intravenous fluids along with diuretics in order to possibly increase toxin excretion is not recommended and should not be practiced.

Urine Alkalinisation

- Urinary alkalinisation is useful in salicylates, phenobarbital, chlorpropamide and 2,4-D intoxication.
- For this, 5% dextrose containing 20–35 mEq/L of bicarbonate is infused at a rate so as to produce a urine pH 7.5–8.5. To prevent hypokalaemia, potassium is added in every second or third bottle.
- Diuresis is not required in most cases (except 2,4-D poisoning) as simple urinary alkalinisation is sufficient to enhance the excretion of these toxins.
- During alkalinisation, monitor vitals of the patient along with input/output, electrolytes and acid–base status.
- It is contraindicated in patients with shock, hypotension, renal failure and congestive heart failure.

Multiple-Dose Activated Charcoal (MDAC)

- When multiple doses of activated charcoal are administered, free charcoal remains in the intestines to bind any toxin that has significant enterohepatic circulation.
- Free toxin in the blood also tends to diffuse out of the blood into the intestines where it binds the charcoal, thereby maintaining the concentration of free toxin in the intestines near zero (gastrointestinal dialysis).
- Depending on the severity of poisoning, the dose is 0.5–1 g/kg body weight every 1–4 hours.
- May be useful in patients with ingestion of carbamazepine, dapsone, phenobarbital, quinine and theophylline.

Dialysis

- Haemodialysis is useful in:
  - Toxins with high water solubility and low molecular weight.
  - Toxin with low volume of distribution.
  - Toxin with low serum protein binding.
  - Toxin not irreversibly bound to the tissues.
- Dialysis is useful in methanol, salicylate, theophylline, ethylene glycol, phenobarbitone and lithium intoxications.

SPECIFIC THERAPY

- If the toxin can be identified, administer specific therapy using antidotes (Table 10.4).

SUPPORTIVE THERAPY

- As antidotes are available only for a few toxins, the treatment of most of the cases with poisoning is largely supportive.
- The aim of the supportive treatment is to preserve the vital organ functions till poison is eliminated

TABLE 10.4 Antidotes

Poison	Antidotes
Cholinesterase inhibitors (organophosphates, carbamates)	• Atropine
Organophosphates	• 2-PAM (controversial role)
Opioids	• Naloxone
Hypoglycaemia induced by toxins	• Dextrose
Tricyclic antidepressants, other sodium channel blockers	• Sodium bicarbonate
Methaemoglobinaemia-producing agents	• Methylene blue
Methanol, ethylene glycol	• Ethanol
Snakebites	• Snake antivenin
Iron	• Desferrioxamine
Lead, arsenic, mercury	• BAL (dimercaprol)
Lead	• Calcium disodium edetate
Mercury, lead, arsenic	• D-penicillamine
Lead, mercury, arsenic	• 2,3-Dimercaptosuccinic acid
Methanol, ethylene glycol	• Fomepizole (4-methylpyrazole)
Paracetamol	• *N*-acetylcysteine
Benzodiazepines	• Flumazenil
β-Blockers, calcium channel blockers	• Glucagon
Cyanide	• Cyanide kit
Isoniazid	• Pyridoxine
Digoxin	• Digoxin-specific Fab fragment
Local anaesthetic-induced systemic toxicity	• Intravenous lipid emulsion
β-Blockers, calcium channel blockers	• High-dose insulin

from the body and the patient resumes normal physiological functions.

- Therefore, support the functions of central nervous system (CNS), cardiopulmonary system and renal system with proper care for coma, seizures, hypotension, arrhythmias, hypoxia and acute renal failure.
- Monitor the fluid, electrolyte and acid–base status closely.
- Venoarterial extracorporeal membrane oxygenation (ECMO) may be used to improve survival in patients with refractory cardiac arrest.

Q. What are the commonly encountered poisonous snakes in your place? Discuss the clinical manifestations, diagnosis and management of snakebites. (IM20.1, IM20.2, IM20.3, IM20.7)

- Though the exact number of snakebites is unknown, an estimated 5.4 million people are bitten globally each year with up to 2.7 million envenoming.
- Around 81,000 to 138,000 people die each year because of snakebites. It is estimated that more than 50,000 people die due to snakebites in India.

TABLE 10.5 Classification of Poisonous Snakes

Family	Common Varieties
• Elapidae	Cobras, kraits, mambas, coral snakes
• Viperidae	Russell's viper, *E. carinatus* (saw-scaled viper)
• Colubridae	Boomslangs, bird snakes
• Crotalidae	Pit vipers, hump-nosed viper, bush master
• Hydrophidae	Sea snakes

- The poisonous snakes of India belong to five families (Table 10.5).

COMMON SNAKES IN INDIA

- In India, the most important species of poisonous snakes are cobra (*Naja naja*), common krait (*Bungarus caeruleus*), Russell's viper (*Daboia russelii*), saw-scaled viper (*Echis carinatus*) and hump-nosed viper (*Hypnale hypnale*) (Fig. 10.1).
- The common krait is black in colour with hexagonal scales on dorsal side and rows of paired white stripes across the body.
- Banded krait is a beautiful snake which has alternating yellow and black stripes.

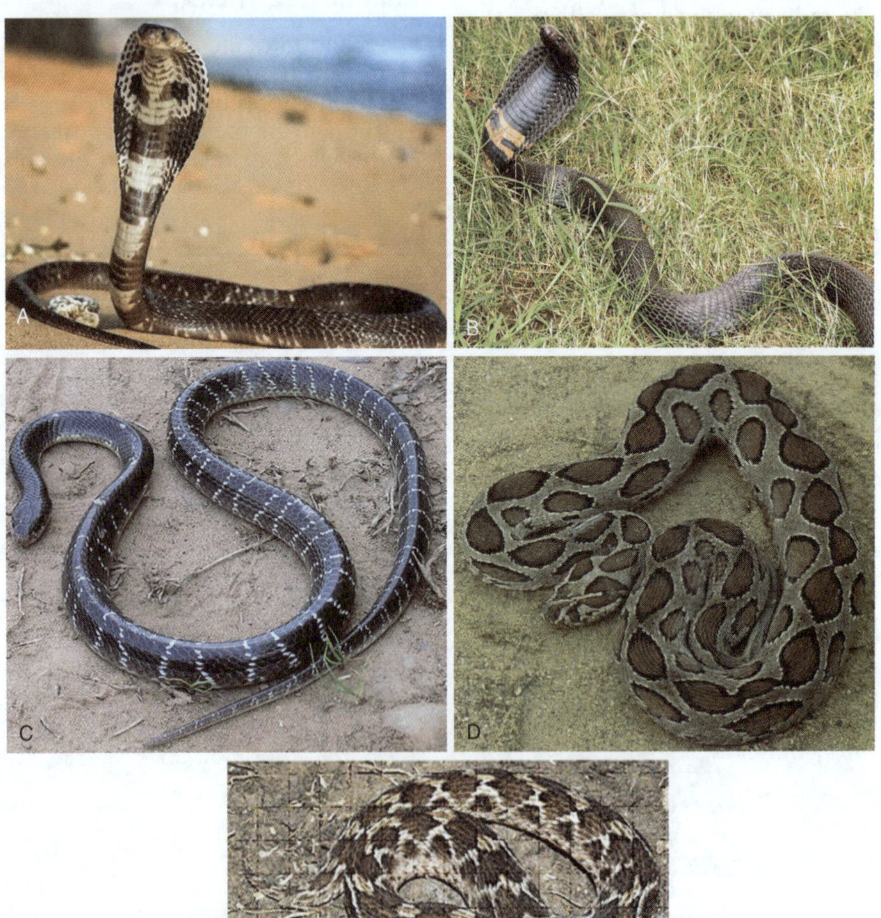

Fig. 10.1 (A) Spectacled cobra, (B) monocellate cobra, (C) common krait, (D) Russell's viper and (E) saw-scaled viper.

TABLE 10.6 Components of Snake Venoms

• Procoagulant enzymes	Major factor in viper venom Stimulate blood clotting Disseminated intravascular coagulation (DIC) Blood becomes incoagulable
• Haemorrhagins	Zinc metalloproteinases Damage endothelial lining of blood vessels Spontaneous systemic bleeding
• Cytolytic or necrotic toxins	Damage cell membranes Increase permeability Produce local swelling and gangrene of bitten part
• Haemolytic and myolytic phospholipase A_2 enzymes	Damage cell membranes, endothelium, skeletal muscle, nerve and red blood cells
• Presynaptic neurotoxins or β-bungarotoxins	Phospholipase A_2 Present in venoms of kraits and Russell's viper Interfere with release of acetylcholine
• Postsynaptic neurotoxins or α-bungarotoxins	Polypeptides Present in venoms of cobra and krait Compete with acetylcholine at the neuromuscular junctions producing curare-like paralysis

- The hood of spectacled cobra bears a binocellate mark on the upper side while monocellate cobra has a single mark.
- Sea snake is sky-blue or black dorsally and white or yellow ventrally. The snake is compressed posteriorly and has a flat tail.
- The fangs of elapids and sea snakes are short and fixed.
- The vipers, on the other hand, have large, mobile fangs which are canalized.
- Russell's viper is brown in colour and has black, chainlike marking on the body.
- Saw-scaled viper has a triangular head bearing a typical arrow mark.
- The hump-nosed viper is a small pit viper with haemotoxic venom. It has large scales on the head as compared to multiple small scales in saw scaled viper.

SNAKE VENOMS

- Venoms are secreted by salivary glands and the duct of glands open well above the tip of the fangs. Due to this reason, a snake may not be able to inject venom even after biting a victim.
- The venom of a given species is usually predominantly neurotoxic (e.g. cobras, kraits and Russell's viper), or necrotising and haematotoxic (e.g. vipers).
- The neurotoxins of Elapidae are rapidly absorbed into bloodstream, whereas the Viperidae venom is taken up more slowly through lymphatics.
- Various components of venoms are listed in Table 10.6.

CLINICAL MANIFESTATIONS

BITES BY ELAPIDAE (COBRAS, KRAITS)

- In general, elapid venoms are best known for their neurotoxic effects.
- Local pain and swelling are frequent in cobra bites. Krait bites are painless and without any local swelling. Fang marks may not be visible with krait bites.
- In krait bites, early symptoms are vomiting and abdominal pain, and occur due to autonomic stimulation.
- Other features in elapid bites include 'heaviness' of eyelids, blurred vision, diplopia, paraesthesia around the mouth, hyperacusis, headache, dizziness, vertigo, hypersalivation, red eyes and 'gooseflesh'.
- Paralysis is first detectable as ptosis and external ophthalmoplegia. Later palate, jaws, tongue, vocal cords, neck muscles and muscles of deglutition become paralysed.
- Respiratory failure may be precipitated by paralysis of intercostal muscles and diaphragm.
- Patients 'spat' at by spitting cobras may develop venom ophthalmia (pain in eye, decreased vision, blepharospasm, conjunctival inflammation and chemosis).
- Cobra bites may also produce cardiovascular involvement producing hypotension and electrocardiogram (ECG) changes.

BITES BY VIPERIDAE (VIPERS)

- In general, the Viperidae venoms are best known for their severe local manifestations and haematotoxic effects.
- There is local swelling which spreads rapidly and may involve the whole limb and adjacent trunk.
- Bruising, blistering and necrosis are very common. Necrosis is particularly common if the envenomation occurs in tight fascial compartments like digits and anterior tibial compartment.
- Haemostatic abnormalities are characteristic. These include persistent bleeding from fang puncture site and venepuncture sites. Spontaneous bleeding is most often detected in the gingival sulci. In addition, epistaxis, haematemesis, cutaneous bleeding, haemoptysis and subconjunctival, retroperitoneal and intracranial haemorrhages can occur.
- Hypotension and shock occur very frequently.
- Direct myocardial involvement is suggested by abnormal ECG or arrhythmias.
- Acute renal failure can occur with Russell's viper, hump-nosed viper and sea snake envenomation. It usually becomes clinically evident by 7 days. Various causes include shock, myoglobinuria, haemolytic uraemic syndrome, direct toxic effect and haemolysis.
- Some species of Russell's viper also produce neuroparalysis. Acute pituitary failure can also occur.

BITES BY HYDROPHIDAE (SEA SNAKES)

- Sea snakes produce myotoxicity that produces muscle pains, muscle weakness and rhabdomyolysis producing myoglobinuria.
- Cardiac involvement can occur due to release of potassium (hyperkalaemia) from necrosed muscles.

SUMMARY OF MANIFESTATIONS OF SNAKEBITES

Flowchart 10.1 summarises manifestations of snakebites.

SYNDROMIC APPROACH

- Given by the WHO and is useful to identify snake especially when the snake has not been identified and only monospecific antivenoms are available (Table 10.7).
- However, overlap of clinical features may occur.

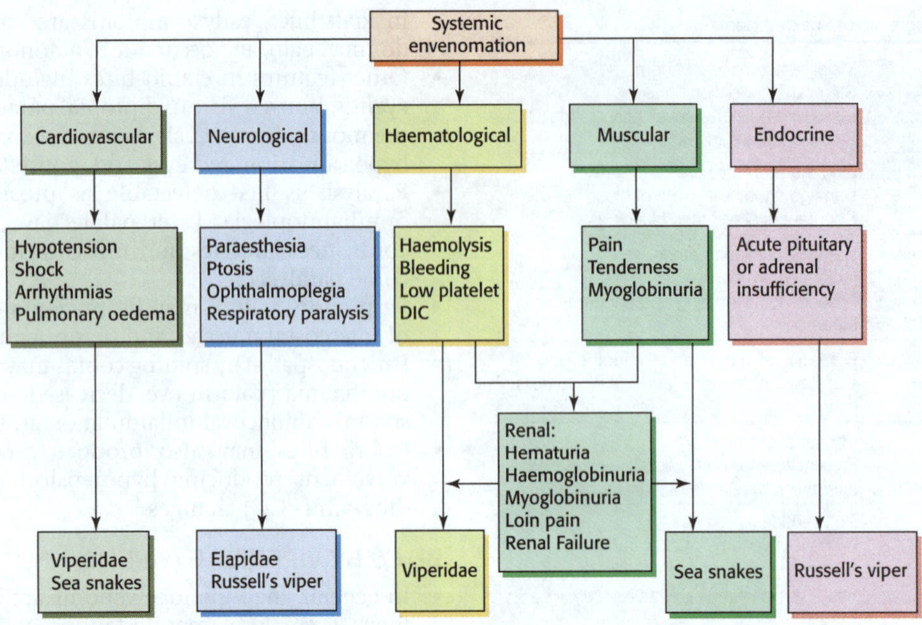

Flowchart 10.1 Summary of Manifestations of Snakebites.

TABLE 10.7 Syndromic Approach to Identify Snake

Syndrome	Clinical Features	Involved Snakes
Syndrome 1	Local envenoming (swelling, etc.) with bleeding/clotting disturbances	All species of Viperidae
Syndrome 2	Local envenoming (swelling, etc.) with bleeding/clotting disturbances, shock or acute kidney injury	Russell's viper, hump-nosed viper
Syndrome 3	Local envenoming (swelling, etc.) with paralysis	Cobra Russell's viper (southern India)
Syndrome 4	Paralysis with minimal or no local envenoming: • Bitten on land while sleeping on the ground with/without abdominal pain • Bitten in the sea	Krait Sea snake
Syndrome 5	Paralysis with dark brown urine and acute kidney injury: • Bitten on land (with bleeding/clotting disturbance) • Bitten in the sea (no bleeding/clotting disturbances)	Russell's viper (southern India) Sea snake

INVESTIGATIONS

- Total leucocyte count exceeding 20,000/mm^3 indicates severe envenomation.
- Anaemia results from bleeding and rarely haemolysis.
- Thrombocytopenia in viper bites.
- Pink plasma and black urine indicate intravascular haemolysis.
- Urine should be examined for red blood cells, red cell casts, protein and myoglobin.
- Twenty-minute whole blood clotting test and clot quality test are useful. For conducting this test, place 5 mL of fresh blood in a clean glass tube and leave it undisturbed for 20 minutes. After 20 minutes, tilt the tube. If blood is still unclotted, venom-induced coagulopathy is diagnosed. If the test is negative, it should be carried out every 30 minutes for 3 hours and then hourly after that.
- Prothrombin time, and tests to detect fibrin degradation products (FDP).
- Renal function should be assessed by blood urea, serum creatinine and electrolytes.
- ECG may show sinus bradycardia, ST–T changes and various degrees of AV blocks.
- Creatine phosphokinase (CPK) is elevated in sea snake bites.
- Specific snake venom antigens may be detected in wound aspirates and body fluids.

MANAGEMENT

- Indian Snakebite Management Protocol gives guidelines on managing a patient with snakebite.

FIRST AID

- Follow the do it 'RIGHT' approach.
  - *R*eassure the patient—70% of all snakebites are from nonvenomous species and only 50% of bites by venomous species actually envenomate the patient.
  - *I*mmobilise the bitten limb using a splint. This reduces absorption of venom.
  - Get to the nearest *H*ospital.
  - *T*ell the doctor about the symptoms.
- Pressure pad immobilisation: A rubber pad approximately 5 cm^2 and 2–3 cm thick is placed directly over the bite site and bound in place with a nonelastic

bandage at a pressure of at least 70 mmHg. If bitten on limb, it is also immobilised.

- Application of tourniquet is controversial. It may be used in case of krait bite if the facilities for administration of antivenom are more than 30–60 minutes away from the location where the patient has been bitten. The tourniquet should be at least 1–1.5 cm wide. It should be applied 5–10 cm proximal to bite area. It should be loose enough to allow one finger to pass beneath without any difficulty. The purpose is to impede lymph flow and not blood flow. However, it may be difficult to identify the snake in the field setting and, therefore, tourniquet is not recommended in the Indian protocol.
- Local incision is not advisable.
- Do not apply ice locally for relieving the pain as it can damage the exposed nerves and vessels.
- The level of swelling should be marked on the skin every 15 minutes.
- If the snake has been killed, handle the dead snake carefully as there is a risk of a second bite. Decapitated snake heads can 'bite' up to 1 hour after death of snake due to reflex action.

HOSPITAL TREATMENT

- Maintain circulation, airway and breathing.
- Clean the site of bite and elevate it to reduce local oedema.
- Send blood for various investigations.
- Examine the patient to look for features of envenomation.
  - Extent of local swelling and local oozing of blood.
  - Evidence of compartment syndrome (local tenseness, tenderness, absence of pulsation and muscle weakness).
  - Examine for enlarged and tender lymph nodes draining the limb.
  - Check blood pressure in both supine and standing positions.
  - Assess the pulse rate and respiratory rate.
  - Examine skin and mucous membranes for any evidence of bleeding. The earliest evidence of bleeding may be in the form of gum bleeding and, therefore, always examine the oral cavity.
  - Examine nervous system for any signs of toxicity:
    - Ask the patient to look up and observe whether the upper lids retract fully.
    - Ask about diplopia and test eye movements for evidence of early external ophthalmoplegia.
    - Check the size and reaction of the pupils.
    - Assess other muscles innervated by the cranial nerves (facial muscles, tongue, gag reflex, etc.).
    - Look for any secretions in the pharynx. Difficulty in swallowing indicates bulbar involvement.
    - Assess the muscles flexing the neck; if paralysed, the head falls backwards when the patient in supine position is asked to lift the head ('broken neck sign').
    - Assess strength of respiratory muscles by single breath count. Observe paradoxical movements of abdomen with respiration (abdomen expands rather than chest on inspiration).

Antivenom Treatment

- The general indications for antivenom are given in the Box 10.2.
- Monospecific (monovalent) antivenom is ideal if the biting species is known. However, it is not available in India.
- Polyspecific (polyvalent) antivenom available in India is effective against the four common varieties of snakes, that is cobra, common krait, Russell's viper and saw-scaled viper. It is ineffective against hump-nosed viper. It is prepared from the equines hyperimmunised with venom.
- Skin sensitivity test is unreliable and is, therefore, not recommended.
- Prophylactic subcutaneous adrenaline (0.25 mg) reduces the frequency and severity of early antivenom reactions and its routine use is recommended.
- Required dose of antisnake venom (ASV) is added in normal saline and is infused over 30–60 minutes. Keep adrenaline loaded to treat any reaction to antivenin.
- Dose is 60 mL for saw-scaled viper and 100 mL for others. It is same for both children and adults.
- In the case of haemotoxic bites, a repeat ASV dose is indicated if the bleeding continues after 6 hours or the whole blood clotting time is still more than 20 minutes after 6 hours. This is because liver requires 6 hours to restore clotting factors and additional ASV before this period is not required. A third dose may be required after another 6 hours in some cases.
- For neurotoxic or cardiotoxic features, a repeat dose is indicated if neurological or cardiac features persist or worsen after 1–2 hours.
- Antivenom can cause two types of reactions: an early (anaphylactoid) reaction and a late (serum sickness–type) reaction. The early (anaphylactoid) reaction is characterised by itching, urticaria, cough, nausea, vomiting, fever and tachycardia. Some may develop hypotension, bronchospasm and angioneurotic oedema. This is treated with adrenaline 0.5–1 mL subcutaneously (may be repeated), chlorpheniramine maleate 10 mg intravenously and hydrocortisone 100 mg intravenously.

Cholinergics

- Cholinergic agents are useful in patients with neurotoxic features, particularly cobra bite.

BOX 10.2 Indications for Antivenom

SIGNS OF SYSTEMIC ENVENOMATION

- Impaired consciousness
- Neurotoxicity
- Hypotension and shock, abnormal ECG and other evidences of cardiovascular dysfunction
- Haemostatic abnormalities such as spontaneous systemic bleeding and evidence of coagulopathy
- Generalised rhabdomyolysis
- Evidence of intravascular haemolysis
- Evidence of renal failure such as oliguria, uraemia, raised serum creatinine and hyperkalaemia

SIGNS OF LOCAL ENVENOMATION

- Local swelling involving more than half of the bitten limb or swelling of fingers and toes
- Rapid extension of swelling (e.g. beyond the wrist or ankle within a few hours of bites on the hands or feet)
- Painful enlargement of lymph nodes draining bitten limb

BOX 10.3 DO NOTs in Snakebite

- Local incision and suction of wound
- Application of ice packs and potassium permanganate
- Cauterisation of wound
- Application of tight constriction bands impeding arterial flow
- Infiltration of antivenom locally

- Neostigmine in a dose of 0.5–2.5 mg is administered intravenously every 1–3 hours up to 10 mg/24 hours along with atropine (to reduce cholinergic effects of neostigmine).

Supportive Therapy

- Respiratory paralysis should be treated by artificial ventilation.
- Hypotension and shock should be treated with fresh whole blood or fresh frozen plasma, noradrenaline, dopamine and hydrocortisone.
- Oliguria and renal failure should be treated conservatively failing which dialysis should be done.
- Fasciotomy may be required for compartment syndrome but it should be done only after correction of haemostatic abnormalities.
- Antibiotics are recommended for bite wounds that are necrotic or that have been tampered with. Otherwise, prophylactic antibiotics are not indicated.
- All patients should receive antitetanus prophylaxis.
- At a later stage, some patients may require surgical debridement and skin grafting.
- Haemostatic disturbances should be treated with fresh whole blood or fresh frozen plasma, cryoprecipitates or platelet concentrates.
- Box 10.3 mentions certain actions which should not be done in patients with snakebites.

Q. Explain toxicity caused by scorpion stings. (IM20.8)

- The poisonous scorpions of India include the red scorpion (*Mesobuthus*) and the black scorpion (*Palamnaeus*).
- The glands in the terminal segment of the tail produce venom that is injected by a stinger.

PATHOGENESIS

- Most important toxins in scorpion venom are α-toxins that bind to a specific site on the voltage-gated sodium channel.
- This inhibits inactivation of sodium channel resulting in prolonged depolarisation and, hence, neuronal excitation.
- Neuronal excitation stimulates both sympathetic and parasympathetic systems.
- In addition, α-toxins cause massive endogenous release of the epinephrine and norepinephrine.

CLINICAL FEATURES

- Most stings are minor. The clinical features of envenomation develop within 2–12 hours of sting by a poisonous scorpion.

LOCAL FEATURES

- Sting may be followed by the onset of intense pain at the site within several minutes. Often there is intense pain with mild palpation or tapping over the site (the 'tap test'). Pain or numbness may radiate up the extremity.

SYSTEMIC FEATURES

- Systemic features reflect sympathetic, parasympathetic and neuromuscular excitation.
- Initial features are due to transient cholinergic hyperactivity. This produces restlessness, anxiety, vomiting, profuse sweating, salivation, sensation of tongue thickening, dysphagia, bradycardia, hypotension and priapism.
- These are followed by sustained adrenergic hyperactivity resulting in hypertension, tachycardia, chest discomfort, cold extremities, pulmonary oedema and myocardial failure. Hypertension occurs within 6 hours of sting while pulmonary oedema occurs within 2–56 hours after being stung.
- In late stages, hypotension and shock develop.
- Electrocardiographic features suggestive of myocarditis may be present.

MANAGEMENT

- Mild analgesics for relieving pain.
- Tetanus vaccine according to the immune status of the patient.
- Monitor for cardiac rhythm, conduction disturbances and oxygen saturation.
- If signs of respiratory failure occur, intubate the patient.
- Correction of fluid deficit; avoid large amount of fluids without proper monitoring because of the risk of pulmonary oedema.
- Prazosin (0.25–0.5 mg every 4–6 hours) to control hypertension. It is an antidote for scorpion stings. An alternative is to give nifedipine; however, it should be avoided in the presence of tachycardia and impending congestive heart failure.
- Dopamine infusion for hypotension.
- Prazosin and furosemide to control pulmonary oedema associated with normal or high blood pressure.
- Glucose–insulin infusion may be beneficial in systemic envenomation.
- Serotherapy (use of scorpion antivenin) is useful and can be added to prazosin.

Q. Discuss the clinical manifestations, diagnosis and management of organophosphorus and carbamate poisoning. (IM 21.3)

- Most common cause of acute poisoning in India.
- Common organophosphorus compounds are malathion, parathion, dichlorvos, diazinon and chlorothion.
- Common carbamate insecticides include carbaryl, aldicarb and propoxur.

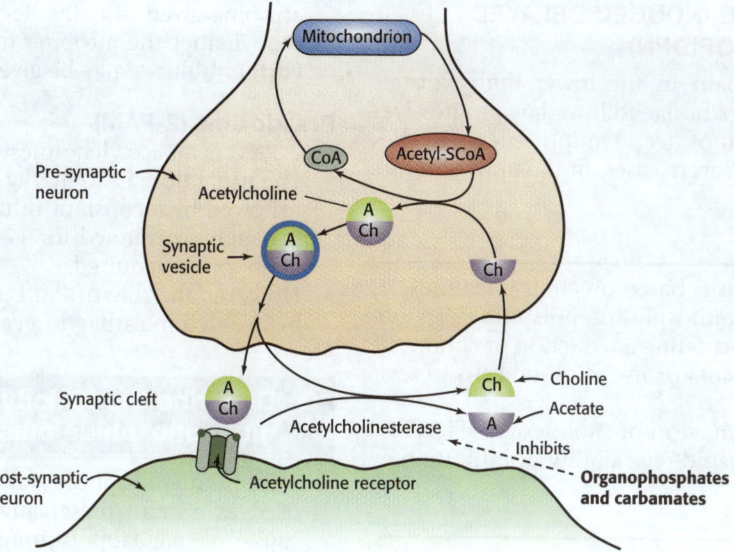

Fig. 10.2 Mechanism of action of organophosphates and carbamates.

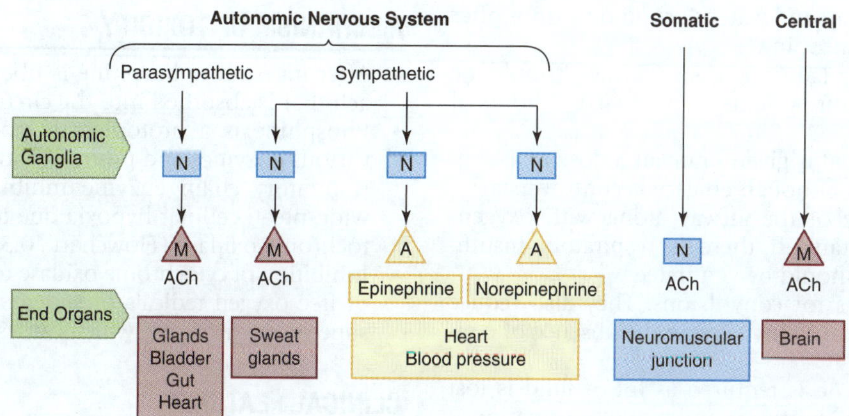

Flowchart 10.2 Location of Muscarinic (M) Receptors and Nicotinic (N) Receptors. Ach, Acetylcholine.

PATHOGENESIS

- Normally, acetylcholine released at synaptic junction is inactivated by the enzyme acetylcholinesterase, which terminates its action.
- Organophosphorus and carbamate insecticides inhibit acetylcholinesterase (Fig. 10.2).
- This results in accumulation of acetylcholine at muscarinic and nicotinic synapses which produces various manifestations (Flowchart 10.2).
- Organophosphorus compounds inhibit acetylcholinesterase irreversibly while carbamates inhibit it reversibly.

CLINICAL FEATURES

- Organophosphorus compounds produce muscarinic, nicotinic and CNS effects. Carbamates produce a similar clinical picture but of shorter duration and lower order of toxicity.

ACUTE CHOLINERGIC CRISIS

- Usually lasts for 48–72 hours.

Muscarinic Manifestations

- DUMBELS (refer page 745).

Nicotinic Manifestations

- Twitching, fasciculations, weakness, diminished respiratory effort, hypertension and tachycardia.

CNS Manifestations

- Anxiety, restlessness, tremors, convulsions, confusion, weakness and coma.

ECG Changes

- Sinus tachycardia most common.
- Others include QT interval prolongation, ST–T changes and ventricular premature contractions.

INTERMEDIATE SYNDROME

- Syndrome of muscular paralysis occurs within 24–96 hours after ingestion of an organophosphate and following treatment of acute cholinergic syndrome.
- Muscle weakness affects predominantly neck flexors, proximal limb muscles, those supplied by cranial nerves and respiratory muscles.

ORGANOPHOSPHATE-INDUCED DELAYED POLYNEUROPATHY (OPIDPN)

- Cramping muscle pain in the lower limbs, distal numbness and paraesthesiae followed by progressive weakness, depression of deep tendon reflexes in the lower limbs and, in severe cases, in the upper limbs.

DIAGNOSIS

- Most often, diagnosis is based on clinical features.
- Diagnosis of organophosphorus poisoning can be confirmed by demonstrating a reduction of cholinesterase activity in plasma or in red blood cells to less than 50% of normal.
- With carbamates, reduction of cholinesterase level is rare because of the rapid reversibility of inhibition.

MANAGEMENT

GENERAL MEASURES

- Remove the patient from site of exposure and wash the skin with soap and water. It should be done after initial doses of atropine.
- In the case of ingestion, gastric lavage should be done if the patient presents within first 1–2 hours of ingestion.
- Activated charcoal is given orally at a dose of 1–2 g/kg body weight, although efficacy is controversial.
- Meticulous care of the airway along with oxygenation is important. If there is respiratory insufficiency, patient should be ventilated.
- Benzodiazepines for convulsions. They also reduce morbidity and mortality even in the absence of convulsions.
- Intravenous saline is required as lot of fluid is lost due to sweating, diarrhoea and frequent urination.

SPECIFIC MEASURES

Atropine

- Atropine is the main antidote. If the initial assessment reveals significant cholinergic features (miosis, excessive sweating, poor air entry due to bronchorrhoea and bronchospasm, bradycardia and hypotension), then atropine is required.
- Atropine is administered at a dose of 1.8–3 mg intravenously. Five minutes after giving atropine, check the five markers of cholinergic poisoning. A uniform improvement in most of the five parameters is required and not the improvement in just one.
- If after 5 minutes a consistent improvement across the five parameters has not occurred, then more atropine is required. Double the dose of atropine every time and continue to double each time when there is no adequate response.
- Target end points for atropine therapy (atropinisation) are the following: clear chest on auscultation with no wheeze, heart rate >80 beats/minute, pupils no longer pinpoint, dry axillae and systolic blood pressure >90 mmHg. Pupil size and heart rate alone should not be used as end points.
- Once atropinised, set up an infusion of atropine at an hourly dose of 10%–20% of the total dose of atropine given initially. Review every 15 minutes to see whether the atropine infusion rate is adequate. Further boluses may be given if required.

Pralidoxime (2-PAM)

- 2-PAM is an acetylcholinesterase reactivator.
- The usual dose is 30 mg/kg initially over 20 minutes followed by a constant infusion at 9 mg/kg/hour. It is usually continued for 12–24 hours after atropine is no longer required.
- However, the role of PAM is controversial. It should be avoided in carbaryl (a carbamate) ingestion.

Q. Describe the toxicity caused by aluminium phosphide poisoning. (IM 21.3)

- Aluminium phosphide (AlP), a solid fumigant widely used as a grain preservative, is one of the leading causes of suicidal poisoning in northern India.
- It is available in pellet as well as in powder form.

MECHANISM OF TOXICITY

- After ingestion, phosphine is liberated in the stomach that is absorbed into the circulation.
- Phosphine is a protoplasmic poison that inhibits various enzymes and protein synthesis. It is a potent respiratory chain enzyme inhibitor that produces widespread cellular hypoxia due to inhibition of cytochrome oxidase (Flowchart 10.3).
- Inhibition of cytochrome oxidase results in generation of free oxygen radicals or superoxide that stimulates superoxide dismutase which causes cellular damage.

CLINICAL FEATURES

- The fatal dose of an unexposed pellet or powder of AlP is 150–500 mg.
- Clinical manifestations develop within 30 minutes of ingestion.
- Initial features include retrosternal burning, epigastric discomfort and recurrent vomiting and diarrhoea. There is fishy smell from breath.
- Within the next 6–8 hours, patients develop systemic features most prominently related to cardiovascular and respiratory systems.

CARDIOVASCULAR FEATURES

- Important cardiovascular features are hypotension, shock, tachycardia or bradycardia and arrhythmias.
- Shock occurs because of cardiotoxicity, recurrent vomiting and widespread vascular injury.
- A few patients may develop congestive heart failure due to myocardial depression.
- The ECG changes include arrhythmias, intraventricular conduction blocks, ST depression and T inversion, ST elevation and various blocks.

RESPIRATORY FEATURES

- The respiratory features include cough, dyspnoea, cyanosis, pulmonary oedema and ARDS that usually occur after 6–36 hours of ingestion.

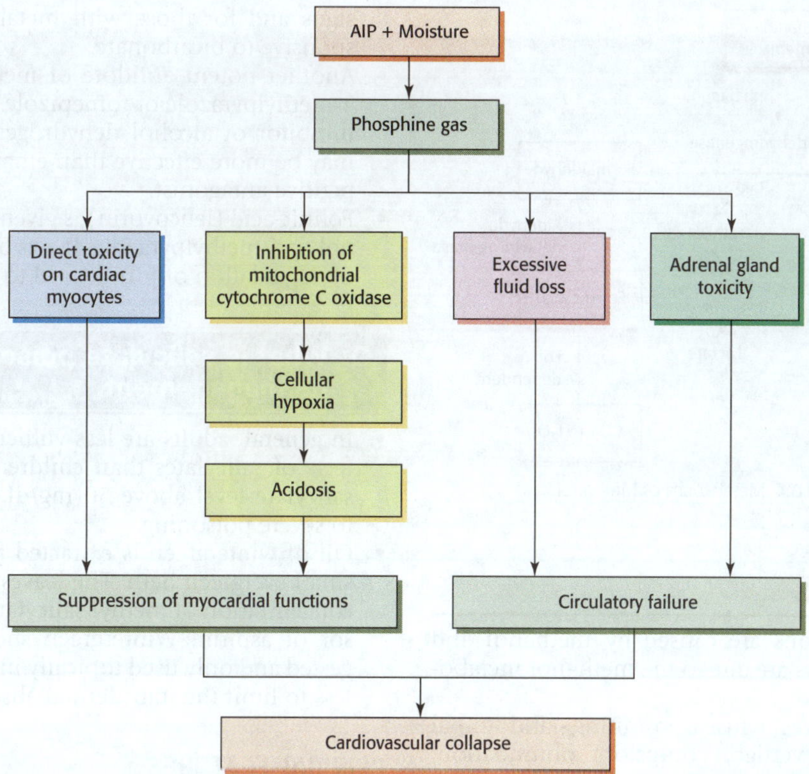

Flowchart 10.3 Various Mechanisms of the Cardiovascular Effects of Aluminium Phosphide Poisoning. AlP, Aluminium Phosphide.

METABOLIC FEATURES

- Hypomagnesaemia or hypermagnesaemia and metabolic acidosis are common.

MISCELLANEOUS

- Other features include liver damage indicated by elevated transaminases and bilirubin, renal failure and pericarditis.

DIAGNOSIS

- Diagnosis of AlP poisoning is made by typical features of poisoning along with fishy smell in the breath and vomitus.
- Confirmation can be done by silver nitrate test on lavage fluid or on breath.

MANAGEMENT

- If patient presents early after ingesting AlP, perform a gastric lavage using potassium permanganate in 1:10,000 dilution. It oxidises phosphine to nontoxic phosphates. However, its role is controversial.
- Activated charcoal also adsorbs phosphine. Vegetable *ghee* may also be useful as it reduces production of phosphine in stomach.
- Adequate ventilation and urine output help to maintain adequate excretion of phosphine.
- Supportive care is the most important step in the management.
  - Monitor the central venous pressure and if possible the pulmonary arterial wedge pressure.
  - Infuse large volumes of saline to maintain the systolic pressure above 90 mmHg. Four to six litres of saline may be required in the first few hours.
  - Infuse bicarbonate to correct acidosis that is quite severe in most cases.
  - Initiate norepinephrine or dopamine if blood pressure is not maintained with saline.
  - If required, add dobutamine.
- Role of magnesium sulphate in reducing toxicity of phosphine remains controversial but most clinicians use it.

Q. Write a short note on the toxicity caused by methanol (methyl alcohol) poisoning. (IM 21.4)

- This occurs when industrial spirit (methylated) is consumed or when the supply of liquor is adulterated with methyl alcohol.
- Methanol is a mild CNS depressant.
- Methanol as such is not a toxic agent. However, its metabolites—formaldehyde and formic acid—are responsible for its toxicity.
- The enzyme responsible for the conversion of methanol to formaldehyde is alcohol dehydrogenase while aldehyde dehydrogenase, formaldehyde dehydrogenase and other enzymes convert formaldehyde to formic acid (Flowchart 10.4).
- Oxidation of methanol is much slower than that of ethanol. In the presence of both ethanol and methanol, the former is preferentially metabolised by alcohol dehydrogenase resulting in a reduced toxicity of methanol.

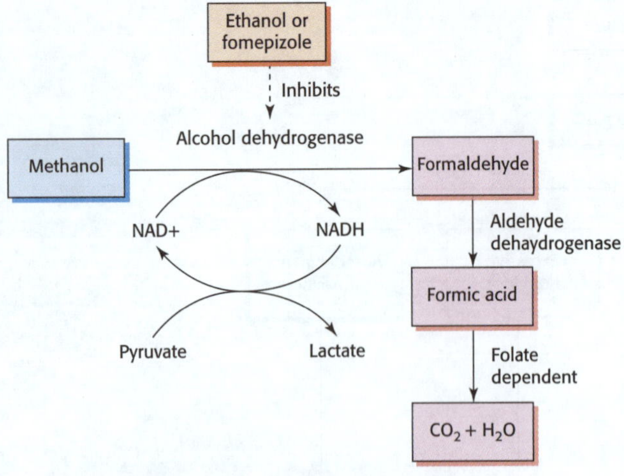

Flowchart 10.4 Metabolism of Methanol.

CLINICAL FEATURES

- Early manifestations are caused by methanol and late manifestations are due to the methanol metabolite formic acid.
- Methanol produces nausea, vomiting, abdominal pain, headache, vertigo, confusion, obtundation, convulsions and coma.
- Late manifestations of formic acid are metabolic acidosis and retinal injury. The ophthalmological manifestations include clouding and diminished vision, dancing and flashing spots, dilated or fixed pupils, hyperaemia of the optic disc, retinal oedema and blindness.
- Other manifestations are rapid breathing due to metabolic acidosis, myocardial depression, bradycardia, shock and anuria.
- An uncommon complication is putaminal necrosis which presents with rigidity, tremor, masked faces and monotonous speech.

DIAGNOSIS

- Diagnosis is confirmed by the measurement of serum methanol level, which is usually more than 20 mg/dL.
- Methanol-derived formic acidosis can be confirmed by a large anion gap, low serum bicarbonate and elevated serum formate levels.
- The osmolal gap is elevated (>10) due to methanol.

MANAGEMENT

- Gastrointestinal decontamination in early stages.
- Correction of systemic acidosis with sodium bicarbonate.
- Ethanol therapy is indicated in patients with visual symptoms or methanol level exceeding 20 mg/dL. Ethanol competitively inhibits alcohol dehydrogenase which reduces conversion of methanol to formic acid.
- Haemodialysis is indicated for patients with methanol level exceeding 50 mg/dL, for those with visual signs and for those with metabolic acidosis unresponsive to bicarbonate.
- Another potent antidote of methanol poisoning is 4-methylpyrazole or fomepizole. It is a direct, potent inhibitor of alcohol dehydrogenase and, therefore, may be more effective than ethanol which is a competitive antagonist.
- Folinic acid (leucovorin) is given in addition to ethanol or 4-methylpyrazole. It acts by increasing the rate of degradation of formic acid to carbon dioxide.

Q. What is salicylate poisoning? Explain its management. (IM21.4)

- In general, adults are less vulnerable to the toxic effects of salicylates than children. In adults, plasma salicylate level above 50 mg/dL indicates moderate to severe poisoning.
- Oil of wintergreen is extracted from the leaves of a small evergreen herb. The leaves contain a very high concentration of methyl salicylate, which is a precursor of aspirin. Wintergreen should NEVER be ingested and only used topically in dilutions of 25% or less to limit the transdermal absorption.

CLINICAL FEATURES

- The earliest signs and symptoms of salicylate toxicity develop within 1–2 hours of ingestion and include nausea, vomiting, sweating and tinnitus.
- These are followed by early CNS features like tachypnoea, hyperactivity, agitation, delirium and hallucinations.
- Later the patient may develop coma, seizures and pulmonary oedema.
- The initial respiratory alkalosis is followed later by metabolic acidosis. Marked acidosis is regarded as a very serious feature as it may herald sudden respiratory or cardiac arrest.
- A marked increase in body temperature is indicative of severe toxicity.
- Development of respiratory acidosis indicates ARDS.
- Acute poisoning also produces GI symptoms and blood level correlates with toxicity.
- In chronic poisoning, GI features are less severe while CNS features including tinnitus are prominent. Blood levels do not correlate with symptoms in chronic poisoning.
- Hypoglycaemia and hypokalaemia are frequent. Hypokalaemia occurs due to intracellular shift produced by respiratory alkalosis as well as due to increased renal excretion of potassium.

MANAGEMENT

- General measures including gastric lavage and activated charcoal.
- Maintain intravascular volume by intravenous fluids.
- Alkalinisation of urine in moderate or severe poisoning.
- Correction of hypoglycaemia and hypokalaemia.
- Haemodialysis may be required in severe cases.

Q. Describe paracetamol poisoning. (IM21.4)

PATHOGENESIS

- In overdose, toxicity is not due to paracetamol but due to one of its metabolites, *N*-acetyl-*para*-benzoquinone imine (NAPQI) which causes liver injury.
- Normally, about 90% of paracetamol undergoes hepatic conjugation with glucuronide and sulphate to form inactive metabolites. Only about 5%–15% is oxidized by cytochrome P450 to NAPQI.
- After therapeutic use of paracetamol, supply of glutathione far exceeds that required to detoxify NAPQI.
- However, after overdose, the rate and quantity of NAPQI formation exceed supply of reduced glutathione. This results in accumulation of hepatotoxic NAPQI.
- Nephrotoxicity may be caused by local production of NAPQI.

TOXIC DOSE

- Ingestion of 150–200 mg/kg or 10 g in adults as a single dose.
- A 4-hour blood level of paracetamol more than 150 mg/L is potentially toxic.

CLINICAL FEATURES

- The clinical course of acute paracetamol toxicity can be divided into four stages (Table 10.8).

LABORATORY TESTS

- Liver function, kidney functions and coagulation profile.
- Blood level for paracetamol (to be taken only after 4 hours of ingestion).

MODIFIED RUMACK–MATTHEW NOMOGRAM

- Indicates the risk of hepatotoxicity after acute exposure.
- In this nomogram, paracetamol concentration is plotted against time since ingestion.
- A 4-hour paracetamol concentration >150 μg/mL (150 mg/L) indicates possibility of hepatotoxicity.

TREATMENT

- Gastric lavage and activated charcoal in early presentation.

N-ACETYLCYSTEINE (NAC)

- Antidote for paracetamol.
- Prevents binding of NAPQI to hepatic macromolecules and also restores glutathione stores.
- Can be administered intravenously as well as orally. IV dosage is 150 mg/kg over 60 minutes, followed by 50 mg/kg over next 4 hours and then 100 mg/kg over next 16 hours. Oral loading dose is 140 mg/kg followed by 70 mg/kg every 4 hours for a total of 18 doses over 72 hours.

Q. Describe the toxicity caused by mushroom poisoning.

- Among the many types of mushrooms, only a small number are poisonous. In general, mushroom poisoning that has its onset within 3 hours of ingestion is not likely to involve a deadly mushroom.

AMANITA PHALLOIDES MUSHROOM

- Majority of the deaths due to mushroom poisoning result from ingestion of *Amanita phalloides* ('death cap'). It contains two types of toxins, both of which are heat stable and survive cooking:
  1. 'Phallotoxins' causing severe gastroenteritis within 6–12 hours of ingestion.
  2. 'Amatoxins' causing delayed liver and renal tubular damage with presentation 2–4 days after ingestion.

MANAGEMENT

- The mushroom eaten should be identified, ideally by an expert.
- Toxins have been found in the duodenal aspirate as long as 36 hours after ingestion. Therefore, a gastric lavage may be performed even in late phases of poisoning. Repeated doses of activated charcoal are useful.
- Initial treatment consists of maintenance of fluid and electrolyte balance.
- The value of thioctic acid, a Krebs cycle coenzyme, is doubtful.
- Penicillin and silymarin inhibit uptake of amatoxin by hepatocytes and their use has been associated with reduced morbidity and mortality. *N*-Acetylcysteine may also be useful.
- Otherwise management is supportive and includes treatment of hepatic and renal failure.

TABLE 10.8 Stages of Paracetamol Poisoning

Stage	Clinical Features	Laboratory Features
Stage 1 (first 24 hours)	Anorexia, nausea, vomiting	Hypokalaemia
Stage 2 (2–3 days)	Improvement in anorexia, vomiting Abdominal pain Hepatic tenderness	Elevated SGOT/PT Elevated bilirubin ↑ PT if severe
Stage 3 (3–4 days)	Recurrence of anorexia, vomiting Encephalopathy Anuria Jaundice	Hepatic failure Metabolic acidosis Coagulopathy Renal failure Pancreatitis
Stage 4 (after 5 days)	Clinical improvement (7–8 days) or deterioration to multiple organ dysfunction and death	Improvement or continued deterioration

MUSHROOMS PRODUCING PSYCHOGENIC FEATURES

- Psychogenic features are produced by two groups of mushrooms: *Amanita muscaria* and *Psilocybe*.
- *A. muscaria* contains a toxin known as ibotenic acid which is a glutamate and GABA agonist. It produces delirium, hallucinations and seizures but no hepatotoxicity.
- *Psilocybe* contains a toxin known as psilocybin which produces nausea, euphoria, ataxia and hallucinations.
- Treatment is supportive.

OTHER MUSHROOMS

- False morel (*Gyromitra*) contains a toxin known as gyromitrin which on hydrolysis forms monomethylhydrazine. It reacts with pyridoxine resulting in reduced formation of GABA.
- The toxicity is similar to INH toxicity with metabolic acidosis, coma and seizures.
- Treatment is supportive and the antidote is pyridoxine.

Q. Discuss the clinical features, laboratory features and treatment in case of oleander poisoning. (IM21.2)

- Oleander plants include yellow oleander (*Thevetia peruviana*) and pink oleander (*Nerium oleander*).
- Oleander plants contain glycosides that resemble digitoxin, a cardiac glycoside.
- All parts contain the toxin but the maximum amount is in the seeds.

CLINICAL FEATURES

- Symptoms of poisoning generally start within 2–3 hours of ingestion.
- Gastrointestinal irritation produces nausea, vomiting, diarrhoea and abdominal pain.
- Other features include dizziness, pupillary dilatation, tingling and numbness, restlessness, bradycardia, arrhythmias, hypotension, nervous system toxicity and abdominal cramps.
- Electrocardiographic features are sinus bradycardia, AV blocks, ST segment depression, inversion of T waves, AV dissociation, ventricular ectopics and, in severe cases, ventricular tachycardia and fibrillation.

LABORATORY FEATURES

- Hyperkalaemia and acidosis.
- Estimation of digoxin using radioimmunoassay (cross-reactivity of oleander glycosides with digoxin).

TREATMENT

- Correction of fluid, electrolyte and acid–base disturbances.
- Gastric lavage.
- Repeated dose of activated charcoal.
- Atropine and pacing for bradycardia-related arrhythmias.
- Lidocaine for ventricular tachyarrhythmias.
- Digoxin-specific Fab antibody fragments in life-threatening oleander poisoning.

Q. Write briefly on datura poisoning, explaining clinical features and management. (IM21.2)

- *Datura stramonium* (jimson seed) produces anticholinergic syndrome.
- All the parts of this plant are poisonous but seeds and fruit are the most toxic.
- The most popular mode of poisoning is by mixing the seeds in sweets and giving to others with the purpose of thefts.
- The active toxic agents include atropine and scopolamine.
- Atropine and related compounds block acetylcholine at the receptor sites of postganglionic synapses of the cholinergic nerves.
- Other related plant is *Atropa belladonna* (deadly nightshade).

CLINICAL FEATURES

- Symptoms of toxicity usually appear within 30 minutes of ingestion and last for 24–48 hours.
- Classically, in addition to manifesting tachycardia, the features are described as 'hot as a hare' (hyperthermia due to cutaneous vasodilatation and anhidrosis), 'blind as a bat' (ciliary muscle paralysis and mydriasis), 'dry as a bone' (anhidrosis and dryness of mouth), 'full as a flask' (urinary retention), 'red as a beet' (cutaneous vasodilatation causing flushing) and 'mad as a hatter' (CNS arousal, agitation, delirium and hallucinations).
- Other features include cardiac arrhythmias and reduced or absent bowel sounds. In fatal cases, stupor, coma and convulsions occur. Death occurs due to respiratory paralysis or cardiovascular collapse.

MANAGEMENT

- Gastric lavage and support of various vital organs.
- Activated charcoal is helpful as it adsorbs the alkaloids.
- Urinary catheterisation.
- Control of hyperthermia by external cooling and benzodiazepines.
- Benzodiazepines are effective in the treatment of agitation and seizures. Avoid phenothiazines to control agitation.
- Physostigmine, a cholinesterase inhibitor, which increases the levels of acetylcholine at receptor sites, may be used in patients with severe CNS features or arrhythmias.

Q. Briefly discuss corrosive poisoning. (IM21.3)

- Corrosive ingestions are commonplace in clinical practice, with presentations ranging from superficial burns to life-threatening oesophageal and gastric ruptures. The intention may be suicidal (common in adults) or accidental (common in children).
- Corrosive ingestions include both acid and alkali substances, and comprise mostly of household items because of easy accessibility (Table 10.9).

TABLE 10.9 Common Corrosive Agents

Corrosive Agent	Use
Hydrochloric acid	Metal cleaner, toilet cleaner, soldering fluxes
Hydrofluoric acid	Rust remover, petroleum industry, glass etching, jewellery cleaners
Sulphuric acid	Automobile batteries, toilet cleaner, explosives, fertilizer
Sodium hydroxide	Industrial chemical, drain cleaner
Potassium hydroxide	Drain cleaner, batteries
Sodium hypochlorite	Bleach
Phenol	Antiseptic, floor cleaner

PATHOPHYSIOLOGY

- The mechanism of injury is different in acids and alkalis.
- Acids denature proteins through coagulation necrosis. The resultant coagulum prevents the acid from reaching deeper tissues, and this limits the damage. These agents are less viscous reaching the stomach quickly, thus affecting the stomach more than the oesophagus.
    - Hydrofluoric acid is a weak acid but has severe systemic effects due to fluoride ions which cause life-threatening electrolyte disturbances like hypocalcaemia and hyperkalaemia.
- Alkalis cause saponification of fats leading to tissue damage via liquefaction necrosis. This allows deeper penetration into tissues resulting in more damage.

CLINICAL PRESENTATION

- The manifestations of corrosive ingestions are variable. The severity can vary from mild superficial ulcerations to life-threatening perforations.
- Table 10.10 lists manifestations of corrosive exposure.

HYDROFLUORIC ACID

- Dermal exposure produces severe pain due to deep cutaneous injury. It is absorbed and produces severe systemic effects, particularly hypocalcaemia, and in some cases hyperkalaemia.
- If more than 2% of the body surface area is burnt with high concentration of hydrofluoric acid, life-threatening systemic toxicity should be expected.

MANAGEMENT

- For skin exposure, the skin is irrigated thoroughly with water. When ocular exposure is suspected, immediate irrigation of the eyes should be done with copious amount of water for at least 15–30 minutes, followed by an ophthalmologist referral.
- Inspect oropharynx for signs of injury and drooling. Note any change in quality of voice. Auscultate neck and chest for stridor. Presence of these features indicate a possibility of airway injury and need for an early intubation.
- Blind nasotracheal intubation is contraindicated as this may cause further damage to the already injured mucosa.
- Charcoal and lavage are contraindicated. However, for mercuric chloride ingestion, a lavage may be done in early presentations as systemic toxicity is significant with it. For hydrofluoric acid, milk may be given after ingestion to limit gut injury. Magnesium citrate is given to reduce systemic toxicity. For other caustic ingestions, dilution and neutralising agents are contraindicated.
- Intravenous fluids are given to maintain the hydration status and correct dyselectrolytaemia.
- Gastric acid suppression with intravenous proton pump inhibitors is to be done.
- Parenteral analgesics are needed to relieve the pain of severe oral and oesophageal injuries.
- Corticosteroids are not recommended because of the lack of demonstrable efficacy.
- An upright chest X-ray should be done to exclude air under diaphragm. Also, look for any evidence of pneumomediastinum or mediastinal widening (suggestive of an oesophageal perforation).
- A computed tomography of the chest and abdomen is the investigation of choice in patients with corrosive ingestion. It identifies patients with transmural necrosis who would need emergency surgery. It can be done even in critically ill patients in whom endoscopy would be difficult.
- Endoscopy is important to find out the extent of damage and it should be done between 6–48 hours after ingestion. Endoscopy done within 6 hours may not reveal the full extent of injury. It should be avoided after 48 hours because of increased risk of perforation. The endoscopy evaluates the extent of oesophageal and gastric damage and helps in guiding management.

TABLE 10.10 Manifestations of Corrosive Ingestions

Acute	Delayed
Cutaneous/ocular/oral pain	Oesophageal strictures
Oedema of tongue, airway	Dysphagia, odynophagia
Perforation of bowel tract	Gastric outlet obstruction
Chemical pneumonitis	Fistula formation
Peritonitis, mediastinitis	Corneal opacification
Sepsis	Oesophageal malignancy
Electrolyte imbalance	

HYDROFLUORIC ACID

- Skin exposure should be treated with calcium gluconate gel or intraarterial infusion of calcium gluconate. Calcium binds with fluoride ion and relieves the pain. Repeated application of calcium gluconate is required to reduce pain and to reduce development of severe hypocalcaemia.

Q. What do you understand by the terms bioterrorism and chemical terrorism?

Q. What are the common chemical and biological agents used in terrorism?

- Bioterrorism is intentional release of biological agents to cause illness or death in humans, animals or plants. These agents may be bacteria, viruses or toxins. They may be naturally occurring or modified by terrorists to increase their pathogenicity, capability to spread in various environmental conditions or resistance to drugs.

TABLE 10.11 Common Chemicals That May Be Used in Terrorism

Asphyxiants	Vesicants
Blood • Hydrogen cyanide • Hydrogen sulphide **Choking or irritants** • Phosgene • Chlorine • Sulphur dioxide • Nitrogen dioxide **Opioids** • Fentanyl • Carfentanil • Remifentanil	• Mustard gas • Lewisite **Nerve agents** • Tabun • Sarin • Soman • VX **Riot-controlling agents** • Chloroacetophenone (CN) • Chlorobenzylidene malononitrile (CS) or tear gas • Bromobenzyl cyanide (CA)

TABLE 10.12 Common Biological Agents that may be used in Terrorism

Category A (diseases that pose a risk to national security, are easily transmitted, have high morbidity and mortality, would have a major public health impact and cause panic and require special public health preparedness)	
• Anthrax • Smallpox • Plague	• Tularaemia • Botulism • Viral haemorrhagic fevers (caused by Marburg, Ebola, Lassa and Machupo viruses)
Category B (diseases with lower morbidity and mortality and more difficult to disseminate)	
• Abrin toxin and ricin toxin • Glanders • Psittacosis	• Brucellosis • Melioidosis • Q fever
Category C (diseases that have the potential to cause significant morbidity and mortality and are emerging pathogens that could be engineered for mass dispersion)	
• H1N1 influenza • Hantavirus pulmonary syndrome	• Nipah virus infection • Severe acute respiratory syndrome (SARS)-CoV

- Chemical terrorism is intentional release of chemical agents to cause illness or death in humans, animals or plants.
- Common chemicals that may be used for terrorism are listed in Table 10.11.
- Common biological agents that may be used in terrorism are listed in Table 10.12.

Q. What are the clues to chemical and biological terrorism?

CLUES TO CHEMICAL TERRORISM (Box 10.4)

BOX 10.4 Clues to Chemical Terrorism

- Any unusual increase in the number of people seeking care especially with respiratory, neurological, dermatological or gastrointestinal symptoms
- Any clustering of symptoms or unusual age distribution (e.g. chemical exposure in children)
- Any unusual clustering of patients in time or location (e.g. persons who attended the same public event; subways)
- Location of release not consistent with a chemical's use
- Simultaneous impact to human, animal and plant populations
- Unprotected rescuers becoming victims themselves

CLUES TO BIOTERRORISM (Box 10.5)

BOX 10.5 Clues to Bioterrorism

- Single case of a disease caused by an uncommon agent (e.g. smallpox, inhalational or cutaneous anthrax and pneumonic plague)
- Large number of persons with similar diseases
- Large number of persons with unexplained deaths
- High morbidity and mortality in association with a common disease
- Failure of patients with a common disease to respond to usual therapy
- Unusual, atypical or genetically engineered strain of an agent
- Agent resistant to most antibiotics
- Disease with an unusual geographic distribution
- Sudden increase in occurrence of a disease, otherwise stable (e.g. plague and tularaemia)
- Atypical disease transmission through aerosols or water
- Unusual illness that affects a large population
- Unusual pattern of death or illness among animals
- Simultaneous clusters of similar illness in noncontiguous areas

Q. How will you recognise and treat patients exposed to a chemical terrorist attack?

- Table 10.13 gives various chemical agents, their mechanisms of toxicities, clinical features and management in case of a terrorist attack.

Q. Discuss physics of radiation.

Q. Describe acute radiation syndrome.

RADIATION PHYSICS

- Radiation energy includes nonionising radiation (e.g. radio waves and microwaves) and ionising radiation.
- Ionising radiation includes alpha and beta particles, positrons, neutrons and gamma rays and X-rays.
- Grey (Gy) or rad is the unit for measuring absorbed dose of radiation.

ALPHA PARTICLES

- Contain two protons and two neutrons.
- Unable to penetrate outer layers of skin; can be shielded with a piece of paper.
- Harmful only after ingestion or inhalation.

BETA PARTICLES

- Contain single electron.
- Can penetrate about 8 mm on skin exposure and cause serious burns.

POSITRONS

- Positively charged beta particles and used in positron emission tomography.

NEUTRONS

- Uncharged particles.
- Require helium or water for shielding.

TABLE 10.13 Chemicals, their Mechanisms of Toxicities, Clinical Features and Management

Agent	Mechanism of Toxicity	Clinical Features	Examples	Management
• Nerve agents	• Inactivate acetylcholinesterase (ACh) enzyme, causing muscarinic, nicotinic and CNS effects	• Mild to moderate toxicity • Miosis • Blurred vision • Rhinorrhoea • Headache • Sweating • Vomiting, diarrhoea • Muscle fasciculations • Severe toxicity • Additional features include seizures and loss of consciousness	• Sarin • Soman • Tabun • VX	• Decontamination • Suction and oxygen • Atropine • Reverses muscarinic features • 2 mg IV; repeat every 5 minutes, titrate until effective • IM in the field • Pralidoxime (2-PAM) • Reactivates ACh • Reverses nicotinic and muscarinic features • 600–1800 mg IM or 1–2 g IV over 20–30 minutes • Repeated doses as required • Diazepam to prevent/control seizures
• Asphyxiants a. Blood asphyxiants	• Bind with iron in cytochrome a_3 preventing intracellular oxygen utilisation	• Mild to moderate toxicity • Giddiness • Palpitations • Dizziness • Nausea, vomiting • Headache • Increase in rate and depth of breathing (hyperventilation) • Drowsiness • Metabolic acidosis • Hypotension • 'Pink' skin colour • Severe toxicity • Immediate loss of consciousness, convulsions and death within 1–15 minutes	• Hydrogen cyanide • Hydrogen sulphide	• 100% oxygen by face mask • Intubation with 100% FiO_2 if indicated • Amyl nitrite via inhalation, one ampoule every 5 minutes • Sodium nitrite (300 mg IV over 5–10 minutes) • Sodium thiosulphate in cyanide poisoning only (12.5 g IV)
b. Choking agents or irritants	• Acids or acid-forming agents that react with cytoplasmic proteins and destroy cell structure	• Shortness of breath • Chest tightness • Wheezing • Laryngeal spasm • Mucosal and dermal irritation • Pulmonary oedema • ARDS	• Chlorine • Phosgene • Chloropicrin • Nitrogen dioxide • Sulphur dioxide	• Management of secretions • Oxygen • High-dose steroids (value controversial) • Treat pulmonary oedema with PEEP[a] to maintain PO_2 above 60 mmHg
c. Vesicants or blister agents	• *Mustard:* Forms metabolites that bind to enzymes, proteins and other cellular components • *Lewisite:* Binds to thiol groups in many enzymes • *Phosgene oxime:* Mechanism unknown but corrosive action like strong acids	• Burning, itching or red skin • Prominent tearing and burning of eyes • Shortness of breath • Nausea, vomiting • Skin erythema and blistering • Watery, swollen eyes • Upper airway sloughing with pulmonary oedema	• Mustard • Lewisite • Phosgene oxime	• Mustard and phosgene oxime have no specific antidotes • For lewisite, British anti-Lewisite (BAL or dimercaprol) IM • Thermal burn therapy • Rupture blisters as they contain toxin • Supportive care

[a]Positive end-expiratory pressure.

GAMMA RAYS AND X-RAYS

- High-energy rays which can travel several metres and penetrate deep into tissues.
- Can cause systemic effects.

ACUTE RADIATION SYNDROME

- It occurs after an acute exposure of whole body to substantial ionising radiation.
- Exposure to 1–2 Gy of radiation can produce it while exposure to 10 Gy of radiation is usually fatal.
- Acute radiation syndrome develops in four phases: prodromal, latent, manifest and recovery/death phase.
- Features and management of acute radiation syndrome are presented in Table 10.14.

Q. How is body temperature maintained?

- Body temperature or the core temperature is dependent on the balance between heat production and heat loss.
  - Core temperature refers to the deep body temperature in the internal environment of the body,

TABLE 10.14 Features and Management of Acute Radiation Syndrome

Phase	Features	Remarks	Treatment
Prodrome	• Transient autonomic nervous system response characterised by nausea, vomiting, anorexia, abdominal cramps and diarrhoea • May have hypotension, sweating and fatigue	• Sooner onset and more severe with greater dose • With exposure to 1–3 Gy, onset within 12 hours • With exposure to 10 Gy, onset within 5–15 minutes	• Paracetamol and opioids for abdominal pain • Antiemetics • Fluid replacement • Haemoglobin, TLC, DLC, absolute lymphocyte count and platelet counts every 6 hours for 24–48 hours and then 12–24 hourly • HLA typing if prodrome occurs within 2–3 hours of exposure (indicating possibility of haematopoietic failure)
Latent phase	• Asymptomatic	• Shorter duration with larger doses • May last for 1–3 weeks with exposure <4 Gy • Lasts for only a few hours with exposure >15 Gy	• Continue monitoring including investigations
Manifest phase			
Haematopoietic syndrome	• Prodrome phase for about 48 hours • Latent phase of 1–3 weeks • Pancytopaenia, infections, haemorrhage	• First system to be affected if exposure >1.5 Gy • Damage to bone marrow and circulating cells, particularly lymphocytes • Platelet, neutrophils and red cells also affected • Most deaths occur due to infections and haemorrhage	• Administration of blood products • Antibiotics, antifungals and antivirals to control infections • Colony-stimulating factors • Romiplostim (a thrombopoietin receptor agonist) • Stem cell or bone marrow transplant
Gastrointestinal syndrome	• Prodrome of nausea, vomiting diarrhoea within hours of exposure • Latency for about 1 week • Recurrence of severe nausea, vomiting, diarrhoea, abdominal pain	• Exposure to >6 Gy results in death of GI mucosa including stem cells which causes impaired mucosal integrity resulting in massive fluid and electrolyte losses and translocation of intestinal flora into blood • Death is due to infection, dehydration and electrolyte imbalance	• Fluid and electrolyte replacement • Antibiotics
Cardiovascular and CNS syndrome	• Immediate hypotension, nausea, vomiting, bloody diarrhoea • Disorientation, ataxia, tremors, seizures, coma	• Exposure to >30 Gy uniformly fatal • Exposure to >100 Gy results in death in a few hours • Significant cerebral oedema due to vascular damage	• Symptomatic only • No recovery is expected

that is the abdominal, thoracic and cranial cavities. From a measurement perspective, it refers to the temperature of venous blood returning to the heart. Practically, it is measured by checking lower oesophageal or rectal temperature.

- Heat generation occurs due to various exothermic metabolic processes and absorption of heat from the environment. Muscles are important in heat production and shivering can increase the heat production several times.
- Loss of heat from the body occurs in several ways including conduction, convection, evaporation and radiation. Varying the amount of blood flow through the skin capillaries helps in controlling heat loss from the skin. When heat needs to be conserved, the sympathetic stimulation leads to vasoconstriction that reduces heat transfer from the body to the skin. Evaporation of sweat is an important method of heat loss.
- The ultimate control of body temperature between 97°F and 99°F (36.1°C and 37.2°C) is done by preoptic hypothalamic centres that control the heat loss and heat production.
- During heat stress, hypothalamus signals for dilatation of cutaneous blood vessels and an increase in sweat production in order to adjust heat loss.
- During cold exposure, hypothalamus signals for constriction of cutaneous blood vessels, minimises sweat production and increases metabolic heat production (shivering and nonshivering thermogenesis).

Q. Discuss various heat-related illnesses.

- High environmental temperatures may result in heat syndromes that include heat rash (miliaria), heat cramps, heat oedema, heat exhaustion, exertional heat injury and heat stroke.
- These syndromes occur primarily at high environmental temperatures (>32°C or 90°F) and at high relative humidity.
- Various predisposing factors are listed in Table 10.15.

TABLE 10.15 Predisposing Factors for Heat-Related Illnesses

Environment Factors	Age
• High temperature • High relative humidity	• Infants • Elderly patients
Drugs/Toxins	**Occupation**
• Anticholinergic agents • Phenothiazines • Cyclic antidepressants • Monoamine oxidase inhibitors (MAOI) • Lysergic acid diethylamide (LSD) • Amphetamine • Lithium intoxication • Diuretics • Cocaine • Antihistamines • β-Blockers	• Athletes • Labourers • Military personnel **Miscellaneous** • Use of alcohol • Mental illnesses • Heavy clothing • Hyperthyroidism

HEAT RASH (MILIARIA)

- Occurs due to vasodilation of skin vessels with obstructed sweat ducts/pores from macerated stratum corneum.
- Presents with eruption of red papules or pustules, primarily on neck, upper extremities, trunk and groin. Skin covered by clothing is most often affected.
- The rash typically resolves after moving to a cooler environment, removing excess clothing and drying the skin. Topical emollients should be avoided.

HEAT CRAMPS

- Most benign heat disorder, generally associated with strenuous physical activity.
- Pathogenesis: Direct exposure to sun is not required.
  - Loss of sodium in the sweat coupled with inadequate sodium replacement results in hyponatraemia that is thought to produce cramps through interference with calcium-dependent muscle relaxation.
  - Hyperventilation producing respiratory alkalosis and mild hypokalaemia may be a contributory factor.
- *Clinical features:*
  - Patients complain of painful spasm of skeletal muscles, both of extremities and of abdomen several hours after exertion.
  - Usually the cramps occur in the muscles that have been subjected to excessive exercise.
  - The body temperature does not rise and the sweating is normal or excessive.
- *Laboratory studies:*
  - Mild hyponatraemia, hypokalaemia and respiratory alkalosis.
- *Treatment:*
  - Rest in a cool environment.
  - Replacement of sodium, potassium and water.
  - Avoid massage of the involved limbs as it generates heat.
- *Prevention:*
  - Liberal ingestion of sodium and water.

HEAT OEDEMA

- It manifests by ankle and wrist swelling occurring in the first few days of heat exposure. It may be pitting in a few patients.
- The oedema resolves within a few days of acclimatisation.

EXERTIONAL HEAT INJURY OR HEAT SYNCOPE

- It occurs in persons who exert in hot and humid environment. It is common in long-distance runners who run without adequate hydration and acclimatisation.
- *Clinical features:*
  - This disorder is characterised by headache, piloerection, chills, hyperventilation, nausea, vomiting, muscular incoordination and incoherent speech.
  - The patients sweat freely and the body temperature is elevated but usually not as high as that seen with heat stroke.
  - Some patients may develop syncope. It occurs due to volume depletion, peripheral vasodilation and decreased vasomotor tone.
  - Examination shows a diaphoretic patient with tachycardia and hypotension.
- *Laboratory features:*
  - Hypernatraemia, abnormal liver and muscle enzymes, hypocalcaemia, hypophosphataemia and hypoglycaemia.
  - Some patients also develop thrombocytopenia, disseminated intravascular coagulation (DIC) and rhabdomyolysis.
- *Treatment:*
  - The patient should be placed in a supine position in a cool place covered with wet cold sheets so as to lower the temperature below 100.4°F (38°C).
  - Massage of extremities is helpful in increasing flow of blood from the core to the periphery.
  - Infuse 5% dextrose in N/2 saline.

HEAT EXHAUSTION

- Heat exhaustion is common in elderly patients and occurs due to fluid and electrolyte losses coupled with inadequate replacement.
- *Clinical features:*
  - It is characterised by weakness, anxiety, fatigue, vertigo, thirst, anorexia, nausea, vomiting, headache, faintness, hyperventilation, muscular incoordination, agitation and confusion.
  - The skin is cold and clammy, the pupils are dilated, the pulse rate is rapid, the blood pressure is low and the body temperature is normal or mildly elevated.
  - The boundary between heat exhaustion and heat stroke is ill defined; usually, the absence of signs and symptoms of severe CNS damage and core temperature below 40°C differentiate between the two.
  - Hepatic transaminases are normal in heat exhaustion.

- *Treatment:*
  - The patient should be moved to a cool area and given salt and water.
  - If severe volume depletion is present, intravenous fluids are given.
  - If temperature is markedly elevated or there is reduced mentation, treatment of heat stroke should be instituted.

HEAT STROKE

- Heat stroke is a true medical emergency that is characterised by hyperthermia (core temperature ≥40°C) and neurological symptoms.
- Heat stroke is of two types: exertional (increased endogenous heat production) and classic (impairment of heat dissipation).
- *Exertional heat stroke:*
  - It occurs in healthy, young individuals, usually during the period of acclimatisation, who exert in hot environment. Typical patients are athletes and military recruits.
  - The patient develops hyperthermia and loss of consciousness.
  - The patient sweats freely.
  - Complications include DIC, rhabdomyolysis, renal failure and lactic acidosis.
- *Classic heat stroke:*
  - It occurs more often in elderly persons with underlying predisposing conditions during hot weather. These predisposing conditions impair thermoregulation, prevent removal from a hot environment or interfere with access to hydration or attempts at cooling. Common examples include cardiovascular diseases, neurological or psychiatric disorders, obesity, physical disability, extremes of age, use of alcohol or cocaine and use of drugs such as anticholinergic agents or diuretics.
  - Some persons develop unconsciousness without any premonitory features.
  - Others may have headache, hyperventilation, vertigo, faintness, ataxia, confusion and abdominal distress before losing consciousness.
  - Examination shows hyperthermia with a core temperature more than 106°F (41.1°C) and in some cases may be as high as 112°F (44.3°C). Core temperature is measured using either an oesophageal or a rectal thermometer.
  - Most of the patients do not sweat and the skin is dry.
  - Other features include tachycardia, cardiac arrhythmias, low blood pressure, rapid respiration, flaccid muscles, decreased deep tendon reflexes and lethargy, stupor or coma depending on the severity.
  - The pupils may be fixed and dilated.
  - Complications in the form of lactic acidosis, DIC, rhabdomyolysis and renal failure are uncommon as compared to exertional heat stroke.
- Laboratory investigations show leucocytosis, proteinuria, elevated blood urea, respiratory alkalosis followed by metabolic acidosis (lactic acidosis), normokalaemia or hypokalaemia, hypocalcaemia, hypophosphataemia, ST–T wave changes in the ECG, thrombocytopenia, coagulopathy and DIC.
- Table 10.16 compares classic heat stroke with exertional heat stroke.

TREATMENT

- Similar for both types of heat stroke.
- Maintenance of airway, breathing and circulation.
- Measurement of rectal temperature.
- IV line and oxygen administration.
- Blood for various investigations.
- The patient should be totally disrobed.
- Application of ice on lateral aspects of the trunk, neck, axillae and groins.
- Evaporative cooling involves the removal of clothing, spraying tepid water over the patient, and facilitating evaporation and convection with the use of a fan.
- Immersing the patient in cold water (8°C–14°C) or ice-cold water (2°C–5°C) is equally or possibly

TABLE 10.16 Comparison of Classic Heat Stroke Versus Exertional Heat Stroke

Feature	Classic Heat Stroke	Exertional Heat Stroke
Age group	Very young and elderly	Adults
Weather conditions	During heat waves	Temperate or hot
Concurrent activity	Sedentary	Sustained or heavy exertion
Health status	Ill or on medications	Healthy
Mechanism	Absorption of environmental heat	Excessive heat production
Sweating	Usually absent	Usually present
Rhabdomyolysis	Uncommon	Common
Liver enzymes	Mild elevation	Marked elevation
DIC	Mild	Severe
Renal failure	Uncommon	Relatively more common
Calcium	Normal	Hypocalcaemia
Potassium	Normal	Hyperkalaemia
Phosphate	Hypophosphataemia	Hyperphosphataemia
Blood glucose	Normal or high	Often low

more effective but is more cumbersome than the methods described above.
- Cold fluids intravenously.
- Additional methods of lowering the body temperature that have been tried with varying success include ice water gastric lavage and enemas, and ice water peritoneal dialysis.
- Other methods include endovascular cooling and extracorporeal membrane oxygenation (ECMO).
- The goal is to reduce the core temperature to 100 °F–102 °F (37.8 °C–38.9 °C) within 30–60 minutes.
- Antipyretic agents such as aspirin and paracetamol are ineffective; additionally, antipyretics aggravate coagulopathy and liver injury in patients with heat stroke.

PREVENTION

- Exertion should be limited when temperature and humidity are high.
- Activities in direct sunlight should be avoided.
- Loose clothes should be worn during summers.
- Adequate hydration should be maintained before and during exertion.

Q. What are the various causes of altered level of consciousness and hyperthermia?

- Causes of altered level of consciousness and hyperthermia are given in Table 10.17.

TABLE 10.17 Causes of Altered Level of Consciousness and Hyperthermia

Intrinsic Causes	Extrinsic Causes
• CNS injury • Thyroid storm • Infection (including cerebral malaria, meningitis, encephalitis and brain abscess) • Phaeochromocytoma • Systemic infections (e.g. sepsis)	• Anticholinergic poisoning • Drug ingestion (e.g. MAO inhibitors, amphetamines and phencyclidine) • Heat stroke • Serotonin syndrome • Salicylate overdose • Neuroleptic malignant syndrome (NMS)

Q. Discuss briefly the various causes of hyperthermia.

CAUSES (Table 10.18)

TABLE 10.18 Causes of Hyperthermia

• Anticholinergic syndrome	• Neuroleptic malignant syndrome
• High fever due to infections (systemic and CNS infection)	• Drug interactions with MAO inhibitors
• Heat stroke	• Serotonin syndrome
• Malignant hyperthermia	• Phaeochromocytoma

MALIGNANT HYPERTHERMIA

- Malignant hyperthermia is characterised by a rapid increase in temperature in response to inhalational anaesthetics (like halothane, cyclopropane and ether) or muscle relaxants (like succinylcholine).
- It is an inherited disorder with inheritance varying from autosomal dominant to autosomal recessive mode.

CLINICAL FEATURES

- Reduced muscle relaxation occurs during induction of anaesthesia and fasciculations occur when succinylcholine is administered. Some patients develop trismus during intubation.
- If the patient is not monitored carefully, sudden rise in temperature occurs resulting in a hot and dry skin.
- Other features include cardiac arrhythmia, muscle rigidity, hypotension and cyanosis.
- Complications include massive swelling of skeletal muscles, pulmonary oedema, DIC and acute renal failure.

King Syndrome

- It is the autosomal recessive form of malignant hyperthermia. It is associated with a number of congenital malformations including short stature, undescended testes, thoracic kyphosis, webbed neck, winged scapulae, low-set ears and antimongoloid obliquity of palpebral fissures of eyes.

LABORATORY FEATURES

- Respiratory and metabolic acidosis, hyperkalaemia and hypermagnesaemia.

TREATMENT

- Whenever malignant hyperthermia is suspected, surgery should be stopped and inhalational anaesthetic is withdrawn.
- Oxygen is administered and external cooling is started.
- Urine output is maintained by infusing fluids.
- Cardiac rhythm should be monitored for any arrhythmias.
- Specific treatment includes intravenous dantrolene in a dose of 1 mg/kg that is continued until improvement occurs or a dose of 10 mg/kg is reached.

NEUROLEPTIC MALIGNANT SYNDROME (NMS)

- It is usually associated with therapeutic use of neuroleptic drugs like phenothiazines, butyrophenones and thioxanthines. Other drugs which can rarely produce NMS include prochlorperazine, metoclopramide and domperidone.
- The onset of NMS is not related to the duration of exposure to the agent or to the dose.

CLINICAL FEATURES

- NMS typically develops over a period of 24–72 hours and lasts for 5–10 days.
- The typical features are hyperthermia, hypertonia of muscles, rigidity, fluctuating levels of consciousness and instability of autonomic nervous system.

- Autonomic features include pallor, sweating, fluctuating blood pressure, tachycardia, urinary incontinence and cardiac arrhythmias.
- Death may occur between 3 and 30 days and is due to respiratory failure, cardiovascular collapse, renal failure and cardiac arrhythmias.

LABORATORY FEATURES

- Leucocytosis with shift to the left is common (less common in serotonin syndrome).
- Elevated liver enzymes and creatine kinase (less frequent in serotonin syndrome).
- Myoglobinuria and acute renal failure.
- Low serum iron.

TREATMENT

- Management focuses on withdrawal of the neuroleptic agent and meticulous supportive care that includes aggressive hydration and reduction of body temperature.
- Dantrolene and bromocriptine (2.5–10 mg TID) have produced variable results.

ANTICHOLINERGIC SYNDROME

- It occurs in overdose with various agents (including neuroleptics) having anticholinergic properties.
- It is usually associated with peripheral features of anticholinergic poisoning that include tachycardia, dry, flushed skin, dry mouth, dilated pupils, reduced bowel sounds, urinary retention and cardiac arrhythmias.
- The patients are often hyperthermic and are disoriented, delirious and confused.
- Details under 'datura poisoning' on page 758.

SEROTONIN SYNDROME

- Serotonin syndrome occurs due to an excess of serotonin in the CNS. The syndrome typically occurs with the coadministration of two serotonergic agents especially if the dose of one is escalated. It can also occur with monotherapy in susceptible patients and with overdose. The drug combination most commonly associated with severe reactions is that of MAOI and selective serotonin reuptake inhibitors (SSRIs). Other drugs include pethidine, linezolid and dextromethorphan.

CLINICAL FEATURES

- Onset of serotonin syndrome is rapid (within hours) with CNS, neuromuscular and autonomic features.
- Change in mental status—agitation, delirium, restlessness, disorientation, anxiety, lethargy, seizures and hallucinations.
- Autonomic dysfunction—diaphoresis, hypertension, hyperthermia, vomiting, tachycardia, dilated pupils, unreactive pupils, diarrhoea and abdominal pain.
- Neuromuscular excitability—myoclonus, clonus, tremor, muscle rigidity, hyperreflexia and nystagmus.
- Others—diarrhoea, nausea and vomiting (rarely seen in NMS), rhabdomyolysis, acute renal failure, DIC and circulatory failure.
- Unlike NMS, serotonin syndrome has rapid onset and is associated with hyperkinesia. Myoclonus is more common in serotonin syndrome as compared to NMS.

TREATMENT

- Stop all serotonergic drugs.
- Supportive care including supplemental oxygen, intravenous fluids and cardiac monitoring.
- Benzodiazepines for agitation.
- Cyproheptadine is useful in some patients.
- Esmolol for autonomic instability.
- Control of hyperthermia.

Q. Define hypothermia. Discuss the clinical features and management of a patient with hypothermia.

- Hypothermia is defined as a core temperature less than 35°C (95°F).
- Hypothermia is further classified into primary and secondary.
  - Primary or accidental hypothermia is usually acute and occurs in healthy individuals after acute exposure to low temperatures.
  - Secondary hypothermia is usually slow in onset and occurs in people with underlying predisposing illnesses (Table 10.19).

STAGING OF ACCIDENTAL HYPOTHERMIA

- Table 10.20 gives staging of a patient with accidental hypothermia.

TABLE 10.19 Predisposing Factors for Hypothermia

Individual Factors	Drug/Toxin Overdose
• Old age • Infants and young children • Chronic alcoholics • Immobilisation for a long time • Anorexia nervosa • Malnutrition **Exposure to cold (accidental or environmental)** **CNS disorders** • Stroke • Head injury • Tumour • Wernicke's encephalopathy	• Phenothiazines • Antidepressants • Barbiturates • Alcohol **Endocrine causes** • Hypopituitarism • Hypothyroidism • Hypoadrenalism • Hypoglycaemia **Miscellaneous** • Sepsis • Massive transfusion with cold blood • Shock due to any cause • Burns

TABLE 10.20 Staging of Accidental Hypothermia

Stage	Clinical Findings	Core Temperature (If Available)
I	Conscious, shivering	32°C–35°C (90°F–95°F)
II	Impaired consciousness; may or may not be shivering	28°C to <32°C (82°F to <90°F)
III	Unconscious; vital signs present	<28°C–24°C (<82°F–75.2°F)
IV	Apparent death; vital signs absent	Variable; generally 13.7°C–24°C (75.2°F–56.7°F)

CLINICAL FEATURES

- Patients with mild hypothermia develop tachypnoea, tachycardia, ataxia, dysarthria, impaired judgement, shivering and diuresis (known as cold diuresis and occurs due to decreased release of antidiuretic hormone by the hypothalamus as well as initial increased renal blood flow from peripheral vasoconstriction).
- In moderate hypothermia, patient develops bradycardia, hypoventilation, CNS depression, hyporeflexia and loss of shivering. Paradoxical undressing may be observed and is due to feeling of warmth produced by peripheral vasoconstriction. Atrial fibrillation and other arrhythmias may occur and the ECG may contain Osborn J waves (positive deflection at the termination of the QRS complex with associated J-point elevation (Fig. 10.3); may also be seen in patients with subarachnoid haemorrhage and cerebral ischaemia).
- Severe hypothermia can lead to pulmonary oedema, oliguria, coma, hypotension, severe bradycardia, ventricular tachycardia and fibrillation and asystole.

DIAGNOSIS

- A low-reading thermometer is required to determine core temperature (generally rectal or oesophageal temperature is taken).
- Arterial blood gas analysis may show metabolic and respiratory acidosis.
- Coagulopathy.

TREATMENT

- Stabilisation of airway, breathing and circulation.
- Avoid rough movements of the patient as hypothermic heart is very sensitive to movement and rough handling may precipitate arrhythmias, including ventricular fibrillation (VF).
- Cardiac arrest due to ventricular arrhythmias and asystole may be refractory to conventional CPR until the patient has been rewarmed. American Heart Association recommends that hypothermic patients in cardiac arrest should receive defibrillation and pharmacological therapy as per ACLS guidelines. On the other hand, the European Resuscitation Council recommends that if VF persists after three shocks, further attempts should be delayed until the core temperature is >30 °C. It also recommends to withhold adrenaline if the core temperature is <30 °C.
- CPR should not be abandoned unless the patient has been rewarmed to 34 °C to 35 °C. It is recommended to stop CPR and declare the patient dead if the serum potassium concentration exceeds 12 mEq/L.
- Volume resuscitation:
  - Hypotension is expected in moderate and severe hypothermia due to cold diuresis. Rewarming also reverses the peripheral vasoconstriction, which may lead to hypotension.
  - Multiple large-bore intravenous lines should be established and warm normal saline should be started. Ringer's lactate should be avoided as hepatic metabolism of lactate is impaired in hypothermic patients.
  - While administering large volume of fluids intravenously, care should be taken to avoid pulmonary oedema as many patients have reduced cardiac output.
- Rewarming:
  - Passive external rewarming is the method of choice for mild hypothermia. After wet clothing is removed, the patient is covered with blankets. The resulting reduction in heat loss combines with

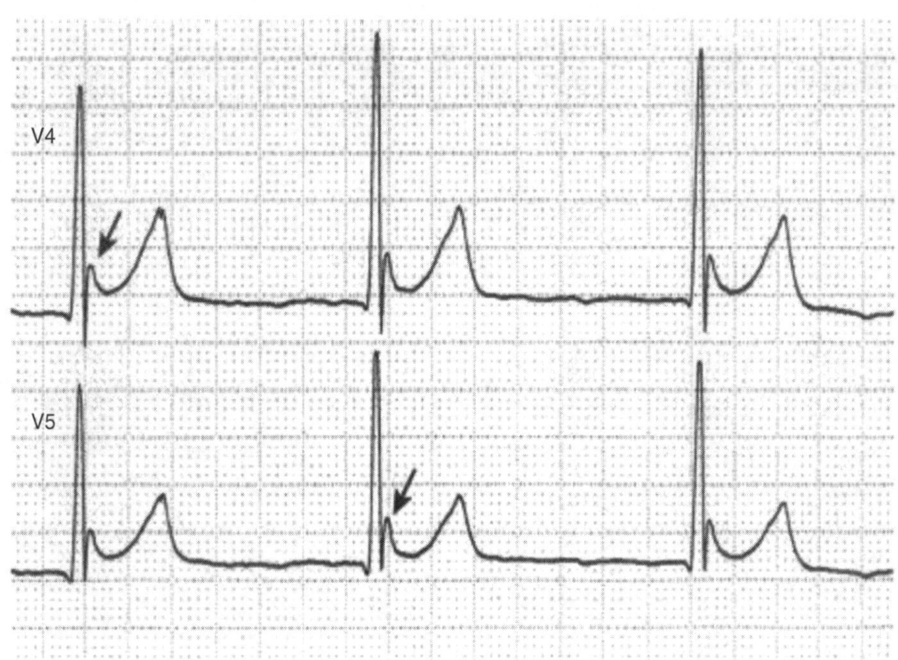

Fig. 10.3 Osborn J waves in lateral leads in moderate hypothermia.

the patient's intrinsic heat production to produce rewarming.

- Active external rewarming includes application of warm blankets, heating pads, heat from radiant heaters or forced warm air through blanket, either singly or in combination. These methods are indicated for moderate to severe hypothermia.
  - A risk of active external rewarming is core temperature afterdrop. This complication occurs when the extremities and trunk are warmed simultaneously. Cold, acidotic blood which has pooled in the vasoconstricted extremities of the hypothermic patient returns to the core circulation causing a drop in temperature and pH. This phenomenon may explain fatal dysrhythmias which sometimes occur during rewarming. Core temperature afterdrop can be avoided by rewarming the trunk before the extremities.
- Active internal rewarming can be combined with active external rewarming in moderate to severe hypothermia. Various techniques include warm humidified oxygen, warm intravenous fluids (at 39°C–41°C), bladder or gastric irrigation with warm saline, pleural and peritoneal irrigation with warm saline, continuous arteriovenous rewarming, haemodialysis, ECMO and cardiopulmonary bypass.

11 Nutritional Factors in Disease

Q. Give a brief account of calcium, vitamin D, parathyroid hormone and calcitonin.

CALCIUM

- Calcium salts (hydroxyapatite) are present in the cellular matrix that provides the hard structure of the bones and teeth—99% of total body calcium is thus present in the skeleton. The human body of an adult contains about 1200 g of calcium. Calcium absorption from the intestines is dependent on vitamin D and parathyroid hormone (PTH).
- Sources of calcium and recommended intake are given in Table 11.1.

VITAMIN D

- Vitamin D is a fat-soluble vitamin having the basic biochemical structure as that of cholesterol. Two chemical forms are present.

TABLE 11.1 Sources of Calcium and Recommended Daily Intake

Dietary Sources of Calcium	Recommended Intake of Calcium
• Milk and milk products (cheese and yoghurt) • Shell fish and fish eaten with bone	• Children—500–600 mg/day • Adolescents—700–800 mg/day • Postmenopausal females—1000 mg/day • Pregnancy and lactation—1200 mg/day

ERGOCALCIFEROL (VITAMIN D_2)

- This is manufactured by the action of ultraviolet light on ergosterol present in fungi. It is not present in humans. It is often used for therapeutic purposes.

CHOLECALCIFEROL (VITAMIN D_3)

- Naturally occurring form of vitamin D; also known as vitamin D_3.
- Formed in the skin by the action of ultraviolet light on 7-dehydrocholesterol.
- Cholecalciferol is converted in the liver to 25-hydroxycholecalciferol [$25(OH)D_3$] or calcidiol, which is further hydroxylated in the kidney to active vitamin D, 1-α,25-dihydroxycholecalciferol [$1,25(OH)_2D_3$] or calcitriol (Flowchart 11.1). The enzyme, $25(OH)D_3$-1-α-hydroxylase, required for

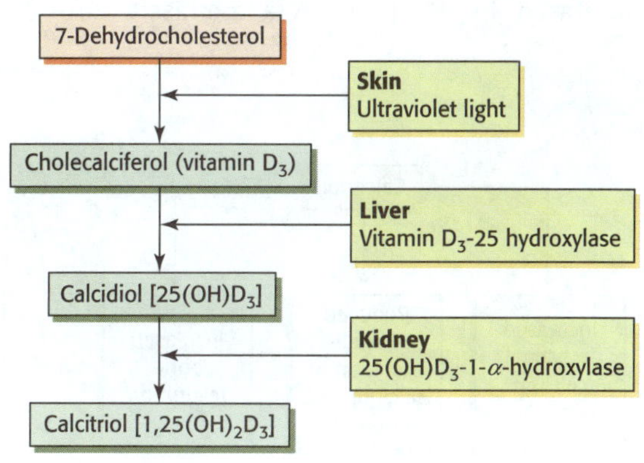

Flowchart 11.1 Production of Calcitriol.

TABLE 11.2 Effects of Calcitriol

• **Intestines** • Increased calcium absorption • Increased phosphorus absorption • Decreased magnesium absorption • **Parathyroid glands** • Decreased PTH synthesis • Decreased PTH secretion	• **Bone** • Release of calcium by acting on osteoblasts which in turn activates osteoclasts • At high doses, increased osteoclastic bone • **Kidney** • Autoregulation of calcitriol production by the kidney • Increased reabsorption of calcium (minor effect)

conversion is present mainly in proximal tubules of kidneys; it has also been described in macrophages and thymic-derived lymphocytes which may explain hypercalcaemia in granulomatous diseases such as active pulmonary sarcoidosis and tuberculosis, and in lymphomas.

- Fibroblast growth factor-23 inhibits renal production of 1,25-dihydroxycholecalciferol by limiting 25(OH)D_3-1-α-hydroxylase activity in the renal proximal tubule and by simultaneously increasing expression of 24-alpha-hydroxylase activity and production of 24,25-dihydroxyvitamin D (an inactive metabolite).
- The function of active vitamin D includes induction of a specific transport protein in the enterocyte to increase calcium absorption. It also increases phosphate absorption though the gut (Table 11.2).
- Dietary sources of vitamin D are fish and cod liver oil, eggs, liver and fatty fish.

PARATHYROID HORMONE

- PTH is secreted by parathyroid glands in response to low serum calcium levels. It raises calcium levels by:
  - Accelerating osteoclastic bone resorption, which occurs within minutes.
  - Increasing renal tubular reabsorption of calcium, which occurs within minutes after PTH secretion increases.
  - Increasing 1,25-dihydroxycholecalciferol formation which raises serum calcium by increased intestinal absorption; it occurs a day or more after PTH secretion increases.
- The increase in calcium in response to the effects mediated by PTH acts via a classic endocrine feedback loop on the calcium-sensing receptors on parathyroid glands, thereby decreasing secretion of PTH.
- Fibroblast growth factor-23 and calcitriol also inhibit PTH synthesis and secretion.
- PTH causes phosphate loss through kidneys producing hypophosphataemia.

CALCITONIN

- It is secreted by the parafollicular C cells of thyroid.
- Its release is stimulated by increase in blood calcium level.
- It is a weak inhibitor of osteoclast activation and opposes the effects of PTH on the kidneys, thereby promoting calcium and phosphate excretion.

CHEMICALS INVOLVED IN BONE FORMATION (Table 11.3)

TABLE 11.3 Functions of Chemicals Involved in Bone Formation

Chemical	Function
• Calcitonin	• Bone—inhibits resorption • Intestine—inhibits calcium and phosphorus absorption • Kidney—increases calcium excretion, inhibits production of calcitriol
• Calcitriol	• Bone—release of calcium by acting on osteoblasts which in turn activate osteoclasts • Intestine—increases calcium and phosphorus absorption • Kidney—autoregulation of calcitriol production by the kidney; increases reabsorption of calcium (minor effect) • Parathyroid gland—negative feedback to decrease secretion of PTH
• PTH	• Bone—mobilises calcium and phosphorus • Intestine—indirectly increases calcium and phosphorus absorption by increasing calcitriol • Kidney—increases calcitriol, increases calcium reabsorption, decreases phosphorus reabsorption

SUMMARY OF ACTIONS OF CALCITRIOL AND PTH (Flowchart 11.2)

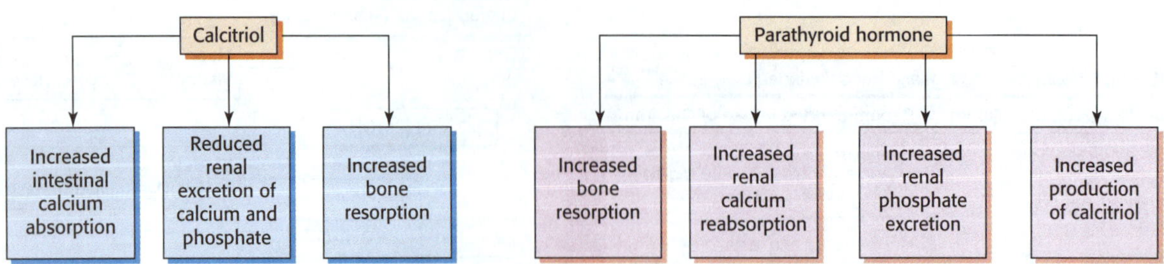

Flowchart 11.2 Summary of Actions of Calcitriol and Parathyroid Hormone.

Q. Write briefly on clinical features, investigations, treatment and prevention of rickets. (IM23.3), (PE 12.7)

- Deficiency of vitamin D in a growing child before the epiphyses have fused results in failure of growing bone to mineralise. This leads to rickets.

CLASSIFICATION OF RICKETS (Box 11.1)

BOX 11.1 Classification of Rickets

- Calciopaenic rickets—due to inability to maintain serum calcium levels in the normal range leading to secondary hyperparathyroidism and hypophosphataemia
- Phosphopaenic rickets—due to a primary inability to maintain serum phosphate levels in the normal range owing to impaired renal phosphate reabsorption or reduced gastrointestinal phosphate absorption
- Rickets associated with a direct inhibition of mineralisation at growth plate

CAUSES OF RICKETS (Table 11.4)

- Dark-skinned persons require more sunlight exposure than others to produce the same amount of vitamin D because melanin acts as a neutral filter and absorbs solar radiation.

TABLE 11.4 Causes of Rickets

Calciopaenic Rickets	
• Reduced calcium intake or absorption	• Nutritional deficiency • Malabsorption states (e.g. coeliac disease and intestinal resection)
• Vitamin D-associated	• Nutritional deficiency • Inadequate sunlight exposure • Malabsorption states (e.g. obstructive jaundice) • 25-hydroxylase deficiency—vitamin D-dependent rickets type 1B • 1-α-hydroxylase deficiency—vitamin D-dependent rickets type 1A due to inherited disorder or due to renal diseases (renal rickets) • Hereditary 1,25(OH)$_2$D$_3$-resistant rickets—vitamin D-dependent rickets type 2 due to mutation of VDR on intestinal cells • Increased degradation of vitamin D—anticonvulsants like phenytoin, phenobarbitone and carbamazepine
Phosphopaenic Rickets	
• Dietary phosphate deficiency or impaired bioavailability	• Breast-fed very low birthweight infants, excessive use of phosphate binders, gastrointestinal surgery
• Increased renal phosphate loss	• X-linked hypophosphataemia (familial hypophosphataemic rickets), tumour-induced rickets
Rickets Due to Direct Inhibition of Mineralisation	
	• Hereditary hypophosphatasia (deficiency of alkaline phosphatase) • Treatment with etidronate (first-generation bisphosphonate) • Fluoride excess

- Hereditary vitamin D-dependent rickets, type 1A (also known as pseudovitamin D deficiency rickets) is secondary to a defect in the gene that codes for the production of renal 25(OH)D$_3$-1-α-hydroxylase. It is an autosomal recessive disorder. This enzyme deficiency can also occur due to renal diseases.
- Vitamin D-dependent rickets, type 2 (or hereditary vitamin D-resistant rickets) is a rare autosomal recessive disorder caused by mutations in the vitamin D receptor (VDR) on intestine cells. It results in failure of vitamin D-dependent calcium absorption that in turn produces hypocalcaemia and rickets. Alopecia is common in this condition. This form of rickets does not respond to vitamin D treatment. Elevated level of circulating calcitriol differentiates this type from type 1.
- Familial hypophosphataemic rickets also produces vitamin D-resistant rickets refractory to vitamin D treatment. Renal wasting of phosphorus at the proximal tubule level results in hypophosphataemia. Normal levels of calcitriol are found in this disorder.
- In rickets secondary to malignancy, the most common pathophysiology is tumour secretion of fibroblast growth factor 23, which causes renal phosphate wasting and impaired calcitriol production (paraneoplastic manifestation).

CLINICAL FEATURES

- Commonly infants younger than 6 months present with hypocalcaemic tetany or seizures, whereas older children present with failure to thrive or skeletal deformities.
- Infantile tetany—due to low serum ionised calcium, resulting in epileptic fits and vocal cord spasm (high-pitched distressing cry).
- Infant appears well nourished but is restless, fretful and pale with flabby muscles.
- Prone to respiratory and gastrointestinal infections.
- Retardation of skeletal growth leads to failure to sit, stand, crawl and walk at the normal ages.
- Poor dentition and late eruption.
- Craniotabes with 'egg shell crackling' feeling (soft skull bones). The skull has small, round, unossified areas in the membranous part.
- Enlargement of the epiphyses at the lower end of radius, femur, tibia and fibula.
- 'Rickety rosary' (enlargement of costochondral junctions visible as beading along the anterolateral aspects of the chest) (Fig. 11.1) and pigeon-shaped chest (pectus carinatum).
- Harrison's groove or sulcus at the lower margin of the thorax caused by muscular pull of diaphragmatic attachments to the lower ribs.
- Frontal bossing of skull.
- Delayed closure of anterior fontanelle.
- Kyphosis, genu valgum (knock knees) and/or genu varum (bow legs).
- Pelvic abnormalities—triradiate pelvis.
- Delayed eruption of the teeth with enamel hypoplasia.
- Adolescents may present with bone pain and proximal muscle weakness.
- Rarely heart failure may develop due to cardiomyopathy.

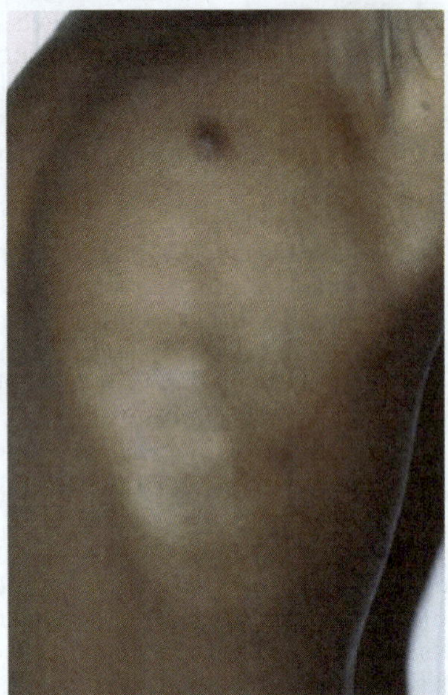

Fig. 11.1 Rickety rosary. (Courtesy: T. Thacher, MD)

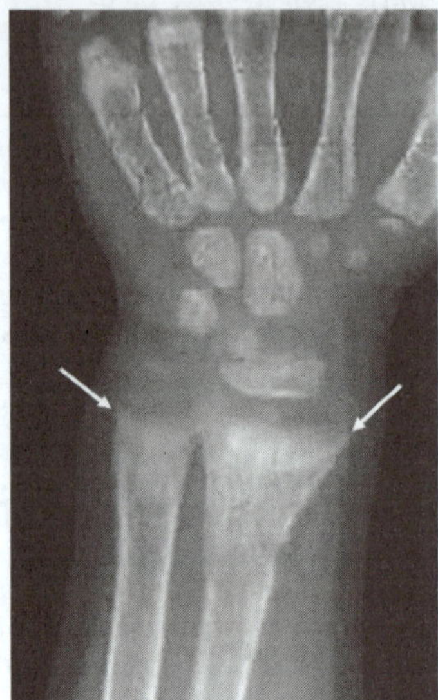

Fig. 11.2 Radiograph of wrist showing metaphyseal cupping and splaying.

INVESTIGATIONS

- Wrist radiography—lower ends of the shaft of radius and ulna become splayed, and epiphyseal surfaces appear fuzzy and ill defined (Fig. 11.2). Unossified zone between shaft and radial epiphysis is widened ('saucer' deformity).
- In calciopaenic rickets, serum calcium is low or normal, PTH levels are increased leading to decreased renal tubular reabsorption of phosphate and low serum phosphate levels. Serum alkaline phosphatase levels are markedly elevated due to the high PTH causing increased bone turnover.
- In phosphopaenic rickets, calcium level is normal, serum phosphate low and serum levels of PTH and 25(OH)D_3 are normal. Serum alkaline phosphatase is only modestly raised.
- Levels of plasma 25-hydroxyvitamin D_3 are low in vitamin D deficiency and elevated in dietary calcium deficiency.

TREATMENT

- Correction of underlying cause.
- Supplementation of calcium and vitamin D.
- For nutritional deficiency of vitamin D, ergocalciferol, 150,000–600,000 IU orally or intramuscularly as a single dose. Another option is to give ergocalciferol in a dose of 2000–6000 IU every day. Cholecalciferol can be given in place of ergocalciferol in a dose of 60,000 IU orally every week or 2000–6000 IU every day.
- For type 1 vitamin D-dependent rickets, calcitriol is required; patient will not respond to high doses of cholecalciferol.
- For type 2 vitamin D-dependent rickets, high doses of calcitriol and calcium may be tried.
- Familial hypophosphataemic rickets is treated with oral phosphorus and calcitriol.
- In phosphopaenic rickets, vitamin D and phosphate are required. Burosumab, a monoclonal antibody against fibroblast growth factor-23, can be used in X-linked hypophosphataemic rickets if the child is not responsive to usual treatment.

PREVENTION

- Adequate intake of vitamin D (1000–5000 IU/day).
- Adequate sunlight exposure (from 30 minutes to 2 hours/week for infants).

Q. Describe hypervitaminosis D.

- Chronic ingestion of large doses of vitamin D (50–100 times the normal physiological requirement, i.e. more than 50,000–100,000 IU/day) causes certain toxic symptoms and hypercalcaemia. It often occurs due to excessive dosages or too frequent dosing intervals of vitamin D administered for osteoporosis, hypoparathyroidism, hypophosphataemia, osteomalacia or renal osteodystrophy.
- Occasionally, vitamin D intoxication and hypercalcaemia can occur due to endogenous excessive production, for example granulomatous diseases.

SYMPTOMS

- Features are related to hypercalcaemia (Table 11.5).

DIAGNOSIS

- Increased serum level of 25(OH)vitamin D (>150 ng/mL).
- Hypercalcaemia.
- Very low or undetectable PTH.

TREATMENT

- Discontinue vitamin D supplementation.

TABLE 11.5 Clinical Features of Vitamin D Toxicity

Neuropsychiatric	Confusion, psychosis, stupor, coma
Gastrointestinal	Abdominal pain, vomiting, polydipsia, anorexia, constipation, pancreatitis
Cardiovascular	Hypertension, shortened QT interval, ST segment elevation, bradyarrhythmias, first-degree heart block
Renal	Hypercalciuria, acute kidney injury, dehydration, nephrocalcinosis
Others	Band keratopathy, hearing loss, painful periarticular calcinosis, metastatic arterial calcification

- Isotonic sodium chloride solution to correct dehydration and restore kidney function.
- Loop diuretics can be added once the volume is restored and maintained.
- Glucocorticoids to reduce intestinal calcium absorption.
- Antiresorptive therapy with the use of calcitonin and bisphosphonates.
- Haemodialysis in severe hypercalcaemia and acute kidney injury (AKI).

Q. Discuss the role of vitamin D in various diseases.

- Active form of vitamin D is 1,25-dihydroxyvitamin D.
- Most tissues and cells in humans express vitamin D receptors (VDRs).
- Vitamin D influences genes regulating many key cellular functions including cellular proliferation, differentiation, apoptosis and angiogenesis.
- Serum $25(OH)D_3$ levels most accurately reflect vitamin D status. The cut-offs representing insufficient and deficient $25(OH)D_3$ are variable, but most physicians take vitamin D deficiency as $25(OH)D_3$ levels less than 20 ng/mL and vitamin D insufficiency as $25(OH)D_3$ levels between 21 and 29 ng/mL. Deficiency of vitamin D may lead to several diseases. However, for many of them, robust evidence is not available.

RICKETS AND OSTEOMALACIA

- Refer to pages 771 and 776.

OSTEOPOROSIS

- Strong link between vitamin D deficiency and osteoporosis especially in the elderly.
- Vitamin D deficiency is associated with marked suppression of intestinal calcium absorption and impairment of calcium balance, which results in low bone mineral content and density.

MUSCLE WEAKNESS

- Muscle weakness is a prominent feature of vitamin D deficiency. This can lead to an increased number of falls.

HYPERTENSION

- Growing evidence suggests that vitamin D has an important association with blood pressure.
- $1,25(OH)_2D_3$ may inhibit renin expression in the kidneys and block proliferation of vascular smooth muscle cells, which could influence blood pressure.

CORONARY ARTERY DISEASE

- Many studies support association between low vitamin D levels and increased cardiovascular adverse events.
- Vitamin D deficiency is associated with impaired endothelial function and vascular stiffness, which are known predictors of long-term cardiovascular morbidity and mortality.
- Inflammation has been shown to have a strong role in the pathogenesis of coronary artery disease (CAD). Vitamin D suppresses inflammation via several pathways:
  - Inhibition of prostaglandin and cyclooxygenase-2 pathways.
  - Reduction of matrix metalloproteinase-9.
  - Up-regulation of antiinflammatory cytokine interleukin-10.

CANCER

- Vitamin D is one of the most potent hormones for regulating cell growth.
- It can induce differentiation into normally functioning cells and inhibit proliferation, invasiveness, angiogenesis and metastatic potential.
- The protective relationship between sufficient vitamin D status and lower risk of cancer has been found in many studies particularly with regard to colorectal cancer.

DIABETES

- Vitamin D deficiency inhibits pancreatic secretion and turnover of insulin. This may result in impaired glucose tolerance and frank diabetes.
- Vitamin D increases insulin sensitivity.

TUBERCULOSIS

- Studies have shown that patients with TB have lower $25(OH)D_3$ levels in comparison with those without TB.

ASTHMA

- Lower serum levels of $25(OH)D_3$ may be associated with increased asthma severity and poor asthma control.

OTHER ASSOCIATIONS WITH REDUCED VITAMIN D (NOT PROVEN)

- Increased severity of infectious diseases.
- Reduced immunity.

- Increased frequency of mood disorders.
- Increased frequency of inflammatory bowel disease.
- Increased autoimmunity.
- Increased risk of multiple sclerosis.
- Increased risk of COVID-19 ARDS.

SUMMARY

- A causal association between poor vitamin D status and major diseases has not been established.

Q. What is renal bone disease or chronic kidney disease-mineral and bone disorder? Explain.

Q. Describe renal osteodystrophy.

- Renal or chronic kidney disease-mineral and bone disorder (CKD-MBD) is characterised by several abnormalities (Box 11.2). The term renal osteodystrophy includes only bone abnormalities in patients with CKD and does not include extraskeletal manifestations.

BOX 11.2 Abnormalities in Chronic Kidney Disease-Mineral and Bone Disorders

- Abnormal metabolism of calcium, phosphorus, PTH and/or vitamin D
- Abnormalities in bone turnover, mineralisation, volume linear growth or strength
- Soft tissue calcifications, either vascular or extraosseous

- In chronic renal disease, the diseased kidney fails to synthesise 1,25-dihydroxyvitamin D_3. This results in impairment of calcium absorption from the gut. As the GFR falls, the serum phosphate concentration begins to rise. This phosphate retention in plasma facilitates calcium entry into the bone, thereby contributing to hypocalcaemia. This triggers PTH release resulting in secondary hyperparathyroidism.
- CKD-MBD is caused by (Flowchart 11.3):
  - Disordered vitamin D metabolism (reduced formation of 1,25-dihydroxyvitamin D_3).
  - Renal phosphate retention.
  - Secondary hyperparathyroidism.
  - Chronic metabolic acidosis of renal failure.
  - Excessive faecal loss of calcium.
  - Aluminium toxicity due to absorption of aluminium from antacids used as phosphate binders.
- Even with high serum PTH level, there is a skeletal resistance to its actions; thus, serum calcium level remains low.

TYPES OF RENAL OSTEODYSTROPHY

- Renal osteodystrophy can be divided according to the rate of bone turnover:
  - High bone turnover osteodystrophy seen due to secondary hyperparathyroidism and includes osteitis fibrosa cystica and osteosclerosis.
  - Low bone turnover osteodystrophy occurs with low PTH level. There is impaired mineralisation activity with decreased number of osteoblasts

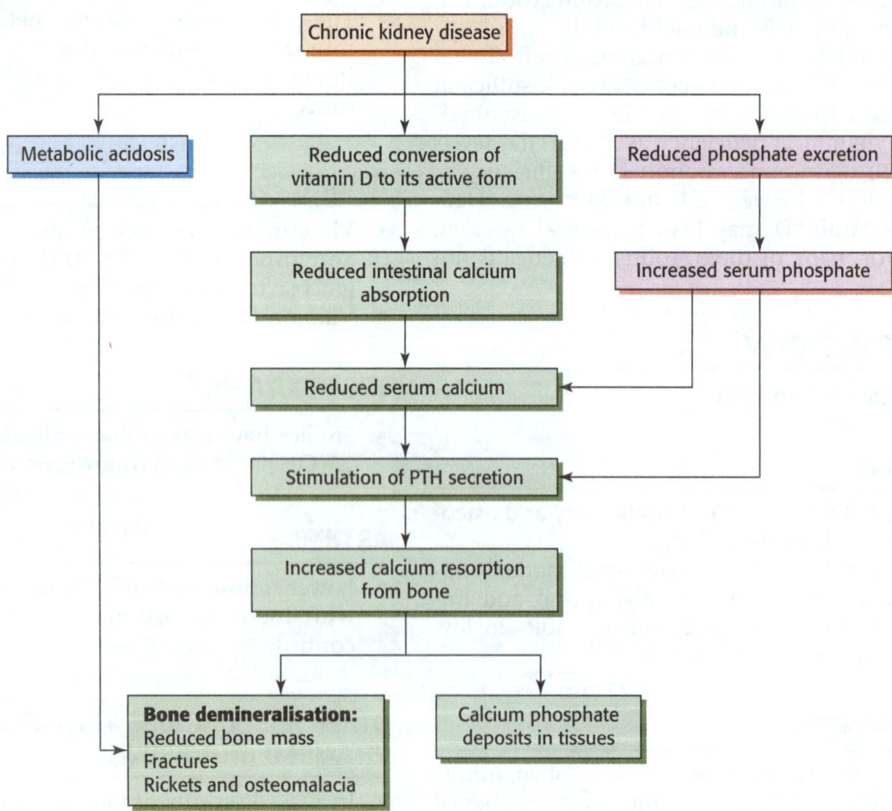

Flowchart 11.3 Pathogenesis of Renal Osteodystrophy.

and osteoclasts. Various entities include rickets or osteomalacia, aluminium-related bone disease and adynamic bone disease (ABD). ABD occurs due to excessive suppression of PTH by the use of calcium-based phosphate binders, vitamin D or following parathyroidectomy and in patients on dialysis. Mortality is increased because of enhanced cardiovascular calcification.
  - Mixed type osteodystrophy is osteitis fibrosa and osteomalacia with impaired mineralisation. The serum PTH level is high.
- In children—renal rickets or renal dwarf occurs due to impaired bone growth.
- In adults—osteomalacia.

CLINICAL FEATURES

- Most patients with renal osteodystrophy are asymptomatic.
- Some patients present with symptoms of an acute arthritis (pain, swelling, erythema, warmth and decreased range of motion).
- Bone pain is rare and is seen usually with osteomalacia and ABD.
- Skeletal deformities (e.g. genu valgum), more common in uraemic children.
- Pathological fractures can occur in some cases.
- These patients may have calciphylaxis that includes both soft tissue and vascular calcifications, including coronary artery calcification. This occurs when calcium × phosphate >70 mg/dL.

INVESTIGATIONS

- Serial assessments of phosphate, calcium and PTH levels.
- Bone mineral density (BMD) in patients with CKD-MBD and/or risk factors for osteoporosis (to assess fracture risk).
- Bone biopsy if knowledge of the type of renal osteodystrophy will impact treatment decisions.

RADIOGRAPHIC FINDINGS

- The classic radiographic finding of secondary hyperparathyroidism is subperiosteal bone resorption and erosions (Fig. 11.3). The earliest findings usually occur on the radial aspect of the middle phalanges, but can progress to include proximal tibia, distal clavicle, radius and ulna and humeral and femoral necks. These lesions are due to osteitis fibrosa cystica.
- Brown tumours may be seen on plain film as radiolucent, cystic regions, often within cortical bone. These lesions are again due to osteitis fibrosa cystica.
- Osteosclerosis is typically seen in the vertebrae, with a striped appearance on lateral spine films demonstrating alternating areas of radiopacity and radiolucency ('rugger jersey spine') (Fig. 11.4).
- Skull radiograph may show mixed lytic and blastic areas—'salt and pepper' appearance (Fig. 11.5).
- Osteopaenia.
- Findings of osteomalacia in adults.

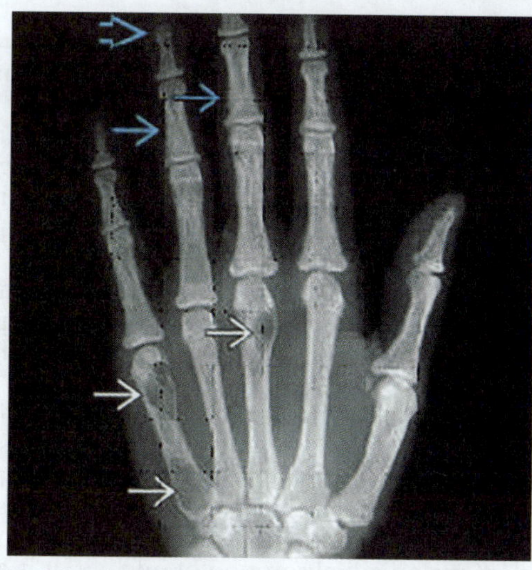

Fig. 11.3 Subperiosteal bone resorption (blue arrows) and multiple lucent lesions (white arrows) of osteitis fibrosa cystica (brown tumour).

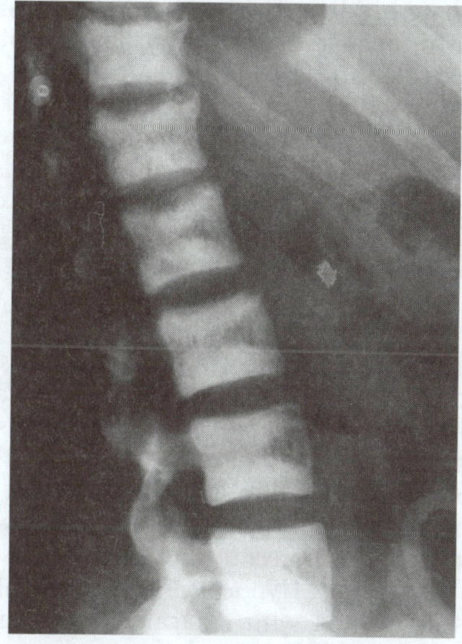

Fig. 11.4 Rugger jersey spine in renal osteodystrophy

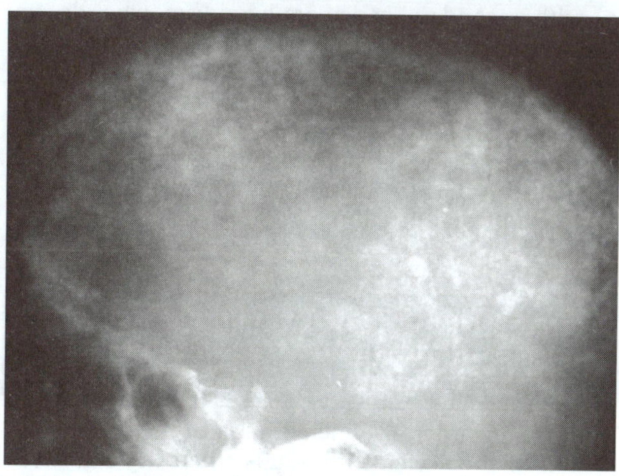

Fig. 11.5 'Salt and pepper' appearance on skull radiograph.

TREATMENT

- The current approach seeks to maintain calcium and phosphate in the normal range.
- Lowering phosphate is done initially by dietary restriction of phosphate intake to 800–1000 mg/day. Foods rich in phosphate are dairy products, meat, fish, sausages, legumes, nuts and chocolates.
- Agents commonly used in the management of renal osteodystrophy include calcium tablets, vitamin D supplements (in the form of calcitriol) and phosphate binders such as calcium carbonate or calcium acetate.
  - Use of calcitriol also enhances the absorption of calcium and phosphorus from the gut. This may lead to hypercalcaemia and elevated phosphate levels that are detrimental to vascular tissues.
- Vitamin D analogues like paricalcitol that has minimal effects on gut absorption of calcium. It is an active analogue based on vitamin D_2 structure (19-nor-1,25-dihydroxyvitamin D_2) that suppresses PTH secretion but has minimal effect on serum level of calcium and phosphate.
- Phosphate binders: The three main classes of phosphate binders are aluminium-based phosphate binders, calcium-based phosphate binders and non-calcium-based phosphate binders.
  - The long-term use of aluminium-based phosphate binders has been limited by its associated side effects such as aluminium-induced osteomalacia and encephalopathy.
  - Use of calcium-containing phosphate binders (calcium carbonate and calcium acetate) may lead to calcium overload.
  - Calcium-free phosphate binders include sevelamer hydrochloride, lanthanum carbonate, magnesium citrate and ferric citrate.
- Calcimimetics (e.g. cinacalcet) decrease the secretion of serum PTH through stimulation of calcium-sensing receptors in the parathyroid gland, which reduces renal osteodystrophy. These are used in patients on dialysis. Hypocalcaemia is one of the side effects associated with cinacalcet and thus regular measurement of serum calcium and phosphate is indicated.
- Parathyroidectomy is recommended for patients with secondary hyperparathyroidism who do not respond to medical therapy.
- The initial approach to treatment of ABD is to allow PTH secretion to rise. This can be achieved by using non-calcium-based phosphate binders, decreasing or stopping active vitamin D analogues and, for patients on dialysis, possibly by using a low-dialysate calcium concentration.

Q. Discuss the causes, clinical features, investigations and treatment in case of osteomalacia. (IM23.3), (OR 7.1)

- It is a disorder of mineralisation of the organic matrix of the skeleton in adults when the epiphyseal growth plates have closed. This produces increased unmineralised matrix. In contrast, in rickets, the growing skeleton is involved.

AETIOLOGY

- A number of disorders can produce osteomalacia, primarily through alteration in vitamin D nutrition or metabolism or because of phosphate wasting (Table 11.6).

CLINICAL FEATURES

- Bone pains and muscle weakness.
- Pain in the hip may produce antalgic gait.
- Proximal muscle weakness produces waddling gait and may mimic a primary muscle disease.
- Fractures of bones with mild trauma.
- Muscle spasms, cramps, a positive Chvostek's sign, tingling/numbness.
- Collapse of vertebrae produces local pain and deformity.
- Deformities due to softening of skeleton and include kyphosis, coxa vara, pigeon chest and triradiate pelvis with a narrow pubic arch.

INVESTIGATIONS

- Serum findings in vitamin D deficiency include the following:
  - Low or normal serum calcium (secondary hyperparathyroidism causes release of calcium from bone and increased resorption of calcium by the kidney; this maintains normal serum calcium in most patients).
  - Low serum phosphorus.
  - Elevated serum alkaline phosphatase.
  - Reduced urinary excretion of calcium.
  - Low serum 25-hydroxyvitamin D_3 levels (<20 ng/mL).
  - Elevated PTH levels.
- Radiological features:
  - Reduced bone density (osteopaenia).
  - Epiphyseal growth plate is increased in thickness, cupped and hazy at the metaphyseal border.
  - Presence of nontraumatic fractures.

TABLE 11.6 Aetiology of Osteomalacia

Nutritional Abnormalities	Acidosis
• Dietary deficiency of vitamin D • Parenteral nutrition **Malabsorption** • Tropical sprue • Coeliac disease • Hepatobiliary diseases • Pancreatic insufficiency **Disorders of vitamin D metabolism** • Vitamin D dependency type 1 and type 2 • Use of anticonvulsants • Chronic renal failure	• Distal renal tubular acidosis (type I) • Ureterosigmoidostomy **Phosphate depletion** • Use of nonabsorbable antacids • X-linked hypophosphataemia • Tumour-associated osteomalacia **Miscellaneous** • Multiple myeloma • Nephrotic syndrome • Lead poisoning • Inadequate sun exposure • Obesity

- Radiolucent, 2–5 mm wide bands with sclerotic borders called pseudofractures (Looser's zones) are seen (Fig. 11.6). They are often bilateral and symmetric and lie perpendicular to the cortical margins of bones. They are usually found at femoral neck, on the medial part of the femoral shaft and in the pubic and ischial rami. They occur due to erosion of bone produced by arterial pulsations.
- Cortical thinning due to secondary hyperparathyroidism.
- Loss of radiological distinctness of vertebral body trabeculae followed by concavity of the vertebral bodies (codfish vertebrae) (Fig. 11.7).

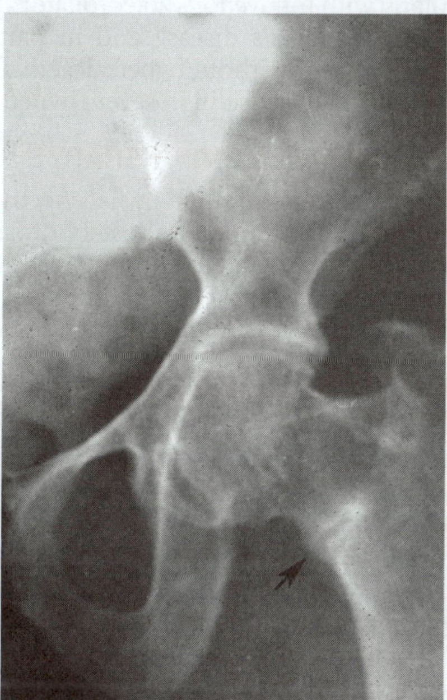

Fig. 11.6 Pseudofracture of the femoral neck.

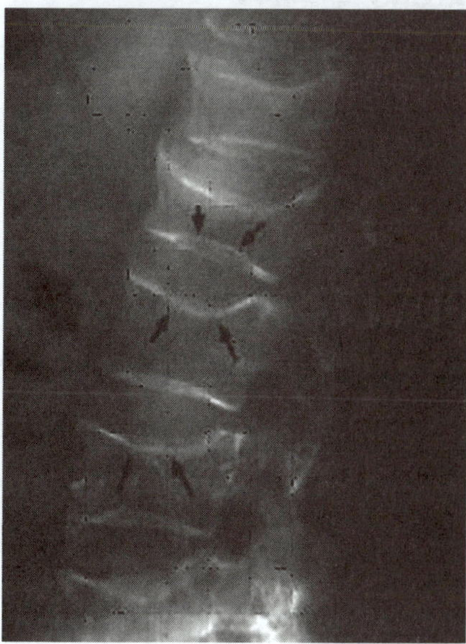

Fig. 11.7 Codfish vertebrae.

- Bone scan may be normal or may show discrete foci of increased radionuclide uptake.
- BMD as assessed by dual-energy X-ray absorptiometry (DEXA) is reduced at spine, hip and forearm, with the greatest deficits at the cortical-rich bone in the forearms.

TREATMENT

- Dietary deficiency is corrected by 1000–4000 IU of vitamin D_2 (ergocalciferol) or vitamin D_3 (cholecalciferol) for 3 months followed by lower doses as maintenance.
- Patients with osteomalacia due to malabsorption require 50,000–100,000 IU of vitamin D along with calcium supplementation. Small doses of calcitriol (0.5–1 μg daily) are also effective.
- In chronic renal failure, calcitriol is required with weekly monitoring of serum calcium.

Q. Discuss briefly the clinical features, investigations and treatment of osteoporosis. (IM24.8), (PH 1.36)

- Osteoporosis is characterised by a reduction in the mass of bone per unit volume (osteopaenia) to a level below that required for adequate mechanical support function. There is no abnormality in the ratio of the mineral to organic phase of bone matrix.
- Osteoporosis is also defined operationally as a bone density that falls 2.5 standard deviation below the mean for a 30-year-old normal reference in that population (also known as *T* score of 2.5).

COMMON DISORDERS ASSOCIATED WITH OSTEOPOROSIS

- Some of the common disorders associated with osteoporosis are shown in Table 11.7.

TABLE 11.7 Common Disorders Associated with Osteoporosis

Nutritional and GI disorders • Malnutrition • Malabsorption syndromes • Severe liver disease **Endocrine disorders** • Cushing's syndrome • Thyrotoxicosis • Hyperparathyroidism • Acromegaly • Hypogonadism **Rheumatological disorders** • Rheumatoid arthritis • Ankylosing spondylitis	**Inherited disorders** • Osteogenesis imperfecta • Marfan's syndrome • Haemochromatosis • Porphyria **Drugs** • Chronic steroid therapy • Chronic phenytoin therapy • Chronic heparin therapy • Antiretroviral drugs • Calcineurin inhibitors (tacrolimus and cyclosporin) • Aromatase inhibitors (anastrozole and letrozole) **Miscellaneous** • Immobilisation • Postmenopausal • Pregnancy and lactation • 'Senile' osteoporosis

CLINICAL FEATURES

- Fracture is the only cause of symptoms in osteoporosis that produces sudden pain. Common sites of fractures include spine, hip and wrist joints. Vertebral fractures can occur without any pain also.
- Vertebral and wrist fractures can occur much before hip fractures.

LABORATORY INVESTIGATIONS

- These include serum calcium, alkaline phosphatase, urinary calcium and other relevant investigations for the suspected underlying cause. Most often, serum calcium, phosphorus and alkaline phosphatase are normal.
- Urinary levels of cross-linked N-telopeptides of type I collagen (NTx) indicate the rate of bone breakdown or turnover. Urine NTx >40 nmol/L indicates excessive bone turnover and is a feature of osteoporosis.
- Radiographs of spine and pelvis:
    - Reduced cortical thickness of bones.
    - Increased radiolucency of bones.
    - Vertebrae show 'codfish' appearance.
    - Collapse of vertebral body with kyphosis.
- Measurement of bone density:
    - Quantitative CT scan.
    - Quantitative ultrasound.
    - DEXA scan for bone mineral density (BMD).

TREATMENT

- Diet should include at least 1 g of calcium and 800–1000 IU of vitamin D daily. Additional supplementation may be done to maintain bone and muscle strength.
- Ensure adequate weight-bearing exercises.
- Smoking and alcohol should be stopped.
- Reduce falls by taking care of home safety and personal precautions.
- If steroids are required for chronic use, add calcium, vitamin D and bisphosphonates.

BISPHOSPHONATES

- Most effective agents for reducing osteoporotic fractures.
- Typically combined with calcium and vitamin D.
- Bisphosphonates suppress osteoclast-mediated bone resorption. They also accelerate osteoclast apoptosis.
- Include alendronate, risedronate, ibandronate and zoledronic acid or zoledronate.
- Indicated for the treatment of osteoporosis in postmenopausal females and corticosteroid-induced osteoporosis.
- Alendronate, risedronate and zoledronic acid reduce the development of both hip and vertebral fractures while ibandronate does not reduce hip fractures.
- Alendronate also indicated in males with osteoporosis.
- Food reduces the absorption of bisphosphonates; therefore, these agents should be taken at least 30 minutes before the first food. Tablets should be swallowed with 200–300 mL of water. To reduce the risk of gastro-oesophageal irritation, patients should remain upright for at least 30 minutes after dosing.
- Dose:
    - Risedronate: 5 mg orally once a day or 35 mg orally once a week.
    - Alendronate: 10 mg orally once a day or 70 mg orally once a week.
    - Ibandronate: 150 mg once a month.
    - Zoledronic acid: 5 mg intravenously once in a year.
    - Pamidronate: 90 mg intravenously once a month.
- Main side effect is gastrointestinal upset. An important complication is osteonecrosis of jaw. Other adverse effects include bone, joint and/or muscle pains. Zoledronic acid may result in flu-like symptoms and fever. Other rare complications include atrial fibrillation (particularly with intravenous zoledronate) and uveitis.
- Also useful in Paget's disease and in painful bone metastasis (with or without hypercalcaemia). Intravenous pamidronate is useful in severe hypercalcaemia.

HORMONE REPLACEMENT THERAPY

- Hormone replacement therapy is effective for the prevention of postmenopausal osteoporosis.
- However, it is associated with increased risks of breast cancer, CAD, stroke and pulmonary thromboembolism. Hence, it is not recommended.

RECOMBINANT HUMAN PARATHYROID HORMONE

- PTH increases the rate of bone remodelling and results in a positive remodelling balance, leading to thicker osteons.
- Teriparatide, a recombinant human PTH, is approved for the treatment of postmenopausal osteoporosis for a period of maximum of 2 years (except in patients with CKD).
- Dose is 20 μg subcutaneously once a day.
- Another agent is abaloparatide, which is a PTH-related protein.

SELECTIVE OESTROGEN RECEPTOR MODULATORS

- Raloxifene is indicated for the prevention and treatment of postmenopausal osteoporosis.
- Dose is 60 mg orally once a day.
- Increased risk of thromboembolism.

SALMON CALCITONIN

- Inhibits bone resorption by acting directly on osteoclasts.
- Indicated for the treatment of osteoporosis if patient is intolerant to other agents.
- Available in both injectable and intranasal spray preparations.
- Dose is 200 IU intranasally once a day (alternating nostrils daily) or 100 units subcutaneously or intramuscularly every other day.

STRONTIUM RANELATE

- Strontium ranelate is a dual-action bone agent that has proven efficacy in the prevention of both vertebral and nonvertebral fractures in patients older than 80 years.

- It stimulates the proliferation of osteoblasts and inhibits the proliferation of osteoclasts.
- Therefore, it increases BMD by forming new bone.
- Dose is 2 g orally daily and is used in patients in whom bisphosphonate and other treatments have failed.
- May increase the risk of myocardial infarction, severe skin reactions and thromboembolism.

DENOSUMAB

- A fully human monoclonal antibody to receptor activator of nuclear factor kappa-B ligand (RANKL), an osteoclast-differentiating factor.
- Inhibits osteoclast formation, thus decreasing bone resorption.

ROMOSOZUMAB

- A humanised monoclonal antibody that binds sclerostin and inhibits its action. Inhibition of sclerostin by romosozumab has been shown to both increase bone formation and decrease bone resorption, resulting in a strong anabolic action on bone.
- Approved for use in postmenopausal women with severe osteoporosis who are at high risk of fracture.

Q. Write a brief note on corticosteroid-induced osteoporosis.

- Oral corticosteroid therapy using more than 5 mg of prednisolone (or equivalent) daily for more than 3 months can lead to a reduction in BMD and an increase in the risk of fractures.

PATHOGENESIS

- Suppression of osteoblast function resulting in decreased bone formation (primary effect).
- Suppression of intestinal calcium absorption.
- Reduced renal tubular calcium reabsorption with increased urinary calcium excretion.
- Renal and intestinal losses of calcium result in the development of secondary hyperparathyroidism that produces increase in bone resorption and bone turnover.
- Increased sensitivity of bone cells to PTH.
- Apoptosis of osteoblasts and osteocytes.

PREVENTION AND TREATMENT

- Bisphosphonates.
- Vitamin D:
  - Active forms of vitamin D (alfacalcidol, 1-α-hydroxyvitamin D_3 and calcitriol) and nonactive forms (cholecalciferol and ergocalciferol) prevent bone mass loss in chronic corticosteroid users.
  - However, the use of nonactive forms may not reduce the incidence of fractures.
- Fluorides.
- Calcium carbonate (1000 mg/day) in combination with vitamin D.
- Calcitonin.
- Oestrogens.
- Teriparatide (a recombinant PTH) for severe osteoporosis.

Q. Write a brief note on scurvy. (IM23.3)

- This is caused by ascorbic acid deficiency (vitamin C) that results in defective formation of collagen in connective tissue. There is failure of hydroxylation of proline to hydroxyproline.

TYPES OF SCURVY

- Adult scurvy.
- Infantile scurvy.

CLINICAL FEATURES

ADULT SCURVY (Box 11.3)

BOX 11.3 Clinical Features of Adult Scurvy

- Swollen and spongy gums—'scurvy buds'
- Scorbutic gingiva—gingivitis, loosening of teeth and bleeding gums
- Perifollicular hyperkeratotic papules
- Perifollicular haemorrhages
- Deformed 'corkscrew' hair projects out of a follicle (Fig. 11.8)
- Petechial haemorrhages, ecchymoses, epistaxis and gastrointestinal bleeding
- Nail—splinter haemorrhages and koilonychia
- Haemorrhage into muscles of arms and legs with secondary phlebothrombosis
- Haemorrhages into joints
- Poor wound healing

INFANTILE SCURVY (Box 11.4)

BOX 11.4 Clinical Features of Infantile Scurvy

- Subperiosteal haemorrhage into shafts of long bones
- 'Scorbutic rosary' denotes enlargement of costochondral junctions
- Purpura or ecchymotic skin lesions
- Gingival changes
- Retrobulbar, subarachnoid and intracerebral haemorrhages
- Anorexia and lassitude
- Painful limbs giving rise to 'pseudoparalysis'

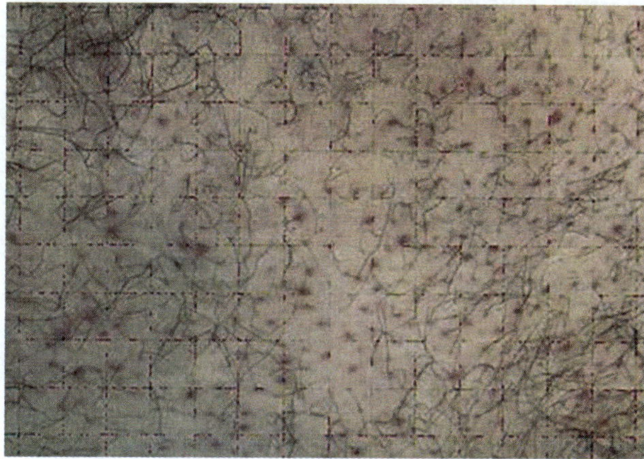

Fig. 11.8 'Corkscrew' hair and perifollicular haemorrhages.

MANAGEMENT

- Consumption of citrus fruits and vegetables. Important food sources of vitamin C are citrus fruits, tomatoes, potatoes, cauliflower, broccoli, strawberries, cabbage and spinach.
- Vitamin C 500 mg daily initially.

Q. Discuss beriberi/vitamin B_1 (thiamine) deficiency. (IM23.3)

SOURCES

- Primarily found in foods such as yeast, legumes, pork, brown rice and cereals made from whole grains. Thiamine is very low in white ('polished' rice) or milled white cereals including wheat flour because the processing removes thiamine.
- Cooking and baking some foods as well as pasteurisation can destroy thiamine.
- Milk products, fruits and vegetables are poor sources of thiamine.

ACTIONS

- Vitamin B_1 is essential for the coenzyme thiamine pyrophosphate. It is required:
  - For decarboxylation of pyruvate (glycolytic pathway) to acetyl-CoA (Krebs cycle).
  - For transketolase in the hexose monophosphate (HMP/pentose) shunt pathway.
  - For decarboxylation of α-ketoglutarate to succinate (Krebs cycle).

DEFICIENCY

- Thiamine deficiency, therefore, results in the following abnormalities:
  - Defective aerobic cellular glucose utilisation.
  - Pyruvic acid and lactic acid accumulation that produces vasodilatation and increased cardiac output.

CLINICAL SYNDROMES OF THIAMINE DEFICIENCY

- Wet beriberi—a high-cardiac-output failure.
- Dry beriberi—a type of peripheral neuropathy.
- Wernicke's encephalopathy.
- Korsakoff's psychosis.

WET BERIBERI

- Oriental or wet beriberi is caused by eating diets in which most of the calories are derived from polished and highly milled rice.
- Oedema—caused by the metabolites like pyruvate and lactate which cause extreme peripheral vasodilatation and leakage of fluid through capillaries.
- Beriberi heart disease (Box 11.5).

BOX 11.5 Features of Beriberi Heart Disease

- Peripheral vasodilatation
- High-cardiac-output state with warm extremities
- Biventricular failure
- Retention of sodium and water
- Extreme tachycardia
- Venous congestive state characterised by raised JVP and tender hepatomegaly
- Hyperdynamic circulation with a rapid circulation time
- Dyspnoea and cardiovascular collapse
- Marked cardiomegaly

Biochemical Tests

- Measurement of blood thiamine, pyruvate and lactate levels.
- Whole blood or erythrocyte transketolase activity.

Management

- Complete bed rest.
- One hundred milligram thiamine IM for the first 7 days, and then 10 mg/day orally for several months.

DRY BERIBERI

- Nutritional polyneuropathy is characterised by symmetric impairment of sensory, motor and reflex functions that affect the distal segments of limbs more severely than the proximal ones.
- Histology—noninflammatory degeneration of myelin sheaths (demyelination).
- There are three types of nervous system involvement in beriberi:
  - Peripheral neuropathy.
  - Cerebral beriberi, that is Wernicke's encephalopathy.
  - Korsakoff's syndrome.

Q. Describe Wernicke's encephalopathy. (IM23.3)

- Wernicke's encephalopathy is an acute neuropsychiatric condition due to an initially reversible biochemical brain lesion caused by depletion of vitamin B_1 (thiamine).

CAUSES (Box 11.6)

BOX 11.6 Causes of Wernicke's Encephalopathy

- Chronic alcohol use
- Protein–calorie malnutrition from malabsorption or forced/self-imposed inadequate diet
- Patients with protracted vomiting
- Carbohydrate loading (intravenous or oral) when thiamine stores are minimal
- Chronic renal failure
- Hyperalimentation, AIDS and drug misuse
- Weight-reducing surgery (e.g. gastric bypass surgery)
- Genetic abnormality of transketolase enzyme

CLINICAL FEATURES

- Mental disturbances:
  - Progressive depression of the state of consciousness.
  - Global confusional apathetic state, profound listlessness, inattentiveness and disorientation.
- Paralysis of eye movements:
  - Sixth nerve palsy and diplopia.
  - Nystagmus.
  - Internuclear ophthalmoplegia.
- Ataxia of gait—this affects stance and gait predominantly.

MANAGEMENT

- Wernicke's disease represents a medical emergency, and its recognition demands immediate administration of thiamine. Dose is 100 mg intravenously or intramuscularly every day for 7 days followed by oral thiamine. There is prompt reversibility within hours of administration of thiamine, especially the ocular signs and later the ataxia.
- Magnesium is often required as it is a cofactor required for normal functioning of thiamine-dependent enzymes.
- Intravenous glucose solutions should not be given particularly in malnourished patients as they may exhaust the patient's reserve of thiamine and either precipitate Wernicke's disease in a previously unaffected patient or cause a rapid worsening of an early form of the disease.

Q. What is Korsakoff's psychosis? (IM23.3)

- This thiamine deficiency–induced metabolic central nervous system disease predominantly affects memory. This is characterised by confabulation and defect in retentive memory (severe defect in storing new information and learning).
- It may follow Wernicke's encephalopathy or can develop on its own.
- Symptoms include:
  - Apathy, drowsiness and global confusion.
  - Confabulation.
  - Amnesic state characterised by large gaps in memory (both antegrade and retrograde memory loss).
- Korsakoff's psychosis is the psychic component of Wernicke's encephalopathy. When both the ocular ataxic and amnesic symptoms can be recognised, the disease is designated as Wernicke–Korsakoff syndrome.
- Treatment includes parenteral thiamine (100 mg IM daily for 7 days). The outcome of Korsakoff's psychosis varies. Complete or almost complete recovery occurs in less than 20% of patients. The recovery is gradual and incomplete in the remainder of patients.

Q. Write briefly on the clinical features and management of niacin deficiency (pellagra). (IM23.3)

- Pellagra (meaning 'raw' skin) is a metabolic encephalopathy caused by niacin (nicotinamide) deficiency.

CAUSES (Box 11.7)

BOX 11.7 Causes of Niacin Deficiency

- Inadequate intake—malnutrition, maize diet, jowar (sorghum) diet, chronic alcoholism, anorexia nervosa
- Malabsorption—refer before
- Drug-induced—6-mercaptopurine, 5-fluorouracil, azathioprine, carbamazepine, isoniazid, phenytoin and phenobarbitone
- Carcinoid syndrome
- Hartnup disease

CLINICAL FEATURES

1. Dermatitis
2. Diarrhoea
3. Dementia

} 3Ds

- Early mental symptoms include:
  - Insomnia.
  - Fatigue.
  - Anxiety, nervousness and irritability.
  - Depressive symptoms.
  - Dementia features.
- Spinal cord affection.
  - Involvement of the posterior and lateral columns.
  - Spastic paretic syndrome characterised by spastic weakness of legs, with absent abdominal and increased tendon reflexes, clonus and extensor plantar responses.
- Skin manifestations:
  - Symmetric erythema over body parts exposed to sunlight, especially neck (Casal's necklace or collar rash).
  - Dermatitis:
    - A. Acute dermatitis characterised by vesiculation, cracking, exudation, crusting and ulceration.
    - B. Chronic dermatitis characterised by bilateral symmetrical roughening, thickening and brown pigmentation of skin limited to sun-exposed areas (Fig. 11.9). Dermatitis over the sun-exposed area of the neck is classically described as 'Casal's necklace'.
- Alimentary tract involvement:
  - Anorexia, nausea, dysphagia, glossitis, angular stomatitis, cheilosis and diarrhoea.

MANAGEMENT

- Oral 100 mg nicotinamide every 6 hours.
- Nutritious diet and high-protein diet.
- Supplementation of other vitamin B complex with iron and folic acid.

Q. Give a brief account of fluorosis.

- This occurs when water fluoride content is high (>3 to 5 ppm). It can also be due to ingestion of fluoride-containing toothpaste or mouthwashes.

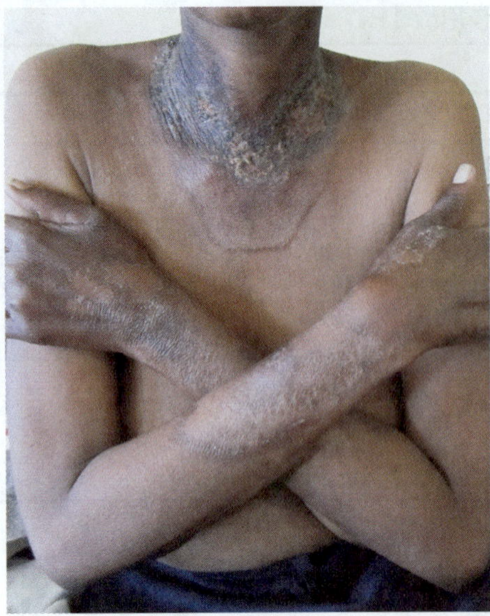

Fig. 11.9 Dermatitis in a patient with pellagra.(Courtesy: Michelle Weir, MD).

- It is estimated that more than 62 million people in India suffer from dental, skeletal and nonskeletal fluorosis. The most seriously affected states are Andhra Pradesh, Rajasthan and Gujarat.

CLINICAL FEATURES

- Dental fluorosis:
  - Mottling of teeth where the enamel loses its lustre, becomes rough, pigmented, pitted and brittle (fluorotic teeth) (Fig. 11.10).
  - Later, the teeth become hard and brittle.
- Skeletal fluorosis:
  - Sclerosis of bones especially of spine, pelvis and limbs.
  - Ligamental calcification, calcification of interosseous membrane and calcification of tendinous insertions.
  - In early stages, pain in bones and joints, muscle weakness and stiffness of joints.
  - Later, osteoporosis.
  - Finally, vertebrae fuse.

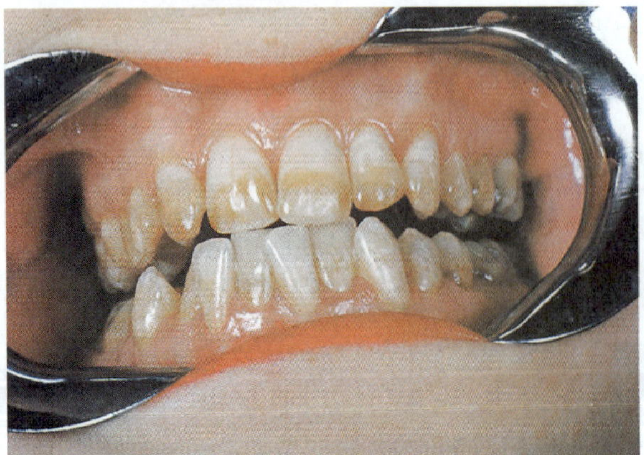

Fig. 11.10 Dental fluorosis (From: Ibsen OAC, Phelan JA. Oral Pathology for Dental Hygienists. 7th ed. Philadelphia: Elsevier; 2018).

  - Movement of the ribs is also reduced and the chest becomes barrel shaped causing difficulty in breathing.
  - Further, the immobilisation of joints leads to development of flexion deformities at hips, knees and other joints making the patient confined to bed.
  - Neurological complications related to skeletal fluorosis are those of radiculomyelopathy.
- Weakness, anaemia, weight loss and brittle bones.

CLINICAL DIAGNOSIS OF SKELETAL FLUOROSIS

- In the initial evaluation, UNICEF's three physical tests should be carried out to assess pain in major joints:
  - Coin test: The patient is asked to lift a coin from the floor. A patient with fluorosis cannot lift without bending the knees.
  - Chin test: The patient is asked to touch chest with chin. If the patient has pain and is not able to do it, this suggests fluorosis.
  - Stretch test: The patient is asked to abduct shoulders, flex elbow and touch back of head. Inability to do so indicates the presence of fluorosis.

TREATMENT

- There is no established cure for fluorosis. Aim is to reduce disability and improve quality of life.
  - Supplementation of calcium and vitamin D.
  - Correction of deformities.
  - Decompression of spine in case of compressive myelopathy.
  - Cosmetic dental treatment.

PREVENTION

- Prevention and control via consuming safe drinking water (defluoridation) is the best approach to deal with fluorosis.

NATIONAL PROGRAMME FOR PREVENTION AND CONTROL OF FLUOROSIS

- National Program for Prevention and Control of Fluorosis (NPPCF) was started in 2008–09 to tackle fluorosis as a public health problem. It was initiated under Ministry of Health and Family Welfare, Government of India.
- Under it, 195 districts of 29 states with high fluoride content in drinking water are covered.
- The strategy of programme includes:
  - Surveillance of fluorosis in the community.
  - Regular screening of dental fluorosis in schools every 3 months.
  - Full health check-up for skeletal changes in endemic areas every 6 months.
  - Capacity building in the form of training and man power support.
  - Diagnostic facilities in the form of laboratory support and equipment including ion meter to monitor the fluoride content in water and urinary levels.
  - Management of fluorosis cases by providing for corrective surgeries and rehabilitation.
  - Health education for the prevention and control of fluorosis cases.

Q. Describe angular stomatitis.

- This refers to cracking of the epithelium at the edges of the lips. Angular stomatitis may be caused by:
  - Iron-deficiency anaemia.
  - Riboflavin deficiency.
  - Pyridoxine (B_6) deficiency.
  - Niacin deficiency.
  - Herpes labialis at the angle of mouth.
- Angular stomatitis is associated with cheilosis in niacin deficiency and pellagra.

Q. Write a short note on definition, causes, risk factors and treatment of obesity. (IM14.1, IM14.11, IM14.13, IM14.14, IM14.2, IM14.5)

- Defined as a chronic, multifactorial, neurobehavioural disease, wherein an increase in body fat promotes adipose tissue dysfunction and abnormal fat mass physical forces, resulting in adverse metabolic, biomechanical and psychosocial health consequences.
- In Asians, obesity is measured by the parameters mentioned in the Box 11.8.

CAUSES (Table 11.8)

GENETIC FACTORS

Melanocortin 4 Receptor Deficiency

- Autosomal dominant or recessive.
- Most common known genetic defect predisposing to obesity.
- Features:
  - Hyperphagia and obesity early in childhood.
  - Increase in BMD ('big boned').
  - Accelerated linear growth.

TABLE 11.8 Causes of Obesity

Simple Obesity	Secondary Obesity
• Physical inactivity • Eating habits • Psychological factors (overeating may be a symptom of depression, anxiety and frustration) • Genetic factors—Prader–Willi syndrome, melanocortin 4 receptor deficiency, Albright's hereditary osteodystrophy, leptin deficiency, leptin receptor deficiency, POMC deficiency	• Hypothyroidism • Cushing's syndrome • Hypothalamic disorders • Diabetes mellitus • Pickwickian syndrome • Laurence–Moon–Biedl syndrome • Medications—valproic acid, carbamazepine, gabapentin, antidepressants, corticosteroids, antipsychotics, lithium, antidiabetics (insulins, sulphonylureas, thiazolidinediones), clozapine, olanzapine

Leptin

- Leptin is a hormone produced by cells of adipose tissue. It controls food intake and energy expenditure. It acts on leptin receptors (expressed in specific regions of the hypothalamus) to activate and regulate mRNA expression of key hypothalamic neuropeptides (e.g. pro-opiomelanocortin [POMC]).
- A defect in leptin gene or its receptor may produce obesity.
- Of obese persons, some have a low level of leptin in the blood while majority have high leptin levels indicating peripheral resistance to its actions.
- Defective leptin gene or leptin receptor may be responsible for only a minority of patients with obesity.

Prader–Willi Syndrome

- Occurs due to loss of function of a portion of chromosome 15; not inherited.
- Hyperphagia with short stature and obesity, hypotonia, small hands/feet, behavioural disturbances, intellectual impairment, narrow forehead, almond-shaped eyes and triangular mouth.
- Often with fair skin and light-coloured hair.

BOX 11.8 Definitions of Obesity (for Asian Indians)

Criteria	Definition	Reference Values
• Body mass index (BMI)	• Defined as person's weight (kilograms) divided by the square of person's height (metres)	• Normal—BMI 18–22.9 kg/m^2 • Underweight—BMI <18 kg/m^2 • Overweight—BMI 23–24.9 kg/m^2 • Obesity—BMI ≥25 kg/m^2
• Ideal body weight for height	• Calculated by multiplying square of height (meters) by 22.5	• Overweight—more than 10% of ideal body weight • Obesity—more than 20% of ideal body weight • Underweight—less than 20% of ideal body weight
• Skin-fold thickness	• Estimated by using special calipers over triceps, biceps, subscapular and suprailiac regions	• Normal triceps skin-fold thickness in males—12.5 mm • Normal triceps skin-fold thickness in females—16.5 mm
• Waist circumference	• Waist measurement using a flexible tape placed on a horizontal plane at the level of the iliac crest as seen from the anterior view	• Abdominal obesity—waist circumference >80 cm in females and >90 cm in males
• Waist to hip ratio (not very useful)	• Ratio of waist circumference and hip circumference (maximum measurement over buttocks)	• Normal—<0.8 in females and <0.9 in males • Abdominal obesity—>0.8 in females and >0.9 in males

Albright's Hereditary Osteodystrophy

- Characterised by obesity, short stature, shortened fourth metacarpals and other bones of the hands and feet, dental hypoplasia, soft tissue calcifications, hypocalcaemia, hyperphosphataemia.

RISKS ASSOCIATED WITH OBESITY

- Obesity is associated with a number of risks. These are shown in Table 11.9.

TABLE 11.9 Risks Associated With Obesity

Cardiovascular • CAD • Hypertension • Heart failure and cor pulmonale • Deep vein thrombosis • Varicose veins **Pulmonary** • Obstructive sleep apnoea • Pickwickian syndrome **Neurological** • Stroke • Pseudotumour cerebri **Musculoskeletal** • Osteoarthritis	**Endocrine** • Diabetes mellitus • Insulin resistance • Dyslipidaemias **Gastrointestinal and hepatic** • Gastro-oesophageal reflux • Cholelithiasis • Fatty liver **Malignancies** • Increased risk of breast, endometrial and colon cancers **Others** • Depression • Gout • Nephrolithiasis

TREATMENT

GOALS

- Attempt initially to reduce weight by approximately 10% from baseline. Further weight reduction is attempted after initial success.
- Reduce weight at a rate of about 0.5–1 kg/week for 6 months.

DIETARY THERAPY

Low-Fat Diet

- Encourage low-calorie diets with low fat. The reduction is usually to the tune of about 500 cal/day.
- Reducing fat alone without reducing total calories is not sufficient.
  - Low-fat diets have a lower energy density than high-fat diets and as humans respond mostly to volume of food eaten rather than calories, this should lead to a lower energy intake.
  - Low-fat diets also have higher fibre content and this may also enhance satiety.
- Unfortunately, many patients cannot maintain low-fat diet for a long time.

Very Low Carbohydrate Diet or Atkins Diet

- Use of a very low carbohydrate diet but with normal or high saturated fats.
- Found to produce loss of weight equivalent to that produced by a low-fat diet but there are no data beyond 1 year.
- These diets work by reducing caloric intake by removing a wide range of carbohydrate-rich foods.
- LDL cholesterol may rise by about 2%–3%.
- May induce precipitation of gout if history of gout present.

High-Protein Diet

- It makes use of the increased satiating effect of protein with reduction in carbohydrate. Fat is kept low at 30%.
- These high-protein–low-carbohydrate diets induce fat burning and mild ketosis which results in suppression of hunger and promotion of satiety.
- Patients with impaired renal function have a greater decline in renal function with a greater protein intake.
- High dietary protein intake increases urinary calcium excretion with potential risk for bone loss and calcium stone formation.
- Increased risk of colorectal cancer if increased amount of red meat is consumed.

Very Low-Calorie Diet

- Diets with energy levels between 200 and 800 kcal/day are called 'very low-calorie diets'.
- Not found to be superior to conventional diets for long-term weight loss.
- Side effects include hair loss, thinning of skin and increased incidence of gallstones.

PHYSICAL EXERCISE

- It reduces abdominal fat and increases cardiorespiratory fitness.
- Moderate exercise should be done for 30–45 minutes/day and 3–5 days/week.

BEHAVIOUR MODIFICATION

- It is a useful adjunct to diet and physical exercise.
- Patients often require motivation to lose weight.

PHARMACOTHERAPY

- Dietary therapy, physical exercise and behaviour modification should be considered before using drugs.
- Drugs may be used if BMI $\geq$30 kg/m^2.
- Drugs may also be used if BMI is 27–30 kg/m^2 and the patient has an increased risk:
  - Asian ethnicity.
  - Overweight/obesity-related disease likely to improve with weight loss such as type 2 diabetes, obstructive sleep apnoea and dyslipidaemia.
- The patient should be monitored for safety throughout.
- If patient has not lost at least 5% of his/her body weight by week 12 of using drugs, consider for discontinuation.

Sibutramine

- Centrally acting noradrenaline and serotonin uptake inhibitor.
- Suppresses appetite.
- Along with lifestyle modification, provides a mean weight loss of approximately 4.5 kg at 1 year.
- Side effects include dry mouth, constipation, headache and insomnia.

- Produces a dose-related increase in heart rate and may increase blood pressure and cardiovascular events.
- Withdrawn due to cardiovascular effects.

Orlistat

- Binds to intestinal and pancreatic lipases in the gut, reducing absorption of dietary triglycerides, cholesterol and fat-soluble vitamins.
- Dose 120 mg three times per day with meals.
- Produces favourable changes in total cholesterol, LDL cholesterol levels, free fatty acids, HbA1c and insulin sensitivity.
- Side effects include oily stools, faecal urgency, diarrhoea, flatulence, faecal incontinence, bloating and abdominal pain that can be minimised by a low-fat diet.
- Fat malabsorption increases the risk of vitamin D, E and β-carotene deficiency. Daily fat-soluble vitamin supplementation is recommended that should be taken between meals.

Rimonabant

- Endocannabinoid receptor CB1 blocking drug that has both central and peripheral actions to reduce weight and weight-related metabolic factors such as increasing adiponectin and reducing circulating free fatty acids.
- Side effects include nausea, diarrhoea, anxiety and depression (including increased suicidal risk).
- Withdrawn due to serious side effects.

Lorcaserin

- Acts by activating serotonin 2C receptor in the brain, which results in increased satiety and decreased hunger.
- Dose is 10 mg twice a day.
- Cautions should be taken in patients who are taking serotonergic medications. This can lead to serotonin syndrome. In diabetic patients, hypoglycaemia may occur.
- Side effects include headache, fatigue, nausea, dry mouth, dizziness and constipation. It also increases risks of certain cancers.
- Withdrawn due to serious side effects.

Phentermine–Topiramate

- Topiramate is contraindicated in pregnancy; hence, it is recommended that pregnancy testing is done before starting the medication and then every month to ensure that patients are not pregnant while taking the medication.
- The combination worsens depression and suicidal ideation; it can also cause mood disorders, anxiety and insomnia.

Others

- Four sympathomimetic agents are approved for short-term use. These are phentermine, diethylpropion, benzphetamine and phendimetrazine. These agents produce a modest weight loss benefit by causing early satiety. These are contraindicated in patients with coronary heart disease, hypertension and hyperthyroidism, and in patients with a history of drug abuse.
- Liraglutide subcutaneously, starting with 0.6 mg/day and gradually increased to 3 mg/day, may be used. It can produce hypoglycaemia.
- Semaglutide subcutaneously, 2.4 mg once a week in adults with obesity with at least one weight-related condition (such as high blood pressure, type 2 diabetes or high cholesterol).
- Naltrexone–bupropion combination can produce 5%–10% weight loss. Bupropion activates POMC, a neuropeptide that appears to decrease appetite by affecting hypothalamic functions. Naltrexone inhibits the appetite-enhancing effects of beta-endorphin caused by cannabinoid-1 receptor activation.
- Setmelanotide is approved for use in obesity due to three rare genetic conditions: POMC deficiency, proprotein subtilisin/kexin type 1 (PCSK1) deficiency, and leptin receptor (LEPR) deficiency.
- Lisdexamfetamine dimesylate may be used to treat binge-eating disorder.
- Fluoxetine may be used to treat bulimia nervosa.

BARIATRIC SURGERY

- Useful in patients with BMI ≥40 kg/m^2 when other methods have failed, and in patients with BMI ≥35 kg/m^2 who have identifiable medical, physical or psychosocial problems associated with their obesity.
- Perioperative mortality varies from 0.05% to 0.5% depending on the method used.
- Various options include:
  - Jaw wiring (rarely done).
  - Jejunoileal shunt:
    - Produces significant long-term adverse events such as dehydration, electrolyte imbalance, calcium oxalate renal stones, cirrhosis and protein–calorie malnutrition.
    - Rarely done presently.
  - Gastroplasty or vertical sleeve gastrectomy.
  - Gastric bypass by retrocolic gastrojejunostomy (Roux-en-Y gastric bypass).
  - Laparoscopic adjustable gastric banding:
    - Involves laparoscopic placement of an inflatable silicone band at the very top of the stomach leaving a small gastric pouch that fills quickly and empties slowly. This induces a sense of satiety after consuming smaller amounts of food and a feeling of not being hungry.
    - The balloon of the band is connected to a subcutaneous access port. This allows adding or removing fluid to the system, control of how tight the band is and, therefore, how much food can be consumed.
    - Safest, least invasive and most effective procedure.
  - Liposuction:
    - Results in a significant reduction in fat mass and weight; however, it does not improve insulin sensitivity or risk factors for coronary heart disease.

ELECTRICAL STIMULATION (VAGAL BLOCKADE) SYSTEMS

- These systems deliver small electrical pulses to block transmission of nerve signals in the vagus nerve, which suppresses neural communication between the brain and the stomach.
- These systems consist of both implanted and external components, and include rechargeable pulse generator implanted in the abdomen, which delivers

electrical signals to electrodes placed on the trunks of the vagus nerve.

HYDROGELS

- Hydrogels are orally administered products, taken twice daily before meals, which expand in the stomach and intestines to create a sensation of satiety.
- They are not systemically absorbed, and are eliminated through the faeces.

MCQs

IM23.3

1. A 23-year-old woman with anorexia nervosa was admitted acutely after assessment by the community eating disorders team for a period of planned nasogastric feeding. She had had no meaningful nutritional intake for >4 weeks, and her BMI had reduced to 11.2 kg/m^2. There was evidence of postural hypotension, hypokalaemia and hypophosphataemia. These were corrected intravenously. She also received intravenous dextrose. She was started on nasogastric feeding as recommended by the dietitian. After 24 hours, she became confused and ataxic and developed diplopia. What is the most likely diagnosis?
   A. Cerebral oedema
   B. Hypoglycaemia
   C. Nonepileptiform attack
   D. Septicaemia
   E. Wernicke's encephalopathy

Ans: E. Wernicke's encephalopathy

Wernicke's encephalopathy is the presence of neurological symptoms caused by a deficiency of thiamine, in this case, resulting from the provision of intravenous dextrose and nasogastric feeding without thiamine replacement. It presents with neurocognitive manifestations, classically the triad of ophthalmoplegia (producing diplopia), ataxia and confusion. Thiamine deficiency is common in severely malnourished individuals; it is difficult to test for and therefore clinicians should have a high index of suspicion and a low threshold to administer thiamine before commencing nutrition support.

IM23.4

2. A 35-year-old man undergoes a craniotomy and evacuation of an extradural haematoma following a severe head injury. Postoperatively, he is transferred to the Intensive Care Unit intubated for continued ventilation and sedation. What is the most appropriate nutritional regimen?
   A. Nil by mouth and IV fluids
   B. Nasogastric (NG) feeding
   C. Percutaneous endoscopic gastrostomy (PEG) feeding
   D. Elemental diet
   E. Total parenteral nutrition (TPN)

Ans: B. Nasogastric (NG) feeding

Nasogastric feeding is required immediately, as the patient has an intact gastrointestinal tract. Enteral feeding is preferable as it helps to maintain the mucosal integrity of the gut. In the context of trauma, the patient's metabolic demands are massively increased.

IM23.4

3. A 29-year-old patient with a diagnosis of Crohn's disease undergoes an emergency laparotomy, adhesiolysis and multilevel small bowel resection. Prior to surgery, she continued her steroids and immunosuppression. Several days postoperatively, a high-output small bowel fistula erupts through the midline laparotomy wound. A water-soluble contrast study confirms this to be a high jejunal fistula. What is the most appropriate nutritional regimen?
   A. Nil by mouth and IV fluids
   B. Nasogastric (NG) feeding
   C. Percutaneous endoscopic gastrostomy (PEG) feeding
   D. Elemental diet
   E. Total parenteral nutrition (TPN)

Ans: E. Total parenteral nutrition (TPN)

TPN is intravenous nutrition, which is administered through a large central vein, due to the irritant and osmotic nature of the feed. This patient requires TPN. The history of Crohn's disease and the emergency nature of the procedure suggests the patient was not nutritionally optimised preoperatively. This patient is likely to require long-term TPN to allow the fistula to heal and should therefore have a tunnelled central venous catheter, such as a Hickman line.

IM23.4

4. A 73-year-old woman underwent a Hartmann's procedure for perforated diverticular disease and faecal peritonitis. Ten days following her procedure, her stoma is yet to function and she has not passed any wind through her stoma. Her nasogastric aspirate is large and she fails to absorb her feeds. She has a right internal jugular central single lumen central venous catheter inserted at the time of surgery through which she receives antibiotics. Examination revealed a soft, nontender, distended abdomen, with a pink and healthy end colostomy. There were no audible bowel sounds on auscultation. She is to be started on total parenteral nutrition (TPN).
   From the following list, select the most appropriate method of delivery for total parenteral nutrition:
   A. Large bore peripheral intravenous catheter
   B. Existing central venous catheter
   C. Dedicated lumen from newly inserted central venous catheter
   D. Nasogastric feeding tube
   E. Nasojejunal feeding tube

Ans: C. Dedicated lumen from newly inserted central venous catheter

A dedicated line (long term: i.e. Hickmann line) (short term: i.e. single or multilumen central venous access) should be used in the delivery of TPN. The principle complication of TPN use is line sepsis, and all measures should be taken to prevent this, including replacing old lines and changing them if line sepsis is suspected.

12 Psychiatry

Q. Give a brief account on psychosis. (PS16.1)

- Presence of mental state where appreciation of reality is impaired, as evidenced by the presence of psychotic symptoms such as delusions, hallucinations, mood disturbance and bizarre behaviour.
- Includes schizophrenia and mood disorders.

CLINICAL FEATURES (Box 12.1)

BOX 12.1 Clinical Features of Psychosis

- Positive symptoms
  - Delusions and hallucinations
  - Formal thought disorder
- Negative symptoms
  - Flat affect
  - Poverty of thought
  - Lack of motivation
  - Social withdrawal
- Cognitive symptoms
  - Distractibility
  - Impaired working memory
  - Impaired executive function
- Mood symptoms
  - Depression
  - Elevation (mania)
- Anxiety/panic/perplexity
- Aggression/hostility/suicidal behaviour

HALLUCINATIONS

- Hallucinations mean wakeful sensory experiences of content that is not actually present.
- Auditory hallucinations: Hearing voices of people talking to the patient even when there is no one nearby.
- Thought insertion: Feeling that thoughts are being put into patient's mind.
- Thought withdrawal: Feeling that thoughts are being taken out of patient's mind.
- Thought broadcasting: Feeling that other people are aware of patient's thoughts.
- Other types of hallucinations are visual, tactile, olfactory and gustatory.

DELUSIONS

- Delusions are false beliefs that are maintained despite obvious evidence to contrary.
- Delusion of control or passivity: Feeling of under the control or influence of an outside force.

- Delusions of reference: Feeling that programmes on television or radio hold special meaning for the patient.
- Delusions of persecution: Feeling that patient is being singled out for special treatment or there is a conspiracy against the patient.
- Erotomanic delusions: Feeling that others are in love with him.
- Delusions of grandeur: Feeling special with unusual abilities or power.
- Delusions of guilt: Feeling that the patient has sinned or has done something deserving punishment.
- Nihilistic delusions: Belief that oneself, a part of one's body or the real world does not exist or has been destroyed.

OTHER CAUSES OF PSYCHOTIC SYMPTOMS

- Psychosis is a common feature of many neurologic, neurodevelopmental and medical conditions (Box 12.2).

BOX 12.2 Other Causes of Psychotic Symptoms

- Substance abuse/withdrawal—amphetamines/stimulants, hallucinogens, cannabis, alcohol
- CNS infections—HIV, herpes simplex
- Neurodegenerative diseases—Huntington's disease, Alzheimer's disease, dementia with Lewy bodies, Parkinson's disease
- Noninfectious, nondegenerative CNS diseases—cerebral trauma, cerebrovascular disease, brain tumours, temporal lobe epilepsy
- Endocrine diseases—Cushing's disease, use of steroids, thyrotoxicosis, hyperparathyroidism, adrenal insufficiency
- Systemic lupus erythematosus
- Metabolic diseases—Wilson's disease, hepatic encephalopathy, uraemic encephalopathy
- Delirium
- Vitamin B_{12} deficiency

INVESTIGATIONS (Box 12.3)

BOX 12.3 Investigations in a Patient with Psychosis

- Complete blood count
- Electrolytes
- Renal and liver function tests
- Thyroid function tests
- HIV
- Vitamin B_{12} level
- Antinuclear antibodies
- CT and MRI brain (if indicated)
- EEG (if indicated)
- Lumbar puncture (if indicated)

TREATMENT

- For most causes of psychosis, initial treatment is with an antipsychotic medication. Most often, second-generation antipsychotics should be used. For severe agitation, first-generation antipsychotics are preferred.
- Patients with psychosis due to central nervous system (CNS) stimulant intoxication should be treated initially with benzodiazepines

Q. Discuss the aetiology, clinical manifestations and management of schizophrenia. (PS16.1, PS5.1, PS5.2, PS5.3)

Q. Write a short note on positive symptoms of schizophrenia and first-rank symptoms of schizophrenia.

- Schizophrenia is a group of disorders characterised by perturbations in language, perception, cognition and behaviour.

AETIOLOGY

- A number of factors have been identified that predispose to, precipitate or sustain schizophrenia:
  - Schizophrenia can be transmitted genetically.
  - Family environment can influence the course of the illness. A highly emotional family environment contributes to relapses.
  - Psychological stresses like adverse life events.
  - A viral vector or early developmental abnormalities in some cases.
  - Some cases of schizophrenia are associated with increased cerebral ventricular size indicating that schizophrenia is accompanied by brain atrophy.
  - Schizophrenia syndrome can be associated with temporal lobe epilepsy, Huntington's chorea, cerebral tumours and demyelinating diseases. This is known as symptomatic schizophrenia.
  - Schizophrenia is associated with a functional overactivity in the dopaminergic neuronal systems in the mesolimbic and mesocortical areas.

TYPES

- There are four major types of schizophrenic disorders—catatonic, disorganised, paranoid and undifferentiated.
- Schizophrenic patients may also be classified as type I or type II.
  - Type I patients have a predominance of 'positive' symptoms, normal ventricular size and a good response to antipsychotic drugs.
  - Type II patients have a predominance of 'negative' symptoms, increased ventricular size and a poor response to antipsychotic drugs.

CLINICAL FEATURES

- Clinical manifestations can be considered under four headings; the first-rank symptoms (which strongly suggest a diagnosis of schizophrenia), other positive symptoms of lower diagnostic significance, the negative symptoms and cognitive symptoms (Table 12.1). The first two groups of symptoms together form the positive symptoms.
- The relative risk for suicide is increased by 12 times. Approximately 5% of people with schizophrenia commit suicide over their lifetime. However, major contributor for mortality is increased cardiovascular

TABLE 12.1 Clinical Features of Schizophrenia

Positive Symptoms			
First-Rank Symptoms	**Other Positive Symptoms**	**Negative Symptoms**	**Cognitive Symptoms**
• Auditory hallucinations • Thought insertion • Thought broadcasting • Passivity feeling (actions felt to be influenced by external agents) • Delusional perception (believes that a normal percept has a special meaning for him or her)	• Catatonia • Thought disorder • Neologisms • Delusions—grandiose, paranoid, sexual or religious • Visual, tactile, olfactory or gustatory hallucinations	• Social withdrawal • Poverty of speech (alogia) • Flatness of affect • Anhedonia (inability to feel pleasure in normally pleasurable activities)	• Impaired visual learning and memory • Impaired verbal learning and memory • Impaired verbal comprehension

risk. The causes of this increase in mortality include smoking and other lifestyle factors, suboptimal treatment of physical disorders, and side effects of pharmacological treatment (especially cardiometabolic outcomes).

DIAGNOSIS

- Diagnosis is based on criteria given by Diagnostic and Statistical Manual of Mental Disorders, Fifth Edition (DSM-5) (Box 12.4).

MANAGEMENT

ANTIPSYCHOTIC DRUGS

- It was conventional to start with chlorpromazine 100 mg thrice daily, gradually building up the dose to a maximum of 1500 mg daily or until symptoms subsided. However, newer (second-generation) antipsychotic drugs are equally effective but better tolerated. These include clozapine, risperidone and olanzapine. They act on D_2 as well as 5-HT_{2A} serotonin receptors.
- First-generation antipsychotic drugs (also known as neuroleptics) block D_2 groups of dopamine receptors. This results in high incidence of extrapyramidal features particularly with older drugs. They also block adrenergic and cholinergic receptors and cause a number of side effects. A rare adverse effect is neuroleptic malignant syndrome.
- Newer antipsychotics (e.g. clozapine, risperidone and olanzapine) mainly act on D_2 receptors but bind loosely.

BOX 12.4 Diagnostic Criteria for Schizophrenia (DSM-V)

A. Two (or more) of the following present for a significant portion of time during a 1-month period (or less if successfully treated) and at least one of these must be 1, 2 or 3:
1. Delusions
2. Hallucinations
3. Disorganised speech
4. Grossly disorganised or catatonic behaviour
5. Negative symptoms

B. For a significant portion of the time since the onset of the disturbance, level of functioning in one or more major areas, such as work, interpersonal relations or self-care, is markedly below the level achieved prior to the onset.

C. Continuous signs of the disturbance persist for at least 6 months.

- These agents are effective against the positive symptoms but not against negative symptoms and cognitive dysfunction.

PSYCHOSOCIAL MEASURES

- These patients do best in an environment that has a regular and predictable routine. Positive symptoms are exacerbated in highly charged emotional situations while negative symptoms are induced in environments that are understimulating.
- Cognitive behavioural therapy is indicated in all patients.

Q. What are affective disorders (mood disorders)? How do you classify them?

Q. What are the clues to bipolar disorders? (PS7.2)

- The affective (mood) disorders are characterised by a disturbance of mood, either depression or mania or both.

CLASSIFICATION OF MOOD DISORDERS

- The term unipolar disorder is used when recurrences always take a depressive form.
- The term bipolar disorder is used when recurrences are both manic and depressive.
- The affective (mood) disorders can be classified as primary and secondary.
  - The term primary affective disorder is used when the affective episodes (mania or depression) are not secondary to any other psychiatric or physical illness.
  - The term secondary affective disorder is used when the affective episodes are secondary to another psychiatric or physical illness.

CLASSIFICATION OF BIPOLAR DISORDERS (Box 12.5)

BOX 12.5 Classification of Bipolar Disorders

BIPOLAR I DISORDER
- At least one lifetime episode of mania and usually (but not necessarily) episodes of depression.
- May also include episodes of hypomania.

BIPOLAR II DISORDER
- Episodes of both hypomania and depression. No manic episodes.

CLUES TO BIPOLAR DISORDERS (Box 12.6)

BOX 12.6 Clues to Bipolar Disorders

- Feeling energized and 'wired'
- Excessively seeking stimulation
- Needing less sleep or hypersomnia
- Irritable if stopped from carrying out ideas
- Disinhibited
- Offensive or insensitive to the needs of others
- Prior episodes of depression or attempted suicide
- Drug or alcohol abuse
- Spending money in an unusual manner or inappropriately
- Indiscreet and disregarding social boundaries
- Having poor self-regulation
- Making excessively creative and grandiose plans
- Having difficulty in discussing issues rationally or maturely
- Reporting enhanced sensory experiences
- Loss of pleasure in life
- Loss of interest in oneself and others

Q. Discuss the clinical manifestations and management of depression. (PS16.1, PS6.2)

- Depressive disorders are characterised by persistent low mood, loss of interest and enjoyment and reduced energy. They often impair day-to-day functioning.
- Major depressive disorder is characterised by one or more major depressive episodes (i.e. at least 2 weeks of depressed mood or loss of interest accompanied by at least four additional symptoms of depression as mentioned below).

CLINICAL FEATURES

PSYCHOLOGICAL

- Depressed (dysphoric) mood is the most characteristic feature. There may be diurnal variation of the mood, the depressed mood being worst in the early morning or in the evening.
- Loss of pleasure in life and loss of interest in oneself and others.
- Low self-esteem and ideas of hopelessness and worthlessness.
- Self-blame and feelings of excessive or inappropriate guilt.
- Psychotic features (e.g. hallucinations and delusions) may be present; such a condition is known as psychotic depression.

SOMATIC

- Sleep disturbance may occur as initial insomnia, early morning wakening or hypersomnia.
- Fatigue, headache and various other pains.
- Anorexia, weight loss or weight gain and constipation.
- Poor concentration, psychomotor retardation and reduced libido.

UNIPOLAR MAJOR DEPRESSION WITH PSYCHOTIC FEATURES

- Patients who have suffered at least one major depressive episode and have no history of mania or hypomania, and have delusions and hallucinations.

DIAGNOSIS (Box 12.7)

BOX 12.7 Diagnosis of Depression (DSM-5)

1. Depressed mood most of the day nearly every day as indicated by either subjective report (e.g. feels sad, empty and hopeless) or observations made by others (e.g. appears tearful) (dysphoria)
2. Markedly diminished interest or pleasure in all or almost all activities most of the day nearly every day (anhedonia)
3. Significant weight loss when not dieting or weight gain (e.g. a change of more than 5% of body weight in a month), or decrease or increase in appetite nearly every day
4. Loss of energy or fatigue nearly every day
5. Loss of confidence or self-esteem
6. Recurrent thoughts of death or suicide or any suicidal behaviour
7. Diminished ability to think or concentrate or indecisiveness nearly every day
8. Unreasonable feelings of self-reproach or excessive or inappropriate guilt nearly every day
9. Psychomotor agitation or retardation nearly every day
10. Insomnia or hypersomnia nearly every day

Note: 1. Symptoms 1 and/or 2 and any four others must be present for at least 2 weeks.
2. Symptoms not caused by a medical condition, a substance or a bereavement.
3. The symptoms cause clinically significant distress or impairment in social, occupational or other important areas of functioning.

MANAGEMENT

- In acute bipolar depression, a mood stabiliser either alone or in combination with an antidepressant is effective. Mood stabilisers with proven antidepressant effects in bipolar depression include lithium, valproate, lamotrigine, quetiapine, lurasidone and olanzapine.
- For patients with bipolar major depression who are treated with an antidepressant, an antimanic drug such as lithium, valproate or a second-generation antipsychotic such as quetiapine, lurasidone or olanzapine should be concurrently prescribed. This will reduce the likelihood of switching from depression to mania.
- A tricyclic antidepressant (e.g. amitriptyline) drug was the first choice previously. In those who did not respond to this, a monoamine oxidase inhibitor (MAOI—tranylcypromine, phenelzine and selegiline) was tried.
- However, at present, selective serotonin reuptake inhibitors (SSRIs) have replaced tricyclic antidepressants as the drugs of choice in the treatment of depressive disorders. These agents are better tolerated and are relatively safer if taken in overdose. SSRIs include fluoxetine, sertraline, fluvoxamine and citalopram.
- Another group of antidepressants is serotonin–norepinephrine reuptake inhibitors (SNRI—venlafaxine, desvenlafaxine, duloxetine and milnacipran).
- Other classes of antidepressants include atypical antidepressants (bupropion and mirtazapine), tetracyclics (mianserin) and serotonin modulators (nefazodone, trazodone, vilazodone and vortioxetine).

- Patients with unipolar major depression with psychotic features are treated with a combination of antidepressants and antipsychotics. If response is inadequate, electroconvulsive therapy (ECT) is added.
- Cognitive therapy in combination with antidepressants may be beneficial in some cases.
- ECT is indicated in selected situations—for example in those with a high risk of suicide, depressive stupor, psychotic symptoms and when antidepressants have been ineffective.

Q. What are the clinical manifestations of mania? Give a broad outline of the management. (PS7.2, PS7.4)

Q. Define hypomania.

CLINICAL FEATURES OF MANIA

- The mood is elevated and expansile with a feeling of well-being.
- High confidence and self-esteem with grandiose ideas.
- Highly energetic with increased motor activity.
- Patient is more talkative than usual with a pressure to keep talking.
- Thoughts come rapidly and jump from one topic to another (flight of ideas).
- Increased appetite and decreased need for sleep.
- Sexual promiscuity may occur.

HYPOMANIA

- Episodes of pathologically elevated (and/or irritable) mood for at least several days in duration.
- Associated characteristic symptoms and behavioural change indicative of disinhibition, poor judgement, grandiosity and increased speed of thoughts, speech and behaviour.
- Distinctly different from the individual's normal functioning.
- No marked functional impairment, psychotic features or hospitalisation.

DIAGNOSIS OF MANIA AND HYPOMANIA (Box 12.8)

BOX 12.8 Diagnosis of Mania and Hypomania (DSM-5)

1. Abnormally and persistently elevated, expansive or irritable mood
2. Distractibility
3. Indiscretions (e.g. shopping sprees and dangerous sexual activities)
4. Grandiosity or inflated self-esteem
5. Fast thoughts or flight of ideas
6. Activity—increase in goal-directed activity
7. Sleep—decrease in the need for sleep
8. Talkativeness or pressured speech

Note: 1. Symptoms 1 and any three others must be present for at least 4 days in hypomania and for 7 days in mania.
2. The episode is severe (mania)/not severe (hypomania) enough to cause marked impairment in social or occupational functioning or to necessitate hospitalisation.
3. The episode is not attributable to the physiological effects of a substance (e.g. a drug of abuse, a medication or other treatment).

MANAGEMENT

- Manic attacks can be suppressed with lithium, valproate or divalproex (a stable coordination compound of sodium valproate and valproic acid), carbamazepine or atypical antipsychotic (e.g. olanzapine, aripiprazole, quetiapine or risperidone).
- Also, add neuroleptic drugs (haloperidol and chlorpromazine) or benzodiazepines to calm or sedate the mood until the mood stabiliser agent takes effect (about 1 week).
- Electroconvulsive therapy (ECT) in resistant cases.
- Lithium carbonate and carbamazepine are useful prophylactically.

Q. How do you classify anxiety disorders? Give a brief account of treatment of anxiety disorders. (PS8.2, PS8.4)

Q. Describe panic disorder.

Q. Discuss generalised anxiety disorder.

Q. What is post-traumatic stress disorder (PTSD)?

Q. How do you classify phobic disorders? Give a brief account of these disorders.

- Anxiety disorder is characterised by excessive and persistent worrying that causes significant distress or impairment, and often associated with somatic features.

CLASSIFICATION OF ANXIETY DISORDERS

- Broadly, anxiety disorders are classified into anxiety states and phobic disorders (Table 12.2).

PANIC DISORDER

- There are recurrent attacks of severe anxiety and fear that are sudden and unpredictable. During attacks, physical symptoms are prominent and include palpitations, chest pain, breathlessness, sweating, chills, nausea, trembling, fear of dying or losing control, numbness and feeling of detachment. These last for 10–15 minutes.
- May be accompanied by agoraphobia, an avoidance of situations where a person may feel trapped and unable to escape. At present, it is classified as a phobic disorder.

TABLE 12.2 Classification of Anxiety Disorders

Anxiety States	Phobic Disorders
• Panic disorder • Generalised anxiety disorder • Post-traumatic stress disorder (PTSD) • Separation anxiety disorder • Selective mutism • Illness anxiety disorder • Acute procedure anxiety	• Agoraphobia • Social phobia • Simple phobia • Specific phobia

- In between attacks, the patient is free of anxiety.
- There is a higher likelihood of suicide attempts among people with panic disorder compared with the general population.

GENERALISED ANXIETY DISORDER

- Characterised by anxiety and excessive worry (e.g. about finances, family, health and the future) which are difficult to control, cause significant distress and impairment, and occur on more days than not for at least 6 months.
- Patients have persistent, excessive and/or unrealistic worry associated with three or more of other features including muscle tension, impaired concentration, irritability, fatiguability, restlessness and insomnia. Complaints of tachycardia, dyspnoea and palpitations are rare.
- Patients typically respond positively to the question, 'Do you worry excessively about minor matters?'
- Associated with poor cardiovascular health, coronary heart disease and increased cardiovascular mortality.
- At times, symptoms of anxiety are prominent in psychiatric disorders such as depressive illness and schizophrenia. Additionally, many physical illnesses like hyperthyroidism, phaeochromocytoma, hypoglycaemia, alcohol withdrawal and temporal lobe epilepsy can mimic anxiety disorders. Hence, these conditions should be excluded before making a diagnosis of generalised anxiety disorder.

POST-TRAUMATIC STRESS DISORDER

- Post-traumatic stress disorder (PTSD) is characterised by recurrent bouts of severe anxiety accompanied by vivid reminiscences (or 'flashbacks') of the initial traumatic event.
- PTSD stems from exposure to a traumatic event (e.g. a military experience, a physical or sexual assault, a motor vehicle accident, a natural disaster) that involved actual or threatened death or serious injury to oneself or others.
- Typically, patients reexperience the traumatic event (e.g. nightmares and flashbacks), engage in avoidance of stimuli associated with the sentinel trauma (e.g. impaired recall of events related to the trauma) and experience increased autonomic reactivity (e.g. hypervigilance, irritability, insomnia and heightened startle response).
- PTSD is classified as either acute or chronic (or delayed). In acute PTSD, onset of symptoms begins within 6 months of trauma or the duration of symptoms is less than 6 months. In chronic (or delayed) PTSD, symptoms start more than 6 months after trauma (delayed) or persist for more than 6 months (chronic).

SEPARATION ANXIETY DISORDER

- There is unrealistic, persistent fear or anxiety about separation from, or loss of attachment figure (such as family members), or adverse events occurring to them.
- The symptoms include nightmares and physical symptoms.
- Although the symptoms develop in childhood, they can be expressed throughout adulthood as well.

SELECTIVE MUTISM

- There is consistent failure to speak in situations for which there is an expectation to speak, even though the individual speaks in other circumstances, can speak, and comprehends the spoken language.
- The disorder is more likely to be seen in young children than in adolescents and adults.

ILLNESS ANXIETY DISORDER

- There is excessive concern about having or developing a serious, undiagnosed general medical disease.

ACUTE PROCEDURE ANXIETY

- There is an excessive fear of medical, dental or surgical procedures which results in acute distress or interference with completing necessary procedures.

PHOBIC DISORDERS

- Phobic disorders comprise a group of disorders having in common persistently recurring, irrational severe anxiety of specific objects, activities or situations with secondary avoidance behaviour of the phobic stimulus.
- Agoraphobia: The individual has marked fear of and thus avoids being alone or being in public places—for example crowds, tunnels and bridges.
- Social phobias (social anxiety disorder): These are persistent irrational fears and the need to avoid any situation where one might be exposed to scrutiny by others and potentially be embarrassed or humiliated. Even the possibility of such a situation evokes an anticipatory anxiety. The individual is aware that this fear is excessive.
- Simple phobia: The individual experiences significant distress when confronted with the phobic stimulus or even the possibility of confrontation with the phobic stimulus. The individual may experience symptoms identical to those of panic attacks. Common examples include fear of heights (acrophobia), fear of closed spaces (claustrophobia) and fear of animals.
- Specific phobia: Characterised by clinically significant fear of a particular object or situation that typically leads to avoidance behaviour. Phobic fears include animals, insects, heights, water, enclosed places, driving, flying, seeing blood, getting an injection and choking or vomiting.

TREATMENT

- Use of an SSRI which increases the availability of serotonin which is thought to be reduced in anxiety disorders.
- Use of a selective serotonin–norepinephrine reuptake inhibitor (e.g. venlafaxine).
- Other useful drugs include buspirone and pregabalin.
- Anxiolytic agents such as benzodiazepines (e.g. lorazepam, alprazolam and clonazepam) can be used as a

temporary adjunct to aid in minimising anxiety, in particular when starting a medication therapy. Their long-term use should be avoided since it may lead to tolerance and increased risk of abuse or dependence.
- Benzodiazepines are the first-line treatment for specific phobias and can be taken on 'as and when required' basis.
- Cognitive behavioural therapy that involves addressing cognitive distortions, psychoeducation, breathing exercises, progressive muscle relaxation and progressive exposure.

Q. Discuss briefly about obsessive-compulsive disorder.

- Previously grouped under anxiety disorders.
- Obsessions are persistent intrusive thoughts. Compulsions are intrusive behaviours (e.g. repeated checking to be assured that the door was locked, repeated hand washing and extreme neatness) or mental acts (e.g. praying and repeating words silently). Attempts made to ignore or suppress the obsessive thought are usually not successful. Obsessions are unwanted and cause marked distress or anxiety in most individuals. The individual attempts to ignore, avoid or suppress obsessions or to neutralise them with another thought or action (e.g. performing a compulsion).
- The compulsive act is performed with a sense of subjective compulsion coupled with a desire to resist the compulsion. The individual generally recognises the senselessness of the behaviour and does not derive pleasure from carrying out the activity, although it provides a release of tension.

TREATMENT

- Cognitive behavioural therapy.
- Pharmacotherapy:
  - SSRIs including fluoxetine, fluvoxamine and citalopram. Higher doses are required to treat obsessive-compulsive disorder (OCD) than depression.
  - Tricyclic antidepressants, particularly clomipramine.
- Neuromodulation (in resistant cases):
  - Transcranial direct current stimulation (tDCS).
  - Repetitive transcranial magnetic stimulation (rTMS).
  - Deep brain stimulation (DBS).

Q. Write a short note on conversion disorder and dissociation disorder.

Q. Give a brief description of hysteria. (PS10.1, PS10.2, PS10.4)

Q. Explain hysterical amnesia and Briquet's syndrome (somatisation disorder) in brief.

- Hysteria is a syndrome characterised by a loss or distortion of neurological function, not fully explained by organic disease. The patient develops symptoms and signs of illness (mental, physical or both) for some real or imagined gain without really being fully aware of the underlying motive. The term hysteria is no longer used and is now replaced with conversion disorder.
- Conversion disorder is protean in manifestation and may simulate any disease. In psychoanalytic terms, it has been seen as a maladaptive way of coping with an unresolved psychological conflict, that is by becoming ill. The patient thus derives primary gain by relieving the conflict and secondary gain by obtaining sympathy and attention from others or by avoiding everyday responsibilities.

CLINICAL FEATURES

- Two main variants of neurologic symptoms in the absence of underlying pathology are conversion disorder and dissociation disorder, although latter is now included under conversion disorder.

CONVERSION DISORDER

- The symptoms mimic lesions of the motor or sensory nervous system. There is apparent unconcern (la belle indifference) even in the face of gross physical disability. Common presentations are gait disturbances, loss of function in limbs, aphonia, pseudoseizures (psychogenic nonepileptic seizures), sensory loss and blindness. The symptoms are not feigned.
- Diagnosis is based on positive clinical findings which indicate the symptom is incongruent with anatomy, physiology or known diseases, or is inconsistent at different times.
- Diagnostic criteria for conversion disorder are given in Box 12.9 while Table 12.3 gives clues suggesting motor weakness due to a conversion disorder.

DISSOCIATION DISORDER

- Dissociation disorder is now included under the category of conversion disorder in which the patient has a feeling of disconnection from one's own body (depersonalisation) or from one's environment (derealization).
- There can be dissociated motor loss, sensory loss, convulsions or amnesia. Amnesia usually develops acutely. The memory loss is patchy and inconsistent. A characteristic feature is a loss of personal identity so that the patient is unable to recall his/her name, address or other personal and family details. Amnesia occurs to escape from intolerable anxiety and distress about some problem or difficulty or situation in which the patient finds himself/herself.

BOX 12.9 Diagnostic Criteria for Conversion Disorder (DSM-5)

1. One or more symptoms of altered voluntary motor or sensory function.
2. Clinical findings demonstrate incompatibility between the symptom and recognised neurological conditions.
3. Symptom or deficit is not better explained by another medical or mental disorder.
4. Symptom or deficit causes significant distress or psychosocial impairment, or warrants medical evaluation.

TABLE 12.3 Clues Suggesting Motor Weakness Due to Conversion Disorder

Variable strength	Resistance applied by patient varies as the examiner applies different levels of force
Hoover's sign	The examiner keeps his hand below the heel of normal leg and asks the patient to lift the 'weak' leg. If the examiner does not feel the normal leg's heel pushing down as the patient tries to lift the 'weak' leg, this suggests functional weakness
Co-contraction	When asked to flex the elbow, both biceps and triceps are activated
Nonpyramidal pattern of hemiparesis	Pyramidal weakness indicates that the extensors are weaker than flexors in the upper limb and flexors are weaker than extensors in the lower limb
Absence of extensor plantar response	Despite hemiparesis, plantar reflex is flexor

BRIQUET'S SYNDROME

- Briquet's syndrome (somatisation disorder or somatic symptom disorder) is a chronic condition almost entirely confined to females, which begins before the age of 30. The cardinal features are multiple and recurrent somatic complaints affecting many organ systems which are accompanied by excessive thoughts, feelings and/or behaviours related to the somatic symptoms and for which medical attention is sought.
- Health care concerns are rarely alleviated despite high utilisation of medical care. Reassurance and explanation by physicians that the symptoms are not caused by a serious medical condition provide only temporary relief or are viewed as signs that the clinician does not understand the patient's symptoms.

TREATMENT

- First-line treatment is educating the patient about illness.
- Second-line therapy is cognitive behaviour therapy.
- Comorbid anxiety or depressive disorders should be treated concurrently.
- Physical therapy for motor conversion symptoms by encouraging normal movements and teaching patients to suppress abnormal movements.
- Resistant cases are treated with antidepressants such as SSRIs.

Q. Describe Munchausen's syndrome.

- This is a factitious disorder imposed on self and is named after the German Baron von Munchausen who was legendary for his inventive lying.
- The disorder is commonly seen in males. The patient changes his name frequently, and usually has a record of various medical reports with a history of 'doctor shopping'.
- He fabricates a convincing history and presents to the doctor with dramatic symptoms of a medical emergency even in the absence of obvious external rewards.
- He usually seeks medical attention at night when junior doctors or residents are on duty.
- He persuades an inexperienced doctor or internee to undertake complicated investigations or even exploratory surgery.
- Abdomen may show a 'surgical battlefield'—that is several scar marks due to previous operations.
- Patients may feign illnesses by several means:
  - Exaggerating or fabricating their symptoms.
  - Exacerbating or inducing signs, physiologic disturbances or illnesses (e.g. ingesting or injecting medications such as anticoagulants, insulin, laxatives; applying or injecting contaminants such as faeces or sputum; delaying wound healing via self-contamination or intentional dehiscence).
  - Aggravating existing illness by not adhering to medical treatment (e.g. precipitating seizures by omitting antiepileptic drugs).
  - Tampering with medical tests or laboratory specimens.

Q. Discuss common psychiatric emergencies (PS17.1, PS17.2)

- A psychiatric emergency is defined as an acute disturbance in thought, behaviour, mood or social relationship, which requires immediate intervention as defined by the patient, family or social unit.
- Some of the commonly encountered psychiatric emergencies are listed in Box 12.10.
- The first priority in a psychiatric emergency is ensuring the safety of the patient and others.
- Initial assessment should consist of a thorough history and physical examination to rule out underlying medical causes.

ACUTE PSYCHOSIS/ACUTE AGITATION

- Acute agitation can be due to acute psychosis, delirium, drug withdrawal or overdose.
- Psychosis is a syndrome that can result from a wide range of psychiatric conditions including schizophrenia, depression or bipolar disorders.
- It is important to differentiate acute psychosis from delirium, which is often due to a medical condition (see page 323).
- Symptoms of acute psychosis include delusions, hallucinations, disorganised speech and disorganised behaviour.

BOX 12.10 Commonly Encountered Psychiatric Emergencies

- Acute psychosis/acute agitation
- Acute panic attack
- Acute catatonic state
- Acute mania
- Suicidal ideation
- Conversion reaction

- An acute onset of psychosis suggests a medical cause, whereas a history of chronic psychotic symptoms without any significant change suggests a primary psychotic disorder.

HISTORY

- Obtain information from the relatives who brought the patient to the hospital.
- In receptive patients, ask questions regarding psychotic symptoms:
  - Does the patient hear voices?
  - Does he hear other people talking about him?
  - Does he feel that people harass him or read his thoughts?
- Assess for suicidal and homicidal thoughts and behaviour.
- Review the patient's medical history, and recent and past use of drugs, illicit drugs and use of herbal medicines.
- Review the family history.

EXAMINATION

- Perform a complete physical examination including general appearance, vital signs, signs of trauma, hydration status and neurologic signs.
- Assess the patient's behaviour, level of consciousness, cognitive functions, mood and affect, and thought process.
- Perform specific organ systems' examination particularly looking for signs of infection, hepatic dysfunction, trauma and cardiac disease.
- Perform a systematic mental status examination. The most widely used mental status instrument is the Mini-Mental Status Examination (MMSE).

LABORATORY INVESTIGATIONS

- Obtain blood counts, electrolytes, glucose, urea and bilirubin.
- A urine drug screen or blood alcohol level may be useful in assessing for intoxication and specific substance abuse in selected patients.
- Get a computed tomography (CT) head if there is any doubt of head injury.
- Consider lumbar puncture in selected patients (if meningitis or subarachnoid haemorrhage is suspected).

DIFFERENTIAL DIAGNOSIS

- First, determine whether the patient's symptoms are truly psychotic and whether the onset is acute or chronic. Symptoms of delirium may include illusions and hallucinations but the impairment of attention, altered level of consciousness and fluctuating mental status are not typical of primary psychotic syndrome.
- Patients with primary psychosis are usually alert and their cognitive abilities are relatively intact. Patients with delirium (secondary psychosis) typically have impaired orientation, memory and intellectual ability.
- Clinical clues that suggest an organic (secondary) psychosis include the following:
  - Atypical age of onset (age <13 years or >40 years).
  - Sudden onset within hours.
  - Lack of personal or family history of psychiatric illness.
  - Disorientation or reduced consciousness.
  - History of substance abuse or toxin exposure.
  - Visual hallucinations.
  - Recent memory loss.
  - Fluctuating course.
  - Abnormal vital signs or physical examination.
- If secondary psychosis is present, determine whether delirium is present.
- If the patient appears to have a secondary psychosis, but is not delirious, consider dementia. Slow onset and progression of profound memory loss and global cognitive defects suggest an underlying dementia.

MANAGEMENT

- Verbal de-escalation is the first step in acutely agitated patient. De-escalation is defined as a combination of both verbal and nonverbal strategies intended to assist the patient with calming down to cooperate with their evaluation and treatment. Patients who are able to make eye contact and engage in any form of conversation are more likely to be de-escalated.
- If clinically indicated, administer medications to reduce agitation of the patient. Haloperidol (1–5 mg every 4 hours) and diazepam (5–10 mg every hour) are the two agents widely used for this purpose. The oral route is preferred over the intramuscular route if the patient can cooperate and tolerate their administration. Atypical antipsychotics like olanzapine and risperidone are also useful agents to control acute agitation.
- Physical restraints are the last options to restrain the agitated patient. If possible, five trained individuals need to apply the physical restraints with one person at each extremity and one person at the head of the bed, being careful to avoid bodily injury due to excessive use of force or compromise the patient's ability to breathe. Extremity restraints are tethered to the side of the bed and not the side rails preferably with one arm upward and the other downward. The legs need to be tied to the opposite side of the bed to minimise the patient's ability to kick the staff.
- Call a psychiatrist for further management.

ACUTE MANIA

- Many patients with mania have bipolar affective disorder, alternating between episodes of mania and depression.
- Illicit drug use, especially stimulants, may cause a clinical picture of mania.

CLINICAL FEATURES

- Patients have an infectious, inappropriate euphoria coupled with hyperactivity and talkativeness.
- Patients are routinely awake all hours of the night and may go for extended periods of time without a significant amount of sleep.
- Other features include flight of ideas, decreased ability to concentrate on a task, inappropriate laughing, increased uninterrupted speech and grandiose delusions.
- In addition, patients may be dehydrated or have an electrolyte or nutritional disorder secondary to decreased consumption of food and water.

MANAGEMENT

- Evaluate patients for toxicity from drugs used to treat mania, such as lithium.
- Reducing the environmental stimuli in the emergency department is important. Place the patient in a safe and quiet room after ensuring that he or she has no objects that may be used to cause harm.
- If the patient continues to be agitated, medical management with lorazepam or diazepam, or haloperidol is appropriate.

ACUTE PANIC ATTACK

- Acute panic reaction occurs spontaneously and is always rapid in onset.
- It can be associated with a number of psychiatric disorders:
  - Psychotic patients may panic in response to hallucinations experienced by them.
  - Depression can be associated with panic attacks.
  - Many patients with anxiety disorder may panic when confronted with something they fear.
  - Besides, panic attacks are characteristic of a psychiatric illness known as panic disorder.

CLINICAL FEATURES

- Panic attack is associated with a sudden rush of fear accompanied by a sense of impending doom and features associated with increased autonomic activity.
- Autonomic features include tachycardia, palpitations, atypical chest pain, trembling, sweating, dyspnoea, subjective weakness of limbs, flushes and chills, dry mouth, choking sensation, dizziness and fear of losing control.

DIAGNOSIS

- While evaluating a patient with acute panic, rule out other medical emergencies including myocardial ischaemia, syncope and stroke.
- The quality of the somatic complaints in panic attack is quite different from those due to organic disorder. For example, in panic attack, the chest pain is usually diffuse and mild, the weakness of limbs is generalised and subjective, and the true syncope and vertigo are unusual.
- Consider several other factors while diagnosing a panic attack. These are as follows:
  - A panicking patient typically has an overwhelming concern about the possibility of losing control during the attack. He also has a fear of dying.
  - A panic disorder rarely starts in the late adulthood.
  - If a patient tries to avoid certain situations (agoraphobia) because of fear of experiencing the symptoms, a diagnosis of panic attack is likely. These patients feel better at home or near their friends and family members.
  - A panic attack usually occurs if there is a recent or anticipated major life event.
  - The family history is usually positive for panic disorders and other anxiety disorders.

MANAGEMENT

- By the time patients reach emergency department, acute features decrease in severity in most cases. Most commonly, they present with post-panic anxiety.
- The first goal of treatment is to reduce acute anxiety, which will also help in proper evaluation of the patient.
- Acute drug therapy is usually not required.
- Psychological intervention is important in alleviating the marked autonomic features.
- Explain clearly to the patient that what he is anticipating is not correct. For example, if a patient is having chest pain, inform him that his examination and the ECG are normal, and there is nothing to worry.
- It is also important to explain to the patient that the features of anxiety do not indicate insanity.
- If severe anxiety persists despite these measures, give diazepam orally.

ACUTE CATATONIC STATES

- Catatonia is a symptom complex usually associated with variety of psychiatric disorders including mood disorders and schizophrenia. It can also occur in drug-induced states or a variety of organic psychiatric disorders as well.

CLINICAL FEATURES

- Patient can be either in stupor or excitement accompanied by behavioural disturbances that include mutism, posturing, rigidity and grimacing. Cataplexy mutism—that is not responding orally though it seems patient is otherwise conscious and alert, is a common catatonic symptom.
- 'Posturing' indicates patient's ability to keep the limbs in odd postures, that is if the physician keeps the limbs in odd postures, the patient usually maintains them in awkward position for long time. Further, the patient may sit and stand in odd postures for long time. This is known as cataplexy.
- Catatonic 'stupor' like in other altered states of consciousness, is to be differentiated from organic disease states, conversion reaction (hysterical stupor) or malingering. Patient in stupor usually lies with his eyes open, apparently unseeing. His skin is pale frequently marred by acne and has an oily or greasy appearance.

- Patient's pulse is usually rapid (90–120/min) and the blood pressure may be elevated. Respiration is normal or rapid. Body temperature is often elevated by 1 °C to 1.5 °C above normal. They may not blink to visual threat, but have normal pupillary responses. Some patients keep their eyes tightly closed.
- Incontinence of urine and stools may occur in a few patients.

DIAGNOSIS

- Diagnosis is essentially based on clinical history. Ingestion of certain drugs and alcohol may also produce simular features. It needs to be differentiated from neuroleptic malignant syndrome, encephalitis and nonconvulsive status epilepticus.
- EEG is commonly useful to differentiate between organic and psychogenic causes.

TREATMENT

- Treatment depends on the diagnosis and requires evaluation by a psychiatrist.
- Use appropriate antidepressants and antipsychotics apart.

CONVERSION REACTION

- Conversion reaction describes a psychogenic or nonphysiologic loss or disorder of neurologic functioning—in motor/sensory/special senses or altered consciousness. These features are not under voluntary control.
- Do not classify patients with conversion reaction as 'cracks' or 'psychiatric'.

CLINICAL FEATURES

- Common presentations include hyperventilation, repeated altered conscious states, motor weakness or seizures (pseudoseizure).
- These symptoms are often preceded by an acute psychological stress.
- It may be difficult to differentiate between conversion disorder and malingering especially when the patient becomes chronic and has a long history.

DIAGNOSIS

- Diagnosis of conversion disorder depends on demonstrating that the patient's symptoms are not due to an organic malfunction. Inconsistency in findings on repeated examinations is a clue to this diagnosis.
- Consider conversion disorder if the patient presents with neurological features that do not follow the neuroanatomic pattern:
    - Acute onset of sensory loss in a sharp glove-and-stocking pattern in all the limbs.
    - Complete paralysis on one side of the body with sensory loss but with preservation of deep tendon reflexes and flexor plantar response.
    - Complete paralysis on one side with inability to turn the head to the same side indicating contralateral sternocleidomastoid muscle paralysis.
    - Pseudoseizures which are often associated with fluttering of eyelids, violent thrashing of limbs and dramatic vocalisation throughout seizure episode. These seizures last for a long time. There is no tongue biting or incontinence of stools and urine during the seizure.
    - In patients who are comatose due to a conversion reaction, the cold-calorie test reveals both the fast and slow components of nystagmus. Patients with a cortical lesion but an intact brainstem show only tonic deviation of the eyes.

MANAGEMENT

- Handle the patient with respect. Do not tell him that he is faking an illness.
- Inform the patient that though the symptoms are bothersome, there is no serious underlying illness.
- Tell the patient that the symptoms will improve gradually over the next few hours.
- Do not use a strong noxious stimulus like ammonia inhalation in these patients.
- Educate the patient about illness.
- Physical therapy for motor conversion symptoms by encouraging normal movements and teaching patients to suppress abnormal movements.
- Call a psychiatrist if the symptoms do not resolve over a period of observation.

SUICIDAL IDEATION

- As per the data from National Crime Records Bureau, poisoning is the most common mode of committing suicide in India.
- Risk factors for suicide are given in Box 12.11.

MANAGEMENT

- The management of the suicidal patient begins with placing the patient in a safe setting. Suicidal patients may use shoelaces, belts, keys and other common objects to inflict self-harm; therefore, their belongings should be searched to remove any possible concealed weapon.
- Suicidal patients should also be placed in a designated room where they are clearly visible and where there are no scalpels, needles or any other medical supplies that could be used to inflict harm.
- In the setting of depression, interpersonal psychotherapy and cognitive behaviour therapy are appropriate. Additionally, cognitive behavioural therapy can decrease hopelessness and suicide attempts among patients in the outpatient setting.

BOX 12.11 Risk Factors for Suicide

- Gender (men more than women)
- Age >60 years
- Widowed or divorced
- Living alone
- Unemployed
- Financial problems
- A recent adverse event
- Clinical depression
- Schizophrenia
- Substance abuse
- History of suicide attempts or ideation
- Feelings of hopelessness

- ECT has proved useful in patients with suicidal ideation regardless of psychiatric diagnosis. It can even be used safely in pregnant women. ECT, however, is not enough for long-term maintenance. Thus, ECT should be done in combination with pharmacologic strategies.
- The pharmacologic treatment of the patient with suicidal ideation depends on the psychiatric diagnosis. When using an antidepressant, it is preferable to use one with little risk of lethality by means of an acute overdose. For this reason, SSRIs or newer agents are preferable.

Q. Discuss briefly about anorexia nervosa. (PE 6.6)

Q. Write a short note on refeeding syndrome.

ANOREXIA NERVOSA

- Anorexia nervosa is an eating disorder defined by the restriction of energy intake relative to requirements, leading to a significantly low body weight.

AETIOLOGY

- The aetiology of anorexia nervosa and bulimia nervosa is unknown and probably multifactorial.
- Environmental influences include societal idealisations about weight and body shape. Parenting style, household stress and parental discord may be contributory.
- Genetic factors leading to abnormal neurotransmitter systems involving serotonin and dopamine.
- Possible roles of hormones such as ghrelin, leptin and oxytocin.

CLINICAL FEATURES

- Usually occurs in adolescents and more common in females.
- Onset often associated with emotional stressors, particularly conflicts with parents about independence and sexual conflicts.

Symptoms

- Restricted food intake which is low in calories with avoidance of high-calorie foods because of intense fear of gaining weight.
- Increased exercises despite bad weather, illness or injury.
- Self-induced vomiting (purging).
- Use of laxatives, diuretics and enemas.
- Significant amount of time spent examining and denigrating self for perceived signs of weight gain.
- Denial of emaciated condition.
- Excessive interest in food-related activities other than eating.
- In females who have attained menarche, amenorrhoea persisting for at least three cycles.
- Features suggesting obsessive-compulsive disorder and depression.

Subtypes of Anorexia Nervosa

- Restrictive type—during the past 3 months, the individual has not engaged in recurrent episodes of binge eating or purging behaviour; weight loss is accomplished primarily through dieting, fasting and/or excessive exercise.
- Binge-eating/purging type—during the past 3 months, the individual has engaged in recurrent episodes of binge eating or purging behaviour in terms of self-induced vomiting or the misuse of laxatives, diuretics or enemas.

Signs

- Signs of malnutrition—emaciation, bradycardia, hypotension, lanugo (fine hair on trunk) and oedema.
- Signs of purging—eroded dental enamel, scarring of fingers due to self-gagging to induce vomiting, parotid abscess and dental caries (due to keeping food in mouth for long periods).
- Signs of medical complications related to restricted food intake, starvation and purging.

DIAGNOSIS

- Restriction of energy intake relative to requirements leading to a significantly low body weight in the context of age, sex and height.
- Intense fear of gaining weight or becoming fat, or persistent behaviour that interferes with weight gain, even though at a significantly low weight.
- Distortion of body image so that patients regard themselves as fat even when they appear grossly underweight.

INVESTIGATIONS

- Table 12.4 lists some of the laboratory abnormalities seen in patients with anorexia nervosa.

TABLE 12.4 Investigations for Anorexia Nervosa

Laboratory Features of Malnutrition	Laboratory Features of Purging	Endocrine Features
• Normocytic, normochromic anaemia • Electrolyte disturbances • Elevated liver enzymes	• Metabolic alkalosis (due to self-induced vomiting) • Hypochloraemia • Hypokalaemia • Metabolic acidosis (due to laxative use) • Hypophosphataemia	• Reduced gonadotropin levels • Low oestrogen levels • Low testosterone levels • Elevated growth hormone and plasma cortisol levels • Low T3, normal T4 and TSH • Increased levels of corticotrophin in CSF

COMPLICATIONS (Table 12.5)

TABLE 12.5 Complications of Anorexia Nervosa

Gastrointestinal and Hepatic
• Dysphagia (due to weakened and uncoordinated pharyngeal muscles) • Aspiration pneumonia (due to dysphagia) • Acute gastric dilatation • Superior mesenteric artery syndrome (loss of fatty tissue pad which normally maintains the angle between superior mesenteric artery and aorta; this results in extrinsic compression of third portion of the duodenum by superior mesenteric artery) • Rectal prolapse and haemorrhoids (due to laxative abuse) • Elevated liver enzymes, hypoglycaemia, acute hepatic failure
Cardiac
• Sudden death • Cardiac arrhythmias • Mitral valve prolapse • Pericardial effusion
Haematological
• Anaemia, leucopenia, thrombocytopenia
Musculoskeletal
• Osteoporosis • Fractures • Sarcopaenia
Endocrine
• Amenorrhoea
Refeeding Syndrome
• Occurs during feeding of severely malnourished patient

CLINICAL COURSE

- Anorexia nervosa is a chronic illness.
- Favourable outcome in 60%–70% of cases at 5–7 years of follow-up.
- Long-term mortality in hospitalised patients is about 10%.

TREATMENT

- Correction of significant complications related to purging and starvation.
- Correction of other complications.
- Slow refeeding (either enteral or parenteral), starting with 1200 to 1400 kcal/day and increase the number of calories every second day by 200 kcal until the necessary intake is achieved.
- Calcium and vitamin D supplementation.
- Behavioural therapy with rewards or punishment based on absolute weight and not on eating behaviour.
- Family therapy to reduce conflicts.
- Antidepressants if underlying depression is present; otherwise their role is doubtful.

REFEEDING SYNDROME

- Carries a risk of mortality.
- Can occur when oral feeding is resumed in a severely malnourished patient, especially if the parenteral route is used.
- It occurs as a consequence of marked shifts in fluid and electrolyte distribution, particularly phosphate, from extracellular to intracellular space.
- With refeeding, availability of glucose reactivates the metabolism resulting in a high demand of phosphates (for the production of ATP) and thiamine (a cofactor in glucose metabolism).
- Rapid intracellular passage of phosphates, potassium and magnesium may cause abrupt reductions of these ions in the blood; in particular, reduced phosphates interfere with the phosphorylation of the energetic compounds and may cause cellular hypoxia and death.
- Due to antinatriuretic effect of insulin, extracellular fluid volume increases.
- The refeeding syndrome is defined by a pentad of life-threatening complications including rhabdomyolysis, heart failure, respiratory failure, haemolysis and seizures. Other features include oedema, muscle weakness, cramps, lethargy, nausea, vomiting and constipation, cardiac arrhythmias, hypotension, thrombocytopenia, renal failure, delirium and coma.
- Warning signs of refeeding syndrome include weight increase (>1.5 kg/week), tachycardia and/or pedal oedema.
- It can be generally treated with oral potassium phosphate tablets, but when more severe (i.e. serum phosphate level <2 mg/dL), intravenous potassium phosphorous can be administered. Correction of other electrolyte abnormalities is also essential.

PREVENTION

- It is advisable to proceed with haemodynamic rebalance before the start of refeeding, preventive correction of electrolyte imbalances and very gradual refeeding with close monitoring of the clinical–metabolic parameters.
- Start from 20–25 kcal/kg/day with a progressive gradual increase in every 3–4 days by about 5 kcal/kg/day.
- Supplementation with phosphates, magnesium, potassium and vitamins B_1, B_6 and B_{12}.

Q. Write a short note on bulimia nervosa. (PE 6.6)

- Bulimia nervosa involves uncontrolled eating of an abnormally large amount of food in a short period, followed by compensatory behaviours such as self-induced vomiting, laxative abuse and/or excessive exercise.

AETIOLOGY

- Similar to those for anorexia nervosa.
- Sexual assault or abuse is an additional risk factor.

CLINICAL FEATURES

- Onset usually in late adolescence or early adulthood; more common in females.
- Often follows a period of dietary restriction.

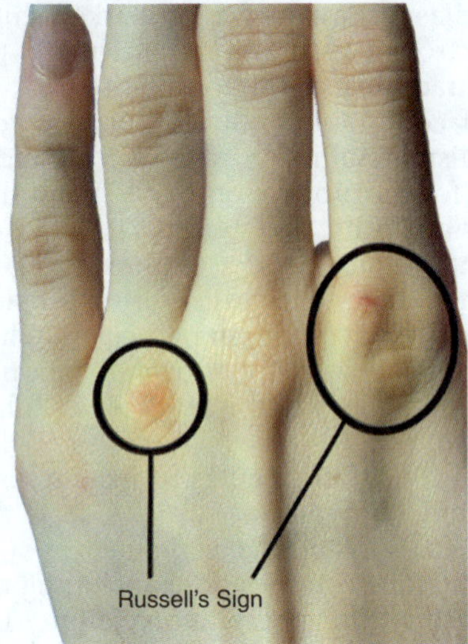

Fig. 12.1 Russell's sign (calluses on the knuckles resulting from repeated self-induced vomiting).

- Associated problems may include anxiety, mood disturbances, substance abuse and impulsivity (kleptomania).
- Suicide rates higher than those in general population.

SYMPTOMS

- Recurrent episodes of binge eating.
- Obsession with dieting but followed by binge eating of high-calorie food.
- Binge eating is associated with emotional stress and followed by feelings of guilt, self-recrimination and compensatory behaviour.
- Self-castigation for mild weight gain or binges.
- Attempts to conceal binge eating or purging.
- Weight maintained.

SIGNS

- Calluses on dorsal aspect of hands—Russell's sign (due to self-induced vomiting) (Fig. 12.1).
- Dental erosion, dental caries and oesophageal erosions due to purging.
- Lanugo hair.
- Enlarged parotid glands (due to parotid inflammation caused by gastric acid and enzymes), bradycardia, hypotension and cardiac arrhythmias (due to hypokalaemia).

DIAGNOSTIC CRITERIA (Box 12.12)

BOX 12.12 Diagnostic Criteria for Bulimia Nervosa

1. Recurrent episodes of binge eating characterised by eating an objectively large amount of food and a sense of loss of control over eating during the episodes.
2. Recurrent inappropriate compensatory behaviour in order to prevent weight gain (e.g. self-induced vomiting, use of laxatives, enemas or diuretics).
3. Binge eating and inappropriate compensatory behaviour occur at least once a week for 3 months.
4. Self-evaluation is unduly influenced by body shape and weight.

COURSE

- Prognosis is better than that of anorexia nervosa.
- Favourable prognostic indicators include younger age at onset, higher social class and comorbid borderline personality.

TREATMENT

- Antidepressants, particularly SSRIs.
- Cognitive behavioural therapy.
- Psychodynamic psychotherapy in patients with borderline personality disorder.

Q. How do you differentiate between anorexia nervosa and bulimia nervosa?

- Table 12.6 differentiates anorexia nervosa from bulimia nervosa.

Q. What are the common symptoms and signs of substance abuse or substance use disorders? List down the investigations required. (PS4.1, PS4.2, PS4.3, PS4.4)

- Substance abuse or substance use disorder is defined as psychological dependence and heavy consumption of a substance despite social and occupational problems.
- Substance dependence is defined as similar impairment with increased tolerance or presence of physical signs on withdrawal of substance.
- The substances most commonly abused are alcohol, benzodiazepines (e.g. diazepam and alprazolam), opioids (e.g. heroin), barbiturates, nicotine (smoking), caffeine, marijuana (cannabis), cocaine, amphetamines, glue, etc.
- Common features suggesting substance abuse are shown in Table 12.7.
- Acute presentation may be due to overdose, withdrawal or accident injuries.

TABLE 12.6 Differentiating Between Anorexia Nervosa and Bulimia Nervosa

Anorexia Nervosa	Bulimia Nervosa
• Patients are thin or emaciated	• Patients usually have normal weight
• Patients prefer to eat less or starve	• Patients eat heavy meals followed by purging
• Denies abnormal eating behaviour	• Recognises abnormal eating behaviour
• Preoccupation with losing more and more weight	• Preoccupation with attaining an 'ideal' but unrealistic weight
• Believes one is fat even when one is really underweight or emaciated	• May be overly focussed on weight and appearance
• May result in amenorrhoea, osteoporosis and infertility	• May result in damage to teeth, oesophagus and parotid glands

TABLE 12.7 Common Symptoms and Signs Suggesting Substance Abuse

Symptoms	Signs
• Frequent absences from school or work	• Tremors
• History of frequent trauma	• Odour of alcohol on breath
• Depression or anxiety	• Conjunctival injection
• Epigastric distress, diarrhoea	• Labile hypertension
• Sexual dysfunction	• Tachycardia
• Sleep disorders	• Tender hepatomegaly

TABLE 12.8 Complications of Substance Use Disorders

- Cardiovascular:
  - Hypertension
  - Cardiomyopathy
  - Endocarditis
  - Heart failure
- Gastrointestinal:
  - Pancreatitis
  - Chronic liver disease
  - Cirrhosis of liver
- Renal:
  - Chronic kidney disease
- Haematologic:
  - Anaemia
  - Hypoplasia of bone marrow
- CNS:
  - Dementia
  - Cerebral vasculitis
  - Stroke
  - Traumatic brain injury
- Pulmonary:
  - Bronchospasm
  - Chronic obstructive lung disease
  - Hypersensitivity pneumonitis
  - Pneumothorax
  - Pneumomediastinum
- Infections:
  - Hepatitis B and C
  - HIV
  - Tuberculosis

COMPLICATIONS OF SUBSTANCE USE DISORDERS

- These depend on the route of administration and type of substance (Table 12.8).

DIAGNOSIS (Box 12.13)

BOX 12.13 Diagnostic Criteria for Substance Abuse (DSM-5)

1. Often taken in larger amounts or over a longer period than was intended.
2. A persistent desire or unsuccessful efforts to cut down or control use.
3. A great deal of time is spent in activities necessary to obtain, use or recover from the substance's effect.
4. Craving or a strong desire or urge to use the substance.
5. Recurrent use resulting in a failure to fulfil major role obligations at work, school or home.
6. Continued use despite having persistent or recurrent social or interpersonal problems caused by it.
7. Important social, occupational or recreational activities are given up or reduced.
8. Recurrent use in situations in which it is physically hazardous.
9. Continued use despite knowledge of having a persistent or recurrent physical or psychological problem that is likely to have been caused or exacerbated by the substance.
10. Tolerance as defined by either of the following:
    a. A need for markedly increased amounts of substance to achieve desired effect.
    b. A markedly diminished effect with continued use of the same amount of substance.
11. Withdrawal.

Note: Severity is mild if two to three criteria are met, moderate if four to five criteria are met and severe if six or more criteria are met.

LABORATORY INVESTIGATIONS

- A urine screen for substances of abuse. However, they may be falsely positive or negative.
- The most useful investigations to confirm alcohol abuse are:
  - Gamma-glutamyl transpeptidase (GGT) is commonly used but its elevation has low sensitivity and specificity for alcohol abuse. Also elevated in obese persons.
  - An AST:ALT ratio of 2:1 is indicative of alcohol-induced liver disease.
  - Elevated mean corpuscular volume, but is less sensitive than GGT.
  - Elevated carbohydrate deficient transferrin level is highly specific in the absence of liver disease.
  - Other markers of alcohol use include ethyl glucuronide, ethyl sulphate, phosphatidylethanol and fatty acid ethyl esters.

MANAGEMENT

- Individuals with opioid use disorder, alcohol use disorder and benzodiazepine use disorder who experience or are at significant risk to experience withdrawal upon stopping use should undergo medically supervised withdrawal. Medically supervised withdrawal generally uses agonists or other medications that provide symptomatic relief.
- Fluids, vitamins and thiamine are adequate for mild alcohol withdrawal while benzodiazepines are required for severe alcohol withdrawal.
- Buprenorphine is used for opioid withdrawal.

Q. Give a brief account of alcohol dependence.

Q. Give a brief account of alcohol use disorder.

(PS4.1, PS4.2, PS4.3, PS4.4, PS4.6)

- A chronic disorder caused by genetic, psychosocial and environmental factors.
- Alcohol abuse and alcohol dependence are combined into one entity known as alcohol use disorder.
- Risky alcohol use refers to consumption of an amount of alcohol which puts an individual at risk for health consequences.

PHYSICAL EXAMINATION

- Look for the following complications related to alcohol intake:
  1. Mental state: Intoxication or withdrawal features, depression.
  2. Neurological: Cognitive decline, cerebellar degeneration, peripheral neuropathy, Wernicke's encephalopathy, subdural haematoma.
  3. Cardiovascular: Atrial fibrillation ('holiday heart'), cardiomyopathy.
  4. Gastrointestinal: Liver and pancreatic disease (acute and chronic).
  5. Respiratory: Aspiration pneumonia.

DIAGNOSTIC CRITERIA

At least two of the features mentioned in Box 12.14 indicate alcohol use disorder.

Box 12.14 Alcohol Use Disorder: Diagnostic Criteria

1. Drinking larger amounts or over longer periods than intended.
2. Desire or unsuccessful attempts to cut down or control alcohol use.
3. A great deal of time spent obtaining, using or recovering from alcohol.
4. Craving, or a strong desire or urge to use alcohol.
5. Failure to fulfil major role obligations as a result of alcohol use.
6. Continued drinking despite social or interpersonal problems.
7. Diminished social, occupational or recreational activities due to drinking.
8. Recurrent alcohol use in physically hazardous situations.
9. Continued drinking despite physical or psychological problems.
10. Tolerance as evidenced by a markedly diminished effect.
11. Withdrawal syndrome or drinking to prevent withdrawal.

LABORATORY INVESTIGATIONS

- See above (under 'Substance Abuse' on page 801).

TREATMENT

- Two phases: detoxification and rehabilitation.

DETOXIFICATION

- Deals with acute withdrawal symptoms and therefore requires use of medications.
- Approved medications include naltrexone, disulfiram and acamprosate.

Disulfiram

- Alcohol is converted to acetaldehyde by alcohol dehydrogenase, which is further broken down by the enzyme acetaldehyde dehydrogenase. Disulfiram acts as a deterrent to drinking by inhibiting the enzyme aldehyde dehydrogenase, thereby increasing the levels of toxic substance acetaldehyde in the body.
- If the patient consumes alcohol while on disulfiram, acetaldehyde accumulates that leads to flushing, palpitations, nausea, faintness and in some cases, cardiac arrhythmias and collapse.
- Initial dose is 250 mg/day that can be increased to a maximum of 500 mg after a few days.
- Side effects include drowsiness, metallic taste, skin rash, headache, peripheral neuropathy, optic neuritis, mood change, impotence, seizure and hepatotoxicity. Severe adverse reactions are rare and include myocardial infarction, congestive heart failure, respiratory depression, convulsions and death.
- Should not be given to patients with serious active liver disease or cardiovascular disorders, to pregnant females or to patients with suicidal tendencies.
- It also interferes with the metabolism of other drugs, most notably tricyclic antidepressants, MAOI, heparin and some anticonvulsants.
- Other drugs which act like disulfiram include metronidazole, cefoperazone, chloramphenicol, nitrofurantoin, isosorbide dinitrate, etc.

Naltrexone

- A mu-opioid receptor antagonist that reduces the feelings of cravings. It also reduces the severity of relapse particularly over a short term.
- Dose is 50–100 mg/day in a single dose.
- Also available as intramuscular injection (dose is 380 mg/month).
- Side effects include nausea, vomiting, headache, dizziness, fatigue, anxiety, insomnia, tiredness and joint or muscle pain.
- Long-term opioid therapy for chronic pain or heroin dependence is a contraindication for naltrexone because the drug could precipitate severe withdrawal syndrome.
- Also contraindicated in patients with liver disease. Liver function tests should be done every month in the initial few months of treatment.

Acamprosate

- Normalises the dysregulation of *N*-methyl-D-aspartate–mediated glutamatergic excitation that occurs in alcohol withdrawal and early abstinence. This reduces cravings.
- Dose is 1998 mg/day if weight >60 kg and 1332 mg/day if weight <60 kg. Available in 333-mg enteric-coated tablet and is to be given thrice a day.
- Side effects include diarrhoea, pruritus, skin rash, altered libido, dizziness and headache.
- Use cautiously in patients with renal impairment.

REHABILITATION

- Helps to prevent relapse and development of lifestyle compatible with long-term abstinence.
- Requires psychotherapeutic interventions.

Q. Discuss alcohol withdrawal in brief.

- Alcohol withdrawal in a chronic alcoholic person is characterised by sudden exhibition of CNS excitation.

CLINICAL FEATURES

- These develop 6–48 hours after the reduction of ethanol intake and may last for 2–7 days.

MINOR WITHDRAWAL SYMPTOMS

- Minor withdrawal symptoms include insomnia, tremors (the shakes), hyperreflexia, mild anxiety, gastrointestinal upset, headache, diaphoresis, tachycardia, palpitations, hypertension and anorexia. These features resolve within 24–48 hours.

ALCOHOLIC HALLUCINOSIS

- This refers to hallucinations that develop within 12–24 hours of abstinence and resolve within 48–72 hours.
- Hallucinations are usually visual, although auditory and tactile phenomena may also occur. In contrast to

delirium tremens, alcoholic hallucinosis is not associated with clouding of the sensorium.

WITHDRAWAL SEIZURES

- Withdrawal-associated seizures or 'rum fits' are generalised tonic–clonic convulsions that usually occur within 7–48 hours after the last drink, but may occur only after 2 hours of abstinence. Seizures have little or no postictal period.
- Withdrawal seizures are usually single but may occur as a brief flurry of seizures over a short period. Recurrent or prolonged seizures or status epilepticus are generally not consistent with withdrawal-associated seizures and should prompt an investigation for possible structural or infectious aetiologies.
- Approximately 3% of chronic alcoholics have withdrawal-associated seizures and of those patients, 3% develop status epilepticus.
- Approximately one-third of patients who develop delirium tremens have a preceding alcohol withdrawal seizure.

DELIRIUM TREMENS

- It typically begins between 48 and 96 hours after the last drink and lasts 1–5 days. If early alcohol withdrawal features are not treated, about 5% of patients will progress to delirium tremens.
- Clinical features include hallucinations, disorientation, delirium, tachycardia, hypertension, low-grade fever (sometimes high-grade), agitation, diaphoresis, dilated pupils and occasionally seizures.
- Patients may be dehydrated as a result of diaphoresis, hyperthermia, vomiting and tachypnoea.
- Hypokalaemia, hypomagnesaemia and hypophosphataemia are common. Arterial blood gas shows respiratory alkalosis.
- Death occurs in 5% of cases and is usually due to arrhythmias, pneumonia or electrolyte imbalance.

DIFFERENTIAL DIAGNOSIS

- The alcohol withdrawal syndrome can be confused with several conditions like encephalitis, drug-induced psychosis, hypoglycaemia (alcohol-induced), anticholinergic intoxication and withdrawal of sedative-hypnotics.
- Opioid withdrawal is associated with a normal mental status, no fever and infrequent seizures.
- Withdrawals associated with barbiturates and benzodiazepines usually progress slowly and the frequency of seizures is higher that tend to appear later, generally around seventh day compared to around second day in alcohol withdrawal.

MANAGEMENT

- Always consider a possibility of associated conditions like pneumonia, GI bleed, liver failure, pancreatitis, electrolyte imbalance, neurological injury, hypothermia or hyperthermia, and trauma.
- Maintain airway and breathing.
- Administer thiamine and glucose intravenously after withdrawing appropriate blood samples in patients with altered sensorium.
- In mild cases of withdrawal, provide supportive care in the form of reassurance and nursing care with frequent monitoring of vital signs. Fluid and electrolyte imbalance should be corrected.
- β-Blockers help in reducing anxiety and tremors.
- Benzodiazepines (diazepam and lorazepam) are required in patients with moderate to severe withdrawal. These are also useful in controlling seizures. If seizures do not respond to benzodiazepines, phenobarbitone or propofol may be used.
- Haloperidol for uncontrolled agitation or hallucinations.
- The utility of magnesium in patients with alcohol-related seizures is controversial. Antiepileptics like phenytoin, valproic acid and levetiracetam are of little use in treating or preventing alcohol withdrawal seizures.

Q. Describe ethanol content in various alcoholic beverages.

Q. Briefly discuss alcohol intoxication.

- Ethanol content of various alcoholic beverages is expressed by volume per cent or proof (Table 12.9).
- Proof is twice the volume per cent of ethanol.

ACUTE INTOXICATION

- Initially, alcohol produces excitement which with increasing blood levels progresses to loss of restraint, behavioural changes, slurring of speech, ataxia, drowsiness, coma and finally death (Table 12.10).

TABLE 12.9 Ethanol Content of Various Alcoholic Beverages

Type of Beverage	Ethanol Content (Volume %)
• Light beer	4–6
• Heavy beer	6–12
• Wine	8–20 (varies according to type of wine)
• Whiskey, brandy, tequila, gin	40–45
• Rum	40–60

Note: To calculate weight in grams, multiply the volume of ethanol in a beverage by 0.79 (approximate specific gravity of ethanol).

TABLE 12.10 Clinical Features of Alcohol Intoxication

Blood Ethanol Level (mg/dL)	Clinical Features
• <25	Feeling of warmth
• 25–50	Euphoria, talkativeness, decreased inhibition
• 50–100	Incoordination, impaired comprehension, increased reaction time
• 100–250	Disoriented, confusion, staggering gait, ataxia, slurring of speech, nystagmus
• 250–400	Comatose, hypothermia, hypotension, incontinence of urine
• >400	Respiratory depression, death

Note: 1. The correlation between blood levels and clinical features is variable with some people tolerating higher levels while others developing severe intoxication at lower levels.
2. Patient with significant metabolic acidosis or significant hypotension should be evaluated for additional causes of these features.

INVESTIGATIONS

- Blood alcohol level.
- Breath alcohol level is a good option if blood level cannot be measured. Expired has a good correlation with the blood alcohol levels.
- Serum electrolytes, glucose and blood gas analysis.
- Osmolality is elevated and osmolar gap is high (>10 mOsm/L).
- CT head if head injury is suspected.

TREATMENT (Box 12.15)

BOX 12.15 Treatment of Alcohol Intoxication

1. Airway assessment and protection.
2. Observation of respiratory and cardiovascular functions.
3. Prevention of aspiration.
4. Mechanical ventilation, if necessary.
5. Intravenous fluids to correct volume depletion.
6. Correction of hypoglycaemia and electrolyte imbalances.
7. Administration of thiamine.
8. Antiemetic drugs.
9. Sedation (if agitated, violent) using haloperidol, one of the benzodiazepines or ketamine.
10. If patient remains comatose over a few hours, consider other diagnoses like head injury and meningitis.

Q. Describe smoking and its health risks.

Q. Name the drugs useful to reduce nicotine dependence.

CONTENTS OF CIGARETTE SMOKE

- More than 4000 substances in cigarette smoke. Some of the common ones are shown in Table 12.11.
- Mainstream smoke—smoke emerging from mouth of a person during puffing.
- Sidestream smoke—smoke emitting between puffs at the burning end and from mouth end. Contains more carcinogens compared to mainstream smoke.

TABLE 12.11 Common Contents of Cigarette Smoke

Category	Components
• Carcinogens	Tar Polynuclear aromatic hydrocarbons *N*-Nitrosonornicotine Benzopyrene Trace metals—nickel, arsenic, polonium, etc. Nitrosamine Hydrazine Vinyl chloride
• Cocarcinogens	Phenol Cresol Catechol
• Addicting agent	Nicotine
• Other	Carbon monoxide

SMOKING INDEX AND PACK-YEARS

- Smoking index is the number of cigarettes per day multiplied by total duration of smoking in years. If a person smokes 10 cigarettes/day for the past 15 years, his/her smoking index is 150.
  - Smoking index <100—light smoker.
  - Smoking index 100–300—moderate smoker.
  - Smoking index >300—heavy smoker.
- Pack-years is number of packs of cigarettes per day multiplied by total duration of smoking in years (1 pack = 20 cigarettes).
  - Risk of developing lung cancer is 40-fold in persons with pack-years of 40.

PASSIVE SMOKING

- Also known as second-hand smoking, involuntary smoking and environmental tobacco smoke exposure.
- Occurs when smoke from one person's burning tobacco product, that is sidestream smoke or exhaled smoke, is inhaled by others.
- Passive smoking increases the risk of cancers, coronary artery disease (CAD), respiratory illnesses and death.

SMOKELESS TOBACCO

- This includes chewing or snuffing tobacco.
- Contains more nicotine than cigarettes and is, therefore, addicting.
- Important risks include oral cancer, loosening of teeth and decay of exposed tooth roots.
- Can also cause systemic effects including increased incidence of oesophageal and pancreatic cancers as well as CAD and stroke.

PHARMACOLOGY OF SMOKE

- Nicotine is the main toxic substance producing acute effects as well as dependence.
- Inhalation of nicotine produces:
  - Increase in both systolic and diastolic blood pressures.
  - Increase in heart rate.
  - Increase in force of myocardial contraction.
  - Increase in excitability of myocardium.
  - Increase in myocardial oxygen consumption.
  - Peripheral vasoconstriction.
- Inhalation of carbon monoxide leads to polycythaemia and CNS impairment.
- Carcinogens increase the occurrence of several cancers.
- Smoking impairs ciliary movement in respiratory tract, inhibits function of alveolar macrophages and produces hyperplasia and hypertrophy of mucus-secreting glands. The airway resistance is increased due to smooth muscle contraction via stimulation of submucosal irritant receptors. It also inhibits antiproteinases and stimulates neutrophils to release proteolytic enzymes.

BOX 12.16 Health Effects of Chronic Smoking

- Cancers
  - Lung
  - Oral cavity
  - Larynx
  - Oesophagus
  - Stomach
  - Urinary bladder
  - Kidney
  - Colon
  - Cervix
  - Acute myeloid leukaemia
- CAD
- Strokes
- Chronic obstructive lung disease
- Aortic aneurysm
- Peripheral vascular disease
- Periodontitis
- Infertility

HEALTH EFFECTS OF CHRONIC SMOKING (Box 12.16)

- All forms of tobacco smoking including cigarettes, cigars, pipes, bidis and hookahs can produce ill health effects and addiction.
- Cigar and pipe smokers tend to inhale less smoke than cigarette smokers, so their risk of lung cancer is lower but is still several times higher than the risk for nonsmokers.
- Occurrence of carcinoma of oral cavity, larynx and oesophagus is same with cigar, pipe and cigarette.
- There is no evidence that 'low-tar' cigarettes produce less ill effect in humans.

SMOKING AND CARDIOVASCULAR DISEASE

- Major risk factors for CAD include smoking, hypertension and hypercholesterolaemia. Presence of all three risk factors increases risk of CAD eight-fold.
- Deaths due to CAD are 60% higher in smokers compared to nonsmokers.
- People younger than 40 years are five times more likely to have a heart attack if they smoke.
- Sudden death is two to four times more common in smokers.
- Females who smoke are also predisposed to CAD.
- Cerebrovascular accidents are more common in smokers.
- Peripheral vascular diseases are more common in smokers.

SMOKING AND RESPIRATORY DISEASES

- Chronic obstructive lung disease is about 10–20 times greater in smokers.
- Male smokers have 4-fold to 25-fold higher mortality due to chronic obstructive lung disease than nonsmokers.
- Increased incidence of influenza infection in smokers.
- Cancers of larynx and lung common in smokers.

SMOKING AND GASTROINTESTINAL TRACT

- Smoking produces discolouration of teeth and reduced taste and smell.
- Peptic ulcers (both gastric and duodenal) are more common. Also impairs ulcer healing.
- Increased prevalence of cancers of oral cavity, oesophagus, stomach, colon and pancreas.

SMOKING AND PREGNANCY

- Smoking reduces chances of conception.
- Smoking during pregnancy produces intrauterine growth retardation leading to reduced weight of newborn.
- Rates of spontaneous abortion, intrauterine foetal death and sudden infant death higher in smokers.

NICOTINE WITHDRAWAL

- Withdrawal symptoms in chronic users begin to appear approximately 30 minutes after every dose.
- Features include confusion, restlessness, anxiety, insomnia, dizziness, depression, feelings of frustration and anger, nightmares, poor concentration, headache and increased appetite.

SMOKING CESSATION

- Behavioural counselling.
- Nicotine replacement therapy:
  - Use of nicotine patches, nicotine gums, lozenges and nasal sprays.
  - Contraindicated in unstable CAD, untreated peptic ulcer disease, recent MI and recent stroke.
  - Method of gum use.
    - Chew slowly until a strong taste or tingling sensation felt.
    - Stop chewing and place the gum between cheek and gums.
    - Chew again when intensity of tingling decreases.
    - Repeat this cycle of 'park and chew' for about 30 minutes or until tingling sensation subsides.
- Bupropion:
  - An antidepressant that is chemically unrelated to tricyclic antidepressants or SSRIs.
  - The mechanism of action is unknown; however, it is a noncompetitive antagonist of nicotine receptors and inhibits reuptake of dopamine, noradrenaline and serotonin in CNS.
  - Dose is 75–150 mg twice a day.
  - Side effects include dry mouth, insomnia and skin rash.
  - Rarely, it can precipitate seizures.
- Varenicline:
  - A partial agonist at the $\alpha4\beta2$ nicotinic acetylcholine receptor.
  - It is possibly more effective than nicotine and bupropion.
  - Contraindicated in pregnancy and lactation.
  - Side effects include nausea, insomnia, abnormal dreams, neuropsychiatric symptoms (agitation, depressed mood and suicidal ideation), visual disturbances and alteration in consciousness.
- Other medicines:
  - Clonidine and nortriptyline.
- Electronic cigarettes:
  - A battery-powered vaporiser which contains nicotine derived from tobacco plant and gives the feeling of smoking a cigarette.
  - Have a heating element which vaporises the liquid solution containing nicotine and other substances some of which are toxic.

TABLE 12.12 Antipsychotic Drugs

Generation	Drug	Usual Dose (mg/day)
First-generation (typical) antipsychotics	Haloperidol	5–30
	Chlorpromazine	100–1500
	Perphenazine	12–24
	Thioridazine	50–800
	Trifluoperazine	5–30
	Fluphenazine	5–15
	Droperidol	5–10[a]
	Flupenthixol	40–200[b]
	Pimozide	4–30
	Loxapine	20–80
Second-generation (atypical) antipsychotics	Sulpiride	600–1800
	Clozapine	200–600
	Quetiapine	300–600
	Risperidone	2–6
	Olanzapine	10–30
	Ziprasidone	20–160; 20[a]
	Aripiprazole	10–30
	Paliperidone	6–12
	Asenapine	10–20[c]
	Lurasidone	40–80

[a]Milligram intramuscularly.
[b]Milligram fortnightly intramuscularly.
[c]Milligram sublingually.

- They possibly reduce various health effects of cigarette smoking.
- However, potential risks of e-cigarettes, how much nicotine or other potentially harmful chemicals are being inhaled during use, and whether there are any benefits associated with using them are not clear and hence not recommended.
- Another complication is e-cigarette or vaping-associated lung injury (EVALI) (see page 199).

Q. What are the commonly used antipsychotic drugs, their uses and adverse effects? (PS14.5, PS18.1, PS3.10, PS5.5)

- The antipsychotic drugs are used in schizophrenia, mania and acute delirium.
- Commonly used antipsychotic drugs are listed in Table 12.12.
- Atypical antipsychotics produce less extrapyramidal side effects as compared to typical ones.

ADVERSE EFFECTS (Box 12.17)

BOX 12.17 Adverse Effects of Antipsychotic Drugs

- Sedation
- Weight gain
- Anticholinergic features (dry mouth, urinary hesitancy, constipation, blurred vision, delirium)
- QTc interval prolongation particularly with ziprasidone
- Hypotension (due to alpha-adrenergic blockade)
- Galactorrhoea, amenorrhoea
- Extrapyramidal reactions like torticollis, dystonia, akathisia (inability to sit still); tardive dyskinesia (repetitive involuntary movements) with prolonged use
- Neuroleptic malignant syndrome
- Elevation in lipid levels
- Insulin resistance

Q. What are the commonly used antidepressant drugs? What are their important side effects? What are their other indications? (PS10.6, PS14.5, PS18.1, PS3.10, PS6.4, PS6.6, PS8.6)

- Antidepressant drugs are useful in depressive illness, OCDs and phobic disorders.
- Various classes of antidepressant drugs are listed in Table 12.13.

Q. Write a short note on lithium carbonate. (PS18.1, PS3.10)

INDICATIONS

- Drug of choice for bipolar disorder, as both treatment and maintenance therapy.
- Used as an adjunctive medication in patients with unipolar disorder (depression) who have inadequately responded to an antidepressant.
- Also useful as an adjunct to antipsychotic agents in patients with schizophrenia.
- Toxic effects occur with serum concentrations ≥1.5 mEq/L.

DOSE

- Initial dose is 300 mg/day.
- Increased every 1 or 2 days depending on response as well as tolerance to a target dose of 900 mg/day.
- Therapeutic blood levels are 0.5–1 mEq/L.

SIDE EFFECTS

- Nausea, vomiting, headache and weight gain.
- Tremors, drowsiness, ataxia, confusion, lethargy, memory impairment, slurred speech and convulsions.
- Hyperreflexia and myoclonus.
- Prolongation of QRS interval and cardiac arrhythmias.
- Nephrogenic diabetes insipidus producing polyuria and polydipsia.
- Renal failure.
- Hypothyroidism.
- Serotonin syndrome, particularly when used in combination with other serotonergic agents.

CAUTION

- Drugs like thiazide diuretics, NSAIDs and ACE inhibitors reduce renal excretion of lithium and should be avoided, if possible.
- Avoid dehydration as it can lead to lithium toxicity.

Q. Discuss electroconvulsive therapy (ECT). (PS18.2)

- Involves the administration of high-voltage, brief and direct current impulses to the head to induce seizures in brain while the patient is anaesthetised

TABLE 12.13 Antidepressant Drugs

Group	Drug	Usual Dose (mg/day)	Important Adverse Effects
• Tricyclics	Amitriptyline Imipramine Dothiepin Clomipramine Amoxapine Desipramine Nortriptyline	75–150 75–150 75–150 75–150 25–300 25–300 50–150	Dry mouth, constipation, blurred vision, sedation, weight gain, postural hypotension, cardiac arrhythmias
• Selective serotonin reuptake inhibitors (SSRIs)	Fluoxetine Fluvoxamine Sertraline Citalopram Escitalopram Paroxetine	20–60 100–200 50–200 10–60 5–30 10–50	Nausea, insomnia, increased risk of fractures and GI bleed, serotonin syndrome
• Tetracyclics	Mianserin	30–90	Constipation, dry mouth, drowsiness, headache, dizziness
• Atypical antidepressants	Bupropion Mirtazapine	300–450 15–45	Nausea, vomiting, dry mouth, constipation, dizziness, weight gain
• MAOI (rarely used)	Phenelzine Tranylcypromine	60–90 20–40	Hypertensive crisis, serotonin syndrome, drug interactions
• Serotonin-norepinephrine reuptake inhibitors	Venlafaxine Duloxetine Milnacipran	75–300 60–120 100–200	Nausea, sweating, dizziness, constipation, sexual dysfunction, serotonin syndrome
• Serotonin modulators	Nefazodone Trazodone Vilazodone	50–600 100–600 10–40	Nausea, drowsiness, dry mouth, dizziness, constipation, hepatotoxicity (nefazodone), priapism (trazodone)

(usually methohexital) and paralysed (usually succinylcholine). Electrodes can be placed bilaterally or unilaterally over the nondominant hemisphere.

- ECT is safe with few side effects. Headache, postictal confusion and a short retrograde and anterograde amnesia can occur. It can occasionally produce cardiac events (bradycardia or tachycardia, hypertension, cardiac arrhythmias and cardiac ischaemia), aspiration pneumonia, fractures and dental and tongue injuries.
- ECT is mainly useful in depressive illness but also in selected cases of mania, acute schizophrenia, catatonia and neuroleptic malignant syndrome.
- Benzodiazepines should be tapered and discontinued whenever possible before ECT because of their anticonvulsant properties. These drugs can increase seizure threshold, shorten seizure duration and decrease the intensity of the ECT seizure.
- Common indications of ECT in depressive illness are given in Box 12.18.

BOX 12.18 Indications for ECT in Depressive Illness

- Severe depression with paranoid or nihilistic delusions
- High suicidal risk where quick response is needed
- Failure to respond to a tricyclic and an alternative antidepressant
- Depressive stupor
- Inability to tolerate the side effects of antidepressants
- Malnutrition in patients with refusal to take food secondary to depressive illness

BOX 12.19 Sleep Disorders

- Insomnia
- Sleep-related breathing disorders
- Central disorders of hypersomnolence
- Circadian rhythm disorders
- Parasomnias
- Sleep-related movement disorders

Q. Discuss briefly the common sleep disorders.

- Various sleep disorders are given in Box 12.19.
- Sleep-related breathing disorders include obstructive sleep apnoea, central sleep apnoea and sleep-related hypoventilation.

INSOMNIA

- Inability to sleep or maintain sleep despite the patient having adequate opportunity and circumstances to sleep, when associated with impairment of daytime functioning or mood symptoms.
- Insomnia should be at least three times per week over a duration of three or more months.
- Patients may complain of difficulty falling asleep (sleep-onset insomnia) or difficulty remaining asleep (sleep-maintenance insomnia) with frequent nocturnal awakenings or early morning awakenings associated with nonrestorative sleep.
- Insomnia can heighten the perception of pain and may be associated with development of endocrine disturbances. It also has an association with increased risk for hypertension or cardiovascular disease. Insufficient

sleep can lead to increased risk for motor vehicle accidents and occupational errors.

CAUSES

- Primary (idiopathic).
- Depression, anxiety or somatoform disorder.
- Medication or substance use including stimulants, corticosteroids, caffeine, alcohol, etc.
- Medical conditions including chronic pain, chronic obstructive pulmonary disease, asthma, menopause, nocturia and neurological disorders (e.g. Alzheimer's disease, Parkinson's disease, painful neuropathies, stroke and brain tumour).

TREATMENT

- Cognitive behavioural therapy.
- Pharmacological therapy:
  - Triazolam, zolpidem, suvorexant (an orexin antagonist) and ramelteon (a melatonin receptor agonist) for sleep-onset insomnia.
  - Estazolam and eszopiclone for sleep-maintenance insomnia.
  - Zaleplon and sustained-release zolpidem for both sleep-onset and sleep-maintenance insomnia.

CENTRAL DISORDERS OF HYPERSOMNOLENCE

- Includes those disorders in which the primary complaint is daytime sleepiness that is not due to another sleep disorder, including disturbed sleep or misaligned circadian rhythms.

NARCOLEPSY TYPE 1

- It is excessive daytime sleep that a patient cannot resist.

Diagnosis

- Severe excessive daytime sleepiness occurring almost daily for at least 3 months that interferes with functioning.
- Rapid eye movement (REM) intrusion phenomena that includes:
  - Cataplexy—sudden self-limited episodes of loss of muscle tone when patient is awake, which is usually triggered by laughter or other strong emotions.
  - Hypnagogic hallucinations—vivid and often frightening perceptual hallucinatory experiences which occur during the transition between waking and sleep.
  - Sleep paralysis—occurs as the patient transitions from sleep to waking and consists of episodes up to several minutes in duration of inability to move and occasionally feeling unable to breathe despite being awake.
- Electrographic evidence:
  - An abnormal multiple sleep latency test (MSLT) done during day with a sleep latency of 8 minutes or less.
  - At least two sleep-onset REM periods (SOREMPs) within 15 minutes of sleep onset on polysomnography (normally REM sleep occurs 60–90 minutes after onset of sleep).
- Low concentration of hypocretin-1 in cerebrospinal fluid in some patients.

Treatment

- One or two well-timed, 20-minute naps will often improve sleepiness.
- Modafinil, a wakefulness-promoting drug, is useful. It has low addiction potential. Side effects include headache, nausea, dry mouth, anorexia and diarrhoea.
- Solriamfetol, an oral selective dopamine and norepinephrine reuptake inhibitor is useful as it has wake-promoting effects.
- Pitolisant is an oral histamine H_3 receptor inverse agonist that improves daytime sleepiness and reduces cataplexy.
- Sodium oxybate, a sodium salt of γ-hydroxybutyrate, is administered at night to help consolidate REM sleep and increase slow-wave sleep. It significantly reduces daytime sleepiness and also improves cataplexy.
- Others: Selegiline (a monoamine oxidase-B inhibitor), clomipramine, fluoxetine and venlafaxine.

NARCOLEPSY TYPE 2

- Criteria are as those for narcolepsy type 1 but cataplexy and low hypocretin-1 in cerebrospinal fluid are not seen.

IDIOPATHIC HYPERSOMNIA

- Sleepiness with an MSLT showing a mean sleep latency of <8 minutes with fewer than two SOREMPs on the MSLT.
- Absence of cataplexy or hypocretin-1 deficiency.

CIRCADIAN RHYTHM SLEEP DISORDERS

- Chronic or recurring sleep disturbances (insomnia or hypersomnia) are because of misalignment between their endogenous circadian timing and external influences.
- Common types:
  - Delayed sleep phase type—sleep and wake times are later than desired, often resulting in daytime sleepiness when conventional waking times are enforced.
  - Advanced sleep phase type—sleep and wake times are earlier than desired.
  - Jet lag—transient symptoms of difficulty falling asleep at the appropriate time and daytime sleepiness following rapid travel across two or more time zones altering the timing of exogenous light stimuli.
  - Shift-work disorder—an inability to obtain sufficient sleep during the day and difficulty remaining awake at night resulting from night work. Can also affect day workers whose early morning shifts require very early rise times.

DIAGNOSIS

- Based on history and a sleep diary.
- Actigraphy—based on a wrist-mounted motion detector worn as an outpatient for at least 7 days that can help to quantify time spent asleep.

TREATMENT

- Bright light therapy—exposure to bright light, around 2500 lux, for 2–3 hours in the mornings for delayed sleep phase type of circadian rhythm disorders and in the evening for advanced sleep–wake phase disorder.

- Chronotherapy—useful in delayed sleep phase type of circadian rhythm disorders; patient delays sleep 3 hours every 2 days until he/she adjusts to the conventional sleep and wake time.
- Melatonin—administered in the afternoon or evening in patients with delayed sleep phase.
- Melatonin-receptor agonists include circadin, tasimelteon, ramelteon and agomelatine.
- For jet lag:
  - Behavioural strategies (good sleep hygiene, shifting sleep and wake times gradually before travel to conform to the destination's time zone and avoiding bright light exposure before bedtime).
  - Melatonin administered before bedtime in the new time zone.

PARASOMNIAS

- Undesirable physical events (complex movements and behaviours) or experiences (emotions, perceptions and dreams) which occur during entry into sleep, within sleep or during arousals from sleep.
- Represent CNS activation and intrusion of wakefulness into sleep, producing nonvolitional motor, emotional or autonomic activity.
- Non-REM sleep parasomnias are disorders of arousal and include confusional arousals (sudden arousals associated with confusion and disorientation), sleep walking (arousal with complex motor behaviour like walking or running), sleep-related eating disorder (arousal with involuntary eating or drinking) and sleep terrors. Sleep terrors are dramatic sudden arousals from non-REM sleep with associated screaming, fear and increased autonomic activity; patients may be disoriented and unresponsive to the environment, and typically do not remember the event afterward.
- REM sleep–associated parasomnias include nightmares and behaviour disorders. Nightmares are recurrent, disturbing dreams that typically occur towards the end of night and are not associated with autonomic activity or amnesia. Behaviour disorders consist of abnormal persistence of muscle tone during REM sleep permitting vigorous movements while dreaming. Sleep behaviours can include screaming, punching and kicking for up to several minutes, sometimes resulting in injury to the patient or bed partner. Polysomnography shows anomalous increase in muscle tone on electromyogram during REM sleep.

TREATMENT

- Avoid serotonin reuptake inhibitors, MAO inhibitors, caffeine or alcohol.
- Remove dangerous objects from the sleep environment.
- Drugs include clonazepam, tricyclic antidepressants, dopamine agonists or levodopa, carbamazepine and melatonin.

SLEEP-RELATED MOVEMENT DISORDERS

- Include restless leg syndrome and periodic limb movement disorder.

RESTLESS LEG SYNDROME

- An overwhelming urge to move legs usually accompanied by an uncomfortable sensation.
- May disrupt sleep initiation.
- Rest or inactivity exacerbates the urge to move the legs.
- Physical activity temporarily relieves the urge to move the legs.
- Symptoms more prominent in the evening or nighttime that may disrupt sleep initiation.
- May be secondary to pregnancy, end-stage renal disease, iron or folate deficiency, peripheral neuropathy, radiculopathy, rheumatoid arthritis or fibromyalgia.
- Certain drugs like antihistamines, dopamine receptor antagonists and antidepressants (with the exception of bupropion) may exacerbate it.
- First-line drugs for treatment are non-ergot-derived dopamine agonists (ropinirole and pramipexole) and ergot-derived dopamine agonists (pergolide and cabergoline). Others include gabapentin, benzodiazepines, clonidine or opiates. Iron treatment is required in presence of serum ferritin <300 mg/L.

PERIODIC LIMB MOVEMENT DISORDER

- Symptoms include repetitive, stereotyped limb movements occurring in non-REM sleep typically involving the lower limbs.
- Occurs every 20–30 seconds.
- Movements often disrupt sleep and lead to daytime sleepiness.
- Treatment is similar to that for restless leg syndrome.

MCQs

1. A 72-year-old man was brought to the Emergency Department by ambulance with a 2-day history of confusion and aggression towards his wife. He had a 2-year history of increasing forgetfulness, had recently failed to remember the names of his grandchildren and had twice got lost when outside the house. He had also had occasional falls. On examination, he was aggressive towards the staff and difficult to examine. His pulse rate was 98 beats/minute, blood pressure 130/70 mmHg, temperature 35.4°C, blood glucose 190 mg/dL and oxygen saturation 96% on air. What is the most likely cause for his presentation?
   A. Sudden, stepwise progression of vascular dementia
   B. Delirium related to a chronic subdural haematoma
   C. Development of delusional features in a patient with Lewy body dementia
   D. Delirium related to an intercurrent infection
   E. Development of disinhibition from fronto-temporal lobe dementia

Ans: D. Delirium related to an intercurrent infection

Although all answers are possible explanations for the presentation described, with the limited information given and no other collateral history or previous investigations available, the safest assumption is that the patient has delirium, possibly on a background of dementia and/or depression.

IM24.3

2. A 75-year-old man is brought to the Emergency Department by his concerned family. Over the past 2 days, he has become confused and disorientated, particularly at night. He appears disheveled and agitated. His daughter reports he has been 'chesty' and bringing up green sputum since the beginning of the week. The patient believes the nurses are policewomen and he appears to be having hallucinations. What is the likely diagnosis?
   A. Severe depressive episode
   B. Generalised anxiety disorder
   C. Delirium
   D. Schizophrenia
   E. Dementia

Ans: C. Delirium

Delirium can be defined as an acute deterioration in mental status from a previously stable baseline. The disorder is usually due to a definable medical condition, drug withdrawal or intoxication that can be elicited from the history, examination or investigation. Here the patient has signs of respiratory tract infection, therefore providing a likely organic cause for delirium. Delirium is often worst at night with a tendency to fluctuate during the course of the day.

13 Oncology

Q. What are tumour markers? Classify them and give examples. (IM13.12)

- A tumour marker is a biochemical substance elaborated by a particular type of malignancy.
- These markers can be normal endogenous products that are produced at a greater rate in cancer cells or products of newly switched-on genes that remained quiescent in the normal cells.
- Can be present in blood, urine or other body fluids, and in tumours and other tissues.
- Assays of such markers may be of great help in a number of ways (Box 13.1).
- Successful use of chemotherapy is associated with disappearance of the abnormal tumour marker.
- Unfortunately, none of the available markers are completely specific for a malignancy. They may be elevated in some benign diseases as well.

CLASSIFICATION

- Classification of tumour markers is given in Table 13.1.

Q. Discuss alpha-foetoprotein briefly.

- This oncofoetal antigen is a glycoprotein produced by the liver, gastrointestinal tract epithelium and yolk sac of foetus during gestation. The α-foetoprotein (AFP) gene is almost completely repressed in fully matured foetus leading to its disappearance soon after birth.
- Although abundant in foetal blood, its concentration is below 15 ng/mL after birth.
- In the prenatal period, amniotic fluid AFP is elevated in open spina bifida, anencephaly and atresia of oesophagus.
- The serum levels are elevated in:
  - Seventy per cent of patients with hepatocellular carcinoma (HCC) in whom very high levels ranging between 500 ng/mL and 5 mg/mL are noted. However, it is not used as the primary surveillance test for HCC because of low sensitivity and specificity.
  - Nonseminomatous testicular cancer (e.g. embryonal carcinoma, teratomas, choriocarcinoma and yolk sac carcinoma), germ cell tumours of ovaries and extragonadal germ cell tumours.
  - Neoplasms of gastrointestinal tract including gastric cancer.
- Minimally elevated levels of AFP may be seen in patients with acute or chronic hepatitis and ataxia telangiectasia.
- AFP is also elevated up to 500 ng/mL in maternal serum during normal pregnancy.
- HCC patients with a high AFP concentration (≥400 ng/mL) tend to have greater tumour size, bilobar involvement, portal vein thrombosis and a lower median survival rate.

BOX 13.1 Uses of Tumour Markers

- Screening of high-risk individuals for the presence of malignancy
- Diagnosis of malignancy
- Monitoring effectiveness of therapy and regression of tumour
- Early detection of recurrence
- Immunodetection of metastatic sites

TABLE 13.1 Classification of Tumour Markers

Class	Associated Conditions
Oncofoetal antigens	
• AFP	HCC Nonseminomatous testicular cancer Germ cell tumour of ovary Extragonadal germ cell tumours Neoplasms of gastrointestinal tract Hepatitis Ataxia telangiectasia Pregnancy
• Carcinoembryonic antigen (CEA)	Colonic malignancies *Other neoplasms:* Stomach, pancreas, lung and breast *Benign conditions:* Cigarette smoking, peptic ulcer disease, inflammatory bowel disease, pancreatitis, hypothyroidism, cirrhosis and biliary obstruction
Glycoprotein antigens or carbohydrate antigens	
• CA 125 (cancer antigen 125)	Ovarian adenocarcinoma *Other neoplasms*: Breast, colon, stomach, oesophagus, biliary tract, pancreas, lung (adenocarcinoma) and endometrium *Benign conditions*: Tuberculosis, benign ovarian tumours, ascites or pleural effusion
• CA 19-9	Pancreatic cancers *Other neoplasms*: Bladder and stomach cancers
• CA 15-3	Breast carcinoma *Other neoplasms*: Pancreatic, lung, ovarian, colorectal and liver *Benign conditions*: Ovarian cysts, benign liver or breast diseases
Hormones	
• Beta-human chorionic gonadotrophin	Germ cell tumours of testes and ovaries, trophoblastic tumours
• Calcitonin	Medullary thyroid carcinoma
• Catecholamines	Phaeochromocytoma
• Other hormones	Ectopic production by tumours (paraneoplastic)
Enzymes	
• Prostate acid phosphatase (PAP)	Prostatic carcinoma
• Alkaline phosphatase (ALP)	HCC, metastatic deposits in liver *Other neoplasms*: Ovarian, gastrointestinal, lung and Hodgkin's lymphoma
• Neurone-specific enolase (NSE)	Small-cell carcinoma of lung, neuroblastoma
• Tartrate-resistant acid phosphatase	Hairy cell leukaemia
Receptors	
• Oestrogen and progesterone (ER and PR)	Breast cancer (useful for hormonal therapy)
• HER-2/neu	Breast cancer (co-receptor for epidermal growth factor; useful for targeted therapy like trastuzumab)
Proteins	
• Prostate-specific antigen (PSA)	Prostatic carcinoma *Benign conditions:* Prostatitis, benign prostatic hypertrophy, prostatic trauma and after ejaculation
• β-2-Microglobulin	Multiple myeloma *Other neoplasms*: Chronic lymphocytic leukaemia, some lymphomas *Benign conditions*: Kidney disease and hepatitis
• S-100	Melanoma
• Chromogranin A	NETs (e.g. carcinoids, neuroblastoma and small cell lung cancer) *Benign conditions*: Use of proton-pump inhibitors
• p53 Mutated protein	Lung cancer
Genetic markers (gene changes)	
• *BCR-ABL1* mutation	Chronic myeloid leukaemia
• *EGFR* mutation (epidermal growth factor receptor)	Non-small cell lung cancer

Q. Discuss briefly the classification of chemotherapeutic agents.

Q. Discuss briefly about mechanisms of action of various chemotherapeutic agents.

CLASSIFICATION OF CHEMOTHERAPEUTIC AGENTS (Table 13.2)

- Alkylating agents:
  - Cell-cycle phase-nonspecific agents that substitute an alkyl group for a hydrogen atom; results in cross-linking of DNA strands and interference with replication of DNA and transcription of RNA.
  - Cyclophosphamide and ifosfamide require activation in liver.
- Antitumour antibiotics:
  - Inhibit cell division by binding to DNA; interfere with RNA transcription. Bleomycin and anthracyclines also generate free radicals.
- Topoisomerase inhibitors:
  - Inhibit topoisomerase I or II resulting in reduced DNA replication and/or increased DNA degradation.
- Antimetabolites:
  - Interfere with nucleic acid synthesis by substituting drug for purines or pyrimidines necessary for normal cellular function.

TABLE 13.2 Chemotherapeutics Agents: Classification

Class/Agents

(A) **Alkylating agents**
- *Oxazaphosphorines*
  - Cyclophosphamide
  - Ifosfamide
- *Nitrogen mustards*
  - Busulfan
  - Chlorambucil
  - Melphalan
  - Bendamustine
- *Platinum-based*
  - Carboplatin
  - Cisplatin
  - Oxaliplatin
- *Hydrazine*
  - Temozolomide
- *Nitrosourea*
  - Carmustine
  - Lomustine
- *Others*
  - Dacarbazine
  - Mechlorethamine
  - Thiotepa

(B) **Antitumour antibiotics**
- *Anthracyclines*
  - Daunorubicin
  - Doxorubicin
  - Epirubicin
  - Idarubicin
  - Mitoxantrone
- *Others*
  - Bleomycin
  - Dactinomycin
  - Mitomycin-C
  - Plicamycin

(C) **Mitotic inhibitors**
- *Vinca alkaloids*
  - Vinblastine
  - Vincristine
  - Vinorelbine
- *Taxanes*
  - Docetaxel
  - Paclitaxel

(D) **Topoisomerase inhibitors**
- *Topoisomerase I inhibitors*
  - Irinotecan
  - Topotecan
- *Topoisomerase II inhibitors*
  - Etoposide
  - Teniposide

(E) **Antimetabolites**
- *Folic acid analogues*
  - Methotrexate
  - Pemetrexed
- *Nucleoside analogues*
  - Gemcitabine
- *Purine analogues*
  - Cladribine
  - Fludarabine
  - 6-Mercaptopurine
  - Pentostatin
  - Thioguanine
- *Pyrimidine analogues*
  - Azacytidine
  - Capecitabine
  - Cytarabine
  - 5-Fluorouracil
- *Substituted urea*
  - Hydroxyurea

(F) **Hormones/hormone modifiers**
- *Adrenocorticoids*
  - Glucocorticoids
- *Androgens*
  - Fluoxymesterone
- *Antiandrogens*
  - Flutamide
  - Nilutamide
- *Antioestrogens*
  - Tamoxifen
  - Haloxitene
- *Aromatase inhibitor*
  - Anastrozole
  - Letrozole
- *Oestrogens*
  - Diethylstilbestrol
- *Progestins*
  - Megestrol acetate
  - Medroxyprogesterone
- *Luteinising hormone–releasing hormone analogues*
  - Goserelin
  - Leuprolide
- *Antioestrogen receptor downregulator*
  - Fulvestrant
- *Somatostatin analogues*
  - Octreotide

(G) **Biological response modifiers**
- *Cytokines*
  - Interferon
  - Interleukin
- *Retinoid*
  - Tretinoin
- *Monoclonal antibody*
  - Alemtuzumab
  - Rituximab
  - Tositumomab
  - Trastuzumab
- *Tyrosine kinase inhibitors*
  - Dasatinib
  - Erlotinib
  - Gefitinib
  - Imatinib mesylate
  - Lapatinib
  - Sorafenib
  - Sunitinib
  - Vandetanib

(H) **Miscellaneous agents**
- *Bisphosphonates*
  - Pamidronate
  - Zoledronic acid
- *Enzymes*
  - L-Asparaginase
  - Procarbazine
- *Others*
  - Arsenic trioxide
  - Bortezomib
  - Lenalidomide
  - Thalidomide

- Hormones/hormone modifiers:
  - Alter cellular metabolism by changing body hormonal milieu for unfavourable tumour growth.
- Vinca alkaloids:
  - Bind and destroy tubulin in microtubules resulting in mitotic arrest in metaphase.
- Taxanes:
  - Stabilise microtubules resulting in reduced mitotic spindles and mitotic arrest in metaphase.
- Tyrosine kinase inhibitors:
  - Prevent phosphorylation and activation of multiple proteins by tyrosine kinases resulting in cell dysfunction and death.
- Miscellaneous agents:
  - Act by a variety of mechanisms.
- Biological response modifiers:
  - Modify host's response to tumours.

Q. What do you understand by adjuvant and neoadjuvant chemotherapy?

ADJUVANT CHEMOTHERAPY

- After surgical removal of a malignancy or after radiotherapy, there may still be some malignant cells left behind.
- When chemotherapeutic drugs are used to kill those remaining malignant cells, it is called adjuvant chemotherapy.

NEOADJUVANT CHEMOTHERAPY

- It indicates the use of chemotherapy before principal treatment using surgery or radiotherapy.
- Administering chemotherapy first can shrink a large malignant tumour, making it easier to remove with surgery or allowing it to be treated more easily with radiation.

Q. Write a short note on immune checkpoint inhibitors.

- An important function of the immune system is its ability to differentiate between normal cells in the body and those it sees as 'foreign'. This lets the immune system attacks the foreign cells while leaving the normal cells alone.
- To do this, it uses 'checkpoints'. Immune checkpoints are molecules on certain immune cells that need to be activated (or inactivated) to start an immune response.
- Cancer cells may find ways to use these checkpoints to avoid being attacked by the immune system.
- Drugs that target these checkpoints are being used to treat several cancers. These drugs are called checkpoint inhibitors.
- Programmed death receptor 1 (PD-1) is a checkpoint protein on T cells. It prevents attacking the cells by binding to programmed death receptor-ligand 1 (PD-L1), a protein found on some normal cells. Some cancer cells have large amounts of PD-L1, which helps them avoid an immune attack.
- Another checkpoint protein on some T cells is cytotoxic T-lymphocyte-associated protein 4 (CTLA-4).
- Monoclonal antibodies that target either PD-1 or PD-L1 can block this binding and boost the immune response against cancer cells.
- Some of the PD-1 inhibitors include pembrolizumab, nivolumab and cemiplimab.
- PD-L1 inhibitors include atezolizumab, avelumab and durvalumab.
- Ipilimumab is a monoclonal antibody that attaches to CTLA-4, thereby boosting body's immune response against cancer cells. This drug is used to treat advanced melanoma of the skin.

ADVERSE EFFECTS

- These include diarrhoea, skin rashes and pneumonitis.
- Immune-related adverse events are also seen in some patients and can range from mild rash to severe colitis to life-threatening myocarditis.
- Some patients may develop type 1 diabetes mellitus and thyroiditis.

Q. Write a brief note on chimeric antigen receptor T-cell therapy.

- Chimeric antigen receptor (CAR) T-cell therapy is used to change T cells so that they can destroy cancer cells. The therapy works by changing genes of T cells and, therefore, is called immunotherapy or gene therapy.
- T cells are taken from the patient's blood (leukapheresis) and are changed in the lab by adding a gene for a man-made receptor (called a CAR). This helps them better identify specific cancer cell antigens. The CAR T cells are then given back to the patient (Fig. 13.1).
- Since different cancers have different antigens, each CAR is made for a specific cancer's antigen. For example, in certain kinds of B-cell leukaemia or lymphoma, the cancer cells have an antigen called CD19. The CAR T-cell therapies to treat these cancers are made to attach to the CD19 antigen and will not work for a cancer that does not have the CD19 antigen.
- An advantage is that CAR T cells can remain stable for several years in the body as long-term memory cells. This feature allows them to recognise and kill cancer cells encountered in the circulation in the case of relapse.
- Examples of CAR T cells include tisagenlecleucel, axicabtagene ciloleucel, brexucabtagene autoleucel, lisocabtagene maraleucel and idecabtagene vicleucel.

ADVERSE EFFECTS

- An important adverse effect is occurrence of cytokine release syndrome. It occurs due to release of large amounts of cytokines from CAR T cells. Various features include high fever and chills, dyspnoea, vomiting, diarrhoea, dizziness, palpitations and syncope
- Another important adverse effect is immune effector cell-associated neurotoxicity syndrome. It develops 3–10 days after treatment and is characterised by confusion and behavioural changes, visual and auditory hallucinations, speech alterations, apraxia, headache, fatigue, tremors, seizures, coma and death.

Q. Write a brief note on cyclophosphamide.

- This is a nucleophilic alkylating agent that inhibits the DNA synthesis by cross-linking DNA.

USES (Box 13.2)

Box 13.2 Uses of Cyclophosphamide

- Autoimmune disorders—SLE (lupus nephritis), rheumatoid arthritis, granulomatosis with polyangiitis (Wegener's granulomatosis), PAN and other systemic vasculitis
- Lymphomas
- Leukaemias
- Other tumours—carcinoma of breast, Ewing's sarcoma, gestational trophoblastic tumours
- Conditioning before stem cell transplantation
- Frequently relapsing steroid-sensitive nephrotic syndrome
- Idiopathic membranous glomerulonephritis

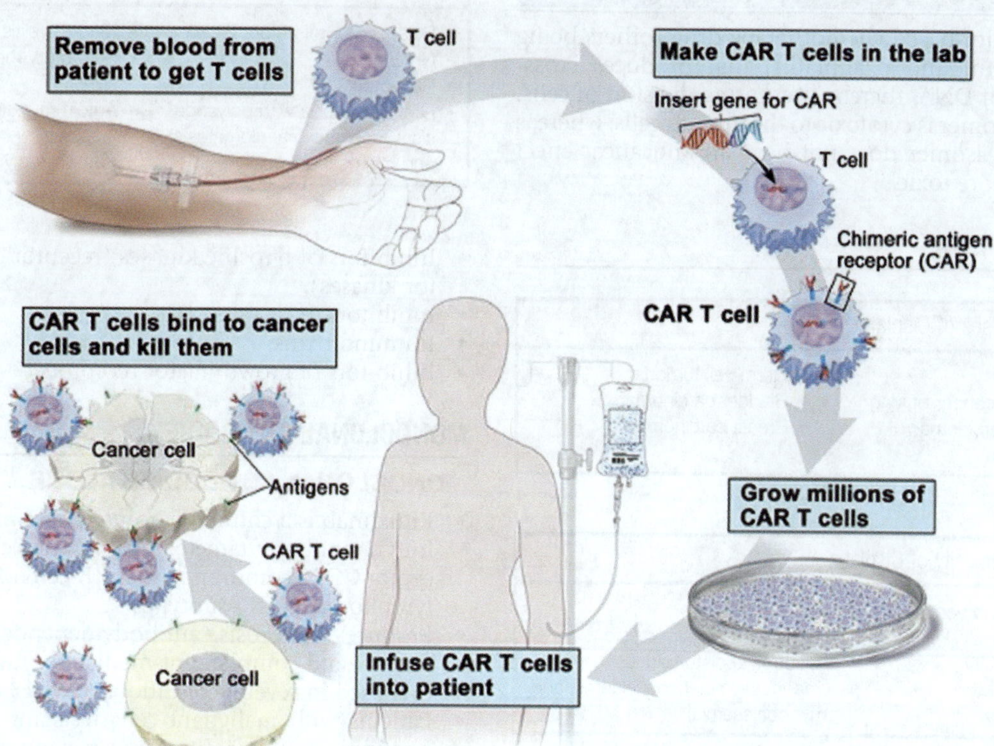

Fig. 13.1 Chimeric antigen receptor T-cells (Source: National Institute of Medicine, NIH).

Box 13.3 Toxicity of Cyclophosphamide

- Alopecia
- Bone marrow depression resulting in cytopenias
- Hepatotoxicity.
- Sterility
- Amenorrhoea
- Cystitis and bladder carcinoma
- Syndrome of inappropriate antidiuretic hormone secretion (SIADH)

TOXICITY (Box 13.3)

- Incidence of cystitis can be reduced by adequate hydration.
- Severe cystitis can be treated by mercaptoethane sulphonate. It can also be used to prevent the occurrence of cystitis.

Q. Give a brief account of uses and toxicity of methotrexate.

- This is a folic acid antagonist which functions as an antimetabolite. It is a competitive inhibitor of folate reductase enzyme, and, therefore, it inhibits DNA synthesis and consequently cell replication.

USES (Box 13.4)

Box 13.4 Uses of Methotrexate

- Choriocarcinoma
- Acute lymphoblastic leukaemia
- Burkitt's lymphoma
- Primary central nervous system lymphoma
- Osteosarcoma
- Rheumatoid arthritis and other connective tissue disorders
- Psoriasis
- Unruptured ectopic pregnancy (low risk)

TOXICITY (Box 13.5)

- Folinic acid (citrovorum factor) is used to antagonise the toxicity of methotrexate.

Box 13.5 Toxicity of Methotrexate

- Hepatotoxicity, hepatic fibrosis (chronic use)
- Bone marrow suppression
- Megaloblastic anaemia
- Ulcerative enteritis, ulcerative dermatitis
- Pulmonary fibrosis
- Nephrotoxicity (in high doses)
- Neurologic toxicity (somnolence, confusion, seizures)

Q. Write a short note on cisplatin.

- A platinum-based chemotherapy drug (others being carboplatin and oxaliplatin) that produces cross-linking of DNA, thereby preventing division of cells.
- The *cis* isomer is cytotoxic to the tumour cells, whereas the *trans* isomer does not have an anticancer effect and is more toxic.

USES (Box 13.6)

Box 13.6 Uses of Cisplatin

- Sarcomas
- Small cell cancer of lung
- Ovarian carcinoma
- Lymphoma
- Germ cell tumours
- Bladder carcinoma
- Breast carcinoma

Box 13.7 Toxicity of Cisplatin

- Nausea and vomiting
- Nephrotoxicity
- Neurotoxicity (sensorimotor)
- Ototoxicity
- Alopecia
- Bone marrow suppression
- Electrolyte disturbances (hypomagnesaemia, hypokalaemia and hypocalcaemia)

TOXICITY (Box 13.7)

- Nephrotoxicity may be reduced by the use of mannitol with forced hydration.
- Carboplatin is less nephrotoxic than cisplatin and is less likely to cause tinnitus and hearing loss, but it has greater myelosuppressant actions.

Q. What is meant by targeted therapy in cancer patients? Explain the various types of targeted therapies.

- Conventional chemotherapy, although directed towards certain macromolecules or enzymes, typically does not discriminate effectively between rapidly dividing normal cells (e.g. bone marrow and gastrointestinal tract) and tumour cells. This leads to partial response and several side effects.
- Targeted therapy interferes with molecular targets that have a role in tumour growth or progression.
- These targets are usually located in tumour cells. Some targeted agents may target other cells that may affect the tumour cells; for example antiangiogenic agents may target endothelial cells.
- Targeted therapies, therefore, have a high specificity towards tumour cells, providing a broader therapeutic window with less toxicity.
- These agents are often used in combination with cytotoxic chemotherapy or radiation to produce additive or synergistic activity.

COMMON TYPES OF TARGETED THERAPIES

- Monoclonal antibodies.

BOX 13.8 Uses of Rituximab

- Relapsed or refractory B-cell NHL
- Refractory ITP
- Granulomatosis with polyangiitis (Wegener's granulomatosis) and microscopic polyangiitis)
- Neuromyelitis optica
- Refractory rheumatoid arthritis
- Autoimmune haemolytic anaemia
- Pemphigus vulgaris

- Inhibitors of tyrosine kinases (receptor or nonreceptor kinases).
- Inhibitors of proteasomes.
- Immunotoxins.
- Inhibitors of growth factor receptors.

MONOCLONAL ANTIBODIES

MONOCLONAL ANTIBODIES ALONE

- Rituximab is a chimeric monoclonal immunoglobulin G1 antibody targeted against the cell surface receptor CD20 common in many B-cell non-Hodgkin's lymphoma (NHL) subtypes.
- Produces apoptosis, antibody-dependent cell cytotoxicity and complement-mediated cytotoxicity.
- It is used in several conditions (Box 13.8).
- Patients with malignant cells resistant to apoptosis and patients whose immune systems will not perform antibody-dependent or complement-dependent cytotoxicity may be resistant.

Side Effects of Rituximab (Box 13.9)

BOX 13.9 Side Effects of Rituximab

- Urticaria, angio-oedema, anaphylaxis
- Progressive multifocal leukoencephalopa-thy
- Toxic epidermal necrosis
- Tumour lysis syndrome
- Infections
- Reactivation of hepatitis B virus

RADIOIMMUNOTHERAPY

- A strategy to optimise the efficacy of anti-CD20 monoclonal antibody therapy as it is not dependent on the mechanism cited above for killing the cells.
- Prepared by combining the antibody with a radioconjugate, yttrium-90 or iodine-131 (e.g. ibritumomab combined with yttrium-90) so as to deliver cytotoxic radiation to a target cell.
- However, radioimmunotherapy is limited by the potency of the radionuclide and the small number of radionuclide molecules that can be added to each monoclonal antibody molecule. Patients often develop dose-limiting toxicity to the bone marrow because of nonspecific uptake of antibodies and have an incomplete response.
- Used in refractory NHL.

CONJUGATE OF MONOCLONAL ANTIBODY

- This involves conjugating chemotherapy molecules to monoclonal antibodies.

- Examples include gemtuzumab ozogamicin, a conjugate of an anti-CD33 monoclonal antibody, and calicheamicin, which is approved for acute myelogenous leukaemia.

BIOSIMILAR MONOCLONAL ANTIBODIES

- Biosimilar monoclonal antibodies are highly similar to the reference monoclonal antibodies in terms of clinical potency and toxicity but may have slight differences in components that do not appear to affect their clinical efficacy and toxicity.
- Biosimilar monoclonal antibodies are named as the reference drug plus a four-letter suffix that consists of four unique and meaningless lowercase letters. As an example, a biosimilar for infliximab is named infliximab-dyyb.

TYROSINE KINASES AND THEIR INHIBITORS

- Tyrosine kinases are activated by either growth factors or mutation of genes.
- Activated forms of tyrosine kinases can produce several effects:
  - Increase in tumour cell proliferation and growth.
  - Antiapoptotic effects.
  - Promote angiogenesis and metastasis.

NONRECEPTOR TYROSINE KINASE INHIBITORS

- Imatinib inhibits nonreceptor tyrosine kinase *BCR–ABL*. Useful in several haematological malignancies, particularly chronic myeloid leukaemia.
- Another agent is baricitinib which is JAK1/2 inhibitor and is useful in resistant cases of rheumatoid arthritis.
- Other JAK (Janus kinase) inhibitors include ruxolitinib (useful in polycythaemia vera), tofacitinib (indicated in rheumatoid arthritis, ulcerative colitis, psoriatic arthritis and ankylosing spondylitis) and upadacitinib (indicated in rheumatoid arthritis and severe ulcerative colitis).

RECEPTOR TYROSINE KINASE INHIBITORS

- These target epidermal growth factor receptors (EGFRs), vascular endothelial growth factor receptors (VEGFRs) and platelet-derived growth factor receptors (PDGFRs).
  - Gefitinib, erlotinib and lapatinib act on EGFR.
  - Vatalanib and semaxanib target VEGFR.
  - Leflunomide targets PDGFR.
  - Pemigatinib targets fibroblast growth factor receptor 2 (FGFR2).

PROTEASOME INHIBITORS

- Proteasome is an organelle responsible for the physiological degradation and recycling of cellular proteins that regulate cell cycle progression.
- A variety of cancer cells are more sensitive than normal cells to inhibition of proteasomes.
- Bortezomib, a proteasome inhibitor, is useful for the treatment of relapsed/refractory multiple myeloma patients. It is also used in mantle cell lymphoma.

IMMUNOTOXINS

- Contain a toxin along with an antibody or growth factor that binds specifically to target cells.
- Immunotoxin binds to the target cell, internalised and then the enzymatic fragment of the toxin kills the cell by inhibiting protein synthesis.
- Various plant and bacterial toxins can be used. These include truncated diphtheria toxin, *Pseudomonas* toxin A, anthrax toxin and plant toxins including ricin and gelonin. The immunotoxins in clinical use are human interleukin-2 combined with truncated diphtheria toxin (for refractory cutaneous T-cell lymphoma), human interleukin-3 combined with truncated diphtheria toxin (refractory blastic plasmacytoid dendritic cell neoplasm) and anti-CD22 with *Pseudomonas* exotoxin A (refractory hairy cell leukaemia).

Q. Write a brief note on the role of positron emission tomography in oncology.

- In oncology, positron emission tomography (PET) is used for screening, for preliminary diagnosis, to establish the extent and distribution of disease and for biopsy guidance, staging, prognostication, therapeutic planning, judging response to therapy and relapse of malignancy.
- PET provides information about the functional and metabolic changes associated with cancer.
- PET scanning requires use of molecules that are labelled with radionuclides. In clinical practice, the principal radioisotope used is the positron-emitting 18F-fluorodeoxyglucose (18F-FDG), which is a glucose analogue labelled with 18F. It has a short half-life and is produced in cyclotrons.
  - FDG is injected intravenously and is transported from the plasma to the cells by glucose transporters (GLUT 1 and GLUT 4).
  - It then undergoes phosphorylation within the cell by the enzyme hexokinase and is converted to FDG-6-phosphate, which can normally be metabolised further by glucose-6-phosphatase.
- Cancer cells demonstrate increased anaerobic glycolysis and reduced levels of glucose-6-phosphatase, thus limiting further metabolism of the tracer (FDG-6-phosphate) in cancer cells. In addition to elevated glycolysis, tumours often have increased expression of glucose transporters (GLUTs).
- Increased 18F-FDG uptake shows up as a bright spot on the PET scan. Tissues with higher glucose uptake and utilisation like brain, liver and kidneys also show bright spot (Warnburg effect).
- PET–computed tomography (CT) combines the functional information from a PET scan with the anatomical information from a CT scan. It can pinpoint the exact location of abnormal activity.
- PET has been found to be useful in several malignancies including melanoma, lymphoma, lung cancer, oesophageal cancer, head and neck cancer, breast cancer and thyroid cancer.
- FDG uptake may occur in various types of active inflammation and infections and is not specific for

cancer. Thus, it is not used for the initial diagnosis of cancer, but is useful in monitoring cancer cell viability and for the diagnosis and detection of recurrence of cancer.
- 68-Gallium DOTA PET scan is used to detect primary and metastatic neuroendocrine tumours (NETs).
- PET is also useful in diagnosing certain cardiovascular and neurological diseases because it highlights areas with increased, diminished or no metabolic activity. Some of the conditions include Alzheimer's disease, Parkinson's disease, detection of viable myocardium and localisation of epileptogenic focus prior to surgery in patients with medically refractory epilepsy.
- PET is also positive in patients with granulomatous diseases like tuberculosis and sarcoidosis. It is also used in patients with fever of unknown origin when other investigations are nondiagnostic.

FALSE-NEGATIVE RESULTS

- Tumours with slow growth and low metabolism, for example some cases of well-differentiated adenocarcinomas and carcinoid tumours.
- Small tumours less than 7 mm in diameter may not be detected.
- Hyperglycaemia decreases intracellular FDG uptake because the FDG and glucose compete for the same cell surface receptor.

Q. Enumerate emergency conditions related to tumours.

Q. Describe febrile neutropenia.

Q. Write briefly on the clinical features and treatment of tumour lysis syndrome.

- Various emergencies related to malignancies are listed in Box 13.10.

FEBRILE NEUTROPENIA

- A major complication of cancer chemotherapy.
- Defined as an oral temperature >38.3°C or two consecutive readings of >38°C over 1 hour and an absolute neutrophil count <500 or <1000/mm³ with predicted decline to less than 500/mm³ within the next 2 days.

BOX 13.10 Oncological Emergencies

ONCOLOGICAL EMERGENCIES

Metabolic
- TLS
- Hypercalcaemia
- SIADH

Haematological
- Febrile neutropenia
- Thrombocytopenia
- Hyperviscosity syndrome
- Hyperleukocytosis and leukostasis
- DIC

Anatomical
- Superior vena cava syndrome
- Epidural spinal cord compression
- Cardiac tamponade
- Malignant pleural effusion

CLINICAL EXAMINATION AND INVESTIGATIONS

- An initial assessment of circulatory and respiratory function with vigorous resuscitation.
- Careful examination for potential foci of infection.
- Signs and symptoms of infection in neutropenic patients can be minimal particularly in those receiving corticosteroids.
- Before antibiotic therapy, send two sets of blood cultures from a peripheral vein and any indwelling venous catheters. In addition, sample sputum, urine, skin swabs and stool specimens if clinically indicated.
- Send serum for *Aspergillus* galactomannan antigen and beta-D-glucan in some high-risk patients.
- Radiographic investigations including chest radiograph and CT scan, if indicated.

MANAGEMENT

- Intravenous broad-spectrum antibiotics (e.g. ceftazidime, meropenem or imipenem and piperacillin/tazobactam or cefepime) with or without an aminoglycoside.
- Gram-positive coverage should be added in patients with any of the following findings: haemodynamic instability, pneumonia, positive blood cultures for Gram-positive bacteria while awaiting susceptibility results, suspected central venous catheter-related infection, skin or soft tissue infection and severe mucositis in patients who were receiving prophylaxis with a fluoroquinolone.
- An antifungal agent may be added if fever persists for 4 days.
- Granulocyte colony-stimulating factor (G-CSF) may be given in patients with pneumonia, hypotension or organ dysfunction, or a patient on a regimen that is known to cause prolonged neutropenia. However, efficacy is modest.
- In some low-risk patients (haemodynamically stable, who do not have acute leukaemia or evidence of organ failure, who do not have pneumonia, an indwelling central venous catheter or severe soft tissue infection), oral antibiotics (combination of a quinolone and amoxicillin/clavulanate) may be given. Another method of risk stratification is the use of Multinational Association of Supportive Care in Cancer (MASCC) score.
- Management is summarised in Flowchart 13.1.

PREVENTION

- Prophylactic fluoroquinolones (levofloxacin or ciprofloxacin) for high-risk and intermediate-risk groups, which largely comprise patients receiving high-dose chemotherapy and those with haematological malignancy in which the anticipated duration of neutropenia is longer than 7 days.
- For most solid tumours undergoing standard outpatient cyclical chemotherapy in which the anticipated duration of neutropenia is less than 7 days, prophylactic fluoroquinolones are not recommended because of the risk of microbial resistance.

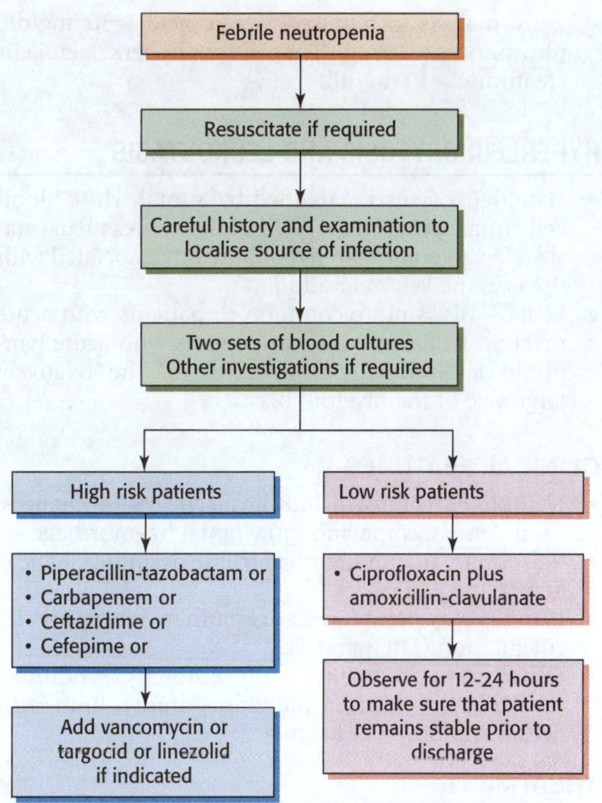

Flowchart 13.1 Management of a Patient With Febrile Neutropenia.

- G-CSF:
  - May be used prophylactically in patients with some types of malignancies receiving chemotherapy in whom risk of neutropenia is greater than 20% (primary prophylaxis).
  - May be used as a secondary prophylactic agent in patients who experience a neutropenic complication from a prior cycle of chemotherapy, if reduced dose intensity might compromise treatment outcome.

TUMOUR LYSIS SYNDROME

- Occurs 1–5 days post-chemotherapy and is due to rapid release of intracellular contents and nucleic acids. It can also occur following radiotherapy and biologic therapy.
- The syndrome is most common in lymphoma and leukaemia.
- Spontaneous lysis in the absence of treatment may occur in rapidly proliferating tumours, especially Burkitt's lymphoma, large T-cell lymphoma and acute lymphocytic leukaemia.
- Risk factors include large tumour burden, high growth fraction, increased pretreatment lactate dehydrogenase (LDH) or uric acid, or pre-existing renal insufficiency.

PATHOPHYSIOLOGY (Flowchart 13.2)

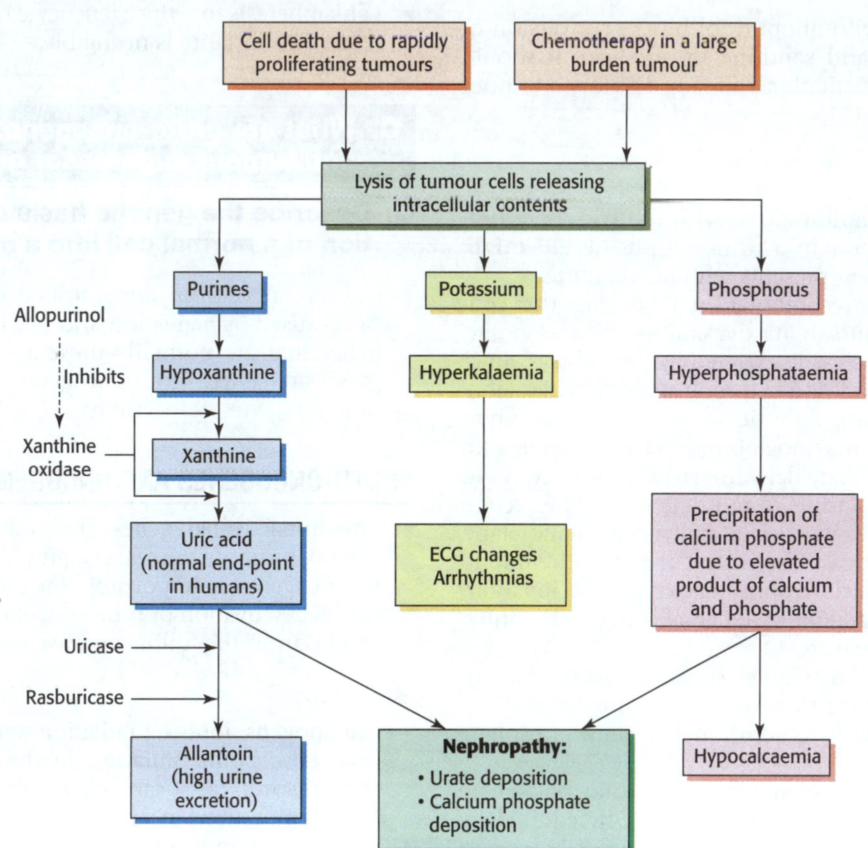

Flowchart 13.2 Pathophysiology of Tumour Lysis Syndrome.

CLINICAL FEATURES

- Lysis of malignant cells causes several metabolic disturbances. Hyperuricaemia produces acute renal failure; hyperkalaemia leads to cardiac arrhythmias; hyperphosphataemia produces acute renal failure as well as vomiting, diarrhoea, lethargy and seizures and hypocalcaemia results in seizures, muscle cramps, tetany and arrhythmia.

DIAGNOSIS (Table 13.3)

TABLE 13.3 Cairo–Bishop Criteria for Diagnosis of Tumour Lysis Syndrome

Laboratory Criteria[a]	Clinical Criteria[b]
• Calcium ≤7 mg/dL or 25% decrease from baseline • Phosphorus ≥4.5 mg/dL or 25% increase from baseline • Potassium ≥6 mEq/L or 25% increase from baseline • Uric acid ≥8 mg/dL or 25% increase from baseline	• Acute kidney injury (defined as serum creatinine >1.5 times upper limit of normal for patient's age and sex) • Cardiac arrhythmias or sudden death • Seizures

[a]≥2 in 24-hour period within 3 days before or 7 days after the initiation of chemotherapy.
[b]Presence of laboratory criteria plus one of clinical criteria indicates clinical TLS.

PREVENTION

- It is important to prevent this syndrome by adequate hydration and diuresis before, during and after chemotherapy.
- Pretreatment with allopurinol blocks conversion of hypoxanthine and xanthine to uric acid. It should not be given if patient has already developed tumour lysis syndrome (TLS).

TREATMENT

- Aggressive hydration along with diuretics is recommended to maintain a urine output of 100 mL/h, unless the patient presents with renal failure.
- Rasburicase is a recombinant urate oxidase that converts uric acid into an inactive and soluble metabolite, allantoin, that is easily excreted by the kidneys. Since hydrogen peroxide is a by-product of uric acid catabolism to allantoin, rasburicase can cause haemolytic anaemia or methaemoglobinaemia in patients with glucose-6-phosphate dehydrogenase deficiency.
- Alkalinisation of urine to promote uric acid excretion is controversial as it may worsen hypocalcaemic tetany. It may also increase the risk of nephropathy due to xanthine and calcium phosphate crystal precipitation.
- Manage life-threatening hyperkalaemia with antihyperkalaemic measures.
- For hypocalcaemia, infuse lowest possible dose of calcium gluconate to relieve symptoms because excess calcium leads to additional calcium phosphate precipitation.
- Manage hyperphosphataemia with oral phosphate binder (aluminium hydroxide) and if required by administering intravenous hypertonic dextrose and insulin.
- Early dialysis is required if uric acid >10 mg/dL, phosphorus >10 mg/dL, persistent hyperkalaemia or creatinine >10 mg/dL.

HYPERLEUKOCYTOSIS AND LEUKOSTASIS

- Hyperleukocytosis is defined by a total white blood cell count greater than 100,000/L, whereas leukostasis refers to end-organ hypoperfusion associated with the extreme WBC elevation.
- Leukostasis is more common in patients with acute myeloid leukaemia than in patients with acute lymphoid leukaemia (ALL) because of the relatively large size of the myeloid blasts.

CLINICAL FEATURES

- Neurologic features include headache, vision changes, focal deficits, coma and intracranial haemorrhage.
- Pulmonary manifestations include dyspnoea, hypoxaemia and ARDS.
- Patients may present with disseminated intravascular coagulation (DIC) and TLS.
- Other features include acute coronary syndrome, cardiac arrhythmias, acute kidney injury, limb ischaemia and bowel ischaemia.

TREATMENT

- Fluid resuscitation with isotonic saline to reduce viscosity and increase urine output.
- Induction chemotherapy or hydroxyurea to reduce leucocyte count.
- Leukapheresis to reduce leucocyte count although its effect on mortality is negligible.

Q. What are proto-oncogene, oncogene and tumour suppressor genes?

Q. Describe the genetic basis of transformation of a normal cell into a malignant cell.

- Cancers arise from uncontrolled cellular proliferation caused by activation and inactivation of certain genes that are normally present in the cells. These genes are called proto-oncogenes and tumour suppression genes, respectively.

PROTO-ONCOGENES AND ONCOGENES

- The nonactivated genes are proto-oncogenes that usually promote normal cell growth. Their activation to oncogenes is responsible for the development of cancers. Activation of proto-oncogenes to oncogenes can occur in the following ways.

MUTATIONS

- Carcinogens, ionising radiation and ultraviolet light can cause point mutation in the proto-oncogenes that in some cases can activate them to oncogenes. Not all mutations in a proto-oncogene cause cancers.
- Since mutation in a single allele of a proto-oncogene can lead to cellular transformation, such mutations

are considered dominant. An example is *ras* mutation, which may lead to pancreatic, lung and colorectal cancers.

CHROMOSOMAL TRANSLOCATION

- If during a cell division two chromosomes translocate (i.e. part of one chromosome attaches to the other), it is possible that part of a proto-oncogene gets translocated to another chromosome and fuses with the gene present on that chromosome. This may result in inappropriate expression of the gene.
- An example is the development of Philadelphia chromosome in patients with chronic myeloid leukaemia. This chromosome arises from a translocation between the long arms of chromosomes 9 and 22. Consequently, the *ABL* gene on chromosome 9 gets joined to the *BCR* gene on chromosome 22. The resultant fused gene is thought to cause the leukaemic transformation.

VIRAL STIMULATION

- The viral DNA may integrate within a proto-oncogene resulting in its transformation.
- Alternatively, the virus may incorporate the proto-oncogene into its genome, and later when this virus infects another person, this oncogene is transferred to the new host. For example, the Rous sarcoma virus of chickens was found to induce cancers because it carried the *ras* oncogene.

TUMOUR SUPPRESSOR GENES

- These genes restrict the abnormal proliferation of cells and induce repair or self-death (apoptosis).
- Mutations of these genes may cause abnormal proliferation of cells and development of cancers. Mutation of both the genes (present on a pair of chromosome) is required for their inactivation and is, therefore, recessive at the level of an individual cell.
- The first tumour suppressor gene described was *RB* gene. Mutation in this gene may produce retinoblastoma.
- Other important tumour suppressor genes are *p53*, *BRCA1* and *BRCA2*. As many as 50% of human tumours have mutated *p53* gene. *BRAC1* and *BRAC2* are seen in breast and ovarian malignancies.

Q. Describe apoptosis.

- Necrotic cell death occurs when external factors (e.g. hypoxia and toxins) produce disintegration of cells. Characteristically, there is an influx of water and ions that results in swelling and rupture of cellular organelles. Lysis of cells releases lysosomal enzymes and other mediators that induce acute inflammatory responses.
- In apoptosis, physiological cell death occurs through activation of genes. The features of apoptosis are as follows:
  - Chromatin aggregation with nuclear and cytoplasmic condensation into distinct membrane-bound vesicles (apoptotic bodies). Organelles remain intact.
  - Cell 'blebs' (intact membrane vesicles) on the surface. No inflammatory response.
  - Phagocytosis by surrounding cells and macrophages.
- Apoptosis is essential part of life. It plays a role in tissue formation during embryogenesis, wound healing, metabolic processes and control of abnormal cells with oncogenic potential.
- Inhibition of apoptosis is responsible for the development of cancer. For example, *p53* tumour suppressor gene activates apoptosis while *ras* oncoproteins inhibit apoptosis.
- This phenomenon is also essential for the effects of chemotherapy and radiotherapy in cancer patients.

MCQs

IM13.12

1. A 40-year-old man presents with a neck lump. He has a past medical history of excision of a phaeochromocytoma. His mother also had 'these sorts of tumours'. Which of the following tumour markers would it be most appropriate to test this patient for?
   A. Calcitonin
   B. Alpha-fetoprotein (AFP)
   C. CA 125
   D. Prostate-specific antigen (PSA)
   E. Human chorionic gonadotropin (βHCG)

Ans: A. Calcitonin

Medullary cancer of the thyroid is associated with multiple endocrine neoplasia type 2 (MEN2).

IM13.12

2. A 50-year-old woman presents with a mole on her back that has recently been weeping pus. She thinks it may have grown slightly too. On examination, the mole is irregular in shape and is variegated in colour. Which of the following tumour markers would it be most appropriate to test this patient for?
   A. Neuron-specific enolase
   B. Prostate-specific antigen (PSA)
   C. S100
   D. CA 125
   E. Human chorionic gonadotropin (βHCG)

Ans: C. S100

S100 protein is a cancer biomarker. S100B is present in malignant melanoma.

IM13.12

3. A 55-year-old woman presents with left flank pain and a distended abdomen. On examination, there is positive shifting dullness and fluid thrill. A pregnancy test is negative. Which of the following tumour markers would it be most appropriate to test this patient for?
   A. Calcitonin
   B. Alpha-fetoprotein (AFP)
   C. Carcinoembryonic antigen (CEA)
   D. CA 125
   E. Human chorionic gonadotropin (βHCG)

Ans: D. CA 125

Ovarian cancers are positive for CA 125.

IM7.1

4. A 45-year-old man presents with painful necrotic ulceration of his left shin. Two weeks previously, it had started as a small papular lesion that he thought was an insect bite. His past medical history includes a panproctocolectomy and ileo-anal pouch formation for ulcerative colitis. On examination there is a 4 × 4 cm, deep ulcer on the anterior left shin. What is the most likely diagnosis?
   A. Erythema nodosum
   B. Neuropathic ulcer
   C. Pyoderma gangrenosum
   D. Venous ulcer
   E. Marjolin's ulcer

Ans: C. Pyoderma gangrenosum

An autoimmune condition which leads to deep chronic ulceration of the skin, most commonly on the lower limbs. Pyoderma gangrenosum is associated with underlying medical conditions such as inflammatory bowel disease, rheumatoid arthritis and multiple myeloma.

IM13.14

5. A 32-year-old woman has a routine blood test as part of a life insurance medical. She has no medical history and has been well except for mild lethargy during the last few weeks. Her blood shows Hb 12 g/dL, platelets 150 × 10^9/L and white blood count 75 × 10^9/L (less than 1% blasts, numerous promyelocytes, myelocytes, metamyelocytes, band forms and mature neutrophils). FISH analysis shows t(9;22) with BCR-ABL fusion. She is informed of the diagnosis of chronic phase chronic myeloid leukaemia (CML). Which of the following is the most appropriate initial therapy?
   A. Hydroxycarbamide
   B. Interferon
   C. Leukapheresis
   D. Tyrosine kinase inhibitor (imatinib)
   E. Watch and wait

Ans: D. Tyrosine kinase inhibitor (imatinib)

This treatment has revolutionised CML management. There are now several oral tyrosine kinase inhibitors which are generally well tolerated and effective. They work by inhibiting the BCR-ABL fusion protein.

IM22.5

6. A 76-year-old man has come to the Emergency Department complaining of a 4-day history of haemoptysis. On investigation, chest X-ray showed a 2 cm opacity at the right middle zone. He has a history of hypertension controlled on amlodipine. Blood test showed serum sodium 130 mmol/L (normal 135–145). Initial haematology and clinical chemistry tests are otherwise normal. What is the likely cause of his hyponatraemia?
   A. ACTH secretion by a lung tumour
   B. ADH secretion by a lung tumour
   C. Underlying hypertension
   D. Amlodipine treatment
   E. VIP secretion by a lung tumour

Ans: B. ADH secretion by a lung tumour

Paraneoplastic syndrome can result in ADH secretion and cause hyponatraemia.

14 Genetics and Diseases

Q. Write a short note on chromosomes. (AN 73.1)

- Present in the nucleus of cells.
- Made up of double-stranded, helical deoxyribonucleic acid (DNA).
- The DNA molecule is complexed with histones and nonhistone proteins to form a deoxyribonucleoprotein fibre called chromatin. Chromatin is the basic unit of a chromosome structure.
- DNA is made up of nucleic acids that are composed of molecules of nucleotides.
- Each nucleotide has three components:
  - Nitrogenous bases:
    - Purines—adenine (A) and guanine (G).
    - Pyrimidines—cytosine (C) and thymine (T).
  - Sugar moiety—deoxyribose.
  - Phosphate molecules.
- Adenine pairs with thymine and cytosine with guanine to form a base pair.
- A sequence of three bases forms a codon that codes for an amino acid.
- Each chromosome consists of a single, enormously long and linear DNA molecule associated with proteins that fold and pack DNA into a more compact structure. The complex of DNA and protein is called chromatin.
- Human somatic cell contains a set of 46 chromosomes. Two of these chromosomes determine the sex of the individuals and are known as sex chromosomes (X and Y). The remaining 44 chromosomes are known as autosomes. The two sex chromosomes of the female are X chromosomes (XX). Y chromosome is morphologically smaller than X chromosome. Male sex is determined by XY chromosomes.
- With the exception of germ cells (sperm and eggs) and highly specialised cells that lack DNA entirely (such as red blood cell), each human cell contains two copies of each chromosome, one inherited from the mother and one from the father; the maternal and paternal chromosomes of a pair are called homologous chromosomes. The only non-homologous chromosome pairs are the sex chromosomes in males, where a Y chromosome is inherited from the father and an X chromosome from the mother.
- Arrangement of chromosomes in pairs in decreasing order of size is known as karyotype of chromosomes and is numbered 1–22. The 23rd pair is the sex-determining (X and Y) chromosomes.
- A karyotype is obtained from peripheral blood lymphocytes using various stains. A more rapid method is by fluorescence in situ hybridisation (FISH).
- The chromosomes have a centromere, which appears like a narrow waist. It is located between the two arms of the chromosome.
- Each chromosome has a short arm known as '*p*' arm ('petite' arm) and a long arm known as '*q*' arm ('queue' arm).
- Depending on the location of the centromere relative to the two arms, human chromosomes are classified as 'metacentric', where the centromere is more or less in the middle of the chromosome, 'submetacentric', where the centromere is somewhat offset from the centre or 'acrocentric', where the centromere is significantly offset from the centre, with only a very short '*p*' arm.
- Since there are 46 chromosomes in a normal individual, males have 46XY chromosomal pattern while females have 46XX.
- Deletion or addition of a chromosome is shown as a '+' or '−' sign. For example, Down's syndrome has one extra autosomal chromosome and a male is represented as 47XY, +21 (indicating one extra chromosome number 21).

- If a part of one arm is missing, it is indicated as 46XY, 5p– (indicating deletion of short arm of chromosome number 5 as occurs in cri-du-chat syndrome).
- Mitochondria have a distinct genome consisting of 16,589 base pairs. The mitochondrial genome encodes 37 genes, including 13 proteins. Mitochondria are transmitted only in the ovum and as such, all mitochondrial DNA is maternally inherited. Many of these are involved in mitochondrial respiration and the electron transport chain.

Q. Describe human genome.

Q. Give a brief account of Human Genome Project.

- A genome is an organism's complete set of DNA including all of its genes. Each genome contains all the information needed to build and maintain that organism.
- The human genome is the genome of *Homo sapiens*, which is composed of 46 distinct chromosomes (22 pairs of autosomal chromosomes + XX or XY chromosomes).
- The Human Genome Project (HGP) was an international effort, which began in 1990. The project was planned to last 15 years, but rapid technological advances had accelerated the completion to 2003.
- Its main aim was to decode a total of approximately 3 billion DNA base pairs containing estimated 20,000–25,000 genes.
- It has produced a reference sequence of the human genome which is used worldwide in biomedical sciences.
- The human genome is much more gene-sparse than was initially predicted at the outset of the HGP, with only about 1.5% of the total length serving as protein-coding exons, and the rest of the genome comprised by introns or so-called junk DNA or noncoding genes. Noncoding genes code for other RNA types such as microRNAs (miRNAs) and small nucleolar RNAs (snRNAs), with functional properties that do not require translation to protein.
- All humans have unique gene sequences; therefore, the data published by the HGP do not represent the exact sequence of each and every individual's genome. It is the combined genome of a small number of anonymous donors.
- About 99.9% of information in the estimated 20,000 human genes is identical from one person to the next. The small differences in the remaining 0.1% of genes present in the human cells are the key to each individual.

POTENTIAL BENEFITS OF HUMAN GENOME PROJECT

- Molecular medicine:
  - Improved diagnosis of disease.
  - Earlier detection of genetic predispositions to disease.
  - Gene therapy.
  - Pharmacogenomics ('custom drugs' to target specific genetic composition so as to get best drug response with minimal side effects).
- Energy and environmental applications:
  - Use microbial genomics research to create new energy sources (biofuels).
  - Use microbial genomics research to develop environmental monitoring techniques to detect pollutants.
- Risk assessment:
  - Assess health damage caused by radiation exposure.
  - Assess health damage caused by exposure to mutagenic chemicals and cancer-causing toxins.
- DNA forensics (identification):
  - Identify potential suspects whose DNA may match evidence left at crime scenes.
  - Exonerate persons wrongly accused of crimes.
  - Establish paternity and other family relationships.
  - Match organ donors with recipients in transplant programmes.
- Cancer genomics:
  - Genomic changes in tumour cells (biomarkers) can define diagnostic subtypes, predict tumour behaviour, prognosis and drug response and enable monitoring for early recurrence of disease.
  - Development of targeted drugs that switch off mutated oncogenes (e.g. *BRAF* inhibitors such as vemurafenib used in metastatic melanoma or *EGFR* inhibitors such as erlotinib used in advanced lung cancer).

ETHICAL, LEGAL AND SOCIAL ISSUES OF HUMAN GENOME

- Privacy and fairness in the use of genetic information which includes the potential for genetic discrimination in employment and insurance.
- Integration of new genetic technologies (e.g. genetic testing) into the practice of clinical medicine.
- Ethical issues surrounding the design and conduct of genetic research in people.
- Education of healthcare professionals, policy makers, students and public about genetics and the complex issues that result from genomic research.

Q. Give a brief account of proteomics.

Q. Describe proteome.

- Proteomics is the study of the interactions, function, composition and structures of proteins and their cellular activities.
- The word 'proteome' is derived from proteins expressed by a genome, and it refers to all the proteins produced by an organism, much like the genome is the entire set of genes. The human body may contain more than 2 million different proteins, each having different functions.
- Study of proteomics is important since proteins and not the genomes are the functioning units.
- However, the task of studying the proteome involves the sheer number of proteins that need to be identified. Another challenge is that amino acids—the base units of proteins—are very small. Each amino acid is made from anywhere between 7 and

24 atoms. This is far beyond the reach of even the most powerful microscopes.

- It is more complicated than genomics because an organism's genome is more or less constant, whereas proteomes differ from cell to cell and from time to time. Many proteins also are subjected to a wide variety of chemical modifications after translation.

TYPES OF PROTEOMICS

EXPRESSION PROTEOMICS

- Expression proteomics is used to study the qualitative and quantitative expression of total proteins in normal and diseased cells. This helps in making us understand the protein that is responsible for the diseased state or the protein that is expressed due to disease. The protein may be overexpressed or underexpressed in diseased cells. Identification of these proteins will give valuable information about molecular biology of tumour formation, diagnostic markers and therapeutic targets.

STRUCTURAL PROTEOMICS

- Structural proteomics helps to understand three-dimensional shape and structural complexities of functional proteins. Structural proteomics can give detailed information about the structure and function of protein complexes present in a specific cellular organelle in diseased cells.

FUNCTIONAL PROTEOMICS

- Functional proteomics is used to understand the protein functions as well as molecular mechanisms within the cell that depend on the identification of the interacting protein partners (protein–protein interaction).

APPLICATIONS

- Proteomic technologies will play an important role in drug discovery, diagnostics and molecular medicine because of the link between genes, proteins and disease. As more and more defective proteins causing particular diseases are found, new drugs will be developed to either alter the shape of a defective protein or mimic a missing one.

Q. Explain pharmacogenetics.

Q. Describe pharmacogenomics.

Q. What is precision medicine?

- There is significant variability in the response to pharmacologic agents among various people despite administration of same dose of a drug. Part of this difference can be explained by drug–drug interactions, drug–food interactions, sex, age, and renal and hepatic functions. However, difference in genetic factors also play a major role.
- Study of interaction between genetics and therapeutic drugs is variously called pharmacogenetics or pharmacogenomics.
  - Pharmacogenomics refers to the role of various components of the genome on response to a drug. These components of genome include genetic sequence variations, structural changes in chromosomes (e.g. translocations), epigenetic variations (e.g. changes in gene methylation) and variation in the expression profile of genes (changes in messenger RNA levels or noncoding RNA).
  - Pharmacogenetics is a subcategory of pharmacogenomics which indicates the role of genetic variation on response to a drug. This term is used to refer to a specific DNA polymorphism or coding variant rather than epigenetic or other changes in the genome.
  - In clinical practice, both terms are used interchangeably.
- Precision medicine is an approach for disease treatment and prevention that takes into account individual variability in genes (pharmacogenetics), environment and lifestyle for each person.
- Broad categories under which pharmacogenetics alters response to drug include:
  - Drug pharmacokinetics (absorption, distribution, metabolism and elimination) affecting plasma drug concentration.
    - For example, activity of cytochrome oxidase may be dependent on genetic variation. This may contribute to either diminished or absent metabolism, or excessive metabolism of a compound.
    - Another example is the enzyme thiopurine S-methyltransferase (TPMT) which is responsible for metabolism of thiopurines (e.g., azathioprine and 6-mercaptopurine). Polymorphisms in the TPMT gene can result in decreased activity of the enzyme and an increased risk of treatment-related leucopenia.
    - CYP2C19 carriers who are intermediate metabolisers for clopidogrel will have reduced antiplatelet action, although routine screening is not recommended.
  - Drug pharmacodynamics affecting binding of the drug to its receptor.
    - An example of a genetic variant that influences pharmacodynamics is the effect of polymorphisms in the gene encoding vitamin K epoxide reductase complex subunit 1 (VKORC1) on response to the anticoagulant warfarin. VKORC1 is responsible for the conversion of vitamin K-epoxide to vitamin K, which is the rate-limiting step in the physiological process of vitamin K recycling and the primary therapeutic target for warfarin.
  - Idiosyncratic reaction to a drug increasing likelihood of hypersensitivity reaction to it.
    - Examples include HLA-B*1502 and carbamazepine hypersensitivity, and HLA-B*5701 and abacavir hypersensitivity.
  - Targeted drug therapy against certain cancers which have specific genetic defects related to their pathogenesis.

POTENTIAL BENEFITS OF PHARMACOGENOMICS (Box 14.1)

Box 14.1. Potential Benefits of Pharmacogenomics

- More powerful medicines—therapy more targeted to specific diseases
- Better, safer drugs the first time based on patient's genetic profile
- More accurate methods of determining appropriate drug dosages—instead of dosages based on weight and age, they will be based on a person's genetics; how well the body processes the medicine and the time it takes to metabolise it
- Introduction of drugs at most appropriate stage of disease
- Better vaccines—vaccines made of genetic material, either DNA or RNA, promise all the benefits of existing vaccines without the risks
- Improvements in the drug discovery and approval process—pharmaceutical companies will be able to discover potential therapies more easily using genome targets; the cost and risk of clinical trials will be reduced by targeting only those persons capable of responding to a drug
- Decrease in the overall cost of health care—related to decreases in the number of adverse drug reactions, number of failed drug trials, time it takes to get a drug approved, length of time patients are on medication, number of medications patients must take to find an effective therapy, etc.

Q. Write a short note on epigenetics.

- It is a study of heritable changes in gene expression that are not due to changes in DNA sequence.
- This term is used to refer to features such as chromatin and DNA modifications that are stable over rounds of cell division but do not involve changes in the underlying DNA sequence of the organism. In other words, epigenetics refers to variability in gene expression, heritable through mitosis and potentially meiosis without any underlying modification in the actual genetic sequence.
- Every nucleated cell in the body contains the same DNA sequence. Despite that, cells from different tissues behave very differently. These differences are due to additional layers of regulation that determine which genes are expressed to create a cell-specific phenotype. Epigenetic regulation, which can increase or decrease the expression of genes without altering genomic sequence, contributes to this cell-type-specific variation. Thus, epigenetic changes play a role in the process of cellular differentiation, allowing cells to maintain different characteristics despite containing the same genomic material.
- Pivotal processes involved in epigenetic changes include modifications in histones (methylation or demethylation, and acetylation or deacetylation) and DNA modifications (methylation or demethylation of DNA base).
- Clinical applications:
  - Epigenetic tumour markers (e.g. septin-9 DNA hypermethylation for detecting colorectal cancer).
  - Epigenetic therapeutic agents:
    - DNA methylation inhibitors (e.g. azacitidine and decitabine are used in the treatment of myelodysplastic syndromes and progressive lymphoma).
    - Histone deacetylase inhibitors (e.g. panobinostat and vorinostat are used in the treatment of multiple myeloma and cutaneous T-cell lymphoma).

Q. Discuss the various types of chromosomal aberrations. (AN 75.1)

- Chromosomal aberrations may be summarised as follows:
  - Autosomal abnormalities.
  - Sex-linked abnormalities.
- Both autosomal and sex-linked abnormalities may be due to:
  - Numerical abnormalities (number of chromosomes different from normal).
  - Structural abnormalities (change in structure of a chromosome due to addition or deletion of a part of it).

NUMERICAL ABNORMALITIES OF AUTOSOMAL CHROMOSOMES

- Polyploidy—one whole set of chromosomes (i.e. 23 chromosomes) is gained ($3n$—triploidy, $4n$—tetraploidy; normal pattern is $2n$). This is not compatible with life.
- Aneuploidy—one or more chromosomes are either gained or lost.
  - Monosomy—loss of one chromosome (instead of the typical two in humans) from a pair of autosomes ($2n - 1$). This is lethal in males.
  - Trisomy—addition of an extra autosome chromosome ($2n + 1$), for example:
    (i) Down's syndrome (trisomy 21; 47XY, +21).
    (ii) Patau's syndrome (trisomy 13; 47XY, +13).
    (iii) Edwards' syndrome (trisomy 18; 47XY, +18).

NUMERICAL ABNORMALITIES OF SEX CHROMOSOMES

- More common than numerical abnormalities of autosomal chromosomes (except Down's syndrome).
- Occurs due to failure of homologous chromosomes to separate in one of the cycles of meiosis during spermatogenesis or oogenesis. This is known as non-disjunction.
- Monosomy is seen with Turner's syndrome (45X or 45XO).
- Presence of more than one X chromosomes produces higher risk of mental retardation (e.g. Klinefelter's syndrome—47XXY).
- Presence of more than one Y chromosome (e.g. 47XYY) results in tall males with aggressive behaviour.

STRUCTURAL ABNORMALITIES OF CHROMOSOMES (Fig. 14.1)

- Deletion—loss of part of a chromosome (e.g. loss of short arm of chromosome number 5 produces cri-du-chat syndrome; 46XY, 5p−).

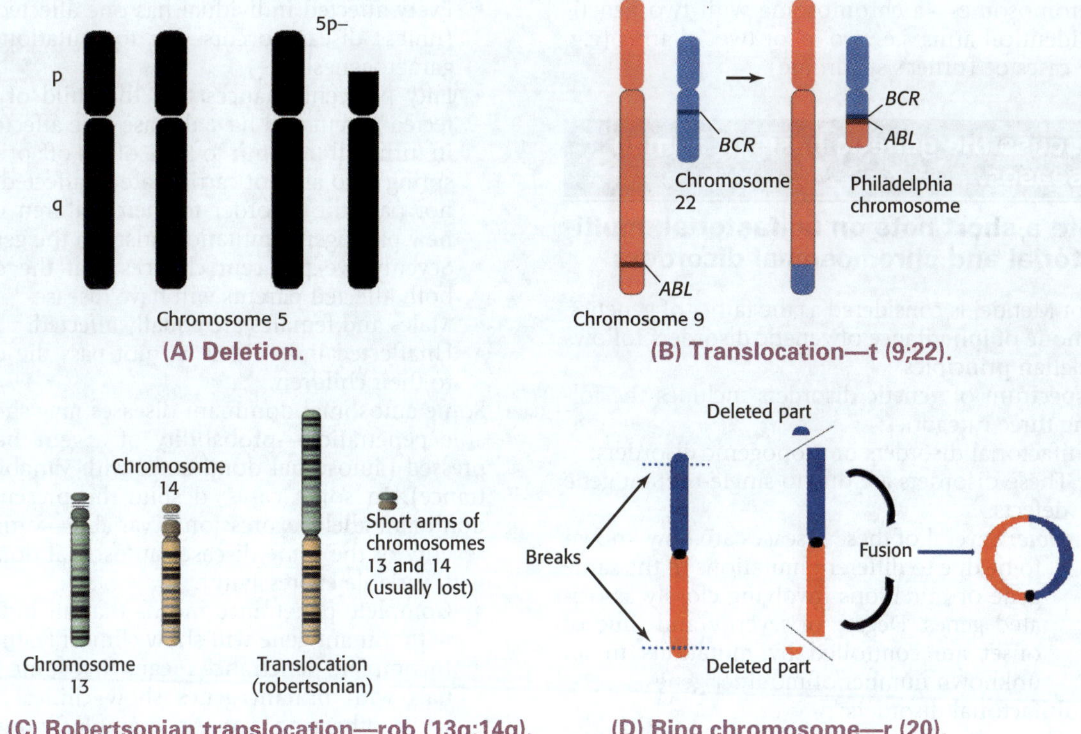

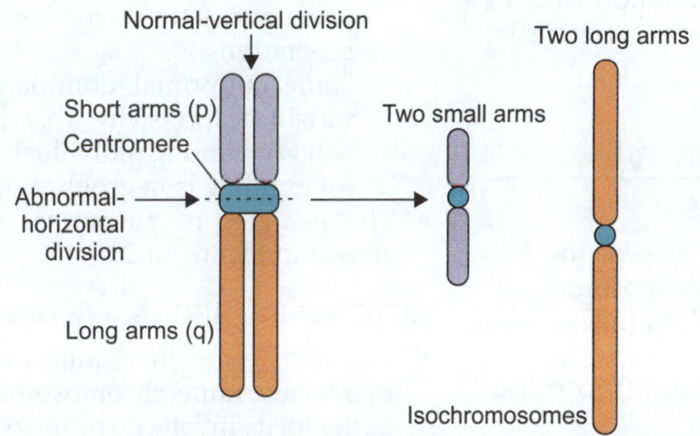

(E) Isochromosomes—i (p) and i (q).

Fig. 14.1 Types of structural abnormalities of chromosomes. (*Source*: (A) https://ghr.nlm.nih.gov/art/large/chromosome-5p-deletion-in-cri-du-chat-syndrome.jpeg; (B) https://en.wikipedia.org/wiki/File:Schematic_of_the_Philadelphia_Chromosome.svg; (C) Mosby's Medical Dictionary, 9th edition. © 2009, Elsevier and (D) https://ghr.nlm.nih.gov/art/large/chromosome-5pdeletion-in-cri-du-chat-syndrome.jpeg).

- Reciprocal translocation—exchange of segments between two nonhomologous chromosomes, that is recombination of two unrelated genes to form new genetic information (e.g. Down's syndrome in a small proportion of patients due to translocation of segments of chromosomes 21 and 14; Philadelphia chromosome due to translocation between chromosomes 9 and 22).
- Robertsonian translocation is a type of translocation caused by breaks of two acrocentric chromosomes (i.e. chromosomes 13, 14, 15, 21 and 22) at or near the centromeres with subsequent fusion of long arms. This produces one large chromosome and one extremely small chromosome; the latter is often lost with little effect because it contains very few genes which are also present on other acrocentric chromosomes. The resulting karyotype contains only 45 chromosomes. The most common Robertsonian translocation involves chromosomes 13 and 14. Robertsonian translocations involving chromosome 21 during gametogenesis have a higher risk of having a child with Down syndrome.
- Ring chromosomes—fusion of the two ends of the same chromosome; there is loss of genetic material at the ends of the chromosome prior to the fusion. It is denoted by symbol 'r' (e.g. ring chromosome 20 is associated with epilepsy).

- Isochromosomes—a chromosome with two genetically identical arms, i.e. two 'p' or two 'q' arms (e.g. some cases of Turner's syndrome).

Q. Discuss the genetic basis of human diseases.

Q. Write a short note on unifactorial, multifactorial and chromosomal disorders.

- Gregor Mendel is considered as the father of genetics.
- The mode of inheritance of genetic disorders follows Mendelian principles.
- The spectrum of genetic disorders includes the following three categories:
  - Unifactorial disorders or monogenic disorders:
    - These disorders are due to single-mutant gene defects.
      Note: Several of these diseases are now known to be due to different mutations in the same gene or mutations involving closely associated genes. Degree of severity and time of onset are controlled by mutations in an unknown number of modifier genes.
  - Multifactorial disorders:
    - These disorders are caused by an interaction of genetic and environmental factors.
  - Chromosomal disorders:
    - These disorders result from an abnormality of number or structure of chromosomes (discussed above).

UNIFACTORIAL DISORDERS (Flowchart 14.1)

AUTOSOMAL DOMINANT DISEASES

- Disorders generally manifest when one of the two homologous (paired) autosomal chromosomes carries a mutant gene at the locus involved (allele).
- Characterised by:
  - Vertical transmission (parent to child) to subsequent generations.
  - Every affected individual has one affected parent (unless disease occurs due to mutation during gametogenesis).
  - Fifty per cent chances that the child of one affected parent will have disease. The affected child in turn will transmit to 50% of his offspring. Offspring who are not carriers are unaffected and do not pass the disorder to their children unless a new pathogenic mutation arises in the germline.
  - Seventy-five per cent chances that the child of both affected parents will have disease.
  - Males and females are equally affected.
  - Unaffected individuals do not pass the disorder to their children.
- Some autosomal dominant diseases may show variable penetration—probability of a gene being expressed (autosomal dominance with variable penetrance). In some cases, despite the presence of a dominant allele, expression is variable—variation in severity of the same disease (autosomal dominance with variable expressivity).
  - Complete penetrance means that all individuals with mutant gene will show clinical features.
  - Incomplete penetrance means that some individuals with mutant genes show clinical features while others do not. An example is retinoblastoma (*RB*) gene where about 10% of individuals with this gene do not develop the disease.
  - Sometimes, the gene is not expressed at all (nonpenetrance) that explains apparent skipping of generations.
  - Some autosomal dominant diseases may show variable expressivity, that is severity of disorder will vary among individuals carrying mutant gene. An example is neurofibromatosis type 1.
- The pedigree of autosomal dominant diseases is shown in Figure 14.2.

AUTOSOMAL RECESSIVE DISEASES

- Disorders generally manifest when both the homologous autosome chromosomes carry mutant genes at the locus involved (homozygous state).

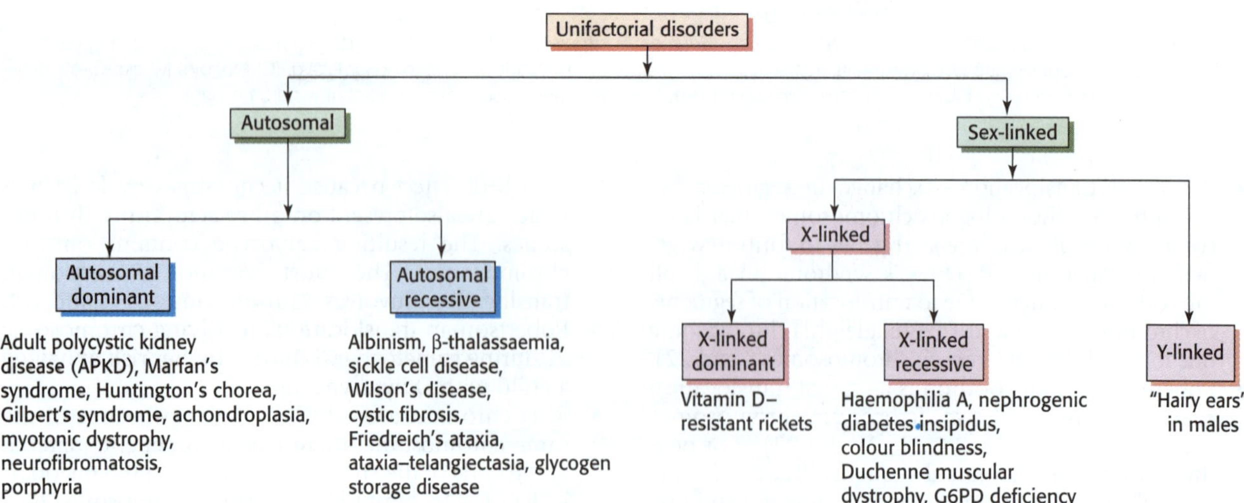

Flowchart 14.1 Unifactorial Disorders.

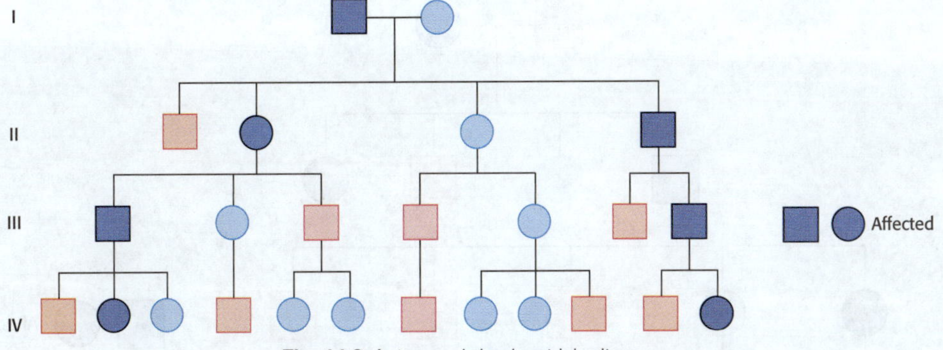

Fig. 14.2 Autosomal dominant inheritance.

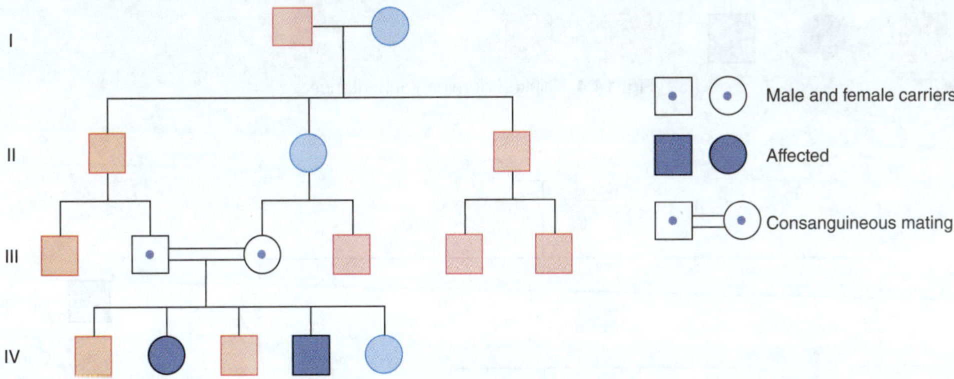

Fig. 14.3 Autosomal recessive inheritance.

- Diseases generally are not manifested when only one mutant allele is present (i.e. in heterozygous or carrier state).
- Characterised by:
  - Males and females are equally likely to be affected, though some traits exhibit different expression in males and females (e.g. hypospadias in males and ovarian cancer in females).
  - Disease present in multiple members of kindred in the same generation with no affected members in other generations (horizontal transmission).
  - Birth of an affected child establishes both parents as carriers of a single copy of the gene mutation.
  - Chance of a second affected child in the sibship is one in four or 25% in each pregnancy. Fifty per cent are heterozygotes (clinically normal) and 25% are normal without any mutant gene.
  - Rarely seen in previous or subsequent generation of the family unless there is consanguinity or a high gene frequency.
- Almost all inborn errors of metabolism are autosomal recessive disorders.
- In some cases, the affected individual may be a compound heterozygote, having inherited two different variants in the same gene on opposite alleles.
- The pedigree of autosomal recessive diseases is shown in Figure 14.3.

X-LINKED DOMINANT DISEASES

- Mutant gene on X chromosome.
- Characterised by:
  - No carriers as the disease will manifest even if single chromosome has abnormal gene.
  - The trait is never passed from father to son as the son's 'normal' X chromosome is from mother.
  - All daughters of an affected father are diseased as the daughter gets abnormal X from the father.
  - If mother is affected and father is normal, 50% of both sons and daughters are affected.
  - In general, males are more severely affected than females. The trait may be lethal in males.
- The pedigree of X-linked dominant diseases is shown in Fig. 14.4.

X-LINKED RECESSIVE DISEASES

- Mutant gene on X chromosome.
- In males, one copy of mutant gene is required for manifestations of disease while in females, both copies of mutant gene are required.
- Characterised by:
  - As with any X-linked trait, the disease is never passed from father to son.
  - Usually, manifests only in males. In many diseases, males do not survive.
  - All affected males in a family are related through their mothers.
  - Trait or disease is typically passed from an affected grandfather through his carrier daughters to half of his grandsons.
  - Mothers are always carriers and all their sons are affected.
- Very rarely, a female can develop the disease. This may occur due to:
  - Female also having Turner's syndrome (XO) where only one X chromosome is present.
  - Presence of testicular feminisation syndrome.

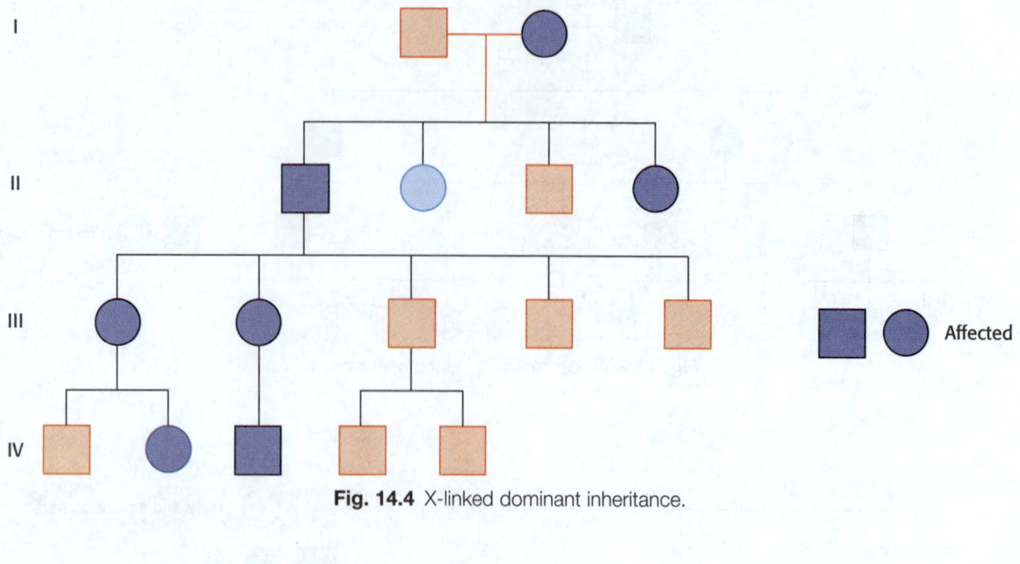

Fig. 14.4 X-linked dominant inheritance.

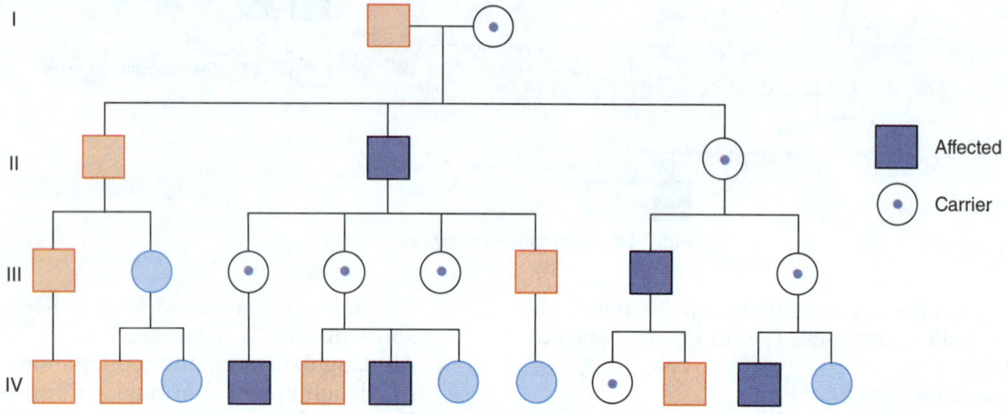

Fig. 14.5 X-linked recessive inheritance (with males surviving to reproduce).

- Normal father with mutation in X chromosome and a carrier female.
- Affected father and carrier mother.
- Inactivation of normal X chromosome in most cells (Lyon hypothesis).

- The pedigrees of X-linked recessive diseases are shown in Figs. 14.5 and 14.6.

Y-LINKED DISEASES

- Characterised by:
  - Only males are affected.
  - An affected male transmits the trait to all his sons but not to his daughters.
  - Most Y-linked mutant genes produce infertility and, therefore, it is rare to see familial transmission of a Y-linked disorder. A benign Y-linked disease is hypertrichosis of the ears.

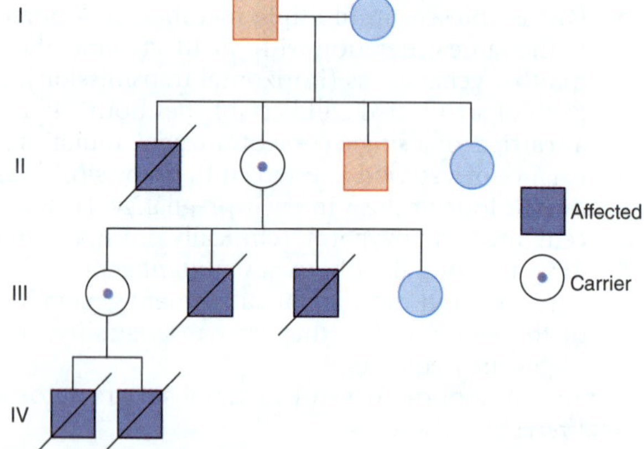

Fig. 14.6 X-linked recessive inheritance (with males not surviving to reproduce; a diagonal line through the symbol for an individual denotes that the individual has died).

MITOCHONDRIAL INHERITANCE

- The mitochondrial genome of all individuals is derived from the mother only.
- Mitochondrial DNA contains 37 genes that encode proteins involved in oxidative phosphorylation, transfer RNAs and ribosomal RNAs.
- Various mitochondrial disorders include MELAS (*mi*tochondrial *e*ncephalomyopathy, *l*actic *a*cidosis and *s*troke-like episodes), MERRF (*m*yoclonus, *e*pilepsy associated with *r*agged *r*ed *f*ibres) and Kearns–Sayre syndrome (ophthalmoplegia, pigmentary retinopathy and cardiomyopathy).

MULTIFACTORIAL DISORDERS (Flowchart 14.2)

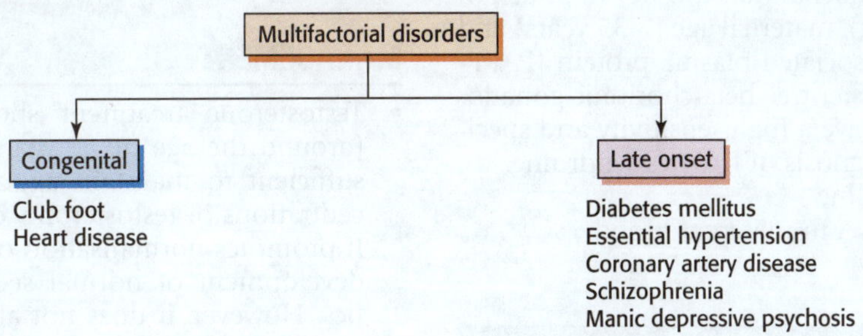

Flowchart 14.2 Multifactorial Disorders.

CHROMOSOMAL DISORDERS

- Chromosomal disorders may be classified in two ways (Flowchart 14.3).

Q. Describe Down's syndrome. (PE 32.1)

- The term Mongolism is not used at present.
- It is an autosomal abnormality where the number of the autosomes present is affected (autosomal imbalance).
  - Extra chromosome 21 (trisomy 21) due to nondisjunction (failure of homologous chromosomes to separate) during meiosis (95%).
  - One per cent mosaicism—two different cell lines are present; one has normal chromosomal constitution, whereas the other has an extra chromosome 21.
  - Four per cent due to Robertsonian translocation (instead of extra separate chromosome 21, it gets translocated to another chromosome).
- Incidence—1:700 of live births.
- Significant relationship with increasing maternal age with incidence as high as 1:100 live births in mothers older than 40 years.

CLINICAL FEATURES (Table 14.1)

TABLE 14.1 Clinical Features of Down's Syndrome

Structure/ System Involved	Features
• Craniofacial and musculoskeletal	Flat nasal bridge, flat face, brachycephaly, malformed large ears Widely spaced eyes (hypertelorism), upward, slanting eyes with epicanthic folds (almond-shaped eyes), Brushfield's spot on iris Protruding furrowed tongue (scrotal tongue) Broad and short neck Simian crease single palmar flexion crease (50% of cases) Short stature Hypotonia Increased space between first and second toes ('sandal' gap) Increased frequency of sleep apnoea syndrome
• Brain	Mental retardation, attention-deficit hyperactivity disorder, autism
• Heart	Atrial septal defect, ventricular septal defect, tetralogy of Fallot, endocardial cushion defects
• Gastrointestinal tract	Oesophageal/duodenal atresia, imperforate anus
• Reproductive	Males are sterile
• Endocrine	Hypothyroidism, type 1 diabetes mellitus
• Bone marrow	Increased incidence of acute leukaemia

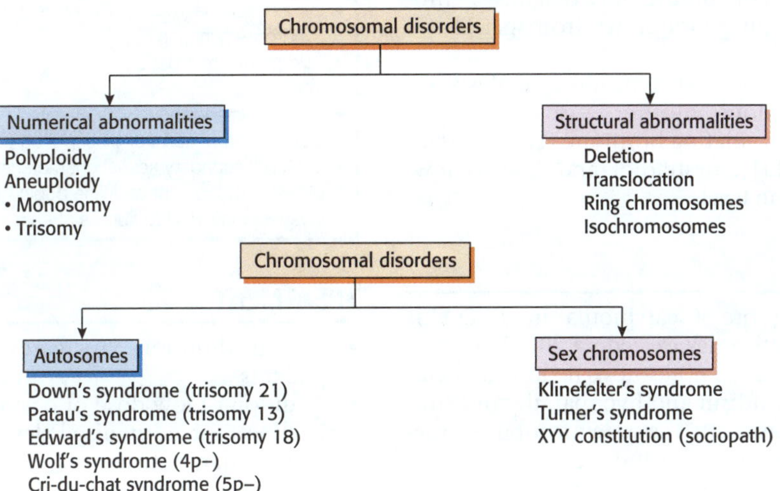

Flowchart 14.3 Chromosomal Disorders.

PRENATAL DIAGNOSIS

- First trimester foetal nuchal translucency (a pouch of fluid behind the neck), maternal age (>35 years) and bi-test (pregnancy-associated plasma protein [PAPP-A] with second trimester free beta-chorionic gonadotropin [beta-hCG]) have a high sensitivity and specificity for prenatal diagnosis of Down's syndrome.
- Chorionic villi sampling.
- Analysis of foetal DNA in maternal blood.
- Amniocentesis.

Q. Briefly outline the clinical features, diagnosis, complications and management of Klinefelter's syndrome. (PE 32.11, PE 32.12, PE 32.13)

- Most common chromosomal disorder.
- Sex chromosomal abnormality.
- Due to nondisjunction of X chromosome during meiosis.
- Males are affected and they have an extra X chromosome.
- Most common karyotype is XXY.
- Other karyotypes include XXXY/XXXXY/XXYY.
- Advanced maternal age is a critical risk factor for this disorder.

CLINICAL FEATURES (Box 14.2)

BOX 14.2 Clinical Features of Klinefelter's Syndrome

- Sterility (azoospermia), small testes and penis
- Gynaecomastia
- Tall and thin with relatively long legs (eunuchoid body proportions)
- Sparse facial, body and sexual hair
- High-pitched, deep voice
- Mental retardation

DIAGNOSIS

- Extra X chromosome may be detected as a Barr body on buccal smears. For confirmatory diagnosis, chromosome analysis on lymphocytes from peripheral blood is used.
- For prenatal diagnosis, chromosome analysis on amniocytes or chorionic villi.
- Elevated follicle-stimulating hormone (FSH), luteinising hormone (LH), oestradiol and low to low-normal testosterone level.

COMPLICATIONS

- Risk of acquiring breast carcinoma in 47XXY is increased with relative risk exceeding 200 times.
- Associated endocrine complications include diabetes mellitus, hypothyroidism and hypoparathyroidism.
- Autoimmune diseases, such as systemic lupus erythematosus, Sjögren's syndrome and rheumatoid arthritis, are more common with frequencies similar to those found in females.
- Development of varicose veins and leg ulcers.
- Decreased bone density.

MANAGEMENT

- Testosterone treatment should begin at puberty (around the age of 12 years), in increasing dosage sufficient to maintain age-appropriate serum concentrations of testosterone, oestradiol, FSH and LH. It promotes normalisation of body proportions and development of normal secondary sex characteristics. However, it does not affect infertility, gynaecomastia and small testes. It also reduces long-term complications of osteoporosis, autoimmune disease and breast cancer.
- Early speech therapy.
- Physical therapy for hypotonia or delayed motor skills.

Q. Discuss briefly about Turner's syndrome. (PE 32.6, 32.7, 32.8, 32.9)

- Sex chromosomal abnormality.
- Due to nondisjunction of X chromosome during meiosis.
- Females are affected where there is a deletion of X chromosome.
- Genetic constitution, hence becomes 45XO.
- In some cases, a combination of monosomy X and normal cells (45X/46XX) is present; it is known as mosaic Turner's syndrome.
- Not related to maternal age and usually not discovered before puberty when patient fails to develop secondary sexual characters.

CLINICAL FEATURES (Box 14.3)

BOX 14.3 Clinical Features of Turner's Syndrome

- Short stature
- Webbed neck and low posterior hairline
- Broad chest with widely spaced nipples—'shield chest'
- Increased carrying angle at the elbows (cubitus valgus)
- Lymphoedema (most common reason to screen for Turner's syndrome during infancy)
- Mild mental retardation
- Infertility
- Primary amenorrhoea with elevated FSH
- Coarctation of aorta or bicuspid aortic valve; aortic dissection
- Lack of secondary sexual characteristics including inadequate breast development and little pubic hair
- Ovaries converted to fibrous streaks

TREATMENT

- Growth hormone increases the height in these patients.
- Addition of low dose of oestrogen is also beneficial. It allows for normalised development of secondary sexual characteristics, as well as uterine and bone mineral development.
- Surgical correction of congenital heart diseases.

BOX 14.4 Features of Mental Retardation

• Slowness in motor development	• Inability to learn
• Poor school progress	• Behavioural abnormalities like dull or silly behaviour
• Dull, apathetic, underactive person	• Aberrant types of behaviour (autism or hyperkinetism)
• Personality disorders • Social or language disorders	• Associated neurological problems like motor or sensory handicaps, seizures, blindness, deafness, chorea, choreoathetosis

Q. Explain mental retardation. (PS 15.1, 15.2, 15.3, 15.4)

Q. Explain intellectual disability.

- At present, the term intellectual disability is used rather than mental retardation.
- Here the mental insufficiency is characterised by limitation in adaptive behaviour and intellectual functioning.
- A wide variation in point prevalence of intellectual disability has been reported from India varying from around 1 to 32 per 1000 population, depending on the case definition, methodology and population selected.

FEATURES

- Various features are given in Box 14.4.
- Frequently, individuals with intellectual disability are able to function well in early childhood, with limitations not becoming apparent until they are challenged with learning upon entering school.

CAUSES (Table 14.2)

TABLE 14.2 Causes of Mental Retardation

• Genetic disorders	Down's syndrome and fragile X syndrome
• Environmental causes	*Prenatal* exposure to alcohol (foetal alcohol syndrome), lead, mercury, hydantoin, valproate and radiation *Intrauterine infections* like congenital rubella syndrome, cytomegalovirus and other infections *Perinatal* causes like preterm birth, hypoxia, infection, birth trauma and intracranial haemorrhage *Postnatal* causes like exposure to toxins, alcohol and heavy metals
• CNS diseases	Hydrocephalus or microcephaly, cerebral palsy, posttraumatic, postmeningitic and postencephalitic states, birth trauma, kernicterus
• Metabolic diseases	Cretinism, phenylketonuria, mucopolysaccharidoses
• Others	Trauma

TABLE 14.3 Mental Retardation by IQ Range

• Mild	50–55 to ,70
• Moderate	35–40 to 50–55
• Severe	20–25 to 35–40
• Profound	Below 20–25

DEGREE OF MENTAL RETARDATION

- Degree of mental retardation is assessed by intelligence quotient (IQ) testing (Table 14.3).
  IQ = mental age/chronological age.

EVALUATION

- Evaluating a person with intellectual disability is a three-step process:
  - Assess intelligence quotient.
  - Assess behaviour and emotional skills.
  - Assess the impact of the individual's limitations on his ability to manage activities of daily living.

APPROACH TO MANAGEMENT

- Periodic dental examination, age-appropriate cancer screening and immunisations.
- Appropriate testing for sexually transmitted diseases including HIV infection.
- Early diagnosis and treatment of associated mental illnesses.
- Treatment of associated serious disorders. These conditions include seizures, cerebral palsy (control of spasticity, bone demineralisation and decubitus ulcers), dysphagia and constipation.
- Behaviour disorders like head-banging, hand-biting and excessive self-rubbing and scratching are common and require multidisciplinary approach for management.
- Patient-centric interventions:
  - The tasks taught to the individual should enable him to function well in day-to-day tasks. Each individual first needs training in self-care (toilet control, bathing, eating, dressing and grooming), motor skills (especially eye–hand coordination skills) and receptive and expressive language abilities. Later, the children can be recommended for academics or functional academics, finally leading to vocational training, gainful occupation and independent living skills.
  - Genetic counselling is essential as two-thirds of cases have genetic aetiologies and helps in knowing risk of recurrence in subsequent pregnancy.
  - Parents and families should be given proper information regarding the nature, needs and management of intelligence disability and its comorbidities in simple language.

Q. Discuss the prevention of genetic diseases.

- Premarital carrier screening to identify heterozygous individuals for a recessive disease who are asymptomatic.

- Genetic counselling—helping people understand and adapt to the medical and psychological implications of genetic contributions to diseases.
  - Genetic counsellors work as part of a health care team, providing information and support to families affected by or at risk of a genetic disorder. They help to identify families at possible risk of a genetic disorder, gather and analyse family history and inheritance patterns, calculate risks of recurrence, and provide information about genetic testing and related procedures.
  - The most common indications for genetic counselling include advanced maternal age, family history of a genetic condition and suspected diagnosis of a genetic condition.
- Detection of genetic association—that is markers by:
  - Restriction fragment length polymorphism.
  - Polymerase chain reaction (PCR) techniques.
  - Microarrays, FISH and high-resolution chromosome analysis.
- Antenatal diagnosis:
  - Amniocentesis.
  - Biochemical studies in maternal blood.
  - Maternal blood to analyse foetal DNA.
  - Transcervical chorionic villous biopsy (chorionic villous sampling).
- Preimplantation diagnosis:
  - Preimplantation testing is performed for couples at high risk for genetic conditions for which the disease-causing variant has already been identified in the parent(s).
  - In vitro fertilisation of the ovum and culture to blastomere stage. One cell is then studied by PCR or gene probe technique to detect genetic markers of diseases.

Q. Give a brief account of gene therapy.

- Genetic disorders are caused when the genes are altered so that the encoded proteins are unable to carry out their normal functions. Similarly, cancers are caused when oncogenes are activated or tumour suppressor genes are inactivated.
- Gene therapy is a technique for correcting defective genes responsible for disease development by using genetic material.
- Besides monogenic disorders, such as cystic fibrosis, haemophilia, muscular dystrophy and sickle cell anaemia, it is also a potential therapy in more complex disorders such as cardiovascular diseases, diseases of nervous system, autoimmune diseases, congenital immunodeficiency diseases and cancer.

FORMS

- Germ-line gene therapy refers to modification of the germ-line cells which results in permanent genetic changes that are passed to the future generations. It is not accepted at present due to ethical reasons.
- Somatic cell gene therapy refers to genetic modification of different somatic cells. Its therapeutic effect ends with the person receiving it and is not passed on to the future generations. This can be achieved by the following ways:
  - Insertion of a normal gene into a nonspecific location within the genome to replace a nonfunctional gene.
  - Repair of defective gene through selective reverse mutation.
  - Swapping an abnormal gene for a normal gene (homologous recombination).
  - Alteration of the regulation of an abnormal gene.
- Gene therapy can also be a tool for the treatment of nongenetic and polygenic disorders by delivering genes that stimulate immune response, suicidal genes inducing cell death, genes modifying cellular information or developmental programme or genes producing a therapeutic protein with specific functions.
- In cancers, gene therapy can be in various forms including use of cancer vaccines (immunotherapy), target viruses to cancer cells for lysis and death (oncolysis) and introduce genes into the cancer cells that cause death or restore normal cellular phenotype (gene transfer).
- Gene doping—transfer of cells or genetic elements (e.g. DNA and RNA) or the use of pharmacological or biological agents that alter gene expression with the potential to enhance athletic performance. It is a prohibited method for improving performance.

APPROACHES

- Two different approaches:
  - In 'ex vivo' gene therapy, specific cells are isolated and purified from a patient, genetically modified and reinfused.
  - In 'in vivo' gene therapy, genes are directly transferred into the tissue of patients using a vector. This is most often used technique.
    - A 'normal' gene is inserted into the genome to replace the disease-causing gene. A carrier molecule called a vector is used to deliver the therapeutic gene to the patient's target cells. Currently, the most common vector is a virus, other being plasmids. Commonly used viruses include retroviruses (e.g. Moloney murine leukaemia virus), adenoviruses, adeno-associated viruses and lentivirus. Lentivirus-derived vectors are promising because they can infect both dividing and nondividing cells.
    - Unlike wild-type viruses, these vectors are engineered by deleting the essential genes that allow replication, assembling or infection.
    - In the next step, target cells such as the patient's liver or lung cells are infected with the viral vector. The vector then unloads its genetic material containing the therapeutic human gene into the target cell.
    - Generation of a functional protein product from the therapeutic gene restores the target cell to a normal state.
    - Besides virus-mediated gene delivery systems, the nonviral options for gene delivery include:
      - Direct inoculation of therapeutic gene into target cells—naked DNA (limited value).

- Use of liposomes to carry the therapeutic gene to target cells.
- Use of plasmids to carry the therapeutic gene to target cells.

LIMITATIONS OF VECTORS

- The main limitation of adenoviral vectors is the B-cell-mediated and T-cell-mediated inflammatory responses resulting from an early activation of immune cells. Majority of the human population has been exposed to adenoviral infection and thus has antibodies against different serotypes.
- Other disadvantages of adenoviruses are their short-term expression and difficult or limited transduction of the cells.
- Important limitations of retroviral vectors include low vector titre, low transfection efficiency in in vitro experiments, particle instability and inability to transduce nondividing postmitotic cells. Therefore, the retroviral vectors are more suitable for ex vivo gene therapy.

RISKS

- Potential for vectors producing disease by recombining with other viruses or getting activated by genes of host.
- May induce cancers when the vector and the genes to be transferred act together on a nearby proto-oncogene present in host.
- Genes that have been transferred (transgenes) can produce some risks after a long latency. Continuous, lifelong exposure to transgenes or vectors increases the probability of subtle toxic properties becoming manifest over the long term.
- Immune overreactions can occur producing serious effects including autoimmunity and death.
- Leukaemia has been reported in treated patients.

THERAPEUTIC APPLICATIONS

- At present, gene therapy is approved for very few diseases.
  - Axicabtagene ciloleucel—a chimeric antigen receptor-T-cell (CAR-T) therapy to treat adult patients with certain types of large B-cell lymphoma who have not responded to or who have relapsed after at least two other kinds of treatment. Patient's T cells are collected and genetically modified to include a new gene that targets and kills the lymphoma cells.
  - Tisagenlecleucel—another CAR-T therapy to treat certain category of patients with B-cell acute lymphocytic leukaemia.
  - Voretigene neparvovec-rzyl for treating some patients with congenital retinal degenerative disorder, Leber's congenital amaurosis 2.
- Onasemnogene abeparvovec-xioi for treating children below the age of 2 years with spinal muscular atrophy.
- Idecabtagene vicleucel, CAR-T-cell-based therapy for adult patients with multiple myeloma who have not responded to, or whose disease has relapsed after at least four prior lines of therapy.
- Trials are going on for using gene therapy in the treatment of various genetic disorders, cancers, infectious diseases, and other diseases like Alzheimer's disease and atherosclerosis.

15 Disturbances in Water, Electrolyte and Acid–Base Balance

Q. Give an account of the normal distribution of water in the body of an average adult male.

- Body water accounts for about 60% of the total body weight in males and 50% in females. Thus, a healthy 65-kg male has about 40 L of water.
- The body water can be divided into two main compartments:
  - Extracellular compartment that contains 25%–40% of total water. This is called extracellular fluid (ECF).
  - Intracellular compartment that contains 60%–75% of total water. This is called intracellular fluid (ICF).
- The extracellular compartment can be further divided into:
  - Vascular compartment.
  - Interstitial compartment in a ratio of 1:3.
- The distribution of body water in a 65-kg male can be represented as given in the Flowchart 15.1.

Q. Define ions, anions and cations. Name the important anions and cations in the human body.

- Ion is an atom or group of atoms with an electrical charge.

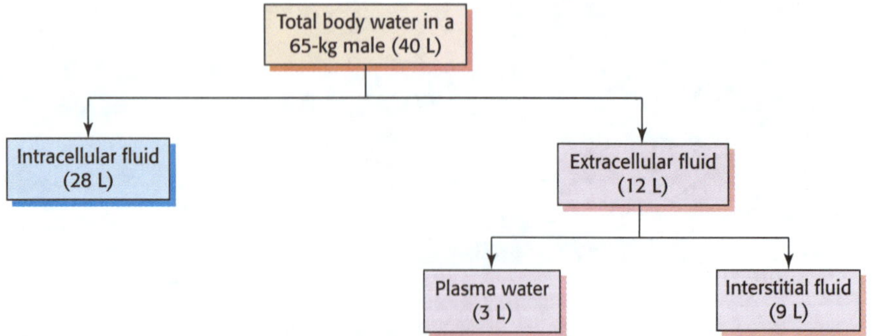

Flowchart 15.1 Distribution of Body Water in a 65-kg Male.

TABLE 15.1 Values of Various Electrolytes and Other Parameters in Blood

Investigation	Normal Range	Investigation	Normal Range
• Sodium (serum)	136–145 mmol/L	• Magnesium (serum)	2–3 mg/dL
• Potassium (serum)	3.5–5 mmol/L	• pH of blood	7.38–7.44
• Chloride (serum)	98–106 mmol/L	• Bicarbonate (blood)	22–26 mmol/L
• Calcium (plasma)	9–10.5 mg/dL	• Osmolality (serum)	285–295 mOsm/kg water
• Phosphorus (serum)	3–4.5 mg/dL		

- Anion is a negatively charged ion. Examples of anions are bicarbonate (HCO_3^-), chloride (Cl^-), phosphates, sulphates, organic acids and proteins.
- Cation is a positively charged ion. Examples of cations are sodium (Na^+), potassium (K^+), calcium (Ca^{2+}) and magnesium (Mg^{2+}).

Q. What are the principal electrolytes in the fluid compartments?

Q. Specify the range of normal values of common electrolytes, pH and osmolality of blood.

- Sodium (Na^+) and chloride (Cl^-) are the principal electrolytes in the ECF compartment.
- Potassium (K^+) and phosphate are the principal electrolytes in the ICF compartment.
- Normal values of various electrolytes and other parameters are given in Table 15.1.
- Osmolality is measured by an instrument called osmometer.
- Osmolarity (mOsm/L) can also be calculated by the following formula:

$$2 \times \text{sodium} + \frac{\text{blood urea nitrogen (mg/dL)}}{2.8} + \frac{\text{blood glucose (mg/dL)}}{18}$$

Q. What do you understand by anion gap? Enumerate a few conditions associated with increased anion gap.

- Anion gap or delta (Δ) denotes the concentration of the unmeasured anions in the plasma—namely phosphates, sulphates, organic acids and protein anions.
- The following formula can be used to calculate the anion gap:

$$\text{Anion gap} = Na^+ - (Cl^- + HCO_3^-)$$

- The normal anion gap is 10–12 mmol/L.
- An increased anion gap is usually seen in some forms of metabolic acidosis. A few examples are given in Box 15.1 and can be remembered by the mnemonic MUDPILES.
- Reduced anion gap is seen in lithium and bromide intoxications, and multiple myeloma.

BOX 15.1 Causes of Elevated Anion Gap

- **M**etformin, **m**ethanol poisoning
- **U**raemic acidosis
- **D**iabetic ketoacidosis
- **P**aracetamol poisoning
- **I**ron, **I**soniazid poisoning
- **L**actic acidosis
- **E**thylene glycol poisoning
- **S**alicylate poisoning

Q. Describe the causes, clinical features, laboratory features and treatment of volume depletion.

- It represents combined water and sodium deficits particularly from extracellular space.
- The term 'dehydration' should be used to define relatively pure water deficit (hypernatraemia).
- Symptoms of pure water loss arise from the effects of increased osmolality and reflect the cellular responses to hypertonicity: confusion, thirst, impaired sensorium and, in more extreme cases, coma or seizures. In contrast, clinical symptoms of volume depletion are a result of the haemodynamic effects of the reduction in intravascular volume and usually do not involve neurological changes.

CAUSES (Table 15.2)

TABLE 15.2 Causes of Volume Depletion

Extrarenal Losses	Renal Losses

• GI losses
  • Vomiting
  • Diarrhoea
  • Gastric aspiration
• Sequestration in the abdomen
  • Peritonitis
  • Intestinal obstruction
• Loss from skin
  • Excessive sweating
  • Burns
• Severe haemorrhage
	• Excessive use of diuretics
	  • Osmotic diuresis
	  • Glycosuria as seen in uncontrolled diabetes
	  • Excessive use of mannitol
	• Renal diseases
	  • Salt-wasting tubular diseases
	  • Diuretic phase of acute renal failure
	  • Chronic renal failure
	• Deficiency of mineralocorticoids
	  • Addison's disease

CLINICAL FEATURES

- The important clinical findings of volume depletion are fatigue, postural dizziness, muscle cramps, dry skin and mucous membranes, reduced or absent tears, reduced skin turgor, tachycardia, shock, delayed

capillary refill (>2 seconds), depressed fontanelles (in infants) and altered mental status.
- In patients with extrarenal losses, the urine output is reduced.
- In massive fluid loss, abdominal pain and chest pain can occur due to mesenteric and coronary ischaemia, respectively.
- Features may also be due to associated loss of electrolytes. These include:
  - Muscle weakness, polyuria and polydipsia due to hypokalaemia
  - Tachypnoea due to acidosis
  - Lethargy, confusion, seizures and coma due to hyponatraemia or hypernatraemia.

DEGREE OF VOLUME LOSS (Table 15.3)

TABLE 15.3 Degree of Volume Depletion

Features	Mild	Moderate	Severe
• Thirst	Drinks normally, not thirsty	Thirsty	Drinks poorly
• Pulse	Normal	Increased (100–120/minute)	>120/minute, thready
• Blood pressure	Normal	Normal to low	Low; unrecordable
• Capillary refill	Normal	2–3 seconds	>3 seconds
• Skin turgor	Fold of pinched skin returns to normal immediately	Takes 1–2 seconds to return to normal	Takes >2 seconds to return to normal
• Mucous membranes (test mouth with a clean finger)	Moist	Dry	Extremely dry
• Eyes	Normal	Normal to mildly sunken	Sunken
• Tears	Normal	Reduced	Absent
• Urine output	Normal	Reduced	Little or none
• Fontanelle (in infants)	Flat	Soft	Depressed
• Estimated fluid loss	<50 mL/kg	50–90 mL/kg	>100 mL/kg

LABORATORY FEATURES

- Sodium concentration is normal, reduced or elevated depending on the proportion of loss between water and sodium.
- Blood urea is often raised particularly in severe volume depletion. This leads to elevated urea/creatinine ratio to more than 40:1.
- Urinary sodium is important in differentiating renal from extrarenal losses. In renal and adrenal causes, urinary sodium is usually more than 20 mEq/L while it is less than 10 mEq/L in extrarenal losses.
- Mild metabolic acidosis is common and occurs due to following mechanisms: (i) bicarbonate loss in stool, (ii) ketone production from starvation, (iii) lactic acid production from decreased tissue perfusion and (iv) reduced renal perfusion leading to decreased glomerular filtration rate which, in turn, leads to decreased hydrogen ion excretion. On the other hand, patients with recurrent vomiting will often have metabolic alkalosis.
- Ultrasound imaging is useful in initial differential diagnosis of hypotension when cause is not obvious on clinical evaluation (RUSH protocol—Rapid Ultrasound for Shock and Hypotension).

TREATMENT

- Mild-to-moderate volume depletion is often due to gastroenteritis. This should be corrected by increasing oral intake of sodium and water, usually in the form of an oral rehydration solution.
- In severe cases, administer 1–2 L of intravenous fluids, usually as normal saline or Ringer's lactate as rapidly as possible in an attempt to restore tissue perfusion. Clinical parameters including heart rate, blood pressure, urine output, skin turgor, mucus membrane integrity and mental status should be continuously followed during fluid replacement to assess the efficacy of volume replacement.
- Volume restoration is sufficient to correct metabolic acidosis as it increases the excretion of hydrogen ions in the urine.

CHOICE OF INTRAVENOUS FLUID REPLACEMENT

- For patients with shock due to volume depletion, replacement can be done by three categories of fluids: crystalloids (normal saline, balanced solutions including Ringer's lactate and others), colloids (albumin, starch, dextran and gelatin) and blood products.
- When volume depletion is due to blood loss, blood components should be replaced as soon as feasible following initial resuscitation with fluids.
- When severe volume depletion is not due to bleeding, crystalloids are usually preferred over colloids. Among the crystalloids, normal saline is the most commonly used solution for initial management as balanced solutions have not been shown to be superior to normal saline particularly when volumes less than 2 L are infused.

- Since normal saline is hyperchloraemic to plasma, infusion of large volume may produce hyperchloraemic metabolic acidosis.

Q. What is hyponatraemia? Discuss its pathophysiology, causes, clinical features and treatment. (IM 22.5)

- Hyponatraemia indicates that the body fluids are diluted by excess of water relative to total solute and is defined as serum sodium <135 mEq/L.

PATHOPHYSIOLOGY

- Most often, hyponatraemia is associated with a low serum osmolality (<280 mOsm/kg—hypotonicity) caused by either retention of water or loss of sodium.
- In some cases, hyponatraemia occurs due to the accumulation of solutes in the ECF (mannitol and glucose) where the osmolality is increased (>295 mOsm/kg).
- Isotonic hyponatraemia (serum osmolarity of 280–295 mOsm/kg) occurs with hypertriglyceridaemia, hyperglobulinaemia and hyperproteinaemia (>10 g/dL).
- Normally, a slight reduction in serum sodium results in suppression of antidiuretic hormone (ADH) due to reduction in osmolality that causes excretion of dilute urine, thereby normalising sodium. However, maintenance of hyponatraemia occurs because of the following factors:
  - Excessive ingestion of water.
  - Reduced excretion of water by the kidneys due to renal failure.
  - Reduced excretion of water by kidneys due to inappropriate release of ADH (syndrome of inappropriate antidiuretic hormone secretion [SIADH]) or increased sensitivity to ADH.
  - Reduced renal excretion of water due to slow urine flow in the collecting tubules. This may occur if there is enhanced proximal tubular reabsorption of salt and water (as in congestive heart failure [CHF] and cirrhosis of liver) that limits delivery of urine to the collecting tubules and because the volume is low, urine flows so slowly that it gets further concentrated without ADH requirement.

EFFECTS OF HYPONATRAEMIA ON BRAIN

- Within minutes after the development of hypotonicity, water enters the brain causing its swelling and reduced osmolality.
- The brain volume is partially restored within a few hours due to loss of electrolytes from the brain cells. This is the rapid adaptation.
- Within the next several days, the brain volume is normalised due to loss of organic compounds from the brain cells. This is the slow adaptation.
- Due to loss of solutes, the brain osmolality is low. Slow correction of hypotonicity produces gradual rise in brain osmolality without any risk. However, rapid correction of hyponatraemia produces loss of brain water resulting in brain damage.

CAUSES (Table 15.4)

TABLE 15.4 Causes of Hyponatraemia

Hyponatraemia with Low Osmolality	Hyponatraemia with Raised Osmolality

• Reduced effective blood volume
• Increased ECF volume (oedema states)
  • CHF
  • Nephrotic syndrome
  • Cirrhosis of liver
• Reduced ECF volume (no oedema)
  • Renal loss of sodium (diuretics, ketonuria, Addison's disease)
  • Extrarenal sodium loss (sweating, vomiting, diarrhoea, peritonitis, pancreatitis)
• Normal or increased effective blood volume
  • Syndrome of inappropriate secretion of ADH (SIADH)
  • Primary polydipsia
  • Chronic renal failure
  • Hypothyroidism
	• Hyperglycaemia
	• Mannitol administration
	Hyponatraemia with Normal Osmolality
	• Hypertriglyceridaemia
	• Hyperproteinaemia (e.g. multiple myeloma and intravenous administration of immunoglobulin)

CLINICAL FEATURES

- Hyponatraemia per se does not produce any significant clinical features. It causes decrease in cellular osmolality that is responsible for various features.
- These include muscle cramps, weakness and fatigue, mental confusion, disorientation, coma and convulsions.
- Speed of development and severity of hyponatraemia determine its clinical significance.

DIFFERENTIAL DIAGNOSIS (Flowchart 15.2)

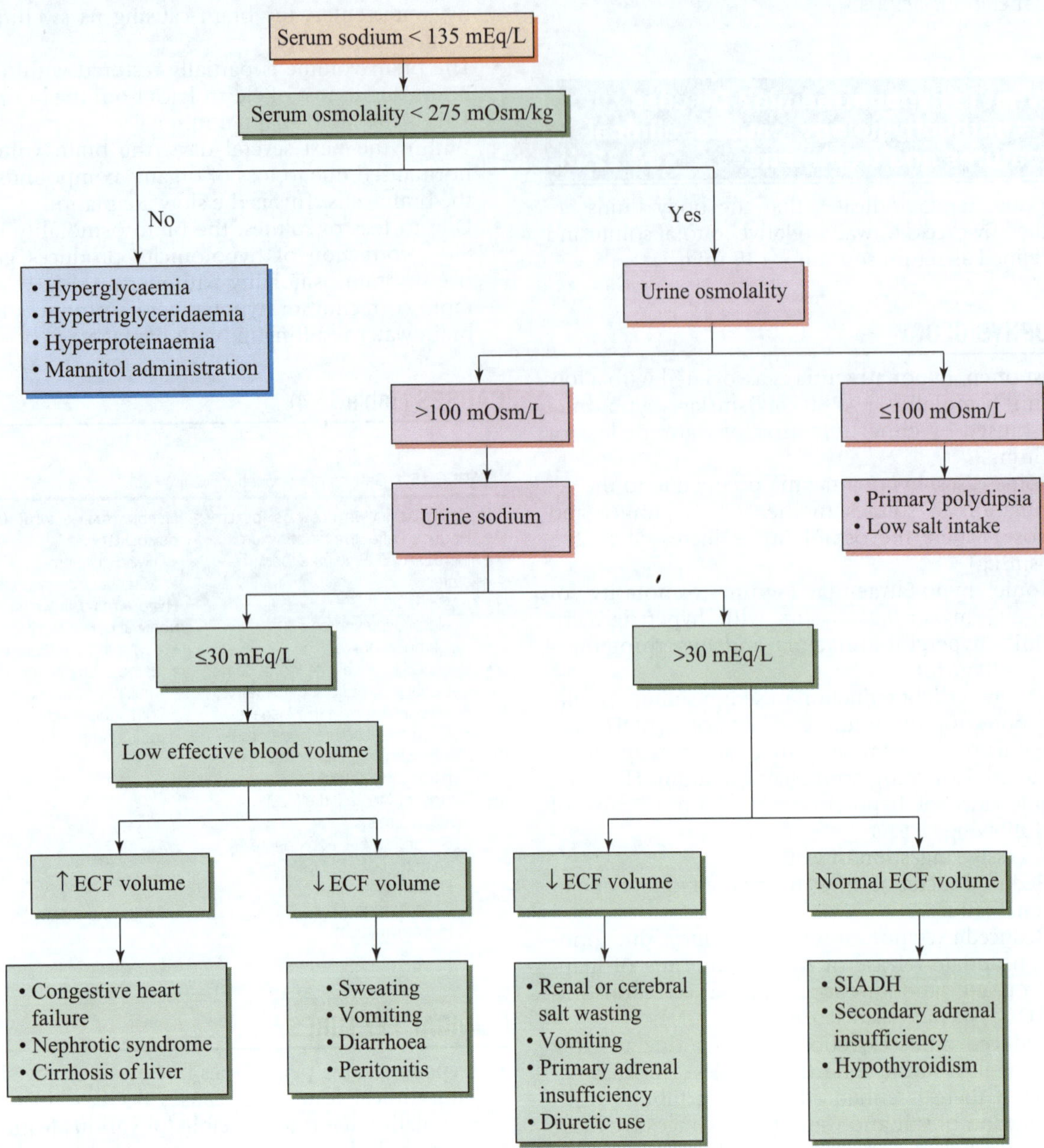

Flowchart 15.2 Differential Diagnosis of Hyponatraemia.

TREATMENT

- The most important dangers of rapid correction of hyponatraemia are vascular overload, shrinkage of brain (if the brain volume has already been normalised through the loss of organic acids) and central pontine myelinolysis (CPM). The latter is characterised by quadriplegia (secondary to corticospinal tract involvement) with dysarthria and dysphagia (secondary to corticobulbar fibre involvement) with varying levels of consciousness. Some patients may develop extrapontine myelinolysis (EPM) characterised by mutism, parkinsonism, dystonia and catatonia. The term osmotic demyelination syndrome includes both CPM and EPM.
- The rate of correction of hyponatraemia in a symptomatic patient should be around 0.6 mEq/L/hour. In severely symptomatic patients, it can be 4–6 mEq/L over 2–4 hours but total correction in a day should not exceed 8–10 mEq/L. This is achieved using hypertonic 3% saline.
- When slow correction of hyponatraemia in a volume-expanded subject is desired, it is best to restrict salt and fluids and add loop diuretics. In patients with CHF, vaptans may be added.

- In patients with normal effective blood volume, fluid restriction is the mainstay of treatment. Vaptans may be added if required.
- In patients with reduced ECF volume, priority is to restore intravascular volume by infusing normal saline.

HYPERTONIC SALINE

- For severely symptomatic hyponatraemia in the form of seizures, altered mental status or coma, 3% hypertonic saline solution (sodium concentration = 513 mEq/L) is required and 100 mL is given over a period of 10–15 minutes. If symptoms persist, additional two boluses of 100 mL are given, each over 10 minutes. The goal of therapy is to rapidly increase the serum sodium by 4 to 6 mEq/L over a period of a few hours.
- For moderately symptomatic patients who require hypertonic saline, infusion rate should not exceed 1–1.5 mL/kg/hour and it should not be generally given for more than 3–4 hours. A total of 1.2 mL/kg of hypertonic saline will raise sodium by about 1 mEq/L.
  - For patients with chronic hyponatraemia (>48 hours), the rate of correction should not exceed 0.5 mEq/L/hour.
  - For acute cases, the rate of correction may be 1 mEq/L/hour initially.
- Sodium levels are rechecked hourly until sodium has increased by 4–6 mEq/L.

VASOPRESSIN V2-RECEPTOR ANTAGONISTS (VAPTANS)

- Vasopressin V2-receptor antagonists promote aquaresis—excretion of electrolyte-free water. These include tolvaptan, conivaptan, satavaptan and lixivaptan.
- Found to be useful in chronic euvolaemic hyponatraemia not responsive to fluid restriction; also useful in CHF.
- Side effects include increased urine flow and thirst, and dry mouth; can produce liver toxicity.
- Intravenous agent is conivaptan that can be used in euvolaemic or hypervolaemic patients with hyponatraemia. It is both V1 and V2-receptor antagonists.
- Tolvaptan is also approved for the treatment of rapidly progressive autosomal dominant polycystic kidney disease in adults.

Q. Give a brief account of syndrome of inappropriate antidiuretic hormone secretion. (IM 22.5)

- Also known as syndrome of inappropriate antidiuresis (SIAD).
- Hypotonicity of the ECF normally shuts off the secretion of ADH. In SIADH, the secretion of ADH may continue 'inappropriately' despite hypotonicity of the ECF. Therefore, hyponatraemia occurs due to excessive water retention.
- The cardinal features of SIADH are given in Box 15.2.

BOX 15.2 Features of SIADH

- Plasma osmolality <270 mOsm/kg
- Evidence of inappropriate urinary concentration (urine osmolality >100 mOsm/kg)
- Clinical euvolaemia
- Serum urea and creatinine are normal or low
- Elevated plasma sodium (>30 mmol/L) with normal salt intake
- Hypothyroidism and hypoadrenalism excluded

CAUSES (Table 15.5)

TABLE 15.5 Causes of SIADH

• Pulmonary causes	Small cell carcinoma, pneumonia, tuberculosis, COPD, acute respiratory failure
• CNS causes	Meningitis, encephalitis, tumours, head injury, stroke, subdural haematoma, brain abscess, subarachnoid haemorrhage, head trauma, Guillain–Barré syndrome
• Drugs	Chlorpropamide, tolbutamide, vincristine, cyclophosphamide, carbamazepine, clozapine, phenothiazines, tricyclic antidepressants, SSRIs, amiodarone
• Others	Head and neck cancers, postoperative state, HIV infection

CLINICAL FEATURES

- Clinical features include nausea, irritability, confusion, seizures and coma. There is no oedema.

TREATMENT

- The underlying cause should be corrected.
- Fluid intake should be restricted to 500–1000 mL/day.
- Demeclocycline (ADH antagonist) may be given at a dose of 600–1200 mg/day. Other useful agents include vaptans, lithium and urea.
- Slow infusion of hypertonic saline and frusemide may be rarely required in severe hyponatraemia.
- Isotonic saline should not be administered to correct hyponatraemia. Water will be retained because of the persistent action of ADH while sodium is excreted in the urine, worsening hyponatraemia.
- Rapid correction of slow-onset hyponatraemia may produce central pontine myelinolysis.

Q. Describe primary water depletion or hypernatraemia or dehydration. (IM 22.6)

- An elevation in the serum sodium concentration >145 mEq/L.

PATHOPHYSIOLOGY

- Hypernatraemia is much less common than hyponatraemia because even a small increase in the serum sodium concentration is a potent stimulus to thirst.

- Elevated sodium concentration develops in those patients who are unable to experience thirst or are unable to gain access to water.

EFFECTS OF HYPERNATRAEMIA ON BRAIN

- Within minutes after the development of hypertonicity, brain cells lose water causing shrinkage of the brain and an increase in osmolality.
- Rapid adaptation occurs within a few hours as electrolytes enter the brain cells causing partial increase in brain volume.
- Over several days, the brain volume becomes normal due to intracellular accumulation of organic compounds.
- Slow correction of the hypertonic state does not induce cerebral oedema as the accumulated solutes are gradually shifted out of the brain cells.
- In contrast, rapid correction may result in cerebral oedema as brain uptakes water from the relatively hypotonic ECF.

CAUSES (Table 15.6)

TABLE 15.6 Causes of Hypernatraemia

• Decreased intake	Coma, depression, inability to swallow, severe dementia
• Increased loss from skin	Fever, hyperthyroidism, hot environment, burns
• Increased respiratory loss	Hyperventilation
• Increased loss in urine	Diabetes insipidus (central and nephrogenic), medullary cystic disease, recovery from acute tubular necrosis, intravenous diuretics
• Increased GI losses	Severe diarrhoea, prolonged vomiting
• Iatrogenic	Inadvertent administration of hypertonic saline, administration of hypertonic sodium bicarbonate solution in patients with metabolic acidosis

CLINICAL FEATURES AND INVESTIGATIONS

- Clinical features of hypernatraemia are due to increased osmolality and are same as those of diabetic hyperosmolar state.
- Various clinical features and relevant investigations are listed in Table 15.7.

URINE OSMOLALITY

- Urine osmolality should be measured in all patients with hypernatraemia as it may help determine the underlying aetiology (Table 15.8).

MANAGEMENT

- In patients with gradual onset of water depletion over more than 2 days, correction should be done slowly as rapid lowering of sodium produces shift of water from ECF into brain cells. The rate of correction should not exceed 0.7 mEq/L/hour and not to exceed 8–10 mEq/L/day.

TABLE 15.7 Clinical Features and Investigations in Hypernatraemia

Clinical Features	Investigations
• Marked thirst	• Haematocrit usually >50%
• Muscle weakness, rigidity	• Raised blood urea levels
• Dry mouth	• Raised plasma sodium
• Mental confusion, coma, seizures	• Urine specific gravity >1.010
• Intracranial haemorrhage (in acute hypernatraemia)	• Polyuria and urine specific gravity <1.010 in diabetes insipidus
• Tachycardia and low systolic blood pressure	• Urine osmolality

TABLE 15.8 Aetiology of Hypernatraemia Based on Urine Osmolality

Urine Osmolality	Possible Aetiology
Lower than plasma (<150 mOsm/kg)	Diabetes insipidus
Higher than plasma (>500 mOsm/kg)	Increased GI, skin or respiratory losses
Nearly same as plasma	Increased losses in urine

- In patients with acute onset, symptomatic hyponatraemia, rate of correction can be 1 mEq/L/hour for the first 4–6 hours.
- When hypernatraemia is associated with hypotension due to volume depletion, the initial solution should be isotonic saline so as to increase the ECF volume. However, if neurological features are also present, therapy should be started with N/2 saline.
- Calculation of free water deficit:
  - Free water deficit is calculated as follows:

$$\text{Total body water} \times \left(\frac{\text{Plasma sodium concentration}}{140}\right) - 1$$

  - In general, 50% of this calculated deficit is given over the first 24 hours and the remaining over the next 24 hours. Insensible losses (10 mL/kg/day) and urine output are added to it.
- As a rough guide, Box 15.3 shows the requirement of fluids in a 65-kg person.
- Relief of thirst, urine output more than 1500 mL/24 hours and normal plasma sodium levels indicate adequate correction.

BOX 15.3 Requirement of Fluids in a 65-kg Person With Hypernatraemia

Severity	Fluid and Route of Administration	Quantity and Time for Replacement
• Mild depletion (1–2 L deficit)	Water by mouth or 5% glucose IV	2 L, over 6–12 hours
• Moderate (2–4 L deficit)	5% glucose IV	2–4 L, over 24 hours
• Severe (4–10 L deficit)	0.9% NaCl IV 5% dextrose IV 5% dextrose IV	1 L, over 1 hour 3 L, over 2 hours 4 L, over 24–48 hours

Q. What are the common causes of generalised oedema?

Q. Discuss the mechanism of oedema formation. How will you differentiate between cardiac, renal and hepatic oedema?

- Sodium and water excess results in a state of generalised oedema.
- Various causes of oedema are shown in Box 15.4.

PATHOGENESIS

- Oedema occurs when there is an imbalance between forces causing filtration of fluid and those causing absorption of fluid resulting in net filtration.

BOX 15.4 Causes of Generalised Oedema

• CHF • Nephrotic syndrome • Hepatic cirrhosis • Acute glomerulonephritis • Hypothyroidism	• Acute kidney injury • Chronic kidney disease • Pregnancy • Protein-losing enteropathy • Chronic venous insufficiency	• Severe malnutrition • Drugs—oestrogens, NSAIDs, corticosteroids, vasodilators, calcium channel blockers (e.g. amlodipine), pioglitazone, insulins

Note: Amlodipine generally produces pedal oedema.

- It may be due to an elevation in capillary hydraulic pressure, an increase in capillary permeability or an increase in interstitial oncotic pressure, or due to a reduction in plasma oncotic pressure.
- Kidneys have a central role in maintaining body fluid homoeostasis. They control ECF volume by adjusting sodium and water excretion.
- ADH, which is secreted in response to stimuli such as changes in blood volume, tonicity and blood pressure, is the primary regulator of body water.
- Effective arterial blood volume (EABV) correlates with ECF volume. It is sensed by volume homoeostatic mechanisms that change renal sodium reabsorption.
- In healthy persons, sodium loading increases ECF volume and EABV resulting in prompt natriuresis and restoration of normal volumes.
- In persons who are volume depleted, EABV and ECF volume are reduced which activates renin–angiotensin–aldosterone system resulting in renal sodium retention and restoration of normal blood volume.
- In oedematous states, there is reduction in EABV which activates sympathetic nervous system, renin–angiotensin–aldosterone axis and ADH secretion. Because of these compensatory mechanisms, oedema persists.
- Pathogenesis of oedema in the commonly encountered clinical conditions like CHF, nephrotic syndrome and hepatic cirrhosis is discussed.

PATHOGENESIS OF OEDEMA IN HEART FAILURE (CARDIAC OEDEMA) (Flowchart 15.3)

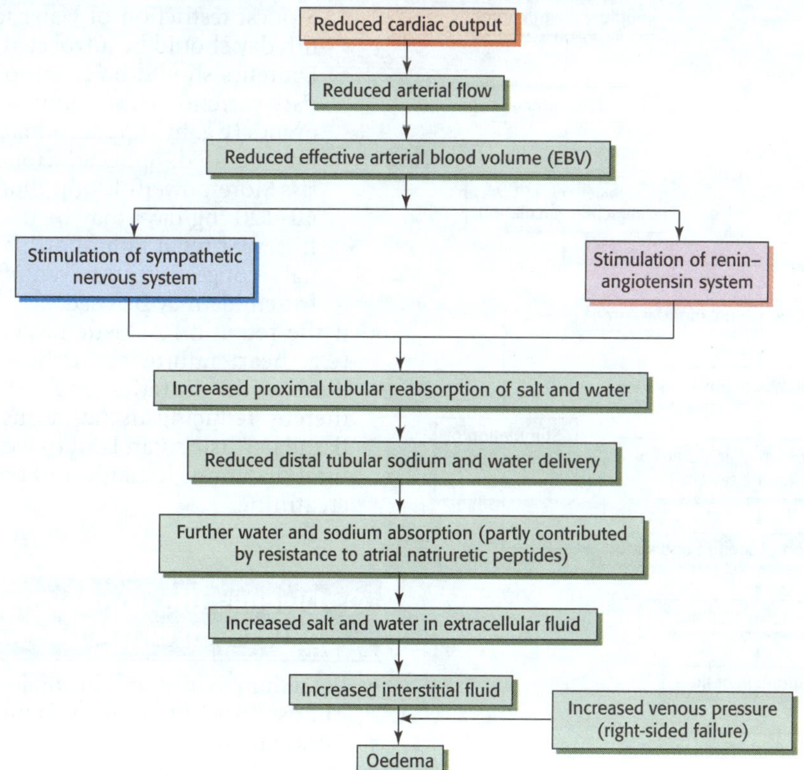

Flowchart 15.3 Pathogenesis of Oedema in Heart Failure.

PATHOGENESIS OF OEDEMA IN NEPHROTIC SYNDROME (RENAL OEDEMA) (Flowchart 15.4)

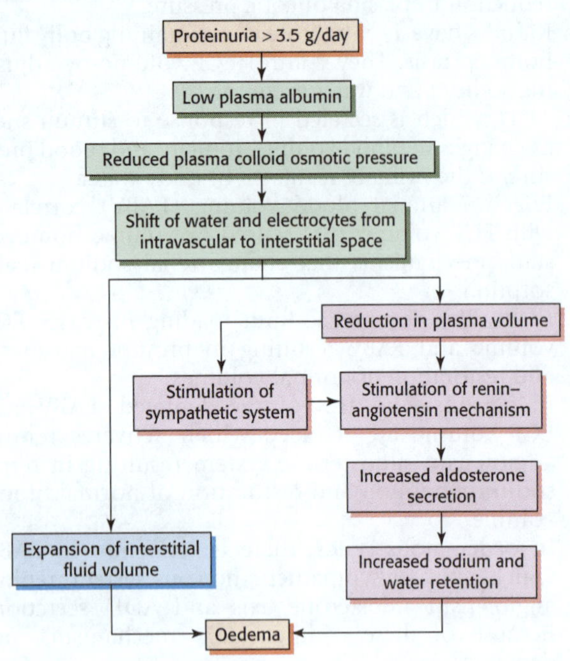

Flowchart 15.4 Pathogenesis of Oedema in Nephrotic Syndrome.

PATHOGENESIS OF OEDEMA IN HEPATIC CIRRHOSIS (HEPATIC OEDEMA) (Flowchart 15.5)

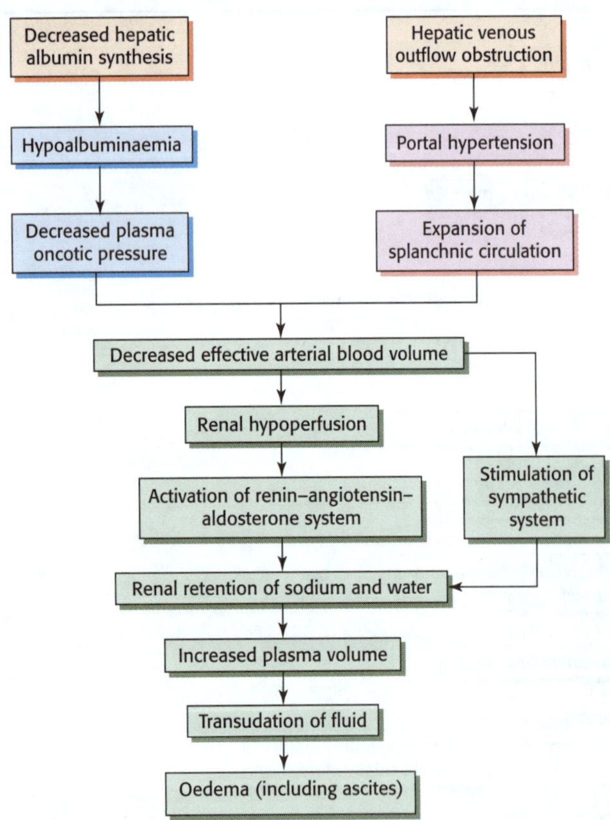

Flowchart 15.5 Pathogenesis of Oedema in Cirrhosis of Liver.

Note: Ascites in cirrhosis of liver can also occur secondary to hepatic lymph weeping from the surface of the liver as a result of obstruction of the lymphatics by distorted hepatic architecture.

CLINICAL FEATURES

- Cardiac oedema accumulates over dependent parts. In ambulant patients, it occurs symmetrically in the legs, particularly in the pretibial region and around the ankles. It is less in the morning and more towards the evening. Oedema is sacral in bedridden patients.
- Oedema of renal origin is classically identified by puffiness of the face, particularly around the periorbital region.
- In oedema of hepatic origin, the accumulation of fluid is predominantly manifested as ascites.

MANAGEMENT

- Treatment may be divided into primary and secondary.
- Primary treatment is directed at eliminating the cause of the problem, for example improvement of cardiac function and correction of hypoalbuminaemia.
- Secondary treatment is mainly concerned with correcting the salt and water overload. They include the following measures:
  - Restriction in sodium intake—dietary sodium should be restricted to about 50–100 mmol/day. A 'no added salt diet', allowing salt only in cooking, with no addition of salt at table and avoidance of salty food is generally satisfactory.
  - Modest restriction of water intake to about 1000 mL/day should be advocated.
  - Diuretics should be given to increase rate of urinary excretion of sodium and water. Thiazide diuretics (e.g. hydrochlorothiazide 50–100 mg/day) may be used. Spironolactone is useful in cirrhosis. More powerful loop diuretics (e.g. frusemide 40–120 mg/day) may be used in severe oedema. In severe renal failure or life-threatening pulmonary congestion, intravenous nitroglycerine and frusemide may be used.
- If the retention of oedema fluid is compensatory (e.g. heart failure or cirrhosis), removal of this fluid with diuretics may diminish the EABV, thereby reducing tissue perfusion. The decline in tissue perfusion can lead to weakness, fatigue, postural dizziness, lethargy and rise in serum urea and creatinine.

Q. Discuss the normal physiology of potassium in the body.

- Potassium is one of the major electrolytes of ICF. Almost 98% of potassium is present in ICF.
- Concentration in ECF varies between 3.5 and 5 mEq/L.
- Potassium is abundant in meat, oranges, lemon, grapes, bananas and dry fruits.

PHYSIOLOGY

- Potassium is the principal intracellular cation (ICF concentration is 150–160 mEq/L) and the concentration gradient between ECF and ICF is maintained by the Na^+–K^+-stimulated ATPase system.
- ECF potassium greatly influences the neuromuscular function, as the latter is dependent on the ratio of ICF to ECF potassium. As ECF potassium concentration is low, a small change in ECF potassium produces large change in this ratio and hence influences the excitability of the tissue. On the other hand, only a large change in ICF potassium is required to change the ratio significantly.
- For a loss or gain of 100–200 mEq, the plasma potassium reduces or increases by 1 mEq/L, respectively.
- An acute potassium load is actively taken by the tissue but within a few hours, renal excretion of potassium increases. Because of this reason, sustained hyperkalaemia is rarely produced by increased ingestion of potassium.
- On the other hand, renal response of conserving potassium is sluggish when potassium intake is reduced. Excretion does not fall to minimal levels for 1–2 weeks and during this period of gradual renal adaptation, around 200 mEq of potassium may be lost from the body.
- Renal excretion of potassium is mainly by secretion at the level of distal tubules and collecting ducts as filtered potassium is almost completely reabsorbed proximally. This secretion is influenced by aldosterone levels, distal tubular urine flow rate, acid–base status and potassium concentration of tubular cells.
  - In hyperkalaemia, potassium secretion is stimulated directly due to increased potassium concentration in the tubular cell and indirectly by increased aldosterone secretion.
  - Administration of loop diuretics enhances distal fluid flow that increases potassium secretion.
  - Acidosis reduces tubular secretion of potassium while alkalosis stimulates it.
- Metabolic changes influence the distribution of potassium in the body. Acidosis causes shift of potassium from ICF to ECF while alkalosis produces opposite effect.
- Insulin produces shift of potassium into ICF.

Q. What are the causes of hypokalaemia? Give a brief account of the clinical features, ECG manifestations and management of hypokalaemia. (IM 22.7)

- Hypokalaemia is defined as serum potassium <3.5 mEq/L.

CAUSES (Table 15.9)

- Common drugs producing hypokalaemia include thiazides, loop diuretics and amphotericin B.

TABLE 15.9 Causes of Hypokalaemia

• Loss from GI tract	Vomiting, diarrhoea, fistulae, villous adenoma, ureterosigmoidostomy, intestinal obstruction, laxatives
• Loss in urine	Primary and secondary hyperaldosteronism, Cushing's syndrome, renal tubular acidosis, diuretics, hypomagnesaemia, drugs, Fanconi's syndrome
• Intracellular shift of K^+	Alkalosis, high-dose insulin, periodic paralysis, beta-agonists (salbutamol, terbutaline)
• Reduced intake	Diet containing inadequate K^+, potassium-free IV fluids

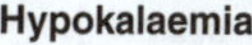

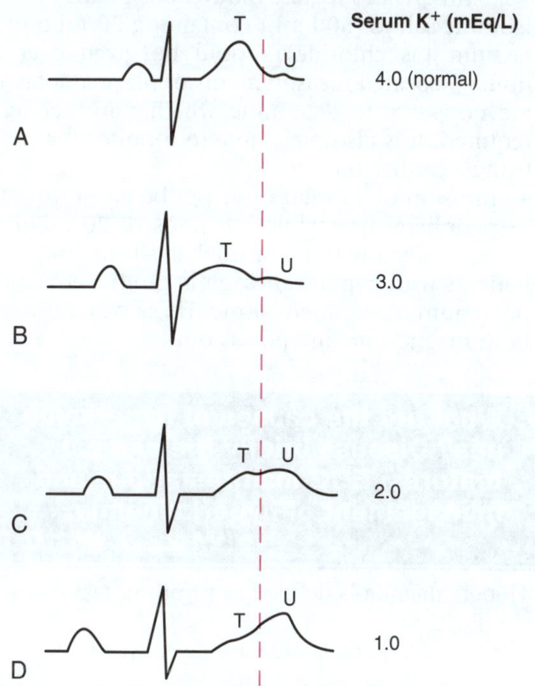

Fig. 15.1 (A–D) Waveforms comparing amplitude of T and U waves with decrease in serum potassium concentrations.

CLINICAL FEATURES

- Generalised muscle weakness and depression of tendon reflexes.
- Paralytic ileus.
- Rhabdomyolysis.
- ECG changes of hypokalaemia include flattening and inversion of T waves, sagging of the ST segment and appearance of U wave. T waves may disappear, leading to apparent prolongation of QT interval (actually QU interval) (Fig. 15.1).
- Atrial and ventricular arrhythmias may occur especially in patients receiving digitalis.
- Death may occur due to respiratory paralysis or cardiac arrest.

TREATMENT

- Treatment must be directed at correcting the hypokalaemia and eliminating the cause of potassium loss.

- Potassium supplementation can be given orally or intravenously in the form of potassium chloride (KCl).
- Patients with mild hypokalaemia with potassium between 3 and 3.5 mEq/L are usually asymptomatic and do not require urgent treatment. These patients should be advised to take a diet rich in potassium.
- Patients with moderate hypokalaemia with potassium between 2.5 and 3 mEq/L should receive oral potassium in a dose of 60–80 mEq/day in divided doses (20 mL of potassium chloride oral solution contains 15 mEq of potassium).
- If a patient cannot tolerate oral potassium or gastrointestinal (GI) losses are massive, intravenous potassium supplementation is required. Patients with symptomatic moderate or severe hypokalaemia with potassium <2.5 mEq/L also require intravenous potassium.
- Isotonic saline (500 mL) containing 20 mEq of potassium (as chloride) should be given over 2–3 hours. Repeated measurements of plasma potassium are necessary to determine whether further KCl is required. It is also preferable to monitor the patient using a cardiac monitor.
  - Infusion of 10 mEq/hour can be given through a peripheral line while infusions of 20 mEq/hour are preferably given through a central line.
- Patients with hypomagnesaemia can be refractory to potassium replacement alone. These patients require both magnesium and potassium.

Q. What are the causes of hyperkalaemia? Discuss briefly the clinical features, ECG manifestations and management of hyperkalaemia. (IM 22.8, IM 10.18)

- Hyperkalaemia is defined as serum potassium above 5 mEq/L.
- Causes of hyperkalaemia are given in Table 15.10.

CLINICAL FEATURES

- The common clinical features include cardiac arrhythmias, muscular weakness progressing to flaccid paralysis and respiratory embarrassment.

TABLE 15.10 Causes of Hyperkalaemia

• Impaired excretion	Acute kidney injury, severe chronic kidney disease, Addison's disease, hypoaldosteronism, type 4 renal tubular acidosis, mineralocorticoid receptor antagonists (spironolactone, eplerenone), potassium-sparing diuretics (amiloride, triamterene), angiotensin-converting enzyme inhibitors, angiotensin receptor blockers, NSAIDs, cyclosporin, tacrolimus, heparin
• Excessive intake	Intravenous fluids containing K^+, high K^+ foods
• Tissue breakdown	Haemolysis, rhabdomyolysis, crush injury, burns, tumour lysis syndrome
• Shift of K^+ out of cell	Acidosis, insulin deficiency, hyperkalaemic periodic paralysis, β-blockers, digitalis poisoning, succinylcholine
• Pseudohyperkalaemia	Haemolysed blood sample, marked thrombocytosis

- Electrocardiographic manifestations of hyperkalaemia are (Fig. 15.2):
  - Tall, peaked T waves.
  - Prolongation of PR interval.
  - Reduced height of P wave.
  - Prolongation of QRS complex.
  - 'Sine wave' pattern.
- Terminally ventricular fibrillation and standstill may occur.

MANAGEMENT

- Identification and elimination of the underlying causes.
- When there are marked ECG changes, 10 mL of 10% calcium gluconate solution is given intravenously slowly over 2–5 minutes. It stabilises the myocardial cell membrane reducing the risk of arrhythmias.
- Intravenous administration of glucose along with insulin encourages shift of potassium from extracellular compartment to intracellular compartment.
  - Fifty millilitres of 50% glucose plus 10 units of soluble (plain) insulin may be given intravenously as a bolus.
  - Alternatively, in moderate hyperkalaemia, 500 mL of 20% glucose plus 10 units of soluble insulin may be given as an infusion over 3–6 hours.
- Intravenous administration of 50–100 mL of 8.4% sodium bicarbonate is useful in renal failure patients with hyperkalaemia and acidosis.
- Nebulisation of β-agonists (salbutamol and terbutaline) also can reduce potassium levels by producing shift of potassium to intracellular compartment. Dose of salbutamol is 10–20 mg over 10 minutes and can be repeated every 2–6 hours.
- Loop diuretics are used commonly in the management of hyperkalaemia, particularly in patients with volume overload associated with heart failure.
- Cation exchange resins such as sodium polystyrene sulphonate are helpful in the removal of K^+. The resins can be given orally or as enema. A serious side effect is colonic necrosis. Other resins are sodium zirconium cyclosilicate (traps potassium in the intestine and exchanges it for sodium and hydrogen) and patiromer (binds potassium in exchange for calcium in the colon).
- If these measures fail, haemodialysis is indicated.

SUMMARY OF MANAGEMENT OF HYPERKALAEMIA

- Table 15.11 summarises the treatment of hyperkalaemia.

Q. Discuss briefly about physiology of acid-base balance.

Q. Describe the various terms used in the assessment of acid–base status of a patient.

NORMAL PHYSIOLOGY

- About 20,000 mmol of carbonic acid (from metabolism of carbohydrates and fats) and 80 mEq of

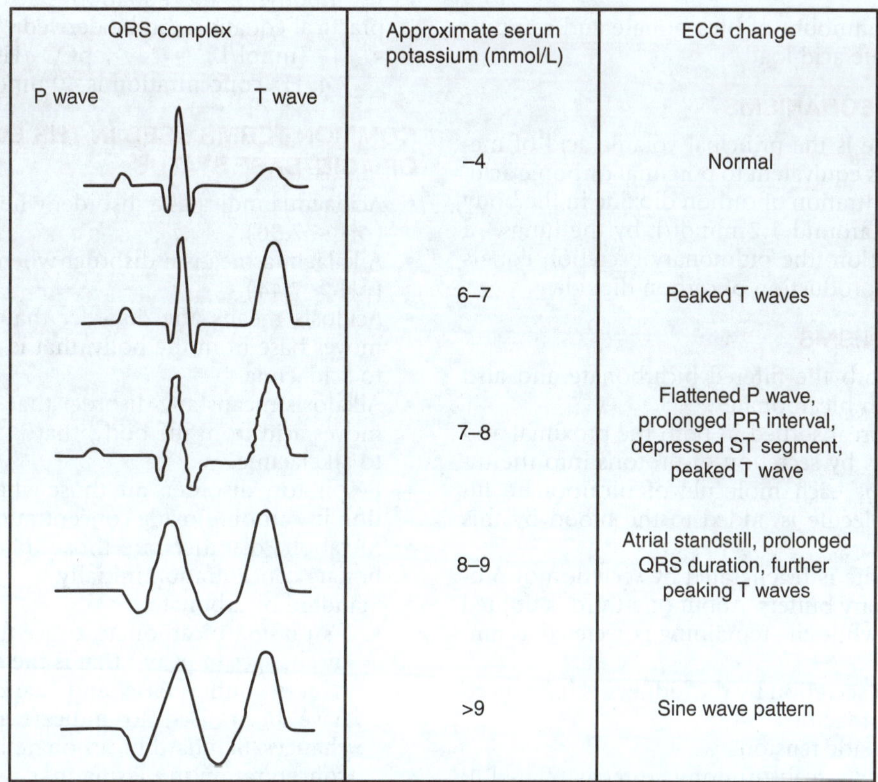

Fig. 15.2 ECG changes in hyperkalaemia.

TABLE 15.11 Summary of Interventions in the Treatment of Hyperkalaemia

Medication/ Intervention	Dosage	Onset	Duration	Comments
• Calcium gluconate	10 mL of 10% solution over 5 minutes	2–3 minutes	30–60 minutes	Stabilises membrane of myocardial cells No effect on serum potassium level
• Hypertonic dextrose with insulin	50 mL of 50% dextrose (25 g) with 10 units of regular insulin IV	15–20 minutes	4–6 hours	Shifts potassium intracellularly
• Sodium bicarbonate	50–100 mEq IV	5–10 minutes	2 hours	Use if patient is acidotic Shifts potassium intracellularly
• Salbutamol	10–20 mg nebulisation over 10 minutes	15–30 minutes	2–3 hours	Shifts potassium intracellularly
• Sodium polystyrene sulphonate	15–30 g orally two to four times a day	1–2 hours	Variable	Exchanges its sodium ions with potassium ions from blood
• Dialysis	—	1–2 minutes after start	Variable	Removes potassium from body

nonvolatile acids (from metabolism of dietary proteins) are produced daily. Despite this, the pH of ECF is maintained between 7.36 and 7.44. The defence against changes in pH is provided by three buffer systems: physiological buffers, pulmonary mechanisms and renal mechanisms.

PHYSIOLOGICAL BUFFERS

Bicarbonate–Carbonic Acid System

- Major physiological buffer.
- Bicarbonate is converted into water and carbon dioxide whenever H^+ ions are added. Carbon dioxide thus liberated is excreted by the lungs.
- Total buffering capacity of this system is about 15 mEq/L, which is sufficient for only 15–20 days. However, kidneys have the ability to regenerate bicarbonate and, therefore, help in maintaining the buffering capacity of the ECF.

Intracellular Proteins

- Haemoglobin is the most important of all intracellular proteins and can buffer large amounts of H^+ ions without disturbing the pH.
- In the red cells, carbon dioxide combines with water to form carbonic acid, which dissociates to produce H^+ ions that are buffered by haemoglobin.

Bone

- Contains large amount of bicarbonate and can buffer parts of acute acid load.

PULMONARY MECHANISMS

- Carbon dioxide is the principal volatile acid of metabolism that is equivalent to potential carbonic acid.
- Normal concentration of carbon dioxide in the body is maintained around 1.2 mmol/L by the lungs. At this concentration, the pulmonary excretion equals the metabolic production of carbon dioxide.

RENAL MECHANISMS

- Kidneys reabsorb the filtered bicarbonate and also regenerate fresh bicarbonate.
- Bicarbonate is reabsorbed in both the proximal and distal segments by secretion of protons into the tubular fluid. For each molecule of bicarbonate filtered, one molecule is added to the blood by this mechanism.
- New bicarbonate is regenerated by secretion of protons onto urinary buffers. About one-third is titrated to phosphate while the remaining is secreted as ammonium.
- Rate of proton secretion by the kidneys is influenced by a number of factors:
  - Carbon dioxide tension:
    - Bicarbonate reabsorption is directly related to the ECF carbon dioxide tension. Hypercapnia stimulates and hypocapnia inhibits renal bicarbonate reabsorption.
  - ECF volume:
    - Contraction of extracellular volume enhances renal bicarbonate reabsorption.
  - Aldosterone levels:
    - Hyperaldosteronism stimulates bicarbonate reabsorption by the kidneys and can lead to alkalosis.
  - Body potassium stores:
    - Severe hyperkalaemia produces increased H^+ secretion and, therefore, produces alkalosis due to increased bicarbonate reabsorption.

EVALUATION OF ACID–BASE STATUS

- This is based on changes in the bicarbonate–carbonic acid system, and is described by the Henderson–Hasselbalch equation:

$$pH = pK_a \times \log \frac{\text{bicarbonate}}{\text{carbonic acid}}$$

  - pK_a is the dissociation constant and for carbonic acid–bicarbonate system, it is 6.1.
  - Carbonic acid can be expressed as dissolved carbon dioxide and equals $\alpha \times pCO_2$, where α represents solubility coefficient and equals 0.031 mmol/L/mmHg of CO_2. At a pCO_2 of 40 mmHg, carbonic acid will be 1.2 mmol/L.
- The arterial blood gas analysers measure the pH and pCO_2 and bicarbonate concentration is calculated using the above-mentioned formula.
- By modifying the equation stated above, a more practical equation can be derived:
  - H^+ (nmol/L) $= 24 \times pCO_2/HCO_3$ (at a pH of 7.4, H^+ concentration is 40 nmol/L).

COMMON TERMS USED IN THE EVALUATION OF ACID–BASE STATUS

- Acidaemia indicates a disorder where pH is deceased ($pH < 7.36$).
- Alkalaemia means a disorder where pH is increased ($pH > 7.44$).
- Acidosis means any disorder that adds acid or removes base from the body, that is processes leading to acidaemia.
- Alkalosis means any disorder that adds alkali or removes acid from the body, that is processes leading to alkalaemia.
- Respiratory disorders are those where there is alteration in carbon dioxide concentration initially.
- Metabolic disorders are those that affect the bicarbonate concentration initially.
- Standard bicarbonate:
  - As plasma bicarbonate concentration is affected by changes in pCO_2, that is the respiratory disturbances, buffer base and standard bicarbonate have been used to indicate purely metabolic changes. Standard bicarbonate is the bicarbonate concentration in plasma in a completely oxygenated blood sample equilibrated with a pCO_2 of 40 mmHg at 37°C. A standard bicarbonate value below 24 mmol/L indicates metabolic acidosis and above 24 mmol/L metabolic alkalosis.
- Buffer base:
  - Represents the total equivalent concentration of all anionic (basic) buffer components of the blood, namely haemoglobin, bicarbonate, plasma proteins and phosphates. It is normally 48 mmol/L.
- Base excess or base deficit:
  - Base excess indicates the deviation of base buffer from its normal value. It can also be defined as the number of millimoles of strong acid that is needed to adjust the pH to 7.4 when blood is equilibrated at a pCO_2 of 40 mmHg. It is calculated from pH, pCO_2 and haemoglobin. An increase in the amount of buffer base is termed base excess while a decrease may be referred to as a base deficit or negative base excess.

Q. Discuss the causes, clinical features and management of metabolic acidosis. (IM 22.9)

- Metabolic acidosis is characterised by a reduction in plasma bicarbonate and a consequent rise in hydrogen ion concentration. The partial pressure of carbon dioxide is reduced secondarily by hyperventilation.
- Anion gap is due to the presence of unmeasured anions like albumin, sulphates, phosphates and organic acids. Increased accumulation of these unmeasured anions leads to acidosis with raised anion gap. In some patients of acidosis, there is an exchange of bicarbonate with chloride leading to loss of bicarbonate

and hyperchloraemia. This leads to a normal anion gap with acidosis.

COMPENSATION

- Compensation to metabolic acidosis is by hyperventilation, which produces hypocapnia.
- Winters' equation can be used to calculate expected carbon dioxide value:
  Expected carbon dioxide = $1.5 \times [HCO_3] + 8 \pm 2$.
- A simpler method is that for every 1 mEq/L fall in bicarbonate, carbon dioxide falls by 1 mmHg.

CAUSES (Table 15.12)

TABLE 15.12 Causes of Metabolic Acidosis

Increased anion gap:
• Severe renal failure
• Increased production of organic acids
• Diabetic ketoacidosis
• Alcoholic ketosis
• Starvation ketosis
• Poisonings: Methanol, salicylates, ethylene glycol, iron, isoniazid, paracetamol, metformin, carbon monoxide, cyanide (latter two cause severe lactic acidosis)
• Increased lactic acid production
• Cardiorespiratory arrest
• Convulsions
• Shock
• Septicaemia
• Liver failure
Normal anion gap (hyperchloraemia):
• Diarrhoea (loss of alkali)
• Laxative overuse
• Potassium-sparing diuretics (renal tubular dysfunction)
• Renal tubular acidosis (type 1, type 2 and type 4)
• Ureterosigmoidostomy
• Ingestion of toxin (ammonium chloride, toluene)
• Infusion of large volumes of normal saline

CLINICAL FEATURES

- In severe cases, there is deep sighing respiration (Kussmaul breathing or 'air hunger').
- Peripheral vasodilatation and reduction in cardiac output may result in a fall in blood pressure.
- Severe acidosis may be associated with drowsiness, confusion and coma.
- Serum bicarbonate is low, blood pH is low and partial pressure of carbon dioxide is low.

DELTA–DELTA GAP

- Calculate delta–delta gap, if metabolic acidosis with an elevated anion gap is present.
- It distinguishes between a pure anion gap metabolic acidosis and a mixed acid–base disorder with both anion gap and nonanion gap acidosis.
- Delta–delta gap is calculated as follows:
  - Delta–delta gap = delta anion gap − delta bicarbonate.
    (Delta anion gap is rise in anion gap from 12; delta bicarbonate is fall in bicarbonate from 24.)
- In a pure anion gap metabolic acidosis, delta–delta gap should be approximately zero.
- If delta–delta gap is significantly positive (more than +6), there is a metabolic alkalosis in addition to the anion gap metabolic acidosis.
- If delta–delta gap is significantly negative (less than −6), there is a concomitant nonanion gap metabolic acidosis.

OSMOLAR GAP

- If high anion gap metabolic acidosis is present, calculate serum osmolar gap (normal <10).
  Serum osmolar gap = measured serum osmolality − calculated serum osmolarity.
  Calculated serum osmolality = 2 × serum Na^+ + glucose/18 + blood urea nitrogen/2.8.

TREATMENT

- Main aim of treatment is to correct the underlying disorder.
- Sodium bicarbonate may be given in severe acidosis (pH <7.1 and bicarbonate <6 mEq/L). Complications of sodium bicarbonate therapy include hypernatraemia, hyperosmolality, hypervolaemia and intracellular acidosis (due to intracellular diffusion of carbon dioxide).
- In renal failure with metabolic acidosis, dialysis may be necessary.
- Normal anion gap metabolic acidosis often responds to bicarbonate therapy.

Q. Give a brief account of metabolic alkalosis. (IM 22.10)

- Metabolic alkalosis is characterised by increased plasma bicarbonate, a fall in hydrogen ion concentration and a small compensatory rise in partial pressure of carbon dioxide.

COMPENSATION

- For every 1 mEq/L rise in bicarbonate, there is a 0.6 mmHg rise in carbon dioxide.

CAUSES (Table 15.13)

TABLE 15.13 Causes Metabolic Alkalosis

Chloride-Responsive or ECF volume Contraction (Urine Cl^- <10 mEq/L)	Chloride-Resistant or ECF Volume Expansion (Urine Cl^- >20 mEq/L)
• Vomiting • Gastric drainage • Diuretic use • Posthypercapnia • Bartter's syndrome • Gitelman's syndrome	• Mineralocorticoid excess—primary and secondary hyperaldosteronism, Cushing's syndrome, use of glucocorticoids, liquorice ingestion **Others** • Excessive alkali ingestion

CLINICAL FEATURES

- Specific clinical disturbances are rare. Acute alkalosis may induce tetany due to increased neuromuscular activity caused by fall in ionised fraction of calcium. Features include tetany, seizures and cardiac arrhythmias.

TREATMENT

- The underlying causes should be corrected.
- Normal saline administration is useful in chloride-responsive metabolic alkalosis.
- Potassium chloride supplementation is necessary in cases of alkalosis associated with hypokalaemia.
- If hypervolaemic, potassium supplementation along with diuretics, which increase bicarbonate excretion are useful. These diuretics include acetazolamide and spironolactone.

Q. Discuss respiratory acidosis. (IM 22.11)

- Respiratory acidosis occurs when the alveolar ventilation fails to keep pace with the rate of carbon dioxide production. As a result, the partial pressure of carbon dioxide rises, the hydrogen ion concentration increases and there is a compensatory rise in bicarbonate levels.
- Acute respiratory acidosis is found in acute type 2 respiratory failure. Here, the partial pressure of carbon dioxide is high and partial pressure of oxygen is low.

COMPENSATION

- In acute respiratory acidosis, for every 10 mmHg rise in pCO_2, HCO_3 rises by 1 mEq/L. Bicarbonate generally does not rise above 30 mEq/L.
- In chronic respiratory acidosis, for every 10 mmHg rise in pCO_2, HCO_3 rises by 3.5 mEq/L. Bicarbonate generally does not rise above 45 mEq/L.

CAUSES (Table 15.14)

TABLE 15.14 Causes of Respiratory Acidosis

Acute	Chronic
Disorders of Gas Exchange	
• Severe asthma • Acute exacerbation of obstructive lung disease • Late stages of pulmonary oedema • Foreign body inhalation • Malfunctioning ventilators	• Chronic obstructive lung disease
Disorders of Musculoskeletal System	
• Flail chest • Tension pneumothorax or massive haemothorax • Use of aminoglycosides	• Myasthenia gravis • Poliomyelitis
CNS and Spinal Cord Abnormalities	
• Overdose with opiates and sedatives • Use of general anaesthetic agents • Cardiac arrest • Brainstem and cervical cord lesions	• Central nervous system lesions

CLINICAL FEATURES

- Severe respiratory acidosis is associated with confusion and obtundation. Other features include asterixis, myoclonus and seizures.
- Papilloedema may occur due to raised intracranial pressure secondary to cerebral vasodilatation. Conjunctival suffusion may be present.

TREATMENT

- The underlying causes should be corrected.
- Hypercapnia in chronic respiratory acidosis should be corrected gradually because rapid alkalisation of the cerebrospinal fluid may lead to seizures.
- Rapid infusion of alkali is justified only in prolonged cardiopulmonary arrest.

Q. Discuss respiratory alkalosis and its causes. (IM 22.12)

- This occurs when there is excessive loss of carbon dioxide by hyperventilation of the lungs.
- Partial pressure of carbon dioxide and hydrogen ion concentration fall. Plasma bicarbonate is decreased due to renal compensation.

COMPENSATION

- In acute respiratory alkalosis, for every 10 mmHg rise in pCO_2, HCO_3 falls by 2 mEq/L. Bicarbonate generally does not fall below 18 mEq/L.
- In chronic respiratory acidosis, for every 10 mmHg rise in pCO_2, HCO_3 falls by 5 mEq/L. Bicarbonate generally does not fall below 12 mEq/L.

CAUSES (Table 15.15)

- Causes of chronic respiratory alkalosis include chronic heart failure, severe anaemia, interstitial lung disease, residence at high altitude and hepatic failure.

TABLE 15.15 Causes of Respiratory Alkalosis

Central Mechanisms	Pulmonary Mechanisms
• Anxiety (hyperventilation syndrome) • Fever • CNS infections • Cerebrovascular accident • Metabolic encephalopathy • Septicaemia • Salicylate poisoning • Hepatic failure • Severe anaemia	• Interstitial lung disease • Acute asthma • Pneumonia • CHF • Pulmonary embolism

CLINICAL FEATURES

- In severe respiratory alkalosis, hyperventilation may be present. Sometimes, there may be manifestations of tetany.
- In acute respiratory alkalosis, patients may complain of paraesthesiae, numbness, tingling and light-headedness.

TREATMENT

- Treatment is the elimination of the underlying disorder.
- In acute hyperventilation syndrome due to anxiety, sedation may terminate the attack. 'Paper-bag' rebreathing should not be used because it may lead to hypoxia.

Q. What are primary and compensatory responses to various acid–base disturbances?

PRIMARY AND COMPENSATORY RESPONSES IN VARIOUS ACID–BASE DISORDERS (Table 15.16)

TABLE 15.16 Primary and Compensatory Responses in Various Acid–Base Disorders

Disorder	pH	Primary Response	Compensatory Response
• Metabolic acidosis	Decreased	Decreased HCO_3	Decreased pCO_2
• Metabolic alkalosis	Increased	Increased HCO_3	Increased pCO_2
• Respiratory acidosis	Decreased	Increased CO_2	Increased HCO_3
• Respiratory alkalosis	Increased	Decreased CO_2	Decreased HCO_3

COMPENSATORY RESPONSES IN ACID–BASE DISORDERS (Table 15.17)

TABLE 15.17 Compensatory Responses in Acid–Base Disorders

Disorder	Compensation	Limit of Compensation
• Metabolic acidosis	For every 1 mEq/L fall in HCO_3, pCO_2 falls by 1.2 mmHg[a]	pCO_2 does not fall below 10 mmHg
• Metabolic alkalosis	For every 1 mEq/L rise in HCO_3, pCO_2 rises by 0.6 mmHg	pCO_2 does not rise above 55 mmHg
• Acute respiratory acidosis	For every 10 mmHg rise in pCO_2, HCO_3 rises by 1 mEq/L	HCO_3 does not rise above 30 mEq/L
• Chronic respiratory acidosis	For every 10 mmHg rise in pCO_2, HCO_3 rises by 3.5 mEq/L	HCO_3 does not rise above 45 mEq/L
• Acute respiratory alkalosis	For every 10 mmHg fall in pCO_2, HCO_3 falls by 2 mEq/L	HCO_3 does not fall below 18 mEq/L
• Chronic respiratory alkalosis	For every 10 mmHg fall in pCO_2, HCO_3 falls by 5 mEq/L	HCO_3 does not fall below 12 mEq/L

[a]Winters' equation may also be used to determine expected compensation ($pCO_2 = 1.5 \times$ serum $HCO_3 + 8 \pm 2$).

Q. How will you evaluate acid–base disturbances? (IM 22.13, IM 10.20)

EVALUATION OF ACID–BASE DISORDERS

- Initial steps in the analysis of acid–base disturbances are shown in Flowchart 15.6.

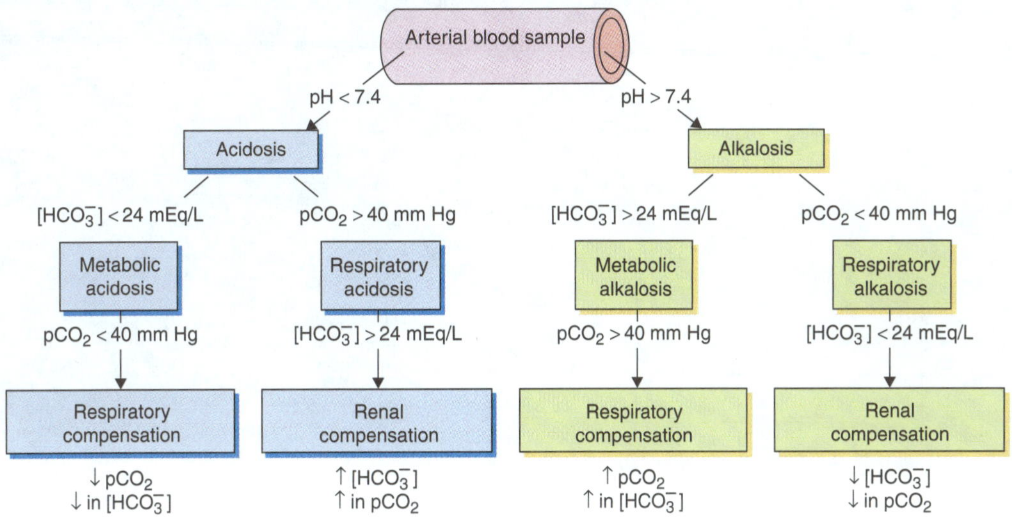

Flowchart 15.6 Approach to Analysis of Primary Acid-Base Disorders.

- Step 1: Check the pH.
  - If $pH < 7.36$, acidosis is present.
  - If $pH > 7.44$, alkalosis is present.
- Step 2: Is primary process metabolic or respiratory? For this, check pCO_2 and HCO_3.
  - If $pH < 7.36$ and $HCO_3 < 24$, metabolic acidosis.
  - If $pH < 7.36$ and $pCO_2 > 40$, respiratory acidosis.
  - If $pH > 7.44$ and $pCO_2 < 40$, respiratory alkalosis.
  - If $pH > 7.44$ and $HCO_3 > 24$, metabolic acidosis.
- Step 3: Choose appropriate compensation for acid–base disorder as shown in the tables above.
- Step 4: Determine whether degree of compensation is appropriate.
  - If it is not, a second acid–base disorder is present, which can be determined on the basis of pCO_2 and HCO_3 levels.
- Step 5: If metabolic acidosis present, calculate the anion gap.
  - If the anion gap is elevated, an elevated gap metabolic acidosis is present.
- Step 6: If high anion gap acidosis, calculate delta-delta gap to determine whether a second metabolic disorder is present.
  - In a simple high anion gap metabolic acidosis, change in anion gap = decrease in bicarbonate, that is delta–delta gap is near zero.
  - If decrease in bicarbonate greater than rise in anion gap (i.e. delta–delta gap is significantly positive), concurrent nonanion gap metabolic acidosis is present.
  - If decrease in bicarbonate less than rise in anion gap (i.e. delta–delta gap is significantly negative), concurrent metabolic alkalosis is present.
- Step 7: Generate a differential diagnosis.

16 Diseases of the Kidneys and Genitourinary System

Q. Describe a nephron with the help of a diagram. What are the functions of the kidney?

STRUCTURE OF A NEPHRON

- A nephron is the functional unit of the kidney. There are approximately 1 million nephrons in each kidney.
- The structure of a nephron is illustrated in Fig. 16.1.

FUNCTIONS OF KIDNEY (Table 16.1)

TABLE 16.1 Functions of Kidney

• Excretory	Excretion of metabolic waste products, drugs
• Regulatory	Control of body fluid volume and composition, maintenance of acid–base balance
• Endocrine	Production of erythropoietin, renin, prostaglandins
• Metabolic	Metabolism of vitamin D

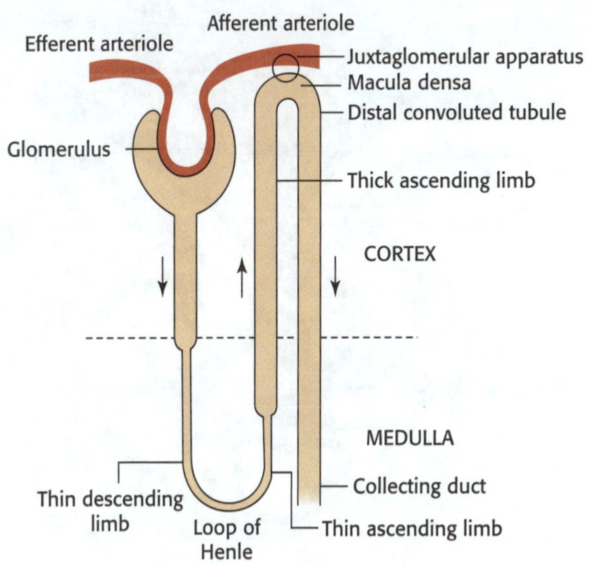

Fig. 16.1 Structure of a nephron.

Q. Write a short note on the juxtaglomerular apparatus.

- The afferent arterioles and the distal convoluted tubules are in contact for a short distance. At this point, the tubular cells become tall and columnar forming the macula densa.
- The wall of the afferent arteriole is thickened by specialised myoepitheloid cells (juxtaglomerular cells, also known as granular cells) that contain large secretory granules of renin.
- The macula densa, the juxtaglomerular cells and the lacis cells (extraglomerular mesangial cells which lie in between) constitute the juxtaglomerular apparatus. A diagrammatic representation of this is shown in Fig. 16.2.
- Cells in the macula densa respond to changes in sodium chloride levels in the distal tubule. An increase in the sodium chloride concentration causes the adjacent afferent arteriole to constrict leading to reduced glomerular filtration rate (tubuloglomerular feedback). An opposite effect occurs when sodium chloride concentration decreases in the distal tubule.

RENIN

- Renin is produced and stored in the juxtaglomerular cells. Its release is controlled by the following factors:
  - Pressure changes in the afferent arteriole.
  - Sympathetic tone.
  - Chloride concentration in the distal convoluted tubule.
  - Local prostaglandin and nitric oxide release.
- Renin acts on angiotensinogen in the blood to form angiotensin I.

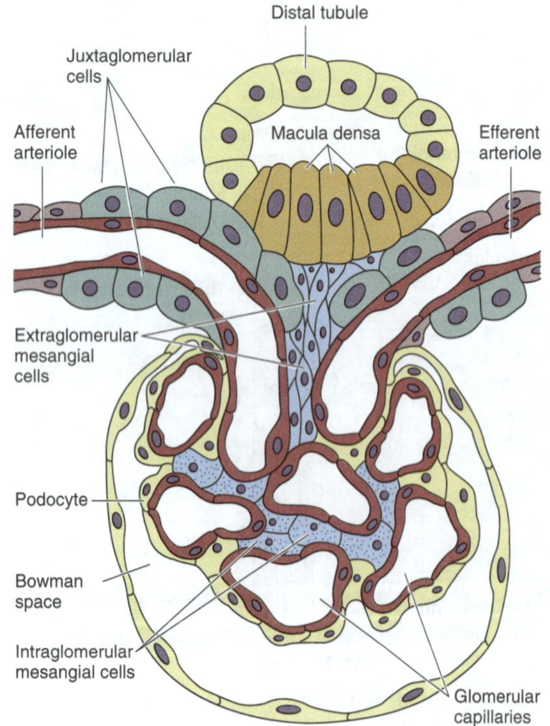

Fig. 16.2 Juxtaglomerular apparatus.

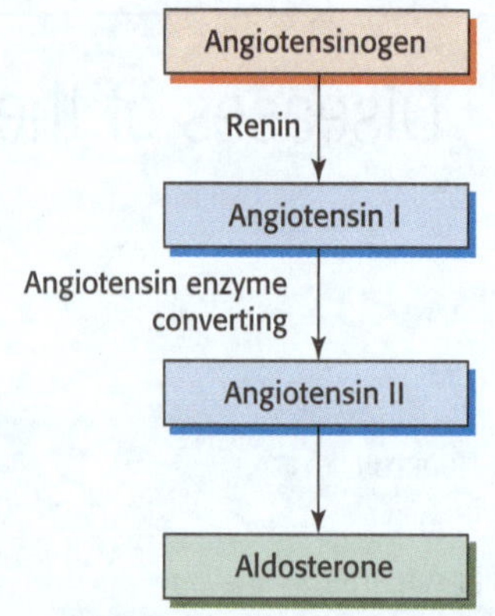

Flowchart 16.1 Renin-Angiotensin System.

- Angiotensin I is converted to angiotensin II by angiotensin-converting enzyme (ACE).
- Angiotensin II is both a vasoconstrictor and an important stimulus for the release of aldosterone by the adrenal cortex (Flowchart 16.1).

Q. What is meant by azotaemia, oliguria and anuria? Enumerate the causes of oliguria and anuria.

- Azotaemia is a term used to denote an increase in the concentration of urea and creatinine in the blood which occurs as a result of a fall in the glomerular filtration rate (GFR).
- Oliguria refers to the production of insufficient urine to enable solute to be excreted in adequate amount and is usually less than 400 mL of urine/day (in an adult of average size). Common causes of oliguria are given in Table 16.2.
- Anuria refers to complete cessation of urine flow. Some authorities define anuria as a daily urinary output less than 100 mL. Anuria more commonly indicates obstruction of the outflow from both kidneys. Causes of anuria are given in Box 16.1. Occasionally, diseases producing oliguria can produce anuria.

Q. What is meant by polyuria? Enumerate the common causes of polyuria.

- The term polyuria denotes persistent increase in urine volume of more than 3 L/day, but this should be qualified to exclude normal individuals who desire a

TABLE 16.2 Common Causes of Oliguria

Pre-renal Factors	Renal Parenchymal Diseases
• Hypovolaemia • Shock • Congestive heart failure • Sepsis • Cirrhosis • Peritonitis • Pancreatitis	• Various causes of acute kidney injury (e.g. acute glomerulonephritis, acute tubular necrosis, acute interstitial nephritis) • Obstructive nephropathy

BOX 16.1 Causes of Anuria

- Bilateral ureteric obstruction
- Prostatic or urethral obstruction
- Bilateral renal stones
- Bilateral renal cortical necrosis
- Bilateral renal arterial or venous occlusion

Note: All causes of oliguria can lead to anuria.

TABLE 16.3 Common Causes of Polyuria

• Osmotic diuresis	Hyperglycaemia, SGLT2 inhibitor use, administration of mannitol, resolving acute kidney injury
• Concentration disorders	Diabetes insipidus, papillary necrosis, diuretic phase of acute tubular necrosis (ATN)
• Drugs	Diuretics, lithium, alcohol, caffeine
• Excessive water intake	Psychogenic polydipsia

large fluid intake and, therefore, form large volumes of urine.
- Common causes of polyuria are listed in Table 16.3.
- Transient polyuria can occur following control of paroxysmal supraventricular tachycardia and relief of bilateral urinary obstruction. It can also occur following cold exposure (cold diuresis) and at high altitude (high-altitude diuresis).

ROLE OF URINE OSMOLALITY IN DIFFERENTIAL DIAGNOSIS

- Patients with a urine osmolality >600 mOsm/kg and normal serum sodium generally have osmotic diuresis as the cause of polyuria.
- Patients with a urine osmolality between 300 and 600 mOsm/kg may have osmotic diuresis or diabetes insipidus.
- Patients with a urine osmolality <300 mOsm/kg generally have diabetes insipidus or primary polydipsia.

Q. What is meant by proteinuria? What is microalbuminuria? What is moderately increased albuminuria? How will you evaluate a patient with proteinuria? (IM 10.8)

Q. Discuss Tamm–Horsfall mucoprotein.

- Pathological proteinuria is the urinary excretion of more than 150 mg of protein/day. Normal adults may excrete up to 150 mg of proteins daily. Pathological proteinuria may be 'mild' (<1.0 g/day), 'moderate' (1.0–3.5 g/day) or 'massive' (>3.5 g/day).
- Isolated proteinuria is proteinuria (non-nephrotic range) without abnormalities in urinary sediment, or reduction in GFR, as well as the absence of hypertension or diabetes mellitus.

TYPES OF PROTEINURIA

- Tubular proteinuria.
  - Occurs in diseases affecting tubulointerstitial component of kidneys (e.g. interstitial nephritis, prolonged use of analgesics, cryoglobulinaemia).
  - Usually has low-molecular-weight proteins (e.g. beta-2 microglobulin, retinol-binding protein).
  - Amount of proteinuria is <2 g/day.
  - Not diagnosed clinically as dipstick for protein is not highly sensitive for the detection of proteins other than albumin.
- Overflow proteinuria.
  - Most commonly associated with increased production of abnormal low-molecular-weight proteins (e.g. light chains in multiple myeloma, myoglobin in rhabdomyolysis, haemoglobin in intravascular haemolysis).
- Glomerular proteinuria.
  - Physiological—associated with fever or heavy exercise.
  - Orthostatic proteinuria—patient has no proteinuria in early morning samples but has low-grade proteinuria at the end of the day. Usually occurs in tall, thin adolescents or adults younger than 30 years.
  - Pathological—associated with glomerular pathologies.
- Postrenal proteinuria.
  - Occurs due to urinary tract infection (UTI), nephrolithiasis and tumours of the urinary tract.

MICROALBUMINURIA OR MODERATELY INCREASED ALBUMINURIA

- Microalbuminuria is more correctly called moderately increased albuminuria. Normal urine contains albumin in a concentration of less than 30 mg/L. Elevation of albumin in the urine from >30 to <300 mg/day (>20 to <200 μg/minute)—microalbuminuria—is so named because conventional dipstick tests cannot detect albumin levels of 30–300 mg/day.
  - Since it is often difficult to obtain 24-hour urine, measurement of urinary albumin concentration (in milligrams) to urinary creatinine concentration (in grams) ratio in an untimed spot urine sample is used in clinical settings (cut-off value >30 mg/g). This is known as albumin to creatinine ratio (ACR).
  - It is known to be an early indicator of diabetic glomerular disease (elevated fractional excretion of magnesium is a more sensitive marker than microalbuminuria in detecting early diabetic nephropathy).
  - It is an established risk marker for the presence of cardiovascular disease (coronary artery disease, peripheral artery disease and stroke) even in normotensive persons and predicts progression of nephropathy when it increases to frank albuminuria (>300 mg/day).
  - Microalbuminuria can be reduced, and progression to overt proteinuria is prevented or retarded by aggressive blood pressure reduction especially

with ACE inhibitors or angiotensin receptor blockers, and control of diabetes.

- Blood pressure levels should be maintained at or below 130/80 mmHg in anyone with diabetes or kidney disease.

TAMM–HORSFALL MUCOPROTEIN

- Tamm–Horsfall mucoprotein (also known as uromodulin) is a urine protein that is a normal constituent of urine. It does not arise from the plasm a but is produced in the thick ascending limb of the loop of Henle and is excreted at a rate of 25 mg/day.
    - Its function is unclear. It may have some immunomodulatory activity and may protect against UTI.
    - It is a constituent of all types of urinary casts. It is implicated in the pathogenesis of cast nephropathy, a form of renal failure associated with multiple myeloma in which intratubular casts occlude the flow of urine.

EVALUATION OF A PATIENT WITH PROTEINURIA (Flowchart 16.2)

Q. Enumerate common causes of haematuria. How will you clinically localise the site of bleeding?

- Haematuria may be macroscopic (visible on gross examination) or microscopic (three or more red blood cells per high-power field or urine dipstick positive).
- The common causes of haematuria are illustrated in Fig. 16.3.
- The following features may help to localise the site of bleeding from the urinary tract:
    - When blood is seen at the start of voiding and then the urine becomes clear, bleeding from the urethra is suggested.
    - When blood is diffusely present throughout the urine, it may suggest bleeding from the bladder or above.
    - Blood only at the end of micturition suggests bleeding from the prostate or bladder base.
    - Haematuria of glomerular origin is described as cola coloured, while haematuria from renal pelvises and lower urinary tract is usually pink or red.
    - Associated pain may indicate UTI, pyelonephritis (costovertebral tenderness) or renal calculus.
    - Family history of haematuria may indicate Alport's syndrome, polycystic kidney disease or sickle cell disease.

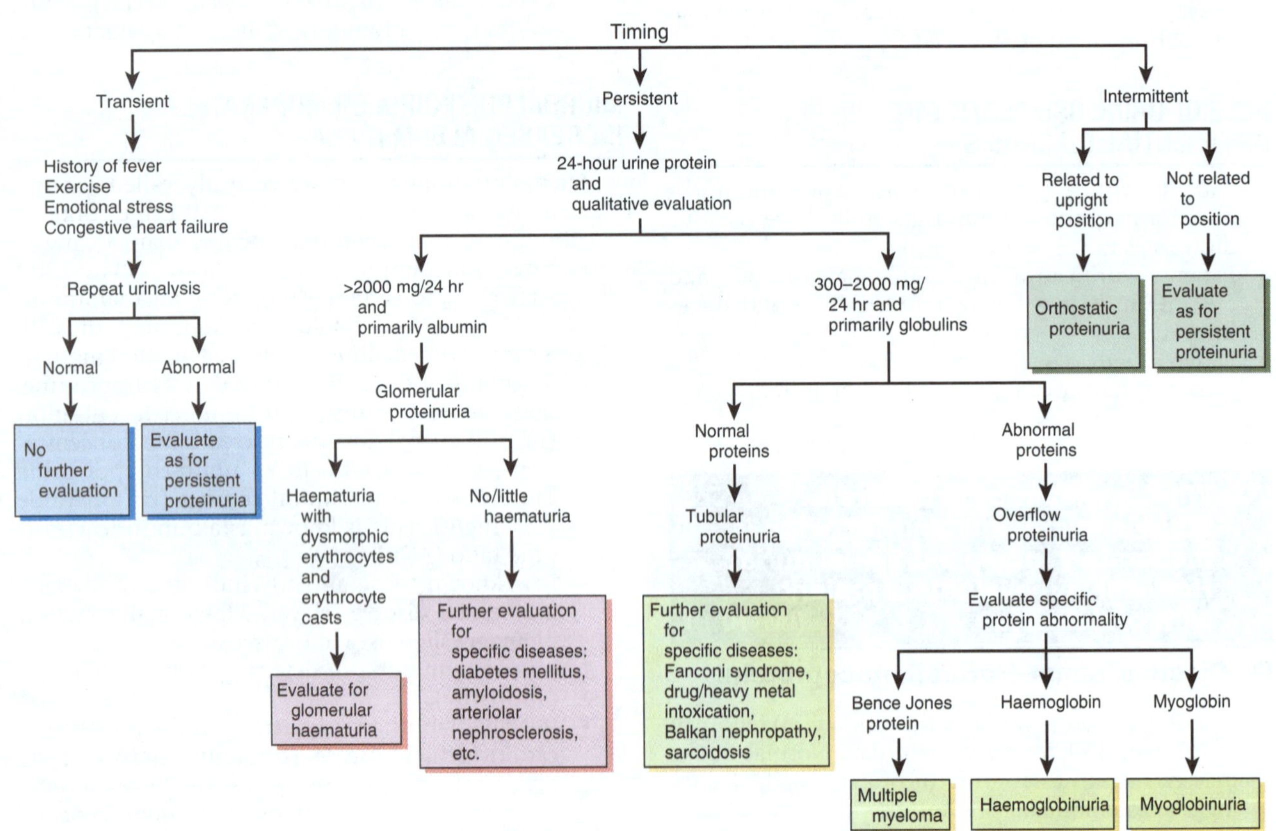

Flowchart 16.2 Evaluation of a Patient with Proteinuria.

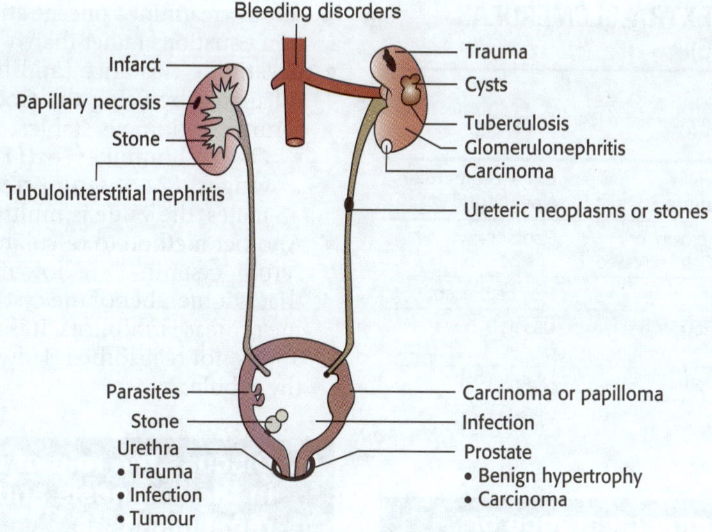

Fig. 16.3 Causes of haematuria.

- The presence of red cell casts in the urine is diagnostic of bleeding from the kidney, most often due to glomerulonephritis.
- Dysmorphic erythrocytes on urine examination are characterised by an irregular outer cell membrane and suggest haematuria of glomerular origin.
- Acanthocytes (ring-formed erythrocytes with one or more membrane protrusions of variable size and shape) represent an early form of dysmorphic erythrocytes and are a marker for haematuria of glomerular origin.
- Erythrocytes of uniform character are classified as isomorphic and suggest haematuria of lower urinary tract origin. Microscopic clots of clumped erythrocytes in urine are also suggestive of lower urinary tract bleeding.

Q. What are the causes of painless haematuria? How will you evaluate such a patient?

CAUSES OF PAINLESS HAEMATURIA

- Causes of painless haematuria are given in Table 16.4.

TABLE 16.4 Causes of Painless Haematuria

• Kidney	Glomerulonephritis, renal stone (may be painless), infective endocarditis, renal tuberculosis, benign familial haematuria, IgA nephropathy, severe acute pyelonephritis, papillary necrosis (more common in diabetes mellitus and sickle cell trait or disease), renal cell carcinoma, microscopic polyangiitis, granulomatosis with polyangiitis (Wegener's granulomatosis), polycystic kidney disease
• Ureter	Neoplasms
• Bladder	Neoplasms, trauma, schistosomiasis
• Prostate	Prostatitis, neoplasms
• Urethra	Trauma

PATIENT'S EVALUATION

HISTORY

- History of recurrent visible haematuria.
- Age over 40 years.
- Current smoker or recent history of smoking.
- History of recurrent UTI or other urological disorders.
- Occupational exposure to chemicals or dyes.
- Previous pelvic irradiation.
- History of excessive analgesic use.
- Treatment with cyclophosphamide.
- Use of anticoagulant and antiplatelet medicines more likely to exacerbate rather than cause, haematuria.
- History to suggest site of bleeding (refer Fig. 16.3 above).

EXAMINATION AND INVESTIGATIONS (Box 16.2)

BOX 16.2 Examination and Investigations in a Patient With Painless Haematuria

- Blood pressure
- Cardiovascular examination
- Abdominal examination and prostatic evaluation
- RBC morphology (assessed by phase contrast microscopy of fresh urine)
- Proteinuria
- Renal function tests
- Platelet count and coagulation studies
- Ultrasound for kidneys, ureters, bladder and prostate
- Urine for acid-fast bacilli
- Urine cytology if risk factors for renal tract cancer present (smoking, analgesic abuse, industrial toxin exposure like aniline, benzidine, aromatic amines, age >40 years, pelvic irradiation, urinary schistosomiasis)
- Autoantibodies (ANA, ANCA)
- Intravenous pyelography
- Cystourethroscopy
- Computed tomography urography, intravenous pyelogram
- Kidney biopsy

GLOMERULAR VERSUS EXTRA-GLOMERULAR HAEMATURIA (Table 16.5)

TABLE 16.5 Differentiating Glomerular From Extra-Glomerular Haematuria

Feature	Glomerular Haematuria	Extra-Glomerular Haematuria
Colour of urine (if haematuria is gross)	Smoky brown, or 'Coca-Cola' coloured	Red or pink
Clots in urine	No	May be present
Proteinuria	Often >500 mg/day	Usually <500 mg/day
Urinary RBCs	Dysmorphic	Normal
Urinary RBC casts	Present	Absent

Q. Describe creatinine clearance or renal clearance. (IM 10.17)

- GFR gives the level of renal function. The GFR for an average adult is about 125 mL/minute.
- Most often, GFR is estimated by measuring renal clearance of certain substances like creatinine, known as creatinine clearance.
- Renal clearance is measured by using the following formula:

$$C = UV/P$$

where C is the renal clearance, U is the urinary concentration of any substance, P is the plasma concentration of the same substance and V is the minute volume of urine.

- The polysaccharide inulin has been found to pass freely through the glomerular capillary wall. Inulin is neither absorbed nor excreted by the tubules and, hence, the quantity of inulin excreted in urine (UV) is identical with the amount filtered by the glomeruli. Therefore, the renal clearance of inulin can be used to estimate the GFR.
- In clinical practice, the measurement of creatinine clearance which approximates to that of inulin indicates the GFR.
- An estimate of GFR (eGFR) utilising creatinine clearance is obtained by measuring the creatinine in a 24-hour urine sample, the plasma concentration of creatinine, and substituting the measured values in the above formula. However, due to creatinine excretion via renal tubular secretion, the measurement of creatinine clearance using the above formula tends to overestimate the true level of GFR.
- Limitation of eGFR using creatinine clearance includes errors in urine collection and increase in both creatinine secretion and extrarenal creatinine degradation as the GFR falls. Therefore, GFR is often estimated from serum creatinine concentration using derived estimation equations rather than a timed urine collection.
- Creatinine clearance (and hence eGFR) can also be calculated by using the Cockcroft–Gault formula if serum creatinine is stable:
  - Cl_{Cr} (mL/minute) = [(140 − age) × ideal body weight]/[72 × serum creatinine (mg/dL)] (for females, the value is multiplied by 0.85)
- Another method to calculate GFR is measurement of serum cystatin C, a low-molecular-weight protein that is a member of the cystatin superfamily of cysteine protease inhibitors. It is filtered at the glomerulus and is not reabsorbed. However, it is metabolised in the tubules.

Q. Discuss the role of ultrasonography in the diagnosis and management of renal diseases. (IM 10.19)

- This is the method of choice for assessing overall renal size and distinguishing solid tumours from cysts.
- Renal ultrasound can demonstrate dilatation of the pelvicalyceal system (hydronephrosis) which may be due to obstruction.
- Perinephric abscess, haematomas or calculi may be demonstrated.
- Useful in differentiating a simple, benign renal cyst from a more complex cyst.
- Renal biopsy and cyst puncture can be done under ultrasound screening.
- It is an excellent screening test for polycystic kidney disease.
- Useful in diagnosing nephrocalcinosis.
- In malignant renal tumours, renal ultrasound can give additional information regarding extension of the tumour to renal veins, vena cava, lymph nodes or liver.
- The prostate size and bladder capacity can also be assessed.
- Doppler ultrasonography can be used to evaluate for renal artery stenosis and renal vein thrombosis.

Q. Give a brief account on acute glomerulonephritis or acute nephritic syndrome.

Q. Discuss the aetiology, pathogenesis, clinical features, diagnosis, complications and management of acute post-streptococcal glomerulonephritis.

- The term glomerulonephritis signifies glomerular inflammation in which there is an immunologically mediated injury to the glomeruli.

AETIOLOGY (Table 16.6)

TABLE 16.6 Aetiology of Acute Glomerulonephritis

• Infectious diseases (postinfectious glomerulonephritis)	Poststreptococcal glomerulonephritis (PSGN), infective endocarditis, syphilis, mumps, measles, hepatitis B, infectious mononucleosis, Epstein–Barr virus infection, malaria, HIV-associated nephropathy
• Multisystem diseases	Systemic lupus erythematosus, Goodpasture's syndrome (anti-GBM antibody disease), Henoch–Schönlein purpura, microscopic polyangiitis, granulomatosis with polyangiitis (Wegener's granulomatosis), sickle cell nephropathy
• Primary glomerular diseases	Diffuse proliferative glomerulonephritis, IgA nephropathy, mesangiocapillary glomerulonephritis, crescentic glomerulonephritis, membranous glomerulonephritis, focal segmental glomerulosclerosis
• Miscellaneous	Malignancy, eclampsia, D-penicillamine, nonsteroidal antiinflammatory drugs, captopril, heroin, mitomycin C, cocaine

PATHOGENESIS

- Two chief pathogenetic mechanisms are recognised:
  - Deposition of antigen–antibody complexes (immune complexes) in the glomeruli can result in glomerular disease.
  - Deposition of an antibody in the glomerular basement membrane which then reacts with an antigen in the basement membrane causing glomerulonephritis.
- Normally, the immune complexes formed in the body are removed by the host's reticuloendothelial system. Impaired ability on the part of the host to clear the immune complexes may result in their deposition in the glomerular capillary walls.
- The antigen involved in the immune complex formation may be exogenous (e.g. bacteria such as streptococci as in poststreptococcal glomerulonephritis [PSGN]) or endogenous (e.g. antibodies to host DNA in patients with SLE). The immune complexes and antibodies against a glomerular antigen may trigger injury by the following mechanisms:
  - Complement activation.
  - Fibrin deposition.
  - Platelet aggregation.
  - Release of cytokines and free oxygen radicals.

CLINICAL FEATURES

- Acute nephritic syndrome is characterised by the acute onset of the features shown in Box 16.3.
- Asymptomatic patients are primarily characterised by microscopic haematuria.

POSTSTREPTOCOCCAL GLOMERULONEPHRITIS

- One of the common causes of acute nephritic syndrome is acute PSGN caused by immune complex deposits.

BOX 16.3 Clinical Features of Acute Nephritic Syndrome

- Haematuria
- Oliguria
- Oedema
- Hypertension
- Red blood cell casts in urine
- Proteinuria
- Uraemia

- PSGN occurs after a pharyngeal or cutaneous infection with nephritogenic strains of group A β-haemolytic *Streptococcus pyogenes*.
- Nephritogenic *S. pyogenes* strains of throat infection are 12, 4 and 1, whereas nephritogenic strains of skin infection are M types 49, 42, 2, 57 and 60.
- Can occur following epidemics of infection or sporadic infections.
- There is a latent period between the streptococcal infection and the onset of nephritis. Following pharyngeal infection, the latent period is about 6–21 days. Cutaneous infections are associated with a longer latent period of about 3–6 weeks.
- Children are commonly affected.
- PSGN is commonly associated with poor personal hygiene, overcrowding and skin diseases like scabies.
- Onset is often abrupt with puffiness of face, oliguria, smoky urine or reddish urine, hypertension and oedema.
- The oedema of acute glomerulonephritis tends to appear initially in areas of low tissue pressure (periorbital areas) but subsequently progresses to involve dependent portions of the body and may lead to ascites and/or pleural effusion.

INVESTIGATIONS

- Investigations in acute PSGN are given in Box 16.4.

TREATMENT

- Treatment of acute PSGN is supportive. Clinical manifestations typically begin to improve 1 to 2 weeks after disease onset and renal function usually returns to baseline levels within 4 weeks.
- The measures include rest, salt restriction, loop diuretics and antihypertensives.
- Antihypertensive agents include calcium channel blockers. Angiotensin converting enzyme inhibitors are avoided as they may further worsen renal function and cause hyperkalaemia.
- Antibiotics are given for presumed throat infection as this may result in a milder form of nephritis. Further, treatment of a carrier state may prevent spread to other household members.
- Dialysis is required in severe oliguria, fluid overload and hyperkalaemia.
- Steroids and cytotoxic drugs are of no value.

BOX 16.4 Investigations in Acute Poststreptococcal Glomerulonephritis

Investigations	Positive Findings
• Urine microscopy	Red cells (particularly dysmorphic—i.e. distorted and fragmented red cells), red cell casts
• Cultures	Throat swab and swab from inflamed skin may grow group A β-haemolytic streptococci
• Antistreptolysin-O (ASO) titre	Elevated after pharyngeal infection
• Anti-DNase B antibodies	Elevated after skin infection
• C3 and CH50 level (complement activity)	Reduced in majority
• Urinary protein	Increased
• Urea and creatinine	May be elevated
• Renal biopsy	Features of glomerulonephritis

COMPLICATIONS

- Complications include pulmonary oedema, hypertensive encephalopathy and renal failure.

PROGNOSIS

- Majority of children and adults with the epidemic form of PSGN have an excellent prognosis. However, some patients develop persistent urine abnormalities or hypertension.
- Conversely, up to 60% of adults with sporadic infections experience progressive irreversible renal damage.

PREVENTION

- Early eradication of pharyngitis-associated group A streptococci by use of antibiotics protects against glomerulonephritis.

Q. What is IgA nephropathy? Explain in brief.

- Also known as Berger's disease.
- Characterised by predominant IgA deposition in the glomerular mesangium.
- Presents with painless haematuria, generally within 1 to 2 days of upper respiratory infection.
- More common in children and young adults with peak incidence between 15 and 30 years.
- May be detected on routine urine examination (microscopic haematuria).
- Occasionally presents as acute renal failure (ARF) or nephritic syndrome.
- Diagnosis by renal biopsy with immunofluorescence or immunoperoxidase studies for IgA deposits mainly in the mesangium.
- Up to 20% of patients have progressive disease leading eventually to end-stage renal disease. In most such cases, rate of progression of disease is usually very slow. Clinical features that mark a poor prognosis include moderate to severe degrees of proteinuria, renal insufficiency at the time of renal biopsy, hypertension and tubulointerstitial fibrosis on kidney biopsy.
- Complete remission uncommon.
- Henoch–Schönlein purpura is a systemic disease which may have mesangial IgA deposition. It is more common during childhood as compared to IgA nephropathy.
- No specific therapy is available. Aggressive therapy is not warranted in patients who are not likely to have progressive disease or who have diffuse glomerulosclerosis on biopsy or those who have stage 4 or 5 chronic kidney disease (CKD).
  - Therapeutic options include ACE inhibitors or angiotensin receptor blockers if >1 g/day proteinuria is present; also for control of hypertension.
  - A 6-month course of corticosteroids may be tried in patients with persistent proteinuria >1 g/day despite 3–6 months of supportive care and blood pressure control if GFR is more than 50 mL/minute.
  - A slow-release oral preparation of budesonide has been approved for use in patients with eGFR >45 mL/minute/1.73 m^2 and persistent proteinuria despite 6 months of optimised ACE inhibitor therapy. It reduces production of aberrantly galactosylated IgA1 in gut, which has been implicated in the pathogenesis of IgA nephropathy.
  - Use of immunosuppressives is controversial. Cyclophosphamide may be added to steroids if patient has rapidly progressive glomerulonephritis (RPGN) or crescentic glomerulonephritis.

Q. Briefly outline the causes, clinical features, investigations and treatment of rapidly progressive glomerulonephritis.

Q. Describe crescentic glomerulonephritis.

- RPGN is defined as any glomerular disease characterised by extensive crescents (usually >50%) as the principal histological finding and by a rapid loss of renal function (usually a 50% decline in the GFR within 3 months).
- A crescent is the accumulation of cells and extracellular material in the urinary space of a glomerulus. The cells are parietal and visceral epithelium as well as monocytes and other blood cells.
- RPGN is classified pathologically into three categories:
  - Antiglomerular basement membrane (anti-GBM) antibody disease—linear deposits of antibodies on immunofluorescence.
  - Immune-complex disease—granular deposits of immune complexes on immunofluorescence.
  - Pauci-immune disease (generally antineutrophil cytoplasmic antibody positive—ANCA positive)—little or no deposits on immunofluorescence.

16

CAUSES (Table 16.7)

TABLE 16.7 Causes of Rapidly Progressive Glomerulonephritis

Anti-GBM Antibody	Immune Complex
• Goodpasture's syndrome • Anti-GBM disease (only kidney involvement) **Pauci-Immune** • Granulomatosis with polyangiitis (Wegener's granulomatosis) • Microscopic polyangiitis • Renal-limited necrotising crescentic glomerulonephritis • Eosinophilic granulomatosis with polyangiitis (Churg–Strauss syndrome)	• Postinfectious GN • Lupus nephritis • Henoch–Schönlein purpura • Mixed cryoglobulinaemia • Primary renal disease • IgA nephropathy • Membranoproliferative glomerulonephritis • Idiopathic

CLINICAL FEATURES

- Presents with moderate proteinuria, haematuria, oliguria, oedema and uraemia.
- Patients with anti-GBM antibody disease, granulomatosis with polyangiitis and microscopic polyangiitis may also have pulmonary haemorrhage and haemoptysis due to pulmonary involvement ('pulmonary-renal syndrome'). The bleeding may occur over a prolonged period, leading to anaemia and iron deficiency.

INVESTIGATIONS

- Leucocytosis and anaemia.
- Blood urea and serum creatinine levels usually elevated.
- Urinalysis shows modest proteinuria (1–4 g/day), microscopic haematuria, and RBC and WBC casts.
- Complement levels (C3 and C4) may be decreased in patients with immune-complex-mediated RPGN.
- Circulating anti-GBM antibodies in Goodpasture's syndrome.
- ANCA in patients with pauci-immune RPGN.
- Serum cryoglobulin levels may be elevated in cryoglobulinaemias.
- Abdominal ultrasound shows normal-sized kidneys.
- Chest X-ray in patients with Goodpasture's syndrome and vasculitides may show diffuse opacities if pulmonary haemorrhage occurs.
- Kidney biopsy shows crescents.

TREATMENT

- Supportive therapy:
  - Control of infection.
  - Control of volume status (dialysis if required).
- Specific therapy:
  - Methylprednisolone pulses of 500–1000 mg/day for 3 days along with oral or IV cyclophosphamide.
  - Immunosuppressive therapy (e.g. cyclophosphamide, azathioprine, mycophenolate).
  - Treatment of choice in anti-GBM antibody disease is plasmapheresis combined with prednisolone and cyclophosphamide.
  - Infliximab and rituximab in ANCA-associated GN not responding to other treatment.

BOX 16.5 Abnormalities in Nephrotic Syndrome

- Proteinuria (>3.5 g in 24 hours)
- Hypoalbuminaemia
- Generalised oedema
- Hyperlipidaemia

Q. Discuss the aetiology, pathogenesis, clinical features, diagnosis and management of nephrotic syndrome.

- The nephrotic syndrome is characterised by the abnormalities given in Box 16.5.

PATHOGENESIS

- In nephrotic syndrome, the permeability of the glomerular capillary wall is increased by glomerular inflammation, change in the surface electrical charge and an alteration in the pore size. These result in excessive leakage of plasma proteins across the glomerular capillary wall into the urine leading to hypoalbuminaemia.
- The decreased concentration of albumin in the blood leads to a decrease in plasma colloid oncotic pressure resulting in a disturbance in the Starling forces acting across peripheral capillaries. Intravascular fluid migrates into the interstitial tissue and causes oedema.
- The hypovolaemia also triggers the renin–angiotensin–aldosterone system. This causes increased reabsorption of sodium and water by the kidney resulting in oedema.
- The low plasma colloid oncotic pressure also appears to stimulate hepatic lipoprotein synthesis. Hence, hyperlipidaemia (elevations of total plasma cholesterol, triglyceride, very low density lipoprotein and low-density lipoprotein) is also associated with nephrotic syndrome. It increases the risk of atherosclerosis and cardiovascular disease.

CONSEQUENCES OF PROTEIN LOSS

- Hypoalbuminaemia can lead to oedema and increased susceptibility to infections. Oedema is most marked in periorbital regions and dependent part of body. Hypoalbuminaemia may also produce pleural effusion and ascites. Subungual oedema may manifest as parallel transverse white lines in the fingernail beds (Muehrcke's lines—Fig. 16.4).
- Urinary losses of plasma proteins like thyroxine-binding globulin can cause abnormalities in thyroid function tests.
- Deficiency of antithrombin III (due to urine loss) may produce a hypercoagulable state and renal vein thrombosis. Other reasons for hypercoagulable state in nephrotic syndrome include altered activity and levels of proteins C and S, increased hepatic synthesis of fibrinogen and increased platelet aggregation.
  - In adults, most thromboses are venous, while in children arterial thromboses are more common.
  - Patient with acute renal vein thrombosis can present with sudden onset of flank or abdominal pain,

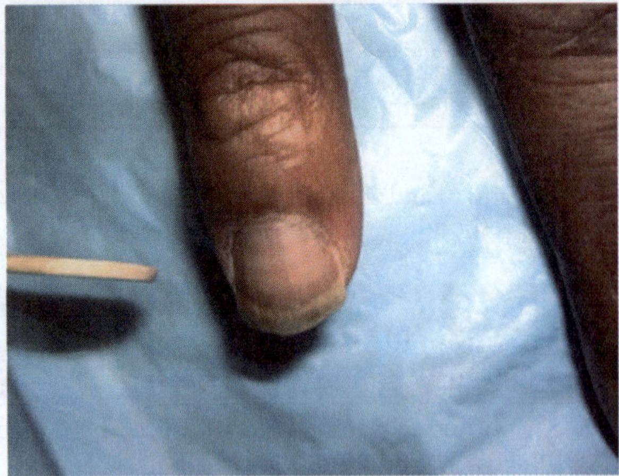

Fig. 16.4 Muehrcke's lines.

gross haematuria and an acute decline in renal function, but most patients are asymptomatic.
  - Other consequences of hypercoagulable state include pulmonary embolism, myocardial infarction and stroke.
- Loss of globulins in urine may result in severe IgG deficiency leading to spontaneous bacterial peritonitis.
- Loss of cholecalciferol-binding protein may lead to vitamin D deficiency state.
- Loss of transferrin may result in microcytic hypochromic anaemia.
- Loss of metal-binding proteins may result in trace metal deficiency, for example zinc and copper.
- Loss of drug-binding proteins results in altered drug pharmacokinetics.
- Severe hypoalbuminaemia may produce hypovolaemia and at times, acute kidney injury.

CAUSES OF NEPHROTIC SYNDROME (Table 16.8)

MINIMAL CHANGE DISEASE

- Most common cause of nephrotic syndrome in children (80%); responsible for 20% of all cases in adults.
- Normal-appearing glomeruli on light microscopy of a renal biopsy specimen.

TABLE 16.8 Causes of Nephrotic Syndrome

Primary (Idiopathic)	
• Idiopathic glomerular diseases like minimal change disease, membranous nephropathy, mesangial proliferative glomerulonephritis, focal and segmental glomerulosclerosis (FSGS), IgA nephropathy, mesangiocapillary glomerulonephritis	
Secondary	
• Infections	Bacterial endocarditis, malaria, syphilis, hepatitis B, leprosy, HIV infection
• Connective tissue diseases	SLE, rheumatoid arthritis
• Neoplasms	Hodgkin's lymphoma, carcinomas, leukaemias
• Drugs and toxins	Penicillamine, captopril, gold, mercury, contaminated heroin
• Metabolic	Diabetes mellitus, amyloidosis

- Effacement of foot processes of epithelial cells on electron microscopy.

FOCAL AND SEGMENTAL GLOMERULOSCLEROSIS (FSGS)

- Accounts for one-third of cases of nephrotic syndrome in adults.
- Characterised histologically by sclerosis that involves some glomeruli (focal) and only part of the capillary tuft (segmental).
- May be idiopathic or develop secondary to HIV infection, heroin use, sickle cell disease, obesity, reflux nephropathy and chronic glomerular hyperfiltration from a solitary kidney.
- Patients usually present with nephrotic-range proteinuria, hypertension, renal insufficiency and occasionally haematuria.

MEMBRANOUS NEPHROPATHY (MN)

- One of the most common primary renal causes of nephrotic syndrome in adults.
- Characterised by diffuse thickening of glomerular capillary wall.
- Idiopathic MN is an autoimmune disease with circulating IgG4 antibodies against the M-type phospholipase A2 receptor (PLA2R) in 70%–80% of cases.
- Secondary causes in about 20%–30% of cases that include systemic lupus erythematosus, hepatitis B, malignancy or drug induced (e.g. chronic gold or penicillamine drug therapy).
- Male predominance.
- Incidence usually peaks between ages 30 and 50 years.
- Approximately 75% of patients present with nephrotic range proteinuria and 50% present with microscopic haematuria.

INVESTIGATIONS

- Investigations in nephrotic syndrome include a 24-hour urinary protein estimation and estimation of serum albumin and serum cholesterol concentrations.
- Red cells and red cell casts may be present in the urine. However, in minimal change disease, RBCs and red cell casts are not present.
- Renal biopsy may be required to make a histological diagnosis.
- For suspected secondary causes, appropriate investigations are required.

MANAGEMENT

- Treatment of nephrotic syndrome involves three steps:
  - Measures to reduce proteinuria.
  - Measures to control complications of nephrotic syndrome.
  - Treatment of underlying cause.

MEASURES TO REDUCE PROTEINURIA

- These are required if immunosuppressive drugs and other specific measures against the underlying cause do not benefit the patient.

- ACE inhibitors or angiotensin receptor blockers reduce proteinuria and also slow the rate of progression of renal failure by lowering the intraglomerular pressure. This also prevents development of haemodynamically mediated FSGS.
- NSAIDs also reduce proteinuria in some patients but their use must be weighed against the risk of producing acute kidney injury, hyperkalaemia, and salt and water retention.

MEASURES TO CONTROL COMPLICATIONS OF NEPHROTIC SYNDROME

- Oedema should be controlled by salt restriction, rest and judicious use of diuretics. The weight loss should not exceed 1 kg/day. Aggressive diuresis may precipitate acute kidney injury due to reduction in intravascular volume.
- In severe cases, intravenous salt-poor albumin may be used as a temporary measure to reduce oedema. However, most of infused albumin will be excreted by the kidneys in 24–48 hours.
- Dietary proteins should be about 0.8–1.0 g/kg as excessive proteins in the diet may hasten the progression of renal disease. However, malnutrition should be prevented.
- Hypertension should be treated with ACE inhibitors or angiotensin receptor blockers. Addition of a mineralocorticoid receptor antagonist further improves control of blood pressure and proteinuria.
- Vitamin D supplementation in patients with biochemical evidence of vitamin D deficiency.
- Hyperlipidaemia should be controlled with dietary restrictions and lipid-lowering drugs.
- Anticoagulants are indicated in patients with deep venous thrombosis or arterial thrombosis. Prophylactic anticoagulants are indicated in membranous nephropathy if serum albumin is 2.0–2.5 g/dL with proteinuria of >10 g/day and BMI >35 kg/m^2.
- Early detection and treatment of infections. Prevention of pneumococcal infections by vaccination.

MEASURES TO TREAT THE UNDERLYING DISEASE

Minimal Change Disease

- Children with nephrotic syndrome due to minimal change disease require initial treatment with corticosteroids in the form of daily prednisolone at a dose of 60 mg/m^2 (1.5 mg/kg body weight in adults) for 4 weeks. This is followed by alternate-day prednisolone at a dose of 35 mg/m^2 (1 mg/kg in adults) for 4 additional weeks. Children who respond within the first 4 weeks of steroid treatment are termed 'steroid responsive'. Those who relapse on withdrawal of steroid are termed 'steroid dependent'. Such relapses are retreated with the same initial regimen but with more gradual withdrawal of prednisolone. Some patients may require low maintenance doses (5–10 mg/day) for 3–6 months.
- Patients who have frequent relapses or develop unacceptable corticosteroid side effects may be benefitted by a brief course of cyclophosphamide (2 mg/kg/day) for 6 weeks. However, for patients who are steroid resistant, calcineurin inhibitors (tacrolimus preferred over cyclosporin) are recommended as first line agents. In patients with no response to therapy with calcineurin inhibitors, treatment with either rituximab or mycophenolate mofetil is recommended.
- Prognosis of patients with minimal change disease is excellent, though it has a characteristic remitting and relapsing course.

Focal and Segmental Glomerulosclerosis

- Steroids may be beneficial in only 20%–30% of cases.
- Cyclophosphamide, tacrolimus and cyclosporin may be of some benefit in steroid-resistant cases. Rituximab may also be useful.

Membranous Nephropathy

- Spontaneous remission may occur in 40% of cases.
- Another 30%–40% of cases remit and relapse repeatedly.
- Rest 10%–20% of patients develop progressive renal failure. Steroids alone are not useful. Cyclophosphamide, cyclosporin and chlorambucil in combination with steroids may retard the progression in this subset of patients. Rituximab may also be useful.

Q. Discuss the aetiopathogenesis, clinical features, investigations and management of urinary tract infection.

Q. Give a brief account of vesicoureteric reflux.

- UTI may be anatomically subdivided into lower tract infections (urethritis, prostatitis and cystitis) and upper tract infections (pyelonephritis and perinephric abscess).
- UTI is associated with multiplication of organisms in the urinary tract and is defined by the presence of more than 10^5 organisms/mL in the midstream sample of urine (MSU). This is denoted as 'significant bacteriuria'. The clinical presentation of UTI may be as follows:
    - Asymptomatic bacteriuria:
        - Presence of bacteriuria (>10^5/mL on two occasions in women and on one occasion in men) indicating UTI but without symptoms. In a single catheterised sample, bacterial growth may be as low as 10^2/mL to be considered representing true bacteriuria in both men and women.
        - Commonly seen in pregnancy and in patients with spinal cord injuries.
    - Symptomatic:
        - Acute urethritis and cystitis.
        - Acute prostatitis.
        - Acute pyelonephritis.
        - Sepsis and septic shock.

AETIOLOGY

- Common microorganisms involved in UTIs are *Escherichia coli* (80% of cases), *Proteus, Klebsiella, Enterobacter, Pseudomonas, Serratia, Chlamydia trachomatis* and *Neisseria gonorrhoeae* (sexually transmitted).

- About one-third of females with dysuria and frequency have either insignificant number of bacteria in midstream cultures or completely sterile cultures. This subset of patients has been defined as having acute urethral syndrome. The syndrome is often due to infection with usual organisms (where culture reveals only 10^2–10^4 bacteria) or with unusual organisms (*N. gonorrhoeae, C. trachomatis*).

PATHOGENESIS

- Bacteria gain access to the bladder via the urethra in the vast majority of cases. Ascent of bacteria from the bladder may then follow which results in parenchymal infections.
- In a minority of patients, pyelonephritis can occur due to haematogenous spread of bacteria.
- Females are more prone to the development of cystitis due to several reasons:
  - Short urethra (4 cm).
  - Gram-negative enteric organisms residing near the anal region colonise the periurethral region.
  - Absence of bactericidal prostatic secretions.
  - Sexual intercourse facilitates entry of introital bacteria into the bladder.
- Susceptibility factor—that is the uroepithelium of these patients has more surface receptors to which adherent strains of *E. coli* become attached.
- Whether bladder infection ensures depends on certain factors:
  - Flushing and dilutional effects of micturition and voiding.
  - Direct antibacterial properties of urine and the bladder mucosa.
  - Size of inoculum.
  - Bacterial virulence factors.
- There are a number of other factors involved in the pathogenesis of UTI:
  - Pregnancy is associated with an increased incidence of UTI. During pregnancy, ureteral tone is decreased (progestational activity), ureteral peristalsis is decreased and there is a transient incompetence of the vesicoureteral valves. All these factors favour the development of UTI.
  - Any impediment to the free flow of urine as with tumours, strictures, calculi, prostatic hypertrophy and posterior urethral valves favours the development of UTI.
  - Instrumentation of urinary tract like catheterisation, urethral dilatation and cystoscopy.
  - Vesicoureteric reflux. This condition is defined as reflux of urine from the bladder cavity up into the ureters. It occurs during voiding or with elevated bladder pressure. As a fluid connection exists between the bladder and kidney, there is retrograde bacterial spread resulting in acute pyelonephritis. Vesicoureteric reflux can be confirmed radiographically when retrograde movement of radiopaque material can be demonstrated (micturating cystourethrography [MCU]).
  - Associated disorders that impair defence mechanisms like diabetes mellitus favour the development of UTI.
- Neurogenic bladder dysfunction that occurs with spinal cord injuries, tabes dorsalis and multiple sclerosis also predisposes to UTI.

CLINICAL FEATURES

- Fever with chills and rigors.
- Frequency of micturition.
- Dysuria or scalding micturition.
- Urgency.
- Haematuria.
- Suprapubic pain resulting from cystitis.
- Strangury results from cystitis. After the bladder has been emptied, there may be an intense desire to pass more urine due to detrusor spasm.
- Flank pain due to pyelonephritis.
- Urine is cloudy with an unpleasant odour.

UNCOMPLICATED URINARY TRACT INFECTION

- Includes cystitis or urethritis due to bacterial colonisation of the bladder or urethra.
- Patients do not have abnormal urinary tract.
- Affects females much more than males.
- Characterised by burning on urination and frequent urination without fever or flank pain.
- Rare sequelae.

COMPLICATED URINARY TRACT INFECTION

- Infection whether localised to the lower or upper tract and associated with an underlying condition that increases the risk of failing therapy is called complicated infection. It often involves renal parenchyma (pyelonephritis) or prostate (prostatitis).
- Features suggesting complicated UTIs include:
  - Fever ≥100°F
  - Presence of chills and/or rigors
  - Flank pain or renal angle tenderness
- Infections in men are often considered complicated, particularly if they have pelvic or perineal pain which can suggest accompanying prostatitis.
- May be difficult to treat with relapses after treatment common.
- Sequelae like sepsis, metastatic abscesses and renal failure are common.
- Underlying conditions often present in complicated UTIs are listed in Box 16.6.

INVESTIGATIONS

- Dipstick tests are often used to detect nitrite (a metabolic product of typical pathogens of the urinary

BOX 16.6 Underlying Conditions in Complicated Urinary Tract Infections

- Diabetes
- Pregnancy
- Hospital-acquired infection
- Renal failure
- Urinary tract obstruction
- Presence of an indwelling urethral catheter, stent, nephrostomy tube
- Recent urinary tract instrumentation
- Functional or anatomic abnormality of the urinary tract
- Immunosuppressed patient

BOX 16.7 Causes of Sterile Pyuria

- Partially treated UTI
- Calculi in urinary tract
- Urinary tuberculosis
- Infection with other organisms (e.g. *Chlamydia, Corynebacterium*)
- Bladder tumours
- Chemical cystitis
- Prostatitis
- Interstitial nephritis
- Appendicitis

tract) and leucocyte esterase (a marker of inflammation). Presence of either of them increases the possibility of UTI.

- A freshly voided midstream urine specimen obtained by a 'clean-catch' technique should be examined for leucocytes, leucocyte casts and red cells. Suprapubic aspiration of bladder avoids a contaminated urine sample but is rarely required.
- Gram staining and bacterial colony count.
- Culture and sensitivity. Causes of sterile pyuria are mentioned in Box 16.7.

SPECIAL INVESTIGATIONS

- Rectal examination to assess the prostate.
- Prostatic massage followed by urine culture if suspicion of prostatitis.
- Cystoscopy in suspected bladder lesions.
- Renal ultrasonography to identify obstruction, cysts and calculi.
- Intravenous urography (IVU), including a postvoid film of bladder to identify physiological and anatomical abnormalities of urinary tract.
- MCU to identify and quantitate vesicoureteric reflux and disturbed bladder emptying.
- Dimercaptosuccinic acid (DMSA) renal scan for pyelonephritis.
- In females with recurrent UTI, pelvic examination is mandatory to exclude cystocele, rectocele and uterovaginal prolapse.

TREATMENT

- Fluid intake more than 2 L/day to initiate water diuresis so as to maintain a high rate of urine flow.
- If patient has a stone, catheter or other obstructions, no antibiotics unless symptomatic.
- Regular complete bladder emptying.
- Alkalinisation of urine.
- Urinary analgesics (e.g. phenazopyridine) and antispasmodics (e.g. hyoscyamine) for detrusor spasm.
- Antibiotic therapy:
  - The choice of antibiotic depends on the organism isolated.
  - The commonly employed antibiotics include cotrimoxazole (one double-strength tablet twice a day), ampicillin or amoxicillin (500 mg 8 hourly), cephalosporins, nitrofurantoin (100 mg 12 hourly) and quinolones (ciprofloxacin, levofloxacin but not moxifloxacin). Antibiotics are given for a period of 3 days in uncomplicated infections (nitrofurantoin for 7 days) and for 7–10 days in complicated infections.
  - Fosfomycin 3 g as a single dose is effective in uncomplicated infections. However, due to fear of rapid development of resistance, its use as a single agent may be avoided.
  - For complicated infection, parenteral antibiotics preferable to oral ones. These antibiotics include ceftriaxone, piperacillin–tazobactam and meropenem. Aminoglycosides may be used for Gram-negative infections.
  - Chlamydial infection is treated with tetracycline 500 mg QID.
- In females, maintenance of adequate perineal hygiene, emptying the bladder before and after intercourse, and application of 0.5% cetrimide cream to periurethral area before intercourse reduces the incidence of UTIs.
- Double micturition should be practised if reflux is present.
- Asymptomatic bacteriuria should be treated if a patient is pregnant or is being planned for a urological surgery. Treatment of asymptomatic bacteriuria in pregnant women decreases the occurrence of pyelonephritis which may also cause damage to the child (low birth weight). Treatment is not required in premenopausal, nonpregnant women, diabetic patients, renal transplant patients, elderly or patients with spinal cord injury or indwelling urethral catheters.

Q. Discuss the clinical features, investigations and management of acute pyelonephritis.

- Acute pyelonephritis is an infection of the upper urinary tract. The renal pelvis is acutely inflamed and there is often coincident cystitis. Small cortical abscesses and linear streaks of pus in the medulla may be present.
- Progression of upper urinary tract infection to emphysematous pyelonephritis, renal abscesses, perinephric abscess or papillary necrosis indicates complicated acute pyelonephritis.

CLINICAL FEATURES

- There is commonly sudden onset of pain in one or both loins (costovertebral or renal angles) which may radiate to the iliac fossa and suprapubic area.
- Frequent passage of small amount of scalding, cloudy urine with urgency and dysuria due to associated cystitis (in nearly 80% of cases).
- Fever with chills and rigors may occur.
- Tenderness and guarding are usually present in the renal angle.
- In the presence of obstruction (stone, tumour, bladder neck obstruction, enlarged prostate), acute pyelonephritis can be extremely severe and may progress to renal abscess.
- Rarely, may be complicated by papillary necrosis particularly in patients with underlying diabetes, sickle cell disease or analgesic nephropathy.

- Emphysematous pyelonephritis is a severe infection of the renal parenchyma that causes gas accumulation in the tissues. It most often occurs in persons with diabetes mellitus and presents like acute pyelonephritis but with a fulminating course.

INVESTIGATIONS

- Peripheral blood leucocytosis is a characteristic feature.
- Microscopic examination of urine shows numerous pus cells, WBC casts and organisms, some red cells and epithelial cells.
- Culture of MSU may grow the organism.
- Investigations to exclude anatomical abnormalities of the urinary tract are required when the diagnosis is uncertain, patient has severe presentations when obstruction or abscess must be expeditiously excluded, or if there is inadequate response or rapid recurrence following appropriate therapy.
  - Ultrasound studies are used most frequently but are relatively insensitive.
  - Computerised tomography (CT) is the imaging modality of choice if ultrasound is normal. It will identify calculi, gas, haemorrhage, obstruction, renal enlargement and inflammatory masses.
  - IVU is rarely required at present.
  - A radionuclide scan (where the radionuclide agent is injected into bladder through suprapubic route) may be performed to detect reflux.
  - DMSA renal scan performed within 2 days can help in diagnosing acute pyelonephritis. However, a scan done 4–6 months after an acute episode is more important to detect renal parenchymal damage in the form of renal scarring.

MANAGEMENT

- In mildly ill patients (those with minimal nausea, no vomiting, stable medical conditions), oral cotrimoxazole, amoxicillin–clavulanate and quinolones (e.g. ciprofloxacin), all active against *E. coli*, are effective following a short observation period, intravenous fluids and oral/parenteral antibiotic therapy in the emergency department. Nitrofurantoin and oral fosfomycin attain adequate concentrations only in the urine and thus should be avoided.
- Severe cases require intravenous amoxicillin–clavulanate plus aminoglycoside, or a cephalosporin (e.g. ceftriaxone, cefepime), or piperacillin–tazobactam or meropenem for 10–14 days.

Q. Give an account of the aetiopathogenesis, clinical features, investigations and management of chronic pyelonephritis (reflux nephropathy).

- Chronic pyelonephritis (also called reflux nephropathy) refers to chronic interstitial nephritis that occurs as a result of recurrent UTIs, commonly due to severe vesicoureteric reflux in children.

AETIOPATHOGENESIS

- Reflux of urine from the bladder into the ureter during voiding is normally prevented because the ureter passes through the vesical wall obliquely and is therefore occluded during contraction of the bladder. Abnormalities of the intramural ureter allow reflux to occur and organisms from the bladder to reach the kidney.
- Vesicoureteric reflux is commonly congenital but can be due to obstructive lesions at the bladder neck. It may be unilateral or bilateral. Reflux diminishes as the child grows and usually disappears.
- When UTI occurs in the presence of obstruction or stasis, permanent renal damage may result in any age group.
- The most important morphological changes in the kidney are the presence of coarse scars. Each scar is associated with contraction of the related papilla and dilatation of the corresponding calyx.

CLINICAL FEATURES

- Clinical features may include lassitude, vague ill health or symptoms of uraemia or hypertension. Other symptoms include frequency of micturition, dysuria and aching lumbar pain. Pyuria may be present.

INVESTIGATIONS

- Culture of the urine is mandatory. *E. coli* is the most common organism. Other agents include *Proteus*, *Pseudomonas aeruginosa* and staphylococci.
- Ultrasound of kidneys.
- Intravenous urogram shows the diagnostic features. There is localised contraction of the renal substance associated with clubbing of the adjacent calyces.
- A micturating cystourethrogram (MCU) will disclose vesicoureteric reflux. This has been replaced by radionuclide cystography scan in many centres.
- DMSA scan more accurate than IVU in evaluating the presence of renal lesions subsequent to UTI in the face of reflux.
- Imaging studies such as CT and MRI are necessary to show evidence of scarred, shrunken kidneys.
- Cystoscopy and urography may help to identify any abnormality causing obstruction to the flow of urine.

MANAGEMENT

- Attempts should be made to correct abnormalities of the urinary tract including malformations. Calculi should be removed.
- Appropriate antibiotics should be given for 7 days.
- If the infection cannot be eradicated, suppressive therapy may be required with trimethoprim (100 mg at bedtime) or nitrofurantoin (50 mg at bedtime) for several months.
- Complete emptying of the bladder should be ensured. If reflux is present, 'double micturition' is practised. The patient is advised to empty the bladder and then again attempt to empty a second time, approximately 10–15 minutes later.
- Control of hypertension is essential.

TABLE 16.9 Causes of Acute Tubulointerstitial Nephropathy

• Infections	Acute pyelonephritis, systemic infections
• Drugs	Analgesics (NSAIDs), antimicrobials (beta-lactams, sulphonamides), diuretics, anticonvulsants, allopurinol, proton-pump inhibitors, cancer immunotherapy agents (immune checkpoint inhibitors)
• Metabolic	Acute oxalate nephropathy, acute acid nephropathy, acute nephrocalcinosis
• Immunological	Renal transplant rejection, SLE, Sjögren's syndrome, sarcoidosis, IgG4 tubulointerstitial nephropathy
• Others	Plasma cell dyscrasias, myeloproliferative disorders, heat stroke, irradiation

- Surgery is indicated if the vesicoureteric reflux persists. Most cases of childhood reflux tend to disappear spontaneously.

Q. Write a short note on acute tubulointerstitial nephropathy or nephritis.

- Tubulointerstitial nephropathy or nephritis is an inflammatory disease affecting primarily tubules and interstitium of kidneys.
- It is a relatively common cause of both acute kidney injury and CKD.
- Common causes of acute tubulointerstitial nephropathy are given in Table 16.9.

CLINICAL FEATURES

DRUG-INDUCED ACUTE TUBULOINTERSTITIAL NEPHROPATHY

- Acute kidney injury may occur within a few hours to weeks after the start of a drug.
- Nonspecific symptoms are common and include generalised malaise, fatigue, weakness and anorexia.
- In many patients, renal involvement is preceded by fever, skin rash and eosinophilia.
- Urine shows microscopic haematuria, leucocytes, WBC casts, renal tubular epithelial cells and proteinuria.
- Eosinophilia (>50% of leucocytes) is a sensitive marker of drug-induced nephropathy.
- Heavy proteinuria may be seen in some cases of NSAIDs-induced acute tubulointerstitial nephropathy.
- Ultrasound shows large swollen kidneys which are often echogenic due to the inflammatory interstitial infiltrates and interstitial oedema.
- Histological features of interstitial immune infiltrate, eosinophils and tubulitis are characteristic.
- Treatment includes cessation of drug and corticosteroids (either orally or intravenous pulses of methylprednisolone).

Q. Write a short note on analgesic nephropathy.

- Prolonged use of analgesics (NSAIDs, paracetamol, phenacetin–paracetamol combination) leads to this type of chronic tubulointerstitial nephropathy.
- Patients often have a history of chronic headache or low back pain that leads to the analgesic use.
- Analgesic nephropathy is characterised by chronic tubulointerstitial disease (producing CKD) and papillary necrosis.
- Usually, patients have no symptoms, and the disease is incidentally detected by laboratory studies that are performed for an unrelated problem and show an elevated creatinine or abnormal urinalysis.
- Episodes of papillary necrosis manifest as gross haematuria with flank pain occasionally accompanied by obstruction.
- Some patients have a history of recurrent UTIs.
- Laboratory investigations show elevated serum creatinine levels. Urinalysis shows haematuria, sterile pyuria and mild proteinuria (<1.5 g/day). Anaemia may be disproportionate to degree of CKD.
- Imaging (X-ray, ultrasound and CT scan) often show shrunken, irregular kidneys with calcification of renal papillae.
- Renal function stabilises in most patients with mild reduction in GFR (GFR between 30 and 89 mL/minute/1.73 m^2) when analgesic consumption is discontinued. However, if renal disease is already advanced, then progression generally occurs even in the absence of drug intake.
- Analgesic nephropathy may be complicated by development of urinary tract malignancy. Therefore, any new haematuria should be investigated to exclude malignancy as its cause.

Q. How do you define and classify chronic kidney disease? What are the risk factors for development of chronic kidney disease? (IM 10.1, IM 10.6)

- CKD is defined as abnormalities of kidney structure or function present for >3 months, with implications for health.
- Criteria for defining CKD are shown in Box 16.8.

BOX 16.8 Criteria for CKD

- Glomerular filtration rate (GFR) of <60 mL/minute/1.73 m^2 for 3 months or more with or without kidney damage

Or

- Kidney damage for 3 or more months with or without decreased GFR as evidenced by any of the following:
  - Urinary albumin excretion rate 30–300 mg/day or urinary albumin 30–300 mg/g excretion of creatinine
  - Urinary albumin excretion rate >300 mg/day or urinary albumin >300 mg/g excretion of creatinine
  - Persistent haematuria (where other causes such as urological conditions have been excluded)
  - Urine sediment abnormalities (e.g. red or white blood cell casts)
  - Electrolyte abnormalities due to tubular disorders
  - Pathological abnormalities (e.g. renal biopsy showing glomerular, vascular or tubulointerstitial disease)
  - Radiological abnormalities (e.g. scarring, hydronephrosis or polycystic kidneys on renal ultrasound scan)
  - History of renal transplantation

PROGRESSION

- Major outcomes of CKD include progression to kidney failure, complications from decreased kidney function and development of cardiovascular disease.
- Cardiovascular events are more common than renal failure.
- Because of the older age at onset for many forms of CKD and the slow rate of decline in kidney function, decreased kidney function is far more common than kidney failure.
- Kidney failure is defined as a GFR <15 mL/minute/1.73 m^2, usually accompanied by signs and symptoms of uraemia, or as the need for initiation of kidney replacement therapy (dialysis or transplantation) for management of the complications of a decreased GFR (the term 'end-stage renal disease' [ESRD] is used when renal replacement therapy is required).
- Therapeutic interventions in the earlier stages may prevent or reduce some of these complications including progression to kidney failure.

STAGES

- CKD is classified based on its cause, six GFR categories (G stages) and three albuminuria categories (A stages) as given by Kidney Disease: Improving Global Outcomes (KDIGO) guidelines (Table 16.10).
- Patients with GFR category of G1 or G2 along with albuminuria category of A1 have low risk of progression of CKD.

RISK FACTORS FOR DEVELOPING CKD

- Risk factors for developing CKD are given in Table 16.11.

TABLE 16.10 Stages of Chronic Kidney Disease Based on Glomerular Filtration Rate and Albuminuria

GFR Stage	Description	GFR (mL/minute/1.73 m^2)	
• G1	Slight kidney damage with normal or increased filtration	>90	
• G2	Mild decrease in kidney function	60–89	
• G3a	Mild to moderate decrease in kidney function	45–59	
• G3b	Moderate to severe decrease in kidney function	30–44	
• G4	Severe decrease in kidney function	15–29	
• G5	Kidney failure (often requires dialysis or transplantation)	<15 (add D if treated by dialysis)	
Albuminuria Categories	**Description**	**Albuminuria (mg/24 hours)**	**Albumin to Creatinine Ratio (mg/g)**
• A1	Normal to mildly increased	<30	<30
• A2	Moderately increased	30–300	30–300
• A3	Severely increased	>300	>300

TABLE 16.11 Risk Factors for Developing Chronic Kidney Disease

Factors	Examples
• Increased susceptibility to kidney damage	Older age, family history of chronic kidney disease (CKD), low birth weight, low income or educational level
• Factors initiating kidney damage	Diabetes mellitus, hypertension, autoimmune diseases, systemic infections, UTIs, urinary stones, obstruction of lower urinary tract, drug toxicity
• Worsening kidney damage	Higher level of proteinuria, higher blood pressure level, poor glycaemic control in diabetes, smoking
• Increased morbidity and mortality in kidney failure	Anaemia, low serum albumin level, late referral for dialysis

Q. Discuss the aetiology, clinical features, investigations, diagnosis and management of chronic kidney disease (CKD) or chronic renal failure (CRF) or chronic kidney failure. (IM10.15, IM10.24, IM10.26, IM10.27, IM10.5, IM10.7, IM10.9)

Q. Describe renal osteodystrophy.

- CKD is defined as abnormalities of kidney structure or function present for >3 months, with implications for health.
- CRF or kidney failure is defined as irreversible deterioration in renal function over 3 months with GFR <15/minute/1.73 m^2.
- Common causes of CKD are given in Box 16.9.

CLINICAL FEATURES

- Many patients in early stages of CKD are asymptomatic. Symptoms generally develop when GFR falls below 30 mL/minute/1.73 m^2.
- Anorexia, nausea and vomiting are usually attributed to the formation of ammonia from urea in the upper gastrointestinal tract.
- Anaemia in CKD is normochromic and normocytic in type and is primarily due to reduced erythropoietin production by the kidney. The causes of anaemia in CKD are given in Box 16.10.
- The term renal osteodystrophy embraces various forms of bone disease that develop in CKD. Renal

BOX 16.9 Causes of Chronic Kidney Disease

- Primary or secondary glomerulonephritis (see the list under 'acute glomerulonephritis')
- Diabetic nephropathy
- Hypertensive nephrosclerosis
- Polycystic kidney disease
- Chronic pyelonephritis
- Tubulointerstitial diseases
- Analgesic nephropathy
- Vesicoureteric reflux
- Renal tuberculosis
- Nephrocalcinosis
- Obstructive uropathy

BOX 16.10 Causes of Anaemia in CKD

- Decreased erythropoiesis due to reduced availability of erythropoietin
- Reduced dietary intake due to anorexia
- Impaired intestinal iron absorption and reduced iron mobilisation from body stores (due to increased hepcidin caused by chronic inflammation)
- Anaemia of chronic disease
- Uraemic toxin depression on marrow precursor cells
- Reduced red cell survival
- Increased blood loss due to poor platelet function and capillary fragility
- Blood loss during haemodialysis

osteodystrophy includes osteomalacia, hyperparathyroid bone disease (osteitis fibrosa), osteoporosis and osteosclerosis. Osteomalacia results from the failure of the kidney to produce 1,25-dihydroxycholecalciferol which causes decreased intestinal absorption of calcium. This leads to reduction in calcification of bone. The low plasma calcium stimulates the parathyroid gland resulting in secondary hyperparathyroidism. In some patients, tertiary autonomous hyperparathyroidism develops. Osteoporosis is probably related to malnutrition. Osteosclerosis literally means 'hardening of bone' and may be a direct result of excess parathyroid hormone. Alternate bands of sclerotic and porotic bone in the vertebrae produce the characteristic 'rugger jersey spine' in the radiograph (also refer to page 774, Chapter 11).
- Generalised myopathy is due to a combination of poor nutrition, hyperparathyroidism and vitamin D deficiency.
- Neuropathy may be motor, sensory (characterised by restless leg or burning feet) or autonomic.
- Endocrine abnormalities include amenorrhoea in females and loss of libido in both sexes.
- Pericarditis is a common cardiovascular complication in untreated end-stage renal failure.
- Hypertension develops in approximately 80% of patients with CRF.
- Metabolic acidosis is a common accompaniment of CRF.
- Electrolyte abnormalities, particularly hyperkalaemia, hypocalcaemia and hyperphosphataemia.
- Patients with CKD have increased susceptibility to infections due to impaired cellular and humoral immunity.
- In addition, uraemia can affect the lung ('uraemic lung') and brain ('uraemic encephalopathy').
- Frequently, patients complain of pruritus, often intractable.
- An increased tendency to bleeding is present due primarily to impaired platelet function.
- Dialysis dementia and dialysis disequilibrium are dialysis-related complications.
- Various features of CKD are shown in Fig. 16.5.

INVESTIGATIONS

- Important urinary abnormalities include a fixed specific gravity around 1.010 (isosthenuria) and the presence of broad casts.

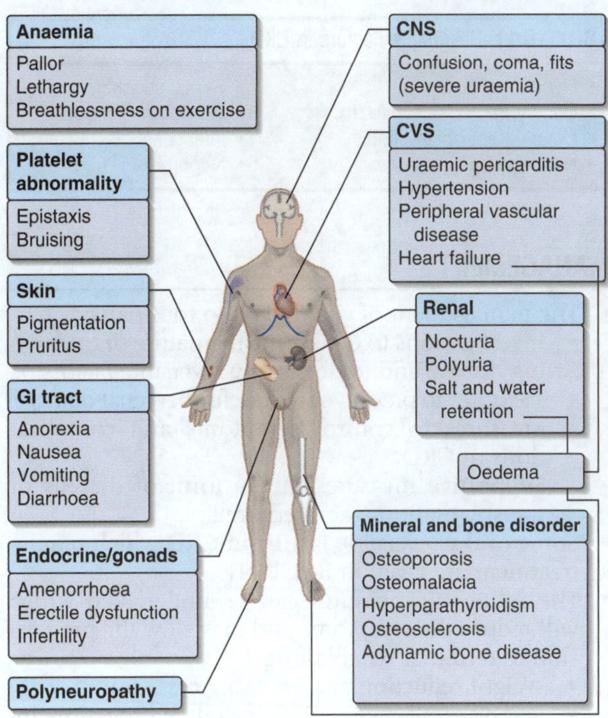

Fig. 16.5 Signs and symptoms of CKD.

- White cells in the urine usually indicate infection but may also occur in renal tuberculosis and papillary necrosis.
- Eosinophils in the urine indicate allergic tubulointerstitial disease while red cell casts suggest glomerulonephritis.
- The common haematological abnormality is a normochromic normocytic anaemia.
- The most consistent biochemical abnormalities are elevated levels of blood urea and creatinine. The level of serum creatinine correlates with the degree of renal impairment. Other biochemical abnormalities include hypocalcaemia, hyperphosphataemia, hyperuricaemia and hyperkalaemia. Bicarbonate levels are reduced.
- Creatinine clearance is important to assess the severity of renal failure.
- A plain radiograph of the abdomen may be useful in determining the kidney size and in the evaluation of obstructive uropathy.
- Renal ultrasound typically shows shrunken kidneys. In diabetic glomerulosclerosis, amyloidosis, polycystic kidney diseases, bilateral hydronephrosis and myeloma kidney, the kidneys may be of normal size.
- CT is useful in some patients with suspected obstructive nephropathy.
- Transcutaneous renal biopsy is of value in establishing the diagnosis in selected cases, particularly in cases associated with normal-sized kidneys, with the possible exception of diabetic glomerulosclerosis. It is particularly useful if renal functions are deteriorating rapidly.

BOX 16.11 Reversible Factors in CKD

- Hypertension
- Urinary tract infection (UTI)
- Urinary tract obstruction
- Haemorrhage
- Septic shock
- Cardiogenic shock
- Infections
- Nephrotoxic drugs

MANAGEMENT

- The management of CRF falls into four parts:
  - Investigations to determine the nature of underlying disease and to detect any reversible factors.
  - Measures to prevent or reduce further renal damage.
  - Measures to control symptoms and complications of CKD.
  - Supportive measures in the form of dialysis or transplantation when required.
- Some of the reversible factors in CKD which require treatment are given in Box 16.11.
- The following measures can be undertaken which will reduce the symptoms and may slow the progression to terminal renal failure:
  - Weight reduction and smoking cessation.
  - Review of all medications including drug–drug interactions as well as potential adverse effect on kidney function or complications. Avoid exposure to gadolinium contrast in patients with CKD stages 4 and 5 because it increases risk for nephrogenic systemic fibrosis.
  - Control of hypertension: The blood pressure should be reduced to less than 130/80 mmHg. If creatinine is below 5 mg/dL, ACE inhibitors or angiotensin-II receptor blockers are the drugs of choice. The 2021 KDIGO guideline recommends a target systolic BP of less than 120 mmHg, if tolerated, in patients with CKD, with and without diabetes, and not receiving dialysis. Other classes of antihypertensive agents (e.g. calcium channel blockers, thiazides, beta-blockers) can be combined with ACE inhibitors or angiotensin-II receptor antagonists if target BP is not achieved with these first-line agents.
  - DASH diet (dietary approaches to stop hypertension), which is high in fruits, vegetables and dairy foods containing little total saturated fat and cholesterol. However, DASH diet is recommended only for patients with a GFR >60 mL/minute/1.73 m^2 (stage 1 or 2 CKD) because it contains more protein, potassium and phosphorous than recommended for patients with stage 3 or 4 CKD. For stages 4 and 5, low-protein diet of 0.6 g/kg body weight is recommended.
  - Avoidance of high-potassium foods.
  - Lowering of salt intake to below 2 g of sodium/day (equivalent to <5 g of common salt/day). However, patients with salt-losing nephropathy (tubulointerstitial disease) require a high-salt intake.
  - Control of diabetes (HbA1c <7.0). Treatment with sodium–glucose co-transporter 2 (SGLT-2) inhibitors may reduce the risk of kidney disease progression in patients with type 2 diabetes.
  - Hypocalcaemia and hyperphosphataemia should be treated aggressively. Hypocalcaemia requires treatment with calcitriol or alphacalcidol (1-α-hydroxyvitamin D_3) or paricalcitol (19-nor-1,25-dihydroxyvitamin D_3) and calcium supplementation. Vitamin D supplementation reduces cardiovascular mortality in ESRD patients. Serum calcium should be monitored frequently to avoid hypercalcaemia. Oral calcium carbonate also reduces the bioavailability of dietary phosphates.
  - Phosphate binders:
    - Previously, aluminium hydroxide was used to bind phosphates in the gut. However, aluminium toxicity was common in these patients.
    - Calcium carbonate and calcium acetate; serum calcium should be monitored.
    - Sevelamer carbonate, an anion-exchange resin.
    - Lanthanum carbonate, a nonaluminium, noncalcium phosphate-binding agent (higher incidence of side effects).
  - Treating hyperparathyroidism:
    - Use of calcium carbonate or acetate.
    - Use of vitamin D analogues.
    - Use of calcimimetics which suppress secretion of parathyroid hormone by sensitising the parathyroid calcium receptor to serum calcium. This results in fall of PTH secretion. Cinacalcet has been approved for use in patients on dialysis.
  - Metabolic acidosis should be corrected with calcium carbonate, and, if required, with small doses of sodium bicarbonate.
  - Hyperkalaemia usually responds to dietary restrictions. Some patients require addition of potassium-exchange resins (sodium polystyrene sulphonate, sodium zirconium cyclosilicate and patiromer).
  - Anaemia should be corrected by appropriate addition of iron, folate and vitamin B_{12} if required. In nondialysis patients, iron can be given orally, although intravenous iron is more effective. If iron replacement alone is not sufficient, erythropoietin (or darbepoetin alpha) should be added. Blood pressure should be carefully monitored during erythropoietin therapy. Goal of iron therapy is to maintain adequate iron stores (transferrin saturation >30% and serum ferritin levels >500 ng/mL) with a target haemoglobin of 11 to 12 g/dL. Haemoglobin >13 g/dL has been shown to be associated with increased incidence of cardiovascular mortality.
- Uraemic pruritus may respond to gabapentin.
- Active uraemic bleed may require administration of desmopressin (dDAVP), cryoprecipitate, oestrogen and initiation of dialysis.
- Hyperlipidaemia should be treated with diet control and drugs.
- If conservative measures are inadequate, haemodialysis may be needed.
- Kidney transplantation offers the possibility of restoring normal kidney functions.
- Indications for urgent dialysis:
  - Severe hyperkalaemia.
  - Pulmonary oedema or severe fluid overload.
  - Severe metabolic acidosis.
  - Uraemic pericarditis.
  - Uraemic encephalopathy.
  - Toxicity with a dialysable poison (methanol, salicylate, phenobarbital).

TABLE 16.12 Renal Replacement Therapies

• Dialysis	• Clearance of small molecules and toxins using diffusion across a membrane
• Haemodialysis	• Dialysis with clearance across a synthetic membrane by diffusion
• Peritoneal dialysis	• Dialysis with clearance across a native membrane (peritoneum)
• Ultrafiltration	• Fluid removal across a semipermeable membrane during dialysis by convection (solutes are moved under pressure across a membrane)
• Haemofiltration	• Continuous dialysis therapy in which large amounts of fluid are removed from blood by convection with concurrent reinfusion of an electrolytic solution
• Haemodiafiltration	• Combination of haemodialysis and haemofiltration
• Continuous renal replacement therapies	• Include haemofiltration and haemodiafiltration

Q. What are the renal replacement therapies available?

- Renal replacement therapies are listed in Table 16.12.

Q. Write a note on haemodialysis.

Q. Write a short note on dialysis in critically ill patients.

- In principle, haemodialysis allows accumulated uraemic toxins (e.g. urea and creatinine) and electrolytes (e.g. potassium) to diffuse across a semipermeable membrane from the blood, where they are in high concentrations, to the dialysate fluid on the other side of the membrane.
- Blood is circulated through an artificial kidney. The artificial kidney consists of a blood compartment and a dialysis fluid compartment separated by a semipermeable membrane. As the blood and the dialysis fluid move on either side of the membrane, diffusion of electrolytes and low-molecular-weight substances occurs.
- The dialyser membrane can be made up of four types of materials: cellulose, cellulose acetate, cellulosynthetic and synthetic (polysulphone, polyacrylonitrile). Synthetic membrane is preferred as it causes very little complement activation.
- Each session of haemodialysis usually lasts for 4 to 5 hours. Two or three sittings per week may be necessary (intermittent haemodialysis).
- For long-term dialysis, access to the bloodstream is ensured by the creation of an arteriovenous fistula, usually in the forearm. Another option is by interposing a piece of synthetic material between native artery and native vein (graft).

COMPLICATIONS

- The major complication is hypotension during dialysis. Factors that contribute to hypotension include:
  - Excessive removal of extracellular fluid.
  - Shift of fluid into intracellular compartment due to rapid reduction in urea in the extracellular compartment.
  - Abnormalities of venous tone.
  - Autonomic neuropathy.
  - Acetate toxicity that causes vasodilatation.
- Other complications include muscle cramps, anaphylactoid reaction to the dialyser, air embolism, infections, haemolysis, uraemic pericarditis (dialysis associated) and pulmonary oedema.
- Dialysis disequilibrium syndrome occurs following a dialysis session and is characterised by nausea, vomiting, restlessness, headache, hypertension, myoclonic jerks and, in severe case, seizures and coma. This is due to rapid changes in plasma osmolality that produces cerebral oedema. Management is supportive.
- Patients on long-term haemodialysis may develop dialysis dementia. It is characterised by speech dyspraxia, myoclonic jerks, dementia, seizures and, later, death. Aluminium toxicity is the most important factor in the pathogenesis of this disorder. Some viral infection may also play a role in this.
- The rate of death from cardiac disease is higher in patients on haemodialysis as compared to in patients on peritoneal dialysis or after renal transplantation.
- Other complications seen in patients on dialysis include Wernicke's encephalopathy and central pontine myelinolysis (due to rapid correction of hyponatraemia).

ACUTE DIALYSIS IN CRITICALLY ILL PATIENTS

- Continuous renal replacement therapy (CRRT) modalities and sustained (or slow) low-efficiency daily dialysis (SLEDD) are used in critically ill patients who are unable to tolerate large fluid shifts and hypotension that frequently accompany standard haemodialysis.
- Allows slow and isotonic fluid removal resulting in excellent haemodynamic tolerance even in patients with shock or severe fluid overload.
- Since dialysis is continuous, volume removal and correction of metabolic abnormalities can be modified at any time, allowing for rapid adjustments in critically ill patients.
- Several CRRT modalities are available. The most common is continuous venovenous haemodiafiltration, which combines convective and diffusive clearance through a dialyser with reinfusion of electrolyte-rich solutions.
- CRRT is the dialysis modality of choice in patients with ARF combined with haemodynamic instability, cerebral oedema, severe fluid overload and hepatic encephalopathy.
- 'Hybrid' or SLEDD combines the advantages of intermittent haemodialysis with those of CRRT. In this technique, classic dialysis hardware is used at low blood and dialysate flow rates for a prolonged period of time (6–12 hours/day). It offers more haemodynamic stability, better correction of hypervolaemia and more adequate solute removal compared with intermittent haemodialysis.

Q. Write a short note on peritoneal dialysis.

- In peritoneal dialysis, the peritoneum of the patient acts as a semipermeable membrane across which diffusion of water and solutes takes place.
- A plastic or silicone catheter is placed into the peritoneal cavity through the anterior abdominal wall. Dialysate (2 L) is instilled into the peritoneal space. Water, urea, creatinine and other toxins pass across the peritoneal membrane into the dialysate. The fluid is removed by gravity after 30–60 minutes and the same procedure is repeated several times. This is called intermittent peritoneal dialysis. It is chiefly used in acute kidney injury (AKI) if haemodialysis is not available.
- The main complication is the occurrence of peritonitis and infections around the catheter site. Abdominal pain may be absent in peritoneal dialysis-associated peritonitis. Some patients may develop pleural effusion due to preexisting pleuroperitoneal communication.
- There are other forms of peritoneal dialysis that are useful for chronic dialysis.

CONTINUOUS AMBULATORY PERITONEAL DIALYSIS (CAPD)

- Here, the dwelling time of fluid is long so that only three to five cycles are done in a day. The patient infuses 1.5–3 L of dialysate in the peritoneal cavity. The solution is allowed to remain for more than 4 hours during the day and 8–12 hours at night. This technique is useful for maintenance of dialysis in patients with CKD.

AUTOMATED PERITONEAL DIALYSIS

- Here, a cycler is used to perform multiple overnight exchanges resulting in multiple short dwells. It includes the following types of peritoneal dialysis:
  - Continuous cycling peritoneal dialysis (CCPD): Here, a cycler delivers three or more overnight exchanges, usually with a fewer exchanges during day time.
  - Nightly intermittent peritoneal dialysis (NIPD): Here, a cycler delivers three to six overnight exchanges, usually with no dwelling during the day.
  - Tidal dialysis: Here, a residual volume of dialysate is left in the peritoneal cavity with continuous cycling of smaller volumes in and out.

Q. Write a short note on renal transplantation.

- Successful renal transplantation offers the potential for complete rehabilitation in advanced CRF.
- The donor is most often a living related person. With the acceptance of the concept of brain death in India, an increasing number of cadaveric transplants are being performed at present.
- Living donors should be healthy with the same ABO blood group as the recipient. He/she should be free of hypertension, diabetes or malignant disease (except possibly those with neoplasms originating in the CNS).
- The donor's HLA is matched with that of the recipient. It is preferable to have an HLA-identical donor. Class I antigens (HLA-A, HLA-B and HLA-C) are detected by a lymphocyte assay and class II (HLA-DR) by mixed lymphocyte culture. If an HLA-identical donor is not available, haplo-identical (half-identical) living donor is required for long survival of the graft.
- Presensitisation (presence of antibodies against donor ABO and class I antigens) is detected by a crossmatch, which if positive is a contraindication for transplantation.

CONTRAINDICATIONS (Box 16.12)

BOX 16.12 Contraindications of Renal Transplantation

Absolute Contraindications	Relative Contraindications
• Reversible renal involvement	• Iliofemoral occlusive disease
• Disseminated or untreated cancer	• Diabetes mellitus
• Severe psychiatric disease	• Severe bladder or urethral abnormalities
• Persistent substance abuse	• Elderly age group
• Severe mental retardation	• Chronic liver disease
• Unreconstructable coronary artery disease	• Treated malignancy
• Refractory congestive heart failure	
• Active infection	
• Active glomerulonephritis	
• Previous sensitisation to donor tissue	

SURGICAL PROCEDURE

- The recipient receives a haemodialysis before transplantation to ensure a relatively normal metabolic state.
- The donor kidney is placed in an extraperitoneal pouch in the iliac fossa of the recipient (heterotopic kidney transplantation). The renal artery and vein are anastomosed to the recipient's iliac vessels. The donor ureter is implanted into the bladder.
- The recipient's own kidneys are left undisturbed.

IMMUNOSUPPRESSIVE THERAPY

- Current immunosuppressive therapy varies from centre to centre. A combination of drugs is often used to prevent rejection.
- Commonly used immunosuppressants include steroids, calcineurin inhibitors (e.g. cyclosporin, tacrolimus) and antiproliferative agents (e.g. azathioprine, mycophenolate mofetil). In addition, antilymphocyte or antithymocyte globulin is used for induction intraoperatively. Basiliximab (antibody against interleukin-2 receptor) may also be used for induction if antithymocyte globulin is not available.

COMPLICATIONS

- Despite prophylaxis with immunosuppressants begun just before or at the time of transplantation, most recipients undergo one or more rejection episodes.

- Hyperacute rejection:
  - A complement-mediated response in recipients with preexisting antibodies to the donor (e.g. anti-ABO blood-type antibodies). Complement activation within the graft is followed by endothelial necrosis, platelet deposition and local coagulation.
  - Occurs within minutes, and the transplant must be immediately removed to prevent a severe systemic inflammatory response and generalised clotting.
- Acute rejection:
  - Mediated by T cells; sometimes also by antibodies.
  - Acute rejection is suggested by deterioration of renal function, hypertension, weight gain, tenderness and swelling of the graft, fever, and appearance in the urine protein, lymphocytes and renal tubular cells. It generally occurs within 12 months of transplantation but can also occur late in patients who are nonadherent to their immunosuppression regimen.
  - A kidney allograft ultrasound with Doppler may reveal perinephric fluid collections (e.g. lymphocoele, urinary leak), urinary obstruction, or transplant renal artery stenosis. Other causes of renal allograft dysfunction include pyelonephritis, hypovolaemia, nephrotoxic medications and calcineurin inhibitor nephrotoxicity.
  - If the diagnosis is unclear, percutaneous needle biopsy is performed for histopathological evaluation of tissue.
  - Treatment of acute rejection involves the use of additional immunosuppressants including intravenous pulses of methylprednisolone and anti-lymphocyte antibody.
  - Antibody-mediated rejection is less likely to respond to steroids and can be treated with plasma exchange (to remove the antibody) and intravenous immunoglobulin.
- Chronic rejection:
  - Some patients suffer irreversible chronic graft rejection.
  - Can be antibody mediated or T-cell mediated.
- Other complications:
  - Drug toxicity including adverse effects of prednisolone.
  - Infections.
  - Recurrent underlying renal disease (e.g. hyperoxaluria, IgA nephropathy).
  - In addition, the incidence of malignancy in renal allograft recipients is increased.

Q. Discuss briefly the pathogenesis, clinical features, investigations and management of acute kidney injury. (IM 10.1, 10.15. 10.17, IM 10.2, IM 10.25, IM 10.3, IM 10.4)

Q. Give a brief account of acute kidney disease.

DEFINITION

- AKI is defined as a rapid, potentially reversible deterioration in renal function sufficient to result in accumulation of nitrogenous wastes in the body (uraemia) (Box 16.13).
- Presently, the term AKI is used in place of acute renal failure (ARF). The conventionally used term ARF is often used in reference to the subset of patients with a need for acute dialysis support.
- The term acute kidney disease (AKD) is used when AKI persists beyond 7 days till 3 months. The term AKD is also used if GFR <60 mL/minute/1.73 m^2 or GFR decreases by ≥35% over baseline within less than 3 months period. If the abnormalities persist beyond 3 months, it is called CKD.
- RIFLE criteria are used to classify severity of AKI. The acronym RIFLE stands for the increasing severity classes (Risk, Injury and Failure) and the two outcome classes (Loss and End-stage kidney disease). The three severity grades are defined on the basis of changes in serum creatinine or urine output where the worst of each criterion is used. Also, two outcome criteria are defined by duration of loss of kidney function, 4 weeks and 3 months, respectively (Table 16.13).
- As per Acute Kidney Injury Network (AKIN) classification, AKI is classified into three stages:
  - Stage 1 is same as risk category of RIFLE with the addition of increase in serum creatinine by 0.3 mg/dL.
  - Stages 2 and 3 are same as injury and failure categories of RIFLE.

BOX 16.13 Definition of Acute Kidney Injury

- An increase in serum creatinine of ≥0.3 mg/dL within 48 hours *or*
- An increase in serum creatinine of ≥1.5 times baseline, which is known or presumed to have occurred within the prior 7 days *or*
- Urine volume <0.5 mL/kg/hour for more than 6 hours

AETIOPATHOGENESIS

- The kidneys receive approximately 25% of the cardiac output at rest.

TABLE 16.13 RIFLE Criteria for Classification of Acute Kidney Injury

Criteria	Definition
• **R**isk	Increased creatinine 1.5–2 times baseline *Or* Urine output <0.5 mL/kg/hour × 6 hours
• **I**njury	Increased creatinine two to three times baseline *Or* Urine output <0.5 mL/kg/hour × 12 hours
• **F**ailure	Increased creatinine >3 times baseline or creatinine ≥4 mg/dL (acute rise of ≥0.5 mg/dL) *Or* Urine output <0.3 mL/kg/hour × 24 hours *Or* Anuria × 12 hours
• **L**oss	Persistent AKI = complete loss of renal function >4 weeks requiring dialysis
• **E**nd-stage kidney disease	End-stage kidney disease (>3 months) requiring dialysis

- In prerenal AKI, the kidneys are inadequately perfused (due to diminished cardiac output), and the GFR is greatly diminished resulting in oliguria (urine output <400 mL/day).
- Renal causes of AKI result from intrinsic diseases of the kidneys themselves, namely glomerular, tubulointerstitial or vascular diseases. In acute tubular necrosis (ATN), a diminution in the supply of oxygen and nutrients to the tubular cells results in ischaemia and necrosis of the tubular cells. Fortunately, the tubular cells can regenerate when the causative factors are removed.
- Postrenal AKI is caused by obstruction of the urinary tract at any point in its course.

CAUSES (Table 16.14)

TABLE 16.14 Causes of Acute Kidney Injury

Prerenal Causes	
• Hypovolaemia	Haemorrhage including antepartum and postpartum haemorrhage, severe vomiting including hyperemesis gravidarum, diarrhoea, loss of plasma as in burns, pancreatitis, excess of diuretics, diabetic ketoacidosis
• Reduced cardiac output	Heart failure, septic shock
• Renal vessel diseases	Renal artery obstruction
• Drugs	ACE inhibitors, NSAIDs
Renal Causes	
• Glomerular diseases	Glomerulonephritis (rapidly progressive GN, acute GN, others)
• Vascular diseases	Vasculitis, renal artery occlusion
• Acute tubulointerstitial nephritis	Drugs (cephalosporins, sulphonamides, NSAIDs, rifampicin) infections
• ATN	Renal ischaemia due to any cause, transfusion reactions, malaria (rhabdomyolysis), crush injury, heavy metals, septic abortion, drugs (contrast agents, aminoglycosides)
• Multiple mechanisms	Sepsis, snake bite (vipers), SARS-CoV-2 infection, hepatorenal syndrome
Postrenal Causes	
• Extrarenal obstruction	Prostatic enlargement, urethral stenosis, tumours, calculi
• Intrarenal obstruction	Uric acid crystals, sloughed papillae, drugs (e.g. acyclovir, methotrexate, indinavir), haemoglobinuria, myoglobinuria

CLINICAL FEATURES

- In AKI due to a prerenal disorder, the clinical features are those of the causal condition together with those of rapidly developing uraemia. Patients often present with a low blood pressure, poor peripheral perfusion and a falling urine output.
- ATN is the most important cause of AKI due to intrinsic renal disease. The clinical course in ATN can be divided into an oliguric phase, a maintenance phase and a diuretic phase.
  - In the oliguric phase, the patient may develop symptoms due to fluid overload and azotaemia. Fluid overload causes elevated jugular venous pressure, pedal oedema, ascites and pulmonary oedema. Hyperkalaemia occurs commonly during this phase. The oliguric phase usually lasts an average of 10–14 days but may vary from a few hours to as long as 4 weeks.
  - In the maintenance phase, which lasts for days to weeks, the GFR reaches its nadir and the urine output remains low.
  - With the onset of the diuretic phase, the urine output progressively increases. In a few days, the patient develops polyuria. During this phase, the tubular concentrating capacity is defective and uncontrolled loss of water and electrolytes may lead to dehydration, hyponatraemia and hypokalaemia. Eventually, the renal concentration capacity improves and urine volume decreases to normal.
- Not all patients with ATN develop oliguric failure. As many as 40% of the patients may have normal urine output. This is called nonoliguric AKI. The electrolyte disturbances are less in these patients.
- Patients with glomerulonephritis typically have hypertension, proteinuria and haematuria.
- Patients with drug-induced acute tubulointerstitial nephritis may present with fever, skin rash and arthralgias.
- AKI due to bilateral postrenal obstruction commonly causes anuria. The patient may give a history of loin pain, haematuria, renal colic or difficulty in micturition.
- Patients with AKI due to any cause may also have symptoms related to uraemia. These include anorexia, nausea, vomiting, pruritus, mental state changes, seizures and dyspnoea due to fluid overload. Important physical findings include asterixis, myoclonus, pericardial rub, and evidence of fluid overload in the form of oedema, elevated JVP and crepitations.
- Presence of anuria (urine <100 mL/day) indicates obstructive uropathy, bilateral renal cortical necrosis, RPGN (some cases) and acute bilateral renal artery or vein occlusion.

INVESTIGATIONS

CREATININE

- Elevated blood urea and creatinine levels are the most consistent findings. In prerenal AKI, there is a disproportionate elevation of urea in relation to creatinine.
- However, rise in creatinine is an unreliable indicator of early renal injury due to several reasons:
  - Serum creatinine is influenced by several nonrenal factors such as age, gender, muscle mass, medications, hydration status, nutrition status and tubular secretion.
  - Greater than 50% of kidney function must be lost before serum creatinine rises.
  - It does not reflect true GFR as several hours to days must elapse before a new equilibrium between presumably steady-state production and decreased excretion of creatinine is established.
- Therefore, several interventions which can prevent and/or treat early AKI cannot be instituted if diagnosis is based solely on creatinine levels.

NEWER MARKERS

- Novel biomarkers for AKI that can diagnose early cases include neutrophil gelatinase-associated lipocalin (NGAL), kidney injury molecule-1 (KIM-1), interleukin-18 (IL-18) and cystatin C.

OTHER INVESTIGATIONS

- Other biochemical abnormalities include hyperkalaemia, hypocalcaemia, hyperphosphataemia and hyperuricaemia.
- Urine analysis may show red cells, red cell casts and proteinuria in glomerulonephritis. In ATN, urinalysis shows epithelial cells and coarsely granular casts with mild proteinuria.
- In allergic interstitial nephritis, the urine shows white cells, red cells and eosinophils.
- In acute tubulointerstitial nephritis, proteinuria, glycosuria, aminoaciduria and potassium wasting can occur due to tubular dysfunction.
- Electrocardiogram may reveal evidences of hyperkalaemia.
- Chest radiograph may show evidences of pulmonary oedema and pleural effusion.
- Prerenal AKI characteristically shows a high urine osmolality (>500 mOsm/kg), low urinary sodium (<20 mmol/L) and a high urine creatinine/plasma creatinine ratio (>40).
- In patients suspected to have RPGN, systemic causes like granulomatosis with polyangiitis (Wegener's granulomatosis) must be excluded by appropriate investigations (cANCA). A kidney biopsy is also indicated in these patients.
- Renal imaging by plain abdominal radiography and ultrasonography may be of value in the evaluation of postrenal AKI.

LABORATORY ABNORMALITIES IN DIFFERENTIAL DIAGNOSIS OF AKI (Table 16.15)

TABLE 16.15 Laboratory Abnormalities in Differential Diagnosis of Acute Kidney Injury

	Prerenal	Renal	Postrenal
• Urine specific gravity	>1.025	~1.010	—
• Urine osmolality (mOsm/kg)	>500	<350	400
• Urine sediments	Scanty	Active	Scanty
• Urine sodium (mEq/L)	<20	>40	>40
• Fractional excretion of sodium (FE_{Na})[a]	<1	>1[b]	>4
• Urine/plasma creatinine	>40	<20	<20
• Fractional excretion of urea (FE_{Urea})[c]	<35%	>50%	—

[a]*Fractional excretion of sodium* (FE_{Na}) is the percentage of the sodium filtered by the kidney which is excreted in the urine. It is calculated as follows:
(Urinary sodium × serum creatinine)/(serum sodium × urinary creatinine) × 100

[b]May be <1% in early stages of glomerulonephritis and vascular disorders.

[c]*Fractional excretion of urea* (FE_{Urea}) is the percentage urea filtered by the kidneys which is excreted in the urine. It is calculated as follows:
(Urinary urea × serum creatinine)/(serum urea × urinary creatinine) × 100

COMPLICATIONS OF AKI (Table 16.16)

TABLE 16.16 Complication of Acute Kidney Injury

• Metabolic	Hyperkalaemia, hypocalcaemia, hyponatraemia or hypernatraemia, hyperphosphataemia, hyperuricaemia, metabolic acidosis
• Cardiovascular	Arrhythmias, pulmonary oedema, pericarditis, pericardial effusion, cardiac tamponade
• Neurological	Seizures, encephalopathy
• Gastrointestinal	Vomiting, haemorrhage
• Haematological	Anaemia, bleeding
• Others	Infections (pneumonia, UTI), chronic kidney disease

MANAGEMENT

- Therapy for AKI is directed at correcting fluid and electrolyte abnormalities, treating the underlying cause and preventing complications including nutritional deficiencies.
- An attempt should be made to identify the cause of AKI and to correct it, if possible.
- Administer a challenge of fluid intravenously in patients with clinical history consistent with fluid loss (such as vomiting and diarrhoea) and physical examination consistent with hypovolaemia (hypotension and tachycardia).
- Emergency treatment should be started for hyperkalaemia (K^+ >6 mmol/L) to prevent life-threatening complications.
- Acidosis should be treated with intravenous or oral bicarbonate if serum bicarbonate level is <15 mEq/L.
- Drugs such as loop diuretics, mannitol and dopamine have been used to increase urine output and reduce the duration of renal failure but they have been shown to be of no value.
- Patients who present with severe pulmonary oedema usually require haemodialysis.
- After correction of fluid deficit, maintain a daily fluid intake equal to the volume of the urine output plus 400–500 mL to balance the insensible loss.
- Dietary proteins should be restricted to about 40 g/day. Attempts can be made to suppress endogenous protein catabolism to a minimum by giving as much energy as possible in the form of carbohydrates and fats. Salt should also be restricted.
- Nephrotoxic drugs should be avoided.
- Patients with drug-induced acute tubulointerstitial nephritis usually recover after stopping the offending drug. At times, a short course of steroids may help.
- Patients with RPGN are treated with corticosteroids and cyclophosphamide.
- If conservative measures fail, haemodialysis may be required. The usual indications of haemodialysis in AKI are given in Box 16.14.

BOX 16.14 Indication of Haemodialysis in Acute Kidney Injury

- Symptomatic uraemia with high blood urea
- Serum creatinine >8 mg/dL
- Resistant hyperkalaemia
- Uraemic pericarditis
- Refractory pulmonary oedema
- Severe metabolic acidosis
- Uraemic encephalopathy

APPROACH TO ACUTE KIDNEY INJURY (Flowchart 16.3)

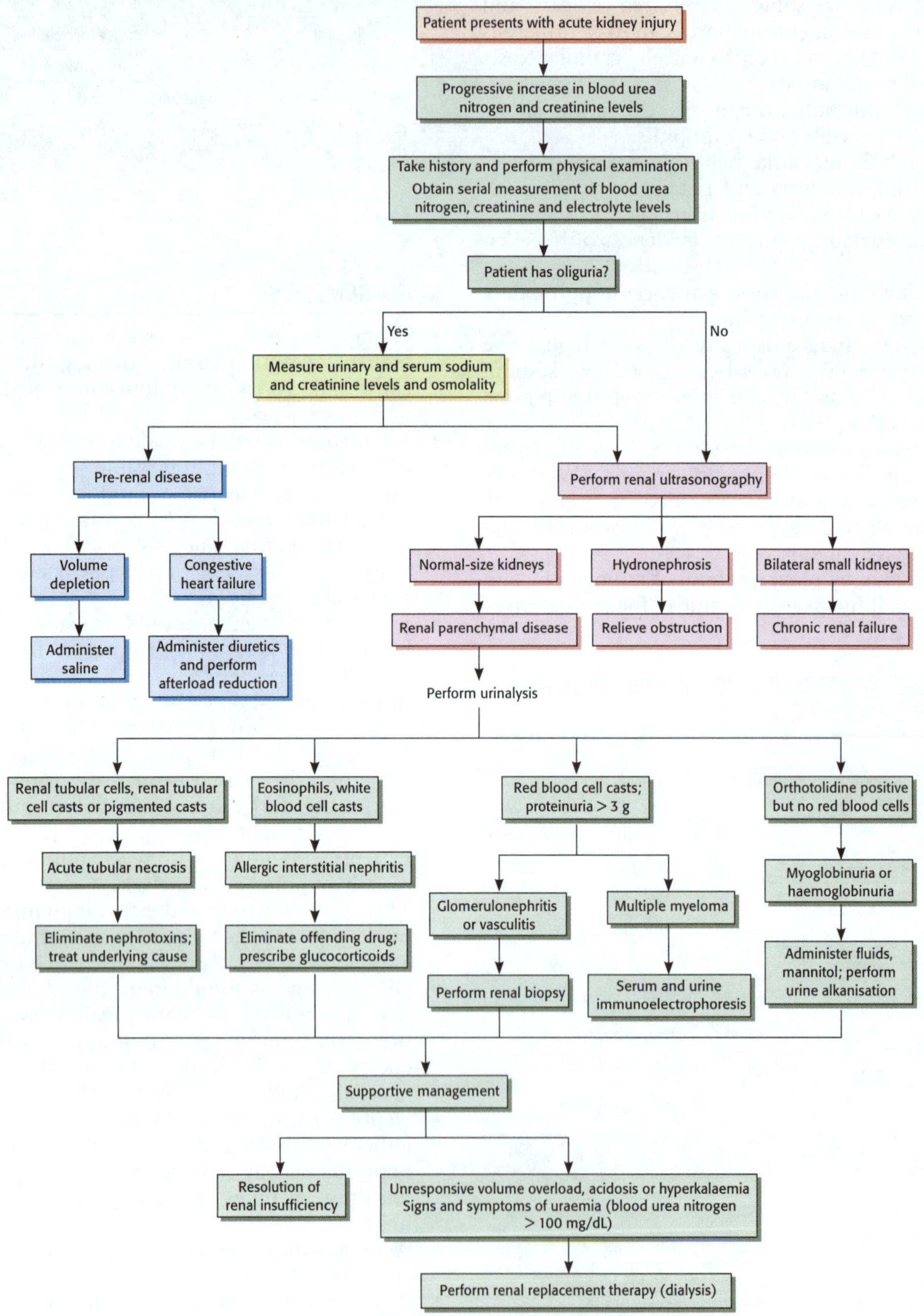

Flowchart 16.3 Algorithm for the Diagnosis and Treatment of Acute Kidney Injury. (*Source*: Adapted with permission from Smith MC. Acute renal failure. In: Resnick MI, Elder JS, Spirnak JP, eds. Critical Decisions in Urology. 3rd ed. Hamilton, Ont., Canada: BC Decker, Inc.; 2004:61.)

TABLE 16.17 Acute Kidney Injury/Acute Kidney Disease Versus Chronic Kidney Disease

Parameter	Acute Kidney Injury/Disease	Chronic Kidney Disease
Duration	Short duration (<3 months)	Longer duration (>3 months)
Precipitating event	Often present	Often have co-morbid condition like diabetes, hypertension
Blood pressure	Normal or high	Usually high
Anaemia	Uncommon	Common
Calcium	Usually normal	Usually low
Creatinine	Rapidly increasing	Stable or very slow rise
Renal size on ultrasound	Normal	Small (normal or large with diabetes, hydronephrosis, polycystic kidney disease, amyloidosis)
Renal osteodystrophy	Absent	Present
Peripheral neuropathy	Absent	Present

Q. How will you differentiate acute kidney injury/disease from chronic kidney disease? (IM 10.1)

- The differentiating points between AKI and CKD are given in Table 16.17.

Q. Describe renal tubular acidosis.

- Renal tubular acidosis (RTA) is a medical condition in which kidneys fail to excrete acids leading to accumulation of acid in the body. This leads to normal anion-gap (hyperchloraemic) metabolic acidosis. The function of kidneys is otherwise normal.
- May occur due to:
  - Failure to reabsorb sufficient bicarbonate ions from the filtrate in the proximal tubule.
  - Impaired secretion of hydrogen ions into the distal tubule.
  - Impaired sodium reabsorption in distal tubule or collecting duct resulting in reduced secretion of both potassium and hydrogen ions.
- Four types of RTA are:
  - Type 1 RTA or distal tubular RTA
  - Type 2 RTA or proximal RTA
  - Type 3 RTA or mixed RTA
  - Type 4 RTA or hypoaldosteronism hyperkalaemic RTA

TYPE 1 RTA OR DISTAL TUBULAR RTA

- Most common type of RTA.
- Occurs due to failure of hydrogen ion secretion by distal tubular cells that leads to a failure to acidify the urine to a pH <5.5 despite metabolic acidosis.
- Various causes are listed in Box 16.15.

BOX 16.15 Causes of Type 1 RTA

- Hereditary
- Autoimmune diseases, particularly Sjögren's syndrome
- Cirrhosis of liver
- Nephrocalcinosis producing damage of cortical collecting duct
- Renal transplantation rejection
- Sickle cell anaemia
- Drugs and toxins, including ifosfamide, toluene, lithium, trimethoprim, amphotericin B
- Chronic urinary tract obstruction

CONSEQUENCES

- Variable metabolic acidosis.
- Hypokalaemia.
- Urinary calculus formation due to hypercalciuria, hypocitraturia and alkaline urine. Stones can produce haematuria and pain.
- Nephrocalcinosis (deposition of calcium in the substance of the kidney).
- Bone demineralisation (causing rickets in children and osteomalacia in adults).

DIAGNOSIS

- Urinary pH >5.5 in the presence of systemic acidosis (serum bicarbonate <20 mEq/L).
- In mild cases, oral ammonium chloride test to produce acid load. Urinary ammonium excretion is minimal or absent.

TREATMENT

- Correction of the acidosis with oral sodium bicarbonate or sodium citrate that reverses bone demineralisation. The goal of alkali therapy is to achieve a normal serum bicarbonate concentration (22–24 mEq/L). Most cases require 1 to 2 mEq/kg of bicarbonate per day.
- Potassium citrate in case of hypokalaemia, stone formation and nephrocalcinosis.
- Thiazide diuretics which cause volume contraction and increase proximal bicarbonate reabsorption are useful.

TYPE 2 RTA OR PROXIMAL TUBULAR RTA

- Caused by a failure of the proximal tubular cells to reabsorb filtered bicarbonate from the urine leading to urinary bicarbonate wasting and subsequent acidosis.
- Acidosis less severe than type 1 RTA and urinary pH is often below 5.3.
- Various causes are listed in Box 16.16.

CONSEQUENCES

- Usually associated with a generalised dysfunction of the proximal tubular cells (Fanconi's syndrome) where there is also phosphaturia, glycosuria, aminoaciduria, uricosuria and tubular proteinuria.
- Due to phosphate wasting, bone demineralisation occurs.
- Hypokalaemia occurs due to potassium loss in urine.

BOX 16.16 Causes of Type 2 RTA

- Cystinosis
- Galactosaemia
- Glycogen storage disease (type I)
- Hereditary fructose intolerance
- Wilson's disease
- Amyloidosis
- Multiple myeloma, monoclonal gammopathy
- Drugs and toxins (e.g. antiretroviral drugs, aminoglycosides, topiramate, valproate, ifosfamide, lead, cadmium)

TREATMENT

- As patients have bicarbonate wasting, large doses of bicarbonate (10–15 mEq/kg/day) are required.
- The alkali dose requirement can be reduced by diminishing the bicarbonate wasting with a thiazide diuretic.
- Potassium supplementation often required as bicarbonate loss potentiates hypokalaemia.

TYPE 3 RTA

- Previously used to designate a rare and transient mixed type 1 RTA and type 2 RTA. Presently, this term is used to describe a genetic defect in type 2 carbonic anhydrase in both proximal and distal tubular cells as well as in bone.
- Produces:
  - Proximal RTA.
  - Distal RTA.
  - Osteopetrosis.
  - Cerebral calcification and mental impairment.
- Treatment is similar to that for type 1 and type 2 RTAs. There is no treatment for osteopetrosis or cerebral calcification.

TYPE 4 RTA

- Most common type of RTA.
- Associated with a mild metabolic acidosis (normal anion gap) due to a reduction in distal tubular ammonium excretion, which is secondary to hypoaldosteronism.
- Measured urinary acidification is normal.
- Hyperkalaemia common.
- Various causes are listed in Table 16.18.

TABLE 16.18 Causes of Type 4 RTA

Primary Aldosterone Deficiency	Hyporeninaemic Hypoaldosteronism	Aldosterone Resistance
• Primary adrenal insufficiency • Congenital adrenal hyperplasia • Aldosterone synthase deficiency • Potassium-sparing diuretics	• Renal dysfunction, most commonly diabetic nephropathy • HIV infection • ACE inhibitors or angiotensin-II receptor blockers • NSAIDs • Cyclosporin	• Drugs (amiloride, spironolactone, trimethoprim, pentamidine) • Pseudohypoaldosteronism

TREATMENT

- Aldosterone deficiency treated with a mineralocorticoid (such as fludrocortisone) as well as possibly a glucocorticoid for cortisol deficiency, if present.
- Hyporeninaemic hypoaldosteronism is amenable to fludrocortisone treatment but the accompanying hypertension and oedema often require a thiazide or loop diuretic. Diuretics are also required to control hyperkalaemia.

Q. Write a short note on polycystic kidney disease.

- There are two types of polycystic kidney disease:
  - The rare infantile polycystic kidney disease is an autosomal recessive disorder, which is usually fatal. It is associated with biliary dysgenesis resulting in congenital hepatic fibrosis plus intrahepatic bile duct dilatation (Caroli's disease). Isolated infantile polycystic kidney disease patients may survive till adulthood but require renal replacement therapy.
  - The more common adult polycystic kidney disease is an autosomal dominant disorder (autosomal dominant polycystic kidney disease—ADPKD). The cortex and medulla of both kidneys are usually filled with thin-walled, spherical cysts that enlarge and compress the intervening renal tissue, thereby interfering with renal function (Fig. 16.6).
- ADPKD may be associated with hepatic cysts in more than 75% of cases (adult hepatorenal polycystic disease).
- ADPKD is caused by mutations of either *PKD1* or *PKD2* gene.
- Clinical presentation may be at any age from the second decade. Presenting manifestations include hypertension, acute loin pain and haematuria resulting

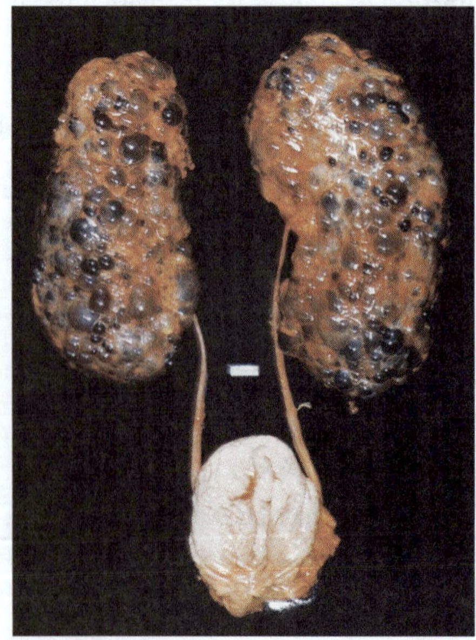

Fig. 16.6 Autosomal dominant polycystic kidney disease showing markedly enlarged kidneys with numerous cysts.

from haemorrhage into a cyst or renal calculus, vague abdominal discomfort due to increased size of the kidneys, and symptoms of uraemia and UTI (pyelonephritis and renal cyst infection).

- Polycythaemia (due to increased erythropoietin production), mitral valve prolapse, mitral regurgitation, aortic regurgitation and abdominal hernias are common accompaniments.
- Berry aneurysms of the cerebral vessels are common (10%–30%) associations, and may result in subarachnoid haemorrhage.
- Patients may present with features of chronic kidney disease.
- Physical examination commonly reveals large irregular kidneys.
- Abdominal ultrasound is the investigation of choice. IVU (rarely done) may demonstrate the characteristic 'drooping water-lily sign'. MRI is more sensitive than ultrasound to detect small cysts.
- Treatment includes control of hypertension (target blood pressure <110/75 mmHg), control of pain, treatment of infection and renal replacement therapy by dialysis or transplantation, if required. Tolvaptan (vasopressin receptor antagonist) slows the decline in renal function even if the baseline GFR is significantly reduced (eGFR >25 mL/minute/1.73 m^2).
- Screening of adult family members helps to detect this condition.

Q. Describe renal tuberculosis.

Q. Briefly outline the clinical features, investigations and treatment of tuberculosis of the urinary tract.

- Tuberculosis of the urinary tract arises as a bloodborne infection from a distant focus.
- Box 16.17 lists various types of tuberculous kidney while Table 16.19 gives stages of kidney tuberculosis.

CLINICAL FEATURES

- Males are more affected than females (2:1) and the right kidney is more commonly affected than the left.
- Manifestations include a dull ache in the renal angle, frequency of micturition, constitutional symptoms like fever and weight loss, low backache, haematuria and painful micturition in tuberculous cystitis.
- Physical examination may reveal an enlarged palpable kidney and tenderness in the renal angle.
- Tuberculosis can also involve prostate, seminal vesicles, vas deferens and epididymis.

BOX 16.17 Types of Tuberculous Kidney

- Tuberculous papillary ulcer
- Cavernous form
- Hydronephrosis
- Pyonephrosis
- Tuberculous perinephric abscess
- Caseous (putty) kidney
- Miliary

TABLE 16.19 Stages of Kidney Tuberculosis (KTB)

KTB Stage	Description	Features
• KTB-Stage 1	• Involvement of kidney parenchyma • Nondestructive form	• Most often, asymptomatic • Intravenous urography (IVU) normal • Urinalysis is often normal in children, but low-level leucocyturia may be found in adults • Full recovery with treatment
• KTB-Stage 2	• TB papillitis • Mildly destructive form	• Antitubercular treatment • Reconstructive surgery for complications only • Post-TB pyelonephritis common
• KTB-Stage 3	• Cavernous KTB • Destructive form	• Surgery required in most cases
• KTB-Stage 4	• Polycavernous KTB • Widespread destructive form	• Fistulas may form secondary to pyonephrosis • Surgery is necessary, often nephrectomy • Self-recovery possible by total calcification of a kidney (auto-amputation of the kidney)

INVESTIGATIONS

- 'Sterile pyuria' is characteristic. Though the urine contains pus cells, it fails to grow any organism on routine culture.
- Urine should be examined for tubercle bacilli. Five early morning consecutive samples should be examined, as there is intermittent excretion of tubercle bacilli. Alternatively, a 24-hour urine collection may be examined for acid-fast bacillus (AFB).
- PCR on urine samples for mycobacteria.
- Culture of the urine may grow tubercle bacilli.
- Automated real-time nucleic acid amplification technology for rapid and simultaneous detection of tuberculosis and rifampicin resistance (e.g. GeneXpert MTB/RIF).
- Plain KUB radiograph may show calcification in the renal parenchyma and ureteric calcification.
- IVU may show irregular contour of the kidney, hydrocalyx, displacement of adjacent calyces by the abscess and a small contracted bladder ('systolic or thimble' bladder). Radiographic features of ureteric involvement may include segmental ureteric strictures, segmental dilatations ('corkscrew' ureter), or shortened rigid ureter ('pipe-stem' ureter).
- Ultrasound may show dilated calyces, hydronephrosis, calcification and small abscesses.
- Cystoscopy may reveal the characteristic 'golf hole' appearance of the ureteric orifice due to sclerosing periureteritis.
- Chest radiograph should be done routinely to exclude active or previous pulmonary tuberculosis.
- Patients with suggestive radiographic findings and negative urine studies warrant fine-needle aspiration of the pathologic tissue, kidney biopsy or bladder

biopsy for mycobacterial culture and histopathology examination.

TREATMENT

- Antituberculous chemotherapy is similar to that for pulmonary tuberculosis. However, important differences exist regarding second-line agents.
  - Streptomycin and kanamycin are not recommended because these drugs provoke a transformation from TB inflammation to fibrosis.
- Ofloxacin and levofloxacin are the only fluoroquinolones suitable to treat urological TB. Moxifloxacin is a respiratory fluoroquinolone that is not optimal for urological TB.
- Surgical treatment may be required in selected cases. In patients with ureteral stricture and hydronephrosis, early stenting or percutaneous nephrostomy is beneficial in the setting of obstructive nephropathy. Some patients may require nephrectomy, dilatation or reconstruction of ureteral stricture or bladder diversion.

17 Diseases due to Infections

Q. Define pyrexia of unknown origin. Discuss briefly your approach to a case of pyrexia of unknown origin or fever of unknown origin. (IM 4.8)

DEFINITION

- The classic definition of pyrexia of unknown origin (PUO) is a fever of at least 3 weeks' duration with daily temperature elevation above 101°F and remaining undiagnosed after 1 week of intensive study in the hospital.
- However, with the availability of several investigations on outpatient basis and the appearance of several immunodeficiency diseases, PUO has been classified into four types (Table 17.1).

AETIOLOGY

- Patients with classic PUO usually do not have rare diseases, but suffer from common diseases with atypical presentations (Table 17.2):
  - Forty per cent of cases—infections.
  - Twenty per cent of cases—neoplasms (primary or metastatic).
  - Twenty per cent of cases—connective tissue (CT) diseases.
  - Ten per cent of cases—miscellaneous disorders.
  - Ten per cent of cases—undiagnosed.
- In neutropenic patients, infections include perianal infections, aspergillosis and candidaemia.
- In nosocomial PUO, causes include catheter infections, urinary tract infections, septic thrombophlebitis and drug fever.
- In HIV patients, tuberculosis and other infections are common.

TABLE 17.1 Classification of Pyrexia of Unknown Origin

Type of PUO	Definition
• Classic PUO	Fever of at least 3 weeks' duration with temperature recorded as more than 101°F (38.3°C) on several occasions, and the cause is not found despite three outpatient visits or 3 days of hospitalisation or 7 days of 'intelligent' ambulatory investigations
• Nosocomial PUO	A temperature of more than 38.3°C (101°F) developing on several occasions in a hospitalised patient who is receiving acute care and in whom infection is not manifest or incubating on admission; it is also mandatory that the cause of fever is not found on 3 days of investigations including at least 2 days' incubation of cultures
• Neutropenic PUO	A temperature of more than 38.3°C (101°F) developing on several occasions in a patient whose neutrophil count is below 500/mL or is expected to fall to that level in 1 or 2 days; it is also mandatory that the cause of fever is not found on 3 days of investigations including at least 2 days' incubation of cultures
• HIV-associated PUO	A temperature of more than 38.3°C (101°F) developing on several occasions over a period of more than 4 weeks for outpatients or more than 3 days for hospitalised patients with HIV infection; it is also mandatory that the cause of fever is not found on 3 days of investigations including at least 2 days' incubation of cultures

TABLE 17.2 Common Causes of Prolonged Fever

• Infections	Tuberculosis, malaria, typhoid, infective endocarditis, urinary tract infections, scrub typhus, intrarenal and perinephric abscesses, pyogenic and amoebic liver abscesses, subphrenic abscess, retroperitoneal abscess, PIDs, HIV infection, histoplasmosis, brucellosis
• Neoplasms	Lymphomas, leukaemias, gastrointestinal malignancies, metastatic tumours of liver, hypernephroma, atrial myxomas
• CT disorders	Systemic lupus erythematosus, rheumatoid arthritis, temporal arteritis, polymyalgia rheumatica, polyarteritis nodosa (PAN), adult-onset Still's disease
• Miscellaneous	Drug fevers (sulphonamides, aminoglycosides, penicillins), multiple pulmonary thromboembolism, haemolytic anaemias, thyroiditis, granulomatous hepatitis, rheumatic fever, cyclic neutropenia
• Psychogenic fevers	Habitual hyperthermia, factitious fever, fabricated fever
• Periodic fevers	Familial Mediterranean fever (polyserositis)

- In general population, a single pathology is the norm, while in HIV patients, about 20% have two or more simultaneous causes of PUO.

DIAGNOSTIC APPROACH TO PUO

- Most pyrexias of 'unknown origin' are atypical or obscure presentations of common diseases rather than due to obscure diseases.
- 'There is no substitute for observing the patient, talking to him/her and thinking about him/her'.
- History should be reviewed with particular emphasis on family history, occupational history and history of recent travel.
- Various points in history and examination, which need to be stressed, are shown in Table 17.3.

LABORATORY TESTS (Box 17.1)

- Procalcitonin (PCT) and C-reactive protein may indicate underlying bacterial infection.

TREATMENT

- Treatment of underlying causes detected after investigations.

TABLE 17.3 Important Points in History and Examinations in a Patient With PUO

History	Examination
• Night sweats • Weight loss • Headache, reduced vision, seizures • Unilateral headache, jaw claudication • Haemoptysis • Altered bowel habits • Occupation • Travel • Recreational activities • Injecting drug use • Medications	• Skin rash • Lymphadenopathy • Stigmata of infective endocarditis • Clubbing • Needle puncture marks suggesting drug injection • Hepatosplenomegaly • Cardiac murmurs • Respiratory examination • Eyes: Uveitis, optic fundus (choroid tubercles, Roth spot, haemorrhage, papilloedema) • Tenderness over temporal arteries • Signs of meningitis, focal neurological deficits, mononeuritis multiplex, sensorimotor neuropathy

BOX 17.1 Laboratory Tests in a Patient With PUO

- CBC, haemoglobin
- Peripheral smear for malaria
- Liver and kidney function tests
- ESR, CRP, PCT
- HBV, HCV, HIV
- Urine microscopy and cultures
- Blood cultures (both anaerobic and aerobic)
- Examination of the stool for ova, parasites and occult blood
- ANA, RF, ANCA, ferritin
- Thyroid function tests
- Paul–Bunnell test and Brucella agglutination test
- Mantoux test and fungal skin tests
- Chest X-ray
- Ultrasound abdomen and pelvis
- Chest and abdominal CT
- Echocardiography
- Radionuclide scintigraphy (67-gallium citrate scintigraphy, ^{111}In-labelled leucocyte scintigraphy and ^{18}F-fluorodeoxyglucose positron emission tomography)
- Bone marrow biopsy, liver biopsy and lymph node biopsy
- Diagnostic surgical procedures like peritoneoscopy, laparoscopy (rarely required)

- Empirical broad-spectrum antibiotics.
- Empirical antitubercular treatment.
- Rheumatic fever and Still's disease respond dramatically to aspirin and non-steroidal anti-inflammatory drugs (NSAIDs).
- Temporal arteritis and polymyalgia rheumatic respond to glucocorticoids dramatically.

APPROACH TO A PATIENT WITH PUO (Flowchart 17.1)

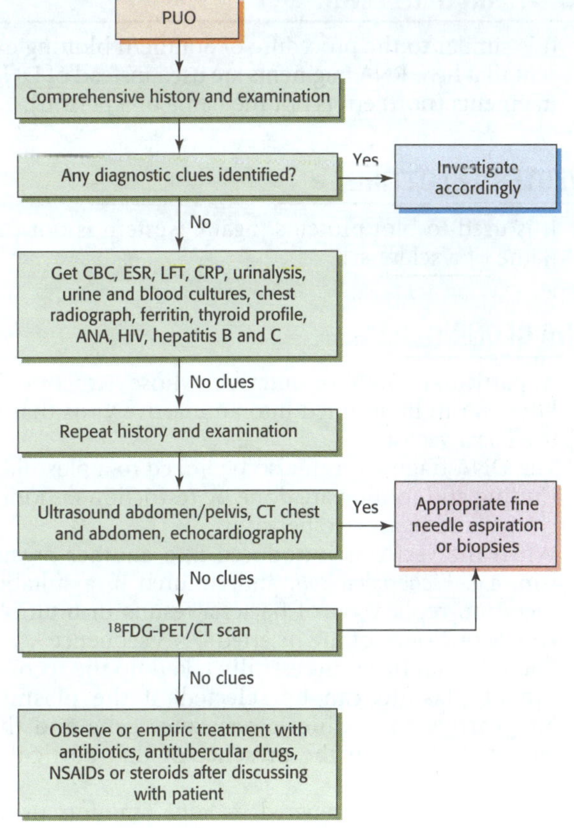

Flowchart 17.1 Approach to a Patient With PUO.

Q. What are the serological methods in infectious diseases?

Q. Describe various immunoassays.

- Serological method typically detects proteins, be it an antibody or an antigen in serum.
- The term 'immunoassay' is a broad term used for a biochemical test that measures the concentration of a substance in a biological liquid, typically serum or urine, using the reaction of an antibody or antibodies to its antigen.

ELISA

- The enzyme-linked immunosorbent assay (ELISA) is a serological technique used mainly to detect the presence of an antibody or an antigen in a sample.
- Enzyme immunoassay (EIA) is a synonym for the ELISA.
- Performing an ELISA involves at least one antibody with specificity for a particular antigen.
- The sample with an unknown amount of antigen (or antibody) is immobilised on a solid support (usually a polystyrene microtitre plate) either non-specifically (via adsorption to the surface) or specifically (via capture by another antibody specific to the same antigen in a 'sandwich' ELISA).
- After the antigen is immobilised, the detection antibody is added, forming a complex with the antigen. The detection antibody can be covalently linked to an enzyme or can itself be detected by a secondary antibody that is linked to an enzyme through bioconjugation.
- Between each step, the plate is typically washed with a mild detergent solution to remove any proteins or antibodies that are not specifically bound.
- After the final wash step, the plate is developed by adding an enzymatic substrate to produce a visible signal that indicates the quantity of antigen in the sample.

IMMUNOFLUORESCENT ANTIBODY

- This method is based on tagging an antibody with fluorescein isothiocyanate and demonstrating antibody-virus complex or viral antigens within or on the surface of the cells by examining the preparation under ultraviolet illumination.
- Since many viruses cannot be cultured, this technique is useful for diagnosing viral infections.

IMMUNOHISTOCHEMISTRY

- Immunohistochemistry (IHC) refers to the process of localising proteins in cells of a tissue section exploiting the principle of antibodies binding specifically to antigens in biological tissues. It takes its name from the roots 'immuno', in reference to antibodies used in the procedure, and 'histo', meaning tissue.
- Immunohistochemical staining is widely used in the diagnosis and treatment of cancer, but it is also of use in infectious diseases as several antigens of microorganisms can be detected in tissues.

IMMUNODIFFUSION

- Immunodiffusion is a diagnostic test that involves diffusion of antibody-containing sample through a substance such as agar.

IMMUNOELECTROPHORESIS

- Electrophoresis of a determined antigen mixture in an agarose gel allows the separation of different proteins along the gel slide and then the lateral diffusion in the gel of an immune serum or a monoclonal antibody is noted.
- If some antibodies are specific to one of the antigens, the precipitation of the antigen–antibody complexes produces a precipitation arc.
- This method is very useful to determine the number of antigens recognised against a particular mixture of antigen (e.g. crude parasite extracts).

Q. What are the various molecular methods used in the diagnosis of infectious diseases? (IM 25.8)

- Most often, these methods are used to identify a nucleic acid, either DNA or RNA.
- In the past two decades, techniques of molecular biology have been extensively used in various fields of infectious diseases. These include:
  - Epidemiology of infectious diseases (to determine whether a single strain of a microbe is responsible for most of the cases in an epidemic).
  - Diagnosis of infectious diseases.
  - Identification of new species or organisms.
  - Prevention of infectious diseases.
- Molecular tests provide several advantages over serological tests. They detect the microbe instead of a serological history of the infection and are usually able to detect the presence of a microbe much earlier in the course of an infection. However, false-positive results may occur due to sample contamination.
- Various techniques used in molecular biology are described in the subsequent text.

RESTRICTION ENZYMES AND GEL ELECTROPHORESIS

- The DNA can be cut into a number of fragments by the enzymes called restriction enzymes. These enzymes are obtained from bacteria.
- Restriction enzymes recognise specific DNA sequences and cut the double-stranded DNA at these sites only.
- Depending on the enzyme used, DNA is thus cut into small fragments with great reproducibility.
- This fragmented DNA can be separated according to the size and charge into fragments using electrophoresis on a gel matrix.
- DNA is added at one end of the gel and current is applied across it. The small fragments of DNA move towards the anode.
- Fragment sizes can be determined by running the fragments of known size on the same gel.

SOUTHERN BLOTTING AND DNA PROBES

- DNA probe is a piece of single-stranded DNA that can be labelled with a radioactive isotope (^{32}P) or a fluorescent signal (biotin and digoxigenin-11-UTP).
- After electrophoresis on a gel, the separated DNA fragments are transferred to a blotting paper.
- A DNA probe is used to indicate whether a particular fragment is present in the DNA or not. DNA probe will bind to a complementary (homologous) DNA.
- Radioactivity is detected by radioactive technique, while fluorescence is detected by a UV lamp.
- As the structure of probe is known, the structure of complementary strand of DNA is easily identified.
- This is the basis of Southern blotting (after E.M. Southern who described the procedure first).

DNA MICROARRAY

- It is the reverse of DNA probes in which known DNA (large oligonucleotides or complementary DNA) is immobilised on a glass slide and the unknown DNA is labelled to make a probe.
- A microarray is so-called because it can comprise 20,000 or more different known DNAs, each DNA being spotted onto glass slides to form the array.

NORTHERN BLOTTING

- It is similar to the procedure of Southern blotting except that here RNA fragments are used instead of DNA fragments (northern is not the name of a person).

WESTERN BLOTTING

- It is used to blot proteins (again, western is not the name of a scientist).

DNA CLONING

- A particular DNA of interest, whose structure is known, can be inserted into an inactive virus that is used as a vector.
- The DNA fragment can also be linked to a plasmid.
- Cutting and joining are done by restriction endonucleases and ligases, respectively.
- When the vector is introduced into another organism, e.g. *Escherichia coli*, and cultured in a suitable medium, replication of bacteria results in multiple copies or clones of the inserted DNA sequence.
- Bacteria that have successfully taken up the recombinant plasmid can be selected, if the plasmid also carries an antibiotic resistance gene and the culture is done in the presence of that particular antibiotic.
- Insulin has been prepared in large amounts using this method.

POLYMERASE CHAIN REACTION (PCR)

- It is a method to amplify a minute amount of DNA within a few hours.
- The double-stranded DNA is denatured by heat into single-stranded DNA.
- DNA primers of interest are added along with the four basic deoxynucleotides and the solution is cooled. This results in binding of DNA probes to their target DNA.
- DNA polymerase is used to extend the primers in opposite directions using target DNA as a template.
- This cycle is repeated several times that results in production of millions of copies of the original DNA.
- Used in medical and biological research laboratories for a variety of tasks, such as sequencing of genes, diagnosis of hereditary diseases, identification of genetic fingerprints (used in forensics and paternity testing), detection and diagnosis of infectious diseases and creation of transgenic organisms.
- In reverse transcriptase PCR (RT-PCR), RNA from the sample is converted to DNA using a retrovirus reverse transcriptase polymerase and the DNA is amplified by PCR.
- In real-time PCR, the rate of DNA amplification is monitored as an indication of the initial concentration of sample DNA.

Q. Discuss sepsis and septic shock. (IM 4.7)

Q. Discuss early goal-directed therapy for sepsis and septic shock. (IM 4.7)

- Initial sepsis definitions were developed in 1991 (sepsis-1) with a subsequent update in the sepsis definitions in 2001 (sepsis-2) that simply expanded the list of signs and symptoms of sepsis to reflect clinical bedside experience.
- The initial definitions included sepsis (systemic inflammatory response syndrome and suspected infection), severe sepsis (sepsis and organ dysfunction) and septic shock (sepsis and hypotension despite adequate fluid resuscitation).
- In 2016, new definitions of sepsis and septic shock were proposed (sepsis-3):
  - Sepsis is a life-threatening organ dysfunction caused by a dysregulated host response to infection.
  - Septic shock is a subset of sepsis with circulatory and cellular/metabolic dysfunction associated with a higher risk of mortality. Despite adequate fluid resuscitation, patients have hypotension requiring vasopressors to maintain a mean arterial blood pressure above 65 mmHg and have an elevated serum lactate concentration of more than 2 mmol/L.
- Clinical criteria for sepsis include suspected or documented infection and an acute increase of two or more Sequential Organ Failure Assessment (SOFA) points as a proxy for organ dysfunction.
- Since SOFA is a complicated score, quick SOFA (qSOFA) score has been used to identify sepsis (Box 17.2). A qSOFA score of two or more identifies a patient at greater risk of poor outcome. However, 2021 guidelines do not recommend the use of qSOFA as a single screening tool for sepsis.

BOX 17.2 Quick Sequential Organ Failure Assessment Score

- Respiratory rate ≥22/minute
- Altered mentation
- Systolic blood pressure ≤100 mmHg

PATHOGENESIS

- In response to infection, highly conserved microbial pathogen-associated molecular patterns are recognised by pattern recognition receptors including Toll-like receptors on the cells of the innate immune system. This interaction triggers the release of both proinflammatory and antiinflammatory mediators. Cytokines, such as tumour necrosis factor-α (TNF-α), interleukin-1, interleukin-2, interleukin-6, interleukin-8 and others, which cause neutrophil–endothelial cell adhesion, activate the complement and clotting cascades, and can lead to the generation of microthrombi.
- Tissue hypoxia, mitochondrial dysfunction and apoptosis are all thought to be important mediators of sepsis-induced organ dysfunction.

CLINICAL FEATURES

- The clinical presentation of sepsis depends on the site of the infection as well as the host response.
- Common features include malaise, fever, tachycardia and tachypnoea. Hypotension may be present.
- The skin can be mottled and the capillary refill time prolonged.
- Other presentations include impaired gas exchange (even when the focus of infection is outside the chest) and oliguria.
- Altered mental status can occur without the focus of infection in the brain (sepsis-associated encephalopathy).

SEPSIS-ASSOCIATED ENCEPHALOPATHY

- It is a state of diffuse cerebral dysfunction caused by inflammatory response of the body to various infections; the infection does not affect the central nervous system (CNS) directly.
- Common features include disturbed cognitive functions and consciousness, lack of concentration, personality changes and depression. Uncommon features include flapping tremors, rigidity and focal and generalised seizures.
- Diagnosis is a challenge. It is usually a diagnosis of exclusion as conditions such as drug use, electrolyte disturbances and primary CNS disorders have to be ruled out before the final diagnosis is made. Ancillary diagnostic studies include CT and MRI brain, EEG and lumbar puncture.

SUMMARY OF CLINICAL FEATURES OF SEPSIS (Fig. 17.1)

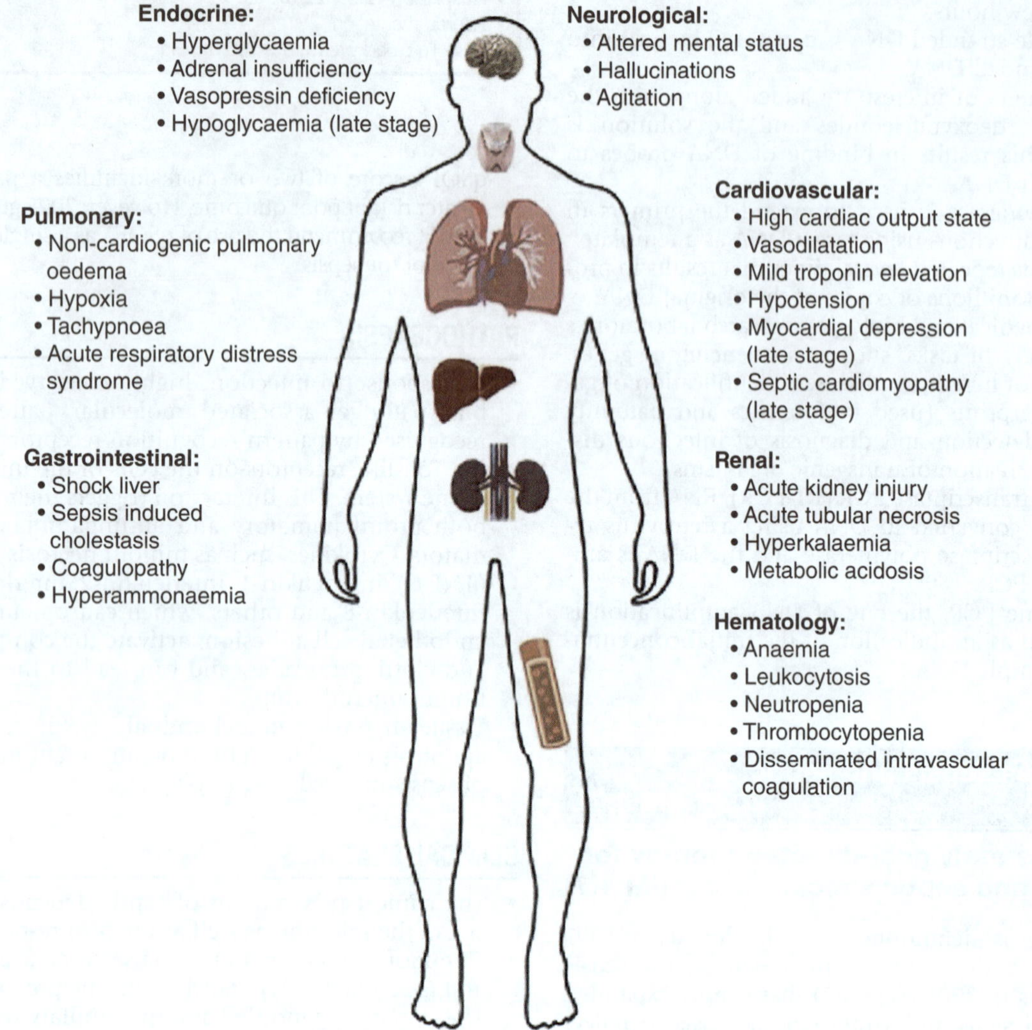

Fig. 17.1 Clinical features of sepsis.(Couretsy: Font MD, Thyagarajan B, Khanna AK. Sepsis and Septic Shock - Basics of diagnosis, pathophysiology and clinical decision making. Med Clin North Am. 2020 Jul;104(4):573-585).

LABORATORY TESTS

- Lactate levels.
- White blood cell count (leucocytosis or leucopenia).
- Urine examination, blood urea/creatinine, liver enzyme.
- Increases in plasma C-reactive protein or PCT concentrations.
- Coagulation profile.
- Other tests are carried out based on suspected focus of infections.

PROCALCITONIN

- PCT is the precursor of the hormone calcitonin.
- Normal level in adults is less than 0.05 μg/L. A level of 0.5–1 μg/L is suggestive of infection while a level above 1 μg/L is highly suggestive of systemic bacterial infection.
- PCT measurement aids in the diagnosis of sepsis. It also helps in guiding and monitoring antibiotic therapy. Most compelling evidence for PCT use is in adults with respiratory tract infections and in the critically ill in whom safety and efficacy of PCT-guided antibiotic therapy has been shown.
- Raised PCT can also be seen following recent major surgery, severe trauma, severe burns and prolonged cardiogenic shock. However, in the absence of infection, these patients should have decreasing PCT levels on subsequent measurements. It can also be elevated in some other infections (e.g. fungal and malaria) which can activate the release of cytokines.

PRESEPSIN

- Presepsin is a new biomarker and has been found to be useful for early diagnosis of bacterial sepsis.

- It may also be useful in guiding antimicrobial therapy.
- However, its exact role still needs to be defined.

MANAGEMENT

- The Surviving Sepsis Campaign (SSC) is an international effort to increase awareness and improve outcomes in severe sepsis.
- The SSC guidelines for the management of severe sepsis and septic shock were first published in 2004 with an update in 2008, 2012, 2016 and 2021 in the form of bundles of care. A care bundle is a group of evidence-based interventions which when performed together have a better outcome than if performed individually.
- The SSC bundles have been changed from the 3-hour and 6-hour bundles to a single '1-hour bundle' with the explicit intention of beginning resuscitation and management immediately.
- More than 1 hour may be required for resuscitation to be completed, but initiation of resuscitation and treatment, such as obtaining blood for measuring lactate and blood cultures, administration of fluids and antibiotics, and, in the case of life-threatening hypotension, initiation of vasopressor therapy, are all begun immediately (Box 17.3).

ADMINISTER INTRAVENOUS FLUID

- Begin initial fluid resuscitation immediately on recognising a patient with sepsis and/or hypotension and elevated lactate, and completed within 3 hours of recognition.
- Administer a minimum of 30 mL/kg of intravenous crystalloid fluid within the first 3 hours. Fluid therapy should be administered in well-defined (e.g. 500 mL), rapidly infused boluses.
- Use either normal saline or balanced salt solutions (e.g. Ringer's lactate). There is some evidence of increased risk of acute kidney injury with normal saline.
- There is no clear benefit of using colloids compared with crystalloids. However, colloids like albumin may be used when patients require large volumes of crystalloids. In such cases, avoid hydroxyethyl starches or gelatin.
- Following initial fluid resuscitation, guide further fluids by frequent reassessment of haemodynamic status. Reassess by a thorough clinical examination and evaluation of available physiological variables (heart rate, blood pressure, capillary refill time, arterial oxygen saturation, respiratory rate, temperature and urine output) as well as other methods (respiratory variation in inferior vena cava diameter, pulse pressure variation and stroke volume variation).

BOX 17.3 One-Hour Bundle for Sepsis/Septic Shock

- Measure lactate level. Remeasure in 3–4 hours if initial lactate is >2 mmol/L.
- Obtain blood cultures prior to administration of antibiotics.
- Administer broad-spectrum antibiotics within 1 hour of recognition of sepsis or septic shock.
- Administer 30 mL/kg crystalloid within first 3 hours for hypotension or lactate ≥4 mmol/L.
- Apply vasopressors if patient is hypotensive during or after fluid resuscitation to maintain MAP ≥65 mmHg.

MEASURE LACTATE LEVEL

- While serum lactate is not a direct measure of tissue perfusion, it can serve as a surrogate, as increases may represent tissue hypoxia or accelerated aerobic glycolysis driven by excess beta-adrenergic stimulation.
- A significant reduction in mortality occurs with lactate-guided resuscitation.
- If initial lactate is elevated (>2 mmol/L), remeasure it within 2–4 hours to guide resuscitation. A 10% reduction in lactate may indicate effective resuscitation although this may not be true in all patients.

OBTAIN APPROPRIATE MICROBIOLOGICAL CULTURES PRIOR TO ANTIBIOTICS

- Sterilisation of cultures can occur within minutes of the first dose of an appropriate antimicrobial. Therefore, obtain relevant cultures from all sites considered to be potential sources of infection if it results in no substantial delay in the start of antimicrobials (1 hour may be considered to be no substantial delay in the initiation of antimicrobial therapy while cultures are being obtained).
- Appropriate blood cultures include at least two sets (aerobic and anaerobic).

ADMINISTER BROAD-SPECTRUM ANTIBIOTICS

- Start empirical broad-spectrum therapy with one or more intravenous antimicrobials to cover all likely pathogens (including bacterial and potentially fungal or viral coverage) as soon as possible.
- Antibiotics should be administered as soon as possible. Do not delay administration of appropriate antibiotic therapy by more than 1 hour in order to obtain blood and other cultures.
- The choice of empirical antimicrobial therapy depends on the patient's history, clinical status and local epidemiological factors.
- Key patient factors include site of infection, concomitant underlying diseases, chronic organ failures, indwelling devices, presence of immunosuppression and receipt of antimicrobials within the previous 3 months.
- Patient's location at the time of acquiring infection (i.e. community, chronic care institution and acute care hospital), local pathogen prevalence and the susceptibility patterns of those common local pathogens in both the community and hospital must be factored while choosing antibiotics.
- Administer a broad-spectrum antibiotic in the beginning. It means the use of one or more antimicrobial agents with the specific intent of broadening the range of potential pathogens covered (e.g. piperacillin/tazobactam, vancomycin and if indicated, anidulafungin; each is used to cover a different group of pathogens).

- Consider addition of empirical antifungal agent if patient has significant risk of invasive *Candida* infections (e.g. immunocompromised status, prolonged invasive vascular devices, total parenteral nutrition, necrotising pancreatitis, prolonged administration of broad-spectrum antibiotics and prolonged hospital/ICU admission).
- In contrast to broad-spectrum coverage, combination therapy is the use of multiple antibiotics (having different mechanisms of action) with the specific intent of covering the known or suspected pathogen(s) with more than one antibiotic so as to accelerate pathogen clearance rather than to broaden antimicrobial coverage. The additional agents include aminoglycosides or fluoroquinolones for Gram-negative bacteria, and vancomycin or teicoplanin for suspected methicillin-resistant *Staphylococcus aureus* (MRSA) infection.
- However, combination therapy against a single pathogen is not recommended as a routine treatment of neutropenic sepsis. This does not preclude the use of multidrug therapy (MDT) for the purpose of broadening the spectrum of antimicrobial treatment.
- Narrow down empirical antimicrobial therapy once pathogen is identified and its sensitivity pattern becomes known. Discontinue antibiotics if a decision is made that the patient does not have infection.
- Additionally, if combination therapy is initially used for septic shock, de-escalate within the first few days in response to clinical improvement and/or evidence of infection resolution.
- Duration of therapy is 7–10 days for most of the infections. Longer courses are appropriate in patients who have a slow clinical response, undrainable foci of infection, bacteraemia with *S. aureus* and some fungal and viral infections.

ADMINISTER VASOPRESSORS

- Urgent restoration of an adequate perfusion pressure to the vital organs is a key part of resuscitation.
- If blood pressure is not restored after initial fluid resuscitation, then commence vasopressors within the first hour to achieve mean arterial pressure (MAP) of ≥65 mmHg.
- Noradrenaline is the first vasopressor to be used in hypotensive patients.
- If an additional vasopressor is required, add either vasopressin (up to 0.03 unit/minute) or adrenalin to noradrenalin with the intent of raising MAP to target.
- Dopamine may be used as an alternative vasopressor agent to noradrenalin only in highly selected patients (e.g. patients with low risk of tachyarrhythmias and absolute or relative bradycardia).
- Do not administer low-dose dopamine for renal protection.
- Add dobutamine in patients who show evidence of persistent hypoperfusion despite adequate fluid loading and the use of vasopressor agents.

SOURCE CONTROL

- Identify or exclude as rapidly as possible a specific anatomic diagnosis of infection requiring emergent source control.
- If such a source is identified (e.g. an abscess or an infected device), implement source control interventions as soon as medically and logistically practical.
- Remove promptly any intravascular access device (after another vascular access has been established) if that is a possible source of sepsis.

OTHER MEASURES

Corticosteroids

- Routine use of intravenous hydrocortisone is not recommended to treat septic shock patients if adequate fluid resuscitation and vasopressor therapy are able to restore haemodynamic stability.
- If haemodynamic stability is not achievable, administer IV hydrocortisone at a dose of 50 mg 6 hourly for 3–7 days.

Blood Products

- Administer RBC transfusion only when haemoglobin concentration decreases to <7 g/dL in adults in the absence of myocardial ischaemia, severe hypoxaemia or acute haemorrhage. Goal is to keep it between 7 and 9 g/dL.
- Erythropoietin is not recommended for the treatment of anaemia associated with sepsis.
- Fresh frozen plasma to correct clotting abnormalities is not recommended in the absence of bleeding or planned invasive procedures.
- Prophylactic platelet transfusion is required when platelet counts are <10,000/mm^3 in the absence of apparent bleeding or when counts are <20,000/mm^3 if the patient has a significant risk of bleeding. Higher platelet counts (≥50,000/mm^3) are advised for active bleeding, surgery or invasive procedures.

Blood Glucose

- Keep blood glucose between 110 and 180 mg/dL. Higher blood glucose should be controlled with insulin infusion.
- Check blood glucose every 1–2 hours until glucose values and insulin infusion rates are stable, and then every 4 hours.

Venous Thromboembolism Prophylaxis

- Give pharmacological prophylaxis using low-molecular-weight heparin (preferred agent) or unfractionated heparin.
- Use mechanical prophylaxis with intermittent pneumatic compression and/or graduated compression stockings when heparin is contraindicated.

Stress Ulcer Prophylaxis

- Administer stress ulcer prophylaxis using either proton pump inhibitors or histamine-2 receptor antagonists to those with risk factors for gastrointestinal bleeding (e.g. pre-existing liver disease, need for renal replacement therapy and higher organ failure scores).

Other Agents

- Immunoglobulins, antithrombin, selenium, arginine, glutamine and vitamin C are not recommended in patients with sepsis or septic shock.

Nutrition

- Enteral feeding should be preferred over administration of early parenteral nutrition alone wherever feasible.

Mechanical Ventilation

- If a patient requires mechanical ventilation due to acute respiratory distress syndrome (ARDS), adjust ventilatory settings as follows:
  - A target tidal volume of 6 mL/kg predicted body weight.
  - An upper limit for plateau pressures of 30 cm H_2O.
  - Use of higher positive end-expiratory pressure (PEEP) over lower PEEP to avoid extensive lung collapse at end expiration.
  - Allow $PaCO_2$ to increase above normal, if needed, to minimise plateau pressures and tidal volumes.
  - Consider using the prone position for ARDS patients requiring potentially injurious levels of FiO_2 or plateau pressure, provided they are not put at risk from positional changes.
  - Maintain mechanically ventilated patients in a semi-recumbent position (head of the bed raised to 45 degrees) unless contraindicated.
  - Do not use a pulmonary artery catheter for the routine monitoring of patients with ARDS.
  - Use a conservative fluid strategy for patients with established ARDS who do not have evidence of tissue hypoperfusion.
  - Avoid the use of high-frequency oscillatory ventilation.

Q. Discuss the aetiology, clinical features, complications and prevention of measles (rubella).

- Measles is caused by a paramyxovirus (RNA virus) infection.
- One-third of all measles-related deaths worldwide occur in India.
- Mode of spread is by droplet infection and the virus infects epithelial cells of the nose and conjunctivae.
- Incubation period is of about 10 days.
- Period of infectivity is from 4 days before to 2 days after the onset of rash. People with compromised immunity can continue to shed virus for the entire duration of illness.

CLINICAL FEATURES

CATARRHAL STAGE

- The patient is highly infective during this stage.
- Febrile onset with nasal catarrh, sneezing, conjunctival redness, watering of eyes, photophobia, conjunctivitis, malaise, irritability and cough.

Koplik's Spots (Fig. 17.2)

- Koplik's spots are small, red and irregular lesions on the buccal mucosa with blue-white centres (enanthem). They appear 1–2 days before the onset of the maculopapular rash and disappear 1–2 days after the appearance of the rash. They are best seen at the opening of the parotid duct (upper second molar tooth). The lesions consist of vesicle formation and epithelial necrosis.

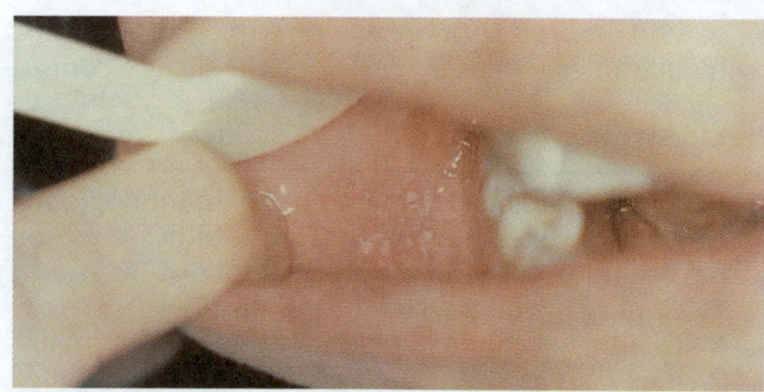

Fig. 17.2 Koplik's spots.

BOX 17.4 Complications of Measles

• Bronchiolitis, bronchitis	• Myocarditis
• Interstitial giant cell pneumonia	• Hepatitis
• Bronchopneumonia, bacterial pneumonia	• Enteritis
• Conjunctivitis, keratitis, corneal ulcers, blindness	• Acute glomerulonephritis
• Subacute sclerosing panencephalitis (SSPE), acute demyelinating encephalomyelitis, measles inclusion body encephalitis	• Thrombocytopenia

EXANTHEMATOUS STAGE

- Red and maculopapular rashes are first seen over the back of the ears and forehead, later spreading downwards over the face, neck, trunk and feet. The rash may also have some petechiae.
- The malaise and fever subside as the rash fades that takes 4–5 days.

COMPLICATIONS (Box 17.4)

- CNS complications may occur early (acute postinfectious measles encephalitis) or after years of viral persistence (subacute sclerosing panencephalitis [SSPE]).
- Signs and symptoms of SSPE appear an average of 7 years after the initial infection and include personality changes, myoclonic seizures and motor disturbances followed by coma and death. Measles virus antibodies are raised in the cerebrospinal fluid (CSF).

TREATMENT

- It is supportive and includes antipyretics, fluids and treatment of bacterial superinfections.
- Administration of vitamin A to children with measles may reduce morbidity and mortality. WHO recommends administration of once-daily doses of 200,000 IU of vitamin A for two consecutive days to all children with measles older than 1 year. Dose is 50,000 IU once a day for two days for infants below the age of 6 months and 100,000 IU once a day for two days for infants between 6–11 months of age.

- In SSPE, use of isoprinosine, ribavirin and intraventricular interferon-α may prolong the disease course.

PREVENTION

- *Passive immunisation*: Human normal immunoglobulin may be given intramuscularly. Indications for passive immunisation are given as follows:
  - Contacts younger than 12 months.
  - Debilitated children, especially those with a malignant disease.
  - Pregnant females.
  - Patients with active tuberculosis.
  - Immunodeficient patients and those with malignant diseases.
- *Active immunisation:*
  - Two doses of live attenuated measles virus are given as a subcutaneous injection at 9–12 months of age and then at 16–24 months of age. This vaccination can offer protection for at least 15 years. It can be given simultaneously in combination with rubella and mumps vaccines (MMR vaccine) or with rubella (measles–rubella [MR] vaccine). Vaccination within 72 hours of exposure is the intervention of choice for susceptible individuals older than 12 months. Measles vaccination is contraindicated in certain conditions (Box 17.5).
  - India resolved to eliminate measles and control rubella/congenital rubella syndrome by 2020. In this direction, the Ministry of Health and Family Welfare initiated MR vaccination campaign in the age group of 9 months to less than 15 years in a phased manner across the nation with the aim of vaccinating over 95% of children with two doses in all the districts. However, the target could not be achieved. India has vaccinated over 324 million children against measles and rubella between 2017 and 2020 through the measles–rubella vaccination campaign. Over the last 6 months of 2021, India achieved the global standard of non-measles, non-rubella discard rate of 2 per 100,000 population for the first time ever.

Q. Give a brief account of rubella (German measles, '3-day measles'), expanded rubella syndrome and congenital rubella or rubella syndrome.

- Rubella is caused by a togavirus infection, an RNA virus.
- Mode of spread is by droplet infection.
- Incubation period is about 18 days.
- The prodromal or catarrhal stage is characterised by malaise, headache, fever, mild conjunctivitis and lymphadenopathy (suboccipital).
- The exanthematous stage is characterised by pink macular rashes first appearing behind the ears and on the forehead, later spreading downwards to the trunk and extremities. The rashes typically last 3 days. Although the distribution of the rubella rash is similar to that of measles, the spread is much more rapid and the rash does not darken or coalesce. An enanthem on the soft palate (Forchheimer spots) may be seen.
- There may be associated polyarthritis and generalised lymphadenopathy that may persist for 2 weeks or more.
- Important complications include postinfectious encephalitis, thrombocytopenia, spontaneous abortion and congenital rubella syndrome.

CONGENITAL RUBELLA OR RUBELLA SYNDROME

- Congenital rubella results from the transplacental transmission of the virus to the foetus from an infected mother. The highest risk is during the first trimester of pregnancy and the risk is limited to first 16 weeks of pregnancy with almost negligible risk after 20 weeks of pregnancy.
- Congenital malformations associated with congenital rubella syndrome are listed in Table 17.4.

EXPANDED RUBELLA SYNDROME

- Expanded rubella syndrome additionally includes the manifestations listed in Box 17.6.

PREVENTION

- Active immunisation can be given with rubella vaccine. This is a live attenuated vaccine.
- The aim of vaccination is to decrease the frequency of infection in the population and, thus, decrease the chance of susceptible pregnant females being exposed to the infection.
- It should be given to all children at the age of 9–12 months along with mumps and measles vaccine (MMR vaccine) with a second dose at 16–24 months.

BOX 17.5 Contraindications to Measles Vaccine

- Pregnant females
- Patients with untreated tuberculosis
- Patients with leukaemias and lymphomas
- Immunocompromised patients (children with asymptomatic HIV infection can receive the vaccine)

TABLE 17.4 Congenital Malformations Associated With Rubella Syndrome

• Congenital heart diseases	Patent ductus arteriosus, ventricular septal defect, pulmonic stenosis
• Ophthalmic diseases	Corneal clouding, cataracts, chorioretinitis, microphthalmia, blindness
• Deafness	
• Mental retardation	
• Microcephaly	

BOX 17.6 Additional Manifestations of Expanded Rubella Syndrome

• Hepatosplenomegaly	• Myocarditis
• Thrombocytopenic purpura	• Interstitial pneumonia
• Intrauterine growth retardation	• Humoral and cellular immunodeficiency

- Measles-rubella (MR) vaccination campaign is to administer one dose of vaccine to children in the age group of 9 months to less than 15 years.
- Rubella vaccine must never be given to pregnant females or to those who may become pregnant within 3 months of immunisation, because of the high risk of vaccine virus-induced foetal damage. It is also contraindicated in patients with immune deficiency diseases and those who are taking immunosuppressive drugs.

Q. Discuss the clinical manifestations, complications and prevention of mumps.

- Mumps is caused by a paramyxovirus, an RNA virus.
- Mode of spread is by droplet infection.
- Incubation period is about 15–20 days.

CLINICAL FEATURES

- Prodromal symptoms consist of malaise, anorexia, feverishness and tenderness at the angle of the jaw. This is followed by typical parotitis. Parotitis is bilateral in two-thirds of the cases and remains confined to one side in the remainder. The chief complaints are pain, and difficulty in eating, swallowing and talking. The parotid duct (orifice of Stensen) may be red and swollen. Trismus may result from parotitis.

COMPLICATIONS

- Epididymo-orchitis, oophoritis.
- Pancreatitis.
- Encephalomyelitis, mumps meningitis.
- Mumps myocarditis.
- Thrombocytopenic purpura.
- Hearing loss.

PREVENTION

- Mumps vaccine is given at the age of 15 months along with measles and rubella vaccines (MMR vaccine).

Q. What are the common herpes viruses infecting humans? Enumerate the diseases caused by them.

- There are eight herpes viruses infecting humans. These have double-stranded DNA. The viruses and the diseases caused by them are briefed in the Table 17.5.

TABLE 17.5 Diseases Caused by Herpes Viruses

Virus	Diseases
• Herpes simplex virus	
• Type 1	Herpes labialis, keratoconjunctivitis, dendritic corneal ulcer, pulp space infections (whitlows), encephalitis with temporal lobe involvement, genital herpes (40%), pneumonitis, tracheobronchitis, ulcerative stomatitis, oesophagitis
• Type 2	Genital herpes (60%), neonatal infections
• Varicella-zoster virus	Chickenpox, herpes-zoster (shingles)
• Epstein–Barr virus (EBV)	Infectious mononucleosis, Burkitt's lymphoma, nasopharyngeal carcinoma, Hodgkin's lymphoma, hairy leucoplakia in AIDS patients, lymphoproliferative disorders (e.g. haemophagocytic lymphohistiocytosis, lymphomatoid granulomatosis, X-linked lymphoproliferative disease)
• Cytomegalovirus	Congenital infections (intrauterine growth retardation), perinatal infections, infections in the immunocompromised patients (pneumonitis, retinitis)
• Human herpes virus 6	Exanthem subitum or roseola (sixth disease)
• Human herpes virus 7	Exanthem subitum or roseola (sixth disease)
• Human herpes virus 8	Kaposi's sarcoma, multicentric Castleman's disease

Q. Discuss the aetiology, clinical features, investigations, complications and treatment of infectious mononucleosis (glandular fever).

AETIOLOGY

- Caused by Epstein–Barr virus (EBV), a herpes virus that infects and replicates in B lymphocytes and oropharyngeal epithelial cells. Transmission is largely by salivary contact, e.g. kissing.
- Oral shedding persists for a median duration of approximately 6 months after the onset of illness, although some patients may shed virus intermittently for decades.
- Peak incidence in 14–16 years for young females and 16–18 years for young males.
- Incubation period is 7–10 days.
- Subclinical infection is very common.

CLINICAL FEATURES

- Constitutional symptoms, especially fever.
- Severe pharyngitis and tonsillitis.
- Lymphadenopathy (particularly posterior cervical lymph node and posterior auricular enlargement but sometimes generalised) which may be tender.
- Hepatosplenomegaly.
- Petechial rashes on palate.
- Maculopapular rash.
- Ampicillin or amoxicillin induces maculopapular eruptions in more than 90% of patients.

INVESTIGATIONS

- Peripheral blood lymphocytosis (>50% lymphocytes) with atypical lymphocytes (>10%) (Fig. 17.3).
- Elevated liver enzymes.

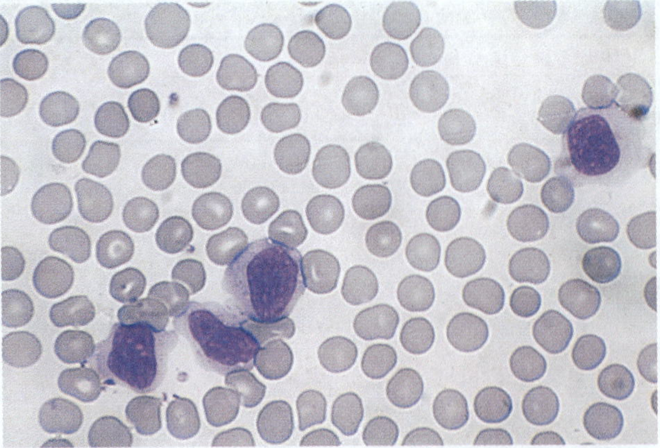

Fig. 17.3 Atypical lymphocytes in infectious mononucleosis.

- Circulating heterophile antibodies are directed against viral antigens that cross-react with antigens found in phylogenetically unrelated species (e.g. sheep and horse red cells). Heterophile antibody tests are negative in 25% of patients during the first week of infection and in 5%–10% of patients during or after the second week. Can be detected by:
    - Positive monospot test (rapid screening test)—horse red cells agglutinate on exposure to heterophile antibodies.
    - Positive Paul–Bunnell test—sheep red blood cells agglutinate in the presence of heterophile antibodies.
- Viral serological tests specific for EBV may be positive.
    - IgM and IgG antibodies against viral capsid antigens (anti-VCA) are usually present at the onset of clinical illness because of the long incubation period.
    - Antibodies to EBV early antigen (anti-EA) are present at the onset of clinical illness.
    - Antibodies to Epstein–Barr nuclear antigen (anti-EBNA) begin to appear 6–12 weeks after the onset of symptoms and persist throughout life; their presence early in the course of an illness effectively excludes acute EBV infection.
- Serological evolution of EBV antibodies is shown in Figure 17.4.

COMPLICATIONS (Box 17.7)

BOX 17.7 Complications of Infectious Mononucleosis

- Chronic fatigue syndrome
- Haemolytic anaemia and thrombocytopenia
- Aplastic anaemia, thrombotic thrombocytopenic purpura or haemolytic-uraemic syndrome and DIC
- Glomerulonephritis, interstitial nephritis
- Hepatitis
- Myocarditis, pericarditis
- Splenic rupture
- Neurological complications, e.g. meningoencephalitis, transverse myelitis and Guillain–Barré (GB) syndrome
- Airway obstruction due to severe pharyngeal oedema
- Chronic active EBV infection (fever, lymphadenopathy, splenomegaly, hepatitis, haemophagocytic lymphohistiocytosis)

TREATMENT

- Infectious mononucleosis is usually a self-limiting disease requiring no specific treatment.
- Symptomatic treatment includes rest, acetaminophen, etc.
- Corticosteroids are indicated in certain specific complications (meningitis, encephalitis, severe haemolysis and severe pharyngeal oedema).

Q. Discuss the clinical manifestations, complications and management of chickenpox.

- Chickenpox is caused by primary infection with varicella-zoster virus, also known as human herpes virus 3. Following primary infection, virus remains latent; afterwards, reactivation gives rise to herpes zoster.
- Mode of transmission is by droplet infection from the upper respiratory tract or by direct cutaneous contact with vesicle fluid from skin lesions.
- The incubation period is about 14–21 days.
- The disease is contagious from 2 days before appearance of rash till pustules disappear.

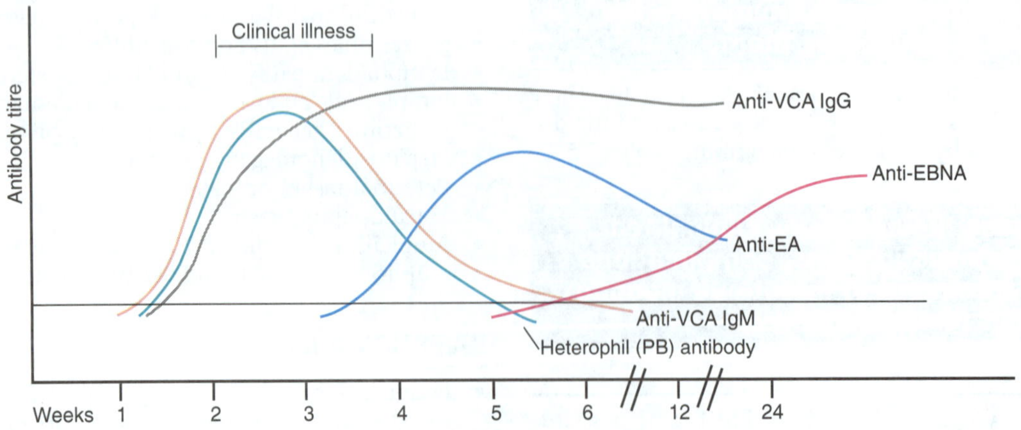

Fig. 17.4 Evolution of antibodies in Epstein–Barr virus infection.

CLINICAL FEATURES

- The characteristic rash first appears on the trunk on the second day of illness and then the face, and finally on the limbs. The lesions are maximum on the trunk and minimum on the periphery of the limbs.
- The characteristic lesions appear as macules and progress to papules, vesicles and pustules. The lesions finally dry up to form scabs.
- The lesions appear in crops so that lesions at all stages of development are seen in any area at the same time.
- New vesicle formation generally stops within 4 days, and most lesions have fully crusted by day 6. Crusts tend to fall off within about 1 to 2 weeks.
- Low-grade fever is often present, although it may be high-grade in some patients.
- In immunocompromised patients, the lesions are haemorrhagic and are numerous. Dissemination to other organs is quite frequent.

COMPLICATIONS (Box 17.8)

BOX 17.8 Complications of Chickenpox

• Myocarditis	• Meningitic, encephalitis
• Hepatitis	• Acute glomerulonephritis
• Corneal lesions	• Interstitial pneumonia
• Bleeding diathesis	• Arthritis, osteomyelitis
• Perinatal varicella	• Congenital varicella
• Cerebellar ataxia	• Reye's syndrome with aspirin use

DIAGNOSIS

- Mainly clinical.
- A Tzanck smear of vesicular fluid demonstrates multinucleated giant cells and epithelial cells with eosinophilic intranuclear inclusion bodies.
- Isolation of virus through culture of vesicular fluid.
- Direct immunofluorescence test to detect virus is easier than culture.
- PCR is to identify viral gene.

MANAGEMENT

- No treatment is required in majority of children.
- Symptomatic treatment includes antihistamines and local calamine lotion.
- Acyclovir (15 mg/kg five times a day for 7 days) can be used in adults, pregnant women or immunocompromised patients. It reduces complications of chickenpox, particularly if given within 24 hours. In immunocompromised patients, acyclovir is generally given intravenously. Other drugs that can be used include valaciclovir (1000 mg TID) and famciclovir (500 mg TID).
- In healthy children, use of antiviral agents may reduce the duration of disease when given within 24 hours of symptoms. However, since the disease is generally self-limiting and symptoms can be controlled and reduced with supportive therapy, antivirals are often not given in children unless they are immunocompromised or on long-term salicylate therapy when Reye's syndrome may develop.
- Secondary bacterial infection is treated with local antiseptic or systemic antibiotics like cloxacillin.

PROPHYLAXIS

- A live attenuated vaccine is available for the prevention of chickenpox in immunocompetent children and adults who are at a high risk of infection. It should not be given to pregnant or immunocompromised patients.
  - For children <4 years, one dose is given after the age of 12 months.
  - For children ≥ 4 years, adolescents and adults, two doses at least 1 month apart.
  - Active immunisation with vaccine within 3–5 days of exposure can prevent infection among exposed persons or reduce disease severity in those who do become ill.
- Passive prophylaxis using purified human varicella-zoster immune globulin may be given to immunocompromised persons, neonates or pregnant women with history of significant exposure within the past 10 days. It should also be given prophylactically to an infant whose mother develops chickenpox up to 5 days before delivery or if the mother develops chickenpox up to 2 days after delivery.

Q. Discuss briefly about human papillomaviruses.

- Human papillomaviruses (HPVs) are double-stranded DNA tumour viruses with strong tropism to stratified squamous epithelial cells of skin and mucous membranes.
- Do not cause viraemia or death of infected epithelial cells.
- Most commonly cause benign papillomas and warts.
- Some types of HPV are oncogenic that can cause anogenital tumours.
- Genital HPV is divided into high-risk and low-risk types—high-risk genital types are associated with intraepithelial neoplasias that can develop into invasive carcinomas; low-risk genital types are responsible for condylomata acuminata and low-grade cervical dysplasias with a low risk of development of invasive carcinoma.
- Infection usually occurs via direct skin or mucous membrane contact. Autoinoculation is another means of spread of HPV infection. Anogenital HPV infections are usually transmitted sexually and are often detected at several sites simultaneously (multifocal infection).
- Most important risk factor in transmission of genital HPV is the number of sexual partners.
- Incubation period for genital HPV infection varies from weeks to months.

- Majority of infections are subclinical. Further, 80% of infection resolves spontaneously within 12 months.
- Diseases produced by HPVs are listed in Table 17.6.

DIAGNOSIS

- Based on clinical presentation.
- May require biopsy to confirm dysplasia or carcinoma.
- Acetic acid: Subclinical HPV infections can be visualised after application of 3%–5% acetic acid with a cotton swab; whitening of HPV-positive lesions occurs in 5 minutes.
- Endoscopic evaluation (colposcopy and proctoscopy) to visualise condyloma, dysplasia and carcinomas.
- Molecular methods (including PCR) to detect viral DNA (e.g. Hybrid Capture 2 DNA test).

TABLE 17.6 Diseases Produced by HPV

Disease	Description
• Verrucae plantaris	Usually involve hands and feet (verrucae palmares, verrucae plantaris) Skin-coloured papules Flat or dome-shaped papules Surface rough and hyperkeratotic Usually asymptomatic; however, at pressure sites, endophytic growth can be very painful
• Verrucae planae	Flat, reddish or skin-coloured papules Mainly involve face, hands or distal forearms
• Periungual warts	Present at nail fold; often painful
• Skin cancers (squamous cell carcinoma and basal cell carcinoma)	May act synergistically with ultraviolet light Usually not caused by high-risk HPV
• Condylomata acuminate (genital warts)	Caused by low-risk HPV Can occur on the external or internal genitalia, perianally, in the anal canal, perineum Multiple, flat or raised exophytic papillomas (Fig. 17.5A and B) May be pedicled or broad based Usually self-limited
• Anogenital malignancies	Caused by high-risk HPV
• Intraepithelial neoplasms	Can involve cervix (50% due to HPV-16), vulva, vagina, anus and penis
• Penile carcinoma	—
• Cervical carcinoma	HPV cause about 70% of all cervical carcinomas Squamous cell carcinoma more common than adenocarcinoma of cervix
• Vulval and vaginal carcinomas	—
• Others	
• Oral lesions	May be asymptomatic or cause papilloma
• Head and neck cancers	Usually involve oropharynx, tonsils, base of tongue and soft palate

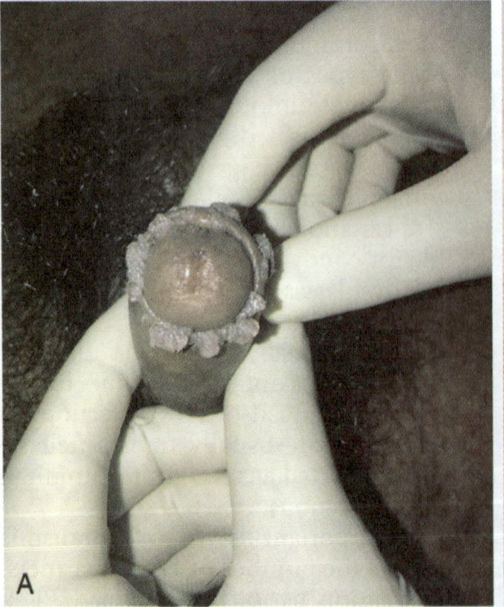

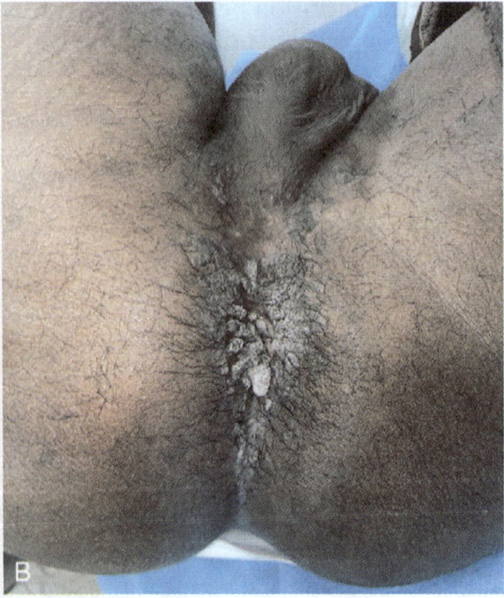

Fig. 17.5 (A) Penile warts. (B) Perianal warts (condyloma acuminatum).

THERAPY

- No specific antiviral agent is available.
- Verrucae:
  - Keratolysis: After mechanical removal of the mass with a sharp knife, verrucae resolve under application of salicylic acid:lactic acid:collodion (1:1:4). Vaseline is applied to the surrounding skin to protect it from chemical corrosion.
  - Cryotherapy: Cryotherapy using liquid nitrogen is used to freeze warts.
- Anogenital warts:
  - Podophyllotoxin: It produces death of infected cells. It is applied twice a day for three consecutive days in cycles consisting of several weeks. Serious systemic side effects can occur if it is applied to larger surface areas and absorbed systemically. Use during pregnancy is contraindicated.
  - Imiquimod: Imiquimod induces the production of antiviral cytokines such as interferon and TNF-α. A 5% cream is applied thrice weekly for up to 4 months.
  - Sinecatechins: Sinecatechins ointment is a partially purified fraction of the water extract of green tea leaves from *Camellia sinensis* and is available in 10% and 15% formulations. It is applied thrice daily for 8–16 weeks.
  - Ablation by surgery, laser and electrocauterisation.
  - Cryotherapy using liquid nitrogen.
  - Trichloroacetic acid: Topical application of 50%–90% of trichloroacetic acid leads to coagulation of cell protein with subsequent cell death.
  - 5-Fluorouracil applied as cream.

HPV VACCINES

- HPV immunisation is not effective in clearing HPV infection, genital warts or cervical intraepithelial neoplasia that is already present.
- Three commercially available HPV vaccines: Quadrivalent vaccine, bivalent vaccine and nonavalent vaccine.
- Can prevent about 70% of cervical dysplasias and cancers when given in girls aged 9–13 years.
- HPV vaccines are available in India but are not included in national vaccination programme due to some unfounded concerns of deaths in trials conducted in 2010.
- In September 2022, India's first indigenously developed quadrivalent HPV vaccine was launched.

Q. How do you classify arboviruses? Enumerate the major clinical syndromes caused by arboviruses.

- Arboviruses are viruses that are maintained in nature through biological transmission between susceptible vertebrate hosts by haematophagous arthropods (arthropod-borne diseases). They multiply and produce viraemia in the vertebrates, multiply in the tissues of arthropods and are passed on to new vertebrates by the bites of arthropods after a period of extrinsic incubation.
- Arboviruses belong to several families. Important families and the diseases caused are listed in Table 17.7.

TABLE 17.7 Important Families of Arboviruses and Diseases Produced by Them

Family	Common Diseases
• Arenaviridae	Lymphocytic choriomeningitis Lassa fever
• Bunyaviridae	California encephalitis Sandfly fever Congo-Crimean haemorrhagic fever Hantaan fever (HFRS)
• Filoviridae	Marburg disease Ebola disease
• Flaviviridae	**Mosquito-borne** Yellow fever Dengue fever Japanese encephalitis Zika disease West Nile encephalitis St. Louis encephalitis **Tick-borne** Kyasanur forest disease (KFD) Tick-borne encephalitis
• Togaviridae	Sindbis disease Chikungunya disease Eastern equine encephalitis Western equine encephalitis

TABLE 17.8 Major Syndromes Produced by Arboviruses

Fever, Arthralgia, Myalgia, Rash Syndrome	Haemorrhagic Fever	Encephalitis/ Aseptic Meningitis
• Chikungunya • Sandfly fever • Dengue fever • Lymphocytic choriomeningitis	• Yellow fever • Kyasanur forest disease (KFD) • Dengue haemorrhagic fever (DHF) and dengue shock syndrome (DSS) • Haemorrhagic fever with renal syndrome (HFRS) • Congo-Crimean haemorrhagic fever • Ebola disease • Marburg disease	• Eastern equine encephalitis • Western equine encephalitis • Japanese encephalitis • West Nile encephalitis • St. Louis encephalitis

MAJOR CLINICAL SYNDROMES

- Based on the major symptoms produced by an arbovirus, the major clinical syndromes are listed in Table 17.8.

Q. Describe classic dengue (breakbone fever), dengue haemorrhagic fever (DHF) and dengue shock syndrome (DSS). (IM 4.3)

Q. Discuss dengue with and without warning features and describe also severe dengue. (IM 4.3)

- An estimated 50 million dengue infections occur annually. More than 100,000 cases are reported from

India every year though these numbers appear to be gross underestimate of actual prevalence.
- Caused by four distinct subgroups of dengue viruses, types 1, 2, 3 and 4 (DEN-1 to DEN-4) which are RNA viruses.
- The genome of DEN virus encodes different gene products: C (capsid), prM (matrix), E (envelope) and seven non-structural (NS) proteins. NS1 protein is secreted in plasma and is useful in early diagnosis.
- Dengue infection of humans occurs from bites of female *Aedes aegypti* mosquitoes. Some cases develop after the bites from *Aedes albopictus* mosquitoes.
- The mosquito feeds during the day and has a propensity for man-made habitats containing water.

SPECTRUM OF DENGUE VIRUS INFECTIONS

- Figure 17.6 gives spectrum of dengue virus infections.

CLASSIFICATION OF DENGUE INFECTION

- Presently, WHO classifies dengue viral infections into non-severe dengue (with and without warning signs) and severe dengue (Table 17.9). However, it should be kept in mind that even dengue patients without warning signs may develop severe dengue.

PATHOGENESIS OF SEVERE DENGUE

- Occurs in persons who were infected with one serotype of dengue virus previously and therefore have antibodies against that particular serotype.
- A second infection by a different serotype causes immunological enhancement of antibody acquired from a previous infection.
- Antibody–virus complex taken up by macrophages.
- Production of vascular permeability factors by macrophages.
- These vascular permeability factors induce plasma leakage, resulting in haemorrhage and, ultimately, shock.

CLINICAL FEATURES

- After the incubation period of 5–8 days, the illness begins abruptly and is followed by the three phases—febrile, critical and recovery.

FEBRILE PHASE

- Patients typically develop high-grade fever suddenly that usually lasts for 2–7 days.
- Often accompanied by facial flushing, skin erythema, generalised body ache, myalgia, arthralgia, severe backache ('breakbone' fever), retro-orbital pain and headache.
- Skin rash is common and can range from a mild erythema to a pruritic, macular rash.
- Sore throat, injected pharynx and conjunctival injection in some patients.
- Anorexia, nausea and vomiting.
- High fever may cause febrile seizures in children.
- In some cases, temperature may decrease to nearly normal after 3–4 days and other symptoms disappear; this remission lasts for 2 days and is followed by return of fever and other symptoms. This is known as 'saddleback fever'.

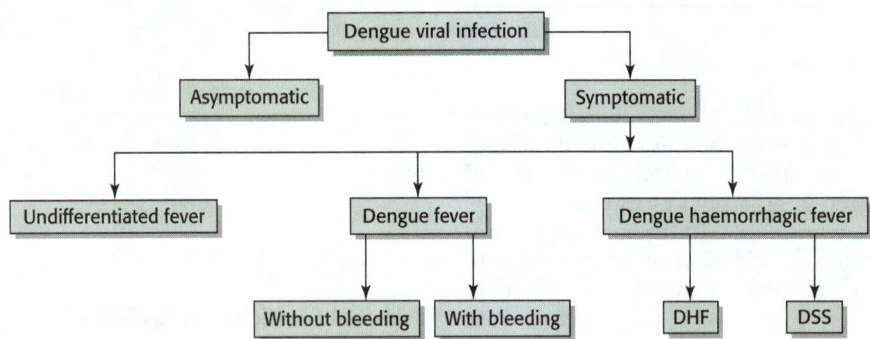

Fig. 17.6 Spectrum of dengue virus infections. DHF = Dengue haemorrhagic fever; DSS = Dengue shock syndrome.

TABLE 17.9 Classification of Dengue

Non-severe Dengue Without Warning Signs	Non-severe Dengue With Warning Signs	Severe Dengue

Probable Dengue
• Live in/travel to endemic area
• Fever and two of the fol-lowing criteria:
  • Nausea and vomiting
  • Rash
  • Aches and pains
  • Tourniquet test positive
  • Leucopenia
  • No warning sign
Laboratory-Confirmed Dengue
• See under 'Diagnosis'
	Presence of Warning Signs
	• Abdominal pain or tenderness
	• Persistent vomiting
	• Clinical fluid accumulation
	• Mucosal bleed
	• Lethargy and restlessness
	• Liver enlargement >2 cm
	• Laboratory: Increase in haematocrit concurrent with rapid decrease in platelet count
		• Severe plasma leakage leading to:
		  • Shock (DSS)
		  • Fluid accumulation with respiratory distress
		• Severe bleeding
		  • As evaluated by clinician
		• Severe organ involvement
		  • Liver: AST or ALT ≥1000
		  • CNS: Impaired consciousness
		  • Involvement of heart and other organs

BOX 17.9 Tourniquet Test

- Apply blood pressure cuff and mark a circle with an area of about 2.5 cm^2 (roughly the size of diaphragm of stethoscope).
- Inflate the cuff to a point midway between the systolic and diastolic pressures for 5 minutes.
- A test is considered positive when 20 or more petechiae appear in the circle.

- Tenderness upon pressure on eyeball.
- A positive tourniquet test may be present (Box 17.9).
- Mild haemorrhagic manifestations like petechiae and mucosal membrane bleeding may be seen.
- Liver is often enlarged and tender.
- These features occur in both severe and non-severe dengue cases. Therefore, monitoring for warning signs and other clinical parameters is crucial for recognising progression to critical phase.
- Earliest laboratory abnormality is a progressive decrease in total white cell count, which should alert the physician to a high probability of dengue.
- Majority of patients will improve after the febrile stage. However, about 5% will progress to the critical phase.

CRITICAL PHASE

- Around the time of defervescence of fever, an increase in capillary permeability along with increasing haematocrit levels may occur. This marks the beginning of critical phase. The degree of increase above the baseline haematocrit often reflects the severity of plasma leakage.
- The period of clinically significant plasma leakage usually lasts for 24–48 hours.
- Progressive leucopenia followed by a rapid decrease in platelet count usually precedes plasma leakage.
- Patients without an increase in capillary permeability will improve while those with increased capillary permeability may become worse as a result of lost plasma volume.
- Pleural effusion and ascites may be detectable.
- Shock occurs when a critical volume of plasma is lost through leakage. It is often preceded by warning signs.
- Body temperature may be subnormal when shock occurs.
- With prolonged shock, organ hypoperfusion results in progressive organ impairment, metabolic acidosis and disseminated intravascular coagulation (DIC). This in turn leads to severe haemorrhage causing the haematocrit to decrease in severe shock.
- Instead of leucopenia usually seen during this phase of dengue, leucocytosis may occur in patients with severe bleeding.
- Severe organ impairment such as severe hepatitis, encephalitis, myocarditis and severe bleeding may also develop without obvious plasma leakage or shock.
- Those who improve after defervescence are said to have non-severe dengue.
- Cases of dengue with warning signs usually recover with early rehydration. However, some cases will deteriorate to severe dengue.

RECOVERY PHASE

- If the patient survives the 24-hour to 48-hour critical phase, a gradual reabsorption of extravascular fluid takes place in the following 48–72 hours.
- General well-being improves, appetite returns, gastrointestinal symptoms abate, haemodynamic status stabilises and diuresis ensues.
- Some patients may have a rash of 'isles of white in the sea of red'.
- Some patients may experience pruritus, particularly on hands and feet.
- Bradycardia and ECG changes are common during this stage.
- The haematocrit stabilises or may be lower due to dilutional effect of reabsorbed fluid.
- White blood cell count usually starts to rise soon after defervescence but recovery of platelet count is typically later than that of white blood cell count.
- Respiratory distress from massive pleural effusion and ascites will occur at any time if excessive intravenous fluids have been administered.

SEVERE DENGUE

- Defined by one or more of the following:
  1. Plasma leakage that may lead to shock (dengue shock) and/or fluid accumulation, with or without respiratory distress
  2. Severe bleeding
  3. Severe organ impairment
- Increasing vascular permeability results in shock. It usually takes place around defervescence, usually on day 4 or 5 (range days 3–7) of illness, usually preceded by warning signs.
- During the initial stage of shock, compensatory mechanisms produce tachycardia and peripheral vasoconstriction with reduced skin perfusion resulting in cold extremities and delayed capillary refill time. Diastolic pressure rises towards the systolic pressure and the pulse pressure narrows (≤20 mmHg) as the peripheral vascular resistance increases.
- Patients in dengue shock often remain conscious and lucid.
- Later, patient decompensates and both systolic and diastolic pressures disappear abruptly.
- Prolonged hypotensive shock may lead to multiorgan failure.
- Hypotension is usually associated with major bleeding as shock in combination with thrombocytopenia, hypoxia and acidosis can lead to DIC.
- Unusual manifestations include acute liver failure, encephalopathy and cardiomyopathy.
- Most deaths from dengue occur in patients with profound shock, particularly if it is complicated by fluid overload.
- Box 17.10 summarises the features of severe dengue.

EXPANDED DENGUE SYNDROME (EDS)

- EDS is a term announced by the WHO in 2011 to cover the uncommon expressions of dengue involving severe damage to the liver, kidneys, bone marrow, heart or brain (Table 17.10).

BOX 17.10 Severe Dengue—Summary

Should be considered if a patient from an area of dengue risk presents with fever of 2–7 days plus any of the following features:

- Evidence of plasma leakage
  - High or progressively rising haematocrit
  - Pleural effusions or ascites
  - Circulatory compromise or shock (tachycardia, cold and clammy extremities, capillary refill time >3 seconds, weak or undetectable pulse, narrow pulse pressure or in late shock, unrecordable blood pressure)
- Significant bleeding
- Altered level of consciousness (lethargy or restlessness, coma, convulsions)
- Severe gastrointestinal involvement (persistent vomiting, increasing or intense abdominal pain, jaundice)
- Severe organ impairment (acute liver failure, acute renal failure, encephalopathy or encephalitis, cardiomyopathy)

TABLE 17.10 Expanded Dengue Syndrome

Neurological	Encephalopathy, encephalitis, intracranial haemorrhage, mononeuropathies, polyneuropathies, Guillain–Barré syndrome, transverse myelitis
Cardiac	Conduction abnormalities, myocarditis, pericarditis
Pulmonary	Pleural effusion, ARDS, pulmonary haemorrhage, pneumonitis
Liver, gallbladder and pancreas	Hepatitis, acute hepatic failure, acalculous cholecystitis, acute pancreatitis
Renal	Acute kidney injury, proteinuria, IgA nephropathy, glomerulonephritis, haemolytic uraemic syndrome
Haematologic	Haemophagocytic lymphohistiocytosis, Idiopathic thrombocytopenic purpura, DIC

- Certain high-risk groups such as pregnant women, infants, elderly persons and immunocompromised individuals are particularly susceptible to developing EDS.

DIAGNOSIS

- Leucopenia, thrombocytopenia and elevated liver enzymes.
- Isolation of virus from the blood (within first 5 days of onset of clinical features).
- Serum NS1 antigen is highly specific and is positive early in the course of illness.
- Molecular methods like RT-PCR or nucleic acid sequence-based amplification (NASBA) to detect viral RNA.
- Rising viral IgM antibody titres (start after 5 days of onset).
- In patients with severe dengue, chest radiograph to look for pleural effusion, and ultrasound abdomen for ascites and gallbladder wall thickening.

OVERVIEW OF MANAGEMENT

- At the first contact, patients should be rapidly screened in order to identify those with severe dengue (who require immediate emergency treatment to avert death), those with warning signs (who should be given priority while waiting in the queue so that they can be assessed and treated without delay) and non-urgent cases. Therefore, the following should be done at the first level of health care:
  - Recognising that the febrile patient could have dengue.
  - Managing patients in early febrile phase of dengue.
  - Recognising early stage of plasma leakage or critical phase and initiating fluid therapy.
  - Recognising patients with warning signs who need to be referred for admission and/or intravenous fluid therapy to a secondary healthcare facility.
  - Recognising and managing severe plasma leakage and shock, severe bleeding and severe organ impairment promptly and adequately.
- During the early febrile phase, it is often not possible to predict clinically whether a patient with dengue will progress to severe disease. Therefore, patients should have daily outpatient healthcare assessments for disease progression with careful checking for manifestations of severe dengue and warning signs.

STEPWISE MANAGEMENT

STEP I—OVERALL ASSESSMENT (Table 17.11)

TABLE 17.11 Step I—Overall Assessment of Patient With Suspected Dengue

History	Examination	Investigations
• Date of onset of fever/illness • Quantity of oral intake • Warning signs • Diarrhoea • Change in mental state, seizure, dizziness • Urine output • Coexisting conditions	• Mental state • Hydration status • Haemodynamic status • Tachypnoea, acidotic breathing • Pleural effusion • Abdominal tenderness, hepatomegaly, ascites • Rash and bleeding manifestations • Tourniquet test	• Full blood count • Haematocrit (in early febrile phase, establishes baseline haematocrit) (decreasing white blood cell count makes dengue very likely; rapid decrease in platelet count in parallel with a rising haematocrit compared to the baseline is suggestive of progress to the plasma leakage/critical phase of the disease)

STEP II—DIAGNOSIS, ASSESSMENT OF DISEASE PHASE AND SEVERITY

- On the basis of step I, determine whether the disease is likely to be dengue, which phase it is in (febrile, critical or recovery), whether there are warning signs, the hydration and haemodynamic status of the patient and whether the patient requires admission.

STEP III—TREATMENT

- Depending on the clinical manifestations and other circumstances, patients may be sent home (Group A), be referred for in-hospital management (Group B) or require emergency treatment and urgent referral (Group C).

Treatment of Group A Patients

- These are patients who are able to tolerate adequate volumes of oral fluids and pass urine at least once every 6 hours, and do not have any of the warning signs particularly when fever subsides.
- These patients should be reviewed daily for disease progression (decreasing white blood cell count, defervescence and warning signs) until they are out of the critical period.
- Those with stable haematocrit can be sent home and are advised to return immediately if they develop any of the warning signs. They are advised to adhere to the following action plan:
    - Oral intake of oral rehydration solution, fruit juice and other fluids containing electrolytes and sugar to replace losses from fever and vomiting.
    - Paracetamol for high fever, if the patient is uncomfortable.
    - Tepid sponging bath, if fever is high.
    - Avoid use of NSAIDs as these drugs may aggravate gastritis or bleeding. Aspirin may also be associated with Reye's syndrome.
    - To be brought to hospital immediately if any of the following occur: no clinical improvement, deterioration around the time of defervescence, severe abdominal pain, persistent vomiting, cold and clammy extremities, lethargy or restlessness, bleeding (e.g. black stools or coffee-ground vomiting) and not passing urine for more than 4–6 hours.
- Patients should be monitored daily for temperature pattern, volume of fluid intake, urine output, warning signs, signs of plasma leakage and bleeding, haematocrit and white blood cell and platelet counts.
- Oral rehydration fluid to be given is calculated based on the weight of the patient (Table 17.12).

Treatment of Group B Patients

- These patients should be referred for in-hospital management. These include patients with warning signs, those with coexisting conditions that may make dengue or its management more complicated (such as pregnancy, infancy, old age, obesity, diabetes mellitus, renal failure and chronic haemolytic diseases) and those with certain social circumstances (such as living alone, or living far from a health facility without reliable means of transport).
- If a patient has dengue with warning signs, action plan should be as follows:
    - Obtain a reference haematocrit before fluid therapy.
    - Give only isotonic solutions such as normal saline or Ringer's lactate.
    - Start with 5–7 mL/kg/hour for 1–2 hours, then reduce to 3–5 mL/kg/hour for 2–4 hours and then reduce to 2–3 mL/kg/hour or less according to the clinical response.
    - Reassess clinical status and repeat haematocrit.
    - If haematocrit remains the same or rises only minimally, continue with the same rate (2–3 mL/kg/hour) for another 2–4 hours.
    - If vital signs are worsening and haematocrit is rising rapidly, increase the rate to 5–10 mL/kg/hour for 1–2 hours.
    - Reassess clinical status, repeat haematocrit and review fluid infusion rates accordingly.
    - Give minimum intravenous fluid volume required to maintain good perfusion and urine output of about 0.5 mL/kg/hour.
    - Intravenous fluids are usually needed for only 24–48 hours.
    - Reduce intravenous fluids gradually when rate of plasma leakage decreases towards the end of critical phase as indicated by urine output and/or oral fluid intake, or haematocrit decreasing below the baseline value in a stable patient.
- The volume of maintenance fluids is shown in Box 17.11.

Treatment of Group C Patients

- Patients with severe dengue require emergency treatment and urgent referral when they are in the critical phase of disease.
- Plasma losses should be replaced immediately and rapidly with isotonic crystalloid solution or, in the case of hypotensive shock, with colloids.
- If possible, obtain haematocrit levels before and after fluid resuscitation.
- The action plan for treating patients with compensated shock is as follows:
    - Start intravenous fluid resuscitation with isotonic crystalloid solutions at 5–10 mL/kg/hour over 1 hour. Then reassess the patient's condition (vital signs, capillary refill time, haematocrit and urine output).
    - If the patient's condition improves, intravenous fluids should be gradually reduced to 5–7 mL/kg/hour for 1–2 hours, then to 3–5 mL/kg/hour for 2–4 hours, then to 2–3 mL/kg/hour and then reduced further.
    - If vital signs are still unstable, check haematocrit after the first bolus. If haematocrit increases or is still high (>50%), repeat a second bolus of crystalloid solution at 10–20 mL/kg/hour for 1 hour. After this second bolus, if there is improvement, reduce the rate to 7–10 mL/kg/hour for 1–2 hours, and then continue to reduce as above. If haematocrit decreases compared to the initial reference haematocrit (<40% in children and

TABLE 17.12 Calculation of Oral Rehydration Solution Using Weight

Body Weight (kg)	ORS to be given (mL/kg/day)
• 3–10	100
• 10–20	75
• 20–30	50–60
• 30–60	40–50

BOX 17.11 Maintenance of Intravenous Fluids

- Normal maintenance fluid per hour can be calculated on the basis of the following formula:
    - 4 mL/kg/hour for the first 10 kg ideal body weight
    - +2 mL/kg/hour for the next 10 kg ideal body weight
    - +1 mL/kg/hour for subsequent kilogram ideal body weight

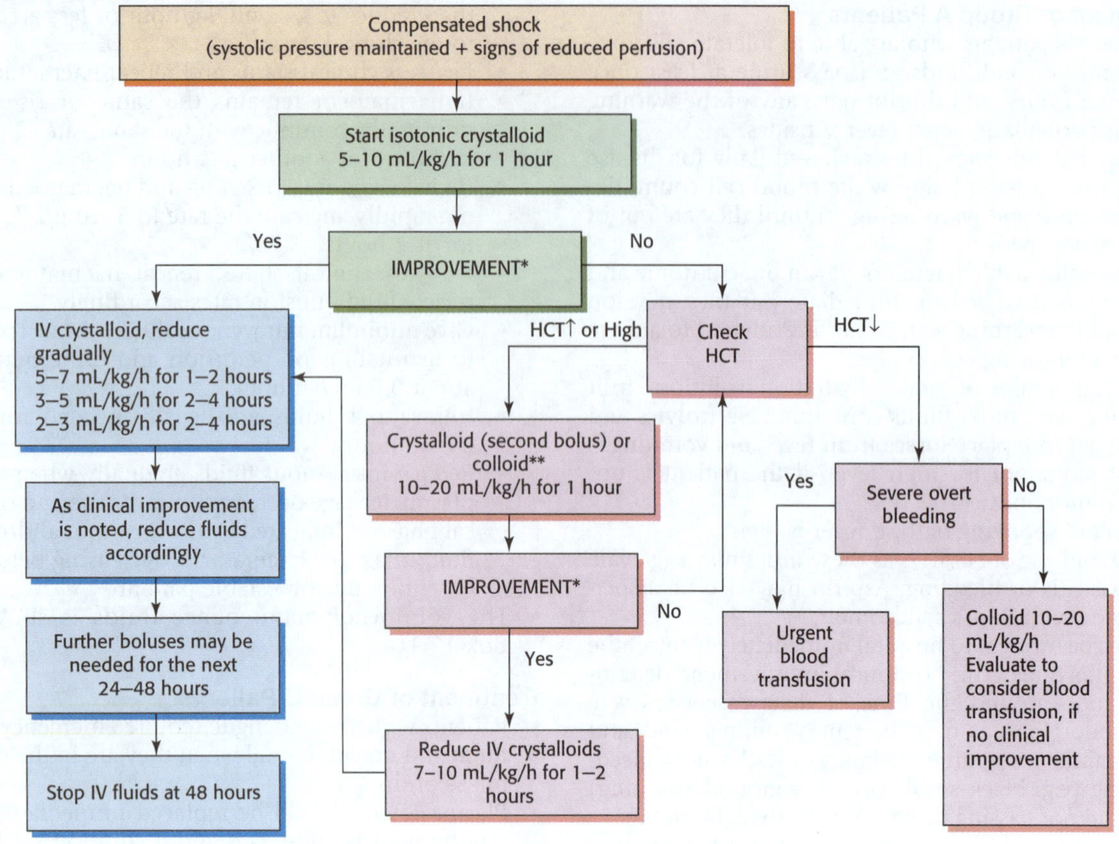

Flowchart 17.2 Management of Severe Dengue With Compensated Shock. IV, intravenous; HCT, haematocrit; ↑ increased; ↓ decreased. (*Source:* World Health Organization. *Handbook for Clinical Management of Dengue*, Figure 5, Page 29, 2012.)

adult females, <45% in adult males), this indicates bleeding and the need to cross-match and transfuse blood as soon as possible.
  - Action plan for patients with compensated shock is shown in Flowchart 17.2.
- The action plan for patients with hypotensive shock is as follows:
  - Initiate intravenous fluid resuscitation with crystalloid or colloid solution at 20 mL/kg as a bolus given over 15 minutes.
  - If the patient's condition improves, give a crystalloid/colloid infusion of 10 mL/kg/hour for 1 hour. Then continue with crystalloid infusion and gradually reduce to 5–7 mL/kg/hour for 1–2 hours, then to 3–5 mL/kg/hour for 2–4 hours and then to 2–3 mL/kg/hour or less, which can be maintained for up to 24–48 hours.
  - If vital signs are still unstable, review haematocrit obtained before the first bolus. If haematocrit was low, this indicates bleeding and the need to transfuse blood as soon as possible.
  - If haematocrit was high compared to baseline value, give intravenous colloid at 10–20 mL/kg as a second bolus over 30 minutes to 1 hour. After second bolus, reassess the patient. If condition improves, reduce the rate to 7–10 mL/kg/hour for 1–2 hours, and then change back to crystalloid solution and reduce the rate of infusion as mentioned above.
  - If condition is still unstable, repeat haematocrit after second bolus. If haematocrit decreases compared to the previous value, this indicates bleeding and the need to transfuse blood. If haematocrit increases compared to previous value, continue colloid solutions at 10–20 mL/kg as a third bolus over 1 hour.
  - A decrease in haematocrit together with stable haemodynamic status and adequate urine output indicates haemodilution; in this case, intravenous fluids must be discontinued immediately to avoid pulmonary oedema.
  - Action plan for patients with shock is shown in Flowchart 17.3.

Treatment of Haemorrhagic Complications

- Mucosal bleeding may occur in any patient with dengue, but if the patient remains stable with fluids, it should be considered as minor.
- In patients with profound thrombocytopenia, ensure strict bed rest and protect from trauma to reduce the risk of bleeding. Do not give intramuscular injections to avoid haematoma.

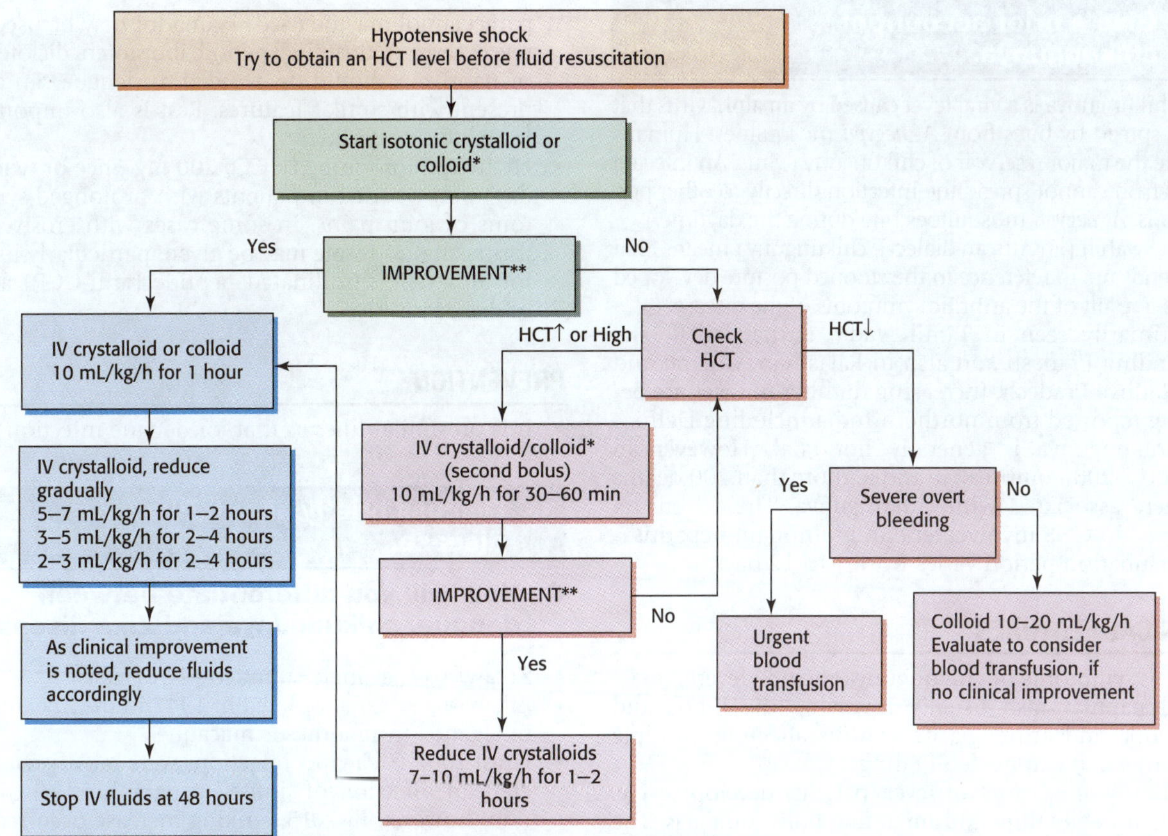

Flowchart 17.3 Management of Severe Dengue With Shock. IV, intravenous; HCT, haematocrit; ↑ increased; ↓ decreased. (*Source:* World Health Organization. *Handbook for Clinical Management of Dengue*, Figure 7, Page 32, 2012.)

- Prophylactic platelet transfusions for severe thrombocytopenia in otherwise haemodynamically stable patients have not been shown to be effective.
- Patients at risk of major bleeding are those who have prolonged/refractory shock, have hypotensive shock and renal or liver failure and/or severe and persistent metabolic acidosis, are given NSAIDs, have pre-existing peptic ulcer disease, are on anticoagulant therapy or have any form of trauma, including intramuscular injection.
- The action plan for the treatment of haemorrhagic complications is as follows:
  - Give 5–10 mL/kg of fresh packed red cells or 10–20 mL/kg of fresh whole blood. Fresh blood is required as stored blood loses 2,3-DPG, low levels of which impede oxygen-releasing capacity of haemoglobin, resulting in functional tissue hypoxia.
  - A good clinical response includes improving haemodynamic status and acid–base balance.
  - There is little evidence to support the practice of transfusing platelet concentrates and/or fresh frozen plasma for severe bleeding.
  - Note that haemoglobin of <7 g/dL as a trigger for blood transfusion, as recommended in the SSC guidelines, is not applicable to severe dengue with shock.

PREVENTION OF DENGUE INFECTION

- Preventive measures are directed towards elimination of adult mosquitoes and their larvae.
- During epidemics, aerial spraying/fogging with malathion is recommended for the control of adult mosquitoes.
- Mosquito repellents to prevent bites.
- Covering body with full clothes to prevent bites.
- Larval control measures include source reduction and use of larvicides. As *A. aegypti* mosquitoes breed in and around human dwellings and flourish in fresh water, stagnation of water in the coolers, flowerpots, bathroom, kitchen, terrace, lawn and other open places should be avoided.
- Another larval control measure is the introduction of larvivorous fish, namely *Gambusia*, in water tanks and other water sources.
- Currently, there is no antiviral drug against dengue viral infections. A tetravalent vaccine (chimeric yellow fever–dengue–tetravalent dengue vaccine [CYD-TDV]) is being used in persons between 9 and 45 years of age in some countries/areas where seroprevalence of dengue infection >70%. However, it might increase the risk of severe disease in people who have never been exposed to the virus. Vaccine is given in three doses at 0, 6 and 12 months.

Q. Give a brief account of chikungunya. (IM 4.3)

- Chikungunya is a viral fever caused by an alphavirus that is spread by bites from *A. aegypti* mosquitoes. Humans are the major reservoir of chikungunya virus. An infected person cannot spread the infection directly to other persons. *A. aegypti* mosquitoes bite during the daytime.
- In Swahili (an African dialect), chikungunya means 'that bends up' in reference to the stooped posture developed as a result of the arthritic symptoms of the disease.
- Primarily seen in Tamil Nadu, Karnataka, Kerala, Andhra Pradesh and also in Rajasthan, Gujarat and Madhya Pradesh. Increasing number of cases are being reported from northern India including Delhi.
- Chikungunya is generally not fatal. However, in 2005–2006 outbreak in India, more than 200 deaths were associated with chikungunya. These were related to CNS involvement and fulminant hepatitis.
- Incubation period varies from 1 to 12 days.

CLINICAL FEATURES

- The symptoms of chikungunya include fever, a maculopapular rash usually involving the limbs and trunk, and arthralgia or arthritis affecting multiple joints that can be debilitating.
- Shortly after onset of fever, patients develop severe, often debilitating and migrating polyarthralgias. The joint pains are usually symmetric and occur most commonly in wrists, elbows, fingers, knees and ankles but can also affect more proximal joints. Swelling of joints due to tenosynovitis can be seen in some cases.
- Skin involvement is present in about 40%–50% of cases and consists of a pruritic maculopapular rash predominating on the thorax, facial oedema, a bullous rash with pronounced sloughing (mainly in children) and localised petechiae.
- Other symptoms include headache, conjunctival injection and slight photophobia.
- Bleeding from skin (petechiae) and epistaxis may occur in some patients but bleeding from internal organs is unusual. Some patients may develop pedal oedema.
- The fever usually lasts for 2–5 days and abruptly comes down. Other symptoms, particularly joint pains, headache and an extreme degree of prostration, last for a variable period, usually for about 7–10 days. However, in many patients, joint pains may last for as long as 6 months or may persist for several years. This is more common in elderly patients.

DIAGNOSIS

- Thrombocytopenia may occur but is uncommon.
- Diagnosis is based on demonstrating antibodies using ELISA method.
- In early stages, viral isolation confirms the diagnosis.
- Molecular methods include RT-PCR to detect structural genes in the blood sample.

TREATMENT

- The treatment is symptomatic as there is no specific treatment for chikungunya. For arthralgias and arthritis, paracetamol may be used. Tramadol may be used in severe cases. In the initial period, ibuprofen, diclofenac or naproxen should be avoided as dengue can also present with similar features. Rest is also important to reduce morbidity.
- Hydroxychloroquine (HCQ, 200 mg once or twice a day) may be tried in patients with prolonged symptoms of joint pains. In some cases with erosive arthritis, methotrexate may be given, particularly if test for anticyclic citrullinated peptide (anti-CCP) antibodies is positive.

PREVENTION

- It is on similar lines as that for dengue infection.

Q. Discuss briefly about Zika virus disease.

Q. How will you differentiate between dengue, chikungunya and Zika disease?

- Zika virus is a single-stranded RNA *Flavivirus*.
- Zika virus was first isolated in 1947 in the Zika forest in Uganda from a rhesus macaque.
- Until 2007, Zika virus infections were mostly considered an infection of limited geographical distribution; however, in 2015, striking increase occurred in Brazil. The outbreak then spread to other countries in South, Central and North America.
- The infections were associated with a significant increase in the number of microcephaly and Guillain–Barré syndrome cases in the infected regions, and this led to the declaration of a Public Health Emergency of International Concern (PHEIC) by WHO in early 2016.
- Over the year, it has been reported from several parts of India, particularly Ahmedabad district.
- Primarily transmitted to humans through *Aedes* spp. mosquitoes. Zika can also be passed from mother to child during pregnancy or spread through sexual contact, organ transplantation or blood transfusion.

CLINICAL FEATURES

- Zika has an incubation period ranging from 3 to 12 days.
- Only approximately 20% of individuals experience symptoms during Zika infection. These include mild fever (37.8°C–38.5°C), arthralgias predominantly of small joints of hands and feet, headache, myalgia, non-purulent conjunctivitis and retro-orbital pain.
- Skin manifestations are seen in majority and are characterised by a pruritic maculopapular rash predominantly localised to the trunk and extremities, followed by the face. Palms and soles may be affected and the palate may show petechiae.
- Fever is not a hallmark sign of this infection. The maculopapular rash is more sensitive for detecting Zika.
- Rare clinical manifestations include thrombocytopenia, facial oedema, uveitis, transient hearing

impairment, myocarditis, pericarditis and haematospermia.

- An increase in the number of Guillain–Barré cases has been reported following Zika infection.
- In pregnant females, infection during first trimester can produce microcephaly. Other CNS effects on foetus include calcifications at the cortical-subcortical junction, and ventriculomegaly and/or hydrocephalus.
- Zika infection may produce meningitis and meningoencephalitis.
- The virus can persist in the male genital tract and men infected with Zika can present with genitourinary symptoms such as haematospermia, prostatitis, painful ejaculation, penile discharge and oligospermia.

DIAGNOSIS

- Virus isolation (from blood, urine, semen, saliva).
- Antigen detection in tissues obtained during autopsy (e.g. brain, placenta).
- Viral RNA detection with molecular assays (RT-PCR).
- Anti-Zika virus antibody detection by different serological assays (e.g. complement fixation, haemagglutination inhibition, immunofluorescence assay (IFA), ELISA and capture ELISA).

TREATMENT

- No effective antiviral treatments are available for Zika virus infection.
- Management consists of rest and symptomatic treatment. Aspirin and other NSAIDs should be avoided until other viral infections have been ruled out.

DIFFERENTIATING DENGUE, CHIKUNGUNYA AND ZIKA INFECTION (Table 17.13)

Q. Write a short note on Ebola.

- Ebola virus (EV) belongs to the *Filoviridae* family and is an enveloped single-stranded RNA virus.
- EV was named after a river in North-Western Zaire, now the Democratic Republic of the Congo, where the first documented outbreak emerged in 1976.
- The illness caused by EV infection in humans was formerly known as Ebola haemorrhagic fever. In the recent outbreaks, the manifestations of haemorrhagic fever among the infected individuals were rare. As a result, the name of the illness has now changed to Ebola virus disease (EVD).
- From 2014 to 2016, West Africa (Guinea, Sierra Leone and Liberia) faced the largest-ever recorded outbreak of EVD, with 28,616 total cases and at least 11,300 fatalities.
- In early 2019 also, Ebola outbreak has been reported from the Democratic Republic of the Congo. In February 2021, a small outbreak was reported in Guinea and the Democratic Republic of the Congo (DRC). Another small outbreak was reported in April 2022.
- The WHO declares an outbreak is over when no confirmed or probable cases are detected for a period of 42 days.

TRANSMISSION

- Bats are thought to be the primary asymptomatic reservoirs for EVs.
- EV is transmitted by contact with the body fluids of an infected individual. Human blood, urine, saliva, sweat, faeces, vomit, breast milk and semen of an individual with EVD are considered potentially infectious.
- The semen of recently recovered individuals may be infectious for several months after recovery from EVD.

TABLE 17.13 Differentiating Dengue, Chikungunya and Zika Infection

Feature	Dengue	Chikungunya	Zika
Vector	*Aedes* spp.	*Aedes* spp.	*Aedes* spp.
Incubation period (days)	5–8	1–12	3–12
Sexual transmission	–	–	+
Asymptomatic cases	6%–80%	<25%	>80%
High-grade fever (≥39°C)	Majority	Majority	Minority
Skin rash	+	++	+++
Arthralgias/myalgias	+/++	+++	++
Arthritis	±	+++	+
Bleeding	++	±	–
Leucopenia	++/+++	++/+++	+
Thrombocytopenia	++/+++	±	–
Guillain–Barré syndrome	±	±	+
Microcephaly (after infection during pregnancy)	–	–	+
Chronic arthritis	–	+	–

- In addition, any physical object that has been contaminated by body fluids from an EVD-infected individual can transmit the virus.

PATHOPHYSIOLOGY

- It has been proposed that EV enters through skin microabrasions and infects macrophages and other antigen-presenting cells in the dermal and subdermal tissues.
- The infected immune cells then migrate to local lymph nodes and then to the vascular system resulting in infection of endothelial cells.
- EV induces release of proinflammatory mediators such as cytokines that cause dysregulation of the immune system.
- Released cytokines produce vasodilatation and disturb the vasculature system integrity resulting in increased vascular permeability, DIC and multiple organ failure.

CLINICAL FEATURES

- Incubation period ranges from 2 to 21 days.
- Early symptoms include high fever, fatigue, malaise and muscle aches, although about 20% of cases may present without fever.
- In addition, patients may present with multiple infections simultaneously, including viral pathogens, malaria parasites and bacteraemia from translocated gut bacteria.
- Once EV infection is established, the predilection of filoviruses for gastrointestinal tract (GIT) leads to life-threatening dehydration from cholera-like diarrhoea of 5–10 L/day. Emesis is also common. These GIT features persist for 5–7 days.
- Rapid intravascular volume depletion coupled with poor absorption of nutrients leads to electrolyte imbalance and acid–base disorders, which can lead to hypoperfusion, shock and multiorgan failure including liver and kidney failure.
- Symptoms improve in approximately 40% of patients around day 10 of illness and nearly all patients alive at day 13 ultimately survive.
- Maculopapular rash is seen in nearly 50% of cases which in some cases may become purpuric or petechial.
- Overall, haemorrhage is uncommon in recent outbreaks and is a manifestation of late disease. Haemorrhagic manifestations were quite common in previous outbreaks.

LABORATORY FEATURES

- The laboratory abnormalities include leucopenia, thrombocytopenia and elevated INR.
- Mildly elevated bilirubin with transaminitis.
- Marked elevation of creatinine kinase and serum lactate.
- Other findings include hyponatraemia, hypocalcaemia, hypomagnesaemia and hypoalbuminaemia.

DIAGNOSTIC TESTS

- The most commonly used diagnostic tests are RT-PCR blood tests or oral swabs to detect EV RNA.
- Filoviral antigen and nucleic acid are detectable in blood samples from as early as day 1 and at least to day 10 of symptomatic illness.

TREATMENT

- The first step in the management of suspected cases is appropriate isolation in Ebola treatment centres (ETCs) with strict infection control measures by trained teams followed by screening all contacts of the suspected case.
- Once suspected of or diagnosed with EVD, early and aggressive supportive care is the mainstay of EVD management.
- Patients usually require 5–10 L of intravenous fluids daily to maintain circulating blood volume in the setting of ongoing gastrointestinal loss.
- Monitoring and aggressive correction of potassium levels, acid–base disturbances and other electrolyte abnormalities can help prevent life-threatening arrhythmias and metabolic complications.
- Transfusion of blood products for patients with coagulopathy and bleeding.
- Treatment of concomitant infections is important to improve survival.

SPECIFIC TREATMENT

- ZMapp is an antibody cocktail based on blood products developed from EVD survivors. It showed some efficacy during the 2014–2016 epidemic.
- Atoltivimab, maftivimab and odesivimab is the triple monoclonal antibody product that has been approved by the US Food and Drug Administration (FDA) for use in EVD. This combination of three monoclonal antibodies targets three non-overlapping epitopes on the EV surface glycoprotein.
- Another approved monoclonal antibody is ansuvimab, which was isolated from a survivor of EVD.
- Plasma from convalescent donors may also be beneficial although results of trials are controversial.

PREVENTION

- Extreme care should be taken when caring for EVD patients and handling waste exposed to the virus. Only those healthcare providers who have been trained in the use of personal protective equipment (PPE) should care for potentially infected patients.
- In addition to PPE, soap and water hand-washing and alcohol hand gel should be practiced as both of them disrupt the lipid membrane of filoviruses and interrupt transmission.
- rVSV-ZEBOV vaccine (recombinant vesicular stomatitis virus–Zaire Ebola virus) is approved for prophylaxis and should be administered in an outbreak setting to protect persons at high risk of contracting EV.

Q. Write a brief note on aetiology, transmission and pathogenesis of severe acute respiratory syndrome coronavirus 2 (SARS-CoV-2) disease or coronavirus disease 2019 (COVID-19).

- Coronavirus disease 2019 (COVID-19) is a novel viral illness caused by severe acute respiratory syndrome coronavirus 2 or SARS-CoV-2, which is a single-stranded RNA virus.
- The first series of cases were reported in December 2019 from Hubei Province in Wuhan, China. The virus quickly spread throughout China and by middle of January 2020, became a serious epidemic. In February 2020, it was announced as a global health emergency by the World Health Organization (WHO) and in March, COVID-19 was formally announced a pandemic.
- As of November 24, 2022, more than 636 million cases of COVID-19 have been reported globally with more than 6.6 million deaths.
- From India, more than 44.6 million cases have been reported with 0.53 million deaths.

AETIOLOGY

- The coronaviruses are group of viruses that are covered by spike proteins and look like a 'crown' (corona means a crown), hence the name coronavirus.
- There are seven types of coronaviruses that infect humans. Four of the coronaviruses have low pathogenicity and are endemic to humans; they cause mild flu infections. The remaining three are SARS-CoV-1 which caused the SARS in China in 2002, MERS-CoV which caused the Middle East respiratory syndrome in middle east countries in 2012, and SARS-CoV-2 which is the causative agent for COVID-19.
- The SARS-CoV-2 virus is thought to have evolved in bats and pangolins before infecting humans.
- There are four structural proteins in the SARS-CoV-2 virus—S or spike protein, E or envelope protein, M or membrane protein and N or nucleocapsid protein.
  - Spike protein has the main function of attaching the virus to the membrane of the host cell through the angiotensin-converting enzyme (ACE-2) receptor. The spike protein binds to ACE-2 receptor with greater affinity than the SARS-CoV-1 virus, which may be the reason for the highly infectious nature of this virus.
  - M and E proteins are important in viral assembly and the release of virus from the host cell. These proteins help the virus gain access to the host cell.
  - The N protein has bound single-stranded RNA and inhibits host cell defence mechanisms and assists in the replication of viral RNA (Fig. 17.7).

VARIANTS

- Like other viruses, the SARS-CoV-2 has evolved over time. Several variants of concern have been notified from across the world.
- Variants of concern have been identified based on the enhanced viral replication, transmissibility, spread across the world or severity of clinical manifestations in population.
- The alpha variant was the first reported variant of concern from United Kingdom and it was reported to have increased transmissibility and disease severity when compared to the wild-type virus.
- The delta variant (B.1.617.2) was first reported from India and is more transmissible when compared to alpha variant. The disease severity also was higher with the delta variant with severe pulmonary features like acute respiratory failure and vascular involvement.
- The omicron variant (B.1.1.529) was first reported from Botswana and South Africa. This variant has increased transmissibility but reduced severity when compared to delta variant. It has replaced delta variant in India.

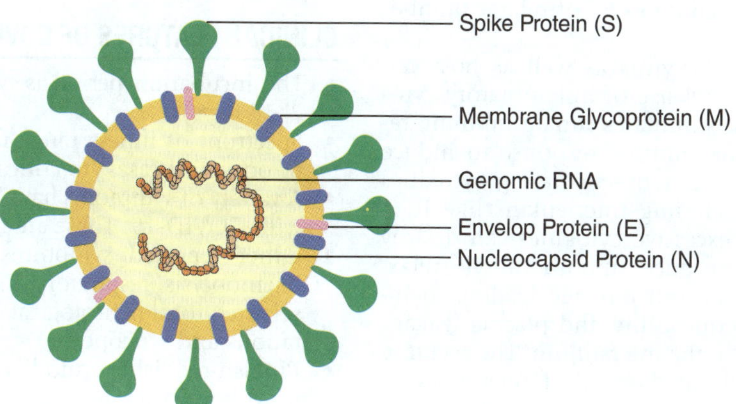

Fig. 17.7 Structure of SARS-corona virus 2.

TRANSMISSION

- The mode of transmission of COVID-19 is primarily human-to-human through droplets, fomites and airborne.
- The droplets thought to be the spread mainly within 2 m when the infected human talks, coughs or sneezes. The droplets may remain active on the surface for several hours to days. On touching the droplets on surface by hand and subsequently touching face, nose or mouth, one may also spread the infection.
- Airborne transmission is seen when the virus particles remain suspended in air for a longer period of time, sometimes hours and spread longer distances in air. It is not clear to what extent this mode of transmission contributed to the spread of the pandemic. In clinical care setting, airborne transmission (in the form of aerosol) can also be seen. This is mostly seen in resuscitation areas within emergency departments and critical care where aerosol-generating procedures are being performed namely intubation, high flow oxygenation, nebulisation and suctioning.

PATHOGENESIS

- The lungs have two types of cells: type 1 pneumocytes (assist in gas exchange) and type 2 pneumocytes (produce surfactant).
- The single-stranded RNA coronavirus attaches to the ACE-2 receptors on the surface of type 2 pneumocytes using its surface spike proteins.
- The virus then enters the cell either by direct mechanism or endocytosis and using the host cell ribosome, makes several viral polypeptides or protein molecules.
- The polypeptides are further cleaved by proteinases enzymes to form different structural components of the virus like capsids and spikes.
- The virus also uses the RNA-dependent RNA polymerase (RdRp) to synthesize more RNA molecules. This combination of RNA molecules and reformed polypeptides creates newer virus particles which are released by exocytic secretory process from the affected cells in large numbers and infect other pneumocytes. Hence the virus uses the host cell machinery, the endoplasmic reticulum and Golgi apparatus to its advantage and replicates to form large number of viral particles.
- On the other side, the virus as well as host cell death stimulates the release of inflammatory cytokines which in turn stimulates innate immune response and adaptive immune response to induce the excessive production of circulating cytokines (cytokine storm) including interleukins like IL-1, IL-6 and TNF. The excessive cytokines can destroy epithelial cells or produce smooth muscle relaxation and endothelial cell damage leading to increased capillary permeability and plasma leakage around alveoli and in the interstitium. The accumulation of fluid leads to damage of pneumocytes, reduction in surfactant production and alveolar collapse, producing ARDS.
- In addition, cytokine storm can produce macrophage activation syndrome and intravascular coagulation. These events together produce ARDS, multiple organ dysfunction syndromes or death (Fig. 17.8).
- One other aspect in COVID-19 disease has been its infliction on blood coagulation. COVID-19 is as much a vascular disease as it is a pulmonary disease. It effects coagulopathy by a multitude of mechanisms which lead to hypercoagulation in COVID-19.
- The virus directly and through complement activation (C5b-9 and IL-6) causes injury to the endothelium, which plays a central role in coagulopathy.
- In addition, the hypercoagulable state is due to elevated factors VIII, fibrinogen and von Willebrand factor.
- Prolonged immobilization of critically ill COVID-19 patients also promotes coagulopathy leading to a systemic multiorgan prothrombotic state including the involvement of the lungs which are already affected as discussed above (Flowchart 17.4).
- On blood tests, one must look for elevated D-dimer and fibrinogen levels, thrombocytopenia, prothrombin time/INR, which are slightly elevated, while activated partial thromboplastin clotting time is reduced.
- Thromboelastography (TEG) has been used to diagnose the coagulopathy of COVID-19. A decreased reaction time (R time) consistent with early thrombin burst formation, shortened clot formation time (K time) consistent with increased fibrin generation, increased maximum amplitude (MA) consistent with greater clot strength and reduced clot lysis time in 30 minutes (LY30) consistent with reduced fibrinolysis are the common findings in COVID-19 coagulopathy.

Q. Describe the clinical features of COVID-19.

Q. Write a short note on multisystem inflammatory syndrome of children (MIS-C).

- The period of infectivity is 2–3 days before the onset of symptoms till about 7–10 days of illness, with maximum infectivity early in the course of illness.

CLINICAL FEATURES OF COVID-19

- The incubation period is typically 5–7 days (range 2–14 days).
- Spectrum of illness range from asymptomatic state (~one-third cases) to critically ill.
- A variety of symptoms have been reported in patients with COVID-19. These are listed in Box 17.12.
- Other reported symptoms include expectoration, haemoptysis, respiratory distress, altered sensorium, seizures, focal neurological deficits, chest pain, palpitations and syncope.
- Pinkish-reddish 'pernio-like' lesions on toes (COVID toes) have been described in toes of young patients (Fig. 17.9). These can turn bluish-purple over time.

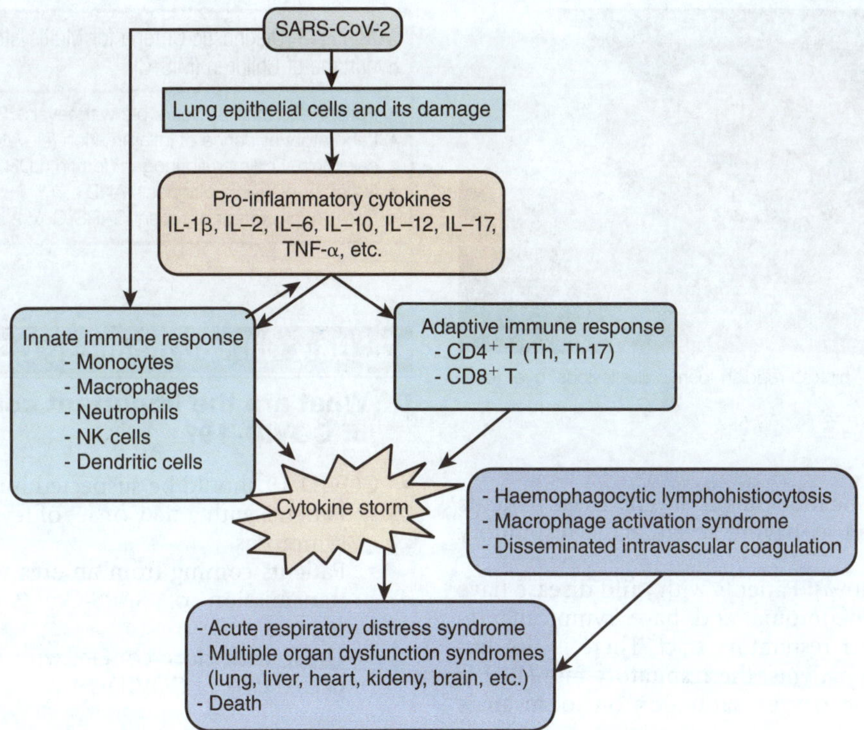

Fig. 17.8 Pathogenesis of cytokine storm in COVID-19.

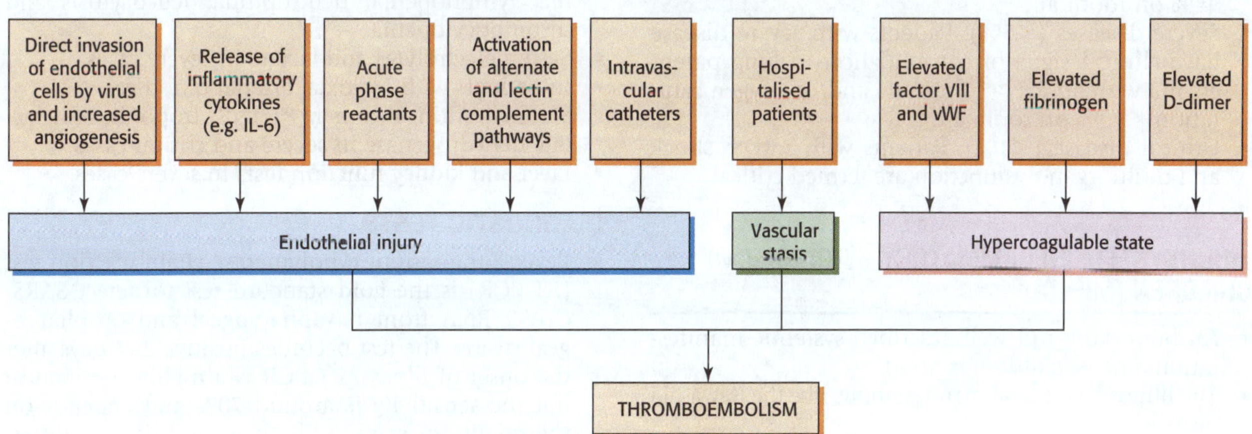

Flowchart 17.4 Pathogenesis of Coagulopathy in COVID-19.

BOX 17.12 Symptoms of COVID-19

• Fever or chills	• Loss of taste
• Dry cough	• Loss of smell
• Sore throat	• Congestion or runny nose
• Shortness of breath	• Nausea or vomiting
• Fatigue	• Diarrhoea
• Body aches	• Skin rash
• Headache	• Red eyes

- Children may also develop hyperinflammatory syndrome known as paediatric inflammatory multisystem syndrome (PIMS) or multisystem inflammatory syndrome in children (MIS-C). It presents with features of typical or atypical Kawasaki disease.

SEVERITY OF COVID-19

- COVID-19 is classified into mild, moderate, severe and critical disease.
- Once the patient develops dyspnoea, hypoxia or more than 50% of the lung involvement on imaging,

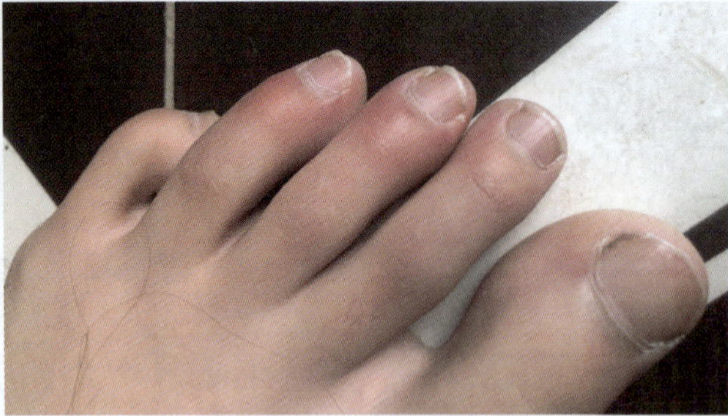

Fig. 17.9 COVID toes—pinkish-reddish 'pernio-like lesions' over toes.

the disease will be moderate to severe. These patients are also labelled as having severe acute respiratory illness (SARI).

- Mild disease (80%): Patients with mild disease have no or mild pneumonia and have symptoms restricted to upper respiratory tract. There is no dyspnoea in these patients, the respiratory rate (RR) is <24/minute and oxygen saturation on room air is >94%.
- Moderate disease (15%): Patients with moderate disease have pneumonia and present with dyspnoea, respiratory rate between 24 and 30/minute and/or hypoxia with oxygen saturation between 90% and 94% on room air.
- Severe diseases (<5%): Patients with severe disease have clinical signs of consolidation in lung parenchyma with an RR >30/minute and/or oxygen saturation <90% on room air.
- Critical disease (<1%): Patients with ARDS, shock and multiorgan dysfunction are termed critical.

MULTISYSTEM INFLAMMATORY SYNDROME OF CHILDREN (MIS-C)

- An important and well-described systemic manifestation among children is MIS-C.
- The illness has several manifestations like the Kawasaki disease.
- These patients present with persistent fever, abdominal pain, vomiting, diarrhoea, skin rash, mucocutaneous lesions, and in severe cases, hypotension and shock. Some patients go on to develop myocarditis, cardiac dysfunction and acute kidney injury.
- Diagnostic criteria for MIS-C are given in Box 17.13.

TREATMENT

- Fluid resuscitation, inotropic support for patients in shock.
- Respiratory support with oxygen and ventilation.
- Intravenous immunoglobulin and steroids to prevent progression of inflammation.
- Low-dose aspirin has commonly been used to prevent coronary artery involvement.
- Prophylaxis against thrombosis using enoxaparin or warfarin is often used in these patients.

BOX 17.13 Diagnostic Criteria for Multisystem Inflammatory Syndrome of Children (MIS-C)

- Patient less than 21 years old with fever ≥38°C AND
- Laboratory evidence of inflammation (elevated CRP, ESR, procalcitonin, D-dimer, fibrinogen, ferritin, LDH, IL-6 etc.) AND
- No other plausible diagnosis AND
- Positive for current or recent SARS-CoV-2 infection

Q. How will you diagnose COVID-19?

Q. What are the important complications of COVID-19?

- COVID-19 should be suspected in:
  - Patients with a new onset of fever and respiratory symptoms.
  - Patients coming from an area where community transmission of SARS-CoV-2 has been documented.
  - Those with close contact with confirmed or suspected case of COVID-19.

DIAGNOSIS

LABORATORY TESTS

- Complete blood count (CBC) to look for leucopenia, lymphopenia, neutrophilia, leucocytosis and thrombocytopenia.
- Serum electrolytes and lactate in severe cases.
- In patients with hypoxia, arterial blood gas.
- Serum ferritin, D-dimer, PT/INR, troponin and lactate dehydrogenase in severe and critical cases.
- Liver and kidney function tests in severe cases.

DIAGNOSTIC TESTS

- Reverse-transcription polymerase chain reaction test (RT-PCR) is the gold standard test to detect SARS-CoV-2 RNA from nasopharyngeal and oropharyngeal swabs. The test becomes positive 2–7 days after the onset of illness. RT-PCR is a highly specific test but the sensitivity is around 70% and depends on the quality of sample obtained and day of illness. Hence, a positive RT-PCR test confirms COVID-19; however, a negative test does not rule it out. If the clinician still suspects COVID-19, the test may be repeated in 24–48 hours. Repeating within 24 hours is not recommended.
- Cartridge-based nucleic acid amplification test (CBNAAT) is also a PCR test with faster turn over time compared to RT-PCR. It is as sensitive as RT-PCR.
- Rapid antigen test (RAT) is a point-of-care test that is conducted on samples obtained from nasopharyngeal swabs. The result is available within 10–15 minutes. A positive test is confirmatory while a negative test needs to be confirmed by RT-PCR or CBNAAT.

IMAGING

- Imaging is not routinely recommended in screening or confirming diagnosis of COVID-19. A patient who is suspected of COVID-19 and has mild symptoms does not require any imaging.

- Patients of moderate and severe disease with suspected or confirmed COVID-19 should get a chest X-ray first. CT chest is indicated in patients who have suspected/confirmed COVID-19 with worsening respiratory failure.

Chest Radiograph

- The classical chest X-ray image shows multifocal, ground-glass opacities in peripheral regions of both lungs. Spontaneous pneumothorax, though uncommon, may be seen in a few patients.

Chest Computed Tomogram

- The chest CT findings are more sensitive for COVID. The most common findings are ground-glass opacities, multifocal consolidations and thickening of the interstitial space. The ground-glass opacities are early changes in the lungs; they are bilateral and are located in peripheral lung segments. These are followed by 'crazy paving pattern' or septal thickening in interlobar and interlobular areas. This pattern is followed by solid white consolidations usually in multifocal distribution. The consolidations are followed by 'reverse halo sign' which means a central ground-glass pattern surrounded by opacity. Although not diagnostic, these CT findings are typical of COVID-19 chest infection.
- Isolated lobar consolidations, discrete small nodules, lung cavitation and pleural effusions are atypical features and do not suggest COVID-19 infection.
- Radiological scoring system was developed to standardize COVID-19 reporting of chest CT scans. This has been popularised as CORADS or COVID-19 Reporting and Data Systems. The objective of this score is to identify the level of suspicion of COVID-19 infection. CORADS score is from 0 to 6.
- Another score, the chest CT severity score, was developed to grade the severity of COVID-19 infection. It is based on the extent of involvement of each of the five lobes. This score has a maximum score of 25, with 5 being the maximum score from each lobe of the lung. In order to give a CT severity score, the radiologist analyses each lobe and scores it depending on the level of involvement. A lobar involvement of less than 5% would give a score of 1 to that lobe. Similarly, involvement of 5%–25% of the lobe scores 2, 25%–50% scores 3, 50%–75% scores 4 and more than 75% scores 5.
- The radiological appearance can suspect COVID-19. However, due to overlapping patterns in other viral pneumonias, influenza infection, cryptogenic organizing pneumonia and drug reactions, a definite diagnosis cannot be established unless patient already is confirmed COVID-19 by molecular testing.

Ultrasound

- Point-of-care ultrasound or POCUS is a non-invasive, real time, bedside tool that is an easily available imaging modality. It shows scattered/confluent 'B' lines, pleural shredding/thickening/irregularity and various sizes of consolidations in patients with COVID-19 pneumonia.

TABLE 17.14 Complications of COVID-19

Respiratory	Arterial/venous thromboembolism
• ARDS	• Deep vein thrombosis
Cardiac	• Pulmonary embolism
• Myocarditis	• Peripheral embolisation
• Arrhythmias	• Mesenteric ischaemia
• Heart failure	Others
• Myocardial infarction	• Acute kidney injury
Neurological	• Hepatitis
• Stroke	• Sepsis and septic shock
• Intracranial bleed	• Multiorgan failure
• Seizures	• Invasive fungal infections including mucormycosis
• Encephalopathy	
• Guillain–Barré syndrome	

COMPLICATIONS

- Complications of COVID-19 are listed in Table 17.14.

Q. How will you manage a patient of COVID-19?

Q. What are the vaccines available for COVID-19?

- Management of COVID-19 patients is described below based on the severity of the disease.

MANAGEMENT OF MILD CASES

- Mild cases can be isolated at home or at COVID Care Centre depending on the availability of resources. Patients should be counselled about signs and symptoms of complications that should prompt urgent care. Patients with risk factors for severe illness (e.g. immunocompromised patients, patients with age >60 years, cardiovascular disease, diabetes, hypertension, chronic liver/lung or kidney disease, cerebrovascular disease and obesity) should be monitored closely, given the possible risk of deterioration.
- If possible, oxygen saturation should be monitored every 4–6 hours. Patients may have 'silent hypoxia' or hypoxia without any dyspnoea or tachypnoea.
- Symptomatic treatment includes antipyretic (paracetamol) for fever and pain, adequate nutrition and appropriate rehydration.
- There is no role of hydroxychloroquine (HCQ) ivermectin, vitamin C, azithromycin, favipiravir or lopinavir–ritonavir in any case of COVID-19.
- Inhalational budesonide can be used (800 mcg via inhaler twice daily for 5–7 days), if fever or cough persist beyond 5 days of disease onset.
- Molnupiravir (a small-molecule ribonucleoside prodrug of N-hydroxycytidine) has been found useful in mild to moderate, non-hospitalised, unvaccinated cases having an underlying comorbidity. Dose is four tablets (total 800 mg) twice daily for five days. It is to be started within 5 days of symptom onset.

- Nirmatrelvir and ritonavir combination is recommended for patients with non-severe COVID-19 who are at the highest risk of developing severe disease and hospitalisation, such as unvaccinated, older or immunosuppressed patients.
- Healthcare workers who assess patients with suspected/proved COVID-19 cases should ideally be in full PPE. Otherwise, N95 mask and gloves are must.

MANAGEMENT OF MODERATE CASES

- Hospital admission; however, those without any risk factors can be isolated at home with frequent oxygen saturation monitoring and oxygen therapy.

OXYGEN THERAPY

- Administer oxygen with a target oxygen saturation of 94%–96%.
- The devices for administering oxygen include nasal prongs, face mask and masks with non-rebreathing reservoir bag, and are chosen based on increasing oxygen requirement. N95 mask should be applied over the oxygen-administering device.
- High-flow nasal oxygen (HFNO) or non-invasive ventilation (NIV) may be required in case there is no improvement with other devices.
- Awake proning is helpful in maintaining oxygen saturation. Typical protocols include 30–120 minutes in prone position, followed by 30–120 minutes in left lateral decubitus, right lateral decubitus and upright sitting position.

OTHER INTERVENTIONS

- Daily ECG.
- Follow CBC with differential count, absolute lymphocyte count, renal and liver function tests daily and CRP, D-dimer and ferritin every 48–72 hours.
- Administer dexamethasone 6 mg or methylprednisolone 0.5–1 mg/kg IV for 7–10 days or till hospital discharge. Steroids should be used only if oxygen is required to maintain saturation. It is preferable to administer steroids along with remdesivir, but if latter is not available, then steroids can be used alone.
- Remdesivir may be considered if no contraindications to its use are present (AST/ALT >5 times upper limit of normal, severe renal impairment, pregnancy or lactating females, children <12 years of age). Dose is 200 mg IV on day 1 followed by 100 mg IV daily for 5 days. However, its role in reducing mortality and duration of hospital stay is controversial. It may be considered in mild or moderate COVID-19 patients who are at high risk of hospitalisation.
- Tocilizumab (a selective inhibitor of the IL-6 pathway) or baricitinib (a JAK inhibitor) may be considered in addition to dexamethasone, if oxygen requirement is increasing or patient is on mechanical ventilation and inflammatory markers (e.g., CRP, ferritin, LDH and IL-6) or D-dimer are elevated or there is progressively increasing levels of fibrinogen. Active infections and tuberculosis should be ruled out before use. Dose of tocilizumab is 8 mg/kg (maximum 800 mg) given over 1 hour; may be repeated once after 12–24 hours, if needed. Again, its role is controversial.
  - If tocilizumab is not available, sarilumab (another IL-6 inhibitor) may be used.
  - If baricitinib is not available, tofacitinib (another JAK inhibitor) may be used.
  - Cases of severe and disseminated strongyloidiasis have been reported in patients with COVID-19 during treatment with tocilizumab and corticosteroids. Many clinicians initiate empiric treatment with ivermectin for strongyloidiasis in patients from areas where strongyloidiasis is endemic.
- Prophylactic dose of unfractionated heparin or low-molecular weight heparin (e.g. enoxaparin 40 mg/day subcutaneously) should be administered in all hospitalised patients. However, there is some evidence that patients who are on supplemental oxygen (except those on high-frequency nasal cannula [HFNC] or NIV) with a D-dimer level above the normal range and not at increased bleeding risk, may benefit from therapeutic dose of heparin (low-molecular weight or unfractionated heparin).
- Convalescent plasma is of little benefit.
- The US Food and Drug Administration (FDA) has given emergency use authorization for use of monoclonal antibodies directed against the spike protein of virus. These antibodies block the attachment of virus to the human cells. These are approved only for mild-to-moderate cases and include the following:
  - Casirivimab/imdevimab combination (not effective against omicron variant).
  - Bamlanivimab/etesevimab combination.
  - Sotrovimab.

MANAGEMENT OF SEVERE AND CRITICAL CASES

- All such cases should be admitted in ICU.
- Administer supplemental oxygen therapy with oxygen saturation target of at least 92%–94%.
- These patients often require HFNC or NIV for oxygen administration. Patients with $paCO_2$ >50 mmHg, cardiogenic pulmonary oedema, haemodynamic instability, multiorgan failure or abnormal mental status should generally not receive HFNC oxygenation.
- Endotracheal intubation and mechanical ventilation may be required if there is no improvement within an hour of oxygen therapy.
- Extracorporeal membrane oxygenation (ECMO) may be tried in selected patients.
- Drugs include dexamethasone or methylprednisolone, remdesivir and tocilizumab.
- In patients with severe ARDS, prone ventilation for 16–18 hours per day is recommended.
- Manage ARDS and sepsis as per standard guidelines.

CARDIAC ARREST IN COVID-19 PATIENTS

- Suspected/confirmed COVID-19 patients with cardiac arrest should be dealt with caution. During a pandemic, all out-of-hospital cardiac arrests or death on arrival are COVID-19 positive until proven otherwise.
- A tightly fitted oxygen face mask should be placed on the patient. Before starting CPR, a surgical mask can

be placed over the oxygen face mask to minimise virus dispersion. Use of aerosol box/plastic drape will contain aerosols. Bag-mask ventilation should be avoided in COVID-19 patients.

- Use hands-only compressions CPR until the airway is secured with an advanced airway.
- Mechanical CPR device should be preferred over manual CPR.
- Consider a sixth 'H' as a reversible cause of cardiac arrest which is hypomagnesaemia, especially if the patient is on HCQ plus azithromycin.
- Personnel without complete PPE should not be allowed into the resuscitation area.
- Intubation should be done by an expert to ensure quick first-pass success.
- If defibrillator pads are available, use them in place of conventional paddles to minimise exposure.
- COVID 19 patients benefit from a negative fluid balance. If postarrest, the patient is hypotensive, consider early use of vasopressors (e.g. noradrenaline) with careful fluid administration instead of aggressive fluid resuscitation.
- All equipment used during CPR should be put on a separate trolley for cleaning and disinfection.

VACCINES

- Currently four types of vaccines are available against SARS-CoV-2. These are based on inactivated whole virus, protein subunit, viral vector, and nucleic acid (mRNA or DNA). Majority of these vaccines require two doses 4–6 weeks apart (in India, the gap between the two doses is higher), although single-dose vaccine is also available.
- Mild side effects including local pain and redness, fever, myalgias and headache may occur after vaccination.
- Rare complications associated with vaccines include arterial thrombosis and venous thrombosis, Guillain–Barré syndrome and anaphylaxis.

INFECTION CONTROL IN HOSPITAL

- Training of staff: Regular and frequent onsite/online training in infection control should be provided. Videos may be developed and circulated. All cadres of staff must be included in training. A constant vigil and monitoring of infection control compliance should be led by an independent infection control team created within the department with constant feedback mechanism.
- Standard precautions should be taken to prevent further transmission by isolating patients in negative pressure room. Patients and their attendants should wear triple layer surgical mask during hospital stay.
- Healthcare providers should wear appropriate PPE for droplet precautions, including N95 mask, face shields and goggles for eye protection, gown and gloves.
- Contaminated surfaces and objects should be cleaned using freshly prepared 1% sodium hypochlorite solution with a contact time of at least 10 minutes

Q. Give a brief account of Japanese encephalitis.

- It is a zoonotic disease maintaining Japanese encephalitis virus in nature by bird–mosquito–bird and pig–mosquito–pig cycles.
- It is an arboviral infection transmitted by the bites of infected culicine mosquitoes (*Culex tritaeniorhynchus*) that have fed on infected animals (pigs) or birds.
- The disease is particularly common in areas where irrigated rice fields are present.
- Bihar, Uttar Pradesh, Assam, Andhra Pradesh, Karnataka, Tamil Nadu, West Bengal and Odisha are major states of India where Japanese encephalitis is endemic.

CLINICAL FEATURES

- Incubation period is 6–8 days after the bite.
- In endemic areas, the highest age-specific attack rates occur in children of 3–15 years of age because of high background immunity in older individuals. Majority of infections are asymptomatic or may present with fever.
- In some, the illness may present as encephalitis or meningitis.
- Following incubation period, a prodrome of fever, headache, nausea, diarrhoea, vomiting and myalgia occurs lasting for few days (1–5 days) followed by irritability, altered behaviour, convulsions and coma.
- The patient may develop difficulty of speech and other neurological deficits like ocular palsies, hemiplegia, quadriplegia and extrapyramidal signs in the form of dull, flat, mask-like facies with unblinking eyes, cogwheel rigidity, dystonia, choreoathetosis and coarse tremors.

DIAGNOSIS

- Laboratory abnormalities include leucocytosis with neutrophilia.
- CSF shows raised pressure, cell count and proteins. Neutrophils may predominate in early CSF samples but a lymphocytic pleocytosis is typical. CSF protein is moderately elevated in about 50% of cases.
- Serological tests detect antibodies to viral antigens and include virus neutralisation test, haemagglutination inhibition and complement fixation. A significant rise in titre should be seen with paired samples from the acute and convalescent stages. An IgM-capture ELISA may be useful and can detect IgM antibodies in serum and CSF.
- Viral antigens can be detected in CSF by indirect IFA. Viral nucleic acid can be analysed by RT-PCR.
- Virus isolation can be done from CSF.
- Persistent EEG abnormalities are commonly seen, particularly in children.
- MRI scans of brain reveal low-density areas and abnormal signal intensities in the thalamus and basal ganglia.

TREATMENT

- Treatment is entirely symptomatic and includes control of fever, raised intracranial tension and convulsions.

PREVENTION

- Reduction of breeding source of mosquitoes includes water management system, intermittent irrigation and using 'neem' products as fertilisers.
- Reduction in man–mosquito contact by various measures including mosquito repellents, pyrethroid-impregnated curtains and periodical aerial sprays.
- Vaccines in use include purified, formalin-inactivated mouse brain-derived and cell-culture-derived live attenuated. Cell-culture-derived live attenuated vaccine is currently used in India in endemic areas in both children and adults.

Q. Describe rabies and its prevention.

EPIDEMIOLOGY

- Rabies continues to be endemic in India. Nearly, 30,000 people die of rabies every year in India.
- Dog is the most common animal responsible for transmitting rabies. Other animals include foxes, monkeys, cats, mongooses and horses. In India, rats and rabbits have not been shown to transmit rabies.

TRANSMISSION

- Humans are usually infected when virus-laden saliva is inoculated through the skin by the bite of a rabid animal, particularly a wild dog.
- Licks on abraded skin and mucosa (even healthy) by infected animals may produce rabies.
- Others modes of transmission of rabies include drinking unboiled milk (very rare) and eating uncooked meat of infected animals.
- Uncommonly, transmission occurs through inhalation of airborne rabies virus.
- Rarely, human rabies has been reported after corneal transplantation from an infected patient.
- There is a theoretical risk of transmission of rabies through contact with patients since their secretions may contain virus. However, there has never been documentation of transmission by such exposure. Nonetheless, the attending medical personnel must wear gloves, mask and goggles, and if exposed, get immunisation done.

CLINICAL FEATURES OF RABIES IN HUMANS

- Incubation period of rabies is quite variable and can range from 10 days to more than 1 year. Average incubation period is between 20 and 90 days. It tends to be shorter in cases of bites on the face as against those on the limbs.
- The clinical manifestations of rabies can be classified into a prodrome phase, and a furious or paralytic phase. Nearly 80% of patients present with classic (furious) rabies while only 20% develop paralytic rabies. Development of furious or paralytic rabies depends on whether the spinal cord or brain is predominantly infected.

PRODROME PHASE

- It lasts for 1–4 days.
- The patient gets fever, headache, malaise, sore throat, anorexia, nausea and vomiting.
- Paraesthesias, pruritus or fasciculations around the site of bite occur in 50%–80% of cases during this phase.

FURIOUS RABIES

- Patient develops excessive motor activity, agitation, hallucinations, lacrimation, salivation, perspiration, muscle spasms, opisthotonus, seizures and focal deficits.
- Complete lucid intervals are interspersed, which become progressively shorter as the disease progresses.
- Shortly after the beginning of excitement phase, the brainstem dysfunction becomes evident. There may be diplopia, facial palsy and hydrophobia (a combination of inspiratory muscle spasm with or without laryngopharyngeal spasm, associated with terror). Initially, hydrophobia is provoked by attempts to drink water but later, it occurs even on sight of water.
- The same phenomenon occurs on blowing air (aerophobia).
- Gradually, the patient develops dysrhythmias and lapses into coma. Involvement of respiratory centre produces apnoea and death.
- Relative intactness of level of consciousness distinguishes rabies from other viral encephalitis.

PARALYTIC RABIES

- After the usual prodromal features, flaccid paralysis develops, usually in the bitten limb, and then ascends symmetrically or asymmetrically with pain and fasciculations in the affected muscles.
- During the early stages of paralytic rabies, notable signs include myoedema at percussion sites, usually in the region of the chest, deltoid muscle and thigh, and piloerection.
- Death occurs due to the involvement of respiratory muscle.
- Clinical course of paralytic rabies is slower than furious rabies and patients may survive for up to 1 month.

RABIES IN ANIMALS

- In infected animals, two forms of rabies occur: frank rabies and dumb rabies.

FRANK RABIES

- It is characterised by three stages, which last for 4–7 days.
- First stage: The animal experiences personality reversion (may either avoid people or become more friendly than usual), appears distracted and becomes either unusually restless or quiet.
- Second stage: The animal wanders about avoiding familiar persons and becomes excitable. It bites any object in its path and barks repeatedly without any

cause. It develops a perverted appetite and swallows any object. The animal also develops fine tremors followed by muscle contractions.

- Third stage: This stage is characterised by paralysis of muscles, excessive salivation, convulsions and hoarse or inaudible bark. The lower jaw may hang loose, with a protruded tongue. The head may either drop listlessly or remain turned at an abnormal angle. The hind limbs grow weak and the animal is finally unable to support its body.

DUMB RABIES

- In dumb rabies, the animal becomes lethargic and develops tremors followed by complete paralysis. It dies within about 2–3 days.

LABORATORY DIAGNOSIS

POSTMORTEM DIAGNOSIS

Fluorescent Antibody (FA) Technique

- It detects viral antigen and is a rapid and sensitive method for diagnosing rabies. Use of smears from hippocampus and brain stem increases its sensitivity.
- The test is based on microscopic examination, under ultraviolet light, of smears or frozen sections of tissues after treatment with antirabies serum conjugated with fluorescein isothiocyanate.

Field Test

- For the field conditions, rapid rabies enzyme immunodiagnosis (RREID) has been developed. The detection of virus is done without the aid of a microscope. However, this test cannot be used with specimens fixed in formalin.
- It is less sensitive than the FA test.

Virus Isolation

- It is done by inoculating the tissue extract into the mouse brain.
- Diagnosis requires at least 10–15 days. Performing the FA test on the brains of mice within 3–4 days of inoculation can shorten this period.

ANTEMORTEM DIAGNOSIS

Fluorescent Antibody (FA) Test

- Antigen can be detected in corneal impressions or skin biopsies using FA test.
- Corneal impression is taken by touching the central part of the cornea lightly with a microscopic slide.
- Multiple skin biopsies are taken from the nuchal area of the neck, with hair follicles containing the peripheral nerves. Both these specimens are refrigerated immediately after collection till the test is carried out.

ISOLATION OF VIRUS

- Rabies virus can be isolated in cell line from body tissues and fluids, especially saliva and CSF.

MANAGEMENT

IMMEDIATE TREATMENT OF WOUND

- Scrub the wound thoroughly with soap and water. In case of punctured bites, use catheters for irrigation.
- Apply tincture iodine or alcohol liberally.
- Do not cauterise with carbolic acid.
- Avoid suturing:
  - To prevent further trauma which may help in penetration of virus into deeper tissues, keep the punctured wounds and wounds on the extremities open and unsutured.
  - Debride extensive bites on extremities and suture them 24–48 hours later, using minimum number of sutures.
  - In facial bites, close the wound using minimum number of sutures.
  - Infiltrate antirabies serum around the wound, if suturing is necessary.

CLASSIFY EXPOSURE

- Exposures to an animal are classified into three categories (Table 17.15).

ANTIRABIES VACCINE

- Antirabies vaccine is indicated in category II and category III exposures.
- Since the availability of safe vaccines, the previous recommendation of withholding antirabies vaccination and observing the animal for 10 days after the bite is no longer valid as the incubation period of rabies may be as short as 2 weeks. Therefore, a delay in starting the vaccine would result in ineffective neutralising antibody levels at 2 weeks postbite.
- Administer vaccine even if the animal is healthy. If the animal is healthy at day 7, the cell-culture vaccine may be discontinued after the first two doses on day 0 and 3; the animal must be observed for the next 3 days. However, a dose may be given at 28 days so as to complete the 'pre-exposure' prophylaxis. Complete the course of vaccination if the animal develops features of rabies or dies any time during observation.
- Complete antirabies treatment if the animal is untraceable or is wild.
- Since incubation period may be long, administer vaccine and antirabies serum (if indicated) even if the patient presents months after having been bitten.

TABLE 17.15 Categories of Contact/Bite With Animals

Category of Contact/Bite	Type of Contact/Bite
I	• Touching or feeding of animals • Licks on intact skin (no mucous membrane exposure) • Consumption of unboiled milk of the suspected animal
II	• Nibbling of uncovered skin • Minor scratches or abrasions without bleeding • Licks on broken skin with intact dermis
III	• Single or multiple transdermal bites or scratches • Contamination of mucous membrane with saliva of animal

- Two broad types of vaccines include the following:
  - Nervous tissue vaccine (Semple's vaccine)
  - Tissue/cell-culture vaccines:
    - Human diploid cell vaccine (HDCV)
    - Purified chick embryo vaccine (PCEV)
    - Purified Vero cell vaccine (PVCV)
    - Purified duck embryo vaccine (PDEV).

Semple's Vaccine

- It was available at most of the primary health centres previously. However, it has been replaced with safer tissue/cell-culture vaccines.
- It needs to be administered in abdominal wall and carries a high risk of neuroparalytic effects particularly when used for more than 6–7 days.
- Since steroids are required for the treatment of neuroparalytic effects, there is depression of the titres of neutralising antibodies even when cell-culture vaccines are used after that. Therefore, it is recommended that such patients should receive double the normal dose of cell-culture vaccine for the continuation of vaccination.

Tissue/Cell-Culture Vaccines

- The cell-culture vaccines (including HDCV) are safe, need lesser number of injections and have very few adverse effects compared to the nervous tissue vaccine.
- These vaccines are to be administered intramuscularly in the deltoid area; in small children, anterolateral thigh muscle may be used. Never administer these vaccines in the gluteal area.
- Generally, five doses are given for postexposure prophylaxis (on days 0, 3, 7, 14 and 30); however, recent evidence suggests that in immunocompetent patients, fifth dose at 28 days may be omitted.
- The first dose may be doubled where antiserum is indicated, but is not available.

Intradermal Administration of Tissue/Cell-Culture Vaccine

- 0.1 mL each is given at two sites intradermally (either forearm or upper arm) on days 0, 3 and 7, and one dose of 0.1 mL at one site on days 30 and 90.
- The total cost is much less than the standard regimen.
- After administering the initial doses, remaining reconstituted vaccine is stored between 4°C and 8°C and is used as soon as possible (preferably within 48 hours).

ANTIRABIES SERUM/IMMUNOGLOBULINS

- Category III exposures require simultaneous passive immunisation by one of the following:
  - Antirabies horse serum—dose is 40 IU/kg.
  - Equine rabies immunoglobulin (ERIG)—dose is 40 IU/kg.
  - Human rabies immunoglobulins (HRIG)—dose is 20 IU/kg.
  - Rabies human monoclonal antibodies (rDNA)—dose is 3.33 IU/kg.
  - Two rabies murine monoclonal antibodies (docaravimab and miromavimab)—dose is 40 IU/kg.
- Antirabies serum/immunoglobulin may be administered any time after the bite. However, if vaccination was started and it was not given at the beginning of active vaccination, antirabies serum/immunoglobulin can be given only up to seventh day after the first dose of vaccine.
- Administer as much as possible of the recommended dose of antirabies immunoglobulin/serum around the wounds, if anatomically feasible. Administer the remainder dose intramuscularly into the gluteal region.
- Horse antirabies serum can produce severe anaphylaxis. However, it is uncommon with ERIG. However, a skin test (intradermal injection of 1:10 dilution of serum) is recommended with both the preparations. It is not required for HRIG.
- HRIGs can occasionally produce transient tenderness at the site of injection, cutaneous reactions and elevations in temperature. In rare cases, nausea, vomiting, circulatory reactions (tachycardia or bradycardia, hypotension, sweating), flushing, urticaria and dyspnoea can occur.
- The cost of rabies human monoclonal antibodies and rabies murine monoclonal antibodies is about 20% of HRIG.
- Immunoglobulins are safe during pregnancy.
- In a patient with multiple bites, the volume of immunoglobulins may not be enough for local infiltration of all wounds; in such cases, dilute the rabies immunoglobulin in normal saline (one to three times dilution) to provide adequate volume.
- Since human immunoglobulins contain antibodies against several other agents, it is advisable that an interval of at least 3 months should be allowed before vaccination with other parenteral live virus vaccines (e.g. mumps, measles and rubella). However, this is not required for administering the oral vaccines (e.g. polio and typhoid fever), and the vaccines containing inactivated pathogens (influenza) or toxoids (e.g. diphtheria and tetanus).

TETANUS TOXOID

- Administer tetanus toxoid depending upon the immune status of the patient; if immune status is unknown, administer a dose of tetanus toxoid.

ANTIBIOTICS

- Role of antibiotics in preventing wound infection is controversial.
- Many physicians administer broad-spectrum antibiotics to victims of animal bites.
- High-risk wounds include wounds on hands or lower extremities, wounds requiring surgical debridement and wounds involving joints, tendons, ligaments or fractures.
- The antibiotics of choice include oral amoxicillin–clavulanate and first-generation cephalosporins like cephalexin. In penicillin-allergic patients, doxycycline, clindamycin and ciprofloxacin are recommended.

MILWAUKEE PROTOCOL

- Although nearly 100% fatal, very few survivors have been reported with aggressive therapy, known as 'Milwaukee protocol'
- Aggressive therapy combines the use of anti-excitatory (ketamine) and antiviral drugs (ribavirin, amantadine

and interferon-alpha) and intensive care, along with active and passive immunisation.

PRE-EXPOSURE IMMUNISATION

- Pre-exposure immunisation is recommended for persons who are at high risk of exposure. These include laboratory staff working with rabies virus, veterinarians, animal handlers and wildlife officers.
- Three doses (on days 0, 7 and 28) are required for immunisation. Depending upon the antibody response, booster dose is required when the serum antibody level falls below 0.5 IU/mL. If such facilities are not available, a booster dose may be given 1 year after vaccination and then every 3–5 years.

ANIMAL BITE IN PREVIOUSLY VACCINATED PERSON

- Local care of wound is very important even in persons who have received full course of vaccination.
- If the person has been vaccinated with tissue culture vaccines and gets a bite, two booster doses are given on days 0 and 3. Passive immunisation is not required.

Q. Discuss briefly about Nipah virus infection.

- Nipah virus (NiV), a paramyxovirus related to Hendra virus, first emerged in Malaysia in 1998. Malaysia has had no more cases since 1999, but outbreaks continue to occur in Bangladesh and India. In India, first outbreak occurred in 2001 in Siliguri, West Bengal.
- In May 2018, NiV disease outbreak was reported from Kerala, India. There were 21 deaths out of 23 cases (18 laboratory confirmed and 5 suspected). Two patients recovered completely and were discharged from the hospital. The two affected districts were Kozhikode and Malappuram. An isolated case was reported from Kerala in 2021.

TRANSMISSION

- Transmission of NiV acquisition has been by different routes.
    - In Bengali culture, sap harvested from the date palm tree is commonly used for fresh consumption or fermented into alcoholic drinks (toddy, tari or palm wine). A top section of the date palm tree bark is shaved, allowing the sap to ooze overnight into collection pots attached to the trees. Fruit bats, which are natural reservoir of the virus, frequently feed on the shaved bark and often contaminate the sap with saliva, urine and excreta.
    - Other risk factors have included climbing trees (probably contaminated with infected date palm sap) and contact with sick animals. Fruit bats commonly drop partially eaten saliva-laden fruit, which are then eaten by domestic animals foraging for such food.
    - Transmission of NiV to humans may occur after direct contact with infected bats, infected pigs or from other NiV-infected people. The person-to-person transmission may occur from close physical contact, especially by contact with body fluids. During acute disease, NiV is shed in urine as well as respiratory secretions from the mouth and nose.
    - In the Malaysia outbreak, transmission occurred primarily through contact with pigs. Fruits partially eaten by bats may have been dropped or thrown into pigsties and subsequently infected the pigs that consumed the contaminated fruit.

CLINICAL FEATURES

- NiV infection in humans causes a range of clinical presentations, from asymptomatic infection (subclinical) to acute respiratory infection and fatal encephalitis.
- The case fatality rate is estimated at 40%–75%.
- The incubation period in humans ranges from 4 to 45 days, with more than 90% at 2 weeks or less.
- Infected people initially develop influenza-like symptoms of fever, headaches, myalgia, vomiting and sore throat.
- These symptoms are followed by dizziness, drowsiness, altered consciousness, myoclonic jerks, coma and seizures.
- Some patients develop prominent signs of brainstem dysfunction including abnormal doll's eye reflex, pupillary reflexes and vasomotor changes (tachycardia and high blood pressure).
- Cerebellar signs are relatively common.
- Respiratory involvement may produce breathing difficulty and respiratory failure.
- Most people who survive acute encephalitis make a full recovery, but long-term neurological conditions have been reported in survivors.

DIAGNOSIS

- MRI scans of brain often show extensive involvement of the cortex, temporal lobe and pons. Some cases may show multiple small (less than 1 cm in maximum diameter), bilateral abnormalities within the subcortical and deep white matter.
- Diagnosis is confirmed by real-time polymerase chain reaction (RT-PCR) on body fluids and antibody detection via ELISA. NiV RNA can be identified by PCR from respiratory secretions, urine or CSF.

TREATMENT

- Treatment measures are largely supportive and consist of anticonvulsants, treatment of secondary infection and mechanical ventilation.
- Ribavirin has been used with encouraging results.

PREVENTION

- PPE by the healthcare professionals to avoid contact with the secretions.
- Preventive strategies include interventions to prevent farm animals from acquiring NiV by eating fruit contaminated by bats.
- Consumption of contaminated sap should be avoided.

- Physical barriers to prevent bats from accessing and contaminating sap.
- No vaccine is available as yet.

Q. Explain briefly about anthrax.

Q. Describe cutaneous anthrax and malignant pustule.

Q. Write a short note on inhalation anthrax and wool-sorter's disease.

- Anthrax is a zoonotic disease caused by inhaling or ingesting the spores of *Bacillus anthracis*, a Gram-positive, non-motile, aerobic bacteria.
- In males, anthrax is an occupational disease of farmers, butchers and dealers in wool and bone meal. It is an important bioterrorism threat.
- In 1979, accidental release of spores from a military research facility in Sverdlovsk, Russia, resulted in 66 deaths.
- In 2001, following intentional contamination of US post, a total of 11 inhalational anthrax cases and 11 cutaneous anthrax cases were identified, 5 of which were fatal.
- From India, outbreaks of cutaneous anthrax have been reported from Andhra Pradesh, Tamil Nadu, Odisha and Karnataka.

CLINICAL MANIFESTATIONS

- Cutaneous anthrax results from inoculation of spores subcutaneously often as a result of contact with infected animals or animal products. Cuts or abrasions increase susceptibility to cutaneous infection. The lesion begins as an itching papule that enlarges to form a vesicle. The vesicle is filled with serosanguineous fluid and is surrounded by gross oedema ('malignant pustule'). The vesicle dries to form a thick black 'eschar' surrounded by blebs (Fig. 17.10). Systemic symptoms including fever, malaise and headache can occur. Untreated cases of cutaneous anthrax can spread haematogenously, causing systemic illness and toxin production.

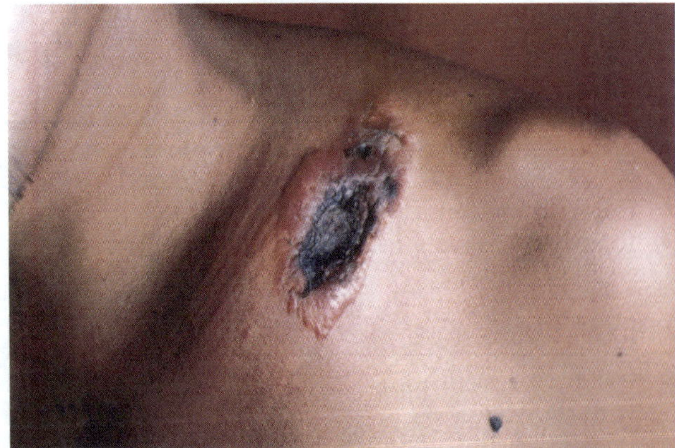

Fig. 17.10 Cutaneous anthrax—eschar. (Courtesy: Thappa DM. Textbook of Dermatology, Venereology and Leprology. 2nd ed. India: Elsevier, 2005, p. 60, Fig. 6.8).

TABLE 17.16 Clinical Features of Inhalation Anthrax

First Stage of Anthrax	Second Stage of Anthrax

• Insidious onset of
  • Malaise
  • Low-grade fever
  • Myalgias
  • Mild cough
  • Retrosternal heaviness
• Lasts for 1–4 days
	• Rapid deterioration with
	  • Haemoptysis
	  • Acute dyspnoea
	  • Cyanosis
	  • Diaphoresis
	  • Fever
	  • Shock
	  • Meningitis, coma
	• Chest X-ray
	  • Mediastinal widening due to haemorrhagic lymphadenopathy
	  • Pleural effusion

- Inhalation anthrax results from inhalation of the spores into the lung leading to 'wool-sorter's disease'. Bioterrorism-related anthrax also occurs due to inhalation of spores. The incubation period is 1–11 days but may be as long as 6 weeks. The disease is characterised by a haemorrhagic bronchopneumonia. Clinical features of inhalation anthrax are shown in Table 17.16.
- Meningeal anthrax (secondary complication of intestinal or inhalation anthrax due to bacteraemic spread) manifests as fulminant meningitis.
- Intestinal anthrax occurs due to eating undercooked meat from an infected animal, which contains vegetative bacterium rather than spores. The disease is divided into two phases: oropharyngeal and lower gastrointestinal. After an incubation period of 3 days, oral or oesophageal ulcers, cervical lymphadenopathy and dysphagia develop. Lower gastrointestinal involvement leads to abdominal pain, vomiting, bloody diarrhoea, abdominal distention and, at times, ascites. Untreated cases can be associated with secondary bacteraemia.

DIAGNOSIS

- A stained smear of fluid taken from the edge of a malignant pustule may demonstrate the organism.
- The organism may also be isolated from stools, laryngeal secretions, sputum and CSF.
- Blood for culture. *B. anthracis* may be cultured in mice, rabbits or guinea pigs.
- Blood for RT-PCR and lethal factor toxin.
- Chest X-ray showing mediastinal widening, bronchopneumonia and pleural effusion (often haemorrhagic).

TREATMENT

- Uncomplicated cutaneous anthrax can be treated with an oral fluoroquinolone (ciprofloxacin, levofloxacin or moxifloxacin) or doxycycline for 10–14 days.
- For inhalational anthrax, a fluoroquinolone (e.g. ciprofloxacin 400 mg BID) plus linezolid or clindamycin (as protein synthesis inhibitor) intravenously is recommended. Linezolid is preferred over clindamycin because it is likely to have better CNS penetration. Penicillin may be used if the organism is known to be sensitive to it. Duration of intravenous treatment is 2 weeks following which oral fluoroquinolone (e.g.

ciprofloxacin 500 mg BID) is given to complete 60 days of treatment.

- For meningitis, a third drug, meropenem, is added.
- Addition of an antitoxin in combination with antibiotic treatment is recommended for any patient with high suspicion of systemic anthrax. Approved antibody-based antitoxin therapies are anthrax immune globulin intravenous (AIGIV), raxibacumab and obiltoxaximab. Raxibacumab and obiltoxaximab are human IgG1 gamma monoclonal antibodies directed against protective antigen of bacterium.
- Glucocorticoids should be considered as adjunctive therapy for patients with anthrax meningitis or cutaneous anthrax with extensive oedema involving the head and neck.

PREVENTION

- Prevention of disease in persons exposed to the spores (postexposure prophylaxis) includes the use of ciprofloxacin (500 mg BID) or doxycycline (100 mg BID) for 60 days.
- In high-risk individuals, long-term prophylaxis is provided by anthrax vaccine adsorbed. Vaccination is also advised along with chemoprophylaxis following aerosolised *B. anthracic* exposure.

Q. Briefly outline the clinical features, treatment and prophylaxis of smallpox.

- The last naturally occurring case of smallpox was reported in 1977. WHO declared the world free of smallpox in 1980. This was possible due to three reasons:
  - Human beings were the only known reservoir for the virus.
  - No asymptomatic carrier state existed.
  - An effective vaccine was available.
- Deliberate introduction of highly contagious smallpox virus via aerosolisation could cause an epidemic of this deadly disease in a few days.
- Caused by variola virus that belongs to the *Orthopoxvirus* genus; the genus also includes monkeypox, vaccinia, cowpox and other viruses. The two variants of variola virus are variola major and variola minor. Variola minor is less virulent than variola major.
- Smallpox is acquired through exposure of the respiratory or oropharyngeal mucosa to viable virions through contaminated aerosols, lesional tissue, body fluids or fomites.

CLINICAL FEATURES

- Incubation period is 12–14 days during which there is viral proliferation within the lymph nodes and subsequent dissemination, thereby seeding other lymphoid tissues throughout the body.
- The period from the development of the mucosal rash up to the 10th day of the cutaneous rash represents the stage at which the disease is most contagious. However, the patient remains contagious till scabs fall off.
- The infection presents abruptly with high fever, headache, backache and malaise.
- Within 2–3 days, the patient develops typical maculopapular rash on the face, forearms, palms, soles and oral mucosa. The rash then spreads to the trunk and legs. Within 48 hours, this centrifugal rash becomes vesicular. In about 4–10 days, the lesions change into pustules. The lesions are deep-seated (in contrast, chickenpox lesions are more superficial).
- All the lesions are at the same stage of development. In contrast, rash in chickenpox is centripetal in nature and at any time skin lesions at various stages of evolution may be seen. In smallpox, eruptions commonly occur on the palms and soles, a highly unusual location for the lesions of chickenpox.
- Within 2–3 weeks, the lesions develop into scabs that detach leaving, at times, scars and hypopigmented lesions.
- Death can occur due to DIC, hypotension and multiorgan failure. When smallpox was prevalent, variola major had a case fatality rate of about 30% and variola minor a case fatality rate of less than 1%.
- Uncommon presentations are flat and haemorrhagic types of lesions. Flat smallpox is associated with soft, flat, confluent or semiconfluent lesions. Haemorrhagic smallpox produces widespread haemorrhages into skin and mucous membranes with a very high case fatality rate.

TREATMENT

- Symptomatic only.
- Two drugs have been approved for the treatment as virus could be used as bioweapon: tecovirimat and brincidofovir.

PROPHYLAXIS

- No effective postexposure therapy is available.

VACCINE

- Vaccine can prevent or reduce the severity of infection, if administered within 4 days of exposure. However, most countries do not have adequate stock of smallpox vaccine.
- The vaccine employs another virus of *Orthopoxvirus* genus, vaccinia and is a live attenuated vaccine.
- Two smallpox vaccines are available: one is a replication-deficient modified vaccinia Ankara (MVA) vaccine and the other is a replication-competent smallpox vaccine.

Contraindications

- Vaccination with replication-competent smallpox vaccine is contraindicated in immunosuppressed people, people with a history of eczema, atopic dermatitis or other inflammatory dermatoses, children younger than 1 year and pregnant persons.
- MVA vaccine is safe even in immunocompromised people and those with skin disorders.

Adverse Effects

- Majority of adverse effects are seen with replication-competent smallpox vaccine.

- An association between vaccination and occurrence of angina and myocardial infarction has been noted in some patients with underlying cardiac disease.
- Myopericarditis may develop due to inflammation of myocardium and pericardium. Clinical features include chest pain, dyspnoea, electrocardiographic changes and elevated levels of cardiac enzymes. NSAIDs are usually effective in treatment.
- Inadvertent inoculation is the most frequent adverse consequence of smallpox vaccination. Vaccinia may spread to other mucocutaneous areas producing lesions if the patient touches the bare vaccination site or resultant lesion and fails to wash hands immediately. This condition typically resolves without significant morbidity.
- Generalised vaccinia occurs if the vaccinia virus enters the circulation leading to focal or widespread vesicular eruption. Occurs 6–9 days after vaccination and subsides on its own.
- Eczema vaccinatum indicates the occurrence of generalised erythema, pruritus and vesicles in patients with active or resolved eczema. It is associated with fever and lymph node enlargement. If a large part of body is involved, dehydration can occur due to fluid exudation. Other complications include secondary infection and septicaemia. The mortality rate may be as high as 40%. Prompt administration of vaccinia immune globulin (VIG) is necessary, if this condition is suspected.
- Postvaccinial encephalopathy and postvaccinial encephalomyelitis may occur in some persons after vaccination.
- Progressive vaccinia occurs in immunosuppressed people. It is suspected if the lesion at the vaccination site continues to increase in size 15 days or more after the procedure. As the lesion increases in size, it often shows central crater and is prone to secondary bacterial infection. Blood-borne viral dissemination often results in the development of new lesions in the skin, organs and bones. Treatment of progressive vaccinia involves VIG and rigorous supportive care.

Q. Describe briefly about monkeypox.

- Monkeypox is a viral zoonotic disease caused by monkeypox virus. It is an enveloped double-stranded DNA virus that belongs to the *Orthopoxvirus* genus of the *Poxviridae* family.
- The disease was first identified in 1958 in monkeys.
- The first human case of monkeypox was reported from the Democratic Republic of the Congo in 1970. Since then, it has been endemic in Central and West Africa.
- In 2022, outbreak of monkeypox has been reported from countries outside West or Central Africa including USA, UK, Belgium, France, Germany and several others. As of 25th November, 2022, more than 81,000 cases of monkeypox were reported worldwide with 55 deaths. Till that time, 17 cases of monkeypox have been reported from India.
- Monkeypox is usually self-limiting but may be severe in some individuals such as children, pregnant women or immunosuppressed persons.

MODE OF TRANSMISSION

- Human-to-human transmission occurs primarily through large respiratory droplets, generally requiring a prolonged close contact. Transmission can also occur through direct contact with lesions and indirect contact with lesion material, such as through contaminated clothing of an infected person.
- The natural reservoir of monkeypox remains unknown. However, African rodents and non-human primates (like monkeys) may harbour the virus and infect people. Animal-to-human transmission may occur by bite or scratch of infected animals like small mammals including rodents (rats, squirrels) and non-human primates (monkeys, apes).

CLINICAL FEATURES

- Incubation period is usually from 6 to 13 days (range 5 to 21 days).
- Period of communicability is 1–2 days before the rash to until all the scabs fall off.
- There is a prodrome of fever, associated with headache, chills, sore throat, myalgias and lymphadenopathy, which may last for 5 days or so. Lymphadenopathy is a distinguishing feature of monkeypox from smallpox and it typically occurs with fever onset, 1 to 2 days before rash onset.
- Skin rash usually begins within 1–3 days of fever onset and lasts for 2–4 weeks.
  - First lesions often develop on tongue and mouth.
  - These are followed by macules starting from face and spreading to arms, legs, palms and soles (centrifugal distribution).
  - The rash develops into papular, vesicular and pustular phase over a period of 5–7 days (Fig. 17.11).
  - The pustules are deep-seated, well-circumscribed and often with umbilication.
  - The lesions heal with hyperpigmented atrophic scars or hypopigmented atrophic scars
- In Africa, monkeypox has been shown to cause death in as many as 1 in 10 persons who contract the disease.

COMPLICATIONS

- Secondary skin infection
- Pneumonia, encephalitis
- Corneal involvement (may lead to loss of vision)

DIAGNOSIS

- PPE should be donned before collecting the specimens. These include coveralls/gowns, N95 mask, face shield or safety goggles, and double pair of gloves.
- Specimens include roof of lesion, fluid present in the vesicle or pustule, and base of lesion. More than one lesion should be sampled, preferably from different locations on the body.
- PCR is done for *Orthopoxvirus* genus on the specimens. If the specimen show positivity for the *Orthopoxvirus*, it should be further confirmed by monkeypox specific conventional PCR or real time PCR for monkeypox DNA.

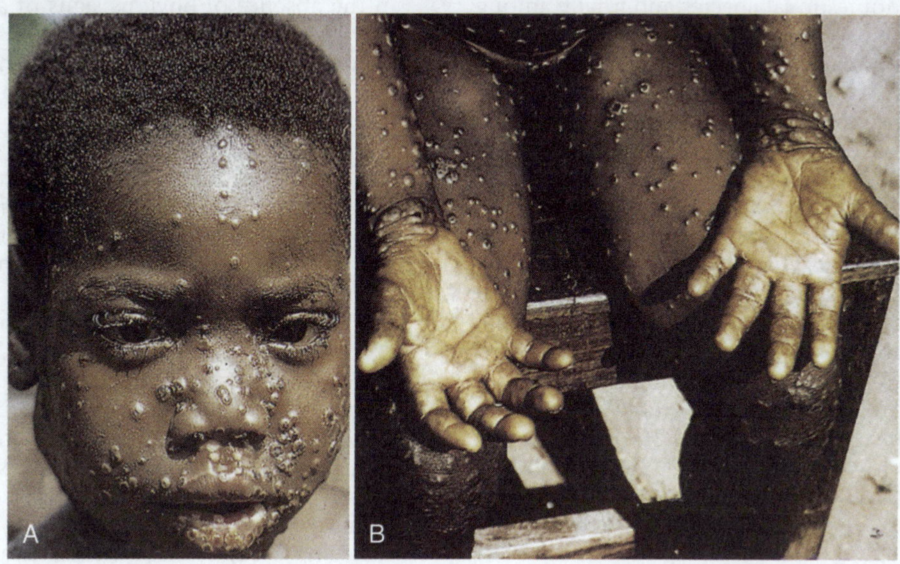

Fig. 17.11 Monkeypox skin lesions. (From Peters W, Pasvol G. Tropical Medicine and Parasitology. 5th ed. New York: Mosby; 2002:238.)

MANAGEMENT

PATIENT ISOLATION

- The patient should be isolated either at home or in a hospital.
- The patient should wear a triple layer mask.
- Skin lesions should be covered to the best extent possible (e.g. long sleeves and long pants) to minimise risk of contact with others.
- Isolation should be continued until all lesions have resolved and scabs have completely fallen off.

PROTECTION OF COMPROMISED SKIN

- Clean with simple antiseptic.
- Cover with light dressing if extensive lesions are present.
- In case of secondary infection, local mupirocin acid may be applied.

REHYDRATION THERAPY

- Encourage ORS or oral fluids; intravenous fluids to be administered, if indicated.

MONITORING OF COMPLICATIONS

- The patient should closely monitor for the appearance of any of the following symptoms during the period of isolation: pain in eye or blurring of vision, shortness of breath, chest pain, altered consciousness, seizure, reduced urine output, poor oral intake and lethargy.

DRUG THERAPY

- Tecovirimat is approved for use in patients with severe disease.

MONITORING EXPOSED HEALTHCARE PROFESSIONALS

- Healthcare worker who has cared for a monkeypox patient should monitor for development of symptoms suggestive of monkeypox infection for 21 days after the last date of care. This includes measurement of temperature at least twice daily for 21 days and evidence of any skin rash.

PREVENTION

- Avoid contact with animals that could harbour the virus.
- Avoid contact with any materials, such as bedding, that has been in contact with a sick person.
- Isolate infected patients from others who could be at risk for infection.
- Practice good hand hygiene after contact with infected animals or humans.
- Use PPE when caring for patients.
- A live attenuated vaccine is approved for the prevention of monkeypox.

Q. Write a brief note on plague.

- Plague, known as 'Black Death', is caused by *Yersinia pestis*, a Gram-negative, non-motile bacillus.
- Historically, three plague pandemics have killed more than 200 million people, including the Black Death epidemic in the 14th century in Europe.
- In India, outbreaks of plague occurred in district Beed, Maharashtra state (bubonic type) and district Surat in Gujarat state (pneumonic type) in September 1994. Subsequently, suspected cases of pneumonic plague were reported from Delhi, Varanasi, Karnataka and other states. In 2002, outbreak of pneumonic plague occurred in Himachal Pradesh. In 2004, outbreak of bubonic plague was reported from Uttarakhand.
- It remains an enzootic infection of rats and other rodents.

- Plague occurs in sylvatic rats that may then spread among more domestic rat species and finally among humans.
- Three types of plague: Bubonic, septicaemic and pneumonic.
- The most common route of infection in humans is after the bite of a plague-infected rat flea. Infection may also occur through direct contact with infected tissues or fluids from sick or dead plague-infected animals, by exposure of humans to respiratory droplets from infected animals, especially cats with plague pneumonia, or by laboratory exposure to plague bacteria. Person-to-person spread of bubonic and septicaemic plague but without secondary pneumonia does not occur. Pneumonic plague is highly contagious.
- *Y. pestis* appears to be a good candidate agent for a bioterrorist attack. The use of an aerosolised form of this agent could cause an explosive outbreak of primary plague pneumonia in the exposed population, or alternatively the bacteria could be used to infect the rodent population and precipitate a secondary outbreak in humans living in poor conditions.

CLINICAL FEATURES

BUBONIC PLAGUE

- The bubonic plague presents 2–8 days after exposure. The features include high fever, chills, malaise, vomiting and acutely swollen painful lymph nodes, usually in the groin or axilla. These are called the buboes that are rarely fluctuant or suppurative (Fig. 17.12A).
- Other manifestations include apathy, confusion, fright, anxiety, oliguria or anuria, tachycardia and hypotension.
- Without specific treatment, complications are common and include secondary septicaemia, secondary pneumonia and meningitis.
- The mortality rate for untreated bubonic plague is 60%.

SEPTICAEMIC PLAGUE

- Septicaemic plague may occur as a complication of untreated bubonic plague or pneumonic plague (secondary septicaemic plague). It can also develop in the absence of obvious signs of any primary disease (primary septicaemic plague).
- Septicaemic plague presents with high fever, chills and malaise, but without any lymph node enlargement. Patients may develop septic shock and DIC with vasculitis, petechiae, purpura and large ecchymoses that can mimic meningococcaemia.
- Gangrene of acral regions, like the tip of the nose or the fingers and toes, due to small artery thrombosis may appear in advanced stages of the disease (Black Death) (Fig. 17.12B).
- Left untreated, the mortality approaches 100%.

PNEUMONIC PLAGUE

- Pneumonic plague may occur by primary respiratory infection or as a complication of the bubonic and septicaemic forms of the disease (secondary pneumonia).
- Primary form occurs within 1–6 days of exposure.
- It begins abruptly with intense headache and malaise, high fever, vomiting, abdominal pain, diarrhoea and marked prostration. Chest pain, cough, dyspnoea and haemoptysis develop thereafter.
- Respiratory failure develops quickly with septic shock and mortality is high. Without antibiotics, the disease is fatal in almost all patients within 2 or 3 days.

DIAGNOSIS

- Leucocyte counts >20,000/mm^3 and/or thrombocytopenia in 50% of cases.
- Smears from blood, sputum, bubo aspirate and CSF may be stained with Gram, Giemsa or Wayson stains to demonstrate bipolar staining coccobacilli (safety pin appearance) (Fig. 17.12C).
- Cultures of various tissue fluids.
- Serological diagnosis is possible but antibodies may not be detectable when the patient first presents.
- Rapid diagnostic test (RDT) based on the F1 antigen in sputum and bubonic aspirate is highly sensitive for diagnosis.

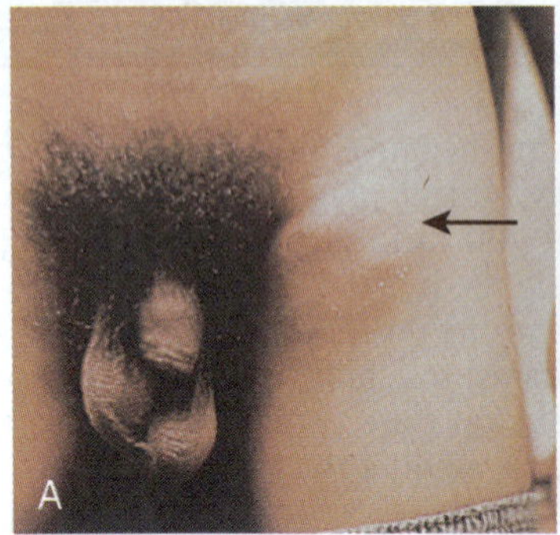

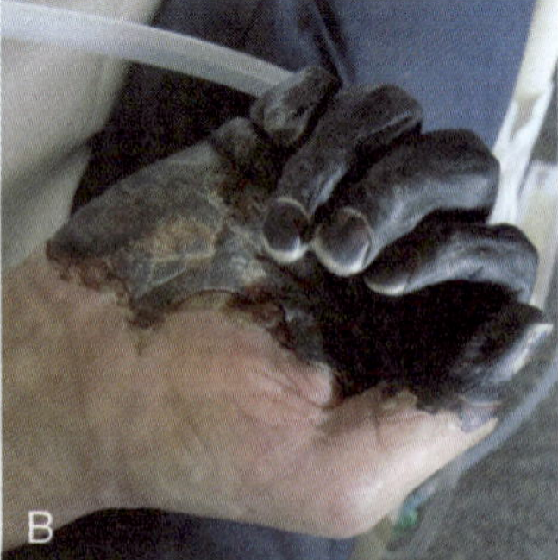

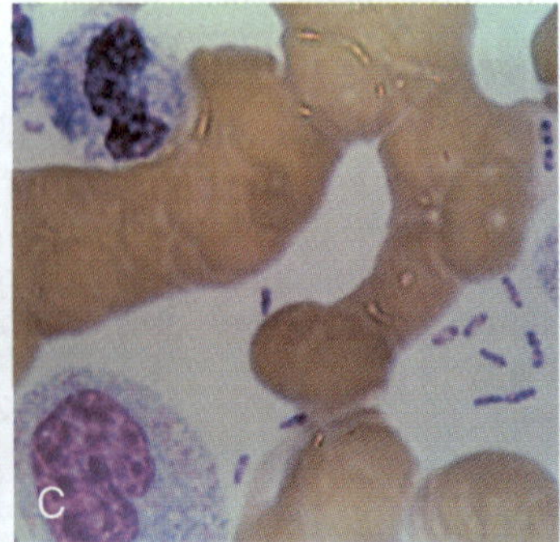

Fig. 17.12 (A) Swollen inguinal lymph nodes in a patient with bubonic plague. (B) Hand of a patient with septicaemic plague showing gangrene of the digits. (C) Wayson-stained blood smear of *Y. pestis* in a patient with septicaemic plague. Note the characteristic bipolar staining of the Gram-negative bacilli. (Courtesy: A from Seidel H, Ball J, Dains, J, Benedict G: Mosby's Guide to Physical Examination, 6th ed, St. Louis, Mosby Elsevier, 2006, p 389; taken from Beeching, Nye, 1996. Bubonic plague. B and C from Goldman L, Schafer A: Goldman's Cecil Medicine, 25th ed, Philadelphia, Elsevier Saunders, 2016, p 1984, 1987 respectively, Figs. 312-1, 312-5, respectively. B courtesy of Centers for Disease Control and Prevention.)

- In patients with pneumonic plague, chest radiograph shows evidence of multilobar consolidation, cavities or bronchopneumonia.
- Septicaemic plague is often associated with laboratory findings of DIC.

TREATMENT

- With prompt use of antibiotics, fatality rate decreases below 5% for bubonic plague and below 10% for septicaemic and pneumonic plague.
- Effective medications include streptomycin (15 mg/kg BID), gentamicin (1.7 mg/kg TID), ciprofloxacin (500 mg BID), ofloxacin (400 mg BID), levofloxacin (500 mg OD) and doxycycline (100 mg BID). Doxycycline is not the first line drug for septicaemic and pneumonic plague. Total duration of treatment is 10 days.
- If infection in the setting of a bioterrorist attack is suspected, a combination of two drugs should be used until susceptibility testing results are available.

PROPHYLAXIS

- Prevention of human-to-human transmission from patients with plague pneumonia can be achieved by implementing standard isolation procedures until at least 4 days of antibiotic treatment have been administered. For the other clinical types of the disease, patients should be isolated for the first 48 hours after the initiation of treatment. Healthcare workers should wear high-efficiency respirators.
- Contacts should receive tetracycline (500 mg QID), doxycycline (100 mg BID), ciprofloxacin (500 mg BID), ofloxacin (400 mg BID) or levofloxacin (500 mg OD) for 7 days.

Q. Write a short note on botulism.

Q. What are the clinical uses of botulinum toxin?

- It is caused by toxins (botulinum) produced by *Clostridium botulinum*, an anaerobic, Gram-positive, spore-forming bacterium. It is the most potent poison known and is lethal at doses as low as 0.05 μg. There are seven types of toxins labelled as A–G. Toxin types A, B, E and rarely F cause human disease.
- Most cases of botulism result from contaminated food being served undercooked; temperature more than 85 °C inactivates the toxin.

PATHOGENESIS

- Botulism occurs from absorption of the toxin through a mucosal surface, with intestinal absorption being much more common than lung and wound intoxication.
- Botulinum neurotoxins, whether ingested, inhaled or produced in the intestine or a wound, enter the circulation and are transported to the peripheral cholinergic nerve terminal, including neuromuscular junctions, postganglionic parasympathetic nerve endings and peripheral ganglia.
- Active neurotoxin is composed of a heavy chain of 100 kDa size which is responsible for binding to the nerve cells and then translocation into the nerve cell, and a light chain which is a 50 kDa fragment and is responsible for intracellular activity. It causes proteolysis of exocytosis apparatus in the nerve cells curtailing the release of acetylcholine at the presynaptic level. This produces neuroparalysis.
- Botulinum toxin binds irreversibly to nerve terminals; therefore, the antitoxin prevents progression of disease rather than reversal. Recovery is a function of new motor neurons restoring connection and innervating paralysed muscles.

CLASSIFICATION

- Food-borne botulism occurs due to ingestion of preformed toxin in contaminated food. It is the most common form of botulism.
- Wound botulism develops from toxin produced by infection of a wound.
- Infantile botulism or intestinal botulism results from ingestion of spores, which, on germination in the gut, produce toxin. Most cases develop in children below 6 months of age. This is the period when intestinal flora has not established. Intestinal botulism involving adults is uncommon but can occur in patients with a history of GI disease, GI surgery or recent antibiotic use.
- Inhalational botulism may occur due to release of aerosolised spores (bioterrorism).

CLINICAL FEATURES

- Incubation period varies from 2 hours to 8 days.

FOOD-BORNE BOTULISM

- Initial presentation includes gastrointestinal symptoms followed rapidly by the involvement of cranial nerves causing ptosis, diplopia, dysphagia and dysarthria.
- This is followed by progressive, descending motor paralysis and then diaphragmatic paralysis and death.
- Parasympathetic dysfunction may occur occasionally which produces dry mouth, paralytic ileus and dilated, non-reactive pupils.
- Fever is absent and patients are alert and oriented, though mild drowsiness may be present.
- Sensory symptoms are absent.

WOUND BOTULISM

- Wound botulism is similar except that GI upset does not occur.

INFANT BOTULISM

- Infant botulism is characterised by onset of constipation, followed by weakness in sucking, crying or swallowing. This is followed by progressive bulbar and extremity muscle weakness.

DIAGNOSIS

- Diagnosis of botulism is based on clinical features.
- Toxin can be demonstrated in blood (food-borne) or stools (infant botulism).
- Culture for organisms from wound.
- Conditions often confused with botulism include GB syndrome, myasthenia gravis, tick paralysis, diphtheria and hypermagnesaemia.

TREATMENT

- Botulism cannot spread from one patient to another person. Hence, standard isolation precautions are sufficient.
- In cases of food-borne botulism, laxatives, enemas or other cathartics can be given, provided no significant ileus is present.
- Most important therapeutic measures include supportive care with assisted ventilation, prevention of secondary infection and administration of equine heptavalent botulinum antitoxin or human botulinum immune globulin (in infant botulism).

CLINICAL APPLICATION OF BOTULINUM TOXIN

- Types A and B have been approved for clinical use.
- The basis of botulinum neurotoxin therapy is the localised inhibition of exocytosis from selected neurons after the toxin has been injected into specific target areas such as muscles.
- Weakness induced by toxin usually lasts for about 3 months. Hence, further injections at regular intervals are required and the interval varies widely depending on the dose and individual susceptibility.
- Useful in many condition (Box 17.14).
- The obvious adverse effects are due to injection of too high a dose or diffusion of the toxin to unintended sites. This may take the form of excessive weakness in the injected muscles or of weakness in muscles adjacent to injected muscles (e.g. dysphagia or dysphonia after injection of neck muscles).

BOX 17.14 Uses of Botulinum Toxin

- Blepharospasm
- Hemifacial spasm
- Strabismus
- Cervical dystonia (torticollis) and other dystonias
- Writer's cramps, tics
- Spasticity
- Focal hyperhidrosis
- Neurogenic bladder
- Cosmetic (removal of frown lines)
- Primary axillary hyperhidrosis
- Achalasia

Q. Write a short note on tularaemia.

- Tularaemia is caused by infection with *Francisella tularensis*, a Gram-negative coccobacillus.

TRANSMISSION

- Tick bites, contact with contaminated animal tissue or fluids, ingestion of contaminated food or water, or inhalation of infectious aerosol droplets (most often a form of bioterrorism) are the modes of transmission.
- Transmission of disease does not occur from human-to-human.

CLINICAL FEATURES

- The various forms include ulceroglandular, glandular, oropharyngeal, oculoglandular, pneumonia and typhoidal.
  - Ulceroglandular and glandular result from percutaneous inoculation such as from an arthropod bite.
  - Oropharyngeal can be caused by ingestion of the bacteria.
  - Pneumonia can be due to inhalation (deliberate release by terrorists).
  - Typhoidal tularaemia is due to septic spread of organisms.
- Ulceroglandular is the most common naturally occurring clinical form of tularaemia. It presents as a tender ulcer and regional lymphadenopathy that develops within days of infection.
- Pneumonic tularaemia has an average incubation period of 3–5 days. It manifests with signs and symptoms similar to those of community-acquired pneumonia followed by septic shock, ARDS and respiratory failure.
- Pharyngeal tularaemia presents with exudative pharyngitis or tonsillitis.
- Typhoidal tularaemia presents with sepsis or chronic febrile illness. Major symptoms include fever, chills, headache, myalgias, sore throat, cough, abdominal pain and diarrhoea.

DIAGNOSIS

- Tularaemia can be diagnosed with the use of culture, although enriched growth medium must be used.
- Immunofluorescence staining, serological testing and PCR can also be used for diagnosis.
- Chest imaging results in tularaemia are non-specific and reveal changes consistent with pneumonia.

TREATMENT

- The drug of choice is streptomycin (1 g IM twice a day).
- Alternatives include gentamicin, ciprofloxacin and doxycycline for 10–14 days.
- Surgical drainage of enlarged nodes in ulceroglandular tularaemia is frequently required for symptomatic relief.

PREVENTION

- Standard precautions are adequate for infection control.
- Postexposure prophylaxis is recommended for all individuals within 24 hours of known airborne exposure. Doxycycline and ciprofloxacin given orally are the preferred agents for a total of 14 days.
- There is no vaccine for tularaemia.

Q. Discuss the clinical manifestations, complications, diagnosis and management of diphtheria.

- Diphtheria is caused by *Corynebacterium diphtheriae*, which is a Gram-positive rod with a Chinese letter configuration on Albert's staining. It produces a powerful exotoxin that damages the heart muscle and the nervous system.
- Despite DPT vaccination in childhood, adults may get diphtheria (also pertussis) due to waning of immunity. Data about diphtheria cases reported to WHO indicate that India accounts for a substantial proportion of global burden of diphtheria; in 2018, India contributed 52.8% of the 16,648 diphtheria cases reported globally.
- The disease is transmitted by droplet infection from active cases or carriers.
- The incubation period is about 1–7 days.
- The infectious period is about 2 weeks from the symptom onset, though some patients can be infective for several weeks.

CLINICAL FEATURES

- The usual presenting manifestations are fever and sore throat.
- The diagnostic feature is the 'wash leather', elevated greyish-green pseudomembrane on the tonsils, with a surrounding area of inflammation (membranous tonsillitis). The membrane is firm and adherent. It is composed of necrotic fibrin, leucocytes, erythrocytes, epithelial cells and organisms.
- There may be swelling of the neck ('bull-neck' appearance) and tender enlargement of cervical lymph nodes.
- Nasal diphtheria is restricted to the nasal mucosa and is characterised by nasal discharge, which is often blood tinged.
- In pharyngeal diphtheria, the diphtheritic membranes are firmly attached to the tonsils or pharynx or both. Later, the soft and hard palates too become covered. In severe cases, there may be accompanying cervical lymphadenopathy and marked oedema of submandibular areas giving rise to the characteristic 'bull-neck' appearance (malignant diphtheria).
- In laryngeal diphtheria, there is involvement of the larynx as a result of extension of the diphtheritic membrane from pharynx. There is a husky voice and a high-pitched cough.
- In cutaneous diphtheria, there are round, deep, 'punched-out' ulcers covered by a grey-yellow or grey-brown membrane. It occurs in individuals with poor hygiene and with burns.

COMPLICATIONS

- Extension of the membrane into larynx and trachea leads to laryngeal obstruction and bronchopulmonary diphtheria.
- Myocarditis can result in arrhythmias, cardiac failure and ECG changes. It often occurs weeks after initial episode of diphtheria.
- Peripheral neuropathy can occur in a 'glove and stocking' distribution.
- Bulbar paralysis results in III, VI, VII, IX and X cranial nerve palsies and diaphragmatic paralysis.
- Encephalitis can occur rarely.

DIAGNOSIS

- The diagnosis is based on the demonstration of the characteristic diphtheritic membrane. However, a variety of other conditions can also cause pseudomembranes. These include infectious mononucleosis, streptococcal pharyngitis, viral exudative pharyngitis, fusospirochaetal infections and acute pharyngeal candidiasis.
- Demonstration of the organisms on methylene blue-stained preparations.
- Culture of the organism on Loeffler's medium.
- Detection of toxin by rapid EIA or PCR.

MANAGEMENT

- Isolation and strict bed rest.
- Antidiphtheritic toxin should be given as early in the course of diphtheria as possible. A delay in administration can be dangerous because toxin once fixed to the tissues can no longer be neutralised. It should be given after an intradermal skin sensitivity test. A dose of 4000–8000 units is given intramuscularly for mild disease, 16,000–32,000 units intramuscularly for moderately severe disease and up to 100,000 units for very severe disease. Antidiphtheritic serum can cause two types of reactions, an immediate anaphylactic reaction and a delayed serum sickness-like reaction. The immediate anaphylactic reaction should be treated with adrenaline and an antihistamine.
- Procaine penicillin is given at a dose of 600,000 units 12 hourly intramuscularly for 14 days to eradicate the organism. Patients allergic to penicillin can be treated with erythromycin (500 mg 6 hourly) or azithromycin.
- Tracheostomy may become necessary for respiratory distress.
- Close contacts should be protected by erythromycin or benzathine penicillin prophylaxis and immunisation.
- Vaccines include DPT (diphtheria, pertussis and tetanus toxins), DT (diphtheria and tetanus toxins), Tdap (tetanus, reduced diphtheria and acellular pertussis) and Td (tetanus and reduced diphtheria toxins). Due to waning immunity to diphtheria (and pertussis), it is advisable to give Td (or Tdap) to adults every 10 years.

Q. Describe the aetiology, clinical features, complications, diagnosis and management of whooping cough.

- Whooping cough is caused by *Bordetella pertussis*, a Gram-negative coccobacillus.
- Mode of spread is by droplet infection.
- Incubation period is about 7–14 days.

CLINICAL FEATURES

- The first stage (catarrhal phase) is characterised by a highly infectious upper respiratory catarrh with rhinitis, conjunctivitis and an unproductive cough. This stage lasts about 1 week.
- The distinctive paroxysmal stage that follows is characterised by severe paroxysmal bouts of coughing that occur during a single expiration. Following a prolonged cough paroxysm, a vigorous inspiration causes the distinctive 'whooping' sound. This sound is common in affected infants and small children due to the relatively small calibre of their trachea; it may also occur in adults. Post-tussive cyanosis, apnoea, syncope or emesis can also occur during the paroxysmal phase. This stage lasts from one to several weeks. Pertussis is most contagious in the catarrhal and early paroxysmal stages.
- The paroxysmal stage is followed by the stage of convalescence during which slow resolution of whoop occurs, although cough may persist for several weeks to months.
- Previously vaccinated adolescents and adults may have less severe paroxysmal symptoms.

COMPLICATIONS (Box 17.15)

BOX 17.15 Complications of Whooping Cough

• Bronchopneumonia	• Rib fracture	• Conjunctival haemorrhage
• Atelectasis	• Encephalitis	• Ulceration of frenum
• Bronchiectasis	• Convulsions	• Prolapse of rectum
• Pneumothorax	• Subdural haematoma	• Hernias

DIAGNOSIS

- Diagnosis is most often clinical.
- Peripheral blood lymphocytosis may be seen in well-established cases.
- The diagnosis can be confirmed by the isolation on culture of *B. pertussis*. A polyester swab of the nasopharynx is more effective than a swab of the throat or anterior nostril. The polyester swab should be inserted into the base of a nostril and left in the posterior pharynx for 10 seconds before withdrawing.
- PCR to detect *B. pertussis*.
- Direct fluorescent antibody test has poor sensitivity and is not recommended.

MANAGEMENT

- Starting antibiotics during catarrhal stage is helpful but during later stages may not reduce duration of disease, though it is helpful in reducing transmission. Azithromycin (for 3 days) and clarithromycin (for 7 days) are antibiotics of choice for treating whooping cough. Erythromycin is no longer recommended because it requires four times daily dosing and is more frequently associated with adverse effects. However, during pregnancy, erythromycin is the drug of choice. Trimethoprim/sulphamethoxazole has been shown to reduce pertussis transmission and is an alternative treatment for patients who are allergic to macrolides.
- A cough suppressant like dextromethorphan can reduce the severity of coughing paroxysms.
- Steroids, antihistamines, β-agonists and immunoglobulins have not been shown to be beneficial.

PREVENTION

- Patients are considered contagious until 3 weeks after the paroxysmal stage ends, if not treated during catarrhal stage. If antibiotics have been given during catarrhal phase, patient is considered infectious until 5 days after starting antibiotics. Therefore, close contacts of patients should receive macrolides, particularly if they are unvaccinated.
- Active immunisation with DPT vaccine is effective in preventing the disease. Immunity begins to decline 4–12 years after vaccination, causing adolescent and adult susceptibility. The vaccine can rarely cause convulsions and neurological damage. Currently approved acellular vaccines produce fewer adverse reactions than whole-cell vaccines and have similar effectiveness. A triple vaccine containing tetanus toxoid, reduced diphtheria toxoid and acellular pertussis (Tdap) is approved for use in adolescents and adults.
- Adults who have not been previously vaccinated against tetanus and diphtheria should receive a series of three vaccines (one Tdap and two Td vaccines). The preferred schedule is a Tdap vaccine dose followed by a Td vaccine dose 4 weeks later and another Td vaccine dose 6–12 months later.

Q. Describe enteric fevers.

Q. Write short notes on typhoid and paratyphoid fevers.

Q. Explain briefly about chronic carrier state in typhoid.

- Enteric fevers include typhoid fever caused by *Salmonella typhi* (also known as *Salmonella enterica* serovar Typhi) and paratyphoid fever caused by *Salmonella paratyphi* A and B (*S. enterica* serovar Paratyphi A, B). A range of clinical syndromes including diarrhoeal disease is caused by a large number of non-typhoidal *Salmonella* serovars; they occasionally can also produce invasive disease.
- Organisms are Gram-negative, flagellate, non-sporulating and facultative anaerobic bacilli.
- These organisms are transmitted by faecal–oral route, usually by carriers, often food handlers, through the contamination of food, milk or water.
- The incubation period of typhoid fever is about 10–14 days (range 3–60 days) but that of paratyphoid is somewhat shorter.

PATHOGENESIS

- The typhoid bacilli reach the small intestine, penetrate the mucosa and enter intestinal lymphatics via Peyer's patches to be carried to the bloodstream. The bacilli are disseminated throughout the body and intracellular multiplication takes place. The organisms re-enter the bloodstream producing bacteraemia when all organs are repeatedly exposed to typhoid bacilli.

CLINICAL FEATURES

- The disease usually presents with fever associated with headache, malaise and chills. A step-like daily increase in temperature to 40 °C–41 °C ('step-ladder' pattern) is seen in some cases. The hallmark of typhoid fever is prolonged, persistent fever, often lasting for 4–8 weeks in untreated patients.
- Early intestinal manifestations include constipation, especially in adults or mild diarrhoea in children, associated with abdominal tenderness.
- Mild hepatosplenomegaly may be present and the liver may be tender.
- There may be bradycardia relative to the height of the fever ('relative bradycardia').
- The characteristic rose spots or 'rose-red spots' may be seen on the chest and abdomen during the first week. These lesions result from bacterial embolism. They are small, 2–4 mm, pale-red macules that blanch on pressure. They usually last only for 2–3 days. *Salmonella* can be cultured from the biopsy of these lesions.
- Often, by the end of first week, constipation is succeeded by diarrhoea and abdominal distension, with tenderness in the right iliac fossa. The stools are characteristically described as 'pea-soup' because faeces are loose and greenish in colour.
- By the end of the second week, patient may become profoundly ill. By the third week, toxaemia increases and patient may pass into coma and die.
- Intestinal complications often occur in the third or fourth week of illness.

COMPLICATIONS (Table 17.17)

TABLE 17.17 Complications of Typhoid

• General	Toxaemia, dehydration, peripheral circulatory failure, DIC
• Gastrointestinal	Perforation of intestine, intestinal haemorrhage
• Neurological	Delirium, psychosis, coma, catatonia, meningitis, encephalopathy, peripheral neuritis, deafness
• Miscellaneous	Myocarditis, endocarditis, pericarditis, pyelonephritis, glomerulonephritis, osteomyelitis, arthritis, periostitis, pneumonia, hepatitis, thrombophlebitis

DIAGNOSIS

- White cell count may show leucopenia with relative lymphocytosis.
- Cultures: The maximum positivity of blood culture is found during the first week of illness. Early in the illness, culture of bone marrow aspirate will yield the organism even after a brief prior antibiotic treatment. Stool and urine cultures become positive in the third week.
- Widal test: This test detects agglutinating antibodies to O, H and Vi antigens of *S. typhi*, and H antigens of *S. paratyphi* A and B. A four-fold rise in antibody titre in paired samples is a good criterion, but of limited practical application.
  - The O antigen is the somatic antigen (lipopolysaccharide cell wall component) of *S. typhi* and is shared by *S. paratyphi* A, *paratyphi* B, other *Salmonella* species and other members of the *Enterobacteriaceae* family. Antibodies against the O antigen are predominantly IgM, rise early in the illness and disappear early. In the absence of recent immunisation, a high titre of O antibodies (=1:320) is useful but not specific for typhoid.
  - The H antigens are flagellar antigens of *S. typhi*, *paratyphi* A and *paratyphi* B. Antibodies to H antigens are both IgM and IgG, rise late in the illness and persist for a longer time. These antibodies also have broad cross-reactivity.
  - The Vi antigen is virulent antigen and Vi antibodies typically rise later, after 3–4 weeks of illness, and are of little use in the early diagnosis.
- Other serological tests:
  - A dot EIA that detects IgG and IgM antibodies against a 50-kDa outer membrane protein distinct from the somatic (O), flagellar (H) or capsular (Vi) antigen of *S. typhi* has a variable specificity and sensitivity.
  - Antigen (Vi) detection using ELISA, counterimmune electrophoresis and coagglutination tests.
- Molecular methods:
  - PCR to detect flagellin, somatic gene and Vi gene.

TREATMENT

- General management includes bed rest, isolation and maintenance of nutrition and fluid intake.
- Antibiotic therapy. Several antibiotics are effective in enteric fever. Various regimens are given in Table 17.18.

TABLE 17.18 Antibiotic Regimens for the Treatment of Enteric Fever

Drug	Dosage and Duration
Chloramphenicol	3–4 g/day till the fever subsides, followed by 2 g/day for a total duration of 14 days
Amoxicillin	4–6 g/day in four divided doses for 14 days
Cotrimoxazole	Trimethoprim 640 mg plus sulphamethoxazole 3200 mg in two divided doses daily for 14 days
Ciprofloxacin	500–750 mg twice daily for 14 days
Ofloxacin	400–800 mg/day for 14 days
Ceftriaxone	75 mg/kg/day for 7–14 days
Cefotaxime	50–75 mg/kg/day for 7–14 days
Cefixime	400 mg twice a day for 10–14 days
Azithromycin	1 g once a day for 5–7 days
Aztreonam	50–100 mg/kg/day for 14 days

- Certain strains of *S. typhi*, particularly in India, are resistant to chloramphenicol, amoxicillin and cotrimoxazole. These patients should be treated with ciprofloxacin. These are called multidrug-resistant strains.
- Even strains that are sensitive to ciprofloxacin in vitro may not respond to ciprofloxacin treatment. These strains are usually resistant to nalidixic acid when tested in vitro (nalidixic acid-resistant *S. typhi* [NARST]). These patients require longer duration of treatment with ciprofloxacin or with ceftriaxone.
- With increasing use of quinolones, many strains isolated have shown susceptibility to traditional first-line antimicrobials.
- A few cases of extensively drug-resistant (XDR) typhoid infection have been reported from India. These cases are resistant to chloramphenicol, ampicillin, trimethoprim/sulphamethoxazole, fluoroquinolones and ceftriaxone. XDR typhoid infection may be treated with a carbapenem (e.g. meropenem) plus azithromycin.
- Corticosteroids. Patients with severe toxaemia, CNS manifestations, shock and DIC should be given intravenous dexamethasone 3 mg/kg as a loading dose, followed by 1 mg/kg every 6 hours for 24 hours.
- The late complications of intestinal perforation and haemorrhage occur in the third or fourth week of illness. The management of these complications depends on the availability of medical facilities and clinical state of the patient.

RELAPSE

- Relapse may occur even with appropriate antimicrobial therapy. It typically occurs 2 to 3 weeks after resolution of fever.
- In relapse, the organism invariably has the same sensitivity pattern as the initial infecting isolate.
- In these cases, repeat antibiotic course is needed.

CARRIER STATE IN TYPHOID

- About 3%–5% of patients become long-term asymptomatic carriers. Many carriers give no history of typhoid fever and probably had an undiagnosed mild infection.
- Chronic carriers are generally older than 50 years, are more commonly found in females and often have gallstones. *S. typhi* reside in the gallbladder and even within the interiors of stones. They intermittently reach the lumen of the intestine and are excreted in the stool, thereby contaminating water or food.
- Have an approximately 8-fold excess risk of developing gallbladder carcinoma than non-carriers and an approximately 200-fold excess risk of developing hepatobiliary carcinoma compared with people who have had acute typhoid and have cleared the infection.
- Chronic carrier state should be treated with ciprofloxacin for 4 weeks. Cholecystectomy may be necessary in some patients.

PREVENTION

- The most important way to prevent typhoid fever is good hygiene, proper sewage disposal and proper water treatment.
- Three vaccines against *S. typhi* infection (do not protect against paratyphoid fever):
    - Ty21a, a live, attenuated *S. typhi* vaccine containing the *S. typhi* strain Ty21a (oral administration in persons older than 6 years; one capsule every other day for three doses). Revaccination is recommended every 3 to 5 years.
    - Vi-polysaccharide (parenteral administration in persons older than 2 years). If continued protection is needed, revaccination is recommended every 2 to 3 years.
    - Typhoid conjugate vaccine (e.g. Vi-tetanus conjugate) for parenteral administration in persons between 6 months and 45 years and is the preferred vaccine.

Q. What are the causes of food poisoning? Discuss briefly the clinical manifestations, diagnosis and management of food poisoning.

- The term 'food poisoning' suggests a food-borne disease outbreak where a cluster of two or more individuals develop similar symptoms following the ingestion of a common food or water. The most common form of 'food poisoning' is gastroenteritis following consumption of food containing preformed toxins or organisms that produce toxin in the gut. It is a likely diagnosis when the onset of gastroenteritis exhibits a strong temporal relationship to a particular meal (refer to 'Diseases of the Gastrointestinal Tract').

CAUSES

- The causes of food poisoning are given in Table 17.19. Based on incubation period, common causes are given in Table 17.20.
- Shiga-producing strain of *E. coli* O157:H7 and O104:H4 (reported from Germany) can result in dysentery and

TABLE 17.19 Causes of Food Poisoning

INFECTIVE
• Toxin-induced
◦ Preformed toxins: *S. aureus*, *B. cereus*, *C. botulinum*
◦ Enterotoxins produced in the intestine: *V. cholerae*, *E. coli* (enterotoxigenic, ETEC), *Clostridium perfringens*, *Clostridium difficile*
• Changes in mucosa
◦ Mucosal alteration without invasion: Rotavirus, Norovirus
◦ Invasion of mucosa with destruction: *Shigella*, *E. coli* (enteroinvasive), *Campylobacter*, *Yersinia enterocolitica*, *Salmonella*, *E. histolytica*, *B. anthracis*
◦ Vascular changes in intestine: Shiga-producing *E. coli* (enterohaemorrhagic)
NON-INFECTIVE
• Allergic: Shellfish, strawberries
• Non-allergic: Scombrotoxin (fish), ciguatoxin (tropical fish), fungi (*Amanita phalloides*), arsenic poisoning

TABLE 17.20 Causes of Food Poisoning Based on Incubation Period

Incubation Period	Cause
1–6 hours	Norovirus *S. aureus* *B. cereus* (vomiting toxin) Scombroid toxins Ciguatoxin Arsenic Mushrooms
6–24 hours	*B. cereus* (diarrhoeal toxin) *C. perfringens* Mushrooms
24–48 hours	*C. botulinum* *E. coli*
2–6 days	*V. cholerae* *Shigella* *Salmonella* (non-typhoidal) *Yersinia* *Campylobacter*

in some patients, haemolytic-uraemic syndrome particularly when antibiotics are given.

- Ciguatera fish poisoning occurs after eating reef fish (tropical fish) contaminated with toxins such as ciguatoxin, which originate from small marine organisms (dinoflagellates). Dinoflagellates are ingested by herbivorous fish in which ciguatoxin is concentrated as it passes up the food chain to large carnivorous fish and finally to humans. Besides features of acute gastroenteritis occurring within 1–3 hours, neurological features also develop over next few hours and include paraesthesias, pain in teeth, metallic taste, blurred vision and cold allodynia (touching cold objects produces pain).
- Scombrotoxin (histamine) poisoning occurs due to ingestion of some fish, which have high histidine content, e.g. tuna and sardine. Histidine is converted into histamine if fish is stored improperly. Features include facial flushing, headache, palpitations, itching, blurred vision, abdominal cramps and diarrhoea. Occasionally, cardiac arrhythmia and hypotension may occur.

CLINICAL FEATURES AND DIAGNOSIS

- Food poisoning presents with vomiting, diarrhoea or both, usually within 48 hours of consumption of the contaminated food or drink. The stools may be bloody and there may be associated crampy abdominal pain and fever.
- Non-infective causes and bacterial toxins that are preformed in the infected food produce symptoms within minutes or hours of a meal, whereas other conditions may not produce symptoms for up to 48 hours.
- Usually, there is a history of simultaneous occurrence of symptoms in more than one member of a household or institution.
- Diagnosis is based on the identification of the specific pathogen by culture of the patient's stool, vomitus or blood or the contaminated food, ELISA to detect antibodies and PCR to detect antigens.

MANAGEMENT

- Non-specific therapy includes oral or intravenous replacement of fluid and electrolyte deficits and loperamide for controlling diarrhoea (only if the patient does not have fever or blood in the stools). Loperamide should be avoided in young children and elderly persons.
- Antibiotics should not be given routinely as they are usually ineffective and frequently exacerbate symptoms. However, antibiotic therapy is indicated in selected cases with features suggestive of cholera or with fever or dysentery, or those with an impaired immune response keeping in mind that antibiotics can precipitate development of haemolytic-uraemic syndrome.

Q. Give a brief description about the aetiology, clinical presentation, diagnosis and management of acute bacillary dysentery.

Q. Discuss the aetiology, pathogenesis, clinical features, diagnosis and complications of amoebic dysentery.

Q. Write a short note on amoebic colitis.

- Dysentery is an acute inflammation of the large intestine (colitis) characterised by diarrhoea with blood and mucus in the stools. It is caused by bacillary and amoebic infections.

BACILLARY DYSENTERY

- Bacillary dysentery results from an acute infection of the intestinal tract by one of the three *Shigella* species—*Shigella dysenteriae, Shigella flexneri* and *Shigella sonnei*.
- These organisms produce an endotoxin as well as an exotoxin (Shiga toxin). The exotoxin has enterotoxin activity causing intestinal secretion and cytotoxic properties directed against intestinal epithelial cells.

CLINICAL FEATURES

- Incubation period is 1–4 days.
- *S. sonnei* produces only mild infection. *S. flexneri* infection is usually more severe while that due to *S. dysenteriae* may be fulminating and cause death within 48 hours.
- Fever and signs of systemic toxicity may be present in severe cases.
- Signs of dehydration and electrolyte disturbances are present in severe cases.
- The dysentery is mild to severe in intensity and is associated with tenesmus and colicky abdominal pain.
- The stools are small in quantity and contain blood, mucus and purulent exudate with little faecal material.
- There may be tenderness over the colon elicited in the left iliac fossa.
- Bowel sounds are hyperactive.

COMPLICATIONS (Table 17.21)

TABLE 17.21 Complications of Bacillary Dysentery

Intestinal	Extraintestinal	Post-infectious
• Rectal prolapse • Toxic megacolon • Intestinal perforation • Intestinal obstruction • Appendicitis	• Volume depletion • Focal infections (e.g. meningitis, osteomyelitis, arthritis) • Sepsis • Seizure • Encephalopathy	• Haemolytic-uraemic syndrome • Reactive arthritis • Irritable bowel syndrome

DIAGNOSIS

- Diagnosis depends on the isolation of the organism from stool cultures.
- Sigmoidoscopy shows that the mucosa is red and swollen. The submucous veins are obscured and mucopus is seen on the surface.
- EIA to detect Shiga toxins in stools.
- PCR for *Shigella* DNA in stools.

MANAGEMENT

- The fluid and electrolyte deficits should be corrected by intravenous fluids in severe cases.
- Loperamide may be used to control diarrhoea in adults who do not have dysentery. It is not recommended in children, and in patients who are debilitated or immunocompromised.
- Infections caused by *S. dysenteriae* and *S. flexneri* should be treated with ciprofloxacin. Second-line agents include azithromycin, cotrimoxazole and ceftriaxone. The benefit of antibiotics for non-dysenteric shigellosis is unknown.

AMOEBIC COLITIS

- Amoebic colitis can occur in two forms: amoebic dysentery and non-dysenteric amoebic colitis.

AMOEBIC DYSENTERY

Pathogenesis

- Amoebic dysentery results from infection of the large intestine by *Entamoeba histolytica*.
- Caused by ingestion of tetra-nucleated cysts that can remain viable for weeks to months. However, these are destroyed in temperature below −5°C or above 40°C.
- After ingestion (faecal–oral transmission), the cysts undergo further nuclear division and eight trophozoites are released in the terminal ileum. The trophozoites are carried to the large intestine where they produce the characteristic 'flask-shaped' amoebic ulcerations. Incubation period is 2–6 weeks.
- Most often, the infection remains subclinical; however, antibody response generally occurs even without local invasion. These asymptomatic patients also need to be treated to prevent transmission to others and occurrence of colitis at a later period.
- A localised granuloma (amoeboma) presenting as a palpable mass in the rectum or causing a filling defect in the colon on radiography is a common complication.
- Amoebae may enter a portal venous radicle and be carried to the liver where they multiply and produce an amoebic liver abscess. They can also travel to lungs and brain.

Clinical Features

- In amoebic dysentery, there is intermittent diarrhoea consisting of one to four, foul-smelling, loose, watery stools that may contain mucus and blood. Flatulence and abdominal cramping are frequent. Fever occurs in some patients.
- Physical examination reveals tender hepatomegaly and tenderness over the caecum (amoebic typhlitis), ascending colon and over the left iliac fossa (amoebic point or Manson–Bahr point).

Complications (Box 17.16)

BOX 17.16 Complications of Amoebic Dysentery

- Massive haemorrhage
- Perforation and peritonitis
- Toxic megacolon in fulminant cases
- Postdysenteric colitis
- Amoebic liver abscess
- Pleuropulmonary amoebiasis
- Amoebic pericarditis
- Cutaneous amoebiasis
- Rectovaginal fistula

Diagnosis

- Stool examination: Microscopic examination of a fresh sample of stool may demonstrate the motile trophozoites. They are about 30 μm in diameter, with a clear ectoplasm and a granular endoplasm, and usually contain red blood cells (haematophagous trophozoites). If a fresh stool specimen cannot be examined immediately, it should be preserved with a fixative such as polyvinyl alcohol or kept cool (4°C).
- Sigmoidoscopy: Sigmoidoscopy may reveal the characteristic 'flask-shaped' ulcers with normal surrounding mucosa. The aspirated material or scrapings from the ulcer or biopsy of the ulcer may demonstrate the trophozoites.
- Amoebic serology: Serological tests (indirect haemagglutination test, ELISA or counter-immunoelectrophoresis) can detect antibodies in the blood. These tests are of more use in extraintestinal amoebiasis.
- Chest radiography and ultrasound for amoebic liver abscess.
- Newer methods include detection of *E. histolytica* antigen or DNA (by PCR) in a stool sample.

NON-DYSENTERIC AMOEBIC COLITIS

- Presents as recurrent bouts of diarrhoea with or without mucus, but no visible blood.

- Stools show *E. histolytica* cysts or non-haematophagous trophozoite (trophozoites with no ingested red blood cells).

TREATMENT OF AMOEBIC COLITIS

- Invasive intestinal amoebiasis is treated with metronidazole 800 mg thrice daily for 7–10 days or tinidazole 2 g daily as a single dose for 3 days. Other options are secnidazole or ornidazole.
- After treatment, diloxanide furoate should be given at a dose of 500 mg thrice daily for 10 days to eliminate luminal cysts. Alternative agents include iodoquinol, nitazoxanide and paromomycin.

Q. How will you differentiate amoebic dysentery from bacillary dysentery on stool examination?

- Differentiating points between amoebic dysentery and bacillary dysentery on stool examination are given in Table 17.22.

TABLE 17.22 Amoebic Dysentery Versus Bacillary Dysentery on Stool Examination

Features	Amoebic Dysentery	Bacillary Dysentery
Macroscopic		
• Frequency	6–8 motions a day	Over 10 motions a day
• Amount	Relatively copious	Relatively small
• Odour	Offensive	Odourless
• Nature	Blood and mucus mixed with faeces	Blood and mucus, no faeces
• Colour	Dark red	Bright red
• Reaction	Acidic	Alkaline
• Consistency	Not adherent to the container	Adherent to the container
Microscopic		
• RBC	In clumps	Discrete or in rouleaux
• Pus cells	Scanty	Numerous
• Macrophages	Very few	Large and numerous
• Eosinophils	Present	Scarce
• Parasites	Trophozoites of *E. histolytica*	Nil
• Bacteria	Nil	Gram-negative bacteria
• Charcot–Leyden crystals	Present	Absent

Q. Explain briefly about brucellosis (abortus fever; Malta fever; undulant fever and Mediterranean fever).

- Brucellosis, a zoonotic disease, is an infection caused by one of the four species: *Brucella melitensis* (goats, sheep and camels), *Brucella abortus* (cattle), *Brucella suis* (pigs) and *Brucella canis* (dogs).
- *Brucella* is a Gram-negative organism.
- The natural reservoir of brucellosis is animals. Human infection most commonly results from ingestion of infected animal tissues or milk products or directly through abraded skin. Inhalational route is also seen in some patients. *Brucella* species are considered class B bioterrorism agents, due to the ease of infection through the inhalation of organisms. Transmission from human-to-human, particularly mother-to-child, has been described rarely.
- *Brucella* bacilli interact with neutrophils and tissue macrophages and spread via lymphatics to the regional lymph nodes, especially axillary, cervical and supraclavicular nodes. The organisms can also spread via bloodstream to other structures like bone marrow, liver, spleen, bones, endocardium, kidneys and testes. There is formation of non-caseating granulomas in these tissues.

MANIFESTATIONS

ACUTE BRUCELLOSIS (<2 MONTHS)

- Acute onset in nearly 50% of cases; also known as undulant fever.
- Incubation period is 2–3 weeks.
- The onset is acute with fever, malaise, chills, fatigue, weakness, backache and myalgia. Patients are anorectic, lose weight and have cough and arthralgias.
- Fever is classically remittent, although continuous and intermittent patterns are also seen.
- Physical findings include splenomegaly (20% of cases), lymphadenopathy (15% of cases) and hepatomegaly (10% of cases). Sacroiliitis may also occur with tenderness on sacroiliac joints.
- A few patients may manifest with localised brucellosis in the form of osteomyelitis, splenic abscess, epididymo-orchitis, pneumonia, pleural effusion, uveitis, meningitis, encephalitis, myelitis and endocarditis.

SUBACUTE BRUCELLOSIS (2–12 MONTHS)

- Similar to acute form, but less severe features.

CHRONIC BRUCELLOSIS (>12 MONTHS)

- Chronic brucellosis is defined as ill health for more than 1 year following onset of brucellosis. These patients may have low-grade fever and neuropsychiatric manifestations. Arthralgia is also common.
- Splenomegaly is often present.
- Others are those seen with localised features of brucellosis. These are more common than in the acute variety.
- Bone and joint complications are the most frequent complications. These include sacroiliitis, spondylitis, peripheral arthritis, osteomyelitis and bursitis.

RELAPSING BRUCELLOSIS

- Symptoms develop again 2–3 months following completion of therapy.

DIAGNOSIS

- Routine blood tests reveal anaemia, leucopenia and thrombocytopenia.

- *Brucella* can be cultured from blood, bone marrow (gold standard) and other involved tissues. For this, biphasic method of Castaneda that uses both a solid medium and a liquid medium in the same container, or automated blood culture system, is required.
- *Brucella* agglutination test—a four-fold rise in titre of agglutinating antibody (IgM and IgG) may be diagnostic.
- PCR to detect *Brucella* antigen in blood and tissues.
- Clinically affected organs and tissues can be biopsied, particularly lymph nodes and liver. Histology reveals non-caseating granulomata.
- Other important tests include ultrasound and CT, bone radiographs, MRI spine and radionuclide bone scans.

TREATMENT

- The treatment of choice is doxycycline 100 mg twice a day for 6 weeks plus streptomycin (1 g twice a day) or gentamicin (1.25–2.5 mg/kg twice a day) for 2–3 weeks. An alternative is to give doxycycline plus rifampicin (10–15 mg/kg as one or two doses per day) for 6 weeks, though it is slightly inferior to doxycycline plus streptomycin combination. Doxycycline is preferred over tetracycline. Doxycycline can be replaced by trimethoprim/sulphamethoxazole in children below 8 years of age.
- Seriously ill patients may be given triple therapy with doxycycline, aminoglycoside and rifampicin with oral medications continued for 3–6 months.
- Spondylitis and endocarditis complications need long treatment courses and possibly surgical treatment.

Q. Write a short note on cholera and cholera sicca.

- Cholera is an acute illness that results from colonisation of the small intestine by *Vibrio cholerae*. The disease is characterised by its epidemic occurrence and explosive, severe diarrhoea with rapid depletion of extracellular fluid and electrolytes.
- The major pathogenic strain has a somatic antigen (O1). It is called serogroup O1. It has two biotypes: classical and El Tor. The El Tor biotype has replaced the classical biotype as the major cause of cholera. Infection with El Tor biotype often causes milder disease, though severe diarrhoea can also occur.
- In 1992, a new serogroup O139 (Bengal serogroup) caused an epidemic in India and is still the major cause of cholera in our country. The clinical features are similar to those of O1 serogroup but the organism may be resistant to cotrimoxazole.
- Infection spreads via the stools or vomitus of patients which may contaminate water or food (faeco-oral route).

PATHOGENESIS

- After ingestion, *V. cholerae* must survive the acidic environment of the stomach and then form colonies of bacteria on the surface of the small intestine.
- An important factor for colonisation is toxin-coregulated pilus (TCP) which also allows the bacteria to resist killing by bile.
- *V. cholerae* produces a powerful enterotoxin that is responsible for the pathophysiological aberrations in cholera. The enterotoxin stimulates adenylate cyclase of the intestinal epithelial cells resulting in secretion of chloride and inhibition of sodium chloride absorption (secretory diarrhoea—high concentrations of sodium, chloride, bicarbonate and potassium). There is no demonstrable damage in the intestinal epithelial cells.
- The pathophysiological defect in cholera is extracellular fluid depletion with resultant hypotension, metabolic acidosis and hypokalaemia.
- In severe cases, massive fluid loss may lead to hypovolaemic shock and acute tubular necrosis resulting in acute kidney injury.

CLINICAL FEATURES

- The incubation period is about 12–48 hours.
- Majority develop mild diarrhoea. Severe cases have explosive onset of watery diarrhoea ('cholera gravis') without pain, colic or tenesmus which follows vomiting (vomiting may be absent). The characteristic 'rice-water' stool consists of clear fluid with flecks of mucus (Fig. 17.13). Several litres of isotonic fluid may be lost within hours leading rapidly to profound shock.
- In extreme cases, there may be signs of severe dehydration. The skin is cold, clammy and wrinkled ('washerwoman' skin) with loss of skin turgor. The blood pressure drops and the pulse becomes rapid and thready. Acidosis from loss of stool bicarbonate as well as lactic acidosis from poor perfusion may result in Kussmaul breathing.
- Occasionally, a very severe form of the disease occurs in which the loss of fluid into the dilated bowel kills the patient before typical gastrointestinal symptoms appear. This is known as 'cholera sicca'.

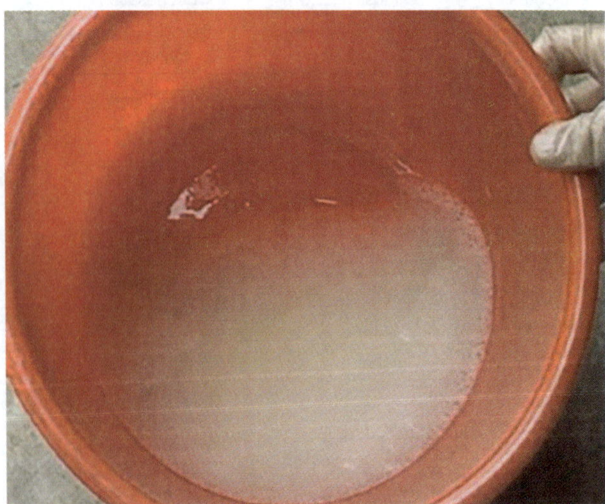

Fig. 17.13 Rice-water stool.

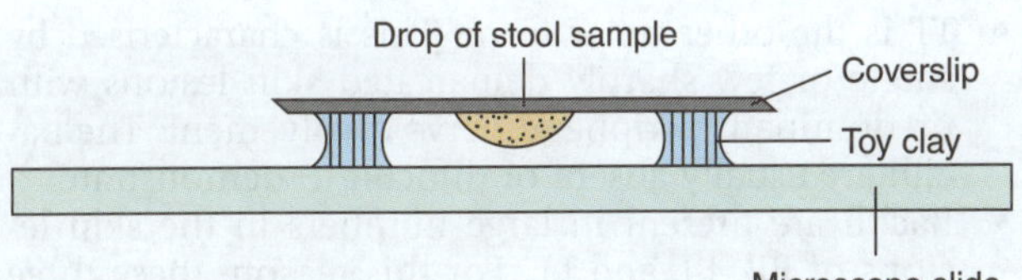

Fig. 17.14 'Hanging-drop' preparation.

DIAGNOSIS

- 'Hanging drop' preparation of the stool (Fig. 17.14) demonstrates the characteristic motile organisms (darting motility or shooting star motility) under dark-field microscopy. *Campylobacter jejuni* may also give similar appearance.
- Culture of the stool or a rectal swab can be used to isolate and identify the organism.
- Immunoassays to detect cholera toxin or *V. cholerae* O1 and O139 lipopolysaccharide directly in stool.

TREATMENT

- Vigorous intravenous fluid and electrolyte therapy should be continued till the patient is haemodynamically stable and vomiting, if present, subsides. Ringer's lactate is an ideal replacement solution. Addition of potassium and sometimes sodium bicarbonate may be required. The initial fluid deficit (generally 100 mL/kg) should be replaced within 3–4 hours of presentation. Replacement of ongoing losses is also crucial.
- Patients with severe cholera may require an average of 200–300 mL/kg of isotonic fluids in the first 24 hours.
- Once the patient is haemodynamically stable, further deficits may be corrected orally. Previously, oral rehydration solution contained commercial salt (NaCl) 3.5 g/L, potassium chloride (1.5 g/L), sodium bicarbonate (2.5 g/L) and glucose (20 g/L). However, presently, a lower-osmolarity solution is recommended in patients with all types of diarrhoea. The composition is sodium chloride (2.6 g/L), potassium chloride (1.5 g/L), trisodium citrate (2.9 g/L) and glucose (13.5 g/L) with an osmolarity of 245 mOsm/L.
- Three days' treatment with tetracycline 500 mg 6 hourly or cotrimoxazole one double-strength tablet daily reduces the duration or excretion of *Vibrio* and the total volume of fluid needed for replacement. However, resistance to cotrimoxazole is common.
- Single-dose doxycycline (300 mg) and tetracycline (2 g) are also effective.
- Other alternative drugs include ciprofloxacin (1 g as single dose or 500 mg twice a day for 3 days), azithromycin (1 g as single dose) and erythromycin (250 mg 6 hourly for 3 days).
- Oral feeding should be resumed as soon as possible after the initial fluid deficit is corrected, and breastfeeding of infants should be encouraged in conjunction with ORS.
- Zinc supplementation in children under 5 years of age may be helpful in reducing severity of diarrhoea. Vitamin A supplementation should also be given once child is stable.

PROPHYLAXIS

- Chemoprophylaxis can be given using tetracycline 500 mg twice a day for 3 days.
- Both live attenuated and bivalent whole-cell killed vaccines are available as oral vaccines.

Q. Discuss the aetiology, clinical features, diagnosis and management of Hansen's disease (leprosy). (DR 9.1, DR 9.5, DR 9.6)

Q. Describe lepra reactions and their management. (DR 9.4)

Q. Write a short note on erythema nodosum leprosum (ENL). (DR 9.4)

DEFINITION

- Leprosy (Hansen's disease) is a chronic granulomatous disease, primarily affecting the peripheral nerves and secondarily involving the skin. The causative organism is *Mycobacterium leprae,* which is an acid–alcohol-fast bacillus.
- The most important mode of spread of *M. leprae* is by droplets from the sneezes of lepromatous patients whose nasal mucosa is heavily infected. The organism may enter the body through the nasal mucosa or by inoculation through the skin. Other rare routes include soil transmission and through insect bites.
- Incubation period is generally 2–6 years.

EPIDEMIOLOGY

- Global leprosy prevalence is 0.84 per 10,000 population.
- Two countries, India and Brazil, account for nearly two-thirds of global burden of leprosy.
- In India, prevalence was much higher (3.3 per 10,000 population) in 2003. However, due to consistent efforts, as of 2020–21, the figure is 0.4 per 10,000 population (leprosy eliminated). A total of 65,147 new cases were detected during the year 2020–21. As of 2019–20, a total of 33 states/union territories have achieved the level of leprosy elimination (prevalence <1 per 10,000 population). However, Chhattisgarh, Dadra and Nagar Haveli, Odisha and Chandigarh still have prevalence rate >1 per 10,000 population.
- Goal is to reduce prevalence in every country to below 1 per 10,000 population (elimination of leprosy).

BACTERIOLOGICAL CONSIDERATIONS

- *M. leprae* is an acid–alcohol-fast bacillus resembling tubercle bacillus. However, it is less acid and alcohol fast than *Mycobacterium tuberculosis*.

- On Ziehl–Neelsen-stained smears or sections, the bacilli are seen singly, in clumps or as globi. Both living and dead bacilli are stained by the Ziehl–Neelsen technique. The living bacilli appear as uniformly stained rods ('solid staining'). The dead bacilli are irregularly stained, either appearing 'fragmented' or 'granular'.
- It appears to survive better at a temperature close to 30°C rather than 37°C. Hence, it affects the skin, peripheral nerves, the mucosa of the upper airways and other tissues such as bone and some viscera.
- *M. leprae* can be grown in mice and the armadillo, but not in artificial media. Local multiplication of the organism in the footpads of mice is a useful technique for studies.
- Bacterial index (BI) is the density of bacilli in the smears. It includes both living and dead bacilli.
- Morphological index (MI) is the percentage of living bacilli calculated after examining 200 red-staining elements lying singly. This is a more sensitive index for bacteriological improvement.
- SFG index is based on the appearance of bacilli—'S' for solid, 'F' for fragmented and 'G' for granular.

CLINICOPATHOLOGICAL CLASSIFICATION

- In the early stage, the disease may be indeterminate and may spontaneously remit or develop into overt leprosy.
- The determinate form of the disease may be classified as tuberculoid (TT), borderline or dimorphic and lepromatous (LL). This forms a spectrum with diminishing host resistance. Resistance is highest in TT and diminishes through borderline spectrum, and is lowest in LL. The borderline group is further subdivided into borderline tuberculoid (BT), borderline (BB) and borderline lepromatous (BL) classes (Fig. 17.15).
- LL is one of the polar forms. This is characterised by extensive, diffuse and bilaterally symmetric skin lesions that contain numerous bacilli. The peripheral nerves are better preserved than in the tuberculoid form.
- TT is the other polar form. This is characterised by single or few sharply demarcated skin lesions with predominant peripheral nerve involvement. The bacilli are usually absent or difficult to demonstrate.
- Bacilli are present in large numbers in the skin lesions of BB, BL and LL. For this reason, these three groups are referred to as multibacillary (MB).
- BT, TT and indeterminate (I) classes are grouped together as paucibacillary (PB) leprosy.

WHO CLASSIFICATION OF LEPROSY

- An additional classification by the World Health Organization is based on the number of skin lesions.
- PB case is a case of leprosy with one to five skin lesions, without demonstrated presence of bacilli in a skin smear.
- MB case is a case of leprosy with more than five skin lesions; or with nerve involvement (pure neuritis, or any number of skin lesions and neuritis); or with the demonstrated presence of bacilli in a slit-skin smear irrespective of the number of skin lesions.

CLINICAL FEATURES

TUBERCULOID LEPROSY

- Skin involvement: The early manifestation is a hypopigmented macule that is sharply demarcated and hypoaesthetic. Later, the lesions become larger, and the margins are elevated and circinate or gyrate. The lesions show peripheral spread and central healing. Fully developed lesions are anaesthetic, with loss of sweat glands and hair follicles.
- Nerve involvement: Nerve involvement occurs early and is usually asymmetric. Involved nerves are thickened and palpable. A routine examination should include palpation of the ulnar, peroneal (lateral popliteal) and greater auricular nerves (Fig. 17.16) as they are frequently involved. The other nerves that are involved are depicted in Fig. 17.17.
- At times, TT may present with only nerve involvement with no skin lesions (neural leprosy or pure neuritic leprosy).

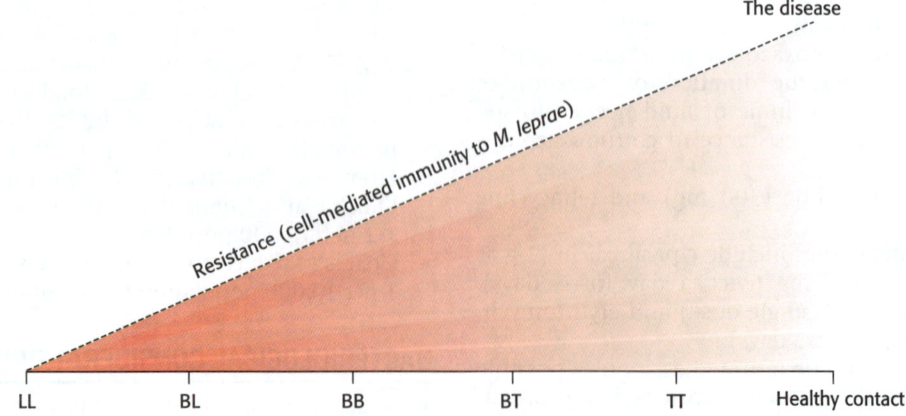

Fig. 17.15 Clinicopathological classification of leprosy. BB, borderline leprosy; BL, borderline lepromatous leprosy; BT, borderline tuberculoid leprosy; LL, lepromatous leprosy; TT, tuberculoid leprosy.

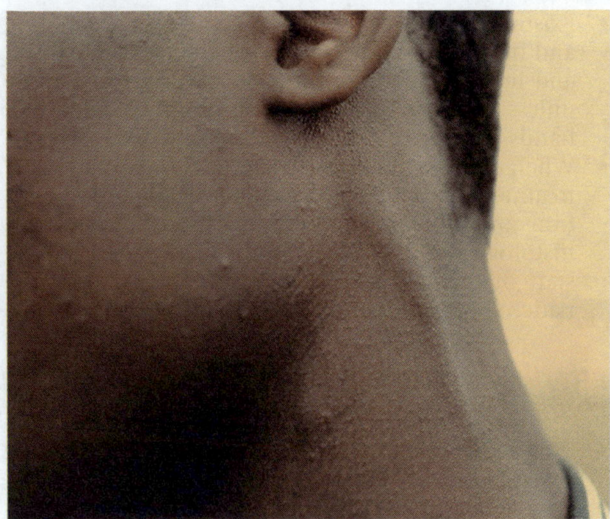

Fig. 17.16 Greater auricular nerve thickening in a patient with tuberculoid leprosy. (From: Walsh DS, Meyers WM. Leprosy. In: Guerrant R, Walker D, Weller P, eds. Tropical Infectious Diseases: Principles, Pathogens and Practice. 3rd ed. Edinburgh: Saunders; 2011: 253–260.)

- Sensory nerve involvement results in sensory dysfunctions like glove and stocking anaesthesia (more common in LL), chronic non-healing plantar ulcers and repeated injuries to hands and feet.
- Motor nerve involvement results in a variety of abnormalities. There is muscle weakness, wasting and later paralysis, followed by contractures.
  - Ulnar nerve—claw hand or 'main en griffe'.
  - Median nerve—ape hand or 'main de singe'.
  - Lateral popliteal nerve—foot drop.
  - Posterior tibial nerve—claw toes or hammer toes.
- Autonomic involvement results in anhidrosis or hyperhidrosis.
- Cranial nerve involvement: Facial nerve (seventh cranial nerve) is commonly involved resulting in facial paralysis, lagophthalmos, exposure keratitis and corneal ulcerations leading to blindness. Trigeminal nerve (fifth cranial nerve) involvement may occur early with the loss of corneal reflex.

LEPROMATOUS LEPROSY

- Nasal symptoms: These are early symptoms of LL. They include anosmia, nasal stuffiness, crust formation and blood-stained nasal discharge.
- Skin involvement: The skin lesions are macules, nodules, plaques or papules. The macules are often hypopigmented. The borders of the lesions are ill defined, and the centres indurated, raised and convex ('inverted saucer' appearance). There is also diffuse infiltration between the lesions. The sites of predilection are face (cheeks, nose and eyebrows), ears, wrists, elbows, buttocks and knees. Thickening and nodulation of ears and loss of lateral eyebrows are early manifestations. With advanced disease, the skin of the face and forehead becomes thickened and corrugated ('leonine facies') (Fig. 17.18).
- Nerve involvement: Involvement of major nerve trunks is less prominent in LL, but a 'glove and stocking' anaesthesia is common in advanced disease. Mononeuritis multiplex can also occur.
- Bone involvement occurs in hands, feet and skull. There is slow atrophy and absorption of distal phalanges leading to shortening of fingers. In the feet, phalanges, metatarsals and tarsal bones are involved. In the skull, there is atrophy of the anterior nasal spine (contributing to nasal collapse) and atrophy of

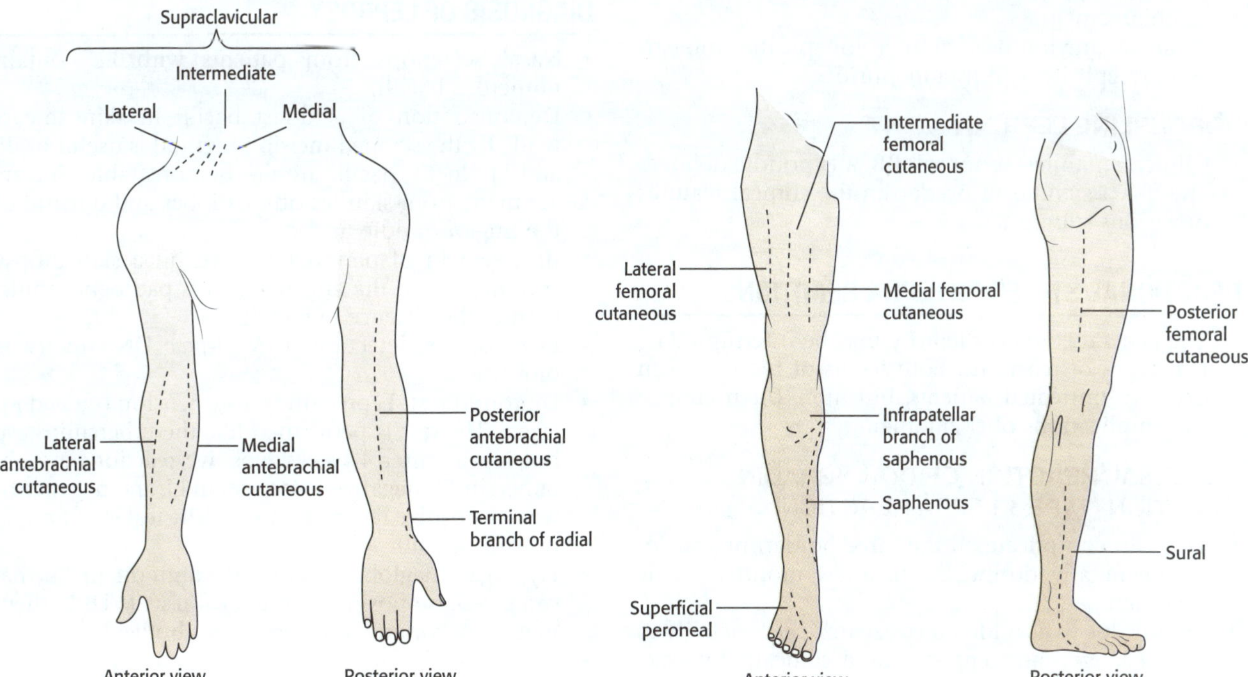

Fig. 17.17 (A) Sensory nerves of arms. (B) Sensory nerves of legs.

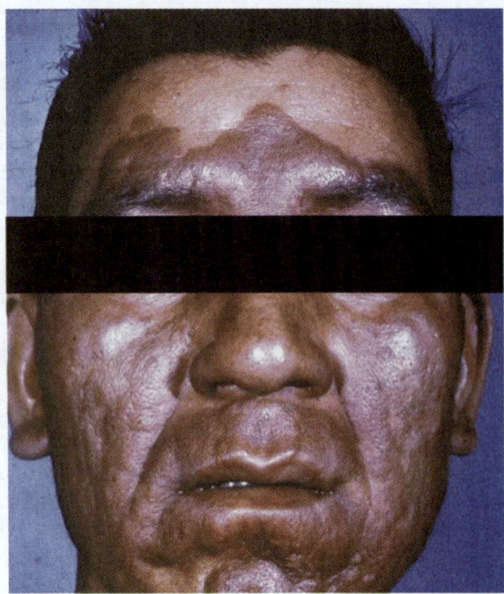

Fig. 17.18 Leonine facies.

maxillary alveolar process (contributing to loosening and loss of upper incisors). These two skull changes are together called 'facies leprosa'.

- Other manifestations:
  - Bilateral oedema of legs and ankles.
  - Swollen and broad nose, septal perforation and nasal collapse leading to saddle nose.
  - The upper incisor teeth may loosen and fall off.
  - Laryngitis, palatal perforation and hoarseness of voice.
  - Involvement of the anterior chamber of the eye results in keratitis and iridocyclitis.
  - Testicular atrophy, impotence, infertility and gynaecomastia.
  - Painless inguinal and axillary lymph nodal enlargement.
  - Renal amyloidosis, glomerulonephritis, interstitial nephritis and pyelonephritis.

BORDERLINE LEPROSY

- Clinical manifestations of BB are poorly defined. There is a significant overlap in the clinical features of various subtypes.

REACTIONAL STATES OR LEPRA REACTIONS

- The general course of leprosy may be interrupted by two types of reactions. Both forms of reactions can occur in untreated patients, but more often emerge as complications of chemotherapy.

REVERSAL REACTION OR DOWNGRADING REACTION (TYPE 1 LEPRA REACTION)

- This can complicate all the three borderline categories, generally during the first few months of the treatment.
- Occurs due to a sudden increase in T-cell reactivity to mycobacterial antigens expressed clinically by exacerbation of skin and nerve trunk inflammation, leading to sensory and motor alterations.
- Existing skin lesions develop erythema and swelling and new lesions may appear. The nerves are painful and tender and nerve function may be lost rapidly unless the reaction is treated promptly. Oedema of hands and feet is common.
- When type 1 lepra reaction precedes the initiation of treatment of leprosy, it is called downgrading reaction and the patient becomes more lepromatous histologically. When the reaction occurs after the start of therapy, it is termed reversal reaction; the patient becomes more tuberculoid.

ERYTHEMA NODOSUM LEPROSUM (TYPE 2 LEPRA REACTION)

- This occurs in patients with BL or LL often during the second year of the treatment.
- Occurs due to widespread immune complex deposition and overproduction of TNF-α.
- Tender and inflamed subcutaneous nodules develop, usually in crops. Each nodule lasts for 1 or 2 weeks, but new crops may appear. Severe reactions may be accompanied by low-grade fever, lymphadenopathy and arthralgias. In addition, iritis, orchitis, myositis, neuritis and oedema can occur.
- Most people have acute multiple episodes of erythema nodosum leprosum (ENL) or chronic ENL. Chronic ENL is defined as an episode lasting for more than 6 months. This could include single and multiple episodes. Few people experience a single acute episode of ENL.
- After completion of treatment, people may still have episodes of ENL for several years because they have persisting mycobacterial antigens despite successful antibacterial treatment.

DIAGNOSIS OF LEPROSY

- Nasal secretions from patients with LL contain numerous bacilli.
- Demonstration of acid-fast bacilli in skin smears made by the scraped incision method is useful in BL and LL. In TT, bacilli are not demonstrable. Smears are made from skin lesions, earlobes and dorsum of the ring or middle finger.
- Involvement of peripheral nerves in a skin biopsy specimen from the affected area is pathognomonic, even in the absence of bacilli.
- PCR for the detection of *M. leprae* DNA in tissue biopsies.
- Lepromin test: Lepromin is a suspension of dead *M. leprae*. The test is performed like the tuberculin test, but is read after 4 weeks. Positive reactions are obtained in TT, negative responses in LL and negative or weakly positive responses in BB. The test is of limited diagnostic value.
- Hypergammaglobulinaemia is common in LL that can give false-positive serological tests (VDRL, rheumatoid factor and antinuclear antibodies).
- IgM antibodies to phenolic glycolipid-1 (PGL-1) are present in 95% of LL but in only 60% of TT. These antibodies may also be present in normal persons.

TREATMENT

- The main drugs available for the treatment of leprosy are dapsone (100 mg), rifampicin (600 mg) and clofazimine (100 mg).
- The side effects of dapsone include haemolysis, agranulocytosis, hepatitis and exfoliative dermatitis.
- The major side effects of clofazimine are restricted to the skin and intestinal tract. They include reddish skin pigmentation, ichthyosis, diarrhoea and cramping abdominal pain.
- Three other drugs—ofloxacin, minocycline and clarithromycin—have also been found to be effective against leprosy, particularly when drug-resistance is suspected.
- Recommended regimens are given in the Box 17.17. The duration of treatment is 1 year for MB and 6 months for PB.

DAPSONE RESISTANCE

- This is treated either by clofazimine alone or by combination treatment with ethionamide 500 mg daily and rifampicin given on the first 2 days of each month.

TREATMENT OF REACTIONAL STATES

- During reactional states, the chemotherapy for leprosy is maintained in addition to the antiinflammatory drugs.
- *Type 1 lepra reaction (reversal reaction).* Mild cases are treated with aspirin 600 mg 6 hourly. Severe cases are treated with prednisone 40–80 mg daily, reducing gradually over 3–9 months.
- *Type 2 lepra reaction (ENL).* Mild cases are treated with aspirin 600 mg 6 hourly. Severe cases are treated with prednisone (1 mg/kg/day). In patients not responding to steroids, clofazimine (300 mg/day) or thalidomide (100 mg four times daily) should be added to prednisone. The doses are reduced slowly over 1–3 months. Eye involvement is treated with 1% hydrocortisone drops or ointment and 1% atropine drops.

NATIONAL PROGRAMME

- The National Leprosy Control Programme was launched by the Government of India in 1955 based on dapsone monotherapy.
- MDT came into wide use from 1982 and the Programme was redesignated as the National Leprosy Eradication Programme (NLEP) in 1983.
- The Programme was expanded with World Bank assistance and the first phase of the World Bank-supported National Leprosy Elimination Project started in 1993–1994 and ended in March 2000. The second phase of the World Bank-supported National Leprosy Elimination Project started on 1 April 2001 for a period of 3 years with the objective to achieve elimination of leprosy as a public health problem by 2005, thereby reducing the caseload to less than 1 per 10,000 population. During the second National Leprosy Elimination Project, the NLEP was decentralised to states/districts and leprosy services were integrated with general health-care system. Free MDT is now available at all subcentres, PHCs and government hospitals and dispensaries on all working days.
- More recently, the NLEP has adopted a three-pronged approach of leprosy case detection campaign (LCDC) in highly endemic districts, focused leprosy awareness campaign using ASHAs and multipurpose health workers in areas where new cases are detected, and area-specific plans for case detection in hard-to-reach areas. It was felt that the major cause of hidden cases is low voluntary reporting in the community due to a lack of awareness as well as the continuing fear, stigma and discrimination against leprosy. The *Sparsh* Leprosy Awareness Campaign (SLAC) was launched on 30 January 2017 and is a programme intended to promote awareness and address the issues of stigma and discrimination.

BOX 17.17 Treatment Regimens for MB and PB Leprosy

TREATMENT OF MULTIBACILLARY (MB) LEPROSY

- Dapsone 100 mg daily (self-administered).
- Clofazimine 50 mg daily (self-administered) plus 300 mg once a month (supervised).
- Rifampicin 600 mg once a month (supervised).

TREATMENT OF PAUCIBACILLARY (PB) LEPROSY

- Dapsone 100 mg daily.
- Rifampicin 600 mg once a month (supervised).
- The duration of treatment is 6 months and the patient should be followed up for 5 years.

PROPHYLAXIS

- Postexposure chemoprophylaxis is advocated to close contacts of new, untreated cases. Chemoprophylaxis with a single-dose rifampicin (SDR) has a 57% overall risk reduction in preventing the development of leprosy for household contacts during the first 2 years after its administration.
- MIP vaccine: The NLEP has introduced the *Mycobacterium indicus pranii* (MIP) vaccine in a project mode in India from the year 2016. MIP vaccine has been shown to have both immunotherapeutic and immunoprophylactic effects in MB leprosy patients.

Q. Explain in brief about leptospirosis.

Q. Write a short note on Weil's syndrome.

AETIOLOGY

- *Leptospira* consists of two species: *Leptospira interrogans*, which is pathogenic, and *Leptospira biflexa*, which is saprophytic. The term leptospirosis describes an infection with any of the subtypes or subgroups of *L. interrogans*.
- The organism is a tightly coiled Gram-negative spirochaete with one axial filament.

EPIDEMIOLOGY

- Leptospirosis is the most widespread zoonosis in the world.
- Reservoirs of infection include rodents, skunks, foxes, domestic livestock and dogs. Many animals exhibit a prolonged urinary shedding of the organism.
- Human infection can occur either by direct contact with urine or tissue of an infected animal or indirectly through contaminated water, soil or vegetation. Transmission may occur through cuts, mucous membranes (nasopharynx, conjunctiva and vagina) and possibly unabraded skin.
- The mechanism by which leptospirae cause tissue damage is not very clear. Early in the disease, tissue damage results from a direct toxic damage due to leptospirae. Later in the illness, damage is the consequence of immune response to leptospiral antigens. Damage to blood vessels is common that leads to vasculitis.

CLINICAL FEATURES

- Most natural infections appear 7–14 days after the exposure.
- Commonly encountered clinical manifestations are fever, headache, myalgia, conjunctival suffusion, gastrointestinal symptoms like nausea, vomiting and abdominal pain, cough, pharyngitis, lymphadenopathy, hepatomegaly and skin rashes.
  - The fever is usually high grade with chills and rigors.
  - Headache is severe and is retro-orbital or occipital.
  - Severe myalgias occur in most patients, the muscles of the thighs and lumbar areas being most prominently involved. Myalgia is accompanied by severe muscle tenderness and cutaneous hyperaesthesia (causalgia).
  - Conjunctival suffusion is very helpful in detecting the disease. It is not conjunctivitis, but rather a pericorneal reddening or hyperaemia.
- Less commonly encountered manifestations are splenomegaly, uveitis and diarrhoea.
- The features last for 4–9 days.
- In many cases, the first phase (leptospiraemic phase) is followed by a period of apparent recovery, after which the symptoms worsen again for another 2–5 days (immune phase). During the second phase, meningitis and iridocyclitis are more common.
  - The initial 'first phase' or 'leptospiraemic phase' is so named because leptospirae are present in the blood and CSF during this phase.
  - The subsequent 'second phase' or 'immune phase' is so named because of the presence of leptospiral antibodies in the blood, the disappearance of leptospirae from the blood and the onset of urine cultures positive for the organism.
- Presence of headache, fever, neck stiffness or pain due to myalgias may suggest meningitis. The CSF is usually acellular in the first 7 days of illness, although the organisms may be seen. With the onset of antibodies in the serum, aseptic meningitis occurs in 90% of patients, with an abnormal CSF (see 'Investigations').

WEIL'S SYNDROME

- Weil's syndrome is not a specific subgroup of leptospirosis; it is simply severe leptospirosis.
- Can develop as the second phase of a biphasic illness or as a progressive illness.
- The overall picture in Weil's syndrome is striking and is characterised by intense jaundice, mental status changes, haemorrhage, purpura or petechiae and renal insufficiency.
  - The first manifestation of severe disease is usually jaundice that develops between the fifth and ninth days. Jaundice does not seem to be due to hepatocellular damage, but seems to be more related to the cholestasis of sepsis.
  - Renal insufficiency may develop concomitantly or later, with progressive oliguria and renal failure from acute tubular necrosis.
  - Haemorrhagic manifestations are common and include purpura and petechiae appearing on oral, vaginal or conjunctival mucosa. Other haemorrhagic manifestations include epistaxis, haemoptysis, gastrointestinal bleeding, haemorrhage into adrenal glands and subarachnoid haemorrhage.

INVESTIGATIONS

- Urinary findings early in the illness include microscopic haematuria, pyuria and proteinuria.
- Total leucocyte count may vary, but neutrophilia of more than 70% is very frequent.
- Anaemia may occur due to intravascular haemolysis, azotaemia and blood loss from haemorrhage.
- Hyponatraemia is common.
- Thrombocytopenia and raised erythrocyte sedimentation rate (ESR).
- Liver function tests reveal an elevation of AST and ALT up to five times normal, conjugated hyperbilirubinaemia and raised alkaline phosphatase. Marked elevations of bilirubin with mildly elevated transaminases are characteristic features of Weil's syndrome.
- Elevation of blood urea nitrogen (BUN) and hyperkalaemia occur with renal failure.
- Coagulation studies may show a prolongation of prothrombin time that is reversible with vitamin K.
- Levels of creatine phosphokinase (CPK) are elevated in 50% of patients in the first week of illness. This is helpful in differentiating the disease from viral hepatitis.
- Chest radiograph may show patchy bronchopneumonia and a small pleural effusion.
- Electrocardiographic abnormalities include bradycardia, low voltage and non-specific ST–T wave changes.
- CSF may be abnormal in up to 90% of cases after 7 days of illness. The cell counts are raised (but $<500/mm^3$) with a neutrophil predominance. Proteins may be normal or elevated while glucose remains normal. In the presence of severe jaundice, xanthochromia can develop.
- The tightly coiled spirochaete in the urine or blood may be visualised by phase contrast or dark-field microscopy.

- IgM antibodies may be detected in blood in the second phase of illness using microscopic agglutination test (MAT).
- Demonstration of *Leptospira* antigen by radioimmunoassay or ELISA.
- The diagnosis can be confirmed by culture (on Fletcher's medium) of the blood in the first week of illness or of the urine thereafter. However, this is a tedious process.
- Detection of bacterial DNA by PCR in various clinical samples.

TREATMENT

- A variety of antimicrobial agents have been found to be effective in vitro, but the recommended drugs are given as follows:
  - Intravenous penicillin (1.5 million units 6 hourly) or ampicillin (1 g 6 hourly) for 7 days is beneficial, even when the treatment is started after the fifth day of illness.
  - Doxycycline (100 mg orally twice daily for 7 days) or azithromycin (500 mg once a day for 3 days), when started within 4 days of onset of symptoms, is also effective in mild cases.
  - Ceftriaxone (1–2 g twice a day) in severe cases.
- A Jarisch–Herxheimer reaction may occur following antibiotic treatment and is due to an acute inflammatory response following clearance of spirochaetes from the circulation. The patient will develop fever, chills, rigors and hypotension.
- Renal failure and jaundice require meticulous attention of fluid and electrolyte therapy. Renal failure may require dialysis. Exchange transfusion may be beneficial in severe hyperbilirubinaemia.
- Anaemia and thrombocytopenia may require blood component transfusion.

Q. Write a brief note on rickettsial diseases.

Q. Describe briefly various rickettsial infections.

- Rickettsia are obligate intracellular, non-motile, Gram-negative bacteria which cannot be propagated in cell-free media.
- Rickettsial infections (except Q fever) are zoonotic (in animals) with occasional transmission to humans by arthropods.
- These organisms replicate within the endothelial cells and smooth muscles of capillaries, arterioles and venules producing vasculitis.
- Most of these infections present with fever, myalgias and skin rash.
- An eschar is a characteristic lesion in some rickettsial infections and develops at the site of inoculation.
- Table 17.23 gives features of various rickettsial diseases including causative agents, vectors and clinical features.

TABLE 17.23 Various Rickettsial Diseases

Disease	Agent	Vector	Reservoir	Clinical Features
Typhus Group				
Epidemic typhus	*Rickettsia prowazekii*	Louse	Humans	• Fever, myalgias, headache, rash over body (sparing palms, soles and face); sometimes petechiae, confusion, drowsiness • Coma, seizures and focal neurological signs
Murine or endemic typhus	*Rickettsia typhi*	Flea	Rodents	• Fever, myalgias, headache, rash over body (sparing palms, soles and face)
Scrub typhus	*O. tsutsugamushi*	Mite	Rodents	• See subsequent text
Spotted Fever Group				
Indian tick typhus	*Rickettsia conorii*	Tick	Rodents, dogs	• Fever, headache, rash appearing on wrists and ankles first, eschar
Rocky Mountain spotted fever	*Rickettsia rickettsii*	Tick	Rodents, dogs	• Fever, headache, macular rash later becoming purpuric, rash appearing on wrists and ankles first with involvement of palms and soles • Complications include encephalitis, ARDS, myocarditis, coagulopathy, gastrointestinal bleeding • Hyponatraemia and abnormal liver function tests common
Rickettsial pox	*Rickettsia akari*	Mite	Mice	• Mild illness with fever, headache, myalgias, maculopapular and vesicular rash, eschar
Others				
Q fever	*Coxiella burnetii*	No	Cattle, sheep, goat	• Fever, headache, myalgias, pneumonia, endocarditis
Trench fever	*Bartonella quintana*	Louse	Human	• Fever, malaise, headache, bone pains, rash, splenomegaly • Bacteraemia, endocarditis

Q. Discuss briefly about scrub typhus.

- A mite-borne disease caused by *Orientia tsutsugamushi*, a Gram-negative coccobacillus.
- It is endemic in several parts of India.
- Disease is acquired from the bite of the larval stage of infected trombiculid mites (chiggers). These chiggers maintain the infection in successive generations via transovarial transmission. They live on the waist-high grass growing in previously cleared jungle around villages and plantations. Chiggers have also been found on many rodent vectors.
- Outbreaks are generally reported towards the end of the rainy season and the beginning of winter months (July–November).

CLINICAL FEATURES

- Incubation period is 7–21 days (median 12 days).
- The severity of infection can range from mild signs and symptoms to multiorgan failure and death.
- Most scrub typhus cases are mild and characterised by acute-onset fever, myalgia, generalised painful lymphadenopathy, maculopapular rash and splenomegaly.
- In untreated patients, fever typically lasts for long periods (9–19 days).
- Rash is non-pruritic, macular or maculopapular. It begins on the abdomen and spreads to the extremities and face. Petechiae are uncommon.
- Unproductive cough is common while some patients present with bilateral infiltrates resembling atypical pneumonia.
- Eschar is variably seen in 20%–90% of cases, typically on torso, axilla or groin, and may be diagnostic. It appears as a painless papule at the site of the infecting chigger bite. Subsequent central necrosis then occurs, which in turn leads to the formation of a characteristic eschar with a black crust (Fig. 17.19). One or multiple eschars may develop before the onset of systemic symptoms. Eschars may be overlooked if a careful clinical examination is not performed.
- Conjunctival suffusion can also occur.

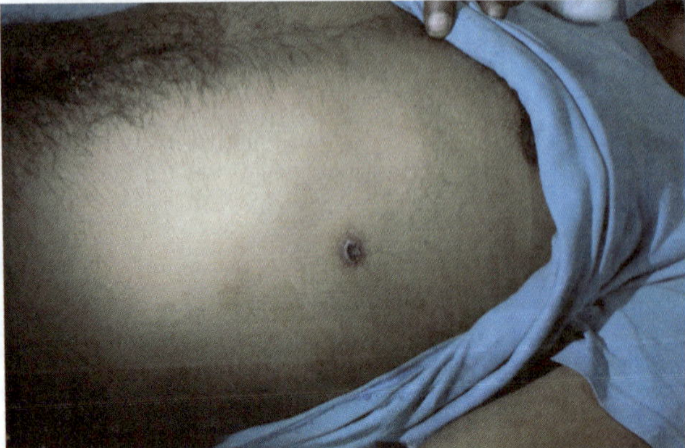

Fig. 17.19 Typical eschar.

- Bone pain and bleeding manifestations are rare and should prompt other diagnosis like dengue.
- Severe clinical features include multiorgan dysfunction, meningoencephalitis, coma, neurological deficits, myocarditis and pulmonary involvement (including ARDS).
- Mortality rates can be up to 25%.

LABORATORY INVESTIGATIONS

- Thrombocytopenia and elevation in liver enzymes, bilirubin and creatinine are common.
- Indirect fluorescent antibody (IFA) test remains the mainstay of serological diagnosis. A four-fold increase between acute-phase and convalescent-phase antibody titres is required to make a diagnosis.
- Indirect immunoperoxidase test has been accepted as an alternative standard assay by the World Health Organization to diagnose rickettsial diseases (particularly for scrub typhus).
- Biopsy of eschar or skin rash may show lymphohistiocytic vasculitis.
- PCR to detect RNA in blood is not routinely available.

TREATMENT

- Doxycycline (100 mg twice a day) or chloramphenicol (250–500 mg every 6 hours) for 7 days can be used to treat scrub typhus.
- An alternative drug is azithromycin.

Q. What is candidiasis (moniliasis)?

- Infection of skin or mucous membranes (e.g. oral cavity and vagina) is called moniliasis.
- *Candida albicans* is the most common cause of candidiasis.
- Invasive candidiasis can also be due to non-*albicans Candida* species (e.g. *Candida glabrata*). Some of these are resistant to fluconazole.
- Local overgrowth of *Candida*:
  - Oral or oropharyngeal candidiasis (thrush) commonly seen with the use of broad-spectrum antibiotics, xerostomia, immune dysfunction (e.g. diabetes, immunosuppressive therapy and HIV infection), radiation to head and neck or presence of removable prostheses (e.g. dentures) or use of inhaled corticosteroids. Furthermore, about one in four patients with lichen planus will have superimposed candidiasis. It presents as white plaques on the buccal mucosa, palate, tongue or the oropharynx. The usual symptoms of oropharyngeal candidiasis are a cottony feeling in the mouth, loss of taste, and sometimes pain on eating and swallowing. Diagnosis is confirmed by scraping the lesions and performing a potassium hydroxide (KOH) preparation on the scrapings. Budding yeasts with or without pseudohyphae are seen.
  - Vaginal candidiasis occurs more commonly in diabetics and HIV infection; also occurs with the

use of oral contraceptives, antibiotics and glucocorticoids. Presenting features include itching, whitish discharge and dyspareunia. Examination shows vulvar and vaginal erythema along with curd-like discharge.
- Cutaneous candidiasis presenting as intertriginous infection, paronychia, balanitis, pruritus ani, vulval candidiasis (in diabetic females) and scrotal candidiasis.
- Chronic mucocutaneous candidiasis occurs in immunocompromised patients with leukaemias, lymphomas and AIDS as well as in autosomal recessive polyglandular autoimmune syndrome type I. Clinical features include severe, recurrent thrush, onychomycosis, vaginitis and chronic skin lesions (hyperkeratotic, crusted appearance on the face, scalp and hands).
- Oesophageal candidiasis is most common in patients with HIV infection and haematologic malignancies. It presents as dysphagia and pain on swallowing. The pain is localised to the retrosternal area. Diagnosis is usually made during endoscopy when white mucosal plaque-like lesions are noted.
- Candidiasis of the urinary tract presents with bladder thrush.

- Invasive candidiasis:
  - Invasive candidiasis usually occurs in immunocompromised patients, particularly those with neutropenia or transplant recipients receiving glucocorticoids. Other risk factors include use of chemotherapeutic agents, especially those associated with extensive gastrointestinal mucosal damage, broad-spectrum antibiotics and central venous catheters.
  - Haematogenous dissemination of *Candida* (invasive candidiasis or candidaemia) presenting with retinal abscesses extending into vitreous humour, pulmonary candidiasis, endocarditis, pyelonephritis, chronic meningitis and arthritis

TREATMENT

- Topical application of antifungal agents like nystatin, clotrimazole or miconazole for vulvovaginitis.
- Swallowing nystatin suspension or sucking on clotrimazole troches for oesophageal candidiasis.
- Systemic antifungal agents: Ketoconazole (200–400 mg/day), fluconazole (200 mg/day), itraconazole (100 mg/day [200 mg/day in oesophageal candidiasis]), voriconazole (400–600 mg/day) or posaconazole. For vulvovaginitis, azoles are given for 1–3 days. For oesophageal candidiasis, therapy is extended for 3 weeks or 2 weeks after the symptoms subside, whichever is longer.
- Severe systemic infections may require intravenous fluconazole (6 mg/kg/day) or amphotericin B for at least 2 weeks after cultures become negative. Echinocandins include caspofungin, micafungin and anidulafungin. These agents have limited toxicity, are safe in the presence of renal or hepatic impairment, have minimal drug interactions and, importantly, have broad-spectrum activity against most *Candida* spp.

Q. Discuss briefly about β-lactamases.

Q. Write a short note on New Delhi metallo-β-lactamase (NDM-1).

β-LACTAMASES

- Production of β-lactamases is the most important contributing factor to β-lactam antibiotic resistance in Gram-negative bacteria.
- β-Lactamases are bacterial enzymes that inactivate β-lactam antibacterials by hydrolysis, which results in ineffective compounds. They are not effective against higher generation cephalosporins, e.g. cefotaxime, ceftazidime, ceftriaxone or cefepime.
- Several serine active β-lactamases inhibitors (clavulanic acid, sulbactam and tazobactam) in combination with β-lactams have been in use to reduce resistance due to presence of β-lactamases.

EXTENDED-SPECTRUM β-LACTAMASES (ESBLS)

- Several isolates of Enterobacteriaceae and *Pseudomonas* produce newer β-lactamases. These enzymes include plasmid-mediated cephamycinases, ESBLs and carbapenem-hydrolysing enzymes or carbapenemases.
- The ESBLs are a group of enzymes that have the ability to hydrolyse and cause resistance to the oxyimino-cephalosporins (cefotaxime, ceftazidime, ceftriaxone, cefuroxime and cefepime) and monobactams (aztreonam), but not the cephamycins (cefoxitin and cefotetan) or carbapenems (imipenem, meropenem, doripenem and ertapenem).
- These enzymes are also inhibited by classical β-lactamase inhibitors such as clavulanic acid, sulbactam and tazobactam.
- ESBLs are often located on large plasmids that also harbour genes for resistance to other antimicrobial classes that include resistance to aminoglycosides and cotrimoxazole. This complicates antimicrobial selection, especially in patients with serious infections.
- Antimicrobials that are regularly used for empirical therapy of serious community-onset infections such as the third-generation cephalosporins (e.g. cefotaxime and ceftriaxone) are often not effective against ESBL-producing bacteria.
- As a result of these major concerns, the carbapenems including imipenem, meropenem, doripenem and ertapenem have become widely recognised as the drug class of first choice for the treatment of serious infections due to ESBL-producing bacteria. Piperacillin/tazobactam is also useful for the treatment of some infections with ESBL-producing pathogens although it may be less effective than carbapenems. Tigecycline has shown excellent activity against ESBL-producing *E. coli* isolates.

NEW DELHI METALLO-β-LACTAMASE

- It is a novel metallo-β-lactamase (MBL) coded by a novel gene *bla* (NDM-1) in *Enterobacteriaceae*. It is a carbapenemase β-lactamase enzyme.

- It was first reported in a Swedish patient, a diabetic male who returned to Sweden after having received treatment at a hospital in New Delhi for gluteal abscess in December 2009. Since the immediate previous treatment was traced to New Delhi, it was named NDM-1.
- Subsequently, organisms in the *Enterobacteriaceae* family containing this genetic element have been found widely throughout India, Pakistan and Bangladesh, and also in Britain and many other countries.
- MBLs are enzymes that mediate resistance to almost all β-lactam agents (except monobactams, e.g. aztreonam) including carbapenems. Many MBLs producing *Enterobacteriaceae* additionally carry ESBLs or other resistant determinants that confer resistance to aztreonam.
- Strains carrying this gene demonstrate multidrug resistance, being susceptible only to tigecycline, colistin and fosfomycin.
- To date, there have been 13 variants of NDM that have been identified: NDM-1 to NDM-14 (NDM-11 was not assigned to any unique variant).

Q. Explain briefly about community-associated methicillin-resistant *Staphylococcus aureus* (CA-MRSA).

- First recognised in the mid-1990s.
- Refers to strains of MRSA seen in patients presenting with infections in the community or presenting to the hospitals for the first time (Box 17.18).
- Typical patients include previously healthy people, often younger, those involved in close contact activities, e.g. sports teams or military service, especially those resulting in skin abrasions.
- Tend to produce aggressive skin and soft tissue infections, necrotising pneumonia, osteomyelitis, septic shock and bacteraemia.
- In mild cases, oral treatment with clindamycin, doxycycline, cotrimoxazole or linezolid is useful. Fluoroquinolones should not be used to treat skin and soft tissue infections due to MRSA.
- In severe cases, intravenous vancomycin, teicoplanin, linezolid, tigecycline and daptomycin (not for pneumonia) are also beneficial.

BOX 17.18 Diagnosis of Community-Associated MRSA

- Infection occurs in the outpatient setting, or a positive culture for MRSA is identified within 48 hours after admission to the hospital
- There is no medical history of MRSA infection or colonisation
- There is no medical history in the past year of hospitalisation, admission to a nursing home, dialysis or surgery
- There are no permanent indwelling catheters or medical devices that pass through the skin into the body

Q. Discuss briefly the life cycle of malarial parasite.

Q. Briefly outline stable malaria and unstable malaria.

Q. Discuss the aetiology, epidemiology, clinical features, complications, investigations and management of malaria. (IM 4.6)

- Malaria is a protozoan disease transmitted by the bite of female *Anopheles* mosquitoes.
- Four species of the genus *Plasmodium* infect humans. These are *Plasmodium falciparum*, *Plasmodium vivax*, *Plasmodium ovale* and *Plasmodium malariae*. A comparison of the developmental characteristics of these species is given in Table 17.24.
- Rarely, *Plasmodium knowlesi* may cause human infection.
- *P. falciparum* causes the most severe forms of the disease. *P. vivax* infection is the most common in India.

LIFE CYCLE OF PARASITE

- Human infection begins when a female *Anopheles* mosquito inoculates the sporozoites from its salivary gland during a blood meal. They are rapidly carried via the bloodstream to the liver where they enter the hepatocytes.
- In the hepatocyte, during phase of asexual reproduction (intrahepatic or pre-erythrocytic schizogony), a single sporozoite produces thousands of merozoites. The swollen hepatocyte bursts, discharging these merozoites into the bloodstream.
- In *P. vivax* and *P. ovale* infections, a proportion of the intrahepatic forms enter a cryptobiotic phase in which they are termed hypnozoites. They may lie dormant for months before starting to divide. These sleeping forms are the cause of the relapses that characterise infection with these two species.
- In *P. falciparum* and *P. malariae* infections, there is no cryptobiotic phase and therefore relapses from the liver do not occur.
- After the entry into the bloodstream, merozoites rapidly invade erythrocytes. Inside the erythrocyte,

TABLE 17.24 Comparison of Developmental Characteristics of Various Species of Malaria

Features	*P. falciparum*	*P. vivax*	*P. ovale*	*P. malariae*
• Erythrocytic cycle	48 hours	48 hours	48 hours	72 hours
• Red cells parasitised	All	Reticulocytes	Reticulocytes	Mature erythrocytes
• Relapse	No	Yes	Yes	No
• Drug resistance	Yes	No	No	No

asexual division occurs and the parasites develop through 'ring' forms to trophozoites and finally to schizonts containing daughter merozoites. The duration of this erythrocytic cycle is 48 hours for *falciparum*, *vivax* and *ovale*, but 72 hours for *malariae*. These daughter merozoites are released into the bloodstream by erythrocyte rupture. Each of these daughter merozoites is capable of invading a new erythrocyte and repeating the cycle.

- A minor proportion of the merozoites within erythrocytes can undergo a different pathway of development into male and female gametocytes. The gametocytes are ingested by the mosquito during a blood meal. The male and female gametocytes fuse in the insect's midgut to form a zygote. This matures to form an ookinete which penetrates the gut wall and forms an oocyst. The oocyst expands by asexual division giving rise to sporozoites that migrate to the insect's salivary gland. During the blood meal, these sporozoites are inoculated into the next human, thus completing the life cycle.
- Life cycle of malaria parasite is shown in Fig. 17.20.

EPIDEMIOLOGY AND RESISTANCE AGAINST MALARIA

- Malaria occurs throughout most of the tropical regions of the world.
- Annual parasite index is defined as the number of confirmed new cases of malaria registered in a year per 1000 individuals under surveillance, for a given country, territory or geographic area.
- In India, annual parasite index has come down from 2.12 per 1000 in 2001 to 0.14 in 2020.
- Data from India shows that a total 190,000 cases of malaria were recorded in the year 2020 of which 120,000 were due to *P. falciparum*.
- Stable malaria: In areas where there is intense malaria transmission, the people are infected repeatedly throughout their lives, starting from childhood. By the time of adulthood, the immunity is high and malaria infections are largely asymptomatic. This is termed 'stable malaria'. The predominant organism in these areas is *P. falciparum*.
- Unstable malaria: In areas where malaria transmission is low, the immunity is low and symptomatic disease occurs at all ages. This is termed 'unstable malaria'. The predominant organism is *P. vivax*.
- *P. falciparum* does not grow well in red cells that contain haemoglobin F, C or, especially, haemoglobin S heterozygotes (AS) are protected against the lethal complications of malaria.
- Attachment of merozoites to red cells is mediated via a specific receptor on the surface of the cells. In the case of *P. vivax*, this receptor is related to the Duffy blood group antigen (Fy^a or Fy^b). If a person is Duffy-negative (as most of the West African population is), he/she will be resistant to infection by *P. vivax*.
- Chloroquine resistance is quite common in the north-eastern part of India as well as states of Andhra Pradesh, Chhattisgarh, Jharkhand, Madhya Pradesh and Odisha. Many strains of *P. falciparum* are resistant to chloroquine as well as combination of sulphadoxine and pyrimethamine (multiple drug resistance).

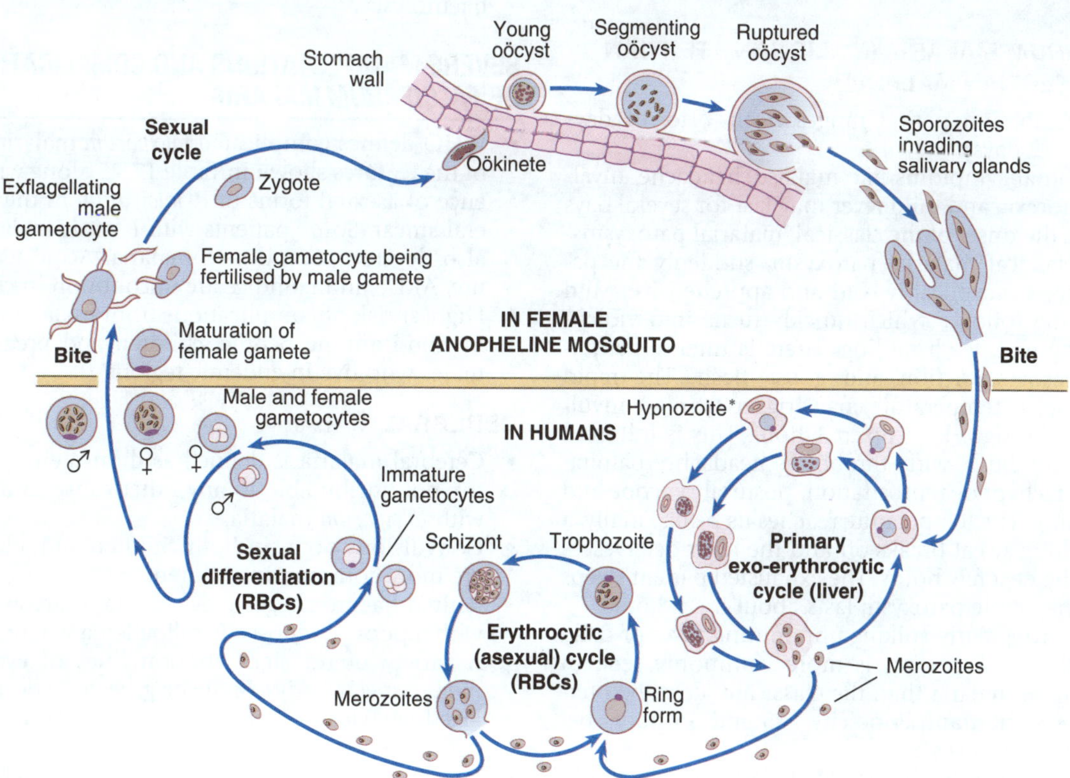

Fig. 17.20 Life cycle of malaria parasite (hypnozoites (*) are present only in *P. vivax* and *P. ovale* infections).

CLINICAL FEATURES

VIVAX, OVALE AND *MALARIAE* MALARIAS

- Incubation period for *P. vivax* is 12–17 days, for *P. ovale*, it is 15–18 days and for *P. malariae*, it is 18–40 days.
- Prodromal symptoms are more severe with *P. malariae* infections.
- These 'benign' malarias also present with paroxysmal feverish symptoms. In *vivax* and *ovale* malaria infections, the characteristic tertian interval (48-hour interval between fever spikes or fever on alternate days) may be seen. In *P. malariae* infections, the quartan interval (72-hour interval between spikes or fever every third day) may be seen.
- Patients suffering from *vivax* malaria may become anaemic, thrombocytopenic and mildly jaundiced with tender hepatosplenomegaly. Splenic rupture is more common with *vivax* malaria.
- The acute symptoms of *ovale* and *malariae* malarias may be as severe as those of *vivax* infection, but anaemia is less severe and the risk of splenic rupture is lower.
- *P. malariae* infections are associated with gross splenomegaly, but splenic rupture is less common. *P. malariae* causes glomerulonephritis and an immune complex nephropathy resulting in nephrotic syndrome.
- *Vivax* and *ovale* malarias have a persistent hepatic cycle that may give rise to relapses. *P. malariae* does not relapse, but a persisting undetectable parasitaemia may cause repeated exacerbations.
- Occasionally, *vivax* malaria can produce complications similar to those of *falciparum* malaria. This has been increasingly reported from India.

FALCIPARUM MALARIA (MALIGNANT TERTIAN OR SUBTERTIAN MALARIA)

- The incubation period ranges from 7 to 14 days (mean 12 days).
- Prodromal symptoms like malaise, headache, myalgia, anorexia and mild fever may last for several days before the onset of the classical 'malarial paroxysms'.
- In a classical malarial paroxysm, suddenly the patient feels inexplicably cold and apprehensive. Mild shivering follows, which quickly turns into violent shaking with teeth rattling. There is intense peripheral vasoconstriction and goose flesh. The rapid increase in temperature may trigger febrile convulsions. The rigor lasts up to 1 hour. This is followed by a hot flush with throbbing headache, palpitations, tachypnoea, prostration, postural syncope and vomiting. The temperature reaches its peak. Finally, a drenching sweat breaks off and the fever defervesces over the next few hours. The exhausted patient sleeps off. The whole paroxysm lasts about 8–12 hours.
- A high irregularly spiking unremitting fever or daily (quotidian) paroxysm is more commonly seen in *falciparum* malaria than the classically described tertian or subtertian periodicity (48 and 36 hours between fever spikes).
- The patient with *falciparum* malaria usually looks severely ill with 'typhoid' facies.
- The patient is often anaemic and jaundiced with moderate tender enlargement of the spleen and liver.
- Neurological complications of *falciparum* malaria can manifest as acute headache, irritability, agitation, seizures, psychosis and impaired consciousness.

JAUNDICE IN MALARIA

- Occurs due to severe haemolysis and hepatic involvement (malarial hepatopathy).
- The parasite, especially *P. falciparum*, infects a large number of cells that are then destroyed in the spleen, resulting in haemolytic anaemia. This is characterised by elevated serum bilirubin (dominant unconjugated fraction), without any significant elevation of the liver enzymes.
- 'Malarial hepatitis' or malarial hepatopathy:
  - This term is commonly used to describe hepatocytic dysfunction in severe and complicated malaria; however, actual inflammation of the liver parenchyma is almost never seen.
  - Occurs due to sequestration of the parasite-infested red blood cells in the capillaries (due to adherence to endothelial cells as well as rosette formation) and causes clogging of the capillaries in the hepatic microvasculature.
  - Characterised by a rise in serum conjugated bilirubin along with the rise in serum glutamate pyruvate transaminase levels to more than three times the upper limit of normal. Prothrombin time is usually normal.
- Some cases have superimposed hepatitis viral infections (e.g. hepatitis E) to produce jaundice and hepatic function derangement.
- DIC can also contribute to liver dysfunction and haemolysis.

SEVERE MANIFESTATIONS AND COMPLICATIONS OF *FALCIPARUM* MALARIA

- WHO defines complicated *falciparum* malaria as one of the features shown in Table 17.25 along with presence of asexual forms of *P. falciparum* in the peripheral smear. Some patients with *P. vivax* malaria may also develop complicated malaria. Acute renal failure, ARDS and jaundice are uncommon in children.
- Highest risk of complications from malaria is found in non-immune people, children and pregnant females who live in endemic regions.

CEREBRAL MALARIA

- Cerebral malaria is defined as diffuse encephalopathy not attributable to any other cause in a patient with *falciparum* malaria.
- Convulsions occur in both children and adults, but are more common in children.
- Retinal haemorrhages may occur and are associated with a poor prognosis. Papilloedema is rare.
- A variety of transient abnormalities of eye movement, especially dysconjugate gaze, have been noted.
- Fixed jaw closure and tooth grinding (bruxism) are common.
- Pouting may occur or a pout reflex may be elicited by stroking the sides of the mouth.

TABLE 17.25 Criteria for Severe and Complicated Malaria

Complication	Definition
• Cerebral malaria	Impaired consciousness, unarousable coma not attributable to any other cause (coma should persist for at least 30 minutes if seizures occur)
• Repeated generalised convulsions	Two convulsions within 24 hours
• Severe anaemia	Haemoglobin concentration <5 g/dL or haematocrit <15%
• Renal failure	Serum creatinine >3 mg/dL, oliguria
• Respiratory distress	Pulmonary oedema
• Hypoglycaemia	Blood glucose <40 mg/dL
• Circulatory collapse or shock	Systolic BP <90 mmHg, rapid thready pulse
• DIC	Bleeding from different sites of the body
• Acidosis	pH <7.25, lactate >5 mmol/L
• Blackwater fever	Macroscopic haemoglobinuria (cola-coloured urine), acute kidney injury
• Jaundice	Bilirubin >3 mg/dL
• Hyperparasitaemia	>5% of erythrocytes infested by parasites

- The most common neurological signs in adults are those of a symmetrical upper motor neuron lesion. The abdominal reflexes are invariably absent.
- Motor abnormalities like decerebrate rigidity, decorticate rigidity and opisthotonus occur.
- Neuropsychiatric manifestations, cerebellar signs, extrapyramidal syndromes and multiple cranial nerve involvement are common in Indian patients.
- Residual neurological sequelae occur in about 5% of adults and 10% of children. These include hemiplegia, cortical blindness, aphasia and ataxia and occur more frequently in patients with prolonged coma, protracted convulsions, severe anaemia and biphasic clinical course.
- Bad prognostic signs include prolonged impaired consciousness, respiratory failure, renal failure, jaundice and hypoglycaemia.
- The CSF pressure is usually normal. The fluid is clear with less than 10 cells/μL; CSF lactic acid and protein levels are elevated.

ANAEMIA

- Anaemia is common in severe malaria. It is often associated with secondary bacterial infection, retinal haemorrhages and pregnancy. Various causes of anaemia are listed in Box 17.19.

BOX 17.19 Causes of Anaemia in Malaria

- Haemolysis of infected and uninfected erythrocytes
- Dyserythropoiesis
- Splenomegaly causing erythrocyte sequestration and haemodilution
- Depletion of folate stores
- Haemorrhage due to DIC

RENAL FAILURE

- Renal failure or acute kidney injury usually occurs in adults. There is a progressive oliguria eventually leading to anuria. It results from acute tubular necrosis. The serum creatinine and urea levels progressively increase.
- It is usually reversible.

HYPOGLYCAEMIA

- Hypoglycaemia is a frequent complication of *falciparum* malaria. It occurs in three different groups of patients:
  - Patients with severe disease, especially young children.
  - Patients treated with quinine or quinidine.
  - Pregnant females, either on admission or following quinine treatment.
- In malaria, hypoglycaemia can occur due to various mechanisms:
  - Failure of hepatic gluconeogenesis.
  - Increased consumption of glucose by host and parasite.
  - Treatment with quinine or quinidine results in stimulation of pancreas to secrete insulin. The resulting hyperinsulinaemia causes hypoglycaemia.

FLUID, ELECTROLYTE AND ACID–BASE DISTURBANCES

- Hypovolaemia manifests as low jugular venous pressure, postural hypotension, oliguria and high urine specific gravity. This may be accompanied by signs of dehydration.
- Acidotic breathing may be seen in severely ill patients in shock, hypoglycaemia, hyperparasitaemia and renal failure.
- Lactic acidosis is a common complication and both blood and CSF lactic acid levels are elevated.

PULMONARY OEDEMA

- This is a grave complication of severe malaria and it carries a high mortality.
- It may appear several days after treatment for malaria has been started and at a time when the patient's general condition is improving.
- Pulmonary oedema is associated with hyperparasitaemia, renal failure, pregnancy, hypoglycaemia and lactic acidosis.

CIRCULATORY COLLAPSE ('ALGID MALARIA')

- Some patients present in a state of collapse with a systolic blood pressure less than 80 mmHg in the supine position. They have cold, clammy and cyanotic skin, constricted peripheral veins and a rapid feeble pulse.
- This clinical picture is often associated with a complicating Gram-negative septicaemia. Possible sites of infection should be sought—e.g. lung, urinary tract, meninges, IV puncture sites and IV lines.
- Circulatory collapse is also seen in patients with pulmonary oedema, metabolic acidosis, massive gastrointestinal haemorrhage, dehydration and hypovolaemia.

SPONTANEOUS BLEEDING AND DISSEMINATED INTRAVASCULAR COAGULATION

- DIC complicated by clinically significant bleeding occurs commonly in non-immune patients. Clinical manifestations include haematemesis or melaena, bleeding gums, epistaxis, petechiae and subconjunctival haemorrhages.
- Thrombocytopenia is common (but is unrelated to DIC); however, it is usually not associated with bleeding. The platelet count usually returns to normal after successful treatment of the malaria.

HYPERPYREXIA

- This is more common in children and is associated with convulsions, delirium and coma.
- Hyperpyrexia (body temperature >42°C) may cause permanent severe neurological sequelae.

HYPERPARASITAEMIA

- Hyperparasitaemia is associated with severe disease. This is more common in non-immune patients with high parasite densities (>5%).
- In highly endemic areas, patients can tolerate high parasite densities (20%–30%) often without clinical symptoms.

MALARIAL HAEMOGLOBINURIA AND BLACKWATER FEVER

- Malaria haemoglobinuria is uncommon and is usually associated with hyperparasitaemia and/or severe disease. It may or may not be accompanied by renal failure.
- Patients with glucose-6-phosphate dehydrogenase (G6PD) deficiency and some other erythrocyte enzyme deficiencies may develop vascular haemolysis and haemoglobinuria when treated with oxidant drugs such as primaquine.
- Blackwater fever typically occurs in non-immune patients with chronic *falciparum* malaria, taking antimalarials (especially quinine) irregularly. It occurs more commonly in patients with G6PD deficiency. Blackwater fever is accompanied by mild or absent fever, scanty or absent parasitaemia, dark or black urine (due to haemoglobinuria) and acute renal injury. It occurs due to haemolysis of both parasitised and non-parasitised erythrocytes. The condition carries a poor prognosis, but is very rare now.

INVESTIGATIONS

MICROSCOPY

- Diagnosis of malaria rests on the demonstration of asexual forms of the parasites in peripheral blood smears stained with one of the Romanowsky stains (Wright, Field, Leishman or Giemsa). Both thin and thick smears should be examined. Parasites should be counted in relation to the total white cell count (on thick films when the parasitaemia is relatively low) or erythrocytes (on thin films).
- Sometimes, no parasites can be found in peripheral blood smears from patients with malaria even in severe infections. This is explained by partial antimalarial treatment or by sequestration of parasitised cells in deep vascular beds. In these cases, examination of smears of bone marrow aspirate reveals parasites or malaria pigment.
- An alternative and probably more sensitive test than the peripheral smear is the quantitative buffy coat (QBC) analysis. In this test, the centrifuged buffy coat is stained with a fluorochrome (e.g. acridine orange) that 'lights up' malarial parasites when viewed under UV light.

IMMUNODIAGNOSIS

- Malarial antibodies can be deleted by serological techniques like immunofluorescent assay (IFA) or ELISA; however, these tests are not specific and are not done routinely.

OTHER LABORATORY FINDINGS

- A number of simple, sensitive and specific antibody-based rapid diagnostic tests (RDTs) have been developed for identifying parasitic enzymes and proteins. Examples include detection of *P. falciparum*-specific histidine-rich protein-2 (PfHRP-2) and *Plasmodium* lactate dehydrogenase antigens (common to all *Plasmodium* species) in finger prick blood samples. HRP-2 can remain positive up to 2–4 weeks after the parasites disappear from blood. Very high *falciparum* parasitaemia can produce negative results due to the prozone effect. Monitoring parasite clearance and parasitic load is not possible with these immunological methods. There is also some cross-reactivity with rheumatoid factor.
  - If the initial RDT is negative in patients with manifestations compatible with severe malaria, a second RDT should be performed 6–12 hours later, and if negative, malaria is extremely unlikely.
  - RDTs have poor sensitivity for detecting *P. malariae* and *P. ovale*.
- PCR testing for parasite messenger RNA or DNA.
- Normochromic normocytic anaemia, thrombocytopenia and raised ESR.
- Total leucocyte count is low to normal but neutrophil leucocytosis may be seen in severe infections.
- Plasma viscosity and C-reactive protein levels are high.
- Prothrombin time and partial thromboplastin time may be prolonged in severe infections. Antithrombin III levels are reduced.
- In complicated malaria, there may be metabolic acidosis and low plasma concentrations of glucose, sodium, bicarbonate, calcium, magnesium and albumin. Lactate, BUN, creatinine, muscle and liver enzymes, bilirubin and gamma globulin levels may be elevated.
- Neuroimaging in patients with cerebral malaria may demonstrate brain swelling, cortical infarcts and hyperintense areas in white matter.

MANAGEMENT

MANAGEMENT OF UNCOMPLICATED MALARIA

P. vivax Malaria

- Most cases of *vivax* malaria are sensitive to chloroquine. Some may be resistant to sulphadoxine/pyrimethamine.

- Chloroquine is the drug of choice. It is given at a dose of 600 mg base (four tablets) stat, followed by 600 mg base (four tablets) on the second day, followed by 300 mg base (two tablets) on the third day. Chloroquine-resistant *P. vivax* strains are being reported from India.
- If *P. falciparum* is negative using rapid tests or no tests are available, cases showing signs and symptoms of malaria without any other obvious cause for fever should be considered as 'clinical malaria'. These should be treated with chloroquine in full therapeutic dose of 25 mg/kg body weight over 3 days.
- Artemisinin-based combination therapies (ACTs) are as effective as chloroquine in *P. vivax*.

P. falciparum Malaria

- Chloroquine resistance in *falciparum* malaria is common and, therefore, WHO recommends combination therapy for *P. falciparum* malaria.
- In India, chloroquine resistance is high in north-eastern states, Andhra Pradesh, Chhattisgarh, Jharkhand, Madhya Pradesh and Odisha.
- Artemisinin derivatives produce faster relief of clinical symptoms and faster clearance of parasites from the blood than other antimalarial drugs. When used as monotherapy, short half-life of artemisinin derivatives means that patients must take the drug for at least 7 days. Failure to complete the course due to rapid improvement in clinical symptoms can lead to high levels of treatment failure or development of resistance. Therefore, artemisinin derivatives are given with another longer-acting drug. This is known as ACT (artemisin-based combination therapy). These combinations can then be taken for shorter durations than artemisinin alone.
- Various treatment regimens for *P. falciparum* are given in Table 17.26.
- A new drug launched by India is arterolane maleate (150 mg) plus piperaquine phosphate (750 mg), which is effective against *P. falciparum*. Dose is one tablet once a day for 3 days.

TABLE 17.26 Treatment of Uncomplicated *P. falciparum* Malaria

Drugs	Comments
• Artesunate 200 mg + sulphadoxine/pyrimethamine (1500 mg/75 mg) on day 1 and then artesunate 200 mg on days 2 and 3	Recommended under National Malaria Eradication Programme Can be given in second and third trimesters of pregnancy
• Artemether (80 mg) + lumefantrine (480 mg) twice a day for 3 days	Recommended under National Malaria Eradication Programme for the north-eastern region due to resistance to partner drug sulphadoxine–pyrimethamine Can be given in second and third trimesters of pregnancy
• Artesunate + mefloquine (15 mg/kg followed by 10 mg/kg after 8 hours)	Alternate combination Avoid in pregnancy
• Quinine 600 mg TDS for 5 days + sulphadoxine/pyrimethamine (1500 mg/75 mg) on day 3	Can be used during first trimester of pregnancy
• Quinine 600 mg TDS + clindamycin 600 mg BD for 7 days	Safest regimen during first trimester of pregnancy
• Quinine 600 mg TDS for 5 days + doxycycline 100 mg BID for 7 days	Can be used if allergic to sulphadoxine and artesunate Do not use in pregnancy
• Artesunate 200 mg + amodiaquine 600 mg once a day for 3 days	Alternate combination
• Dihydroartemisinin 200 mg + piperaquine 1600 mg once a day for 3 days	Alternate combination

MANAGEMENT OF COMPLICATED *FALCIPARUM* MALARIA

- Maintenance of airway, anticonvulsant therapy and nursing care.
- Control high fever, hypoglycaemia, seizures and anaemia.

Specific Drug Therapy

- Chloroquine:
  - With chloroquine resistance being reported from most parts of India, quinine or artemisinin derivatives are the first-line drug for cerebral malaria. Both are rapidly acting drugs and are combined with slower-acting drugs for complete cure.
- Quinine:
  - Quinine is the drug of choice in the first trimester of pregnancy.
  - Important adverse and toxic effects include hypoglycaemia, hypotension, nausea, vomiting and blindness. Therefore, blood glucose should be monitored.
  - A loading dose of quinine should not be used if the patient has received quinine, quinidine or mefloquine within the preceding 12 hours.
  - There has been decline in response rate over years to quinine. Also, fever clearance takes more time than artemisinin derivatives. In addition, high frequency of adverse effects is seen. Hence, quinine is not preferred by many physicians as a first-line agent.
- Artemisinin derivatives:
  - Derivatives of Chinese drug, qinghaosu.
  - Artesunate or artemether.
  - Clear the parasitaemia rapidly and can be used as first line or after failure of quinine.
  - Patients receiving artemisinin derivatives should get full course of oral ACT. However, ACT containing mefloquine should be avoided in cerebral malaria due to neuropsychiatric complications.
- Other drugs:
  - Use of steroids and mannitol is not recommended.
  - Treatment of cerebral malaria is shown in Table 17.27.

RADICAL CURE OF MALARIA DUE TO *PLASMODIUM VIVAX* AND *PLASMODIUM OVALE*

- Primaquine is given at a dose of 15 mg daily for 14 days. It destroys the hypnozoite phase in the liver.
- Primaquine may cause haemolysis in patients with G6PD deficiency and cyanosis due to the formation of methaemoglobin in red cells. It is also contraindicated in pregnant women and infants.

TABLE 17.27 Antimalarials for Complicated Malaria

Initial Treatment	Treatment After Patient is Able to Tolerate Oral Treatment
• Artesunate: Three doses of 2.4 mg/kg (120 mg in adults) intravenously at 0, 12 and 24 hours and then 2.4 mg/kg once a day (maximum duration 6 days if IV treatment required)	Oral artesunate + sulphadoxine/pyrimethamine *or* Oral artesunate + amodiaquine for 3 days Avoid mefloquine combination
• Artemether 3.2 mg/kg (160 mg in adults) IM followed by 1.6 mg/kg daily (maximum duration 6 days if IV treatment required)	Oral artemether + lumefantrine for 3 days Avoid mefloquine combination
• Quinine: 20 mg/kg in 5% dextrose over 4 hours followed by 10 mg/kg infusion (over 4 hours) every 8 hours starting 8 hours after beginning of initial dose	Oral ACT for 3 days or Oral quinine in a dose of 10 mg/kg three times a day for total course of 7 days plus doxycycline 3 mg/kg/day for 7 days Replace doxycycline with clindamycin (10 mg/kg 12 hourly for 7 days) in pregnant women and children

- In people with G6PD deficiency, consider preventing relapse by giving primaquine base at 0.75 mg/kg once a week for 8 weeks, with close medical supervision for potential primaquine-induced haemolysis.
- In 2018, tafenoquine as a single dose of 300 mg has been approved for radical cure of *P. vivax* infection.

PREVENTION OF TRANSMISSION OF *PLASMODIUM FALCIPARUM*

- None of the drugs used to kill *P. falciparum* is gametocidal and, hence the patient acts as a reservoir for transmission of parasite to mosquito.
- To prevent this, the patient should receive primaquine in a single dose of 45 mg on day 2 of the treatment.

CLASSIFICATION OF RESPONSES TO TREATMENT (Box 17.20)

BOX 17.20 Classification of Responses to Antimalarial Treatment

EARLY TREATMENT FAILURE (ETF)

- Danger signs or severe malaria on day 1, 2 or 3, in the presence of parasitaemia
- Parasitaemia on day 2 higher than on day 0, irrespective of axillary temperature
- Parasitaemia on day 3 with axillary temperature ≥37.5°C
- Parasitaemia on day 3 ≥25% of count on day 0

LATE CLINICAL FAILURE (LCF)

- Danger signs or severe malaria in the presence of parasitaemia on any day between day 4 and day 28 in patients who did not previously meet any of the criteria of early treatment failure
- Presence of parasitaemia on any day between day 4 and day 28 with axillary temperature ≥37.5°C in patients who did not previously meet any of the criteria of early treatment failure

LATE PARASITOLOGICAL FAILURE (LPF)

- Presence of parasitaemia on any day between day 7 and day 28 with axillary temperature <37.5°C in patients who did not previously meet any of the criteria of early treatment failure or late clinical failure

ADEQUATE CLINICAL AND PARASITOLOGICAL RESPONSE (ACPR)

- Absence of parasitaemia on day 28, irrespective of axillary temperature, in patients who did not previously meet any of the criteria of early treatment failure, late clinical failure or late parasitological failure

CHEMOPROPHYLAXIS OF MALARIA

- For short-term chemoprophylaxis (less than 6 weeks), doxycycline in a dose of 100 mg daily. It should be started 2 days before travel and continued for 4 weeks after leaving the malarious area.
- For long-term chemoprophylaxis (more than 6 weeks), mefloquine in a dose of 5 mg/kg (up to 250 mg) weekly. It should be administered 2 weeks before, during and 4 weeks after leaving the area.

MALARIA VACCINE

- The World Health Organization has approved a malaria vaccine RTS,S/AS01 (RTS,S) among children in regions with moderate to high *P. falciparum* malaria transmission.
- RTS,S/AS01 malaria vaccine should be provided in a schedule of four doses in children from 5 months of age for the reduction of malaria disease and burden.
- It produces a significant reduction (30%) in deadly severe malaria.

Q. Describe tropical splenomegaly syndrome (TSS) or hyperreactive malarial splenomegaly (HMS).

- Seen in areas hyperendemic for malaria.

AETIOLOGY

- It is a response to exaggerated immune response to repeated attacks of malaria. There is increased production of IgM antibodies to suppressor ($CD8^+$) T-lymphocytes that leads to increased and uninhibited IgM production by B cells and formation of cryoglobulins and immune complexes. This immunological process stimulates hyperplasia of the reticuloendothelial system resulting in splenomegaly.
- Typically, these patients have only low levels of parasites in the blood.

CLINICAL FEATURES

- Clinical presentation is with massive splenomegaly, hepatomegaly and occasionally low-grade fever.
- Vulnerability to respiratory and skin infections and splenic rupture is increased.

- Some cases may evolve into a malignant lymphoproliferative disorder, particularly CLL.

DIAGNOSIS OF TSS

- High levels of antimalarial antibodies in blood. IgM levels are markedly raised (up to 20 times).
- Anaemia or pancytopaenia due to hypersplenism and volume expansion.
- Light microscopic examination of liver biopsy shows sinusoidal lymphocytosis.
- Immunofluorescence microscopy of liver biopsy shows IgM aggregates phagocytosed by RE cells.
- Malarial parasites may be rarely present in peripheral blood. Parasite nucleic acids can also be detectable by PCR.

DIAGNOSTIC CRITERIA (Box 17.21)

BOX 17.21 Diagnostic Criteria for Hyperreactive Malarial Splenomegaly

- Gross splenomegaly ≥10 cm below costal margin in adults for which no other cause can be found
- Elevated serum IgM level two standard deviations or more above the local mean
- Clinical and immunologic responses to antimalarial therapy
- Regression of splenomegaly by 40% by 6 months after start of therapy
- High antibody levels of *Plasmodium* species (≥1:800)

TREATMENT

- Prolonged administration of antimalarials is required. This removes the antigenic stimulus provided by repeated malarial infection and allows the immune system to return to normal.
  - Proguanil 100 mg daily lifelong or chloroquine 300 mg base every week.
  - Folic acid 5 mg daily.
  - Splenectomy carries an appreciable risk of mortality and so should only be considered in presence of massive splenomegaly unresponsive to medical management.

Q. Discuss about amoebic liver abscess.

Q. How do you differentiate amoebic liver abscess from pyogenic liver abscess?

- Involvement of liver by *E. histolytica* produces amoebic liver abscess. The term amoebic hepatitis is not used at present.

PATHOGENESIS

- The trophozoites of *E. histolytica* are carried as emboli by the radicles of the portal vein from the base of an amoebic ulcer in the large intestine. The capillary system of the liver acts as an efficient filter and holds these parasites. They multiply in large number and cause coagulation necrosis of the liver and abscess formation.
- In majority, the abscess is single and confined to the posterosuperior aspect of the right lobe of the liver. This is because the right lobe receives most of the blood draining the right colon through the 'streaming' effect in portal vein flow.

CLINICAL MANIFESTATIONS

- Acute or insidious onset of fever, sweats, weight loss, chills and rigors. There may be pain in the right hypochondrium resulting from stretching of the liver capsule.
- Diaphragmatic irritation may give rise to referred pain in the right shoulder.
- Clinical examination may reveal enlargement and tenderness of the liver, upward extension of the liver dullness on percussion, point tenderness in the posterolateral portion of a lower right intercostal space (intercostal tenderness) and bulging of the intercostal spaces.

COMPLICATIONS (Box 17.22)

BOX 17.22 Complications of Amoebic Liver Abscess

- Spontaneous external rupture may result in 'granuloma cutis'.
- Direct extension into lung may result in amoebic lung abscess.
- Rupture into a bronchus leads to expectoration of large amounts of the typical 'anchovy sauce' pus.
- Rupture into pleural space may result in massive pleural effusion.
- Left lobe abscess may rupture into pericardium resulting in pericarditis and rarely cardiac tamponade.
- Rupture into peritoneal cavity may result in peritonitis.
- Compression of inferior vena cava producing pedal oedema.
- Hepatic vein or portal vein thrombosis.
- Rarely, metastatic brain abscess, splenic abscess and rupture into stomach.

INVESTIGATIONS

- Polymorphonuclear leucocytosis is a characteristic feature.
- Liver function tests may be abnormal.
  - The most consistent abnormality is an elevation of alkaline phosphatase.
  - The level of SGOT (aspartate aminotransaminase) reflects the severity of the disease.
  - Jaundice is uncommon and when present, implies a grave prognosis.
- Chest radiograph commonly shows raised dome of the diaphragm on the right side. Other findings include right-sided pleural effusion and right basal pneumonitis.
- Ultrasonic scanning of liver is very useful in establishing the diagnosis and localisation of the abscess. The defect in liver usually persists for several months after the complete recovery of the patient.

- Isotope liver scans and computed tomography have better sensitivity than ultrasound.
- Serological tests ('amoebic serology') are positive in more than 90% of the patients.
- Aspiration:
  - Needle aspiration yields the characteristic 'anchovy sauce' or 'chocolate' pus, which consists of liquefied necrotic liver tissue. It is usually thick in consistency, yellow or green in colour and characteristically odourless. The pus does not contain polymorphonuclear leucocytes. As the parasites are localised in the cyst wall, they may be demonstrated in the terminal portion of the aspirate or, at times, by a needle biopsy of the cyst wall.
  - Antigen detection or PCR on liver abscess pus

TREATMENT

- Metronidazole 800 mg thrice daily orally for 7–10 days or tinidazole 2 g daily as a single dose for 5 days is usually effective. Severe cases may require intravenous metronidazole (500 mg 8 hourly).
- Chloroquine may be given at a dose of 300 mg twice daily for 2 days followed by 150 mg twice daily for 19 more days. It is generally given to a patient who does not show adequate response to metronidazole.
- Emetine and dehydroemetine have a direct lethal action on the trophozoites of *E. histolytica*. However, these agents are very toxic and therefore are rarely used at present. Their toxicity includes cardiac arrhythmias, precordial pain, muscle weakness, vomiting and diarrhoea. Dehydroemetine is less toxic than emetine.
- Therapeutic aspiration of the pus may be required with large abscesses (>5 cm), those threatening to burst and when the response to chemotherapy is not prompt.
- After treatment, diloxanide furoate should be given at a dose of 500 mg thrice daily for 10 days to eliminate intestinal luminal cysts.

ROLE OF PERCUTANEOUS DRAINAGE

- This involves placing a large-bore catheter into the abscess. Even multiple abscesses can be drained.
- Percutaneous drainage is generally performed after a therapeutic aspiration has failed and is indicated when:
  - Volume of abscess is large and there is risk of spontaneous rupture (especially left lobe abscesses).
  - Actual rupture has occurred (drainage of both abscess and extraneous collection).
  - There is lack of response to medical therapy after 3–5 days with clinical signs of persistent sepsis or enlarging abscess or persistent symptoms.
  - Abscess with thin rim of hepatic parenchyma (<10 mm) around it.
- Percutaneous catheter drainage is preferred over percutaneous needle aspiration, particularly in larger abscess (>10 cm), subcapsular location or high risk for rupture.

DIFFERENTIATION BETWEEN AMOEBIC AND PYOGENIC LIVER ABSCESSES (Table 17.28)

TABLE 17.28 Differentiation Between Amoebic and Pyogenic Liver Abscesses

Parameter	Amoebic Liver Abscess	Pyogenic Liver Abscess
• History	History of diarrhoea or dysentery	History of diabetes mellitus, diverticulitis, gallstones, colonic cancer
• Onset	More likely to be acute	Subacute
• Age	Younger patients (20–40 years)	Older patients (60–70 years)
• Male:female ratio	10:1	1.5:1
• Leucocytosis with left shift	Usually absent	Usually present
• Serum bilirubin	Normal to mildly elevated	Usually elevated
• Number of abscesses	Often single (80%)	Often multiple (50%)
• Organisms in aspirated pus	*E. histolytica*	Bacteria
• Amoebic serology	Positive	Negative

Q. Write a note on leishmaniasis.

- Leishmaniasis denotes disease caused by any of the number of species of protozoa in the genus *Leishmania*. There are four major clinical syndromes described:
  - Visceral leishmaniasis (kala-azar)—caused by *Leishmania donovani*.
  - Cutaneous leishmaniasis of the Old World—caused by *Leishmania major* and *Leishmania tropica*; cutaneous leishmaniasis of the New World—caused by *Leishmania mexicana* and *Leishmania amazonensis*.
  - Mucocutaneous leishmaniasis (espundia)—caused by *Leishmania braziliensis*.
  - Diffuse cutaneous leishmaniasis—caused by *L. mexicana* and *Leishmania aethiopica*.

Q. Give a brief account of kala-azar or visceral leishmaniasis.

AETIOLOGY

- Kala-azar (visceral leishmaniasis) is a generalised visceral infection by the organism *L. donovani*. It affects the monocytes and macrophages of liver, spleen, bone marrow and lymph nodes.
- The flagellated forms (promastigotes) of the organism develop within the female sandflies (*Phlebotomus argentipes*), which transmits the disease to humans.
- In humans, the organism is seen in the cells of monocyte-macrophage system as oval bodies known as amastigotes (Leishman-Donovan bodies [LD bodies]).

EPIDEMIOLOGY

- Endemic in several countries; of all kala-azar cases, more than 90% are from India, Bangladesh, southern Sudan, Nepal and Brazil.
- Kala-azar is endemic in several parts of India. Most cases occur in the states of Bihar, Jharkhand, West Bengal and eastern parts of Uttar Pradesh.
  - There were three large-scale outbreaks, peaking in 1978, 1992 and 2007.
  - With sustained efforts, number of cases of kala-azar have gradually reduced. In 2021, around 1350 cases of kala-azar were reported with 28 deaths.
  - The aim is to eliminate kala-azar as a public health problem which is defined as incidence <1 per 10,000 population at the subdistrict level.
  - The main components of National Kala-Azar Elimination Programme comprise rapid diagnosis followed by effective treatment, integrated vector management including indoor residual spraying, and systematic disease surveillance under the auspices of the National Vector-Borne Disease Control Programme (NVBDCP).
- Sporadic cases have been reported from several other parts of India.
- HIV-infected patients are predisposed to kala-azar.

CLINICAL FEATURES

- Incubation period is usually 2–6 months, but can range from a few weeks to several years.
- Onset is often insidious although a few patients may have subacute onset.
- Some patients present with a low-grade fever, whereas others present with a high-grade, intermittent fever showing a double rise of temperature in 24 hours ('camel hump fever').
- Anaemia, lymphadenopathy (the latter is more common in patients from West Bengal and rarely seen in patients from Bihar).
- Massive splenomegaly and hepatomegaly.
- Generalised hyperpigmentation, particularly over face, is common (kala-azar means 'black fever').
- In advanced stages, patients develop marked cachexia and oedema.

COMPLICATIONS

- Complications include repeated infections (including tuberculosis and malaria), malnutrition and cancrum oris.

INVESTIGATIONS

- Anaemia, granulocytopenia and thrombocytopenia.
- Low serum albumin and high serum globulin, especially IgG.
- Mild elevation in bilirubin, AST/ALT and alkaline phosphatase.
- Demonstration of amastigotes (LD bodies) in stained smears of aspirates of bone marrow, liver, spleen, lymph nodes or buffy coat of peripheral blood. Bone marrow is positive in 50%–70% of cases while splenic aspirate is positive in 70%–90% of cases.
- Culture of the aspiration in the Novy–MacNeal–Nicolle (NNN) medium for the organism.

IMMUNODIAGNOSTIC TESTS

- These are less invasive and are useful in community surveillance studies.
- The skin test to demonstrate delayed-type hypersensitivity (Leishmanin skin test or Montenegro test) is positive only in patients with cured kala-azar.
- Increased production of immunoglobulins—Napier's aldehyde test and Chopra's antimony test (non-specific).
- Specific antibody detection can be done by several methods. Complement fixation test, indirect haemagglutination test, IFA test and countercurrent immunoelectrophoresis have poor sensitivity and specificity. On the other hand, direct agglutination test (DAT) is a simple, quick, cheap and specific test that can be applied in the field conditions. Another antibody detection test is based on using recombinant K39 antigen-impregnated nitrocellulose strips that has shown excellent results in field setting and can be used on both blood and urine (immune-chromatographic test). The drawback of these tests is that they remain positive for more than 5 years after complete cure of the patient.
- Antigen detection by reverse Western blotting, dot EIA and latex agglutination test.
- DNA detection by PCR.

POST-KALA-AZAR DERMAL LEISHMANIASIS

- Recovery may be followed by post-kala-azar dermal leishmaniasis (PKDL).
- It occurs in about 10% of cases several months or even years after successful treatment of kala-azar.
- In 15%–20% of PKDL cases, no preceding history of kala-azar is available, suggestive of subclinical infection.
- Contributes to spread of infection to sandflies by providing reservoir of infection.
- It presents with hypopigmented macules, papules or nodules. Three types of skin lesions can occur in varying combinations:
  - Erythematous indurated lesions on the butterfly area of face.
  - Multiple symmetrical hypopigmented macules with irregular margins that may coalesce, having generalised distribution to the extremities and trunk.
  - Combination of papules, nodules and plaques.
- Diagnosis is by demonstration of parasite in the slit smear or by culture of the dermal tissue.

TREATMENT

- Blood transfusions to correct anaemia and antibiotics for treatment of intercurrent bacterial infections.

PENTAVALENT ANTIMONIALS

- Pentavalent antimonials (sodium stibogluconate, meglumine) have been the mainstay of antileishmanial therapy for the past several decades. The dose is 20 mg/kg for 40 days. However, a large number of patients fail to respond due to parasitic resistance. Important side effects include myalgias, abdominal pain, abnormalities of liver enzymes, T-wave abnormalities and, in rare cases, death from cardiac causes.

- For PKDL, prolonged treatment for 3–4 months is required.

PENTAMIDINE

- Pentamidine in a dose of 3–4 mg/kg on alternate days for 5–25 weeks was recommended as a second-line drug in patients who failed to respond to antimony. However, its effectiveness has reduced over the years with cure rates of only 70%–80% reported in recent years. Important side effects are hypoglycaemia and induction of diabetes mellitus.

AMPHOTERICIN B

- At present, amphotericin B deoxycholate is recommended either as the primary drug of choice or as a second-line drug in patients unresponsive to antimonials. It is almost 100% curative. Dose is 0.75–1 mg/kg/day given on alternate days for 15–20 doses. Side effects include fever with chills, hypokalaemia and renal impairment. Some of these side effects can be reduced by using lipid preparations of amphotericin B, but these formulations are very costly. These include liposomal amphotericin B, amphotericin B lipid complex and amphotericin B colloidal dispersion.
- Liposomal amphotericin B at a single dose of 10 mg/kg has been shown to be as effective as 15 days of conventional amphotericin B. Under National Kala-Azar Elimination Programme, liposomal amphotericin B in a single dose of 10 mg/kg is recommended as the first-line agent. It may be combined with 7–14 days of oral miltefosine, particularly in patients with underlying HIV infection.

MILTEFOSINE

- Miltefosine has shown excellent results and is the first highly effective, oral drug for treating visceral leishmaniasis as well as PKDL.
- Dose is 50 mg once a day if weight is less than 25 kg and 50 mg twice a day if weight is more than 25 kg. Duration of treatment is 4 weeks.
- Toxic effects include gastrointestinal symptoms such as vomiting and diarrhoea and, occasionally, reversible hepatotoxicity and nephrotoxicity.
- Should not be used in children younger than 2 years, HIV-positive patients, pregnant and lactating women and women of reproductive age who refuse to use contraceptives during the treatment period and 2 months after completion of treatment.

PAROMOMYCIN

- Paromomycin (aminosidine) is a highly effective and safe drug that needs to be given intramuscularly in a dose of 11 mg/kg of base/day for 21 days. It can be combined with miltefosine as recommended under National Kala-Azar Elimination Programme.

TREATMENT OF POST-KALA-AZAR DERMAL LEISHMANIASIS

- Liposomal amphotericin B in a dose of 5 mg/kg per day by infusion two times per week for 3 weeks for a total dose of 30 mg/kg or
- Miltefosine, 100 mg orally per day for 12 weeks or
- Amphotericin B deoxycholate, 1 mg/kg over 4 months for 60–80 doses.

Q. Discuss the aetiology, clinical manifestations, diagnosis and management of toxoplasmosis.

Q. Describe briefly about congenital toxoplasmosis.

- Toxoplasmosis is caused by the protozoan *Toxoplasma gondii* and is a common infection in immunocompromised persons.
- Acute infection is usually asymptomatic, and once acquired, parasites remain in human tissues lifelong.

TRANSMISSION

- Humans are the intermediate hosts while cat is the definitive host.
- Ingestion of oocysts from contaminated soil or bradyzoites from undercooked meat, contaminated vegetables or water.
- Transplacental transmission results in congenital toxoplasmosis.
- Occasionally, blood-borne transmission.

CLINICAL MANIFESTATIONS

INFECTION IN IMMUNOCOMPETENT HOST

- Most often, acute toxoplasmosis is asymptomatic.
- In symptomatic patients, the most common presentation is cervical lymphadenopathy. Some cases have generalised lymph node enlargement, which can persist for several weeks.
- Other features include fever, malaise and myalgias.
- Uncommon features are skin rash and confusion.
- Myocarditis, encephalitis, pneumonia and polymyositis occur rarely.
- Symptoms usually resolve within a few weeks without treatment.

OCULAR INFECTION

- Most cases of ocular involvement (chorioretinitis) occur after congenital infection or in immunocompromised patients, though it can also occur in immunocompetent persons.
- Blurred vision, scotomas, photophobia and eye pain.
- Loss of vision.
- Episodic flare-ups can occur.
- Examination shows grey-white foci of retinal necrosis with adjacent choroiditis, vasculitis, haemorrhage and vitreitis.
- Anterior uveitis may also be seen.

INFECTION IN IMMUNOCOMPROMISED HOST

- The infection in immunosuppressed patients is usually due to reactivation of latent infection.
- Most common involvement is of the CNS.
- Encephalopathy, meningoencephalitis, seizures, headache and focal neurological deficits are common.
- Pneumonitis (presents with fever, dyspnoea with reticulonodular infiltrates on chest radiograph) and ocular involvement are also common.

CONGENITAL TOXOPLASMOSIS

- Cerebral manifestations like hydrocephalus or microcephaly, convulsions, tremors, paralysis.
- Patches of calcification in the brain on radiograph.
- CSF may be xanthochromic with increased protein and mononuclear cells.
- Microphthalmos, nystagmus, chorioretinitis and blindness.
- Hepatomegaly, jaundice, thrombocytopenia and purpura may also occur.
- Demonstration of antitoxoplasma IgA and IgE in cord serum or in serum from the newborn is diagnostic of congenital disease.

DIAGNOSIS

- Minimal lymphocytosis, elevated ESR and mild increase in liver enzymes.
- Antibodies are detectable in the blood. A rise in titre of IgM antibodies indicates acute infection. However, most cases of toxoplasmosis in immunocompromised patients are due to reactivation where there is no rise in IgM antibody. Hence, IgG antibodies are used for presumptive diagnosis.
- PCR for *Toxoplasma* DNA in blood, CSF, aqueous humour and bronchoalveolar lavage.
- Biopsy material from a lymph node may be inoculated into mice or may show characteristic histological changes and any of the three infectious stages: tachyzoites in groups, bradyzoites (tissue cysts) or sporozoites within oocysts.
- *Toxoplasma* encephalitis:
  - CSF may be normal or shows mild increase in cells and protein.
  - IgG antibodies to *Toxoplasma*.
  - Markedly elevated LDH in patients with disseminated toxoplasmosis and pulmonary disease.
  - CT scan of head shows multiple contrast-enhancing ring lesions.
  - MRI is more sensitive than CT scan in picking the lesions.
  - Single-photon emission computed tomography (SPECT) is an important tool for differentiating CNS lymphoma from toxoplasmic encephalitis.

MANAGEMENT

- A combination of sulphadiazine (1 g 6 hourly) and pyrimethamine in a loading dose of 200 mg followed by 50–75 mg daily, both for 4–6 weeks, along with leucovorin. In patients sensitive to sulphonamides, clindamycin or azithromycin can be used.
- Steroids are added for ocular toxoplasmosis.
- If there is definite evidence of foetal infection based on PCR and evidence of intracranial abnormalities on foetal ultrasound, termination of pregnancy should be considered. For others, spiramycin is given if gestation age is <18 weeks, and sulphadiazine–pyrimethamine combination if gestation age is >18 weeks. Ultrasound follow-up should include examination of the foetus every 4 weeks, with a focus on brain, eye and growth assessment.

Q. Write a short note on taeniasis solium and cysticercosis.

Q. Briefly explain neurocysticercosis.

- *Taenia solium*, the pork tapeworm, inhabits the intestinal lumen of humans, its only definitive host. Pigs are the usual intermediate hosts. Humans acquire the infection following eating of undercooked pork containing cysticerci.
- When human tissue is invaded by the larval form, the condition is referred to as cysticercosis. Human cysticercosis results from swallowing of ova shed in the stool of a human tapeworm carrier or gaining access to the human stomach by regurgitation from the person's own adult worm. The larvae are liberated from eggs in the stomach, penetrate the intestinal mucosa and are carried to many parts of the body where they develop and form cysticerci. The common locations are subcutaneous tissue, skeletal muscles, eyes and brain. Humans with cysticercosis are intermediate or dead-end hosts.
- Ingestion of infected pork causes only adult tapeworm infestation because infected pork contains the larval cysts that develop into adult worms in human intestine but does not contain the eggs that cause cysticercosis.

CLINICAL FEATURES

- Presence of adult worm in the intestine is generally asymptomatic. Some may have nausea, anorexia, epigastric pain or urticaria.
- In cysticercosis, superficially placed cysts may be palpable under the skin or mucosa as pea-like ovoid bodies.
- The dead larvae may invoke marked tissue response with muscular pain, weakness, fever and eosinophilia.
- Neurocysticercosis results from brain cysts. It may manifest as meningoencephalitis, epilepsy, personality changes, staggering gait, space-occupying lesion, stroke (due to inflammatory changes in the wall of intracranial arteries located in the vicinity of cysticerci) or hydrocephalus.

DIAGNOSIS

- Eggs and proglottids in stool. Eggs are round with a double-walled, radially striated membrane and measure 30–40 μm.

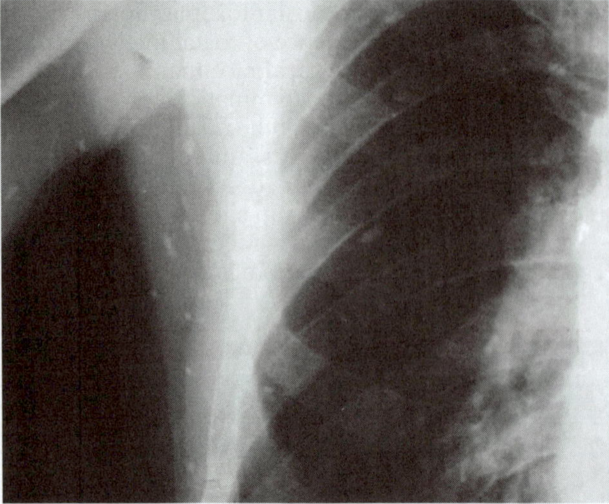

Fig. 17.21 Chest radiograph shows 'rice-grain' calcifications over the right hemithorax and proximal arm.

- ELISA for the detection of *T. solium* antigens in stools.
- Soft tissue radiographs may show calcified cysts (cigar-shaped or rice-grain calcification) in muscles (Fig. 17.21).
- CT scan of the brain may show calcified spots, solid nodules, cystic lesions containing a scolex or hydrocephalus.
- CT scan is more sensitive than MRI in identifying calcified lesions, while MRI is better for identifying cystic lesions and enhancement.
- CSF shows mononuclear pleocytosis and presence of eosinophils.
- In CSF and blood, specific enzyme-linked immunoelectrodiffusion transfer blot (EITB) using lentil lectin-purified glycoproteins is highly sensitive and specific.
- Histological examination of the excised subcutaneous nodule can establish a specific diagnosis.

TREATMENT

- For removal of the adult worm in the intestine, niclosamide (2 g as a single dose), praziquantel (PZQ) (10 mg/kg as a single dose) or albendazole may be used.
- Neurocysticercosis should be treated on the following lines:
    - Albendazole 15 mg/kg/day in two divided doses for 2 weeks is the drug of choice for one to two cysts.
    - If the number of cysts is >2, PZQ can be used orally in a dose of 50 mg/kg/day in three divided doses for 10–14 days along with albendazole. Efficacy of a single-day course of 50 mg/kg is good in patients with a single cyst or low cyst burdens, but it is less efficacious in those with heavier cyst burdens.
    - Prednisolone 10 mg 8 hourly is given for 14 days, starting 1 day before the albendazole or PZQ.
    - Antiepileptic drugs should be given until the reaction in the brain has subsided.
    - Operative intervention may be required for internal hydrocephalus.

Q. Discuss briefly about hydatid disease.

- Hydatid disease is a tissue infection of humans caused by the larval stage of *Echinococcus granulosus*. Canines (especially dogs) are the definitive hosts for *E. granulosus*. Sheep and cattle are the common intermediate hosts. Hence, this form of disease has its highest incidence in countries where sheep and cattle raising is carried out and population of dogs is high. Humans are infected accidentally.
- The adult *E. granulosus* is a small worm measuring 5 mm in length that resides in the jejunum of canines for 5–20 months. In addition to the scolex and neck, it has three proglottides. The gravid segment splits to release eggs that are ingested by an appropriate intermediate host. The embryos escape from the eggs, penetrate the intestinal mucosa and enter the portal circulation. Most are filtered out by the liver and lungs, but some escape into general circulation to involve brain, kidney and other tissues. Those larvae develop into hydatid cysts. When the hydatid cyst is ingested by a canine, the life cycle is complete.
- The hydatid cysts are unilocular, fluid-filled, distended cysts with an external pericyst, a middle laminated layer and an internal germinal layer. Brood capsules and second- and third-generation daughter cysts develop from the germinal layer. 'Hydatid sand' found in the cyst consists of scolices liberated from the ruptured brood capsules. The hydatid fluid is highly antigenic.
- Alveolar hydatid disease caused by *Echinococcus multilocularis* is extremely rare in India. Cure is possible only with early detection and complete surgical excision.

CLINICAL FEATURES

- Humans may ingest the eggs while handling a dog or drinking contaminated water. Usually, a latent period of 5–20 years occurs before diagnosis.
- In 75% of the patients with hydatid disease, the right lobe of the liver is involved and it contains a single cyst. These hepatic lesions often present as palpable masses or abdominal pain.
    - Obstruction of bile duct may result in obstructive jaundice.
    - Intrabiliary extrusion of calcified hepatic cysts can present with recurrent cholecystitis.
    - Rupture of a hydatid into the bile duct, peritoneal cavity, lung, pleura or bronchus may produce fever, pruritus, urticarial rash or an anaphylactoid reaction that may be fatal.
- A pulmonary hydatid may rupture producing cough, chest pain or haemoptysis. Pleural rupture can cause pneumothorax, pleural effusion or empyema. Secondary bacterial infection of the cyst can manifest as a pulmonary abscess.
- CNS involvement may produce epilepsy or blindness.
- The disease can rarely involve heart, kidneys, spleen, ovary and thyroid.

DIAGNOSIS

- Routine radiographs may pick up hydatid cysts. Pulmonary lesions are seen as round, irregular masses of uniform density. The 'meniscus sign' or 'crescent sign' is characterised by the presence of air between the pericyst and the laminated membrane (Fig. 17.22). The 'water lily sign' represents an endocyst floating in a partially fluid-filled cyst (Fig. 17.23). Occasionally, a chest radiograph may show smooth rim of calcified hepatic cyst.
- CT scan and ultrasonography can detect the hydatid lesions by showing scolices and daughter cysts.
- The skin test (Casoni's test) may be positive (not routinely available).
- Complement fixation, immunofluorescent tests and ELISA to detect antibodies are positive in 70%–90% of cases.

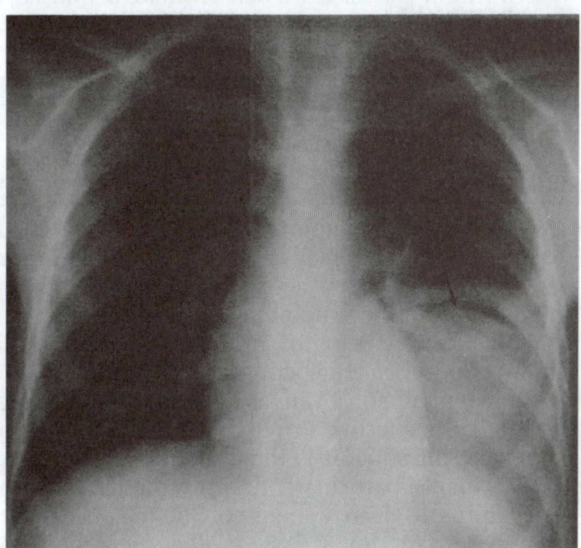

Fig. 17.22 Meniscus sign.

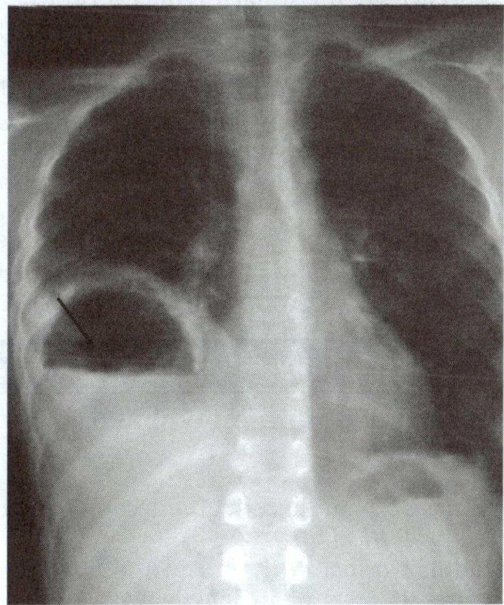

Fig. 17.23 'Water lily' sign.

- Specific echinococcal antigens by immunoblot assays for confirmation (rarely required).
- Percutaneous aspiration may rarely be required to confirm the diagnosis by demonstrating the presence of protoscolices, hooklets or hydatid membranes. The risk of complications is very low.

TREATMENT

- Surgical excision of the cysts is the treatment of choice for some types of cysts (e.g. cysts >10 cm, ruptured cyst, cysts with biliary fistulae, cysts compressing vital structures, cysts with secondary infection or haemorrhage and cysts with many daughter vesicles)
- In inoperable cases, albendazole (7.5 mg/kg twice daily) should be given for 1–3 months.
- In selected cases, *p*ercutaneous puncture, *a*spiration, *i*njection of scolicidal agents (e.g. 95% ethanol or hypertonic saline) and *r*easpiration (PAIR) can be done. It is followed by albendazole treatment for 1 month.

Q. Write a short note on enterobiasis, pinworm infection or threadworm infection.

- Enterobiasis is an intestinal infection of humans caused by *Enterobius vermicularis*. The adult female averages 10 mm in length and the male 3 mm. They are seen in the caecum, appendix and the adjacent parts of the colon. The gravid female migrates through the anal canal at night, deposits her eggs on the perianal skin and dies. As many as 15,000 eggs may be laid in one night. These eggs are ingested and the larvae are released in the small intestine. The larvae migrate down the bowel lumen to reach the caecum and develop into adult worms.

CLINICAL FEATURES

- Humans are usually infected by the direct transfer of eggs from the anus to the mouth by way of contaminated fingers. 'Retroinfection' occurs when the eggs hatch in the perianal area and the larvae migrate back into the bowel lumen.
- The most common symptom is perianal itching (pruritus ani), especially at night, being related to the migration of the gravid female. Secondary bacterial infections can result if excoriation is severe
- Other symptoms include irritability, insomnia and enuresis.
- Occasionally, the worm burden is so high that patient may get abdominal pain, nausea and vomiting.
- Migration of adult worm into the female genital tract may result in vaginal discharge, salpingitis and endometritis.

DIAGNOSIS

- Directly visualising the worms in the perineal area.
- Stool examination for eggs (positive in only 5%–10% of cases). Eggs are flattened on one side, giving them a characteristic 'bean-shaped' appearance.

- 'Cellophane tape test':
  - This test consists of touching cellophane tape to the perianal area several times, removing it and examining the tape under direct microscopy for eggs.
  - The test should be conducted right after awakening on at least three consecutive days.
  - This technique can increase the sensitivity to roughly 90%.

TREATMENT

- Two highly satisfactory drugs are available. Pyrantel pamoate given in an oral dose of 11 mg/kg is the treatment of choice. It is repeated once after 2 weeks. Alternatively, a single oral dose of mebendazole 100 mg or albendazole 400 mg may also be given; both are repeated once after 2 weeks.
- Where infection constantly recurs in a family, each member should be treated with mebendazole 100 mg twice daily for 3 days and repeated after 2 weeks. During this period, all night clothes and bed linen are laundered and fingernails must be scrubbed before meals.

Q. What are soil-transmitted helminth infections?

Q. Give a brief account of ascariasis or roundworm infection.

- Helminths transmitted through contaminated soil are known as soil-transmitted helminths (STH). These include:
  - *Ascaris lumbricoides*.
  - *Trichuris trichiura*.
  - *Ancylostoma duodenale* and *Necator americanus*.
  - *Strongyloides stercoralis*.
- Ascariasis is an infection of humans caused by *A. lumbricoides*. The pale yellow worm is 20–35 cm long.
- Humans are infected by eating food contaminated with mature ova which hatch in the duodenum to release the larvae. The larvae migrate through the wall and are carried by bloodstream or lymphatics to the lungs. From the lungs, the larvae ascend the bronchial tree, trachea and epiglottis and are swallowed. These then mature in the small intestine to become adult worms.

CLINICAL FEATURES

- *Ascaris* bronchopneumonia characterised by fever, cough, dyspnoea, wheeze, eosinophilic leucocytosis and migratory pulmonary infiltrates may occur during the stage of larval migration through the lungs (Loffler's syndrome).
- The adult worm may be vomited or passed in the stool.
- Heavy infections may be associated with abdominal pain and malabsorption of fat, protein, carbohydrate and vitamins.
- Bolus of worms may result in volvulus, intussusception or intestinal obstruction.
- The adult worms may migrate into appendix, bile ducts or pancreatic ducts, causing appendicitis, cholangitis, liver abscess or pancreatitis.

DIAGNOSIS

- During larval migration through the lungs, chest radiograph may reveal patchy pulmonary infiltrates.
- Diagnosis is by demonstrating typical eggs in the stools either on direct examination or following concentration techniques. The eggs are oval-shaped. The fertilised eggs have a bile-stained albuminous mammillated coat while unfertilised eggs lack this coat.
- In heavily infected patients, large collections of worms may be detectable on plain radiograph of the abdomen as a mass which produces contrast against the gas in the bowel ('whirlpool' effect).
- CT may demonstrate worms in the bowel. Imaging the worm in cross-section demonstrates a 'bull's-eye' appearance.
- Ultrasonography for demonstration of hepatobiliary or pancreatic ascariasis. In some cases, the worms demonstrate curling movements.

TREATMENT

- *Ascaris* bronchopneumonia is treated symptomatically. Severe cases may require steroids. However, *Strongyloides* infection needs to be excluded by sputum and stool examination as administration of steroids in the setting of *Strongyloides* infection can induce *Strongyloides* hyperinfection syndrome.
- Pyrantel pamoate given as a single oral dose of 11 mg/kg is effective in removing the adult worms from the intestine. It is the drug of choice in pregnant patients, particularly in first trimester.
- Mebendazole given at a dose of 500 mg once or 100 mg twice daily for 3 days or albendazole 400 mg (one dose) is also effective.
- The older agent, piperazine citrate is a bit less effective and slightly more toxic. It may still be useful for cases in which intestinal or biliary obstruction is suspected since the drug paralyses worms, aiding expulsion.
- For intestinal obstruction, a conservative dual strategy of 'starve worms, hydrate patient' is followed by keeping the affected patient nil orally and giving intravenous fluid to avoid dehydration. Additional use of hypertonic saline enema may facilitate disentanglement of worms. Once bowel motility is restored, anthelminthic therapy should be administered.

Q. Describe briefly about trichuriasis.

Q. Write a short note on whipworm infection.

- Trichuriasis is an intestinal infection of humans caused by *T, trichiura*.
- The adult worms are found in the large intestine. They are 30–50 mm in length, with anterior two-thirds as a thread and posterior one-third as stouter,

giving them a whip-like appearance ('whipworm'). The female produces the eggs that are passed in the stool. The eggs must incubate at least 3 weeks in the soil before they become infective. The ingested eggs hatch in the small intestine and release the larvae. The larvae migrate to the large intestine (mostly caecum) where they mature into adult worms.

CLINICAL FEATURES

- Petechiae are seen at worm attachment sites in the intestine. On an average, the patient loses 0.005 mL blood/worm/day.
- Most infections are asymptomatic.
- The clinical manifestations include growth retardation, persistent diarrhoea, anaemia and abdominal pain. Nocturnal diarrhoea is common.
- *Trichuris* dysentery syndrome is a more serious manifestation of heavy whipworm infection resulting in chronic dysentery and rectal prolapse. Triad of rectal prolapse, clubbing of fingers and chronic diarrhoea is considered pathognomonic of trichuriasis in endemic areas.

DIAGNOSIS

- Diagnosis is by demonstration of eggs in stools. The eggs have a characteristic barrel shape with smooth thick wall and a hyaline plug at each end.
- Proctoscopy or colonoscopy can frequently demonstrate adult worms protruding from the bowel mucosa.

TREATMENT

- Mebendazole given at a dose of 100 mg twice daily for 3 days or albendazole 400 mg once a day for 3 days is the treatment of choice. The dose may have to be repeated in patients with heavy infections.

Q. Describe ancylostomiasis or hookworm disease.

- Hookworm disease is a symptomatic infection caused by *A. duodenale* or *N. americanus*. It is one of the main causes of anaemia in the tropics.
- *A. duodenale* or Old World hookworm is found in Europe, Africa, China, Japan, India and the Pacific islands. *N. americanus* or New World hookworm is found in Americas and the Caribbean.
- *A. duodenale* adult worms are about 1 cm long and inhabit the upper part of the human small intestine where they attach to the mucosa by means of the mouth parts and suck blood. Each adult extracts about 0.15–0.5 mL blood daily. The adults migrate within the small intestine and each site of attachment persists temporarily as a bleeding point. Following fertilisation, the female liberates about 20,000 eggs/day that are passed in the stool.
- *N. americanus* is smaller in size, deposits fewer eggs and sucks less blood (0.03 mL/worm/day).
- The life cycles of the hookworms are similar. The eggs in the soil develop into rhabditiform larvae and later filariform larvae that penetrate the skin to enter vessels that carry them to the lungs. Approximately 8 to 21 days following infection, the larvae leave the alveolar capillaries, enter the alveoli, ascend the respiratory tree, enter the pharynx and are swallowed. In the intestine, they develop into adult worms.

CLINICAL FEATURES

- Itching dermatitis ('ground itch dermatitis') occurs at the site of entry of the larvae. The lesions are maximum on the feet, particularly between the toes. Less often, serpiginous tracks of intracutaneous larval migration can be seen.
- The larval migration through the lungs is usually asymptomatic but may cause cough with blood-tinged sputum, fever and patchy pulmonary consolidation.
- A variety of gastrointestinal symptoms are common. These include vague epigastric discomfort or typical ulcer pain, abdominal distension, pica, vomiting, and small, frequent loose stools.
- The major clinical manifestations of hookworm disease are those of iron-deficiency anaemia and hypoalbuminaemia consequent to chronic intestinal blood loss.
- Young children often have extreme anaemia, with cardiac insufficiency and anasarca.
- Older children may show retarded physical, mental and sexual development.
- In adults, there may be lassitude, dyspnoea, palpitation, tachycardia, constipation and pallor of skin and mucous membranes.

DIAGNOSIS

- The characteristic eggs can be demonstrated in the stool by microscopic examination. The eggs of both worms are 60–70 μm in length and bounded by an ovoid transparent hyaline membrane; they contain two to eight cell divisions.
- The stools seldom contain gross blood but tests for occult blood are usually positive.
- A peripheral blood eosinophilia as high as 70%–80% may be seen in some cases.
- Haemoglobin level is usually low and anaemia is characteristically hypochromic and microcytic.
- Hypoalbuminaemia is a common finding in severe disease.
- PCR test to detect DNA of hookworm is a highly sensitive test.

TREATMENT

- Improvement of nutrition with a high-protein diet.
- Anaemia should be treated with oral iron or blood transfusions. Mild anaemia usually responds to oral iron therapy. Severe anaemia is often associated with anasarca and this should be treated carefully with blood transfusions.
- The drugs currently favoured for the treatment of hookworms are mebendazole, albendazole and pyrantel pamoate. Mebendazole is given at a dose of

100 mg twice daily for 3 days. Albendazole requires a single dose of 400 mg. Pyrantel pamoate is given as a single oral dose of 11 mg/kg. Confirm eradication with follow-up stool examination 2 weeks after discontinuation of the treatment. Ivermectin has poor efficacy against hookworm and is not recommended.

Q. Explain briefly about cutaneous larva migrans (creeping eruption).

- Cutaneous larva migrans are creeping eruptions caused by the filariform larvae of *Ancylostoma braziliense* and *Ancylostoma caninum* whose eggs are found in dog and cat faeces. *S. stercoralis* may also produce creeping eruptions known as larva currens (reflecting fast movement of *Strongyloides* larva).
- It is endemic in Caribbean islands, Africa, South America, South East Asia and coastal parts of India.
- The larvae that are present in soil penetrate the intact skin to enter the epidermis The larvae lack collagenase necessary to break through the basement membrane, though occasionally, larvae may enter the subcutaneous tissue. In the skin, they cause multiple, intensely pruritic, serpiginous reddish-brown tracks that progress forwards (Fig. 17.24). At the anterior end of the eruption, the larva is present and a bleb may form.
- The main affected areas are the dorsum and sole of the feet, buttocks, pelvic waist, legs and shoulders.
- Dermoscopy may show translucent, brown, structureless areas corresponding to the larval bodies, and red-dotted vessels corresponding to an empty burrow.
- Infestation is usually self-limited that can persist for a few days to months, but rarely for years.
- Loeffler's syndrome (transient migratory pulmonary infiltrates, peripheral blood eosinophilia and sputum eosinophilia) is observed in some cases of larva migrans.

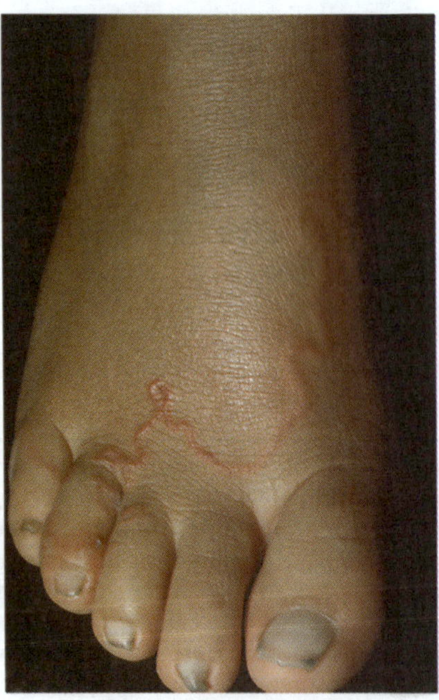

Fig. 17.24 Cutaneous larva migrans.

TREATMENT

- Ivermectin is the drug of choice. Dose is 150–200 μg/kg for 1 or 2 days.
- Alternative drug is albendazole (400 mg once a day for 3 days).
- Local application of 15% thiabendazole cream for 7 days is as effective as ivermectin.
- Antihistamines may be of value in intense itching.

Q. Discuss the clinical features, diagnosis and treatment of strongyloidiasis.

- Strongyloidiasis is an intestinal infection of humans caused by *S. stercoralis*.
- The adult worms are tiny and measure 2 mm in length. They reside in the upper part of jejunum. The adult female lays eggs in the mucosa of jejunum. The eggs hatch and release the rhabditiform larvae, which are passed in the stools. In the soil, the rhabditiform larvae develop into the infective filariform larvae. The filariform larvae penetrate the skin of humans and are carried by bloodstream to the lungs. In the lungs, they ascend the respiratory tree, enter the pharynx and are swallowed. On reaching the jejunum, these larvae mature into the adult worms. This cycle is known as the direct host–soil–host cycle.
- In the indirect cycle, the rhabditiform larvae develop into free-living adult worms that reside in the soil. These free-living adults reproduce sexually to produce filariform larvae that initiate a new human cycle.
- In the autoinfection cycle, the rhabditiform larvae develop into filariform larvae before they are passed in the stool. They may then invade the intestinal mucosa (internal autoinfection) or perianal skin (external autoinfection) of the same host without first going through a soil phase.
- In HIV infection, patients taking corticosteroids, or patients with an immunocompromising condition, autoinfection can lead to tremendously increased number of worms ('hyperinfection').

CLINICAL FEATURES

- The larval migration through skin may produce itchy rashes (ground itch).
- The larval migration through lungs may produce cough, dyspnoea, haemoptysis and bronchospasm.
- The adult worms in the intestine may produce abdominal pain, bloating, diarrhoea or constipation, steatorrhoea and weight loss.
- Autoinfection may cause urticarial wheals across abdomen and buttocks (larva currens).
- *Strongyloides* hyperinfection occurs when patients chronically infected with *S. stercoralis* become immunosuppressed, or if immunosuppressed patients develop autoinfection. The clinical features are attributable to increased larval migration within the organs normally involved in the autoinfection cycle (i.e. GIT, lungs and skin).
- When hyperinfection involves organs and tissues outside those in the autoinfection cycle, it is called

disseminated strongyloidiasis. The infection may involve liver, pancreas, kidneys, muscles, heart and brain. Bacterial and fungal infections often occur because of leakage of gut flora from the bowel damaged by moving larvae. The enteric bacteria are also carried by invasive larvae on their outer surfaces that can result in sepsis, meningitis and pneumonia.

DIAGNOSIS

- Stool examination for larvae (at least three samples).
- Eosinophilia in some patients.
- Examination of duodenal aspirate for larvae.
- ELISA for detecting IgG antibody to filariform larvae of *S. stercoralis*.
- In patients with disseminated infection, stool, sputum and blood examination for larvae. Blood cultures should be done to exclude sepsis.

TREATMENT

- The drug of choice is ivermectin (200 μg/kg/day) for 2 days. In immunocompromised patients, the course is repeated after 2 weeks.
- An alternative but less effective drug is albendazole, given orally at a dose of 400 mg twice daily for 7 days.
- In disseminated systemic infections, both ivermectin and albendazole should be given and continued until stool or sputum samples are negative for 2 weeks. Broad-spectrum antibiotics to cover Gram-negative bacteria should also be given.

Q. Describe briefly about lymphatic filariasis and bancroftian filariasis.

- Filariasis is a group of disorders caused by infection with thread-like nematodes belonging to the family *Filariidae*. They invade lymphatics, and subcutaneous and deep tissues of humans. Filariasis includes the following conditions:
  - Lymphatic filariasis caused by *Wuchereria bancrofti* and *Brugia malayi*.
  - Loiasis caused by *Loa loa*.
  - Onchocerciasis (river blindness) caused by *Onchocerca volvulus*.

LYMPHATIC FILARIASIS

PATHOGENESIS

- Lymphatic filariasis is caused by *W. bancrofti* (bancroftian filariasis) and *B. malayi*. In India, 99.4% of infections are caused by *W. bancrofti* and rest by *B. malayi*.
- These nematodes are conveyed to humans by the bites of infected mosquitoes of a number of different species, the most common being *Culex fatigans* in *W. bancrofti* infection and *Mansonioides* in *B. malayi* infections.
- The adult worms live in the lymphatics of humans. The females produce microfilariae that circulate in large numbers in the peripheral blood at night. In the mosquito, the ingested microfilariae develop into infective larvae.
- In humans, the microfilariae are present chiefly in the capillaries of the lungs and cause pulmonary eosinophilia. The presence of adult worms in the lymphatics causes allergic lymphangitis. Recurrent episodes of allergic lymphangitis lead to intermittent lymphatic obstruction (obliterative lymphangitis) and transient lymphoedema, which may later become permanent in the leg (elephantiasis), arm, genitalia or breast. Increased lymphatic pressure may cause retrograde flow of lymph or rupture of lymphatics causing chyluria, chylous ascites and chylous pleural effusion.
- Filarial nematodes contain endosymbiotic bacteria, *Wolbachia*. These are essential in worm fertility and survival. Doxycycline depletes *Wolbachia* from the worms and leads to long-term worm sterility and macrofilaricidal activity.

CLINICAL FEATURES

Acute Manifestations

Acute Dermato-Adeno-Lymphangitis (ADLA)

- It occurs in both early and late stages of the disease progression.
- Associated with fever and chills.
- Affected area, usually in the extremities, is extremely painful, warm, red, swollen and tender.
- Draining lymph nodes in the groin or axilla become swollen and tender.
- There may be lymphangitis, lymphadenitis, cellulitis or abscess.
- Entry of bacteria through the lesions of the affected parts responsible.
- Recurrent attacks are responsible for persistence and progression of lymphoedema leading to elephantiasis.

Acute Filarial Lymphangitis

- It is caused by immune response to spontaneous or drug-induced (diethylcarbamazine [DEC]) destruction of adult worms.
- Presents with sudden onset of fever and painful lymphadenopathy. Retrograde lymphangitis (spread of inflammation distally from the lymph node) is frequently observed. It manifests as pain, tenderness and erythema along the course of inflamed lymphatics.
- The inguinal lymph nodes may become enlarged, painful and tender.
- Acute inflammation generally resolves in 4–7 days. Recurrences typically occur one to four times per year.

Acute Epididymo-Orchitis and Funiculitis

- Characterised by severe pain, tenderness and swelling of scrotum, usually with fever and rigor.
- Testes, epididymis or the spermatic cord may become swollen and extremely tender.
- Also precipitated by secondary infections.

Tropical Pulmonary Eosinophilia

- Discussed on page 958.

Chronic Stage

- Characterised by permanent lymphoedema ('elephantiasis') of legs, scrotal oedema, hydrocele, chylous ascites, chylous pleural effusion and chyluria.
- In early disease, pitting oedema develops. However, later, chronic inflammation leads to brawny, nonpitting oedema.

INVESTIGATIONS

- In the early stages of lymphangitis, there may be peripheral blood eosinophilia. Microfilariae are not seen in the peripheral blood.
- By about 1 year from the time of infection, microfilariae can be demonstrated in the peripheral blood at night (10 PM to 2 AM).
- Microfilariae are usually present in the hydrocele fluid that may occasionally contain an adult worm.
- 'DEC provocation test' involves the administration of 100 mg DEC (diethylcarbamazine) that usually produces positive blood specimens within 30–60 minutes.
- Calcified filariae may sometimes be demonstrable by radiography.
- Serological tests demonstrating antibodies against filarial antigens are non-specific.
- Circulating filarial antigen detection by ELISA or immunochromatic method is highly sensitive and specific for *W. bancrofti*.
- PCR for DNA detection.
- Radionuclide lymphoscintigraphy to detect widespread lymphatic abnormalities.
- High-frequency ultrasound in conjunction with Doppler techniques may result in the identification of motile adult worms within dilated lymphatics. Live adult worms have a distinctive pattern of continuous motion within the lymphatic vessels described as 'filarial dance sign'.

TREATMENT

- DEC 6 mg/kg as a single dose except in tropical pulmonary eosinophilia where the dose is 6 mg/kg in three divided doses for 12–21 days. It kills microfilariae and adult worms.
- Ivermectin is effective in killing microfilariae but not the adult worms. However, it is useful in patients with concomitant onchocerciasis as DEC is contraindicated in such patients due to the potential for severe adverse events related to killing of *O. volvulus* microfilariae in the eye. DEC is administered a month after ivermectin.
- Doxycycline 200 mg/day for 4 weeks plus ivermectin as a single dose (200 μg/kg).
- Antihistamines and corticosteroids may be necessary to control allergic phenomena.
- Surgery may be of use in established elephantiasis.

CONTROL

- Mass drug administration of DEC 6 mg/kg as single dose along with 400 mg of albendazole once in a year in highly endemic areas.
- Administration of triple drug combination (DEC, albendazole and ivermectin) started in some districts of India since 2018 as triple drug combination and is superior to double drug combination.

Q. Give a brief account of tropical pulmonary eosinophilia.

- This represents an atypical host response to various filariae including *W. bancrofti* and *B. malayi*. It is caused by an immune hyper-responsiveness to microfilariae trapped in the lungs. When the microfilariae are destroyed in lung microcirculation, the antigens are released which initiate an immediate IgE-mediated reaction. The eosinophilic inflammatory reaction, over time, progresses to granuloma formation and fibrosis. In children, there may be marked enlargement of lymph nodes and spleen (Meyers–Kouwenaar syndrome), whereas in adults, cough, nocturnal bronchospasm and miliary pulmonary infiltrates are seen (Weingarten's syndrome or tropical pulmonary eosinophilia).
- Can progress to interstitial fibrosis.

DIAGNOSIS

- History of prolonged residence in an endemic area.
- Lack of microfilariae in the peripheral blood despite repeated examinations.
- Peripheral blood eosinophilia in excess of 3000/μL.
- High titres of filarial antibodies.
- IgE levels of at least 1000 units/mL.
- Chest radiograph shows diffuse interstitial lesions and/or military opacities (usually most prominent in the lower lung fields).
- Pulmonary function tests typically demonstrate a predominantly restrictive pattern together with mild to moderate airway obstruction.
- Bronchoalveolar lavage reveals an intense eosinophilic alveolitis.

TREATMENT

- Therapeutic response to DEC occurs within 7–10 days of initiating therapy (the drug is continued for 2–3 weeks).
- Corticosteroids are sometimes used to reduce inflammation. Strongyloidiasis should be ruled out before starting corticosteroids due to the risk of dissemination of infection.
- Bronchodilators are required for initial few days to weeks for bronchospasm.

Q. Write a short note on gonorrhoea. (DR 10.10)

Q. What is acute gonococcal urethritis? (DR 10.10)

- Gonorrhoea, a sexually transmitted disease (STD), is due to the Gram-negative diplococcus, *Neisseria gonorrhoeae*, which infects columnar epithelium of urethra, endocervix, rectum, pharynx and conjunctivae.
- Although it usually remains localised to initial sites of infection, it can ascend to genital tract to cause

pelvic inflammatory disease (PID) in females and epididymo-orchitis and prostatitis in males. Dissemination can result in bacteraemia.
- Transmission is by genital–genital, genital–anorectal, orogenital or oroanal contact or by mother-to-child transmission at birth.
- Gonococcal infection increases the risk of sexually transmitted HIV infection.

CLINICAL FEATURES

- In men, predominant presentation is of acute urethritis ('clap'). Incubation period is 2–7 days following exposure. Symptoms are urethral discharge and dysuria. On examination, there may be mucopurulent urethral discharge which may be accompanied by erythema of the urethral meatus.
- In women, symptoms relate to endocervical and urethral infection and include increased or altered vaginal discharge, intermenstrual bleeding, dysuria and menorrhagia.
- Asymptomatic genital tract infection occurs up to 50% of women.
- Rectal and pharyngeal infections are usually asymptomatic.
- Gonococcal bacteraemia (disseminated gonococcaemia) on uncommon and presents with skin lesions (mainly on extremities), fever, arthralgia, acute arthritis and tenosynovitis. Skin lesions initially appear as small vesicles that subsequently become pustules and develop a haemorrhagic base. Gonococcal arthritis is asymmetric and migratory. Some patients may develop purulent arthritis. Uncommon manifestations are endocarditis, myopericarditis, meningitis and osteomyelitis.
- Acute perihepatitis (Fitz–Hugh–Curtis syndrome) is a rare complication of PID and is thought to occur through direct extension of *N. gonorrhoeae* from fallopian tube to liver capsule and peritoneum along the paracolic gutters. Patients present with sharp, pleuritic right upper quadrant pain.
- In neonates, perinatal transmission of gonorrhoea may produce ophthalmia neonatorum. If left untreated, it can lead to severe eye complications or disseminated infection.

DIAGNOSIS

- Sterile pyuria—i.e. leucocyturia that accompanies a negative urine culture report.
- Gram stain and culture of urethral, genital, rectal, pharyngeal or ocular secretions.
  - When collecting specimens in males with urethritis, any discharge present at the meatus can be easily recovered for examination. If no discharge is present at the meatus, urethral material must be recovered by inserting and rotating a small swab 2–3 cm into the urethra.
  - Nucleic acid amplification tests (NAATs) are generally more sensitive than culture. They can be used on urine samples and on swabs from endocervix, urethra, rectum and pharynx.
  - Antigen detection by fluorescein-conjugated monoclonal antibodies and direct fluorescence microscopy.
  - Enzyme-linked immunoassays for the detection of gonococcal antigen.
  - Blood cultures in disseminated disease.

TREATMENT

- Penicillin, tetracycline, ampicillin and quinolone resistance is quite frequent and hence, should not be used to treat gonococcal infections.
- One of the following regimens is recommended at present:
  - Ceftriaxone[a] 500 mg intramuscularly (single dose)—preferred drug.
  - Cefixime[a] 400 mg orally (single dose). However, it has a lower response rate compared with ceftriaxone when used for non-genital sites.
  - Spectinomycin 2 g intramuscularly (single dose).
- If quinolone and azithromycin resistance is not a problem:
  - Ciprofloxacin 500 mg orally (single dose).
  - Ofloxacin 400 mg orally (single dose).
  - Levofloxacin 250 mg orally (single dose).
  - Azithromycin 2 g orally (single dose).
- For epididymo-orchitis and pelvic inflammatory disease, doxycycline 100 mg twice daily for 14 days along with one dose of ceftriaxone or ciprofloxacin.
- For disseminated gonococcal infection, ceftriaxone 1 g once a day or cefotaxime 1 g every 8 hours or spectinomycin 2 g every 12 hours for 7 days.
- Coinfection with *Chlamydia trachomatis* is common in young, heterosexual patients with gonorrhoea. Treatment for gonorrhoea should routinely be accompanied by effective treatment for *Chlamydia* infection (azithromycin 1 g as a single dose or doxycycline 100 mg twice a day for 7 days).

Q. Discuss clinical features and treatment of chancroid. (DR 10.6, DR 10.8)

Q. Explain briefly about bubo.

- Chancroid or soft chancre is an acute sexually transmitted infection characterised by painful genital ulcerations associated with inflammatory inguinal adenopathy. The responsible organism is *Haemophilus ducreyi*.
- Coinfection with *Treponema pallidum* and Herpes simplex in 10% of cases.

CLINICAL FEATURES

- Incubation period is usually 3–10 days.
- A small inflammatory papule appears on the external genitalia which ulcerates within 2–3 days to give rise to the chancroidal ulcer. The classic chancroidal

[a]Due to increasing resistance, may be combined with doxycycline 100 mg BID for 7 days.

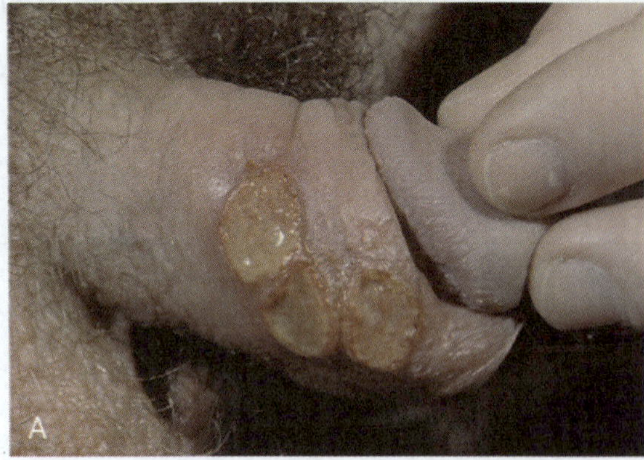

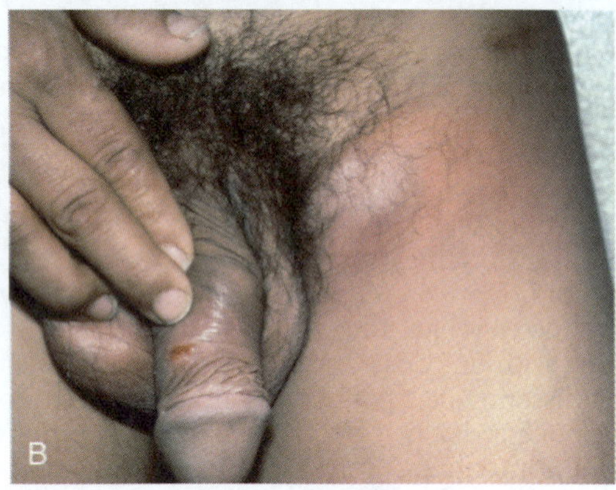

Fig. 17.25 (A) Chancroid ulcer. (B) Chancroid ulcer on penis with left inguinal bubo.

ulcer is superficial. The edge is ragged and undermined. The ulcer base is covered by a necrotic exudate (Fig. 17.25A). Chancroidal ulcer is painful and not indurated.

- In men, most lesions involve the prepuce, corona or glans penis. In women, labia, vaginal introitus and perianal areas are most commonly affected.
- Acute, painful, tender, inflammatory inguinal adenopathy occurs (usually unilateral). The involved nodes become matted, forming a unilocular suppurative bubo (Fig. 17.25B). The overlying skin may rupture forming a single deep ulcer.
- Women may present with more subtle symptoms such as dysuria, vaginal discharge or dyspareunia.
- Constitutional symptoms such as fever or rash are usually absent.
- Diagnosis is based on the isolation of *H. ducreyi* from an ulcer or bubo which appear as Gram-negative, slender rod or coccobacillus in a chain, the so-called 'school of fish' pattern.

TREATMENT

- Resistance to chloramphenicol, tetracyclines, ampicillin and sulphonamides is common.
- Effective regimens include:
  - Ceftriaxone 250 mg intramuscularly as a single dose.
  - Azithromycin 1 g as a single dose.
  - Ciprofloxacin 500 mg twice a day for 3 days.
- Lymphadenitis usually takes about 2 weeks to resolve. Repeated needle aspiration with or without incision and drainage may be required if fluctuant lymphadenitis does not resolve.
- Sex partners of patients with chancroid should be examined and treated regardless of whether symptoms of the disease are present, if they had sexual contact with the patient during the 10 days preceding the patient's onset of symptoms.

Q. What are the various infections produced by *Chlamydia*?

Q. Write a short note on lymphogranuloma venereum (LGV). (DR 10.6, DR 10.8)

- Most of the infections caused by *C. trachomatis* infection are sexually transmitted.

CLINICAL FEATURES

- Majority are asymptomatic.
- Trachoma.
- Urethritis, epididymitis, prostatitis, cervicitis and salpingitis.
- Untreated infection can cause infertility in women and reactive arthritis in both sexes.
- Most women with *C. trachomatis* infection are typically asymptomatic; they are therefore more likely to develop complications from undiagnosed *Chlamydia* infection such as PID, infertility or ectopic pregnancy.
- Lymphogranuloma venereum (LGV) is a typical manifestation of *C. trachomatis* (L1, L2, and L3 serovars).
  - Primary genital lesion occurs from 3 days to 3 weeks after exposure. It is small, painless vesicle or non-indurated ulcer or papule located on the external genitalia. These lesions heal within a few days. These ulcers are often missed due to their small size and lack of pain.
  - Inguinal syndrome is characterised by painful inguinal lymphadenopathy beginning 2–6 weeks after presumed exposure. The inguinal lymphadenopathy is usually unilateral. The nodes are initially discrete that later become matted, fluctuant and suppurative. The overlying skin becomes fixed, inflamed and thinned. Finally, multiple draining fistulae develop. Extensive enlargement of inguinal lymph nodes above and below the inguinal ligament can occur ('groove sign of Greenblatt') (Fig. 17.26).
  - Anorectal involvement produces symptoms of proctocolitis with rectal discharge, anal pain, constipation, fever and/or tenesmus.
  - Constitutional symptoms include fever, chills, headache, anorexia, meningismus, myalgias and arthralgias.

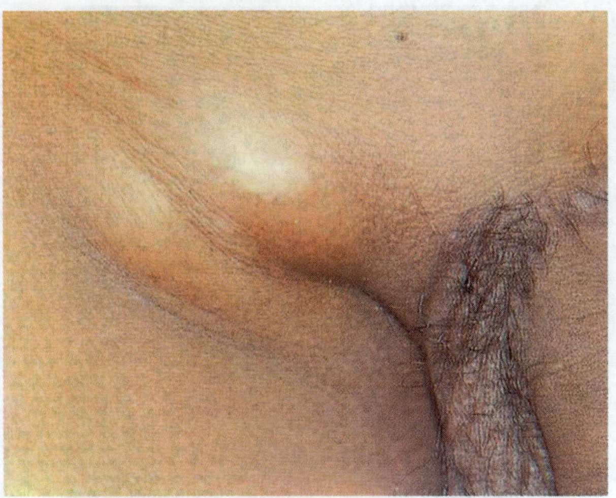

Fig. 17.26 Lymphogranuloma venereum—'groove sign'.

DIAGNOSIS

- Isolation of the LGV strain of *Chlamydia* from aspirated bubo pus, rectum, urethra, endocervix or from other infected tissue.
- Frei skin test is of little value.
- Serological tests (e.g. microimmunofluorescence test and complement fixation test) to detect antibodies.
- Direct immunofluorescent antibody test to identify antigens associated with the bacteria in the smear.
- Nucleic acid probes and PCR to detect antigens.

TREATMENT

- Azithromycin 1 g as a single dose or doxycycline 100 mg BID for 7 days.
- For LGV, doxycycline 100 mg BID for 3 weeks or azithromycin 1 g once a week for 3 weeks or erythromycin 500 mg QID for 3 weeks.
- Fluctuant buboes should be aspirated with a syringe and needle.

Q. Discuss granuloma inguinale (donovanosis). (DR 10.6, DR 10.8)

- Granuloma inguinale is a genital ulcerative disease caused by the intracellular Gram-negative bacterium *Klebsiella granulomatis* (previously known as *Calymmatobacterium granulomatis*).

CLINICAL FEATURES

- Incubation period is 7–90 days.
- Presents as painless, progressive ulcerative lesions without regional lymphadenopathy.
- The lesions are highly vascular ('beefy red appearance') and bleed easily on contact. However, the clinical presentation can also include hypertrophic, necrotic or sclerotic variants.
- The causative organism is difficult to culture and diagnosis requires visualisation of dark-staining Donovan bodies on tissue crush preparation or biopsy using Wright stain.

TREATMENT

- Treatment stops the progression of lesions, although prolonged therapy may be required to permit granulation and re-epithelialisation of the ulcers.
- Treatment with antibiotics is required for at least 3 weeks. Effective regimens include:
  - Doxycycline 100 mg orally twice a day.
  - Trimethoprim-sulphamethoxazole one double-strength (800 mg/160 mg) tablet orally twice a day.
  - Ciprofloxacin 750 mg orally twice a day.
  - Erythromycin base 500 mg orally four times a day.
  - Azithromycin 1 g orally once per week.

Q. Give a brief account of syphilis. (DR 10.1, DR 10.3, DR 10.4)

Q. Describe condylomata lata, mucous patches and snail track ulcers.

- Syphilis is a chronic systemic infection caused by spirochete *T pallidum* and is usually sexually transmitted. Most cases are acquired by sexual contact with infectious lesions—i.e. the chancre, mucous patch, skin rash or condylomata lata. It may spread by kissing or touching a person who has active lesions on the lips, oral cavity, breasts or genitals. It may be transmitted through other non-sexual modes also—i.e. blood transfusion or infection in utero.
- *T. pallidum* can rapidly penetrate intact mucous membranes or abraded skin. Within a few hours, the organism enters the lymphatics and bloodstream to produce systemic infection. The primary lesion appears at the site of inoculation. The generalised parenchymal, constitutional and mucocutaneous manifestations of secondary syphilis usually appear about 6–8 weeks after healing of the chancre.

CLASSIFICATION (Table 17.29)

TABLE 17.29 Syphilis: Classification

Acquired Syphilis	Congenital Syphilis
• Primary syphilis	• Early
• Secondary syphilis	• Late
• Latent syphilis	• Stigmata
• Late syphilis (tertiary, quaternary)	

PRIMARY SYPHILIS

- The median incubation period before the chancre appears is 21 days (range 3–90 days).
- Primary chancre begins as a single painless papule that rapidly becomes an ulcerated and indurated lesion ('hard chancre'). The chancre is usually located on the penis in heterosexual males (Fig. 17.27). In homosexual males, it may be seen in the anal canal,

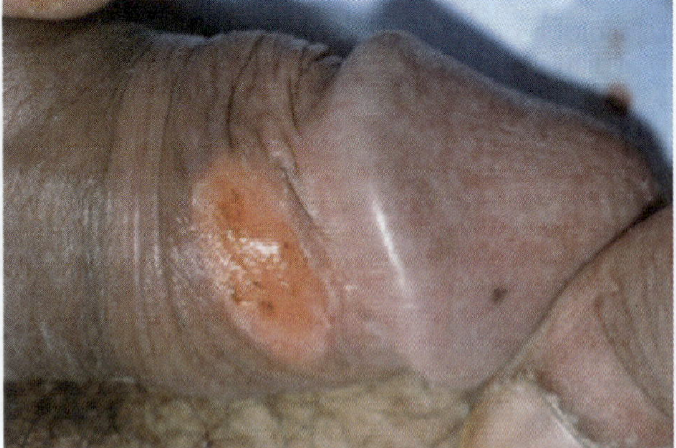

Fig. 17.27 Primary chancre of syphilis. (From: James WD, Berger TG, Elston DM: Andrews' Diseases of the Skin: Clinical Dermatology, Philadelphia, Elsevier, 2006)

rectum or within the mouth. In females, the common primary sites are the cervix and the labia.

- Regional lymphadenopathy usually accompanies the primary lesion, appearing within 1 week of the onset of the lesion. The nodes are firm, rubbery, non-suppurative, painless and non-tender. External genital and anal chancres produce bilateral inguinal lymphadenopathy. Chancres of cervix and vagina result in iliac or perirectal adenopathy.
- The primary chancre usually heals within 4–6 weeks (even without treatment), but the lymphadenopathy may persist for months.
- Primary syphilis in HIV-positive patients is often symptomless and these patients frequently present with secondary or latent infection.

SECONDARY SYPHILIS

- Secondary syphilis develops 6–8 weeks after the appearance of the primary chancre. It starts with symptoms of generalised infection like malaise, headache and low-grade fever. The four cardinal signs of secondary syphilis are:
  - Skin rashes (75%).
  - Generalised lymphadenopathy (50%).
  - Condylomata lata (10%).
  - Mucous patches (30%).
- Skin rashes start as macular lesions on the trunk and proximal limbs, progressing to a generalised papular rash (Fig. 17.28). These lesions may progress to necrotic ulcers which frequently involve the palms and soles.
- Generalised, firm, non-tender lymphadenopathy occurs in about 50% of cases. Involvement of epitrochlear lymph nodes is common.
- In warm, moist, intertriginous areas including the perianal area, vulva, scrotum and inner thighs, papules enlarge and become eroded to produce broad, moist, pink or grey-white highly infectious lesions called condylomata lata (Fig. 17.29).
- Mucous patches occur on the lips, oral mucosa, tongue, palate, pharynx, vulva, vagina or glans penis. The typical mucous patch is a superficial mucosal erosion surrounded by a red serpiginous periphery and is usually painless (Fig. 17.30). Sometimes they may coalesce to form 'snail track' ulcers.

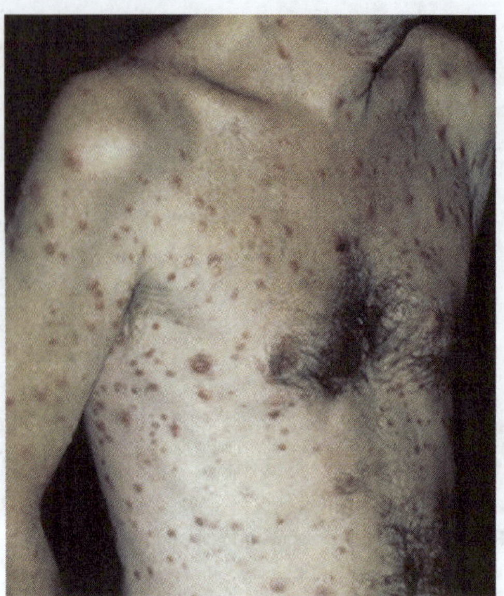

Fig. 17.28 Skin rash in secondary syphilis.

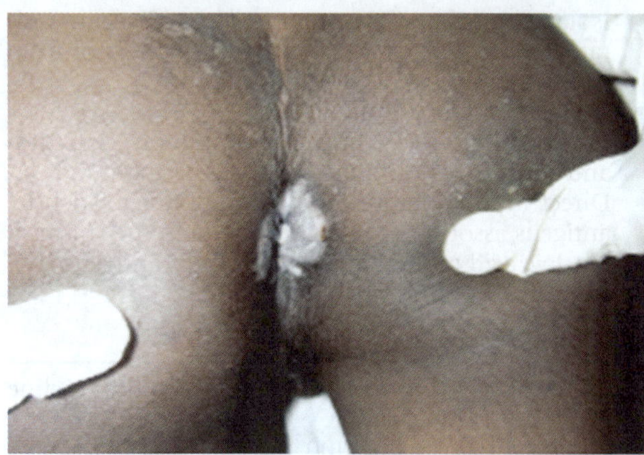

Fig. 17.29 Typical perianal greyish-white plaque (condylomata lata) in secondary syphilis.

- 'Moth-eaten' alopecia is occasionally seen and may involve scalp, eyebrows or beard.
- Other less common manifestations of secondary syphilis include meningitis, hepatitis, nephropathy (proteinuria, nephrotic syndrome or haemorrhagic glomerulonephritis), gastrointestinal involvement, ocular involvement (anterior uveitis, choroiditis, interstitial keratitis, retinal vasculitis, retinitis, optic neuritis, dacryoadenitis or scleritis), arthritis and periostitis.
- After several months, the secondary syphilis resolves to be followed by a latent period.

LATENT SYPHILIS

- 'Early latent' syphilis encompasses the first year after infection (according to the Centers for Disease Control and Prevention [CDC]) or first 2 years after infection

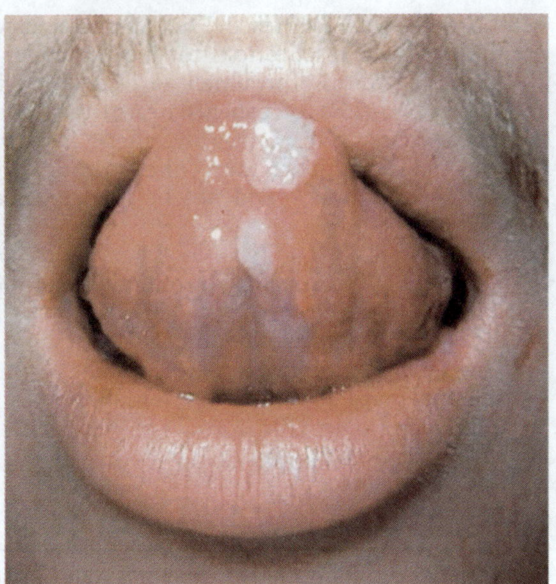

Fig. 17.30 Mucous patches of secondary syphilis.

(according to the World Health Organization [WHO]), while 'late latent' syphilis begins at the first year after infection (according to CDC) or >2 years after infection (according to WHO). A diagnosis of latent syphilis is established based on:

- Positive specific treponemal antibody test for syphilis.
- Normal CSF examination.
- Absence of clinical manifestations of syphilis on physical examination and chest film.
- History of primary or secondary lesions.
- History of exposure to syphilis.

- Patients with early latent syphilis may have transmitted *T. pallidum* to their sexual partners through lesions that were recently active but are no longer present. Patients with late latent disease are not considered infectious to their recent sexual contacts.
- Pregnant females with latent syphilis may infect the foetus in utero up to 4 years after infection.
- About 70% of untreated patients never develop features of late syphilis; rest 30% of cases go on to develop late syphilis.

LATE SYPHILIS

ASYMPTOMATIC LATE NEUROSYPHILIS

- The patient does not have any symptoms or signs.
- The CSF shows mononuclear pleocytosis and increased protein.
- Venereal Disease Research Laboratory (VDRL) test is positive.
- Patients are at risk of developing symptomatic neurosyphilis and therefore, this condition requires treatment.

TERTIARY (BENIGN GUMMATOUS) SYPHILIS

- This takes 10 or more years to develop and affects skin, subcutaneous tissues, mucous membranes, submucosa, liver, spleen and bones, causing organomegaly and infiltrative or destructive lesions, as well as perforation of affected structures. The characteristic feature is a granulomatous lesion called a gumma.

QUATERNARY SYPHILIS

- Quaternary syphilis includes cardiovascular syphilis and neurosyphilis.
- The manifestations of cardiovascular syphilis (e.g. aortitis) are discussed under 'Diseases of the Cardiovascular System' and of neurosyphilis (e.g. meningovascular syphilis and tabes dorsalis) under 'Diseases of the Nervous System'.

CONGENITAL SYPHILIS

EARLY CONGENITAL SYPHILIS

- Manifestations appear within the first 2 years of life, most often between 2 and 10 weeks of age. They resemble features of secondary syphilis.
- Rhinitis with blood-stained mucous or 'snuffles'.
- Mucocutaneous lesions including bullae, vesicles, mucous patches and condylomata lata.
- Bone involvement in the form of osteochondritis, osteitis and periostitis. Parrot pseudoparalysis occurs due to painful epiphysitis causing reluctance to move. Abnormal long-bone radiographs are common. Abnormalities are usually bilateral, symmetric and polyostotic; femur, humerus and tibia are the most frequently involved bones. Hepatosplenomegaly, generalised lymphadenopathy, anaemia, jaundice and thrombocytopenia are the important symptoms of early congenital syphilis.

LATE CONGENITAL SYPHILIS

- Occurs after 2 years of age.
- Remains subclinical in 50%–60% of cases.
- Manifestations are related to scarring or persistent inflammation from early infection and are characterised by gumma formation in various tissues.
- Various stigmata of congenital syphilis are present (Box 17.23). Hutchinson teeth (centrally notched, widely spaced upper central incisors—Fig. 17.31), interstitial keratitis and sensorineural hearing loss are known as Hutchinson triad.
- Cardiovascular involvement is rare.

BOX 17.23 Stigmata of Congenital Syphilis

• Hutchinson's teeth	• Interstitial keratitis
• Mulberry molars (extra cusps on first molars)	• Clutton's joints (painless arthritis of the knees)
• Frontal bossing	• Sensorineural deafness
• Saddle nose	• Neurosyphilis
• Destruction of palate	• Gummatous periostitis
• Sabre chin (anterior tibial bowing)	• Rhagades (perioral fissures)

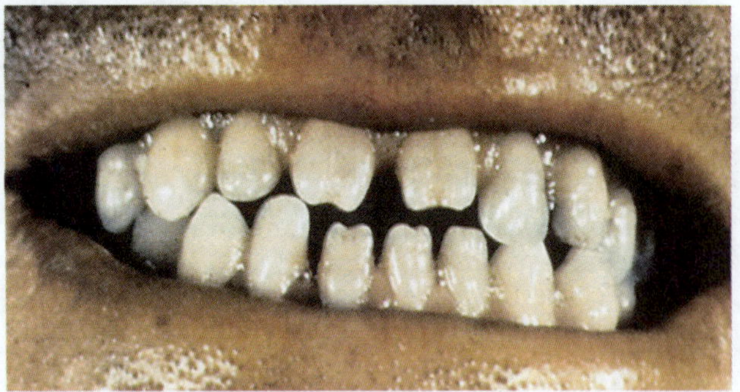

Fig. 17.31 Congenital syphilis—Hutchinson teeth.

DIAGNOSIS

- In primary and secondary stages, *T. pallidum* may be demonstrable in the infectious lesions by dark-field microscopy that shows a drifting rotary motion (corkscrew).
- Direct fluorescent antibody *T. pallidum* (DFA-TP) test can detect *T. pallidum* in fixed smears prepared from suspect lesions.
- Demonstration of *T. pallidum* in tissues by appropriate stains.

SEROLOGICAL TESTS

Non-treponemal Tests

- Used for screening.
- Measure both IgG and IgM antiphospholipid antibodies formed by the host in response to lipoidal material released by damaged host cells and lipid from the cell surfaces of the treponeme itself.
- Non-treponemal test antibody titres usually correlate with disease activity and results should be reported quantitatively. A four-fold change in titre is considered necessary to demonstrate a clinically significant difference between two non-treponemal test results that were obtained using the same serological test.
- Non-treponemal tests usually become non-reactive with time after treatment; however, in some patients (e.g. HIV positive), these antibodies can persist at a low titre for a long period of time.
- A nontreponemal serological test should be obtained just before initiating therapy (ideally, on the first day of treatment) to establish the pretreatment titre. This test is critical to establishing the adequacy of posttreatment serological response. A four-fold decline in the non-treponemal titre is considered to be an acceptable response to syphilis therapy.
- False positives may occur due to pregnancy and autoimmune disorders.
- The tests are:
  - VDRL test.
  - Rapid plasma reagin (RPR) test.

Treponemal Tests

- Used for confirmation. However, newer versions of these tests have become cheaper, and are easy to perform. As a result, these tests are increasingly used as an initial screening test for syphilis rather than as confirmatory tests. A positive result is then confirmed with a non-treponemal test (reverse screening).
- Most patients who have reactive treponemal tests will continue to have reactive tests for the remainder of their lives regardless of treatment or disease activity. However, 15%–25% of patients treated during the primary stage revert to non-reactive after 2–3 years.
- Treponemal test antibody titres correlate poorly with disease activity and should not be used to assess treatment response.
- Various tests are:
  - Fluorescent treponemal antibody-absorption (FTA-ABS) test.
  - *T. pallidum* haemagglutination (TPHA) test.
  - *T. pallidum* immobilisation (TPI) test.
  - Microhaemagglutination test for antibodies to *T. pallidum* (MHA-TP).
  - Immunocapture assay.

MANAGEMENT (Table 17.30)

- In primary, secondary and early latent syphilis, penicillin-allergic patients should receive tetracycline or doxycycline for 2 weeks. In late latent, gummatous and cardiovascular syphilis, these drugs should be given for 4 weeks. Another option is penicillin desensitisation.
- Ceftriaxone may also be used in a dose of 1–2 g once a day for 10–14 days. Azithromycin in a single dose of 2 g is also effective except in men having sex with men and during pregnancy.
- Patients with gummatous or cardiovascular syphilis should have a CSF examination prior to initiation of therapy to exclude neurosyphilis.
- A four-fold decrease in non-treponemal titres at 3–6 months is considered a satisfactory treatment response in all stages of syphilis.

TABLE 17.30 Syphilis: Management

Stage	Drug	Regimen
• Primary	Procaine penicillin	600,000 units IM once daily for 12 days
	Tetracycline	500 mg orally four times daily for 14 days
	Doxycycline	100 mg orally two times daily for 14 days
	Benzathine penicillin	2.4 million units IM single dose (1.2 million units in each buttock)
• Secondary	Procaine penicillin	600,000 units IM once daily for 14 days
	Benzathine penicillin	2.4 million units IM single dose
• Early latent	Benzathine penicillin	2.4 million units IM single dose
• Late latent/ tertiary	Benzathine penicillin	2.4 million units IM weekly for 3 weeks
• Cardiovascular	Benzathine penicillin	2.4 million units IM weekly for 3 weeks
• Neurosyphilis	Crystalline penicillin	18–24 million units/day for 10–14 days
	Procaine penicillin *plus* Probenecid	2.4 million units/day IM for 10–14 day *plus* 500 mg QID for 10–14 days

- For neurosyphilis, follow-up should include lumbar puncture with CSF evaluation repeated every 6 months until the cell count is normal. If the cell count has not decreased after 6 months, retreatment should be considered.

JARISCH–HERXHEIMER REACTION

- The Jarisch–Herxheimer reaction occurs most often among patients who have early syphilis.
- Develops due to massive release of endotoxins and cytokines.
- It is an acute febrile reaction frequently accompanied by headache, myalgia and other symptoms that usually occurs within the first 24 hours after any therapy for syphilis. Uncommon manifestations include meningitis, respiratory distress, renal dysfunction, hepatic dysfunction, mental status changes, stroke and seizures.
- It may induce early labour or cause foetal distress in pregnant females. This concern should not prevent or delay therapy.
- NSAIDs and other antipyretics may be used to control the reaction but they have not been proven to prevent it.

Q. Give a differential diagnosis of genital ulcers. (DR 10.9)

- Various causes of genital ulcers include the following:
  - Herpes simplex virus types 1 and 2
  - *T. pallidum* (causative agent for syphilis)
  - *C. trachomatis* (causative agent for LGV)
  - *H. ducreyi* (causative agent for chancroid)
  - *K. granulomatis* (causative organism for donovanosis)
  - HIV infection (uncommon)
  - Behçet syndrome
- Table 17.31 gives the differential diagnosis of infectious causes of genital ulcers.

Q. Tabulate the recommendations on adult immunisation.

- Table 17.32 gives recommendations on adult immunisation.

TABLE 17.31 Infectious Causes of Genital Ulcers

Condition	Incubation Period	Type of Ulcer	Presence of Pain	Inguinal Lymphadenopathy
Herpes simplex	2–7 days	Multiple small, grouped vesicles coalescing and forming shallow ulcers	Painful	Mild, tender bilateral
Syphilis	3–90 days	Indurated, smooth borders, relatively clean base; often single; usually heals spontaneously	Most often painless	Firm, rubbery, discrete nodes; not tender
Lymphogranuloma venereum	3–21 days	Small and shallow ulcers; usually not seen as they heal rapidly; associated proctocolitis with fistulas and strictures	Painless	Tender lymph nodes; painful; groove sign; often bilateral
Chancroid	3–10 days	Multiple, irregular, ulcers with exudative base; not indurated	Painful	Painful, suppurative, inguinal lymph nodes in 50% of cases; usually unilateral
Donovanosis	7–90 days	Beefy red, bleeding ulcers	Painless	No

TABLE 17.32 Recommendations on Adult Immunisation

Vaccine	Schedule	Comments
Hepatitis A	• Hepatitis A vaccine: 0, 6–12 months • Combined hepatitis A and B vaccine: 0, 1 and 6 months	• Indicated in high-risk conditions, e.g. persons with chronic liver disease or those infected with other hepatitis viruses, men who have sex with men, persons who use illegal drugs and food handlers
Hepatitis B	• Hepatitis B vaccine: 0, 1 and 6 months	• Recombinant vaccine • Postexposure: Adults with percutaneous or mucosal exposure to blood and patients with sexual exposure • Pre-exposure: Adults at high risk (intravenous drug users, household contacts of persons with chronic hepatitis B virus infection, inmates and staff of institutions with long-term care facilities); persons at risk for occupational exposure to HBV (such as dialysis staff, laboratory staff dealing with blood samples, blood bank staff, doctors and nurses working in emergency and intensive care units, operation theatres); patients with HIV infection, chronic liver disease, chronic kidney disease; patients with diseases where multiple blood transfusions are required such as haemophilia, aplastic anaemia, leukaemia

Continued

TABLE 17.32 Recommendations on Adult Immunisation—cont'd

Vaccine	Schedule	Comments
Pneumococcal	• Polysaccharide pneumococcal vaccine (PPV-23)—single dose; revaccination after 5 years • Pneumococcal conjugate vaccine (PCV-13)—one dose only	• Conflicting evidence whether PPV-23 can prevent pneumococcal non-bacteraemic pneumonia • PPV-23 covers 23 strains while PCV-13 covers 13 strains • PPV-23 and PCV-13 approved for immunocompetent persons older than 65 years • PPV-23 and PCV-13 also for persons younger than 65 years with CKD, HIV, cancer, CSF leak, asplenia or splenectomy; those on steroid and immunosuppressants • PPV-23 only (not PCV-13) in persons younger than 65 years who have chronic cardiac or pulmonary disease (including asthma), chronic liver disease, alcoholism or diabetes, or who smoke cigarettes • Persons older than 65 years who never received pneumococcal vaccine should receive one dose of PCV-13 followed by one dose of PPV-23 1 year later • Persons older than 65 years who had already received one dose of PPV-23 should receive one dose of PCV-13 at least 1 year after the last dose of PPV-23 • PPV-23 should be given every 5 years
Influenza	• Trivalent and quadrivalent, killed vaccine, one dose intramuscularly every year (should contain prevalent strains)	• All adults older than 50 years of age • Otherwise in high-risk persons, e.g. those with COPD, CKD, cardiac or liver diseases, diabetes, haematological diseases, pregnancy, healthcare personnel
Meningococcal	• Quadrivalent vaccine (contains antigens A, C, Y and W135) • Bivalent vaccine (contains antigens A and C) • Single dose during outbreaks; two doses 2 months apart for others	• During outbreaks to be given to healthcare workers, laboratory workers and close contacts of cases • Also given to Haj pilgrims, military recruits • Persons with splenectomy, terminal complement component deficiency, HIV
Rabies	• Pre-exposure: three doses at 0, 7 and 28 days • See 'Rabies' for postexposure schedule • Available as both intradermal and intramuscular vaccines	• High-risk persons, e.g. veterinarians, laboratory personnel working with rabies virus, medical and paramedical personnel treating rabies patients, dog catchers, forest staff, zookeepers
HPVs	• Age group 9–14 years: Two doses at an interval of 6 months • Age >15 years: Three doses at 0, 1 and 6 months	• To reduce incidence of cervical carcinoma, for both males and females between the ages of 9 and 26 years
Tetanus, diphtheria and pertussis	• For children older than 6 years: Acellular pertussis vaccine (DTaP) • For those older than 10 years: Tetanus toxoid, reduced diphtheria toxoid and acellular pertussis vaccine (Tdap) • For adults: Tetanus toxoid and reduced diphtheria toxoid (Td) or Tdap	• Tdap for the second booster at 5 and 10–15 years (after primary immunisation and first booster with DPT in children) • For adults between 18 and 64 years who have completed their primary vaccination schedule, a booster dose of Td vaccine is indicated once every 10 years till the age of 65 years; one dose of Tdap vaccine may be administered in place of Td vaccine • For adults older than 18 years who have not received prior vaccination, three doses of Td vaccine are indicated; two doses are administered at least 4 weeks apart, and the third dose 6–12 months after the second dose; Tdap vaccine can substitute any one of the Td doses • Pregnant women who have received the Td vaccination more than 10 years ago should receive one dose of Td vaccine in the second or third trimester of pregnancy • Pregnant women who have received Td vaccination during the preceding 10 years should receive one dose of Tdap in the immediate postpartum period if the last dose of Td was administered more than 2 years ago • For pregnant women who have never received previous vaccination, three doses of Td vaccine are indicated; in the second or third trimester of pregnancy, two doses are administered at least 4 weeks apart, and the third dose is given 6–12 months after the second dose • Tdap contraindicated if history of encephalopathy not attributable to an identifiable cause occurred within 7 days following DTP, DTaP or Tdap
Haemophilus influenzae	• *H. influenzae* B (HiB) conjugate vaccine: One dose	• A part of primary immunisation in children • Adults at high risk, e.g. asplenia, HIV, haematological malignancies, corticosteroid use, CSF leak, diabetes, immunosuppression, cancer
Typhoid	• Live Ty21a vaccine: Three doses orally on alternate days; to be repeated every 3 years • Vi polysaccharide vaccine: Single dose subcutaneously or IM with revaccination every 3 years • Typhoid conjugate vaccine (e.g. Vi-tetanus conjugate): Single dose intramuscularly in individuals aged between 6 months and 45 years; may be repeated every 3–7 years	• During an outbreak, entire community at risk should be vaccinated • Ty21a should not be used during pregnancy, in transplant recipients and in persons taking antibiotics

TABLE 17.32 Recommendations on Adult Immunisation—cont'd

Vaccine	Schedule	Comments
Japanese encephalitis	• Mouse brain-derived inactivated vaccine (not used in India at present) • Cell-cultured, live attenuated vaccine currently used in India as a single subcutaneous dose (booster may be given after 1 year)	• Primarily useful in the paediatric age in endemic areas and during an outbreak • Also being used in adults, though efficacy is not clear
Varicella	• Live attenuated varicella-zoster vaccine: In adults, two doses subcutaneously 4–8 weeks apart	• Used in people older than 13 years who never had chickenpox • For those already immunised, booster dose is not needed if titres are adequate • In resource-limited countries, at least the females in reproductive age group, people at high risk for exposure to varicella (e.g. healthcare workers, household contacts) should be vaccinated • Should not be given to persons with HIV (with $CD4^+$ <200/μL), and those receiving high-dose steroids
Measles, mumps, rubella	• Live attenuated, MMR vaccine: Single dose subcutaneously	• Recommended in all adults • Contraindicated in pregnancy and immunocompromised states

Box 17.24 Vaccines Recommended for Healthcare Workers

- Hepatitis A
- Hepatitis B
- Tdap
- Varicella
- Influenza
- Pneumococcal
- Typhoid
- MMR
- Meningococcal

- Box 17.24 depicts vaccines recommended for healthcare workers.

18 Endocrine and Metabolic Diseases

Q. Describe the anatomy of pituitary gland.

- The pituitary gland is located in sella turcica, bridged over by diaphragma sellae.
- It is related to sphenoidal air sinuses below, optic chiasma above and cavernous sinuses laterally.
- The gland is composed of two lobes, the anterior lobe (adenohypophysis) and the posterior lobe (neurohypophysis).
- The pituitary gland is connected to hypothalamus by the infundibular stalk that carries portal vessels carrying blood from hypothalamus to the anterior lobe, and nerve fibres to the posterior lobe.
- Hypothalamus has paraventricular and supraoptic nuclei which produce two hormones: oxytocin and vasopressin or antidiuretic hormone (ADH). These hormones are carried by the nerve fibres to the posterior lobe of pituitary from where these two hormones are released into blood.
- Conventional staining demonstrates three types of cells in the anterior lobe: acidophils, basophils and chromophobes.
- Electron microscopically, five distinct types of cells can be identified in the anterior pituitary that secrete six different hormones. These are somatotrophs secreting growth hormone (GH), lactotrophs secreting prolactin (PRL), thyrotrophs secreting thyroid-stimulating hormone (TSH), gonadotrophs secreting follicle-stimulating hormone (FSH) and luteinising hormone (LH), and corticotrophs secreting adrenocorticotrophic hormone (ACTH) (Fig. 18.1).

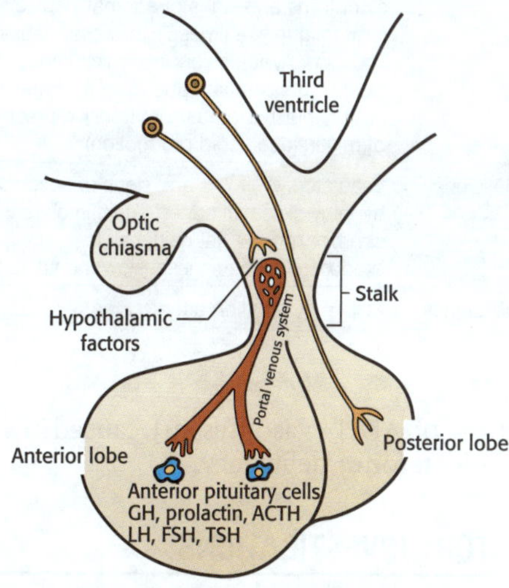

Fig. 18.1 Pituitary gland.

Q. Enumerate the pituitary hormones. Give their principal actions.

- Various hormones secreted by pituitary gland and their principal actions are listed in Table 18.1.

TABLE 18.1 Pituitary Hormones and Their Principal Actions

Hormone	Actions
Anterior pituitary hormones	
• Thyroid-stimulating hormone (TSH)	Stimulates the production of thyroxine (T_4) and triiodothyronine (T_3)
• Luteinising hormone (LH), follicle-stimulating hormone (FSH)	In males, both FSH and LH are necessary for spermatogenesis In males, FSH stimulates Sertoli's cells to secrete androgen-binding protein (ABP), transferrin, plasminogen activator and inhibin In males, LH stimulates Leydig's cells to produce testosterone In females, FSH promotes growth and development of ovarian follicles during the follicular phase of menstrual cycle In females, the mid-cycle peak of LH (LH surge) induces ovulation In females, both FSH and LH are necessary for the development of corpus luteum during the luteal phase of menstrual cycle
• Growth hormone (GH)	Promotes growth
• Prolactin (PRL)	Exerts its main effects on the breasts, stimulating lactation
• Adrenocorticotrophic hormone (ACTH)	Controls cortisol release from adrenal cortex and skin pigmentation
Posterior pituitary hormones	
• Arginine vasopressin (AVP)	Promotes reabsorption of water by renal tubules
• Oxytocin	Promotes uterine contraction and expression of milk from the breasts

Q. What are the hypothalamic hormones influencing the anterior pituitary? Give their principal effects. (IM12.3)

- Various hypothalamic hormones influencing the anterior pituitary and their principal actions are given in Fig. 18.2.
- In addition, GH secretion is influenced by multiple other peptides including ghrelin which is produced both in the hypothalamus and in the stomach. It stimulates release of growth hormone–releasing hormone (GHRH).

Q. Give a brief account of hyposecretion of anterior pituitary (hypopituitarism and panhypopituitarism).

- Hypopituitarism is the partial or complete deficiency of one or more anterior pituitary hormone secretion and may result from pituitary or hypothalamic disease.

AETIOLOGY

- Various causes of hypopituitarism are given in Table 18.2.

CLINICAL FEATURES

- Patients may be asymptomatic or present with symptoms related to hormone deficiency or a mass lesion.
- Involvement of hypothalamus can affect secretion of one or more of the hypothalamic hormones that

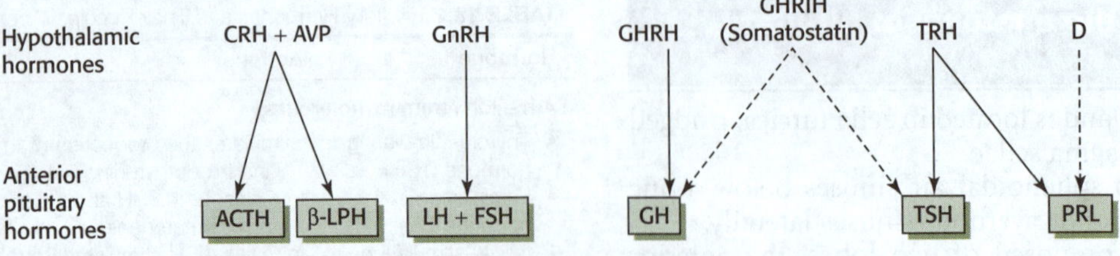

Note:

1. **GHRIH (Somatostatin) is now called somatostatin or somatotropin release-inhibiting factor (SRIF). Growth hormone produces its main effects via insulin-like growth factor-1 (IGF-1) secreted by liver.**
2. **β-Lipotropin (β-LPH) is a hormone produced by the cleavage of pro-opiomelanocortin (POMC). The anterior pituitary gland produces the prohormone POMC, which undergoes cleavage to adrenocorticotropin (ACTH) and β-lipotropin.**

Fig. 18.2 Effects of hypothalamic hormones on pituitary gland. Hypothalamic hormones stimulating anterior pituitary (⟶). Hypothalamic hormones inhibiting anterior pituitary (--➤). AVP, arginine vasopressin; CRH, corticotrophin-releasing hormone; D, dopamine or prolactin release inhibitory factor; GHRH, growth hormone–releasing hormone; GHRIH, growth hormone release inhibitory hormone or somatostatin; GnRH, gonadotrophin-releasing hormone; β-LPH, β-lipotropic pituitary hormone; TRH, thyrotrophin-releasing hormone.

TABLE 18.2 Aetiology of Hypopituitarism

• Congenital hypothalamic diseases	Deficiencies of GnRH (Kallmann's syndrome), TRH, GHRH
• Acquired hypothalamic diseases	Craniopharyngioma, sarcoidosis, tuberculosis, Langerhans' cell histiocytosis (histiocytosis X), surgery, radiotherapy, metastatic tumours, head trauma
• Pituitary diseases	Pituitary adenoma, postpartum necrosis (Sheehan's syndrome), autoimmune (lymphocytic hypophysitis), surgery, radiotherapy, haemorrhage (pituitary apoplexy), empty sella syndrome, haemochromatosis, snake bite (particularly Russell's viper)

influence secretion of corresponding pituitary hormones. Hypothalamic disorders can also diminish the secretion of vasopressin resulting in diabetes insipidus.

- When hypopituitarism is secondary to pituitary tumours, symptoms related to mass effects (e.g. headache, visual impairment, diplopia, electrolyte alterations and disorders of the autonomic nervous system produced by hypothalamic involvement) may be present.
- With progressive lesion (e.g. nonfunctioning pituitary tumours), there is a sequential loss of hormone secretion. Ultimately the patient goes into coma resulting from hypoglycaemia, water intoxication and hypothermia.
- Features of various hormonal deficiencies are given in Table 18.3.
- Lactotroph cells, unlike any other pituitary cell lines, receive predominantly inhibitory signals from the hypothalamus; this inhibitory control explains increase in PRL levels that result from either hypothalamic damage or hypothalamic–pituitary disconnection. However, when pituitary itself is damaged, PRL levels fall.
- Compared to primary adrenal insufficiency, ACTH deficiency generally does not cause salt wasting, volume contraction and hyperkalaemia because it does not result in clinically important deficiency of aldosterone. Furthermore, ACTH deficiency results in pallor of skin and not hyperpigmentation. However, hyponatraemia can occur due to inappropriate secretion of ADH (vasopressin) caused by cortisol (not aldosterone) deficiency.

TABLE 18.3 Features of Various Hormonal Deficiencies

• GH deficiency	Earliest to occur but no significant symptoms in adults. May produce an increased risk of fracture, a deranged cardiovascular risk profile (deposition of visceral fat, increased LDL and reduced HDL) and a decreased quality of life. In children, lower final height, decreased lean body mass and higher fat mass.
• LH deficiency	Leads to loss of libido and impotence in males, and oligomenorrhoea or amenorrhoea, vaginal atrophy and hot flushes in females. Later, in males, there may be gynaecomastia and decreased frequency of shaving. In both sexes, infertility and osteoporosis occur, axillary and pubic hair becomes sparse, and the skin becomes finer and wrinkled.
• ACTH deficiency	Leads to cortisol deficiency resulting in symptoms and signs of adrenal insufficiency (e.g. fatigue, weakness, dizziness, nausea, vomiting, hypotension, hypoglycaemia, weight loss) with skin pallor due to lack of melanin and *normal* plasma potassium (relative preservation of mineralocorticoid production).
• TSH deficiency	Leads to symptoms and signs of secondary hypothyroidism (tiredness, cold intolerance, constipation, weight gain, hair loss, dry skin, bradycardia, hoarseness, slow mental processes).
• PRL deficiency	Failure of lactation after delivery.

LABORATORY INVESTIGATIONS

- Demonstration of low levels of trophic pituitary hormones in the setting of low-target hormones. However, sometimes, levels of trophic hormones may be normal.
  - Low free T_4 (fT_4) with low or inappropriately normal TSH.
  - Low early morning cortisol with low or inappropriately normal ACTH.
  - Low testosterone without elevation of gonadotrophins (LH and FSH).

- Low IGF-1 (insulin-like growth factor-1) level (an indicator of GH deficiency).
- Provocation tests may be required to assess pituitary reserve. These include the following:
  - GH response to insulin-induced hypoglycaemia, l-dopa or combination of arginine and GHRH. Insulin-induced hypoglycaemia (also known as insulin tolerance test) is considered the gold standard test.
  - PRL level fails to rise after thyrotrophin-releasing hormone (TRH).
  - Adrenocorticotrophic hormone (ACTH) response as assessed by measuring cortisol response to insulin-induced hypoglycaemia, corticotrophin-releasing hormone (CRH) or metyrapone.
  - Thyroid stimulating hormone (TSH) response to TRH.

MANAGEMENT

- ACTH deficiency is treated with cortisol (same as hydrocortisone) 20 mg in the morning and 10 mg in the evening or prednisolone 5 mg in the morning and 2.5 mg in the evening. Doses should be at least doubled during acute illness and administered without delay by intramuscular or intravenous injection in patients who are vomiting. Unlike the situation in primary adrenal insufficiency, mineralocorticoid replacement is not necessary in hypopituitarism.
- TSH deficiency is treated with T_4 0.1–0.15 mg daily with the aim of maintaining fT_4 in the upper quartile of normal range. T_4 should not be administered until adrenal function has been evaluated and either found to be normal or treated. In a patient with co-existing hypothyroidism and hypoadrenalism, treatment with T_4 alone may increase the clearance of already deficient cortisol.
- Gonadotrophin deficiency is treated with sex hormone (testosterone or oestrogen–progestin) replacement based on the age and sex of the patient. Men and women who wish to be fertile should be given gonadotrophins.
- Children with GH deficiency should be treated with recombinant human GH. However, it is not recommended in adults due to high cost and need for daily injections.
- For prolactin deficiency, no treatment is currently available.

Q. Discuss the differential diagnosis, investigations and management of short stature or dwarfism.

- Dwarfism is defined as a height that is more than two standard deviations below the mean for age and sex within a population.
- Most cases are due to normal variants in growth (familial short stature and constitutional delay of growth and puberty) which are normal, nonpathologic variants of growth.

DIFFERENTIAL DIAGNOSIS OF SHORT STATURE

- Various causes of short stature and their associated features are shown in Table 18.4.

TABLE 18.4 Differential Diagnosis of Short Stature

• Familial (genetic) short stature	Born adequate size for gestational age, followed by low-normal growth velocity throughout life
• Constitutional delay of growth and puberty	Growth deceleration during the first 2 years followed by a normal growth velocity, with acceleration late in adolescence, leading to a final height that is close to the target height; delayed puberty, near-normal adult height
• GH deficiency	Frontal bossing, central obesity, high-pitched voice
• Hypothyroidism	Dry skin, coarse hair, immature facies
• Cushing's syndrome	Central obesity, striae, hypertension
• Gonadal dysgenesis	Webbed neck, multiple pigmented naevi, shield chest, delayed sexual development
• Pseudohypo-parathyroidism	Moon facies and obesity, short metacarpals, mental retardation
• Bone–cartilage dysplasia	Abnormal proportions, macrocephaly
• Russell–Silver dwarfism	Small at birth, pointed facies, asymmetry
• Other causes	Turner's syndrome, intrauterine growth retardation, premature birth, cyanotic congenital heart diseases, chronic liver, pulmonary or kidney disease, undernutrition, rickets, malabsorption, uncontrolled type 1 diabetes mellitus, idiopathic

TABLE 18.5 Laboratory Investigations in Short Stature

Screening Test	Disorder
• Bone age	Familial short stature (bone age is consistent with their chronological age), constitutional delay (bone age is delayed compared to chronological age), hypothyroidism, GH deficiency
• Lateral skull film	Craniopharyngioma or other central nervous system lesions
• Serum calcium	Pseudohypoparathyroidism
• Serum phosphate	Vitamin D-resistant rickets
• Serum bicarbonate	Renal tubular acidosis
• Blood urea nitrogen (BUN), liver function tests	Renal disease, liver disease
• Calcium, alkaline phosphatase, iron, ferritin, albumin	Malabsorption syndrome
• Complete blood count	Anaemia, nutritional disorder
• ESR	Inflammatory bowel disease
• Chromosomal karyotype	Gonadal dysgenesis or other abnormalities
• Serum thyroxine, TSH	Hypothyroidism
• Insulin like growth factor-1 and insulin-like growth factor binding protein-3 (IGFBP-3)	GH deficiency
• Antiendomysial antibodies, antitissue transglutaminase antibodies	Coeliac disease

LABORATORY INVESTIGATIONS

- The goal of laboratory evaluation is to identify the subset of patients with pathologic causes of short stature.
- Various laboratory investigations required in a patient with short stature are shown in Table 18.5.

DIAGNOSTIC ALGORITHM (Flowchart 18.1)

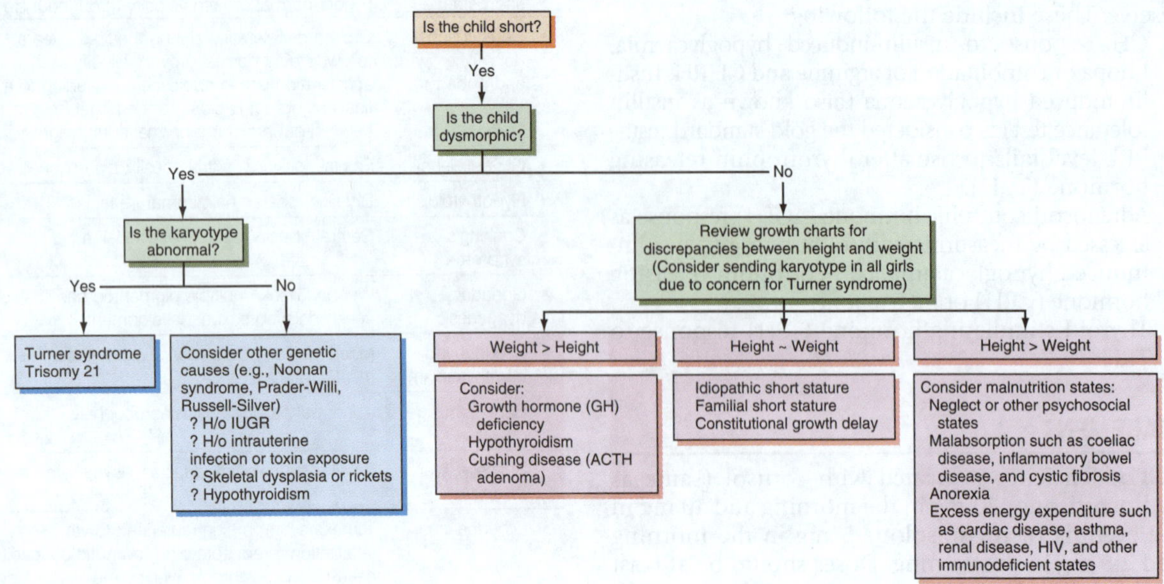

Flowchart 18.1 Differential Diagnosis of Short Stature.

TREATMENT

- Treatment of underlying cause.
- GH may be of some benefit in children with idiopathic dwarfism whose epiphyses are open.

Q. Describe Sheehan's syndrome.

- Sheehan's syndrome results from infarction of anterior pituitary gland due to significant blood loss during postpartum period. Rarely, pituitary infarction can occur following Russell's viper bite.
- Postpartum pituitary infarction occurs because the enlarged pituitary gland of pregnancy is more vulnerable to ischaemia of postpartum haemorrhage and systemic hypotension.

PATHOPHYSIOLOGY

- The blood supply of the anterior pituitary gland is a relatively low-pressure system. This makes the anterior pituitary cells susceptible to ischaemia, particularly following significant haemorrhage.
- On the other hand, blood supply of posterior pituitary gland is under higher pressure than the anterior pituitary, and is therefore, usually not affected by shock.

CLINICAL FEATURES

- Failure to lactate (agalactorrhoea) is the earliest symptom.
- Another typical symptom is failure to regain menstruation after delivery and breast involution.
- Other symptoms of hypopituitarism appear over months or years, though some patients present acutely.
- Features of hypothyroidism include fatigue, bradycardia, hypotension, weight gain, constipation, cold intolerance and loss of axillary and pubic hair.
- Adrenal insufficiency can result in fatigue and weight loss.
- Uncommonly, it can present acutely with circulatory collapse, severe hyponatraemia, diabetes insipidus, hypoglycaemia, congestive cardiac failure and psychosis, finally leading to coma and death.

DIAGNOSIS

- Diagnosis is same as that for hypopituitarism (refer page 970). MRI may show hypertrophic pituitary in early stages, but, later, atrophic pituitary and empty sella develop. It also excludes a pituitary mass.

TREATMENT

- Treatment is substitution of deficient hormones.

Q. What is pituitary apoplexy?

- A rare but potentially life-threatening clinical syndrome resulting from acute haemorrhage or infarction of the pituitary gland.
- It is associated with a variety of precipitating factors which include head trauma, surgery, pregnancy, medication and use of anticoagulants.
- Presents with a sudden onset of headache (which can have a thunderclap character), vomiting, visual disturbances (visual acuity impairment and visual field impairment), diplopia (due to pressure on the oculomotor nerves), decreased consciousness and hypopituitarism.

- If extra and suprasellar adenoma expansions involve the internal carotid arteries, patients may develop focal neurologic deficits secondary to brain ischaemia and infarction.
- Extension of the haemorrhage to the subarachnoid space may result in meningeal signs and changes in the level of consciousness.
- Sudden onset of ACTH deficiency can cause life-threatening hypotension.
- It usually occurs in presence of a pituitary adenoma.
- MRI confirms the presence of a sellar mass with haemorrhagic/ischaemic components within the tumour.
- Initial management consists of careful monitoring of fluid and electrolyte balance coupled with immediate replacement of deficient hormones, in particular corticosteroids.
- Surgical decompression may be required in those with progressive neuro-ophthalmic signs.

Q. What are the common pituitary tumours? Discuss briefly their clinical manifestations, investigations and management.

- Pituitary tumours may be microadenomas (less than 10 mm diameter) or macroadenomas (more than 10 mm diameter).
- They may be functional or non-functional. Some functional tumours may produce more than one hormone. Most non-functional tumours are gonadotroph cell adenomas and do produce intact gonadotrophins or their glycoprotein subunits. Non-functional tumours found incidentally during MRI/CT examination or at autopsy are known as pituitary incidentalomas.

COMMON PITUITARY TUMOURS

- Pituitary adenomas are the most common pituitary tumours. Box 18.1 lists the common pituitary tumours.
- Prolactinomas account for up to 30% of all pituitary adenomas and nearly 50% of functional adenomas.

CLINICAL FEATURES

- Due to hypofunction by pressure on surrounding normal pituitary tissue (see hypopituitarism, page 969).

BOX 18.1 Common Pituitary Tumours

- Lactotroph adenoma (prolactinoma)
- Somatotroph adenoma
- Thyrotroph adenoma
- Corticotroph adenoma
- Gonadotroph adenoma
- Multiple endocrine neoplasia type 1 (MEN1), which includes parathyroid, pancreatic and pituitary (usually prolactinoma) tumours
- Plurihormonal and double adenoma (often lactotroph and somatotroph adenoma)
- Pituitary carcinoma
- Craniopharyngioma
- Metastatic tumours

- Due to involvement of neighbouring structures.
  - Dura—headache (commonest).
  - Optic chiasma, nerve or tract—visual field defects, loss of acuity and optic atrophy.
  - Cavernous sinus—III, IV and VI nerve palsies resulting in diplopia and strabismus; facial numbness.
  - Hypothalamus—obesity, disturbances of sleep, thirst, appetite and temperature regulation, and diabetes insipidus (DI).
  - Miscellaneous—anosmia (frontal lobe involvement), headache, vomiting, papilloedema (raised intracranial tension).
  - Occasionally, bleeding into tumour (pituitary apoplexy).
- Due to secretion of hormones.
  - GH—acromegaly or gigantism.
  - PRL—amenorrhoea, impotence and occasionally galactorrhoea.
  - ACTH—Cushing's syndrome.
  - TSH—hyperthyroidism.
  - Gonadotrophins—majority of gonadotroph adenomas are clinically silent; rarely present with precocious puberty, amenorrhoea or oligomenorrhoea.

INVESTIGATIONS

- Plain radiograph of the pituitary fossa may show one or more of the following abnormalities:
  - Enlargement of sella turcica.
  - Erosion of clinoid process.
  - Suprasellar calcification.
  - Double floor of the sella.
- CT scan with contrast enhancement—more sensitive than MRI for bony erosions and presence of calcification.
- Magnetic resonance imaging (before and after gadolinium)—more sensitive than CT scan for defining the soft tissue tumour.
- Visual field plotting can identify the site of lesion in some cases:
  - Bitemporal hemianopia—optic chiasma.
  - Unilateral loss of acuity or scotoma—optic nerve.
  - Homonymous hemianopia—optic tract.
- Functional assessment of the gland—for example hormonal assays.
  - Hormonal assays—PRL, IGF-1, 24-hour urinary cortisol, FSH, LH and thyroid function tests.

TREATMENT

- Except for prolactinomas, management of other pituitary tumours includes surgery as a first-line treatment.
- Drug therapy with dopamine agonists like bromocriptine and cabergoline is effective in prolactinomas. This can shrink the tumour and possibly avoid surgery.
- Somatostatin analogues including lanreotide, octreotide and pasireotide are considered first-line medical therapy for GH-producing tumours if surgery is not possible. Other drug includes pegvisomant which is a GH receptor antagonist.

- Trans-sphenoidal or transfrontal surgery enables removal of the tumour.
- Radiotherapy can suppress the tumour growth and reduce its secretory capacity. It is indicated in patients with clinically relevant tumour growth despite surgery in non-functioning tumours, or surgery and standard medical treatment in functioning tumours. This can be achieved by external radiotherapy (fractionated), implantation of yttrium in pituitary fossa, gamma knife or a modified linear accelerator. Gamma knife (stereotactic radiosurgery) involves precise delivery of large, single, high-energy dose directly to the tumour under stereotactic surgery.
- Temozolomide is first-line chemotherapeutic agent for aggressive and malignant pituitary tumours where surgery and radiation fail and tumour progresses.

Q. Describe the clinical features, diagnosis and management of acromegaly.

AETIOLOGY

- GH hypersecretion occurring in adult life after epiphyseal closure results in acromegaly (excess before epiphysis closure results in gigantism).
- Pituitary tumour (somatotroph pituitary adenoma) is the most common cause. Some adenomas are mixed that secrete GH as well as PRL.
- Rare causes include excessive GH secretion from pancreatic islet cell tumour, or excessive secretion of GH-releasing hormone from hypothalamic lesions, bronchial carcinoid and small cell lung carcinoma.

CLINICAL FEATURES

- Clinical features of acromegaly are shown in Table 18.6.

TABLE 18.6 Clinical Features of Acromegaly

• Soft tissue changes	Thickening of skin, increased skin tags, acanthosis nigricans, increased sweat and sebum resulting in moist and oily skin, enlargement of lips, nose and tongue, increased heel pad thickness (normal <23 mm in men and 21.5 mm in women—Fig. 18.3A), visceral enlargement—for example thyroid, heart and liver, carpal tunnel syndrome, myopathy, sleep apnoea, Raynaud's phenomenon
• Bone changes	Large spade-like hands, large feet, prognathism, prominent supraorbital ridges, large frontal sinuses, wide spacing of the teeth, arthropathy, kyphosis, osteoporosis, 'arrow-head' distal phalanges on radiograph (Fig. 18.3B)
• Metabolic effects	Glucose intolerance or clinical diabetes mellitus, hypertriglyceridaemia, decreased HDL-cholesterol, hypercalciuria
• Pressure effects	Refer pituitary tumour (page 973)
• Cardiac effects	Coronary heart disease, cardiomyopathy, hypertension, left ventricular hypertrophy, valvulopathy (aortic and mitral regurgitation), heart failure, arrhythmias
• Others	Increased risk of colonic polyps and carcinoma, increased risk of thyroid nodule and carcinoma

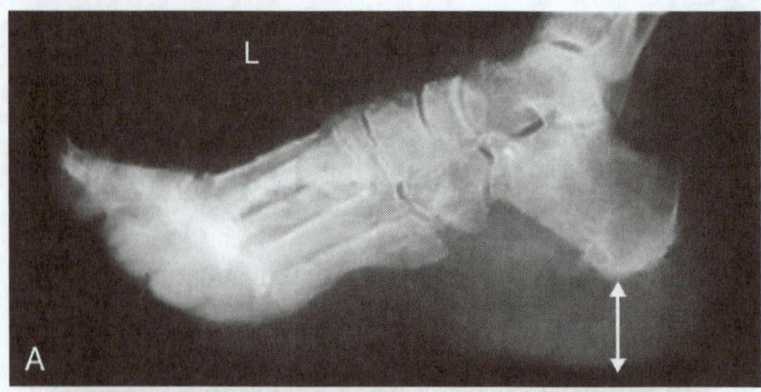

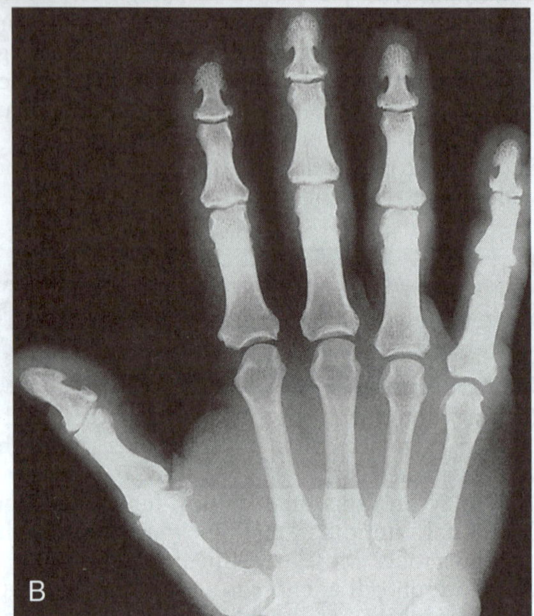

Fig. 18.3 (A) Increased heel pad thickness in a patient of acromegaly. (B) 'Arrow-head' (tufting) distal phalanges with increased soft tissue.

INVESTIGATIONS

- Investigations of pituitary tumour (refer pituitary tumours, page 973).
- Other radiological investigations:
  - Skull radiograph shows thickening of calvarium, enlargement of sinuses and enlargement of jaw.
  - Radiograph of hands shows 'arrow-head' tufting of distal phalanges and increased width of intraarticular cartilages.
  - Radiograph of feet shows increased thickness of heel pad >22 mm.
- Elevated IGF-1 levels.
- GH levels are measured during an oral glucose tolerance test (OGTT). A failure of suppression or a paradoxical rise of GH indicates acromegaly.
- A few patients also have elevated levels of PRL due to cosecretion from the tumours (page 973).
- Additional endocrine assessment includes baseline testing of corticotroph, thyrotroph and gonadotroph function by measurements of plasma cortisol, TSH and free T_4, FSH, LH, oestradiol or testosterone.

TREATMENT

SURGERY

- Transsphenoidal surgical removal of adenoma is the treatment of choice.

MEDICAL THERAPY

- Primary treatment with drugs is indicated in:
  - Those with no risk of visual impairment from the tumour.
  - Those who are poor candidates for surgery; those who decline surgery.
  - Those with tumours unlikely to be controlled by surgery.
  - Those who require the preservation of intact pituitary function (especially fertility).
- Various drugs are as follows:
  - Bromocriptine or cabergoline (dopamine receptor agonists) are useful in those with mildly elevated IGF-1.
  - Octreotide, lanreotide or pasireotide (somatostatin analogues). Somatostatin analogues are more effective than dopamine agonists and act on pituitary somatostatin receptors to produce inhibition of GH and IGF-1.
  - Pegvisomant, a GH receptor antagonist, blocks peripheral IGF-1 action in almost all patients, and is indicated in patients who are inadequately controlled with other modalities or in patients experiencing clinically significant drug side effects. Tumour size should be monitored at intervals as the therapy is directed at blocking peripheral GH receptors and not at treating the pituitary tumour.

RADIOTHERAPY

- External radiotherapy in patients not candidates for surgical therapy and in whom medical therapy fails.
- Radiosurgery (gamma knife, cyber knife).

OTHERS

- Treatment of diabetes, hypertension and hyperlipidaemia.

Q. Discuss prolactinoma and hyperprolactinaemia. Write briefly on their causes, clinical features, investigations and treatment.

- Prolactinoma is a pituitary tumour producing PRL. Most of them are microadenomas.
- Hyperprolactinaemia means elevated levels of plasma PRL.

CAUSES

- Various causes of hyperprolactinaemia are listed in Table 18.7.

TABLE 18.7 Causes of Hyperprolactinaemia

• Physiological—for example pregnancy, lactation, sleep, stress • Pituitary tumours—for example prolactinomas • Hypothalamic and pituitary stalk diseases • Primary hypothyroidism • Acromegaly	• Chronic renal failure • Cirrhosis of the liver • Drugs—for example dopamine receptor blockers (antipsychotics e.g. phenothiazines, haloperidol, risperidone; tricyclic antidepressants; selective serotonin reuptake inhibitors; metoclopramide; domperidone), dopamine synthesis inhibitors (α-methyldopa), reserpine, opiates, cimetidine, oestrogens, verapamil

CLINICAL FEATURES

- Galactorrhoea and osteoporosis (secondary to hypogonadism) in both sexes; galactorrhoea uncommon in postmenopausal females.
- Amenorrhoea, oligomenorrhoea decreased libido and infertility in premenopausal females.
- Loss of libido, impotence, infertility and gynaecomastia in males; galactorrhoea less common than in premenopausal females.
- A sufficiently large macroadenoma is usually associated with visual field defects and compression of other parts of pituitary (see 'pituitary tumours'). This is more common in postmenopausal women as they generally do not have galactorrhoea.

INVESTIGATIONS

- Raised plasma PRL levels but exclude other causes of elevated PRL levels.
- Study of pituitary anatomy and assessment of the other pituitary functions (refer 'pituitary tumours', page 973).
- Up to 50% of patients with GH-secreting tumours also have hyperprolactinaemia. Therefore, it is important to exclude this condition by IGF-1 measurement.

TREATMENT

- Bromocriptine (2.5 mg thrice daily) or cabergoline; both are dopamine agonists. These agents reduce the secretion of PRL as well as size of tumour. Cabergoline is preferred to bromocriptine.
- Transsphenoidal removal, if dopamine agonists do not help or there is a large, invasive tumour.
- External radiotherapy is rarely required. It may be considered in cases resistant to medical treatment and poor response to surgery.
- Asymptomatic patients who do not require restoration of pregnancy should be monitored regularly and given oestrogens/progesterone to prevent bone loss.

Q. Give a brief account of diabetes insipidus. (PM8.4)

- DI is a metabolic disorder characterised by an absolute or relative inability to concentrate urine resulting in the production of large quantities of dilute urine.
- DI can be divided into the following types:
  - Deficient production of ADH.
    - Primary deficiency (also called neurogenic, pituitary, hypothalamic, cranial or central DI)

occurs due to agenesis or destruction of neurohypophysis.
  - Secondary deficiency occurs due to inhibition of ADH secretion (primary polydipsia).
- Deficient action of ADH (nephrogenic DI).
- Transient DI of pregnancy or gestational DI (produced by accelerated metabolism of vasopressin).

AETIOLOGY

- Various causes of DI are given in Table 18.8.

PATHOPHYSIOLOGY

- Plasma volume and osmolality are maintained within a narrow range by an integrated neurohumoral system coordinating the balance between fluid intake and renal water loss.
- The key regulator of renal water loss, vasopressin or ADH, is synthesised in hypothalamus from where it is carried by neurons to posterior pituitary for release in circulation.
- Plasma osmolality is sensed by osmoreceptors present in the hypothalamus which regulate ADH synthesis and release.
- ADH release is also regulated by circulating volume and blood pressure which can lead to ADH release at plasma osmolality below the standard osmolar threshold of around 290 mOsm/kg.
- ADH acts on type-2 ADH or vasopressin receptors present on the distal collecting duct cells of kidneys, increasing water permeability through the increased synthesis of aquaporin-2 water channels.

TABLE 18.8 Aetiology of Diabetes Insipidus

Primary Deficiency of ADH	Secondary Deficiency of ADH

• Severe head injury
• Pituitary surgery
• Neoplasms
  • Craniopharyngioma
  • Pituitary adenoma
  • Meningioma
  • Metastatic
  • Lymphoma, leukaemias
• Granulomas
  • Sarcoidosis
  • Langerhans' cell histiocytosis
• Infections
  • Chronic meningitis
  • Viral encephalitis
• Inflammatory
  • Hypophysitis
  • Granulomatosis with polyangiitis (Wegener's granulomatosis)
• Vascular
  • Sheehan's syndrome
  • Hypoxic encephalopathy
  • Subarachnoid haemorrhage involving anterior communicating artery
• Drugs
  • Phenytoin
  • Temozolomide
• Genetic defects (autosomal dominant or recessive, X-linked)
• Idiopathic
	• Psychogenic polydipsia
	• Dipsogenic polydipsia (abnormal thirst)
	• Iatrogenic
	Nephrogenic diabetes insipidus
	• Drugs
	  • Lithium
	  • Demeclocycline
	  • Amphotericin B
	  • Aminoglycosides
	  • Cisplatin
	  • Rifampicin
	• Metabolic
	  • Hypercalcaemia
	  • Hypokalaemia
	• Chronic kidney disease
	• Obstructive uropathy
	• Amyloidosis
	• Vascular causes
	  • Sickle cell anaemia
	  • Acute tubular necrosis
	• Genetic
	• Idiopathic

- Central DI results from impaired production, transportation or release of ADH while nephrogenic DI results from impairment of ability of renal collecting ducts to respond to ADH.
- Both central and nephrogenic DI are characterised by impaired renal water reabsorption resulting in production of excessive, hypotonic urine, which is accompanied by significant thirst and polydipsia, as central osmoreceptors and peripheral baroreceptors stimulate thirst to maintain circulating volume and osmolar status.

CLINICAL FEATURES

- Polyuria, excessive thirst and polydipsia (with predilection for cold drinks) are the cardinal manifestations of DI.
- Daily urine output >50 mL/kg/day and may reach as high as 10–15 L.
- Other features include restlessness, altered sensorium and seizures (due to hypernatraemia) and tachycardia and hypotension (due to intravascular volume loss).
- In traumatic DI, triphasic response may be seen: initial polyuria, prolonged antidiuresis and final polyuria.
- In cases with sellar or parasellar mass leading to DI, evidence of hypopituitarism may be present.

DIAGNOSIS

- The urine is clear and of low specific gravity.
- A reduced urine osmolality <300 mOsm/kg in conjunction with high serum osmolality >290 mOsm/kg strongly suggests DI. However, in primary polydipsia, plasma osmolality may be lower than urinary osmolality.
- A low plasma sodium concentration (less than 137 mEq/L) with a low urine osmolality is usually indicative of primary polydipsia.
- Borderline high serum sodium (143–150 mEq/L) indicates water loss in central or nephrogenic DI.
- Water deprivation test (see below).
- Another recent test is hypertonic saline infusion and copeptin (a precursor of ADH) measurement.
- MRI of pituitary and hypothalamus.
- Anterior pituitary function tests for associated hypopituitarism.

DIAGNOSIS OF DIABETES INSIPIDUS BY WATER DEPRIVATION TEST

- Patients are deprived of all fluids for 16–18 hours or until a 3% loss of their body weight is reached.
- Serum osmolality, urine volume and urine osmolality are measured hourly.
- Plasma sodium and weight of patient should be monitored closely during the test.
- Failure to concentrate urine appropriately is confirmed by a final urine osmolality <300 mOsm/kg with corresponding plasma osmolality >290 mOsm/kg.
- If DI is confirmed by failure to concentrate urine, desmopressin is given subcutaneously. Serum and urine osmolality, and urine volume are measured hourly over the next 4 hours.
- In patients with central DI, the kidneys respond to desmopressin with a reduction in urine output and

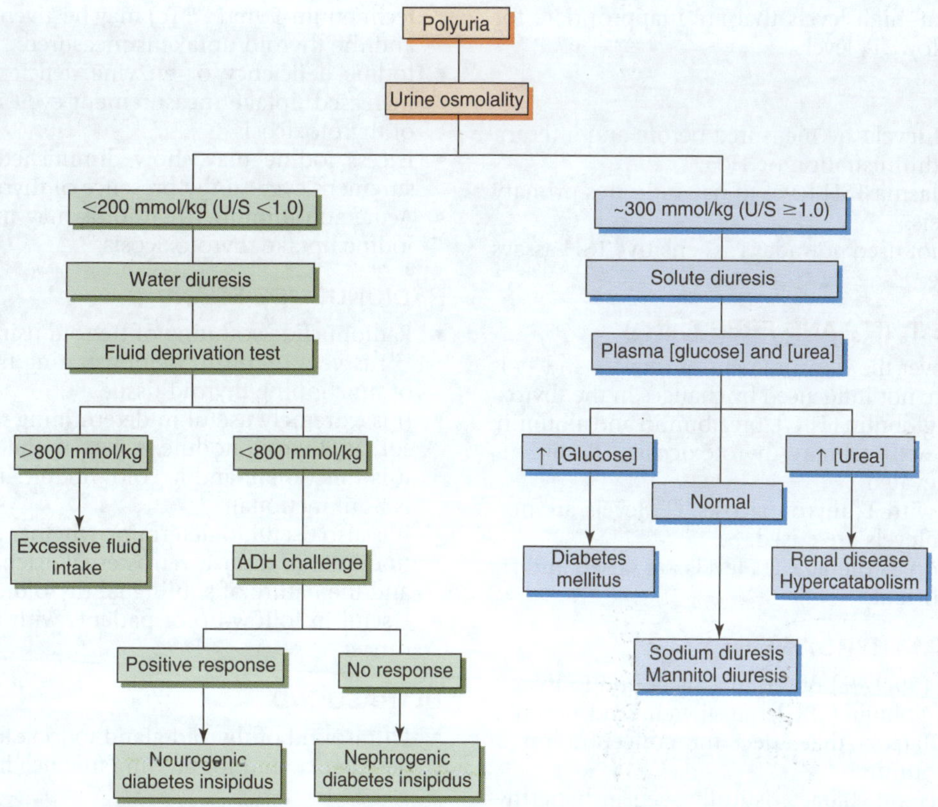

Flowchart 18.2 Approach to a Patient with Polyuria. U/S, urine to serum osmolality (Redrawn from: Walmsley RN, White GH: A guide to diagnostic clinical chemistry, Melbourne, 1983, Blackwell Science.)

an increase in urine osmolality to >800 mOsm/kg. In patients with nephrogenic DI, there is a lack of response to desmopressin, with little or no increase in urine osmolality.

- In dipsogenic polydipsia, urinary osmolality rises appropriately during fluid restriction.

APPROACH TO A PATIENT WITH POLYURIA

- Flowchart 18.2 shows approach to a patient with polyuria.

TREATMENT

- Desmopressin [1-deamino-8-d-arginine vasopressin (DDAVP)] 10–20 μg intranasally once or twice a day. It is also available in oral and subcutaneous formulations.
- Chlorpropamide enhances the renal responsiveness to vasopressin. Hypoglycaemia can be a problem.
- Carbamazepine enhances the renal responsiveness to vasopressin. It also enhances ADH release. Clofibrate also increases ADH release.
- Thiazide diuretics (e.g. hydrochlorothiazide) are the only effective drugs for nephrogenic DI. Hypovolaemia induced by them increases proximal sodium and water reabsorption, thereby diminishing water delivery to ADH-sensitive sites in the collecting tubules and reducing urine output.
- NSAIDs (particularly indomethacin) are also effective as they inhibit renal prostaglandin synthesis. Normally, prostaglandins antagonise the action of ADH.
- Nephrogenic DI patients are treated with low-salt, low-protein diet, thiazide diuretics and NSAIDs. If response is not adequate, desmopressin in high doses may be tried.

Q. What are the various thyroid function tests? Explain. (IM12.3, IM12.4)

- The hormones secreted by thyroid gland are T_3, T_4 and calcitonin.

THYROID FUNCTION TESTS

SERUM THYROID-STIMULATING HORMONE

- Measured by immunoradiometric assays (TSH IRMAs) or chemiluminometric assays.
- Normal values: 0.4–5.0 mU/L.
- Most sensitive index of thyroid function.
- Suppressed levels indicate primary thyrotoxicosis while elevated levels indicate primary hypothyroidism.
- Besides primary thyroid disease, TSH levels may also vary in certain other conditions. Therefore, TSH value should always be interpreted along with T_4 assay. These conditions include the following:
    - Severe nonthyroidal illness (sick euthyroid syndrome).
    - TSH-secreting pituitary tumours.
    - First trimester of pregnancy (low TSH).
    - High doses of corticosteroids (low TSH).
    - Secondary hypothyroidism caused by hypothalamic–pituitary disease may produce low, normal

or normal–high levels that are inappropriate for the very low fT_4 level.

TRH TEST

- Plasma TSH levels are measured before and after intravenous administration or TRH.
- Failure of plasma TSH level to rise indicates primary thyrotoxicosis.
- This test is not used nowadays as sensitive TSH assays are available.

SERUM FREE T_3 (fT_3) AND FREE T_4 (fT_4)

- Advantage over the measurement of total T_3 and T_4 is that these are not influenced by changes in the thyroxine binding globulin (TBG), prealbumin and albumin.
- In patients with primary thyrotoxicosis, fT_3 and fT_4 levels are elevated.
- In patients with T_3 thyrotoxicosis, fT_4 levels are normal and fT_3 levels are raised.
- In patients on T_4 therapy, fT_4 levels are raised and fT_3 levels are normal.

TOTAL SERUM THYROXINE (tT_4)

- Virtually all (99.97%) of serum T_4 is bound to thyroxine-binding globulin (TBG), transthyretin and albumin.
- Altered by factors that affect the concentration of TBG and albumin.
- Raised levels are characteristically seen in hyperthyroidism; also during pregnancy, oestrogen therapy, tamoxifen use and as a congenital anomaly.
- Depressed levels are characteristically seen in hypothyroidism; also with nephrotic syndrome, androgen therapy, liver failure, or drugs like salicylates, sulphonylureas and phenytoin.

TOTAL SERUM TRIIODOTHYRONINE (tT_3)

- T_3 is less tightly bound to TBG and transthyretin but more tightly bound to albumin than T_4.
- Subject to the same limitations as for tT_4 in relation to TBG and albumin.

REVERSE T_3 (rT_3)

- rT_3 is principally an inactive product of T_4 degradation in peripheral tissues. It is also secreted by the thyroid gland but the amounts are insignificant.
- Elevated in subjects with high TBG.
- Normal in hypothyroid patients treated with thyroxine, indicating that peripheral T_4 metabolism is an important source of circulating rT_3.

THYROGLOBULIN

- Serum thyroglobulin (Tg) levels are increased in all types of thyrotoxicosis except thyrotoxicosis factitia. Levels of Tg are also used to follow-up a patient with thyroid cancer.

UPTAKE OF RADIOACTIVE IODINE OR TECHNETIUM

- Overactive gland synthesising excess T_3 has an increased uptake of iodine. The increased uptake is demonstrated by giving an oral tracer dose of ^{131}I or ^{121}I and measuring the thyroid uptake after 4 hours, using a counter over the neck. Alternatively, technetium-99m (^{99m}Tc) may be given intravenously and the thyroid uptake is measured.
- Iodine deficiency or enzyme deficiency may show increased uptake measurement even in the absence of thyrotoxicosis.
- Excess iodine may show diminished uptake measurement even in the presence of thyrotoxicosis.
- Acute autoimmune thyroiditis may manifest as low iodine uptake thyrotoxicosis.

RADIONUCLIDE SCAN

- Radionuclide scanning of thyroid using ^{131}I, ^{99m}Tc or ^{121}I is very useful in demonstrating the distribution of functioning thyroid tissue.
- It is extremely useful in determining the activity of a solitary thyroid nodule. A 'hot' nodule indicates that it is functional, and a 'cold' nodule indicates that it is nonfunctional.
- It is also useful to determine whether a goitre is multinodular or diffuse, retrosternal extension of thyroid and the nature of sublingual thyroid.
- Useful in follow-up of patients with treated thyroid cancer.

ULTRASOUND

- Ultrasound of thyroid gland to look for nodules and vascularity, and for guiding fine needle aspiration.

THYROID ANTIBODY TESTS

- In autoimmune thyroiditis, antibodies against thyroid peroxidase (TPO) and Tg are present. These antibodies may also occur in normal population but these persons are at a high risk of developing thyroid disease late in life.
- Anti-TPO antibodies may be useful to predict the likelihood of progression to permanent overt hypothyroidism in patients with subclinical hypothyroidism.
- TSH-receptor antibody (TRAb), previously known as thyroid-stimulating immunoglobulins (TSI), is present in Graves' disease. These antibodies stimulate TSH receptors.

TESTS TO DETERMINE AETIOLOGY OF THYROID DISEASE

- Calcitonin, secreted by parafollicular (C) cells, is increased in medullary thyroid carcinoma.
- Fine needle aspiration cytology of thyroid nodule.

Q. Discuss the aetiology, clinical features, investigations and management of hyperthyroidism. (IM12.11, IM12.13, IM12.15)

Q. Discuss the pathogenesis, clinical features, investigations and management of Graves' disease. (IM12.1, IM12.13, IM12.15)

CAUSES OF HYPERTHYROIDISM

- Various causes of hyperthyroidism are given in Box 18.2.

BOX 18.2 Causes of Hyperthyroidism

- Graves' disease
- Multinodular goitre
- Solitary thyroid nodule (toxic adenoma)
- Excess pituitary secretion of TSH
- Drugs (amiodarone, excess of iodine, excess intake of thyroxine)
- Hydatidiform mole
- Choriocarcinoma
- Struma ovarii (functioning thyroid tissue in an ovarian neoplasm)
- Carcinoma of thyroid with bony metastasis
- Hashimoto's thyroiditis and other thyroiditis (initial stages)

PATHOGENESIS

GRAVES' DISEASE

- TSI or TRAb are IgG antibodies directed against the TSH receptors on the follicular cell, which stimulate thyroid hormone production and goitre formation.
- The ophthalmopathy and dermatopathy associated with Graves' disease are due to immunologically mediated activation of fibroblasts in the extraocular muscles and skin, with accumulation of glycosaminoglycans, leading to trapping of water and oedema initially. Later, fibroblasts produce fibrosis.
- Genetic factors are significant in a minority of cases. HLA-DR3 is the best-documented risk factor.
- Viral or bacterial infections may trigger hyperthyroidism. *Escherichia coli* and *Yersinia enterocolitica* possess cell membrane TSH receptors. The antibodies produced against these organisms cross-react with the TSH receptors, triggering the disease.
- Another immunoglobulin, a blocking antibody against TSH receptor, finally results in thyroid failure in late stages.

TREATMENT-INDUCED HYPERTHYROIDISM

- Iodine-induced hyperthyroidism can occur after intake of excess iodine in the diet, exposure to radiographic contrast media or medications.
- It generally occurs in patients with an underlying autonomously functioning thyroid gland (caused, e.g. by a nodule, multinodular goitre or Graves' disease). It can also occur in patients with endemic goitre who are treated with iodine. This is known as Jod–Basedow phenomenon.
- It is characterised by suppressed serum TSH level with normal circulating thyroid hormone levels.
- Paradoxically, excess uptake of iodine by the thyroid may inhibit thyroid hormone synthesis (Wolff–Chaikoff effect). Thus, iodide toxicity can eventually cause iodide goitre, hypothyroidism or myxoedema.
- The antiarrhythmic drug amiodarone has 37% iodine content with high tissue penetration and a half-life of months. The elemental iodine load of about 9 mg/day from a 200-mg tablet can precipitate hyperthyroidism if there is preexisting goitre (type I: amiodarone-induced hyperthyroidism), while the drug itself causes thyroiditis in 5%–10% of users, typically after about 2 years of therapy (type II: amiodarone-induced hyperthyroidism) that can later on lead to hypothyroidism.

TABLE 18.9 Clinical Features of Thyrotoxicosis

• Thyroid	• Diffuse or nodular enlargement; may be normal in size
• Gastrointestinal	• Weight loss, increased appetite, vomiting, increased stool frequency, diarrhoea, steatorrhoea, dysphagia due to goitre
• Cardiorespiratory	• Exertional dyspnoea, exacerbation of asthma, palpitations, angina, sinus tachycardia, atrial fibrillation, wide pulse pressure, cardiac failure, cardiomyopathy
• Neuromuscular	• Nervousness, irritability, emotional lability, psychosis, fine tremors, hyper-reflexia, ill-sustained clonus, muscle weakness, proximal myopathy, bulbar myopathy
• Dermatological	• Increased sweating, pruritus, palmar erythema, spider naevi, onycholysis, alopecia, hyperpigmentation
• Reproductive	• Menstrual disturbances (amenorrhoea or oligomenorrhoea), infertility, repeated abortions, loss of libido, impotence
• Miscellaneous	• Heat intolerance, fatigue, apathy, gynaecomastia, thirst, lid lag, lid retraction, osteoporosis, nocturia, impaired glucose tolerance

- Factitial hyperthyroidism is caused by intentional or accidental ingestion of excess amounts of thyroid hormone. Some patients may take thyroid preparations to achieve weight loss.

CLINICAL FEATURES OF THYROTOXICOSIS

- Clinical features of thyrotoxicosis are given in Table 18.9.
- Patients with painless thyroiditis may have no thyroid enlargement. Thyromegaly is also absent in exogenous hyperthyroidism and struma ovarii.
- Elderly patients with hyperthyroidism present with anorexia, apathy, and dominant cardiovascular and myopathic features. Younger patients with hyperthyroidism present with dominant neurological manifestations.
- A rare presentation of thyrotoxicosis is periodic paralysis which is often precipitated by exercise, fasting or a high carbohydrate meal. Hypokalaemia is frequently seen.

GRAVES' DISEASE

- In addition to above-mentioned features, Graves' disease is distinguished from other forms of hyperthyroidism by the presence of diffuse thyroid enlargement with or without bruit, ophthalmopathy and pretibial myxoedema.
- Vitiligo, finger clubbing and lymphadenopathy are common in Graves' disease.

OPHTHALMOPATHY (EYE SIGNS)

- It is present in 50% of the patients when first seen, but may precede Graves' disease by many years (exophthalmic goitre) or may develop even after successful treatment of Graves' disease.

- Pathogenesis of ophthalmopathy is not well understood. There is an increase in the bulk of orbital contents with a rise in retrobulbar pressure. This results in exophthalmos and optic nerve compression (congestive ophthalmopathy). Ocular myopathy is also seen.
- Symptoms include excessive lacrimation, grittiness, redness, diminution of visual acuity and diplopia.
- Signs include exophthalmos, corneal ulcers, chemosis, ophthalmoplegia, lid lag, lid retraction, visual field defects and papilloedema.
- Riesman's sign or Snellen–Riesman sign is bruit over the closed eye heard with bell of a stethoscope during systole.
- Majority do not require any treatment. Various symptomatic measures include the following:
  - Methylcellulose eye drops for grittiness.
  - Tinted glasses to reduce lacrimation.
  - Lateral tarsorrhaphy for corneal ulcers.
  - Persistent diplopia is treated by surgical correction of extraocular muscles.
  - Papilloedema, loss of visual acuity and visual field defect require emergency treatment with prednisolone. If there is no response, orbital decompression should be done.

PRETIBIAL MYXOEDEMA

- This is an infiltrative dermopathy typically affecting the anterior aspect of the leg extending on to the dorsum of the foot. Rarely, face and arms are affected.
- There are raised pinkish or purplish plaques that may be itchy (Fig. 18.4). The skin may have a peau d'orange appearance with coarse hair.
- Pretibial myxoedema may be treated with local injections of triamcinolone or application of betamethasone ointment.

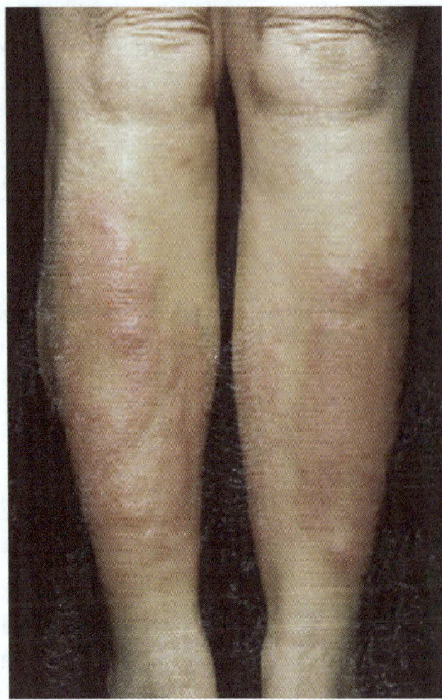

Fig. 18.4 Pretibial myxoedema.

OTHER DISORDERS ASSOCIATED WITH GRAVES' DISEASE

- Autoimmune disorders:
  - Endocrine: Addison's disease, type 1 diabetes mellitus (DM), primary gonadal failure, hypophysitis, Hashimoto's thyroiditis.
  - Nonendocrine: Coeliac disease, vitiligo, alopecia areata, myasthenia gravis, pernicious anaemia, immune thrombocytopenic purpura, rheumatoid arthritis.
- Others:
  - Hypokalaemic periodic paralysis, mitral valve prolapse.

SUBCLINICAL THYROTOXICOSIS

- Causes atrial fibrillation in people older than 60 years as well as bone loss in postmenopausal women.
- Serum levels of free T_4 and triiodothyronine are within the broad range of normal, but serum concentration of TSH is subnormal, often <0.1 mU/L.

MULTINODULAR GOITRE

- A toxic multinodular goitre (Plummer's disease) has at least two autonomously functioning nodules that secrete excess thyroid hormone.
- On RAIU scan, the nodules appear 'hot' with increased uptake of radioactive iodine when the remainder of the thyroid gland is suppressed.

INVESTIGATIONS

- TSH levels are very low or undetectable. This is the primary test performed, and if normal, virtually excludes thyrotoxicosis.
- Serum T_3 and T_4 levels are elevated in the majority. T_3 thyrotoxicosis is characterised by elevated levels of T_3 and normal levels of T_4. T_4 thyrotoxicosis is characterised by elevated levels of T_4 and normal levels of T_3. It occurs due to inhibition of peripheral conversion of T_4 to T_3 (as seen with amiodarone- and iodine-induced hyperthyroidism or concurrent nonthyroidal illness).
- Absent TSH response following intravenous TRH.
- ^{131}I uptake by the thyroid gland may be increased. However, it will be reduced or absent in thyroiditis, exogenous thyroxine, struma ovarii and metastatic follicular thyroid carcinoma.
- Elevated levels of antibodies to TPO.
- Measurement of TRAb may be useful in Graves' disease.
- Minor LFT abnormalities, mild hypercalcaemia and glycosuria may be present in few.
- Flowchart 18.3 shows an algorithm to evaluate a patient with thyrotoxicosis.

MANAGEMENT OF HYPERTHYROIDISM OF GRAVES' DISEASE

- There are three methods of treatment:
  1. Antithyroid drugs with initial supplementation of a β-blocker.

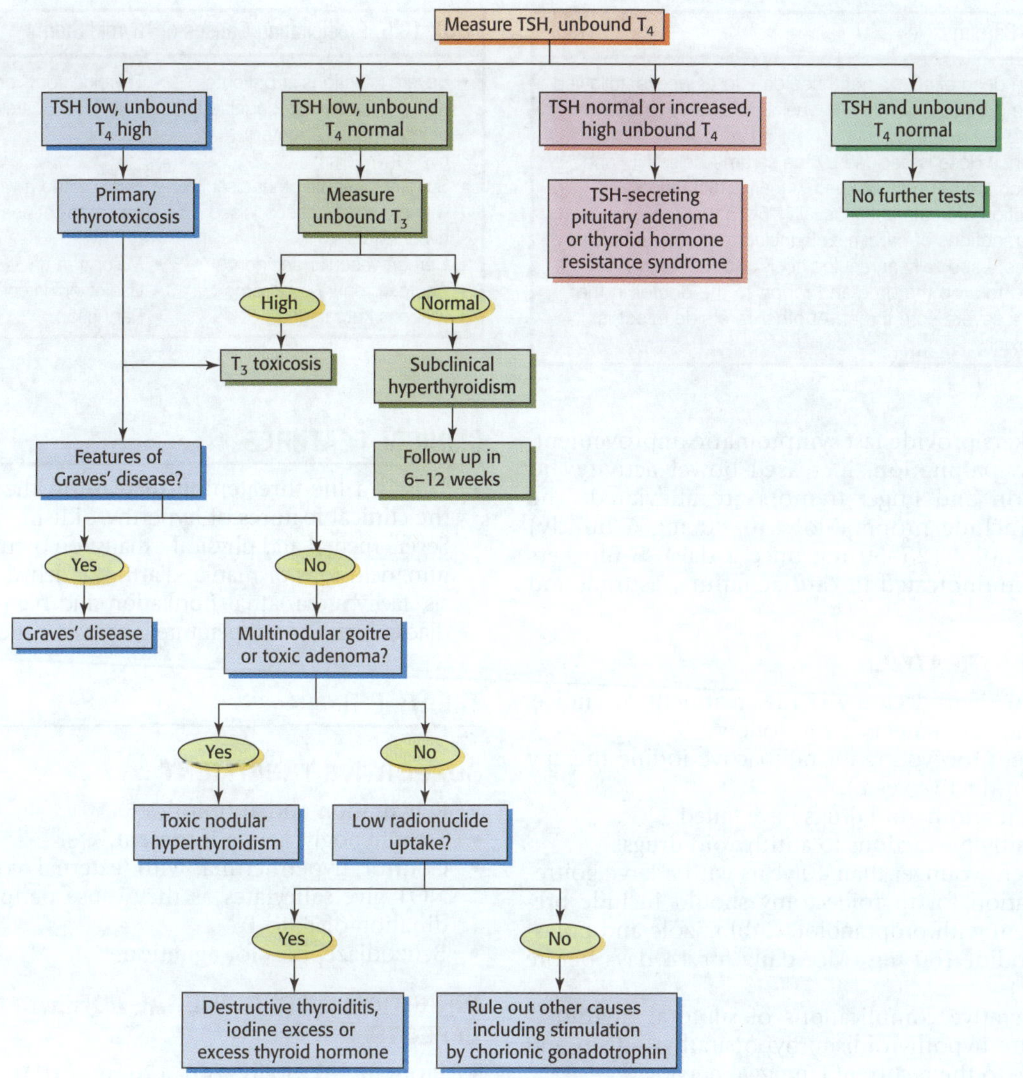

Flowchart 18.3 Evaluation of Thyrotoxicosis. (Source: *J.L. Jameson, A.S. Fauci, D.L. Kasper, et al.:* Harrison's Principles of Internal Medicine, *20th Edition, Chapter 377: Hyperthyroidism, McGraw-Hill Education.*)

BOX 18.3 Antithyroid Drugs

- Carbimazole
- Methimazole
- Propylthiouracil
- Lithium
- Potassium perchlorate
- Potassium iodide

2. Surgical treatment.
3. Radioactive iodine.

ANTITHYROID DRUGS (Box 18.3)

- Antithyroid drugs are often considered the primary therapy in pregnancy, in children and adolescents, and for patients who have severe Graves' eye disease.
- Potassium perchlorate reduces the uptake of iodine. Methimazole, carbimazole and thiouracil group prevent the organic binding of iodine to tyrosine in Tg by interfering with TPO. Carbimazole has an additional immunosuppressive action. Propylthiouracil also inhibits conversion of T_4 into T_3 at peripheral level and, therefore, is more useful in severe thyrotoxicosis.
- Propylthiouracil is preferred in first trimester of pregnancy because of more significant teratogenic effects of methimazole. It can cause severe liver injury and is not recommended for routine use.
- Potassium perchlorate is more toxic and induces red cell aplasia. It is used only as temporary measure in iodine-induced thyrotoxicosis (e.g. amiodarone induced) or when no other therapy is acceptable.
- Potassium iodide (five drops TID) is indicated only in the preparation for thyroidectomy and treatment of thyrotoxic crisis. Iodide decreases T_4 and T_3 synthesis by inhibiting iodide oxidation and organification, the Wolff–Chaikoff effect. It also blocks the release of T_4 and T_3 by inhibiting Tg proteolysis.
- The most commonly used antithyroid drug in India is carbimazole (Box 18.4).

BOX 18.4 Carbimazole

- Given at a dose of 10–15 mg thrice daily for 3 weeks, followed by 5–10 mg thrice daily for 4–8 weeks, followed by a maintenance of 5–20 mg daily.
- Maintenance dose is decided by the serum levels of T_4 and TSH, which are to be maintained in the normal range.
- Total duration of treatment is usually 15–18 months.
- Adverse reactions of carbimazole include rashes and blood dyscrasias, especially agranulocytosis. So, patients are instructed to stop the drug and report to the doctor in the event of a severe sore throat. Another rare side effect is hepatotoxicity.

BOX 18.5 Precipitating Causes of Thyroid Storm

- Severe infections in patients with previously unrecognised or inadequately treated hyperthyroidism
- Surgery for some other disability with previously unrecognised hyperthyroidism
- Cerebrovascular accident
- Acute coronary syndrome
- Diabetic ketoacidosis
- Thyroidectomy or ^{131}I therapy in an inadequately prepared patient
- Rapid withdrawal of antithyroid medications
- Major trauma
- Use of iodine contrast agents
- Parturition

- β-Blockers provide fast symptomatic improvement. Anxiety, palpitation, increased bowel activity, lid retraction and finger tremors are alleviated. The drugs include propranolol (40–80 mg 6 hourly) and atenolol (25–50 mg once a day). β-Blockers are contraindicated in cardiac failure, asthma and diabetes.

SURGICAL TREATMENT

- Subtotal thyroidectomy is the treatment of choice. Indications of surgery are as follows:
  - Patient too young for radioactive iodine therapy (reproductive years).
  - When antithyroid drugs have failed.
  - Sensitivity reactions to antithyroid drugs.
  - Patient younger than 40 years with a large goitre.
- Preparation for thyroidectomy should include pretreatment with propranolol, carbimazole and potassium iodide (60 mg twice daily for 14 days before surgery).
- Postoperative complications of subtotal thyroidectomy are hypothyroidism, hypoparathyroidism and damage to the recurrent laryngeal nerve.

RADIOACTIVE IODINE

- Indications of radioactive iodine therapy include the following:
  - Patients older than 40 years.
  - Young patients with a short lifespan due to some other reason.
  - Young patients who are sterilised.
- Absolutely contraindicated in pregnancy and breastfeeding.
- The only complication is hypothyroidism in the ensuing years. During the lag period, treat the patient with propranolol and carbimazole in severe cases.
- No evidence to suggest an increased risk of thyroid cancer and leukaemia after radioiodine therapy in adults, but data are not available for children.

Q. Describe hyperthyroid crisis, thyrotoxic crisis or thyroid storm.

PRECIPITATING CAUSES

- Precipitating causes of thyrotoxic crisis or thyroid storm are given in Box 18.5.

CLINICAL FEATURES

- This is a life-threatening increase in the severity of the clinical features of hyperthyroidism.
- Severe mental and physical exhaustion occur with delirium, delusions or mania, diarrhoea, dehydration, ketosis, tachycardia, atrial fibrillation and high-output cardiac failure. The temperature is characteristically raised.

TREATMENT

SUPPORTIVE TREATMENT

- Rehydration and antibiotics.
- Treat hypoglycaemia if present.
- Control hyperthermia with external cooling. DO NOT give salicylates as they cause peripheral deiodination of T_4 to T_3.
- Benzodiazepines for agitation.

INHIBITION OF PERIPHERAL ADRENERGIC EFFECTS

- Propranolol orally (40–120 mg TID) or intravenously (1 to 2 mg every 15 minutes till desired effect is achieved). It also blocks peripheral conversion of T_4 to T_3.
- In presence of mild heart failure, a short acting betablocker, esmolol may be administered with a loading dose of 250–500 μg/kg followed by 50–100 μg/kg/minute. It does not have any effect on peripheral conversion of T_4 to T_3.

INHIBITION OF THYROID HORMONE SYNTHESIS

- Propylthiouracil 800–1200 mg orally followed by 200 mg every 4–6 hours or methimazole 40–100 mg orally followed by 20 mg every 4–6 hours.

INHIBITION OF THYROID HORMONE RELEASE

- Lugol's iodine 10 drops TID or sodium ipodate (oral cholecystographic agent containing iodine) 0.5–3 g daily or intravenous iopanoic acid 1 g every 8 hours or lithium carbonate in a dose of 300 mg QID.
- These drugs should be given only about 1 hour after propylthiouracil or methimazole.
- Lithium also inhibits thyroid hormone synthesis and release.

PREVENTING PERIPHERAL CONVERSION OF T_4 TO T_3

- Intravenous hydrocortisone 300 mg initially followed by 100–200 mg every 6 hours. Glucocorticoids also treat possible relative adrenal insufficiency.
- Propylthiouracil and propranolol also reduce this conversion to some extent.

PREVENTING REABSORPTION OR REMOVAL OF THYROID HORMONES

- Cholestyramine breaks enterohepatic circulation of thyroid hormones thereby reducing reabsorption. It is given in a dose of 4 g every 6 hours.
- If propylthiouracil and methimazole are contraindicated, thyroid hormone can be removed by plasmapheresis, charcoal haemoperfusion and plasma exchange and one of these measures may be used if patient fails to respond to other therapeutic modalities.

TREATING PRECIPITATING CONDITION

- Search for precipitating conditions and provide appropriate treatment.

Q. Describe the aetiology, clinical features, diagnosis and management of primary hypothyroidism/ Hashimoto's thyroiditis. (IM12.1, IM12.11)

Q. What is myxoedema?

- The term myxoedema indicates severe hypothyroidism in which there is accumulation of hydrophilic mucopolysaccharides in the ground substance of the dermis and other tissues, leading to thickening of the facial features and doughy induration of the skin.

CLASSIFICATION OF HYPOTHYROIDISM

- Primary hypothyroidism—due to a cause within the thyroid gland itself.
- Secondary hypothyroidism—due to failure of TSH production following pituitary or hypothalamic disease.

COMMON CAUSES OF PRIMARY HYPOTHYROIDISM (Box 18.6)

BOX 18.6 Common Causes of Primary Hypothyroidism

• Hashimoto's thyroiditis	• Dyshormonogenesis
• Iodine deficiency (and excess)	• Drugs (PAS, lithium, amiodarone, antithyroid drugs, interferon-alpha, sunitinib)
• ^{131}I therapy	• External irradiation of neck for lymphoma or cancer
• Thyroidectomy	• Infiltrative disorders (amyloidosis, sarcoidosis, haemochromatosis)

HASHIMOTO'S THYROIDITIS

- Also known as spontaneous atrophic hypothyroidism; it is the most common cause of primary hypothyroidism.
- This is an organ-specific autoimmune disorder with lymphoid infiltration of thyroid leading to fibrosis and atrophy.
- TRAb are present that block the effects of endogenous TSH.
- May be seen in some patients of Graves' disease treated with antithyroid drugs 10–20 years earlier.
- High risk of developing type 1 DM, pernicious anaemia and Addison's disease.

IODINE DEFICIENCY

- Iodine deficiency is the most common cause of hypothyroidism (and goitre) worldwide.

IODINE EXCESS

- Inhibits iodide organification and synthesis of T_4 and T_3 (Wolff–Chaikoff effect). Most people quickly escape from this effect. However, patients with abnormal thyroid glands can become hypothyroid if given iodine for more than a few days. Patients at risk for iodine-induced hypothyroidism include those with chronic autoimmune thyroiditis, partial thyroidectomy, a history of radioiodine therapy and subacute thyroiditis.

CLINICAL FEATURES (Table 18.10)

- Delayed relaxation of tendon reflexes is a common feature. Other causes include anorexia nervosa, advanced age, peripheral oedema, hypothermia, peripheral arterial disease and pregnancy.
- Myxoedema facies is a peculiar facial appearance due to periorbital puffiness resulting from myxoedema, scanty eyebrows, facial pallor due to vasoconstriction and anaemia, a lemon-yellow tint of the skin due to carotenaemia (caused by reduced conversion of carotene to vitamin A), purplish lips and malar flush.

TABLE 18.10 Clinical Features of Hypothyroidism

• Thyroid	Enlargement of the gland
• Gastrointestinal	Decreased appetite, constipation, ileus, ascites
• Cardiorespiratory	Angina, bradycardia, hypertension, cardiac failure, pericardial effusion, pleural effusion, obstructive sleep apnoea, QT interval prolongation
• Neuromuscular	Aches and pains, muscle stiffness, delayed relaxation of tendon reflexes (Woltman's sign), carpal tunnel syndrome, deafness, depression, psychosis, cerebellar ataxia, myotonia
• Dermatological	Myxoedema (nonpitting oedema of the skin of hands, feet and eyelids), dry, flaky skin and hair, alopecia, loss of lateral third of eyebrow, vitiligo, purplish lips and malar flush, carotenaemia, erythema ab igne (localised areas of reticulated erythema and hyperpigmentation), xanthelasmas
• Reproductive	Menorrhagia, infertility, galactorrhoea, impotence
• Haematological	Macrocytosis, anaemia
• Miscellaneous	Tiredness, somnolence, cold intolerance, hypothermia, hoarseness of voice, low-pitched voice, slurred speech, macroglossia, weight gain, hyponatraemia, hypoglycaemia

INVESTIGATIONS

- Serum T_4 levels are low and TSH levels are high.
- Thyroid peroxidase antibodies (TPOAb) to look for autoimmune hypothyroidism and to decide requirement of treatment in cases of mild or subclinical hypothyroidism.
- Serum cholesterol and triglyceride (TG) levels are raised.
- Serum lactate dehydrogenase (LDH) and creatine kinase (CK) levels are raised.
- Serum sodium levels may be low.
- Electrocardiogram demonstrates sinus bradycardia, low-voltage QRS complexes and ST–T wave abnormalities.
- Chest radiograph may show enlarged cardiac shadow due to pericardial effusion.

SUBCLINICAL HYPOTHYROIDISM

- It is a milder degree of thyroid failure characterised by mild to moderate increase in serum TSH but with T_4 values still within normal range.
- Antithyroid antibodies can be detected in 80% of these patients.
- Progression from subclinical to overt hypothyroidism occurs in 5%–18% of persons with subclinical hypothyroidism per year.
- Patients have risk of cardiovascular disease including diastolic dysfunction, hypertension and increased low density lipoprotein (LDL).
- Levothyroxine therapy should be started if TSH >10.0 mIU/L or the patient is a woman who wishes to conceive or is pregnant, while therapy needs to be individualised if TSH <10.0 mIU/L.

EVALUATION OF HYPOTHYROIDISM (Flowchart 18.4)

TREATMENT

- Hypothyroidism is treated with T_4. It is usually given at a dose of 50 μg/day for 3 weeks, followed by 100 μg/day for 3 weeks, followed by a maintenance dose of 150 μg/day. The correct dose of T_4 is that which restores serum TSH to below 3 mU/L. It should be given on empty stomach in the morning.
- In elderly patients and those with ischaemic heart disease, T_4 is started at a lower dose of 12.5–25 μg/day.
- In a few patients with ischaemic heart disease, angina may develop or worsen with T_4 therapy. They should be treated with β-blockers and vasodilators, or CABG, or balloon angioplasty. This allows full replacement dosage of T_4.

Q. Describe myxoedema coma and myxoedema madness.

- Myxoedema coma is a rare complication of hypothyroidism, seen usually in elderly patients.
- More than 90% of cases occur during the winter months.
- The usual precipitating causes are infections, drugs (amiodarone, anaesthetic agents, barbiturates, β-blockers, diuretics, lithium, narcotics, phenothiazines, antidepressants), cardiac failure, hyponatraemia, exposure to cold, hypoxia, hypercapnia, myocardial infarction, cerebrovascular accident and gastrointestinal bleed.
- Patients with myxoedema coma usually have longstanding hypothyroidism, although it may not have been previously diagnosed.

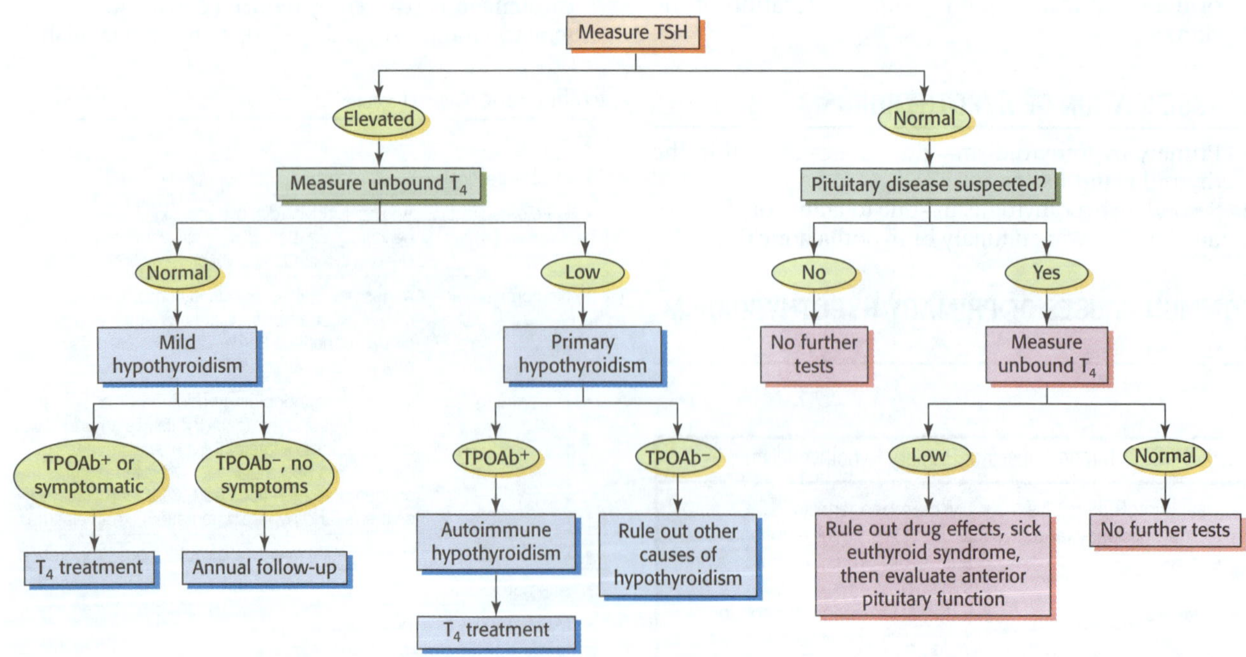

Flowchart 18.4 Evaluation of Hypothyroidism. (Source: *J.L. Jameson, A.S. Fauci, D.L. Kasper, et al.:* Harrison's Principles of Internal Medicine, *20th Edition, Chapter 376: Hypothyroidism, McGraw-Hill Education.)*

- Patients present with hypothermia, bradycardia and neuropsychiatric manifestations. They develop psychosis with delusions and hallucinations ('myxoedema madness'), progressing to depressed level of consciousness, convulsions and coma ('myxoedema coma').
- Metabolic abnormalities include hyponatraemia and hypoglycaemia.
- Arterial blood gases often reveal respiratory acidosis, hypoxia and hypercapnia.
- The cerebrospinal fluid pressure is low and protein content may be elevated.

MANAGEMENT

SUPPORTIVE CARE

- Includes gentle warming of the patient with blankets, broad-spectrum antibiotics, high-flow oxygen and, if required, assisted ventilation.
- Correction of hyponatraemia and hypoglycaemia.
- Hydrocortisone (100 mg intravenously 8 hourly) is required due to increased metabolic stress.

THYROID HORMONE REPLACEMENT

- Any patient with suspected myxoedema coma should be treated presumptively with thyroid hormone. As T_3 is more biologically active than T_4, most physicians recommend intravenous T_3 (20 μg 8 hourly). However, parenteral T_3 is not easily available. Therefore, intravenous T_4, initially 100–150 μg and then 75–100 μg daily, is recommended. If intravenous formulation is not available, T_4 may be administered orally in a dose of 300 μg stat followed by 100–300 μg daily.

TREAT PRECIPITATING CAUSES

- Identify and treat the precipitating cause.

Q. Briefly outline the neuropsychiatric manifestations of hypothyroidism.

- Neuropsychiatric manifestations of hypothyroidism are listed in Box 18.7.

BOX 18.7 Neuropsychiatric Manifestations of Hypothyroidism

• Muscle aches, pains and stiffness	• Hypothermia
• Carpal tunnel syndrome	• Cerebellar ataxia
• Myxoedema madness	• Cerebral cortical degeneration
• Myxoedema coma	• Deafness
• Delayed relaxation of deep tendon reflexes	• Myotonia
• Mental retardation (in cretinism)	• Depression, psychosis

Q. Give a brief account of sick euthyroid syndrome.

- Also known as nonthyroidal illness syndrome; it refers to abnormal findings on thyroid function tests in patients with severe illnesses not caused by primary thyroid or pituitary dysfunction. Therefore, routine testing of thyroid function should be avoided in acutely ill patients unless a thyroid disorder is strongly suspected.
- Conditions associated with sick euthyroid syndrome include malnutrition, anorexia nervosa, trauma, major surgery, myocardial infarction, chronic renal failure, diabetic ketoacidosis (DKA), cirrhosis, hypothermia and sepsis.
- Most common pattern of abnormality is low levels of total and free T_3, with normal T_4 and TSH (low T_3 syndrome). Peripheral conversion of T_4 to T_3 is reduced leading to increase in rT_3. There is reduced clearance of rT_3 in these patients that is the major cause of raised rT_3. In true hypothyroidism, rT_3 will be low.
- In severe illness, total T_4 may also fall (low T_4 syndrome). This indicates a poor prognosis. This is partly related to altered binding to TBG. Therefore free T_4 is normal. TSH levels fluctuate from low to high. However, if TSH >20 mU/L or is undetectable, euthyroid sick syndrome is less likely to be the cause.
- No role for levothyroxine treatment in sick euthyroid syndrome.
- Thyroid function tests should be repeated 6 weeks after hospitalisation to exclude overt thyroid dysfunction.

Q. What are the causes of thyroiditis?

- The term thyroiditis encompasses a heterogeneous group of disorders characterised by thyroid inflammation.

CAUSES OF THYROIDITIS (Table 18.11)

TABLE 18.11 Causes of Thyroiditis

• Acute	Bacterial infections (e.g. staphylococcal, streptococcal), fungal infections (*Aspergillus*, *Candida*, *Histoplasma*), radiation (e.g. thyroiditis after radioiodine treatment), amiodarone
• Subacute	Viral or granulomatous (de Quervain's thyroiditis), mycobacterial infection, postpartum thyroiditis
• Chronic	Autoimmune (Hashimoto's thyroiditis, Graves' disease), Riedel's thyroiditis, parasitic infections

Q. Describe subacute granulomatous thyroiditis (de Quervain's thyroiditis).

- Virus-induced (coxsackie, mumps, adenovirus, H1N1) inflammation of thyroid gland results in release of colloid and its contents (thyroglobulin) into the bloodstream. Thyroglobulin (Tg) is degraded by serum proteases into T_4 and T_3.

- A prodrome of flu-like illness 1–3 weeks before onset of thyroiditis.
- Thyroiditis is characterised by systemic symptoms of hyperthyroidism (e.g. tachycardia, sweating, tremors, diarrhoea, heat intolerance) and pain in the region of thyroid gland radiating to the angle of jaw and ears. Pain is made worse by swallowing, coughing and movement of the neck.
- The thyroid gland is enlarged and tender.
- ESR, CRP and serum Tg are raised in most patients.
- Thyroid radionuclide uptake is reduced or absent.
- Thyroid histology shows thyroid follicle destruction, infiltrates of mononuclear cells and characteristic multinucleated giant cell granulomas.
- Initially there is hyperthyroidism (with elevated T_3 and T_4 and depressed TSH), which is followed by a period of hypothyroidism, and finally full recovery in 4–6 months. In less than 5% of cases, hypothyroidism may persist.
- Treated with aspirin or other nonsteroidal antiinflammatory drugs, prednisolone (in severe disease) and propranolol.
    - Aspirin in high doses should be avoided as it causes thyroid hormone to be displaced from serum plasma proteins, increasing free thyroid hormone.
    - Antithyroid medications such as propylthiouracil and carbimazole are ineffective in reducing thyroid hormone levels because thyrotoxicosis is caused by release of preformed hormone as thyroglobulin.
- Therapy for hyperthyroidism is not often needed because symptoms are mild and short-lived.

Q. What is Hashimoto's thyroiditis? Discuss briefly its investigations and treatment. (IM12.1)

Q. Give a brief account of chronic autoimmune thyroiditis. (IM12.1)

- Also called chronic lymphocytic or autoimmune thyroiditis.
- It is an autoimmune condition characterised by high titres of circulating antibodies to TPO and Tg.
- It is the commonest cause of goitrous hypothyroidism.
- Common in middle-aged females (female to male ratio of 7:1), and is often associated with ulcerative colitis or type 1 DM.
- Pathologically there is lymphocytic infiltration, fibrosis and follicular cell hyperplasia of thyroid.
- Most patients are asymptomatic, though some may complain of a feeling of tightness or fullness in the neck; however, neck pain and tenderness are rare.
- Diffuse enlargement of thyroid with a characteristic firm or rubbery consistency is typical. Occasionally, it may produce local symptoms due to the compression of the anatomical structures of the neck (e.g. dysphonia due to involvement of recurrent laryngeal nerve, dyspnoea and stridor due to compression of trachea and dysphagia due to compression of oesophagus).
- A few patients may have transient features of thyrotoxicosis in initial stages (Hashitoxicosis).
- Twenty-five per cent of these patients present with hypothyroidism; the rest are at a higher risk of developing it later.
- It is one of the components of type 2 autoimmune polyglandular syndrome.
- Hashimoto's encephalopathy is one of the most relevant clinical variants. The symptoms include subacute cognitive deterioration, myoclonus, change in behaviour and seizures. This condition responds to corticosteroids.
- Non-Hodgkin primary thyroid lymphoma has a strong association with Hashimoto's thyroiditis.

INVESTIGATIONS

- Thyroid function tests suggest hypothyroidism.
- Serum contains antibodies to TPO and Tg.
- Antinuclear antibodies (ANA) may be positive in the young.
- Ultrasound of thyroid shows reduced echogenicity, heterogeneity hypervascularity and presence of hypoechoic micronodules with echogenic rim.
- Fine needle aspiration cytology from thyroid shows lymphocytes and macrophages.

TREATMENT

- Thyroxine (150–200 µg/day) is effective in hypothyroidism, and can also bring about goitre shrinkage.

Q. Classify goitre.

Q. Briefly outline the clinical features, investigations and treatment of endemic goitre. (IM12.1)

Q. What is Jod–Basedow phenomenon?

Q. Describe briefly the National Iodine Deficiency Disorders Control Programme. (IM12.12)

- Goitre is the enlargement of thyroid gland.

CLASSIFICATION (Table 18.12)

TABLE 18.12 Classification of Goitre

Diffuse Goitre	Nodular Goitre
• Simple goitre—physiological (puberty, pregnancy), iodine deficiency (endemic goitre) • Toxic goitre—Graves' disease • Autoimmune/inflammatory goitre—Hashimoto's thyroiditis, subacute thyroiditis • Dyshormonogenesis goitrogens—lithium, sulphonylureas, amiodarone, cassava root, cauliflower • Elevated TSH production—pituitary adenoma	• Multinodular goitre (Plummer's disease) • Solitary nodular goitre • Riedel's thyroiditis • Neoplastic—thyroid adenoma, thyroid carcinoma

ENDEMIC GOITRE

- When iodine deficiency manifests as diffuse goitre in a particular geographic region where more than 5% of the population is affected, it is called endemic goitre.
- These endemic belts are characterised by:
  - A daily iodine intake of less than 50 μg (normal recommendation is 100 μg/day in children).
  - Very low iodine content in drinking water.
  - Deficient dietary sources of iodine like sea-fish, milk and eggs.
- Occasionally, goitre may be due to ingestion of goitrogens (e.g. cassava roots, cabbage, cauliflower).
- Goitre is one of the several disorders that occur due to iodine deficiency. Other disorders include mental and physical retardation, deaf mutism, cretinism, stillbirths, abortions. All the disorders are categorised under a term 'iodine deficiency disorders' (IDD). In India, of 414 districts surveyed in all the 29 states and 7 UTs, 337 districts are endemic for goitre, that is where the prevalence of endemic goitre is more than 5% (as per year 2014 to 2015).

CLINICAL FEATURES

- Endemic goitre manifests clinically as a diffuse enlargement of the thyroid with a patient in euthyroid state in the initial stage. This is known as simple goitre.
- The goitre is initially diffused but eventually becomes nodular because the cells in some thyroid follicles proliferate more than others.
- In children and adults, endemic goitre may be associated with features of hypothyroidism and mental retardation. In older adults, autonomous growth and function of nodules may occur which results in toxic goitre and hyperthyroidism if iodine deficiency is not extremely severe.
- Large goitre may compress surrounding structures like trachea, oesophagus, blood vessels and nerves.
- Occasionally, goitre may be substernal. Pemberton's manoeuvre can be used to exacerbate obstructive symptoms produced by a large substernal goitre. In this manoeuvre, the patient holds his arms vertically above the head for 1 minute. The test is considered positive if the neck veins become more distended or if the patient develops facial plethora, cyanosis or if other compressive features increase (dysphagia, dyspnoea or stridor).

Cretinism

- Iodine deficiency during pregnancy causes severe hormone-induced physiological damage to foetus and newborn resulting in cretinism (stunting, deaf-mutism, malformed limbs, spastic motor disorders, goitre, as well as mental impairment).

INVESTIGATIONS

- Plasma inorganic iodide levels are low.
- Urinary iodide excretion is low (<50 μg/day).
- Serum T_4 is normal; T_3 may be normal or elevated (due to enhanced conversion of T_4 to T_3).
- TSH may be normal or mildly elevated suggesting increased sensitivity to TSH.

TREATMENT

- Iodine replacement in early cases.
- Suppressive therapy with T_4.

PREVENTIVE MEASURES

- Fortification of common salt with iodine.
- Intramuscular injection of 3 to 4 mL of iodised oil once in 2 years.

JOD–BASEDOW PHENOMENON

- 'Jod–Basedow phenomenon' is the development of acute hyperthyroidism following iodine replacement. It is due to enhanced thyroid hormone production by autonomous nodules that may be present in some cases.

WOLFF–CHAIKOFF EFFECT

- Excessive iodine ingestion during pregnancy, particularly third trimester, may also have adverse effects on foetal thyroid function. Sudden exposure to excess serum iodide inhibits organification of iodide, thereby diminishing hormone biosynthesis; this phenomenon is called the Wolff–Chaikoff effect.

NATIONAL IODINE DEFICIENCY DISORDERS CONTROL PROGRAMME (NIDDCP)

GOALS

- To bring the prevalence of iodine deficiency disorders to below 5% in the country.
- To ensure 100% consumption of adequately iodated salt (15 ppm) at the household level.

OBJECTIVES

- Surveys to assess the magnitude of iodine deficiency disorders in the districts.
- Supply of iodated salt in place of common salt.
- Resurveys to assess iodine deficiency disorders and the impact of iodated salt after every 5 years in the districts.
- Laboratory monitoring of iodated salt and urinary iodine excretion.
- Health education and publicity.

POLICY

- In 1984, the Government of India took a policy decision to iodate the entire edible salt in the country by 1992. The programme started in 1986 in a phased manner. The annual production of iodated salt in our country is more than 65 lakh metric tons.

Q. Classify hyperparathyroidism.

Q. Discuss the clinical features, investigations and management of primary hyperparathyroidism.

CLASSIFICATION AND AETIOLOGY OF HYPERPARATHYROIDISM (Table 18.13)

TABLE 18.13 Classification and Causes of Hyperparathyroidism

• Primary hyperparathyroidism	Autonomous secretion of PTH by parathyroid. Serum calcium and PTH are raised. Causes—single adenoma (90%), multiple adenomata, nodular hyperplasia and carcinoma; rarely lithium and thiazides.
• Secondary hyperparathyroidism	Parathyroid hyperplasia with increased PTH secretion in an attempt to compensate for prolonged hypocalcaemia. Serum calcium is low and PTH is raised. Causes—chronic renal failure, malabsorption, osteomalacia and rickets (vitamin D deficiency).
• Tertiary hyperparathyroidism	Adenoma formation and autonomous PTH secretion occurring in cases of secondary hyperparathyroidism. Serum calcium and PTH are raised.

CLINICAL FEATURES

- More than 70% of patients are diagnosed by incidental finding of hypercalcaemia.
- Classical features described as 'moans (neuropsychiatric features), bones (arthritis, osteomalacia, osteitis), stones (renal stones, uraemia) and abdominal groans (abdominal pain, constipation, vomiting)' are present in a minority of patients. Various features are listed in Table 18.14.
- Primary hyperparathyroidism, secondary to a parathyroid adenoma, may be a part of multiple endocrine neoplasia syndrome.
  - MEN1 (Werner's syndrome) consists of tumours of the pituitary, pancreas and parathyroid glands. Other abnormalities often seen include Zollinger–Ellison syndrome.
  - MEN2A is characterised by phaeochromocytoma and medullary carcinoma of thyroid as well as hyperparathyroidism.
  - MEN2B (previously called MEN3) has additional multiple neuromas but hyperparathyroidism is not present.
  - MEN4 is characterised by parathyroid adenoma and anterior pituitary adenoma along with neuroendocrine tumours (pulmonary, gastrointestinal, pancreatic) and tumours of the reproductive tract, adrenal glands and kidneys.

TABLE 18.14 Clinical Features of Hyperparathyroidism

Gastrointestinal manifestations: • Anorexia, nausea, vomiting • Bowel hypomotility and constipation • Peptic ulcer disease • Pancreatitis **Renal manifestations:** • Polyuria and polydipsia • Recurrent calculus formation • Nephrocalcinosis—deposition of calcium salts in the renal parenchyma • Impairment of renal function • Nephrogenic diabetes insipidus • Renal tubular acidosis **Neurological manifestations:** • Weakness, tiredness, proximal myopathy • Drowsiness, poor concentration, memory loss and depression • Stupor, coma	**Skeletal manifestations:** • Bone pain, osteopenia, osteoporosis, fractures and deformity due to osteitis fibrosa cystica • Localised bone swelling, especially of the mandible • Degenerative arthritis and attacks of acute pseudogout, especially of the knee joints due to chondrocalcinosis affecting the menisci **Other manifestations:** • Corneal calcification, best seen by slit-lamp examination • Calcification of arterial walls and soft tissues of hand • Hypertension • Shortening of QT interval

INVESTIGATIONS

- Biochemical abnormalities.
  - Raised serum calcium and raised intact parathyroid hormone (PTH) (or normal PTH despite elevated calcium).
  - During blood drawing, venous stasis should be avoided to ensure accurate results.
  - Serum calcium concentrations should be corrected to the prevailing serum albumin concentration. The total calcium level can be corrected for low albumin levels by adding 0.8 mg/dL to the total serum calcium level for every 1.0 g/dL by which the serum albumin concentration is lower than 4 g/dL.
  - Serum 25-hydroxyvitamin D levels should be checked initially because presence of vitamin D deficiency can result in elevated PTH levels.
  - Serum phosphate is usually low.
  - Serum alkaline phosphatase may be raised depending on the degree of bone involvement.
- Urine.
  - Hypercalciuria (>300 mg/24 hours) in 30% of cases. In familial hypocalciuric hypercalcaemia, urinary calcium is less than 100 mg/24 hours.
  - Increased markers of bone resorption (urinary pyridinoline, deoxypyridinoline and *N*-telopeptide of collagen).
- ECG showing features of hypercalcaemia.
  - Shortened QT interval.
  - Cardiac arrhythmias (rare).
- Radiological abnormalities.
  - Osteitis fibrosa cystica is the pathognomonic skeletal feature evident by routine skeletal radiograph. These features include demineralisation and subperiosteal erosions/resorption of phalanges, most marked on the radial side of the middle phalanx, subperiosteal resorption of the distal phalanges (Fig. 18.5), 'pepper–pot' or 'salt-and-pepper' appearance of the skull on the lateral view (Fig. 18.6), tapering of the distal clavicle, bone cysts and brown tumours (osteolytic lesions in bones) (Fig. 18.7A and B).
  - Nephrocalcinosis—scattered opacities within the renal outline.
  - Soft tissue calcification (e.g. arterial wall).
  - Fractures.
- Dual-energy X-ray absorptiometry (DEXA) and CT scan show reduced bone density.
- Investigations for localisation of the tumour.
  - High-resolution ultrasonography.
  - Selective neck vein catheterisation with PTH measurements.
  - CT scanning and subtraction imaging.
  - Scintigraphy with technetium-99m sestamibi.

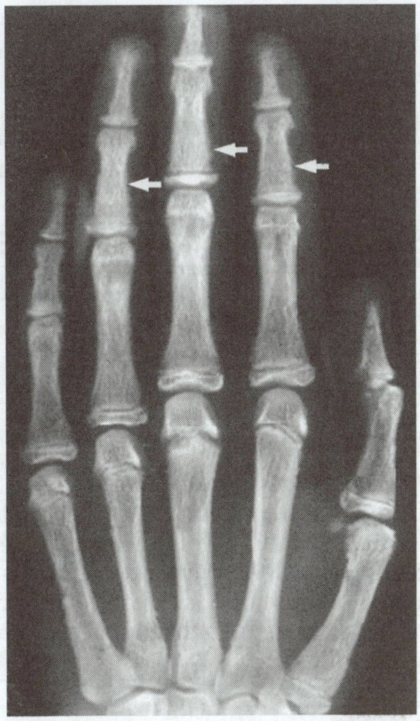

Fig. 18.5 Hyperparathyroidism. Subperiosteal bone resorption can be seen, predominantly involving the radial margins of the middle phalanges of the second, third and fourth digits (arrows) with resorption of terminal tufts.

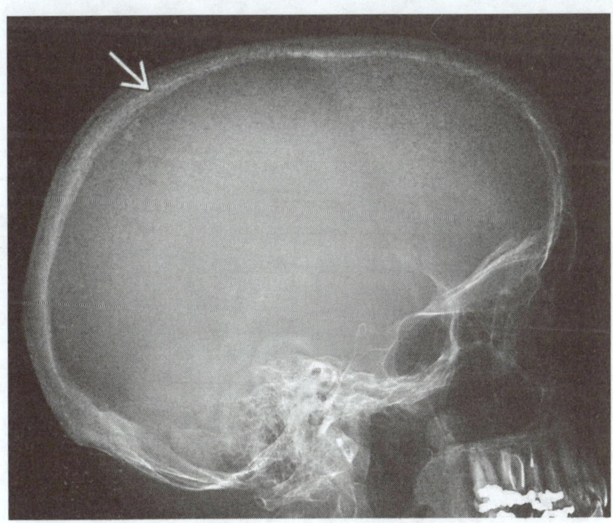

Fig. 18.6 Hyperparathyroidism. Characteristic salt-and-pepper skull.

TREATMENT

- Treatment of hypercalcaemia (see below).
- Adenoma is treated by surgical removal.
- Hyperplasia is treated by removal of all four glands and transplantation of some of the excised tissue to the forearm or by removing three glands and part of fourth gland.

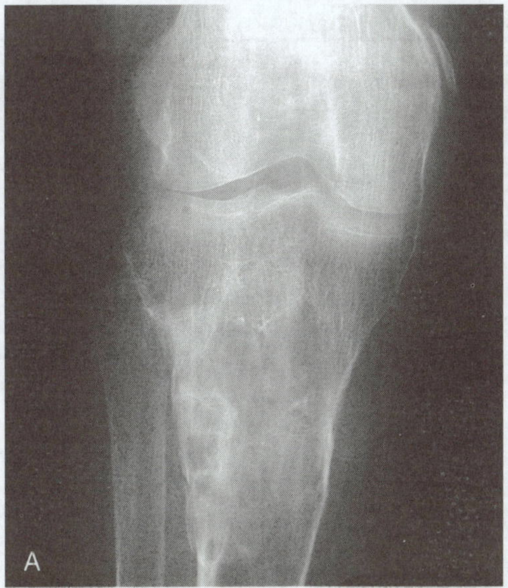

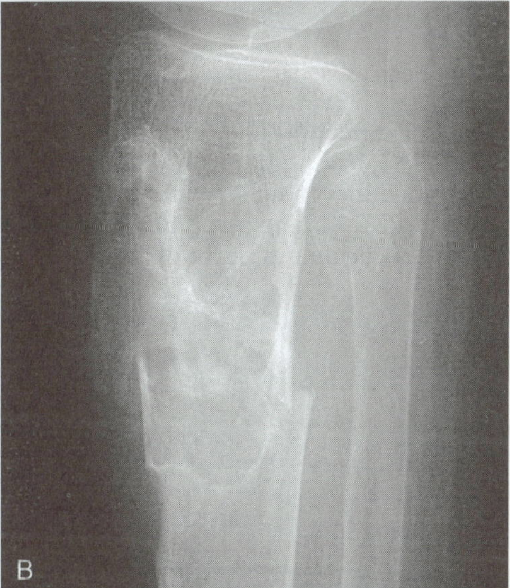

Fig. 18.7 (A and B) Pathologic fracture of right proximal tibia through 'brown tumour' of hyperparathyroidism.

Q. What are the causes of hypercalcaemia? Outline the management of hypercalcaemia.

- Parathyroid hormone (PTH), 1,25-dihydroxyvitamin D_3 (calcitriol) and calcitonin control calcium homeostasis in the body.
- Normal serum calcium levels are 8–10 mg/dL (2.0–2.5 mmol/L).
- Normal ionised calcium levels are 4 to 5.6 mg/dL (1–1.4 mmol/L).
- Hypercalcaemia is considered mild if the total serum calcium level is between 10.5 and 12 mg/dL (2.6 to 3 mmol/L) while levels above 14 mg/dL indicate severe hypercalcaemia.

CAUSES

- Various causes of hypercalcaemia are given in Table 18.15.

TABLE 18.15 Causes of Hypercalcaemia

Parathyroid hormone related (normal or elevated PTH):	Vitamin D related (low PTH):
• Primary hyperparathyroidism • Tertiary hyperparathyroidism • Lithium therapy • Familial hypocalciuric hypercalcaemia • Multiple endocrine neoplasia syndromes	• Vitamin D intoxication • Granulomatous diseases (sarcoidosis, tuberculosis, berylliosis) • Idiopathic hypercalcaemia of infancy
Malignancy related (low PTH):	**High bone turnover:**

• Humoral-mediated (e.g. PTH-related peptide)
  • Squamous cell carcinomas (e.g. lung, head and neck, oesophageal, cervical, colonic)
  • Renal carcinoma
  • Breast carcinoma
  • Ovarian carcinoma
• Local osteolysis mediated
• Breast carcinoma (metastatic)
• Multiple myeloma
• Lymphoma
	• Immobilisation
	• Hyperthyroidism
	Associated with renal failure:
	• Secondary hyperparathyroidism
	• Aluminium intoxication
	Miscellaneous:
	• Milk–alkali syndrome
	• Thiazide diuretics

- Lithium decreases parathyroid gland sensitivity to calcium.
- Familial hypocalciuric hypercalcaemia is due to a mutation in calcium-sensing receptor in parathyroid glands and kidneys.
- In milk-alkali syndrome, associated metabolic alkalosis enhances calcium reabsorption from renal tubules.
- Thiazide diuretics directly enhance active calcium reabsorption in the distal tubule.

CLINICAL FEATURES

- Discussed under 'Hyperparathyroidism', page 988.

DIAGNOSTIC APPROACH TO HYPERCALCAEMIA

- Algorithm for the diagnosis of hypercalcaemia is shown in Flowchart 18.5.

MANAGEMENT

MILD HYPERCALCAEMIA (<12 MG/DL)

- Avoid factors aggravating hypercalcaemia (e.g. thiazide diuretics, lithium, volume depletion, bed rest).
- Simple oral hydration along with increased salt intake is sufficient. Many hypercalcaemic patients are dehydrated because of poor intake, vomiting, confusion or hypercalcaemia-related defects in renal concentrating ability.

SEVERE HYPERCALCAEMIA

- Forced diuresis with isotonic saline at an initial rate of 200–300 mL/hour and then adjusted to maintain a urine output at 100–150 mL/hour. Sodium, potassium and magnesium should be supplemented. Saline acts

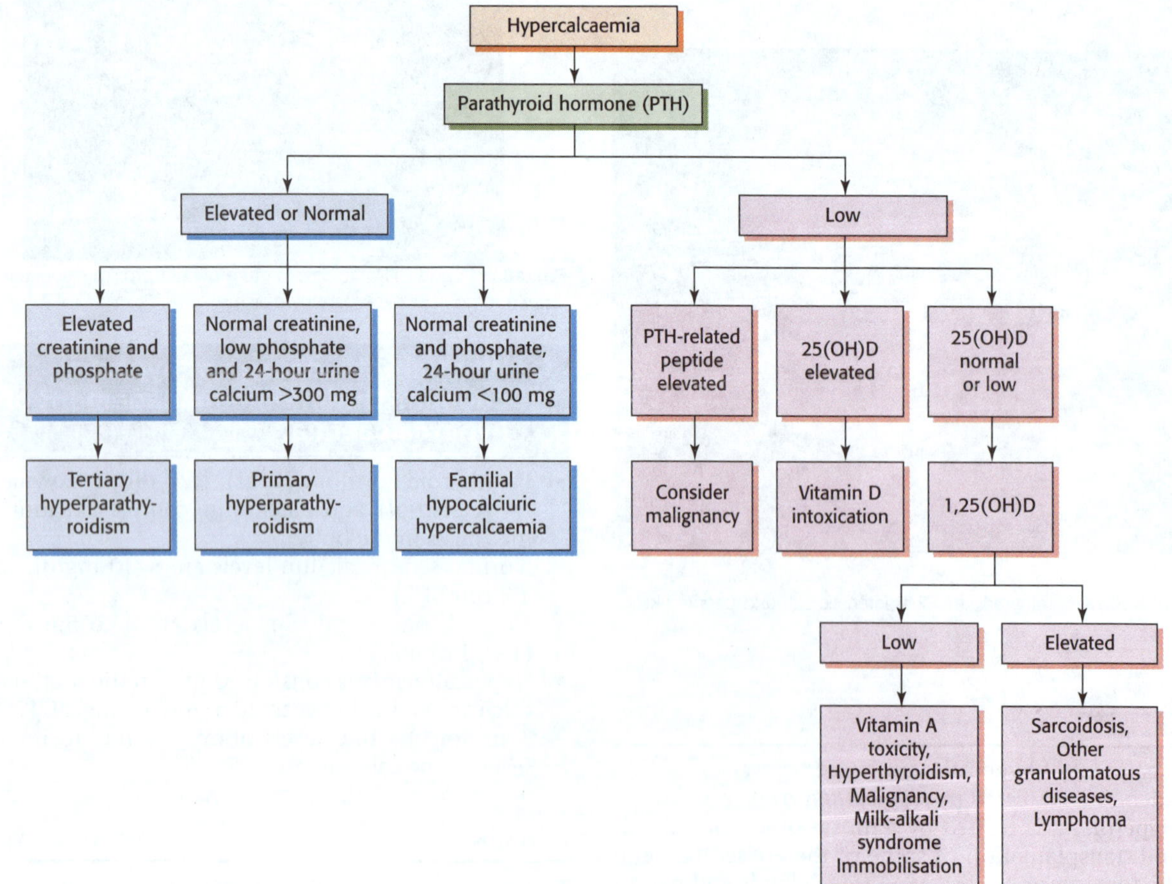

Flowchart 18.5 Approach to a Patient with Hypercalcaemia.

by decreasing concomitant reabsorption of sodium and calcium in both the proximal and distal renal tubules, and enhancing urinary calcium excretion by increasing glomerular filtration rate.

- Diuretics like furosemide 40–160 mg/day (after correction of volume deficit) to maintain urine output particularly in patients with CKD or heart failure.
- Intravenous bisphosphonates (pamidronate, zoledronic acid, ibandronate) are useful in malignancy-associated hypercalcaemia. These agents inhibit osteoclast action, thereby reducing bone resorption. Most commonly used agent is pamidronate in a dose of 60–90 mg intravenously over 4 hours. Effect of bisphosphonates on serum calcium concentrations is apparent after 24–48 hours.
- Salmon calcitonin 200–400 IU subcutaneously 8 hourly for 24 hours. It inhibits bone resorption and augments renal excretion of calcium. It is used in severe hypercalcaemia refractory to other measures.
- Most often saline infusion is combined with calcitonin and a bisphosphonate.
- Prednisolone 5–15 mg 6 hourly orally or hydrocortisone 50–100 mg IV 6 hourly. Steroids inhibit vitamin D conversion to calcitriol and are useful in vitamin D intoxication, lymphoma and granulomatous diseases where intestinal absorption of calcium is increased due to increased endogenous calcitriol production.
- Others:
    - Mithramycin 10–25 μg/kg intravenously over 6 hours for 3–8 days if bisphosphonates cannot be given.
    - Calcimimetics (e.g. cinacalcet) reduce serum calcium in patients with severe hypercalcaemia due to parathyroid carcinoma and in haemodialysis patients with secondary hyperparathyroidism and an elevated calcium–phosphorus product.
    - Denosumab (a RANK ligand inhibitor monoclonal antibody which reduces bone resorption) in patients refractory to bisphosphonates or where they are contraindicated (e.g. CKD).
    - Haemodialysis with a low-calcium bath.

Q. Give a brief account of the causes and general management of hypoparathyroidism.

CAUSES

- Postoperative hypoparathyroidism (thyroidectomy, parathyroidectomy, radical neck dissection).
- Genetic hypoparathyroidism (abnormal parathyroid gland development, abnormal PTH synthesis).
- Idiopathic hypoparathyroidism.
- Postradiation.
- Destruction or invasion due to tumour.
- Infiltration by iron or copper.
- DiGeorge's syndrome (asymptomatic hypocalcaemia due to hypoparathyroidism along with thymic hypoplasia with immunodeficiency and congenital heart defects).
- Autoimmune polyendocrinopathy type 1 (chronic mucocutaneous candidiasis, hypoparathyroidism and autoimmune adrenal failure).
- Autoimmune hypoparathyroidism.
- Kearns–Sayre syndrome due to deletions in the mitochondrial genome (hypoparathyroidism, encephalopathy and stroke-like episodes).
- Pseudohypoparathyroidism (inherited disorder with resistance of target organs to PTH; PTH is high).

CLINICAL FEATURES

- The common clinical manifestation is tetany, irrespective of the cause (see below).
- Chronic hypoparathyroidism may lead to basal ganglia calcifications, cataracts and dental abnormalities.
    - Basal ganglia calcification may be asymptomatic or may produce parkinsonism and other movement disorders like dystonia, hemiballismus, choreoathetosis and oculogyric crises.
    - Dental abnormalities occur when hypocalcaemia is present during early development. They include dental hypoplasia, failure of tooth eruption, defective enamel and root formation, and abraded carious teeth.
- Chronic hypocalcaemia may produce dry, coarse skin with coarse, brittle and sparse hair. The nails become brittle with characteristic transverse grooves.
- Pseudohypoparathyroidism is of three types with type 1A being the most common. It is an autosomal dominant disorder. Additional features in type 1A include short stature, rounded face, shortened fourth metacarpals and other bones of the hands and feet, obesity, dental hypoplasia, and soft tissue calcifications and ossifications. These developmental and skeletal defects are collectively termed Albright's hereditary osteodystrophy.
- Pseudopseudohypoparathyroidism is a condition which has normal PTH, calcium and phosphorus but with Albright's hereditary osteodystrophy.

DIAGNOSIS

- Characteristically serum calcium is low, serum phosphate is high and PTH is low or inappropriately normal.
- Serum 25-hydroxyvitamin D is normal, while 1,25-dihydroxyvitamin D is normal or low.

TREATMENT

- In the acute phase, calcium is given intravenously as for tetany.
- Substitution therapy is provided by 1-α-hydroxycholecalciferol (alphacalcidol) or 1,25-dihydroxycholecalciferol (calcitriol), both at a dose of 0.25–2 μg/day.
- In the long term, thiazide diuretics are useful as they enhance renal calcium reabsorption and increase serum calcium.
- Recombinant human PTH can be used as an adjunct for the treatment of adults with hypoparathyroidism who are not well controlled with calcium and vitamin D.

Q. Discuss hypocalcaemia.

Q. What are the causes of tetany? Give the clinical picture and management of tetany.

Q. Explain briefly Trousseau's sign and Chvostek's sign.

CAUSES OF TETANY AND HYPOCALCAEMIA

- Tetany is caused by an increased excitability of peripheral nerves due to hypocalcaemia or alkalosis or hypomagnesaemia.
- Alkalosis enhances binding of calcium to albumin, thereby reducing ionised calcium.
- Hypomagnesaemia induces hypocalcaemia both by inducing resistance to PTH and by diminishing its secretion.
- Various causes of hypocalcaemia and tetany are listed in Table 18.16.

CLINICAL FEATURES

- In children, the characteristic triad of tetany is carpopedal spasm, stridor and convulsions. In 'carpal spasm', the metacarpophalangeal joints are flexed, the interphalangeal joints are extended and there is opposition of the thumb (main d'accoucheur).
- In adults, there is tingling in the hands, feet and around the mouth (circumoral paraesthesia).
- Latent tetany may be present when signs of overt tetany are lacking. It is recognised by eliciting two signs:
  - Trousseau's sign—inflation of sphygmomanometer cuff on the upper arm to more than systolic pressure is followed by the characteristic carpal spasm within 3 minutes.
  - Chvostek's sign—tapping over the branches of facial nerve as they emerge from the parotid gland produces twitching of the facial muscles.
- Severe hypocalcaemia may result in life-threatening seizures, refractory heart failure, laryngospasm or papilloedema.
- Cardiac findings may include a prolonged QT interval, hypotension, heart failure and arrhythmia.
- Chronic hypocalcaemia may produce dry, coarse skin with coarse, brittle and sparse hair. The nails become brittle with characteristic transverse grooves.

TABLE 18.16 Causes of Hypocalcaemia and Tetany

Due to hypocalcaemia:	Due to alkalosis producing hypocalcaemia:
• Malabsorption • Hypoparathyroidism due to any cause • Vitamin D deficiency • Vitamin D resistance • Acute pancreatitis • Chronic kidney disease • Massive transfusion (citrated blood) • Tumour lysis syndrome • Drugs inhibiting bone resorption (bisphosphonates, calcitonin, denosumab) • Calcium chelators (EDTA, foscarnet)	• Repeated vomiting or aspiration of gastric juice • Excessive intake of oral alkalis • Hyperventilation—for example conversion disorder • Primary hyperaldosteronism **Due to hypomagnesaemia producing hypocalcaemia**

TREATMENT

CONTROL OF TETANY

- Slow intravenous injection of 10–20 mL of 10% solution of calcium gluconate over 10 minutes is effective. This may be followed by 10 mL infusion over next 8 hours.
  - Ten millilitres of 10% calcium gluconate solution = 1 g calcium gluconate = 93 mg or 4.65 mEq calcium.
- If tetany is not relieved, administration of magnesium (1 to 2 g magnesium sulphate every 6 hours IV or IM) may be required. Frequent monitoring of serum magnesium, and serum total calcium or ionised calcium is recommended.

CORRECTION OF ALKALOSIS

- Persistent vomiting is treated with intravenous isotonic saline and potassium.
- In alkali excess, its withdrawal and, if necessary, ammonium chloride 2 g 4 hourly orally will control tetany.
- Hysterical hyperventilation may be controlled by reassuring the patient and, if required, by using benzodiazepines.

CHRONIC HYPOCALCAEMIA

- Oral calcium (500–1000 mg twice a day) with vitamin D.

TREATMENT OF HYPOPARATHYROIDISM

- See page 991.

Q. Mention the hormones secreted by the adrenal gland.

- Adrenal gland has an inner medulla and an outer cortex. The adrenal cortex is divided into three zones: zona glomerulosa, zona fasciculata and zona reticularis.
- Hormones secreted by adrenal gland are shown in Table 18.17.
- Glucocorticoid and mineralocorticoid are collectively known as corticosteroids. However, the term corticosteroid is often used only for glucocorticoid.

TABLE 18.17 Hormones Secreted by Adrenal Gland

Site	Class	Hormone
• Adrenal cortex		
• Zona glomerulosa	Mineralocorticoid	Aldosterone
• Zona fasciculate	Glucocorticoid	Cortisol
• Zona reticularis	Androgens	Dehydroepiandrosterone sulphate, dehydroepiandrosterone, androstenedione
• Adrenal medulla	Catecholamines	Adrenaline, noradrenaline

Q. Discuss the causes, clinical features, investigations and management of Cushing's syndrome.

Q. Write a short note on Cushing's disease.

- Cushing's syndrome is defined as the symptoms and signs associated with corticosteroid excess of long duration.
- Cushing's disease is corticosteroid excess due to pituitary-dependent bilateral adrenal hyperplasia. The pituitary tumours in Cushing's disease are usually microadenomas (<10 mm in size) that generally do not cause symptoms by local mass effect. Macroadenomas are uncommon in these patients. These tumours generally retain some negative feedback responsiveness to high doses of glucocorticoids. It is usually sporadic but may be associated with multiple endocrine neoplasia type 1.

CAUSES OF CUSHING'S SYNDROME (Table 18.18)

TABLE 18.18 Causes of Cushing's Syndrome

ACTH Dependent	ACTH Independent
• Cushing's disease	• Iatrogenic (use of corticosteroids)
• Ectopic ACTH syndromo (tumours)	• Adrenal adenoma
• Iatrogenic (ACTH therapy)	• Adrenal carcinoma
• Ectopic corticotrophin-releasing hormone syndrome (rare)	• Micronodular adrenal hyperplasia (rare)
• Macronodular adrenal hyperplasia (initial stages)	• Macronodular adrenal hyperplasia (rare)

- Cushing's syndrome of pituitary origin (Cushing's disease) is more common in females.
- Ectopic ACTH syndrome, usually due to small cell carcinoma of lung, is more common in males. Other tumours include carcinoid of thymus, pancreatic carcinoma and bronchial adenoma. Ectopic sources of ACTH are generally not responsive to negative feedback with high doses of glucocorticoids.
- Excluding iatrogenic group, pituitary-dependent Cushing's disease is the most common cause of Cushing's syndrome (80%).

CLINICAL FEATURES

- The symptoms and signs of Cushing's syndrome are shown in Tables 18.19 and 18.20, respectively.

TABLE 18.19 Symptoms of Cushing's Syndrome

Symptom	Cause
• Weight gain	Accumulation of fat and retention of fluid
• Hirsutism	Increased adrenal androgen secretion
• Back pain	Osteoporosis and vertebral compression fractures
• Muscle weakness	Proximal myopathy and hypokalaemia
• Oligomenorrhoea, amenorrhoea and impotence	Gonadal dysfunction
• Easy bruisability	Loss of subcutaneous connective tissue
• Hyperpigmentation	Ectopic ACTH secretion
• Depression, irritability, psychosis	

TABLE 18.20 Signs of Cushing's Syndrome

Sign	Cause/Description
• Central obesity ('lemon on match-stick')	Centripetal distribution of fat
• Buffalo hump	Fat accumulation at the lower part of neck
• Plethoric appearance	Thinning of the skin
• Moon face	Rounded plethoric appearance
• Bruising	Thinning of blood vessels from collagen breakdown
• Purplish striae over abdomen, buttocks and thighs	Thinning of the skin from collagen breakdown
• Hypertension	Increase in plasma volume and sodium retention
• Proximal myopathy	Loss of protein in muscle
• Skin infections	Tinea versicolor
• Onychomycosis	Fungal infection of nails
• Recurrent infections	Glucocorticoid-induced inhibition of immunity

- Risk of coronary artery disease, stroke and venous thrombosis higher than in general population.
- Impaired glucose tolerance due to increased gluconeogenesis, stimulation of lipolysis and proteolysis, and potentiation of glucagon effect.
- Hypercoagulability.

FEATURES OF CUSHING'S SYNDROME DUE TO ECTOPIC ADRENOCORTICOTROPHIC HORMONE SECRETION

- Hypokalaemic alkalosis.
- Skin pigmentation.

INVESTIGATIONS IN CUSHING'S SYNDROME

HORMONAL STUDIES

- Hormonal studies are done in a stepwise manner. Studies are aimed at the diagnosis of Cushing's syndrome and establishing its cause.

Tests Establishing the Presence of Cushing's Syndrome

- Plasma cortisol levels—in normal persons, measurement of plasma cortisol levels at 8 a.m. and 12 midnight will show the lowest levels at 12 midnight. In Cushing's syndrome, this circadian rhythm is lost and the cortisol levels remain the same throughout the day. A midnight level below 1.8 μg/dL is normal, and has a high sensitivity for excluding Cushing's syndrome.
- Twenty-four-hour urinary free cortisol (UFC) excretion is raised in Cushing's syndrome (normal value <90 μg/24 hours). Milder elevations of UFC can be found in conditions such as chronic anxiety, depression, polycystic ovary and alcoholism, all of which are also known as pseudo-Cushing's states.
- Overnight dexamethasone suppression test—the patient takes 1 mg dexamethasone at 11 p.m. and the plasma cortisol is measured at 8 a.m. the following day. Normal value is less than 1.8 μg/dL. In Cushing's syndrome, cortisol levels are not suppressed. The test may be falsely positive in alcoholics or obese patients.

BOX 18.8 Conditions Causing an Apparent Lack of Cortisol Suppression

- Reduced dexamethasone absorption
- Drugs enhancing hepatic dexamethasone metabolism (barbiturates, phenytoin, carbamazepine, rifampicin, meprobamate, aminoglutethimide, methaqualone)
- Increased concentration of cortisol-binding globulin (oestrogen treatment, pregnancy)
- Pseudo-Cushing's states (anxiety, obesity, alcoholic)

- Low-dose dexamethasone suppression test (LDDST)—if UFC or overnight dexamethasone suppression tests are borderline, then this test is performed. The patient is administered 0.5 mg dexamethasone 6 hourly for 2 days. Twenty-four-hour urine is collected from second day and plasma is collected for cortisol on third day. If the UFC falls below 10 μg/24 hours or plasma cortisol is below 1.8 μg/dL, it excludes the diagnosis of Cushing's syndrome. Several conditions can cause lack of cortisol suppression (Box 18.8).
- Late-night salivary cortisol—cortisol concentration in saliva is highly correlated with free plasma cortisol, independent of salivary flow rates, and stable at room temperature for 1 week.

Tests Establishing the Cause of Cushing's Syndrome

- Plasma ACTH level at 8 a.m.
  - Low ACTH (<10 pg/mL) suggests adrenal tumours, macronodular adrenal hyperplasia or exogenous steroid administration.
  - Normal levels (10–20 pg/mL) suggest ACTH-dependent (pituitary or ectopic) or adrenal cause.
  - ACTH values >20 pg/mL suggest either pituitary-dependent disease or ectopic ACTH syndrome.
- Thin-section CT of adrenals if ACTH is low.
  - This can reveal adrenal hyperplasia, adrenal adenoma and carcinoma.
- High-dose dexamethasone suppression test (HDDST) if ACTH is normal or elevated.
  - In this test, 2 mg dexamethasone is administered 6 hourly for 2 days. Twenty-four-hour urine is collected from second day and plasma is collected for cortisol on third day. If the UFC falls below 10 μg/24 hours or plasma cortisol is below 1.8 μg/dL, it indicates suppression of axis and is considered a positive test. This test is positive in pituitary-dependent disease. It is negative in ectopic ACTH syndrome and adrenal tumours.
- ACTH/cortisol response to corticotrophin-releasing hormone (CRH).
  - Increased levels in pituitary-dependent disease.
  - Unchanged levels in ectopic ACTH syndrome and adrenal tumours.
- Desmopressin stimulation test.
  - Desmopressin also stimulates ACTH release in most patients with Cushing's disease and usually induces a response similar to that of CRH.
- Bilateral inferior petrosal sinus sampling (BIPSS) for ACTH before and after CRH stimulation.
- CT/MRI head.

OTHER INVESTIGATIONS

- Blood sugar, cholesterol and LDL may be elevated. Frank's diabetes may occur in 25%–50% of patients.
- Plasma potassium levels.
  - Normal in pituitary-dependent disease and adrenal tumours.
  - Low (<3.5 mmol/L) in ectopic ACTH syndrome.
- Plain radiograph of the skull to look for enlargement of sella turcica.
- Radiograph of chest to detect bronchogenic carcinoma.
- CT scan of anterior mediastinum and upper abdomen including pancreas and scintigraphy with ^{111}In-octreotide to rule out tumours.
- Flowchart 18.6 summarises the approach to evaluation of a patient with suspected Cushing's syndrome.

MANAGEMENT

ADRENAL TUMOURS

- Metyrapone, osilodrostat, etomidate or ketoconazole can reduce cortisol overproduction by blocking its production.
- Mifepristone, a glucocorticoid receptor antagonist, blocks the effect of cortisol at the receptor level and may be used to control hyperglycaemia.
- Adrenal adenomas are removed surgically. Replacement therapy with prednisolone is given postoperatively till the contralateral adrenal, hypothalamus and pituitary recover.
- Adrenal carcinomas are resected surgically. The tumour bed is irradiated and the patient is given the adrenolytic drug, *o,p′*-DDD (mitotane).

CUSHING'S DISEASE

- Pasireotide is a somatostatin analogue that selectively targets somatostatin receptors in corticotroph pituitary adenomas and is sometimes used to medically treat mild Cushing's disease.
- Metyrapone, osilodrostat or ketoconazole may be given during the preparation for surgery to reduce the synthesis of cortisol.
- Mifepristone if surgery is not possible.
- Transsphenoidal surgical removal of the adenoma is the treatment of choice.
- If no tumour is found, radical hypophysectomy is done.
- If surgery is delayed, contraindicated or unsuccessful, adrenal enzyme inhibitors are the most commonly used drugs. Drugs reducing ACTH release from the pituitary tumour such as cabergoline or pasireotide may also be used.
- Radiotherapy and radiosurgery for the treatment of recurrent or residual ACTH-secreting tumours.
- If the diagnosis is uncertain, bilateral adrenalectomy is done. This should be followed by pituitary irradiation to prevent the development of Nelson's syndrome.
- Following successful adrenalectomy, prednisolone and fludrocortisone should be given postoperatively for a variable length of time.

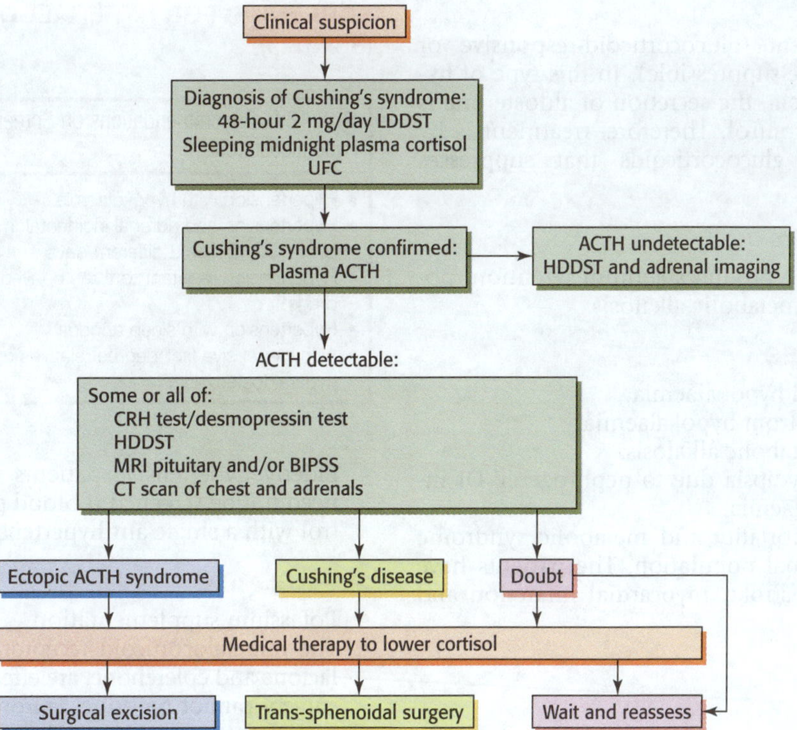

Flowchart 18.6 Differential Diagnosis of Cushing's Syndrome. LDDST, low-dose dexamethasone suppression test; UFC, urinary free cortisol; HDDST, high-dose dexamethasone supression test; BIPSS, bilateral inferior petrosal sinus sampling (Source: *J. Newell-Price, P. Trainer, M. Besser, A. Grossman, et al.: The diagnosis and differential diagnosis of Cushing's syndrome and pseudo-Cushing's states.* Endocrine Reviews *19(5): 647–672, Fig. 3, Copyright 1998 by The Endocrine Society.)*

ECTOPIC ADRENOCORTICOTROPHIC HORMONE SYNDROME

- Benign tumours like bronchial carcinoid should be removed.
- Malignant tumours are treated with radiotherapy and chemotherapy.
- Recurrence may be treated with metyrapone, ketoconazole or etomidate either alone or in combination. These drugs reduce cortisol production.

OTHERS

- Mifepristone is approved to control hyperglycaemia secondary to hypercortisolism in adults with endogenous Cushing's syndrome and type 2 diabetes or glucose intolerance who have failed surgery or are not candidates for surgery.

Q. What is Nelson's syndrome?

- Develops in patients with Cushing's disease (pituitary-dependent bilateral adrenal hyperplasia) treated by bilateral adrenalectomy with no definitive treatment for pituitary adenoma.
- Characterised by an enlarging pituitary tumour with very high levels of ACTH in the blood producing hyperpigmentation of skin. Enlarging pituitary tumour can cause headache, visual field defects and, sometimes, cranial nerve palsies. Other features due to mass effect include panhypopituitarism and diabetes insipidus.
- Rarely seen as bilateral adrenalectomy is nowadays an uncommon primary treatment for pituitary tumours.
- Treatment includes trans-sphenoidal or transcranial surgery and radiotherapy.
- Medical treatment in patients unfit for surgery or radiotherapy include temozolomide and octreotide.

Q. Discuss the aetiology, clinical features, diagnosis and management of primary hyperaldosteronism.

Q. Describe Conn's syndrome.

- Overproduction of the hormone aldosterone is called hyperaldosteronism.
  - Primary hyperaldosteronism is due to an abnormality in the zona glomerulosa of the adrenal gland.
  - Secondary hyperaldosteronism results from the stimulation of aldosterone secretion by angiotensin II following activation of renin–angiotensin system.

PRIMARY HYPERALDOSTERONISM

AETIOLOGY

- Adenoma (Conn's syndrome).
- Bilateral zona glomerulosa hyperplasia.

- Idiopathic.
- ACTH-dependent (glucocorticoid-responsive or dexamethasone-suppressible). In this type of hyperaldosteronism, the secretion of aldosterone is under ACTH control. Therefore, treatment is by administering glucocorticoids that suppresses ACTH release.

PATHOPHYSIOLOGY

- Excess aldosterone produces sodium retention, potassium loss and metabolic alkalosis.

CLINICAL FEATURES

- Hypertension and hypokalaemia.
- Muscle weakness from hypokalaemia.
- Tetany due to metabolic alkalosis.
- Polyuria and polydipsia due to nephrogenic DI induced by hypokalaemia.
- Cardiovascular mortality and metabolic syndrome higher than normal population. The patients have increased risk of stroke, myocardial infarction and atrial fibrillation.

INVESTIGATIONS

Diagnosis

- Hypokalaemia.
- Elevated urinary potassium (>30 mEq/day during hypokalaemia is inappropriate).
- Plasma aldosterone concentration (PAC) is elevated (>15 ng/dL).
- Plasma renin activity (PRA) is suppressed (<1 ng/mL/hour).
- PAC:PRA ratio is the accepted screening test for primary hyperaldosteronism. A level above 20 is considered abnormal when plasma aldosterone is measured in nanograms per decilitre and PRA is measured in nanograms per millilitre per hour.
- Confirmatory tests include oral salt loading test, saline infusion test, frusemide test and captopril test.
  - Suppression of aldosterone below 8.5 ng/dL with salt loading (2 L 0.9% saline infused over 4 hours) rules out primary hyperaldosteronism.
  - In frusemide test, 40 mg frusemide is given IV with patient in upright posture for 2 hours. PRA <2 ng/mL/hour confirms the diagnosis.
  - Oral captopril does not produce any significant decrease in PAC in primary hyperaldosteronism.

Differential Diagnosis

- CT/MRI scanning can detect adenoma and hyperplasia.
- Adrenal vein catheterisation.
  - Unilateral hypersecretion of aldosterone is seen in adenoma.
  - Bilateral hypersecretion of aldosterone is seen in hyperplasia.
- Dexamethasone suppression.
  - Lowers plasma aldosterone transiently in adenoma.
  - Prolonged suppression in glucocorticoid-sensitive hyperaldosteronism.
- Scanning of the adrenal with selenium-75-cholesterol can detect an adenoma.

SCREENING FOR HYPERALDOSTERONISM (Box 18.9)

BOX 18.9 Recommendations on Screening for Primary Hyperaldosteronism

- Hypertension with hypokalaemia
- Hypertension and adrenal incidentaloma
- BP >150/100 on 3 different days
- Hypertension resistant to three conventional antihypertensive drugs
- Hypertension with sleep apnoea
- All hypertensive first-degree relatives of patients with primary hyperaldosteronism

- Elderly hypertensive patients with normokalaemia need not be screened if blood pressure is under control with a single antihypertensive agent.

MANAGEMENT

- Potassium supplementation.
- The mineralocorticoid receptor antagonists, spironolactone and eplerenone, are effective in patients where surgery cannot be done. Spironolactone may require high doses (up to 400 mg/day). A few patients develop gynaecomastia with spironolactone; the incidence is lower with eplerenone. Another option is to give amiloride (10–40 mg/day).
- Unilateral adrenalectomy may be done in an adenoma.
- Angiotensin receptor blockers may be given for control of hypertension. These agents also reduce the ill-effects of excessive aldosterone on various tissues. ACE inhibitors may also be given to control blood pressure.

Q. Give a brief account of secondary hyperaldosteronism.

- Secondary hyperaldosteronism results from aldosterone excess mediated through the renin–angiotensin system.

CONDITIONS CAUSING SECONDARY HYPERALDOSTERONISM (Table 18.21)

TABLE 18.21 Causes of Secondary Hyperaldosteronism

• Physiological	Salt depletion from inadequate intake or excessive loss through kidney or gastrointestinal tract; pregnancy (causes oestrogen-induced increase in plasma renin substrate)
• Pathological	Excessive diuretic therapy, nephrotic syndrome, cirrhosis with ascites, congestive heart failure, Bartter's syndrome, accelerated or malignant phase of hypertension, severe renal artery stenosis

BARTTER'S SYNDROME

- A group of autosomal recessive disorders of the renal tubules causing excessive loss of sodium, potassium and chloride.

- Characterised by hypokalaemia, hypochloraemic metabolic alkalosis, elevated aldosterone excretion, hyperreninaemia, hypercalciuria and normal blood pressure.
- Clinical features include polyuria, dehydration, failure to thrive, growth retardation and a history of polyhydramnios with premature birth.

INVESTIGATIONS

- Hypokalaemia.
- PAC is elevated.
- PRA is elevated.
- PAC:PRA ratio is <10.

MANAGEMENT

- Salt depletion is treated with intravenous saline.
- Congestive heart failure is treated with spironolactone and ACE inhibitors.
- Bartter's syndrome is treated with spironolactone and indomethacin.
- Accelerated or malignant hypertension is treated with antihypertensive drugs.
- Renovascular disease is treated with ACE inhibitors, but definitive therapy is angioplasty or surgical correction.
- If excessive diuretic therapy (e.g. thiazide) is the cause, it should be substituted or supplemented with one of the potassium-sparing diuretics like spironolactone, amiloride or triamterene.

Q. How do you classify adrenocortical insufficiency?

Q. Write a short note on Addison's disease.

CLASSIFICATION AND CAUSES (Table 18.22)

TABLE 18.22 Classification and Causes of Adrenocortical Insufficiency

Primary Causes (Adrenal Causes)	Secondary Causes (Interference With ACTH Release)	Tertiary Causes (Interference With CRH Release)
• Addison's disease • Congenital or acquired enzyme defects	• Pituitary diseases	• Hypothalamic diseases • Withdrawal of glucocorticoid therapy

ADDISON'S DISEASE

- Indicates adrenocortical insufficiency due to destruction or dysfunction of entire adrenal cortex. Approximately 90% of the adrenal cortex needs to be destroyed to produce adrenal insufficiency.
- Various causes of Addison's disease are listed in Table 18.23.

CLINICAL FEATURES

- Clinical features of Addison's disease result from glucocorticoid deficiency, mineralocorticoid deficiency, androgen deficiency and ACTH excess.

TABLE 18.23 Causes of Addison's Disease

• **Autoimmune adrenalitis**
• **Infectious adrenalitis**
  • Tuberculosis
  • Fungal (histoplasmosis)
• **Adrenal haemorrhage**
  • Waterhouse–Friderichsen syndrome
  • Anticoagulation therapy
  • Trauma (external or by invasive procedures)
• **Adrenal infarction (due to thrombosis)**
  • Systemic lupus erythematosus
  • Polyarteritis nodosa
  • Antiphospholipid syndrome
• **Trauma**
• **Adrenoleukodystrophy**
	• **Metastases in the adrenal**
	  • Lung, breast, stomach carcinomas
	  • Lymphoma
	• **Drug induced**
	  • Adrenolytic therapy (e.g. mitotane)
	  • Other agents (ketoconazole, metyrapone, etomidate, rifampicin, cyproterone acetate)
	• **Genetic**
	  • Congenital adrenal hyperplasia
	• **Others**
	  • Bilateral adrenalectomy
	  • Amyloidosis
	  • Haemochromatosis
	  • Sarcoidosis
	  • Autoimmune polyglandular syndrome types 1 and 2

- The cardinal features of Addison's disease are hypotension, pigmentation and previous history of acute adrenal crisis following stress, or slow recovery from illness.
- Glucocorticoid deficiency results in malaise, weakness, weight loss, anorexia, nausea, vomiting, diarrhoea or constipation, postural hypotension and hypoglycaemia.
- Mineralocorticoid deficiency manifests as hypotension. Many patients have salt craving.
- ACTH excess results in pigmentation of exposed areas, pressure areas like elbows, knees and knuckles, palmar creases (Fig. 18.8), mucous membranes (Fig. 18.9), conjunctivae and recently acquired scars. Other areas where pigmentation can occur include perineum, axillae and areolae of breasts. It occurs due to increased production of proopiomelanocortin, a prohormone that is cleaved into biologically active hormones ACTH and melanocyte-stimulating hormone.
- Androgen deficiency results in diminution of body hair, especially in females, and usually occurs with a secondary cause of adrenal insufficiency.

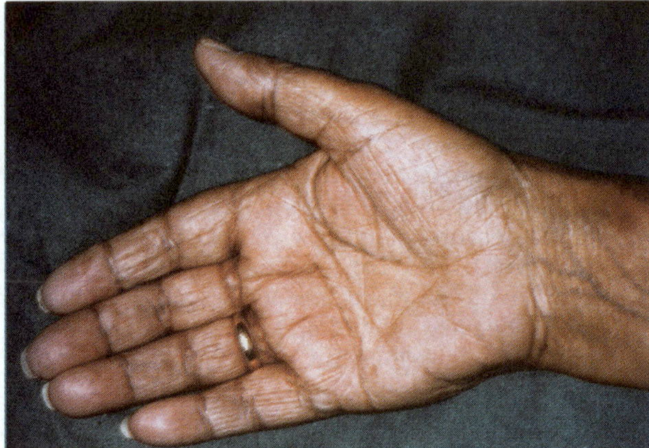

Fig. 18.8 Palmar crease pigmentation.

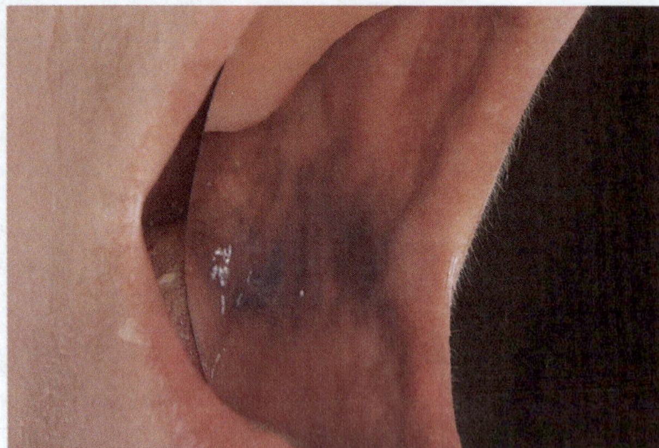

Fig. 18.9 Pigmentation of the buccal mucosa.

- A number of autoimmune diseases may be associated with Addison's disease.
  - The association of primary adrenal insufficiency, chronic autoimmune thyroiditis (Hashimoto's thyroiditis) and type 1 DM is known as type 2a polyglandular autoimmune syndrome. Primary hypogonadism (particularly ovarian failure) is common. The association of Addison's disease and Hashimoto's thyroiditis is known as Schmidt's syndrome.
  - The combination of adrenal insufficiency, hypoparathyroidism and chronic mucocutaneous candidiasis constitutes type 1 polyglandular autoimmune syndrome.
- Secondary adrenal insufficiency is also associated with severe cortisol deficiency, but patient has no pigmentation and only mild mineralocorticoid deficiency.

INVESTIGATIONS

- Elevated blood urea, hyponatraemia and hyperkalaemia.
- Low blood sugar levels.
- Mild anaemia, mild eosinophilia.
- Plasma cortisol measured between 8 and 9 a.m. <3 µg/dL suggests adrenal insufficiency while a level >19 µg/dL excludes it.
- ACTH stimulation test—there is failure of plasma cortisol to rise beyond 19 µg/dL following administration of 250 µg of synthetic ACTH.
- Plasma ACTH levels are elevated (>100 pg/mL) in primary adrenal insufficiency.
- Plasma renin activity (PRA) is high and plasma aldosterone levels are low or normal.
- Plasma dehydroepiandrosterone (DHEA) and DHEA sulphate (DHEAS) concentrations are low.
- In tuberculous adrenalitis, chest radiograph may show evidences of pulmonary tuberculosis. Plain radiograph of abdomen, CT scan and MRI scan may show adrenal calcification.
- Adrenal and other organ-specific antibodies (e.g. adrenal cortex antibodies, 21-hydroxylase antibodies) may be detected in the serum in autoimmune adrenalitis.
- CT-directed percutaneous fine needle aspiration of enlarged adrenal glands.

MANAGEMENT

- Patients with Addison's disease require lifelong glucocorticoid and mineralocorticoid replacement therapy.
- Cortisone is given at a dose of 20 mg on getting up in the morning and 10 mg in the evening at 6 p.m. Alternatively, prednisolone is given in a dose of 5 mg in the morning and 2.5 mg in the evening.
- Fludrocortisone (mineralocorticoid) 0.05–0.1 mg daily in patients with primary adrenal insufficiency. Excessive mineralocorticoid replacement causes hypertension, hypokalaemia and oedema.
- Addison's disease due to tuberculous adrenalitis should be treated with antituberculous chemotherapy.
- During periods of stress and infections, the patient should be told to increase doses of prednisolone two to three times for 3 days (3 × 3 rule).
- Patients with secondary adrenal insufficiency should be evaluated for other pituitary hormone deficiencies and accordingly managed.
- Every patient should be advised to carry a card mentioning diagnosis, and daily medications and doses.

Q. Describe adrenal crisis.

- Adrenal crisis (acute adrenal insufficiency) can occur in a patient with primary adrenal insufficiency who has a serious infection or other acute stress.
- It can also occur after bilateral adrenal infarction or bilateral adrenal haemorrhage.
- Adrenal haemorrhage and often death has been associated with meningococcaemia (Waterhouse–Friderichsen syndrome).
- It is rare in patients with secondary adrenal insufficiency.

CLINICAL FEATURES

- The predominant manifestation of adrenal crisis is shock, but the patients often have nonspecific symptoms such as anorexia, nausea, vomiting, abdominal pain, weakness, fatigue and lethargy. Confusion or coma can also occur.
- Two other common features are abdominal tenderness and fever.
- Patients with long-standing adrenal insufficiency who present in crisis may be hyperpigmented (due to chronic ACTH hypersecretion) and have weight loss, serum electrolyte abnormalities and other manifestations of chronic adrenal insufficiency.
- Loss of mineralocorticoid activity is associated with development of hypotension, hyponatraemia and hyperkalaemia.

MANAGEMENT

- Initiate therapy as soon as acute adrenal crisis is suspected.
- Correct hypovolaemia and sodium depletion with normal saline.
- Add 5% dextrose solution if the patient is hypoglycaemic.
- Administer hydrocortisone in a dose of 100 mg 6 hourly and taper it over 24–48 hours to a maintenance dose once the underlying stress resolves.

Q. What is the present role of steroid therapy?

Q. Discuss the use and side effects of steroids.

Q. What are the complications of corticosteroid therapy?

Q. How can you minimise the side effects of corticosteroid?

EQUIVALENT DOSES OF GLUCOCORTICOIDS (ANTIINFLAMMATORY POTENCY)

- Equivalent doses of glucocorticoids in terms of antiinflammatory potency are given in Box 18.10.
- Prednisolone has only 25% of mineralocorticoid activity as compared to hydrocortisone while dexamethasone and betamethasone have negligible mineralocorticoid activity.

COMMON INDICATIONS OF STEROIDS

- Bronchial asthma, COPD, raised intracranial tension, cerebral oedema, rheumatoid arthritis, SLE, other connective tissue diseases, nephrotic syndrome, adrenal insufficiency, septic shock, leukaemia, lymphoma, as an adjunct in chemotherapy for malignancies, myocarditis, rheumatic fever, demyelinating diseases, tuberculosis of pericardium and tuberculous meningitis, inflammatory bowel disease, postorgan transplant, transplant rejection, graft versus host diseases, autoimmune haemolytic anaemia, idiopathic thrombocytopenic purpura.

COMMON CONTRAINDICATIONS OF STEROIDS (RELATIVE)

- Active tuberculosis, peptic ulcer, bleeding tendencies, diabetes, uncontrolled hypertension, any active infection, etc.

BOX 18.10 Equivalent Doses of Glucocorticoids (Antiinflammatory Potency)

- Hydrocortisone (cortisol)—20 mg
- Cortisone acetate—25 mg
- Prednisolone—5 mg
- Methylprednisolone—4 mg
- Betamethasone—0.60 mg
- Dexamethasone—0.75 mg

SIDE EFFECTS OF GLUCOCORTICOID THERAPY (Table 18.24)

TABLE 18.24 Side Effects of Glucocorticoids

Endocrine
- Glucose intolerance or Frank's diabetes mellitus
- Cushingoid features
- Growth retardation
- Hypothalamic–pituitary–adrenal axis suppression
- Menstrual irregularities
- Adrenal crisis

Cardiovascular
- Hypertension
- Fluid retention and oedema
- Accelerated atherosclerosis
- Ischaemic heart disease
- Atrial fibrillation and flutter
- Venous thromboembolism

Gastrointestinal
- Gastric erosion, peptic ulceration
- Masked perforation
- Upper GI bleed
- Pancreatitis

Immune system
- Increased susceptibility to infections
- Reactivation of latent tuberculosis
- Impaired wound healing

Musculoskeletal
- Osteoporosis
- Fractures
- Avascular necrosis of hip
- Myopathy

Skin
- Acne
- Hirsutism
- Striae
- Ecchymosis

Eye
- Cataract
- Glaucoma

Metabolic
- Weight gain
- Hyperlipidaemia
- Hypokalaemia

Neuropsychiatric
- Depression
- Psychosis
- Insomnia
- Pseudotumour cerebri

SUPPRESSION OF HYPOTHALAMIC–PITUITARY–ADRENAL AXIS

- Occurs with high-dose therapy.
- This makes it difficult to withdraw steroids.
- Can be minimised by giving steroids as a single morning dose or better, on alternate days.

MEASURES TO REDUCE THE SIDE EFFECTS (Box 18.11)

BOX 18.11 Various Measures to Reduce Side Effects of Glucocorticoids

- Giving the lowest possible dose
- Giving on alternate days rather than daily
- Giving as a single dose rather than in divided doses
- Giving in the morning rather than at any other time
- Giving for the shortest possible duration
- Giving for established indications only
- Exercise programme to reduce myopathy and osteoporosis
- Giving only under medical supervision
- Monitoring caloric intake to prevent weight gain
- Reducing sodium intake
- Using H_2 receptor blockers or proton-pump inhibitors
- Providing high calcium intake and vitamin D
- Using biphosphonates

Q. Write briefly on Waterhouse–Friderichsen syndrome.

- Waterhouse–Friderichsen syndrome is characterised by acute haemorrhagic destruction of both the adrenal glands, usually associated with fulminant meningococcal sepsis. It is characterised by vasomotor collapse and shock.

- Onset is abrupt and profound prostration occurs within a few hours. Petechiae, purpuric lesions and haemorrhage into the skin occur.
- Early in the preshock stage, there is generalised vasoconstriction and the patient looks alert and pale, with circumoral cyanosis and cold extremities.
- In the shock stage, coma develops, cardiac output falls and blood pressure drops. If untreated, patient dies of cardiac and/or respiratory failure.
- Treatment includes appropriate antibiotics, intravenous fluids, vasopressors and steroids.

Q. Give a brief account of phaeochromocytoma.

- Phaeochromocytoma is a tumour of the chromaffin tissue of adrenal medulla that secretes catecholamines (adrenaline and noradrenaline).
- Paraganglioma is an extra-adrenal tumour that arises from both sympathetic and parasympathetic paraganglia located anywhere from the base of the skull to the pelvis.
- Ninety per cent of the tumours arise from the adrenal medulla (phaeochromocytoma) while 10% are paragangliomas.
- Ninety per cent of phaeochromocytomas are unilateral, while 10% are in bilateral adrenals.
- Ninety per cent are benign while 10% are malignant.
- Neurofibromatosis type 1 is associated with an increased incidence of phaeochromocytoma.
- Phaeochromocytoma is seen in up to 50% of patients with multiple endocrine neoplasia type 2 (MEN2) and in 10%–20% of patients with von Hippel–Lindau syndrome.

CLINICAL FEATURES

- The classic triad of symptoms in patients with a phaeochromocytoma consists of episodic headache, sweating and tachycardia. However, it is seen in a minority of patients only.
- Patients may present with paroxysmal hypertension associated with or without episodes of pallor or flushing, palpitations, sweating, headache and anxiety (fear of death). However, sustained hypertension is more common than paroxysmal hypertension.
- Gastrointestinal symptoms include abdominal pain, vomiting, constipation and weight loss.
- Other features include orthostatic hypotension (due to low plasma volume), visual blurring, papilloedema, weight loss, polyuria and polydipsia.
- Glucose intolerance.
- Complications of hypertension like stroke, myocardial infarction, cardiomyopathy (can also occur due to catecholamine excess) and left ventricular failure.
- Rarely, secondary erythrocytosis due to overproduction of erythropoietin.
- May be associated with MEN2.

INVESTIGATIONS

- Twenty-four-hour urine vanillylmandelic acid (VMA) is raised (less sensitive and specific compared to other tests).
- Twenty-four-hour urine metanephrines and normetanephrines are raised.
- Twenty-four-hour urine-free catecholamines are raised.
- Plasma noradrenaline and adrenaline levels, and plasma-free metanephrines are raised.
- Chromogranin A (a major secretory protein present in the soluble matrix of chromaffin granules) is elevated.
- Provocative (glucagon provocation test), suppressive (clonidine suppression test) and adrenolytic (phentolamine test) tests are rarely required.
- CT scan to localise tumour.
- Scintigraphy to localise tumour.
  - ^{123}I-labelled meta-iodobenzylguanidine (MIBG) scintigraphy.
  - Somatostatin receptor scintigraphy using ^{111}indium-labelled diethylenetriaminepentaacetic acid octreotide scan.
- [^{18}F]fluorodihydroxyphenylalanine (DOPA) or 68-Ga DOTATATE PET scan.

MANAGEMENT

- Excision of the tumour after medical preparation (controlling hypertension and tachycardia, and expansion of contracted blood volume by high sodium diet).
- If excision is not possible, long-term treatment with combined α- and β-adrenoreceptor blocking drugs (phenoxybenzamine and propranolol) is advocated. β-Blockers should never be given alone because blockade of vasodilatory peripheral β-adrenergic receptors with unopposed α-adrenergic receptor stimulation can lead to a further elevation in blood pressure. β-Blockers should be started at least 2 to 3 days after α-adrenoreceptor blocking drugs. Other α-adrenoreceptor blocking drugs include prazosin, terazosin or doxazosin. Labetalol has both α- and β-adrenoreceptor blocking properties and can be used.
- Treatment options for hypertensive crisis include sodium nitroprusside, phentolamine or nicardipine.

Q. What is impotence? Discuss briefly.

- Male sexual dysfunction is termed impotence. It may manifest in various ways like loss of desire, inability to obtain and maintain erection, premature ejaculation, absence of emission and inability to achieve orgasm.
- Erectile impotence or dysfunction (inability to achieve or maintain an erection sufficient for sexual performance) could be of various causes but majority are due to psychological causes. In every case of erectile impotence or dysfunction, it is mandatory to rule out the organic causes given in Box 18.12.

BOX 18.12 Organic Causes of Erectile Impotence or Dysfunction

- Endocrine causes—for example hypogonadism, hyperprolactinaemia, hypothyroidism, hyperthyroidism, diabetes mellitus
- Drugs—for example antihistamines, antihypertensives (thiazides, clonidine, methyldopa), anticholinergics, antidepressants, antipsychotics, tranquillisers, alcohol, spironolactone, ketoconazole, cimetidine
- Penile diseases—cavernous fibrosis, penile fracture
- Neurological diseases—stroke, spinal cord injury, multiple sclerosis, Parkinson's disease, Alzheimer's disease, prostate surgery
- Vascular disease—for example cardiovascular disease, hypertension, diabetes mellitus, hyperlipidaemia, smoking, Leriche's syndrome

TABLE 18.25 Organic Versus Psychogenic Erectile Dysfunction

Organic Erectile Dysfunction	Psychogenic Erectile Dysfunction
• Gradual in onset	• Usually acute in onset
• Usually present in all sexual scenarios (i.e. with partner, nocturnal erections, self-stimulation)	• Usually varies in sexual situations
• Follows a constant clinical course	• Variable in its course
• Poor noncoital erections	• Preserved noncoital erections
• Leads to secondary psychosexual problems	• Preexisting psychosexual disorder is often present

DIFFERENTIAL DIAGNOSIS (Table 18.25)

- A meticulous clinical examination is required to exclude a neurological cause of erectile impotence.

INVESTIGATIONS

- Fasting blood glucose and HbA1c.
- TSH.
- If required (e.g. suppressed libido), serum testosterone. If low, FSH, LH and prolactin.

TREATMENT OF ERECTILE DYSFUNCTION

- Treatment of cardiovascular risk factors such as smoking, obesity, hypertension and dyslipidaemia.
- Psychosocial interventions.
- Treatment of underlying disorder.
- Testosterone for hypogonadism.
- Use of phosphodiesterase-5 inhibitors (e.g. sildenafil, vardenafil, tadalafil and avanafil).
- If above fail, vacuum devices, penile self-injectable drugs, intraurethral alprostadil and intracavernosal alprostadil or a combination of papaverine and phentolamine.
- Surgical implantation of a penile prosthesis.

Q. Describe the classification and causes of diabetes mellitus. (IM11.1)

- Diabetes mellitus is a clinical syndrome characterised by hyperglycaemia due to absolute or relative deficiency of insulin, or both (i.e. defects in insulin secretion, insulin action or both).

AETIOLOGICAL CLASSIFICATION (Table 18.26)

- The two broad categories of DM are designated type 1 and type 2.
- In type 1 DM, there is absolute insulin deficiency. Type 1 is subdivided into two groups: type 1A due to cell-mediated autoimmune destruction of β-cells and type 1B (idiopathic type 1 DM) where β-cell destruction occurs due to unknown cause. It most often occurs in younger patients but nearly 10% of patients older than 30 years have this type of DM.
- In type 2 DM, there are variable degrees of insulin resistance, impaired insulin secretion and increased glucose production. It also occurs due to several genetic and metabolic syndromes. Some children have type 2 DM.
- Maturity onset of diabetes in the young (MODY) is characterised by autosomal dominant inheritance, early onset of diabetes, impairment of insulin secretion and lack of autoantibodies.

TABLE 18.26 Classification of Diabetes Mellitus

Type 1 diabetes mellitus:
- Type 1A (immune-mediated)
- Type 1B (idiopathic)

Type 2 diabetes mellitus

Other specific types of diabetes mellitus:
- Genetic defects of β-cell function [maturity-onset diabetes of the young (MODY)]
- Genetic defects in insulin action (e.g. type A insulin resistance, lipoatrophic diabetes)
- Diseases of exocrine pancreas (pancreatitis, pancreatectomy, pancreatic neoplasm, haemochromatosis, fibrocalculous pancreatopathy, cystic fibrosis)
- Other endocrine diseases (acromegaly, Cushing's syndrome, glucagonoma, phaeochromocytoma, hyperthyroidism)
- Infections (congenital rubella, cytomegalovirus)
- Drug/toxin-induced (vacor, glucocorticoids, pentamidine, diazoxide, thyroxine, β agonists, thiazides, protease inhibitors, α-interferon, nicotinic acid)
- Insulin receptor defects or insulin receptor antibodies
- Other genetic syndromes—Down's syndrome, Klinefelter's syndrome, Turner's syndrome, myotonic dystrophy, porphyria, Friedreich's ataxia, Wolfram's or DIDMOAD (diabetes insipidus, diabetes mellitus, optic atrophy and deafness) syndrome

Gestational diabetes mellitus (GDM)

Q. Briefly outline the pathogenesis of diabetes mellitus. (IM11.2, IM11.3, IM11.4)

PATHOGENESIS OF TYPE 1A DIABETES MELLITUS

- Type 1 diabetes appears when more than 90% of β-cells of pancreas are destroyed by an autoimmune process. The pathogenetic sequence is given as follows.
- First, genetic susceptibility to the disease must be present. About 95% of patients with type 1 DM have HLADR3 and/or DR4. Despite this, most individuals with type 1 DM do not have a first-degree relative with diabetes.
- Second, an environmental event (commonly viral infection) initiates the process in genetically susceptible individuals.
- Third step in the sequence is an inflammatory response in the pancreas called 'insulitis'. There is infiltration of the islets with activated T lymphocytes.
- Fourth step is the activation of autoimmunity. There is an alteration of the surface of the β-cell such that it is no longer recognised as 'self', but is seen by the immune system as a foreign cell or 'non-self'.
- Fifth step is the development of an immune response. Though islet cell antibodies (ICA) and several other autoantibodies are present in most patients, they are not involved in destructive process. Instead, activated T lymphocytes present in the islets release cytokines (tumour necrosis factor-α, interferon-γ and interleukin-1) that destroy β-cells. $CD8^+$ cell-induced cytotoxicity and apoptosis are also involved. This results in an immune attack on β-cells with resultant destruction of β-cells. When more than 90% of β-cells are destroyed, diabetes appears. α-Cells remain intact.
- Flowchart 18.7 gives the pathogenesis of type 1 DM.
- The events that trigger the transition from glucose intolerance to frank diabetes are often associated with increased insulin requirements that might occur during stress, infection or puberty. Thus, following initial development of frank DM, many patients become euglycaemic without need of insulin for some time. This is called 'honeymoon phase'. This generally lasts for a few months after which the patient develops Frank's DM again.
- Markers of immune destruction of the β-cells include islet cell autoantibodies, autoantibodies to insulin, autoantibodies to glutamic acid decarboxylase (GAD65), autoantibodies to the tyrosine phosphatases IA-2 and IA-2β, and autoantibodies to ZnT8 (zinc transporter 8). One and usually more of these autoantibodies are present in 85%–90% of individuals when fasting hyperglycaemia is initially detected.
- The disease also has strong HLA associations with linkage to the HLA DR4-DQ8 and HLA DR3-DQ2 genes. The risk of type 1 diabetes in children with an affected family member is 5%.
- These patients are also prone to other autoimmune disorders such as Graves' disease, Hashimoto's thyroiditis, Addison's disease, vitiligo, coeliac sprue, autoimmune hepatitis, myasthenia gravis and pernicious anaemia.

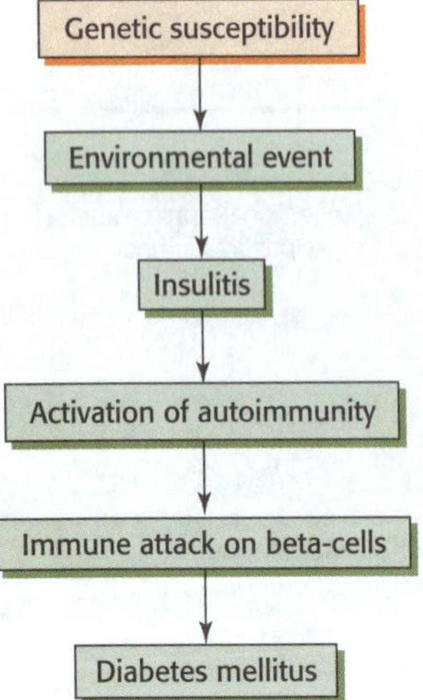

Flowchart 18.7 Pathogenesis of Type 1A Diabetes Mellitus.

IDIOPATHIC TYPE 1 DIABETES MELLITUS

- This form of diabetes is strongly inherited, lacks immunological evidence for β-cell autoimmunity and is not HLA associated.

PATHOGENESIS OF TYPE 2 DIABETES MELLITUS

- In contrast to type 1 DM, in type 2 DM, no HLA relationship has been identified and autoimmune mechanisms are not operative.
- Genetic influence is much more powerful in type 2 DM than in type 1 DM.
- Pancreatic β-cell mass is intact in type 2 DM, in contrast to the situation with type 1 DM. The α-cell population is increased.
- Certain factors need to be considered in the pathogenesis of type 2 diabetes. They are as follows:
  - Type 2 DM is associated with increased hepatic production of glucose, resistance to the action of insulin and impaired insulin secretion. Insulin resistance may be due to any one of three general causes: an abnormal insulin molecule, an excessive amount of circulating antagonists and target defects. The last is the most common cause of insulin resistance in type 2 DM.
  - The defects in the receptors present in target tissues are generally at the postreceptor level.
  - Reduced utilisation of glucose by peripheral tissues (mostly skeletal muscles) results in postprandial hyperglycaemia while increased hepatic glucose output produces fasting hyperglycaemia.
  - In the early stages, glucose tolerance remains normal despite insulin resistance. This is due to compensatory increase in insulin secretion by β-cells. As insulin resistance and compensatory hyperinsulinaemia progress, the β-cells become unable to sustain this hypersecretion. This results

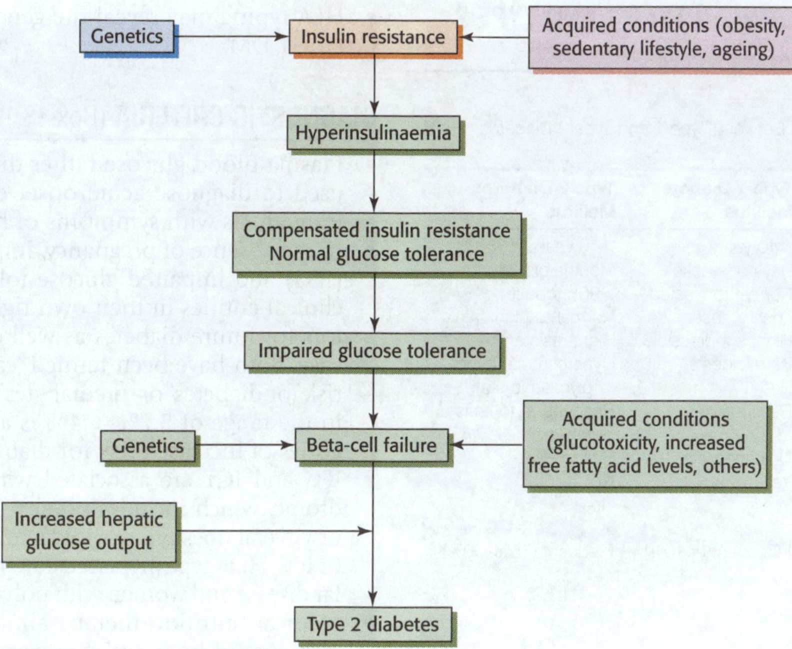

Flowchart 18.8 Pathogenesis of Type 2 Diabetes Mellitus.

in impaired glucose tolerance and later Frank's DM. Ultimately, β-cell failure develops.

- Overeating, especially when combined with obesity and underactivity, is associated with the development of type 2 DM.
- Ageing is an important risk factor for type 2 DM.
- In females who are genetically predisposed, pregnancy may be associated with the development of hyperglycaemia. It may or may not disappear following pregnancy. Repeated pregnancies may increase the likelihood of developing permanent diabetes, particularly in obese females.
- In type 2 DM, there is deposition of amyloid in pancreatic islets that is accompanied by atrophy of islet epithelial cells.

- Pathogenesis of type 2 DM is summarised in Flowchart 18.8.

Q. What are the clinical features of diabetes mellitus?

Q. Describe potential diabetes and latent diabetes.

- Typically, the clinical features of type 1 and type 2 DM are distinctive.

TYPE 1 DIABETES MELLITUS

- Usually begins before the age of 40.
- Body habitus is normal to wasted.
- The onset of symptoms may be abrupt, with polyuria, polydipsia, polyphagia and weight loss developing over days or weeks.
- Some cases may present as ketoacidosis during an intercurrent illness or following surgery.
- Occasionally, an initial episode of ketoacidosis is followed by a symptom-free interval ('honeymoon period') during which no treatment is required.
- Characteristically, the plasma insulin is low or unmeasurable. Glucagon levels are elevated but suppressible with insulin.

TYPE 2 DIABETES MELLITUS

- Usually begins after the age of 40.
- The typical patient is obese.
- The symptoms begin gradually, over a period of months to years. Frequently, hyperglycaemia is detected in an asymptomatic person on a routine examination. Many patients will present with one of the chronic complications of diabetes and on investigations are found to be diabetic.
- Depressed immune status may result in flare-ups of pulmonary tuberculosis, nonhealing of wounds, recurrent styes, candidal pruritus vulvae, balanitis and recurrent urinary tract infections.
- These patients usually do not develop ketoacidosis. In the decompensated state, they are susceptible to the syndrome of hyperosmolar hyperglycaemic state (hyperosmolar nonketotic coma).
- The plasma insulin levels are normal to high. Glucagon levels are elevated and are resistant to suppression by insulin.

DIFFERENTIATION BETWEEN TYPE 1 AND TYPE 2 DIABETES MELLITUS (Table 18.27)

TABLE 18.27 Comparison Between Type 1 and Type 2 Diabetes Mellitus

Feature	Type 1 Diabetes Mellitus	Type 2 Diabetes Mellitus
• Age of onset	<40 years	>40 years
• Duration of symptoms	Days or weeks	Months or years
• Body habitus	Normal to wasted	>90% obese
• Plasma insulin	Low to absent	Normal to high
• Plasma glucagon	High, suppressible	High, resistant
• Acute complication	Ketoacidosis	Hyperosmolar hyperglycaemic state
• Insulin therapy	Responsive	Responsive to resistant
• Sulphonylurea therapy	Unresponsive	Responsive
• Autoantibodies	Yes	No
• Other autoimmune diseases	Yes	No
• Family history of diabetes	Infrequent (<10%)	Frequent (75%–90%)

POTENTIAL DIABETICS

- Potential diabetics are persons with a normal glucose tolerance test who have an increased risk of developing diabetes for genetic reasons. Examples are as follows:
  - Children of two diabetic parents.
  - Sibling of a diabetic.
  - Nondiabetic member of a pair of monozygotic twins where the other is a diabetic.

LATENT DIABETICS

- Latent diabetics are persons in whom the glucose tolerance test is normal but who are known to have given an abnormal result under conditions imposing a burden on the pancreatic cells—for example during pregnancy, infection, severe stress (physical or mental), during treatment with corticosteroids, thiazide diuretics or other diabetogenic drugs, or when overweight.

Q. Discuss briefly the diagnosis of diabetes mellitus. (IM11.11)

Q. Explain what is impaired fasting glucose.

Q. Write briefly on impaired glucose tolerance.

- Diabetes may present with polyuria, polydipsia, polyphagia and significant weight loss despite polyphagia.
- Some patients may present with depressed immune status or end-organ involvement—for example retinopathy, nephropathy or neuropathy.
- Urine examination may show glycosuria with or without ketonuria.
- Glycosylated haemoglobin (HbA1c) levels may be elevated (normal <6%).
- HLA typing may reveal the genetic predisposition in type 1 DM.

DIAGNOSTIC CRITERIA (Box 18.13)

- Plasma blood glucose rather than HbA1c should be used to diagnose acute onset of type 1 diabetes in individuals with symptoms of hyperglycaemia.
- In the absence of pregnancy, impaired fasting glucose (IFG) and impaired glucose tolerance (IGT) are not clinical entities in their own right but rather risk factors for future diabetes as well as cardiovascular disease. Both have been termed 'categories of increased risk for diabetes' or 'prediabetes'. Additionally, HbA1c in the range of 5.7%–6.4% is also included in 'categories of increased risk for diabetes'.
- IFG and IGT are associated with the metabolic syndrome, which includes obesity (especially abdominal or visceral obesity), dyslipidaemia of the high-TG and/or low-HDL type, hypertension, history of cardiovascular disease and women with polycystic ovary syndrome.
- Medical nutrition therapy aimed at producing 5%–10% loss of body weight, exercise and certain pharmacological agents (acarbose, metformin) have been variably demonstrated to prevent or delay the development of diabetes in people with IGT.
- At the time of diagnosis, assess the patient completely, particularly blood pressure, possible diabetes complications such as neurological and foot examinations, lipid profile, urine microalbumin: creatinine ratio and an ophthalmological assessment to evaluate for retinopathy.

BOX 18.13 Diagnostic Criteria for Diabetes Mellitus

Diabetes mellitus

- Symptoms of diabetes plus random plasma glucose >200 mg/dL (symptoms of diabetes plus random whole blood glucose >175 mg/dL)
  OR
- Fasting plasma glucose ≥125 mg/dL (fasting whole blood glucose ≥110 mg/dL)
  OR
- Two-hour plasma glucose ≥200 mg/dL during an oral glucose tolerance test (OGTT) (whole blood ≥175 mg/dL during an oral 75 g glucose tolerance test)
  OR
- Glycated haemoglobin (HbA1c) ≥6.5%

Impaired fasting glucose (IFG)

- Fasting plasma glucose ≥100 but <125 mg/dL (whole blood glucose ≥88 but <110 mg/dL)

Impaired glucose tolerance (IGT)

- Plasma glucose between 140 and 200 mg/dL 2 hours after oral glucose load (whole blood glucose between 125 and 175 mg/dL 2 hours after oral glucose load)

Normal glucose levels

- Fasting plasma glucose <100 mg/dL (whole blood glucose <88 mg/dL)
- Two-hour postprandial or postoral glucose tolerance test plasma glucose <140 mg/dL (whole blood glucose <125 mg/dL)

- C-peptide is a by-product formed when proinsulin is processed to insulin. Therefore, its levels reflect insulin production. In type 1 DM, levels of C-peptide are very low (<0.2 nanomol/L) or undetectable indicating absence of insulin secretion from pancreas.
- The goal of treatment is to achieve HbA1c ≤6.5% or HbA1c >6.5% if lower target cannot be achieved without adverse outcomes.

Q. Write briefly on Benedict's test.

Q. Describe renal glycosuria and Marble's criteria for diagnosis of renal glycosuria.

Q. What is meant by alimentary (lag storage) glycosuria?

Q. Discuss the differential diagnosis of glycosuria.

BENEDICT'S TEST

- Benedict's qualitative reagent contains copper sulphate, sodium potassium citrate or tartrate (Rochelle salt) and sodium carbonate.
- Principle:
  - When a reducing sugar solution is heated with Benedict's solution, the reducing sugar under alkaline conditions tautomerises to form enediols. The enediols are unstable and decompose to yield short-chain aldehydes. Short-chain aldehydes are powerful reducing agents that reduce the cupric ions to cuprous ions.
- Procedure:
  - To 5 mL Benedict's qualitative reagent, 8–10 drops of protein-free urine are added and the mixture is boiled for 2 minutes and allowed to cool. If a reducing substance is present, a precipitate will appear, varying from light green turbidity to a red precipitate. If the reducing substance is glucose, the test gives approximately quantitative results.
    - Light green turbidity—0.1 to 0.5 g sugar/dL urine.
    - Green precipitate—0.5 to 1.0 g sugar/dL urine.
    - Yellow precipitate—1.0 to 2.0 g sugar/dL urine.
    - Red precipitate—≥2.0 g sugar/dL urine.

DIFFERENTIAL DIAGNOSIS OF GLYCOSURIA

- When glycosuria (melituria) is found, it should be determined whether it is secondary to hyperglycaemia (DM) or nondiabetic glycosuria. Glycosuria generally occurs when blood glucose level exceeds the renal glucose threshold of 180 mg/dL, although in some cases with diabetes, renal threshold is increased.
- Use of sodium–glucose cotransporter 2 (SGLT2) inhibitors (e.g. dapagliflozin) also produces glycosuria.
- Nondiabetic melituria occurs in a number of conditions, the most important being renal glycosuria and alimentary (lag storage) glycosuria.

RENAL GLYCOSURIA

- Diagnosis of renal glycosuria is based on the Marble's criteria.
  - Glycosuria in the absence of hyperglycaemia.
  - Constant glycosuria (10–100 g/day) with little fluctuation related to diet.
  - Normal OGTT.
  - Normal plasma insulin levels.
  - Identification of urinary reducing substance as glucose.
  - Normal storage and utilisation of carbohydrates.

ALIMENTARY (LAG STORAGE) GLYCOSURIA

- Here, there is a transient abnormal rise in blood glucose level following a meal and the concentration exceeds the normal renal threshold. During this time, glucose spills into the urine. This may occur in the following conditions:
  - Following gastric surgery with rapid gastric emptying time.
  - Some normal people.
  - Hyperthyroidism.
  - Hepatic diseases.

Q. Give a brief account of oral glucose tolerance test. (IM11.11)

- The patient, who should have been taking an unrestricted carbohydrate diet for at least 3 days or more prior to the test, fasts overnight (at least 8 hours).
- The patient should rest for at least half an hour before starting the test and refrain from smoking during the test.
- A sample of blood is drawn to estimate the fasting glucose level.
- A glucose load of 75 g dissolved in 300 mL of water is given orally.
- Blood samples are withdrawn at half-hourly intervals for 2 hours (0.5, 1, 1.5, 2 hours) and glucose levels are estimated.

Q. Discuss briefly the dietary management of diabetes mellitus.

Q. Describe medical nutrition therapy in diabetes.

- People with diabetes should receive individualised lifestyle interventions which include dietary advice (medical nutrition treatment) as needed to achieve treatment goals, exercise and weight reduction.
- Medical nutrition therapy is the process by which the dietary plan is tailored for people with diabetes, based on medical, lifestyle and personal factors.
- Medical nutrition diet and physical exercise activate cellular mechanisms which protect by improving mitochondrial function, reducing generation of radicals and improving efficacy of insulin.
- Regular exercise (30–60 minutes of moderate-intensity aerobic exercises per day) is beneficial in type 2 diabetes, independent of weight loss.

- The preparation of a dietary regimen for a diabetic can be considered under three steps.

FIRST STEP

- This involves the estimation of the total daily caloric requirement of the individual patient. This must be estimated after considering a number of variable factors like age, sex, actual weight, desirable weight, activity and occupation of the patient. However, an approximate total daily caloric requirement can be calculated as follows:
  - Sedentary individuals—30 kcal/kg/day.
  - Moderately active individual—35 kcal/kg/day.
  - Heavily active individuals—40 kcal/kg/day.

SECOND STEP

- This involves allocation of the calories in a proper proportion to carbohydrate, protein and fat. The recommended proportion of calories to be derived from each of them is given as follows:
  - Carbohydrate—50% to 65%.
  - Protein—10% to 20%.
  - Total fat—25% to 30%.
    - Saturated fat—≤7%.
    - Polyunsaturated fat—≤10%.
    - Monounsaturated fat—10% to 15%.
- However, a few more important factors need be considered at this stage. They are as follows:
  - The minimal protein requirement for a good nutritious diet is about 0.9–1.0 g/kg/day.
  - The carbohydrates should be taken in the form of starches and other complex sugars. Rapidly absorbed simple sugars like glucose and even sucrose should generally be avoided.
  - Use of non-caloric sweeteners (non-nutritive sweeteners) like acesulfame potassium, aspartame, neotame, saccharin and sucralose is acceptable over a short period but overall, people are encouraged to decrease both sweetened and nonnutritive sweeteners and beverages and use other alternatives, with an emphasis on water intake.
  - Fish oils containing omega-3 fatty acids have been reported to be beneficial as antiatherogenic.
  - A high-fibre diet is beneficial as it has an antiatherogenic effect mediated through lowering of blood lipids.

THIRD STEP

- This involves distribution of the calories throughout the day. This is particularly important in insulin-requiring diabetics to avoid hypoglycaemia. Different distributions may be required for different lifestyles. However, a typical pattern of distribution of calories is as follows:
  - Twenty per cent of the total calories—for breakfast.
  - Thirty-five per cent of the total calories—for lunch.
  - Thirty per cent of the total calories—for dinner.
  - Fifteen per cent of the total calories—for late-evening feed.

Q. What are oral antidiabetic drugs? Discuss their mechanism of actions and indications. (IM11.16)

- Oral antidiabetic drugs (previously called hypoglycaemic drugs) fall into different categories as shown in Box 18.14.

SULPHONYLUREAS

MECHANISM OF ACTION

- Sulphonylureas are insulin secretagogues, that is they stimulate insulin secretion by blocking the opening of ATP-sensitive potassium channels on the β-islet cells. This produces depolarisation of the membrane leading to an influx of calcium. These events result in an increased production of insulin by the β-cells.
- Contrary to previously held belief, they do not increase insulin sensitivity and, therefore, should be avoided in type 1 DM.

INDICATIONS

- Sulphonylureas are effective in the treatment of non-obese patients with type 2 DM who fail to respond to dietary measures alone.

COMPARATIVE FEATURES

- Comparative features of various sulphonylureas are given in Table 18.28.

SPECIAL POINTS

- The first-generation sulphonylureas like chlorpropamide have longer half-life, greater incidence of hypoglycaemia and more frequent drug interactions

BOX 18.14 Oral Antidiabetic Drugs

- Sulphonylureas
- Meglitinides
- Biguanides
- α-Glucosidase inhibitors
- Thiazolidinediones
- Incretin-based therapy
- Sodium–glucose cotransporter 2 (SGLT2) inhibitors
- Other drugs

TABLE 18.28 Comparative Features of Sulphonylureas

Drug	Daily Dose (mg)	Doses/Day	Half-Life (Hours)	Metabolism/Excretion
First generation				
• Acetohexamide	500–1500	1 to 2	5	Liver/kidney
• Chlorpropamide	100–500	1	36	Kidney
• Tolbutamide	500–3000	2 to 3	4	Liver
• Tolazamide	100–750	1 to 2	7	Liver
Second generation				
• Glibenclamide	2.5–20	1 to 2	12	Liver/kidney
• Gliclazide	40–320	1 to 2	10–12	Liver/kidney
• Glipizide	2.5–30	1 to 2	3.5	Liver/kidney
• Glyburide	1.25–20	1 to 2	12–14	Liver/kidney
• Glimepiride	1–8	1	5–8	Liver/kidney

compared to the second-generation sulphonylureas. Therefore, second-generation drugs are preferred.
- They increase the insulin secretion acutely and hence, should be taken shortly before a meal.
- As these drugs are metabolised in liver and then excreted through kidneys, they should be avoided in the presence of significant renal or liver dysfunction.
- Common side effects include hypoglycaemia (which may be prolonged) and weight gain (due to increased insulin levels and control of DM).
- Hypoglycaemia occurring with sulphonylureas (particularly chlorpropamide and glibenclamide) tends to be severe and prolonged.
- In patients with significant renal disease, it is preferable to use tolbutamide or tolazamide, as these agents are exclusively metabolised by the liver.
- Chlorpropamide has a long biological half-life of about 36 hours and, hence, has the advantage that it can be given as a single dose at breakfast. However, it has significant side effects like prolonged and severe hypoglycaemia, cholestatic jaundice, SIADH, skin rashes and a disulfiram-like reaction in patients after taking alcohol.
- Some sulphonylureas have significant interactions with other medications such as warfarin, aspirin, ketoconazole and alcohol.
- Some patients do not respond to sulphonylureas, and these are termed 'primary treatment failures'. Some patients respond initially to sulphonylureas, but then cease to respond in the next 1 or 2 years. These are termed 'secondary treatment failures'. Dietary noncompliance is the most common cause of secondary treatment failure.

MEGLITINIDES

- These drugs also act on ATP-sensitive potassium channel to increase insulin secretion.
- Examples include repaglinide and nateglinide.
- Because of their short half-lives, these drugs are given immediately before each meal to reduce meal-related glucose excursions.
- Dose of repaglinide is 0.5–4 mg TID while that of nateglinide is 60–120 mg TID.
- They should be avoided in presence of significant liver dysfunction as well as in combination with sulphonylureas.

BIGUANIDES

- Metformin is the only drug used in this group (the other agent, phenformin, is no longer used because of associated side effects).

MECHANISM OF ACTION

- The main effect is to reduce the hepatic glucose production.
- Minor effect is to improve the peripheral glucose utilisation.

INDICATIONS

- Metformin is the preferred initial pharmacological agent for the treatment of type 2 diabetes, particularly obese patients who do not respond to dietary measures and weight reduction.
- If diabetes is not controlled with metformin, other agents including insulin may be added.

SPECIAL POINTS

- It reduces the fasting blood glucose and insulin levels, promotes modest weight loss and improves the lipid profile (reduction in fasting TG levels and LDL).
- It is started at a dose of 500 mg twice daily and gradually increased to a maximum of 1 g thrice daily. Sustained-release preparations are also available and need to be given once or twice a day.
- Its main side effect is acidosis that can be prevented if it is not used in some situations like presence of renal impairment (creatinine >1.4 mg/dL), heart failure, liver disease, severe hypoxia or preexisting acidosis.
- Other side effects are anorexia, diarrhoea and metallic taste in mouth.
- Long-term use of metformin may be associated with vitamin B_{12} deficiency.
- As it is not an insulin secretagogue, it is not usually associated with hypoglycaemia.

α-GLUCOSIDASE INHIBITORS

- This group includes acarbose, miglitol and voglibose.

MECHANISM OF ACTION

- α-Glucosidase is an enzyme located on the brush border of the intestine. It is required for the breakdown of disaccharides to form single sugars before carbohydrates can be absorbed. Acarbose and other agents inhibit the α-glucosidase enzymes. This leads to poor absorption of carbohydrates, thereby causing reduced rise in postprandial blood glucose.

INDICATIONS

- These agents are useful in managing patients who develop significant postprandial hyperglycaemia but otherwise have relatively well-controlled blood glucose levels.

SPECIAL POINTS

- Dose of both acarbose and miglitol is 25 mg with evening meal first. This can be gradually increased to 50 mg with each meal. Dose of voglibose is 0.2–0.3 mg with each meal.
- These agents are poorly tolerated because of fermentation of unabsorbed carbohydrates in the large intestine. This produces diarrhoea, flatulence and abdominal distension. However, increased disaccharide concentration leads to the induction of α-glucosidase enzymes (disaccharidases) in the jejunum and ileum. Eventually, this induction of new enzymes results in a slower, smoother absorption of disaccharides. The slower absorption is still effective in reducing postprandial glucose levels but with fewer malabsorptive symptoms. Therefore, α-glucosidase inhibitors must

be started at a very low dose, with small increments over time.

- The blood levels of sulphonylureas may increase if administered simultaneously.
- These agents do not cause hypoglycaemia.
- They do not undergo renal excretion, so they are safe in patients with a modest elevation of serum creatinine. However, these agents should be avoided if creatinine >2.0 mg/dL and also in inflammatory bowel disease.

THIAZOLIDINEDIONES

- This group includes pioglitazone. Rosiglitazone, the other agent, has been withdrawn due to increased incidence of acute myocardial infarction and cardiovascular deaths in patients using it.

MECHANISM OF ACTION

- Pioglitazone binds to peroxisome proliferator-activated receptor (PPAR-γ), a nuclear receptor that regulates transcription of genes involved in lipid metabolism and insulin action. This promotes adipocyte differentiation and reduced insulin resistance in skeletal muscles.
- Due to reduction in insulin resistance, it increases peripheral glucose utilisation. It may also reduce hepatic glucose production.

SPECIAL POINTS

- Dose of pioglitazone is 15–45 mg/day.
- Can be combined with metformin and sulphonylureas.
- Maximum effect may be seen only after 3 to 4 weeks.
- Liver functions should be monitored periodically as liver dysfunction may develop.
- Important side effects include weight gain (due to water retention as well as increase in adiposity) and mild rise in LDL. High density lipoprotein (HDL) levels may increase.
- Contraindicated in liver disease and congestive cardiac failure.
- May produce fluid retention, cardiac insufficiency and increased propensity to bone fractures.

INCRETIN-BASED THERAPY

- Incretin hormones, primarily glucagon-like peptide 1 (GLP-1) and glucose-dependent insulinotropic polypeptide (GIP), are polypeptide hormones synthesised in gut. GIP and GLP-1 are secreted by enteroendocrine K-cells in the proximal gut and L-cells in the distal gut, respectively. These act on their receptors present on islet cells to stimulate insulin secretion in response to food. This potentiation of insulin secretion by the gut is referred to as the *in*testinal se*cret*ion of *in*sulin or incretin effect—increase in insulin is markedly greater in response to an oral than to an intravenous glucose challenge.
- In addition, they enhance β-cell proliferation and promote resistance to apoptosis.
- GLP-1 also lowers plasma glucose levels through inhibition of glucagon secretion, deceleration of gastric emptying and inhibition of food intake. It also provides cardioprotective and vasodilatory effects.
- Insulin modulatory properties of GIP are attenuated in patients with type 2 diabetes; hence, in clinical practice, only GLP-1 analogues are used.
- GLP-1 as well as GIP are rapidly degraded in the circulation by dipeptidyl peptidase IV.
- Various analogues of GLP-1 and inhibitors of dipeptidyl peptidase IV have been developed. These are known as incretin mimetics.

GLUCAGON-LIKE PEPTIDE-1 ANALOGUES

- Exenatide, liraglutide, dulaglutide, lixisenatide, semaglutide and albiglutide have been approved for use in combination with metformin, a sulphonylurea or a thiazolidinedione. They produce weight loss.
- These analogues need to be given parenterally.
- Preferred among patients with established atherosclerotic cardiovascular disease.
- Risk of hypoglycaemia is low.
- Adverse effects include nausea, diarrhoea and rarely pancreatitis.

DIPEPTIDYL PEPTIDASE IV INHIBITOR

- An alternative approach to the use of GLP-1 analogues is to inhibit dipeptidyl peptidase IV to conserve endogenous GLP-1.
- Vildagliptin, sitagliptin, saxagliptin, linagliptin and alogliptin are oral agents for use in type 2 DM either as monotherapy or with other agents. Risk of hypoglycaemia is low.
- Side effects include nausea, diarrhoea, headache, upper respiratory symptoms and possible risk for pancreatitis.

SODIUM–GLUCOSE COTRANSPORTER 2 INHIBITORS

- SGLT2 inhibitors like dapagliflozin, empagliflozin, ertugliflozin and canagliflozin reduce renal glucose resorption and thus cause glycosuria and a resulting insulin-independent reduction in blood glucose as well as weight loss.
- SGLT2 inhibitors do not confer any risk of hypoglycaemia but produce increased incidence of genital infections.
- Preferred among patients with established atherosclerotic cardiovascular disease and heart failure.
- Canagliflozin has been shown to reduce the risk of kidney failure and cardiovascular events in type 2 diabetic patients.
- Adverse effects include a higher rate of genital infections (including necrotising fasciitis), diabetic ketoacidosis, acute kidney injury, fracture and increased risk of amputation.

OTHERS

- Pramlintide, a synthetic form of pancreatic hormone amylin, should be injected before each meal. Amylin

is a hormone cosecreted with insulin and regulates glucose influx through the suppression of glucagon and slowing of gastric emptying. The most common side effects are nausea and hypoglycaemia.
- Bile acid sequestrant (e.g. colesevelam).
- Dopamine-2 agonist (e.g. bromocriptine).

Q. Describe briefly the role of insulin in the management of diabetes. (IM11.16)

Q. How do you classify insulins? Give a brief account of the commonly used insulins. (IM11.16)

Q. Discuss briefly about pancreatic transplantation.

- Insulin is required for treatment of all patients with type 1 DM and many patients with type 2 DM. The goals of insulin therapy are as follows:
  - Normal growth and development in children.
  - Normal pregnancy, delivery and conceptus in females.
  - Minimal interference with psychological adjustment.
  - Acceptable glycaemic control with minimal hypoglycaemia.
  - Prevention of complications.
- Insulin can be administered with an insulin syringe or a pen or by a pump.
- Insulin should be injected into subcutaneous tissue, not intramuscularly. Recommended sites for insulin injection include abdomen, thigh, buttock and upper arm.

GENERAL INDICATIONS FOR INSULIN THERAPY (Box 18.15)

BOX 18.15 Indications for Insulin Therapy

- Type 1 DM
- Diabetic ketoacidosis (DKA)
- Hyperosmolar hyperglycaemic state
- Stress of surgery, infections and trauma
- Diabetes during pregnancy
- Nonobese type 2 DM unresponsive to oral drugs
- Postrenal transplantation diabetic patients

INSULIN PREPARATIONS

- Insulin preparations can be classified in different ways:
  - Based on source as bovine, porcine and human insulins.
  - Based on purity as conventional, single-peak and monocomponent insulins.
  - Based on time course of action as rapid-, intermediate- and long-acting insulins.
  - Based on strength as 40 and 100 units/mL.
  - Newer insulin analogues.

PURIFICATION OF PORCINE INSULIN

CRYSTALLISATION

- Processing of conventional porcine insulin on gel chromatography reveals the impurities as three peaks—'a', 'b' and 'c' peaks.
  - The 'a' peak is due to pancreatic proteins of high molecular weight (>12,000).
  - The 'b' peak is due to proinsulin and intermediates.
  - The 'c' peak is due to insulin fragments (derivatives) and pancreatic hormones (glucagon, somatostatin and pancreatic polypeptides).
- Crystallisation removes the 'a' peak to a large extent and results in an insulin preparation of conventional purity. As this conventional insulin contains significant contaminants (proinsulin), it is highly immunogenic and can result in the development of antiinsulin antibodies.

GEL FILTRATION

- Insulin processed by gel chromatography results in a preparation known as 'single-peak' insulin (highly purified insulin).

ION EXCHANGE CHROMATOGRAPHY

- Insulin purified by ion exchange chromatography results in the purest insulin preparation. This insulin preparation is hence known as monocomponent insulin.
- The advantages of monocomponent insulin are that it is less immunogenic and causes less lipodystrophy and insulin resistance.
- The indications for monocomponent insulin are as follows:
  - Allergic reaction to conventional insulin.
  - Treatment of insulin resistance.
  - Treatment of lipodystrophy.
  - In pregnancy, to prevent transplacental transfer of antibodies, which can damage the foetal pancreas.
  - Liver disease.
  - As a short-term therapy to tide over surgery.

HUMAN INSULIN

- Human insulin differs from porcine insulin by one amino acid residue and from bovine insulin by three amino acid residues. The changes in the amino acid residues of these three insulins are given in Box 18.16.

BOX 18.16 Position of Amino Acids in Human, Porcine and Bovine Insulins

	Amino Acid Position		
	A8	**A10**	**B30**
• Human	Threonine	Isoleucine	Threonine
• Porcine	Threonine	Isoleucine	Alanine
• Bovine	Alanine	Valine	Alanine

- Bovine insulin is more immunogenic than porcine insulin that is more immunogenic than human insulin. As the amino acid sequence of human insulin is known, it can be completely synthesised step by step. There are two types of human insulins:
  - Semisynthetic human insulin—This is an enzymatically modified pork insulin. The monocomponent porcine insulin is enzymatically de-alaninated from the B30 position, which is then replaced by threonine to make the structure identical to human insulin.
  - Highly purified human insulin is now available as a product of recombinant DNA biosynthesis.
- Human insulin is more rapidly absorbed and has a shorter duration of action compared to porcine or bovine regular insulin.
- Presently, the cost of human insulin is nearly the same as that of animal insulin. Therefore, many physicians are using it as the initial choice in diabetics requiring insulin.

PROPERTIES OF VARIOUS INSULIN PREPARATIONS

- The commonly used insulin preparations are classified based on their time of action into rapid-, intermediate- and long-acting insulins (Table 18.29).

INSULIN ANALOGUES

- These analogues are useful in patients who get repeated episodes of hypoglycaemia or show hyperglycaemia during some part of the day while on regular insulins.
- Insulin analogues have been prepared by modifying human insulin.
- Various preparations which are available are shown in Table 18.30.

TABLE 18.29 Properties of Various Insulin Preparations Based on Time of Action

Class	Type	Peak Effect (Hours)	Duration of Action (Hours)
• Rapid	Regular (crystalline, soluble, plain)	2–4	6–8
	Semilente	2–6	10–12
• Intermediate	Isophane (NPH)	6–12	18–24
	Lente	6–12	18–24
• Long acting	Protamine zinc (PZI)	14–24	36
	Ultralente	18–24	36

TABLE 18.30 Various Preparations of Insulin Analogues

Class	Type	Peak Effect (Hours)	Duration of Action (Hours)
• **Short-acting insulin analogues**	Insulin lispro	1–1.5	3–5
	Insulin aspart	0.6–0.9	3–5
	Insulin glulisine	1	3–5
• **Long-acting insulin analogues**	Insulin glargine	None	24
	Insulin detemir	None	24
	Insulin degludec	None	42

INSULIN LISPRO

- It is a human insulin analogue created when the amino acids at positions 28 and 29 on the insulin B-chain are reversed. Like any other human insulin, it is produced by recombinant DNA technology utilising a nonpathogenic strain of *E. coli*.
- It is absorbed faster than regular human insulin and, therefore, has a more rapid onset of glucose-lowering activity (<15 minutes), an earlier peak for glucose lowering (60–90 minutes) and a shorter duration of glucose-lowering activity (<5 hours). Therefore patient needs to take this insulin just before or after meals.
- However, it is equipotent to human regular insulin (i.e. 1 unit of insulin lispro has the same glucose-lowering capacity as 1 unit of regular insulin).
- Because of its short duration of action, it reduces the risk of hypoglycaemia several hours after meals.
- Patients require additional use of longer-acting insulin to maintain glucose control.

INSULIN ASPART AND INSULIN GLULISINE

- These are also short-acting insulin analogues that are similar to lispro.

INSULIN GLARGINE

- It is a human insulin analogue that has a long duration of action (up to 24 hours) and has a pH of 4.
- It differs from human insulin in that there is an amino acid substitution of asparagine with glycine at the 21 position of the α-chain, and two arginines are added at the C-terminal of the β-chain.
- After injection into the subcutaneous tissue, the acid solution becomes neutralised and leads to microprecipitate formation. These microprecipitates release insulin very slowly, which results in a relatively constant concentration and time profile over 24 hours without a pronounced peak. This profile allows for dosing once a day as a basal insulin level.
- It is generally taken at breakfast or at bedtime.
- As insulin glargine is presented in an acidic formulation, its ability to mix with other insulins is limited. This may also possibly account for increased injection pain.

INSULIN DETEMIR

- Insulin detemir is soluble and has a neutral pH.
- It is an acylated derivative of human insulin with protracted action. When injected subcutaneously, insulin detemir binds to albumin via its fatty acid chain leading to a substantial reduction in the free insulin detemir concentration.
- By combining the basal soluble analogue insulin detemir and the rapid-acting analogue insulin aspart or lispro, it may be possible to more closely mimic near-normal insulin profiles, with resulting improvement in glycaemic control compared with more conventional insulin therapy.

INSULIN DEGLUDEC

- It forms soluble multihexamers at the injection site from which monomers slowly separate and are absorbed.

- Has a long duration of action (>40 hours) and reduces variability in plasma concentration with once-daily dosing.

INHALED INSULIN

- Inhaled human insulin powder was introduced in 2006 with much hope. Absorption of insulin was through the alveolar surface in the lungs. It was used with each meal along with single injection of long-acting insulin to provide basal levels of insulin. Side effects included cough, dry mouth, sore throat and shortness of breath, besides hypoglycaemia. Because of adverse effects, clinical efficacy similar to injectable insulin and cost issues, it was withdrawn in 2007.
- In 2014, another preparation of human insulin inhalation powder was approved. It is composed of recombinant human insulin adsorbed onto Technosphere microparticles formed by fumaryl diketopiperazine. It has a rapid onset of action, faster return of action to baseline levels and lower intrapatient variability of insulin action. It is contraindicated in patients with COPD and asthma and is not recommended in patients who smoke or who recently stopped smoking. All patients require spirometry (FEV_1) testing to identify potential lung disease prior to and after starting inhaled insulin therapy.

INSULIN REGIMENS

- Four treatment regimens will be described—that is conventional insulin therapy, multiple subcutaneous injections (MSI), continuous subcutaneous insulin infusion (CSII) and automated insulin delivery.

CONVENTIONAL INSULIN THERAPY

- In conventional insulin therapy, one or two injections a day of intermediate-acting insulin is/are administered, with or without the addition of small amounts of regular insulin.
- Insulin mixtures—here, in addition to the intermediate-acting insulin, small doses of regular insulin are added to achieve better euglycaemic status.
- Split NPH regimen—when the total daily insulin dose exceeds 50 or 60 units, or when diabetic state needs better control, the intermediate-acting insulin (NPH) is given in two doses. Two-thirds of the total dose is given before breakfast (7 to 8 a.m.) and the remaining one-third before dinner (7 to 8 p.m.).

MULTIPLE SUBCUTANEOUS INJECTIONS

- This involves administration of intermediate- or long-acting insulin (e.g. insulin glargine) in the evening as a single dose together with regular insulin prior to each meal. This regimen improves the overall control and may reduce the rate of development of long-term complications. A commonly used schedule is as follows:
    - The total daily dose of insulin is calculated at 0.6–0.7 unit/kg body weight.
    - The 30%–40% of the calculated dose is given at bedtime in the form of an intermediate-acting or long-acting insulin.
    - The 60%–70% of the calculated dose is given in three divided doses as regular insulin (40% before breakfast, 30% before lunch and 30% before dinner).

CONTINUOUS SUBCUTANEOUS INSULIN INFUSION

- This involves the use of a small battery-driven pump as a means of mimicking the physiological basal plus prandial pattern of insulin secretion. The insulin pump is worn externally and connected to a butterfly needle, which is inserted into the anterior abdominal wall.
- About 40% of the total daily dose is given at basal rate, the remainder being administered as preprandial boluses.
- The dangerous complication of this regimen is hypoglycaemia, especially nocturnal, which may be fatal.

AUTOMATED INSULIN DELIVERY

- Consists of three components: an insulin pump, a continuous glucose sensor and an algorithm that determines insulin delivery.
- This provides physiological insulin delivery as insulin delivery can be increased, decreased and suspended based on sensor glucose values.

COMPLICATIONS OF INSULIN THERAPY

- Hypoglycaemia.
- Local allergic reactions at the injection site including local itching, erythematous and indurated lesions, and discrete subcutaneous nodules.
- Rarely, patients may develop systemic reactions, including generalised urticaria and anaphylactic reactions.
- Fat atrophy or fat hypertrophy may develop at the injection sites. Fat atrophy is usually due to impurities in the insulin preparation. Fat hypertrophy is attributed to the local lipogenic effects of the injected insulin.
- Formation of antiinsulin antibodies.

PANCREATIC TRANSPLANTATION

- Other options in patients with type 1 DM include pancreatic transplantation and islet cell transplantation.
- Both are capable of restoring normoglycaemia without exogenous insulin therapy and both have patient survival rates that are consistent with other organ transplantation procedures.

Q. Describe the assessment of metabolic control in diabetes. (IM11.11)

- There are various methods of assessing blood glucose control in diabetic patients. Each method has its own advantages and disadvantages. The commonly employed methods are enumerated in the following text.

URINARY GLUCOSE

- Semiquantitative measurements of urinary glucose and ketones can be obtained before breakfast and once or twice throughout the day. Patients should be instructed to void 30 minutes before obtaining urine sample for glucose determination ('double voiding'), particularly for the morning sample, so that the urinary glucose is more representative of the corresponding blood glucose. Regardless of this, it provides only a rough approximation of blood glucose levels. In addition, factors such as renal threshold, renal blood flow and urine volume greatly affect the meaning of urine glucose measurement (e.g. a raised renal threshold for glucose may mask persistent hyperglycaemia).
- Periodic assessment of 24-hour urinary glucose excretion provides a better estimate of day-long control (less than 5 g/day indicates excellent control).

BLOOD GLUCOSE

- Single random measurements of blood glucose levels are of limited value.
- Estimation of at least two blood glucose values (preprandial glucose and bedtime) must be done to assess the glycaemic control. The targets are as follows:
  - Preprandial whole blood glucose 80–120 mg/dL (capillary plasma 90–130 mg/dL).
  - Peak postprandial whole blood glucose (between 1 and 2 hours after meals) <160 mg/dL (capillary plasma 180 mg/dL).
- The best current method to assess glycaemic control is home- or self-monitoring of blood glucose (SMBG). This requires the patient to assess his/her own blood glucose level daily and to make appropriate adjustments in insulin dosage. The measurements may be done using blood glucose test strips read either visually or with a reflectance meter.

GLYCOSYLATED OR GLYCATED PROTEINS

- Glycosylated haemoglobin (vide infra) can be measured which provides an excellent assessment of the overall state of glycaemic control during the preceding 3 months. In general, the goal is to get a value of less than 7%. A more stringent HbA1c goal of 6.5% may be kept in selected patients (short duration of type 2 diabetes without cardiovascular disease) if this can be achieved without significant hypoglycaemia or other adverse effects of treatment:
  - Some factors can influence HbA1c independent of glycaemia. The most common is any disease that alters red blood cell survival. Since glycation of haemoglobin occurs only as the erythrocyte circulates in blood, haemoglobin in the older erythrocytes is more glycosylated, and haemoglobin in the reticulocyte is less. Total HbA1c reflects the mix of older and younger erythrocytes. Therefore, if the average life of red cells is abnormally short (as in, e.g. haemolytic anaemia), then measured HbA1c will be lower, independent of glycaemia. Conversely, if the average age of circulating erythrocytes is older (e.g. occurs if erythropoiesis is suddenly stopped in an aplastic anaemia), then the older red cell population would have higher HbA1c levels, regardless of glycaemia.
  - In conditions associated with an altered relationship between HbA1c and glucose levels such as hereditary spherocytosis, sickle cell disease, pregnancy (second and third trimesters and the postpartum period), glucose-6-phosphate dehydrogenase deficiency, HIV, haemodialysis, recent blood loss or transfusion, or erythropoietin therapy, only plasma blood glucose criteria should be used to diagnose diabetes.
- Fructosamine assay measures glycation of all serum proteins. Since albumin accounts for most of the protein in blood, the fructosamine, for practical purposes, measures glycated albumin. As albumin has a turnover of about 2 weeks, fructosamine reflects glycaemia over this far shorter period.

BLOOD LIPIDS

- Concentrations of serum cholesterol, TG and HDL measured in the fasting state provide an index of overall metabolic control in diabetic patients.

Q. Discuss briefly glycosylated (glycated) haemoglobin (HbA1c). (IM11.11)

- When haemoglobin from a normal adult is passed through a chromatographic column, it separates into two major components:
  - Haemoglobin A (HbA) comprising 92%–94% of the total haemoglobin.
  - Haemoglobin A1c (HbA1c) consisting of several, fast-moving components, comprising 6%–8% of the total haemoglobin.
- The rate of synthesis of HbA1c depends on the exposure of the red cell to glucose, and, hence, its level increases with hyperglycaemia.
- The percentage of glycosylated haemoglobin (HbA1c) gives an estimate of the diabetic control for the preceding 3-month period.
- The goal in general is to have HbA1c below 7% but for individual patients, it should be as close to normal (<6%) as possible without significant hypoglycaemia.

Q. Enumerate the complications of diabetes. How do you classify them?

- Complications of DM are listed in Table 18.31.

TABLE 18.31 Acute and Chronic Complications of Diabetes Mellitus

Acute Metabolic Complications	Chronic (Long-Term) Complications	
	Microvascular	*Macrovascular*

• Diabetic ketoacidosis (DKA)
• Hyperosmolar hyperglycaemic state (HHS, hyperosmolar nonketotic diabetic coma)
• Hypoglycaemia
• Lactic acidosis
	• Diabetic retinopathy (nonproliferative and proliferative)
	• Cataract
	• Glaucoma
	• Neuropathy
	  ◦ Sensory
	  ◦ Motor
	  ◦ Sensory motor
	  ◦ Autonomic
	• Nephropathy
		• Coronary artery disease
		• Peripheral vascular disease
		• Cerebrovascular disease
		Others
		• Dermatological complications

Q. Discuss the pathogenesis, clinical features, diagnosis, complications and management of diabetic ketoacidosis. (IM11.15, IM11.23, IM11.6, IM11.9)

- DKA is a complication of type 1 DM. It is rare in type 2 DM.
- Precipitating factors of DKA include too little or no insulin intake, new onset type 1 diabetes, infections, severe stress (e.g. physical, emotional), myocardial infarction, stroke, acute pancreatitis and drugs (e.g. thiazides, corticosteroids, clozapine, olanzapine, lithium, cocaine).
- SGLT2 inhibitors, pregnancy, chronic liver disease, starvation and chronic alcohol use can also precipitate DKA with blood glucose below 250 mg/dL (euglycaemic DKA). Management of euglycaemic DKA is similar to DKA except that the initial resuscitation is done with saline along with dextrose.

PATHOGENESIS

- DKA and hyperosmolar hyperglycaemic state (HHS) result from insulin deficiency (absolute or relative) and counter-regulatory hormonal excess (glucagon, catecholamines, cortisol, glucagon and GH).

CONSEQUENCES OF INSULIN DEFICIENCY

- Hyperglycaemia resulting in a hyperosmolar state which induces an osmotic diuresis leading to volume depletion and dehydration.
- Activation of lipolysis in adipose tissue results in release of increased amounts of free fatty acids (FFA) into plasma which are taken up by the liver. The fate of FFA in the liver is discussed below (see 'Consequences of Glucagon Excess').

CONSEQUENCES OF GLUCAGON EXCESS

- Accelerated hepatic gluconeogenesis and impaired peripheral utilisation of glucose both result in severe hyperglycaemia. This hyperglycaemia induces an osmotic diuresis leading to volume depletion and dehydration.
- Activation of ketogenic process results in ketosis and metabolic acidosis. The mechanism is complex and involves the following sequences: the excess glucagon causes a resetting of the hepatic metabolism of FFA. This is achieved through an increased activity of the enzyme, carnitine acyltransferase. The result is that hepatic mitochondria convert FFA to ketone bodies which accumulate in the body fluids. The ketone bodies mainly include acetoacetic acid and β-hydroxybutyric acid, but acetone also in a minor amount.
- The two strong acids, acetoacetic acid and β-hydroxybutyric acid, are responsible for the acidotic state. These acids dissociate completely, releasing hydrogen ions into the body fluids with a resultant fall in pH. The fall in pH is countered by the buffers, especially bicarbonate, which is used up.
- Pathogenesis of DKA and HHS is given in Flowchart 18.9.

CLINICAL FEATURES

- DKA begins with anorexia, nausea, vomiting and increased rate of urine formation.
- Abdominal pain is a dominant symptom.
- Altered consciousness or frank coma may occur in untreated cases.
- Kussmaul's breathing and a fruity odour to the breath due to acetone.
- Signs of volume depletion and dehydration are invariably present which may proceed to vascular collapse and renal failure.
- Body temperature is normal or low in uncomplicated DKA. Fever suggests infection.
- Leucocytosis is a feature of DKA per se and may not indicate infection.

COMPLICATIONS

- Acute gastric dilatation or erosive gastritis, cerebral oedema, hyperkalaemia, hypokalaemia, hypoglycaemia, infections, insulin resistance, myocardial infarction, mucormycosis, ARDS and vascular thrombosis.
- Symptoms and signs of cerebral oedema include onset of headache, gradual deterioration in level of consciousness, seizures, sphincter incontinence, pupillary changes, papilloedema, bradycardia, elevation in blood pressure and respiratory arrest.

INVESTIGATIONS

- Urine examination shows glucose and ketones.
- Plasma glucose levels are raised, often markedly.
- Plasma ketone values are raised.
- Plasma potassium levels are normal or raised in the initial stages despite a total body deficit. This is due to metabolic acidosis which shifts potassium from intracellular compartment to extracellular compartment. The levels drop once the treatment is commenced.
- Plasma sodium levels are usually low particularly if the patient has vomited repeatedly and continued to drink water.

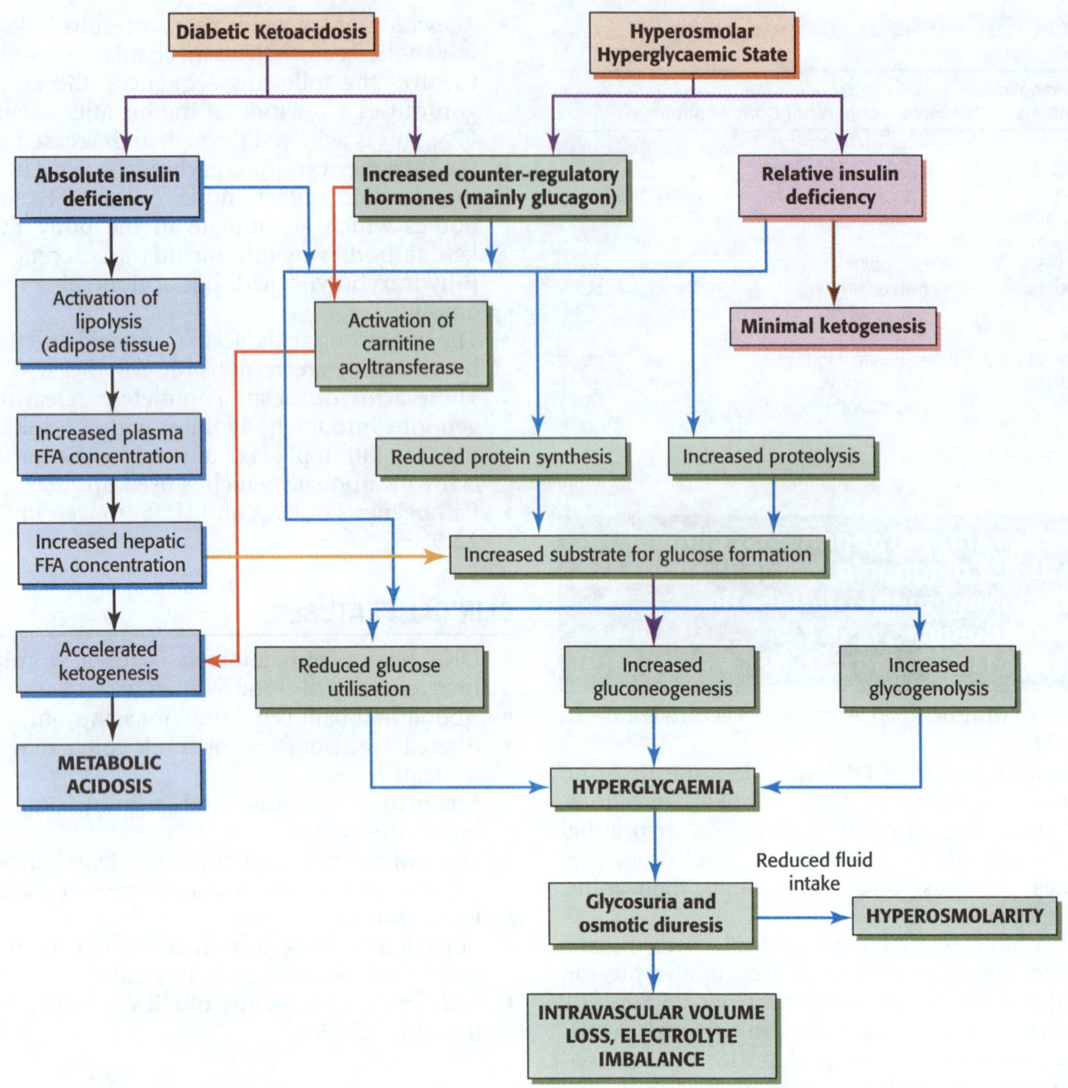

Flowchart 18.9 Pathogenesis of DKA and HHS: Stress, Infection or Insufficient Insulin. FFA, free fatty acid. (Source: *A.E. Kitabchi, G.E. Umpierrez, J.M. Miles, J.N. Fisher: Hyperglycemic crises in adult patients with diabetes.* Diabetes Care. *2009:32(7): 1335–1343.)*

- Serum phosphorus level may be high initially despite a total body deficit.
- Plasma bicarbonate levels are low and a value less than 12 mmol/L indicates severe acidosis.
- The hydrogen ion concentration of the blood is raised and the pH low.
- Blood urea nitrogen (BUN) is usually elevated due to prerenal failure resulting from volume depletion.
- Serum amylase may be raised especially in the presence of pancreatitis.
- The anion gap of >12 mEq/L is usually present in DKA patients.
- Assessment of ketonuria and ketonaemia is usually performed by nitroprusside test which provides semiquantitative assay of acetoacetate and acetone levels. This assay underestimates the severity of ketoacidosis as it does not recognise presence of β-hydroxybutyric acid, the main ketoacid in DKA; acetoacetate may not be elevated until later in the course of the illness.
- Diagnosis criteria for DKA.
    - These are blood glucose >250 mg/dL, arterial pH <7.3, serum bicarbonate <15 mEq/L and moderate degree of ketonaemia and/or ketonuria.

MANAGEMENT

- The patient should be managed with the aid of a flow sheet outlining amounts and timing of insulin and fluids, vital signs, urine output and blood chemistries including glucose, sodium, potassium, bicarbonate, urea and ketones.
- Fluid replacement:
    - The usual fluid deficit in DKA is 3–5 L. It should be replaced intravenously. One to two litres of isotonic saline should be given rapidly intravenously on admission within 1 hour. Additional amounts are determined by urine output and clinical assessment of the fluid state. Generally, additional 1 to 2 L is administered over next 2 hours.

- Intravenous fluid also increases insulin responsiveness by lowering plasma osmolality, reducing vasoconstriction and improving perfusion, and reducing counter-regulatory hormone levels.
- Switch to 0.45% sodium chloride after an initial bolus if the serum corrected sodium is high or normal. The corrected sodium concentration is calculated by adding 2 mEq/L to the serum sodium concentration for each 100 mg/dL increase in glucose above normal. If corrected sodium is less than 135 mEq/L, isotonic saline should be continued at a rate of approximately 250–500 mL/hour.
- When plasma glucose falls to less than 200 mg/dL, 5% glucose–saline solution should be given to prevent cerebral oedema and control ketogenesis (as 5% dextrose allows continued administration of insulin required to shut down ketone body formation).
- If the blood glucose drops below 150 mg/dL despite administration of 5% dextrose–saline, 10% dextrose should be started instead of reducing the dose of insulin.

- Insulin:
  - Insulin is generally started about an hour after IV fluid replacement is started.
  - It should not be started if potassium is less than 3.3 mEq/L as this may lead to further drop in potassium.
  - DKA should be treated with regular insulin intravenously. A reasonable goal is to maintain the plasma glucose level around 200 mg/dL.
  - Most patients can be treated by 'low-dose' insulin schedules in which 8–10 units of regular insulin is infused intravenously each hour. A priming bolus dose is not recommended. Most patients respond to this schedule but some may not, probably due to insulin resistance. They are identified by the persistence of acidosis despite several hours of treatment. For them, larger amounts of insulin should be given. In addition, if the serum glucose does not fall by at least 50 mg/dL in the first hour, insulin infusion rate should be doubled.
- Potassium replacement:
  - The initial potassium level is often high despite a total body deficit because of severe acidosis. With the initiation of therapy, reversal of acidosis and the action of insulin cause a shift of K^+ into the intracellular space. This usually takes 3 to 4 hours when plasma potassium levels drop. Potassium supplementation should commence at this stage.
  - If the admission potassium value is <5.3 mEq/L, potassium should be given early provided urine output is more than 50 mL/hour. This is to prevent hypokalaemia which can predispose to cardiac arrhythmias. Potassium is give at a rate of 20–40 mEq/hour.
  - In severe hypokalaemia (potassium <3.3 mEq/L), insulin is started only after potassium replacement is under way.
  - If initial potassium is more than 5.3 mEq/L, potassium replacement should be delayed till it falls below this level.
  - In view of the phosphate depletion, potassium should be administered initially as phosphate salt rather than as potassium chloride if initial phosphate is below 1 mg/dL. This is especially required if cardiac dysfunction, haemolytic anaemia or respiratory depression develop.
- Bicarbonate therapy:
  - This is indicated only in patients with severe acidosis (pH ≤6.9) especially if hypotension or coma is present. Bicarbonate should be given as an infusion of isotonic sodium bicarbonate (1.4%, i.e. 100 mL of 7.5% sodium bicarbonate is diluted with 400 mL of 5% dextrose or normal saline). The infusion is given over 2 hours and should be stopped when the pH reaches 7.0.
- Prevention of cerebral oedema includes avoidance of excessive hydration and rapid reduction of plasma osmolarity, a gradual decrease in serum glucose, and maintenance of serum glucose between 250 and 300 mg/dL until serum osmolality is normalised and mental status is improved. Mannitol infusion and mechanical ventilation are suggested for treatment of cerebral oedema.
- Initiate oral feeds when nausea and abdominal pain subside. Give a dose of regular insulin along with intermediate acting insulin (NPH) or long acting insulin (glargine or detemir) subcutaneously before stopping intravenous insulin.

PROGNOSIS

- Major causes of death in DKA are myocardial infarction and infection, particularly pneumonia, and cerebral oedema in children.
- Poor prognostic signs at admission include hypotension, azotaemia, deep coma and associated illness.

Q. Briefly outline precipitating factors, clinical features, laboratory findings and management of hyperosmolar hyperglycaemic state. (IM11.15, IM11.24, IM11.6, IM11.9)

Q. Describe hyperosmolar nonketotic diabetic coma.

- The terms 'hyperosmolar hyperglycaemic nonketotic coma', 'hyperosmolar nonketotic diabetic coma' and 'hyperosmolar hyperglycaemic nonketotic state' have been replaced with the term HHS as coma may not be present in all cases, and variable degree of ketosis may be present as determined by the nitroprusside method.
- Usually a complication of type 2 diabetes.
- Characterised by extreme dehydration resulting from a sustained hyperglycaemic diuresis under circumstances in which the patient is unable to drink sufficient water. The biochemical hallmark of the syndrome is extreme hyperglycaemia in the absence of significant ketoacidosis.
- It carries a high mortality rate of more than 50%.

PRECIPITATING FACTORS (Box 18.17)

BOX 18.17 Precipitating Factors for Hyperosmolar Hyperglycaemic State

- Infections
- Cerebrovascular accidents
- Peritoneal dialysis and haemodialysis
- Tube feeding of high-protein formulas
- Parenteral nutrition
- Osmotic agents like mannitol
- Steroids, immunosuppressive agents, phenytoin and diuretics

PATHOGENESIS

- It is similar to DKA but with some differences.
  - Insulin deficiency is relative (both reduced secretion and increased peripheral resistance).
  - Residual insulin produces suppression of lipolysis and ketogenesis and this minimises development of ketoacidosis. However, relative deficiency of insulin is not adequate to control hyperglycaemia.
  - In addition, elevation in glucagon levels is also lower in HHS compared to in DKA and, therefore, lesser ketogenesis occurs.

CLINICAL FEATURES

- Onset is usually more insidious as compared to that of DKA.
- Signs of volume depletion and extreme dehydration are invariably present.
- Central nervous system manifestations include alteration in the level of consciousness ranging from clouded sensorium to coma, convulsions (sometimes Jacksonian in type) and transient hemiplegia.
- Infections, particularly pneumonia and Gram-negative sepsis, are very common.
- Bleeding and acute pancreatitis may accompany the illness.

LABORATORY FINDINGS

- Plasma glucose is markedly elevated, usually around 1000 mg/dL (range 600–2400 mg/dL).
- Serum osmolality is markedly raised.
- Prerenal azotaemia with elevation of BUN and creatinine.
- A mild metabolic acidosis with marginal decrease in plasma bicarbonate (about 20 mmol/L) is present. Marked decrease in plasma bicarbonate ($<$10 mmol/L) indicates lactic acidosis.
- Diagnostic criteria for HHS include plasma glucose more than 600 mg/dL, osmolality more than 330 mOsm/kg and absence of severe ketoacidosis. The blood pH is usually more than 7.3 with bicarbonate more than 18 mEq/L. Approximately 50% of the patients with HHS have an increased anion gap metabolic acidosis as a result of concomitant ketoacidosis and elevated lactate levels.

MANAGEMENT

- *Fluid replacement*: The average fluid deficit is about 10 L that should be corrected intravenously. Initially 2 to 3 L of isotonic (0.9%) saline should be given over 1 to 2 hours. Subsequently, half-strength (0.45%) saline should be used. Once the plasma glucose approaches 300 mg/dL, 5% dextrose–saline solution should be used.
- *Insulin*: Regular insulin should be given as a low-dose intravenous infusion, as for DKA. It should be started after initial bolus of saline has been given. The goal is to keep the plasma glucose around 200 mg/dL. Rapid reductions in glucose levels are undesirable as these can lead to large shifts in water and sodium status resulting from rapid changes in serum osmolality.
- Potassium supplementation is required early, as for DKA.
- Infections should be treated with antibiotics.
- Anticoagulants should be given to prevent thrombosis.
- Flowchart 18.10 gives protocol for management of an adult patient with DKA or HHS.

Q. How will you differentiate between diabetic ketoacidosis and hyperosmolar hyperglycaemic state? (IM11.9)

- Differentiating clinical and laboratory features between DKA and HHS are given in Table 18.32.

Q. Discuss the pathogenesis, clinical features and management of hypoglycaemia. (IM11.14, IM11.15, IM11.22, IM11.6, IM11.9)

- Hypoglycaemia is a dangerous complication, and, in the short run, more serious than hyperglycaemia. Prolonged hypoglycaemia may cause permanent brain damage.

CAUSES (Table 18.33)

- Postprandial or reactive hypoglycaemia occurs within 4 hours after a meal. The blood glucose is below 50 mg/dL and the patient develops symptoms of hypoglycaemia.

PATHOGENESIS

- Protection against hypoglycaemia is normally provided by two mechanisms as plasma glucose concentration falls:
  - Cessation of insulin release.
  - Secretion of counter-regulatory hormones.
- The four counter-regulatory hormones are glucagon, catecholamines (adrenaline and noradrenaline), cortisol and GH. They counter hypoglycaemia by increasing hepatic glucose production and decreasing glucose utilisation by nonhepatic tissues. Glucagon is the primary counter-regulatory hormone while

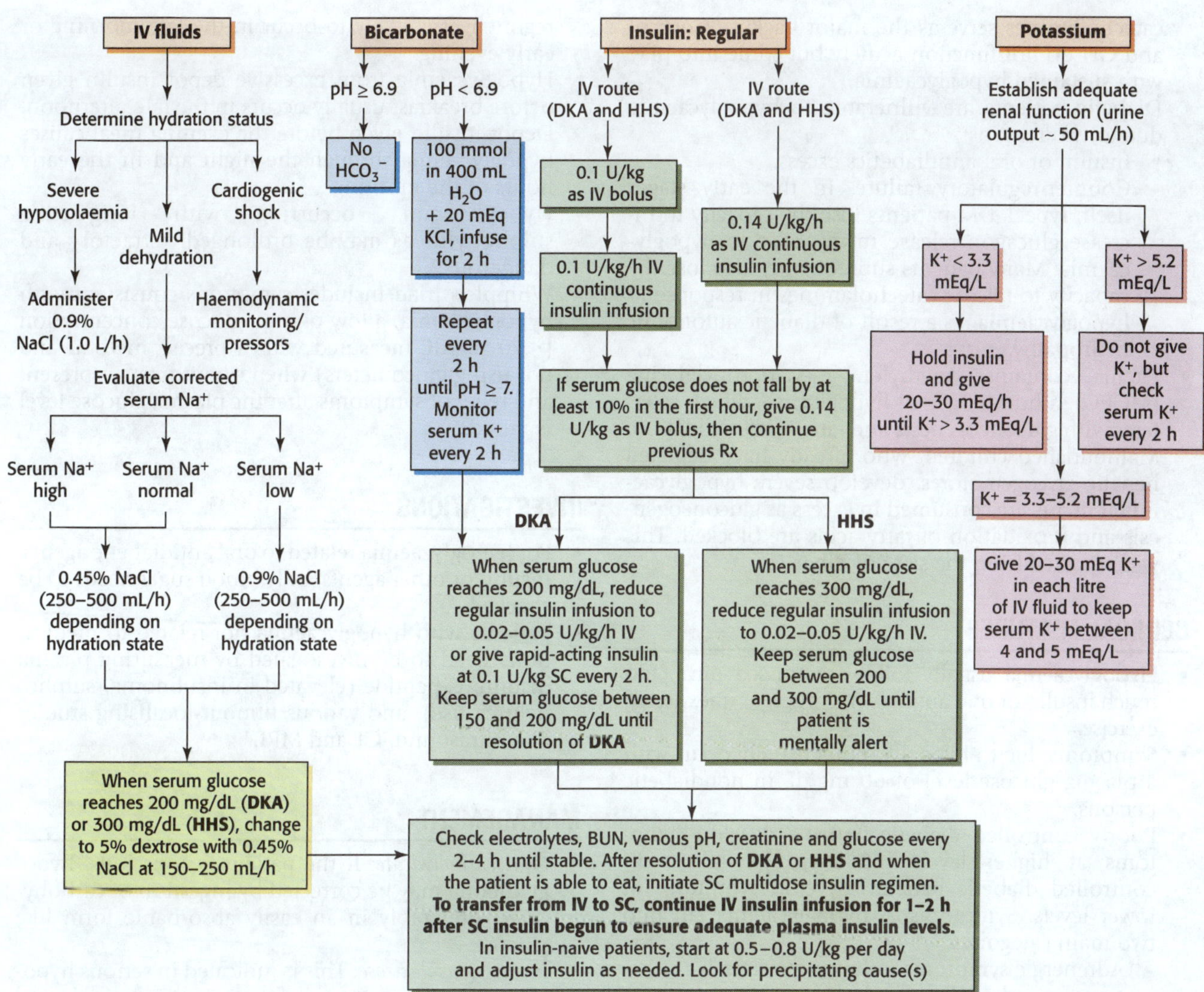

Flowchart 18.10 Protocol for Management of Adult patients with DKA or HHS. Complete initial evaluation. Check capillary glucose and serum/urine ketones to confirm hyperglycaemia and ketonaemia/ketonuria. Obtain blood for metabolic profile. Start IV fluids: 1.0 L of 0.9% NaCl per hour. (Source: *A.E. Kitabchi, G.E. Umpierrez, J.M. Miles, J.N. Ficher: Hyperglycemic crises in adult patients with diabetes.* Diabetes Care. *2009:32(7): 1335–1343.)*

TABLE 18.32 Clinical and Laboratory Features of Diabetic Ketoacidosis and Hyperosmolar Hyperglycaemic State

Features	Diabetic Ketoacidosis	Hyperosmolar Hyperglycaemic State
• Type of diabetes	Type 1 or occasionally type 2	Type 2
• Evolution	Over hours	Over days
• Acetone odour on breath	Yes	No
• Kussmaul's respiration	Yes	No
• Abdominal pain/ tenderness	Yes	No
• Blood glucose	>250 mg/dL	>600 mg/dL
• Serum sodium	Normal or low	Usually high
• Blood/urine ketones	+ + + +	Negative or trace
• Blood pH	<7.3	>7.3
• Serum bicarbonate	<18 mEq/L	>18 mEq/L
• Serum osmolality	Variable	>330 mOsm/kg
• Serum uric acid	Elevated	Normal
• Mortality	5%–10%	20%–30%

TABLE 18.33 Causes of Hypoglycaemia

Drugs:
- Oral antidiabetic agents
- Insulins
- Pentamidine
- Didanosine
- Quinine

Poisoning:
- Alcohol
- Salicylates
- Beta-blockers

Critical illnesses:
- Sepsis (including malaria)
- Cardiac or liver failure

Endocrine:
- Hypoadrenalism
- Hypopituitarism
- Growth hormone deficiency

Tumours:
- Insulinoma

Others:
- Gastric bypass
- Ingestion of excessive amount of litchi in malnourished state
- Postprandial hypoglycaemia

catecholamines serve as the major backup. Cortisol and GH do not function acutely but come into play with sustained hypoglycaemia.

- Diabetic patients are vulnerable to hypoglycaemia due to two reasons:
  - Insulin or oral antidiabetics excess.
  - Counter-regulatory failure. In the early stages itself, type 1 DM patients lose the capacity to increase glucagon release in response to hypoglycaemia. Many patients subsequently also lose the capacity to release catecholamines in response to hypoglycaemia, as a result of diabetic autonomic neuropathy.
- Litchi contains methylene cyclopropylglycine (MCPG), a homologue of hypoglycin A which interferes with gluconeogenesis and fatty acid β-oxidation. Malnourished children, who already have depleted hepatic glycogen stores, develop severe hypoglycaemia if litchis are consumed in excess as gluconeogenesis and β-oxidation of fatty acids are blocked. This was reported from the state of Bihar.

CLINICAL FEATURES

- Hypoglycaemia usually follows a missed meal, too much insulin or oral antidiabetic drugs, or unexpected exercise.
- Symptoms due to hypoglycaemia usually occur with a plasma glucose level of 60 mg/dL in nondiabetic persons.
- Poorly controlled diabetic patients develop symptoms at higher levels (80 mg/dL) while well-controlled diabetic patients develop symptoms at lower levels. Symptoms of hypoglycaemia fall into two main categories:
  - Adrenergic symptoms induced by excessive secretion of adrenaline include sweating, tremor, tachycardia, anxiety and hunger.
  - Central nervous system dysfunction causes dizziness, headache, clouding of vision, blunted mental acuity, loss of fine motor skill, confusion, abnormal behaviour, convulsions and loss of consciousness. Focal deficits including hemiplegia can occur which mimic stroke.
- When hypoglycaemia is of rapid onset (e.g. insulin reactions), adrenergic symptoms predominate. When hypoglycaemia is of gradual onset, manifestations of central nervous system predominate.
- In long-standing diabetics, adrenergic symptoms may not manifest due to severe neuropathy. Consequently, central nervous system manifestations may predominate.
- Indications of daytime hypoglycaemic episodes are sweating, nervousness, tremor and hunger.
- Indications of nocturnal hypoglycaemic episodes during sleep include night sweats, unpleasant dreams and early morning headache. Frequently, nocturnal hypoglycaemic is asymptomatic.
- Hypoglycaemia due to overdosage with unmodified insulin occurs at the time when the insulin has its maximum effect. With the standard twice-daily regimen, it is likely to occur in the late morning or early evening.
- Hypoglycaemia from excessive depot insulin given before breakfast usually occurs in the late afternoon. Depot insulin given before the evening meal causes hypoglycaemia through the night and in the early hours of the morning.
- Hypoglycaemia occurring with long-acting sulphonylureas may be prolonged, refractory and dangerous.
- Whipple's triad includes symptoms consistent with hypoglycaemia, a low plasma glucose concentration (<70 mg/dL measured with a precise method and not using glucometers) when symptoms are present and relief of symptoms after the plasma glucose level is raised.

INVESTIGATIONS

- For hypoglycaemia related to oral antidiabetic agents, insulin or other agents, only blood sugar needs to be checked.
- Patients with hypoglycaemia not related to medications need to be investigated by measuring plasma insulin, C-peptide (elevated in insulinoma, sulphonylurea use), and various tumour-localising studies like ultrasound, CT and MRI.

MANAGEMENT

- *Oral carbohydrate*: If the patient is conscious, hypoglycaemia may be corrected by ingestion of carbohydrate, preferably in an easily absorbable form like glucose.
- *Intravenous dextrose*: This is indicated in serious hypoglycaemia when mental function is impaired, and prolonged hypoglycaemia is anticipated (e.g. with depot insulin and oral sulphonylureas like chlorpropamide). Fifty millilitres of 50% dextrose should be given initially followed by infusion of 5%–10% dextrose. Oral carbohydrate should be administered as soon as the patient is able to eat.
- *Glucagon*: Severe hypoglycaemia may be treated with glucagon 1 mg subcutaneously or intramuscularly, and repeated if necessary after 10 minutes. Glucagon acts by stimulation of hepatic glycogenolysis. It may not be effective in severe and prolonged hypoglycaemia due to depot insulins. It should not be used to treat hypoglycaemia induced by oral antidiabetic drugs. Dasiglucagon, an analogue of glucagon, is approved for severe hypoglycaemia produced by insulin.
- *Octreotide* is effective for patients who develop recurrent hypoglycaemia following dextrose infusion (which stimulates endogenous release of insulin).
- *Other measures*: These are aimed at prevention of recurrence. They include adjustments in the dosage of oral antidiabetic drugs, changing the timing of insulin injections, adjustments in diet and physical activity.

Q. Describe Somogyi's phenomenon and dawn phenomenon.

THE SOMOGYI PHENOMENON

- The Somogyi phenomenon (post-hypoglycaemic hyperglycaemia) refers to rebound hyperglycaemia following an episode of hypoglycaemia, and is due to counter-regulatory hormone release. The rebound hyperglycaemia manifests as morning fasting hyperglycaemia, in response to unrecognised nocturnal hypoglycaemia.
- The significance of the Somogyi phenomenon is that the correction of the morning hyperglycaemia depends on reducing and not increasing the evening dose of intermediate-acting insulin.

CLUES TO THE PRESENCE OF SOMOGYI'S PHENOMENON

- The classical clinical picture is one of worsening diabetic control in the presence of increasing insulin doses and is manifested especially by fasting hyperglycaemia.
- Excessive hunger and weight gain occurring in the context of worsening hyperglycaemia.
- Subtle clinical signs of nocturnal hypoglycaemia, such as mild nocturnal sweating, morning headaches and hypothermia.
- Wide fluctuations in the plasma glucose and urine glucose occurring over short time intervals and not related to meals.
- The Somogyi phenomenon can be confirmed by documenting hypoglycaemia at 3 a.m. and hyperglycaemia in the morning (fasting state).
- The ultimate criterion for the diagnosis of Somogyi's phenomenon is improvement in diabetic control after a decrease in the insulin dose. It is better to replace NPH insulin with insulin glargine or insulin detemir which do not have a peak level.

THE DAWN PHENOMENON

- This phenomenon is closely related to the Somogyi phenomenon in that there is fasting hyperglycaemia, but no hypoglycaemia during the night.
- The mechanism of the dawn phenomenon is thought to be nocturnal surge of GH release as well as increased clearance of insulin in the mornings.
- The dawn phenomenon can be confirmed and differentiated from the Somogyi phenomenon by documenting hyperglycaemia at 3 a.m. and in the morning (fasting state).
- The significance of the dawn phenomenon is that the correction of the fasting hyperglycaemia depends on increasing and not decreasing the insulin. Oral agents may not be adequate to control the dawn phenomenon.
- Better control of morning glucose levels also occurs with exercise in the evening and also by increasing protein to carbohydrate ratio in the evening meal.

Q. Enumerate the differences in coma due to hypoglycaemia and ketoacidosis in type 1 diabetes mellitus.

- Differentiating features between coma due to hypoglycaemia and ketoacidosis are shown in Table 18.34.

TABLE 18.34 Hypoglycaemia Coma Versus Coma With Ketosis

Feature	Hypoglycaemic Coma	Coma With Ketosis
• History	No food; too much insulin or oral antidiabetics; unaccustomed exercise	Too little or no insulin; an infection; digestive disturbance
• Onset	In good previous health; related to last insulin injection or oral antidiabetic	Ill-health for several days
• Symptoms	Of hypoglycaemia	Of glycosuria and dehydration; abdominal pain and vomiting
• Signs	Moist skin and tongue Full pulse Normal or raised blood pressure Shallow or normal breathing Brisk reflexes	Dry skin and tongue Weak pulse Low blood pressure Kussmaul's breathing; acetone smell
• Urine	No ketonuria No glycosuria	Ketonuria Glycosuria
• Blood	Hypoglycaemia Normal plasma bicarbonate	Hyperglycaemia Reduced plasma bicarbonate

Q. How does lactic acidosis occur in a diabetic patient? Briefly outline the clinical setting, manifestations, diagnosis and management of lactic acidosis. (IM11.6)

- Lactic acidosis occurs when lactic acid is produced at accelerated rates due to anaerobic metabolism in skeletal muscles and other tissues. In a diabetic, it usually occurs as a complication of treatment with biguanides, usually with phenformin (not available now) and rarely with metformin. These drugs inhibit hepatic gluconeogenesis from lactate, pyruvate and alanine.
- Clinical manifestations include nausea, vomiting, restlessness, Kussmaul's breathing and alteration in the level of consciousness ranging from stupor to coma.
- Diagnosis is confirmed by a low arterial pH (<7.2), increased anion gap, decreased plasma bicarbonate and a high concentration (>5.0 mmol/L) of lactic acid in the blood.
- Lactic acidosis should be treated with intravenous sodium bicarbonate to raise the plasma pH to above 7.0. Intravenous insulin and glucose are also required.

Q. What are the cardiovascular complications of diabetes? (IM11.18)

- The main cardiovascular complications of diabetes are accelerated atherosclerosis and increased platelet adhesiveness, possibly due to enhanced thromboxane A_2 synthesis and decreased prostacyclin synthesis.
- The atherosclerotic lesions can manifest in a variety of ways:
  - Intermittent claudication, gangrene and impotence.
  - Coronary artery disease leading to ischaemic heart disease, especially silent myocardial infarctions.
  - Cerebrovascular accidents.
- Another effect is development of diabetic cardiomyopathy that is possibly related to direct effects of diabetes on the myocardium. It is not due to hypertension, coronary artery disease or any other known cardiac disease. The patient may have diastolic dysfunction, systolic dysfunction or both.

Q. What are the stages in the development of diabetic nephropathy? (IM11.18)

Q. Describe Kimmelstiel–Wilson lesions.

- Diabetic nephropathy is a leading cause of death and disability in diabetes. It is more common in type 2 DM than in type 1 DM.
- It is typically associated with retinopathy.

PATHOLOGY

- Diabetic nephropathy involves two distinct pathological patterns that may or may not coexist.
  - In the diffuse form that is more common, there is widening of the glomerular basement membrane together with generalised mesangial thickening.
  - In the nodular form, large amounts of PAS-positive material are deposited at the periphery of glomerular tufts, the Kimmelstiel–Wilson lesion.
  - In addition, there may be hyalinisation of afferent and efferent arterioles, 'drops' in Bowman's capsule, fibrin caps and occlusion of glomeruli. Deposition of albumin and other proteins occurs in both glomeruli and tubules.

CLINICAL FEATURES

- The earliest stage is characterised by nephromegaly (enlargement of kidneys) and 'hyperfunction' or 'hyperfiltration' (i.e. increased glomerular filtration).
- The next stage is characterised by moderately increased albuminuria (microalbuminuria) with the urinary excretion of albumin in the range of 30–300 mg/day. Normal persons excrete less than 30 mg/day. At this stage, the disease is probably reversible. Moderately increased albuminuria is also a well-established marker of increased cardiovascular disease risk. Because of the long duration of abnormal glucose metabolism that often precedes diagnosis, patients with type 2 diabetes are more likely to have moderately increased albuminuria (or overt nephropathy) at diagnosis. Thus, patients with type 2 diabetes should be screened at the time of diagnosis and later once a year for the presence of moderately increased albuminuria.
- The next stage is characterised by severely increased albuminuria (macroalbuminuria) with the urinary excretion of albumin more than 300 mg/day. From this stage, the disease is irreversible, and a steady decline in glomerular filtration rate occurs at a rate of about 1 mL/minute/month. The stage of severely increased albuminuria may progress to include all the classic features of the nephrotic syndrome.
- With further progression, azotaemia develops and progression to renal failure and uraemia is inevitable.

DIAGNOSIS OF MODERATELY INCREASED ALBUMINURIA (MICROALBUMINURIA)

- Screening for moderately increased albuminuria can be accomplished in a variety of ways:
  - Measurement of albumin-to-creatinine ratio on a spot urine test. This is obtained most easily and collection errors occur less frequently. A ratio of more than 30 mg albumin/g creatinine is considered elevated on a spot urine test.
  - Albumin from a 24-hour urine collection (urinary albumin >30 mg/24 hours is diagnostic).
- Transient elevations of albuminuria can be caused by exercise, urinary tract infections, hyperglycaemia, febrile illness, severe hypertension or heart failure.

MANAGEMENT

- Stop smoking and control dyslipidaemia.
- Meticulous control of diabetes can reverse microproteinuria in some patients.
- In addition, angiotensin-converting enzyme inhibitors can retard the progression of nephropathy at this stage.
- Aggressive control of hypertension is mandatory as high blood pressure can accelerate nephropathy.
  - The blood pressure should be decreased to less than 130/80 mmHg.
  - ACE inhibitors and angiotensin receptor blockers have proved beneficial in patients with diabetic renal disease and are considered preferred therapy in patients with hypertension and diabetes. These agents slow progression of nephropathy and can be used if creatinine is less than 3 mg/dL.
  - Mineralocorticoid receptor antagonists when added to an ACE inhibitor convey a significant decrease in proteinuria, although they are associated with an increased risk of hyperkalaemia. Further, they are contraindicated in patients with impaired renal function.
  - Other agents that can be used include thiazide diuretics, calcium channel blockers, β-blockers and α-blockers.

- Oral antidiabetic drugs:
  - Metformin should be considered the first-line treatment for all patients with diabetic nephropathy but with the following cautions:
    - It is contraindicated in patients with an estimated GFR (eGFR) <30 mL/minute/1.73 m^2.
    - eGFR should be monitored while taking metformin.
    - Benefits and risks of continuing treatment should be reassessed when eGFR falls below 45 mL/minute/1.73 m^2.
    - It should not be initiated for patients with an eGFR <45 mL/minute/1.73 m^2.
  - If additional drug is required to control diabetes, consider use of a SGLT2 inhibitor (if eGFR >45 mL/minute/1.73 m^2 for empagliflozin and canagliflozin or if eGFR >60 mL/minute/1.73 m^2 for dapagliflozin) or GLP-1 receptor agonist as they may reduce risk of chronic kidney disease progression, cardiovascular events or both.
  - GLP-1 receptor agonists (liraglutide, dulaglutide and semaglutide) also reduce risk of chronic kidney disease progression and can be used even if eGFR is 15 mL/minute/1.73 m^2.
  - Dipeptidyl peptidase-4 (DPP-4) inhibitors may also be reno-protective though the effect is lower than SGLT2 inhibitors. The agents include sitagliptin, saxagliptin and linagliptin. Linagliptin has the advantage that it is not renally cleared and thus a dose adjustment is not necessary.
- Low-protein diets (0.8 g/kg/day) may be beneficial, as there is some evidence suggesting that high-protein diets can accelerate glomerulosclerosis.
- Once the azotaemic phase is reached, the management is similar to that for other forms of chronic renal failure.

Q. Discuss briefly diabetic retinopathy. (IM11.18)

- A 1% decrease in glycated haemoglobin roughly equates to a decreased risk of retinopathy by 40%.
- Puberty and pregnancy are risk factors for diabetic retinopathy in people with type 1 diabetes.
- Implicated pathogenetic mechanisms include accumulation of sorbitol and advanced glycation endproducts, oxidative stress, protein kinase C activation, inflammation, and up regulation of the renin–angiotensin system and vascular endothelial growth factor (VEGF).
- Retinopathic lesions are divided into two large categories, simple (background or nonproliferative) and proliferative (Table 18.35).
- Investigations include fundus examination, optical coherence tomography scanning, fluorescein angiography and B-scan ultrasound.
- Treatment involves tight control of diabetes, hypertension and hyperlipidaemia.
- Diabetic retinopathy is treated by focal or panretinal photocoagulation depending on the extent of involvement.

TABLE 18.35 Lesions of Diabetic Nephropathy

Simple (Background) (Fig. 18.10)	Proliferative (Fig. 18.11)
• Increased capillary permeability	• New vessels
• Capillary closure and dilatation	• Scar (retinitis proliferans)
• Microaneurysms	• Vitreal haemorrhage
• Arteriovenous shunts	• Retinal detachment
• Dilated veins	
• Haemorrhages (dot and blot)	
• Cotton-wool spots	
• Hard exudates	

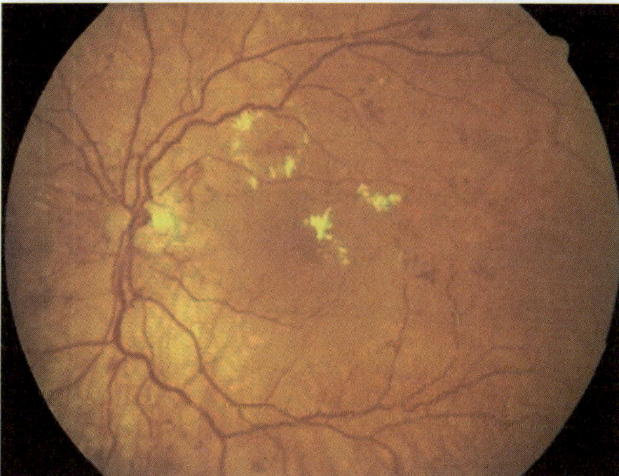

Fig. 18.10 Background diabetic retinopathy showing exudates, microaneurysms and small haemorrhages.

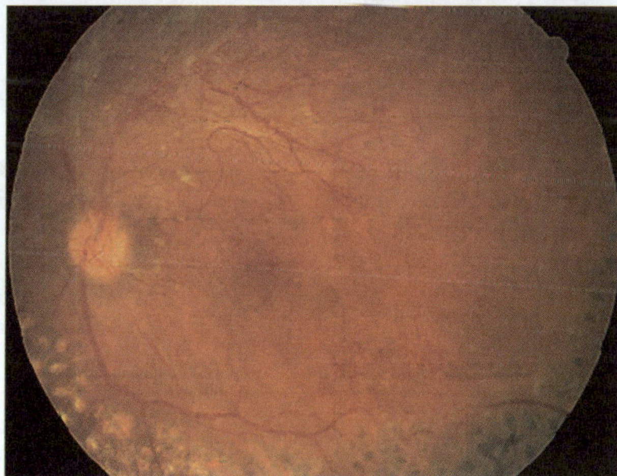

Fig. 18.11 Proliferative diabetic retinopathy with neovascularisation.

- An alternative is intravitreous injections of anti-VEGF monoclonal antibodies like bevacizumab and ranibizumab.
- Diabetic macular oedema refractory to intravitreal anti-VEGF treatment may respond to intravitreal corticosteroid therapy.
- Pars plana vitrectomy is utilised for the treatment of nonresolving vitreal haemorrhage and retinal detachment.

Q. Discuss the classification, clinical manifestations and management of diabetic neuropathy. (IM11.18)

CLASSIFICATION

- Classification of diabetic neuropathy is given in Table 18.36.
- Symmetric neuropathies are due to 'metabolic' abnormalities of the neurons of Schwann's cells, whereas the asymmetric neuropathies are due to vascular occlusion and ischaemia.

DISTAL SYMMETRIC SENSORIMOTOR POLYNEUROPATHY

- This form of diabetic neuropathy can be divided into two types:
  - A relatively asymptomatic form that is diffuse, distal, usually occurring in the lower extremities with a stocking type of distribution. There is numbness, tingling or pins-and-needles sensation often worse at night. This type is generally progressive and irreversible.
  - A painful form presenting with burning or dull-aching sensation or excruciating, lancinating pain. The pain is often worse at night and partially relieved by movement. Hyperaesthesia may be marked.
- The characteristic early physical findings in both forms are loss of vibration sense and deep tendon reflexes (especially ankle jerk). With progression, there may be involvement of other sensations like joint position, touch, pain and temperature, later leading to weakness and wasting of muscles.

ASYMMETRIC NEUROPATHY

- Diabetic mononeuropathies of the cranial nerves usually involve III, VI or IV cranial nerve in order of frequency. Third nerve involvement is characteristically pupil-sparing.
- Mononeuropathies of peripheral nerves manifest as carpal tunnel syndrome, foot drop or wrist drop.
- Radiculopathy is a sensory syndrome in which dysaesthesias and painful hyperaesthesia occur in the anatomic distribution of one or more spinal nerves.
- Diabetic amyotrophy (diabetic proximal neuropathy) is characterised by atrophy and weakness of the muscles of thigh (especially quadriceps) and pelvic girdle. This may be associated with anorexia and depression.

AUTONOMIC NEUROPATHY

- Denervation of sympathetic and parasympathetic systems results in loss of awareness of hypoglycaemia.
- The common manifestations of autonomic neuropathy in diabetes are given in Table 18.37.

DIAGNOSIS

- Clinical examination includes assessment of muscle power, sensations of pinprick and temperature (for small-fibre function), and joint position and vibration (for large-fibre function). Vibration test should be done by a 128-Hz tuning fork.
- Annual 10-g monofilament testing to identify feet at risk for ulceration and amputation. It generates a reproducible stress on buckling and tests the protective sensation. The monofilament is placed on the patient's feet; when there is considerable loss of sensation, the patient will not be able to detect the presence of the filament at buckling.
- Autonomic function tests based on blood pressure and heart rate response to a series of manoeuvres including deep breathing, standing, Valsalva's manoeuvre and sustained isometric muscular strain.
- Nerve conduction studies:
  - Motor nerve conduction, F response and sensory nerve conduction studies are important methods of documentation and follow-up of nerve functions.
  - Motor nerve conduction studies are affected in a small subset (large fibre neuropathies).
  - Entrapment neuropathies result in unilateral nerve conduction velocity (NCV) changes, especially across the entrapped segment of the nerve.

TABLE 18.36 Classification of Diabetic Neuropathy

Symmetric Distal Polyneuropathy	Asymmetric Neuropathy

• Distal symmetrical sensorimotor polyneuropathy
• Painful autonomic neuropathy
• Painful distal neuropathy with weight loss ('diabetic cachexia')
• Insulin neuritis
• Polyneuropathy after ketoacidosis
• Polyneuropathy with glucose impairment
• Chronic inflammatory demyelinating polyneuropathy with diabetes mellitus
	• Cranial mononeuropathy and mononeuropathy multiplex
	• Peripheral mononeuropathy and mononeuropathy multiplex
	  • Median neuropathy at wrist
	  • Ulnar neuropathy at elbow
	  • Peroneal neuropathy at fibular head
	• Radiculoplexoneuropathies
	  • Lumbosacral
	  • Thoracic
	  • Cervical
	• Neuromuscular syndromes (e.g. diabetic amyotrophy)
	Autonomic neuropathy

TABLE 18.37 Manifestations of Diabetic Autonomic Neuropathy

Manifestations of Diabetic Autonomic Neuropathy	
• Cardiovascular	Postural hypotension, resting tachycardia, absence of sinus arrhythmia, abnormal Valsalva's response, QTc interval prolongation, sudden cardiac death
• Gastrointestinal	Oesophageal dysmotility, dysphagia, gastroparesis, nocturnal and postprandial diarrhoea, constipation, anal incontinence
• Genitourinary	Frequency, urgency, nocturia, hesitancy in micturition, weak stream, urinary incontinence, urine retention, erectile dysfunction, retrograde ejaculation
• Secretomotor	Gustatory sweating, nocturnal sweats without hypoglycaemia, anhidrosis
• Vasomotor	Dependent pedal oedema
• Pupillary	Decreased pupil size, resistance to mydriatics

- The commonest abnormality is reduction in the amplitude of motor or sensory action potentials because of axonopathy.
- Pronounced slowing of NCV suggests demyelinating neuropathy, which is rarely associated with diabetes; therefore, pronounced slowing of NCV in a diabetic patient should prompt investigations for an alternative diagnosis.

- Exclude other causes of peripheral neuropathy (e.g. vitamin B_{12} deficiency common after metformin therapy, hypothyroidism, alcoholism).

MANAGEMENT

- Proper care of feet. This includes daily inspection for any wounds, keeping them clean and dry, using proper fitting foot-wear and avoiding any injuries.
- Mononeuropathies and radiculopathies are usually self-limiting and do not require any specific therapy.
- Pain of diabetic neuropathy may be treated with gabapentin or pregabalin. Duloxetine, a potent dual reuptake inhibitor of serotonin and noradrenaline, has been found to be useful. In refractory cases, extended-release tapentadol (a centrally acting agonist of the mu-opioid receptor and noradrenaline reuptake inhibitor) may be used. Other drugs which may be used include phenytoin, carbamazepine, amitriptyline or imipramine. Topical capsaicin may also be useful in reducing pain; it stimulates release and depletion of substance P from sensory nerve fibres. In refractory cases, transcutaneous electrical nerve stimulation (TENS) or percutaneous electrical nerve stimulation (PENS) may be tried.
- Diabetic diarrhoea often responds to diphenoxylate, loperamide or tetracyclines.
- Orthostatic hypotension often responds to sleeping with the head of the bed elevated, avoidance of sudden assumption of the upright position, full-length elastic stockings and increased salt intake. Physical exercise should be encouraged to avoid deconditioning. Pharmacotherapy includes midodrine (an α_1-receptor agonist) and droxidopa (a prodrug of noradrenaline). Rarely, fludrocortisone is required. Other agents which may be useful include erythropoietin, clonidine and octreotide.
- Gastroparesis may be treated with frequent small meals and prokinetic agents (e.g. metoclopramide, domperidone, erythromycin). Intrapyloric botulinum toxin injection may be used in refractory cases.
- Erectile dysfunction may be treated with psychological counselling, sildenafil, vardenafil, tadalafil, prostaglandin E_1 injection, device or prosthesis.

SPECIFIC TREATMENT TO REVERSE NEUROPATHY

- No drug is approved for reversal of diabetic neuropathy.
  - Aldolase reductase inhibitors (e.g. epalrestat) reduce the flux of glucose through polyol pathways, inhibiting accumulation of sorbitol and fructose and preventing reduction of redox potential. However, their use has not been found to be effective.
  - Carnitine may be useful in some patients.
  - Methylcobalamin has also been shown to provide some benefit in patients with diabetic neuropathy.
  - Other agents which have been used but not found to be useful include alpha-lipoic acid and benfotiamine.

Q. What are the dermatological complications of diabetes?

- Dermatological complications of diabetes are listed in Box 18.18.

BOX 18.18 Dermatological Complications of Diabetes Mellitus

- Bacterial infections (e.g. carbuncles, furuncles, necrotising fasciitis, malignant otitis externa)
- Fungal infections (e.g. angular cheilitis, candidal balanitis, candidal paronychia, dermatophytosis)
- Diabetic ulcers (due to peripheral neuropathy and ischaemia)
- Vaginal candidiasis
- Necrobiosis lipoidica diabeticorum
- Diabetic dermopathy (shin spots)
- Acanthosis nigricans
- Xanthomatoses secondary to hyperlipoproteinaemia
- Tight, scleroderma-like waxy skin over the dorsum of the hands in conjunction with joint contractures (in type 1 DM)

Q. What is gestational diabetes mellitus? How will you diagnose it?

Q. Discuss the significance and management of gestational diabetes mellitus.

Q. Describe the O'Sullivan's criteria for the diagnosis of gestational diabetes mellitus.

Q. Describe Carpenter and Coustan criteria for the diagnosis of gestational diabetes mellitus.

- Gestational diabetes mellitus (GDM) was defined as any degree of glucose intolerance that began or was first recognised during pregnancy. The definition was applied whether insulin or only diet modification was used for treatment and whether or not the condition persisted after pregnancy. It did not exclude the possibility that unrecognised glucose intolerance might have antedated or begun concomitantly with the pregnancy.
- Presently, women diagnosed with diabetes by standard diagnostic criteria in the first trimester are classified as having preexisting DM while GDM is diabetes that is first diagnosed in the second or third trimester of pregnancy that is not clearly either preexisting type 1 or type 2 diabetes.
- Furthermore, women with GDM should be screened for diabetes 6–12 weeks postpartum.
- The importance of proper diagnosis can be appreciated as GDM is known to cause increased foetal loss (two to three times greater risk than in general popu-

lation) and congenital malformations like foetal macrosomy. Other risks include polyhydramnios, foetal/neonatal hypertrophic cardiomyopathy, neonatal respiratory problems and neonatal metabolic complications (e.g. hypoglycaemia, hyperbilirubinaemia and hypocalcaemia).

- Furthermore, females with GDM are at increased risk for the development of diabetes after pregnancy.
- Offspring of females with GDM are at increased risk of obesity and diabetes.
- The diagnosis of GDM is based on an OGTT done at 24–28 weeks of gestation in women with moderate to high risk. It is not required in women with low risk of GDM that is defined as presence of all of the criteria given in Box 18.19.

CRITERIA FOR DIAGNOSIS OF GESTATIONAL DIABETES MELLITUS

- A two-step test is most widely used approach for identifying pregnant people with GDM. In the first hour, 50 g oral glucose is administered without regard to time of day and previous meals. If 1 hour plasma glucose is ≥135 mg/dL, second step of 100 g OGTT is performed to confirm diagnosis of GDM.
- A total of 100 g rather than 75 g OGTT is recommended at present as there is an increased turnover of glucose in pregnant state. One hundred grams of glucose is dissolved in 300–400 mL of water and consumed over 5 minutes.
- The first criteria for diagnosing GDM were given by O'Sullivan and were based on whole blood glucose levels. However, as the levels of glucose may vary in whole blood due to uptake by red blood cells, Carpenter and Coustan have given values based on plasma glucose levels (Table 18.38).
- However, guidelines by Maternal Health Division, Ministry of Health & Family Welfare, Government of India recommend the use of 75 g OGTT irrespective of last meal with plasma glucose ≥140 mg/dL at 2 hours for diagnosing GDM. The first testing should be done during first antenatal contact as early as possible in pregnancy. The second testing should be done during 24–28 weeks of pregnancy if the first test is negative. The test is done irrespective of risk for GDM.

BOX 18.19 Criteria for Low Risk of Gestational Diabetes Mellitus

- Age <25 years
- Weight normal before pregnancy
- Member of an ethnic group with a low prevalence of diabetes
- No known diabetes in first-degree relatives
- No history of abnormal glucose tolerance
- No history of poor obstetrical outcome

TABLE 18.38 Criteria for Diagnosis of Gestational Diabetes Mellitus

Time (Hour)	Upper Limit of Normal Values (mg/dL) Whole Blood (O'Sullivan)	Plasma (Carpenter and Coustan)
• 0 (fasting)	85	95
• 1	160	180
• 2	140	155
• 3	125	140

Note: Two or more of these values must be abnormal.

MANAGEMENT

- Management: Oral antidiabetic drugs except metformin and glyburide are contraindicated in GDM. It is best to manage pregnant diabetics meticulously with insulin although some patients may be controlled with metformin or glyburide (after 20 weeks of gestation).

Q. Give a brief account of metabolic syndrome.

Q. Discuss briefly clinical diagnosis, risks and treatment of insulin resistance syndrome (syndrome X).

- Metabolic syndrome (previously known as syndrome X or insulin resistance syndrome) refers to the clustering of risk factors for cardiovascular and type 2 DM and includes abdominal obesity, hyperglycaemia (impaired fasting glucose), dyslipidaemia (high TGs or low HDL) and elevated blood pressure.
- The clinical relevance of metabolic syndrome is that it identifies people who are at increased long-term risk of cardiovascular disease and type 2 diabetes, thus providing an opportunity for preventive lifestyle interventions.
- Another utility of diagnosing metabolic syndrome is the identification of people at high risk of cardiovascular disease beyond low-density lipoprotein-cholesterol levels.
- The underlying defect in this syndrome is insulin resistance.
  - Defined as inability of insulin to produce its numerous actions in spite of unimpaired secretion from the β-cells.
  - Except in a few rare cases involving antibodies against insulin receptor or mutations in the insulin receptor gene, insulin resistance of metabolic syndrome results from impairments in cellular events distal to the interaction between insulin and its surface receptor.
  - Metabolic abnormalities result from interaction between effects of insulin resistance primarily in the muscle and adipose tissue, and adverse impact of compensatory hyperinsulinaemia on other tissues that retain normal insulin sensitivity.
  - Adipose tissue is also considered central in pathogenesis of complications associated with metabolic syndrome. It releases proinflammatory mediators (interleukin-6 and tumour necrosis factor-α) as well as prothrombotic mediator (plasminogen activator inhibitor-1). These may lead to accelerated atherosclerosis due to chronic inflammation and vascular endothelial dysfunction.

CLINICAL DIAGNOSIS

- Presence of at least three of the features given in Box 18.20 are required to make a diagnosis of metabolic syndrome.
- People receiving medical treatment for dyslipidaemia, hypertension or elevated blood glucose are included in the criteria.

BOX 18.20 Clinical Diagnosis

- Abdominal obesity (waist circumference >80 cm in females and >90 cm in males)
- Elevated TG levels (≥150 mg/dL)
- Reduced HDL-cholesterol level (<40 mg/dL in males and <50 mg/dL in females)
- Elevated blood pressure (systolic ≥130 mmHg or diastolic ≥85 mmHg)
- Elevated fasting plasma glucose level (≥100 mg/dL)

ASSOCIATED RISKS (Box 18.21)

BOX 18.21 Risks Associated With Metabolic Syndrome

- Cardiovascular diseases
- Type 2 diabetes mellitus
- Polycystic ovary syndrome
- Nonalcoholic fatty liver disease
- Hyperuricaemia and gout
- Sleep disordered breathing
- Chronic kidney disease
- Erectile dysfunction
- Hepatocellular and intrahepatic cholangiocarcinoma

TREATMENT

- There is currently no sound evidence showing that the treatment of insulin resistance reduces mortality and morbidity in these patients. Nevertheless, treatment of insulin resistance involves lifestyle changes.
- Components of lifestyle changes include the following:
  - Exercise.
  - Hypocaloric diet.
  - Weight reduction.
  - Diet high in fibres.
- Control of diabetes, hypertension and lipid abnormalities by various drugs.
- In the absence of diabetes, oral antidiabetic drugs (e.g. metformin, thiazolidinediones) are not recommended to control insulin resistance.

Q. Write a short note on insulin resistance.

- Defined as subnormal glucose response to endogenous and/or exogenous insulin. An arbitrary figure of insulin requirement of >200 U/day in a diabetic to control blood glucose has been given as definition for insulin resistance.

CAUSES (Box 18.22)

- Stress leads to elevated levels of counter-regulatory hormones—glucagon, cortisol, GH, catecholamines.

BOX 18.22 Causes of Insulin Resistance

- Associated with obesity
- Induced by stress
- Drugs—glucocorticoids, antiretrovirals, oral contraceptives
- Pregnancy
- Associated with lipodystrophy
- Antibodies against insulin
- Type A insulin resistance
- Type B insulin resistance

- Antibodies in titres sufficient to impair insulin action are rare in patients treated with recombinant human insulin,
- In type A insulin resistance, there are genetic defects in insulin-signalling pathways.
- In type B insulin resistance, blocking autoantibodies are present against the insulin receptor.

CLINICAL FEATURES

- Metabolic syndrome.
- Obesity.
- Uncontrolled DM.
- Type A insulin resistance affects young women and is characterised by severe hyperinsulinaemia, along with obesity and features of hyperandrogenism (e.g. polycystic ovarian syndrome).
- Type B insulin resistance usually presents with uncontrolled type 2 DM, although some patients may present with symptoms of hypoglycaemia which develops due to interaction between insulinomimetic antibodies and the insulin receptor.
- Others: acanthosis nigrans, lipoatrophy, lipohypertrophy.

Q. Write a short note on lipodystrophy.

- Lipodystrophy implies redistribution of fat tissue. Lipoatrophy refers to partial or complete decrease of adipose tissue. The terms lipoatrophy and lipodystrophy are used interchangeably in clinical practice.
- Lipodystrophies include three main groups: generalised, partial (extensive, but not generalised) and localised (limited to isolated areas).

CLASSIFICATION OF LIPODYSTROPHIES

- Classification of lipodystrophies is given in Table 18.39.

TABLE 18.39 Classification of Lipodystrophies

Inherited	Acquired

• Congenital generalised lipodystrophy (Fig. 18.12)
• Familial partial lipodystrophy
• Mandibuloacral dysplasia
	• Acquired generalised lipodystrophy
	• Acquired partial lipodystrophy (Fig. 18.13)
	• Lipodystrophy in HIV-infected patients
	• Localised lipodystrophy
	  • Drugs (injectable drugs like insulin, glucocorticoids, methotrexate)
	  • Pressure, trauma
	  • Panniculitis
	• Idiopathic

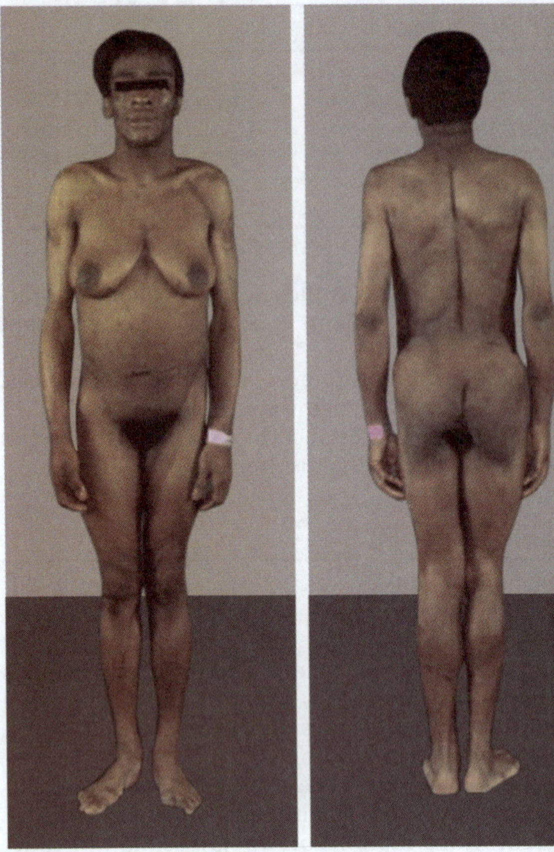

Fig. 18.12 Congenital generalised lipodystrophy. (Note generalised lack of fat and extreme muscularity.)

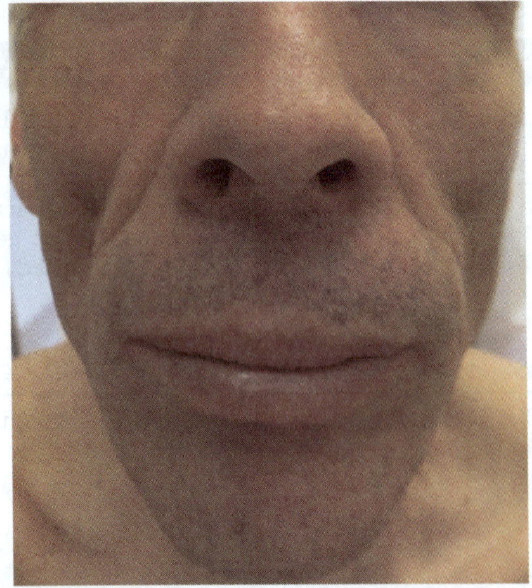

Fig. 18.13 Acquired partial lipodystrophy.

CLINICAL FINDINGS IN GENERALISED LIPODYSTROPHY

- Adipose tissue is almost completely absent from most subcutaneous areas except orbits, mouth, tongue, palms, soles, scalp, perineum and periarticular regions.

BOX 18.23 Clinical Findings in Generalised Lipodystrophy

- Lipodystrophy
- Metabolic disease
- Insulin resistance
- Hyperglycaemia
- Hypertriglyceridaemia
- Lactic acidosis
- Acanthosis nigricans
- Hepatic disease (steatosis, cirrhosis)
- Proteinuria
- Hypertrichosis, hirsutism, polycystic ovarian syndrome
- Muscular hypertrophy
- Mental retardation

- Clinical findings seen in patients with generalised lipodystrophy are summarised in Box 18.23.

TREATMENT

- Low-fat diet.
- Treatment of diabetes, hypertriglyceridaemia.
- Metreleptin (a leptin analogue) in conjunction with diet to treat leptin deficiency in patients with congenital generalised or acquired generalised lipodystrophy. It is not approved for treatment of HIV-associated lipodystrophy.
- Facial reconstruction with free flaps and silicone or other implants to replace adipose tissue.

HIV-ASSOCIATED LIPODYSTROPHY

- Peripheral lipoatrophy, central fat accumulation and lipomatosis.
- Related to use of protease inhibitors and nucleoside reverse transcriptase inhibitors; may occur in treatment-naïve patients also.
- Affected patients frequently show associated metabolic features (e.g. reduced HDL-cholesterol, hypertriglyceridaemia, insulin resistance, type 2 DM and lactic acidosis).
- Usually starts in the first 6–12 months after beginning therapy.
- Commonly encountered patterns of lipodystrophy include the following:
  - Generalised or localised lipoatrophy of face, extremities and buttocks.
  - Lipohypertrophy with generalised or local fat deposition involving abdomen, breasts, and supraclavicular and dorsocervical regions (buffalo hump).
  - A mixed pattern with central adiposity and peripheral lipoatrophy.
- No specific treatment for lipoatrophy has been found to be useful, although several drugs like metformin, pioglitazone and leptin have been tried. Switching from one NRTI such as stavudine or zidovudine to an alternative NRTI such as abacavir or tenofovir may be tried.
- Plastic surgery can be used for severe facial lipoatrophy. This involves autologous fat transplantation and injections of biodegradable or nonbiodegradable gel fillers.
- For abnormal fat deposition (lipohypertrophy), metformin and tesamorelin (a GH-releasing hormone analogue) may be tried.

Q. Discuss the structure of lipoproteins and their transport in body. (IM2.3)

- Cholesterol and TG constitute the lipid particles in the body. These lipids are insoluble in water and are transported in the blood in complexes known as lipoproteins.
- Lipoproteins serve a number of functions including transportation of lipids to various tissues for energy utilisation, lipid deposition, steroid hormone production and bile acid formation.
- Plasma lipoproteins are composed of a core of TG and cholesterol ester, enveloped by a surface coat of phospholipids, unesterified cholesterol and special proteins called apolipoproteins. Apolipoproteins (apo), such as apoB, apoC and apoE, coat lipoprotein particles and are involved in recognition of lipoprotein particles by enzymes that process or remove lipids from the lipoprotein particles.
- The five main classes of lipoproteins are as follows:
  - Chylomicrons carry dietary lipid. Associated apoproteins include A, B-48, C and E.
  - Very low density lipoprotein (VLDL) carries endogenous TGs and to a lesser degree cholesterol. The major apolipoproteins associated with VLDL are B-100, C and E.
  - Intermediate density lipoprotein (IDL) carries cholesterol esters and TG with major apolipoproteins being B-100, C and E.
  - LDL carries cholesterol esters and is associated with apoprotein B-100.
  - HDL also carries cholesterol esters.
- Lipoprotein(a) [Lp(a)] is another lipoprotein particle that in structure is very similar to LDL with the addition of apolipoprotein(a). Lp(a) links lipid metabolism with blood coagulation and is thought to be both atherogenic and thrombogenic. Through this structural similarity to plasminogen, Lp(a) interferes with fibrinolysis by competing with plasminogen binding to plasminogen receptors, fibrinogen and fibrin. This leads to reduced fibrinolysis. Lp(a) also binds to macrophages by a high-affinity receptor that promotes foam cell and plaque formation.
- Small dense LDL particles contain more cholesterol ester and are considered to be more atherogenic than LDL particles. These are the end-products of large VLDL lipolysis. These particles bind less avidly to the LDL receptor, making them more susceptible to oxidative modification and to subsequent uptake by the macrophage receptors.

LIPID TRANSPORT IN BODY

- There are three main pathways responsible for the generation and transport of lipids within the body.

EXOGENOUS (DIETARY) LIPID PATHWAY

- The first step is intestinal absorption of dietary cholesterol and fatty acids.
- In the intestinal epithelial cells, FFA combine with glycerol to form TGs, and cholesterol is esterified by acyl-coenzyme A: cholesterol acyltransferase (ACAT) to form cholesterol esters.
- TG and cholesterol are packaged to form chylomicrons in the epithelial cells of the intestines.
- Chylomicrons are the largest lipoprotein and are rich in TG.
- They are transported in the blood to tissues such as skeletal muscle, fat and liver.
- Lipoprotein lipase (LPL) hydrolyses TG in the chylomicrons into FFA that are oxidised by the muscle cells to generate energy, stored in adipose tissue, oxidised in the liver or used in hepatic VLDL synthesis.
- The end-products of chylomicron metabolism are chylomicron remnants that are cleared from the circulation by hepatic chylomicron remnant receptors.

ENDOGENOUS PATHWAY

- The endogenous pathway involves the liver-synthesising lipoproteins.
- TGs and cholesterol ester are generated by the liver and packaged into VLDL particles and then released into the circulation. Microsomal triglyceride transfer protein (MTP) is an intracellular lipid-transfer protein found in the liver and is essential for the transfer of the lipid molecules (principally TGs) onto apolipoprotein. Abetalipoproteinaemia is a rare genetic disorder in which MTP is absent.
- The TG component of VLDL undergoes hydrolysis by capillary LPL to provide fatty acids to adipose and muscle tissue. The remaining lipid portion is called IDL. IDL is then converted to LDL by enzymatic action of hepatic lipase or is taken up by the liver via the LDL receptor.
- LDL particles carry the majority of the cholesterol in the blood-supplying cholesterol to the cells.
- LDL receptors in peripheral cells or liver bind with LDL and clear it from the blood.
- Peripheral cells utilise LDL cholesterol for cell membrane structure and also the production of hormones.
- In the liver, LDL cholesterol can be converted to bile acids and secreted into the intestinal lumen.
- LDL is an atherogenic lipoprotein particle. Oxidised LDL can enter macrophages through the unregulated scavenger receptor. This pathway can result in excess accumulation of intracellular cholesterol and the formation of foam cells, which contribute to the formation of atheromatous plaques.
- Plasma LDL concentration is regulated by:
  - Altering the synthesis of hydroxy-3-methylglutaryl coenzyme A (HMG-CoA) reductase that controls the rate of cholesterol synthesis in the liver.
  - Suppressing the synthesis of new LDL receptors in the cells.

REVERSE CHOLESTEROL TRANSPORT

- Reverse cholesterol transport refers to the process by which cholesterol is removed from the tissues and returned to the liver.
- HDL is the key lipoprotein involved in reverse cholesterol transport. It is synthesised and catabolised in the liver and intestines.

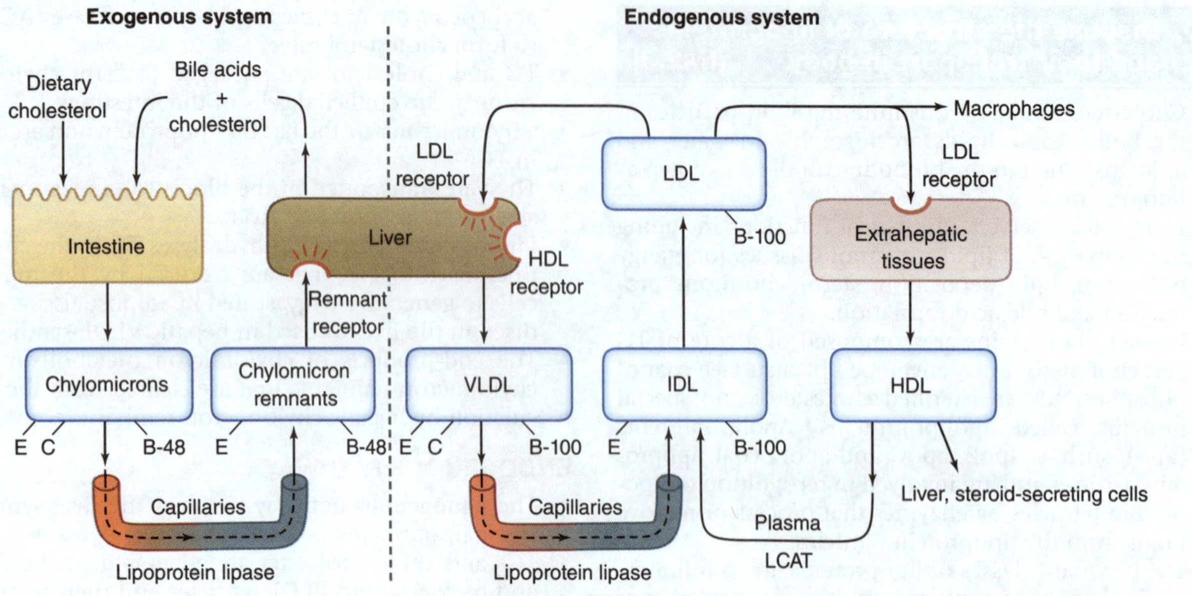

Flowchart 18.11 Lipid Transport.

- It facilitates the transfer of cholesterol from atherogenic lipoproteins (macrophage cholesterol efflux) and peripheral tissues to the liver. A circulating enzyme called lecithin cholesterol acyltransferase (LCAT) promotes the uptake of free cholesterol by HDL by a reaction called esterification. Other actions of HDL include protection against thrombosis and maintenance of endothelial function.

SUMMARY OF LIPID TRANSPORT

- Flowchart 18.11 summarises lipid transport in the body.

Q. Discuss hyperlipidaemias (or dyslipidaemias), their causes and drugs used in their management. (IM2.18)

Q. Classify hyperlipidaemias.

HYPERLIPIDAEMIA

- Hyperlipidaemia or dyslipidaemia refers to an abnormality in the lipid profile, encompassing a variety of disorders relating to elevations in total cholesterol, LDL or TG, or, conversely, lower levels of HDL.
- It is difficult to define hyperlipidaemia by giving a single cut-off value. It may, however, be defined as total cholesterol, LDL-C, triglyceride or lipoprotein(a) levels above the 90th percentile, or HDL-C or apo A-1 levels below the 10th percentile for the general population.

CAUSES

- Primary hyperlipidaemia refers to a genetic defect in the lipid metabolism as a cause of the problem. For example, familial hypercholesterolaemia is a cause of primary hyperlipidaemia. It is characterised by a genetic mutation resulting in impaired clearance of LDL from the circulation due to lack of LDL receptors.
- Secondary hyperlipidaemia refers to hyperlipidaemia secondary to a cause other than the genetic defect (Table 18.40).

CLASSIFICATION

- Fredrickson's classification of hyperlipidaemias is given in Table 18.41.

TABLE 18.40 Causes of Hyperlipidaemia

Primary Hyperlipidaemia (Genetic)	Secondary Hyperlipidaemia
	• Diet rich in saturated fat • Sedentary lifestyle • Diabetes mellitus • Cushing's syndrome • Hypothyroidism • Nephrotic syndrome • Alcohol intake • Obstructive liver disease • Drugs (thiazide diuretics, steroids, oestrogens, protease inhibitors)

TABLE 18.41 Classification of Hyperlipidaemias

Fredrickson's Class	Lipoprotein Abnormality
I	Chylomicrons
IIa	LDL
IIb	LDL and VLDL
III	Remnants of chylomicrons and VLDL
IV	VLDL
V	Chylomicrons and VLDL

CLINICAL FEATURES

- Due to atherosclerosis, patients may develop ischaemic heart disease, peripheral vascular disease or cerebrovascular disease.
- Xanthomas.
  - Planar xanthomas (on hands, elbows, buttocks or knees) have yellow-to-orange colour (Fig. 18.14). Xanthelasmas are a type of planar xanthomas which are seen around the eyelids (Fig. 18.15). Xanthelasmas are not a specific finding of hypercholesterolaemia as they may occur in older patients with normal cholesterol levels.
  - Tuberous xanthomas (on hands, elbows or knees) (Fig. 18.16).
  - Tendon xanthomas (especially on extensor tendons of hands or Achilles tendon) (Fig. 18.17).
- Corneal arcus (gray or white arc visible in the outer part of cornea) particularly in children and young adults (Fig. 18.18).
- Acute pancreatitis with severe hypertriglyceridaemia (TG >1000–2000 mg/dL).
- Other features of hypertriglyceridaemia include xanthoma striata palmaris (orange–yellow discolourations of the palmar creases), tuberous xanthomas, tendon xanthomas and eruptive xanthomas (small nodular papules over the trunk, buttock and thighs).

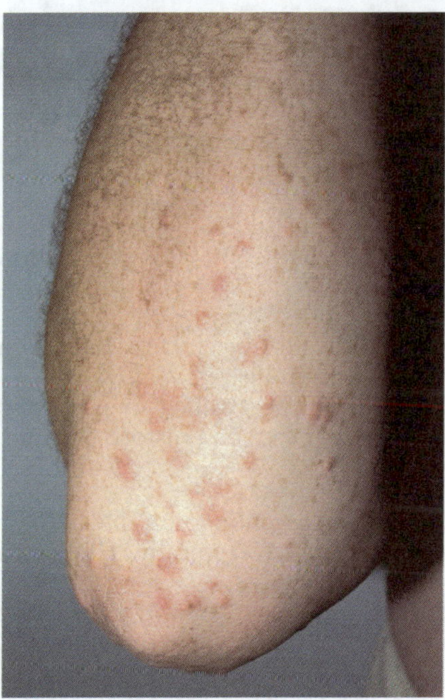

Fig. 18.14 Planar xanthomas.

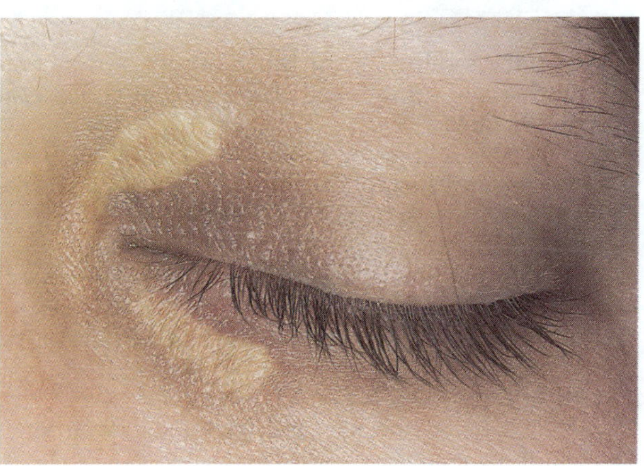

Fig. 18.15 Xanthelasmas of the eyelids.

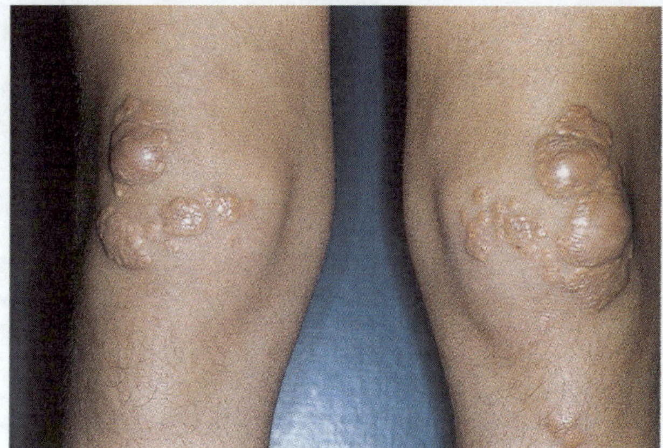

Fig. 18.16 Tuberous xanthomas of the knees.

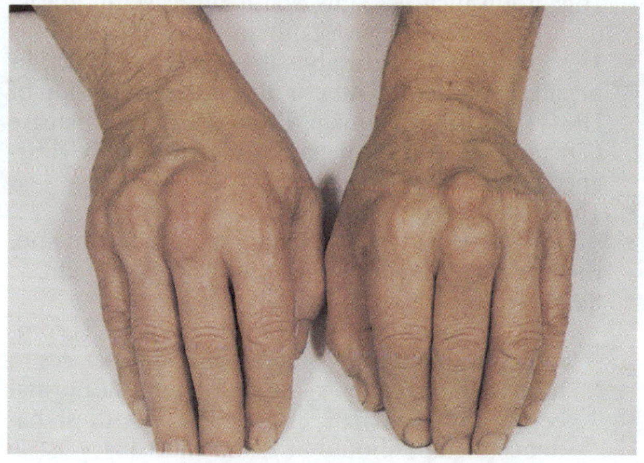

Fig. 18.17 Tendon xanthomas of hands.

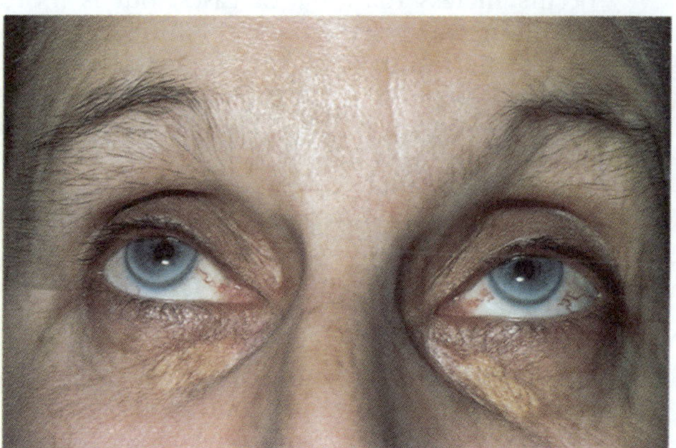

Fig. 18.18 Corneal arcus. (Note xanthelasmas also.)

MANAGEMENT STRATEGIES

THERAPEUTIC LIFESTYLE CHANGES

- Reduced intake of saturated fats (<7% of total calories) and cholesterol (<200 mg/day). Saturated fats (cheese, milk and red meat) are replaced with monounsaturated fats (olive oil, canola oil) and polyunsaturated fats (corn oil, peanut oil). Monounsaturated and polyunsaturated fats should constitute up to 10% and 20% of total calories, respectively.
- Increased intake of soluble fibre (10–25 g/day).
- Weight reduction if overweight or obese.
- Increased physical activity, practically every day.
- These should be tried for 12 weeks before considering the use of drugs.

PHARMACOTHERAPY

- This is used along with therapeutic lifestyle changes.
- First-line pharmacotherapy is the use of statins.
- If the patient is not able to tolerate a statin, a bile acid resin, fibrate or niacin is offered as a substitute.
- Benefits of drug therapy should initially be monitored at 6-week intervals. Once LDL levels are within recommended range, monitoring should be done every 6–12 months.

Statins or HMG-CoA Reductase Inhibitors

- This group includes simvastatin, atorvastatin, lovastatin, pravastatin, pitavastatin and rosuvastatin.
- This group of drugs inhibits the rate-limiting step in hepatic cholesterol synthesis, that is the conversion of HMG-CoA to mevalonate. These drugs also increase LDL receptor levels in hepatocytes and enhance clearance of LDL from circulation.
- These agents reduce LDL by 25%–40%.
- Activity of HMG-CoA is maximum during night and, therefore, statins should be administered at night.
- Side effects:
  - Mild transient elevation of liver enzymes is common but elevation of serum aminotransferases to more than three times the upper limit of normal occurs in less than 2% of patients. In these patients, therapy should be discontinued.
  - Another rare but serious side effect is the occurrence of myopathy manifested by muscle pain and elevation of serum muscle enzymes. This occurs in less than 1% of cases, but is more common when statins are combined with fibrates, niacin or cyclosporin. Factors which increase the risk of myopathy are listed in Table 18.42.

TABLE 18.42 Factors Increasing the Risk of Statin-Induced Myopathy

• Major illness
  • Severe infection
  • Surgery
  • Trauma
  • Hypoxia
  • Hypothermia
  • Uncontrolled seizures
• Chronic illness
  • Debilitation
  • Chronic renal or liver failure
• Endocrine and metabolic disorders
  • Hypothyroidism
  • Hyponatraemia
  • Metabolic acidosis
	• Medications (inhibit CYP3A4)
	  • Fibrates (gemfibrozil more than fenofibrate)
	  • Macrolide antibiotics
	  • Azole antifungals
	  • Calcium channel blockers (verapamil, diltiazem)
	  • Antidepressants (fluoxetine, fluvoxamine)
	  • Warfarin
	  • Cyclosporin
	• Viral infection
	• Others
	  • Concomitant use of recreational drugs
	  • Dose of statin

Bile Acid Sequestrants

- The bile acid sequestrants are cholestyramine, colestipol and colesevelam.
- These agents interfere with the absorption of bile acids from the gut resulting in a compensatory increase in bile acid synthesis.
- The major effect of the bile acid sequestrants is to reduce LDL by 15%–30%, with only modest changes in HDL.
- Side effects:
  - The major side effects are gastrointestinal (GI) distress and decreased absorption of other drugs.
  - These agents elevate TG level; elevated TG (>400 mg/dL) is a contraindication for this class of drugs.

Niacin

- It lowers LDL by 5%–25%. It also significantly lowers TG and raises HDL.
- Side effects:
  - These include flushing, increased blood sugar and uric acid, and GI distress.
  - Its use should be avoided in people who have peptic ulcer disease or a history of gout.

Fibrates

- Gemfibrozil and fenofibrate are able to lower TG and modestly lower LDL. Typically, HDL increases by 10%–15%.
- Side effects:
  - The side effects are restricted mainly to GI disturbance, and these agents should not be used in people with marked hepatic disease.
  - Other side effects include increase in gallstone formation and rarely myopathy.

Ezetimibe

- Ezetimibe localises at the brush border of the small intestine and inhibits the absorption of cholesterol from the diet.
- Specifically, it appears to bind to a critical mediator of cholesterol absorption, the Niemann–Pick C1-like 1 (NPC1L1) protein on the GI tract epithelial cells as well as in hepatocytes.
- In addition to this direct effect, decreased cholesterol absorption leads to an increase in LDL-cholesterol uptake into cells, thus decreasing levels in the blood plasma.
- Side effects:
  - Headache, diarrhoea; rarely elevated liver enzymes and myopathy.

Omega-3 Fatty Acid

- Useful to reduce TG levels.
- Dose is 1 to 2 g/day.

Newer Agents

- Torcetrapib is a cholesteryl ester transfer protein (CETP) inhibitor. CETP is a lipid transfer protein that is secreted by the liver and binds primarily to HDL, greatly facilitating the transfer of cholesteryl esters from HDL to apoB-containing particles such as VLDL, LDL and chylomicrons in exchange for TG. When CETP is inhibited, HDL-C levels rise markedly. However, one trial was halted due to excess number of deaths in torcetrapib group.
- Lomitapide, a MTP inhibitor, is approved for use in adults with homozygous familial hypercholesterolaemia.
- Proprotein convertase subtilisin kexin 9 (PCSK9) inhibitors are another class of drugs which may be used if statins are unable to control LDL or patient is unable to tolerate statins. PCSK9 is a natural protein that binds to and destroys LDL receptors in the liver, thereby preventing them from removing LDL-C from the circulation. The PCSK9 inhibitors block this protein, allowing the receptors to continue clearing LDL-C. This class of drugs includes alirocumab and evolocumab (monoclonal antibodies) which are given subcutaneously.
- Lomitapide is an oral inhibitor of the microsomal triglyceride transport protein (MTP). This blocks hepatic secretion of VLDL and intestinal secretion of chylomicrons. It is indicated in patients with homozygous familial hypercholesterolaemia.
- Bempedoic acid is an ATP citrate lyase inhibitor, which acts by decreasing cholesterol biosynthesis and upregulating LDL receptors. Uric acid levels should be monitored in those taking bempedoic acid as it may increase risk for gout. Additionally, it has been associated with tendon rupture.
- Inclisiran is small interfering RNA (siRNA) therapeutic agent. It is a subcutaneous injection given with an initial dose, then again at 3 months, and then every 6 months.

Other Modalities

- In patients with very high LDL-C (as seen in familial homozygous hypercholesterolaemia), liver transplantation, LDL apheresis or ileal bypass surgery are required to dramatically lower LDL-C levels.

MAJOR EFFECTS OF LIPID-LOWERING DRUGS (Table 18.43)

TABLE 18.43 Main Effects of Drugs Used in Treating Hyperlipidaemia

Agents	Effects on LDL	Effects on HDL	Effects on TG
• Statins	↓↓↓↓	↑	↓↓
• Bile acid resins	↓↓↓	±	None
• Fibrates	↓	↑↑	↓↓↓↓
• Niacin	↓↓	↑↑↑	↓↓↓↓
• Ezetimibe	↓↓	None	None

DOSAGES OF DRUGS USED IN HYPERLIPIDAEMIA (Table 18.44)

TABLE 18.44 Doses of Drugs Used in Hyperlipidaemia

• Statins:	
• Simvastatin	20–80 mg/day
• Atorvastatin	10–80 mg/day
• Lovastatin	20–80 mg/day
• Pravastatin	10–40 mg/day
• Rosuvastatin	5–40 mg/day
• Pitavastatin	2–4 mg/day
• Bile acid resins:	
• Cholestyramine	4–16 g/day in divided doses
• Colestipol	5–30 g/day in divided doses
• Colesevelam	3.75 g/day
• Fibrates:	
• Gemfibrozil	600 mg twice a day
• Fenofibrate	160–200 mg/day (micronised)
• Niacin	1.5–3.0 g/day
• Ezetimibe	5–20 mg/day
• Omega-3 fatty acids	2–4 g/day

Q. Discuss the guidelines on the use of statins.

Q. Discuss the guidelines on management of hypercholesterolaemia.

- The current American College of Cardiology/American Heart Association guidelines on the management of blood cholesterol (2018) are based on LDL-C levels, 10-year atherosclerotic cardiovascular disease (ASCVD) risk and presence of other ASCVD-enhancing risk factors (Box 18.24).
- Clinical ASCVD consists of acute coronary syndrome, history of MI, stable or unstable angina or coronary artery revascularisation, stroke, transient ischaemic attack and peripheral artery disease including aortic aneurysm, all of atherosclerotic origin.
- Calculation of ASCVD risk is based on pooled cohort equation (PCE). It is calculated using age, sex, race, total cholesterol, HDL-C, systolic blood pressure, presence of diabetes, smoking and any treatment for hypertension.
- Individuals are classified based on estimated risk: 10-year ASCVD risk $<5\%$ is low risk, 5%–7.5% is borderline risk, 7.5%–20% is intermediate risk and $\geq 20\%$ is high risk.

BOX 18.24 ASCVD-Enhancing Risk Factors

- Family history of premature ASCVD (men <55 years, women <65 years)
- Persistently elevated LDL-C ≥ 160 mg/dL
- Chronic kidney disease (eGFR 15-59 mL/minute/1.73 m^2)
- Metabolic syndrome
- South Asian ethnicity
- Conditions specific to women (e.g. preeclampsia, premature menopause)
- Inflammatory diseases (e.g. rheumatoid arthritis, HIV, psoriasis)
- Elevated high-sensitivity CRP (>2 mg/L)
- Elevated lipoprotein(a) (>50 mg/dL)

- A healthy lifestyle is recommended for all persons.
- Statin therapy can be high-intensity or medium-intensity. High-intensity statin therapy indicates use of atorvastatin 40–80 mg or rosuvastatin 20–40 mg/day. Medium-intensity statin therapy means atorvastatin 10–20 mg, rosuvastatin 5–10 mg, simvastatin 20–40 mg, pravastatin 40–80 mg, pitavastatin 2–4 mg and lovastatin 40 mg.
    - A moderate-intensity statin generally lowers LDL-C level by 30%–49%, while a high-intensity statin lowers LDL-C level by ≥50%.
- If response to statins is less than anticipated or patients are unable to tolerate a less than recommended intensity of a statin, or who are completely statin intolerant, consider addition or use of non-statin cholesterol-lowering therapy.
- If patient has characteristics predisposing to statin-associated adverse effects or drug–drug interaction is a strong possibility, moderate-intensity statin therapy may be used instead of high-intensity therapy.

RECOMMENDATIONS ON PRIMARY PREVENTION OF ATHEROSCLEROTIC CARDIOVASCULAR DISEASE (Table 18.45)

TABLE 18.45 Primary Prevention of Atherosclerotic Cardiovascular Disease

Category	Recommendations
Persons with severe primary hypercholesterolemia (LDL-C level ≥190 mg/dL)	• Use high-intensity statin therapy without calculating 10-year ASCVD risk • If LDL-C level remains ≥100 mg/dL, add ezetimibe
Patients 40–75 years of age with diabetes mellitus and LDL-C ≥70 mg/dL	• Use moderate-intensity statin therapy without calculating 10-year ASCVD risk • In patients with multiple risk factors or those 50–75 years of age, initiate a high-intensity statin to reduce the LDL-C level by ≥50%
Persons 40–75 years of age without diabetes mellitus and with LDL-C levels ≥70 mg/dL	• If 10-year risk is between 5% and 7.5%, evaluate other risk factors; if present, consider moderate-intensity statin therapy • If 10-year risk is ≥7.5%, use a moderate-intensity statin particularly in presence of other risk factors so as to reduce LDL-C levels by 30%–49% • If 10-year risk is ≥20%, reduce LDL-C levels by ≥50%
Persons 20–39 years of age with moderate hypertriglyceridaemia (triglycerides 175–499 mg/dL)	• Manage lifestyle factors (obesity and metabolic syndrome), secondary factors (diabetes mellitus, chronic liver or kidney disease and/or nephrotic syndrome, hypothyroidism)
In adults 40–75 years of age with hypertriglyceridaemia (triglycerides ≥175 mg/dL)	• If ASCVD risk ≥7.5%, re-evaluate ASCVD risk after lifestyle and secondary factors are taken care of • If ASCVD risk is still elevated, initiate or intensify statin therapy • If triglycerides ≥500 mg/dL (and especially ≥1000 mg/dL), advise a very low-fat diet, avoidance of alcohol and consumption of omega-3 fatty acids, and start fibrate therapy

RECOMMENDATIONS ON SECONDARY PREVENTION OF ATHEROSCLEROTIC CARDIOVASCULAR DISEASE (Table 18.46)

TABLE 18.46 Secondary Prevention of Atherosclerotic Cardiovascular Disease

Category	Recommendations
Patients with clinical ASCVD	• Use high-intensity statin therapy to reduce LDL-C by ≥50%
Patients with very high-risk ASCVD[a]	• Use high-intensity statin therapy and, if required, add ezetimibe to reduce LDL-C below 70 mg/dL • If LDL-C level remains ≥70 mg/dL on maximally tolerated statin and ezetimibe therapy, add a PCSK9 inhibitor

[a]Very high risk includes a history of multiple clinical ASCVD events or one clinical ASCVD event and multiple high-risk conditions.

19 Geriatrics

Q. Describe briefly epidemiology of the elderly population.

Q. Define geriatric medicine and Gerontology.

EPIDEMIOLOGY OF ELDERLY POPULATION

- An elderly person is defined as anyone who has attained the age of 60 years.
- Ageing is a global phenomenon and India is also experiencing growth in the number and proportion of older persons in its population. This is significantly related to improvements in health and medical care system. With longevity and declining fertility rates, the population of older persons is growing faster than the general population globally. This phenomenon is known as population ageing.
- Ageing population has implications for nearly all sectors of society, including labour and financial markets. Aged persons have different emotional, physical and resource needs.
- As populations become increasingly aged, it is more important that the governments design innovative policies and public services specifically targeted to older persons.
- As per UN Report on World Population Ageing, by 2030, persons older than 60 years are expected to outnumber the children under the age of 10 years. In addition, two-thirds of older persons would live in developing countries.
- As per World Health Organization (WHO) report, it is estimated that the number of older people globally is around 1 billion in 2020. By 2050, the world's population of people aged 60 years and older will double (2.1 billion).
- According to the Report of the Technical Group on Population Projections for India and States 2011–2036, there are nearly 138 million elderly persons in India in 2021 comprising of 67 million males and 71 million females. This is further expected to increase by around 56 million elderly persons by 2031.
- In term of proportion of population, in 1961, 5.6% of the population was in the age bracket of 60 years or more. This proportion has increased to 10.1% in 2021 and is further likely to increase to 13.1% in 2031.

GERIATRIC MEDICINE

- It is the branch of medicine that is concerned with diagnosis, treatment and prevention of diseases in older people (60 years or more) and the problems specific to ageing. It is also called Geriatrics.
- Physicians trained in Geriatrics are better equipped to understand the unique needs of older persons compared to internal medicine-trained physicians.

GERONTOLOGY

- Gerontology is a broader term. It is the multidisciplinary study of old persons and the process of ageing. It includes the study of social, cultural, psychological, cognitive and biological aspects of ageing. It deals not only with medical issues but also with several other problems faced by older people. Researchers in the field of Gerontology are diverse and are trained in areas such as physiology, social science, psychology, public health and policy related to older people.

- Thus, Gerontology is multidisciplinary and is concerned with physical, mental and social aspects and implications of ageing. Geriatrics is a medical specialty focused on care and treatment of older persons.

Q. Discuss the process of ageing.

DEFINITION OF AGEING

- Ageing is defined as gradual, insidious and progressive decline in structure and function of an organism which begin to start after the attainment of sexual maturity.
- Ageing results from the impact of accumulation of a wide variety of molecular and cellular damage over time which leads to a gradual decrease in physical and mental capacity, an increasing risk of disease and ultimately death. However, these changes are neither linear nor consistent, and they are only loosely associated with a person's age.

THEORIES OF AGEING

- The term 'senescence' has been used to describe normal process of ageing which means progressive deterioration of bodily functions over time. There are countless biological theories to explain how we age. No single theory can explain the process of ageing. The changes take place not only at a cellular and molecular level, but also on tissues and organ systems.
- According to various theories, all organs in an individual do not age at the same rate, and any single organ does not necessarily age at the same rate in all individuals.
- Theories of ageing can be divided into four: biological, sociological, psychological and spiritual. Of these, biological theories are most relevant.

BIOLOGICAL THEORIES

- The biologic theories try to explain the following aspects:
  - Deleterious effects of ageing leading to decreasing function of the organism which may lead to a complete failure of either an organ or an entire system.
  - Gradually occurring age-related changes that are progressive over time.
  - Intrinsic changes that can affect all members of a species because of chronologic age.
- Biologic theories are subdivided into two main divisions: stochastic and nonstochastic.
  - Stochastic theories explain ageing as events that occur randomly from both internal and external events, and accumulate over time. There is a possibility that these changes can be reversed by some therapeutic measures.
  - Nonstochastic theories view ageing as certain predetermined, timed phenomenon and nothing can change the process of ageing.
- Various biological theories are described in Table 19.1.

SUMMARY OF MECHANISMS OF CELLULAR AGEING

- Flowchart 19.1 summarises various mechanisms of cellular ageing and possible interventions which can counteract it.

TABLE 19.1 Biological Theories of Ageing

Stochastic theories	Error theory	• As a cell ages, changes occur in its DNA and RNA. These can also occur due to exposure to toxins and radiation. This can produce errors in transcription in any step of protein synthesis which would cause production of an enzyme or protein that was not an exact copy of the original. This will eventually lead to either ageing or actual death of a cell. • Studies do show that changes occur in the activity of various enzymes with ageing but have not found that aged cells contain altered or mis-specified proteins. Further, ageing is not accelerated if mis-specified proteins or enzymes are introduced to a cell.
	Free radical theory	• Free radicals are byproducts of metabolic activities within the body. Their production can increase as a result of environmental pollutants such as ozone, pesticides and radiation. Normally, they are neutralised by enzymatic activity or natural antioxidants. If, however, they are not neutralised, they may react with molecules in membranes, in particular of mitochondria, lysosomes, and nucleus (lipid peroxidation). Therefore, these organelles can no longer function as efficiently, and their membranes may become damaged, resulting in increased permeability. • Free radicals may also cause mutations in the DNA and RNA, thereby producing changes in protein production.
	Cross-linkage theory	• With age, some molecules become cross-linked and may impede metabolic processes by obstructing the passage of nutrients and wastes between the intracellular and extracellular compartments. Primarily this involves collagen which results in decreased transport of nutrients and waste products across cell membranes. Eventually, this results in a decrease in the function of the cells. • An example would be the changes associated with ageing skin. • Normally, immune system helps in removing cross-linked molecules but with ageing, immune functions decline. • Elevated blood sugar increases the amount of cross-linking. • There is some in-vitro evidence to support that a combination of exercise and dietary restrictions help to inhibit the cross-linkage process.

TABLE 19.1 Biological Theories of Ageing—cont'd

	Wear and tear theory	• Cells wear out over time because of continued use and this damage exceeds the body's ability to repair itself. • Essentially, the theory indicates that organs and tissues have a preprogrammed amount of energy available to them and eventually wear out when the allotted energy is expended. • Microscopic signs of wear and tear have been found in muscles and nerve cells. • However, increased functional abilities have been shown in individuals who participate in daily exercise, which otherwise should increase wear and tear.
	Membrane theory	• As we grow older, the cell membrane becomes less lipid which impedes its efficiency to conduct normal function. This may result in accumulation of lipofuscin in the skin, brain, heart and lungs. • The cells declining efficiency also means that the essential and regular transfer of sodium and potassium is impaired, thus reducing communication.
	Metabolic theory/ caloric restriction	• All organisms have a finite amount of metabolic lifetime and that organisms with a higher metabolic rate have a shorter lifespan. • Evidence for this theory comes from research that has shown that certain fish, when the water temperature is lowered, live longer than their warm water counterparts. • Extensive experimentation on the effects of caloric restriction on rodents has demonstrated that caloric restriction increases the lifespan and delays the onset of age-dependent diseases.
Nonstochastic theories	Programmed ageing theory or Hayflick's limit theory	• A biological clock controls cell behaviour and lifespan of an individual. • The biological clock for humans was estimated at 110–120 years.
	Immunity theory	• It has been found that as a person ages, the immune system functions less effectively (immunosenescence). The changes that occur with ageing are most apparent in the T-lymphocytes, although changes also occur in the functioning capabilities of B-lymphocytes. • Accompanying these changes is a decrease in the body's defence against foreign pathogens, which manifests itself as an increased incidence of infectious diseases and an increase in the production of autoantibodies, which lead to a propensity to develop autoimmune diseases.
	Neuroendocrine control or pacemaker theory	• There is relationship between the neurologic and the endocrine systems over the lifespan of an individual. The neuroendocrine system regulates and controls many important metabolic activities. • There is a decline, or even a cessation, in many of the components of the neuroendocrine system over the lifespan (e.g. reproductive system). • Another hormone which decreases over time is dehydroepiandrosterone (DHEA). Administration of this hormone to mice increased longevity and bolstered immunity. • Melatonin may have a role as a biological clock as its levels gradually decline just after puberty until old age. In addition, it has powerful antioxidant properties and may enhance immune function.
	Telomere theory	• Telomeres are the regions at the ends of chromosomes that may function as biologic clocks. Each time a cell divides, the telomere becomes shorter; when this shortening reaches some critical point, the cell can no longer divide, and this may contribute to the ageing process.

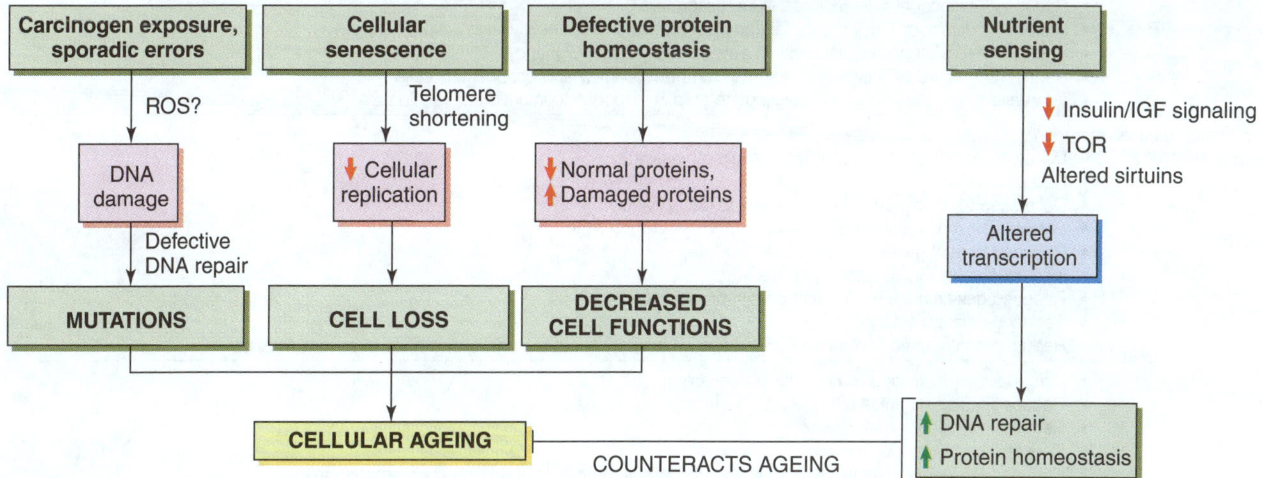

Flowchart 19.1 Mechanisms That Cause and Counteract Cellular Ageing (IGF, insulin-like growth factor; ROS, reactive oxygen species; TOR, target of rapamycin).

Q. Describe the physiological changes which occur in the elderly persons.

- Ageing is characterised by several changes in the homeostasis of body. Almost all the systems show some changes during ageing.
- Table 19.2 describes common physiological changes seen in the elderly people.

TABLE 19.2 Physiological Changes in the Elderly

System	Age-Related Change
Respiratory system	• Reduced number and motility of cilia in respiratory tract (reduced mucous clearance) • Muscle wasting and decrease in muscle mass • Kyphosis due to degenerative changes in thoracic spine and vertebral wedge collapse • Increased dependence on abdominal muscles • Flattening of diaphragm which becomes less efficient (contributes to increase in work of breathing during exercise) • Lungs voluminous and resemble emphysematous lungs • Changes in lung volumes and compliance (lung compliance increased, reduced chest wall compliance, decreased vital capacity, increased residual volume, reduced FEV_1) • Increased physiological dead space • Enlargement of alveolar ducts resulting in a decreased surface area for gas exchange • Increased ventilation/perfusion mismatch (reduced alveolar-arterial oxygen gradient and PaO_2) • Blunted central and peripheral response to low PaO_2 and high $PaCO_2$
Cardiovascular system	• Increased risk of systolic hypertension and coronary artery disease • Left ventricular hypertrophy • Impaired early diastolic filling of left ventricle (diastolic dysfunction) resulting in more dependence on left atrial systole for ventricular filling (this results in S_4 which is normal in people aged 75 years or above) • Calcification of aortic and mitral valves • Reduced maximum heart rate on exertion • Increased supraventricular and ventricular ectopics • Normal resting left ventricular ejection fraction (LVEF) but smaller increases in LVEF in response to exercise • Elevated brain natriuretic peptide (BNP) • Stiffening of arteries including aorta
Haematopoietic system	• Reduced haematopoietic functional reserve (decrease in bone marrow mass and increase in bone marrow fat)—reduced tolerance to chemotherapy • Delayed compensatory haematopoietic response to phlebotomy and hypoxia • Increased responsiveness of platelets to thrombotic stimulators • Reduced bleeding time • Elevated fibrinogen, factor V, factor VII, factor VIII, factor IX, high molecular-weight kininogen and prekallikrein • Elevated fibrin degradation fragments • Elevated plasminogen activator inhibitor 1
Immune system	• Reduced macrophage precursors in bone marrow • Reduced phagocytic activity of neutrophils • Involution of thymus • Reduced number of naïve T cells • Reduced T-helper cells, increased T-suppressor cells • Reduced diversity of T cell repertoire (reduced protection from new viral infections) • Reduced T-regulatory cells (increase in autoimmunity and malignancy) • Reduced numbers of B cells precursors in the bone marrow and peripheral B cells • Decrease in specific immunoglobulins generated in response to infection or vaccination
Gastrointestinal tract	• Gums recede • Decay of teeth, dental caries and incomplete mastication • Reduced saliva production • Decreased food clearance from pharynx to oesophagus • Reduced oesophageal contractions • Reduced tone of gastro-oesophageal sphincter • Increased sensitivity to gastric irritants • Reduced gastric acid, gastric and ghrelin production • Reduced colonic motility • Reduced content of cytochrome P450 in liver which may affect metabolic clearance of several drugs
Neurological system	• Sarcopaenia (decreased muscle mass and strength) • Reduced or absent ankle reflex • Reduced vibration sense • Reduced neural conduction • Progressive sluggishness in the response of the pupils, both to light and on accommodation • Absence or impairment of the conjugate movements of upwards deviations of the eyeballs • Reduced hearing, taste and smell • Shrinkage of brain • Difficulty in learning a new task or language • Blunting of baroreceptor responses (increased risk of postural hypotension) • Blunting of compensatory responses to hypothermia and hyperthermia

TABLE 19.2 Physiological Changes in the Elderly—cont'd

System	Age-Related Change
Urinary system	• Decrease in renal mass • Reduction in functional glomeruli • Decrease in creatinine clearance • Impaired ability to excrete a water load • Decreased hydroxylation of vitamin D • Reduced bladder capacity
Endocrine system	• Impaired glucose tolerance • Impaired growth hormone secretion • Reduced melatonin secretion • In women, oestrogen and prolactin decrease • In men, testosterone decreases
Integumentary	• Wrinkling of skin • Senile purpura • Dry skin • Reduced subcutaneous fat

Q. Briefly describe some of the atypical manifestations of common diseases in elderly individuals.

- Elderly individuals may present with atypical features of common diseases and this may make diagnosis difficult.
- Possible causes of atypical presentations in older adults include the following:
  - Age-related physiologic changes
  - Age-related loss of physiologic reserve
  - Interactions of chronic conditions with acute illnesses
  - Underreporting of symptoms
- Some of these atypical features are shown in Table 19.3.

TABLE 19.3 Atypical Presentations of Common Diseases in Elderly

Condition	Atypical Features
Acute coronary syndrome	• Asymptomatic • Altered mental status • Heart failure • Fatigue • Dyspnoea • Dizziness
Sepsis	• Hypothermia or normal temperature • Altered mental status • Absence of tachycardia • Absence of leucocytosis
Urinary tract infection	• Absence of dysuria • Incontinence • Confusion
Malignancy	• Pathologic fracture • Altered mental status • Fever
Pulmonary embolism	• Syncope • Fever • Fatigue • Altered mental status • Chest pain less frequent • Dyspnoea and hypoxaemia more common

TABLE 19.3 Atypical Presentations of Common Diseases in Elderly—cont'd

Condition	Atypical Features
Hyperthyroidism	• Atrial fibrillation • Heart failure • Anorexia • Constipation (diarrhoea uncommon) • Fatigue • Altered mental status or cognitive decline • Apathy • Agitation
Depression	• Cognitive impairment • Confusion • Apathy • Absence of subjective feeling of depression
Faecal impaction	• Spurious diarrhoea • Urinary incontinence • Chest pain • Dyspnoea • Altered mental status
Acute appendicitis	• Diffuse abdominal pain • Confusion • Urinary urgency • Absence of fever or tachycardia

Q. Discuss comprehensive geriatric assessment. (IM24.2)

Q. What is geriatric syndrome?

DEFINITION OF COMPREHENSIVE GERIATRIC ASSESSMENT

- Comprehensive geriatric assessment (CGA) is defined as a multidisciplinary diagnostic and treatment process that identifies medical, psychosocial and functional problems of a frail older person so as to develop a coordinated and integrated plan to maximise overall health with ageing.
- Health care for the elderly extends beyond the traditional medical management of illnesses. It requires evaluation of multiple issues including physical,

cognitive, affective, social, financial, environmental and spiritual components that influence an elderly's health.
- A systematic evaluation of frail, older persons by a team of health professionals may identify a variety of treatable health problems which may lead to better health outcomes. The team often consists of trained nurses, occupational therapists, physical therapists, social workers, dieticians, psychiatrists, psychologists, dentists, audiologists, opticians, pharmacists, besides geriatricians. However, members are generally included based on the need.

GERIATRIC SYNDROME

- The term 'geriatric syndrome' refers to common health conditions in the elderly which do not fit into distinct organ-based disease categories and often have multifactorial causes. Examples of these conditions include incontinence, malnutrition, falls, cognitive impairment, delirium, gait disorders, sleep disorders.

INDICATIONS FOR REFERRAL FOR COMPREHENSIVE GERIATRIC ASSESSMENT

- CGA is usually initiated through a referral by the clinician caring for the elderly either in the hospital setting or in practice. Indications for referral are given in Box 19.1.

MAJOR DOMAINS OF ASSESSMENT

- Figure 19.1 shows the major domains of CGA.

FUNCTIONAL STATUS

- Functional status indicates ability to perform activities necessary or desirable in daily life. This can be assessed by activities of daily living (ALD) which can be defined at three levels: basic activities of daily living (BADLs), instrumental or intermediate activities of daily living (IADLs) and advanced activities of daily living (AADLs).

Basic Activities of Daily Living

- These are fundamental activities essential for personal care and are basic to independent living.

BOX 19.1 Indications for Referring for Comprehensive Geriatric Assessment

- Age >75 years
- Medical comorbidities such as heart failure or cancer
- Psychosocial disorders such as depression
- Lives alone
- Needs help with basic activities of daily living or instrumental activities of daily living
- Specific geriatric conditions such as dementia, falls or functional disability
- ≥2 admissions to acute care hospital in last 1 year
- Increased home resources to manage medical and functional needs
- Failure to thrive

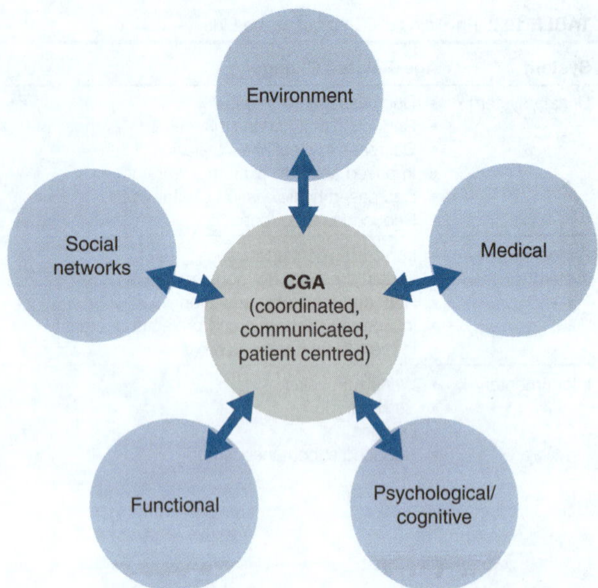

Fig. 19.1 Comprehensive geriatric assessment (CGA): major domains of assessment.

- Loss of these activities places burden on caregivers and is a marker of complete dependence.
- Ask whether person can perform these activities independently, requires some assistance or is completely dependent on caregiver.
- Basic activities of daily living are shown in Fig.19.2 and Table 19.4.

Instrumental Activities of Daily Living

- These are complex tasks which enable older people to live independently and safely.
- These activities are not necessary for basic existence.
- IADLs should be assessed at baseline and then during follow up as loss of these activities is a sign of deterioration.
- IADLs are shown in Figure 19.2 and Table 19.4.

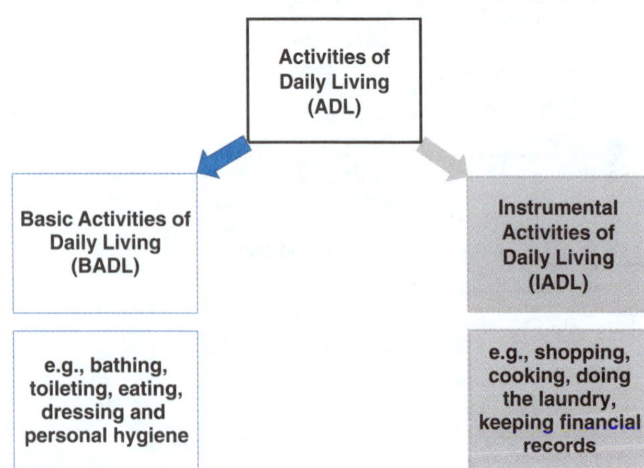

Fig. 19.2 Activities of daily living classified as basic activities of daily living and instrumental activities of daily living.

TABLE 19.4 Basic and Instrumental Activities of Daily Living

Basic Activities of Daily Living (BADLs)	Instrumental Activities of Daily Living (IADLs)
• Bathing • Dressing • Toileting • Maintaining continence • Grooming • Eating • Ambulation	• Driving or using public transportation • Shopping for groceries • Using a telephone • Housekeeping • Doing home repair • Planning and preparing meals • Doing laundry • Taking medications • Financial management

Gait Speed

- In addition to ADLs, gait speed alone predicts functional decline and early mortality in the elderly. Assessing gait speed may identify those people who are at increased risk of fall. Additionally, assessing gait speed may help identify frail patients who might not benefit from treatment of chronic asymptomatic diseases such as hypertension. For example, hypertension in those above the age of 65 years was not associated with increased mortality unless walking speed was ≥0.8 metres/second (measured over 6 metres).

Timed Up and Go Test

- The 'Timed Up and Go Test' (TUGT) can also be a good indicator of overall function, combining an assessment of physical ability—being able to 'get up and go'. This is also a test of cognition relating specifically to following instructions and carrying them out successfully.
- The patient is asked to sit in a chair of knee height. Then he is asked to stand up, walk 3 metres (10 feet) at his normal pace, turn round, return to the chair and sit down.
- Time from when the patient starts to try and stand up to when the patient sits down again is noted. Normal scores are between 7 and 10 seconds for people between 65 and 99. If a patient takes more than 12 seconds, then their mobility may be considered impaired (Fig. 19.3).

Falls

- An assessment of fall risk should be integrated into the history and physical examination of all geriatric patients.

COGNITION

- Many elderly people with cognitive impairment remain undiagnosed. It is important to make an early diagnosis so as to uncover treatable conditions. Initial evaluation should include a thorough history and brief cognition screens. If cognitive impairment is suspected after initial evaluation, detailed assessment is required.

Q. Define diagnostic criteria of dementia or major neurocognitive disorder.

Q. Discuss briefly common causes of dementia or major neurocognitive disorder in older individuals. (IM24.4)

- Dementia or major neurocognitive disorder is a global deterioration of the higher mental functions. It is characterised by problems with memory and at least one other cognitive function (learning, reasoning, language, spatial ability and orientation, and handling complex tasks) which are severe enough to interfere with occupational, domestic or social functioning.

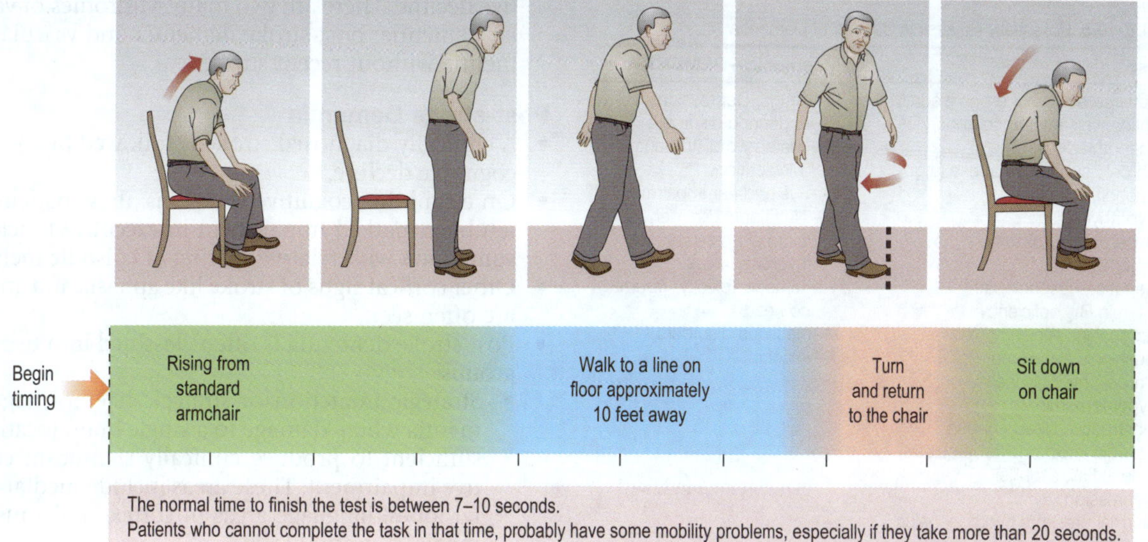

Fig. 19.3 Timed up and go test.

DIAGNOSTIC CRITERIA FOR DEMENTIA

- Dementia is called major neurocognitive disorder under Diagnostic and Statistical Manual of Mental Disorders, Fifth Edition (DSM-5).
- Diagnostic criteria for dementia or major neurocognitive disorder are given in Box 19.2.

CAUSES OF DEMENTIA

- Causes of dementia are listed on page 322.
- Some of the potentially reversible causes of dementia are listed in Table 19.5.

INVESTIGATIONS

- Investigations are carried out to detect a reversible cause of dementia and are listed on page 322.

BOX 19.2 Diagnostic Criteria for Major Neurocognitive Disorder (DSM-5)

- Evidence of significant cognitive decline from a previous level of performance in one or more cognitive domains:
  - Learning and memory
  - Language
  - Executive function
  - Complex attention
  - Perceptual-motor
  - Social cognition
- The cognitive deficits interfere with independence in everyday activities. At a minimum, assistance should be required with complex instrumental activities of daily living, such as paying bills or managing medications
- The cognitive deficits do not occur exclusively in the context of a delirium
- The cognitive deficits are not better explained by another mental disorder (e.g. major depressive disorder, schizophrenia)

TABLE 19.5 Potentially Reversible Causes of Dementia

Causes	Mnemonic—DEMENTIA
• Adverse effects of drugs (sedatives, anticonvulsants, anticholinergics, phenothiazines, others)	D—Drugs, Depression
• Chronic substance abuse (e.g. alcohol)	E—Endocrine disorders
• Hypothyroidism	M—Metabolic disturbances, Medications
• Hyperparathyroidism	E—Eye and ear impairment
• Uraemia	N—Nutritional disorder, Normal pressure hydrocephalus
• Hepatic encephalopathy	T—Tumour, Toxicity, Trauma to head
• Vitamin B_{12} deficiency	I—Infectious disorders
• Adrenal insufficiency	A—Alcohol
• Cushing's syndrome	
• Chronic hypoglycaemia or hyponatraemia	
• Obstructive sleep apnoea	
• Chronic infections (tuberculosis, fungal, HIV, syphilis)	
• Depression	
• Normal pressure hydrocephalus	
• Chronic subdural haematoma	
• Brain tumours	
• Vasculitides	

ALZHEIMER'S DISEASE

- Alzheimer's disease is discussed on page 359.

VASCULAR DEMENTIA

- Vascular dementia refers to any dementia that is primarily caused by cerebrovascular disease or impaired cerebral blood flow.
- It is the second most common form of dementia, the most common being Alzheimer's disease.
- The cerebrovascular disease can be due to any of the causes of ischaemic stroke (e.g. cardioembolism, large artery atherosclerotic disease, cerebral small vessel diseases) or haemorrhagic stroke.

VASCULAR COGNITIVE IMPAIRMENT

- It indicates cognitive impairment caused by cerebrovascular diseases and includes both dementia and mild cognitive impairment.

MIXED DEMENTIA

- Often vascular dementia is only of the aetiologies of dementia. Other aetiologies may either be found at autopsy or clinically (e.g. clinically patient may also meet criteria of Alzheimer's disease).

RISK FACTORS

- Risk factors of cerebrovascular disease are also the risk factors for vascular dementia. These include male sex, advanced age, smoking, diabetes, hypertension, hypercholesterolaemia, sedentary life style, atrial fibrillation.
- Risk factors of stroke-related features are intracerebral haemorrhage, left hemisphere location and multiple or recurrent strokes.
- Post-stroke risk factors include occurrence of incontinence, confusion or seizures.

CLINICAL FEATURES

- The essential feature of vascular dementia is cognitive decline. There are two main syndromes of vascular dementia: post-stroke dementia and vascular dementia without recent stroke.

Post-stroke Dementia

- A clinically diagnosed stroke is followed by stepwise cognitive decline.
- On examining cognitive functions, these patients often have marked impairment in executive functions, sometimes with relative sparing of episodic memory.
- Other cortical signs of stroke like aphasia and apraxia are often seen.
- Post-stroke dementia is often classified into two subgroups:
  - Strategic infarction or strategic haemorrhage dementia where damage to a single brain location is sufficient to produce clinically significant cognitive impairment. These areas include medial frontal lobes, language areas of cortex, thalamus and medial temporal lobes.
  - Multi-infarct or multi-haemorrhage dementia occurs when there is damage to multiple areas of

brain over time which can have cumulative effect to produce dementia.

Vascular Dementia Without Recent Stroke (Binswanger's Disease or Subcortical Ischaemic Vascular Dementia)

- In this type of vascular dementia, there is a progressive or stepwise cognitive decline without a concurrent history of symptomatic stroke, although there is imaging evidence of clinically unrecognised cerebrovascular disease. It occurs due to arteriolosclerotic cerebral small vessel disease or cerebral amyloid angiopathy. On testing cognition, there is prominent impairment in executive function and processing speed.

DIAGNOSIS

- A thorough history, physical examination followed by investigations are required to make a diagnosis of vascular dementia.

History and Physical Examination

- The history should focus on eliciting time course of cognitive decline and its relationship to BADLs and IADLs.
- Previous history of stroke as well as its relation to the onset of cognitive impairment should be noted.
- A cognitive screen should be performed to identify objective evidence of cognitive impairment. Various tools include Mini-Mental State Examination (MMSE), Montreal Cognitive Assessment (MoCA) and others.
- Physical examination should focus on identifying focal neurological deficits and signs, which may suggest presence of cerebral small vessel disease or stroke.
- Based on history and physical examination, the Hachinski's ischaemic score can be calculated to indicate a possibility of vascular stroke (Table 19.6).

Laboratory Tests

- Laboratory tests should be conducted to exclude reversible or contributory causes of dementia (see Table 19.5 for reversible causes of dementia).

Neuroimaging

- Brain imaging should be performed to confirm infarct or haemorrhage in a patient with stroke and also to identify clinically unrecognised cerebrovascular disease. MRI is more sensitive than CT for signs of cerebral small vessel disease including microbleeds.

TABLE 19.6 Hachinski's Ischaemic Score

Feature	Points
Abrupt onset	2
Fluctuating course	2
History of stroke	2
Focal neurologic symptoms	2
Focal neurologic signs	2
Stepwise deterioration	1
Nocturnal confusion	1
Preservation of personality	1
Depression	1
Somatic complaints	1
Emotional incontinence (pseudobulbar affect)	1
Hypertension	1
Associated atherosclerosis	1

A score of ≥7 indicates that a vascular contribution to dementia is likely.

Evaluation for Risk Factors for Stroke

- It is important to look for risk factors of stroke so that measures for reducing them can be taken (secondary prophylaxis).

TREATMENT

Management of Risk Factors

- These include lifestyle modifications, control of diabetes, hypertension and hypercholesterolaemia, and antiplatelet agents.
- Anticoagulants in presence of atrial fibrillation.
- Carotid endarterectomy.

Cholinesterase Inhibitors

- Treatment with a cholinesterase inhibitor drug may be initiated in patients who have progressive cognitive decline that cannot be directly attributed to a fresh stroke. Many of such patients will have concomitant Alzheimer's disease. The drugs include donepezil, galantamine and rivastigmine.

Memantine

- Role of memantine is doubtful.

Q. Write a short note on normal pressure hydrocephalus.

- Normal pressure hydrocephalus (NPH) is a form of communicating hydrocephalus in which the ventricles are pathologically enlarged with normal opening pressure on lumbar puncture.
- It is most common in adults over the age of 60 years.
- Majority of cases are idiopathic although some cases may occur following subarachnoid haemorrhage or meningitis which lead to impaired absorption of CSF (secondary NPH).

PATHOPHYSIOLOGY

- The exact cause of idiopathic NPH is not known. The proposed mechanisms include the following:
  - Congenital hydrocephalus becoming symptomatic later in life (decompensated congenital hydrocephalus).
  - Chronic periventricular ischaemia.
  - Elevated central venous pressure.
  - Reduced CSF absorption.

CLINICAL FEATURES

- The classical triad of NPH is urinary incontinence, gait disturbance and dementia (Adams' triad or Hakim's triad— 'wet, wobbly and wacky').
- Gait difficulty is the most prominent and may be the only clinical feature. Patients walk with small steps with broad base, and have difficulty in turning. At time, they have 'glue-footed' gait.

- Urinary urgency rather than incontinence may be present at early stages.
- Since opening pressure on lumbar puncture is normal, patients do not have headache, vomiting, visual loss or papilloedema (signs of raised intracranial pressure).

NEUROIMAGING

- On CT or MRI, there is enlargement of ventricles in the absence of or out of proportion to sulcal enlargement, with no evidence of obstruction at the level of the third or fourth ventricles. Brain atrophy associated with age produces a proportionate enlargement of both ventricular and sulcal size.

HIGH-VOLUME LUMBAR PUNCTURE

- In this procedure, 30–50 mL of CSF is removed. Improvement in gait within 30–60 minutes suggests a good outcome of ventriculo-peritoneal shunt (VP shunt) as a therapeutic modality.

TREATMENT

- Treatment of NPH is by placing a VP shunt.

Q. Write a short note on depression in an older person. (IM24.5)

- Depression in elderly people is a common problem and is often associated with comorbidity, impaired functioning, excessive use of healthcare resources and increased mortality.
- To compound the issue, depression is underdiagnosed and inadequately/not treated in elderly people.
- It is important to remember that depression is not a normal consequence of ageing. Grief and sadness should not be confused with depression. These are normal reactions after retirement, loss of income or death of a spouse.
- Risk factors for depression in old age are given in Box 19.3.
- Diagnosis as per DSM-5 is discussed on page 790.
- Several screening instruments are available to suspect depression in primary care setting. One of them is the Geriatric Depression Scale (Box 19.4).
- Treatment includes addressing comorbid conditions, psychotherapy (cognitive-behavioral therapy, interpersonal psychotherapy, problem-solving therapy), pharmacotherapy (tricyclic and tetracyclic antidepressants, selective serotonin reuptake inhibitors, serotonin-norepinephrine reuptake inhibitors, atypical antidepressants, serotonin modulators) and close follow up for effectiveness and side effects. Therapy with single drug is preferred in older persons in order to minimise side effects and drug–drug interactions. Electroconvulsive therapy (ECT) is used if response is inadequate with above treatment.

BOX 19.3 Risk Factors for Depression in the Elderly

- Female sex
- Social isolation
- Widowed or divorced
- Nursing home residence
- Lower socioeconomic status
- Comorbid general medical conditions
- Uncontrolled pain
- Insomnia
- Functional impairment
- Cognitive impairment

BOX 19.4 Geriatric Depression Scale

- Are you basically satisfied with your life?
- Do you often get bored?
- Do you often feel helpless?
- Do you prefer to stay at home rather than going out and doing new things?
- Do you feel pretty worthless the way you are now?

Two out of five responses ('no' to question 1 or 'yes' to questions 2 through 5) suggest a diagnosis of depression.

Q. Describe briefly urinary incontinence in the elderly.

Q. Define overactive bladder.

- Urinary incontinence is defined as involuntary urination irrespective of volume. It may vary from dribbling of small amount or urine to almost continuous incontinence.
- Urinary incontinence is not a natural consequence of ageing and is a pathological condition.
- Since it is a social problem, it is usually not mentioned by the elderly person.
- Incidence in the population over 60 years is 15%–30% while this rate reaches 60%–70% in the elderly in nursing homes. It is 1.5–2 times more in women up to 80 years and after that age, it is observed in equal frequency in both sexes.
- Urinary incontinence is often associated with dementia, faecal incontinence, gait disturbances and transfer dependency.

CONSEQUENCES OF INCONTINENCE

- Urinary incontinence often leads to poor hygiene, increased urinary tract infections, pressure sores, sleep disturbance, sexual dysfunction, depression, social isolation, increased risk of fracture, impaired quality of life and increase in the risk of being placed in a nursing home. Many patients limit their social activity.

AETIOLOGY

- Reversible causes of incontinence of urine are listed in Box 19.5.
- Drugs which can produce incontinence of urine are shown in Table 19.7.

BOX 19.5 Reversible Causes of Incontinence of Urine

'DIAPPERS'

D—Delirium
I—Infection (urinary)
A—Atrophic (vaginitis), Alcohol
P—Pharmaceuticals
P—Psychological
E—Endocrine/Excess urine output
R—Restricted mobility
S—Stool impaction

TABLE 19.7 Drugs Producing Incontinence of Urine

Category	Examples	Mechanism
Diuretics	Furosemide, hydrochlorothiazide, chlorothiazide	Polyuria, frequency, urgency
Anticholinergic drugs	Antihistamines, tricyclic antidepressants, some antipsychotics	Urinary retention producing overflow incontinence or faecal impaction
Calcium channel blockers	Verapamil, nifedipine	Urinary retention, nocturnal diuresis resulting from fluid retention
Alpha-adrenergic agonists	Nasal decongestants	Urinary retention with overflow incontinence related to BPH
Alpha-adrenergic antagonists	Prazosin, terazosin, doxazosin	Urethral relaxation
Narcotic analgesics	Opiates	Urinary retention, sedation
Sedatives/ hypnotics	Benzodiazepines	Sedation, immobility

CLASSIFICATION OF INCONTINENCE

URGE INCONTINENCE

- Also known as detrusor hyperactivity or spastic bladder.
- Most common type of incontinence.
- Sudden and compelling desire to pass urine that is difficult to defer and is accompanied by involuntary leakage.
- Causes include benign prostate hypertrophy (BPH), urethritis, neurologic conditions affecting brain (e.g. stroke, normal pressure hydrocephalus, dementia, Parkinson's disease) and some medications.

STRESS INCONTINENCE

- Most common in women.
- It occurs in the absence of bladder contraction and is due to inadequate urethral sphincter function, either from mechanical damage to the urethral sphincter or from physiologic effects that limit sphincter function.
- Commonly occurs when intra-abdominal pressure increases, for example, with coughing, sneezing, laughing or rising quickly.
- Causes include ageing, trauma of childbirth or pelvic surgery, hormonal changes, pelvic radiation, pelvic trauma or neurologic diseases. It can also occur for a few months after prostate surgery.

OVERFLOW INCONTINENCE

- It occurs when urine is retained in the bladder due to incomplete emptying after an attempt to urinate.
- History of sense of incomplete emptying is present.
- Urine retention can lead to damage to kidneys.
- Causes include BPH, urethral stricture, neurologic disorders (e.g. stroke, Parkinson' disease, NPH), neuropathy, cauda equina syndrome and some medications.

POST-VOID DRIBBLING

- It is not truly incontinence. It indicates dribbling of urine retained in the urethra after the bladder has emptied.
- It causes wetness soon after the patient has completed urinating but not at other times.

FUNCTIONAL INCONTINENCE

- Functional incontinence occurs when an individual with normal bladder and urethral function has difficulty getting to the toilet before urination occurs.
- It occurs in those with impaired mobility, impaired cognition or mental confusion.

OVERACTIVE BLADDER

- Overactive bladder is a syndrome characterised by a sudden and compelling need to urinate, a sensation that is difficult to defer.
- It is often associated with urge incontinence, urinary frequency (voiding eight or more times in a 24-hour period) and nocturia (need to wake one or more times per night to void).

EVALUATION FOR URINARY INCONTINENCE

- A focused history is often sufficient to identify the most probable type of urinary incontinence. Medication history is important.
- Physical examination should include rectal examination to assess prostate size and consistency, and abdominal examination after voiding to assess for a palpable bladder or any abdominal mass that could cause pressure on the bladder. In females, per vaginal examination should be carried out to assess for atrophic vaginitis and vaginal prolapse.
- Urinalysis is an important investigation in patients with incontinence.
- Ultrasound helps in looking at prostate size and residual urine volume.

MANAGEMENT

GENERAL MEASURES

Non-pharmacological Measures

- Proper nutrition, avoidance of constipation, weight loss and physical activity are beneficial in improving symptoms.
- Modify amount and timing of fluid intake.
- Avoid bladder stimulants (e.g. caffeine and alcohol).
- Reduce physical barrier to toilet (e.g. having a bedside commode).
- Scheduled voiding of urine.
- Absorbent bladder-protection pads for social situations.
- Pelvic floor (Kegel) muscle training and bladder training.
- Biofeedback.

Pharmacological Measures

- The current recommended treatment for urge incontinence is control of detrusor muscle overactivity through the inhibition of M2 and M3 muscarinic receptors on the bladder using anticholinergic agents. These agents include oxybutynin, tolterodine, solifenacin, darifenacin and fesoterodine.
- Pharmacotherapeutic options for overflow incontinence secondary to BPH include peripheral alpha-adrenergic blockers (AABs), 5-alpha-reductase inhibitors (ARIs) or a combination of the two. AABs include alfuzosin, silodosin and tamsulosin. 5-ARIs are finasteride and dutasteride.

SURGICAL TREATMENT

- For stress incontinence, surgical treatment is required if conservative treatment fails. Women are often treated with sling procedures which are designed to correct sphincter deficiencies and urethral hypermobility.
- For overflow incontinence in men due to BPH, transurethral resection of the prostate should be done.

OTHER MEASURES

- Weighted cone devices attached to vaginal muscles may help women with stress incontinence. These devices are designed to help patients improve pelvic floor tone through active, continuous muscle contractions.
- Vaginal continence pessaries are helpful for various pelvic floor disorders.
- Electrical stimulation to the pelvic floor helps in inhibiting the micturition reflex and improving contraction of the pelvic floor musculature.
- Injection of transurethral bulking agents such as collagen.
- Transurethral collagen denaturation (the Renessa procedure) uses non-ablative radiofrequency to reduce tissue compliance.

SUMMARY OF MANAGEMENT OF URINARY INCONTINENCE

- Flowchart 19.2 summarises assessment and management of urinary incontinence in an elderly person.

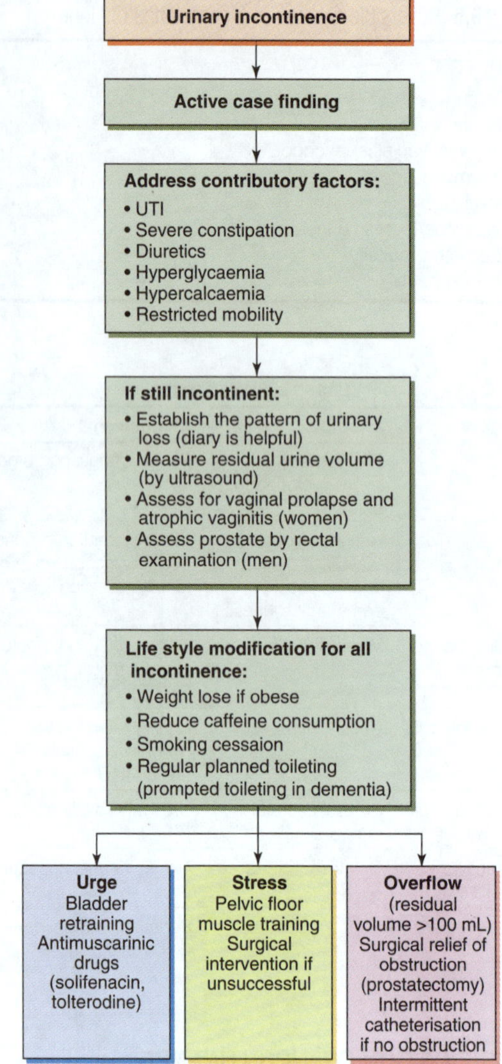

Flowchart 19.2 Approach to Urinary Incontinence. (Based on European Association of Urology Guidelines 2018.)

Q. Describe epidemiology, risk factors, consequences, evaluation and management of falls in the elderly. (IM24.13)

DEFINITION

- An event which results in a person unintentionally and suddenly coming to rest on the ground or on some lower level and not being due to stroke or sustaining violent blow.

EPIDEMIOLOGY

- Falls in older persons occur commonly which may result in injury. However, while treating injuries sustained due to fall, its cause should also be investigated.
- About 30% of individuals over the age of 65 years fall each year while this figure rises to 35% above the age of 85 years. Almost 60% of those with a history of a fall in the previous year will have a subsequent

fall. About 10% of falls result in injury, usually bruises. Significant number of persons also sustain serious injuries including hip fractures, head injury and major lacerations.

RISK FACTORS

- Risk factors for falls in the elderly are given in Table 19.8.
- Medications which predispose to a fall are listed in Table 19.9.

CONSEQUENCES OF FALLS

- Due to falls, there are several effects on the person which are mentioned in Table 19.10.

EVALUATION

- A targeted history and physical examination can identify patients at risk for falling. Try to identify all potential contributing factors by systematic clinical evaluation.
- Goals of evaluation are to identify the following:
  - Reversible physical conditions and environmental factors.
  - Modifiable impairments.
  - Fixed disabilities requiring some degree of compensation.

TABLE 19.8 Risk Factors for Falls in the Elderly

Cause	Examples
Syncope and related causes	Arrhythmias, seizures, acute coronary syndrome, hypoglycaemia, pulmonary embolism
Related to vasodilatation or near-syncope	Dehydration, postural hypotension, medications, haemorrhage, hot bath, sepsis, anaemia
Mechanical causes	Unsafe home conditions (e.g. poor lighting, loose rugs, slippery floor), poor footwear, ankle oedema (legs too heavy to lift)
Auditory or vestibular causes	Reduced hearing, Meniere's disease, benign paroxysmal positional vertigo
Visual causes	Reduced visual acuity, reduced visual field
Carotid sinus	Carotid sinus hypersensitivity
Incontinence	Urge incontinence
Neurological causes	Parkinson's disease, reduced position sense, reduced balance, foot drop, dementia, confusion, medications
Musculoskeletal causes	Arthritis, stiffness of joints, weak muscles, deconditioning due to immobility, frailty
Others	Alcohol, substance use, previous history of fall

TABLE 19.9 Medications Commonly Responsible for Falls in the Elderly

Class	Examples
Antihypertensives	ACE inhibitors, angiotensin receptor blockers, calcium channel blockers, beta-blockers
Diuretics	Hydrochlorothiazide, chlorthalidone, furosemide
Antidepressants	Sertraline, trazodone, amitriptyline, fluoxetine, imipramine
Benzodiazepines	Alprazolam, diazepam, lorazepam, chlordiazepoxide
Antipsychotics	Chlorpromazine, flupentixol, haloperidol, olanzapine, quetiapine, risperidone
Antihistamines	Diphenhydramine, promethazine
Opioids	Morphine, buprenorphine, fentanyl, methadone, oxycodone, tramadol, codeine

TABLE 19.10 Consequences of Falls

Physical problems	• Bruising • Laceration • Fracture • Head injury • Burns (if fall is against a heat convector or radiator) • Dehydration (prolonged lying on ground) • Rhabdomyolysis (prolonged lying on ground) • Death
Mental problems	• Fear of recurrence of fall • Depression • Loss of confidence • Restriction of lifestyle
Immobility	• Reduced activities of daily life • Deconditioning of muscles • Stiffening of joints
Social problems	• Nursing home care • Inability to follow hobbies • Inability to socialise
Financial burden	• Cost of treatment

HISTORY

- The history can be based on the mnemonic 'SPLATT' (Box 19.6).
- In the history, also include risk factors, alcohol intake, medication review and acute illnesses (e.g. dehydration, infection, acute cardiac or neurologic features).

EXAMINATION

- Examine for postural vital signs (pulse and blood pressure), mental state, anaemia, vision, feet and footwear, musculoskeletal abnormalities (e.g. pain, weakness, deformity), cardiovascular features (arrhythmias, heart failure, peripheral oedema), neurological features (focal signs, peripheral neuropathy, proprioception), balance and gait.

DIAGNOSTIC TESTS

- Extensive tests are generally not required.
- Laboratory tests should be guided by history and physical examination.

BOX 19.6 Evaluating a Patient With a History of Fall

- **S**ymptoms before the fall
- **P**revious history of fall
- **L**ocation of fall
- **A**ctivity at the time of fall
- **T**ime when the fall occurred
- **T**rauma sustained after fall

- Radiological imaging may be required if a fracture or head injury is suspected.
- ECG is required if a cardiovascular cause is suspected.

MANAGEMENT

- Multidisciplinary approach is required to manage patients after fall. It mainly involves preventing further falls by targeted interventions to reduce or eliminate risk factors.
- Interventions may be medical, surgical, rehabilitative or environmental (Table 19.11).

TABLE 19.11 Targeted Interventions to Prevent Falls

Intervention	Examples
Postural hypotension	• Elevation of head of bed • Discontinuation of high-risk medications • Use of pressure stockings
Exercise programs	• Strength training • Balance, gait and coordination training
Vision impairment	• Formal assessment of vision • Conditions such as cataracts should be treated
Modification of home environment	• Removal of identified risks • Installation of safety equipment (e.g. grab bars) • Improvement in lighting
Foot and footwear problems	• Treatment of foot problems such as bunions, deformities or ulcers • Appropriate footwear (e.g., low heel, high surface contact)
Gait impairment	• Gait training • Assistive devices • Balance exercises
Multiple medications	• Minimise medications as far as possible • Emphasis on reducing dose if medication cannot be eliminated • Prioritise psychotropic medications for review and discontinuation or reduction
Sedatives	• Education about sleep hygiene • Discontinue sedatives

Q. Discuss frailty in the elderly.

DEFINITION

- Frailty is characterised by a decrease in strength, endurance, physical ability and physiological processes, which result in an increased risk of vulnerability to disease, dependence and death.
- Frail adults are at increased risk of falls, disability, hospitalisation, admission to long-term care and death.

PARADIGMS OF FRAILTY

- Conceptually, frailty can be defined in two forms as illustrated in Fig. 19.4.
  - Physical or phenotypic or syndromic frailty captures specific signs and symptoms of older individuals who are vulnerable to adverse health outcomes. These signs and symptoms include fatigue, low activity, weakness, weight loss and slow walking speed.
  - Deficit accumulation frailty or frailty index is a conceptual framework that identifies the most frail, vulnerable older adults through cumulative comorbidities, social illnesses and disabilities as frail.

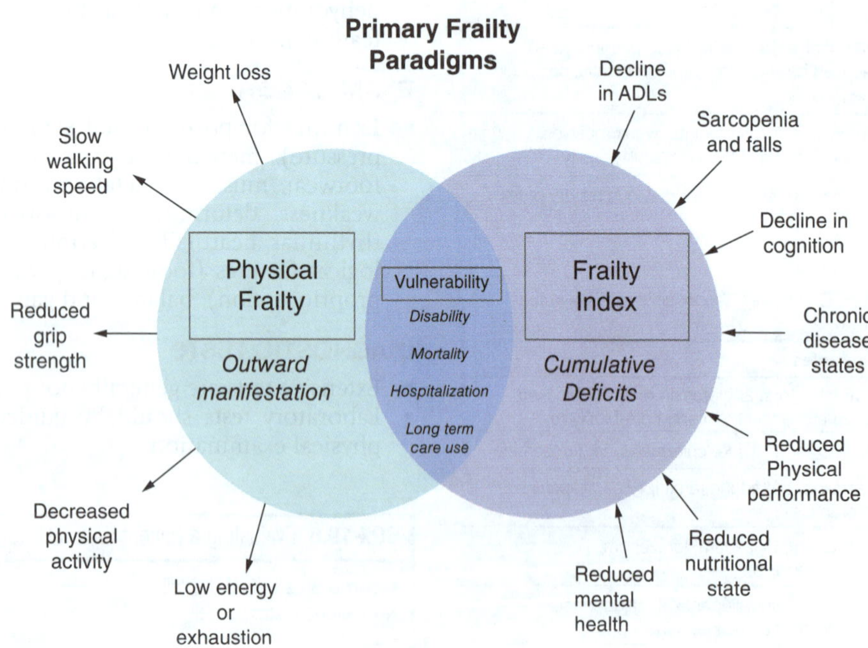

Fig. 19.4 This Venn diagram is a representation of the two major frailty paradigms. Phenotypical or physical frailty is more defined by external manifestations whereas the frailty index views frailty more as an accumulation of deficits. Both share the commonality of increased vulnerability in this population. ADLs, activities of daily living.

PATHOPHYSIOLOGY

- Endocrine, immune and stress responses are important in the development of frailty.

ENDOCRINE SYSTEM

- Decreased growth hormone and insulin-like growth factor-1 (IGF-1) are associated with lower strength and decreased mobility.
- Decreased dehydroepiandrosterone (DHEA) sulphate (normally, it plays a role in maintaining muscle mass and prevents activation of inflammatory pathways) that contribute to muscle decline.
- Increased cortisol levels which may impact skeletal muscle and immune system components.
- Decreased sex steroids may also contribute to frailty.

INFLAMMATION AND IMMUNE SYSTEM

- Levels of IL-6 and CRP are elevated which may impact skeletal muscle, appetite, adaptive immune system function and cognition, and contribute to anaemia.
- Activation of immune system may trigger clotting cascade which has a correlation with frailty.

OTHER STRESS RESPONSES

- Other alterations include altered glucose metabolism, dysregulation of autonomic nervous system and age-related changes in renin-angiotensin system and in mitochondria. These may impact sarcopaenia (progressive loss of skeletal muscle mass, strength and power) and inflammation which are important components of frailty.

SUMMARY OF PATHOPHYSIOLOGY OF FRAILTY

- Pathophysiology of frailty is summarised in Flowchart 19.3.

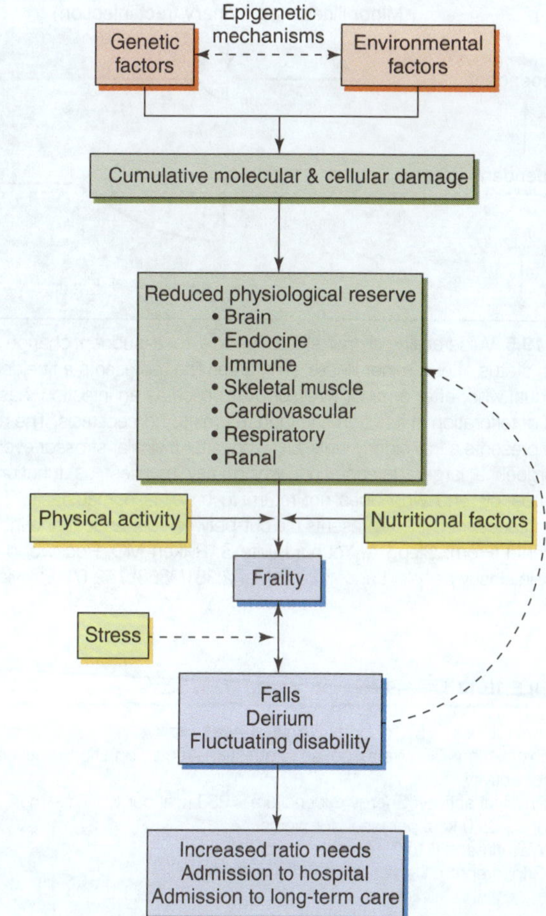

Flowchart 19.3 Pathophysiology of Frailty. (From: Clegg A, Young J, Iliffe S, Rikkert MO, Rockwood K. Frailty in elderly people. Lancet. 2013 Mar 2;381(9868):752-62. Elsevier).

CLINICAL PRESENTATION

NON-SPECIFIC FEATURES

- Extreme fatigue, unexplained weight loss and frequent infections.

FALLS

- Balance and gait impairment are major features of frailty, and are important risk factors for falls.
- 'Hot fall' is related to a minor illness that reduces postural balance below a crucial threshold necessary to maintain gait integrity.
- Spontaneous falls occur in more severe frailty when vital postural systems (vision, balance and strength) are no longer consistent with safe navigation through straightforward environments. These are typically repeated and are closely associated with the psychological reaction of fear of further falls that causes the patient to develop severely impaired mobility.

DELIRIUM

- Delirium is related to reduced integrity of brain function and is independently associated with adverse outcomes.

FLUCTUATING DISABILITY

- Fluctuating disability is day-to-day instability, resulting in patients with 'good', independent days, and 'bad' days on which care is often needed.

EFFECT OF MINOR STRESSOR

- Figure 19.5 demonstrates the effect of minor stressor in the elderly. A frail individual after a minor stressor event, undergoes a larger deterioration, which may manifest as functional dependency, and who does not return to baseline homeostasis.

ASSESSMENT OF FRAILTY

ASSESSMENT OF PHENOTYPIC FRAILTY

- There are several frailty assessment methods of which Fried Phenotype or Fried Frailty Score is most often used.
- Fried Phenotype or Fried Frailty Score has five criteria, each given one point. It classifies older adults as frail (score 3–5), prefrail (score 1 to 2) or nonfrail (score 0) (Table 19.12).

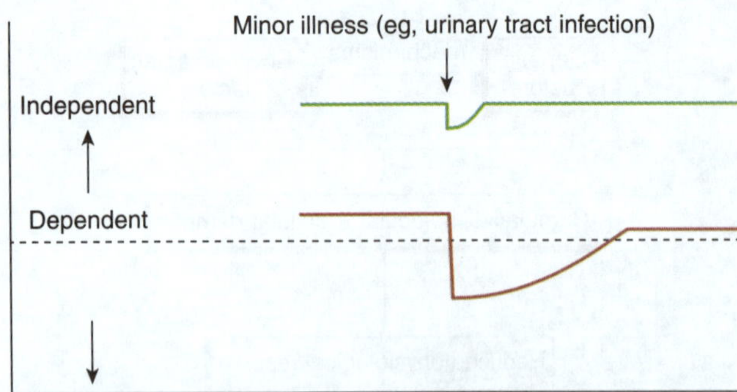

Fig. 19.5 Vulnerability of frail elderly people to a sudden change in health status after a minor illness. (The green line represents a fit elderly individual who, after a minor stressor event such as an infection, has a small deterioration in function and then returns to homeostasis. The red line represents a frail elderly individual who, after a similar stressor event, undergoes a larger deterioration, which may manifest as functional dependency, and who does not return to baseline homeostasis. The horizontal-dashed line represents the cut-between dependent and independent.) (From: Clegg A, Young J, Iliffe S, Rikkert MO, Rockwood K. Frailty in elderly people. Lancet. 2013 Mar 2;381(9868):752-62. Elsevier).

TABLE 19.12 Fried Phenotype or Fried Frailty Score

- Weight loss: ≥5% of body weight in last 1 year
- Exhaustion: Positive response to questions regarding effort required for activity
- Physical activity: Energy expenditure <383 kcal per week for men and <270 kcal per week for women
- Walk time: >6 to 7 seconds to walk 15 feet
- Grip strength: Decreased hand grip strength

ASSESSMENT OF DEFICIT ACCUMULATION FRAILTY OR FRAILTY INDEX

- This is based on the accumulation of illnesses, functional and cognitive declines, and social situations that are added together to calculate frailty. It requires answering 20 or more medical and functional-related questions.

LABORATORY TESTING

- Evaluation of a frail person should include certain laboratory investigations in order to rule out treatable conditions (Box 19.7).

MANAGEMENT

- A variety of interventions are important in the prevention or reduction of frailty (Box 19. 8).

BOX 19.7 Laboratory Investigations in a Frail Elderly

- Complete blood count
- Basic metabolic panel
- Liver biochemical tests including albumin
- Vitamin B_{12}
- Vitamin D
- Thyroid-stimulating hormone

BOX 19.8 Interventions in Frail Elderly

- Exercises improve mobility, enhance performance of activities of daily living (ADLs), improve gait, decrease falls, improve bone mineral density and increase general wellbeing
- Occupational therapy improves ability to perform ADLs
- Nutritional supplementation if weight loss is significant component of frailty; oral nutritional supplements between meals helpful
- Medication review and deprescribing, substituting a therapy with a potentially safer agent, or changing drug dose
- Address acute precipitating illness early

- General use of vitamin D as treatment for frailty is still controversial.
- There is no role of testosterone, growth hormone or DHEA sulphate supplementation.

Q. Write a short note of failure to thrive in the elderly.

- Failure to thrive in the elderly is defined as a syndrome of weight loss, decreased appetite, poor nutrition and inactivity, often accompanied by dehydration, depressive symptoms, impaired immune function and low cholesterol.
- It may be caused by a single disease (e.g. cancer, hypothyroidism) and management involves treatment of that particular disease.
- More often, failure of thrive is due to multiple factors such as medical comorbidities, medications and psychological factors. In these cases, it is important to recognise these factors and treat them so as to improve quality of life.
- Failure to thrive results from interaction of three components: frailty, disability (basic and instrumental activities of daily life) and impaired neuropsychiatric function (mainly dementia and depression).
- The history should be obtained from the patient and their caregivers. In addition to a complete history and review of symptoms, the clinician should explore timing of symptom onset and progression, prescription and over-the-counter medication use, substance abuse, functional status, depression and cognitive issues, and social history. Signs of elder abuse and neglect should be kept in mind.
- A comprehensive medical examination should be done to assess for any underlying cause.
- Laboratory investigations should be based on suspected underlying diseases.
- Management involves treatment of underlying condition and controlling symptoms contributing to failure to thrive. A multidisciplinary team including social worker, dietitian, dentist, and physical, occupational and speech therapists to address symptoms is important in management. Medication side effects should be critically looked for.

Q. Write a short note on drug prescription in the elderly.

Q. Write a short note on polypharmacy.

PROCESS OF PRESCRIPTION

- The process of prescribing a medication is complex and includes several components (Box 19.9).
- If a new symptom develops while the patient has been started on a drug, it should be considered to be drug related until proven otherwise.

BOX 19.9 Process of Prescribing a Drug

- Deciding that a drug is indicated
- Choosing the best among available drugs
- Determining dose, schedule and duration appropriate for the disease and patient's physiologic status
- Monitoring for effectiveness of drug
- Monitoring for toxicity of drug
- Educating the patient about expected side effects of drug

CHALLENGES OF DRUG PRESCRIPTION IN THE ELDERLY

- There are several challenges of prescribing drugs in the elderly:
- Drug trials often exclude older people.
- Approved doses may not be appropriate for older people.
- Age-related changes in pharmacokinetics (absorption, distribution, metabolism and excretion) (Fig. 19.6).
  - An increased volume of distribution may result from the proportional increase in body fat relative to skeletal muscle with ageing. Decreased drug clearance may result from the natural decline in renal function with age. Larger drug storage reservoirs and decreased clearance prolong drug half-lives and lead to increased plasma drug concentrations in older people.
- Age-related changes in pharmacodynamics (physiologic effects of the drug).

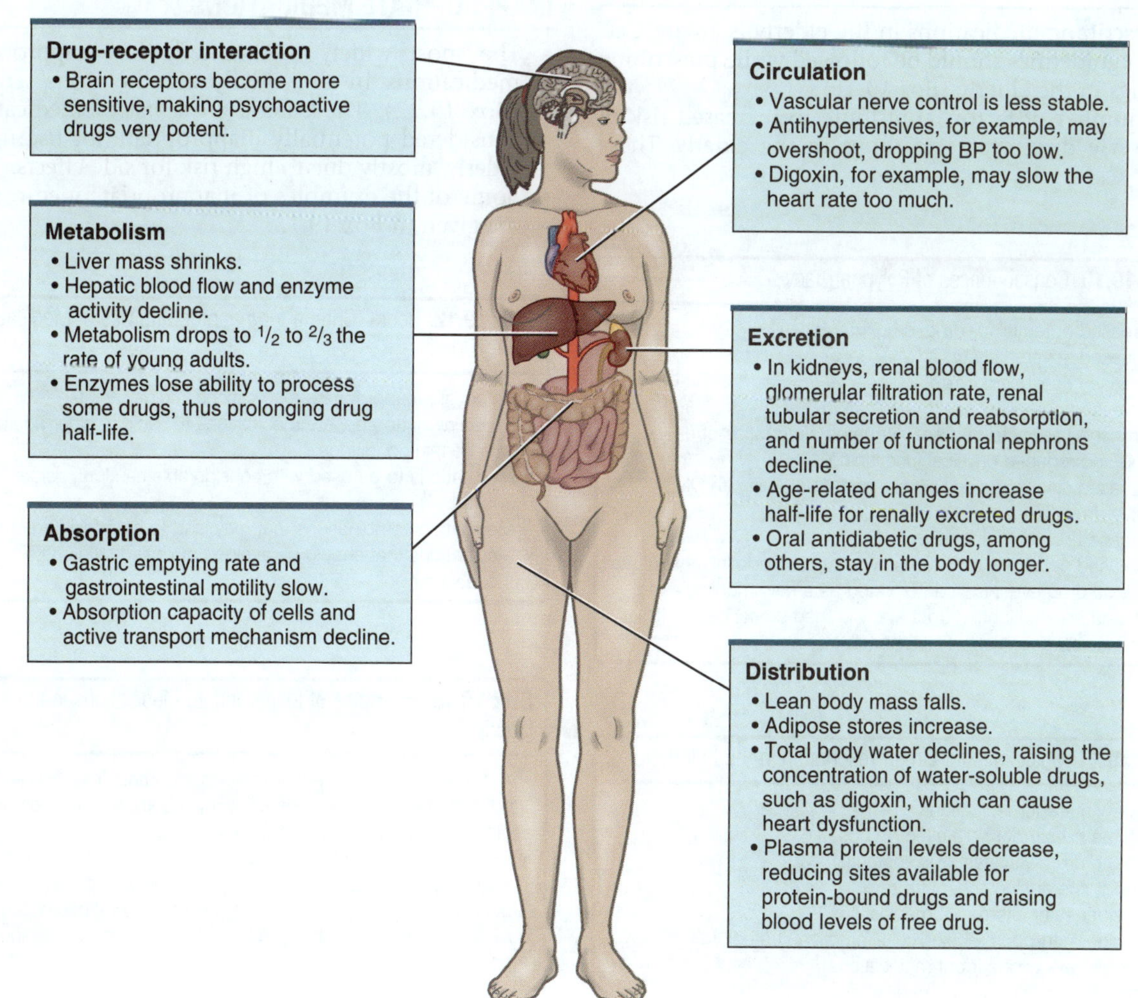

Fig. 19.6 Effects of ageing on pharmacokinetics of drugs.

POLYPHARMACY

- Polypharmacy is defined as administration of ≥5 drugs during a 3-month period. It can be appropriate or problematic.
- While polypharmacy most commonly refers to prescribed medications, it is important to also consider over-the-counter and herbal/supplements used.

APPROPRIATE POLYPHARMACY

- Administration of ≥5 drugs for complex or multiple conditions when drug use has been optimised and where drugs are prescribed according to the best evidence.

PROBLEMATIC POLYPHARMACY

- Administration of ≥5 drugs inappropriately or when intended benefits of drugs are not realised.

CONSEQUENCES OF POLYPHARMACY

- Consequences of polypharmacy are mentioned in Box 19.10.

GUIDELINES FOR DRUG PRESCRIPTION IN THE ELDERLY

- Prescribing medications in the elderly is an art. Certain guidelines should be followed while prescribing drugs in the elderly (Box 19.11).
- A number of factors contribute to increased risk of adverse drug events to drugs in the elderly. These include frailty, comorbidities, memory issues and use of multiple prescribed and nonprescribed medications.

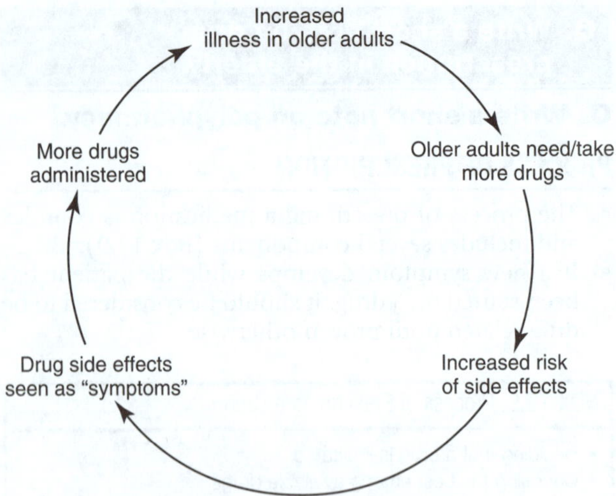

Flowchart 19.4 Vicious Cycle of Drug Administration.

INAPPROPRIATE MEDICATIONS

- The most widely used criteria for inappropriate medications in the elderly are the Beers' criteria (Box 19.12). The criteria are a list of medications considered potentially inappropriate for use in the elderly, mostly due to high risk for side effects.
- Some of the examples of inappropriate medications are given in Box 19.13.

BOX 19.10 Consequences of Polypharmacy

- Increased potential for drug–drug interactions
- Increased adverse effects
- Increased healthcare costs
- Decreased compliance with medications
- Diminished ability to perform instrumental activities of daily living and reduced physical functioning
- Increased risk of falls and subsequent fractures with CNS-active drugs
- Increased risk of malnutrition
- Increased possibility of 'vicious cycle of drug administration' (an adverse drug event is misinterpreted as a new medical condition and an additional drug therapy is then prescribed to 'treat' this medical condition—Flowchart 19.4)

BOX 19.11 Guidelines for Drug Prescription in the Elderly

- Review current medications
- Use the lowest possible effective dose
- Use the drug with least toxic potential
- Simplify the dosing schedule
- Consider safer alternative medications
- Consider non-pharmacological alternative strategies
- Periodic review of current medications
- Discontinue unnecessary medications
- Prescribe beneficial drugs
- Consider adverse drug events for any new symptom

BOX 19.12 Beers' Criteria for Inappropriate Use of Medications in the Elderly

- Potentially inappropriate medications in older adults
- Potentially inappropriate medications to avoid in older adults with certain conditions
- Medications to be used with considerable caution in older adults
- Medication combinations that may lead to harmful interactions
- Medications that should be avoided or dosed differently in those with poor renal function

BOX 19.13 Examples of Inappropriate Medications in the Elderly

- Avoid first generation antihistamines (clearance reduced with advanced age; risk of confusion, dry mouth, constipation and other anticholinergic effects or toxicity)
- Avoid nitrofurantoin for long-term suppression if creatine clearance is less than 30 mL/minute/1.73 m^2 due to potential for pulmonary toxicity, hepatotoxicity and peripheral neuropathy
- Avoid proton pump inhibitors for >8 weeks (unless for high-risk patients, erosive oesophagitis, Barrett's oesophagitis, pathological hypersecretory condition or demonstrated need for maintenance treatment) due to risk of *Clostridium difficile* infection, bone loss and fractures

BOX 19.13 Examples of Inappropriate Medications in the Elderly—cont'd

- Avoid the concurrent use of opioids with either benzodiazepines or gabapentinoids, due to increased risk of overdose and severe sedation-related adverse events
- Use caution when prescribing aspirin for primary prevention of cardiovascular disease in patients age 70 years or older due to increased risk of bleeding
- Use caution when prescribing trimethoprim-sulphamethoxazole in patients who are taking an angiotensin-converting enzyme inhibitor or angiotensin receptor blocker, and who have decreased creatinine clearance so as to avoid hyperkalaemia
- Avoid use of serotonin-norepinephrine reuptake inhibitors in patients with a history of falls or fractures as these agents increase risk of fractures
- Avoid use of sliding-scale short-acting insulin regimens according to blood glucose levels due to the risk of hypoglycaemia unless patients are also on long-acting insulin

Q. Write a short note on nutritional assessment in an older person. (IM24.22)

- Ageing is characterised by diminished organ system reserves of various nutrients. Malnutrition is associated with increased mortality.
- The term malnutrition includes undernutrition as well as overnutrition. However, in common usage, it means undernutrition only.

DIAGNOSTIC CRITERIA FOR MALNUTRITION

- Presence of two out of six criteria listed in Box 19.14 indicates a diagnosis of malnutrition.

SCREENING FOR NUTRITIONAL STATUS

- Screening for nutritional status can be done by assessing weight, weight loss and utilising screening tools.

WEIGHT

- A weight below 80% of the recommended body weight is considered as low body weight.

WEIGHT LOSS

- A weight loss of 2% over a period of 1 month, 5% over 3 months and 10% over 6 months is considered significant.

BOX 19.14 Diagnostic Criteria for Malnutrition

- Insufficient energy intake
- Weight loss
- Loss of muscle mass
- Loss of subcutaneous fat
- Localised or generalised fluid accumulation that may mask weight loss
- Diminished functional status as measured by handgrip strength

SCREENING TOOLS

- Several screening tools are available to identify older adults at risk for poor nutrition. One of the most commonly used tools is Mini Nutritional Assessment. It consists of a global assessment and subjective perception of health, as well as questions specific to diet and a series of body measurements.

CAUSES OF MALNUTRITION

- The most important reasons for malnutrition in the elderly are as follows:
  - Inadequate dietary intake (due to poverty, isolation, depression, malignancy, dementia, edentulism, dysphagia, reduced taste and smell sensitivity, early satiety).
    - Older people who eat in the presence of others consume more than those who eat alone.
  - Anorexia (affected by diseases, dementia, drugs, mood disorders, changes in taste).
  - Sarcopaenia (loss of muscle mass, strength and performance; due to disuse, changing endocrine function, chronic diseases, inflammation, insulin resistance and nutritional deficiencies).
  - Cachexia (due to inflammatory effects of disease including cancer, chronic kidney disease, chronic pulmonary disease, heart failure and others; elevated levels of IL-1, IL-6, and TNF-alpha seen).

EVALUATION OF WEIGHT LOSS

- Evaluation starts with documentation of weight loss followed by evaluation of appetite and dietary intake.
- A complete history including oral symptoms, and physical examination including a complete oral examination are performed.
- Baseline investigations include a basic chemistry profile including glucose and electrolytes, thyroid-stimulating hormone, complete blood count, and C-reactive protein if cachexia is suspected.
- Chest and plain abdomen radiographs may be considered.
- If these are noncontributory, CT chest and abdomen may be required.
- Upper gastrointestinal endoscopy is indicated for patients with early satiety.

EVALUATION OF SARCOPAENIA

- A four-step diagnostic approach is recommended for sarcopaenia:
  1. SARC-F (strength, assistance in walking, rise from chair, climb stairs, falls) questionnaire.
  2. Muscle strength assessment by grip strength or chair stand test.
  3. Confirmation of sarcopaenia via decreased muscle quantity or quality on dual energy X-ray (DXA), CT or MRI.
  4. Severity assessment by physical performance (e.g. locomotion-related whole-body function—as measured by gait speed, timed up and go, short physical performance battery or 400 m walk).

TREATMENT

- Treatment of underlying condition.
- Nutritional repletion to restore the patient to a target weight.
- Role of appetite stimulants is controversial. These agents include megestrol acetate and dronabinol.

Q. Describe elder abuse. (IM24.19)

- WHO defines elder abuse as, 'a single or repeated act, or lack of appropriate action, occurring within any relationship where there is an expectation of trust which causes harm or distress to an older person'.
- Elder abuse is unfortunately common, affecting 5%–10% of community dwelling older adults each year. Nursing home residents are at even higher risk. Abuse leads to increased mortality.

MAJOR TYPES OF ELDER ABUSE

- Abuse includes physical abuse, sexual abuse, neglect, psychological abuse and financial exploitation (Table 19.13).

POTENTIAL RISK FACTORS FOR ELDER ABUSE (Box 19.15)

BOX 19.15 Elder Abuse: Risk Factors

- Female
- Functional dependence or disability
- Poor physical health
- Cognitive impairment
- Low income/socio-economic status
- Social isolation/low social support
- Previous history of family violence
- Previous traumatic event exposure
- Substance use

REASONS FOR ABUSE (Box 19.16)

BOX 19.16 Elder Abuse: Reasons

- Mental illness
- Substance use
- Caregiver stress
- Previous history of family violence
- Financial dependence on older adult
- Lack of social support

INDICATORS OF ELDER ABUSE (Box 19.17)

BOX 19.17 Elder Abuse: Indicators

- Conflicting accounts of events given by older adult and caregiver
- Caregiver interrupts/answers for the older adult
- Delay between occurrence of injury/physical ailment and presentation
- Inconsistencies between an observed injury and associated explanation
- Past history of frequent injuries
- Recurrent visits to the emergency department for similar injuries
- Unexplained malnutrition
- Lack of appropriate hygiene
- Failure of medical condition to improve despite appropriate prescription of treatment
- Older adult seems fearful of or hostile towards caregiver
- Caregiver appears unengaged/inattentive in caring for the older adult
- Caregiver appears frustrated, tired, angry or burdened by the older adult
- Caregiver appears to lack knowledge of the older adult's needs
- Caregiver appears to be ignorant of medical problems or treatments of older adults he/she is directly caring for
- Using multiple physicians and emergency departments for care rather than one primary care physician

TABLE 19.13 Major Forms of Elder Abuse

Type	Definition	Examples
Physical abuse	Intentional use of physical force that may result in bodily injury, physical pain or impairment	• Slapping, hitting, kicking, pushing, burning, pulling hair • Use of physical restraints
Sexual abuse	Any type of sexual contact with an elderly person that is non-consensual or when person is incapable of giving consent	• Sexual assault (rape, sodomy) • Sexually explicit photographing • Unwanted touching • Indecent exposure
Neglect	Refusal or failure to fulfill any part of a person's obligations or duties to an elder, which may result in harm (intentional or unintentional)	• Withholding food, water, clothing, shelter, medications • Failure to ensure elder's personal hygiene or to provide physical aids (e.g. walker, cane, glasses, hearing aids, dentures) • Failure to ensure elder's personal safety • Not taking an elder to his/her doctor's appointments • Not assisting an elder with his/her daily activities which he/she cannot do himself/herself
Psychological and emotional abuse	Intentional infliction of anguish, pain or distress through verbal or nonverbal acts	• Verbal harassment or intimidation • Threats of punishment • Isolating the older person from others
Financial and material exploitation	Illegal or improper use of an older adult's money, property or assets	• Stealing money or belongings • Cashing an older person's cheques without permission and/or forging his or her signature • Coercing an older adult into signing contracts, changing a will, or assigning durable power of attorney against his or her wishes or when the older adult does not possess the mental capacity to do so

PHYSICAL SIGNS SUSPICIOUS FOR POTENTIAL ELDER ABUSE (Box 19.18)

BOX 19.18 Elder Abuse: Physical Signs Suspicious of Abuse

- Bruising in atypical locations (not over bony prominences but on lateral arms, back, face, ears or neck)
- Patterned injuries (bite marks or injury consistent with the shape of a belt buckle, fingertip or other object)
- Wrist or ankle lesions or scars (suggesting inappropriate restraint)
- Burns (particularly stocking/glove pattern suggesting forced immersion or cigarette pattern)
- Multiple fractures or bruises of different ages
- Traumatic alopecia or scalp hematomas
- Subconjunctival, vitreous or retinal ophthalmic haemorrhages
- Intraoral soft tissue injuries

MANAGEMENT

- Treatment initially should focus on correcting the acute presenting problem or injury. However, it is crucial to address the social and psychological components of elder abuse as well. Social interventions may include coordinating home health services, meal delivery, transportation for appointments, helping set up insurance, or connecting the older adult with old age centres.
- If the patient is in immediate danger, it is vital to protect the patient. This action could require the involvement of law enforcement or hospital security.

Q. Discuss briefly about therapies to delay the process of ageing.

- Ageing is a process characterised by numerous pathologies, the sum of which inevitably leads to death and its biology by loss of homeostasis and the accumulation of molecular damage.
- Although advances aiming at curing ageing are being made, none is existing as of now. Research is ongoing to prolong healthy life.

EXPERIMENTAL THERAPIES TO DELAY AGEING

RESTRICTION OF CALORIES

- Restricting calories has been shown to extend lifespan in laboratory animals. This may be related to an increased formation of free radicals within the mitochondria, which causes a secondary induction of increased antioxidant defence capacity. Another postulation is that limited calorie availability may result in optimisation of metabolism. Caloric restriction also induces alterations at hormonal and proteomic levels which may delay ageing.

STEM CELL THERAPIES

- Stem cells have been used experimentally in a large number of conditions. Depletion of stem cells are considered to play a role in ageing. However, there is no evidence to suggest that stem cell therapies will delay ageing process.

RESTRICTION OF ADVANCED GLYCATION END-PRODUCTS

- Intervention studies have demonstrated that high intake of advanced glycation end-products (AGEs) correlates with tissue damage which can be prevented by restriction of dietary AGEs. A number of agents which either block action of AGEs or blocker reactions leading to formation of AGEs have been studied. These agents include aminoguanidine, benfotiamine, aspirin, metformin and inhibitors of the renin-angiotensin system. However, none has been found to delay ageing process.

HORMONAL THERAPIES

- Since patients with deficiencies of growth hormone (GH) and IGF-1 exhibit signs of early ageing, GH has been used as an anti-ageing treatment. Although GH therapy may increase muscle mass and libido, and strengthen the immune system, it can produce several side effects. At present, it is not recommended to delay the ageing.

ANTIOXIDANTS

- Antioxidants help the cells to ward off the bad effects of reactive oxygen species (ROS) on lipids, proteins and nucleic acids. The most common antioxidants include vitamins A, C and E, as well as the co-enzyme Q10. However, no large study has shown any beneficial effect of these antioxidants in delaying ageing process.

TELOMERE-BASED THERAPIES

- A few in vitro studies have shown that telomere extension can increase cell proliferative capacity and reverse tissue degeneration. Some commercial kits are available which can measure telomere length with the aim of estimating biological age of individuals. There is a theoretical possibility of its use in delaying human ageing process. However, telomerase expression has been linked to promotion of tumour growth and cell proliferation.

MISCELLANEOUS THERAPIES

- A few other therapies are being investigated to delay the process of ageing. These include the use of rapamycin (an immunosuppressant), increasing expression of the klotho gene by resveratrol, and supplementation with precursors of the oxidised form of cellular nicotinamide adenine dinucleotide. Perhaps the most futuristic anti-ageing therapy is nanotechnology. An example of use of nanotechnology to delay ageing is the use of capped silica nanoparticles which can selectively release drugs in aged human cells and has enormous potential in the treatment of a myriad of diseases, namely, cancer or Alzheimer's disease.

20 Clinical Pharmacology

Q. Describe adverse drug reactions. (PH 1.7)

Q. Write a short note on pharmacovigilance in India.

DEFINITIONS

- Adverse drug reaction (ADR) is defined as unwanted or harmful reaction to a drug which is unintended, and which occurs at doses normally used for the prophylaxis, diagnosis, or therapy of disease, or for the modification of physiological function.
- ADR is also defined as an undesirable effect, reasonably associated with the use of a drug that may occur as a part of the pharmacological action of a drug or may be unpredictable in its occurrence.
    - Serious adverse reaction is an ADR that results in death, requires hospital admission or prolongation of existing hospital stay, results in persistent or significant disability/incapacity, or is life threatening.
- Adverse drug event (ADE) is any untoward medical occurrence that may be present during treatment with a pharmaceutical product but which does not necessarily have a causal relationship with this treatment.
    - ADRs occur despite appropriate prescribing and dosing, whereas ADEs may also be associated with inappropriate use of the drug or other confounders that occur during drug therapy but are not necessarily caused by the pharmacology of the drug itself.
- Side effect is any unintended effect of a pharmaceutical product occurring at doses normally used by a patient which is related to the pharmacological properties of the drug.
- A medication error is any preventable event that has the potential to lead to inappropriate medication use or patient harm.

MAGNITUDE

- ADRs are one of the leading causes of morbidity and mortality in health care.
- The Institute of Medicine (USA) reported in 2000 that between 44,000 and 98,000 deaths occur annually from medical errors and of these, an estimated 7000 deaths occur due to ADRs.
- Approximately 5% of all hospital admissions are due to ADRs and 5%–10% of hospitalised patients will experience an ADR during their hospital stay.
- In 2008, in Europe, 197,000 deaths per year were attributed to ADRs.

FACTORS AFFECTING OCCURRENCE OF ADVERSE DRUG REACTIONS (Box 20.1)

BOX 20.1 Factors Affecting Occurrence of Adverse Drug Reactions

- Patient characteristics—gender, age, weight, maternity status, creatinine clearance, number of comorbidities, genetic factors
- Drug related—dosage, administration route, number of concomitant drugs
- Social factors—alcohol drinking, race and ethnicity, smoking
- Disease-related factors

CAUSE–EFFECT RELATIONSHIP OF ADVERSE DRUG REACTIONS (Box 20.2)

BOX 20.2 Cause–Effect Relationship of ADR

- Definite—a reaction that follows a reasonable temporal sequence from administration of the drug, and that is confirmed by improvement on stopping the drug (dechallenge), and reappearance of the reaction on repeated exposure (rechallenge)
- Probable—a reaction that follows a reasonable temporal sequence from administration of the drug, that is confirmed by dechallenge and that could not be reasonably explained by the known characteristics of the patient's clinical state
- Possible—a reaction that follows a reasonable temporal sequence from administration of the drug, but that could have been produced by the patient's clinical state or other modes of therapy administered to the patient
- Unlikely—any reaction that does not meet the criteria above

SEVERITY OF ADVESRE DRUG REACTION

- ADRs are classified by severity from minor to severe, as defined in Table 20.1.

CLASSIFICATION OF ADVERSE DRUG REACTIONS

- Different methods can be used to classify ADRs. One of the commonly used classification is shown in Table 20.2.

TYPES OF ADVERSE DRUG REACTIONS

- ADRs may be related to the pharmacologic or pharmacodynamic properties of drugs which can be used to classify the types of reaction that occurs.
  - Idiosyncrasy: An uncharacteristic response of a patient to a drug, usually not occurring on administration. It is genetically determined. Examples include phenobarbitone causing excitement; streptomycin causing deafness with single dose; DRESS (drug reaction with eosinophilia and systemic symptoms) syndrome with various drugs.
  - Hypersensitivity or allergy: A reaction, not explained by the pharmacologic effects of the drug, caused by altered reactivity of the patient and generally considered to be an allergic manifestation. Prior sensitisation is often required. Chemically related drugs may show cross-sensitivity. Drugs can produce four types of hypersensitivity.
    - Type I: Immediate in onset and mediated by IgE and mast cells and/or basophils. Presentation is with urticaria, angioedema, anaphylaxis. Commonly implicated drugs include beta-lactam drugs (penicillins and cephalosporins) and quinolones.
    - Type II: Delayed in onset and caused by antibody-mediated cell destruction. Presentation is with haemolytic anaemia (drugs include cephalosporins, penicillins, NSAIDs, quinine), thrombocytopenia (drugs include heparin, quinine, beta-lactam antibiotics, NSAIDs), and neutropenia (drug includes propylthiouracil).
    - Type III: Delayed in onset and caused by antibody:drug immune complex deposition

TABLE 20.1 Classification Based on Severity: ADR

Severity	Description	Examples
Minor	• No antidote, therapy or prolongation of hospitalisation is required in response to the ADR	• Antidepressants: dry mouth • Antihistamines: mild drowsiness
Moderate	• The management of the ADR requires a change in drug therapy, specific treatment or an increase in hospitalisation by at least 1 day	• Hormonal contraceptives: venous thrombosis • NSAIDs: hypertension, oedema • ACE inhibitor: cough • Opioids: constipation
Severe	• The ADR is potentially life threatening, causing permanent damage or requiring intensive medical care	• ACE inhibitors: angioedema • Azithromycin: Torsades de pointes
Lethal	• The ADR directly or indirectly contributes to the death of the patient	• Acetaminophen overdosage: acute liver failure • Anticoagulants: intracranial haemorrhage

TABLE 20.2 Classification of Adverse Drug Reactions

Type of ADR	Type of Effect	Characteristics	Examples	Management
Type A	Augmented	• Dose related • Low mortality • Predictable • Comprise 80% of all ADRs	• Orthostatic hypotension with antihypertensive medications • Respiratory depression with opioids • Bleeding with warfarin • Sedation with antihistamines • Anticholinergic effects of tricyclic antidepressants	• Dose reduction • Withdrawal of drug if necessary • Evaluation of effects of concomitant therapy
Type B	Bizarre	• Non-dose related • High mortality • Unpredictable • Comprise 10%–15% of all ADRs	• Hypersensitivity reactions such as anaphylaxis to penicillin • Idiosyncratic reactions such as malignant hyperthermia with halothane • Aplastic anaemia caused by chloramphenicol	• Withdrawal of the drug • Avoidance of same drug in the future
Type C	Chronic	• Cumulative dose related • Time related	• Hypothalamic–pituitary–adrenal axis suppression by corticosteroids • Osteonecrosis of jaw with bisphosphates	• Dose reduction • Withdrawal of drug if necessary
Type D	Delayed	• Often dose and time related	• Tardive dyskinesia • Teratogenesis • Carcinogenesis	• Often non-treatable
Type E	End of use	• Related to withdrawal of drug	• Myocardial ischaemia after β-blocker discontinuation • Withdrawal syndrome in opiates or benzodiazepines users	• Slow withdrawal • Reintroduction of the drug
Type F	Failure	• Dose related • Drug interactions related	• Inadequate action of an oral contraceptive if used with an enzyme inducer • Resistance to antimicrobial agents	• Increase of dosage • Evaluation of effects of concomitant therapy and drug interaction

and complement activation. Presentation is with arthralgias, lymphadenopathy and vasculitis. Commonly implicated drugs include antitoxins, penicillins, cephalosporins, sulphonamides, phenytoin and allopurinol.
  - Type IV: Delayed in onset and T cell mediated. Presentation is with contact dermatitis, photosensitivity, Stevens–Johnson syndrome/toxic epidermal necrolysis and DRESS. Implicated drugs include locally applied medications, carbamazepine, abacavir, dapsone and sulphonamides.
- Drug-induced autoimmunity: Drugs can induce autoimmune diseases. For example, SLE can be induced by procainamide, phenytoin, isoniazid and hydralazine.
- Intolerance: A characteristic pharmacologic effect of a drug produced by an unusually small dose so that the usual dose tends to induce a massive overaction. For example, only a few doses of carbamazepine may produce ataxia.
- Drug interaction: An unusual pharmacologic response that could not be explained by the action of a single drug, but was caused by two or more drugs.
- Pharmacologic: A known, inherent pharmacologic effect of a drug, directly related to dose. For example, atropine is used in pre-anaesthesia as antisecretory medication due to its anticholinergic effect.
- Photosensitivity:
  - Phototoxic: In this, drug accumulates in skin where it absorbs light, producing photochemical reaction and tissue damage. For example, tetracyclines can produce skin erythema and blistering on sun exposure.
  - Photoallergic: Drug accumulation in skin stimulates cell-mediated immune response which produces contact dermatitis on sun exposure. For example, griseofulvin and sulphonamides.
- Drug dependence: Patient develops drug craving and withdrawal features.
- Teratogenicity: Drugs used during pregnancy (especially first trimester) produce congenital malformations in the foetus. Examples include thalidomide producing phocomelia, phenytoin producing foetal hydantoin syndrome (microcephaly, hypoplastic distal phalanges, cardiac defects, cleft lip, etc.).
- Carcinogenicity and mutagenicity: Drugs produce mutations and cancers.
- Drug withdrawal reactions: If a drug is used for long duration, withdrawal may produce reactions. For example, withdrawal of beta-blockers may produce hypertension; withdrawal of corticosteroid may produce adrenal insufficiency.

PREVENTING ADVERSE DRUG REACTIONS

- Important steps in preventing or reducing ADRs are the following:
  - Identification of the group of individuals who are probably more susceptible to the adverse effect and accordingly modification in the treatment plan.
  - A patient's medication history helps in identifying any previous ADRs and therefore prevents re-exposure to the drug.
  - Patient's susceptibility helps in making the decision for prescribing the right drug of choice. For this, factors which affect the susceptibility such as age, gender, pregnancy status and racism can help predict the risk of an ADR occurrence. Using right dose, route and frequency based on such factors is important.
- Ensuring that the treatment plan alleviates any possible adverse effects. For example:
  - Co-prescription of folic acid with methotrexate will reduce the incidence of adverse effects associated with folate deficiency.
  - Monitoring electrolytes and renal function when treating with renally active drugs or diuretics.
  - Monitoring INR/PT while prescribing warfarin.
  - Monitoring drug levels, for example use of some antiepileptic agents.
- Avoid and be vigilant of high-risk drugs.
- Discontinue unnecessary drugs.
- Avoid treating side effects with another drug.
- Keep drug interactions in mind while prescribing medications.
- Educating patients about common and serious adverse effects so that they report immediately on noticing them.

PHARMACOVIGILANCE IN INDIA

- Pharmacovigilance is a specific domain of pharmacological sciences that deals with the drug safety information of medicinal products. It is defined as the science and activities relating to the detection, assessment, understanding and prevention of adverse effects or any other possible drug-related problem.
- Taking serious note of thalidomide tragedy, WHO launched a programme for International Drug Monitoring in 1968.
- With technical guidance and support from WHO, the Uppsala Monitoring Centre (UMC), Sweden functions as a WHO-Collaborating Centre and is responsible for International Drug Monitoring.
- In India, the Drugs Controller General of India, Central Drugs Standard Control Organization (CDSCO) is responsible for collecting data on ADRs.
- It is essential that the dug safety information is monitored throughout the lifecycle of a medicine.
- The Individual Case Safety Reports (ICSRs) are one of the important sources of safety data of medicines collected through spontaneous reporting by the healthcare practitioners or patients or relatives of the patients or consumers. The other sources such as manufacturers may also report drug safety information through periodic safety update reports (PSURs)/ other suitable mechanisms to the Drug Regulatory Authorities (DRAs).

- In respect of every new drug approved for marketing in India, the manufacturers of new drugs are bound to submit PSURs to the Central Licensing Authority, that is the Drugs Controller General of India, CDSCO, New Delhi.
- PSURs submission is also a condition for import of new drugs for sale or distribution in India. To facilitate adverse events reporting, Pharmacovigilance Programme of India (PvPI) has initiated requisite training program for skill development for stakeholders including manufacturers, from time to time as well as to create awareness among the stakeholders and educate them in this regard.
- In PvPI, new ADRs are detected as 'signals'. A 'signal' is a possible causal relation between an adverse event and a drug, the relation being previously unknown or incompletely documented.

Q. Discuss drug interactions. (PH 1.8)

DEFINITION

- A measurable modification (in magnitude and/or duration) of the action of one drug by prior or concomitant administration of another substance including prescription, non-prescription drugs, food, alcohol or diagnostic tests.

TYPES OF DRUG INTERACTIONS

- Based on the underlying mechanisms, drug–drug interactions are considered under three broad classes.

PHARMACODYNAMIC INTERACTIONS

- Pharmacodynamic interactions refer to interactions in which the drugs influence the effects of each other directly without any change in concentration.

PHARMACOKINETIC INTERACTIONS

- Pharmacokinetic interactions refer to interactions in which a drug influence the effects of another drug by altering its absorption, distribution, metabolism or excretion.

PHARMACEUTICAL INCOMPATIBILITY

- Pharmaceutical incompatibility means the drugs are not compatible before administration. Example includes incompatibility of calcium gluconate, dopamine, dobutamine and norepinephrine with sodium bicarbonate. These are not true drug interactions.

PHARMACOKINETIC INTERACTIONS

ALTERED GASTROINTESTINAL ABSORPTION

- Altered pH: The non-ionised form of a drug is more lipid soluble and is more readily absorbed from gut than the ionised form. For example, antacids and H2 blockers increase gastric pH which decreases dissolution of ketoconazole as it requires acidic pH. Therefore, there should be a gap of at least 2 hours between these agents.
- Drug-induced mucosal damage: Many chemotherapeutic agents like cyclophosphamide, procarbazine and vincristine damage the gut mucosa which inhibits absorption of several drugs, for example digoxin.
- Altered intestinal bacterial flora: Nearly 40% of orally administered digoxin is metabolised by gut microflora. Therefore, if a patient takes antibiotics simultaneously which destroy intestinal microflora, more of digoxin is absorbed and hence, its toxicity can occur.
- Complexation or chelation: Some drugs form complexes with each other which reduces absorption. Examples include tetracycline and iron, and antacids and ciprofloxacin.
- Altered motility: Metoclopramide hastens gastric emptying and therefore increases absorption of cyclosporin.
- P glycoprotein: Compounds in grapefruit juice and some drugs inhibit the P-glycoprotein drug transporter in the intestinal epithelium and may increase the net absorption of drugs that are normally expelled by the transporter. For example, absorption of digoxin is increased when accompanied by oral administration of verapamil.

ALTERED DISTRIBUTION

Displacing Drug From Protein Binding

- Many drugs are bound to plasma proteins. Several drugs can displace protein-bound drugs increasing levels of free drugs in circulation.
  - Phenytoin and warfarin are highly protein bound (90% and 99%, respectively). Drugs such as aspirin and sulphonamides can displace these protein-bound drugs and produce toxicity.
  - Sulphonamides can displace methotrexate, phenytoin, sulphonylureas and warfarin from binding sites on albumin.

Altered Volume of Distribution

- Changes in drug distribution can occur if one agent alters the size of the physical compartment in which another drug distributes. For example, diuretics, by reducing total body water, can increase plasma levels of aminoglycosides and lithium, possibly enhancing drug toxicities.

ALTERED METABOLISM

- Liver is the major site of metabolism of majority of drugs.
- Cytochrome P450 (CYP450) family of isoenzymes is the major enzyme in phase I metabolism of oxidation. The most common isozyme is CYP3A4, followed by 2C19, 2C9, 1A2, 2E6 and 2D6

Enzyme Induction

- A drug may induce the enzyme that is responsible for metabolism of another drug or even itself. Examples include carbamazepine increases its own metabolism; phenytoin increases hepatic metabolism of theophylline and vice versa; rifampicin increases metabolism of cyclosporin which may lead to transplant rejection; carbamazepine increases metabolism of warfarin.

Enzyme Inhibition

- A drug may inhibit the enzyme that is responsible for metabolism of another drug which leads to increased concentration of the target drug, thereby increasing its toxicity. Examples include inhibition of metabolism of terfenadine by erythromycin which increases cardiotoxicity of terfenadine; inhibition of metabolism of warfarin by erythromycin and clarithromycin (azithromycin shows almost no interactions with the cytochrome P450 system) which leads to increased risk of bleeding; inhibition of metabolism of theophylline by quinolones such as ofloxacin and ciprofloxacin which leads to increased toxicity of theophylline.

ALTERED EXCRETION

Renal Excretion

- Active tubular secretion occurs in proximal tubules. Drug is generally combined with a specific protein before reaching proximal tubule. When a drug has a competitive reactivity to the protein that is responsible for active transport of another drug, it will reduce excretion of that drug and increase its concentration. For example, probenecid decreases tubular secretion of methotrexate.
- Passive tubular reabsorption is by passive diffusion and is regulated by lipid solubility, degree of ionisation and concentration. For example, sodium bicarbonate increases excretion of phenobarbitone and salicylates. Drugs that alter urinary pH can alter the ionisation state of drugs that are weak acids or weak bases, leading to changes in renal tubular reabsorption.

PHARMACODYNAMIC INTERACTIONS

- Pharmacodynamic interactions can occur at different levels. They can occur at the same receptor site located on the cell membrane, in the cytoplasm or in the nucleus. The interactions can occur at a receptor site different from the receptor for the other drug. There can be general interactions due to which the effect of each drug is either enhanced or reduced without any change in the pharmacokinetics of the drugs.
- Pharmacodynamic interactions can be categorised broadly as additive when the effect of two drugs is merely the sum of the effects of each drug, antagonistic when the effect of two drugs is less than the sum of their individual effects and synergistic when the effect of two drugs is greater than the sum of their individual effects. An example of synergistic interaction is combination of amoxicillin and clavulanic acid.
- Beneficial effects can be due to increased efficacy either due to additive effect or synergistic effect. Examples include combinations of antihypertensive drugs, anticonvulsant drugs, synergistic antibiotics and antidiabetic agents.
- Beneficial effects can also be due to antagonistic effects. For example, the effects of neuromuscular blockers including cobra venom are reversed by neostigmine. Toxicities of opioids and benzodiazepines are reduced by naloxone and flumazenil, respectively. Phentolamine is useful in cocaine and amphetamine poisonings by reversing their effects on alpha receptors, thereby controlling severe hypertension.
- The harmful drug interactions can be due to reduced efficacy or increased toxicity (Table 20.3).

TABLE 20.3 Harmful Pharmacodynamic Drug Interactions (Examples)

Drug 1	Drug 2	Effect
ACE inhibitors	NSAIDs	Reduced antihypertensive effect Reduced beneficial effect on heart failure
Beta agonist	Beta antagonist	Worsening of asthma control
Levodopa	Neuroleptics	Reduced efficacy in patients with Parkinson's disease
Warfarin	NSAIDs	Increased bleeding risk
ACE inhibitors	Spironolactone	Hyperkalaemia
Macrolides	Fluoroquinolones	QT interval prolongation
Selective serotonin reuptake inhibitors (SSRIs)	Lithium, tramadol, pethidine	Serotonin syndrome

Q. Write a brief note on prescribing medications in patients with liver disease.

- Liver is a primary site of drug metabolism. Various steps in the drug biotransformation in the liver are uptake by the liver cells, phase I reaction (hydrolysis, hydroxylation, oxidation, reduction, demethylation) and phase II reactions (conjugation).
- These steps of biotransformation are dependent on two factors: hepatic blood flow and metabolic capacity of the liver.
- In patients with liver cirrhosis, drug handling by liver is impaired due to several factors (Table 20.4).

TABLE 20.4 Changes in Drug Handling in Patients With Liver Disease

Pathophysiological Factor	Consequence
Liver cell necrosis (reduced cytochrome metabolic activity)	Reduced first-pass metabolism; increased drug level
Shunting of the blood through portosystemic shunts	Higher serum levels
Reduction in the concentration of drug-binding proteins	Less protein binding leading to increased serum concentration
Ascites	Increased volume of distribution of hydrophilic drugs
Reduced glutathione stores	Increased toxicity
Impaired biliary excretion	Increased serum level
Altered pharmacodynamics	Increased effect of drugs
Associated renal failure	Increased serum level
Portal gastropathy	Reduced or increased absorption

BOX 20.3 Antibiotics to Be Avoided or Used With Caution in Patients With Cirrhosis of Liver

- Chloramphenicol—higher risk of bone marrow suppression due markedly increased half-life
- Erythromycin estolate—causes cholestasis
- Tetracycline—dose-related hepatotoxicity
- Antituberculous therapy in combinations, pyrazinamide (in Child–Pugh C)
- Griseofulvin—contraindicated
- Nalidixic acid
- Nitrofurantoin (prolonged use)

DRUG DOSAGE IN CIRRHOTIC PATIENTS

- Dose adjustment is necessary in cirrhosis but probably not in acute or chronic hepatitis. Cholestatic liver diseases, in particular obstructive jaundice, requires dose adjustment for drugs with a predominantly biliary excretion.
- Though various tests like liver function tests, and scores like Child–Pugh score and Model for End-stage Liver Disease (MELD) score are used for prediction of impaired liver function, no tests can accurately determine drug dosing in patients with liver disease.
- A generally followed dose recommendation is based on Child–Pugh score:
  - Child–Pugh A: Reduce maintenance dose by 50%.
  - Child–Pugh B: Reduce maintenance dose by 75%.
  - Child–Pugh C: Use drugs which have been proven to be safe or where drug level monitoring is available.

ANTIBIOTICS IN CIRRHOSIS

- A list of antibiotics which should be avoided in patients with cirrhosis of liver is given in Box 20.3.

SEDATIVES AND ANALGESICS IN CIRRHOSIS

- Prefer benzodiazepines with minor phase I metabolism such as lorazepam or oxazepam.
- Do not withhold opiates from patients with advanced liver disease but adjust for altered first-pass metabolism and consider overdose in patients with worsening hepatic encephalopathy.
- Avoid analgesic drugs for which no antagonist is available.
- Do not exceed 4 g of paracetamol in chronic liver disease.

Q. How will you prescribe medications in patients with kidney disease?

- Inappropriate dosing in patients with chronic kidney disease (CKD) can cause toxicity or ineffective therapy.
- CKD can affect glomerular blood flow and filtration, tubular secretion and reabsorption, and renal bioactivation and metabolism.
- Drug absorption, bioavailability, protein binding, distribution volume and non-renal clearance (metabolism) also can be altered in patients with CKD.

ALTERED PHARMACOKINETICS

DRUG ABSORPTION

- Absorption of drugs can be reduced by GI disturbances seen in CKD (vomiting, diarrhoea), uraemic gastritis and pancreatitis.
- Oedema of GIT can occur in nephrotic syndrome which can impair absorption.
- Gastric motility is impaired in uraemia.
- Gastric ammonia levels increase in uraemia. This elevates gastric pH, thus affecting absorption of drugs that require acidic pH for absorption (e.g. ferrous sulphate).

DRUG DISTRIBUTION

- In nephrotic syndrome, hypoalbuminaemia is common which leads to reduced protein binding of some drugs, thereby increasing levels of free drugs (e.g. phenytoin).

DRUG ELIMINATION

- With progression of kidney disease, the excretion of drugs and their metabolites decreases.
- The decreased glomerular filtration rate (GFR) does not principally affect the volume of distribution of water soluble, non-protein-bound drugs. Therefore, their initial dose is unchanged in patients with CKD. However, the maintenance dosing needs to be changed, either dose reduction or lengthening the dosing interval, or both.
  - Dose reduction involves reducing each dose while maintaining the normal dosing interval. This approach maintains more constant drug concentrations, but it is associated with a higher risk of toxicities if the dosing interval is inadequate to allow for drug elimination.
  - Second method is to maintain normal doses with extended intervals to allow time for drug elimination before redosing. Lengthening the dosing interval has been associated with a lower risk of toxicities but a higher risk of subtherapeutic drug concentrations, especially towards the end of the dosing interval.
  - Another method is by monitoring plasma drug concentrations over time.

DRUG REMOVAL BY DIALYSIS

- An important consideration in patients with CKD is removal of drugs by dialysis if patient is on it.

EXAMPLES

DRUGS TO BE AVOIDED

- Examples of some of the drugs which should be avoided in patients with CKD are given in Table 20.5.

ANTIHYPERTENSIVES IN CHRONIC KIDNEY DISEASE

- Thiazide diuretics are not recommended if the serum creatinine level is higher than 2.5 mg/dL or if GFR <30 mL/minute/1.73 m^2.

TABLE 20.5 Important Drugs to Be Avoided in Renal Failure

Drug	Glomerular Filtration Rate	Reason
Pethidine	GFR <60	Can cause convulsions
Glimepiride	GFR <60	Can cause hypoglycaemia
Metformin	GFR <60 or creatinine >1.5	Can cause lactic acidosis
Cefepime	GFR <30	Can cause CNS toxicity
Lithium	GFR <60	Can cause neurotoxicity and nephrotoxicity
Spironolactone	GFR <30	Can cause hypokalaemia
Enoxaparin	GFR <60	Can cause haemorrhage
Gentamicin, amikacin	GFR <60	Can cause further nephrotoxicity

- Potassium sparing diuretics should be avoided if GFR is below 30.
- ACE inhibitors and ARBs should be discontinued if serum creatinine rises by more than 30% after their initiation. In general, full dose is given if GFR > 50, 50%–75% of usual dose if GFR is between 10 and 50, and 25%–50% of usual dose if GFR < 10.
- Metoprolol, labetalol and propranolol are excreted through liver and do not require any dose modification. Atenolol, bisoprolol, nadolol and acebutolol require dose modification.
- Calcium channel blockers, alpha-blockers and clonidine do not require dose modification.

Q. Discuss use of drugs in pregnancy.

EFFECTS OF PREGNANCY ON PHARMACOKINETICS OF DRUGS

- Due to the effect of progesterone, gastric emptying time is decreased particularly in the third trimester thus delaying the onset of effect of some drugs.
- During pregnancy, plasma volume increases by 30%–50%, and cardiac output and GFR also increase in similar proportion. These factors contribute to lower circulating concentration of some drugs (especially those excreted by kidney) in a pregnant woman and possibly to subtherapeutic drug levels.
- There is increase in body fat during pregnancy, which increases the volume of distribution of fat-soluble drugs.
- A decrease in plasma albumin concentration during pregnancy increases the volume of distribution for highly protein bound drugs (e.g. anticonvulsants).

CONGENITAL DEFECTS

- Congenital defects are present in 2% to 3% of babies at birth with approximately 1% to 2% of the total associated with drug treatment.
- Malformations may occur during the period of organogenesis or at a later stage by altering the structure or function of organ systems involved.

PRESCRIBING PRINCIPLES IN PREGNANCY (Box 20.4)

BOX 20.4 Principles of Prescribing Drugs in Pregnancy

- Consider whether it is appropriate to try nondrug measures
- Drugs should be prescribed only for clear indications where the benefits (usually for the mother) outweigh the potential risks (usually to the foetus)
- Wherever possible try and avoid all drugs in the first trimester
- Medication should be used in the smallest effective dose for the shortest required duration
- Prescribe medication that has been widely used in pregnancy and has a good safety track record

CATEGORIES OF DRUG USE IN PREGANNCY

- Categories of drug use in pregnancy as given by Food and Drug Administration (FDA) and applicable prior to 2014 are given in Table 20.6.
- In 2014, the FDA published the Pregnancy and Lactation Labeling Final Rule (PLLR), which changed the labelling requirements for the pregnancy and lactation sections for prescription drugs and biological agents. The final rule removed the pregnancy letter categories, and created descriptive subsections for pregnancy exposure and risk, lactation, and effects to reproductive potential for females and males.

TABLE 20.6 Categories of Drug Use in Pregnancy

Category	Description
A	• Adequate, well-controlled studies in pregnant women have not shown an increased risk of foetal abnormalities • Example: Magnesium sulphate, folic acid, vitamin B, vitamin C, vitamin D, thyroxine, iron
B	• Animal studies have revealed no evidence of harm to the foetus; however, there are no adequate and well-controlled studies in pregnant women OR • Animal studies have shown an adverse effect, but adequate and well-controlled studies in pregnant women have failed to demonstrate a risk to the foetus • Example: Methyldopa, metronidazole, erythromycin, azithromycin, amoxicillin-clavulanic acid, meclizine, paracetamol, albendazole, ethambutol, diltiazem, spironolactone, nitrofurantoin, clindamycin, cephalosporins, metformin, sitagliptin, insulins
C	• Animal studies have shown an adverse effect and there are no adequate and well-controlled studies in pregnant women OR • No animal studies have been conducted and there are no adequate and well-controlled studies in pregnant women • Example: Diclofenac, rifampicin, isoniazid, gentamicin, amikacin, fluoroquinolones, salbutamol (oral), sulphamethoxazole/trimethoprim, clarithromycin
D	• Studies, adequate well controlled or observational, in pregnant women have demonstrated a risk to the foetus. However, the benefits of therapy may outweigh the potential risk • Example: Phenytoin, carbamazepine, valproic acid, ACE inhibitors, hydroxyprogestrone, streptomycin, tetracycline
X	• Studies, adequate well controlled or observational, in animals or pregnant women have demonstrated positive evidence of foetal abnormalities. The use of the product is contraindicated in women who are or may become pregnant • Example: Thalidomide, oral contraceptives, misoprostol, androgens, warfarin

DRUGS WITH PROVEN TERATOGENICITY (Table 20.7)

TABLE 20.7 Drugs With Teratogenic Effects

Drug	Effect
ACE inhibitors	• Reduced skull ossification, renal tubular dysgenesis, oligohydramnios, lung hypoplasia
Aminoglycosides	• Deafness, vestibular damage
Androgens	• Masculinisation of female foetus
Carbamazepine	• Neural tube defects
Diethylstilbestrol	• Genitourinary defects in male and female offspring
Lithium	• Cardiovascular defects
Misoprostol	• Moebius' syndrome
Phenytoin	• Growth restriction, CNS defects, cardiac defects
Retinoids	• Cardiovascular and skeletal defects
Thalidomide	• Phocomelia
Valproic acid	• Neural tube defects, dysmorphic features, developmental delay
Warfarin	• Skeletal and CNS defects, Dandy–Walker syndrome

USE OF DRUGS FOR COMMON PROBLEMS DURING PREGNANCY (Table 20.8)

TABLE 20.8 Safe Use of Drugs for Common Problems During Pregnancy

Problem	Safe Drugs
Nausea and vomiting	• Pyridoxine, meclizine, doxylamine, diphenhydramine
Constipation	• Psyllium, isabgol
Diarrhoea	• ORS, bismuth salicylate, loperamide
Muscular pain	• Paracetamol, NSAIDs (avoid in third trimester)
Antispasmodic	• Drotaverine (avoid in first trimester)
Peptic ulcer, gastritis	• Sucralfate, H_2-blockers, lansoprazole
Iron deficiency anaemia	• Iron
Folic acid deficiency	• Folic acid
Asthma	• Inhaled beta-agonists, inhaled corticosteroids; oral corticosteroids can be given if indicated for acute asthma
Urinary tract infection	• Amoxicillin, cefuroxime, cephalexin, nitrofurantoin (avoid in first trimester), fosfomycin
Amoebiasis	• Metronidazole, diloxanide furoate
Malaria	• Chloroquine, quinine (watch for hypoglycaemia), artesunate, clindamycin, mefloquine (avoid in first trimester), sulphadoxine-pyrimethamine (avoid in first trimester), artemether-lumefantrine (avoid in first trimester)
Worm infestation	• Piperazine, pyrantel pamoate, albendazole
Oral fungal infection	• Miconazole, clotrimazole, nystatin
Tuberculosis	• Isoniazid, rifampicin, ethambutol
Hypothyroidism	• Thyroxine
Hyperthyroidism	• Propylthiouracil, methimazole (avoid in first trimester)
Hypertension	• Methyldopa, hydralazine, labetalol
Venous thromboembolism	• Heparin
Diabetes mellitus	• Insulin
Fever	• Paracetamol
Epilepsy	• Carbamazepine in lowest possible dose

Q. Discuss various types of study designs in clinical practice.

- Several types of studies are conducted in clinical practice to find out relevance of risk factors, comparison of diagnostic tests and efficacy of drugs, and other issues. These are detailed in Table 20.9 along with their advantages and disadvantages.

EXAMPLE OF CASE-CONTROL STUDY

- In a study trying to show that people who smoke (the risk factor) are more likely to be diagnosed with lung cancer (the outcome), the cases would be persons with lung cancer, the controls would be persons without lung cancer (not necessarily healthy), and some of each group would be smokers. If a larger proportion of the cases with lung cancers smoke than the controls, that suggests, but does not conclusively prove, that the hypothesis is valid.

EXAMPLE OF COHORT STUDY

- To find out whether smoking causes lung cancer, a cohort should include both smokers (the exposed group) and non-smokers (the unexposed group). Both should be followed for long time to see how many develop lung cancer in each group.

Q. What are the levels of clinical evidence?

LEVELS OF CLINICAL EVIDENCE

- Levels of evidence or hierarchy of evidence are assigned to studies based on methodological quality of their design, validity and applicability to patient care.
- The levels of evidence are given in Table 20.10.

TABLE 20.9 Types of Various Study Designs

Study Design	Description	Advantages	Disadvantages
Meta-analysis	• A way of combining data from many different research studies • It is a statistical process that combines the findings from individual studies	• Increases statistical power through increased sample size • Allows for an objective appraisal of evidence • Resolves uncertainty when studies disagree • Reduces probability of false negative results • Heterogeneity between study results may be explained	• Data from individual trial may not be available and therefore many studies need to be excluded • Selection of studies and data from studies may be biased • Publication bias (many negative studies are not published) • Inclusion and exclusion criteria may not be detailed
Systematic review	• It is a critical assessment and evaluation of all research studies that address a particular clinical issue • The researchers use an organised method of locating, assembling and evaluating a body of literature on a particular topic using a set of specific criteria	• Bias is reduced by the use of a systematic method for selecting studies for the review	• Often more time consuming than other types of review
Randomised controlled trial (RCT)	• In this study, participants are allocated to intervention or control (or placebo) groups randomly	• Best for studying effect of an intervention • Takes care of confounding factors (e.g. age, sex, race) • Patients (single blinded), investigators (double blinded) and evaluators/ statisticians (triple blinded) can be blinded to which groups the patients were randomised	• Expensive • Time consuming • Ethical problems at times
Cross-over study	• A controlled trial in which each participant gets both therapies (therapy A first and then therapy B or vice versa)	• All participants serve as own controls, thus reducing sample size • Blinding is possible	• Washout period required between two therapies to eliminate persisting effect of a therapy • Cannot be used if one therapy has long effect or persisting effect
Cohort study (Fig. 20.1A)	• In this study, data are obtained from groups of participants who have already been exposed or not exposed to the factor of interest	• Best for studying effects of certain risk factors on outcome • Ethically safe • Participants can be matched	• Controls may be difficult to identify • Unidentified confounders may alter results • Blinding is difficult
Case-control study (Fig. 20.1B)	• Observational study in which two existing groups differing in a selected outcome are identified and compared on the basis of some supposed risk attribute • This type of study is often used to identify factors that may contribute to a medical condition by comparing subjects who have that condition/disease (the 'cases') with persons who do not have the condition/disease but are otherwise similar (the 'controls')	• Easy to conduct • Shorter duration • Cheap • Can be conducted in a single institute • Only feasible study for rare disorders or those with long lag between postulated exposure and outcome	• Relies on recall or records to determine exposure • Confounders can bias the results • Selection of control group is difficult
Cross-sectional study	• In this type of study, relationship between diseases/health-related characteristics and other variables of interest are examined as they exist in defined population at one time • Exposure and outcomes are measured at the same time • The study quantifies prevalence, risk or diagnostic test accuracy	• Cheap • Simple • Ethically safe	• Study established only association and not causality • Suffers from recall bias, social desirability bias, researcher's bias • Confounders may be unequally distributed • Group sizes may be unequal

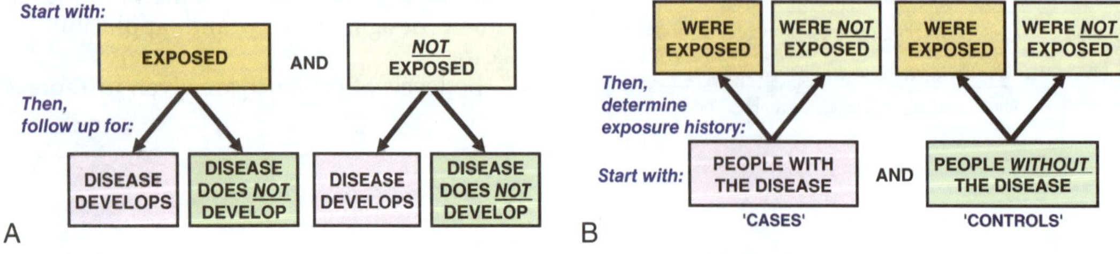

Fig. 20.1 (A) Cohort study. (B) Case-control study.

TABLE 20.10 Levels of Evidence

Level of Evidence (LOE)	Description
Level I	Evidence from systematic review or meta-analysis of all relevant randomised controlled trials (RCTs) or evidence-based guidelines based on systematic reviews of RCTs or three or more RCTs of good quality that have similar results
Level II	Evidence from at least one well-designed randomised controlled trial (e.g. one large multisite RCT)
Level III	Evidence from well-designed controlled trials without randomisation
Level IV	Evidence from well-designed case-control or cohort study
Level V	Evidence from systematic reviews of descriptive and qualitative studies
Level VI	Evidence from a single descriptive or qualitative study
Level VII	Evidence from the opinion of authorities and/or reports of expert committees

CLASS (STRENGTH) OF RECOMMENDATIONS (Table 20.11)

TABLE 20.11 Class (Strength) of Recommendations

Class	Description
Class I	Strong recommendation Is useful/indicated/effective/beneficial Treatment A preferred over treatment B
Class IIa	Moderate recommendation Is reasonable treatment Can be useful/effective/beneficial Reasonable to choose treatment A over treatment B
Class IIb	Weak recommendation May be reasonable May be considered Usefulness/effectiveness unknown/unclear/uncertain/not well established
Class III	No benefit or may be harmful

Q. Write a brief note on various terms used in describing a clinical study.

- A number of terms are used while describing a clinical study. Some of these are briefly described in Table 20.12.

Q. What are the phases of clinical trials? Briefly define them.

- Clinical trials are studies to test new drugs, already approved drugs, devices or other forms of treatments.

TABLE 20.12 Terms Used in Clinical Studies

Term	Description
Placebo	• An inert substance supposed to have no physiological effect on human
Placebo effect	• At times, a placebo can produce some positive response, usually psychological relief of symptoms
Nocebo effect	• Negative expectations of the patient regarding a treatment cause the treatment to have a more negative effect than it otherwise would have (negative of placebo effect). May lead to non-adherence by patient, physician may discontinue what is otherwise an appropriate therapy, or attempts are made to treat these side effects with additional drugs. These non-specific side effects distress patients, add to the burden of their illness and increase the cost of their care
Bias	• Any process at any stage of inference which tends to produce results or conclusions that differ systematically from the truth. Selection bias refers to systematic differences between baseline characteristics of the groups involved in the study
Control group	• Group that serves as a standard for comparison in experimental studies. They are similar in relevant characteristics to the experimental group but do not receive the experimental intervention
Random allocation	• A process involving allocation of study participants into two or more groups (arms) using random number tables. This will eliminate allocation bias and will greatly enhance validity of the study
Blinding	• The participants, the investigators and/or the evaluators are kept unaware (or blinded) of the treatment received by the patient. It eliminates participant bias, investigator bias and evaluator bias
Unblinding	• The process by which the allocation code is broken so that the patient, investigator and/or evaluator becomes aware of the intervention. During ongoing trial, it can be done in case of a serious adverse event
Hawthorne effect	• It is alteration of behaviour by the subjects of a study due to their awareness of being observed. It occurs in both control and treatment group participants and is probably balanced out due to randomisation
Intention to treat analysis	• Strategy for the analysis of randomised controlled trial that compares patients in the groups to which they were originally randomly assigned. Includes all participants once randomised even if they did not participate in the study after that
Lost to follow up	• Study subjects whose outcomes are unknown, for example because they could not or did not wish to attend follow-up visits
Numbers needed to treat	• Number of patients who need to be treated in order to prevent one additional bad outcome

Continued

TABLE 20.12 Terms Used in Clinical Studies—cont'd

Informed consent	• A continuous process involving four main components—providing relevant information about the study (purpose, duration of participation, required procedures/treatments, possible risks/benefits) to potential participants, ensuring the information is easily comprehended by the participants, assuring voluntariness of participation (ability of an individual to judge freely, independently, and in the absence of any coercion or incentive, what is good, right and best for him), and assuring that the participant can withdraw from the trial at any time without any consequence
Adaptive clinical trial	• These trials use existing data to design the trial, and then use interim results to modify the trial as it proceeds. Modifications include dosage, sample size, drug undergoing trial and patient selection criteria
Epidemiological trials	• These trials have the goal of identifying the general causes, patterns or control of diseases in large numbers of people
Institutional Review Board (IRB)	• An IRB (also known as an independent ethics committee—IEC) is a group of doctors, scientists, advocates, researchers and members of the community that has been formally designated to review and monitor all research involving humans. IRBs are in place to provide ethical oversight and to minimise risk to participants

Many clinical trials look at new ways to diagnose or measure the extent of disease. Some even look at ways to prevent diseases from happening. The trials are done on patients.

WHY ARE CLINICAL TRIALS REQUIRED?

- Is the new treatment better than the standard treatment given for this disease? If it is not better, is it as good and cause fewer side effects? Or does it work in some people who are not helped by current treatments?
- Is the new treatment safe?

PHASES OF CLINICAL TRIALS

PRECLINICAL PHASE

- Clinical trials are done only after preclinical findings (laboratory studies) suggest that the new drug or treatment is likely to be safe and will work in people. New treatments for cancers are studied first on cancer cells and then on animals.

CLINICAL PHASE

- Once deemed safe, the trial goes through following phases:

Phase 0

- Phase 0 trials are optional first-in-human trials. Single subtherapeutic doses of the study drug are given to a small number of subjects (typically 10–15) to gather preliminary data on the drug's pharmacodynamics and pharmacokinetics. For the test drug, the trial documents the absorption, distribution, metabolisation and clearance (excretion) of the drug, and the drug's interactions within the body, to confirm that these appear to be as expected.

Phase I

- Phase I studies of a new drug are usually the first that involve small group of people (~20–80). Phase I studies are done to evaluate safety, determine safe dosage range and identify side effects. Disease response is not the main purpose of a phase I study.

Phase II

- If a new treatment is found to be safe in phase I clinical trials, a phase II clinical trial is done on a larger group of patients (~100–300) to confirm effectiveness, monitor side effects and further evaluate safety.

Phase III

- Treatments that have been shown to work in phase II clinical trials must succeed in one more phase before they are approved for general use. Phase III clinical trials compare the safety and effectiveness of the new treatment against the current standard treatment in an even larger group of patients (~1000–3000).

Phase IV

- It is also called postmarketing surveillance and is done after the drug has been marketed. Even after testing a new medicine on thousands of people, all the effects of the treatment may not be known. In phase IV, study continues to collect data about effects in various populations and side effects on long-term use.

Q. Write a short note on CONSORT.

- CONSORT stands for Consolidated Standards of Reporting Trials and encompasses various initiatives developed by the CONSORT Group to alleviate the problems arising from inadequate reporting of randomised controlled trials.
- The main product of CONSORT is the CONSORT Statement which is a minimum set of recommendations for reporting randomised trials.
- CONSORT Statement offers a standard way for authors to prepare reports of trial findings, facilitating

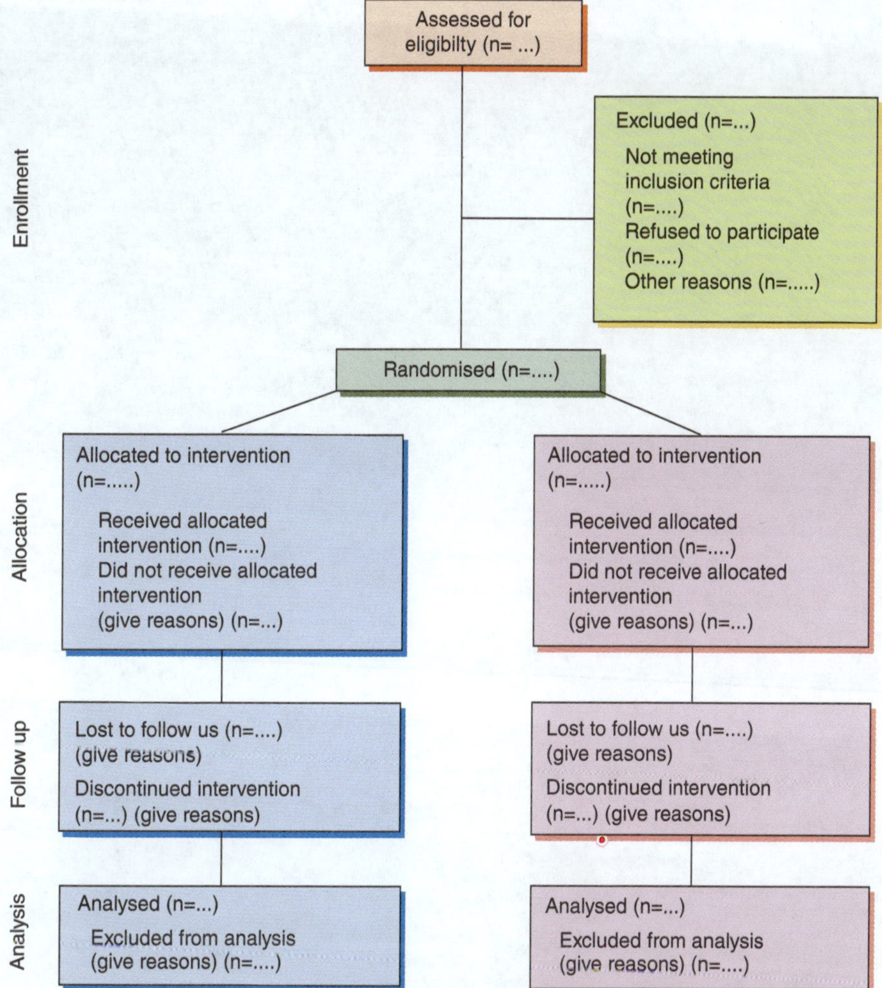

Flowchart 20.1 The Consolidated Standards of Reporting Trials (CONSORT) Flow Diagram.

their complete and transparent reporting, and aiding their critical appraisal and interpretation.

- The CONSORT Statement comprises a 25-item checklist and a flow diagram.
- The checklist items focus on reporting how the trial was designed, analysed and interpreted.
- The flow diagram displays the progress of all participants through the trial (Flowchart 20.1).

Index

D

E

F

G

H

R